Cryptosporidium infection	I
Diarrhea, acute	III
Diarrhea, chronic	III
Diarrhea, chronic in patients with HIV infection, algorithm	III
Diverticular disease	I
Dumping syndrome	I
Dysphagia	III
Dyspepsia	III
Echinococcosis	I
Esophageal tumors	I
Food poisoning, bacterial	I
Gardner's syndrome	I
Gastric cancer	I
Gastritis	I
Gastroesophageal reflux disease (GERD)	I
Giardiasis	I
Gilbert's disease	I
Glossitis	I
Hemochromatosis	I
Hemorrhoids	I
Hepatic encephalopathy	I
Hepatitis A	I
Hepatitis, autoimmune	I
Hepatitis B	I
Hepatitis B prophylaxis	V
Hepatitis C	I
Hepatitis, viral	III
Hepatoma	I
Hepatomegaly algorithm	III
Hepatorenal syndrome	I
Hiatal hernia	I
Hookworm	I
Irritable bowel syndrome (IBS)	I
Jaundice, neonatal, algorithm	III
Jaundice and hepatobiliary disease	III
Lactose intolerance	I
Malabsorption algorithm	III
Mallory-Weiss syndrome	I
Nonalcoholic fatty liver disease	I
Pancreatic cancer, exocrine	I
Pancreatitis, acute	I
Pancreatitis, chronic	I
Peptic ulcer disease	I
Peritonitis	I
Peritonitis, spontaneous bacterial	I
Peutz-Jeghers syndrome	I
Pinworms	I
Portal hypertension	I
Portal vein thrombosis	I
Pruritus ani	I
Pseudomembranous colitis	I
Shigellosis	I
Short-bowel syndrome	I
Tapeworm infestation	I
Tropical sprue	I
Typhoid fever	I
Ulcerative colitis	I
Wilson's disease	I
Whipple's disease	I
Zenker's (pharyngoesophageal diverticulum)	I
Zollinger-Ellison syndrome	I

GYNECOLOGY AND OBSTETRICS

Abruptio placenta	I
Abscess, pelvic	I
Abscess, perirectal	I
Amenorrhea, primary	III
Bleeding, early pregnancy	III
Bleeding, vaginal	III
Breast abscess	I
Breast cancer	I
Breast nipple discharge	III
Breast radiologic evaluation	III
Breast, routine screen or palpable mass evaluation	III
Breastfeeding difficulties	III
Breech birth	I
Cervical cancer	I
Cervical dysplasia	I
Cervical polyps	I
Cervicitis	I
Chancroid	I
Chlamydia genital infections	I
Condyloma acuminatum	I
Contraceptive method selection	III
Contraceptive use, oral, algorithm	III
Contraception	I
Dysfunctional uterine bleeding (DUB)	I
Dysmenorrhea	I
Dyspareunia	I
Dysuria and/or urethral/vaginal discharge	III
Eclampsia	I
Ectopic pregnancy	I
Endometrial cancer	I
Endometriosis	I
Endometritis	I
Fatty liver of pregnancy	I
Fibrocystic breast disease	I
Genital lesions or ulcers algorithm	III
Gonorrhea	I
Granuloma inguinale	I
Herpes simplex genital	I
HEELP syndrome	I
Hirsutism algorithm	III
Hot flashes	I
Hyperemesis gravidarum	I
Hypogonadism	III
Immunizations during pregnancy	V
Incontinence	I
Infertility	III
Lymphogranuloma venereum	I
Mastodynia	I
Meig's syndrome	I
Menopause	I
Ovarian cancer	I
Ovarian tumor, benign	I
Paget's disease of the breast	I
Pelvic inflammatory disease (PID)	I
Pelvic mass algorithm	III
Pelvic pain, reproductive age woman	III
Placenta previa	I
Polycystic ovaries	I
Preeclampsia	I
Premenstrual dysphoric disorder (PMDD)	I
Premenstrual syndrome (PMS)	I
Pruritus vulvae	I
Puberty, delayed, algorithm	III
Puberty, precocious, algorithm	III
Rh incompatibility	I
Sexual dysfunction	III
Sheehan's syndrome	I
Spontaneous miscarriage	I
Syphilis	I
Therapeutic insemination (frozen donor semen)	I
Therapeutic insemination (husband/partner)	I
Toxic shock syndrome	I
Urethritis, gonococcal	I
Urethritis, nongonococcal	I
Urinary tract infection	I
Uterine malignancy	I
Uterine myomas	I
Uterine prolapse	I
Vaginal discharge algorithm	III
Vaginal malignancy	I
Vaginal prolapse	III
Vaginismus	I
Vaginosis, bacterial	I
Vulvar cancer	I
Vulvovaginitis, bacterial	I
Vulvovaginitis, estrogen deficient	I
Vulvovaginitis, fungal	I
Vulvovaginitis, prepubescent	I
Vulvovaginitis, trichomoniasis	I

HEMATOLOGY/ONCOLOGY

Anemia algorithm	I
Anemia, aplastic	I
Anemia, autoimmune hemolytic	I
Anemia, iron deficiency	I
Anemia, macrocytic	III
Anemia, microcytic	III
Anemia, pernicious	I
Anemia, sickle cell	I
Anemia, sideroblastic	I
Anemia with reticulocytosis	III
Antiphospholipid syndrome	I
Astrocytoma	I
Basal cell carcinoma	I
Bladder cancer	I
Bleeding disorder, congenital	III
Bleeding time, prolonged	IV
Bone tumor, primary malignant	I
Brain neoplasm	I
Breast cancer	I
Carcinoid syndrome	I
Cervical cancer	I
Colorectal cancer	I
Craniopharyngioma	I
Disseminated intravascular coagulation (DIC)	I
Endometrial cancer	I
Eosinophilia	IV
Erythrocytosis, acquired	III
Esophageal tumors	I
Felty's syndrome	I
Gastric cancer	I
HELPP syndrome	I
Hemophilia	I
Hemolytic-uremic syndrome	I
Henoch-Schönlein purpura	I
Hepatocellular carcinoma	I
Histiocytosis X	I
Hodgkin's disease	I
Hypercoagulable state	I
Hypereosinophilic syndrome	I
Hypersplenism	I
Idiopathic thrombocytopenic purpura (ITP)	I
Insulinoma	I
Kaposi's sarcoma	I
Lambert-Eaton syndrome	I
Laryngeal carcinoma	I
Lead poisoning	I
Leukemia, acute lymphoblastic (ALL)	I
Leukemia, acute myelogenous (AML)	I
Leukemia, chronic lymphocytic (CLL)	I
Leukemia, chronic myelogenous (CML)	I
Leukemia, hairy cell	I
Leukocytosis, neutrophilic	IV
Lung neoplasm, primary	I
Lymphadenopathy, generalized, algorithm	III
Lymphadenopathy, localized, algorithm	III
Lymphocyte abnormalities in peripheral blood	IV
Lymphoma, non-Hodgkin's	I
Macrocytosis	IV
Meig's syndrome	I
Melanoma	I
Meningioma	I
Mesothelioma	I
Microcytosis and hypochromia	IV
Multiple myeloma	I
Mycosis fungoides	I
Myelodysplastic syndromes (MDS)	I
Nephroblastoma	I
Neutropenia	IV
Neutrophilia	IV
Neuroblastoma	I
Ovarian cancer	I
Ovarian tumor, benign	I
Paget's disease of breast	I
Pancreatic cancer, exocrine	I
Pancreatic islet cell tumors	III
Paroxysmal cold hemoglobinuria	I
Paroxysmal nocturnal hemoglobinuria	I
Pheochromocytoma	I
Pituitary adenoma	I
Polycythemia vera	I
Priapism	I
Prolactinoma	I
Prostate cancer	I
Renal cell adenocarcinoma	I
Reticulocyte count elevation	IV
Retinoblastoma	I
Rh incompatibility	I
Salivary gland neoplasms	I
Shilling test	IV
Splenomegaly, algorithm	III
Squamous cell carcinoma	I

FERRI'S

CLINICAL ADVISOR

Instant Diagnosis and Treatment

FRED F. FERRI, M.D., F.A.C.P.

Clinical Professor
Department of Community Health
Brown Medical School
Providence, Rhode Island

2005 EDITION

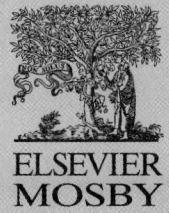

ELSEVIER
MOSBY

ELSEVIER
MOSBY

The Curtis Center
170 S Independence Mall W 300E
Philadelphia, Pennsylvania 19106

NOTICE

Pharmacology is an ever-changing field. Standard safety precautions must be followed, but as
new research and clinical experience broaden our knowledge, changes in treatment and drug
therapy may become necessary or appropriate. Readers are advised to check the most current
product information provided by the manufacturer of each drug to be administered to verify
the recommended dose, the method and duration of administration, and contraindications.
It is the responsibility of the licensed prescriber, relying on experience and knowledge of the
patient, to determine dosages and the best treatment for each individual patient. Neither the
publisher nor the editor assumes any liability for any injury and/or damage to persons or
property arising from this publication.

Previous editions copyrighted 1999, 2000, 2001, 2002, 2003, 2004

International Standard Book Number 0-323-02973-6
International Standard Book Number 0-323-02974-4 (Package)

Publisher: Thomas H. Moore
Associate Editor: Elyse W. O'Grady
Publishing Services Manager: Melissa Lastarria
Project Manager: Joy Moore
Senior Book Designer: Teresa McBryan

Printed in the United States of America

Last digit is the print number: 9   8   7   6   5   4   3   2   1

Section Editors

MICHAEL BENATAR, M.B.CH.B., D.PHIL.
Assistant Professor of Neurology
Department of Neurology
Emory University
Atlanta, Georgia
Section I

GEORGE T. DANAKAS, M.D., F.A.C.O.G.
Clinical Assistant Professor
Department of Obstetrics and Gynecology
State University of New York at Buffalo
Buffalo, New York
Section I

FRED F. FERRI, M.D., F.A.C.P.
Clinical Professor
Department of Community Health
Brown Medical School
Providence, Rhode Island
Sections I-V

JOSEPH R. MASCI, M.D.
Director of Medicine
Elmhurst Hospital Center
Professor of Medicine
Mount Sinai School of Medicine
Elmhurst, New York
Section I

LONNIE R. MERCIER, M.D.
Clinical Instructor
Department of Orthopedic Surgery
Creighton University School of Medicine
Omaha, Nebraska
Section I

PETER PETROPOULOS, M.D., F.A.C.C.
Clinical Assistant Professor
Brown Medical School
Department of Veterans Affairs
Providence, Rhode Island
Section I

IRIS TONG, M.D.
Clinical Assistant Professor
Brown Medical School
Attending Physician
Women's Health Associates
Division of General Internal Medicine
Rhode Island Hospital
Providence, Rhode Island
Section I

TOM J. WACHTEL, M.D.
Physician-in-Charge
Division of Geriatrics
Rhode Island Hospital
Professor of Community Health and Medicine
Brown Medical School
Providence, Rhode Island
Section I

Contributors

SONYA S. ABDEL-RAZEQ, M.D.
Clinical Instructor
Department of Obstetrics and Gynecology/Resident
　Education
State University of New York at Buffalo
Women's and Children's Hospital
Buffalo, New York

PHILIP J. ALIOTTA, M.D., M.S.H.A., F.A.C.S.
Clinical Instructor
Department of Urology
School of Medicine and Biomedical Sciences
State University of New York at Buffalo
Buffalo, New York
Medical Director
Center for Urologic Research of Western New York
Williamsville, New York

GEORGE O. ALONSO, M.D.
Director, Department of Infection Control
Elmhurst Hospital Center
Elmhurst, New York
Assistant Professor, Department of Medicine
Mount Sinai School of Medicine
New York, New York

MEL L. ANDERSON, M.D., F.A.C.P.
Clinical Assistant Professor of Medicine
Brown Medical School
Providence, Rhode Island

ETSUKO AOKI, M.D., PH.D.
Fellow of General Internal Medicine
Rhode Island Hospital
Providence, Rhode Island

VASANTHI ARUMUGAM, M.D.
Assistant Professor, Department of Medicine
Mount Sinai School of Medicine
New York, New York
Attending Physician
Division of Infectious Diseases/Department of Medicine
Elmhurst Hospital Center
Elmhurst, New York

AMAAR ASHRAF, M.D.
Assistant Professor
Department of Medicine
Mount Sinai School of Medicine
New York, New York
Attending Physician
Division of Infectious Diseases
Elmhurst Hospital Center
Elmhurst, New York

SUDEEP KAUR AULAKH, M.D., C.M., F.R.C.P.C.
Associate Professor of Medicine
Albany Medical College
Albany, New York

MICHAEL BENATAR, M.B.CH.B., D.PHIL.
Assistant Professor of Neurology
Department of Neurology
Emory University
Atlanta, Georgia

LYNN BOWLBY, M.D.
Attending Physician
Division of General Internal Medicine
Rhode Island Hospital
Clinical Instructor of Medicine
Brown Medical School
Providence, Rhode Island

WILLIAM F. BOYD, M.D., M.P.H.
Staff Physician
Academic Medical Center
Internal Medicine Inpatient Service
Rhode Island Hospital/The Miriam Hospital
Providence, Rhode Island

MANDEEP K. BRAR, M.D.
Clinical Assistant Professor
Department of Obstetrics and Gynecology
State University of New York at Buffalo
Buffalo, New York

REBECCA S. BRIENZA, M.D., M.P.H.
Assistant Professor
Department of Internal Medicine
Yale University School of Medicine
New Haven, Connecticut

JENNIFER CLARKE, M.D.
Assistant Professor of Medicine and Obstetrics and
　Gynecology
Brown Medical School
Physician, Rhode Island Hospital
Providence, Rhode Island

MARIA A. CORIGLIANO, M.D., F.A.C.O.G.
Clinical Assistant Professor
Department of Obstetrics and Gynecology
State University of New York at Buffalo
Buffalo, New York

KAROLL CORTEZ, M.D.
Fellow in Infectious Disease
Division of Infectious Disease
Rhode Island Hospital
Providence, Rhode Island

JOHN E. CROOM M.D., PH.D.
Clinical Fellow in Neurology
Harvard Medical School
Beth Israel Deaconess Medical Center
Boston, Massachusetts

CLAUDIA L. DADE, M.D.
Attending Physician
Division of Infectious Diseases
Elmhurst Hospital Center
Elmhurst, New York
Instructor in Medicine
Mount Sinai School of Medicine
New York, New York

GEORGE T. DANAKAS, M.D., F.A.C.O.G.
Clinical Assistant Professor
Department of Obstetrics and Gynecology
State University of New York at Buffalo
Buffalo, New York

ALEXANDRA DEGENHARDT, M.D.
Clinical Fellow, Multiple Sclerosis Center
Department of Neurology
Beth Israel Deaconess Medical Center
Boston, Massachusetts

JOSEPH DIAZ, M.D.
Assistant Professor of Medicine
Division of General Internal Medicine
Memorial Hospital of Rhode Island
Brown Medical School
Providence, Rhode Island

CHRISTINE M. DUFFY, M.D., M.P.H.
Fellow, Center for Gerontology and Health Care
   Research
Brown University
Providence, Rhode Island

JEFFREY S. DURMER, M.D., PH.D.
Assistant Professor, Department of Neurology
Director, Emory Sleep Laboratory
Director, Egleston Children's Hospital Sleep Clinic
Emory University School of Medicine
Atlanta, Georgia

JANE V. EASON, M.D.
Attending Physician, Division of Infectious Diseases
Elmhurst Hospital Center
Elmhurst, New York
Instructor in Medicine, Mount Sinai School of Medicine
New York, New York

PEGGY L. EL-MALLAKH, B.S.N., M.S.N.
Lecturer
College of Nursing
University of Louisville
Louisville, Kentucky

RIF S. EL-MALLAKH, M.D.
Associate Professor
Department of Psychiatry and Behavioral Sciences
University of Louisville School of Medicine
Louisville, Kentucky

MARILYN FABBRI, M.D.
Assistant Professor
Department of Medicine
Mount Sinai School of Medicine
New York, New York
Attending Physician
Division of Infectious Diseases/Department of Medicine
Elmhurst Hospital Center
Elmhurst, New York

MARK J. FAGAN, M.D.
Director, Medical Primary Care Unit
Rhode Island Hospital
Associate Professor of Medicine
Brown Medical School
Providence, Rhode Island

GIL FARKASH, M.D.
Assistant Clinical Professor
State University of New York at Buffalo
School of Medicine
Buffalo, New York

FRED F. FERRI, M.D., F.A.C.P.
Clinical Professor
Department of Community Health
Brown Medical School
Providence, Rhode Island

TAMARA G. FONG, M.D., PH.D.
Instructor in Neurology
Beth Israel Deaconess Medical Center
Harvard Medical School
Boston, Massachusetts

GLENN G. FORT, M.D., PH.D.
Clinical Associate Professor of Medicine
Brown Medical School
Chief
Infectious Diseases
Our Lady of Fatima Hospital
North Providence, Rhode Island

TIFFANY B. GENEWICK, M.D.
Clinical Instructor
Department of Obstetrics and Gynecology
State University of New York at Buffalo
Buffalo, New York

DAVID R. GIFFORD, M.D., M.P.H.
Assistant Professor, Division of Geriatrics
Rhode Island Hospital
Assistant Professor of Community Health and Medicine
Brown Medical School
Providence, Rhode Island

GEETHA GOPALAKRISHNAN, M.D.
Assistant Professor of Medicine
Department of Endocrinology
Brown Medical School
Providence, Rhode Island

REBECCA A. GRIFFITH, M.D.
Attending Physician
Department of Medicine
Morristown Memorial Hospital
Morristown, New Jersey

JOSEPH GRILLO, M.D.
Fellow, Infectious Diseases
Roger Williams Medical Center,
Providence, Rhode Island

MICHAEL GRUENTHAL, M.D., PH.D.
Mason C. and Mary D. Rudd Chair of Neurology
University of Louisville School of Medicine
Louisville, Kentucky

MICHELE HALPERN, M.D.
Attending Physician, Division of Infectious Diseases
Sound Shore Medical Center of Westchester
New Rochelle, New York
Clinical Assistant Professor of Medicine
New York Medical College
Valhalla, New York

SAJEEV HANDA, M.D.
Director, Division of Hospitalist Medicine
Rhode Island Hospital
Clinical Instructor of Medicine
Brown Medical School
Providence, Rhode Island

TAYLOR HARRISON, M.D.
Neuromuscular Fellow
Department of Neurology
Emory University
Atlanta, Georgia

SHARON S. HARTMAN, M.D., PH.D.
Clinical Associate
Department of Neurology
Emory University
Atlanta, Georgia

JENNIFER ROH HUR, M.D.
Clinical Instructor
Brown Internal Medicine Residency Program
Brown Medical School
Providence, Rhode Island

RICHARD S. ISAACSON, M.D.
Resident in Neurology
Beth Israel Deaconess Medical Center
Harvard Medical School
Boston, Massachusetts

JENNIFER JEREMIAH, M.D.
Clinical Associate Professor of Medicine
Brown Medical School
Providence, Rhode Island

MICHAEL P. JOHNSON, M.D.
Staff Physician, Division of General Internal Medicine
Rhode Island Hospital
Assistant Professor of Medicine
Brown Medical School
Providence, Rhode Island

WAN J. KIM, M.D.
Clinical Instructor
Department of Obstetrics and Gynecology
State University of New York at Buffalo
Buffalo, New York

MELVYN KOBY, M.D.
Associate Clinical Professor of Medicine
Department of Ophthalmology
University of Louisville School of Medicine
Louisville, Kentucky

DAVID KURSS, M.D., F.A.C.O.G.
Clinical Assistant Professor
Department of Obstetrics and Gynecology
State University of New York at Buffalo
Buffalo, New York

JOSEPH J. LIEBER, M.D.
Associate Director of Medicine
Chief, Medical Consultation Service
Elmhurst Hospital Center
Clinical Associate Professor of Medicine
Mount Sinai School of Medicine
New York, New York

CHUN LIM, M.D., PH.D.
Department of Neurology
Beth Israel Deaconess Medical Center
Boston, Massachusetts

ZEENA LOBO, M.D.
Attending Physician
Division of Infectious Diseases
Elmhurst Hospital Center
Elmhurst, New York

EUGENE J. LOUIE-NG, M.D.
Clinical Instructor
Department of Obstetrics and Gynecology
State University of New York at Buffalo
Buffalo, New York

JOSEPH R. MASCI, M.D.
Director of Medicine
Elmhurst Hospital Center
Elmhurst, New York
Professor of Medicine
Mount Sinai School of Medicine
New York, New York

DANIEL T. MATTSON, M.D., M.SC.(MED.)
Clinical Fellow in Neurology
Beth Israel Deaconess Medical Center
Harvard Medical School
Boston, Massachusetts

MAITREYI MAZUMDAR, M.D., M.P.H.
Clinical Fellow in Neurology
Harvard Medical School
Children's Hospital of Boston
Boston, Massachusetts

KELLY MCGARRY, M.D.
Associate Program Director
General Internal Medicine Residency Program
Rhode Island Hospital
Assistant Professor of Medicine
Brown Medical School
Providence, Rhode Island

LYNN MCNICOLL, M.D.
Assistant Professor of Medicine
Brown Medical School
Geriatrician, Division of Geriatrics
Rhode Island Hospital
Providence, Rhode Island

LONNIE R. MERCIER, M.D.
Clinical Instructor
Department of Orthopedic Surgery
Creighton University School of Medicine
Omaha, Nebraska

DENNIS J. MIKOLICH, M.D.
Chief, Division of Infectious Diseases
VA Medical Center
Clinical Associate Professor of Medicine
Brown Medical School
Providence, Rhode Island

TAKUMA NEMOTO, M.D.
Research Associate Professor of Surgery
State University of New York at Buffalo
Buffalo, New York

JAMES J. NG, M.D.
Staff Physician
The Vancouver Clinic
Vancouver, Washington

GAIL M. O'BRIEN, M.D.
Medical Director
Adult Ambulatory Services
Rhode Island Hospital
Clinical Associate Professor of Medicine
Brown Medical School
Providence, Rhode Island

CAROLYN J. O'CONNOR, M.D.
Internal Medicine
Primary Care of Southbury
Danbury Hospital
Southbury, Connecticut

LAURA OFSTEAD, M.D.
Clinical Assistant Professor
Brown Medical School
Rhode Island Hospital
Providence, Rhode Island

ALEXANDER OLAWAIYE, M.D.
Clinical Instructor
Department of Obstetrics and Gynecology/Resident
  Education
State University of New York at Buffalo
Women's and Children's Hospital
Buffalo, New York

JEANNE M. OLIVA, M.D.
Staff Physician
Division of General Internal Medicine
Rhode Island Hospital
Providence, Rhode Island

MINA B. PANTCHEVA M.D.
Resident
Internal Medicine
Roger Williams Medical Center
Providence, Rhode Island

PETER PETROPOULOS, M.D., F.A.C.C.
Clinical Assistant Professor
Brown Medical School
Department of Veterans Affairs
Providence, Rhode Island

MICHAEL PICCHIONI, M.D.
Attending Physician
Baystate Medical Center
Assistant Professor of Medicine
Tufts University School of Medicine
Springfield, Massachusetts

PAUL A. PIRRAGLIA, M.D. M.P.H.
Assistant Professor of Medicine
Brown University
Rhode Island Hospital
Providence, Rhode Island

MAURICE POLICAR, M.D.
Chief of Infectious Diseases
Elmhurst Hospital Center
Elmhurst, New York
Assistant Professor of Medicine
Mount Sinai School of Medicine
New York, New York

HEMCHAND RAMBERAN, M.D.
Resident, Internal Medicine
Memorial Hospital of Rhode Island
Brown Medical School
Providence, Rhode Island

HARLAN G. RICH, M.D.
Director of Endoscopy
Rhode Island Hospital
Associate Professor of Medicine
Brown Medical School
Providence, Rhode Island

LUTHER K. ROBINSON, M.D.
Associate Professor of Pediatrics
Director, Dysmorphology and Clinical Genetics
State University of New York at Buffalo
Buffalo, New York

SEAN I. SAVITZ, M.D.
Clinical Fellow in Neurology
Harvard Medical School
Chief Resident in Neurology
Beth Israel Deaconess Medical Center
Boston, Massachusetts

JACK L. SCHWARTZWALD, M.D.
Clinical Assistant Professor of Medicine
Brown Medical School
Rhode Island Hospital
Providence, Rhode Island

HARVEY M. SHANIES, M.D., PH.D.
Director of Critical Care Medicine
Vassar Brothers Medical Center
Poughkeepsie, New York

DEBORAH L. SHAPIRO, M.D.
Chief, Division of Rheumatology
Elmhurst Hospital Center
Elmhurst, New York
Clinical Assistant Professor of Medicine
Mount Sinai School of Medicine
New York, New York

U. SHIVRAJ SOHUR, M.D., PH.D.
Clinical Fellow in Neurology
Harvard Medical School
Chief Resident in Neurology
Beth Israel Deaconess Medical Center
Boston, Massachusetts

JENNIFER SOUTHER, M.D.
Attending Physician
Department of Family Practice
Memorial Hospital of Rhode Island
Pawtucket, Rhode Island

ANNE SPAULDING, M.D.
Centers for Disease Control and Prevention
Atlanta, Georgia

MICHELLE STOZEK, M.D.
Clinical Instructor
Brown Medical School
Division of General Internal Medicine
Rhode Island Hospital
Providence, Rhode Island

JULIE ANNE SZUMIGALA, M.D.
Clinical Instructor
Department of Obstetrics and Gynecology
State University of New York at Buffalo
Buffalo, New York

DOMINICK TAMMARO, M.D.
Associate Director, Categorical Internal Medicine
    Residency
Co-Director, Medicine-Pediatrics Residency
Division of General Internal Medicine
Rhode Island Hospital
Associate Professor of Medicine
Brown Medical School
Providence, Rhode Island

PETER E. TANGUAY, M.D.
Ackerly Professor of Child & Adolescent Psychiatry
    (Emeritus)
Department of Psychiatry and Behavioral Sciences
University of Louisville School of Medicine
Louisville, Kentucky

IRIS TONG, M.D.
Clinical Assistant Professor
Brown Medical School
Attending Physician
Women's Health Associates
Division of General Internal Medicine
Rhode Island Hospital
Providence, Rhode Island

EROBOGHENE E. UBOGU, M.B.B.S.(HONS.)
Clinical Neurophysiology Fellow
Department of Neurology
Emory University School of Medicine
Atlanta, Georgia

NICOLE J. ULLRICH, M.D., PH.D.
Clinical Fellow in Neurology/Neurooncology
Children's Hospital Boston
Boston, Massachusetts

TOM J. WACHTEL, M.D.
Physician-in-Charge
Division of Geriatrics
Rhode Island Hospital
Professor of Community Health and Medicine
Brown Medical School
Providence, Rhode Island

DENNIS M. WEPPNER, M.D., F.A.C.O.G.
Associate Professor of Clinical Gynecology/Obstetrics
State University of New York at Buffalo
Clinical Chief
Department of Gynecology/Obstetrics
Millard Fillmore Hospital
Buffalo, New York

LAUREL M. WHITE, M.D.
Clinical Assistant Professor
Department of Obstetrics and Gynecology
Division of Maternal Fetal Medicine
State University of New York at Buffalo
Buffalo, New York

JOHN M. WIECKOWSKI, M.D., PH.D., F.A.C.O.G.
Director
Reproductive Medicine and In Vitro Fertilization
Williamsville, New York

MATTHEW L. WITHIAM-LEITCH, M.D.
Clinical Instructor
Department of Obstetrics and Gynecology
State University of New York at Buffalo
Buffalo, New York

WEN-CHIH WU, M.D.
Assistant Professor of Medicine
Brown Medical School
Cardiologist
Providence VA Medical Center
Providence, Rhode Island

BETH J. WUTZ, M.D.
Clinical Assistant Professor of Medicine
Division of Internal Medicine/Pediatrics
Kajeida Health–Buffalo General Hospital
State University of New York at Buffalo
Buffalo, New York

MADHAVI YERNENI, M.D.
Staff Physician, Academic Medical Center
Miriam Hospital
Pawtucket, Rhode Island

CINDY ZADIKOFF, M.D.
Fellow, Movement Disorders
Morton and Gloria Shulman Movement Disorders
Center
Toronto Western Hospital, Toronto, Ontario

SCOTT J. ZUCCALA, D.O., F.A.C.O.G.
Staff Physician
Mercy Hospital of Buffalo
Buffalo, New York

To
OUR FAMILIES
Their constant support and encouragement
made this book a reality

Preface

This book is intended to be a clear and concise reference for the primary care physician. It is available in clinical text and CD-ROM format. Its user-friendly format was designed to provide a fast and efficient way to identify important clinical information and to offer practical guidance in patient management. The book is divided into five sections and an appendix, each with emphasis and clinical information useful to primary care physicians.

The tremendous success of the previous editions and the enthusiastic comments from numerous colleagues have brought about several positive changes. Each section has been significantly expanded from the first edition, bringing the total number of medical topics covered in this book to more than 1000. Illustrations have been added to several topics to enhance recollection of clinically important facts. A detailed table of contents facilitates identification and retrieval of topics. The use of ICD-9-CM codes in all the topics will expedite claims submission and reimbursement.

Section I describes in detail 680 medical disorders. Several new topics ranging from recently discovered disorders like Severe Respiratory Syndrome (SARS) to frequently encountered problems such as hot flashes have been added to the 2005 edition. Two new section editors have also been added for this edition. Medical topics in this section are arranged alphabetically, and the material in each topic is presented in outline format for ease of retrieval. Key, quick-access information is consistently highlighted, clinical photographs are used to further illustrate selected medical conditions, and relevant ICD-9-CM codes are listed. Most references focus on current peer-reviewed journal articles rather than outdated textbooks and old review articles. Topics in this section use the following structured approach:

1. Basic Information (Definition, Synonyms, ICD-9-CM Codes, Epidemiology and Demographics, Physical Findings and Clinical Presentation, Etiology)
2. Diagnosis (Differential Diagnosis, Workup, Laboratory Tests, Imaging Studies)
3. Treatment (Nonpharmacologic Therapy, Acute General Rx, Chronic Rx, Disposition, Referral)
4. Pearls and Considerations (Comments, References)

Section II includes the differential diagnosis, etiology, and classification of signs and symptoms. This section has been completely revised and expanded to over 300 topics for the 2005 edition. It is a practical section that allows the user investigating a physical complaint or abnormal laboratory value to follow a "workup" leading to a diagnosis. The physician can then easily look up the presumptive diagnosis in Section I for the information specific to that illness.

Section III includes clinical algorithms to guide and expedite the patient's workup and therapy. This section has been significantly expanded for the 2005 edition. Many physicians describe it as particularly valuable in today's managed care environment.

Section IV includes normal laboratory values and interpretation of results of commonly ordered laboratory tests. By providing interpretation of abnormal results, this section facilitates the diagnosis of medical disorders and further adds to the comprehensive, "one stop" nature of our text. For the 2005 edition we have adapted a one-column format for this section and added several new laboratory tests.

Section V focuses on preventive medicine and offers essential guidelines from the U.S. Preventive Services Task Force. Information in this section on clinical preventive services includes recommendations for the periodic health examination, screening for major diseases and disorders, patient counseling, and immunization and chemoprophylaxis recommendations.

The **Appendix** contains common definitions used in Complementary and Alternative Medicine (CAM), a listing of frequently used herbals with documented or suspected risks, and selected resources for complementary/alternative medicine. CAM has gained tremendous popularity over the past decade; however, the gap between allopathy and CAM remains substantive. With the material in this appendix we hope to lessen the current scarcity of exposure of allopathic physicians to the diversity of CAM therapies.

As practicing physicians, we all realize the importance of patient education and the need for clear communication with our patients. Toward that end, the CD-ROM package contains not only the entire book contents with hyperlinks to drug information, but also includes easy-to-use, practical patient instruction sheets, organized alphabetically and covering the majority of the topics in this book. Several new patient instruction sheets have been added to the 2005 edition. These Patient Teaching Guides (PTGs) are available in English and Spanish and can be easily customized and printed from any computer. They are a valuable addition to patient care and are useful to improve physician-patient communication, patient satisfaction, and quality of care. For ease of identification, each clinical topic in Section I of the book with a corresponding patient teaching guide on the CD is marked with a *"PTG"* icon after the topic name in the running head. In addition, the cross-references to the CD are included in the table of contents. The CD-ROM version of Clinical Advisor 2005 also contains several PTGs unrelated to Section I topics.

I believe that we have produced a state-of-the-art information system with significant differences from existing texts. It contains five sections that could be sold separately based on their content, yet are available under a single cover, offering the reader a tremendous value. I hope that the *Clinical Advisor's* user-friendly approach, its numerous unique features, and yearly updates will make our book and CD-ROM, as well as the PDA ancillary, valuable medical references not only to primary care physicians, but also to physicians in other specialties, medical students, and allied health professionals.

Fred F. Ferri, M.D.

Contents

Detailed Contents

SECTION I   DISEASES AND DISORDERS

PTG indicates that a patient teaching guide is available on the companion CD-ROM.

SECTION II DIFFERENTIAL DIAGNOSIS

SECTION III   CLINICAL ALGORITHMS

SECTION IV   LABORATORY TESTS AND INTERPRETATION OF RESULTS

SECTION V   CLINICAL PREVENTIVE SERVICES

APPENDIX   COMPLEMENTARY AND ALTERNATE MEDICINE

ADDITIONAL PTGS ON CD-ROM NOT LINKED TO TOPICS IN SECTION I

Diseases and Disorders

BASIC INFORMATION

DEFINITION

Abruptio placentae is the separation of placenta from the uterine wall before delivery of the fetus. There are three classes of abruption based on maternal and fetal status, including an assessment of uterine contractions, quantity of bleeding, fetal heart rate monitoring, and abnormal coagulation studies (fibrinogen, PT, PTT).

- Grade I: mild vaginal bleeding, uterine irritability, stable vital signs, reassuring fetal heart rate, normal coagulation profile (fibrinogen 450 mg %)
- Grade II: Moderate vaginal bleeding, hypertonic uterine contractions, orthostatic blood pressure measurements, unfavorable fetal status, fibrinogen 150 mg % to 250 mg %
- Grade III: severe bleeding (may be concealed), hypertonic uterine contractions, overt signs of hypovolemic shock, fetal death, thrombocytopenia, fibrinogen <150 mg %

ICD-9CM CODES

641.2 Premature separation of placenta

EPIDEMIOLOGY & DEMOGRAPHICS

INCIDENCE (IN U.S.): 1/86-206 births; incidence by grade: I = 40%, II = 45%, III = 15%; 80% occur before the onset of labor

RISK FACTORS: Hypertension (greatest association), trauma, polyhydramnios, multifetal gestation, smoking, use of crack cocaine, chorioamnionitis, preterm premature rupture of membranes

RECURRENCE RATE: 5% to 17%; with two prior episodes, 25%

PHYSICAL FINDINGS & CLINICAL PRESENTATION

- Triad of uterine bleeding (concealed or per vagina), hypertonic uterine contractions or signs of preterm labor, and evidence of fetal compromise exists.
- More than 80% of cases have external bleeding; 20% of cases have no bleeding but have indirect evidence of abruption, such as failed tocolysis for preterm labor.
- Tetanic uterine contractions are found in only 17% of cases, unless grade II or III abruption.

ETIOLOGY

- Primary etiology: unknown
- Hypertension: found in 40% to 50% of grade III abruptions

- Rapid decompression of uterine cavity, such as is found with polyhydramnios or multifetal gestation
- Blunt external trauma (motor vehicle accident, spousal abuse)

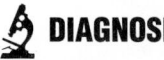 **DIAGNOSIS**

DIFFERENTIAL DIAGNOSIS

Placenta previa, cervical or vaginal trauma, labor, cervical cancer, rupture of membranes. The differential diagnosis of vaginal bleeding in pregnancy is described in Section II.

WORKUP

- Initial assessment should evaluate for the source of bleeding, ruling out placenta previa and associated conditions that contraindicate any type of vaginal examination (e.g., pelvic speculum examination).
- Continuous fetal heart monitoring is indicated for all viable gestations (60% incidence of fetal distress in labor); may show early signs of maternal hypovolemia (late decelerations or fetal tachycardia) before overt maternal vital sign changes.
- Actual amount of blood loss is often greater than initially perceived because of the possibility of concealed retroplacental bleeding and the apparent "normal" vital signs. The relative hypervolemia of pregnancy initially protects the gravida until late in the course of bleeding, when abrupt and sudden cardiovascular collapse can occur without warning.

LABORATORY TESTS

- Baseline Hgb and Hct help quantify blood loss and, even more important, with every four to six determinations can demonstrate significant trends during expectant management.
- Coagulation profile: platelets, fibrinogen, prothrombin, and partial thromboplastin time. DIC can develop with severe abruption. If fibrinogen is <150 mg %, estimated blood loss equals 2000 ml, and if fibrinogen is <100 mg %, consider FFP to prevent further bleeding.
- Type and antibody screen is important to identify Rh-negative patients who may need Rh immune globulin.

IMAGING STUDIES

Ultrasound should include fetal presentation and status, amniotic fluid volume, placental location, as well as any evidence of hematoma (retroplacental, subchorionic, or preplacental).

 TREATMENT

Treatment is dependent on gestational age of the fetus, severity of the abruption, and maternal status. Stabilization of the mother is the first priority.

ACUTE GENERAL Rx

- Initial assessment for signs of maternal hemodynamic compromise or hemorrhagic shock; large-bore intravenous access, with crystalloid fluid resuscitation using a replacement of 3 ml LR solution for every 1 ml estimated blood loss.
- Indwelling Foley catheter to monitor urine output and maternal volume status, with a goal of 30 ml/hr urine output.
- Assess fetal status and gestational age using sonogram and continuous fetal heart rate monitoring.
- Because of the unpredictable nature of abruptions, cross-matched blood should be made available during the initial resuscitation period.

CHRONIC Rx

- In the term fetus or where lung maturity has been documented, delivery is indicated.
- In the preterm fetus or with an immature lung profile, consideration should be given for betamethasone 12.5 mg IM q24h for two doses and then delivery, depending on the severity of the abruption and the likelihood of fetal complications from preterm birth.
- C-section should be reserved for cases of fetal distress or for standard obstetric indications.
- In select cases, such as severe prematurity with a stable mother and mild contractions, magnesium sulfate can be used for tocolysis, 6 g IV loading dose then 3 g/hr maintenance, to allow for course of steroids.

DISPOSITION

Because of the unpredictable nature of abruptions, expectant management should occur only under controlled circumstances.

REFERRAL

Abruptio placentae places mother and fetus in a high-risk situation and should be managed by a qualified obstetrician in a facility with capability for neonatal and maternal resuscitation and ability to perform emergency C-sections.

Author: **Scott J. Zuccala, D.O.**

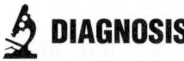 **BASIC INFORMATION**

■ **DEFINITION**
A brain abscess is a focal, intracerebral infection that begins as a localized area of cerebritis and develops into a collection of pus surrounded by a well-vascularized capsule.

ICD-9CM CODES
324.0 Brain abscess

■ **EPIDEMIOLOGY & DEMOGRAPHICS**
- Quite uncommon (occur about 2% as commonly as brain tumors)
- Occur at any age.
- Peak incidences in preadolescence and middle age.
- Most common source of underlying infection: contiguous spread from the paranasal sinuses, middle ear, or teeth.
- Headache is usually localized to the side of the abscess, onset can be gradual or severe; present in 70% of cases.

■ **PHYSICAL FINDINGS & CLINICAL PRESENTATION**
- Classic triad: fever, headache, and focal neurologic deficit are present in 50% of cases.
- Fever is present in only 50% of patients.
- Focal neurologic findings (e.g., seizures, hemiparesis, aphasia, ataxia) depend on the location of the abscess and are seen in 30% to 50% of cases.
- Papilledema is present in 25% of cases.
- Presence of adjacent infections (dental abscess, otitis media, and sinusitis) may be a clue to the underlying diagnosis and should be sought in any suspected case.

- Time course from symptom onset to presentation ranges from hours in fulminant cases to more than 1 mo; 75% present in the first 2 wk.
- The nonspecific presentation of a brain abscess warrants that clinicians maintain a high index of suspicion.

■ **ETIOLOGY**
- Brain abscesses arise from:
  Contiguous infection
  Hematogenous spread from a remote site
- They are classified based on the likely portal of entry:
Likely source of abscess:
A. Contiguous focus or primary infection (55% of all brain abscesses):
  1. Paranasal sinus: occur in frontal lobe; streptococci, *Bacteroides, Haemophilus,* and *Fusobacterium* species
  2. Otitis media/mastoiditis: occur in temporal lobe and cerebellum; streptococci, Enterobacteriaceae, *Bacteroides,* and *Pseudomonas* species
  3. Dental sepsis: occur in frontal lobe; mixed *Fusobacterium, Bacteroides,* and *Streptococcus* species
  4. Penetrating head injury: site of abscess depends on site of wound; *Staphylococcus aureus, Clostridium* species, Enterobacteriaceae species
  5. Postoperative: *Staphylococcus epidermidis* and *S. aureus,* Enterobacteriaceae, and Pseudomonadaceae
B. Hematogenous spread/distant site of infection (25% of all brain abscesses): abscesses most commonly multiple, especially in middle cerebral artery distribution; infecting organisms depend on source.
  1. Congenital heart disease: streptococci, *Haemophilus* species
  2. Endocarditis: *S. aureus,* viridans streptococci
  3. Urinary tract: Enterobacteriaceae, Pseudomonadaceae

  4. Intraabdominal: streptococci, Enterobacteriaceae, anaerobes
  5. Lung: streptococci, *Actinomyces* species, *Fusobacterium* species
  6. Immunocompromised host: *Toxoplasma* species, fungi, Enterobacteriaceae, *Nocardia* species, tuberculosis, listeriosis
C. Cryptogenic (unknown source): 20% of all brain abscesses

DIAGNOSIS

■ **DIFFERENTIAL DIAGNOSIS**
- Other parameningeal infections: subdural empyema, epidural abscess, thrombophlebitis of the major dural venous sinuses and cortical veins
- Embolic strokes in patients with bacterial endocarditis
- Mycotic aneurysms with leakage
- Viral encephalitis (usually resulting from herpes simplex)
- Acute hemorrhagic leukoencephalitis
- Parasitic infections: toxoplasmosis, echinococcosis, cysticercosis
- Metastatic or primary brain tumors
- Cerebral infarction
- CNS vasculitis
- Chronic subdural hematoma

■ **WORKUP**
Physical examination, laboratory tests, and imaging studies

■ **LABORATORY TESTS**
- WBC counts are elevated in 60% of patients.
- ESR is usually elevated, but may be normal.
- Blood cultures are most often negative (10% positive).
- Lumbar puncture is contraindicated in patients with suspected abscess (20% die or suffer neurologic decline).
- The yield of Gram stain and culture of material aspirated at time of surgical drainage approaches 100%.

■ IMAGING STUDIES
- MRI is the diagnostic procedure of choice; provides superior detail compared with CT scan (higher sensitivity and specificity than CT scan, but not always immediately available).
- CT scan (Fig. 1-1) with intravenous contrast is still an excellent test (sensitivity 95% to 99%).
- Serial CT or MRI scanning is recommended to follow the response to therapy.

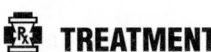 **TREATMENT**

Effective treatment involves a combination of empiric antibiotic therapy and timely excision or aspiration of the abscess.

■ ACUTE GENERAL Rx
- If evidence of edema or mass effect, treatment of elevated intracranial pressure is paramount (includes hyperventilation of the mechanically ventilated patient, dexamethasone, mannitol).
- Medical therapy is never a substitute for surgical intervention to relieve increased intracranial pressure.
- Steroids should be limited to patients with severe cerebral edema or midline shift.

■ MEDICAL Rx
Empiric antibiotic therapy guided by:
- Abscess location
- Suspicion of primary source
- Presence of single or multiple abscesses
- Patient's underlying medical conditions (e.g., HIV, immunocompromised)

Selection of empiric antibiotic therapy:
- Primary infection or contiguous source:
  1. Otitis media/mastoiditis, sinusitis, dental infection: third-generation cephalosporin (cefotaxime 2 g q6h IV or ceftriaxone 2 g q12h IV) plus metronidazole 7.5 mg/kg q6h IV or 15 mg/kg q12h IV
  2. Dental infection: penicillin G 6 million units q6° plus metronidazole
  3. Head trauma or postcranial surgery: third-generation cephalosporin plus metronidazole and nafcillin or vancomycin 1 g q12h IV
- Hematogenous spread (congenital heart disease, endocarditis, urinary tract, lung, intraabdominal): nafcillin or vancomycin plus metronidazole plus third-generation cephalosporin

Duration of antibiotic therapy is unclear. Most recommend parenteral treatment for 4 to 8 wk, with repeated neuroimaging to ensure adequate treatment. (Imaging suggested every wk for first 2 wk of therapy, then every 2 wk until antibiotics finished, and then every 2 to 4 mo for 1 yr to monitor for disease recurrence.)

■ SURGICAL Rx
- Two indications:
  1. Collect specimens for culture and sensitivity
  2. Reduce mass effect
- Stereotactic biopsy or aspirate of the abscess if surgically feasible
- Essential to selection of targeted antimicrobial coverage
- Timing and choice of surgery depends on:
  Primary infection source
  Number and location of the abscesses
  Whether the procedure is diagnostic or therapeutic
  Neurologic status of the patient

■ DISPOSITION
- Prompt diagnostic consideration, early institution of appropriate antimicrobial therapy, and advanced neuroradiologic imaging have reduced the mortality resulting from brain abscesses from 40% to 80% in the preantibiotic era to 10% to 20% at present.
- Morbidity is usually manifest as persistent neurologic sequelae (seizures, intellectual or behavioral impairment, motor deficits) seen in 20% to 60% of patients.

■ REFERRAL
Consultation with a neurosurgeon is mandatory.

REFERENCE
Calfee DP, Wispelwey B: Brain abscess, *Semin Neurol* 20(3):353, 2000.
Author: **Kelly McGarry, M.D.**

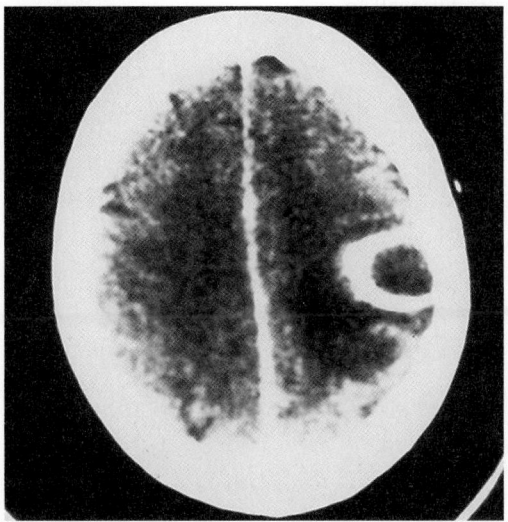

Fig. 1-1   Computed tomography (CT) scan showing a brain abscess. A woman presented to physicians after a focal seizure followed by headache and weakness of the arm. Dental work had been performed several weeks before. CT scan revealed a contrast-enhanced, ringlike mass surrounded by edema. It is not possible on this scan to differentiate tumor from abscess. At surgery a well-encapsulated abscess was encountered. (From Andreoli TE [ed]: *Cecil essentials of medicine,* ed 4, Philadelphia, 1997, WB Saunders.)

BASIC INFORMATION

■ DEFINITION

Breast abscess is an acute inflammatory process resulting in the formation of a collection of pus. Typically there is painful erythematous mass formation in the breast, occasionally with draining through the overlying skin or nipple duct opening.

■ SYNONYMS

Subareolar abscess
Lactational or puerperal abscess

ICD-9CM CODES

6.110 Abscess of the breast
675.0 Abscess of the nipple related to childbirth
675.1 Abscess of the breast related to childbirth

■ EPIDEMIOLOGY & DEMOGRAPHICS

- 10% to 30% of all breast abscesses are lactational.
- Acute mastitis occurs in 2.5% of nursing mothers, with 1 in 15 of these women developing abscess.

■ PHYSICAL FINDINGS & CLINICAL PRESENTATION

Painful erythematous induration involving the part of the breast leading to fluctuant abscess

■ ETIOLOGY

- Lactational abscess: milk stasis and bacterial infection leading to mastitis, then to abscess, with *Staphylococcus aureus* the most common causative agent

- Subareolar abscess:
  1. Central ducts involved, with obstructive nipple duct changes leading to bacterial infection
  2. Cultured organisms mixed, including anaerobes, staphylococci, streptococci, and others

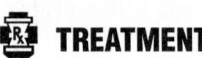 DIAGNOSIS

■ DIFFERENTIAL DIAGNOSIS

- Inflammatory carcinoma
- Advanced carcinoma with erythema, edema, and/or ulceration
- Rarely, tuberculous abscess
- Hydradenitis of breast skin
- Sebaceous cyst with infection

■ WORKUP

- Clinical examination sufficient
- If abscess suspected, referral to surgeon for incision, drainage, and biopsy
- If possible abscess or advanced carcinoma, referral for workup required

■ LABORATORY TESTS

- Perform C&S test of abscess contents.
- If mammogram or ultrasound prevented by discomfort, perform after resolution of abscess if required.

TREATMENT

■ NONPHARMACOLOGIC THERAPY

- Established abscess: incision and drainage, preferably with general anesthesia
- Biopsy of abscess cavity wall to exclude carcinoma

■ ACUTE GENERAL RX

- Antibiotics: the pathogen is generally staphylococci in lactational abscess. Recommended initial antibiotic therapy is with nafcillin or oxacillin 2 g q4h IV or cefazolin 1g q8h IV.
- If acute mastitis is treated early, resolution without drainage is possible.
- Subareolar abscess: broad-spectrum antibiotic treatment and drainage are needed to control acute phase.

■ CHRONIC Rx

Further surgical treatment for recurrences or fistula

■ DISPOSITION

- Lactational abscess: possible to continue breast-feeding without apparent risk of infection to the infant
- Subareolar abscess:
  1. Notorious for recurrence or complication of fistula formation
  2. Patient informed and referred for subsequent care

■ REFERRAL

- If abscess drainage required
- For surgical consultation if subareolar abscess involved

REFERENCES

Schwarz RJ, Shrestha R: Needle aspiration of breast abscesses, *Am J Surg* 182(2):117, 2001.
Tan YM, Yeo A, Chia KH, Wong CY: Breast abscess as the initial presentation of squamous cell of the breast, *Eur J Surg Oncol* 28(1):91, 2002.
Author: Takuma Nemoto, M.D.

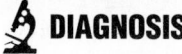
 BASIC INFORMATION

■ **DEFINITION**
Liver abscess is a necrotic infection of the liver usually classified as pyogenic or amebic.

■ **SYNONYMS**
Pyogenic hepatic abscess
Amebic hepatic abscess

ICD-9CM CODES
572.0 Abscess of liver

■ **EPIDEMIOLOGY & DEMOGRAPHICS**
• Worldwide, amebic liver abscess is more common than pyogenic liver abscess.
• In the U.S., pyogenic liver abscess is more common than amebic liver abscess.
• Incidence of pyogenic liver abscess is 8 to 15 cases per 100,000 population.
• Amebic liver abscesses complicate amebic colitis in nearly 10% of cases.
• Most abscesses occur on the right lobe of the liver.
• More common in men than women. Male:female ratio of 2:1.
• Most common in fourth to sixth decade of life.

■ **PHYSICAL FINDINGS & CLINICAL PRESENTATION**
• Fever, chills, and sweats
• Anorexia with weight loss
• Nausea, vomiting, and diarrhea
• Cough with pleuritic chest pain
• Right upper quadrant abdominal pain
• Hepatomegaly
• Splenomegaly
• Jaundice
• Pleural effusions, rales, and friction rubs may be present

■ **ETIOLOGY**
• Pyogenic liver abscess is usually polymicrobial (*E. coli* (33%), *K. pneumoniae* (18%), *Streptococcal Sp* (37%), *P. aeruginosa*, *Proteus*, *Bacteroides* (24%), *Fusobacterium*, *Actinomyces*, gram-positive anaerobes and *S. aureus*).
• Amebic hepatic abscess is caused by the parasite *Entamoeba histolytica*.
• Pyogenic liver abscess occurs from:
  1. Biliary disease with cholangitis (accounts for approximately 21% to 30%)
  2. Gallbladder disease with contiguous spread to the liver
  3. Diverticulitis or appendicitis with spread via the portal circulation
  4. Hematogenous spread via the hepatic artery
  5. Penetrating wounds
  6. Cryptogenic
  7. Infection via portal system (portal pyemia)
  8. No causes found in approximately half of cases
  9. Incidence increased in patients with diabetes and metastatic cancer
• Amebiasis is usually due to fecal-oral contamination and invades the intestinal mucosa gaining entry into the portal system to reach the liver.

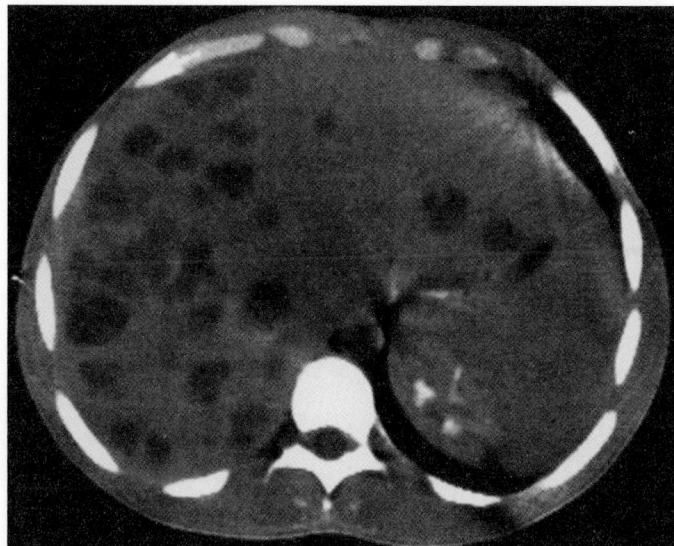

Fig. 1-2 CT scan demonstrating multiple pyogenic liver abscesses in a 25-year-old man. (From Goldman L, Bennett JC [ed]: *Cecil textbook of medicine*, ed 21, Philadelphia, 2000, WB Saunders.)

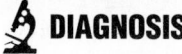 **DIAGNOSIS**

The diagnosis of liver abscess requires a high index of suspicion after a detailed history and physical examination. Imaging studies with diagnostic aspiration confirm the presence of a liver abscess.

■ **DIFFERENTIAL DIAGNOSIS**
• Cholangitis
• Cholecystitis
• Diverticulitis
• Appendicitis
• Perforated viscus
• Mesentery ischemia
• Pulmonary embolism
• Pancreatitis

■ **WORKUP**
• The workup of a liver abscess should focus on differentiating between amebic and pyogenic causes.
• Features suggesting an amebic cause are travel to an endemic area, single abscess rather than multiple abscesses, subacute onset of symptoms, and absence of conditions predisposing to pyogenic liver abscess as highlighted under "Etiology."
• Laboratory studies are not specific but useful as adjunctive tests.
• Imaging studies cannot differentiate between the two, and bacteriologic cultures may be sterile in 50% of the cases.

■ **LABORATORY TESTS**
• CBC showing leukocytosis
• Liver function tests: alkaline phosphatase is most commonly elevated (95% to 100%); AST and ALT elevated in 50% of cases; elevated bilirubin (28% to 30%); decreased albumin
• PT (INR) prolonged (70%)
• Blood cultures positive in 50% of cases
• Aspiration (50% sterile)
• Stool samples for *E. histolytica* trophozoites (positive in 10% to 15% of amebic liver abscess cases)
• Serologic testing for *E. histolytica* does not differentiate acute from old infections

■ **IMAGING STUDIES**
• Chest x-ray examination abnormal in 50% of the cases showing elevated right hemidiaphragm, subdiaphragmatic air fluid levels, pleural effusions, and consolidating infiltrates.
• Ultrasound (80% to 100% sensitivity in detecting abscesses) seen as round or oval hypoechogenic mass.
• CT scans more sensitive in detecting hepatic abscesses and contiguous organ extension (Fig. 1-2). Imaging study of choice.

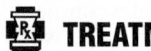
- Most liver abscesses are single; however, multiple liver abscesses are seen with systemic bacteremia.

TREATMENT

■ NONPHARMACOLOGIC THERAPY
- The management of pyogenic liver abscess differs from that of amebic liver abscess.
- Medical management is the cornerstone of therapy in amebic liver abscess, whereas early intervention in the form of surgical therapy or catheter drainage and parenteral antibiotics is the rule in pyogenic liver abscess.

■ ACUTE GENERAL Rx
- Percutaneous drainage under CT or ultrasound guidance is essential in the treatment of pyogenic liver abscesses.
- Aspiration of hepatic amebic abscesses is not required unless there is no response to treatment or a pyogenic cause is being considered.
- Antibiotic treatment for pyogenic liver abscess initially is empirical triple therapy with penicillin, aminoglycoside, and metronidazole.
  1. In severely ill patients, parenteral antibiotics with cefotaxime or piperacillin/tazobactam and metronidazole for 2 wk followed by a 4- to 6-wk PO therapy is recommended.
  2. Clindamycin with an aminoglycoside or imipenem alone are alternative choices.

- Antibiotic coverage for amebic liver abscesses includes:
  1. Metronidazole 750 mg PO tid for 10 days
  2. Dehydroemetine 1 mg/kg/day IM for 5 days followed by chloroquine 1 g/day for 2 days; then 500 mg/day for 2 to 3 wk can be used as an alternative to metronidazole

■ CHRONIC Rx
- If fever persists for 2 wk despite percutaneous drainage and antibiotic therapy as outlined under "Acute General Rx," or if there is failure of aspiration or failure of percutaneous drainage, surgery is indicated.
- In patients with evidence of metastatic disease that is causing biliary obstruction, a gastroenterology consultation for ERCP and stenting should be considered.

■ DISPOSITION
- Most patients with pyogenic liver abscesses defervesce within 2 wk of treatment with antibiotics and drainage.
- Pyogenic liver abscess cure rates using percutaneous drainage and antibiotics have been reported to be between 88% and 100%.
- Mortality of untreated pyogenic liver abscess is nearly 100%.
- Most patients with amebic liver abscesses defervesce within 4 to 5 days of treatment.
- Amebic liver abscess mortality rate is <1% unless complications occur (see under Comments).

■ REFERRAL
Infectious disease, gastroenterology, interventional radiology, and general surgical consultations are recommended in any patient with a single hepatic abscess or multiple abscesses.

PEARLS & CONSIDERATIONS

■ COMMENTS
- Complications of pyogenic and amebic liver abscesses include:
  1. Pleuropulmonary extension resulting in empyema, abscess, and fistula formation
  2. Peritonitis
  3. Purulent pericarditis
  3. Sepsis

REFERENCES

Kar P, Kapoor S, Jain A: Pyogenic liver abscess: aetiology, clinical manifestations and management, *Trop Gastroenterol* 19(4):136, 1998.

Krige JE, Beckingham IJ: ABC of diseases of liver, pancreas, and biliary system, *BMJ* 322(7285):537, 2001.

Liew KVS et al: Pyogenic liver abscess: a tropical centre's experience in management with review of current literature, *Singapore Med J* 41(10):489, 2000.

Sharma MP, Ahuja V: Management of amebic and pyogenic liver abscess, *Indian J Gastroenterol Suppl* 1:C33, 2001.

Authors: **Hemchand Ramberan, M.D., and Peter Petropoulos, M.D.**

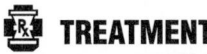
 BASIC INFORMATION

■ **DEFINITION**
A lung abscess is an infection of the lung parenchyma resulting in a necrotic cavity containing pus.

■ **SYNONYMS**
Pulmonary abscess

ICD-9CM CODES
513.0 Abscess of lung

■ **EPIDEMIOLOGY & DEMOGRAPHICS**
• Incidence has decreased over the last 30 years as a result of antibiotic therapy.
• Lung abscess in patients age 50 and over is associated with primary lung neoplasia in 30% of the cases.
• Lung abscesses commonly coexist with empyemas.
• Risk factor population includes patients with:
  1. Alcohol-related problems
  2. Seizure disorders
  3. Cerebrovascular disorders with dysphagia
  4. Drug abuse
  5. Esophageal disorders (e.g., scleroderma, esophageal carcinoma, etc.)
  6. Poor oral hygiene
  7. Obstructive malignant lung disease
  8. Bronchiectasis

■ **PHYSICAL FINDINGS & CLINICAL PRESENTATION**
• Symptoms are generally insidious and prolonged, occurring for weeks to months
• Fever, chills, and sweats
• Cough
• Sputum production (purulent with foul odor)
• Pleuritic chest pain
• Hemoptysis
• Dyspnea
• Malaise, fatigue, and weakness
• Tachycardia and tachypnea
• Dullness to percussion, whispered pectoriloquy, and bronchophony

■ **ETIOLOGY**
• The most important factor predisposing to lung abscess is aspiration.
• Following aspiration as a major predisposing factor is periodontal disease.
• Lung abscess is rare in an edentulous person.
• Approximately 90% of lung abscesses are caused by anaerobic microorganisms (*Bacteroides fragilis, Fusobacterium nucleatum, Peptostreptococcus,* microaerophilic *Streptococcus*).

• In most cases anaerobic infection is mixed with aerobic or facultative anaerobic organisms (*S. aureus, E. coli, K. pneumoniae, P. aeruginosa*).
• Parasitic organisms including Paragonimus westermani and Entamoeba histolytica.
• Fungi including *Aspergillus, Cryptococcus, Histoplasma, Blastomyces,* and *Coccidioides.*
• Immunocompromised hosts may become infected with *Aspergillus,* mycobacteria, *Nocardia,* and *Rhodococcus equi.*

🔬 **DIAGNOSIS**

Lung abscess may be primary or secondary.
• Primary lung abscess refers to infection from normal host organisms within the lung (e.g., aspiration, pneumonia).
• Secondary lung abscess results from other preexisting conditions (e.g., endocarditis, underlying lung cancer, pulmonary emboli).
Lung abscess may be acute or chronic.
• Acute lung abscess is present if symptoms are of less than 4 to 6 wk.
• Chronic lung abscess is present if symptoms are greater than 6 wk.

■ **DIFFERENTIAL DIAGNOSIS**
The differential diagnosis is similar to cavitary lung lesions:
• Bacterial (anaerobic, aerobic, infected bulla, empyema, actinomycosis, tuberculosis)
• Fungal (histoplasmosis, coccidioidomycosis, blastomycosis, aspergillosis, cryptococcosis)
• Parasitic (amebiasis, echinococcosis)
• Malignancy (primary lung carcinoma, metastatic lung disease, lymphoma, Hodgkin's disease)
• Wegener's granulomatosis, sarcoidosis, endocarditis, and septic pulmonary emboli

■ **WORKUP**
• The workup of a patient with lung abscess attempts to elicit a primary or a secondary cause.
• Blood tests are not specific in diagnosing lung abscesses.
• Most diagnoses are made from imaging studies; however, to diagnose a specific cause bacteriologic studies are needed.

■ **LABORATORY TESTS**
• CBC with leukocytosis
• Bacteriologic studies
  1. Sputum Gram stain and culture (commonly contaminated by oral flora)
  2. Percutaneous transtracheal aspiration

  3. Percutaneous transthoracic aspiration
  4. Fiberoptic bronchoscopy using bronchial brushings or bronchoalveolar lavage is the most widely used intervention when trying to obtain diagnostic bacteriologic cultures
• Blood cultures on some occasions may be positive
• If an empyema is present, obtaining empyema fluid via thoracentesis may isolate the organism

■ **IMAGING STUDIES**
• Chest x-ray examination makes the diagnosis of lung abscess showing the cavitary lesion with an air fluid level.
• Lung abscesses are most commonly found in the posterior segment of the right upper lobe.
• Chest CT scan can localize and size the lesion and assist in differentiating lung abscesses from other pathologic processes (e.g., tumor, empyema, infected bulla, etc.) (Fig. 1-3).

℞ **TREATMENT**

■ **NONPHARMACOLOGIC THERAPY**
• Oxygen therapy
• Postural drainage
• Respiratory therapy maneuvers

■ **ACUTE GENERAL Rx**
• Penicillin 1 to 2 million units IV q4h until improvement (e.g., afebrile, decrease in sputum production, etc.) followed by penicillin VK 500 mg PO qid for the next 2 to 3 wk but usually requiring longer 6- to 8-wk courses.
• Metronidazole is given with penicillin at doses of 7.5 mg/kg IV q6h followed by PO 500 mg bid to qid dosing.
• Clindamycin is an alternative choice if concerned about penicillin-resistant organisms. The dose is 600 mg IV q8h until improvement, followed by 300 mg PO q6h.

■ **CHRONIC Rx**
• Bronchoscopy to assist with drainage and/or diagnosis is indicated in patients who fail to respond to antibiotics or if there is suspected underlying malignancy.
• Surgery is indicated on rare occasions (<10%) in patients with complications of lung abscess (see Comments).

■ DISPOSITION
- More than 95% of patients are cured with the use of antibiotics alone.
- Complications of lung abscesses include:
  1. Empyema
  2. Massive hemoptysis
  3. Pneumothorax
  4. Bronchopleural fistula
- Mortality is low in community-acquired lung abscess (2.5%).
- Hospital-acquired lung abscess carries a high mortality rate (65%).

■ REFERRAL
If lung abscess is present, consultation with pulmonary and infectious disease specialist is recommended.

⚙ PEARLS & CONSIDERATIONS

■ COMMENTS
- Complications of lung abscesses include:
  1. Empyema
  2. Bronchopleural fistula
  3. Hepatobronchial fistula
  4. Brain abscess
  5. Bronchiectasis
- Refractory cases are usually the result of:
  1. Large cavity size (>6 cm)
  2. Recurrent aspiration
  3. Thick-walled cavities
  4. Underlying lung carcinoma
  5. Empyema formation
- Necrotizing pneumonia is similar to a lung abscess but differs in size (<2 cm in diameter) and number (usually multiple suppurative cavitary lesions)

REFERENCES
Cassiere HA, Niederman MS: Aspiration pneumonia, lipoid pneumonia, and lung abscess. In Baum GL et al: *Textbook of pulmonary diseases,* ed 6, New York, 1998, Lippincott-Raven.

Finegold SM: Lung abscess. In *Mandell, Douglas, and Bennett's principles and practice of infectious diseases,* ed 5, New York, 2000, Churchill Livingstone.

Hirshberg B, Sklair-Levi M, Nir-Paz R et al: Factors predicting mortality of patients with lung abscess, *Chest* 115:746, 1999.

Mwandumba HC, Beeching NJ: Pyogenic lung infections: factors for predicting clinical outcome of lung abscess and thoracic empyema, *Curr Opin Pulm Med* 6(3):234, 2000.

Rowe S, Cheadle WG: Complications of nosocomial pneumonia in the surgical patient, *Am J Surg* 179(2A suppl):63s, 2000.

Wiedemann HP, Rice TW: Lung abscess and empyema, *Semin Thorac Cardiovasc Surg* 7:119, 1995.

Authors: **Peter Petropoulos, M.D., and Dennis J. Mikolich, M.D.**

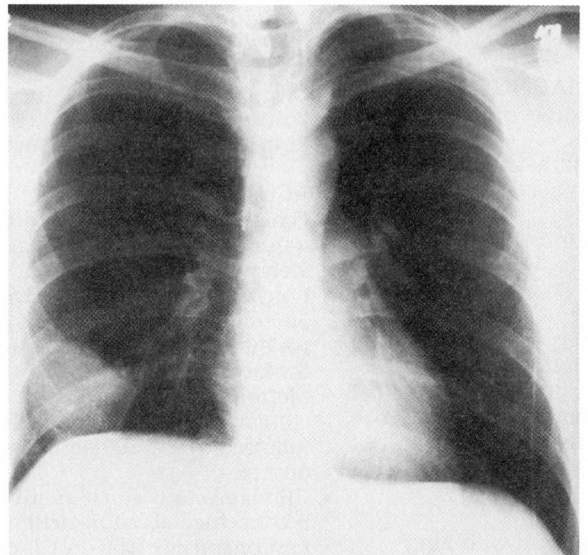
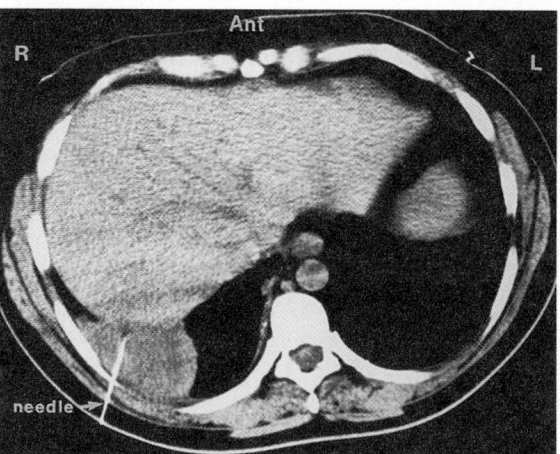

Fig. 1-3 Lung abscess. On a chest radiograph, a lung abscess may look to be a solid rounded lesion **(A),** or, if it has a connection with the bronchus, there may be an air fluid level in a thick-walled cavitary lesion. CT scanning **(B)** can be used to localize the lesion and to place a needle for drainage and aspiration of contents for culture. (From Mettler FA [ed]: *Primary care radiology,* Philadelphia, 2000, WB Saunders.)

BASIC INFORMATION

■ DEFINITION
Pelvic abscess is an acute or chronic infection, most commonly involving the pelvic viscera, initially localized and thus creating its own unique environment, so that treatment and possible cure require specific therapy. There are four categories based on etiologic factors:
- Ascending infection, spreading from cervix through endometrial cavity to adnexa, forming a tuboovarian complex
- Infection occurring in the puerperium, which spreads to the adnexa from the endometrium or myometrium via hematogenous or lymphatic route
- Abscess complicating pelvic surgery
- Involvement of the pelvic viscera secondary to spread from contiguous organs, such as appendicitis or diverticulitis

■ SYNONYMS
Tuboovarian abscess (TOA)
Vaginal cuff abscess

ICD-9CM CODES
614.2 Salpingitis and oophoritis not specified as acute, subacute, or chronic

■ EPIDEMIOLOGY & DEMOGRAPHICS
INCIDENCE:
- 34% of hospitalized patients with PID
- 1% to 2% of patients undergoing hysterectomy, most with vaginal approach
- Peak incidence third to fourth decade
- 25% to 50% are nulliparous
RISK FACTORS: Same risk factors as for PID, although in 30% to 50% of patients there is no prior history of salpingitis before abscess forms.

■ PHYSICAL FINDINGS & CLINICAL PRESENTATION
- Abdominal or pelvic pain (90%)
- Fever or chills (50%)
- Abnormal bleeding (21%)
- Vaginal discharge (28%)
- Nausea (26%)
- Up to 60% to 80% present in the absence of fever or leukocytosis; lack of these findings should not rule out diagnosis

■ ETIOLOGY
- Mixed flora of anaerobes, aerobes, and facultative anaerobes, such as *E. coli, B. fragilis, Prevotella* species, aerobic streptococci, *Peptococcus,* and *Peptostreptococcus.*
- *N. gonorrhoeae* and *Chlamydia* are the major etiologic factors in cervicitis and salpingitis but are rarely found in abscess cavity cultures.

- In elderly patients consider diverticular disease.

DIAGNOSIS

■ DIFFERENTIAL DIAGNOSIS
- Pelvic neoplasms, such as ovarian tumors and leiomyomas
- Inflammatory masses involving adjacent bowel or omentum, such as ruptured appendicitis or diverticulitis
- Pelvic hematomas, as may occur after C-section or hysterectomy
- Section III, Fig. 3-140 describes the diagnostic approach to patients with a pelvic mass; the differential diagnosis of pelvic mass is described in Section II.
- The differential diagnosis of pelvic pain is described in Section II.
- Physical examination
- Sonogram or CT scan: commonly employed because, owing to associated pain and guarding, a suboptimal abdominal or pelvic examination is the rule rather than the exception
- Most common cause of preventable death: physician delay in diagnosis

■ LABORATORY TESTS
- CBC including WBC with differential, Hgb, and Hct
- Aerobic as well as anaerobic cultures of cervix, blood, urine, sputum, peritoneal cavity (if entered), and abscess cavity before starting antibiotics
- Pregnancy test in patients of reproductive age if the possibility of pregnancy exists

■ IMAGING STUDIES
- Sonogram: noninvasive, inexpensive study to confirm diagnosis, estimate size of abscess, and monitor response to therapy; sensitivity >90%
- CT scan: used for both diagnosis and therapy (CT-guided drainage)
  1. Primary focus where sonogram provided insufficient information, as with intraabdominal vs. pelvic abscesses
  2. Success rate with CT-guided abscess drainage: unilocular, 90%; multilocular, 40%

TREATMENT

Major concerns:
1. Desire for future fertility
2. Likelihood of rupture of abscess, with resulting peritonitis, septic shock, and morbid sequelae

■ ACUTE GENERAL Rx
- Decision as to whether patient requires immediate surgery (uncertain diagnosis or suspicion of rupture) or

management with IV antibiotics, reserving surgery for those with inadequate clinical response (e.g., 48 to 72 hr of therapy, with persistent fever or leukocytosis, increasing size of mass, or suspicion of rupture)
- Poor response to medical therapy in those with adnexal masses >8 cm, bilateral disease, or immunocompromise
- Antibiotic combinations:
  1. Clindamycin 900 mg IV q8h or metronidazole 500 mg IV q6-8h plus gentamicin either 5 to 7 mg/kg q24h or 1.5 mg/kg q8h
  2. Alternatives: ampicillin sulbactam 3 g IV q6h or cefoxitin 2 g IV q6h or cefotetan 2 g IV q12h plus doxycycline 100 mg IV q12h
- During medical management, high index of suspicion for acute rupture, such as acute worsening of abdominal pain or new-onset tachycardia and hypotension, mandating immediate surgical intervention after patient stabilization
- Surgical options:
  1. Laparoscopy with drainage and irrigation
  2. Transvaginal colpotomy (abscess must be midline, dissect rectovaginal septum, and be adherent to vaginal fornix)
  3. Laparotomy, including total abdominal hysterectomy with bilateral salpingo-oophorectomy or unilateral salpingo-oophorectomy
  4. Evidence of ruptured TOA = surgical emergency

■ DISPOSITION
- Of patients treated with medical therapy, response in 75%, with a 50% pregnancy rate
- No response in 30% to 40%; can be treated with either CT-guided drainage or surgical intervention, keeping in mind that unilateral adnexectomy may give equal chance of cure vs. hysterectomy, yet preserve reproductive potential

■ REFERRAL
If patient has a TOA, refer to gynecologist.

PEARLS & CONSIDERATIONS

■ COMMENTS
If *Actinomyces* species is isolated from culture, treatment with penicillin is required for an extended period (6 wk to 3 mo).

REFERENCE
Aimakhu CO, Olayemi O, Odukogbe AA: Surgical management of pelvic abscess: laparotomy versus colpotomy, *J Obstet Gynaecol* 23(1):71, 2003.
Author: **Scott J. Zuccala, D.O.**

BASIC INFORMATION

■ DEFINITION

A perirectal abscess is a localized inflammatory process that can be associated with infections of soft tissue and anal glands based on anatomic location. Perianal and perirectal abscesses may be simple or complex, causing suppuration. Infections in these spaces may be classified as superficial perianal or perirectal with involvement in the following anatomic spaces: ischiorectal, intersphincteric, pestianal, and supraelevator (Fig. 1-4).

■ SYNONYMS

Rectal abscess
Perianal abscess
Anorectal abscess

ICD-9CM CODES

566 Perirectal abscess

■ EPIDEMIOLOGY & DEMOGRAPHICS

INCIDENCE (IN U.S.): Commonly encountered
PREDOMINANT SEX: Male > female
PREDOMINANT AGE: All ages
PEAK INCIDENCE: Not seasonal; common
GENETICS: None known

■ PHYSICAL FINDINGS & CLINICAL PRESENTATION

- Localized perirectal or anal pain—often worsened with movement or straining
- Perirectal erythema or cellulitis
- Perirectal mass by inspection or palpation
- Fever and signs of sepsis with deep abscess
- Urinary retention

■ ETIOLOGY

Polymicrobial aerobic and anaerobic bacteria involving one of the anatomic spaces (see Definition), often associated with localized trauma
Microbiology: most bacteria are polymicrobial, mixed enteric and skin flora
Predominant anaerobic bacteria:
- *Bacteroides fragilis*
- *Peptostreptococcus* spp.
- *Prevotella* spp.
- *Fusobacterium* spp.
- *Porphyromonas* spp.
- *Clostridium* spp.
Predominant aerobic bacteria:
- *Staphylococcus aureus*
- *Streptococcus* spp.
- *Escherichia coli*

DIAGNOSIS

Many patients will have predisposing underlying conditions including:
- Malignancy or leukemia
- Immune deficiency
- Diabetes mellitus
- Recent surgery
- Steroid therapy

■ DIFFERENTIAL DIAGNOSIS

- Neutropenic enterocolitis
- Crohn's disease (inflammatory bowel disease)
- Pilonidal disease
- Hidradenitis suppurativa
- Tuberculosis or actinomycosis; Chagas' disease
- Cancerous lesions
- Chronic anal fistula
- Rectovaginal fistula
- Proctitis—often STD-associated, including:
  Syphilis
  Gonococcal
  Chlamydia
  Chancroid
  Condylomata acuminata
- AIDS-associated:
  Kaposi's sarcoma
  Lymphoma
  CMV

■ WORKUP

- Examination of rectal, perirectal/perineal areas
- Rule out necrotic process and crepitance suggesting deep tissue involvement
- Local aerobic and anaerobic culture
- Blood cultures if toxic, febrile, or compromised
- Possible sigmoidoscopy

■ IMAGING STUDIES

Usually not indicated unless extensive disease abscess

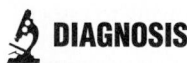 TREATMENT

- Incision and drainage of abscess
- Debridement if necrotic tissue
- Rule out need for fistulectomy
- Local wound care—packing
- Sitz baths
Antibiotic treatment: Directed toward coverage for mixed skins and enteric flora

Outpatient—oral:	Amoxicillin clavulanic acid (Augmentin) Ciprofloxacin plus metronidazole or clindamycin
Inpatient—intravenous:	Ampicillin/ sulbactam (Unasyn) Cefotetan Piperacillin/ Tazobactam Imipenem

REFERENCES

Nelson RL et al: Prevalence of benign anorectal disease in a randomly selected population, *Dis Colon Rectum* 88:341, 1994.
Nomikos IN: Anorectal abscesses: need for accurate anatomical localization of the disease, *Clin Anat* 10:239, 1997.
Author: **Dennis J. Mikolich, M.D.**

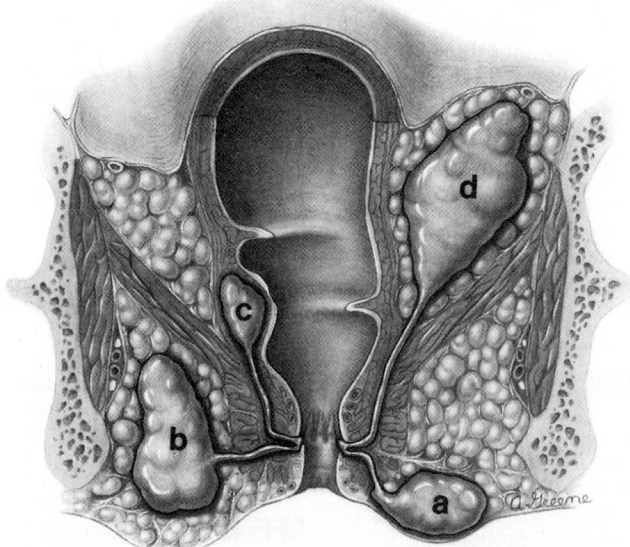

Fig. 1-4 Common sites of anorectal abscesses: perianal *(a)*, ischiorectal *(b)*, intersphincteric *(c)*, and supralevator *(d)*.(From Noble J [ed]: *Textbook of primary care medicine*, ed 2, St Louis, 1996, Mosby.)

BASIC INFORMATION

■ DEFINITION

Child abuse refers to the intentional maltreatment by a caregiver of any child under the age of 18 yr. Four categories are generally defined:
1. Neglect: failure to provide basic needs such as food, shelter, supervision
2. Physical abuse: infliction of bodily injury or harm
3. Sexual abuse: passive or active use or exposure of children to sexual acts
4. Emotional abuse: humiliating, coercive behavior that retards a child's psychologic development

■ SYNONYMS

Child maltreatment
Child neglect
Sexual abuse
"Shaken baby syndrome"
"Battered child syndrome"

ICD-9CM CODES

995.5 Child maltreatment syndrome

■ EPIDEMIOLOGY & DEMOGRAPHICS

INCIDENCE (IN U.S.):
- 1.2 cases/100,000 persons/yr (70% physical abuse, 25% sexual abuse, 5% neglect)
- Death rate: 1000 to 4000 children/yr
- 10% of emergency injuries for children <5 yr of age
- 2.3% of children with any life-threatening event

PREVALENCE (IN U.S.): More than 5% of children <18 yr of age
PREDOMINANT SEX: Females may be at a slightly greater risk.
PREDOMINANT AGE:
- Incidence of all forms of abuse increases with age; teenagers are at twice the risk of infants.
- Risk of death is much higher in children <5 yr.
- Of the 1000 to 4000 annual deaths attributable to abuse, 80% are in children <5 yr, and 40% are in children <1 yr of age. For children <6 mo of age, abuse is the second-leading cause of death (sudden infant death is first).

PEAK INCIDENCE:
- Approximately one third before the age of 1 yr, one third between 1 yr and 6 yr, and one third above age 6 yr
- Handicapped children at a much greater risk throughout childhood

GENETICS:
- No genetic factors are known.
- Sexual abuse is equally distributed throughout all socioeconomic groups, but physical abuse and neglect are more prevalent in lower socioeconomic groups, because abuse increases with severe stress, family violence, and substance abuse.
- Approximately 30% of abused children will abuse their children.

■ PHYSICAL FINDINGS & CLINICAL PRESENTATION

- Presence of multiple injuries of various ages, particularly in the setting of a discrepancy in the history and severity of injury
- Injuries of childhood usually on bony prominences; soft tissue injuries more commonly inflicted by others (Fig. 1-5)
- Burns occur in 10% of abused children; usually result from cigarettes or immersion of buttocks or extremities in scalding hot water
- Retinal hemorrhage diagnostic for "shaken baby syndrome," because it occurs with head injury or sudden compression of the chest (Purtscher's retinopathy)
- Subdural bleeding exceedingly rare in children unless child has suffered shaking or significant head trauma
- Presence of sperm or acid phosphatase in the vaginal vault diagnostic of intercourse within 72 hr and indicates sexual abuse of female child
- Sexually transmitted diseases in a child highly suggestive of sexual abuse
- Disruption of normal genital anatomy often associated with recurrent sexual abuse (e.g., a lax anal sphincter, thickening or darkening of labial skin, significantly enlarged hymen opening)

MARKS from INSTRUMENTS

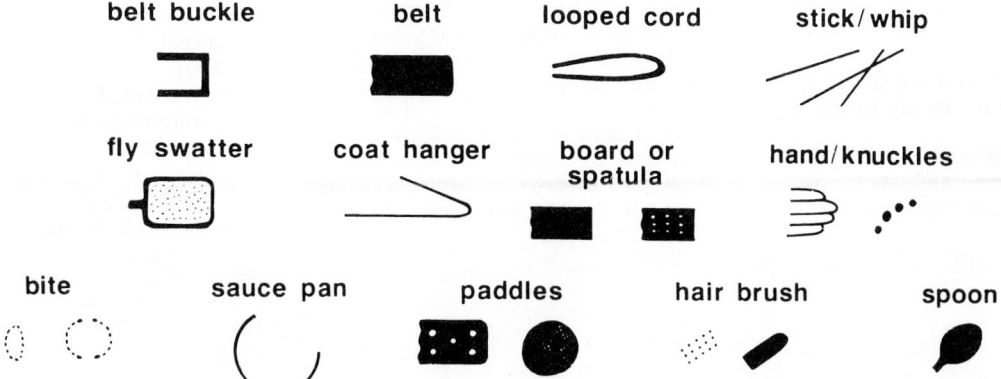

Fig. 1-5 A variety of instruments may be used to inflict injury on a child. Often the choice of an instrument is a matter of convenience. Marks tend to silhouette or outline the shape of the instrument. The possibility of intentional trauma should prompt a high degree of suspicion when injuries to a child are geometric, paired, mirrored, of various ages or types, or on relatively protected parts of the body. Early recognition of intentional trauma is important to provide therapy and prevent escalation to more serious injury. (From Behrman RE: *Nelson textbook of pediatrics,* Philadelphia, 1996, WB Saunders.)

ETIOLOGY

- Sexual abuse of girls: passive mother and domineering father (or stepfather)
- Physical abuse: severe psychosocial stressors such as poverty, unemployment, drug abuse, or marital discord
- History of abuse in the parent or the presence of violence in the family of origin: may predispose to child abuse
- Neglect associated with similar factors, particularly if child's birth was unplanned

DIAGNOSIS

DIFFERENTIAL DIAGNOSIS

Distinction from accidental injuries is crucial.

WORKUP

- History from the child, caregivers, and other individuals living in the home to reconstruct events and determine any inconsistency or implausibility in the story (Caution is required not to taint the history with the way in which it is obtained or the interviewer's own bias.)
- Physical examination to determine developmental parameters (height, weight) and to document extent and age of bruises
- Examinations for sexual abuse performed within the first 72 hr to be conducted by a rape-crisis team
- Section III, Fig. 3-1 describes the management of suspected child abuse

LABORATORY TESTS

- Examine fluids in the vaginal vault for sperm and acid phosphatase if intercourse was believed to have occurred within 72 hr.
- Culture oral, vaginal, and anal orifices for sexually transmitted diseases.
- Do bleeding studies if bruising is thought to be secondary to clotting abnormality.
- Examine nutritional, hematopoietic, and endocrine parameters for patients with neglect or failure to thrive.

IMAGING STUDIES

- For children ages 2 to 5 yr: obtain a bone survey (skull, thorax, pelvis, spine, arms, and legs).
- In children older than 5 yr: obtain more focused x-rays.
- Do brain imaging if head trauma or shaking is suspected.
- Take color photographs of skin lesions if legal action is anticipated. (NOTE: Parental consent is not required for photos documenting suspected child abuse.)

TREATMENT

NONPHARMACOLOGIC THERAPY

- Gear initial interventions toward stabilizing the injuries and preventing further abuse.
- Contact Child Protective Services. (NOTE: Physicians are mandated to report suspected abuse.)
- Where hospitalization is not required, arrange for emergency foster care if possible.
- If a child is returned to abusive environment, 5% mortality rate and 35% severe injury rate is to be expected.

ACUTE GENERAL Rx

Pharmacologic intervention is limited to that required to stabilize the injuries.

CHRONIC Rx

- Treatment in abusive families is generally poor. A review of several studies including some 3000 families found that a third of abusive parents will continue abuse while in treatment and half may revert to abuse at end of treatment.
- Separation of child via foster care may be traumatic to the child.
- Preventive programs for young single mothers at high risk are thought more effective than other interventions.
- Treatment of sexual abusers is marred by a high recurrence rate.
- In <5% of cases the abuse is related to a psychotic illness that can be treated directly.

DISPOSITION

- Victims of abuse and neglect may die or suffer lifelong emotional or physical disability.
- Abused children are more aggressive and have greater interpersonal difficulties. As adults they suffer from depression, anxiety, and substance abuse at twice the rate of the general population, and 30% are likely to abuse their children. Risk for suicide attempt is 2-5 times that of general population.
- Victims of sexual abuse will experience problems with sexual identity and function. Of women with borderline personality disorder, 60% have suffered physical or sexual abuse.

REFERRAL

- The physician is mandated to report suspected abuse to Child Protective Services.
- Rape-crisis teams exist in most urban areas and are usually better prepared to deal with issues of sexual abuse.
- People at high risk may benefit from prophylactic counseling.
- Most abused children need some therapy to cope with abuse and resulting separation from the family of origin.

REFERENCES

Coury DL: Recognition of child abuse: notes from the field, *Arch Pediatr Adolesc Med* 154:9, 2000.

Dube SR et al: Childhood abuse, household dysfunction, and risk of attempted suicide throughout the life span, *JAMA* 286:2089, 2001.

Jenny C, Roesler T: Caring for survivors of childhood sexual abuse in medical practice, *Med Health R I* 86:376, 2003.

Lahoh SL et al: Evaluating the child for sexual abuse, *Am Fam Physician* 63:883, 2001.

Pitetti RD et al: Prevalence of retinal hemorrhages and child abuse in children who present with an apparent life-threatening event, *Pediatrics* 110:557, 2002.

Author: **Rif S. El-Mallakh, M.D.**

BASIC INFORMATION

■ **DEFINITION**

Drug abuse is a recurring pattern of harmful use of a substance despite adverse consequences of the substance in work, school, relationships, the legal system, or personal health. This may occur concurrently with or independently from *substance dependence,* in which there is the presence of physiologic tolerance, discontinuation-induced withdrawal, or inability to willfully control rate or discontinue substance.

■ **SYNONYMS**

Substance abuse
Addiction

ICD-9CM CODES

Defined by specific substance F10-F19 (DSM-IV code is also defined by specific substance 291-292, 303-305).

■ **EPIDEMIOLOGY & DEMOGRAPHICS**

INCIDENCE (IN U.S.): For alcohol the incidence is 7%/yr.
PREVALENCE (IN U.S.):
• For alcohol: lifetime
• For cocaine abuse: lifetime prevalence is 0.2%
• For marijuana abuse: lifetime prevalence is 4%
• For amphetamine abuse: lifetime prevalence is 2%
• For hallucinogens: rate is 0.3%
• For opiates: rate is 0.7%
• For nicotine: lifetime prevalence of dependence is 20%
• For MDMA (3,4-methylene-dioxymethamphetamine, or ecstasy): college student rate is 4.7%

PREDOMINANT SEX:
• Males abuse substances more frequently than females.
• The rates of male:female substance abusers are as follows:
Alcohol 5:1
Opiates 3-4:1
Amphetamines 3-4:1
Hallucinogens 2:1
Marijuana 1-2:1
Cocaine 1:1
PREDOMINANT AGE:
• Problematic use of substances may begin in early life (8 to 10 yr).
• The mean age of onset of problem drinking is about 25 yr for men and 30 yr for women.
PEAK INCIDENCE:
• For most substances: 18 to 30 yr of age
• Men: average >20 yr of heavy drinking
• Women: average 15 yr of heavy drinking
GENETICS
• There is evidence of a nonspecific genetic factor.
• Vulnerability to alcohol abuse is increased in Asians with the alcohol dehydrogenase type 2 isozyme and the aldehyde dehydrogenase type 2 isozyme.

■ **PHYSICAL FINDINGS & CLINICAL PRESENTATION**
• Abuse of several substances generally occurs together (e.g., alcohol abuse is often found in association with abuse of or dependence on nicotine).
• Symptoms of anxiety, depression, insomnia, cognitive and memory dysfunction, and emotional/behavioral dyscontrol are frequent.

• Alcohol and cocaine abuse are specifically associated with violence and accidents (e.g., more than half of all murderers *and* their victims are intoxicated at the time of the crime).

■ **ETIOLOGY**

Two models of addiction: (1) Conditioning—substance use paired with enforcing and triggering stimuli, and (2) Homeostatic—either preexisting abnormalities or drug-induced abnormalities lead to initial or continued use of the drug.

🔬 **DIAGNOSIS**

■ **DIFFERENTIAL DIAGNOSIS**
• Psychiatric disorders such as depression, mania, social phobia, or other anxiety disorders that coexist or occur as a consequence of substance abuse
• Cannot diagnose these disorders accurately in the setting of active substance abuse (Table 1-1)

■ **WORKUP**
• The history is crucial for diagnosis of any substance abuse disorder; because of frequent denial and poor insight into problem substance abuse, collateral information from family, friends, and co-workers is often helpful.
• Observation of problematic behavior during intoxication or withdrawal is diagnostic.
• Physical examination findings are limited and not diagnostic (e.g., needle scars from repeated intravenous injections, rhinorrhea secondary to intranasal cocaine).

TABLE 1-1   **Diagnostic Criteria for Dependence and Drug Abuse**

DEPENDENCE (>3 NEEDED)	ABUSE (>1 FOR 12 MO)
1. Tolerance	1. Recurrent substance use resulting in failure to fulfill major role obligations at work, school, or home
2. Withdrawal	2. Recurrent substance use in situations in which it is physically hazardous
3. The substance is often taken in larger amounts over a longer period than intended	3. Recurrent substance-related legal problems
4. Any unsuccessful effort or a persistent desire to cut down or control substance use	4. Continued substance use despite having persistent or recurrent social or interpersonal problems caused or exacerbated by the effects of the substance
5. A great deal of time is spent in activities necessary to obtain the substance or recover from its effects	Never met criteria for dependence
6. Important social, occupational, or recreational activities given up or reduced because of substance use	
7. Continued substance use despite knowledge of having had persistent or recurrent physical or psychological problems that are likely to be caused or exacerbated by the substance	

From Goldman L, Bennett JC (eds): *Cecil textbook of medicine,* ed 21, Philadelphia, 2000, WB Saunders.

■ **LABORATORY TESTS**

Most helpful tests: toxicology screen or blood alcohol level

■ **IMAGING STUDIES**

- Not helpful in routine diagnosis and management of substance abuse, but possibly useful in the management of sequelae of substance abuse (e.g., head CT scan to evaluate the alcohol abuse–associated increased risk of subdural hematomas or increased evidence of cerebral atrophy)
- Liver ultrasound to evaluate for alcohol-related fatty changes
- Two-dimensional echo for intravenous drug use–associated valvular lesions

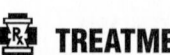 **TREATMENT**

■ **NONPHARMACOLOGIC THERAPY**

- Relapse prevention by avoidance of trigger stimuli or by uncoupling trigger stimuli from substance ingestion
- Self-help groups such as Alcoholics Anonymous, Narcotics Anonymous, and Al-Anon
- Nonpharmacologic strategies have greatest documented efficacy

■ **ACUTE GENERAL Rx**

- Acute interventions are usually confined to safe withdrawal in the setting of dependence.
- Benzodiazepines are safe and effective in acute alcohol withdrawal.
- Anticonvulsants, particularly carbamazepine, are used effectively in Europe.
- β-Blockers and clonidine should be avoided in alcohol withdrawal, because they mask markers of the severity of the withdrawal (blood pressure and pulse rate).
- Clonidine alleviates the discomfort of opiate and nicotine withdrawal.
- Nicotine patches and gum reduce withdrawal symptoms.

■ **CHRONIC Rx**

- Few agents are useful in prevention of substance abuse relapse.
- Disulfiram (Antabuse) workup and metronidazole (Flagyl): possible interaction with alcohol causes physical discomfort.
- Naltrexone helps reduce craving for alcohol.
- Adjunctive use of antidepressants or lithium is helpful when substance use is associated with anxiety and mood symptoms.
- Methadone replacement is used in opiate abuse/dependence (controversial).

■ **DISPOSITION**

- Substance abuse is a chronic relapsing illness.
- The goal of treatment is always abstinence, but success of treatment is measured by return of function and increasing duration between relapses.
- When substance abuse is complicated by another psychiatric illness, prognosis for both conditions is quite poor.
- Abuse of one substance increases likelihood for abuse of other substances.

■ **REFERRAL**

- Always refer to self-help groups (AA, NA) for patient, Al-Anon for significant others.
- Intensive substance abuse treatment is nearly always indicated in substance-dependent individuals.
- Individuals with coexisting primary psychiatric illness and substance abuse nearly always require the care of a psychiatrist.

REFERENCES

Fiellin DA, O'Connor P: Office-based treatment of opioid-dependent patients. *N Engl J Med* 347:817, 2002.

Strote J, Lee JE, Wechsler H: Increasing MDMA use among college students: results of a rational survey, *J Adolesc Health* 30:64, 2002.

Author: **Rif S. El-Mallakh, M.D.**

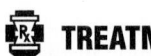

 BASIC INFORMATION

■ DEFINITION

Geriatric abuse is the willful infliction of physical pain or injury; emotional pain, injury, humiliation, or intimidation; exploitation or misappropriation of money or property; or neglect by the designated caregiver of nutritional hygiene or medical needs (Box 1-1).

■ SYNONYMS

Elder abuse
Battered elder syndrome

ICD-9CM CODES

995.81 Adult maltreatment syndrome

■ EPIDEMIOLOGY & DEMOGRAPHICS

INCIDENCE (IN U.S.): Unknown
PREVALENCE (IN U.S.):
- 3.2% in a large study in Boston.
- Estimated up to 10% of individuals >65 yr of age.
- Only 15% of elder abuse comes to the attention of authorities.
- Most (>60%) abuse is committed by one spouse against another.
- Approximately 25% of abuse is committed by an adult child of the victim who is living in the same home and is usually financially dependent on the victim.

PREDOMINANT SEX:
- Women thought to be at greater risk

PREDOMINANT AGE: Risk increases as level of disability, not age, increases
PEAK INCIDENCE: >80 yr old

■ PHYSICAL FINDINGS & CLINICAL PRESENTATION

- Physical abuse with multiple injuries at various stages with implausible or inconsistent descriptions of their origins; injuries are usually to head, neck, chest, breast, abdomen
- Extreme fear, hypervigilance, or withdrawal
- Torn or blood-stained underwear or new onset of a sexually transmitted disease signaling sexual abuse
- Toxicologic evidence of unprescribed medications

■ ETIOLOGY

- Relatives with mental illness or substance abuse
- Excessive dependence on the elderly individual for financial, housing, and other necessities
- A history of violence, particularly within the family

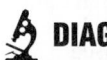 **DIAGNOSIS**

■ DIFFERENTIAL DIAGNOSIS

Risk increases as the elder's level of disability increases. Consequently, poor hygiene, poor nutrition, confusion, psychosis in the setting of dementia, and poor compliance with prescribed treatments may all occur without ongoing abuse.

■ WORKUP

- Interview patient separately from the suspected abuser.
- Build trust; patients may be reticent.
- Ask direct questions.
- Be aware that physical findings are usually unexplained injuries or burns.

■ LABORATORY TESTS

- Toxicology screens or therapeutic drug monitoring
- If sexual abuse suspected, screening for sexually transmitted diseases

■ IMAGING STUDIES

X-rays as indicated

TREATMENT

■ NONPHARMACOLOGIC THERAPY

- Reporting abuse to Adult Protective Services is mandatory in most states. This also provides the physician access to specialized personnel who can aid in evaluation and disposition.
- Separate patient and abuser.
- If the burden of care underlies the abuse, refer to respite services.

■ ACUTE GENERAL RX

As indicated for injury or pain relief

■ CHRONIC RX

If the patient's level of disability does not allow for independent living, institutionalization may be required.

■ REFERRAL

Referral to Adult Protective Services is mandatory in 42 states.

REFERENCES

Campbell J et al: Intimate partner violence and physical health consequences, *Arch Intern Med* 162:1157, 2002.
Gundersen L: Intimate-partner violence: the need for primary prevention in the community, *Ann Intern Med* 136:637, 2002.
Ramsay J et al: Should health professionals screen women for domestic violence? Systematic review, *BMJ* 325:314, 2002.
Author: **Rif S. El-Mallakh, M.D.**

BOX 1-1 Types of Geriatric Abuse

Physical abuse
    Assault
    Rough handling
    Burns
    Sexual abuse
    Unreasonable physical confinement
Physical neglect
    Dehydration
    Malnutrition
    Poor hygiene
    Inappropriate or soiled clothing
    Medications given improperly
    Lack of medical care
Psychological abuse
    Verbal or emotional abuse
    Threats
    Isolation/confinement
Material abuse
    Withholding finances
    Misuse of funds
    Theft
    Withholding means for daily living

From Bosker G et al: *Geriatric emergency medicine*, St Louis, 1990, Mosby.

BASIC INFORMATION

■ DEFINITION
Acetaminophen poisoning is a disorder manifested by hepatic necrosis, jaundice, somnolence, and potential death if not treated appropriately. Pathologically there is hepatic necrosis.

■ SYNONYMS
Paracetamol poisoning

ICD-9CM CODES
965.4 Acetaminophen poisoning

■ EPIDEMIOLOGY & DEMOGRAPHICS
• Potentially toxic ingestions of acetaminophen-containing medications exceed 100,000 cases annually.
• Death rate is approximately 1/1000 persons. Nearly 50% of exposures occur in children <6 yr.
• Hepatic necrosis is most likely to occur in people who are chronically malnourished, who regularly abuse alcohol, and who are using other potentially hepatotoxic medications.

■ PHYSICAL FINDINGS & CLINICAL PRESENTATION
• The physical examination may vary depending on the number of hours lapsed from the ingestion of acetaminophen.
• Initially, symptoms may be mild or absent and may consist of diaphoresis, malaise, nausea, and vomiting.
• After the initial 12 to 24 hr, patient may complain of RUQ pain with associated vomiting, diaphoresis, and subsequent somnolence.
• In massive overdoses, jaundice may occur within the initial 72 hr.
• Subsequent coma, somnolence, and confusion follow and can ultimately lead to death if not treated appropriately.

■ ETIOLOGY
The amount of acetaminophen necessary for hepatic toxicity varies with the patient's body size and hepatic function. Using standardized nomograms calculating the acetaminophen plasma level and the number of hours after ingestion, the clinician can determine potential hepatic toxicity.

DIAGNOSIS

■ DIFFERENTIAL DIAGNOSIS
• Liver disease from alcohol abuse or hepatitis
• Ingestion of other hepatotoxic substances

■ WORKUP
Initial workup is aimed at confirming acetaminophen overdose with plasma acetaminophen level and assessment of hepatic damage and potential damage to other organ systems, such as kidneys, pancreas, and heart (see "Laboratory Tests"). An acetaminophen overdose algorithm is described in Section III.

■ LABORATORY TESTS
• Initial laboratory evaluation consists of plasma acetaminophen level with a second level drawn approximately 4 to 6 hr after the initial level. Subsequent levels can be obtained q2-4h until the levels stabilize or decline. These levels can be plotted using the Rumack-Matthew nomogram (see acetaminophen poisoning algorithm in Section III) to calculate potential hepatic toxicity.
• Transaminases (AST, ALT), bilirubin level, PT, BUN, and creatinine should be initially obtained on all patients.
• Serum and urine toxicology screen for other potential toxic substances is also recommended on admission.

TREATMENT

■ NONPHARMACOLOGIC THERAPY
Consultation with Poison Control Center for management recommendations is recommended in patients with large ingestions of acetaminophen and/or ingestion of other toxic substances. A toxic dose of acetaminophen usually exceeds 7.5 g in the adult or 140 mg/kg.

■ ACUTE GENERAL Rx
• Perform gastric lavage and administer activated charcoal if the patient is seen within 1 hr of ingestion or the clinician suspects polydrug ingestion.
• Determine blood levels 4 hr after ingestion; if in the toxic range, start N-acetylcysteine (Mucomyst), 140 mg/kg PO as a loading dose, followed by 70 mg/kg PO q4h for 48 hr. (N-Acetylcysteine therapy should be started within 24 hr of acetaminophen overdose.) If charcoal therapy was initially instituted, lavage the stomach and recover as much charcoal as possible; then instill N-acetylcysteine, increasing the loading dose by 40%.
• Monitor acetaminophen level; use graph to plot possible hepatic toxicity.
• Provide adequate IV hydration (e.g., $D_5 1/2NS$ at 150 ml/hr).
• If acetaminophen level is nontoxic, acetylcysteine therapy may be discontinued.

■ DISPOSITION
Most patients will recover fully without persisting hepatic abnormalities. Hepatic failure is particularly unusual in children <6 yr.

■ REFERRAL
Psychiatric referral is recommended following intentional ingestions.
Author: **Fred F. Ferri, M.D.**

BASIC INFORMATION

■ DEFINITION
Achalasia is a motility disorder of the esophagus characterized by inadequate relaxation of the lower esophageal sphincter (LES) and ineffective peristalsis of esophageal smooth muscle. The result is functional obstruction of the esophagus.

■ SYNONYMS
Esophageal achalasia
Esophageal cardiospasm

ICD-9CM CODES
530.0 Achalasia

■ EPIDEMIOLOGY & DEMOGRAPHICS
- Annual incidence is about 1 in 100,000 persons.
- Although the onset of symptoms may occur at any age, it is more common in persons 30 to 50 yr old.
- Men and women are affected equally.

■ PHYSICAL FINDINGS & CLINICAL PRESENTATION
Symptoms:
- Difficulty belching
- Dysphagia to both solids and liquids
- Chest pain and/or heartburn
- Globus
- Frequent hiccups
- Vomiting of undigested food
- Symptoms of aspiration such as nocturnal cough; possible dyspnea and pneumonia

Physical findings:
- If severe and prolonged, then possible weight loss
- Focal lung examination abnormalities and wheezing also possible

■ ETIOLOGY
- Etiology is poorly understood.
- This motility disorder may be due to autoimmune degeneration of the esophageal myenteric plexus, as association with the HLA class II antigen, DQw1, has been noted.
- Herpes zoster and measles virus have been implicated, but the association has not been confirmed.

DIAGNOSIS

■ DIFFERENTIAL DIAGNOSIS
- Angina
- Bulimia
- Anorexia nervosa
- Gastric bezoar
- Gastritis
- Peptic ulcer disease
- Postvagotomy dysmotility
- Esophageal disease:
  GERD
  Sarcoidosis
  Amyloidosis
  Esophageal stricture
  Esophageal webs and rings
  Scleroderma
  Barrett's esophagus
    Chagas' disease
  Esophagitis
  Diffuse esophageal spasm
- Malignancy:
  Esophageal cancer
    Infiltrating gastric cancer
    Lung cancer
  Lymphoma

■ WORKUP
- Physical examination and laboratory analyses to rule out other causes and assess complications
- Imaging studies and manometry for diagnosis

■ LABORATORY TESTS
- Assessment of nutritional status with albumin and prealbumin if indicated
- CBC, ECG, stress test, stool and emesis for occult blood if diagnosis is in doubt

■ IMAGING STUDIES
Barium swallow with fluoroscopy may demonstrate the following findings:
- Uncoordinated or absent esophageal contractions
- An acutely tapered contrast column ("bird's beak," Fig. 1-6)
- Dilation of the distal (smooth muscle portion) esophagus
- Esophageal air fluid level

Manometry may be indicated if barium swallow is inconclusive. Characteristic abnormalities are as follows:
- Low-amplitude disorganized contractions
- High intraesophageal resting pressure
- High LES pressure
- Inadequate LES relaxation after swallow

Direct visualization by endoscopy can rule out other causes of dysphagia.

TREATMENT

Three modalities of treatment:
- Medical:
  Smooth muscle relaxants including nitrates and calcium channel blockers are effective in up to 70% of patients.
  Botulinum toxin injection will benefit up to 90% of patients but will require repeat injections.
- Mechanical dilation:
  Fixed or pneumatic dilators may benefit up to 90%. Esophageal rupture or perforation is a rare complication that can be managed conservatively in some stable patients.
- Surgical:
  Open and thoracoscopic esophagomyotomy are available and effective (90%). This approach currently offers the most durable symptom relief. About 10% of patients undergoing surgery will have symptomatic reflux disease.

■ DISPOSITION
Prognosis is excellent in patients who respond to therapy. In long-standing disease or inadequately treated disease, there is an increased risk of squamous cell carcinoma. Chronic GERD, as a result of treatment, may be complicated by Barrett's esophagus and malignant transformation.

■ REFERRAL
Choice of and response to therapy will determine referral. Some surgeons may not be facile with thoracoscopic procedures.

REFERENCES
Harris AM et al: Achalasia management, outcome and surveillance in a specialist unit, *Br J Surg* 87(3):364, 2000.
Spiess AE, Kahrilas PJ: Treating achalasia, *JAMA* 280:638, 1998.
Vaezi MF, Richter JE: Practice guidelines: diagnosis and management of achalasia, *Am J Gastroenterol* 94(12):3406, 1999.
Vaezi MF et al: Botulinum toxin versus pneumatic dilatation in the treatment of achalasia: a randomized trial, *Gut* 44:231, 1999.
Author: **James J. Ng, M.D.**

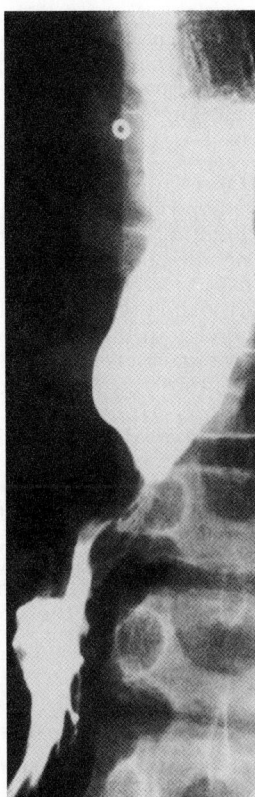

Fig. 1-6 Classic appearance of achalasia of the esophagus. The dilated esophagus ends in a narrow segment. (From Hoekelman R [ed]: *Primary pediatric care,* ed 3, St Louis, 1997, Mosby.)

BASIC INFORMATION

■ DEFINITION

Achilles tendon rupture refers to the loss of continuity of the *tendo Achillis,* usually from attrition.

ICD-9CM CODES
845.09 Achilles tendon rupture

■ EPIDEMIOLOGY & DEMOGRAPHICS
PREDOMINANT AGE: 30 to 55 yr

■ PHYSICAL FINDINGS & CLINICAL PRESENTATION

Injury often occurs during an activity that puts great stress on the tendon. Sudden "pop" is often felt followed by weakness and swelling.

- Patient walks flat-footed and is unable to stand on the ball of the foot.
- Tenderness and hemorrhage are present at the site of injury, and a sulcus is usually palpable but may be obscured by an organizing clot if the examination is delayed.
- Although active plantar flexion is usually lost, some plantar flexion occasionally remains because of the activity of the other posterior compartment muscles.
- Thompson's test is usually positive. Test measures plantar flexion of the foot when the calf is squeezed with the patient kneeling on a chair; normal foot plantarflexes with calf compression, but movement is absent when *tendo Achillis* is ruptured.
- Excessive passive dorsiflexion of the foot is also present on the injured side (Fig. 1-7).

■ ETIOLOGY

- Relative hypovascularity predisposing to tendon rupture in several tendons (Achilles, biceps, and supraspinatus)
- With advancing age, vascular supply to the tendon further compromised
- Repetitive trauma leading to degeneration of this critical area and weakness
- Rupture of *tendo Achillis* usually 2.5 to 5 cm from the insertion of the tendon into the os calcis
- Most common causative event leading to rupture: sudden dorsiflexion of the plantar flexed foot (landing from a height) or sudden pushing off with the weight on the forefoot

DIAGNOSIS

■ DIFFERENTIAL DIAGNOSIS
- Incomplete (partial) *tendo Achillis* rupture
- Partial rupture of gastrocnemius muscle, often medial head (previously thought to be "plantaris tendon rupture")

■ WORKUP
- Clinical diagnosis of *tendo Achillis* rupture is usually obvious.
- If bony injury is suspected, plain roentgenograms are indicated.
- Other studies are usually unnecessary.

TREATMENT

- Early referral is necessary for surgical repair.
- If surgery is contraindicated, a short leg cast applied with the foot in equinus may allow healing.
- In cases of neglected rupture, reconstruction is usually indicated.

■ DISPOSITION
- Prognosis for recovery after surgical repair of the acute rupture is good, but recurrence is not uncommon regardless of treatment.
- *Tendo Achillis* must be protected from excessive activity for up to 1 yr.
- Results of reconstruction for neglected cases are worse than with primary repair.

REFERENCES

Bhandari M et al: Treatment of acute Achilles tendon rupture: a systematic overview and metaanalysis, *Clin Orthop* (400):190, 2002.

Kocher MS et al: Operative versus nonoperative management of acute achilles tendon rupture: expected-value decision analysis, *Am J Sports Med* 30(6):783, 2002.

Maffulli N, Kader D: Tendinopathy of tendo Achillis, *J Bone Joint Surg Br* 84(1):1, 2002.

Mazzone MF, McCue T: Common conditions of the Achilles tendon, *Am Fam Physician* 65(9):1805, 2002.

Moller M et al: Acute rupture of the tendo achilles, *J Bone Joint Surg* 83(B):843, 2001.

Paffey MD, Faraj AA: Acute rupture of tendo Achillis, *J Bone Joint Surg Br* 84(4):620, 2002.

Roberts C, Deliss L: Acute rupture of tendo Achillis, *J Bone Joint Surg Br* 84(4):620, 2002.

Schepsis AA, Jones H, Haas AL: Achilles tendon disorders in athletes, *Am J Sports Med* 30(2):287, 2002.

Wong J, Barrass V, Maffulli N: Quantitative review of operative and nonoperative management of Achilles tendon ruptures, *Am J Sports Med* 30(4):565, 2002.

Author: **Lonnie R. Mercier, M.D.**

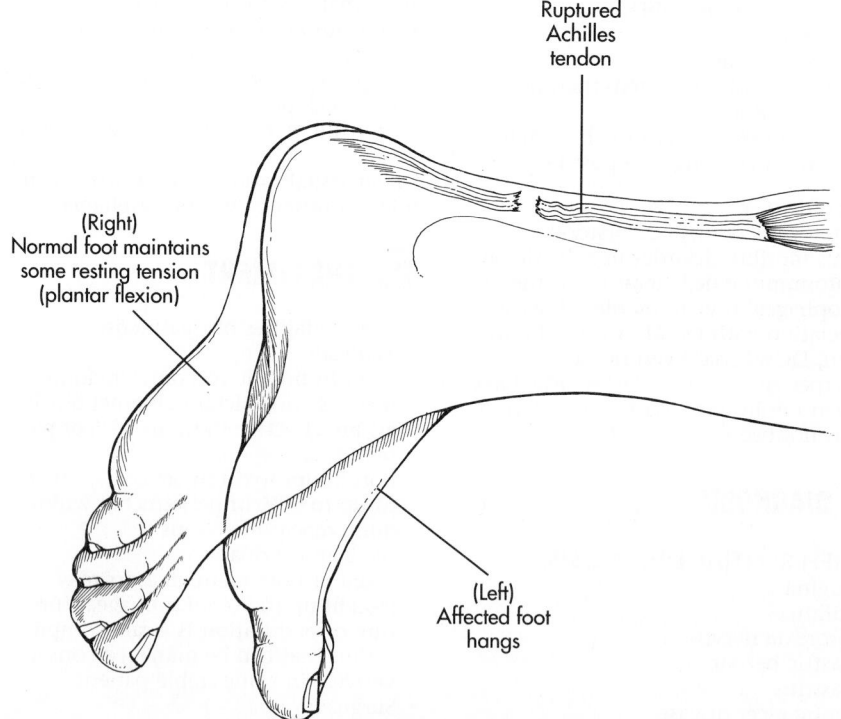

Fig. 1-7   **Observation of Achilles tendon rupture.** The patient is asked to lie prone on the examining table with feet hanging off the end. The intact leg retains inherent plantar flexion, whereas on the injured side, the foot hangs straight down with gravity. (From Scudieri G [ed]: *Sports medicine: principles of primary care,* St Louis, 1997, Mosby.)

BASIC INFORMATION

DEFINITION
Acne vulgaris is a chronic disorder of the pilosebaceous apparatus caused by abnormal desquamation of follicular epithelium leading to obstruction of the pilosebaceous canal, resulting in inflammation and subsequent formation of papules, pustules, nodules, comedones, and scarring.

SYNONYMS
Acne

ICD-9CM CODES
706.1 Acne vulgaris

EPIDEMIOLOGY & DEMOGRAPHICS
- Acne is the most common skin disease in the U.S.
- It is most common in teenagers (highest incidence between ages of 16 and 18 yr).

PHYSICAL FINDINGS & CLINICAL PRESENTATION
- Open comedones (blackheads), closed comedones (whiteheads)
- Greasiness (oily skin)
- Presence of scars from prior acne cysts
- Various stages of development and severity may be present concomitantly
- Common distribution of acne: face, back, and upper chest
- Inflammatory papules, pustules, and ectatic pores

ETIOLOGY
- Overactivity of the sebaceous glands and blockage in the ducts. The obstruction leads to the formation of comedones, which can become inflamed because of overgrowth of *Propionibacterium acnes*.
- Exacerbated by environmental factors (hot, humid, tropical climate), medications (e.g., iodine in cough mixtures, hair greases), industrial exposure to halogenated hydrocarbons.

DIAGNOSIS

DIFFERENTIAL DIAGNOSIS
- Gram-negative folliculitis
- Staphylococcal pyoderma
- Acne rosacea
- Drug eruption
- Sebaceous hyperplasia
- Angiofibromas, basal cell carcinomas, osteoma cutis
- Occupational exposures to oils or grease
- Steroid acne

WORKUP
History and physical examination:
- Inquire about previous treatment
- Careful drug history
- Family history, history of cyclic menstrual flares
- History of use of cosmetics and cleansers
- Oral contraceptive use

LABORATORY TESTS
- Laboratory evaluation is generally not helpful.
- Patients who are candidates for therapy with isotretinoin (Accutane) should have baseline liver enzymes, cholesterol, and triglycerides checked, because this medication may result in elevation of lipids and liver enzymes.
- A negative serum pregnancy test should also be obtained in females 1 wk before initiation of isotretinoin; it is also imperative to maintain effective contraception during and 1 mo after therapy with isotretinoin ends because of its teratogenic effects.

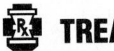

TREATMENT

NONPHARMACOLOGIC THERAPY
- Blue light (ClearLight therapy system) can be used for treatment of moderate inflammatory acne vulgaris. Light in the violet/blue range can cause bacterial death by a photoreaction in which porphyrins react with oxygen to generate reactive oxygen species, which damage the cell membranes of *P. acnes*. Treatment usually consists of 15 min exposures twice weekly for 4 wk.

ACUTE GENERAL Rx
Treatment generally varies with the type of lesions (comedones, papules, pustules, cystic lesions) and the severity of acne.
- Comedones can be treated with tretinoin (Retin-A); it is applied generally once qhs; large open comedones (blackheads) should be expressed.
- Patients should be reevaluated after 4 to 6 wk. Benzoyl peroxide gel (2.5% or 5%) may be added if the comedones become inflamed or form pustules. Topical antibiotics (erythromycin, clindamycin lotions or pads) can also be used in patients with significant inflammation. The combination of 5% benzoyl peroxide and 3% erythromycin (Benzamycin) is highly effective in patients who have a mixture of comedonal and inflammatory acne lesions.
- Pustular acne can be treated with tretinoin and benzoyl peroxide gel applied on alternate evenings; drying agents (sulfacetamide-sulfa lotions [Novacet, Sulfacet]) are also effective when used in combination

with benzoyl peroxide; oral antibiotics (doxycycline 100 mg qd or erythromycin 1 g qd given in 2 to 3 divided doses) are effective in patients with moderate to severe pustular acne; patients not responding well to these antibiotics can be switched over to minocycline 50 to 100 mg bid; however, this medication is more expensive.
- Patients with nodular cystic acne can be treated with systemic agents: antibiotics (erythromycin, tetracycline, doxycycline, minocycline), isotretinoin (Accutane), or oral contraceptives. Periodic intralesional triamcinolone (Kenalog) injections by a dermatologist are also effective. The possibility of endocrinopathy should be considered in patients responding poorly to therapy.
- Isotretinoin is indicated for acne resistant to antibiotic therapy and severe acne; dosage is 0.5 to 1 mg/kg/day in 2 divided doses (maximum of 2 mg/kg/day); duration of therapy is generally 20 wk for a cumulative dose ≥120 mg/kg for severe cystic acne; before using this medication patients should undergo baseline laboratory evaluation (see "Laboratory Tests"). This drug is absolutely contraindicated during pregnancy because of its teratogenicity. It should be used with caution in patients with history of depression.
- Tazarotene (Tazorac), an acetynilic retinoid, is also effective for acne vulgaris; however, it may be more irritating than tretinoin or the retinoid analog adapalene. It is available as a 0.1% gel or cream for treatment of acne.
- Oral contraceptives reduce androgen levels and therefore sebum production. They represent a useful adjunctive therapy for all types of acne in women and adolescent girls.

REFERRAL
Referral for intralesional injection and dermabrasion should be considered in patients with severe acne unresponsive to conventional therapy.

PEARLS & CONSIDERATIONS

COMMENTS
Indications for systemic therapy of acne are:
- Painful deep papules or nodules
- Extensive lesions
- Active acne with severe scarring or hyperpigmentation
- Patient's morale

Patients should be educated that in most cases acne can be controlled but not cured and that at least 4 to 6 wk of initial therapy should be required before significant improvement is noted.
Author: **Fred F. Ferri, M.D.**

BASIC INFORMATION

■ DEFINITION
Acoustic neuroma is a benign proliferation of the Schwann cells that cover the vestibular branch of the eighth cranial nerve (CN VIII). Symptoms are commonly a result of compression of the acoustic branch of CN VIII, the facial nerve (CN VII), and the trigeminal nerve (CN V). The glossopharyngeal nerve (CN IX) and vagus nerve (CN X) are less commonly involved. In extreme cases, compression of the brainstem may lead to obstruction of cerebrospinal fluid (CSF) outflow and elevated intracranial pressure (ICP).

■ SYNONYMS
Vestibular schwannoma

ICD-9CM CODES
225.1 Acoustic neuroma

■ EPIDEMIOLOGY & DEMOGRAPHICS
Annual incidence is about 1 in 100,000 patients per year. There may be a slight female predominance. The tumor most commonly presents in the fifth and sixth decades.

■ PHYSICAL FINDINGS & CLINICAL PRESENTATION
- Most frequently unilateral hearing loss and/or tinnitus. Also balance problems, vertigo, facial pain (trigeminal neuralgia) and weakness, difficulty swallowing, fullness or pain of the involved ear. Headache may occur.
- With elevated ICP, patients may also suffer from vomiting, fever, and visual changes.
- Hearing loss is the most common presenting complaint and is usually high frequency.

■ ETIOLOGY
The etiology is incompletely understood, but long-term exposure to acoustic trauma has been implicated. Bilateral acoustic neuromas may be inherited in an autosomal dominant manner as part of neurofibromatosis type 2. This disease is associated with a defect on chromosome 22q1.

DIAGNOSIS

■ DIFFERENTIAL DIAGNOSIS
Benign positional vertigo, Meniere's disease, trigeminal neuralgia, cerebellar disease, normal-pressure hydrocephalus, presbycusis, glomus tumors, vertebrobasilar insufficiency, ototoxicity from medications, and other tumors: meningioma, glioma, facial nerve schwannoma, cavernous hemangioma, metastatic tumors

■ WORKUP
Physical examination, laboratory analysis, and imaging studies

■ PHYSICAL EXAMINATION
- A detailed neurologic examination with special attention to the cranial nerves is crucial.
- Otoscopic evaluation may help to rule out other causes of hearing loss.

■ LABORATORY TESTS
CSF protein may be elevated.

■ IMAGING STUDIES
- MRI with gadolinium is the preferred test. It can detect tumors as small as 2 mm in diameter.
- CT scan with contrast can detect tumors 1 cm in diameter or larger (Fig. 1-8).

TREATMENT

Treatment decisions should be based on the size of the tumor, rate of growth (older patients tend to have slower-growing tumors), degree of neurologic deficit, life expectancy, age of the patient, and surgical risk.
- Surgery is the definitive treatment. Choice of approach (middle cranial fossa, translabyrinthine, orretromastoid suboccipital) may vary depending on the size of the tumor, amount of residual hearing desired, and degree of surgical risk that can be tolerated. Partial resection is sometimes undertaken to minimize the risk of injury to nearby structures. Intraoperative facial nerve monitoring is recommended.
- Proton beam radiotherapy has been used to treat tumors that are less than 3 cm in diameter. Radiotherapy following partial resection has also been used to minimize complications.
- Observation with MRI every 6 to 12 mo may be appropriate for frail patients with small tumors, but risk of unrecoverable hearing loss may increase if surgery is delayed. Age alone is not a contraindication to surgery.

■ DISPOSITION
Hearing can be preserved at near preoperative levels in more than two thirds of patients with small- to medium-sized tumors.

■ REFERRAL
Prompt referral to an ENT specialist who is facile with all three surgical approaches is recommended.

REFERENCES

Kondziolka D et al: Long-term outcomes after radiosurgery for acoustic neuromas, *N Engl J Med* 339:1426, 1999.

Pitts LH, Jackler RK: Treatment of acoustic neuromas, *N Engl J Med* 339:1471, 1998.

Poen JC et al: Fractionated stereotactic radiosurgery and preservation of hearing in patients with vestibular schwannoma: a preliminary report, *Neurosurgery* 45(6):1299, 1999.

Schmidt RJ et al: The sensitivity of auditory brainstem response testing for the diagnosis of acoustic neuroma, *Arch Otolaryngol Head Neck Surg* 127(1):19, 2001.

Authors: **Paul Pirraglia, M.D., and James J. Ng, M.D.**

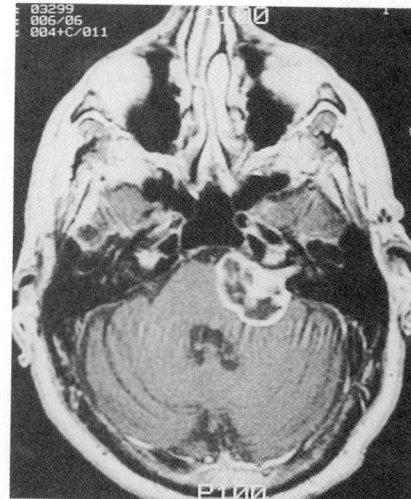

Fig. 1-8 Acoustic schwannoma. Axial, postcontrast-enhanced T1-weighted image demonstrates an inhomogeneously contrast-enhancing mass in the left cerebellopontine angle with extension into the left internal auditory canal. There is associated displacement of the brainstem. (From Specht N [ed]: *Practical guide to diagnostic imaging,* St Louis, 1998, Mosby.)

BASIC INFORMATION

■ DEFINITION
Acquired immunodeficiency syndrome (AIDS) is a disorder caused by infection with the human immunodeficiency virus, type 1 (HIV-1) and marked by progressive deterioration of the cellular immune system, leading to secondary infections or malignancies.

■ SYNONYMS
AIDS

ICD-9CM CODES
042.9 AIDS, unspecified

■ EPIDEMIOLOGY & DEMOGRAPHICS
INCIDENCE (IN U.S.):
- 27.1 cases/100,000 persons
- Varies widely by location
- 85% of cases in large cities

PREVALENCE (IN U.S.): 62 cases/100,000 persons

PREDOMINANT SEX: Males 84%, females 16% (through 1998). 40% of newly reported U.S. cases in 1999 were in females.

PREDOMINANT AGE: 80% between ages 20 and 40 yr

PEAK INCIDENCE: See Incidence

GENETICS:
- Familial disposition: Although there is no proven genetic predisposition, individuals with deletions in the CCR5 gene are immune from infection with macrophage tropic virus (the predominant virus in sexual transmission).
- Congenital infection:
  1. Transmittable from an infected mother to the fetus in utero in as many as 30% of pregnancies.
  2. No specific congenital malformations associated with infection; low birth weight and spontaneous abortion are possible.

- Neonatal infection: transmission possible to the neonate intrapartum or postpartum through breast-feeding.

■ PHYSICAL FINDINGS & CLINICAL PRESENTATION
- Nonspecific findings: fever, weight loss, anorexia
- Specific syndromes:
1. Seen in association with opportunistic infection and malignancies, so-called indicator diseases (see Box 1-2)
2. Most common:
   Respiratory infections (*Pneumocystis carinii* pneumonia, TB, bacterial pneumonia, fungal infection)
   CNS infections (toxoplasmosis, cryptococcal meningitis, TB)
   GI (cryptosporidiosis, isosporiasis, cytomegalovirus); Sections II and III describe organisms associated with diarrhea in patients with AIDS
   Eye infections (cytomegalovirus, toxoplasmosis)
   Kaposi's sarcoma (cutaneous or visceral) or lymphoma (nodal or extranodal)
- Possibly asymptomatic
- Diagnosis of AIDS if T-lymphocyte subset analysis demonstrating CD4 cell count <200 or <14% of total lymphocyte in the presence of proven HIV infection even in the absence of other infections
- The various manifestations of HIV infection are described in Section II

■ ETIOLOGY
- Caused by infection with human immunodeficiency virus, type 1 (HIV-1)
- Transmitted by heterosexual or male homosexual contact, needle-sharing (during IV drug use), transfusion of contaminated blood or blood products, and from infected mother to fetus or neonate as described previously

DIAGNOSIS

■ DIFFERENTIAL DIAGNOSIS
- Other wasting illnesses mimicking the nonspecific features of AIDS:
  1. TB
  2. Neoplasms
  3. Disseminated fungal infection
  4. Malabsorption syndromes
  5. Depression
- Other disorders associated with dementia or demyelination producing encephalopathy, myelopathy, or neuropathy

■ WORKUP
Prompt evaluation of respiratory, CNS, GI complaints

■ LABORATORY TESTS
- HIV antibody testing
- T-lymphocyte subset analysis: performed to determine the degree of immunodeficiency
- Viral load assay: to plan long-term antiviral therapy consider genotype or phenotype sensitivity testing for patients failing therapy
- CSF examination: for meningitis
- Serologic tests for syphilis, hepatitis B, hepatitis C, and toxoplasmosis
- Genotypic resistance testing: used to assess for primary resistance in naïve patients and secondary resistance in patients failing a regimen
- Eye exam: to evaluate for CMV retinitis in patients with CD counts <50 cells/mm^3
- Cryptococcal antigen: part of the evaluation in AIDS patients with CD4 <100 cells/mm^3 who have fever, diffuse pneumonia, or symptoms of meningitis

■ IMAGING STUDIES
- Cerebral CT for encephalopathy or focal CNS complications (e.g., toxoplasmosis, lymphoma)
- Pulmonary gallium scanning to aid in the diagnosis of a *Pneumocystis carinii* pneumonia
- Baseline chest x-ray

TREATMENT

■ NONPHARMACOLOGIC THERAPY
- Maintain adequate caloric intake
- Encourage good oral hygiene, regular dental care

■ ACUTE GENERAL Rx
Acute management of opportunistic infections and malignancies is reviewed elsewhere in this text under specific AIDS-related disorders.

■ CHRONIC Rx
For all HIV-infected patients, particularly those meeting the case definition of AIDS:
- Preventive therapy for *Pneumocystis carinii* pneumonia and TB (see specific chapters elsewhere in this text). With the advent of modern antiretroviral therapy many patients have experienced substantial restoration of cellular immune function. It has become clear that preventive therapy for *Pneumocystis carinii* and *Mycobacterium avium* complex as well as suppressive therapy for cytomegaloviral and cryptococcal infection can often be safely withdrawn if the CD4 cell count rises above 200 for at least 6 months.
- Antiretroviral therapy employs a combination of three or more of the following: nucleoside and nucleotide reverse transcriptase inhibitors (NRTI), protease inhibitors, and non-nucleoside reverse transcriptase inhibitors (NNRTI). The standard antiretroviral regimen for naïve patients includes two NRTIs and either one protease inhibitor or one NNRTI. Ritonavir-boosted protease inhibitors are preferred because of their improved potency and resistance profile. See Tables 1-2 through 1-6, the HIV chapter, and DHHS guidelines for more specifics on antiretroviral therapy (http://www.aidsinfo.nih.gov/guidelines/).
- An approach to evaluating chronic diarrhea in patients with HIV infection, the approach to the acutely ill HIV-infected patient, and the evaluation of respiratory complaints are described in Section III, Fig. 3-91. Approach to a patient with a suspected CNS lesion is also described in Section III.
- Genotypic resistance testing should be strongly considered for any patient failing antiretroviral therapy.

■ REFERRAL
All patients with AIDS: to a physician knowledgeable and experienced in the management of the disease and its complications

REFERENCES
Carpenter C et al: Antiretroviral therapy in adults, updated recommendations of the International AIDS Society-USA Panel, *JAMA* 283:381, 2000.

Henry K: The case for more cautious, patient-focused antiretroviral therapy, *Ann Intern Med* 132(4):307, 2000.

Isada CM: New developments in long-term treatment of HIV: the honeymoon is over, *Cleve Clin J Med* 68(9):804, 2001.

Kaplan JE et al: Epidemiology of human immunodeficiency virus–associated opportunistic infections in the United States in the era of highly active antiretroviral therapy, *Clin Infect Dis* 30(suppl 1):S5, 2000.

Kaplan JE et al: Discontinuing prophylaxis against recurrent opportunistic infections in HIV-infected persons: a victory in the era of HAART, *Ann Intern Med* 137:285, 2002.

Kirk O et al: Safe interruption of maintenance therapy against previous infection with four common HIV-associated opportunistic pathogens during potent antiretroviral therapy, *Ann Intern Med* 137:239, 2002.

Palmer S et al: Tenofovir, adefovir and zidovudine susceptibilities of primary human immunodeficiency virus type 1 isolates with non-B subtypes or nucleoside resistance, *AIDS Res Hum Retroviruses* 17(12):1167, 2001.

Piot P et al: The global impact of HIV/AIDS, *Nature* 410:968, 2001.

Richman DD: HIV chemotherapy, *Nature* 410:995, 2001.

Author: **Joseph R. Masci, M.D.**

BOX 1-2 **Conditions Included in the 1993 AIDS Surveillance I Case Definition**

Bacterial infections, multiple or recurrent*
Candidiasis of bronchi, trachea, or lungs
Candidiasis, esophageal
Cervical cancer, invasive†
Coccidioidomycosis, disseminated or extrapulmonary
Cryptococcosis, extrapulmonary
Cryptosporidiosis, chronic intestinal (>1-mo duration)
Cytomegalovirus disease (other than liver, spleen, or nodes)
Cytomegalovirus retinitis (with loss of vision)
Encephalopathy, HIV related
Herpes simplex, chronic ulcer(s) (>1-mo duration); or bronchitis, pneumonitis, or esophagitis
Histoplasmosis, disseminated or extrapulmonary
Isoporiasis, chronic intestinal (>1-mo duration)
Kaposi's sarcoma

Lymphoid interstitial pneumonia and/or pulmonary lymphoid hyperplasia*
Lymphoma, Burkitt's (or equivalent term)
Lymphoma, primary, of brain
Mycobacterium avium-intracellulare complex or *Mycobacterium kansasii*, disseminated or extrapulmonary
Mycobacterium tuberculosis, any site (pulmonary† or extrapulmonary)
Mycobacterium, other species or unidentified species, disseminated or extrapulmonary
Pneumocystis carinii pneumonia
Pneumonia, recurrent†
Progressive multifocal leukoencephalopathy
Salmonella septicemia, recurrent
Toxoplasmosis of brain
Wasting syndrome of HIV infection

*Children younger than 13 years.
†Added in the 1993 expansion of the AIDS surveillance case definition for adolescents and adults.

TABLE 1-2   Approved Nucleoside Reverse Transcriptase Inhibitors

AGENT	TRADE NAME	ORAL BIOAVAIL-ABILITY (%)	SERUM HALF-LIFE (H)	INTRACELLULAR HALF-LIFE OF TRIPHOSPHATE (H)	ELIMINATION	DOSE*	AVAILABIILITY	MAJOR ADVERSE EFFECTS‡
Zidovudine	Retrovir	63	1.1	3-4	Hepatic glucuronidation Renal excretion	Adults: 200 mg PO q8h or 300 mg PO q12h Pediatric: 90-180 mg/m² PO q6-12h, up to adult dose	300-mg tablets 100-mg capsules 10-mg/ml syrup 10-mg/ml solution for IV infusion	Headache Insomnia Gastrointestinal intolerance Fatigue Anemia Neutropenia Myositis
Didanosine	Videx EC	40	1.5	8-24	Cellular metabolism	Adult ≥60 kg: 400 mg PO qd; buffered tablets or enteric coated capsule 200 mg PO q12h; buffered tablets	25-mg, 50-mg, 100-mg, 150-mg chewable tablets	Diarrhea Abdominal discomfort Nausea Peripheral neuropathy Pancreatitis
					Renal excretion	Adult <60 kg: 250 mg PO qd; buffered tablets or enteric tablets or enteric coated capsule 125 mg PO q12h; buffered tablets Pediatric: 90-150 mg/m² PO q12h of solution up to adult dose	100-mg, 167-mg, 250-mg powder packets 10-mg/ml solution	
Zalcitabine	Hivid	87	1.2	2.6	Renal excretion	Adult: 0.75 mg PO q8h	0.375-mg, 0.75-mg tablets	Peripheral neuropathy Pancreatitis Oral ulcers
Stavudine	Zerit	86	1.1	3	Renal excretion	Adult ≥60 kg: 40 mg PO q12h Adult <60 kg: 30 mg PO q12h Pediatric: 1 mg/kg q12h, up to adult dose	15-mg, 20-mg, 30-mg, 40-mg capsules 1-mg/ml solution	Peripheral neuropathy
Lamivudine	Epivir	86	2.5	11-14	Renal excretion	Adult: 150 mg PO q12h 300mg PO qd Pediatric: 4 mg/kg PO q12h, up to adult dose	150-mg, 300-mg tablets 10-mg/ml solution	Headache Fatigue
Abacavir	Ziagen	83	1.5	3.3	Hepatic glucuronidation and carboxylation	Adult: 300 mg PO q12h Pediatric: 8 mg/kg PO q12h, up to adult dose	300-mg tablets 20-mg/ml solution	Hypersensitivity reaction
Zidovudine + Lamivudine	Combivir†					Adult: One tablet PO q12h	300-mg zidovudine/ 150-mg lamivudine tablet	
Zidovudine + Lamimudine + Abacavir	Trizivir	—	—	—	—	Adult: One tablet PO q12h	300-mg zidovudine/150-mg lamivudine 300-mg abacavir	Hypersensitivity reaction (due to abacavir)

Adapted from Mandell GL: *Mandell, Douglas, and Bennett's principles and practice of infectious diseases*, ed 5, New York, 2000, Churchill Livingstone.
*Neonatal dose may differ significantly from pediatric dose described here.
†Pharmacokinetic properties, adverse effects, and drug interactions are similar to those of lamivudine and zidovudine used separately.
‡All nucleoside reverse transcriptase inhibitors may also be associated with rare occurrence of potentially fatal lactic acidosis and hepatomegaly with steatosis.

TABLE 1-2 Approved Nonnucleoside Reverse Transcriptase Inhibitors—cont'd

AGENT	TRADE NAME	ORAL BIOAVAIL-ABILITY (%)	SERUM HALF-LIFE (H)	ELIMINATION	DOSE*	AVAILABIILITY	MAJOR ADVERSE EFFECTS
Nevirapine	Viramune	>90	>24	Hepatic cytochrome P450	Adult: 200 mg PO qd for 14 d, then 200 mg PO q12h if no rash develops Pediatric: 120 mg/m² PO qd for 14 d then increase to 120-200 mg/m² PO q12h if no rash develops, up to adult dose	200-mg tablets	Rash Elevated hepatic transaminases
Delavirdine	Rescriptor	85	5.8	Hepatic cytochrome P450	Adult: 400 mg PO q8h	100-mg, 200-mg tablets	Rash Dizziness
Efavirenz	Sustiva		>24	Hepatic cytochrome P450	Adult: 600 mg PO qd	50 mg-, 100 mg-, 200 mg, 600-mg capsules	Headache Rash

TABLE 1-3 Approved Protease Inhibitors

AGENT	TRADE NAME	ORAL BIOAVAIL-ABILITY (%)	SERUM HALF-LIFE (H)	ELIMINATION	DOSE*	AVAILABIILITY	MAJOR ADVERSE EFFECTS†
Saquinavir (soft gel capsule)	Fortovase		1-2	Hepatic cyto-chrome P450	Adult: 1200 mg PO q8h	200-mg soft gel capsules	Nausea Diarrhea Abdominal discomfort
Saquinavir (hard capsule)	Invirase	4	1-2	Hepatic cyto-chrome P450	Adult: When used in combination with ritonavir, 400-600 mg PO q12h When used in combination with ritonavir, 1000/100 mg SQV/RTV PO bid or 400/400 mg SQV/RTV PO bid	200-mg hard capsules	Nausea Diarrhea Abdominal discomfort
Ritonavir	Norvir	70	3.2	Hepatic cyto-chrome P450	Adult: 300 mg PO q12h with escalation over 1-2 wk to 600 mg PO q12h Pediatric: 250 mg/m² of solution PO q12h with escalation over 1-2 wk to 400 mg/m² PO q12h, up to adult dose	100-mg capsules 80-mg/ml solution	Nausea, vomiting Diarrhea Abdominal discomfort Circumoral or peripheral paresthesias Fatigue Altered taste Hypercholesterolemia Hypertriglyceridemia Elevated hepatic transaminases
Indinavir	Crixivan	60-65	1.8	Hepatic cyto-chrome P450	Adults: 800 mg PO q8h When used in combination with ritonavir, 400/400 mg or 800/100 mg or 800/200 mg IDV/RTV PO bid	200-mg, 400-mg capsules	Nausea Abdominal discomfort Nephrolithiasis Hyperbilirubinemia Diarrhea
Nelfinavir	Viracept	20-80	3.5-5	Hepatic cyto-chrome P450	Adult: 750 mg PO q8h Pediatric: 20-30 mg/kg q8h, up to adult dose	250-mg tablets 50-mg/g powder	Nausea, vomiting Rash
Amprenavir	Agenerase		9	Hepatic cyto-chrome P450	Adult: Capsule 1200 mg PO q12h When used in combination with ritonavir, 600/100 mg APV/RTV PO q12 or 1200/200 mg APV/RTV PO qd Pediatric: Capsule 20 mg/kg PO q12h or 15 mg/kg PO q8h, up to adult dose; solution 22.5 mg/kg PO q12h or 17 mg/kg PO q8h, up to 2800	50-mg, 150-mg capsules 15 mg/ml solution	
Lopinavir/ ritonavir	Kaletra	Not yet established	5-6	Hepatic cyto-chrome P450	3 capsules 2×/day	Soft-gel capsules 133.3 mg lopinavir 33.3 mg ritonavir	Diarrhea, pancreatitis
Atazanavir	Reyataz	Not yet established	7	Hepatic	400 mg PO qd. When dosed with ritonavir, 300/100 mg ATZ/RTV PO qd	100-mg, 150-mg, 200-mg capsules	Hyperbilirubinemia

Adapted from Mandell GL: *Mandell, Douglas, and Bennett's principles and practice of infectious diseases,* ed 5, New York, 2000, Churchill Livingstone.
*Neonatal dose may differ significantly from pediatric dose described here.
†All protease inhibitors may be associated with hyperglycemia and changes in body fat distribution. They may also be associated with rare episodes of hemorrhage in persons with hemophilia.

TABLE 1-4   Approved Nucleotide Reverse Transcriptase Inhibitor

AGENT	TRADE NAME	ORAL BIO-AVAILABILITY (%)	SERUM HALF-LIFE (H)	ELIMINATION	DOSE	AVAILABILITY	MAJOR ADVERSE EFFECTS
Tenofovir	Viread	25	—	Renal	300 mg/d	300-mg tablet	Nausea, vomiting, diarrhea

TABLE 1-5   Therapy for Opportunistic Infections in Patients with HIV Infection

CLINICAL DISEASE	DRUG	DOSE	ROUTE	INTERVAL	DURATION
Pneumocystis pneumonia	Trimethoprim with sulfamethoxazole	5 mg/kg with 25 mg/kg	PO, IV	q8h	21 d
	or				
	Trimethoprim plus dapsone	300 mg	PO	18h	21 d
	or	100 mg	PO	qd	
	Pentamidine	3-4 mg/kg	IV (IM)	qd	21 d
	or				
	Atovaquone	750 mg	PO	q12h	21 d
	or				
	Clindamycin plus primaquine	300-450 mg	PO, IV	q6h	21 d
	or	15 mg	PO	qd	
	Trimetrexate plus leucovorin	45 mg/m²	IV	q24h	21 d
		20 mg/m²	PO, IV	q6h	
	Prednisone (adjunctive therapy for severe episode)	40 mg	PO	q12h*	21 d
Pneumocystis pneumonia (maintenance)	Trimethoprim plus sulfamethoxazole	1 single- or double-strength tablet	PO	q24h	Lifelong¶
	or				
	Dapsone	100 mg	PO	q24h	Lifelong
Toxoplasmosis	Sulfadiazine plus pyrimethamine plus leucovorin	1-2 g	PO	q6h	Lifelong
		100 mg†	PO	qd	Lifelong
	or	10-25 mg	PO, IV	qd	Lifelong
	Clindamycin plus pyrimethamine	450-600 mg	PO	q6h	Lifelong
		50-100 mg†	PO	qd	Lifelong
Cryptosporidiosis	Paromomycin	1.0 g	PO	bid	Lifelong
Microsporidiosis	Albendazole	400 mg	PO	bid	Lifelong
Isosporiasis	Trimethoprim wih sulfamethoxazole	160 mg	PO, IV	q6h	10 d
	followed by	800 mg			
	Trimethoprim plus sulfamethaxazole	160 mg	PO	bid	14 d
		800 mg			
Candidiasis					
Oral	Fluconazole	100-200 mg	PO, IV	q24h	5-10 d
Esophageal	Fluconazole	100-400 mg	PO, IV	q24h	14-21 d
Vaginal	Fluconazole	150 mg	PO	—	One dose
Coccidioidomycosis (Pulmonary)	Amphotericin B	0.5-1.0 mg/kg	IV	q24h	≥56 d
	followed by				
	Itraconazole	300 mg	PO	bid	3 d
	followed by	200 mg	PO	bid	Lifelong
	Fluconazole	400-800 mg	PO	q24h	Lifelong
Cryptococcal infection	Amphotericin B with flucytosine	0.7 mg/kg with	IV	q24h	≥14 d
	followed by	25 mg/kg	PO	q6h	≥14 d
	Fluconazole	400 mg	PO	q24h	8 wk
	followed by				
	Fluconazole	200 mg	PO	q24h	Lifelong
Histoplasmosis	Amphotericin B	0.5-1.0 mg/kg	IV	q24h	≥28-56 d
	followed by				
	Itraconazole	200 mg	PO	q24h	Lifelong
Herpes simplex	Acyclovir	200 mg	PO	5/d	10-14 d
	or				
	Famciclovir	125-250 mg	PO	q12h	10-14 d
	or				
	Valacyclovir	500 mg	PO	q12h	10-14 d
Varicella-zoster virus					
Dermatomal	Acyclovir	800 mg	PO	5/d	7-10 d
	or				
	Famciclovr	500 mg	PO	q8h	7-10 d
	or				
	Valacyclovir	1000 mg	PO	q8h	7-10 d
Disseminated	Acyclovir	10-12 mg/kg	IV	q8h	7-14 d

From Mandell GL: *Mandell, Douglas, and Bennett's principles and practice of infectious diseases,* ed 5, New York, 2000, Churchill Livingstone.
*Prednisone, 40 mg q12h × 5 d, followed by 20 mg bid × 5 d, followed by 20 mg qd × 11 d.
†Following a single loading dose of pyrimethamine, 200 mg.
‡With probenecid as described in package insert.
§With pyridoxine 50 mg PO qd.
¶For patients who have sustained response to HAART (see text for criteria for discontinuation of maintenance therapy).

TABLE 1-5 Therapy for Opportunistic Infections in Patients with HIV Infection—cont'd

CLINICAL DISEASE	DRUG	DOSE	ROUTE	INTERVAL	DURATION
Cytomegalovirus	Ganciclovir *followed by*	5 mg/kg	IV	q12h	14-21 d
	Ganciclovir *or*	5 mg/kg	IV	q24h	Lifelong¶
	Foscarnet *followed by*	60 mg/kg	IV	q8h	14-21 d
	Foscarnet *or*	90-120 mg/kg	IV	q24h	Lifelong¶
	Ganciclovir implant *or*	—	—	q6-9m	Lifelong¶
	Cidofovir‡ *followed by*	5 mg/kg	IV	qwk	2 wk
		5 mg/kg	IV	q2wk	Lifelong¶
Mycobacterium tuberculosis	Isoniazid§ *and*	300 mg	PO, IM	q24h	At least 6 mo
	Rifampin *and*	600 mg	PO, IV	q24h	At least 6 mo
	Ethambutol *and*	15-25 mg/kg	PO	q24h	Depends on sensitivity
	Pyrazinamide	15-25 mg/kg	PO	q24h	2 mo
Mycobacterium avium complex	Clarithromycin	500 mg	PO	q12h	Lifelong¶
	Ethambutol	15 mg/kg	PO	q24h	Lifelong
Bartonella (Rochalimaea) spp.	Erythromycin *or*	500 mg	PO	q6h	≥12 wk
	Doxycycline	100 mg	PO	q12h	≥12 wk

From Mandell GL: *Mandell, Douglas, and Bennett's principles and practice of infectious diseases,* ed 5, New York, 2000, Churchill Livingstone.
*Prednisone, 40 mg q12h × 5 d, followed by 20 mg bid × 5 d, followed by 20 mg qd ×11 d.
†Following a single loading dose of pyrimethamine, 200 mg.
‡With probenecid as described in package insert.
§With pyridoxine 50 mg PO qd.
¶For patients who have sustained response to HAART (see text for criteria for discontinuation of maintenance therapy).

TABLE 1-6 Prophylaxis for Human Immunodeficiency Virus–Related Opportunistic Infections

PATHOGEN	INDICATION FOR PROPHYLAXIS	FIRST CHOICE	ALTERNATIVES	COMMENTS
Pneumocystis	CD4+ <200/mm³ Persistent unexplained fever Chronic oropharyngeal candidiasis	Trimethoprim-sulfamethoxazole, 1 DS qd or SS	Dapsone, 50 mg qd, + pyrimethamine, 50 mg/wk Dapsone alone (100 mg qd) Aerosolized pentamidine	SS tablets are effective and may be less toxic than DS. Aerosol pentamidine should be delivered by Respirgard nebulizer.
Mycobacterium avium complex	CD4+ <100/mm³	Clarithromycin, 500 mg bid	Azithromycin (1200 mg qwk) Rifabutin, 300 mg qd	Rifabutin increases hepatic metabolism of other drugs.
Toxoplasma	No consensus	Trimethoprim-sulfamethoxazole, 1 DS qd	—	Pyrimethamine alone is not effective.
Mycobacterium tuberculosis	PPD >5 mm "High risk"	Sensitive: Isoniazid, 300 mg × 9 mo Resistant: ?	Rifampin* 600 mg, or Rifabutin* 300 mg, and pyrizinamide (15-25 mg/kg qd × 2 mo)	For resistant strains, two-drug regimens using combinations of rifampin, pyrazinamide, or a quinolone can be considered.
Candida	Multiple recurrences	Fluconazole, 200 mg daily		Include pyridoxine, 500 mg qd for isoniazid-containing regimens. Recommended only if recurrences are severe or frequent.
Herpes simplex	Multiple recurrences	Acyclovir, 200 mg qd 3-4 ×/day Famciclovir, 125 mg PO bid Valacyclovir, 500 mg PD bid	Itraconazole, 100 mg qd —	
Cytomegalovirus	None	—	—	Oral ganciclovir is not recommended currently.
Pneumococcus	All patients	Pneumovax	—	Trimethoprim-sulfamethoxazole, clarithromycin, and azithromycin appear to prevent some disease.
Influenza	All patients	Influenza vaccine	—	—

From Mandell GL: *Mandell, Douglas, and Bennett's principles and practice of infectious diseases,* ed 5, New York, 2000, Churchill Livingstone.
DS, Double strength; *PPD,* purified protein derivative; *SS,* single strength.
*For patients receiving HAART, dose adjustments may be necessary.

BASIC INFORMATION

■ DEFINITION
Acromegaly is a chronic debilitating disease with an insidious onset, resulting from the effects of either hypersecretion of growth hormone (GH) or increased amounts of an insulin-like growth factor I (IGF-I).

■ SYNONYMS
Marie's disease

ICD-9CM CODES
253.0 Acromegaly

■ EPIDEMIOLOGY & DEMOGRAPHICS
INCIDENCE: 3 to 4 new cases/ 1,000,000 persons
PREVALENCE: 50 to 60 cases/1 million persons, with some estimates as high as 90 cases/1 million persons
PREDOMINANT SEX: No sexual predominance
MEAN AGE AT DIAGNOSIS: Males: 40 yr; females: 45 yr
RISK FACTORS
- Increased mortality, primarily from cardiovascular and respiratory causes
- Death in 50% of untreated patients by age 50 yr (twice the rate of the general population)
- Increased prevalence of colon carcinoma and other malignancies

■ PHYSICAL FINDINGS & CLINICAL PRESENTATION
- Coarse features resulting from growth of soft tissue
- Coarse, oily skin
- Hands and feet that are spadelike, fleshy, and moist
- Prognathism, which can give an underbite
- Carpal tunnel syndrome
- Excessive sweating
- Arthralgias and severe osteoarthritis
- History of increased hat, glove, and/or shoe size
- Hypertension
- Skin tags
- Muscle weakness and decreased exercise capacity
- Headache, often severe
- Diabetes mellitus
- Visual field defects

■ ETIOLOGY
Cause is usually a pituitary adenoma, affecting the anterior lobe.

DIAGNOSIS

■ DIFFERENTIAL DIAGNOSIS
Ectopic production of growth hormone–releasing hormone (GHRH) from a carcinoid or other neuroendocrine tumor

■ WORKUP
1. First screening test: measure serum IGF-I level.
   a. Direct measurement of the GH level is not as useful, because it is secreted in a pulsatile fashion and a random level may be falsely normal.
   b. Upper limits of a normal IGF-I level, depending on the assay: >380 ng/ml or 2.5 U/ml.
2. Failure to suppress serum GH to less than 2 ng/ml after 100 g oral glucose is considered conclusive.
   a. Patients may show suppression of GH or a paradoxical response.
   b. Patients will not suppress GH to 2 ng/ml or less (the normal response).
   c. GHRH level >300 ng/ml is indicative of an ectopic source of GH.

■ LABORATORY TESTS
- Elevated serum phosphate
- Elevated urine calcium

■ IMAGING STUDIES
- Imaging studies of choice: MRI of the pituitary and hypothalamus
- CT of the pituitary and hypothalamus used initially

TREATMENT

■ SURGERY
Treatment of choice: transsphenoidal microsurgical adenomectomy
- Surgical failure rate: about 13.3% for microadenomas (tumors <10 mm) and 11.1% for macroadenomas (tumors >10 mm confined to the sella)
- Preoperative IGF-I level: indicator of surgical outcome with higher levels in the surgical failure group

■ RADIOTHERAPY
- Irradiation to reduce further growth of the tumor in most patients
- Major complication: hypopituitarism, which may occur in up to 50% of patients; this complication is more likely in patients who had surgery irradiation

■ MEDICAL Rx
- Indicated when patients have failed surgical therapy, when surgery is contraindicated, and in patients waiting for the effects of radiotherapy to begin
- Octreotide
   1. A somatostatin analog given tid at a dose of 100 μg subcutaneously
   2. Important side effects: biliary sludge and gallstones; nausea, cramps, and steatorrhea; suppression of GH levels to about 5 μg/L in 52% of patients; IGF-I levels normalized to about 53%
   3. Important in the preoperative shrinkage of pituitary tumors and softening of adenomatous tissue
- Bromocriptine
   1. A dopamine analog given at a dosage of 10 to 60 mg PO tid to qid
   2. Less effective than octreotide
   3. Important advantages: less expensive than octreotide and taken orally
   4. Important side effects: orthostatic hypotension, lightheadedness, nausea, constipation, and nasal stuffiness
   5. Suppresses GH levels to <5 μg/L in about 20% of patients; normalizes GH levels in approximately 10%, and shrinks pituitary adenomas in 10% to 20%; IGF-I levels normalized to about 10%
- Pegvisomant is a growth hormone receptor antagonist that has shown promising results in the treatment of acromegaly.

■ CHRONIC Rx
Combination of bromocriptine and octreotide may be synergistic, allowing a lower combination dosage than alone.

■ DISPOSITION
- Patients receiving radiotherapy need long-term follow-up to monitor the potential development of hypopituitarism.
- Continuation of medical therapy should be based on the normalization of IGF-I levels.

REFERENCES
Melmad S et al: Current status and future opportunities for controlling acromegaly, *Pituitary* 5(3):185, 2002.
Trainer PJ et al: Treatment of acromegaly with the growth hormone-receptor antagonist pegvisomant, *N Engl J Med* 342:1172, 2000.
Author: **Beth J. Wutz, M.D.**

BASIC INFORMATION

■ DEFINITION
Actinomycosis is an indolent, slowly progressive infection caused by both anaerobic or microaerophilic bacteria that normally colonize the mouth, vagina, and colon. Actinomycosis is characterized by the formation of painful abscesses, soft tissue infiltration, and draining sinuses.

■ SYNONYMS
Actinomyces infection

ICD-9CM CODES
039.9 Actinomycosis

■ EPIDEMIOLOGY & DEMOGRAPHICS
- Actinomycosis is worldwide in distribution.
- Commonly found as normal flora of the oral cavity (within gingival crevices, tonsillar crypts, periodontal pockets, dental plaques, and carious teeth), pharynx, tracheobronchial tree, gastrointestinal tract, and female urogenital tract.
- Incidence 1:300,000.
- Males infected more often than females 3:1.
- Can occur at any age but commonly seen in midlife.
- Incidence has decreased since the 1950s and is attributed to better oral hygiene and antibiotics.

■ PHYSICAL FINDINGS & CLINICAL PRESENTATION
Actinomycosis can affect any organ. Although not typically considered as opportunistic pathogens, *Actinomyces* species capitalize on tissue injury or mucosal breach to invade adjacent structures in the head and neck regions. As a result, dental infections and oromaxillofacial trauma are common antecedent events. Characteristic manifestations include:
- Cervicofacial disease (most common site):
  1. Occurs in the setting of poor dental hygiene, recent dental surgery, or minor oral trauma
  2. Painful soft tissue swelling commonly seen at the angle of the mandible
  3. Fever, chills, and weight loss
  4. Trismus
  5. Soft tissue facial infection with sinus tract or fistula formation
- Thoracic disease:
  1. Can involve the lungs, pleura, mediastinum, or chest wall.
  2. Presumed secondary to aspiration of *Actinomyces* organisms in patients with poor oral hygiene.
  3. Fever, cough, weight loss, and pleuritic chest pains are common symptoms.
  4. Signs of pneumonia or pleural effusion may be present.
  5. With extension beyond the lungs to mediastinal structures and the chest wall, signs and symptoms of pericarditis, empyema, chest wall sinus drainage, and tracheoesophageal fistula can all occur (Fig. 1-9).

- Abdominal disease:
  1. Occurs most commonly after appendectomy, perforated bowel, diverticulitis, or surgery to the gastrointestinal tract.
  2. Lesions develop most commonly in the ileocecal valve, causing abdominal pain, fever, weight loss, and a palpable mass.
  3. Extension may occur to the liver, causing jaundice and abscess formation.
  4. Sinus tracts to the abdominal wall can occur.
- Pelvic disease:
  1. Commonly occurs by extension from abdominal disease of the ileocecal valve to the right adnexa (80% of cases).
  2. Endometritis.

■ ETIOLOGY
- Actinomycosis is most commonly caused by *Actinomyces israelii*. Other causes are *A. naeslundii*, *A. odontolyticus*, *A. viscosus*, *A. meyeri*, and *A. gerencseriae*.
- *Actinomyces* are gram-positive, non-spore-forming, anaerobic or microaerophilic rods.
- Actinomycosis infections are polymicrobial, usually associated with *Streptococcus*, *Bacteroides*, *Eikenella corrodens*, *Enterococcus*, and *Fusobacterium*.
- Infects individuals only after entry into disrupted mucosa or tissue injury.

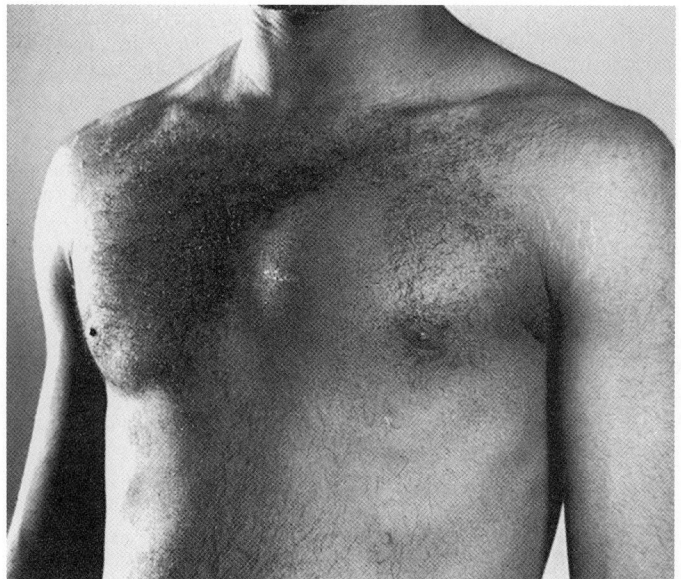

A

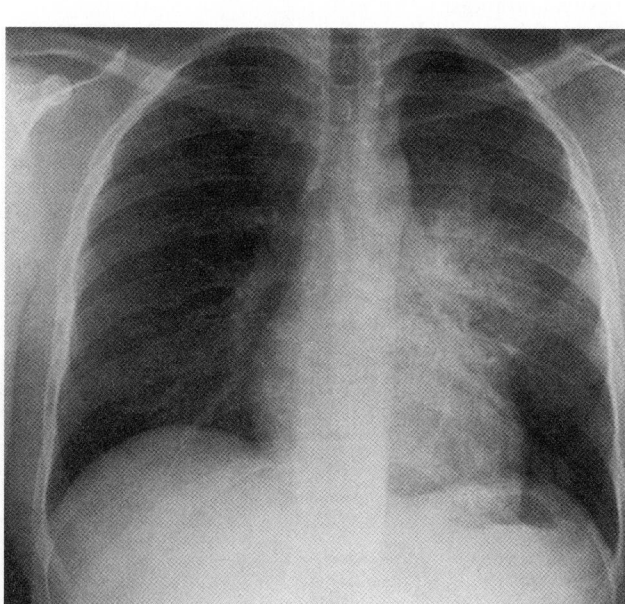

B

Fig. 1-9   Thoracic actinomycosis. A, Initial presentation with a bulging mass lesion in the chest wall with a central sinus tract. **B,** The chest radiograph with the associated pulmonary infiltrate. (From Gorbach SL: *Infectious diseases,* ed 2, Philadelphia, 1998, WB Saunders.)

DIAGNOSIS

Isolating the bacteria in the proper clinical setting makes the diagnosis of actinomycosis.

■ DIFFERENTIAL DIAGNOSIS

Nocardiosis, botryomycosis, chromomycosis, intestinal tuberculosis, ameboma, Crohn's disease, colon cancer, and other causes of acute, subacute, or chronic infections of the lung, abdomen, hepatic, GI, GU, musculoskeletal, and CNS system.

■ WORKUP

The workup includes obtaining specimens either by aspirating abscesses, excising sinus tracts, or tissue biopsies.

■ LABORATORY TESTS

- Isolating "sulfur granules" from tissue specimens or draining sinuses confirms the diagnosis of actinomycosis. *Actinomyces* are noted for forming characteristic sulfur granules in infected tissue but not in vitro. The term *sulfur granule* is a misnomer, reflecting only the yellow color of the granule in pus, because the granules are not composed of any sulfur at all.
  1. Sulfur granules are nests of *Actinomyces* species. Sulfur granules may be macroscopic or microscopic (Fig. 1-10).
  2. Sulfur granules are crushed and stained for identification of *Actinomyces* organisms and may take up to 3 wk to grow in culture media.

■ IMAGING STUDIES

- Imaging studies are useful adjunctive tests in localizing the site and spread of infection.
  1. Chest x-ray examination
  2. CT scan of the head, chest, abdomen, and pelvic areas is useful

TREATMENT

■ NONPHARMACOLOGIC THERAPY

- Incision and drainage of abscesses
- Excision of sinus tract

■ ACUTE GENERAL Rx

- Penicillin 10 to 20 million units per day in 4 divided doses for 4 to 6 wk.
- In penicillin-allergic patients, erythromycin, tetracycline, clindamycin, or cephalosporins (depending on the type of penicillin allergy) are reasonable alternatives.
- Chloramphenicol 50 to 60 mg/kg/day has been used for CNS actinomycosis.

■ CHRONIC Rx

- Following 4 to 6 wk IV penicillin, oral penicillin V 500 mg PO qid for 6 to 12 mo.
- Treatment of associated microorganisms is not needed.

■ DISPOSITION

- Clinical actinomycosis, if not treated, spreads to contiguous tissues and structures ignoring tissue planes. Hematogenous spread, although possible, is rare.

- Actinomycosis is very sensitive to antibiotics but requires chronic long-term treatment to prevent relapse.

■ REFERRAL

If the diagnosis of actinomycosis is suspected, consultation with an infectious disease specialist is suggested. General surgical consultation for excision of sinus tracts and abscess incision and drainage is recommended.

PEARLS & CONSIDERATIONS

■ COMMENTS

- There is no person-to-person transmission of *Actinomyces*.
- Isolation of the organism in an asymptomatic individual does not mean the person has actinomycosis. Active symptoms must be present to make the diagnosis.
- Pelvic actinomycosis has been associated with use of an intrauterine device (IUD).
- Actinomycosis can also involve the CNS, causing multiple brain abscesses.

REFERENCES

Jacobs RF, Schutze GE: Actinomycosis. In Behrman RE (Ed), *Nelson Textbook of Pediatrics*, ed 16, Philadelphia, 2000, WB Saunders, p. 823.

Russo TA: Agents of actinomycosis. In *Mandell, Douglas, and Bennett's principles and practice of infectious diseases*, ed 5, New York, 2000, Churchill Livingstone.

Smego RA, Foglia G: Actinomycosis, *Clin Infect Dis* 26:1255, 1998.

Authors: **Joseph F. Grillo, M.D., and Dennis Mikolich, M.D.**

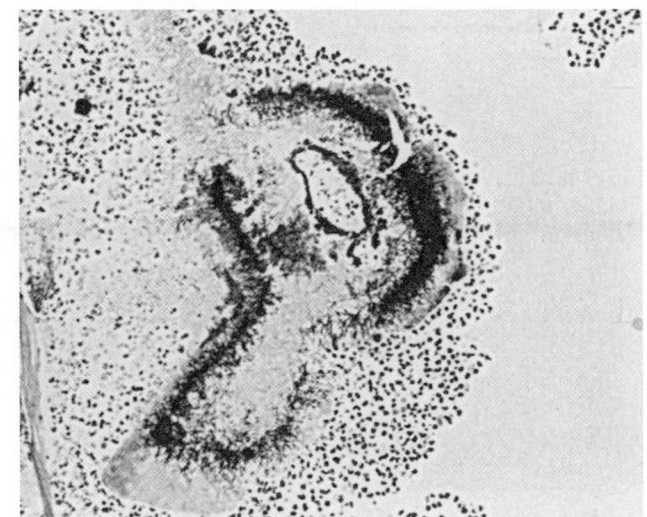
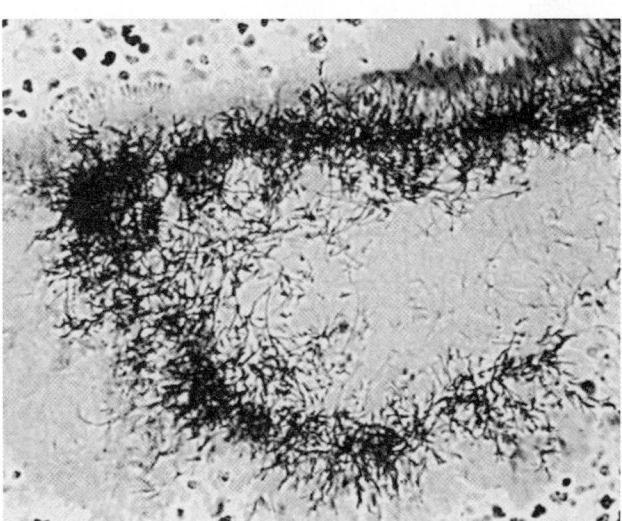

Fig. 1-10 **A,** Actinomycotic sulfur granule surrounded by inflammatory cells (Brown-Brenn stain, ×250). **B,** Increased magnification (×1000) demonstrates the delicate, branched filaments of *Actinomyces*. (From Mandell GL [ed]: *Mandell, Douglas, and Bennett's principles and practice of infectious diseases*, ed 5, New York, 2000, Churchill Livingstone.)

BASIC INFORMATION

■ DEFINITION
Acute respiratory distress syndrome (ARDS) is a form of noncardiogenic pulmonary edema that results from acute damage to the alveoli. It is characterized by acute diffuse infiltrative lung lesions with resulting interstitial and alveolar edema, severe hypoxemia, and respiratory failure. The definition of ARDS includes the following three components:
1. A ratio of Pao_2 to Fio_2 ≤200 regardless of the level of PEEP
2. The detection of bilateral pulmonary infiltrates on frontal chest x-ray
3. Pulmonary artery wedge pressure (PAWP) ≤18 mm Hg or no clinical evidence of elevated left atrial pressure on the basis of chest radiograph or other clinical data

■ SYNONYMS
ARDS
Adult respiratory distress syndrome

ICD-9CM CODES
518.82 Acute respiratory distress syndrome

■ EPIDEMIOLOGY & DEMOGRAPHICS
In the U.S. there are 75,000 to 100,000 ARDS cases/yr.
Incidence is 1.5 to 8.3 cases/100,000/yr.

■ PHYSICAL FINDINGS & CLINICAL PRESENTATION
- Signs and symptoms
  1. Dyspnea
  2. Chest discomfort
  3. Cough
  4. Anxiety
- Physical examination
  1. Tachypnea
  2. Tachycardia
  3. Hypertension
  4. Coarse crepitations of both lungs
  5. Fever may be present if infection is the underlying etiology

■ ETIOLOGY
- Sepsis (>40% of cases)
- Aspiration: near drowning, aspiration of gastric contents (>30% of cases)
- Trauma (>20% of cases)
- Multiple transfusions, blood products
- Drugs (e.g., overdose of morphine, methadone, heroin; reaction to nitrofurantoin)
- Noxious inhalation (e.g., chlorine gas, high O_2 concentration)
- Post-resuscitation
- Cardiopulmonary bypass
- Pneumonia
- Burns
- Pancreatitis
- A history of chronic alcohol abuse significantly increases the risk of developing ARDS in critically ill patients

■ DIAGNOSIS

■ DIFFERENTIAL DIAGNOSIS
- Cardiogenic pulmonary edema
- Viral pneumonitis
- Lymphangitic carcinomatosis

■ WORKUP
The search for an underlying cause should focus on treatable causes (e.g., infections such as sepsis or pneumonia)
- ABGs
- Hemodynamic monitoring
- Bronchoalveolar lavage (selected patients)

■ LABORATORY TESTS
- ABGs:
  1. Initially: varying degrees of hypoxemia, generally resistant to supplemental oxygen
  2. Respiratory alkalosis, decreased Pco_2
  3. Widened alveolar-arterial gradient
  4. Hypercapnia as the disease progresses
- Bronchoalveolar lavage:
  1. The most prominent finding is an increased number of polymorphonucleocytes.
  2. The presence of eosinophilia has therapeutic implications, because these patients respond to corticosteroids.
- Blood and urine cultures

■ IMAGING STUDIES
Chest x-ray examination (Fig. 1-11).
- The initial chest radiogram might be normal in the initial hours after the precipitating event.
- Bilateral interstitial infiltrates are usually seen within 24 hr; they often are more prominent in the bases and periphery.
- "White out" of both lung fields can be seen in advanced stages.

 TREATMENT

■ NONPHARMACOLOGIC THERAPY
Hemodynamic monitoring:
- Hemodynamic monitoring can be used for the initial evaluation of ARDS (in ruling out cardiogenic pulmonary edema) and its subsequent management. Recent studies, however, have shown that clinical management involving the early use of pulmonary artery catheters in patients with ARDS did not significantly affect mortality and morbidity.
- Although no dynamic profile is diagnostic of ARDS, the presence of pulmonary edema, a high cardiac output and a low PAWP is characteristic of ARDS.
- It is important to remember that partially treated intravascular volume overload and flash pulmonary edema can have the hemodynamic features of ARDS; filling pressures can also be elevated by increased intrathoracic pressures or with fluid administration; cardiac function can be depressed by acidosis, hypoxemia, or other factors associated with sepsis.
Ventilatory support: mechanical ventilation is generally necessary to maintain adequate gas exchange (see Section III, Fig. 3-5); assist-control is generally preferred initially with the following ventilator settings:
- Fio_2 1.0 (until a lower value can be used to achieve adequate oxygenation). When possible, minimize oxygen toxicity by maintaining Fio_2 at <60%.
- Tidal volume: Set initial tidal volume at 5-6 ml/kg of body weight. Aim to maintain plateau pressure (Pplat) at <30 mm Hg.
- PEEP 5 cm H_2O or greater (to increase lung volume and keep alveoli open). PEEP should be applied in small increments of 3 to 5 cm H_2O (up to a maximum of 15 cm H_2O) to achieve acceptable arterial saturation (≥ 0.9) with nontoxic FiO_2 values (<0.6) and acceptable airway plateau pressures > 30-35 cm H_2O). It is important to remember that an increase in PEEP may lower cardiac output and, despite improvement in PaO_2, may actually have a negative effect on tissue oxygenation (the major determinants of tissue oxygenation are Hb, percent saturation, and cardiac output).

- Inspiratory flow: 60 L/min.
- Ventilatory rate: high ventilatory rates of 20 to 25 breaths/min are often necessary in patients with ARDS because of their increased physiologic deadspace and smaller lung volumes. Patients must be monitored for excessive intrathoracic gas trapping ("auto-PEEP" or "intrinsic-PEEP") that can depress cardiac output.

■ ACUTE GENERAL Rx

Identify and treat precipitating conditions:

- Blood and urine cultures and trial of antibiotics in presumed sepsis (routine administration of antibiotics in all cases of ARDS is not recommended).
- Prompt repair of bone fractures in patients with major trauma.
- Bowel rest and crystalloid resuscitation in pancreatitis.
- Fluid management: optimal fluid and hemodynamic management of patients with ARDS is patient specific; generally, administration of crystalloids is recommended if a downward trend in pulmonary capillary wedge pressures (PCWP) is associated with diminished cardiac index, resulting in prerenal azotemia, oliguria, and relative tachycardia; on the other hand, if PCWP increases with little or no change in cardiac index, one should begin diuretic therapy and use low-dose dopamine (2 to 4 μg/kg/min) to maintain natriuresis and support adequate renal flow.
- Positioning the patient: changes in position can improve oxygenation by improving the distribution of perfusion to ventilated lung regions; repositioning (lateral decubitus positioning) should be attempted in patients with hypoxemia that is not responsive to other medical interventions. Placing patients with acute respiratory failure in a prone position improves their oxygenation but does not improve their survival.
- Corticosteroids: routine use of corticosteroids in ARDS is not recommended; corticosteroids may be beneficial in patients with many eosinophils in the bronchoalveolar lavage fluid; systemic infections should be ruled out or adequately treated before administration of corticosteroids.

- Nutritional support: nutritional support is necessary to maintain adequate colloid oncotic pressure and intravascular volume.
- Tracheostomy: tracheostomy is warranted in patients requiring >2 wk of mechanical ventilation; discussion regarding tracheostomy should begin with patient (if alert and oriented) and family members/legal guardian, after 5 to 7 days of ventilatory support.
- Some form of DVT prophylaxis is indicated in all patients with ARDS.
- Stress ulcer prophylaxis with sucralfate suspension (via NG tube), or IV proton pump inhibitors (PPIs) or IV H_2 blockers.

■ DISPOSITION

- Prognosis for ARDS varies with the underlying cause. Prognosis is worse in patients with chronic liver disease, nonpulmonary organ dysfunction, sepsis, and advanced age.
- Elevated values of deadspace fraction [$(Paco_2-Peco_2)/Paco_2$] (normal is <0.3) is associated with an increased risk of death.
- Overall mortality varies between 40% and 60%. The majority of deaths are attributable to sepsis or multiorgan dysfunction rather than primary respiratory causes.

■ REFERRAL

Surgical referral for tracheostomy (see "Acute General Rx").

REFERENCES

Ely EW et al: Recovery rate and prognosis in older persons who develop acute lung injury and the acute respiratory distress syndrome, *Ann Intern Med* 136:25, 2002.

Nuckton T et al: Pulmonary dead-space fraction as a risk factor for death in the acute respiratory distress syndrome, *N Engl J Med* 346:1281, 2002.

Richard C et al: Early use of the pulmonary artery catheter and outcomes in patients with shock and acute respiratory distress syndrome, *JAMA* 290:2713, 2003.

Udobi KF et al: Acute respiratory distress syndrome, *Am Fam Physician* 67:315, 2003.

Author: **Fred F. Ferri, M.D.**

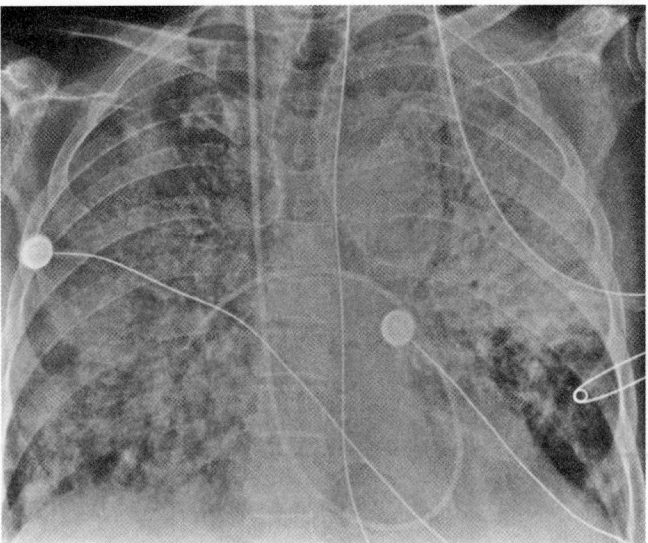

Fig. 1-11   ARDS. AP radiograph in an elderly woman reveals widespread consolidation with air bronchograms. The heart size is normal. There are no pleural effusions. (From McLoud TC: *Thoracic radiology: the requisites,* St Louis, 1998, Mosby.)

BASIC INFORMATION

■ DEFINITION
Addison's disease is characterized by inadequate secretion of corticosteroids resulting from partial or complete destruction of the adrenal glands.

■ SYNONYMS
Primary adrenocortical insufficiency
Adrenal insufficiency

ICD-9CM CODES
255.4 Addison's disease

■ EPIDEMIOLOGY & DEMOGRAPHICS
PREVALENCE: 5 cases/100,000 persons
PREDOMINANT SEX: Female:male ratio of 2:1

■ PHYSICAL FINDINGS & CLINICAL PRESENTATION
• Hyperpigmentation: more prominent in palmar creases, buccal mucosa, pressure points (elbows, knees, knuckles), perianal mucosa, and around areolas of nipples
• Hypotension
• Generalized weakness
• Amenorrhea and loss of axillary hair in females

■ ETIOLOGY
• Autoimmune destruction of the adrenal glands (80% of cases)
• Tuberculosis (15% of cases)
• Carcinomatous destruction of the adrenal glands
• Adrenal hemorrhage (anticoagulants, trauma, coagulopathies, pregnancy, sepsis)
• Adrenal infarction (arteritis, thrombosis)
• AIDS (adrenal insufficiency develops in 30% of patients with AIDS)
• Other: sarcoidosis, amyloidosis, postoperative, fungal infections

DIAGNOSIS

■ DIFFERENTIAL DIAGNOSIS
Sepsis, hypovolemic shock, acute abdomen, apathetic hyperthyroidism in the elderly, myopathies, GI malignancy, major depression, anorexia nervosa, hemochromatosis, salt-losing nephritis, chronic infection

■ WORKUP
• If the clinical picture is highly suggestive of adrenocortical insufficiency, the diagnosis can be made with the rapid ACTH (Cortrosyn) test:
  1. Give 250 μg ACTH by IV push and measure cortisol levels at 0 and 30 min.

  2. Cortisol level <18 μg/dl at 30 or 60 min is suggestive of adrenal insufficiency.
  3. Measure plasma ACTH. A high ACTH level confirms primary adrenal insufficiency.
• Secondary adrenocortical insufficiency (caused by pituitary dysfunction) can be distinguished from primary adrenal insufficiency by the following:
  1. Normal or low plasma ACTH level following rapid ACTH (Cortrosyn test)
  2. Absence of hyperpigmentation
  3. No significant impairment of aldosterone secretion (because aldosterone secretion is under control of the renin-angiotensin system)
  4. Additional evidence of hypopituitarism (e.g., hypogonadism, hypothyroidism)

■ LABORATORY TESTS
• Increased potassium, decreased sodium and chloride
• Decreased glucose
• Increased BUN/creatinine ratio (prerenal azotemia)
• Mild normocytic, normochromic anemia, neutropenia, lymphocytosis, eosinophilia (significant dehydration may mask hyponatremia and anemia)
• PPD and antiadrenal antibodies

■ IMAGING STUDIES
• Chest x-ray examination may reveal a small heart.
• Abdominal x-ray film: adrenal calcifications may be noted if the adrenocortical insufficiency is secondary to TB or fungus.
• Abdominal CT scan: small adrenal glands generally indicate either idiopathic atrophy or long-standing TB, whereas enlarged glands are suggestive of early TB or potentially treatable diseases.

TREATMENT

■ NONPHARMACOLOGIC THERAPY
• Perform periodic monitoring of serum electrolytes, vital signs, and body weight; liberal sodium intake is suggested.
• Periodic measurement of bone density may be helpful in identifying patients at risk for the development of osteoporosis.
Patients should carry a Medic Alert bracelet and an emergency pack containing hydrocortisone 100 mg ampule, syringe, and needle. Patients and partners should be educated on how to give IM injection in case of vomiting or coma.

■ ACUTE GENERAL Rx
Addisonian crisis is an acute complication of adrenal insufficiency characterized by circulatory collapse, dehydration, nausea, vomiting, hypoglycemia, and hyperkalemia.
1. Draw plasma cortisol level; do not delay therapy while waiting for confirming laboratory results.
2. Administer hydrocortisone 50-100 mg IV q6h for 24 hr; if patient shows good clinical response, gradually taper dosage and change to oral maintenance dose (usually prednisone 7.5 mg/day).
3. Provide adequate volume replacement with D_5NS solution until hypotension, dehydration, and hypoglycemia are completely corrected. Large volumes (2 to 3 L) may be necessary in the first 2 to 3 hr to correct the volume deficit and hypoglycemia and to avoid further hyponatremia.
Identify and correct any precipitating factor (e.g., sepsis, hemorrhage).

■ CHRONIC Rx
• Give hydrocortisone 15 to 20 mg PO every morning and 5 to 10 mg in late afternoon or prednisone 5 mg in morning and 2.5 mg hs.
• Give oral fludrocortisone 0.05 mg/day to 0.20 mg/day: this mineralocorticoid is necessary if the patient has primary adrenocortical insufficiency. The dose is adjusted based on the serum sodium level and the presence of postural hypotension or marked orthostasis.
• Instruct patients to increase glucocorticoid replacement in times of stress and to receive parenteral glucocorticoids if diarrhea or vomiting occurs. Typical supplementation varies from 25 mg PO qd of hydrocortisone for minor medical and surgical stress to 50-100 mg IV hydrocortisone every 8 hr for sepsis-induced hypotension or shock.
• The administration of dehydroepiandrosterone 50 mg PO qd improves well-being and sexuality in women with adrenal insufficiency.

REFERENCES
Cooper MS, Stewart PM: Corticosteroid insufficiency in acutely ill patients, *N Engl J Med* 348:727, 2003.
Dorin RI et al: Diagnosis of adrenal insufficiency, *Ann Intern Med* 139:194, 2003.
Author: **Fred F. Ferri, M.D.**

BASIC INFORMATION

■ DEFINITION
In the United States, agoraphobia is considered part of the continuum of panic attacks and panic disorder. In Europe, agoraphobia is conceptualized as a phobic condition independent of panic. A *panic attack* is a relatively brief, sudden episode of intense fear or apprehension, often associated with a sense of impending doom and various uncomfortable and disquieting physical symptoms. *Panic disorder* is diagnosed if at least one panic attack is followed by a significant degree of concern about future attacks or a major change in behavior related to these attacks. Agoraphobia is anxiety about, or avoidance of, places or situations in which the ability to leave suddenly is limited or impossible in the event of having a panic attack.

■ SYNONYMS
Anxiety attacks
Fear attacks

ICD-9CM CODES
F 41.0 Panic disorder without agoraphobia (DSM-IV: 300.01)
F 40.01 Panic disorder with agoraphobia (DSM-IV: 300.01)

■ EPIDEMIOLOGY & DEMOGRAPHICS
INCIDENCE (IN U.S.): 1% 1-mo incidence of panic attacks
PREVALENCE (IN U.S.):
- 15% lifetime prevalence of panic attacks
- Panic disorder much more uncommon, with a lifetime prevalence of 1.5% to 3.5%; chronicity of condition reflected by a similar 1-yr prevalence rate of 1% to 2%
- Agoraphobia relatively rare; 0.3% to 1% lifetime prevalence

PREDOMINANT SEX:
- Women more commonly affected (>85% of clinical population)
- Panic disorder twice as common in women
- Panic disorder with agoraphobia three times as common in women
PREDOMINANT AGE:
- Age of onset earlier in males (24 yr) than females (28 yr)
- Onset after age 45 yr rare
PEAK INCIDENCE:
- Chronic condition with a waxing and waning course
- Bimodal incidence peaks noted, with the first peak between ages 15 and 24 yr and second peak between 35 and 44 yr
GENETICS:
- Risk of developing panic disorder in first-degree relatives of individuals with panic disorder four to seven times that of general population
- Findings in twin studies: about 60% of contributing factors to panic are genetic

■ PHYSICAL FINDINGS & CLINICAL PRESENTATION
- Panic disorder
  1. Present either with a panic attack or with fear and anxiety related to anticipation of a future panic attack
  2. Typical presentation: unexpected, untriggered periods of intense anxiety and fear with associated physiologic changes (e.g., palpitations, sweating, tremulousness, shortness of breath, chest pain, GI distress, faintness, derealization, paresthesia)
  3. Emergency or physician visits often occasioned by physical symptoms

- Agoraphobia
  1. Rare complaints to physician
  2. Activities usually self-limited by avoiding public situations where the patient might experience a panic attack and would be unable to exit readily, such as the following:
  Crowded public areas (stores, public transportation, church)
  Individual interactions (hair dresser, neighborhood meetings)
  3. On exposure to or anticipation of exposure to such situations, significant anxiety occurs
ETIOLOGY
Hypotheses (NOTE: There are sufficient data to support each model.)
1. Central dyscontrol of autonomic arousal (typically localized to the locus ceruleus)
2. Cognitive overreaction to relatively mild physiologic cues
3. Dysfunction of a central suffocation alarm mechanism

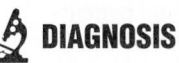

DIAGNOSIS

■ DIFFERENTIAL DIAGNOSIS
- Medical conditions
  1. Arrhythmias
  2. Hyperthyroidism
  3. Hyperparathyroidism
  4. Seizure disorders
  5. Respiratory diseases
  6. Pheochromocytoma
- Therapeutic (theophylline, steroids) and recreational (cocaine, amphetamine, caffeine) drugs and drug withdrawal (alcohol, barbiturates, benzodiazepines)
- Phobias (e.g., specific phobia or social phobia)
- Obsessive-compulsive disorder (cued by exposure to the object of the obsession)
- Posttraumatic stress disorder (cued by recall of a stressor)

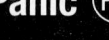
■ WORKUP
- Emergency presentation: cardiac, respiratory, or neurologic symptoms
- History and physical examination to rule out a concomitant medical condition

NOTE Panic disorder and agoraphobia are not diagnoses of exclusion, but exclusion of other conditions is usually required.

■ LABORATORY TESTS
- Thyroid profile
- Electrolyte measures, including calcium
- Toxicology screen
- ECG
- Acute cases: possible monitoring and cardiac enzymes to rule out arrhythmia or ischemia

■ IMAGING STUDIES
- For temporal lobe dysfunction (e.g., temporal lesions or as ictal or interictal manifestation of temporal lobe seizures): brain CT scan or MRI and/or an EEG in some patients
- Holter monitor to rule out occult or episodic arrhythmias
- Chest x-ray examination, ABG, or pulmonary function tests if respiratory compromise suspected

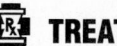 **TREATMENT**

■ NONPHARMACOLOGIC THERAPY
- Psychotherapy: generally very effective; long-term follow-up studies of panic patients suggest that therapy is possibly superior to pharmacologic interventions
- Interpersonal and cognitive-behavioral therapy modalities: most extensively studied

■ ACUTE GENERAL Rx
- Benzodiazepines, particularly alprazolam: very effective in acute setting
- Low-dose alprazolam for patients with rare panic attacks and asymptomatic interattack periods (0.25 to 0.5 mg PO or sublingually prn)

■ CHRONIC Rx
- Because disorder patients, as a group, have a low likelihood of abusing benzodiazepines, uncomplicated cases managed with low-dose benzodiazepines on a schedule or prn
- Preferred pharmacologic agents: antidepressants with a significant serotonin reuptake inhibitory action
- Imipramine quite effective in both panic disorder and agoraphobia
- Newer antidepressants (paroxetine, sertraline, and fluoxetine) quite effective in preventing panic attacks and ameliorating agoraphobia

■ DISPOSITION
- Typical course chronic but with significant waxing and waning (common to have long periods of remission)
- Presence of agoraphobia associated with a more chronic course
- Findings with long-term follow-up studies: 6 to 10 yr after treatment some 30% in remission, 40% to 50% improved with residual symptoms, and the remainder either unchanged or worse

■ REFERRAL
Referral needed if:
- Patients do not respond to a serotonin reuptake inhibitor
- Therapy is the preferred treatment

REFERENCES
Mavissakalian MR, Perel JM: Duration of imipramine therapy and relapse in panic disorder with agoraphobia. *J Clin Psychopharmacol* 22:294, 2002.

Pohl RB et al: Sertraline in the treatment of panic disorder: a double-blind multicenter trial, *Am J Psychiatry* 155:1188, 1998.

Rapaport MH et al: Sertraline treatment of panic disorder: results of a long-term study, *Acta Psychiatr Scand* 104:289, 2001.
Author: **Rif S. El-Mallakh, M.D.**

BASIC INFORMATION

■ DEFINITION

Although it is impossible to define alcoholism precisely, among the commonly used screening instruments for this disorder are the CAGE questionnaire, short Michigan Alcoholism Screening Test (SMAST), National Council on Alcoholism criteria, and DSM-IV-R criteria.

Although not generally included under the topic alcoholism, hazardous or at-risk drinking should also be considered. For men, at-risk drinking is defined as greater than 14 drinks/week or more than 4 drinks/occasion. For women, at-risk drinking is defined as about half that given for men.

■ SYNONYMS

Alcohol abuse
Substance abuse

ICD-9CM CODES

303.9 Alcoholism

■ EPIDEMIOLOGY & DEMOGRAPHICS

INCIDENCE (IN U.S.):
- See "Prevalence."
- 20% achieve abstinence without help, 70% achieve sobriety for 1 yr.

PREVALENCE (IN U.S.): 7% of population 18 yr or older

PREDOMINANT SEX:
- Lifetime risk for males 8% to 10%
- Lifetime risk for females 3% to 5%

PEAK INCIDENCE: 20 to 40 yr

GENETICS: More common with a family history of alcoholism and in patients of Irish, Scandinavian, and Native American descent

■ PHYSICAL FINDINGS & CLINICAL PRESENTATION

- Recurring minor trauma
- GI bleeding
- Pancreatitis
- Liver disease
- Odor of alcohol on breath
- Tremulousness
- Tachycardia
- Peripheral neuropathy
- Recent memory loss
- Table 1-7 describes some alcohol-related medical disorders.

■ ETIOLOGY

- Social and genetic factors important
- Risk factors:
  1. Broken homes
  2. Unemployment
  3. Divorce
  4. Recurrent depression
  5. Addiction to another substance, including tobacco

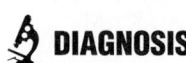 **DIAGNOSIS**

■ WORKUP

- Screening tests (CAGE or SMAST)
- Blood studies (see "Laboratory Tests")

■ LABORATORY TESTS

- γ-Glutamyltransferase (GGTP), generally elevated
- Liver transaminases (ALT, AST), often elevated, may be normal or low in advanced liver disease
- Low albumin level, hypophosphatemia, hypomagnesemia from malnutrition
- CBC reveals elevated mean corpuscular volume (MCV) from toxic effect of alcohol on erythrocyte development on nutritional deficiencies
- Stool for occult blood may be positive secondary to gastritis, or variceal bleeding

■ IMAGING STUDIES

Indicated only if there is a history of trauma. CT or ultrasound of abdomen may reveal fatty liver or cirrhosis in advanced stages.

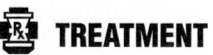 **TREATMENT**

■ NONPHARMACOLOGIC THERAPY

- Complete abstinence
- Depression, if present, should be treated at same time ETOH is withdrawn

---

TABLE 1-7 Alcohol-Related Medical Disorders

AFFECTED ORGAN OR SYSTEM	DISORDERS
Nutrition	Deficiencies of primarily thiamine but also the following: Vitamins: Folate, thiamine, pyridoxine, niacin, riboflavin Minerals: Magnesium, zinc, calcium Protein
Metabolites and electrolytes	Hypoglycemia, ketoacidosis, hyperlipidemia, hyperuricemia, hypomagnesemia, hypophosphatemia
GI tract	Liver: Fatty liver, hepatitis, cirrhosis Gut: Esophagitis, gastritis Pancreatitis
Nervous system	Brain: Hepatic encephalopathy, Wernicke-Korsakoff syndrome, cerebellar degeneration, central pontine myelinolysis, Marchiafava-Bignami disease, cerebral atrophy with dementia Neuromuscular: Neuropathy, myopathy Amblyopia
Cardiovascular	Heart: Arrhythmia, cardiomyopathy Hypertension
Bone marrow	Macrocytosis, anemia, thrombocytopenia, leukopenia
Endocrine	Pseudo-Cushing's syndrome, testicular atrophy, amenorrhea
Other	Traumatic injury Osteopenia Fetal alcohol syndrome

From Goldman L, Bennett JC (eds): *Cecil textbook of medicine,* ed 21, Philadelphia, 2000, WB Saunders.

■ ACUTE GENERAL Rx

Alcohol withdrawal syndrome occurs when a person stops ingesting alcohol after prolonged consumption. It can result in four possible clinical patterns depending on the severity of the patient's alcohol abuse and the time interval from the patient's previous alcohol ingestion. Blood ethanol level decreases by 20 mg/dL/hr in a normal person. Although discussed separately in the text, these alcohol withdrawal states blend together in real life.

1. **Tremulous state:** (early alcohol withdrawal, "impending DTs," "shakes," "jitters")
   a. Time interval: usually occurs 6 to 8 hr after the last drink or 12 to 48 hr after reduction of alcohol intake; becomes most pronounced at 24 to 36 hr
   b. Manifestation: tremors, mild agitation, insomnia, tachycardia; symptoms are relieved by alcohol
   c. Inpatient treatment
      (1) Admit to medical floor (private room); monitor vital signs q4h; institute seizure precautions; maintain adequate sedation.
      (2) Administer lorazepam as follows:
         (a) Day 1: 2 mg PO q4h while awake and not lethargic
         (b) Day 2: 1 mg PO q4h while awake and not lethargic
         (c) Day 3: 0.5 mg PO q4h while awake and not lethargic
         (d) NOTE: Hold sedation for lethargy or abnormal vital or neurologic signs. The preceding doses are only guidelines; it is best to titrate the dose case by case
      (3) In patients with mild to moderate withdrawal and without history of seizures, individualized benzodiazepine administration (rather than a fixed-dose regimen) results in lower benzodiazepine administration and avoids unnecessary sedation. The Clinical Institute Withdrawal Assessment-Alcohol (CIWA-A) scale can be used to measure the severity of alcohol withdrawal. It consists of 10 items: nausea; tremor; autonomic hyperactivity; anxiety; agitation; tactile, visual, and auditory disturbances; headache; and disorientation. The maximum score is 67. When the CIWA-A score is ≥8, patients are usually given 2 to 4 mg of lorazepam hourly.
      (4) β-Adrenergic blockers: β-blockers are useful for controlling BP and tachyarrhythmias. However, they do not prevent progression to more serious symptoms of withdrawal and if used, should not be administered alone but in conjunction with benzodiazepines. β-Blockers should be avoided in patients with contraindications to their use (e.g., bronchospasm, bradycardia, or severe CHF)
      (5) Vitamin replacement: thiamine 100 mg IV or IM for at least 5 days, plus PO multivitamins. The IV administration of glucose can precipitate Wernicke's encephalopathy in alcoholics with thiamine deficiency; therefore thiamine administration should precede IV dextrose
      (6) Hydration PO or IV (high-caloric solution): if IV, glucose with Na^+, K^+, Mg^{2+}, and phosphate replacement prn
      (7) Laboratory studies
         (a) CBC, platelet count, INR
         (b) Electrolytes, glucose, BUN, creatinine
         (c) GGTP, ALT, AST
         (d) Phosphorus and magnesium
         (e) Serum vitamin B_{12} and folic acid (if megaloblastic features in blood smear)
      (8) Diagnostic imaging: generally not necessary; if subdural hematoma is suspected (evidence of trauma, persistent lethargy), a CT scan should be ordered.
      (9) Social rehabilitation: group therapy such as Alcoholics Anonymous; identification and treatment of social and family problems should be initiated during the patient's hospital stay.

2. **Alcoholic hallucinosis**
   a. Manifestations: usually hallucinations are auditory, but occasionally hallucinations are visual, tactile, or olfactory; usually there is no clouding of sensorium as in delirium (clinical presentation may be mistaken for an acute schizophrenic episode). Disordered perceptions become most pronounced after 24 to 36 hr of abstinence.
   b. Treatment: same as for DTs (see Withdrawal seizures).

3. **Withdrawal seizures** ("rum fits")
   a. Time interval: usually occurs 7 to 30 hr after cessation of drinking, with a peak incidence between 13 and 24 hr.
   b. Manifestations: generalized convulsions with loss of consciousness; focal signs are usually absent; consider further investigation with CT scan of head and EEG if clearly indicated (e.g., presence of focal neurologic deficits, prolonged postictal confusion state). In addition, in a febrile patient who is having a seizure or altered mental state, a lumbar puncture is necessary.
   c. Treatment
      (1) Diazepam 2.5 mg/min IV until seizure is controlled (check for respiratory depression or hypotension) may be beneficial for prolonged seizure activity; IV lorazepam 1 to 2 mg every 2 hr can be used in place of diazepam. Generally withdrawal seizures are self-limited and treatment is not required; the use of phenytoin or other anticonvulsants for short-term treatment of alcohol withdrawal seizures is not recommended.
      (2) Thiamine 100 mg IV, followed by IV dextrose, should also be administered.
      (3) Electrolyte imbalances (↑ Mg^{2+}, ↓ K^+, ↑/↓ Na^+, ↓ PO_4^{-3}) that may exacerbate seizures should be corrected.

4. **DTs:**
   a. Time interval: variable; usually occurs within 1 wk after reduction or cessation of heavy alcohol intake and persists for 1 to 3 days. Peak incidence is 72 hr and 96 hr after the cessation of alcohol consumption.
   b. Manifestations: profound confusion, tremors, vivid visual and tactile hallucinations, autonomic hyperactivity; this is the most serious clinical presentation of alcohol withdrawal (mortality is approximately 15% in untreated patients).
   c. Treatment
      (1) Admission to a detoxification unit where patient can be observed closely
      (2) Vital signs q30min (neurologic signs, if necessary)
      (3) Use of lateral decubitus or prone position if restraints are necessary
      (4) NPO: NG tube for abdominal distention may be nec-

essary but should not be routinely used

(5) Laboratory studies: same as for early alcohol withdrawal

(6) Vigorous hydration (4-6 L/day): IV with glucose (Na^+, K^+, PO_4^{-3}, and Mg^{2+} replacement)

(7) Vitamins: thiamine, 100 mg IV qd. The initial dose of thiamine should precede the administration of IV dextrose; multivitamins (may be added to the hydrating solution)

(8) Sedation

   (a) Initially: lorazepam 2 to 5 mg IM/IV repeated prn

   (b) Maintenance (individualized dosage): chlordiazepoxide, 50 to 100 mg PO q4-6h, lorazepam 2 mg PO q4h, or diazepam 5 to 10 mg PO tid; withhold doses or decrease subsequent doses if signs of oversedation are apparent

   (c) Midazolam is also effective for managing DTs. Its rapid onset (sedation within 2 to 4 min of IV injection) and short duration of action (approximately 30 min) make it an ideal agent for titration in continuous infusion.

(9) Treatment of seizures (as previously described)

9. Diagnosis and treatment of concomitant medical, surgical, or psychiatric conditions

■ **CHRONIC Rx**
• See "Referral."
• Pharmacotherapies for alcoholism include the opiate antagonists (naltrexone 50 mg PO qd or nalmefene 10 to 40 mg qd), disulfiram, acamprosate, and SSRIs.

■ **DISPOSITION**
See "Referral."

■ **REFERRAL**
• To Alcoholics Anonymous or Adult Children of Alcoholics
• Family members to Al-Anon or Al-A-Teen
• Many cities have Salvation Army Adult Rehabilitation centers; all patients accepted, regardless of ability to pay

☼ **PEARLS & CONSIDERATIONS**

■ **COMMENTS**
The cure rate for alcoholism is very disappointing, regardless of the modality. Only those who want to be helped will be helped. An effective strategy for the primary care physician is a prominently displayed sign in the office that states, "If you think you consume too much alcoholic beverage, please discuss it with me." Those who do open up the discussion can be given the facts in a nonjudgmental way and often can be helped. All too often, problem drinkers lie on the questionnaire until they face a life-threatening health issue—and even then denial often reigns supreme.

REFERENCES

Beich A et al: Screening in brief intervention trials targeting excessive drinkers in primary care: systematic review and meta-analysis, *BMJ* 327:536, 2003.

Daeppen JB et al: Symptom-triggered vs fixed-schedule doses of benzodiazepine for alcohol withdrawal: a randomized treatment trial, *Arch Intern Med* 162:1117, 2002.

Enoch ME, Goldman D: Problem drinking and alcoholism: diagnosis and treatment, *Am Fam Physician* 65:441, 2002.

Fiellin DA et al: Outpatient management of patients with alcohol problems, *Ann Intern Med* 133:816, 2000.

Fleming MF et al: Brief physician advise for problem drinkers: long-term efficacy and benefit-cost analysis, *Alcohol Clin Exp Res* 26:36, 2002.

Kosten TR, O'Connor PG: Management of drug and alcohol withdrawal, *N Engl J Med* 348:1786, 2003.

Krystal JH et al: Naltrexone in the treatment of alcohol dependence, *N Engl J Med* 345:1734, 2001.

Moyer A et al: Brief interventions for alcohol problems: a meta-analytic review of controlled investigations in treatment-seeking populations, *Addiction* 97:279, 2002.

Nicholas JM et al: The effect of controlled drinking in alcoholic cardiomyopathy, *Ann Intern Med* 136:192, 2002.

O'Connor PG, Schotrenfeld RS: Patients with alcohol problems, *N Engl J Med* 9:592, 1998.

Schneekloth TD et al: Point prevalence of alcoholism in hospitalized patients: continuing challenges of detection, assessment, and diagnosis, *Mayo Clin Proc* 76:460, 2001.

White IR et al: Alcohol consumption and mortality: modelling risks for men and women at different ages, *BMJ* 325:191, 2002.

Author: **Fred F. Ferri, M.D.**

BASIC INFORMATION

■ DEFINITION
Primary aldosteronism is a clinical syndrome characterized by hypokalemia, hypertension, low plasma renin activity (PRA), and excessive aldosterone secretion.

■ SYNONYMS
Hyperaldosteronism
Conn's syndrome

ICD-9CM CODES
255.1 Primary aldosteronism

■ EPIDEMIOLOGY & DEMOGRAPHICS
INCIDENCE/PREVALENCE: 1% to 2% of patients with hypertension; more common in females

■ PHYSICAL FINDINGS & CLINICAL PRESENTATION
- Generally asymptomatic
- If significant hypokalemia is present, possible muscle cramping, weakness, paresthesias
- Hypertension
- Polyuria, polydipsia

■ ETIOLOGY
- Aldosterone-producing adenoma (>60%)
- Idiopathic hyperaldosteronism (>30%)
- Glucocorticoid-suppressible hyperaldosteronism (<1%)
- Aldosterone-producing carcinoma (<1%)

DIAGNOSIS

■ DIFFERENTIAL DIAGNOSIS
- Diuretic use
- Hypokalemia from vomiting, diarrhea
- Renovascular hypertension
- Other endocrine neoplasm (pheochromocytoma, deoxycorticosterone-producing tumor, renin-secreting tumor)

■ WORKUP
In patients with hypokalemia and a low PRA, confirming tests for primary hyperaldosteronism include the following:
- 24-hr urine test for aldosterone and potassium levels (potassium >40 mEq and aldosterone >15 μg).

- Captopril test: administer 25 to 50 mg of captopril (ACE inhibitor) and measure plasma renin and aldosterone levels 1 to 2 hr later. A plasma aldosterone level >15 ng/dl confirms the diagnosis of primary aldosteronism. This test is more expensive and is best reserved for situations in which the 24-hr urine for aldosterone is ambiguous.
- 24-hr urinary tetrahydroaldosterone (<65 μg/24 hr) and saline infusion test (plasma aldosterone >10 ng/dl) can also be used in ambiguous cases.
- The renin-aldosterone stimulation test (posture test) is helpful in differentiating IHA from aldosterone-producing adenoma (APA). Patients with APA have a decrease in aldosterone levels at 4 hr, whereas patients with IHA have an increase in their aldosterone levels.
- As a screening test for primary aldosteronism, an elevated plasma aldosterone-renin ratio (ARR), drawn randomly from patients on antihypertensive drugs, is predictive of primary aldosteronism (positive predictive value 100% in a recent study). ARR is calculated by dividing plasma aldosterone (mg/dl) by plasma renin activity (mg/ml/hour). ARR >100 is considered elevated.
- Bilateral adrenal venous sampling may be done to localize APA when adrenal CT scan is equivocal. In APA, ipsilateral/contralateral aldosterone level is >10:1, and ipsilateral venous aldosterone concentration is very high (>1000 ng/dl).
- A diagnostic evaluation of hypertensive patients with suspected aldosteronism is described in Section III.

■ LABORATORY TESTS
Routine laboratory tests can be suggestive but are not diagnostic of primary aldosteronism. Common abnormalities are:
- Spontaneous hypokalemia or moderately severe hypokalemia while receiving conventional doses of diuretics
- Possible alkalosis and hypernatremia

■ IMAGING STUDIES
- Adrenal CT scans (with 3-mm cuts) may be used to localize neoplasm.

- Adrenal scanning with iodocholesterol (NP-59) or 6-beta-iodomethyl-19-norcholesterol after dexamethasone suppression. The uptake of tracer is increased in those with aldosteronoma and absent in those with idiopathic aldosteronism and adrenal carcinoma.

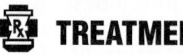 TREATMENT

■ NONPHARMACOLOGIC THERAPY
- Regular monitoring and control of blood pressure
- Low-sodium diet, tobacco avoidance, maintenance of ideal body weight, and regular exercise program

■ ACUTE GENERAL Rx
- Control of blood pressure and hypokalemia with spironolactone, amiloride, or ACE inhibitors
- Surgery (unilateral adrenalectomy) for APA

■ CHRONIC Rx
Chronic medical therapy with spironolactone, amiloride, or ACE inhibitors to control blood pressure and hypokalemia is necessary in all patients with bilateral idiopathic hyperaldosteronism.

■ DISPOSITION
Unilateral adrenalectomy normalizes hypertension and hypokalemia in 70% of patients with APA after 1 yr. After 5 yr, 50% of patients remain normotensive.

■ REFERRAL
Surgical referral for unilateral adrenalectomy following confirmation of unilateral APA or carcinoma

PEARLS & CONSIDERATIONS

■ COMMENTS
Frequent monitoring of blood pressure and electrolytes postoperatively is necessary, because normotension after unilateral adrenalectomy may take up to 4 mo.
Author: **Fred F. Ferri, M.D.**

BASIC INFORMATION

■ DEFINITION

Alpha-1-antitrypsin deficiency is a genetic deficiency of the protease inhibitor, alpha-1-antitrypsin, that results in a predisposition to pulmonary emphysema and hepatic cirrhosis.

■ SYNONYMS

AAT

ICD-9CM CODES

277.6 Alpha-1-antitrypsin deficiency

■ EPIDEMIOLOGY & DEMOGRAPHICS

- Felt to be underrecognized
- Affects approximately 80,000-100,000 Americans (including symptomatic and asymptomatic)
- Accounts for approximately 2% of COPD cases in Americans
- One in 10 individuals of European descent carry one of two mutations that may result in partial alpha-1-antitrypsin deficiency

■ PHYSICAL FINDINGS & CLINICAL PRESENTATION

- Physical findings and clinical presentation are varied and dependent upon phenotype (see etiology)
- Most often affects the lungs but can also involve liver and skin
- Classically associated with early-onset, severe, lower-lobe predominant emphysema; bronchiectasis may also be seen
- Symptoms are similar to "typical" COPD presentation (dyspnea, cough, sputum production).
- Liver involvement includes neonatal hepatitis, cirrhosis in children and adults, and primary carcinoma of the liver
- Panniculitis is the major dermatologic manifestation

■ ETIOLOGY

- Degree of alpha-1-antitrypsin deficiency is dependent on phenotype.
- "MM" represents the normal genotype and is associated with alpha-1-antitrypsin levels in the normal range.
- Mutation most commonly associated with emphysema is Z, with homozygote (ZZ) resulting in approximately 85% deficit in plasma alpha-1-antitrypsin concentrations.
- Development of emphysema is believed to be a result from an imbalance between the proteolytic enzyme, elastase, produced by neutrophils, and alpha-1-antitrypsin, which normally protects lung elastin by inhibiting elastase.

- Deficiency of alpha-1-antitrypsin increases risk of early-onset emphysema, but not all alpha-1-antitrypsin deficient individuals will develop lung disease.
- Smoking increases risk and accelerates onset of COPD.
- Liver disease is caused by pathologic accumulation of alpha-1-antitrypsin in hepatocytes.
- Similar to lung disease, skin involvement is thought to be secondary to unopposed proteolysis in skin.

DIAGNOSIS

■ DIFFERENTIAL DIAGNOSIS

See COPD
See cirrhosis

■ WORKUP

- Suspicion for alpha-1-antitrypsin deficiency usually results from emphysema developing at an early age and with basilar predominance of disease.
- Suspicion for alpha-1-antitrypsin deficiency resulting in liver disease or skin involvement may arise when other more common etiologies are excluded.

■ LABORATORY TESTS

- Serum level of alpha-1-antitrypsin is decreased or not detected in lung disease.
- Investigate possibility of abnormal alleles with genotyping.
- Pulmonary function testing is generally consistent with "typical" COPD.

■ IMAGING STUDIES

- Chest x-ray examination shows characteristic emphysematous changes at lung bases.
- High-resolution chest CT usually confirms the lower-lobe predominant emphysema and may also show significant bronchiectasis.

TREATMENT

■ NONPHARMACOLOGIC THERAPY

- Avoidance of smoking is paramount
- Avoidance of other environmental and occupational exposures that may increase risk of COPD

■ ACUTE GENERAL Rx

Acute exacerbations of COPD secondary to alpha-1-antitrypsin deficiency are treated in a similar fashion to "typical" COPD exacerbations.

■ CHRONIC Rx

- The goal of treatment in alpha-1-antitrypsin deficiency is to increase serum alpha-1-antitrypsin levels above a minimum, "protective" threshold.
- Although there are several therapeutic options under investigation, IV administration of pooled human alpha-1-antitrypsin is currently the only approved method to raise serum alpha-1-antitrypsin levels.
- Organ transplantation for patients with end-stage lung or liver disease is also an option.

■ DISPOSITION

Prognosis of patients with alpha-1-antitrypsin deficiency will depend on phenotype and level of deficiency.

■ REFERRAL

- Pulmonary and hepatology referrals for advanced lung and liver disease, or if replacement therapy is contemplated (e.g., moderate-severe lung disease)
- Lung and liver transplantation in suitable cases

PEARLS & CONSIDERATIONS

- The liver damage arising from the mutation is not from a deficiency in alpha-1-antitrypsin but from a pathologic accumulation of alpha-1-antitrypsin in hepatocytes.
- Consider alpha-1-antitrypsin deficiency in patients presenting with lower-lobe predominant emphysema; in most smokers without alpha-1-antitrypsin deficiency, emphysema predominates in the upper lobes.

REFERENCE

Carell RW, Lomas DA: Alpha-1-antitrypsin deficiency: a model for conformational diseases, *N Engl J Med* 346(1):45, 2002.

Author: **Joseph A. Diaz, M.D.**

BASIC INFORMATION

■ DEFINITION
Altitude sickness refers to a spectrum of illnesses related to hypoxia occurring in people rapidly ascending to high altitudes. Common acute syndromes occurring at high altitudes include acute mountain sickness, high-altitude pulmonary edema, and high-altitude cerebral edema (see Table 1-8).

■ SYNONYMS
Acute mountain sickness (AMS)
High-altitude pulmonary edema (HAPE)
High-altitude cerebral edema (HACE)

ICD-9CM CODES
289 Mountain sickness, acute
993.2 High altitude, effects

■ EPIDEMIOLOGY & DEMOGRAPHICS
- More than 30 million people are at risk of developing altitude sickness.
- Acute mountain sickness is the most common of the altitude diseases.
- In Summit County, Colorado, the incidence of acute mountain sickness was 22% at altitudes of 1850 to 2750 m (7000 to 9000 ft) and 42% at altitudes of 3000 m (10,000 ft).
- Approximately 0.01% of tourists to Colorado ski resorts experience HAPE or HACE.
- Men are 5 times more likely to develop HAPE than women.
- AMS and HACE affect men and women equally.

■ PHYSICAL FINDINGS & CLINICAL PRESENTATION
Acute mountain sickness
- Occurs within hours to a few days after rapid ascent over 8000 ft (2500 m)
- Headache is the most common symptom
- Dizziness and lightheadedness
- Nausea, vomiting, and loss of appetite
- Fatigue
- Sleep disturbance
- AMS can evolve into HAPE and HACE
High-altitude pulmonary edema (Fig. 1-12 and Section III, Fig. 3-88)
- Occurs usually during the second night after rapid ascent over 8000 ft (2500 m)
- Dyspnea at rest
- Dry cough
- Chest tightness
- Tachycardia, tachypnea, rales, cyanosis with pink-tinged frothy sputum

High-altitude cerebral edema
- Usually presents several days after AMS
- Confusion, irritability, drowsiness, stupor, hallucinations
- Headache, nausea, vomiting
- Ataxia, paralysis, and seizures
- Coma and death may develop within hours of the first symptoms

■ ETIOLOGY
- As one ascends to altitudes above sea level, the atmospheric pressure decreases. Although the percentage of oxygen in the air remains the same, the partial pressure of oxygen decreases with altitude.
- Thus the cause of altitude sickness is primarily hypoxia resulting from low partial pressures of oxygen.
- The body responds to low oxygen partial pressures through a process of acclimatization (see "Comments").

DIAGNOSIS
The diagnosis of altitude sickness is made by clinical presentation and physical findings described previously.

■ DIFFERENTIAL DIAGNOSIS
- Dehydration
- Carbon monoxide poisoning
- Hypothermia

TABLE 1-8   High-Altitude Sickness

	ACUTE MOUNTAIN SICKNESS	HIGH-ALTITUDE PULMONARY EDEMA	HIGH-ALTITUDE CEREBRAL EDEMA
Diagnostic findings	Nausea, vomiting, headache, lethargy, sleep disturbance, tinnitus, vertigo	Shortness of breath, tachypnea, tachycardia, cough, variable cyanosis	Headache, mental confusion, delirium, ataxia, hallucination, seizure, focal neurologic signs, coma
Onset	4-6 hr after reaching high altitude	24-96 hr	48-72 hr
Altitude	>8000 ft	8000-14,000 ft	Usually >12,000 ft
Ancillary data (in addition to those indicated for diagnostic evaluation)	ABG Chest x-ray study Electrolytes	ABG Chest x-ray study ECG Bleeding screen	ABG Electrolytes CT head
Differential considerations			
Trauma	Concussion Gastroenteritis	Pulmonary contusion	Head Meningitis
Infection	Respiratory or CNS infection	Pneumonia	Encephalitis
Metabolic		Uremia	Diabetic ketoacidosis Uremia Encephalopathy $\downarrow\uparrow Na^+$, $\uparrow Ca^{++}$
Intoxication	Salicylates	Multiple	Narcotics
Vascular		CHF	Subarachnoid hemorrhage
Management (all respond to descent)			
Admit	Variable	Yes	Yes
Oxygen	Yes	Yes	Yes
Acetazolamide	Prophylactic	Prophylactic	Prophylactic
Bronchodilator	No	Yes	No
Steroids	Controversial	Yes	Yes
Ventilation with PEEP	No	Yes, if severe	Hyperventilation

From Barkin RM, Rosen P: *Emergency pediatrics*, St Louis, 1999, Mosby.
ABG, Arterial blood gas; *CHF*, congestive heart failure; *CNS*, central nervous system; *CT*, computed tomography; *ECG*, electrocardiogram; *PEEP*, peak end-expiratory pressure.

- Infection
- Substance abuse
- Congestive heart failure
- Pulmonary embolism
- Cerebrovascular accident

■ WORKUP
Typically the diagnosis is self-evident after history and physical examination. Laboratory tests and imaging studies help monitor cardiopulmonary and CNS status in patients admitted to the intensive care unit for pulmonary and/or cerebral edema.

■ LABORATORY TESTS
Laboratory tests are not very useful in diagnosing altitude sickness.

■ IMAGING STUDIES
CXR showing Kerley B-lines and patchy edema (see Fig. 1-12)
CT scan of the head showing diffuse or patchy edema

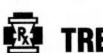 ### TREATMENT

■ NONPHARMACOLOGIC THERAPY
- Stop the ascent to allow acclimatization or start to descend until symptoms have resolved.
- Oxygen 4 to 6 L/min is used for severe AMS, HAPE, and HACE.
- Portable hyperbaric bags are useful if available at the site.
- Avoid dehydration.

■ ACUTE GENERAL Rx
- Aspirin 325 mg PO q6h can be used for headaches in AMS.
- Acetazolamide 125 mg to 250 mg PO bid has been shown to alleviate symptoms of AMS and HAPE.
- Nifedipine 10 mg sublingual followed by long-acting nifedipine 30 mg bid is used for patients with HAPE who cannot descend immediately.
- Dexamethasone 4 mg PO every 6 hr is used in patients with severe AMS, HAPE, and HACE.

■ CHRONIC Rx
- Prevention therapy is the most prudent therapy.
  1. Slow, staged ascent to avoid altitude sickness.
  2. Start the ascent below 8000 ft.
  3. Ascend 1000 ft/day and rest.
  4. Spend two nights at the same altitude every 3 days.
  5. Sleep at lower heights than the altitude climbed ("climb high, sleep low").
  6. Prophylactic therapy with acetazolamide 750 mg daily or dexamethasone 8 to 16 mg daily decreases the risk of developing AMS. The drugs are used until acclimatization occurs.

7. Prophylactic inhalation of a β-adrenergic agonist, salmeterol 125 mcg every 12 hr, or the use of slow-release nifedipine 20 mg bid reduces the risk of HAPE in susceptible individuals.

■ DISPOSITION
- AMS improves over a period of 2 to 3 days.
- HAPE is the most common cause of death among the altitude illnesses.
- More than 60% of patients with HAPE will have recurrence of symptoms on subsequent climbs.
- Neurologic deficits may persist for weeks but eventually resolve. If coma occurs, prognosis is poor.

■ REFERRAL
Cardiology and neurology referrals are made in patients with pulmonary edema and CNS findings, respectively.

☼ PEARLS & CONSIDERATIONS

■ COMMENTS
- Acclimatization is the process whereby the body adapts to hypoxia by optimizing oxygen delivery to cells. Adaptive mechanisms include:
  1. Hyperventilation to increase O_2 in the setting of hypoxia
  2. Tachycardia secondary to hypoxemia
  3. Pulmonary hypertension developed to improve ventilation-perfusion mismatch

  4. Cerebral vasodilation to increase blood flow to the brain
  5. Rise in hemoglobin and hematocrit
- Risk factors for the development of altitude sicknesses are:
  1. Rapid ascent
  2. Strenuous exertion on arrival
  3. Obesity
  4. Previous history of altitude sickness
  5. Male gender
- Physical fitness is not protective against high-altitude illness.
- HAPE is characterized by elevated pulmonary pressures resulting in protein-rich, hemorrhagic exudates into the lung alveoli.

REFERENCES
Dumont L, Mardirosoff C, Tramer MR: Efficacy and harm of pharmacological prevention of acute mountain sickness: quantitative systematic review, *BMJ* 321:267, 2000.

Hachett PH, Roach RC: High-altitude illness, *N Engl J Med* 345:107, 2001.

Hackett P, Rennie D: High altitude pulmonary edema, *JAMA* 287:2275, 2002.

Sartori C et al: Salmeterol for the prevention of high-altitude pulmonary edema, *N Engl J Med* 346:1631, 2002.

Swenson ER et al: Pathogenesis of high-altitude pulmonary edema, *JAMA* 287:2228, 2002.

Author: **Peter Petropoulos, M.D.**

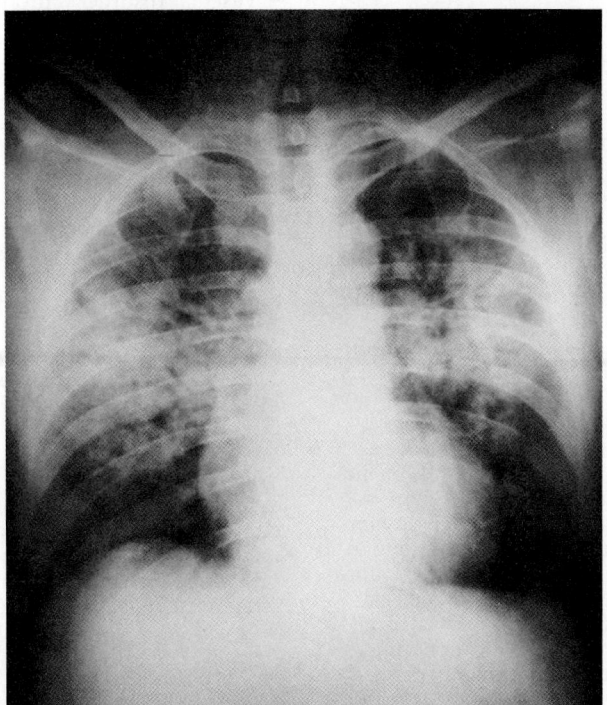

Fig. 1-12   Chest radiograph showing high-altitude pulmonary edema. (From Strauss RH [ed]: *Sports medicine,* ed 2, Philadelphia, 1991, WB Saunders.)

BASIC INFORMATION

■ DEFINITION

Dementia is a syndrome characterized by progressive loss of previously acquired cognitive skills including memory, language, insight, and judgment. Alzheimer's disease (AD) accounts for the majority (50% to 75%) of all cases of dementia.

ICD-9CM CODES
331.0 Alzheimer's disease
290.0 Senile dementia, uncomplicated

■ EPIDEMIOLOGY & DEMOGRAPHICS

INCIDENCE: Risk doubles every 5 yr after the age of 65; above the age of 85 the incidence is about 8%
PREVALENCE: Currently an estimated 4 million Americans have AD; 5% of patients are over the age of 65; 35% to 50% of patients are over the age of 85
PREDOMINANT SEX: Female

■ PHYSICAL FINDINGS & CLINICAL PRESENTATION
- Spouse or other family member, not the patient, often notes insidious memory impairment.
- Patients have difficulties learning and retaining new information, handling complex tasks (e.g., balancing the checkbook), and have impairments in reasoning, judgment, spatial ability and orientation (e.g., difficulty driving, getting lost away from home).
- Atypical presentations include early and severe behavioral changes, focal findings on examination, parkinsonism, hallucinations, falls, or onset of symptoms younger than the age of 65.

DIAGNOSIS

There is no definitive imaging or laboratory test for the diagnosis of dementia; rather, diagnosis is dependent on clinical history, a thorough physical and neurological examination, and use of reliable and valid diagnostic criteria (i.e., DSM-IV or NINDCS-ADRDA) such as the following:
- Loss of memory and one or more additional cognitive abilities, including *aphasia* (disturbance in language), *apraxia* (impaired ability to carry out motor activities despite intact motor function), *agnosia* (failure to recognize or identify objects despite intact sensory function), or disturbance in executive function (e.g., planning, organizing, sequencing, abstracting)

- Impairment in social or occupational functioning that represents a decline from a previous level of functioning and results in significant disability
- Deficits that do not occur exclusively during the course of delirium
- Insidious onset and gradual progression of symptoms
- Cognitive loss documented by neuropsychological tests
- No physical signs, neuroimaging, or laboratory evidence of other diseases that can cause dementia (i.e., metabolic abnormalities, medication or toxin effects, infection, stroke, Parkinson's disease, subdural hematoma, or tumors)
- Deficits do not occur exclusively during the course of a delirium
- The disturbance is not better accounted for by another Axis I disorder

Patients with isolated memory loss who lack functional impairment at home or work do not meet criteria for dementia but may have a mild cognitive impairment (MCI). Identifying patients with MCI is important because patients with MCI may have a slightly higher rate of progression to dementia.

■ DIFFERENTIAL DIAGNOSIS
- Cancer (brain tumor, meningeal neoplasia)
- Infection (AIDS, neurosyphilis, PML)
- Metabolic (EtOH, hypothyroidism, B_{12} deficiency)
- Organ failure (dialysis dementia, Wilson's disease)
- Vascular disorder (chronic SDH)
- Depression

■ WORKUP
History and general physical examination:
- Medication use should always be reviewed for drugs, which may cause mental status changes
- Patients should be screened for depression, because it can sometimes mimic dementia but also often occurs as a coexisting condition and should be treated
- On examination, look for signs of metabolic disturbance, presence of psychiatric features, or focal neurologic deficits

Mental status testing:
Brief mental status testing can be done easily and quickly in the office. Most commonly used is the Folstein Minimental status examination (MMSE). The MMSE is widely available in many reference books and on the Internet. A

MMSE score <24 (scores range from 0 to 30, with lower scores reflecting poorer performance) suggests dementia; however, results must be interpreted with caution. The MMSE is not sensitive enough to detect mild dementia, or dementia in patients with high baseline IQ. Scores may be spuriously low in patients with limited education, poor motor function, African American or Hispanic ethnicity, poor language skills, or impaired vision. If the MMSE is not available, mental status testing should include tests that assess the following cognitive functions:
- *Orientation:* ask the patient to give the day, date, month, year, and place, and to name the current president
- *Attention:* ask patient to recite the months of the year forwards and in reverse
- *Verbal recall:* ask the patient to remember four items; test for recall after a 1- and 5-min delay
- *Language:* ask patient to write and then read a sentence; have the patient name both common and less common objects
- *Visual-Spatial:* ask the patient to draw a clock and to set the hands of the clock at 11:10

Patients with AD typically have trouble with verbal recall, plus visual-spatial and/or language deficits. Attention is usually preserved until the late stages of AD, so consider alternate diagnoses in patients who do poorly on tests of attention.

Patients should be referred for formal neuropsychological testing to confirm screening mental status testing, especially for those patients who have an atypical history and/or clinical presentation, nondiagnostic performance on screening mental status testing, or high baseline IQ. Formal testing may help to differentiate AD from other causes of dementia, such as diffuse Lewy body disease, fronto-temporal dementia, vascular dementia, and pseudodementia.

■ LABORATORY TESTS
- CBC
- Serum electrolytes
- Glucose
- BUN/creatinine
- Liver and thyroid function tests
- Serum vitamin B_{12} and methylmalonic acid
- Syphilis serology, if high clinical suspicion
- Lumbar puncture if history or signs of cancer, suspicion of infectious process, or when the clinical presentation is unusual (i.e., rapid progression of symptoms)

- EEG if there is history of seizures, episodic confusion, rapid clinical decline, or suspicion of Creutzfeldt-Jakob disease
- Measurement of Apolipoprotein E genotyping, CSF tau and amyloid, and functional imaging including positron emission tomography (PET) or scanning proton emission computed tomography (SPECT) are not routinely indicated

■ IMAGING STUDIES
CT scan or MRI to rule out hydrocephalus and mass lesions, including subdural hematoma.

 TREATMENT

■ NONPHARMACOLOGIC THERAPY
- Patient safety, including risks associated with impaired driving, wandering behavior, leaving stoves unattended, and accidents, must be addressed with the patient and family early and appropriate measures implemented.
- Family education and support may help reduce need for skilled nursing facility, and reduce caregiver stress, depression, and burnout.

■ ACUTE GENERAL Rx
None

■ CHRONIC Rx
1. Symptomatic treatment of memory disturbance:
   Cholinesterase inhibitors: this class of medication is FDA-approved for the treatment of mild to moderate AD (MMSE 10-26). Clinical studies have demonstrated small improvements in memory, language, and ability to perform activities of daily living. Medication may also help to reduce symptoms of agitation and aggressiveness. At present there are no data supporting superiority of one cholinesterase inhibitor over another. Common side effects include nausea, diarrhea, and anorexia and may be bothersome enough to require a slower escalation of dosage, or switching to another agent. Benefit in severe AD has not been established
   - Donepezil (Aricept): dose is 5 mg qd for 4 to 6 wk, then increase to 10 mg qd
   - Rivastigmine (Exelon): dose is 1.5 mg bid with food, and then increased as tolerated by 1.5 mg bid until target dose of 3-6 mg bid

- Galantamine (Reminyl): dose is 4 mg bid with food, then increasing by 4 mg bid until target dose of 8-12 mg bid
2. Symptomatic treatment of behavioral disturbances
   - Wandering, hoarding or hiding objects, repetitive questioning, withdrawal, and social inappropriateness often respond to behavioral therapies.
   - Agitation, delusions, or hallucinations:
     ○ Olanzapine (Zyprexa) 2.5 mg qd to bid; may increase by 2.5 mg to maximum dose to 15 mg/day as needed
     ○ Quetiapine (Seroquel) 25 mg bid, increase by 25 mg per day every 2 days as needed, maximum dose 250 mg 3 times daily as needed
   - Depression:
     ○ Citalopram (Celexa): 10 mg qd; may increase to 20 mg after 1-2 wk
     ○ Sertraline (Zoloft): 25-50 mg qd; may increase by 25-50 mg qd every wk to maximum dose of 200 mg qd
     ○ Tricyclic antidepressants are generally avoided because of anticholinergic properties
3. Disease-modifying agents:
   - Vitamin E: 1000 IU given twice daily has been shown to delay progression.
   - Memantine is an NMDA receptor antagonist that has been shown in recent clinical trials to improve symptoms and delay progression in patients with moderate to severe AD. FDA decision on approval is anticipated by end of 2003. Benefits of this drug in combination with cholinesterase inhibitors or in mild to moderate AD are currently being studied.
   - Use of estrogen, NSAIDs, or ginkgo biloba is not routinely recommended.

☼ PEARLS & CONSIDERATIONS

The physician must make a thorough search for the treatable causes of dementia.
Current American Academy of Neurology practice parameters recommend:
- Treat cognitive symptoms of AD with cholinesterase inhibitors and Vitamin E
- Treat agitation, psychosis, and depression

- Encourage caregivers to participate in educational programs and support groups

■ COMMENTS
For additional information for patients, families, and clinicians:
Alzheimer's Association (http://www.alzheimers.org; 800-272-3900)
Alzheimer's Disease Education and Referral Center (http://www.alzheimers.org; 800-438-4380)

REFERENCES
Doody RS, Stevens JC, Beck C, et al: Management of dementia (an evidence-based review): report of the Quality Standards Subcommittee of the American Academy of Neurology, *Neurology* 56:1154, 2001.

DSM-IV: Diagnostic and statistical manual of mental disorders, ed 4, Washington, DC, 1994, American Psychiatric Association.

Folstein MF, Folsein SE, McHugh PR: "Mini-mental state": a practical method for grading the cognitive state of patients for the clinician, *J Psychiatr Res* 12:189, 1975.

Kawas CH: Early Alzheimer's disease, *N Engl J Med* 349(11):1056, 2003.

Knopman DS, DeKosky ST, Cummings JL, et al: Diagnosis of dementia (an evidence-based review): report of the Quality Standards Subcommittee of the American Academy of Neurology, *Neurology* 56:1143, 2001.

McKhann G et al: Clinical diagnosis of Alzheimer's disease: report of the NINCDS-ADRDA work group under the auspices of Department of Health and Human Services Task Force on Alzheimer's disease, *Neurology* 34:939, 1984.

Reisberg B, Doody R, Stoffler A, et al: Memantine in moderate-to-severe Alzheimer's disease, *N Engl J Med* 348:1333, 2003.

Sano M, Ernesto C, Thomas RG, et al: A controlled trial of selegiline, alpha-tocopherol, or both as treatment for Alzheimer's disease, *N Engl J Med* 336:1216, 1997.

Author: **Tamara G. Fong, M.D., Ph.D.**

BASIC INFORMATION

■ DEFINITION

Amaurosis fugax (AF) is a temporary loss of monocular vision caused by transient retinal ischemia. Distinguished from an ischemic optic neuropathy (usually anterior) in which visual loss is permanent.

ICD-9CM CODES

362.34 Amaurosis fugax

■ EPIDEMIOLOGY & DEMOGRAPHICS

INCIDENCE (IN U.S.): An uncommon presentation of carotid artery disease
PEAK INCIDENCE: 55 yr and older

■ PHYSICAL FINDINGS & CLINICAL PRESENTATION

- Onset is sudden, typically lasting seconds to minutes, and often accompanied by scotomas such as a shade or curtain being pulled over the front of the eye (usually downward).
- Vision loss can be complete or quadrantic.
- There are usually no physical findings.
- Acute stage: cholesterol emboli may be seen in retinal artery (Hollenhorst plaque): carotid bruits or other evidence of generalized atherosclerosis.
- If embolus is cardiac in origin, atrial fibrillation is often present.

■ ETIOLOGY

Usually embolic from the internal carotid artery or the heart but may also be due to vasculitis, such as giant cell arteritis (GCA), or hyperviscosity syndromes, such as sickle cell disease, that cause ischemia in the vascular territory of the ophthalmic artery

DIAGNOSIS

■ DIFFERENTIAL DIAGNOSIS

The differential diagnosis of transient monocular visual loss includes the following:

- Retinal migraine: in contrast to amaurosis, the onset of visual loss develops more slowly, usually over a period of 15-20 min.
- Transient visual obscurations (TVOs) occur in the setting of papilledema; intermittent rises in intracranial pressure briefly compromise optic disc perfusion and cause transient visual loss lasting 1-2 s and the episodes may be binocular.
  If the visual loss persists at the time of evaluation (i.e., vision has not yet recovered), then the differential diagnosis should be broadened to include: Anterior ischemic optic neuropathy—arteritic (classically GCA) or nonarteritic
Central retinal vein occlusion

■ WORKUP

Because amaurosis is usually due to emboli, the workup should focus on embolic sources; however, GCA should always be considered as well.

- Careful examination of retina; embolus may be visible and confirm the diagnosis (Fig. 1-13)
- Auscultation of arteries for bruits
- Examination of all pulses and for temporal artery tenderness
- Inquire about symptoms of GCA (scalp tenderness, jaw claudication)
- Examine for signs of hemispheric stroke resulting from ICA disease (contralateral limb and face weakness and/or sensory loss, aphasia, etc.)

■ LABORATORY TESTS

- CBC with ESR and CRP
- Serum chemistries, including lipid profile
- ECG and consider cycling cardiac enzymes
- Hypercoagulable workup is discretionary based on younger age and history

■ IMAGING STUDIES

- Carotid Dopplers followed by MRA or four-vessel angiography as indicated.
- Transthoracic echocardiography (TTE) is indicated to screen for embolization in patients with evidence of heart disease and in patients without an evident source for their transient neurologic deficit. Transesophageal echocardiography (TEE) is more sensitive for detecting cardiac sources of embolization (ventricular mural thrombus, atrial appendage, patent foramen ovale, aortic arch).
- Consider MRI of the brain with diffusion-weighted imaging to look for ischemic injury.

TREATMENT

■ NONPHARMACOLOGIC THERAPY

- Diet (decrease saturated fatty acids and high-cholesterol foods)

- Exercise
- Cessation of tobacco use if AF thought to be atherosclerotic in origin

■ ACUTE GENERAL Rx

- Investigate as an emergency.
- Give aspirin if etiology is presumed embolic.
- If GCA is suspected, start prednisone and refer for temporal artery biopsy within 48 hr (see Section I, "Giant Cell Arteritis").

■ CHRONIC Rx

- Reduce risks by carotid endarterectomy or stent if stenosis >70%.
- Control hypertension and manage vascular risk factors.
- Antiplatelet therapy.
- Consider starting an HMG CoA reductase inhibitor.

■ DISPOSITION

Among patients with >50% carotid stenosis who do not undergo carotid endartectomy, those who present with transient monocular blindness have about a 10% risk of stroke in 3 yr compared with a 20% risk in patients who present with a hemispheric transient ischemic attack (TIA).

■ REFERRAL

- Recommend referral to a neurologist for an evaluation and workup.
- If significant carotid stenosis, consider carotid endarterectomy or carotid stenting for the following:
  1. High-grade (≥70%) stenosis
  2. Multiple TIAs despite medical therapy, in the setting of high-grade or ulcerative disease

REFERENCES

Benauente O et al: Prognosis after transient monocular blindness associated with carotid-artery stenosis, *N Engl J Med* 345:1084, 2001.
Ryan MR, Combs G, Penix L: Preventing stroke in patients with transient ischemic attacks, *Am Fam Physician* 60:2329, 1999.
Author: **Sean I. Savitz, M.D.**

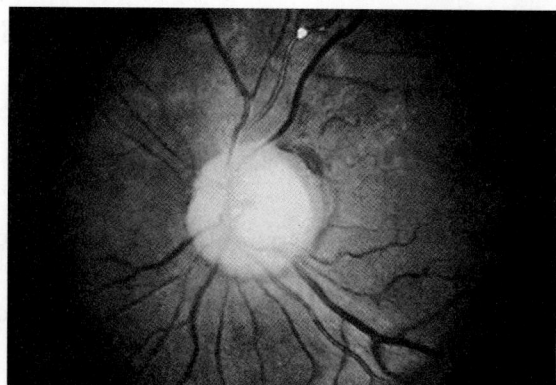

Fig. 1-13 **A cholesterol crystal embolus lodged at an arterial bifurcation.** (From Stein JH [ed]: *Internal medicine*, ed 5, St Louis, 1998, Mosby.)

BASIC INFORMATION

■ DEFINITION
Amblyopia refers to a decrease in vision in one or both eyes in the presence of an otherwise normal ophthalmologic examination.

■ SYNONYMS
Deprivation amblyopia
Occlusion amblyopia
Strabismus amblyopia
Refractive amblyopia
Organic or toxic amblyopias
Lazy eye

ICD-9CM CODES
368.00 Amblyopia

■ EPIDEMIOLOGY & DEMOGRAPHICS
INCIDENCE (IN U.S.): 1% to 4% of the general population
PREVALENCE (IN U.S.): High incidence in premature infants with drug-dependent mothers and in neurologically impaired children
PREDOMINANT SEX: None
PREDOMINANT AGE: Childhood
PEAK INCIDENCE: Childhood

■ PHYSICAL FINDINGS & CLINICAL PRESENTATION
Decreased vision using best refraction in the presence of normal corneal, lens, retinal, and optic nerve appearance (Fig. 1-14)

■ ETIOLOGY
- Visual deprivation
- Strabismus
- Occlusion with patching
- Refractive error organic lesions in the nervous system
- Toxins

DIAGNOSIS

■ DIFFERENTIAL DIAGNOSIS
- Central nervous system (CNS) disease (brainstem)
- Optic nerve disorders
- Corneal or other eye diseases

■ WORKUP
- Complete eye examination
- Motility evaluation

■ LABORATORY TESTS
Usually none

■ IMAGING STUDIES
Usually not necessary unless CNS lesion suspected

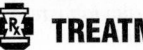

TREATMENT

■ NONPHARMACOLOGIC THERAPY
- Glasses
- Patches, mechanical vs atropine
- Removal of the cause of the amblyopia if possible
- Surgery to align the eyes

■ CHRONIC Rx
Patching or optics, including prisms and atropine

■ DISPOSITION
Immediate patching, alternating eyes daily

■ REFERRAL
To ophthalmologist if vision is compromised

PEARLS & CONSIDERATIONS

■ COMMENTS
The earlier the referral, the better the outcome.

REFERENCES
Donahue SP et al: Screening for amblyopia in preverbal children, *Ophthalmology* 108:1711, 2001.
Holmes JM et al: The amblyopia treatment study visual acuity testing protocol, *Arch Ophthalmol* 119:1345, 2001.
The clinical profile of moderate amblyopia in children younger than 7 years old, *Arch Ophthalmol* 120:281, 2003.
The Pediatric Eye Disease Investigator Group: A randomized trial of atropine vs patching for treatment of moderate amblyopia in children, *JAMA* 287:2145, 2002.
Williams C et al: Amblyopia treatment outcomes after screening before or at age 3 years: follow up from randomized trial, *BMJ* 324:1549, 2002.
Author: **Melvyn Koby, M.D.**

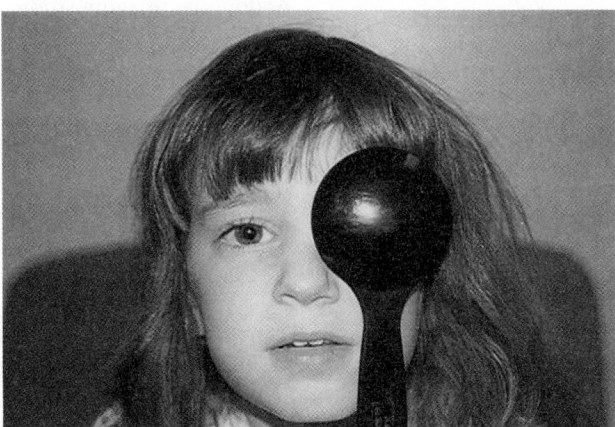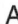

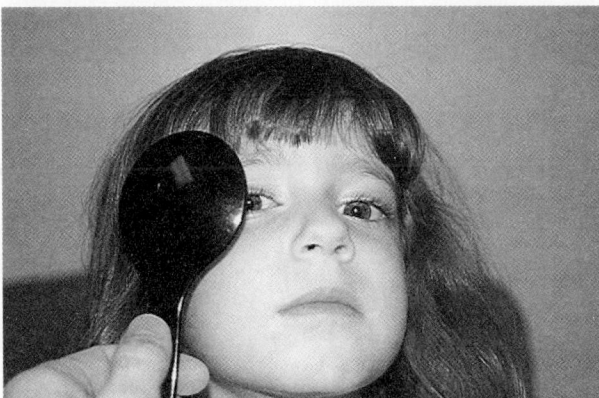

Fig. 1-14   A, This child happily fixes with her right eye and does not object if the left eye is covered. **B,** When the right eye is covered she moves her head away and tries to remove the cover, demonstrating a fixation preference for the right eye and amblyopia of the left eye. (From Hoekelman R [ed]: *Primary pediatric care,* ed 3, St Louis, 1997, Mosby.)

BASIC INFORMATION

■ DEFINITION
Amebiasis is an infection caused by the protozoal parasite *Entamoeba histolytica*. Although primarily an infection of the colon, amebiasis may cause extraintestinal disease, particularly liver abscess.

■ SYNONYMS
Amebic dysentery (when severe intestinal infection)

ICD-9CM CODES
006.9 Amebiasis

■ EPIDEMIOLOGY & DEMOGRAPHICS
INCIDENCE (IN U.S.): Highest in institutionalized patients, sexually active homosexual men
PREVALENCE (IN U.S.): 4% (80% of infections asymptomatic)
PREDOMINANT SEX:
- Equal sex distribution in general
- Striking male predominance of liver abscess

PREDOMINANT AGE: Second through sixth decades
PEAK INCIDENCE: Peaks at age 2 to 3 yr and >40 yr
GENETICS: Infection more likely to be fulminant in young infants

■ PHYSICAL FINDINGS & CLINICAL PRESENTATION
- Often nonspecific
- Approximately 20% of cases symptomatic
  1. Diarrhea, which may be bloody
  2. Abdominal and back pain
- Abdominal tenderness in 83% of severe cases
- Fever in 38% of severe cases
- Hepatomegaly, RUQ tenderness, and fever in almost all patients with liver abscess (may be absent in fulminant cases)

■ ETIOLOGY
- Caused by the protozoal parasite *E. histolytica* (Fig. 1-15)
- Transmission by the fecal-oral route
- Infection usually localized to the large bowel, particularly the cecum where a localized mass lesion (ameboma) may form
- Extraintestinal infection in which the organism invades the bowel mucosa and gains access to the portal circulation

DIAGNOSIS

■ DIFFERENTIAL DIAGNOSIS
- Severe intestinal infection possibly confused with ulcerative colitis or other infectious enterocolitis syndromes, such as those caused by *Shigella, Salmonella, Campylobacter,* or invasive *Escherichia coli*
- In elderly patients: ischemic bowel possibly producing a similar picture

■ WORKUP
- Three stool specimens over a period of 7 to 10 days to exclude the diagnosis (sensitivity 50% to 80%)
- Concentration and staining the specimen with Lugol's iodine or methylene blue to increase the diagnostic yield
- Available culture (rarely necessary in routine cases)

■ LABORATORY TESTS
- Stool examination is generally reliable.
- Mucosal biopsy is occasionally necessary.
- Serum antibody may be detected and is particularly sensitive and specific for extraintestinal infection or severe intestinal disease.
- Aspiration of abscess fluid is used to distinguish amebic from bacterial abscesses.

■ IMAGING STUDIES
Abdominal imaging studies (sonography or CT scan) to diagnose liver abscess

TREATMENT

■ ACUTE GENERAL Rx
- Metronidazole (750 mg PO tid for 10 days) is used in the treatment of mild to severe intestinal infection and amebic liver abscess; it may be administered intravenously when necessary.
- Follow with iodoquinol (650 mg PO tid for 20 days) to eradicate persistent cysts.

- For asymptomatic patients with amebic cysts on stool examination, use iodoquinol or paromomycin (500 mg PO tid for 7 days).
- Avoid antiperistaltic agents in severe intestinal infections to avoid risk of toxic megacolon.
- Liver abscess is generally responsive to medical management but surgical intervention indicated for extension of liver abscess into pericardium or, occasionally, for toxic megacolon.

■ DISPOSITION
Host immunity incomplete and reinfection rate high for patients remaining at risk

■ REFERRAL
- For consultation with infectious diseases specialist for extraintestinal infection or persistent or relapsing intestinal infection
- For surgical consultation:
  1. For toxic megacolon
  2. For impending rupture of or extension of liver abscess into adjacent structures

⚙ PEARLS & CONSIDERATIONS

■ COMMENTS
- Infection with other intestinal parasites, particularly *Giardia lamblia*, may coexist with amebiasis.

REFERENCES
Haque R et al: Amebiasis, *N Engl J Med* 348(16):1565, 2003.
Stanley SL: Protective immunity to amebiasis: new insights and new challenges, *J Infect Dis* 184(4):504, 2001.
Author: **Joseph R. Masci, M.D.**

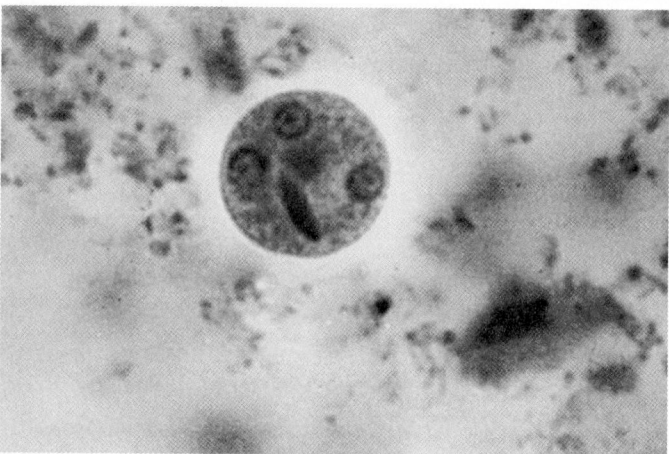

Fig. 1-15 **Mature cyst of *Entamoeba histolytica*.** Three of the four nuclei are seen in the plane of focus of this photomicrograph. (From Mandell GL [ed]: *Mandell, Douglas, and Bennett's principles and practice of infectious diseases*, ed 5, New York, 2000, Churchill Livingstone.)

BASIC INFORMATION

■ DEFINITION

Amyloidosis is a generic term describing the deposition of amyloid fibrils in body tissues. *Amyloid* is an amorphous, eosinophilic material; it is birefringent and usually extracellular. Electron microscopy reveals nonbranching fibrils that are soluble and relatively resistant to proteolytic digestion. There are two major forms of acquired systemic amyloidosis:

- AA, associated with chronic inflammatory diseases (e.g., rheumatoid arthritis) and amyloid deposits in kidneys, liver, and spleen
- AL (formerly known as primary amyloidosis) affecting the kidneys, heart, liver, intestines, skin, peripheral sensory nervous system, spleen, and lungs

ICD-9CM CODES
277.3 Amyloidosis

■ EPIDEMIOLOGY & DEMOGRAPHICS

- Amyloidosis affects primarily males between the ages of 60 and 70 yr.
- There are between 1500 and 3500 new cases annually in the U.S.
- The most common type in the U.S. is immunoglobulin light chain related (AL).

■ PHYSICAL FINDINGS & CLINICAL PRESENTATION

- Findings are variable with organ system involvement. Symmetric polyarthritis, peripheral neuropathy, and carpal tunnel syndrome may be present with joint involvement.
- Signs and symptoms of nephrotic syndrome may be present with renal involvement.
- Fatigue and dyspnea may occur with pulmonary involvement.
- Diarrhea, macroglossia (20% of patients), malabsorption, hepatomegaly, and weight loss may occur with GI involvement.
- Cardiac involvement is common and can lead to predominantly right-sided CHF, JVD, peripheral edema, and hepatomegaly.
- Vascular involvement can result in easy bleeding and periorbital purpura ("raccoon-eyes").

■ ETIOLOGY

In patients with amyloidosis, a soluble circulating protein (serum amyloid P [SAP]) is deposited in tissues as insoluble β-pleated sheets. The source of amyloid protein is a population of monoclonal plasma cells in the bone marrow. There are several chemically documented amyloidoses that can be principally subdivided into:
1. Acquired systemic amyloidosis (immunoglobulin light chain, multiple myeloma, hemodialysis amyloidosis)
2. Heredofamilial systemic (polyneuropathy, familial Mediterranean fever)
3. Organ-limited (Alzheimer's disease)
4. Localized endocrine (pancreatic islet, medullary thyroid carcinoma)

DIAGNOSIS

■ DIFFERENTIAL DIAGNOSIS

Variable, depending on the organ involvement:
- Renal involvement (toxin- or drug-induced necrosis, glomerulonephritis, renal vein thrombosis)
- Interstitial lung disease (sarcoidosis, connective tissue disease, infectious etiologies)
- Restrictive cardiac (endomyocardial fibrosis, viral myocarditis)
- Carpal tunnel (rheumatoid arthritis, hypothyroidism, overuse)
- Mental status changes (multi-infarct dementia)
- Peripheral neuropathy (alcohol abuse, vitamin deficiencies, diabetes mellitus)

■ WORKUP

Diagnostic approach is aimed at demonstration of amyloid deposits in tissues. This may be accomplished with rectal biopsy (positive in >60% of cases). Renal, myocardial, and bone marrow biopsy are other options. Abdominal fat pad biopsy can also be diagnostic; however, its yield is low and it should generally be reserved for evaluation of patients with peripheral neuropathy who also have findings associated with systemic amyloidosis.

■ LABORATORY TESTS

- Initial laboratory evaluation should include CBC, TSH, renal functions studies, ALT, AST, alkaline phosphatase, bilirubin, urinalysis, and serum and urine protein immunoelectrophoresis.
- Various laboratory abnormalities include proteinuria (found in >70% of cases), anemia, renal insufficiency, liver function abnormalities, hypothyroidism (10% to 20% of patients), and elevated monoclonal proteins. The finding of a monoclonal light chain in the serum or urine is very useful for diagnosis.
- DNA analysis is necessary for the diagnosis of hereditary amyloidosis.

■ IMAGING STUDIES

- Chest x-ray may reveal hilar adenopathy and mediastinal adenopathy.
- Two-dimensional Doppler echocardiography to study diagnostic filling is useful to evaluate for cardiac involvement.
- Nuclear imaging with technetium-labeled aprotinin may detect cardiac amyloidosis. SAP scintigraphy has high sensitivity for the detection of amyloid deposits in liver, spleen, kidneys, adrenal glands, and bones.

TREATMENT

■ ACUTE GENERAL Rx

- Therapy is variable, depending on the type of amyloidosis. Amyloidosis associated with plasma cell disorders may be treated with melphalan and prednisone, along with colchicine. Colchicine may also be effective in renal amyloidosis.
- Promising results have been found with the use of a molecule known as CPHPC given IV or SC in amyloidosis. This molecule has been shown effective in reducing circulating levels of SAP.

■ CHRONIC Rx

Renal transplantation is needed in patients with renal amyloidosis. Peritoneal dialysis in place of hemodialysis in patients with renal failure may improve hemodialysis amyloidosis by clearing β-2 microglobulin.

■ DISPOSITION

Prognosis is determined primarily by the presence or absence of cardiac involvement and with the form of amyloidosis:

- In reactive amyloidosis, eradication of the predisposing disease slows and can occasionally reverse the progression of amyloid disease. Survival of 5 to 10 yr after diagnosis is not uncommon.
- Patients with familial amyloidotic polyneuropathy generally have a prolonged course lasting 10 to 15 yr.
- Amyloidosis associated with immunocytic processes carries the worst prognosis (life expectancy <1 yr).
- The progression of amyloidosis associated with renal hemodialysis can be improved with newer dialysis membranes that can pass β-2 microglobulin.
- Median survival in patients with overt CHF is approximately 6 mo, 30 mo without CHF.

REFERENCES

Andrews TR et al: Utility of subcutaneous fat aspiration for diagnosing amyloidosis in patients with isolated peripheral neuropathy, *Mayo Clin Proc* 77:1287, 2002.

Merlini G, Bellotti V: Molecular mechanisms of amyloidosis. *N Engl J Med* 349:583, 2003.

Author: **Fred F. Ferri, M.D.**

BASIC INFORMATION

■ DEFINITION

Amyotrophic lateral sclerosis (ALS) is a progressive, degenerative neuromuscular condition of undetermined etiology affecting corticospinal tracts and anterior horn cells resulting in dysfunction of both upper motor neurons (UMN) and lower motor neurons (LMN), respectively.

ICD-9CM CODES

335.20 Amyotrophic lateral sclerosis

■ EPIDEMIOLOGY & DEMOGRAPHICS

INCIDENCE: 0.5 to 2 cases/100,000 persons. Onset is usually between the ages of 50 and 70 years. The male:female ratio is 2:1.
PREVALENCE: 5 in 100,000 persons

■ PHYSICAL FINDINGS & CLINICAL PRESENTATION

- Lower motor neuron signs (weakness, hypotonia, wasting, fasciculations, hypoflexia or areflexia)
- Upper motor neuron signs (loss of fine motor dexterity, spasticity, extensor plantar responses, hyperreflexia, clonus)
- Preservation of extraocular movements, sensation, bowel and bladder function
- Dysarthria, dysphagia, pseudobulbar affect, frontal lobe dysfunction
- Other presentations of motor neuron disease include progressive muscular atrophy, primary lateral sclerosis, progressive bulbar palsy, progressive pseudobulbar palsy, and ALS-parkinsonism-dementia complex. ALS comprises approximately 90% of adult-onset motor neuron disease.

■ ETIOLOGY

- 90% to 95% of all cases are sporadic; of the familial cases, approximately 20% are associated with a genetic defect in the copper-zinc superoxide dismutase enzyme (SOD1).

DIAGNOSIS

■ DIFFERENTIAL DIAGNOSIS

- Multifocal motor neuropathy with conduction block (MMN)
- Cervical spondylotic myelopathy with polyradiculopathy
- Spinal stenosis with compression of lumbosacral nerve roots
- Chronic inflammatory demyelinating polyneuropathy with CNS lesions

- Syringomyelia
- Syringobulbia
- Foramen magnum tumor
- Spinal muscular atrophy (SMA)
- Late-onset hexosaminidase A deficiency
- Polyglucosan body disease
- Bulbospinal muscular atrophy (Kennedy's disease)
- Monomyelic amyotrophy
- ALS-like syndromes have been reported in the setting of lead intoxication, HIV, hyperparathyroidism, hyperthyroidism, lymphoma, and B_{12} deficiency

■ WORKUP

- EMG and nerve conduction studies
- Lumbar puncture to assess protein, serum GM-1 Ab if MMN suspected
- Assessment of respiratory function (FVC, NIF)

■ LABORATORY TESTS

- B_{12}, thyroid function, PTH, HIV may be considered
- Serum protein and immunofixation electrophoresis
- DNA studies for SMA or bulbospinal atrophy, hexosaminidase levels in pure LMN syndrome
- 24-hour urine for lead if indicated

■ IMAGING STUDIES

- Craniospinal neuroimaging contingent upon clinical scenario
- Modified barium swallow to evaluate aspiration risk

TREATMENT

■ NONPHARMACOLOGIC THERAPY

- Noninvasive positive pressure ventilation improves quality of life and increases tracheostomy-free survival
- PEG placement may prolong life on the order of 1-4 mo
- Nutrition, speech therapy, physical and occupational therapy services
- Suction device for sialorrhea
- Communication may be eased with computerized assistive devices
- Early discussion of living will, recusitation orders, desire for PEG and tracheostomy, potential long-term care options
- Encourage contact with local support groups

■ ACUTE GENERAL Rx

Riluzole (Rilutek), a glutamate antagonist, is the only medication approved to extend tracheostomy-free survival in patients with ALS. Dosage is 50 mg q12h, at least 1 hr before or 2 hr after meals. Shown to prolong survival by 3-6 mo.

■ CHRONIC Rx

- Glycopyrrolate (Robinul) to help with siallorhea
- Relief of spasticity with baclofen, tizanadine, clonazepam
- Treatment of pseudobulbar affect with sertraline (Zoloft), dextromethorphan

■ DISPOSITION

- Mean duration of symptoms is 3 to 5 yr.
- About 20% of patients survive >5 yr.

■ REFERRAL

- Referral to a neurologist experienced in neuromuscular disease is recommended to confirm diagnosis.
- GI referral for PEG placement may be needed, recommended while forced vital capacity (FVC) >50% for optimal safety

PEARLS & CONSIDERATIONS

■ COMMENTS

- Patient education material may be obtained through the following: ALS Association, 21021 Ventura Boulevard, Suite 321, Woodland Hills, CA 91364, phone: (800) 782-4727; or the Muscular Dystrophy Association, 3561 East Sunrise Drive, Tucson, AZ 85718-3204, phone: (800) 572-1717, www.mdausa.org/.

REFERENCES

Bradley WG et al: Current management of ALS: comparison of the ALS CARE Database and the AAN Practice Parameter. The American Academy of Neurology, *Neurology* 57(3):500, 2001.
Miller RG et al: Practice parameter: the care of the patient with amyotrophic lateral sclerosis (an evidence-based review), *Muscle Nerve* 22(8):1104, 1999.
Rowland LP, Shneider NA: Amyotrophic lateral sclerosis, *N Engl J Med* 344:1688, 2001.

Author: **Taylor Harrison, M.D.**

BASIC INFORMATION

■ DEFINITION

An anaerobic infection is caused by one of a group of bacteria that require a reduced oxygen tension for growth.

ICD-9CM CODES

See specific condition.

■ PHYSICAL FINDINGS & CLINICAL PRESENTATION

- May occur at any site, but most are anatomically related to mucosal surfaces
- Should be suspected when there is foul-smelling tissue, soft-tissue gas, necrotic tissue, or abscesses
- Head and neck
  1. Odontogenic infections from dental or soft tissue possibly progressing to periapical abscesses, at times extending to bone
  2. Both anaerobic and aerobic pathogens in chronic sinusitis, chronic mastoiditis, and chronic otitis media
  3. Peritonsillar abscess possible
  4. Complications: deep neck space infections, brain abscesses, mediastinitis
- Pleuropulmonary
  1. May involve anaerobes present in the oropharynx
  2. Aspiration more common in persons with altered mental status or seizures
  3. Anaerobic bacteria more likely in those with gingivitis or periodontitis
  4. Manifestations: necrotizing pneumonia, empyema, lung abscess
- Intraabdominal
  1. Disruption of intestinal integrity leading to infection involving anaerobic bacteria
  2. Bacteria from colonic neoplasm, perforated appendicitis, diverticulitis, or bowel surgery, causing bacteremia, peritonitis, at times intraabdominal abscesses
  3. Resulting infections usually mixed, containing both anaerobes and aerobes
- Female genital tract
  1. Anaerobes in bacterial vaginosis, salpingitis, endometritis, pelvic abscesses, septic abortion; infections tend to be mixed
  2. Possible pelvic thrombophlebitis when resolving pelvic infection is accompanied by new or persistent fever
- Other anaerobic infections
  1. Skin and soft-tissue infection at any site
  2. More commonly associated infections: synergistic gangrene, bite wound infections, infected decubitus ulcers

3. Clinical significance of anaerobes in diabetic foot infections unclear
4. Anaerobic bacteremia uncommon with source usually intraabdominal, followed by female genital tract, pleuropulmonary, and head and neck infections
5. Osteomyelitis especially when associated with decubitus ulcers or vascular insufficiency
6. Facial bone osteomyelitis from adjacent infections of the teeth or sinuses

■ ETIOLOGY

- Most commonly endogenous, arising from bacteria that normally line mucosal surfaces
- Disruption of mucosal barriers resulting from various conditions (trauma, ischemia, surgery, perforation), with infection occurring when organisms gain access to normally sterile sites, causing tissue destruction and abscess formation
- Synergy between different anaerobes or between anaerobes and aerobes important
- Most commonly involved: gram-negative anaerobic bacilli

 DIAGNOSIS

■ WORKUP

- Specimens submitted for culture processed within 30 min
- Large volume of material more likely to have significant growth; swabs less efficient for transporting infected material
- Blood cultures—preferably before antibiotic administration

■ LABORATORY TESTS

- Elevated WBC count, with extremely high WBC counts sometimes seen with pseudomembranous colitis
- Positive stool *C. difficile* toxin assay
- Increased lactate levels in ischemia or perforation
- Possible positive blood or wound cultures, but failure to grow anaerobes in culture may be common, attributed to inadequate culturing techniques and/or fastidious organisms

■ IMAGING STUDIES

- Plain film of an affected area to show gas in tissues, free air resulting from a perforated viscus, or an air/fluid level inside an abscess
- Ultrasound, CT scan, or MRI to reveal abscesses or tissue destruction

 TREATMENT

■ NONPHARMACOLOGIC THERAPY

- Removal of necrotic tissue
- Drainage of abscesses (accomplished by CT scan–guided percutaneous drainage)

■ ACUTE GENERAL Rx

Oral antibiotics with anaerobic activity: clindamycin, metronidazole, and chloramphenicol

- Broader spectrum of activity with amoxicillin/clavulanate
- Penicillin VK in odontogenic infections
- Oral metronidazole for *C. difficile*–associated diarrhea, with oral vancomycin reserved for recurrent or recalcitrant infections

Parenteral antibiotics for more serious illness

- IV clindamycin, metronidazole, and chloramphenicol
- Cephalosporins (anaerobic or mixed infections): cefoxitin and cefotetan
- Extended-spectrum penicillins (e.g., piperacillin) and combination β-lactamase plus β-lactamase inhibitor drugs
  1. Significant anaerobic activity, plus various degrees of broad-spectrum coverage
  2. Include ampicillin/sulbactam, ticarcillin/clavulanate, and piperacillin/tazobactam
- Imipenem: a broad-spectrum agent with extensive anaerobic activity
- Actinomycosis treated with penicillin for 6 to 12 mo
- SMX/TMP and fluoroquinolones: ineffective

 PEARLS & CONSIDERATIONS

■ COMMENTS

- Chloramphenicol is associated with aplastic anemia, although this is an extremely rare complication.
- Imipenem is a possible cause of thrombocytopenia and may lower the seizure threshold, especially in elderly patients with renal insufficiency.

REFERENCE

Ortiz E, Sande MA: Routine use of anaerobic blood cultures: are they still indicated? *Am J Med* 108:445, 2000.
Author: **Maurice Policar, M.D.**

BASIC INFORMATION

■ DEFINITION
A fissure is a tear in the epithelial lining of the anal canal (i.e., from the dentate line to the anal verge).

■ SYNONYMS
Anorectal fissure
Anal ulcer

ICD-9CM CODES
565.0 Anal fissure

■ EPIDEMIOLOGY & DEMOGRAPHICS
- Can occur at any age
- Most common in young and middle-aged adults
- Occurs in men > women
- Women more likely to have anterior fissure than men (10% vs. 1%, respectively)
- Most common cause of rectal bleeding in infants
- Common in women before and after childbirth

■ PHYSICAL FINDINGS & CLINICAL PRESENTATION
With separation of the buttocks will see a tear in the posterior midline or, less frequently, in the anterior midline (Fig. 1-16)
- Acute anal fissure:
  1. Sharp burning or tearing pain exacerbated by bowel movements
  2. Bright-red blood on toilet paper, a streak of blood on the stool or in the water
- Chronic anal fissure:
  1. Pruritus ani
  2. Pain seldom present
  3. Intermittent bleeding
  4. Sentinel tag at the caudal aspect of the fissure, hypertrophied anal papilla at the proximal end
- Underlying disease possible if the fissure:
  1. Is ectopically located
  2. Extends proximal to the dentate line
  3. Is broad-based or deep
  4. Is especially purulent

■ ETIOLOGY
- Most initiated after passage of a large, hard stool
- May result from frequent defecation and diarrhea
- Bacterial infections: TB, syphilis, gonorrhea, chancroid, lymphogranuloma venereum
- Viral infections: herpes simplex virus, cytomegalovirus, human immunodeficiency virus
- Inflammatory bowel disease (IBD): Crohn's disease, ulcerative colitis
- Trauma: surgery (hemorrhoidectomy), foreign bodies, anal intercourse
- Malignancy: carcinoma, lymphoma, Kaposi's sarcoma

DIAGNOSIS

■ DIFFERENTIAL DIAGNOSIS
- Proctalgia fugax
- Thrombosed hemorrhoid

■ WORKUP
- Digital rectal examination after lubricating the entire anus with anesthetic jelly (i.e., 2% lidocaine) and waiting 5 to 10 min
- Anoscopy
- Proctosigmoidoscopy to exclude inflammatory or neoplastic disease
- Biopsy if doubt exists about the etiology of the condition
- All studies done under adequate anesthesia

■ IMAGING STUDIES
- Colonoscopy or barium enema: if diagnosis of IBD or malignancy is suspected
- Small bowel series: occasionally obtained for similar reasons
- Biopsy to reveal caseating granuloma if TB is suspected
- Wet prep with darkfield examination to demonstrate treponemes if syphilis is suspected

TREATMENT

■ NONPHARMACOLOGIC THERAPY
- Sitz baths
- High-fiber diet
- Increased oral fluid intake

■ ACUTE GENERAL Rx
- Bulk-producing agent (e.g., Metamucil)/stool softener
- Local anesthetic jelly (may exacerbate pruritus ani)
- Nitroglycerin ointment
- Suppositories *not* recommended
- Surgery

■ CHRONIC Rx
- Surgery: lateral internal anal sphincterotomy
- Topical glyceryl trinitrate ointment
- Injection of botulinum toxin (an injection into each side of the internal anal sphincter) is effective in healing chronic anal fissures in more than 90% of patients.

■ DISPOSITION
Outpatient surgery

■ REFERRAL
- If fissure does not resolve with conservative therapy in 4 to 6 wk
- If patient prefers surgery for acute fissure
- If patient has chronic fissure

PEARLS & CONSIDERATIONS

■ COMMENTS
HIV-positive patients should be referred to clinicians who are well versed in the myriad infectious and neoplastic conditions that masquerade as anal ulcers in these patients.

REFERENCES
Brisinda G et al: A comparison of injection of botulinum toxin and topical nitroglycerin ointment for the treatment of chronic anal fissure, *N Engl J Med* 341:65, 1999.
Pfenninger JL, Zainea GG: Common anorectal conditions, *Am Fam Physician* 64:77, 2001.
Author: **George T. Danakas, M.D.**

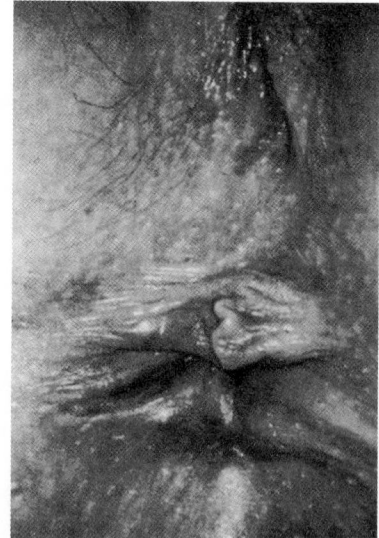

Fig. 1-16 **Lateral anal fissure.** (In Seidel HM et al: *Mosby's guide to physical examination,* ed 3, St Louis, 1995, Mosby. Courtesy Gershon Efron, MD, Sinai Hospital of Baltimore.)

BASIC INFORMATION

■ DEFINITION

Anaphylaxis is a sudden-onset, life-threatening event characterized by bronchial contractions in conjunction with hemodynamic changes. Its clinical presentation may include respiratory, cardiovascular, cutaneous, or gastrointestinal manifestations.

■ SYNONYMS

Anaphylactoid reaction is closely related to anaphylaxis. It is caused by release of mast cells and basophil mediators triggered by non–IgE-mediated events.

ICD-9CM CODES

995.0 Anaphylactic shock
995.60 Anaphylaxis due to food
999.4 Anaphylaxis due to immunization
977.9 Anaphylaxis due to drugs
989.5 Anaphylaxis following stings

■ EPIDEMIOLOGY & DEMOGRAPHICS

INCIDENCE: 20,000 to 50,000 persons/yr in the U.S. Anaphylaxis rates are 0.0004% for food, 0.7% to 10% for penicillin, 0.22% to 1% for radiocontrast media, and 0.5% to 5% after insect stings. It is estimated that 1 in every 3000 inpatients in U.S. hospitals develops an anaphylactic reaction.

■ PHYSICAL FINDINGS & CLINICAL PRESENTATION

- Urticaria, pruritus, skin flushing, angioedema, weakness, dizziness
- Dyspnea, cough, malaise, difficulty swallowing
- Wheezing, tachycardia, diarrhea
- Hypotension, vascular collapse

■ ETIOLOGY

Virtually any substance may induce anaphylaxis in a given individual.
- Commonly implicated medications are antibiotics, insulin, allergen extracts, opiates, vaccines, NSAIDs, contrast media, streptokinase
- Foods and food additives, nuts, egg whites, shellfish, fish, milk, fruits, and berries
- Blood products, plasma, immunoglobulin, cryoprecipitate, whole blood
- Venoms such as snake venom, fire ant venom, bee sting (*Hymenoptera* stings)
- Latex

DIAGNOSIS

■ DIFFERENTIAL DIAGNOSIS

- Endocrine disorders (carcinoid, pheochromocytoma)
- Globus hystericus, anxiety disorder
- Systemic mastocytosis
- Pulmonary embolism, serum sickness, vasovagal reactions
- Severe asthma (the key clinical difference is the abrupt onset of symptoms in anaphylaxis without a history of progressive worsening of symptoms)

■ WORKUP

Workup is aimed mainly at eliminating other conditions that may mimic anaphylaxis (e.g., vasovagal syncope may be differentiated by the presence of bradycardia as opposed to the tachycardia seen in anaphylaxis; the absence of hypoxemia in ABG analysis may be useful to exclude pulmonary embolism or foreign body aspiration).

■ LABORATORY TESTS

- Laboratory evaluation is generally not helpful, because the diagnosis of anaphylaxis is a clinical one.
- ABG analysis may be useful to exclude pulmonary embolism, status asthmaticus, and foreign body aspiration.
- Elevated serum and urine histamine levels can be useful for diagnosis of anaphylaxis, but these tests are not commonly available.

■ IMAGING STUDIES

Generally not helpful.
- Chest x-ray is indicated in patients presenting with acute respiratory compromise.
- Radiologic evaluation for epiglottitis is useful in patients with acute respiratory compromise.
- ECG should be considered in all patients with sudden loss of consciousness or complaints of chest pains or dyspnea and in any elderly patient.

TREATMENT

■ NONPHARMACOLOGIC THERAPY

- IV access should be rapidly established, and intravenous fluids (i.e., saline) should be administered.
- Supplemental oxygen and cardiac monitoring are also recommended.

■ ACUTE GENERAL Rx

- Epinephrine should be rapidly administered as an SC or IM injection at a dose of 0.01 ml/kg of aqueous epinephrine 1:1000 (maximum adult dose 0.3 to 0.5 ml). The dose may be repeated approximately q5-10 min if there is persistence or recurrence of symptoms. Endotracheal epinephrine should be considered if IV access is not possible during life-threatening reactions.
- Administration of H_1- and H_2-receptor antagonists is also recommended in the initial treatment of anaphylaxis.
  1. Administer diphenhydramine 50 to 75 mg IV or IM.
  2. Cimetidine 300 mg IV over 3 to 5 min, or ranitidine 50 mg IV, should be given initially; subsequent doses of H_1- and H_2-blockers can be given orally q6h for 48 hr.
- Corticosteroids are not useful in the acute episode because of their slow onset of action; however, they should be administered in most cases to prevent prolonged or recurrent anaphylaxis. Commonly used agents are hydrocortisone sodium succinate 250 to 500 mg IV q4-6h in adults (4 to 8 mg/kg for children) or methylprednisolone 60 to 125 mg IV in adults (1 to 2 mg/kg in children).
- Aerosolized β-agonists (i.e., albuterol, 2.5 mg, repeat prn 20 min) are useful to control bronchospasm.
- Additional useful agents in specific circumstances: atropine for refractory bradycardia, dopamine for refractory hypotension (despite volume expansion), and glucagon in patients on β-blocking drugs.

PEARLS & CONSIDERATIONS

■ COMMENTS

- Patient education regarding the nature of the illness and preventive measures is recommended. A documented history of previous anaphylactic episodes or known anaphylaxis triggers is the most reliable method of identifying individuals at risk.
- Prescription for prefilled epinephrine syringe (EpiPen) should be given, and the patient should be instructed on the use of this emergency epinephrine kit in case of recurrent anaphylactic episodes.
- Patients should also be advised to carry or wear Medic Alert ID describing substances that have caused anaphylaxis.
- Avoidance of radiologic contrast is also recommended.
- Venom immunotherapy immediately after a sting is effective and recommended for up to 5 yr after the anaphylactic incident.

REFERENCE

Neugut AI et al: Anaphylaxis in the United States, *Arch Intern Med* 161:15, 2001.

Tang AW: A practical guide to anaphylaxis, *Am Fam Physician* 68:1325, 2003.
Author: **Fred F. Ferri, M.D.**

BASIC INFORMATION

■ DEFINITION

Aplastic anemia is a bone marrow failure resulting from a variety of causes and characterized by stem cell destruction or suppression leading to pancytopenia.

■ SYNONYMS

Refractory anemia
Hypoplastic anemia

ICD-9CM CODES
284.9 Aplastic anemia
284.8 Acquired aplastic anemia
284.0 Congenital aplastic anemia

■ EPIDEMIOLOGY & DEMOGRAPHICS
- There is no predominant age or sex for the acquired form.
- The annual incidence of aplastic anemia in the U.S. is 3 to 9 cases/ 1 million persons.

■ PHYSICAL FINDINGS & CLINICAL PRESENTATION
- Skin pallor, ecchymosis, petechiae, retinal hemorrhage
- Possible fever, mouth and tongue ulceration, pharyngitis
- Possible short stature or skeletal and nail anomalies in the congenital form
- Possible audible systolic ejection murmur with profound anemia

■ ETIOLOGY
- In most patients with acquired aplastic anemia, bone marrow failure results from immunologically mediated, active destruction of blood-forming cells by lymphocytes.
- Common etiologic factors in aplastic anemia:
  Toxins (e.g., benzene, insecticides)
  Drugs (e.g., Felbatol, cimetidine, busulfan and other myelosuppressive drugs, gold salts, chloramphenicol, sulfonamides, trimethadione, quinacrine, phenylbutazone)
  Ionizing irradiation
  Infections (e.g., hepatitis C, HIV)
  Idiopathic
  Inherited (Fanconi's anemia)
  Other: immunologic, pregnancy

DIAGNOSIS

■ DIFFERENTIAL DIAGNOSIS
- Bone marrow infiltration from lymphoma, carcinoma, myelofibrosis
- Severe infection
- Hypoplastic acute lymphoblastic leukemia in children

- Hypoplastic myelodysplastic syndrome or hypoplastic acute myeloid leukemia in adults
- Hypersplenism
- Hairy cell leukemia

■ WORKUP
- Diagnostic workup consists primarily of bone marrow aspiration and biopsy and laboratory evaluation (CBC and examination of blood film).
- Bone marrow examination generally reveals paucity or absence of erythropoietic and myelopoietic precursor cells; patients with pure red cell aplasia demonstrate only absence of RBC precursors in the marrow.

■ LABORATORY TESTS
- CBC reveals pancytopenia. Macrocytosis and toxic granulation of neutrophils may also be present. Isolated cytopenias may occur in the early stages.
- Reticulocyte count reveals reticulocytopenia.
- Additional initial laboratory evaluation should include Ham test to exclude paroxysmal nocturnal hemoglobinuria (PNH) and testing for hepatitis C.

■ IMAGING STUDIES
- Chest x-ray examination
- Abdominal sonogram or CT scan to evaluate for splenomegaly
- Radiography of hand and forearm in patients with constitutional anemia
- CT scan of thymus region if thymoma-associated RBC aplasia is suspected

TREATMENT

■ NONPHARMACOLOGIC THERAPY
- Discontinuation of any offending drugs or agents
- Evaluation for bone marrow transplantation

■ ACUTE GENERAL Rx
- Aggressive treatment of neutropenic fevers with parenteral broad-spectrum antibiotics
- Platelet and RBC transfusions prn; however, avoidance of transfusions in patients who are candidates for bone marrow transplantation
- Immunosuppressive therapy with antithymocyte globulin (ATG) and/or cyclosporine (CSP); ATG in combination with prednisone (1 to 2 mg/kg/day initially) to avoid complications of serum sickness

- Transplantation of allogeneic marrow or peripheral blood stem cell transplantation from a histocompatible sibling usually cures the underlying bone marrow failure
- In patients with severe aplastic anemia who are not candidates for allogeneic bone marrow, use of high-dose cyclophosphamide therapy without bone marrow transplantation represents a third treatment option for initial treatment of aplastic anemia.

■ CHRONIC Rx
- Long-term patient monitoring with physical examination and routine laboratory evaluation to screen for relapse.
- ATG with CSP restore hematopoiesis in approximately two thirds of patients; however, recovery of blood cell count is often incomplete, recurrent pancytopenia requires retreatment. In some patients, myelodysplasia is a late complication of immunosuppressive therapy.
- Patients refractory to immunosuppression have a poor long-term outlook and should consider unrelated stem cell transplantation.
- There is little justification for either a therapeutic trial of corticosteroids as primary treatment or for their long-term use to prevent bleeding.

■ DISPOSITION
- Patients with severe aplastic anemia who have marrow transplants before the onset of transfusion-induced sensitization have an excellent probability of long-term survival and normal life; age is a significant factor; the incidence of graft vs. host disease increases with age and is >90% in patients >30 yr of age.
- Following bone marrow transplantation from an HLA-identical sibling, >70% of patients are long-term survivors and can be considered cured.
- Response to immunosuppression in aplastic anemia is independent of age, but treatment is associated with increased mortality in older patients.
- Overall 5-yr survival rate for aplastic anemia is now 70% to 90%.

■ REFERRAL
Hematology referral is indicated in all patients with aplastic anemia.
Author: **Fred F. Ferri, M.D.**

BASIC INFORMATION

■ DEFINITION

Autoimmune hemolytic anemia is anemia secondary to premature destruction of red blood cells caused by the binding of autoantibodies and/or complement to red blood cells.

ICD-9CM CODES

283.0 Autoimmune hemolytic anemia

■ EPIDEMIOLOGY & DEMOGRAPHICS

Autoimmune hemolytic anemia is most common in women <50 yr.

■ PHYSICAL FINDINGS & CLINICAL PRESENTATION

- Pallor
- Tachycardia
- Hepatomegaly, splenomegaly

■ ETIOLOGY

- Warm antibody mediated: IgG (often idiopathic or associated with leukemia, lymphoma, thymoma, myeloma, viral infections, and collagen-vascular disease)
- Cold antibody mediated: IgM and complement in majority of cases (often idiopathic, at times associated with infections, lymphoma, or cold agglutinin disease)
- Drug induced: three major mechanisms:
  1. Antibody directed against Rh complex (e.g., methyldopa)
  2. Antibody directed against RBC-drug complex (hapten induced, e.g., penicillin)
  3. Antibody directed against complex formed by drug and plasma proteins; the drug-plasma protein-antibody complex causes destruction of RBCs (innocent bystander, e.g., quinidine).

DIAGNOSIS

■ DIFFERENTIAL DIAGNOSIS

- Hemolytic anemia caused by membrane defects (paroxysmal nocturnal hemoglobinuria, spur-cell anemia, Wilson's disease)
- Non–immune mediated (microangiopathic hemolytic anemia, hypersplenism, cardiac valve prosthesis, giant cavernous hemangiomas, march hemoglobinuria, physical agents, infections, heavy metals, certain drugs [nitrofurantoin, sulfonamides])

■ WORKUP

Evaluation consists primarily of laboratory evaluation to confirm hemolysis and to exclude other causes of the anemia.

■ LABORATORY TESTS

- Initial laboratory tests: CBC (anemia), reticulocyte count (elevated), liver function studies (elevated indirect bilirubin, LDH), evaluation of peripheral smear, Coombs' test (positive direct Coombs' test indicates presence of antibodies or complement on the surface of RBC, positive indirect Coombs' test implies presence of anti-RBC antibodies freely circulating in the patient's serum), haptoglobin level (decreased)
- IgG antibody and IgM antibody
- Hepatitis serology, ANA

■ IMAGING STUDIES

- Chest x-ray
- CT scan of chest and abdomen to rule out lymphoma should also be considered

TREATMENT

■ NONPHARMACOLOGIC THERAPY

- Discontinuation of any potentially offensive drugs
- Plasmapheresis-exchange transfusion for severe life-threatening cases only
- Avoid cold exposure in patients with cold antibody

■ ACUTE GENERAL Rx

- Prednisone 1 to 2 mg/kg/day in divided doses initially in warm antibody autoimmune hemolytic anemia. Corticosteroids are generally ineffective in cold antibody autoimmune hemolytic anemia
- Splenectomy in patients responding inadequately to corticosteroids when RBC sequestration studies indicate splenic sequestration
- Immunosuppressive drugs and/or immunoglobulins only after both corticosteroids and splenectomy (unless surgery is contraindicated) have failed to produce an adequate remission
- Danazol, usually used in conjunction with corticosteroids (may be useful in warm antibody autoimmune hemolytic anemia)
- Immunosuppressive drugs (azathioprine, cyclophosphamide) may be useful in warm antibody autoimmune hemolytic anemia but are indicated only after both corticosteroids and splenectomy (unless surgery is contraindicated) have failed to produce an adequate remission

■ DISPOSITION

Prognosis is generally good unless anemia is associated with underlying disorder with a poor prognosis (e.g., leukemia, myeloma).

■ REFERRAL

Surgical referral for splenectomy in refractory cases

PEARLS & CONSIDERATIONS

■ COMMENTS

Monitor for potential complications such as thromboembolism or severe anemia with shock.

Author: **Fred F. Ferri, M.D.**

BASIC INFORMATION

■ DEFINITION
Iron deficiency anemia is anemia secondary to inadequate iron supplementation or excessive blood loss.

ICD-9CM CODES
280.9 Iron deficiency anemia
648.2 Iron deficiency anemia complicating pregnancy

■ EPIDEMIOLOGY & DEMOGRAPHICS
- Dietary iron deficiency occurs often in infants as a result of unsupplemented milk diets. It is also commonly seen in women during their reproductive years, as a result of heavy menstrual periods, and during pregnancy (increased demand).
- Iron deficiency is the most common nutritional deficiency worldwide.
- The prevalence of iron deficiency is greatest among toddlers ages 1-2 yr (7%) and adolescents and adult families ages 12-49 yr (9%-16%).

■ PHYSICAL FINDINGS & CLINICAL PRESENTATION
- Most patients have a normal examination.
- Skin pallor and conjunctival pallor may be present.

■ ETIOLOGY
- Blood loss from GI or menstrual bleeding (GU blood loss less often the cause)
- Dietary iron deficiency (rare in adults)
- Poor iron absorption in patients with gastric or small bowel surgery
- Repeated phlebotomy
- Increased requirements (e.g., during pregnancy)
- Other: traumatic hemolysis (abnormally functioning cardiac valves), idiopathic pulmonary hemosiderosis (iron sequestration in pulmonary macrophages), paroxysmal nocturnal hemoglobinuria (intravascular hemolysis)

DIAGNOSIS

■ DIFFERENTIAL DIAGNOSIS
- Anemia of chronic disease
- Sideroblastic anemia
- Thalassemia trait

■ WORKUP
Diagnostic workup consists primarily of laboratory evaluation. Most patients with iron deficiency anemia are asymptomatic in the early stages. With progressive anemia, the major complaints are fatigue, dizziness, exertional dyspnea, pagophagia (ice eating), and pica. Patient's history may also suggest GI blood loss (melena, hematochezia, hemoptysis).

■ LABORATORY TESTS
- Laboratory results vary with the stage of deficiency.
- Absent iron marrow stores and decreased serum ferritin are the initial abnormalities.
- Decreased serum iron and increased TIBC are the next abnormalities.
- Hypochromic microcytic anemia is present with significant iron deficiency.
- Peripheral smear in patients with iron deficiency generally reveals microcytic hypochromic RBCs with a wide area of central pallor, anisocytosis, and poikilocytosis when severe.
- Laboratory abnormalities consistent with iron deficiency are low serum ferritin level, elevated RBC distribution width (RDW) with values generally >15, low MCV, elevated TIBC, and low serum iron.
- The reticulocyte hemoglobin content (CHr) may be a good screening test for iron deficiency. It can be measured on an automated hematology analyzer and represents a relatively inexpensive and fast way to detect iron deficiency.

TREATMENT

■ NONPHARMACOLOGIC THERAPY
Patients should be instructed to consume foods containing large amounts of iron, such as liver, red meat, and legumes.

■ ACUTE GENERAL Rx
- Treatment consists of ferrous sulfate 325 mg PO qd for at least 6 mo. Calcium supplements can decrease iron absorption; therefore, these two medications should be staggered.
- Parenteral iron therapy is reserved for patients with poor tolerance, noncompliance with oral preparations, or malabsorption.
- Transfusion of packed RBCs is indicated in patients with severe symptomatic anemia (e.g., angina) or life-threatening anemia.

■ CHRONIC Rx
Patients should be instructed to continue their iron supplements for at least 6 mo or longer to correct depleted body iron stores.

■ DISPOSITION
Most patients respond rapidly to iron supplementation with improvement in CBC and general well-being. GI side effects from oral iron therapy are common and may require decreased dose to once every other day.

■ REFERRAL
GI referral for evaluation of GI malignancy is recommended in all patients with iron deficiency and suspected GI blood loss.

PEARLS & CONSIDERATIONS

■ COMMENTS
If the diagnosis of iron deficiency anemia is made, it is mandatory to try to locate the suspected site of iron loss.

REFERENCE
Tefferi A: Anemia in adults: a contemporary approach to diagnosis, *Mayo Clin Proc* 78:1274, 2004.
Author: **Fred F. Ferri, M.D.**

BASIC INFORMATION

■ DEFINITION
Pernicious anemia is an autoimmune disease resulting from antibodies against intrinsic factor and gastric parietal cells.

■ SYNONYMS
Megaloblastic anemia resulting from vitamin B_{12} deficiency

ICD-9CM CODES
281.0 Pernicious anemia

■ EPIDEMIOLOGY & DEMOGRAPHICS
- Increased incidence in females and older adults (diagnosis is unusual before age 35 yr)
- The overall prevalence of undiagnosed PA over age 60 yr is 1.9%
- Prevalence is highest in women (2.7%), particularly in black women (4.3%)
- Increased incidence of autoimmune disease (e.g., type 1 DM, Graves' disease, Addison's disease), *Helicobacter pylori* infection

■ PHYSICAL FINDINGS & CLINICAL PRESENTATION
- Mucosal pallor, glossitis
- Peripheral sensory neuropathy with paresthesias initially and absent reflexes in advanced cases
- Loss of joint position sense, pyramidal or long track signs
- Possible splenomegaly and mild hepatomegaly
- Generalized weakness and delirium/dementia

■ ETIOLOGY
- Antigastric parietal cell antibodies in >70% of patients, antiintrinsic factor antibodies in >50% of patients
- Atrophic gastric mucosa

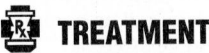 **DIAGNOSIS**

■ DIFFERENTIAL DIAGNOSIS
- Nutritional vitamin B_{12} deficiency
- Malabsorption
- Chronic alcoholism (multifactorial)
- Chronic gastritis related to *H. pylori* infection
- Folic acid deficiency
- Myelodysplasia

■ WORKUP
- The clinical presentation of pernicious anemia varies with the stage. Initially, patients may be asymptomatic. In advanced stages, patients may present with impaired memory, depression, gait disturbances, paresthesias, and complaints of generalized weakness.
- Investigation consists primarily of laboratory evaluation.
- Endoscopy and biopsy for atrophic gastritis may be performed in selected cases.
- Diagnosis is crucial because failure to treat may result in irreversible neurologic deficits.

■ LABORATORY TESTS
- CBC generally reveals macrocytic anemia and leukopenia with hypersegmented neutrophils.
- MCV is generally significantly elevated in the advanced stages.
- Reticulocyte count is low/normal.
- Falsely low serum cobalamin levels can occur in patients with severe folate deficiency, in patients using high doses of ascorbic acid, and when cobalamin levels are measured following nuclear medicine studies (radioactivity interferes with cobalamin RIA measurement).
- Falsely high normal levels in patients with cobalamin deficiency can occur in severe liver disease or chronic granulocytic leukemia.
- The absence of anemia or macrocytosis does not exclude the diagnosis of cobalamin deficiency. Anemia is absent in 20% of patients with cobalamin deficiency, and macrocytosis is absent in >30% of patients at the time of diagnosis. It can be blocked by concurrent iron deficiency or anemia of chronic disease and may be masked by thalassemia trait.
- Schilling test is abnormal in part I; part II corrects to normal after administration of intrinsic factor.
- Laboratory tests used for detecting cobalamin deficiency in patients with normal vitamin B_{12} levels include serum and urinary methylmalonic acid level (elevated), total homocysteine level (elevated), intrinsic factor antibody (positive).
- An increased concentration of plasma methylmalonic acid (P-MMA) does not predict clinical manifestations of vitamin B_{12} deficiency and should not be used as the only marker for diagnosis of B_{12} deficiency.

- Additional laboratory abnormalities can include elevated LDH, direct hyperbilirubinemia, and decreased haptoglobin.

TREATMENT

■ NONPHARMACOLOGIC THERAPY
Avoid folic acid supplementation without proper vitamin B_{12} supplementation.

■ ACUTE GENERAL Rx
Traditional therapy of a cobalamin deficiency consists of IM injections of vitamin B_{12} 1000 μg/wk for the initial 4 to 6 wk followed by 1000 μg/mo IM indefinitely. When hematologic parameters have returned to normal range, intranasal cyanocobalamin may be used in place of IM cyanocobalamin. The initial dose of intranasal cyanocobalamin (Nascobal) is one spray (500 μg) in one nostril once per week. Monitor response and increase dose if serum B_{12} levels decline. Consider return to intramuscular vitamin B_{12} supplementation if decline persists.

■ CHRONIC Rx
Parenteral vitamin B_{12} 1000 μg/mo or intranasal cyanocobalamin 500 μg/wk (see "Acute General Rx") for the remainder of life

■ DISPOSITION
Anemia generally resolves with appropriate treatment. Neurologic deficits, if present at diagnosis, may be permanent.

■ REFERRAL
GI referral for endoscopy upon diagnosis of pernicious anemia and surveillance endoscopy every 5 yr to rule out gastric carcinoma

PEARLS & CONSIDERATIONS

■ COMMENTS
- Patients must understand that therapy is lifelong.
- Self-injection of vitamin B_{12} may be taught in selected patients.
- Oral cobalamin (1000 mcg/day) has been reported as also being effective in mild cases of pernicious anemia because about 1% of an oral dose is absorbed by passive diffusion, a pathway that does not require intrinsic factor.

Author: **Fred F. Ferri, M.D.**

BASIC INFORMATION

DEFINITION

Sideroblastic anemias are blood disorders resulting from defective heme synthesis and are classified as hereditary, acquired, and reversible.

SYNONYMS

- Primary hereditary sideroblastic anemia
- Primary acquired refractory anemia with ringed sideroblasts (RARS)
- Reversible sideroblastic anemias

ICD-9CM CODES

285.0 Sideroblastic anemia

EPIDEMIOLOGY & DEMOGRAPHICS

- Hereditary sideroblastic anemia, being sex-linked, primarily affects males.
- Primary acquired sideroblastic anemia is usually a disease of the elderly.

PHYSICAL FINDINGS & CLINICAL PRESENTATION

The symptoms for sideroblastic anemia are the same for any anemia:
- Symptoms include fatigue, weakness, palpitations, shortness of breath, headaches, irritability, and chest pain.
- Physical findings may include pallor, tachycardia, hepatosplenomegaly, S_3, JVD, and rales.

ETIOLOGY

- The exact cause in many cases of hereditary and primary acquired sideroblastic anemias remains unknown. However, in some cases the underlying molecular defect may involve genes encoding:
  5-aminolevulinate synthase enzyme (ALAS2)
  Mitochondrial iron transporter (ABC7)
  Ferrochelatase
  Cytochrome oxidase
  Mitochondrial proteins (e.g., Pearson Marrow-Pancrease Syndrome)
- Primary hereditary sideroblastic anemia may be inherited as a sex-linked recessive disease.
- Secondary acquired sideroblastic anemia can be caused by alcohol, isoniazid, pyrazinamide, cycloserine, chloramphenicol, and copper deficiency.

DIAGNOSIS

DIFFERENTIAL DIAGNOSIS

- Sideroblastic anemia must be differentiated from other causes of microcytic hypochromic anemia: iron deficiency anemia, thalassemia, anemia of chronic disease, lead poisoning, and blood loss.
- Tissue iron overload from sideroblastic anemia may act similar to hereditary hemochromatosis with liver cirrhosis, diabetes, congestive heart failure, and cardiac arrhythmias.

WORKUP

The diagnostic workup of suspected sideroblastic anemia includes laboratory evaluation and bone marrow aspiration and biopsy.

LABORATORY TESTS

- Sideroblastic anemias are characterized by hypochromic anemia (low Hgb, low Hct, low MCV, high RDW).
- Iron, TIBC, ferritin, free erythrocyte protoporphyrin (FEP), copper, and zinc levels may all assist in the diagnosis of sideroblastic anemias.
- Peripheral smear: dimorphic large and small cells revealing "Pappenheimer bodies" or siderocytes when stained for iron.
- Bone marrow shows the classic ringed sideroblasts not seen in normal bone marrow tissue (Fig. 1-17). The ringed sideroblasts represent iron storage in the mitochondria of normoblasts.

TREATMENT

NONPHARMACOLOGIC THERAPY

- Avoid alcohol.
- Secondary sideroblastic anemia due to isoniazid, pyrazinamide, and cycloserine can expect a full recovery by withdrawing the medication and by the use of vitamin B_6 (50 to 200 mg/day).

ACUTE GENERAL Rx

- Hereditary sideroblastic anemia:
  1. Nearly 35% of patients receiving vitamin B_6 (50 to 200 mg/day) will improve their red blood cell to near normal values.
  2. The remainder of patients will require blood transfusions to treat symptoms of anemia.
- Primary acquired sideroblastic anemia:
  1. Most patients do not respond to vitamin B_6.
  2. Erythropoietin has shown some success in improving the anemia.
  3. Blood transfusions are indicated for patients with symptomatic anemia.

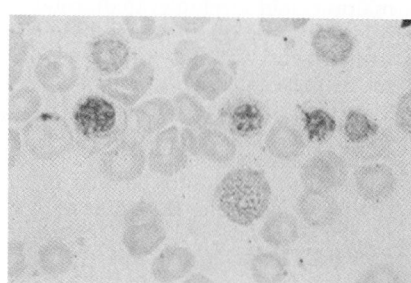

Fig. 1-17   Prussian blue iron stain of the bone marrow shows ringed sideroblasts. (From Goldman L, Bennett JC [eds]: *Cecil textbook of medicine,* ed 21, Philadelphia, 2000, WB Saunders.)

CHRONIC Rx

- Hereditary sideroblastic anemia:
  1. Organ dysfunction resulting from iron overload will require periodic phlebotomies.
  2. In advanced cases, desferrioxamine 40 mg/kg/day IV is given.
- Primary acquired sideroblastic anemia:
  1. As in the hereditary form, periodic phlebotomies are indicated when serum iron levels increase to >500 µg/L and desferrioxamine is used in patients requiring frequent blood transfusions.

DISPOSITION

- Hereditary sideroblastic anemia:
  1. With previously mentioned treatment, prognosis is good for a normal life expectancy.
- Primary acquired sideroblastic anemia:
  1. In patients with anemia alone, life expectancy is normal. In patients dependent on blood transfusions, one can expect morbidity from organ dysfunction.
  2. Some patients with acquired sideroblastic anemia can go on to develop leukemia.

REFERRAL

- Hematology

PEARLS & CONSIDERATIONS

COMMENTS

- Sideroblastic anemia can be thought of as an iron-loading anemia secondary to defective heme synthesis. Protein enzymes necessary for heme synthesis are located in the mitochondria of erythroid cells. A decrease in the activity of these enzymes (D-aminolevulinic acid synthetase, ferrochelatase) impedes protoporphyrin formation and the incorporation of iron into protoporphyrin preventing heme synthesis. Iron continues to be absorbed from the GI tract accumulating in the mitochondria surrounding the nucleus of the normoblast and forming the "ringed sideroblast."
- Vitamin B_6, pyridoxal phosphate, is a required cofactor in heme synthesis, and drugs such as isoniazid, cycloserine, and pyrazinamide can inhibit its function.

REFERENCES

Aleindor T, Bridges KR: Sideroblastic anemias, *Br J Haematol* 116(4):733, 2002.
Bottomley SS: Sideroblastic anemias. In Lee GR, Floerster J, Lukens J et al. (Eds), *Wintrobe's Clinical Hematology,* ed 10, Baltimore, 1999, Williams and Wilkins, p.1022.
Author: Peter Petropoulos, M.D.

BASIC INFORMATION

■ DEFINITION

An abdominal aortic aneurysm is a permanent localized dilation of the abdominal aortic artery to at least 50% when compared with the normal diameter. The normal diameter in men is 2.3 cm, and in women it is 1.9 cm.

■ SYNONYMS

AAA

ICD-9CM CODES

441.4 Aneurysm, abdominal (aorta)
441.3 Ruptured abdominal aortic aneurysm

■ EPIDEMIOLOGY & DEMOGRAPHICS

- The incidence of abdominal aortic aneurysms has been rising from 12.2 cases/100,000 persons in 1951 to 36.2 cases/100,000 persons in 1980.
- The prevalence ranges from 2% to 5% in men >60 yr.
- AAA is predominantly a disease of the elderly, affecting men > women (4:1).
- Rupture of an abdominal aortic aneurysm is the tenth leading cause of death in men >55 yr (15,000 deaths/yr in the U.S.).

■ PHYSICAL FINDINGS & CLINICAL PRESENTATION

- Pulsatile epigastric mass that may or may not be tender.
- Discoloration and pain of the feet if the thrombus within the aneurysm embolizes.
- Shock, hypoperfusion, abdominal distention if rupture occurs.
- Rare presentations include hematemesis or melena with abdominal and back pain in patients with aortoenteric fistulas. Aortocaval fistula produces loud abdominal bruits.

■ ETIOLOGY

Multifactorial
- Atherosclerotic (degenerative or nonspecific)
- Genetic (e.g., Ehlers-Danlos syndrome)
- Trauma
- Cystic medial necrosis (Marfan's syndrome)
- Arteritis, inflammatory
- Mycotic, infected (syphilis)

DIAGNOSIS

■ DIFFERENTIAL DIAGNOSIS

Almost 75% of abdominal aneurysms are asymptomatic and are discovered on routine examination or serendipitously when ordering studies for other complaints. This must be considered in the differential of anyone presenting with abdominal pain or back pain.

■ IMAGING STUDIES

- Abdominal ultrasound is nearly 100% accurate in identifying an aneurysm and estimating the size to within 0.3 to 0.4 cm. It is not very good in estimating the proximal extension to the renal arteries or involvement of the iliac arteries.
- CT scan is recommended for preoperative aneurysm imaging and estimating the size to within 0.3 mm. There are no false-negatives, and the CT scan can localize the proximal extent, detect the integrity of the wall, and rule out rupture.
- Angiography gives detailed arterial anatomy, localizing the aneurysm relative to the renal and visceral arteries. This is the definitive preoperative study for surgeons.
- MRI can also be used, but it is more expensive and not as readily available.

TREATMENT

■ NONPHARMACOLOGIC THERAPY

- Treat atherosclerotic risk factors (diet and exercise for blood pressure, cholesterol, and diabetes, and abstinence from tobacco).
- Definitive treatment depends on the size of the aneurysm (see "Chronic Rx").

■ ACUTE GENERAL Rx

Abdominal aortic rupture is an emergency. Surgery is the only chance for survival.

■ CHRONIC Rx

- Diagnosing, sizing, and repairing the aneurysm in an asymptomatic patient is crucial.
- The most commonly used predictor of rupture is the maximum diameter of the abdominal aortic aneurysm.
- Recent randomized trials found no reduction in mortality from repairing abdominal aortic aneurysms smaller than 5.5 cm in patients at low operative risk.
- For aneurysms 5.5 cm or greater, prosthetic graft replacement is recommended, providing there is no contraindication (e.g., MI within 6 mo, refractory CHF, life expectancy <2 yr, severe residual from CVA).
- For the high-risk patient deemed inoperable for such major surgery, endovascular stent-anchored grafts under local anesthesia have provided an alternative approach.

■ DISPOSITION

- The risk of rupture is 0% per year in aneurysms <4 cm, 0.6%-1%/yr in aneurysms 4.0-5.5 cm, 4.4%/yr in aneurysms 5.5-5.9 cm, 10.2%/yr in aneurysms 6.0-6.9 cm, and 32.5%/yr in aneurysms >7 cm.

- Mortality after rupture is >90%. Of those patients who reach the hospital, it is estimated 50% will survive compared with a 4% mortality rate for elective repair of the nonruptured aorta.

■ REFERRAL

Vascular surgical referral should be made in asymptomatic patients with aneurysms 4 cm or greater or in rapidly expanding aneurysms of 0.7-1 cm/yr, especially if symptoms are present.

PEARLS & CONSIDERATIONS

■ COMMENTS

- Most abdominal aortic aneurysms are infrarenal. Surgical risk is increased in patients with coexisting coronary artery disease, pulmonary disease (Pao_2 <50 mm Hg, FEV_1 <11), liver cirrhosis, and chronic renal failure (Cr >3 mg/dl). Detailed cardiac workup with radionuclide perfusion studies for ischemia and aggressive perioperative hemodynamic monitoring help identify high-risk patients and decrease postoperative complications.
- It is estimated that abdominal aortic aneurysms <5 cm expand at a rate of 0.4 cm/yr.
- The use of the β-blocker propranolol has demonstrated a trend toward fewer surgeries in patients with asymptomatic small abdominal aortic aneurysms (3.0-5.0 cm).

REFERENCES

Lederle FA et al: Rupture rate of large abdominal aortic aneurysms in patients refusing or unfit for elective repair, *JAMA* 287:2968, 2002.

Lederle FA et al: Immediate repair compared with surveillance of small abdominal aortic aneurysms, *N Engl J Med* 346:1437, 2002.

Sparks AR et al: Imaging of abdominal aortic aneurysms, *Am Fam Physician* 65:1565, 2002.

The Propranolol Aneurysm Trial Investigators: Propranolol for small abdominal aortic aneurysms: results of a randomized trial, *J Vasc Surg* 35:72, 2002.

The United Kingdom Small Aneurysm Trial Participants: Long-term outcomes of immediate repair compared with surveillance of small abdominal aortic aneurysms, *N Engl J Med* 346:1445, 2002.

Author: **Peter Petropoulos, M.D.**

BASIC INFORMATION

■ DEFINITION

Angina pectoris is characterized by discomfort that occurs when myocardial oxygen demand exceeds the supply. Myocardial ischemia can be asymptomatic (silent ischemia), particularly in diabetics. Angina can be classified as follows:

1. CHRONIC (STABLE):
   - Usually follows a precipitating event (e.g., climbing stairs, sexual intercourse, a heavy meal, emotional stress, cold weather)
   - Generally same severity as previous attacks; relieved by the customary dose of nitroglycerin
   - Caused by a fixed coronary artery obstruction secondary to atherosclerosis
2. UNSTABLE (REST OR CRESCENDO, CORONARY SYNDROME):
   - Recent onset
   - Increasing severity, duration, or frequency of chronic angina
   - Occurs at rest or with minimal exertion
3. PRINZMETAL'S VARIANT:
   - Occurs at rest
   - Manifests electrocardiographically as episodic ST-segment elevations
   - Caused by coronary artery spasms with or without superimposed coronary artery disease
   - Patients also more likely to develop ventricular arrhythmias
4. MICROVASCULAR ANGINA (SYNDROME X):
   - Refers to patients with normal coronary angiograms and no coronary spasm but chest pain resembling angina and positive exercise test
   - Defective endothelium-dependent dilation in the coronary microcirculation contributing to the altered regulation of myocardial perfusion and the ischemic manifestations in these patients
   - Excellent prognosis
5. OTHER:
Angina due to aortic stenosis and idiopathic hypertrophic subaortic stenosis, cocaine-induced coronary vasoconstriction.

■ FUNCTIONAL CLASSIFICATION

- New York Heart Association Functional Classification of Angina:
  Class I—Angina only with unusually strenuous activity.
  Class II—Angina with slightly more prolonged or rigorous activity than usual.
  Class III—Angina with usual daily activity.
  Class IV—Angina at rest.

- Grading of Angina by the Canadian Cardiovascular Society Classification System:
  Class I—Ordinary physical activity does not cause angina, such as walking, climbing stairs. Angina (occurs) with strenuous, rapid, or prolonged exertion at work or recreation.
  Class II—Slight limitation of ordinary activity. Angina occurs on walking or climbing stairs rapidly; walking uphill; walking or stair climbing after meals, in cold, in wind, or under emotional stress; or only during the few hours after awakening. Angina occurs on walking more than two blocks on the level and climbing more than one flight of ordinary stairs at a normal pace and in normal condition.
  Class III—Marked limitations of ordinary physical activity. Angina occurs on walking one to two blocks on the level and climbing one flight of stairs in normal conditions and at a normal pace.
  Class IV—Inability to carry on any physical activity without discomfort—anginal symptoms may be present at rest.

ICD-9CM CODES
411.1 Angina, stable
413 Angina pectoris
413.1 Prinzmetal's angina
413.9 Angina, unspecified

■ EPIDEMIOLOGY & DEMOGRAPHICS

- Angina is most common in middle-aged and elderly males.
- Females are usually affected after menopause.
- Prevalence of angina pectoris in people older than 30 yr is >3%.
- Within 12 mo of initial diagnosis, 10% to 20% of patients with diagnosis of stable angina progress to MI or unstable angina.

■ PHYSICAL FINDINGS & CLINICAL PRESENTATION

- Although there is significant individual variation, most patients complain of substernal chest pain (pressure, tightness, heaviness, sharp pain, sensation similar to intestinal gas or dysphagia).
- The pain is of short duration (30 sec to 30 min), nonpleuritic, and often accompanied by shortness of breath, nausea, diaphoresis, and numbness or pain in the left arm, jaw, or shoulder.

■ ETIOLOGY

UNCONTROLLABLE RISK FACTORS FOR ANGINA:
- Advanced age
- Male sex
- Genetic predisposition
MODIFIABLE RISK FACTORS FOR ANGINA:
- Smoking (risk is almost double)
- Hypertension (risk is double if systolic blood pressure is >180 mm Hg)
- Hyperlipidemia
- Impaired glucose tolerance or diabetes mellitus
- Obesity (weight >30% over ideal)
- Hypothyroidism
- Left ventricular hypertrophy (LVH)
- Sedentary lifestyle
- Oral contraceptive use
- Cocaine use (Cocaine is used by >5,000,000 Americans regularly and is responsible for >64,000 ER evaluations yearly to rule out myocardial ischemia.)
- Low serum folate levels (Folate is required for conversion of homocysteine to methionine. Hyperhomocysteinemia has a toxic effect on vascular endothelium and interferes with proliferation of arterial wall smooth muscle cells. Folate deficiencies are associated with an increased risk of fatal coronary heart disease.)
- Elevated homocysteine levels
- Elevated levels of highly sensitive C-reactive protein (hs-CRP, cardio CRP)
- Elevated levels of lipoprotein-associated phospholipase A2
- Elevated fibrinogen levels
- Depression
- Vasculitis
- Low level of RBC glutathione peroxidase 1 activity

DIAGNOSIS

■ DIFFERENTIAL DIAGNOSIS

Noncardiac pain mimicking angina may be caused by:
- Pulmonary diseases (pulmonary hypertension, pulmonary embolism, pleurisy, pneumothorax, pneumonia)
- GI disorders (peptic ulcer disease, pancreatitis, esophageal spasm or spontaneous esophageal muscle contraction, esophageal reflux, cholecystitis, cholelithiasis)
- Musculoskeletal conditions (costochondritis, chest wall trauma, cervical arthritis with radiculopathy, muscle strain, myositis)
- Acute aortic dissection
- Herpes zoster

■ WORKUP

- The most important diagnostic factor is the history.
- The physical examination is of little diagnostic help and may be totally normal in many patients, although the presence of an S_4 gallop is suggestive of ischemic chest pain.
- An ECG taken during the acute episode may show transient T-wave inversion or ST-segment depression or elevation, but some patients may have a normal tracing.
- Treadmill exercise tolerance test is useful to identify patients with coronary artery disease who would benefit from cardiac catheterization. Stress echocardiogram or radionuclide testing (e.g., thallium, Persantine, dobutamine) are useful and sensitive in the detection of myocardial ischemia.
- Although invasive, coronary angiography remains the gold standard for the identification of clinically significant coronary artery disease, coronary magnetic resonance angiography can also detect coronary artery disease of the proximal and middle segments. This noninvasive approach, where available, can be used to reliably identify (or rule out) left main coronary artery or three-vessel disease.

■ LABORATORY TESTS

- Initial laboratory tests in patients with chronic stable angina should include hemoglobin, fasting glucose, and fasting lipid panel.
- Cardiac isoenzymes (CK-MB q8h × 2) should be obtained to rule out MI in patients with unstable angina or coronary syndrome.
- Cardiac troponin I and T are specific markers of myocardial necrosis and are useful in evaluating patients with acute chest pain. Elevation of either of these proteins in the setting of an acute coronary syndrome identifies patients with a several-fold increased risk of death in subsequent weeks. Patients with negative troponin assays on arrival in the ER and repeated 4 hr later are at a low level of risk for cardiac events within the following 30 days, and most of these patients can be safely discharged from the ER. Troponin T tests can be false-positive in patients with renal failure, sepsis, rhabdomyolysis, fibrin clots, and heterophile antibodies. The presence of jaundice or the concurrent use of heparin can result in underestimation of troponin.
- Cardio-CRP (hs-CRP)—elevation of cardio-CRP is a strong predictor of cardiovascular events and it adds prognostic information to that conveyed by the Framingham risk score. However, based on current data, it may be premature to adapt widespread assessment of cardio-CRP and of the other markers noted below.
- CD40 ligand, an immunomodulator, is an important contributor to the inflammatory process that leads to atherosclerosis and thrombosis. In patients with unstable coronary artery disease, elevation of soluble CD 40 ligand is useful to identify patients who are at high risk for cardiac events.
- Circulating interleukin-6 (IL-6), a cytokine with both proinflammatory and antiinflammatory effects, is a strong independent marker of increased mortality in unstable coronary artery disease and identifies patients who benefit most from a strategy of early intervention.
- New markers for risk stratification in acute coronary syndromes based on neurohormonal activation and inflammation have recently been identified. A single measurement of B-type natriuretic peptide, a natriuretic and vasodilative peptide regulated by ventricular wall tension and stored mainly in the ventricular myocardium, obtained in the first few days after the onset of ischemic symptoms, provides predictive information for risk stratification in acute coronary syndromes. Pregnancy-associated plasma protein A (PAPP-A), which is found in both men and women, is an activator of insulin-like growth factor I (IGF-I), and may be a marker for unstable plaques. Elevated plasma levels of PAPP-A may identify patients with unstable angina in the absence of elevations of either troponin I or C-reactive protein.
- Plasma myeloperoxidase measurement may be a potentially useful lab test for stratification of patients presenting with chest pain. An elevated single initial measurement of plasma myeloperoxidase in patients presenting with chest pain independently predicts the early risk of MI, and the risk of major adverse events in the following 1 mo and 6 mo periods.

■ IMAGING STUDIES

- Echocardiography is indicated in patients with systolic murmur suggestive of aortic stenosis, mitral valve prolapse, or hypertrophic cardiomyopathy. It is also useful in the detection of ischemia-induced regional wall motion abnormalities or mitral regurgitation. Echocardiography combined with treadmill exercise (stress echo) or pharmacologic stress with dobutamine can be used to detect regional wall abnormalities that occur during myocardial ischemia associated with CAD.
- Coronary angiography is performed to define the location and extent of coronary disease; this is indicated in selected patients who are candidates for CABG surgery or angioplasty.
- Noninvasive methods for assessing myocardial viability to predict which patients will have increased LVEF and improved survival after revascularization include positron-emission tomography, dobutamine echocardiography, and contrast-enhanced MRI. Additional studies are needed to determine the cost effectiveness of these studies in patients with ischemic cardiomyopathy.

■ TREATMENT

■ NONPHARMACOLOGIC THERAPY

- Aggressive modification of preventable risk factors (weight reduction in obese patients, regular aerobic exercise program, correction of folate deficiency, low-cholesterol and low-sodium diet, cessation of tobacco use)
- Diets using nonhydrogenated unsaturated fats as the predominant form of dietary fat, whole grains as the main form of carbohydrates, an abundance of fruits and vegetables, and adequate omega-3-fatty acids are optimal for prevention of coronary heart disease.
- Correction of possible aggravating factors (e.g., anemia, hypertension, diabetes mellitus, hyperlipidemia, thyrotoxicosis, hypothyroidism)

■ ACUTE GENERAL Rx

The major classes of antiischemic agents are nitrates, β-adrenergic blockers, calcium channel blockers, aspirin, and heparin; they can be used alone or in combination.

- Nitrates cause venodilation and relaxation of vascular smooth muscle; the decreased venous return from venodilation decreases diastolic ventricular wall tension (preload) and thereby reduces mechanical activity (and myocardial oxygen consumption) during systole. Relaxation of vascular smooth muscle increases coronary blood flow and reduces systemic pressure. Tolerance to nitrates can be minimized by avoiding sustained blood levels with a daily nitrate-free period (e.g., omission of bedtime dose of oral isosorbide dinitrate or 12 hr on/12 hr off transdermal nitroglycerin therapy). Nitrates are relatively contraindicated in patients with hypertrophic obstructive cardiomyopathy, and should also be avoided in patients with severe aortic stenosis.
- β-Adrenergic blockers achieve their major antianginal effect by reducing heart rate and systolic blood pressure. Absent contraindications, they should be regarded as initial therapy for stable angina for all patients. Their dose should generally be adjusted to reduce the resting heart rate to 50-60 beats/min.
- Calcium channel blockers play a major role in preventing and terminating myocardial ischemia induced by coronary artery spasm. They are particularly effective in treating microvascular angina. Short-acting calcium channel blockers should be avoided. Calcium channel blockers should generally also be avoided after complicated MI (CHF) and in patients with CHF secondary to systolic dysfunction (unless necessary to control heart rate).

- Aspirin: give initial dose of at least 160 mg/day followed by 81 to 325 mg/day. Aspirin inhibits cyclooxygenics and synthesis of thromboxane A_2 and reduces the risk of adverse cardiovascular events by 33% in patients with unstable angina. Patients intolerant to aspirin can be treated with the antiplatelet agent clopidogrel.
- Heparin is useful in patients with unstable angina and reduces the frequency of MI and refractory angina. Patients with unstable angina treated with aspirin plus heparin have a 32% reduction in the risk of MI and death compared with those treated with aspirin alone; therefore, unless heparin is contraindicated, most hospitalized patients with unstable angina should be treated with both aspirin and heparin.
Enoxaparin (low–molecular weight heparin) 1 mg bid SC is as effective as continuous unfractionated heparin in reducing the incidence of unstable angina. It is usually given for 3-8 days, or until coronary revascularization is performed. Longer administration does not provide additional cardiac benefits and may increase risk of hemorrhage.
- Early administration of platelet glycoprotein IIb/IIIa receptor antagonists tirofiban and eptifibatide is useful in unstable angina, in high-risk patients with positive troponin tests, or those undergoing percutaneous revascularization. Abciximab, the first GP IIb/IIa inhibitor, is an important component of percutaneous revascularization. Started in the catheterization lab, it reduces the incidence of ischemic events. Contraindications to the use of GP IIb/IIa inhibitors are: severe hypertension (>180/110), internal bleeding within 30 days, history of intracranial hemorrhage, neoplasm, NVM, aneurysm, CVA within 30 days or history of hemorrhagic CVA, thrombocytopenin (<100 k), acute pericarditis, history or symptoms suggestive of aortic dissection, and major surgical procedures or severe physical trauma within previous month.

■ CHRONIC Rx

Use of lipid-lowering drugs (e.g., statins) is recommended in patients with coronary heart disease and in patients with hyperlipidemia refractory to diet and exercise. Most statins also decrease the level of the inflammatory marker hs-CRP independently of the magnitude of change in lipid parameters.

■ REFERRAL

Surgical therapy:
CABG surgery is recommended for patients with left main coronary disease, for those with symptomatic three-vessel disease, and for those with left ventricular EF <40% and critical (>70% stenosis) in all three major coronary arteries. Surgical therapy improves prognosis, particularly in diabetic patients with multivessel disease.
Minimally invasive direct coronary artery bypass (MIDCAB) is a variation of CABG for patients in whom sternotomy and cardiopulmonary bypass is either contraindicated or unnecessary. In this procedure the left internal mammary is anastomosed to the LAD through a thoracic incision without cardiopulmonary bypass. This operation is generally performed for patients with only single-vessel CAD.
The Port-Access Procedure is another type of minimally invasive technique.

Angioplasty and coronary stents:
Percutaneous coronary intervention (PCI) should be considered for patients with one- or two-vessel disease that does not involve the main left coronary artery and in whom ventricular function is normal or near normal. Patients selected for PCI should also be candidates for CABG. The types of lesions best suited for angioplasty are proximal lesions, noncalcified, concentric, and preferably shorter than 5 mm (should not exceed 10 mm). Approximately 80% of patients show immediate benefit after PCI. The frequency of abrupt closure postangioplasty can be reduced by pretreatment with IV glycoprotein IIb/IIIa receptor inhibitors, which block the final common pathway of platelet aggregation. In patients with clinically documented acute coronary syndrome who are treated with GP IIb/IIa inhibitors, even small elevations in cTmI and cTmT identify high-risk patients who derive a large clinical benefit from an early invasive strategy. Abciximab (ReoPro) and eptifibatide (Integrilin) are approved for use before and during percutaneous coronary interventions. They are expensive (>$1400 per dose of abciximab) and can cause thrombocytopenia in 0.5% to 1% of patients. Platelet counts should be monitored for 24 hours after starting glycoprotein IIb/IIIa inhibitors. Reversal of thrombocytopenia (e.g., patients undergoing emergency CABG) can be achieved with platelet transfusions.

The development of *coronary stents* has broadened the number of patients who can be treated in the cardiac laboratory. Cardiac stents are currently used in nearly 95% of all percutaneous interventional lesions. The rate of restenosis may be reduced by placing a stent electively in primary atheromatous lesions. In patients with symptomatic isolated stenosis of the proximal left anterior descending artery, stenting has advantages over standard coronary angioplasty in that it is associated with both a lower rate of restenosis and a better clinical outcome. The major limitations of stenting are subacute thrombosis, restenosis within the stent, bleeding complications when anticoagulants are used post-stenting, and higher cost ($1500 average unit price). The combination of aspirin and clopidogrel is effective in preventing coronary stent thrombosis. Stents coated with sirolimus have been shown to dramatically reduce the incidence of stent restenosis by inhibiting the growth of endothelium and fibrosis within the lumen of the stent on the short term. Stents coated with paclitaxel, which inhibits cellular replication and reduces proliferation and migration of endothelial smooth muscle cells, are also effective in reducing the incidence of restenosis.

CO2 laser revascularization:
This operation is performed only in selected centers and consists of placing 1-mm laser channels in the heart muscle. It may be indicated in selected Class III or Class IV angina patients who are failing maximum medical therapy and are not amenable to any other PTCA or coronary bypass surgery.

REFERENCES

Aviles RJ et al: Troponin T levels in patients with acute coronary syndromes, with or without renal dysfunction, *N Engl J Med* 346:2047, 2002.

Blankenberg S et al: Glutathione Peroxidase 1 activity and cardiovascular events in patients with coronary artery disease, *N Engl J Med* 349:1605, 2003.

Brennan ML et al: Prognostic value of myeloperoxidase in patients with chest pain, *N Engl J Med* 349:1595, 2003.

Buffon A et al: Widespread coronary inflammation in unstable angina, *N Engl J Med* 347:5, 2002.

Glassman AH et al: Sertraline treatment of major depression in patients with acute MI or unstable angina, *JAMA* 288:701, 2002.

Heeschen C et al: Soluble CD 40 ligand in acute coronary syndromes, *N Engl J Med* 348:1104, 2003.

Hu F, Willet W: Optimal diets for prevention of coronary heart disease, *JAMA* 288:2569, 2002.

Kushner I, Sehgal A: Is high-sensitivity C-Reactive protein an effective screening test for cardiovascular risk? *Arch Intern Med* 162:867, 2002.

Levinson SS, Elin RJ: What is c-reactive protein telling us about coronary artery disease, *Arch Intern Med* 162:389, 2002.

Moses JW et al: Sirolimus-eluting stents versus standard stents in patients with stenosis in a native coronary artery, *N Engl J Med* 349:1315, 2003.

Ridker PM et al: Plasma homocysteine concentration, statin therapy, and the risk of first acute coronary events, *Circulation* 105:1776, 2002.

Ridker PM et al: Comparison of C-reactive protein and low-density lipoprotein cholesterol levels in the prediction of first cardiovascular events, *N Engl J Med* 347:1557, 2002.

Sabatine MS et al: Multimarker approach to risk stratification in non-ST elevation acute coronary syndromes: simultaneous assessment of troponin I, C-reactive protein, and B-type natriuretic peptide, *Circulation* 105:1760, 2002.

Serruys PW et al: Fluvastatin for prevention of cardiac events following successful first percutaneous coronary intervention, *JAMA* 287:3215, 2002.

Author: **Fred F. Ferri, M.D.**

BASIC INFORMATION

■ DEFINITION
- The cutaneous swelling caused by the release of vasoactive mediators is called urticaria and angioedema.
- Urticaria causes edema of the superficial dermis.
- Angioedema involves the deep layers of the dermis and the subcutaneous tissue.

■ SYNONYMS
Angioneurotic edema

ICD-9CM CODES
995.1 Angioedema (allergic)
277.6 Angioedema (hereditary)

■ EPIDEMIOLOGY & DEMOGRAPHICS
- Approximately 20% of the population experiences urticaria and/or angioedema at some time during life.
- Race: No predilection.
- Sex: More occurrences in women than men.
- Angioedema can occur together with urticaria (40%) or alone (20%); the remaining 40% have urticaria alone
- Angioedema commonly occurs after adolescence in the third decade of life.
- Incidence of hereditary angioedema is 1/150,000 persons.

■ PHYSICAL FINDINGS & CLINICAL PRESENTATION
- Angioedema may be acute or chronic.
  1. Acute angioedema is defined as symptoms lasting 6 wk.
  2. Chronic angioedema is defined as symptoms lasting >6 wk.
- Urticaria is commonly known as "hives" and is characterized by:
  1. Pruritus
  2. Palpable
  3. Erythematous
  4. Millimeters to centimeters in size
  5. Multiple in number
  6. Fades within 12 to 24 hr
  7. Reappears at other sites
- Angioedema is characterized by the following:
  1. Nonpruritic
  2. Burning
  3. Not well demarcated
  4. Involves eyelids (Fig. 1-18), lips, tongue, and extremities
  5. Can involve the larynx causing respiratory distress
  6. Resolves slowly

■ ETIOLOGY
- Angioedema, with or without urticaria, is classified as acquired (allergic or idiopathic) or hereditary.
- Angioedema is primarily due to mast cell activation and degranulation with release of vasoactive mediators (e.g., histamine, serotonin, bradykinins) resulting in postcapillary venule inflammation, vascular leakage, and edema in the deep layers of the dermis and subcutaneous tissue.
- Pathologically angioedema has both immunological and nonimmunological mediated mechanisms.
  1. Immunoglobulin E (Ig E)-mediated angioedema may result from antigen exposure (e.g., foods [milk, eggs, peanuts, shell fish, tomatoes, chocolate, sulfites] or drugs [penicillin, aspirin, NSAIDs, phenytoin, sulfonamides]).
  2. Complement-mediated angioedema involving immune complex mechanisms can also lead to mast cell activation that manifests as serum sickness.
  3. Hereditary angioedema is an autosomal dominant disease caused by a deficiency of C1 esterase inhibitor (C1-INH). C1-INH is a protease inhibitor that is normally present in high concentrations in the plasma. C1-INH serves many functions, one of which is to inhibit plasma kallikrein, a protease that cleaves kininogen and releases bradykinin. A deficiency in C1-INH results in excess concentration of kininogen and the subsequent release of kinin mediators.
  4. Acquired angioedema is usually associated with other diseases, most commonly B-cell lymphoproliferative disorders, but may also result from the formation of autoantibodies directed against C1 inhibitor protein.
  5. Other causes of angioedema include infection (e.g., herpes simplex, hepatitis B, coxsackie A and B, streptococcus, candida, ascaris, and strongyloides), insect bites and stings, stress, physical factors (e.g., cold, exercise, pressure, and vibration), connective tissue diseases (e.g., SLE, Henoch-Schönlein purpura), and idiopathic causes.

DIAGNOSIS

A detailed history and physical examination usually establishes the diagnosis of angioedema. Extensive lab testing is of limited value.

■ DIFFERENTIAL DIAGNOSIS
The differential diagnosis of angioedema includes:
1. Cellulitis
2. Hypothyroidism
3. Contact dermatitis
4. Atopic dermatitis
5. Mastocytosis
6. Granulomatous cheilitis
7. Bullous pemphigoid
8. Urticaria pigmentosa
9. Anaphylaxis
10. Erythema multiforme
11. Epiglottitis
12. Peritonsillar abscess

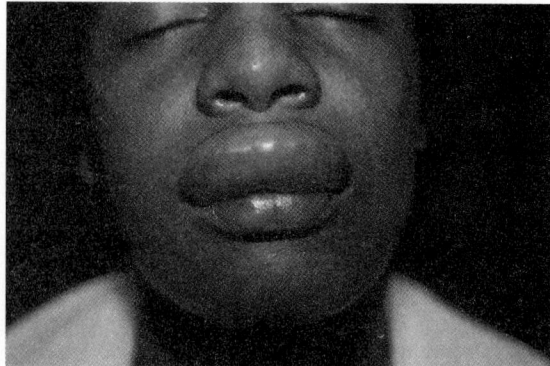

Fig. 1-18 Angioedema of the upper lip, with severe swelling of deeper tissues. (From Goldstein BG, Goldstein AO: *Practical dermatology*, ed 2, St Louis, 1997, Mosby.)

■ WORKUP

- An extensive workup searching for the cause of angioedema is often unrevealing (90%).
- Workup including diagnostic blood tests and allergy testing is performed based on the history and physical examination.

■ LABORATORY TESTS

- CBC, ESR, and urinalysis are sometimes helpful as part of the initial evaluation
- Stools for ova and parasites
- Serology testing
- C4 levels are reduced in acquired and hereditary angioedema. If C4 levels are low, C1-INH levels and activity should be obtained
- Skin and radioallergosorbent (RAST) testing may be done if food allergies are suspected
- Skin biopsy is usually done in patients with chronic angioedema refractory to corticosteroid treatment

℞ TREATMENT

■ NONPHARMACOLOGIC THERAPY

- Eliminate the offending agent
- Avoid triggering factors (e.g., cold, stress)
- Cold compresses to affected areas

■ ACUTE GENERAL Rx

- Acute life-threatening angioedema involving the larynx is treated with:
  1. Epinephrine 0.3 mg in a solution of 1:1000 given SC
  2. Diphenhydramine 25 to 50 mg IV or IM
  3. Cimetidine 300 mg IV or ranitidine 50 mg IV
  4. Methylprednisolone 125 mg IV

- Mainstay therapy in angioedema is H1 antihistamines.
  1. Diphenhydramine 25 to 50 mg q6h
  2. Chlorpheniramine 4 mg q6h
  3. Hydroxyzine 10 to 25 mg q6h
  4. Cetirizine 5 to 10 mg qd
  5. Loratadine 10 mg qd
  6. Fexofenadine 60 mg qd
- H2 antihistamines can be added to H1 antihistamines.
  1. Ranitidine 150 mg bid
  2. Cimetidine 400 mg bid
  3. Famotidine 20 mg bid
- Tricyclic antidepressants
  1. Doxepin 25 to 50 mg qd can be tried.
- Corticosteroids are rarely required for symptomatic relief of acute angioedema.

■ CHRONIC Rx

- Chronic angioedema is treated as described under "Acute General Rx."
- Corticosteroids are used more often in chronic angioedema.
- Prednisone 1 mg/kg/day for 5 days and then tapered over a period of weeks.
- Androgens are used for the treatment of hereditary angioedema.

■ DISPOSITION

- Antihistamines achieve symptomatic relief in more than 80% of patients with angioedema.
- In chronic angioedema, corticosteroids are given in addition to antihistamines.
- A small percentage of people will have recurrence of symptoms after steroid treatment.
- Chronic angioedema can last for months and even years.

■ REFERRAL

Dermatology consultation is recommended in patients with chronic angioedema, hereditary angioedema, and recurring angioedema.

☼ PEARLS & CONSIDERATIONS

■ COMMENTS

- Identifying a cause for angioedema in patients is often difficult and met with frustration.
- Chronic angioedema, unlike acute angioedema, is rarely caused by an allergic reaction.

REFERENCES

Joint Task Force on Practice Parameters: The diagnosis and management of urticaria: a practice parameter. Part I: acute urticaria/angioedema. Part II: chronic urticaria/angioedema, *Ann Allergy Asthma Immunol* 85(6 pt 2):521, 2000.

Kamboj S et al: Hereditary angioedema: a rare but potentially lethal disease, *J La State Med Soc* 154(3):121, 2002.

Kaplan AP: Clinical practice: chronic urticaria and angioedema, *N Engl J Med* 346(3):175, 2002.

Authors: **Peter Petropoulos, M.D., and Mel Anderson, M.D.**

BASIC INFORMATION

■ DEFINITION

Ankle fractures involve the lateral, medial, or posterior malleolus of the ankle and may occur either alone or in some combination. Associated ligamentous injuries are included.

ICD-9CM CODES
824.8 Ankle fracture (malleolus) (closed)
824.2 Lateral malleolus fracture (fibular)
824.0 Medial malleolus fracture (tibial)

■ PHYSICAL FINDINGS & CLINICAL PRESENTATION
- Deformity usually dependent on extent of displacement
- Pain, tenderness, and hemorrhage at the site of injury
- Gentle palpation of ligamentous structures (especially deltoid ligament) to determine the extent of soft tissue injury
- Evaluation of distal neurovascular status; results recorded

■ ETIOLOGY
- The ankle depends on its ligamentous and bony support for stability. The joint, or *mortise,* is an inverted U with the dome of the talus fitting into the medial and lateral malleoli. The posterior margin of the tibia is often called the *third* or *posterior malleolus.*
- Most common ankle fractures are the result of eversion or lateral rotation forces on the talus (in contrast to common sprains, which are caused usually by inversion).

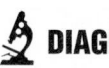 DIAGNOSIS

■ IMAGING STUDIES
Standard AP and lateral views accompanied by an AP taken 15° internally rotated. The last view is taken to properly visualize the mortise.

TREATMENT

All fractures: elevation and ice to control swelling for 48 to 72 hr.

■ ACUTE GENERAL Rx
- Clinical and roentgenographic assessment of the status of the ankle mortise and stability of the injury is mandatory to determine treatment.
- There is potential for displacement if both sides of the joint are significantly injured (e.g., fracture of the lateral malleolus with deltoid ligament injury).

- Deviation of the position of the talus in the mortise could lead to traumatic arthritis.
- If there is no widening of the ankle mortise, many injuries can be safely treated with simple casting without reduction:
  1. Undisplaced or avulsion fractures of either malleolus below the ankle joint line:
     a. Stability of the joint is not compromised and a short leg walking cast or ankle support is sufficient.
     b. Weight bearing is allowed as tolerated.
     c. In 4 to 6 wk, protection may be discontinued.
  2. Isolated undisplaced fractures of the medial, lateral, or posterior malleolus:
     a. Usually stable and require only the application of a short leg walking cast with the ankle in the neutral position or fracture cast boot.
     b. Immobilization should be continued for 8 wk.
     c. Fracture line of lateral malleolus may persist roentgenographically for several months, but immobilization beyond 8 wk is usually unnecessary.
     d. Undisplaced bimalleolar fractures are treated with a long leg cast flexed 30° at the knee to prevent motion and displacement of the fracture fragments. In 4 wk, a short leg walking cast may be applied for an additional 4 wk.
  3. Isolated fractures of the lateral malleolus that are slightly displaced:
     a. May be treated with casting if no medial injury is present.
     b. A below-knee walking cast is applied with ankle in the neutral position and weight bearing is allowed as tolerated.
     c. Six weeks of immobilization is sufficient.
     d. If medial tenderness is present, suggesting deltoid ligament rupture, a carefully molded cast may suffice if weight bearing is not allowed and the patient is followed closely for signs of instability, especially after swelling recedes. If significant widening of the medial ankle mortise (increase in the "medial clear space") develops as a result of lateral displacement of the talus, referral for possible reduction is indicated.
     e. If signs of instability are already present at initial examination (widening of the medial clear space with medial tenderness), referral is indicated.

  4. Undisplaced fracture of the distal fibular epiphysis:
     a. Diagnosed clinically.
     b. There is tenderness over the epiphyseal plate.
     c. Roentgenographic findings are often negative.
     d. A short leg walking cast is applied for 4 wk.
     e. Growth disturbance is rare.
  5. Isolated posterior malleolar fractures involving less than 25% of the joint surface on the lateral roentgenogram:
     Safely treated by applying a short leg walking cast or fracture brace. (Fractures involving >25% of the weight-bearing surface should be referred because of the potential for instability and subsequent traumatic arthritis.)

■ CHRONIC Rx
- Early motion is encouraged through a home exercise program.
- Protection from reinjury is appropriate for 4 to 6 wk following cast or brace removal.
- Temporary increase in lower extremity swelling that frequently occurs after short leg cast removal may benefit from the use of support hose.

■ DISPOSITION
Significant factors involved in the development of traumatic arthritis:
- Amount of joint trauma at the time of injury
- Eventual position of the talus in the mortise
Fracture nonunion is uncommon unless displacement is significant.

■ REFERRAL
Orthopedic consultation for:
- Unstable ankle joint
- Widened ankle mortise
- Posterior malleolar fracture over 25% of joint with incongruity
- Marked displacement of fracture fragment

REFERENCES
Hasselman CT, Vogt MT et al: Foot and ankle fractures in elderly white women: incidence and risk factors, *J Bone Joint Surg* 85:820, 2003.
Kay RM, Matthys GA: Pediatric ankle fractures: evaluation and treatment, *J Am Acad Orthop Surg* 9:268, 2001.
Makwana NK et al: Conservative versus operative treatment for displaced ankle fractures in patients over 55 years of age, *J Bone Joint Surg* 83(B):525, 2001.
Author: **Lonnie R. Mercier, M.D.**

BASIC INFORMATION

■ DEFINITION
An ankle sprain is an injury to the ligamentous support of the ankle. Most (85%) involve the lateral ligament complex (Fig. 1-19). The anterior inferior tibiofibular (AITF) ligament, deltoid ligament, and interosseous membrane may also be injured. Damage to the tibiofibular syndesmosis is sometimes called a *high sprain* because of pain above the ankle.

ICD-9CM CODES
845.00 Sprain, ankle or foot

■ EPIDEMIOLOGY & DEMOGRAPHICS
PREVALENCE: 1 case/10,000 people each day
PREDOMINANT SEX: Varies according to age and level of physical activity

■ PHYSICAL FINDINGS & CLINICAL PRESENTATION
• Often a history of a "pop"
• Variable amounts of tenderness and hemorrhage
• Possible abnormal anterior drawer test (pulling the plantar flexed foot forward to determine if there is any abnormal increase in forward movement of the talus in the ankle mortise) (Fig. 1-20)
• Inversion sprains: tender laterally; syndesmotic injuries: area of tenderness is more anterior and proximal
• Evaluation of motor function (Fig. 1-21)

■ ETIOLOGY
• Lateral injuries usually result from inversion and plantar flexion injuries.
• Eversion and rotational forces may injure the deltoid or AITF ligament or the interosseous membrane.

DIAGNOSIS

■ DIFFERENTIAL DIAGNOSIS
• Fracture of the ankle or foot, particularly involving the distal fibular growth plate in the immature patient
• Avulsion fracture of the fifth metatarsal base

■ WORKUP
• History and clinical examination are usually sufficient to establish the diagnosis.
• Plain radiographs are always needed.

■ IMAGING STUDIES
Roentgenographic evaluation
1. Usually normal but always performed
2. Should include the fifth metatarsal base
3. All minor avulsion fractures noted
Varying opinions on the usefulness of arthrograms, tenograms, and stress films

TREATMENT

■ ACUTE GENERAL Rx
Ankle sprains are often graded I, II, or III, according to severity, with Grade III injury implying complete rupture. The first line of treatment is described by the mnemonic device, *RICE:*
• Rest
• Ice
• Compression
• Elevation
• Varying opinions regarding the initial use of NSAIDs
• In 48 to 72 hr, active range of motion and weight bearing as tolerated
• In 4 to 5 days, exercise against resistance added
• Possible cast immobilization for some patients who require early independent walking; short leg orthoses also available for the same purpose
• Surgery is rarely recommended, even for Grade III sprains; reports of equally satisfactory outcomes with nonsurgical treatment

■ CHRONIC Rx
• Lateral heel and sole wedge to prevent inversion
• Protective taping or bracing during vigorous activities (Fig. 1-22)
• Strengthening exercises

■ DISPOSITION
• Lateral sprains of any severity may cause lingering symptoms for weeks and months.
  1. Some syndesmotic sprains take even longer to heal.
  2. Heterotopic ossification may even develop in the interosseous membrane, but long-term results do not seem to be affected by such ossification.
• Continuing lateral symptoms may require surgical reconstruction, although late traumatic arthritis or chronic instability is rare regardless of treatment.

■ REFERRAL
For orthopedic consultation for cases that fail to respond to conservative treatment

PEARLS & CONSIDERATIONS

■ COMMENTS
If healing seems delayed (more than 6 wk), the following conditions should be considered:
1. Talar dome fracture
2. Reflex sympathetic dystrophy
3. Chronic tendinitis
4. Peroneal tendon subluxation
5. Other occult fracture
6. Peroneal weakness (poor rehabilitation)
7. A "high" (syndesmotic) sprain
Repeat plain roentgenograms, bone scan, or MRI may be indicated.

REFERENCES
Bachman LM, Kolb E et al: Accuracy of Ottawa ankle rules to exclude fractures of the ankle and mid-foot: systematic review, *BMJ* 326:417, 2003.
Judd DB, Kim DH: Foot fractures misdiagnosed as ankle sprains, *Am Fam Physician* 66:785, 2002.
Wolfe M et al: Management of ankle sprains, *Am Fam Physician* 63:83, 2001.
Author: **Lonnie R. Mercier, M.D.**

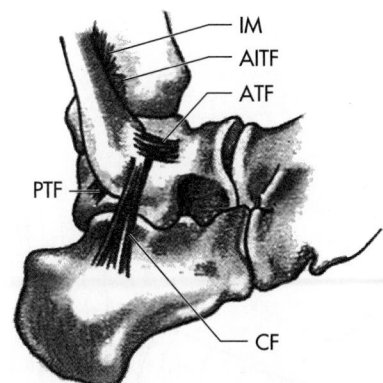

Fig. 1-19 The lateral ankle ligaments, anterior and posterior talofibular *(ATF, PTF)* and calcaneofibular *(CF)*. Also shown are the anterior inferior tibiofibular ligament *(AITF)* and the beginning of the interosseous membrane *(IM)*. (From Mercier LR [ed]: *Practical orthopaedics,* ed 4, St Louis, 1995, Mosby.)

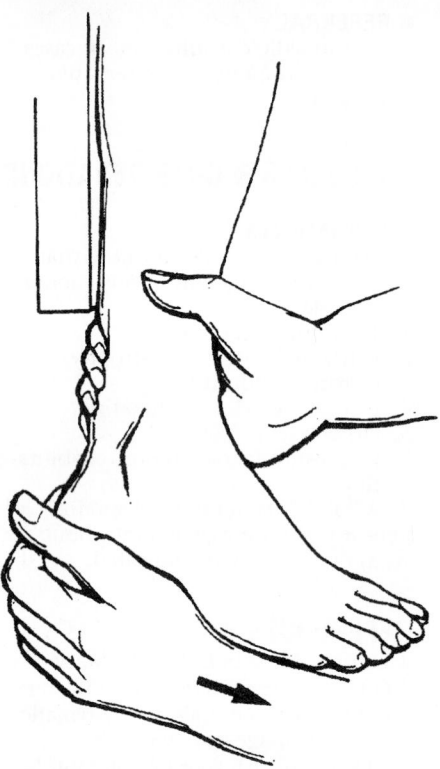

Fig. 1-20 Anterior drawer test of the ankle (tests the integrity of the anterior talofibular ligament). (From Brinker MR, Miller MD: *Fundamentals of orthopaedics,* Philadelphia, 1999, WB Saunders.)

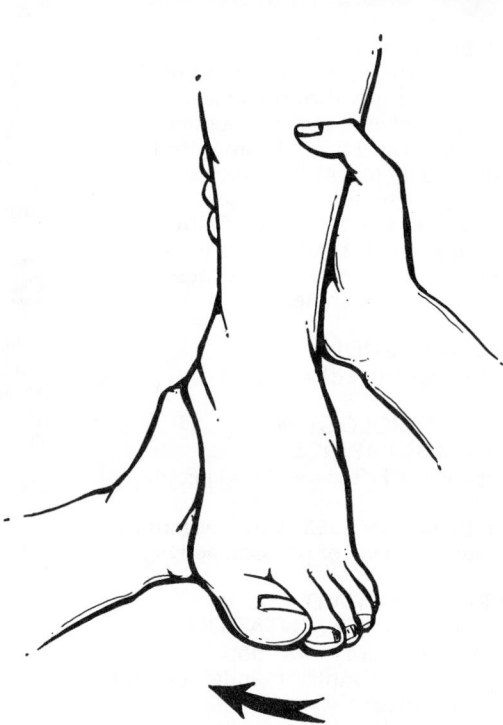

Fig. 1-21 Talar tilt test (inversion stress) of the ankle (tests the integrity of the anterior talofibular ligament and the calcaneofibular ligament). (From Brinker MR, Miller MD: *Fundamentals of orthopaedics,* Philadelphia, 1999, WB Saunders.)

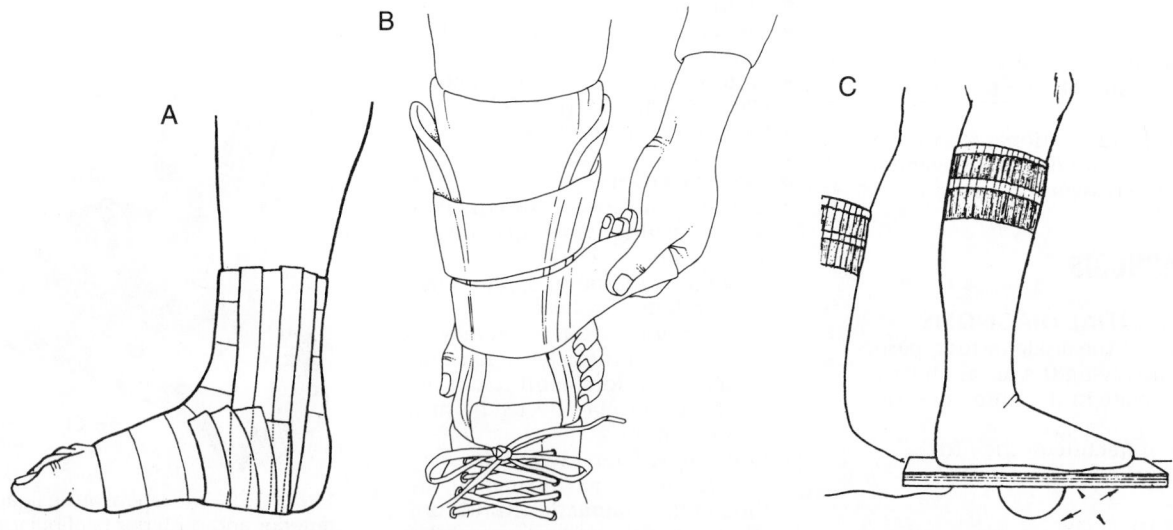

Fig. 1-22 A, The most effective method of supporting most acute ankle sprains is by using an Ace wrap reinforced with 1-in medial and lateral tape strips. The anterior and posterior aspects of the ankle are left free to allow the patient to flex and extend the ankle. The patient is encouraged to bear weight with crutches. **B,** Diagram of an air splint. Straps are adjusted to heel size, the lower straps are wrapped about the ankle, and the side extensions are centered. The splint is then pressurized and straps adjusted until comfortable support and pressure are attained. **C,** As the ankle pain subsides, about the third to fifth day, balancing exercises can begin to allow the patient to regain ankle proprioception and avoid recurrent instability problems. (From Jardon OM, Mathews MS: Orthopedics. In Rakel RE [ed]: *Textbook of family practice,* ed 5, Philadelphia, 1995, WB Saunders.)

BASIC INFORMATION

■ DEFINITION

Ankylosing spondylitis is a chronic inflammatory condition involving the sacroiliac joints and axial skeleton characterized by ankylosis and enthesitis (inflammation at tendon insertions). It is one of a group of several overlapping syndromes, including spondylitis associated with Reiter's syndrome, psoriasis, and IBD. Patients are typically seronegative for the rheumatoid factor, and these disorders are now commonly called *rheumatoid variants* or *seronegative spondyloarthropathies*.

■ SYNONYMS

Marie-Strümpell disease

ICD-9CM CODES

720.0 Ankylosing spondylitis

■ EPIDEMIOLOGY & DEMOGRAPHICS

PREVALENCE: 0.15% of male population (rare in blacks)
PREDOMINANT AGE AT ONSET: 15 to 35 yr
PREDOMINANT SEX: Male:female ratio of 10:1

■ PHYSICAL FINDINGS & CLINICAL PRESENTATION

- Morning stiffness
- Fatigue, weight loss, anorexia, and other systemic complaints in more severe forms
- Bilateral sacroiliac tenderness (sacroiliitis)
- Limited lumbar spine motion (Fig. 1-23)
- Loss of chest expansion measured at the nipple line <2.5 cm, reflecting rib cage involvement

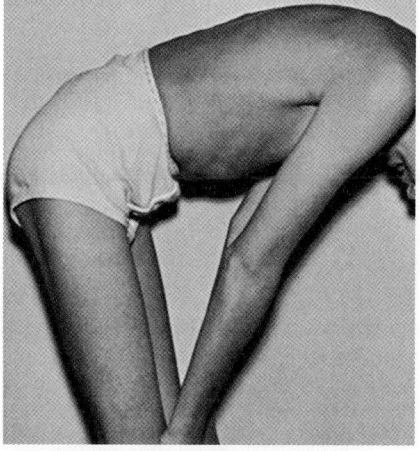

Fig. 1-23 Loss of lumbodorsal spine mobility in a boy with ankylosing spondylitis: the lower spine remains straight when the patient bends forward. (From Behrman RE: *Nelson textbook of pediatrics,* Philadelphia, 1996, WB Saunders.)

- Occasionally, peripheral joint involvement (large joints are more commonly affected)
- Possible extraskeletal manifestations affecting the cardiovascular system (aortic insufficiency, heart block, cardiomegaly), lungs (pulmonary fibrosis), and eye (uveitis)
- Tenderness at tendon insertion sites
- Radiation below the knee is rare

■ ETIOLOGY

Unknown. Genetic factors play an important role.

DIAGNOSIS

■ DIFFERENTIAL DIAGNOSIS

- Other spondyloarthropathies
- A clinical algorithm for the evaluation of back pain is described in Section III.

■ WORKUP

The modified New York criteria are often used for diagnosis:
- Low back pain of at least 3 mo duration improved by exercise and not relieved by rest
- Limitation of lumbar spine movement in sagittal and frontal planes
- Decreased chest expansion below normal values for age and sex
- Bilateral sacroiliitis of minimal grade or greater
- Unilateral sacroiliitis of moderate grade or greater

■ LABORATORY TESTS

- Elevated sedimentation rate, CRP
- Absence of rheumatoid factor and ANA
- Possible mild hyperchromic anemia
- Presence of HLA/B27 antigen in >90% of patients (although this antigen is often present in the general population)

■ IMAGING STUDIES

- Early roentgenographic features are those of bilateral sacroiliitis on plain films.
- Vertebral bodies may become demineralized and a typical "squaring off" occurs.
- With progression, calcification of the annulus fibrosus and paravertebral ligaments develop, giving rise to the so-called bamboo spine appearance.
- End result may be a forward protruding cervical spine and fixed dorsal kyphosis.

TREATMENT

■ NONPHARMACOLOGIC THERAPY

- Exercises primarily to maintain flexibility; general aerobic activity also important

- Postural training
  1. Patients must be instructed to sit in the erect position and to avoid stooping; otherwise, a flexion contracture of the spine may develop, which can become so severe that the patient cannot see forward.
  2. Sleeping should be in the supine position on a firm mattress; pillows should not be placed under the head or knees.

■ CHRONIC Rx

- NSAIDs: indomethacin is often successful in relieving symptoms; newer nonsteroidal agents may be tried as well.
- New research into the use of DMARDs such as tumor necrosis factor antagonists such as etanercept appears promising.

■ DISPOSITION

- Most patients have a normal life span.
- The usual course of the disease is not life-threatening, but death may occur as a result of aortic insufficiency or secondary amyloidosis with renal disease.

■ REFERRAL

- Orthopedic consultation for pain or deformity
- Ophthalmologic consultation for ocular complications
- Rheumatology consultation for uncontrolled symptoms

PEARLS & CONSIDERATIONS

■ COMMENTS

Years may pass between the onset of symptoms and the ultimate diagnosis because of the frequency of nonspecific low back pain from other disorders.

REFERENCES

Braun J, De Keyser F et al: New treatment options in spondyloarthropathies: increasing evidence for significant efficacy of anti-tumor necrosis therapy, *Curr Opin Rheumatol* 13:245, 2001.

Gorman JD et al: Treatment of ankylosing spondylitis by inhibition of tumor necrosis factor alpha, *N Engl J Med* 346:1349, 2002.

Olivieri I et al: Ankylosing spondylitis and undifferentiated spondyloarthropathies: a clinical review and description of a disease subset with older age at onset, *Curr Opin Rheumatol* 13:280, 2001.

Author: **Lonnie R. Mercier, M.D.**

BASIC INFORMATION

■ DEFINITION

A fistula is an inflammatory tract with a secondary (external) opening in the perianal skin and a primary (internal) opening in the anal canal at the dentate line. It originates in an abscess in the intersphincteric space of the anal canal. Fistulas can be classified as follows:

1. Intersphincteric: fistula track passes within the intersphincteric plane to the perianal skin; most common
2. Transsphincteric: fistula track passes from the internal opening, through the internal and external sphincter, and into the ischiorectal fossa to the perianal skin; frequent
3. Suprasphincteric: after passing through the internal sphincter, fistula tract passes above the puborectalis and then tracts downward, lateral to the external sphincter, into the ischiorectal space to the perianal skin; uncommon; if abscess cavity extends cephalad, a supralevator abscess possibly palpable on rectal examination
4. Extrasphincteric: fistula tract passes from the rectum, above the levators, through the levator muscles to the ischiorectal space and perianal skin; rare

With a horseshoe fistula, the tract passes from one ischiorectal fossa to the other behind the rectum.

■ SYNONYMS

Fistula-in-ano

ICD-9CM CODES

565.1 Anal fistula

■ EPIDEMIOLOGY & DEMOGRAPHICS

• Common in all ages
• Occurs equally in men and women
• Associated with constipation
• Pediatric age group: more common in infants; boys > girls

■ PHYSICAL FINDINGS & CLINICAL PRESENTATION

• Acute stage: perianal swelling, pain, and fever
• Chronic stage: history of rectal drainage or bleeding; previous abscess with drainage
• Tender external fistulous opening, with 2 to 3 cm of the anal verge, with purulent or serosanguineous drainage on compression; the greater the distance from the anal margin, the greater the probability of a complicated upward extension
• Goodsall's rule:
  1. Location of the internal opening related to the location of the external opening.
  2. With external opening anterior to an imaginary line drawn horizontally across the midpoint of the anus: fistulous tract runs radially into the anal canal.
  3. With opening posterior to the transanal line: tract is usually curvilinear, entering the anal canal in the posterior midline.
  4. Exception to this rule: an external, anterior opening that is >3 cm from the anus. In this case the tract may curve posteriorly and end in the posterior midline.
• If perianal abscess recurs, presence of a fistula is suggested

■ ETIOLOGY

• Most common: nonspecific cryptoglandular infection (skin or intestinal flora)
• Fistulas more common when intestinal microorganisms are cultured from the anorectal abscess
• Tuberculosis
• Lymphogranuloma venereum
• Actinomycosis
• Inflammatory bowel disease (IBD): Crohn's disease, ulcerative colitis
• Trauma: surgery (episiotomy, prostatectomy), foreign bodies, anal intercourse
• Malignancy: carcinoma, leukemia, lymphoma
• Treatment of malignancy: surgery, radiation

DIAGNOSIS

■ DIFFERENTIAL DIAGNOSIS

• Hidradenitis suppurativa
• Pilonidal sinus
• Bartholin's gland abscess or sinus
• Infected perianal sebaceous cysts

■ WORKUP

• Digital rectal examination:
  1. Assess sphincter tone and voluntary squeeze pressure
  2. Determine the presence of an extraluminal mass
  3. Identify an indurated track
  4. Palpate an internal opening or pit
• Gentle probing of external orifice to avoid creating a false tract; 50% do not have clinically detectable opening
• Anoscopy
• Proctosigmoidoscopy to exclude inflammatory or neoplastic disease
• All studies done under adequate anesthesia

■ LABORATORY TESTS

• CBC
• Rectal biopsy if diagnosis of IBD or malignancy suspected; biopsy of external orifice is useless

■ IMAGING STUDIES

• Colonoscopy or barium enema if:
  1. Diagnosis of IBD or malignancy is suspected
  2. History of recurrent or multiple fistulas
  3. Patient <25 yr old
• Small bowel series: occasionally obtained for reasons similar to above
• Fistulography: unreliable; but may be helpful in complicated fistulas

TREATMENT

■ NONPHARMACOLOGIC THERAPY

Sitz baths

■ ACUTE GENERAL Rx

• Treatment of choice: surgery
• Broad-spectrum antibiotic given if:
  1. Cellulitis present
  2. Patient is immunocompromised
  3. Valvular heart disease present
  4. Prosthetic devices present
• Stool softener/laxative

■ CHRONIC Rx

• Surgery
• Surgical goals are as follows:
  1. Cure the fistula
  2. Prevent recurrence
  3. Preserve sphincter function
  4. Minimize healing time
• Methods for the management of anal fistulas: fistulotomy, setons, rectal advancement flaps, colostomy

■ DISPOSITION

Outpatient surgery

■ REFERRAL

Refer to a surgeon with expertise in this area.

PEARLS & CONSIDERATIONS

■ COMMENTS

• HIV-positive and diabetic patients with perirectal abscesses/fistulas are true surgical emergencies.
• Risk of septicemia, Fournier's gangrene, and other septic complications make immediate drainage imperative.

REFERENCE

Pfenninger JL, Zainea GG: Common anorectal condition, *Am Fam Physician*, 64:22, 2001.
Author: **George T. Danakas, M.D.**

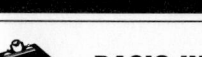

BASIC INFORMATION

■ DEFINITION

Anorexia nervosa is a psychiatric disorder characterized by abnormal eating behavior, severe self-induced weight loss, and a specific psychopathology (see "Workup").

ICD-9CM CODES

307.1 Anorexia nervosa

■ EPIDEMIOLOGY & DEMOGRAPHICS

INCIDENCE/PREVALENCE (IN U.S.):
- Anorexia nervosa occurs in 0.2% to 1.3% of the general population, with an annual incidence of 5 to 10 cases/100,000 persons.
- Participation in activities that promote thinness (athletics, modeling) are associated with a higher incidence of anorexia nervosa.

PREDOMINANT SEX: Female: male ratio is 9:1. Approximately 0.5% to 1% of women between the ages of 15 and 30 yr have anorexia nervosa.

PREDOMINANT AGE: Adolescence to young adulthood is the predominant age. Mean age of onset is 17 yr.

■ PHYSICAL FINDINGS & CLINICAL PRESENTATION

Primary care physicians must be skilled at recognizing this disorder because patients with mild cases usually present with nonspecific symptoms such as asthenia, lack of energy, or dizziness. The physical examination may be normal in the early stages or in mild cases. Patients with moderate to severe anorexia have the following physical characteristics:
- Patient is emaciated and bundled in clothing.
- Skin is dry and has excessive growth of lanugo. Skin may also be yellow-tinged from carotenodermia.
- Brittle nails, thinning scalp hair are present.
- Bradycardia, hypotension, hypothermia, and bradypnea are common.
- Female fat distribution pattern is no longer evident.
- Axillary and pubic hair is preserved.
- Peripheral edema may be present.

■ ETIOLOGY

- Etiology is unknown, but probably multifactorial (sociocultural, psychologic, familial, and genetic factors).
- A history of sexual abuse has been reported in as many as 50% of patients with anorexia nervosa.
- Psychologic factors: anorexics often have an incompletely developed personal identity. They struggle to maintain a sense of control over their environment, they usually have a low self-esteem, and they lack the sense that they are valued and loved for themselves.

DIAGNOSIS

■ DIFFERENTIAL DIAGNOSIS

- Depression with loss of appetite
- Schizophrenia
- Conversion disorder
- Occult carcinoma, lymphoma
- Endocrine disorders: Addison's disease, diabetes mellitus, hypothyroidism or hyperthyroidism, panhypopituitarism
- GI disorders: celiac disease, Crohn's disease, intestinal parasitosis
- Infectious disorders: AIDS, TB
- A clinical algorithm for the evaluation of anorexia is described in Section III, Fig. 3-18

■ WORKUP

- A diagnosis can be made using the following DSM-IV diagnostic criteria for anorexia nervosa:
  1. Refusal to maintain body weight (BW) at or above a minimally normal weight for age and height (e.g., weight loss leading to maintenance of BW <85% of that expected or failure to make expected weight gain during a period of growth, leading to BW <85% of that expected)
  2. Intense fear of gaining weight or becoming fat, even though underweight
  3. Disturbance in the way in which BW or shape is experienced, undue influence of BW or shape on self-evaluation, or denial of the seriousness of the current low BW
  4. In postmenarchal females, amenorrhea, that is, the absence of at least three consecutive menstrual cycles (A woman is considered to have amenorrhea if her periods occur only following hormone, [e.g., estrogen] administration.)

Specify type:
  Restricting type: During the current episode of anorexia nervosa, the person has not regularly engaged in binge-eating or purging behavior (i.e., self-induced vomiting or the misuse of laxatives, diuretics, or enemas).
  Binge-eating/purging type: During the current episode of anorexia nervosa, the person has regularly engaged in binge-eating or purging behavior (i.e., self-induced vomiting or the misuse of laxatives, diuretics, or enemas).
- The SCOFF questionnaire is a useful screening tool used in England for eating disorders. It consists of the following five questions:
  1. Do you make yourself Sick because you feel full?
  2. Have you lost Control over how much you eat?
  3. Have you lost more than One stone (about 6 kg) recently?
  4. Do you believe yourself to be Fat when others say you are thin?
  5. Does Food dominate your life?
- A positive response to two or more questions has a reported sensitivity of 100% for anorexia and bulimia, and an overall specificity of 87.5%.
- Baseline ECG should be performed on all patients with anorexia nervosa. Routine monitoring of patients with prolonged QT interval is necessary; sudden death in these patients is often caused by ventricular arrhythmias related to QT interval prolongation.

■ LABORATORY TESTS

- Endocrine abnormalities:
  1. Decreased FSH, LH, T_4, T_3, estrogens, urinary 17-OH steroids, estrone, and estradiol
  2. Normal free T_4, TSH
  3. Increased cortisol, GH, rT_3, T_3RU
  4. Absence of cyclic surge of LH
- Leukopenia, thrombocytopenia, anemia, reduced ESR, reduced complement levels, and reduced CD4 and CD8 cells may be present.
- Metabolic alkalosis, hypocalcemia, hypokalemia, hypomagnesemia, hypercholesterolemia, and hypophosphatemia may be present.
- Increased plasma β-carotene levels are useful to distinguish these patients from others on starvation diets.

TREATMENT

■ NONPHARMACOLOGIC THERAPY

- A multidisciplinary approach with psychologic, medical, and nutritional support is necessary.
- A goal weight should be set and the patient should be initially monitored at least once a week in the office setting (Box 1-3). The target weight is 100% of ideal BW for teenagers and 90% to 100% for older patients.
- Weight gain should be gradual (1 to 3 lb/wk) to prevent gastric dilation.
- Electrolyte levels should be strictly monitored.
- Mealtime should be a time for social interaction, not confrontation.
- Postprandially, sedentary activities are recommended. The patient's access to a bathroom should be monitored to prevent purging.

■ ACUTE GENERAL Rx

- Criteria to decide on the appropriate initial course of treatment for patients with anorexia nervosa are usually based on the presence of complications, percentage of ideal body weight, and severity of body image distortion.
- Outpatient treatment is adequate for most patients.
- Indications for hospitalization are described in the "Referral" section.
- Medically stable patients who are within 85% of ideal body weight can be followed up by the primary care physician at 3- or 4-wk intervals, which can be lengthened as the patient improves.

- Pharmacologic treatment generally has no role in anorexia nervosa unless major depression or another psychiatric disorder is present. SSRIs can be used to alleviate the depressed mood and moderate obsessive-compulsive behavior in some individuals.

■ CHRONIC Rx

- Psychotherapy continued for years and focused specifically on self-image, family and peer interactions, and relapse prevention is an integral part of a successful recovery.
- Family therapy is also recommended, especially in younger patients.

■ DISPOSITION

- The long-term prognosis is generally poor and marked by recurrent exacerbations. The percentage of patients with anorexia nervosa who fully recover is modest. Most patients continue to suffer from a distorted body image, disordered eating habits, and psychic difficulties.
- Most patients with anorexia nervosa will recover menses within 6 months of reaching 90% of their ideal body weight. It is important to note that patients with anorexia nervosa can become pregnant despite amenorrhea.
- Mortality rates vary from 5% to 20%. Frequent causes of death are electrolyte abnormalities, starvation, or suicide.
- A prolonged QT interval is a marker for risk of sudden death.

■ REFERRAL

Hospitalization should be considered in the following situations:
1. Severe dehydration or electrolyte imbalance
2. ECG abnormalities (prolonged QT interval, arrhythmias)
3. Significant physiologic instability (hypotension, orthostatic changes)
4. Intractable vomiting, purging, or bingeing
5. Patient having suicidal thoughts
6. Weight loss exceeds 30% of ideal BW and is unresponsive to outpatient treatment
7. Rapidly progressing weight loss (>2 lbs in a week)
8. Failure to progress in nutritional rehabilitation in outpatient treatment

REFERENCES

American Psychiatric Association: Practice guideline for the treatment of patients with eating disorders, *Am J Psychiatry* 157(suppl):4, 2000 (revision).

Becker AE et al: Eating disorders, *N Engl J Med* 340:1092, 1999.

Mehler PS: Diagnosis and care of patients with anorexia nervosa in primary care setting, *Ann Intern Med* 134:1048, 2001.

Morgan JF et al: The SCOFF questionnaire: assessment of a new screening tool for eating disorders, *BMJ* 319:1467, 1999.

Author: **Fred F. Ferri, M.D.**

BOX 1-3   Example of Refeeding Protocol

1. Contract with patient for a weight goal. Goal should not exceed 1 to 2 pounds in the first week and 3 to 5 pounds afterward.
2. Begin 800 to 1200 kcal in frequent small meals (to avoid bloating sensation).
3. Increase calories to 1500 to 3000 depending on height and age (consult with nutrition service).
4. Add, as necessary, vitamin and mineral supplements.
5. In severe cases, total parenteral nutrition must be used (starting at 800 to 1200 kcal/day).

From Goldberg RJ (ed): *Practical guide to the care of the psychiatric patient*, ed 2, St Louis, 1998, Mosby.

BASIC INFORMATION

DEFINITION

Anthrax is an acute infectious disease caused by the spore-forming bacterium *Bacillus anthracis*.

ICD-9CM CODES
0.22.0 Cutaneous anthrax
0.22.1 Inhalation anthrax
0.22.2 Gastrointestinal anthrax
022.3 Sepsis from anthrax

EPIDEMIOLOGY & DEMOGRAPHICS

- Anthrax most commonly occurs in hoofed animals and can only incidentally infect humans who come in contact with infected animals or animal products. Between 20,000 and 100,000 cases of cutaneous anthrax occur worldwide annually. In the U.S. the annual incidence was about 130 cases before 2001.
- Until the recent bioterrorism attack in 2001, most cases of anthrax occurred in industrial environments (contaminated raw materials used in manufacturing process) or in agriculture.
- In 2001 there were more than 20 confirmed cases of anthrax resulting from bioterrorism, most of which were associated with handling of contaminated mail. Inhalation anthrax is the most lethal form of anthrax and results from inspiration of 8000-50,000 spores of *Bacillus anthracis*. Before 2001 there had not been a case of inhalation anthrax in the U.S. for 20 years.
- Direct person-to-person spread of anthrax is extremely unlikely, if it occurs at all; therefore, there is no need to immunize or treat contacts of persons ill with anthrax, such as household contacts, friends, or co-workers, unless they also were exposed to the same source of infection.

PHYSICAL FINDINGS & CLINICAL PRESENTATION

Symptoms of disease vary depending on how the disease was contracted, but usually occur within 7 days after exposure. The serious forms of human anthrax are inhalation anthrax, cutaneous anthrax, and intestinal anthrax.

- **Inhalation anthrax** begins with a brief prodrome resembling a viral respiratory illness followed by development of hypoxia and dyspnea, with radiographic evidence of mediastinal widening. Host factors, dose of exposure, and chemoprophylaxis may affect the duration of the incubation period. Initial symptoms include mild fever, muscle aches, and malaise and may progress to respiratory failure and shock; meningitis often develops.
- **Cutaneous anthrax** is characterized by a skin lesion evolving from a papule, through a vesicular stage, to a depressed black eschar. The incubation period ranges from 1-12 days. The lesion is usually painless, but patients also may have fever, malaise, headache, and regional lymphadenopathy. The eschar dries and falls off in 1-2 wk with little scarring.
- **Gastrointestinal anthrax** is characterized by severe abdominal pain followed by fever and signs of septicemia. Bloody diarrhea and signs of acute abdomen may occur. This form of anthrax usually follows after eating raw or undercooked contaminated meat and can have an incubation period of 1-7 days. Gastric ulcers may occur and may be associated with hematemesis. An oropharyngeal and an abdominal form of the disease have been described. Involvement of the pharynx is usually characterized by lesions at the base of the tongue, dysphagia, fever, and regional lymphadenopathy. Lower bowel inflammation typically causes nausea, loss of appetite, and fever followed by abdominal pain, hematemesis, and bloody diarrhea.

ETIOLOGY

The disease is caused by *Bacillus anthracis*, a gram-positive, spore-forming bacillus. It is aerobic, nonmotile, nonhemolytic on sheep's blood agar, and grows readily at temperature of 37° C, forming large colonies with irregularly tapered outgrowths (a Medusa's head appearance). In the host it appears as single organisms or chains of two or three bacilli.

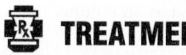 **DIAGNOSIS**

DIFFERENTIAL DIAGNOSIS

- Inhalation anthrax must be distinguished from influenza-like illness (ILI) and tularemia. Most cases of ILI are associated with nasal congestion and rhinorrhea, which are unusual in inhalation anthrax. Additional distinguishing factors are the usual absence of abnormal chest x-ray in ILI (see below).
- Cutaneous anthrax should be distinguished from staphylococcal disease, ecthyma, ecthyma gangrenosum, plague, brown recluse spider bite, and tularemia.
- The differential diagnosis of gastrointestinal anthrax includes viral gastroenteritis, shigellosis, and yersiniosis.

LABORATORY TESTS

- Presumptive identification is based on Gram stain of material from skin lesion, CSF, or blood showing encapsulated gram-positive bacilli.
- Confirmatory tests are performed at specialized labs. Virulent strains grow on nutrient agar in the presence of 5% CO_2. Susceptibility to lysis by gamma phage or DFA staining of cell-wall polysaccharide antigen are also useful confirmatory tests.
- Nasal swab culture to determine inhalation exposure is of limited diagnostic value. A negative result does not exclude the possibility of exposure. It may be used by public health officials to assist in epidemiologic investigations of exposed persons to evaluate the dispersion of spores.
- Serologic testing by enzyme-linked immunosorbent assay (ELISA) can confirm the diagnosis.
- A skin test (Anthracin Test) that detects anthrax cell-mediated immunity is also available in specialized labs.

IMAGING STUDIES

Chest x-ray usually reveals mediastinal widening. Additional findings include infiltrates and pleural effusion.

TREATMENT

NONPHARMACOLOGIC THERAPY

IV hydration and ventilator support may be necessary in inhalation anthrax

ACUTE GENERAL THERAPY

- Most naturally occurring *B. anthracis* strains are sensitive to penicillin. The FDA has approved penicillin, doxycycline, and ciprofloxacin for the treatment of inhalational anthrax infection.
- Table 1-9 describes a treatment protocol for inhalation anthrax.
- Initial postexposure prophylaxis therapy in adults is with ciprofloxacin, 500 mg PO bid or doxycycline 100 mg bid. The total duration of treatment is 60 days.

CHRONIC Rx

None

DISPOSITION

- Case fatality estimates for inhalation anthrax are extremely high (>90%).
- The case fatality rate for cutaneous anthrax is 20% without and <1% with antibiotic treatment.
- The case fatality rate for gastrointestinal anthrax is estimated to be 25% to 60%.

REFERRAL

Consultation with an infectious disease specialist is recommended in all cases of anthrax. Local state authorities should also be notified of suspected cases of anthrax.

☼ PEARLS & CONSIDERATIONS

COMMENTS

- Postexposure prophylaxis: If the exposure to *B. anthracis* is confirmed and anthrax vaccine is available, 3 doses of the vaccine should be given at 0, 2, and 4 wk, and antibiotics should be continued throughout the 4-wk period. If vaccine is not available, antibiotics should be continued for 60 days.
- Preexposure vaccination is limited to groups at risk for repeated exposures to *B. anthracis* spores, such as bioterrorism level-B laboratories and workers who will be making repeated entries into known *B. anthracis* spore-contaminated areas.

- The U.S. anthrax vaccine is an inactivated cellfree product licensed to be given in a 6-dose series.

REFERENCES

Inglesby TV et al: Anthrax as a biological weapon, 2002, *JAMA* 287:2236, 2002.

Hupert N et al: Accuracy of screening for inhalational anthrax after a bioterrorist attack, *Ann Intern Med* 139:337, 2003.

Interim guidelines for investigation of and response to *Bacillus anthracis* exposures, *MMWR* 50:987, 2001.

Post-exposure anthrax prophylaxis, *Med Lett Drugs Ther* 43:91, 2001.

Swartz MN: Recognition and management of anthrax: an update, *N Engl J Med* 345:1621, 2001.

Use of anthrax vaccine for pre-exposure vaccination, *MMWR Morb Mortal Wkly Rep* 51:1024, 2002.

Author: **Fred F. Ferri, M.D.**

TABLE 1-9 Inhalational Anthrax Treatment Protocol[a,b]

CATEGORY	INITIAL THERAPY (INTRAVENOUS)[c,d]	DURATION
Adults	Ciprofloxacin 400 mg every 12 hr[a] **or** Doxycycline 100 mg every 12 hr[f] **and** One or two additional antimicrobials[d]	IV treatment initially.[e] Switch to oral antimicrobial therapy when clinically appropriate: Ciprofloxacin 500 mg PO bid **or** Doxycycline 100 mg PO bid Continue for 60 days (IV and PO combined)[g]
Children	Ciprofloxacin 10-15 mg/kg every 12 hr[h,i] **or** Doxycycline[f,j]: >8 yr and >45 kg: 100 mg every 12 hr >8 yr and ≤45 kg: 2.2 mg/kg every 12 hr ≤8 yr: 2.2 mg/kg every 12 hr **and** One or two additional antimicrobials[d]	IV treatment initially.[e] Switch to oral antimicrobial therapy when clinically appropriate: Ciprofloxacin 10-15 mg/kg PO every 12 hr[i] **or** Doxycycline[j]: >8 yr and >45 kg: 100 mg PO bid >8 yr and ≤45 kg: 2.2 mg/kg PO bid ≤8 yr: 2.2 mg/kg PO bid Continue for 60 days (IV and PO combined)[g]
Pregnant women[k]	Same for nonpregnant adults (the high death rate from the infection outweighs the risk posed by the antimicrobial agent)	IV treatment initially. Switch to oral antimicrobial therapy when clinically appropriate.[b] Oral therapy regimens same for nonpregnant adults
Immunocompromised persons	Same for nonimmunocompromised persons and children	Same for nonimmunocompromised persons and children

MMRW 5:987, 2001.

[a]For gastrointestinal and oropharyngeal anthrax, use regimens recommended for inhalational anthrax.

[b]Ciprofloxacin or doxycycline should be considered an essential part of first-line therapy for inhalational anthrax.

[c]Steroids may be considered as an adjunct therapy for patients with severe edema and for meningitis based on experience with bacterial meningitis of other etiologies.

[d]Other agents with in vitro activity include rifampin, vancomycin, penicillin, ampicillin, chloramphenicol, imipenem, clindamycin, and clarithromycin. Because of concerns of constitutive and inducible beta-lactamases in *Bacillus anthracis,* penicillin and ampicillin should not be used alone. Consultation with an infectious disease specialist is advised.

[e]Initial therapy may be altered based on clinical course of the patient; one or two antimicrobial agents (e.g., ciprofloxacin or doxycycline) may be adequate as the patient improves.

[f]If meningitis is suspected, doxycycline may be less optimal because of poor central nervous system penetration.

[g]Because of the potential persistence of spores after an aerosol exposure, antimicrobial therapy should be continued for 60 days.

[h]If intravenous ciprofloxacin is not available, oral ciprofloxacin may be acceptable because it is rapidly and well absorbed from the gastrointestinal tract with no substantial loss by first-pass metabolism. Maximum serum concentrations are attained 1-2 hours after oral dosing but may not be achieved if vomiting or ileus are present.

[i]In children, ciprofloxacin dosage should not exceed 1 g/day.

[j]The American Academy of Pediatrics recommends treatment of young children with tetracyclines for serious infections (e.g., Rocky Mountain spotted fever).

[k]Although tetracyclines are not recommended during pregnancy, their use may be indicated for life-threatening illness. Adverse effects on developing teeth and bones are dose related; therefore, doxycycline might be used for a short time (7-14 days) before 6 months of gestation.

BASIC INFORMATION

■ DEFINITION

The antiphospholipid antibody syndrome (APS) is characterized by arterial or venous thrombosis and/or pregnancy loss and the presence of antiphospholipid antibodies (aPL). APL are antibodies directed against either phospholipids or proteins bound to anionic phospholipids. Four types of aPL have been characterized:

- False-positive serologic tests for syphilis
- Lupus anticoagulants
- Anticardiolipin antibodies
- Anti-β2 glycoprotein-1 antibodies

The syndrome is referred to as primary APS when it occurs alone and as secondary APS when in association with SLE, other rheumatic disorders, or certain infections or medications (Fig. 1-24). APS can affect all organ systems and includes venous and arterial thrombosis, recurrent fetal losses, and thrombocytopenia.

ICD-9CM CODES
795.79 Antiphospholipid antibody syndrome

■ EPIDEMIOLOGY & DEMOGRAPHICS

- 1% to 5% of healthy subjects have anticardiolipin and lupus anticoagulant antibodies.
- 12% to 30% of patients with systemic lupus erythematosus have anticardiolipin antibodies and 15% to 34% have lupus anticoagulant antibodies.
- Some APS-positive families exist, and HLA studies have suggested associations with HLA DR7, DR4, and Dqw7 plus Drw53.
- Other risk factors: underlying SLE and collagen-vascular diseases; other autoimmune disorders including rheumatoid arthritis, Sjögren's syndrome, Behçet's syndrome, and ITP; drug-induced; and AIDS.
- Most individuals are otherwise healthy and have no underlying medical condition.

- Several studies assessing presence of aPL in patients with cardiovascular and cerebrovascular disease have found a higher than expected prevalence of antibody.

■ PHYSICAL FINDINGS & CLINICAL PRESENTATION (BOX 1-4)

Associated conditions and effects on various systems of APS include:

- **Thrombosis:** patients with APS are at risk for both venous and arterial thromboses, although venous thromboses are more common, occurring as the initial manifestation of APS in approximately 30% of APS patients. Of all patients with venous thrombosis, 5% to 20% have APA. The most common site for deep vein thrombosis is the calf, but thromboses may also occur in the renal, hepatic, axillary, subclavian, vena cava, and retinal veins. The most common site of arterial thrombosis is the cerebral vessels. Other common sites are the coronary, renal, mesenteric arteries, and arterial bypass. Recurrent thrombosis is common with APS

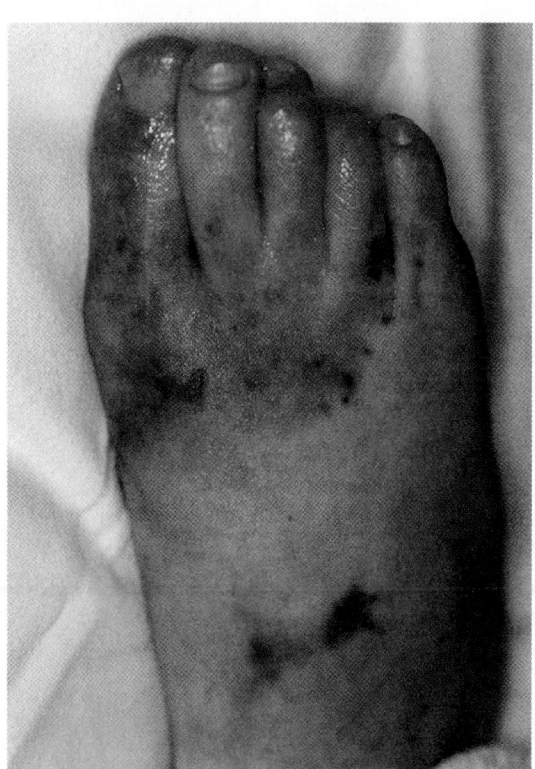

Fig. 1-24 A 12-year-old girl with systemic lupus erythematosus and antiphospholipid antibodies with painful cutaneous vasculitis of the right foot. Arterial thrombosis documented by angiography resulted in cyanosis of the large toe. Symptoms resolved with treatment with heparin and corticosteroids. (From Behrman RE [ed]: *Nelson textbook of pediatrics,* ed 16, Philadelphia, 2000, WB Saunders.)

> ### BOX 1-4 Clinical Manifestations of the Antiphospholipid Antibody Syndrome
>
> **Common**
>
> > Venous thrombosis
> > Arterial thrombosis
> > > Stroke
> > > Extremity gangrene
> > > Visceral infarction
> > Recurrent fetal loss
> > Thrombocytopenia
> > Livedo reticularis
>
> **Uncommon**
>
> > Coombs'-positive hemolysis
> > Valvular heart disease
> > Chorea
> > Nonstroke ischemia syndrome
> > Transverse myelopathy

From Andreoli TE (ed): *Cecil essentials of medicine,* ed 4, Philadelphia, 1997, WB Saunders.

- **Central Nervous System:** stroke, TIA, migraine, multiinfarct dementia, epilepsy, movement disorders, transverse myelopathy, depression, and Guillain-Barré syndrome
- **Pulmonary:** pulmonary embolism and infarction, pulmonary HTN, ARDS, intraalveolar pulmonary hemorrhage, a postpartum syndrome characterized by fever, pleuritic chest pain, dyspnea, and patchy infiltrates with pleural effusion on CXR
- **Cardiology:** Libman-Sacks endocarditis, intracardiac thrombosis, CAD, MI
- **Gastrointestinal:** abd pain, GI bleed secondary to ischemia, splenic or pancreatic infarction, hepatic vein thrombosis, Budd-Chiari syndrome (second most common cause of BCS)
- **Renal:** proteinuria, acute renal failure, HTN, renal infarct, renal artery or vein thrombosis, postpartum hemolytic-uremic syndrome
- **Hematology:** thrombocytopenia, hemolytic anemia
- **Endocrine:** Addison's disease secondary to adrenal hemorrhage and less frequently thrombosis
- **Cutaneous:** livedo reticularis, cutaneous necrosis, skin ulcerations, gangrene of digits
- **Obstetrics:** recurrent spontaneous abortion (secondary to placental vessel thrombosis and ischemia)
- **Catastrophic APS:** widespread thrombotic disease with visceral damage

■ ETIOLOGY
- APL react with negatively charged phospholipids
- Range of possible mechanisms of thrombosis includes effects of aPL on platelet membranes, endothelial cells, and clotting components such as prothrombin, protein C or S
- Recently shown that prephospholipids are not immunogenic and that a binding protein (β_2-glycoprotein I) may be the key immunogen in the APS

DIAGNOSIS

Diagnostic criteria of APS include at least one of the following clinical criteria and at least one of the following laboratory criteria:
- *Clinical:*
  - venous, arterial, or small vessel thrombosis OR
  - morbidity with pregnancy (fetal death at >10 wks gestation OR premature births before 34 wks gestation secondary to eclampsia, preeclampsia, or severe placental insufficiency OR three or more unexplained consecutive spontaneous abortions at <10 wks gestation)
- *Laboratory:*
  - IgG and/or IgM anticardiolipin antibody in medium or high titers OR
  - lupus anticoagulant activity found on two or more occasions, at least 6 wk apart

■ DIFFERENTIAL DIAGNOSIS
- Other hypercoagulable states (inherited or acquired)
- Inherited: ATIII, protein C, S deficiencies, Factor V Leiden, prothrombin gene mutation
- Acquired: heparin-induced thrombopathy, myeloproliferative syndromes, cancer, hyperviscosity
- Homocystinemia
- Nephrotic syndrome

■ WORKUP
History of thrombosis and/or pregnancy loss and laboratory testing

■ LABORATORY TESTS
Laboratory testing indicated in:
- Patient with underlying SLE or collagen-vascular disease with thrombosis
- Patient with recurrent, familial, or juvenile DVT or thrombosis in an unusual location (mesenteric or cerebral)
- Possibly in patients with lupus or lupuslike disorders in high-risk situations (e.g., surgery, prolonged immobilization, pregnancy)
Abnormal tests include:
- False-positive test for syphilis (RPR/VDRL), "false-positive"
- Lupus anticoagulant activity, demonstrated by prolongation of apTT that does not correct with 1:1 mixing study
- Presence of anticardiolipin antibodies (ELISA for anticardiolipin is most sensitive and specific test [>80%])
- Presence of anti β_2-glycoprotein I antibody

■ PROGNOSIS
Limited data on natural history in untreated patients. APS patients are at risk for recurrent thrombosis. Initial arterial thrombosis tends to be followed by arterial events and initial venous thrombosis tends to be followed by venous events. Catastrophic APS is associated with a high mortality rate, approaching 50%. Incidence of developing catastrophic APS is approximately 0.8% among APS patients.

℞ TREATMENT

■ ACUTE GENERAL Rx

- Treatment of APS: Positive aPL and major thrombotic events or recurrent thrombotic events:
  - Initial anticoagulation with heparin, then lifelong warfarin treatment, INR 3-4
    - One prospective analysis (Vianna et al, 1994) comparing intermediate-to-high intensity warfarin therapy (INR>3.0) to low-intensity warfarin (INR<3.0) to aspirin demonstrated that:
      - Aspirin alone appears to be of no benefit for the thrombotic manifestations of APS.
      - Low-intensity warfarin (INR<3.0), with or without low-dose aspirin, reduced the rate of thrombosis from 30%/yr to 23%/yr.
      - High-intensity warfarin (INR>3.0) reduced the risk of thrombosis from 30%/yr to 1.3%/yr.
    - A recent randomized, double blind trial (Crowther et al., 2003) of 114 APS patients who were randomized to receive warfarin therapy to achieve an INR 2.0-3.0 vs. to achieve an INR of 3.0-4.0 demonstrated
      - No difference in thrombosis rate or bleeding events and therefore moderate-intensity warfarin may be appropriate for patients with APS
- Prophylaxis for (+) aPL: Asymptomatic patients with abnormal laboratory results, no previous thrombosis:
- Questionable whether ASA (81 mg) is effective
  - No routine prophylaxis

- Antithrombotic prophylaxis for major surgery, prolonged immobilization, and pregnancy
- Avoid oral contraceptive pills in women with (+) aPL

Pregnant women:
- With positive aPL antibodies, no history of nonplacental thrombotic event (e.g., DVT) or positive aPL antibodies and history of <3 spontaneous abortions:
  - ASA, 81 mg at conception and SQ heparin 10,000 IU q12h at time of documented viable intrauterine pregnancy (approximately 7 wk gestation).
  - A mid-interval PTT should be checked and should be normal or similar to baseline before therapy.
- Who carry a diagnosis of APS and who should already be chronically anticoagulated:
  - Warfarin should be discontinued secondary to its teratogenic effects
- ASA, 81 mg and heparin SQ to PTT of 1.5 to 2 × control value
  - IVIG and prednisone have also been used with success if aspirin and heparin fail.

■ CHRONIC Rx

Cerebral features of lupus may be more related to thrombosis than inflammation, may respond better to anticoagulants than immunosuppression.

REFERENCES

Asherson RA et al: Catastrophic antiphospholipid syndrome: clues to the pathogenesis from a series of 80 patients, *Medicine* (Baltimore) 80:355, 2001.

Bick RL: Syndromes of thrombosis and hypercoagulability: congenital and acquired causes of thrombosis, *Med Clin North Am* 82(3):409, 1998.

Crowther MA et al: A comparison of two intensities of warfarin for the prevention of recurrent thrombosis in patients with the antiphospholipid antibody syndrome, *N Engl J Med* 359(12):1133, 2003.

Espiritu JD et al: Fatal tumor thrombosis due to inferior vena cava leiomyosarcoma in a patient with antiphospholipid antibody syndrome, *Mayo Clin Proc* 77:595, 2002.

Levine JS et al: The antiphospholipid syndrome, *N Engl J Med* 346:752, 2002.

Petri M: Pathogenesis and treatment of the antiphospholipid antibody syndrome, *Med Clin North Am* 81:151, 1997.

Rosove MH et al: Antiphospholipid thrombosis: clinical course after the first thrombotic event in 70 patients, *Ann Intern Med* 117(4):303, 1992.

Ruiz-Irastorza G et al: Bleeding and recurrent thrombosis in definite antiphospholipid syndrome, *Arch Intern Med* 162:1164, 2002.

Vianna JL et al: Comparison of the primary and secondary antiphospholipid syndrome: a European multicenter study of 114 patients, *Am J Med* 96(1):3, 1994.

Wilson WA et al: International consensus statement on preliminary classification criteria for definite antiphospholipid syndrome: report of an international workshop, *Arthritis Rheum* 42:1309, 1999.

Authors: **Iris Tong, M.D., and Rebecca S. Brienza, M.D., M.P.H.**

BASIC INFORMATION

■ DEFINITION

Anxiety may present as a symptom in a wide range of psychiatric and medical conditions. Generalized anxiety disorder (GAD) is a condition in which the individual experiences excessive anxiety, fear, and worry for most of the time, continuously for at least 6 mo. The subjective anxiety must be accompanied by at least three somatic symptoms (e.g., restlessness, irritability, sleep disturbance, muscle tension, difficulty concentrating, or fatigability).

■ SYNONYMS

Anxiety neurosis
Chronic anxiety
GAD

ICD-9CM CODES

F41.1 (DSM-IV Code 300.02)

■ EPIDEMIOLOGY & DEMOGRAPHICS

INCIDENCE (IN U.S.): 31% in 1 yr
PREVALENCE (IN U.S.):
- In general population: 4.1% to 6.6% lifetime
- In primary care setting: 2.9% (It is the most common anxiety disorder in this setting.)

PREDOMINANT SEX: Females are more frequently affected (2:1 ratio), but they present for treatment less frequently (3:2 female:male).
PREDOMINANT AGE:
- 30% of patients report onset of symptoms before age 11 yr.
- 50% of patients have onset before age 18 yr.

PEAK INCIDENCE: Chronic condition with onset in early life
GENETICS: Concordance rates in dizygotic twins and monozygotic twins are not different (0% to 5%), but detailed analysis of 1033 female twin pairs finds that heredity contributes about 30% of the factors that may cause GAD.

■ PHYSICAL FINDINGS & CLINICAL PRESENTATION

- Report of being "anxious" all of their lives
- Excessive worry, usually regarding family, finances, work, or health
- Sleep disturbance, particularly early insomnia
- Muscle tension (typically in the muscles of neck and shoulders)
- Headaches (muscle tension)
- Difficulty concentrating
- Day form of fatigue
- Gastrointestinal symptoms compatible with IBD (one third of patients)

- Physical consequences of anxiety are the driving force for patients seeking medical attention
- Comorbid psychiatric illness (e.g., dysthymia or major depression) and substance abuse (e.g., alcohol abuse) are frequent

■ ETIOLOGY

- There is no clear etiology.
- Several hypotheses centering on neurotransmitter (catecholamines, indolamines) and developmental psychology are used as framework for treatment recommendations.

DIAGNOSIS

■ DIFFERENTIAL DIAGNOSIS

- Wide range of psychiatric and medical conditions; however, for a diagnosis of GAD to be made a person must experience anxiety with coexisting physical symptoms the majority of the time continuously for at least 6 mo
- Cardiovascular and pulmonary disease
- Hyperthyroidism
- Parkinson's disease
- Myasthenia gravis
- Consequence of recreational drug use (e.g., cocaine, amphetamine, and PCP) or withdrawal (e.g., alcohol or benzodiazepines)

■ WORKUP

- History: required for diagnosis
- Physical examination: confirm the patient's physical complaints
- Exclusion of organic basis for the complaints possibly requiring additional workup

TREATMENT

■ NONPHARMACOLOGIC THERAPY

- Cognitive-behavioral therapy
- Relaxation training
- Biofeedback
- Psychodynamic psychotherapy
NOTE: Studies directly comparing medications with psychotherapy are not available, but the general clinical impression is that the psychotherapies are probably superior to pharmacotherapies.

■ ACUTE GENERAL Rx

- Acute treatment is rarely indicated because GAD is a chronic condition.
- Occasionally, patients are in acute distress, requiring physician to respond quickly; benzodiazepines are given under these conditions as drug of choice for both daytime anxiety and initial insomnia.

■ CHRONIC Rx

- Benzodiazepines provide long-term symptom control with only occasional problems with tolerance or abuse; however, rate of relapse after discontinuation of benzodiazepines may be twice the rate after discontinuation of the available nonbenzodiazepine anxiolytic buspirone.
- SSRIs and venlafaxine are also effective in generalized anxiety disorders.
- Buspirone is effective without any potential for tolerance or abuse.
- Tricyclic antidepressants are useful if an element of comorbid depression exists.
- Sedating antidepressants are also useful in ameliorating initial insomnia.
- Trazodone and nefazodone possibly have unique benefits for these patients.

■ DISPOSITION

- This condition is chronic with periodic exacerbations.
- Treatment is given to provide a significant degree of improvement, but symptoms and dysfunction may persist.
- The risk for suicide is higher than general population.

■ REFERRAL

- If the symptoms are refractory to treatment
- If the case is complicated with a comorbid psychiatric condition
- If treatment response is suboptimal with residual dysfunction

REFERENCES

Gorman JM: Treatment of generalized anxiety disorder, *J Clin Psychiatry* 63(suppl 8):17, 2002.
Katz IR et al: Venlafaxine ER as a treatment for generalized anxiety disorder in older adults: pooled analysis of five randomized placebo-controlled clinical trials, *J Am Geriatr Soc* 50:18, 2002.
Khan A et al: Suicide risk in patients with anxiety disorder: a meta-analysis of the FDA database, *J Affect Disord* 68:183, 2002.
Varia I, Rauscher F: Treatment of generalized anxiety disorder with citalopram, *Int Clin Psychopharmacol* 17:103, 2002.
Author: **Rif S. El-Mallakh, M.D.**

BASIC INFORMATION

■ DEFINITION
Aortic dissection occurs when an intimal tear allows blood to dissect between medial layers of the aorta.

■ ICD-9CM CODES
441.00 Aortic dissection
444.01 Aortic dissection, thoracic

■ SYNONYMS
Dissecting aortic aneurysm, unspecified site

■ EPIDEMIOLOGY & DEMOGRAPHICS
PREDOMINANT SEX: Males > females
PEAK INCIDENCE: Ages 60 to 80
RISK FACTORS: Hypertension, atherosclerosis, and family history of aortic aneurysms. Others include inflammatory diseases that cause a vasculitis, disorders of collagen (Marfan syndrome, Ehlers-Danlos syndrome), bicuspid aortic valve, aortic coarctation, Turner's syndrome, crack cocaine, and trauma.

■ CLASSIFICATION
Based on the fact that the majority of aortic dissections originate in the ascending or descending aorta, three major classification systems (Fig. 1-25):
- DeBakey type I ascending and descending aorta
- DeBakey type II ascending aorta
- DeBakey type III descending aorta
- Stanford type A ascending aorta (proximal)
- Stanford type B descending aorta (distal)

■ PHYSICAL FINDINGS & CLINICAL PRESENTATION
- Sudden onset of very severe chest pain, at its peak at onset
- Little radiation to neck, shoulder, or arm
- Sharp, tearing or ripping pain
- Ascending aortic dissection with anterior chest pain
- Descending aortic dissection with back pain
- Most with severe hypertension, 25% with hypotension (SBP <100), which can indicate bleeding, cardiac tamponade, or severe aortic regurgitation
- Pulse and blood pressure differentials common (38%) caused by partial compression of subclavian arteries
- Cardiac and neurological systems are most commonly involved organ systems
- Aortic regurgitation in 18% to 50% of cases of proximal dissection
- Myocardial ischemia caused by coronary artery compression
- Cerebral ischemia/stroke in 5% to 10% of patients

■ ETIOLOGY
- Unknown, risk factors known
- Medial degeneration of aorta appears to be the culprit

DIAGNOSIS

■ DIFFERENTIAL DIAGNOSIS
- Known as the great imitator
- Acute MI needs to be ruled out
- Aortic insufficiency
- Nondissecting aortic aneurysm

■ LABORATORY TESTS
ECG: Helpful to rule out MI, generally nonspecific findings.
Serum biochemical marker: Smooth muscle myosin heavy chain high first 6 hr after onset.

■ IMAGING STUDIES
- Chest x-ray may show widened mediastinum (62%, nonspecific) and displacement of aortic intimal calcium.
- Transesophageal echocardiography, sensitivity 97% to 100%, can detect aortic insufficiency and pericardial effusion; study of choice in unstable patients, but operator dependent.
- MRI, sensitivity 90% to 100%, is the gold standard, but length of test and difficult access not suitable for stable intubated patients. Gives best information for surgeons.

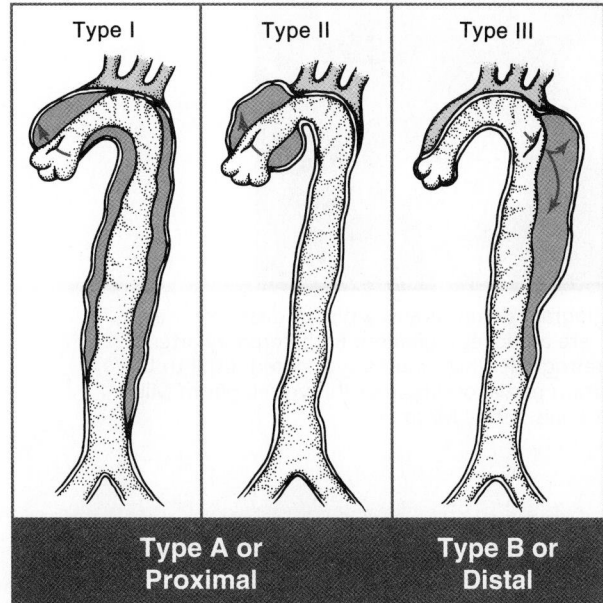

Fig. 1-25 Classification systems for aortic dissection. (From Isselbacher EM, Eagle KA, DeSanctis RW: Disease of the aorta. In Braunwald E [ed]: *Heart disease: a textbook of cardiovascular medicine,* ed 5, Philadelphia, 1997, WB Saunders.)

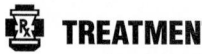
- CT, sensitivity 83% to 100%, involves IV contrast (Fig. 1-26).
- Aortography rarely done now.
- Transthoracic echocardiography has poor sensitivity.

◼ TREATMENT

◼ ACUTE GENERAL Rx
- Admit to ICU for hemodynamic monitoring.
- Decrease contractility and BP with IV
- IV Labetalol can be used instead, 20 mg IV, then 40-80 mg every 10 min.
- IV calcium channel blockers or ACE inhibitors may be used.
- Proximal dissections require emergent surgery.

- Distal dissections are treated medically only unless distal organ involvement or impending rupture occurs.
- Endovascular stent placement is a new treatment, especially for older high-risk surgical patients.

◼ CHRONIC Rx
Chronic aortic dissection (>2 wks) followed with aggressive BP control

◼ DISPOSITION
- Natural history of untreated aortic dissection: 85% mortality within 2 wk.
- Proximal aortic dissection is a surgical emergency. Time is critical; mortality is 1% to 3% per hr.
- Postsurgical repair, patients should be followed with frequent MRI because recurrent aneurysm or dissection common in first 2 yr.
- Overall, in-hospital mortality is 30% in patients with proximal dissections and 10% in patients with distal dissections.

◼ REFERRAL
For ICU management and surgery

REFERENCES

Hagan PG et al: The international registry of acute aortic dissection: new insights into an old disease, *JAMA* 283:897, 2000.

Khan IA et al: Clinical, diagnostic, and management perspectives of aortic dissection, *Chest* 122(1):311, 2002.

Authors: **Lynn Bowlby, M.D., and Mark Fagan, M.D.**

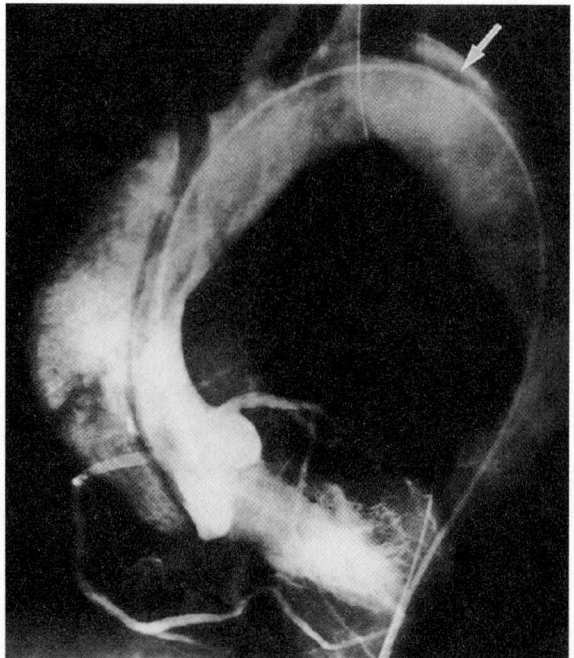

Fig. 1-26 Aortic dissection. An angiogram demonstrates a type-A dissection beginning in the aortic root and causing severe aortic regurgitation. Both coronary arteries fill from the true channel. A separate retrograde dissection entry is noted distal to the origin of the left subclavian artery, causing partial occlusion of this vessel. (From Miller SW: *Cardiac radiology: the requisites,* St Louis, 1996, Mosby.)

BASIC INFORMATION

■ **DEFINITION**

Aortic regurgitation is retrograde blood flow into the left ventricle from the aorta secondary to incompetent aortic valve.

■ **SYNONYMS**

Aortic insufficiency
AI
AR

ICD-9CM CODES
424.1 Aortic valve disorders

■ **EPIDEMIOLOGY & DEMOGRAPHICS**

- The most common cause of isolated severe aortic regurgitation is aortic root dilation.
- Infectious endocarditis is the most frequent cause of acute aortic regurgitation.

■ **PHYSICAL FINDINGS & CLINICAL PRESENTATION**

The clinical presentation varies depending on whether aortic insufficiency is acute or chronic. Chronic aortic insufficiency is well tolerated (except when secondary to infective endocarditis), and the patients remain asymptomatic for years. Common manifestations after significant deterioration of left ventricular function are dyspnea on exertion, syncope, chest pain, and CHF. Acute aortic insufficiency manifests primarily with hypotension caused by a sudden fall in cardiac output. A rapid rise in left ventricular diastolic pressure results in a further decrease in coronary blood flow.

Physical findings in chronic aortic insufficiency include the following:

- Widened pulse pressure (markedly increased systolic blood pressure, decreased diastolic blood pressure) is present.
- Bounding pulses, head "bobbing" with each systole (de Musset's sign) are present; "water hammer" or collapsing pulse (Corrigan's pulse) can be palpated at the wrist or on the femoral arteries ("pistol shot" femorals) and is caused by rapid rise and sudden collapse of the arterial pressure during late systole; capillary pulsations (Quincke's pulse) may occur at the base of the nail beds.
- A to-and-fro "double Duroziez" murmur may be heard over femoral arteries with slight compression.
- Popliteal systolic pressure is increased over brachial systolic pressure ≥40 mm Hg (Hill's sign).
- Cardiac auscultation reveals:
  1. Displacement of cardiac impulse downward and to the patient's left
  2. S_3 heard over the apex

3. Decrescendo, blowing diastolic murmur heard along left sternal border
4. Low-pitched apical diastolic rumble (Austin-Flint murmur) caused by contrast of the aortic regurgitant jet with the left ventricular wall
5. Early systolic apical ejection murmur

In patients with acute aortic insufficiency both the wide pulse pressure and the large stroke volume are absent. A short blowing diastolic murmur may be the only finding on physical examination.

■ **ETIOLOGY**

- Infective endocarditis
- Rheumatic fibrosis
- Trauma with valvular rupture
- Congenital bicuspid aortic valve
- Myxomatous degeneration
- Syphilitic aortitis
- Rheumatic spondylitis
- SLE
- Aortic dissection
- Fenfluramine, dexfenfluramine
- Takayasu's arteritis, granulomatous arteritis

DIAGNOSIS

■ **DIFFERENTIAL DIAGNOSIS**

- Patent ductus arteriosus, pulmonary regurgitation, and other valvular abnormalities
- The differential diagnosis of cardiac murmurs is described in Section II

■ **WORKUP**

- Echocardiogram, chest x-ray, ECG, and cardiac catheterization (selected patients)
- Medical history and physical examination focused on the following clinical manifestations:
  1. Dyspnea on exertion
  2. Syncope
  3. Chest pain
  4. CHF

■ **IMAGING STUDIES**

- Chest x-ray study
  1. Left ventricular hypertrophy (chronic aortic regurgitation)
  2. Aortic dilation
  3. Normal cardiac silhouette with pulmonary edema: possible in patients with acute aortic regurgitation
- ECG: left ventricular hypertrophy
- Echocardiography: coarse diastolic fluttering of the anterior mitral leaflet; LVH in patients with chronic aortic regurgitation
- Cardiac catheterization: assesses degree of left ventricular dysfunction, confirms the presence of a wide pulse pressure, assesses surgical risk, and determines if there is coexistent coronary artery disease

TREATMENT

■ **NONPHARMACOLOGIC THERAPY**

- Avoidance of competitive sports and strenuous activity
- Salt restriction

■ **ACUTE GENERAL Rx**

MEDICAL:

- Digitalis, diuretics, ACE inhibitors, and sodium restriction for CHF; nitroprusside in patients with acute aortic regurgitation
- Long-term vasodilator therapy with ACE inhibitors or nifedipine for reducing or delaying the need for aortic valve replacement in asymptomatic patients with severe aortic regurgitation and normal left ventricular function
- Bacterial endocarditis prophylaxis for surgical and dental procedures

SURGICAL: Reserved for:

- Symptomatic patients with chronic aortic regurgitation despite optimal medical therapy
- Patients with acute aortic regurgitation (i.e., infective endocarditis) producing left ventricular failure
- Evidence of systolic failure:
  1. Echocardiographic fractional shortening <25%
  2. Echocardiographic and diastolic dimension >55 mm
  3. Angiographic ejection fraction <50% or end-systolic volume index (ESVI) >60 ml/m²
- Evidence of diastolic failure:
  1. Pulmonary pressure >45 mm Hg systolic
  2. Left ventricular end-diastolic pressure (LVEDP) >15 mm Hg at catheterization
  3. Pulmonary hypertension detected on examination
- In general, the "55 rule" has been used to determine the timing of surgery: surgery should be performed before EF <55% or end-systolic dimension >55 mm.

■ **DISPOSITION**

Variable depending on underlying condition and left ventricular function; aortic regurgitation (except when secondary to infective endocarditis) is generally well tolerated, and patients remain asymptomatic for years.

■ **REFERRAL**

Surgical referral (see "Acute General Rx" for indications)

PEARLS & CONSIDERATIONS

■ **COMMENTS**

The operative mortality rate for aortic regurgitation is 3% to 5%.
Author: **Fred F. Ferri, M.D.**

I

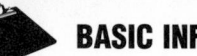

BASIC INFORMATION

■ DEFINITION

Aortic stenosis is obstruction to systolic left ventricular outflow across the aortic valve. Symptoms appear when the valve orifice decreases to <1 cm² (normal orifice is 3 cm²). The stenosis is considered severe when the orifice is <0.5 cm²/m² or the pressure gradient is 50 mm Hg or higher.

■ SYNONYMS

Aortic valvular stenosis
AS

ICD-9CM CODES

424.1 Aortic valvular stenosis

■ EPIDEMIOLOGY & DEMOGRAPHICS

- Aortic stenosis is the most common valve lesion in adults in Western countries.
- Calcific stenosis (most common cause in patients >60 yr old) occurs in 75% of patients.

■ PHYSICAL FINDINGS & CLINICAL PRESENTATION

- Rough, loud systolic diamond-shaped murmur, best heard at base of heart and transmitted into neck vessels; often associated with a thrill or ejection click; may also be heard well at the apex
- Absence or diminished intensity of sound of aortic valve closure (in severe aortic stenosis)
- Late, slow-rising carotid upstroke with decreased amplitude
- Strong apical pulse
- Narrowing of pulse pressure in later stages of aortic stenosis
- Some patients with aortic stenosis experience bleeding into their GI tract or skin. This is caused by an acquired defect in von Willebrandt factor. Aortic valve replacement restores normal hemostasis.

■ ETIOLOGY

- Rheumatic inflammation of aortic valve
- Progressive stenosis of congenital bicuspid valve (found in 1%-2% of population)
- Idiopathic calcification of the aortic valve
- Congenital (major cause of aortic stenosis in patients <30 yr)

DIAGNOSIS

■ DIFFERENTIAL DIAGNOSIS

- Hypertrophic cardiomyopathy
- Mitral regurgitation
- Ventricular septal defect
- Aortic sclerosis. Aortic stenosis is distinguished from aortic sclerosis by the degree of valve impairment. In aortic sclerosis, the valve leaflets are abnormally thickened but obstruction to outflow is minimal.

■ WORKUP

- Echocardiography
- Chest x-ray examination, ECG
- Cardiac catheterization in selected patients (see "Imaging Studies")
- Medical history focusing on symptoms and potential complications:
  1. Angina
  2. Syncope (particularly with exertion)
  3. CHF
  4. GI bleeding: in patients with associated hemorrhagic telangiectasia (AVM)

■ IMAGING STUDIES

- Chest x-ray examination
  1. Poststenotic dilation of the ascending aorta
  2. Calcification of aortic cusps
  3. Pulmonary congestion (in advanced stages of aortic stenosis)
- ECG:
  1. Left ventricular hypertrophy (found in >80% of patients)
  2. ST-T wave changes
  3. Atrial fibrillation: frequent
- Doppler echocardiography: thickening of the left ventricular wall; if the patient has valvular calcifications, multiple echoes may be seen from within the aortic root and there is poor separation of the aortic cusps during systole. Gradient across the valve can be estimated but is less precise than with cardiac catheterization.
- Cardiac catheterization: indicated in symptomatic patients; it confirms the diagnosis and estimates the severity of the disease by measuring the gradient across the valve, allowing calculation of the valve area. It also detects coexisting coronary artery stenosis that may need bypass at the same time as aortic valve replacement.

TREATMENT

■ NONPHARMACOLOGIC THERAPY

- Strenuous activity should be avoided.
- Sodium restriction if CHF is present.

■ GENERAL Rx

MEDICAL:
- Diuretics and sodium restriction are needed if CHF is present; digoxin is used only to control rate of atrial fibrillation.
- ACE inhibitors are relatively contraindicated.
- Calcium channel blocker verapamil may be useful only to control rate of atrial fibrillation.
- Antibiotic prophylaxis is necessary for surgical and dental procedures

SURGICAL:
- Valve replacement is the treatment of choice in symptomatic patients because the 5-yr mortality rate after onset of symptoms is extremely high, even with optimal medical therapy; valve replacement is indicated if cardiac catheterization establishes a pressure gradient >50 mm Hg and valve area <1 cm².
- Balloon aortic valvotomy for adult acquired aortic stenosis is useful only for palliation.

■ DISPOSITION

- 15% to 20% of patients with severe aortic stenosis die before age 20 yr.
- The 5-yr survival rate in adults is 40%.
- The average duration of symptoms before death is as follows: angina, 60 mo; syncope, 36 mo; CHF, 24 mo.
- About 75% of patients with symptomatic aortic stenosis will be dead 3 yr after onset of symptoms unless the aortic valve is replaced.

■ REFERRAL

- Surgical referral for valve replacement in symptomatic patients. However, the presence of moderate or severe valvular calcification, together with a rapid increase in aortic-jet velocity, identifies patients with a very poor prognosis who should be considered for early valve replacement rather than have surgery delayed until symptoms develop.
- Surgical mortality rate for valve replacement is 3% to 5%; however, it varies with patient's age (>8% in patients >75 yr old).
- Balloon valvuloplasty is useful in infants and children or poor surgical candidates who do not have calcified valve apparatus; it can be done as an intermediate procedure to stabilize high-risk patients before surgery.
- When performed in adults who have calcified valves, balloon valvuloplasty is useful only for short-term reduction in severity of aortic stenosis when surgery is contraindicated, because restenosis occurs rapidly.

REFERENCES

Alpert JS: Aortic stenosis, a new face for an old disease, *Arch Intern Med* 163:1769, 2003.

Carabello BA: Aortic stenosis, *N Engl J Med* 346:677, 2002.

Vincentelli A et al: Acquired von Willebrand syndrome in aortic stenosis, *N Engl J Med* 349: 343, 2003.

Author: **Fred F. Ferri, M.D.**

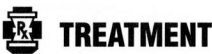

 BASIC INFORMATION

■ **DEFINITION**

Appendicitis is the acute inflammation of the appendix.

ICD-9CM CODES
540.9 Appendicitis
540.0 Appendicitis with generalized peritonitis

■ **EPIDEMIOLOGY & DEMOGRAPHICS**
• Appendicitis occurs in 10% of the population, most commonly between the ages of 10 and 30 yr.
• It is the most common abdominal surgical emergency.
• Incidence of appendicitis has declined over the past 30 yr.
• Male:female ratio is 3:2 until mid-20s; it equalizes after age 30 yr.

■ **PHYSICAL FINDINGS & CLINICAL PRESENTATION**
• Abdominal pain: initially the pain may be epigastric or periumbilical in nearly 50% of patients; it subsequently localizes to the RLQ within 12 to 18 hr. Pain can be found in back or right flank if appendix is retrocecal or in other abdominal locations if there is malrotation of the appendix.
• Pain with right thigh extension (psoas sign), low-grade fever: temperature may be >38° C if there is appendiceal perforation.
• Pain with internal rotation of the flexed right thigh (obturator sign) is present.
• RLQ pain on palpation of the LLQ (Rovsing's sign): physical examination may reveal right-sided tenderness in patients with pelvic appendix.
• Point of maximum tenderness is in the RLQ (McBurney's point).
• Nausea, vomiting, tachycardia, cutaneous hyperesthesias at the level of T12 can be present.

■ **ETIOLOGY**
Obstruction of the appendiceal lumen with subsequent vascular congestion, inflammation, and edema; common causes of obstruction are:
• Fecaliths: 30% to 35% of cases (most common in adults)
• Foreign body: 4% (fruit seeds, pinworms, tapeworms, roundworms, calculi)

• Inflammation: 50% to 60% of cases (submucosal lymphoid hyperplasia [most common etiology in children, teens])
• Neoplasms: 1% (carcinoids, metastatic disease, carcinoma)

DIAGNOSIS

■ **DIFFERENTIAL DIAGNOSIS**
• Intestinal: regional cecal enteritis, incarcerated hernia, cecal diverticulitis, intestinal obstruction, perforated ulcer, perforated cecum, Meckel's diverticulitis
• Reproductive: ectopic pregnancy, ovarian cyst, torsion of ovarian cyst, salpingitis, tuboovarian abscess, Mittelschmerz endometriosis, seminal vesiculitis
• Renal: renal and ureteral calculi, neoplasms, pyelonephritis
• Vascular: leaking aortic aneurysm
• Psoas abscess
• Trauma
• Cholecystitis
• Mesenteric adenitis

■ **WORKUP**
• Patients presenting with RLQ pain, nausea, vomiting, anorexia, and RLQ rebound tenderness should undergo prompt clinical and laboratory evaluation. Imaging studies are generally not necessary in typical appendicitis. They are useful when the diagnosis is uncertain. Laparoscopy may be useful as both a diagnostic and a therapeutic modality.

■ **LABORATORY TESTS**
• CBC with differential reveals leukocytosis with a left shift in 90% of patients with appendicitis. Total WBC count is generally lower than 20,000/mm³. Higher counts may be indicative of perforation. Less than 4% have a normal WBC and differential. A low Hgb and Hct in an older patient should raise suspicion for carcinoma of the cecum.
• Microscopic hematuria and pyuria may occur in <20% of patients.

■ **IMAGING STUDIES**
• Spiral CT of the right lower quadrant of the abdomen has a sensitivity of >90% and an accuracy >94% for acute appendicitis. A distended appendix, periappendiceal inflammation, and a thickened appendiceal wall are indicative of appendicitis.

• Ultrasonography has a sensitivity of 75% to 90% for the diagnosis of acute appendicitis. Ultrasound is useful, especially in younger women when diagnosis is unclear. Normal ultrasonographic findings should not deter surgery if the history and physical examination are indicative of appendicitis.

TREATMENT

■ **NONPHARMACOLOGIC THERAPY**
• NPO
• Do not administer analgesics or antibiotics until the diagnosis is made (may mask signs of peritonitis).

■ **ACUTE GENERAL Rx**
• Urgent appendectomy (laparoscopic or open), correction of fluid and electrolyte imbalance with vigorous IV hydration and electrolyte replacement
• IV antibiotic prophylaxis to cover gram-negative bacilli and anaerobes (ampicillin-sulbactam [Unasyn] 3 g IV q6h or piperacillin-tazobactam [Zosyn] 4.5 g IV q8h in adults)

PEARLS & CONSIDERATIONS

■ **COMMENTS**
• Perforation is common (20% in adult patients). Indicators of perforation are pain lasting >24 hr, leukocytosis >20,000/mm³, temperature >102° F, palpable abdominal mass, and peritoneal findings.
• In general, prognosis is excellent. Mortality is <1% in young adults without complications; however, it exceeds 10% in elderly patients with ruptured appendix.

REFERENCE
Paulson EK et al: Suspected appendicitis, *N Engl J Med* 348:236, 2003.
Author: **Fred F. Ferri, M.D.**

BASIC INFORMATION

■ DEFINITION
The prototype of granulomatous arthritis is tuberculous arthritis. Atypical mycobacteria, sarcoidosis, and sporotrichosis can cause granulomatous involvement of the synovium, but these entities are much less common.

■ SYNONYMS
Tuberculous arthritis
Pott's disease

■ ICD-9CM CODES
711.40 Arthropathy associated with other bacterial disease
730.88 Other infection involving bone

■ EPIDEMIOLOGY & DEMOGRAPHICS
INCIDENCE (IN U.S.): Unknown
PREVALENCE (IN U.S.): Unknown
PREDOMINANT SEX: Male = female
PREDOMINANT AGE: Rare in childhood
PEAK INCIDENCE: No seasonal predilection

■ PHYSICAL FINDINGS
- Often no constitutional symptoms (fever and weight loss)
- Possibly no clinical or radiographic evidence of pulmonary TB
- Spinal infection most often in the thoracic or upper lumbar area, with back pain as the most common symptom
- Considerable local muscle spasm possible
- Kyphosis and neurologic symptoms resulting from spinal cord compression in advanced disease
- Chronic monoarticular arthritis in the peripheral joints
- Single joint involved in 85% of patients
- Pain, swelling, limitation of motion, and joint stiffness less dramatic than in acute bacterial arthritis; possibly present for months to years
- Seen more often in persons from developing countries, elderly patients, and hemodialysis patients

■ ETIOLOGY
- Hematogenous spread of organisms from a distant site of infection or by direct spread from bone
- Most commonly affected area: 50% of cases in the spine; next most commonly affected area: large joints (knee and hip)
- Primary infection beginning in the lungs and spreading to the highly vascular synovium
- Tuberculous osteomyelitis commonly involving an adjacent joint
- In peripheral joints, a granulomatous reaction in the synovium causing joint effusion and eventual destruction of underlying bone
- In the spine, infection of the intervertebral disk spreading to adjacent vertebrae
- Osteomyelitis of vertebrae causing collapse, kyphosis, or gibbous deformity, and possibly paraspinal "cold" abscess

DIAGNOSIS

■ DIFFERENTIAL DIAGNOSIS
- Sarcoidosis
- Fungal arthritis
- Metastatic cancer
- Primary or metastatic synovial tumors

■ WORKUP
- High index of suspicion needed
- Gold standard: synovial biopsy
- Joint aspiration and culture of the synovial fluid performed while awaiting biopsy
- Positive synovial fluid smear for acid-fast bacilli in 20% of cases; positive culture in 80%
- Elevated synovial fluid protein, low glucose
- Considerable variation in synovial fluid WBC count, but values of 10,000 to 20,000 cells/mm³ typical; may be predominantly polymorphonuclear leukocytes
- Usually positive tuberculin skin test
- Anergy in elderly patients or in advanced disease
- In spinal infections, percutaneous or open biopsy to obtain accurate C&S data

■ LABORATORY TESTS
Peripheral WBC count and ESR are elevated but nonspecific.

■ IMAGING STUDIES
- Plain radiographs of the affected joint
  1. Typically demonstrate bony destruction with little new bone formation
  2. Osteopenia and soft tissue swelling in early infections
  3. Later, erosions at the joint margins
  4. In the spine, disk space narrowing with vertebral collapse (wedging) causing characteristic kyphosis
- CT scan: useful in early diagnosis of infections of the spine and to detect paraspinal abscess
- Technetium and gallium scintigraphic scans: may be positive, but do not permit differentiation from inflammation or osteoarthritis

TREATMENT

■ NONPHARMACOLOGIC THERAPY
Encourage range-of-motion exercises of the affected joint to prevent contractures.

■ ACUTE GENERAL Rx
- Combination chemotherapy
  1. If sensitive TB suspected, give isoniazid 5 mg/kg/day (maximum 300 mg/day) plus rifampin 10 mg/kg/day (maximum 600 mg/day) for at least 6 mo and pyrazinamide 15 to 30 mg/kg/day (maximum 2 g/day) for at least the first 2 mo plus ethambutol 15 to 25 mg/kg/day until sensitivity results are available.
  2. Most patients are treated successfully with chemotherapy alone.
  3. Urgent surgical intervention is necessary if spinal cord compression causes neurologic changes.
- Surgical debridement in cases of extensive bone involvement

■ CHRONIC Rx
In long-standing extensive disease, arthrodesis of weight-bearing joints

■ DISPOSITION
Loss of cartilage and destruction of underlying bone if treatment is not initiated promptly

■ REFERRAL
- To a physician experienced in the management of TB
- For consultation with an infectious diseases specialist if drug resistance is suspected or documented
- For neurosurgical and/or orthopedic consultation if neurologic impairment suspected

PEARLS & CONSIDERATIONS

■ COMMENTS
- As TB has become more prevalent in the U.S. in the last 10 to 20 yr, TB arthritis and osteomyelitis have also become more common.

REFERENCES
Emery P et al: Detection of *Mycobacterium tuberculosis* group organisms in human and mouse joint tissue by reverse transcriptase PCR: prevalence in diseased synovial tissue suggests lack of specific association with rheumatoid arthritis, *Infect Immun* 69(30):1821, 2001.

Miyata K, Kanzaki T: Early onset sarcoidosis masquerading as juvenile rheumatoid arthritis, *J Am Acad Dermatol* 43:969, 2001.

Shanahan EM, Hanley SD: Tuberculosis of the wrist, *Arth Rheum* 42(12):2724, 1999.

van de Loo FA et al: Deficiency of NADPH oxidase components p47phox and gp91phox caused granulomatous synovitis and increased connective tissue destruction in experimental arthritis models, *Am J Pathol* 163(4):1525, 2003.
Author: **Deborah L. Shapiro, M.D.**

BASIC INFORMATION

■ DEFINITION

Bacterial arthritis is a highly destructive form of joint disease most often caused by hematogenous spread of organisms from a distant site of infection. Direct penetration of the joint as a result of trauma or surgery and spread from adjacent osteomyelitis may also cause bacterial arthritis. Any joint in the body may be affected. Gonococcal arthritis causes a distinct clinical syndrome and is often considered separately.

■ SYNONYMS

Septic arthritis
Pyogenic arthritis

ICD-9CM CODES

711 Pyogenic arthritis, site unspecified

■ EPIDEMIOLOGY & DEMOGRAPHICS

INCIDENCE (IN U.S.): Unknown
PREVALENCE (IN U.S.): Unknown
PREDOMINANT SEX: Gonococcal arthritis in males
PREDOMINANT AGE: Gonococcal arthritis in sexually active adults
PEAK INCIDENCE:
- Gonococcal arthritis: young adults
- Other bacterial causes: all ages

■ PHYSICAL FINDINGS & CLINICAL PRESENTATION

- Hallmark: acute onset of a swollen, painful joint
- Limited range of motion of the joint
- Effusion, with varying degrees of erythema and increased warmth around the joint
- Single joint affected in 80% to 90% of cases of nongonococcal arthritis
- Gonococcal dermatitis-arthritis syndrome
  1. Typical pattern is a migratory polyarthritis or tenosynovitis
  2. Small pustules on the trunk or extremities
- Febrile patient at presentation
- Most commonly affected joints in adult: knee and hip, but any joint may be involved; in children: hip

■ ETIOLOGY

- Bacteria spread from another locus of infection
  1. Highly vascular synovium is invaded by hematogenously spread bacteria.
  2. WBC enzymes cause necrosis of synovium, cartilage, and bone.
  3. Extensive joint destruction is rapid if infection is not treated with appropriate IV antibiotics and drainage of necrotic material.
- Predisposing factors: rheumatoid arthritis, prosthetic joints, advanced age, immunodeficiency
- The most common nongonococcal organisms are *Staphylococcus aureus*, β-hemolytic streptococci, and gramnegative bacilli.

DIAGNOSIS

■ DIFFERENTIAL DIAGNOSIS

- Gout
- Pseudogout
- Trauma
- Hemarthrosis
- Rheumatic fever
- Adult or juvenile rheumatoid arthritis
- Spondyloarthropathies such as Reiter's syndrome
- Osteomyelitis
- Viral arthritides
- Septic bursitis

■ WORKUP

- Joint aspiration, Gram stain, and culture of the synovial fluid
- Immediate arthrocentesis before other studies are undertaken or antibiotics instituted

■ LABORATORY TESTS

- Joint fluid analysis
  1. Synovial fluid leukocyte count is usually elevated >50,000 cells/mm³ with a differential count of 80% or more polymorphonuclear cells.
  2. Counts are highly variable, with similar findings in gout, pseudogout, or rheumatoid arthritis.
  3. The differential diagnosis of synovial fluid abnormalities is described in Section II.
- Blood cultures
- Culture of possible extraarticular sources of infection
- Elevated peripheral WBC count and ESR (nonspecific)

■ IMAGING STUDIES

- X-ray examination of the affected joint to rule out osteomyelitis
- CT scan for early diagnosis of infections of the spine, hips, and sternoclavicular and sacroiliac joints
- Technetium and gallium scintigraphic scans (positive, but do not permit differentiation of infection from inflammation)
- Indium-labeled WBC scans (less sensitive, but more specific)

TREATMENT

■ NONPHARMACOLOGIC THERAPY

- Affected joints aspirated daily to remove necrotic material and to follow serial WBC counts and cultures
- If no resolution with IV antibiotics and closed drainage: open debridement and lavage, particularly in nongonococcal infections
- Prevention of contractures:
  1. After acute stage of inflammation, range-of-motion exercises of the affected joint
  2. Physical therapy helpful

■ ACUTE GENERAL Rx

- IV antibiotics immediately after joint aspiration and Gram stain of the synovial fluid
- For infections caused by grampositive cocci: penicillinase-resistant penicillin, such as nafcillin (2 g IV q4h), unless there is clinical suspicion of methicillin-resistant *Staphylococcus aureus,* in which case vancomycin (1 g IV q12h)
- Infections caused by gram-negative bacilli: treated with a third-generation cephalosporin or an antipseudomonal penicillin plus an aminoglycoside, pending C&S results
- For suspected gonococcal infection, including young adults when the synovial fluid Gram stain is nondiagnostic: ceftriaxone 1 g IV q24h

■ CHRONIC Rx

See indications for surgical drainage.

■ DISPOSITION

- With prompt treatment, complete resolution is expected.
- Delay in treatment may result in permanent destruction of cartilage and loss of function of the affected joint.

■ REFERRAL

To an orthopedist for open drainage if the infected joint fails to improve on appropriate antibiotics and closed aspiration

PEARLS & CONSIDERATIONS

■ COMMENTS

- Any patient with an acute monoarticular arthritis should undergo an urgent joint aspiration to rule out septic arthritis, even if there is a history of gout.

REFERENCES

Lidgren L et al: Infection and arthritis: infection of prosthetic joints, *Best Pract Clin Rheumatol* 17(2):209, 2003.
McGill PE: Geographically specific infections and arthritis, including rheumatic syndromes associated with certain fungi and parasites, *Brucella* species and *Mycobacterium leprae, Best Pract Res Clin Rheumatol* 17(2): 289, 2003.
Nade S: Septic arthritis, *Best Pract Clin Rheumatol* 17(2):183, 2003.
Author: **Deborah L. Shapiro, M.D.**

■ BASIC INFORMATION

■ DEFINITION
Juvenile rheumatoid arthritis is arthritis beginning before the age of 16 yr.

■ SYNONYMS
Still's disease
Juvenile chronic arthritis
Juvenile polyarthritis

ICD-9CM CODES
714.3 Juvenile chronic polyarthritis

■ EPIDEMIOLOGY & DEMOGRAPHICS
PREVALENCE (IN U.S.): 250,000 to 300,000 cases
PREVALENT SEX: Female:male ratio of 2:1
PREVALENT AGE: Two peak incidences, between ages of 1 and 3 yr and ages 8 and 12 yr.

■ PHYSICAL FINDINGS & CLINICAL PRESENTATION
Usually one of three types:
SYSTEMIC OR ACUTE FEBRILE JUVENILE RHEUMATOID ARTHRITIS (20% OF CASES):
- Characterized by extraarticular manifestations, especially spiking fevers and a typical rash that frequently appears in the evening and may be elicited by gently scratching the skin in susceptible areas (Koebner's phenomenon)
- Possible splenomegaly, generalized lymphadenopathy, pericarditis, and myocarditis
- Often, minimal articular findings overshadowed by systemic symptoms
PAUCIARTICULAR OR OLIGOARTICULAR FORM (50% OF CASES):
- Involves fewer than five joints
- Usually involves the larger joints, such as the knees, elbows, and ankles
- Systemic features often minimal, and only one to three joints usually involved
- Rarely causes impairment but chronic iridocyclitis develops in approximately 30% of cases with this form, and permanent loss of vision will develop in a high percentage of these patients (Fig. 1-27)
- Accelerated growth of the affected limb from chronic hyperemia possibly resulting in a temporary leg length discrepancy that is eventually equalized in most cases on control of the inflammation

POLYARTICULAR JUVENILE RHEUMATOID ARTHRITIS (30% OF CASES):
- Involves five or more joints
- Resembles the adult disease in its symmetric involvement of the small joints of the hands and feet (Fig. 1-28)

- Cervical spine involvement common and may produce marked loss of motion
- Early closure of the ossification centers of the mandible, often producing a markedly receding chin, a characteristic of this form

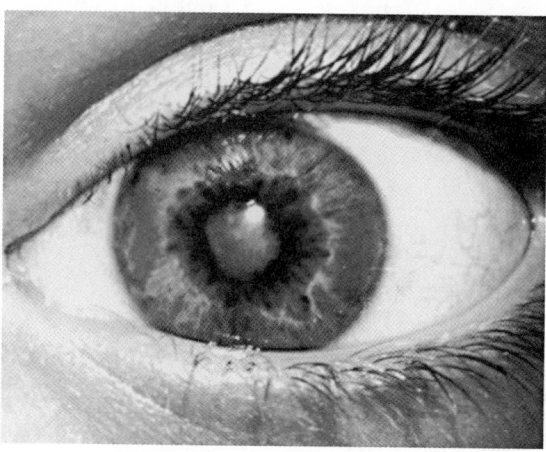

Fig. 1-27 Chronic iridocyclitis of juvenile rheumatoid arthritis. Extensive posterior synechiae have resulted in a small, irregular pupil. There is a well-developed cataract and early band keratopathy at the medial and lateral margins of the cornea. (From Behrman RE [ed]: *Nelson textbook of pediatrics,* ed 16, Philadelphia, 2000, WB Saunders.)

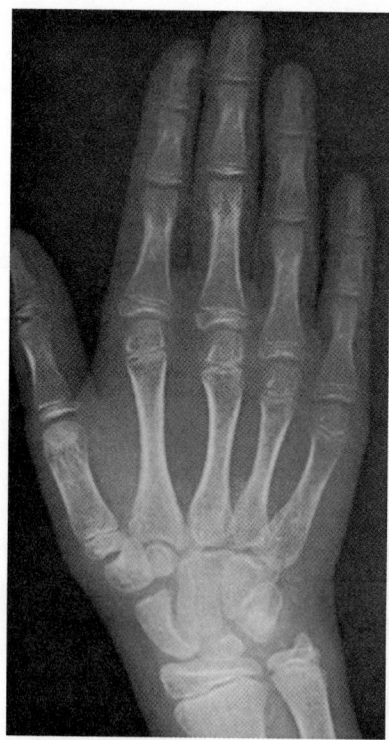 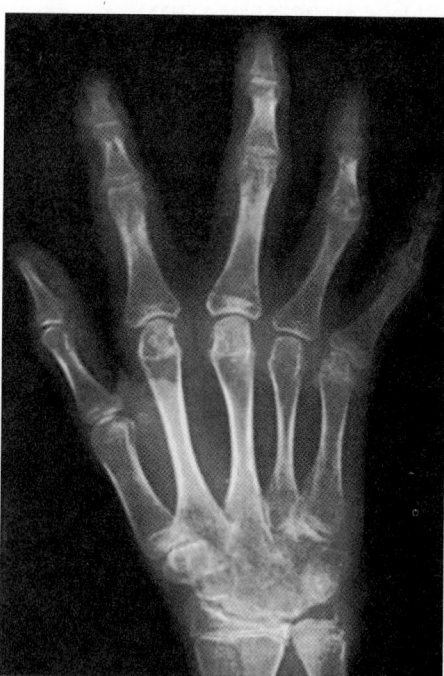

Fig. 1-28 Progression of joint destruction in a girl with rheumatoid factor-positive juvenile rheumatoid arthritis despite doses of corticosteroids sufficient to suppress symptoms in the interval between A and B. **A,** Roentgenogram of the hand at onset. **B,** Roentgenogram 4 years later, showing a loss of articular cartilage and destruction changes in the distal and proximal interphalangeal and metacarpophalangeal joints and destruction and fusion of wrist bones. (From Behrman RE [ed]: *Nelson textbook of pediatrics,* ed 16, Philadelphia, 2000, WB Saunders.)

- Systemic manifestations similar to the febrile variety but not as dramatic

■ ETIOLOGY

Unknown. There is increasing evidence that the inflammation and destruction of bone and cartilage that occurs in many rheumatic diseases are the result of the activation, by some unknown mechanism, of proinflammatory cells that infiltrate the synovium. These cells, in turn, release various substances, such as cytokines and tumor necrosis factor (TNF) alpha, which subsequently cause the pathologic changes typical of this group of diseases. Many of the newer therapeutic agents are directed at the suppression of these final mediators of inflammation.

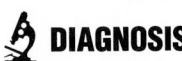

DIAGNOSIS

■ DIFFERENTIAL DIAGNOSIS
- Infectious causes of fever
- SLE
- Rheumatic fever
- Drug reaction
- Serum sickness
- "Viral arthritis"
- Lyme arthritis

■ WORKUP
Initial laboratory and imaging studies are often nonspecific in children with rheumatoid arthritis.

■ LABORATORY TESTS
- Increased ESR
- Low-grade anemia
- Very high peripheral WBC count
- Rheumatoid factor: rarely demonstrable in the serum of children
- Antinuclear antibodies: often found in children with ocular complications

■ IMAGING STUDIES
- Roentgenographic findings are similar to those in adult, with soft tissue swelling and osteoporosis early in the disease.
- Joint destruction is less frequent.
- Bony erosion and cyst formation may be present as a result of synovial hypertrophy.

TREATMENT

■ NONPHARMACOLOGIC THERAPY
Proper management requires close cooperation among primary physician, therapist, rheumatologist, and orthopedist.
- Rest
- Physical and occupational therapy
- Patient and family education
- Proper diet and weight maintenance

■ ACUTE GENERAL Rx
- Aspirin (stopped during childhood viral illnesses to avoid Reye's syndrome)
- Other NSAIDs
- DMARDs and biologic response modifiers (BMRs)
- Intraarticular steroids
- Systemic corticosteroids

■ DISPOSITION
- Complete remission occurs in the majority of patients and may occur at any age.
- 70% to 85% of children regain normal function.
- Mortality rate is 2%.
- Children with a protracted systemic phase of the disease are most at risk for developing serious intercurrent infection and potentially fatal amyloidosis.
- Myocarditis may develop in the systemic form.
- Blindness is the most serious complication of the pauciarticular form; joint deformity is the most serious problem of polyarticular disease.

■ REFERRAL
- Early rheumatology consultation
- For ophthalmology consultation when ocular involvement is suspected (frequent eye examinations, especially in oligoarticular form)
- For orthopedic consultation for corrective surgery

PEARLS & CONSIDERATIONS

■ COMMENTS
Patient information on juvenile rheumatoid arthritis can be obtained from the National Arthritis Foundation, 1330 West Peachtree Street, Atlanta, GA 30309; 800-283-7800.

REFERENCES

Choy EHS, Panayi G: Cytokine pathways and joint inflammation in rheumatoid arthritis, *N Engl J Med* 344:907, 2001.

Gardner GC, Kadel NJ: Ordering and interpreting rheumatologic laboratory tests, *J Am Acad Orthop Surg* 11:600, 2003.

Uremer JM: Rational use of new and existing disease-modifying agents in rheumatoid arthritis, *Ann Intern Med* 134:695, 2001.

Wulffraat NM, Kuis W: Treatment of refractory juvenile idiopathic arthritis, *J Rheumatol* 28:929, 2001.

Author: **Lonnie R. Mercier, M.D.**

BASIC INFORMATION

■ DEFINITION

Psoriatic arthritis is an inflammatory spondyloarthritis occurring in patients with psoriasis who are usually seronegative for rheumatoid factor. It is often included in a class of disorders called *rheumatoid variants* or *seronegative spondyloarthropathies.*

ICD-9CM CODES
696.0 Psoriatic arthritis

■ EPIDEMIOLOGY & DEMOGRAPHICS
PREVALENCE: 5% to 10% of patients with psoriasis (psoriasis affects 1% to 1.5% of general population)
PREVALENT SEX: Males = females
PREVALENT AGE: 30 to 55 yr

■ PHYSICAL FINDINGS & CLINICAL PRESENTATION
- Usually gradual clinical onset
- Asymmetric involvement of scattered joints
- Selective involvement of the DIP joints (described in "classic" cases but present in only 5% of patients; Fig. 1-29)
- Symmetric arthritis similar to RA in 15% of patients
- Possible development of predominant sacroiliitis in a small number of cases
- Advanced form of hand involvement (arthritis mutilans) in some patients
- Dystrophic changes in the nails (pitting, ridging) in many patients with DIP involvement

■ ETIOLOGY
Unknown

DIAGNOSIS

■ DIFFERENTIAL DIAGNOSIS
- Rheumatoid arthritis
- Erosive osteoarthritis
- Gouty arthritis
- Ankylosing spondylitis
- The differential diagnosis of spondyloarthropathies is described in Section II.

■ WORKUP
- Early diagnosis may be difficult to establish because the arthritis may develop before skin lesions appear.
- Laboratory studies show no specific abnormalities in most cases.

■ LABORATORY TESTS
- Slight elevation of ESR
- Possible mild anemia
- Possible HLA-B27 antigen (especially in patients with sacroiliitis)

■ IMAGING STUDIES
- Peripheral joint findings similar to those in rheumatoid arthritis but erosive changes in the distal phalangeal tufts characteristic of psoriatic arthritis
- Bony osteolysis; periosteal new bone formation
- Changes in axial skeleton: sacroiliitis, development of vertebral syndesmophytes (osteophytes) that often bridge adjacent vertebral bodies
- Paravertebral ossification
- Spinal changes: do not have same appearance as ankylosing spondylitis; however, spine abnormalities are less common than sacroiliitis

TREATMENT

■ NONPHARMACOLOGIC THERAPY
- Rest
- Splinting
- Joint protection
- PT

■ ACUTE GENERAL Rx
- NSAIDs
- Occasional intraarticular steroid injections
- DMARDs: rarely are required

■ DISPOSITION
- Different from rheumatoid arthritis in both prognosis and response to treatment
- Generally, mild joint symptoms in psoriatic arthritis
- Disease-free intervals lasting for several years in many patients

■ REFERRAL
Orthopedic consultation for painful joint deformity.

REFERENCES

Crotty JG et al: Interventions for psoriatic arthritis, Cochrane Database System Rev 3: CD 000212, 2000.

Hohkr T, Marker-Hermann E: Psoriatic arthritis: clinical aspects genetics, and the role of T-cells, *Curr Opin Rheumatol* 13:245, 2001.

Patel S et al: Psoriatic arthritis-emerging concepts, *Rheumatology* (Oxford) 40:243, 2001.

Author: **Lonnie R. Mercier, M.D.**

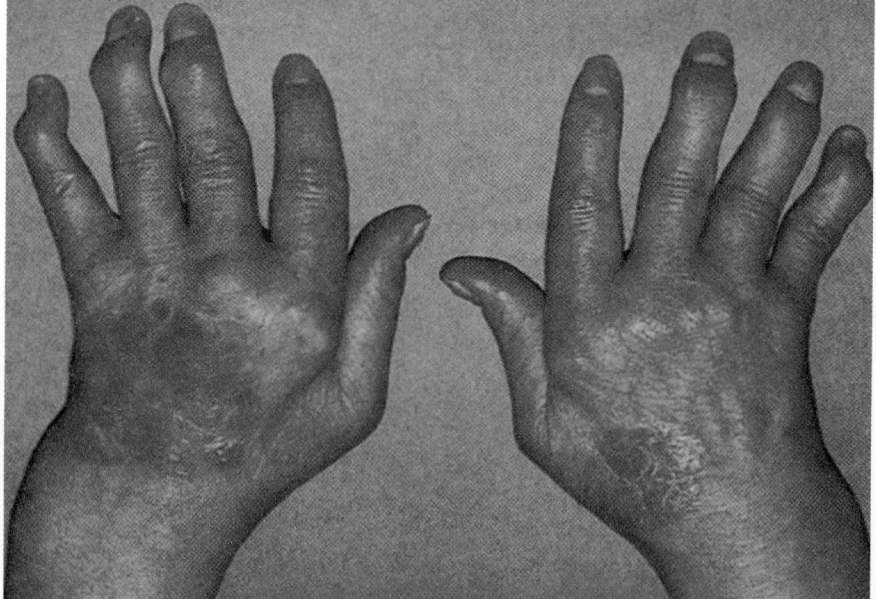

Fig. 1-29   The hands of a woman with symmetric polyarthritis. Initially, this was indistinguishable from rheumatoid disease, but note the distal interphalangeal joint involvement, which is uncommon in rheumatoid arthritis, as well as the skin psoriasis. (From Klippel J, Dieppe P, Ferri F [eds]: *Primary care rheumatology,* London, 1999, Mosby.)

■ BASIC INFORMATION

■ DEFINITION
Rheumatoid arthritis (RA) is a systemic disorder characterized by chronic joint inflammation that most commonly affects peripheral joints. This process results in the development of pannus, a destructive tissue that damages cartilage.

ICD-9CM CODES
714.0 Rheumatoid arthritis

■ EPIDEMIOLOGY & DEMOGRAPHICS
PREVALENCE: 5 cases/1000 adults
PREVALENT AGE: 35 to 45 yr
PREDOMINANT SEX:
• Female:male ratio of 3:1
• After age 50 yr, sex difference less marked

■ PHYSICAL FINDINGS & CLINICAL PRESENTATION
• Usually gradual onset; common prodromal symptoms of weakness, fatigue, and anorexia
• Initial presentation: multiple symmetric joint involvement, most often in the hands and feet, usually MCP, MTP, and PIP joints (Fig. 1-30)
• Joint effusions, tenderness, and restricted motion usually present early in the disease
• Eventual characteristic deformities: subluxations, dislocations, and joint contractures
• Extraarticular findings:
  1. Tendon sheaths and bursae frequently affected by chronic inflammation
  2. Possible tendon rupture
  3. Rheumatoid nodules over bony prominences such as the elbow and shaft of the ulna
  4. Splenomegaly, pericarditis, and vasculitis
  5. Findings of carpal tunnel syndrome resulting from flexor tenosynovitis

■ ETIOLOGY
Unknown. There is increasing evidence that the inflammation and destruction of bone and cartilage that occurs in many rheumatic diseases are the result of the activation by some unknown mechanism of proinflammatory cells that infiltrate the synovium. These cells, in turn, release various substances, such as cytokines and tumor necrosis factor (TNF) alpha, which subsequently cause the pathologic changes typical of this group of diseases. Many of the newer therapeutic agents are directed at the suppression of these final mediators of inflammation.

■ DIAGNOSIS

■ DIFFERENTIAL DIAGNOSIS
• SLE
• Seronegative spondyloarthropathies
• Polymyalgia rheumatica
• Acute rheumatic fever
• Scleroderma

According to the American College of Rheumatology, RA exists when four of seven criteria are present, with criteria 1 to 4 being present for at least 6 wk.
1. Morning stiffness over 1 hr
2. Arthritis in three or more joints with swelling
3. Arthritis of hand joints with swelling
4. Symmetric arthritis
5. Rheumatoid nodules
6. Roentgenographic changes typical of RA
7. Positive serum rheumatoid factor

■ LABORATORY TESTS
• Increase in rheumatoid factor in 80% of cases (rheumatoid factor also present in the normal population)
• Possible mild anemia
• Usually, elevated acute phase reactants (ESR, C-reactive protein)
• Possible mild leukocytosis
• Usually, turbid joint fluid, which forms a poor mucin clot; elevated cell count, with an increase in polymorphonuclear leukocytes

■ IMAGING STUDIES
Plain radiography
• Usually reveals soft-tissue swelling and osteoporosis early (Fig. 1-31)
• Eventually, joint space narrowing, erosion, and deformity visible as a result of continued inflammation and cartilage destruction

■ TREATMENT

■ NONPHARMACOLOGIC THERAPY
Proper management requires close cooperation among primary physician, therapist, rheumatologist, and orthopedist.
• Patient education is important.

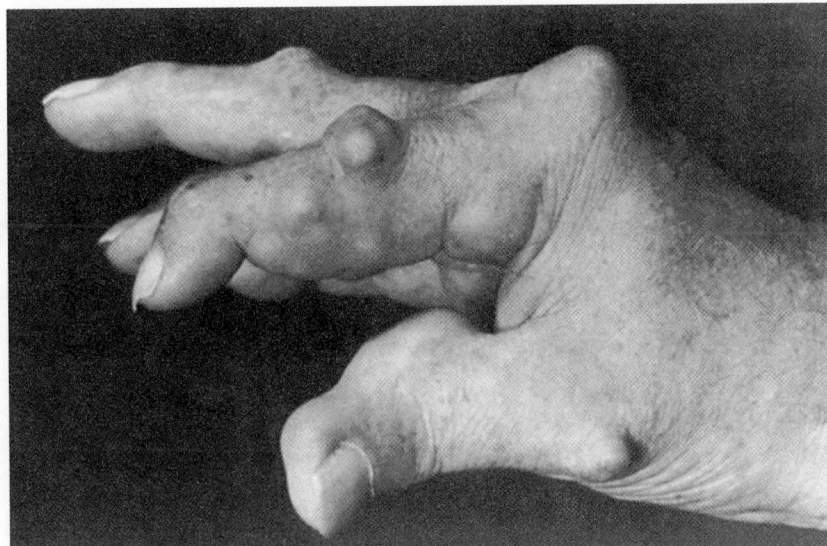

Fig. 1-30 Rheumatoid arthritis. Hand of a 60-year-old man with seropositive rheumatoid arthritis. There are fixed deformities and gross rheumatoid nodules. (From Canoso JJ: *Rheumatology in primary care,* Philadelphia, 1997, WB Saunders.)

- Rest with proper exercise and splinting can prevent or correct joint deformities.
- Maintain proper diet and control obesity.

CHRONIC Rx

- NSAIDs: commonly used as the initial treatment to relieve inflammation (drug of choice for most patients: aspirin, but other NSAIDs also effective)
- Disease-modifying drugs (DMARDs): are traditionally begun when NSAIDs are not effective; current recommendations favor early aggressive treatment with DMARDs, seeking to minimize long-term joint damage. Commonly used agents are methotrexate, cyclosporine, hydroxychloroquine, sulfasalazine, leflunomide, and infliximab. Most of these are associated with potential toxicity and require close monitoring. They are also usually slow-acting drugs that require more than 8 wk to become effective (see Table 1-10)
- Oral prednisone
- Intrasynovial steroid injections
- Etanercept (Enbrel), a tumor necrosis factor α-blocker, is indicated in moderately to severely active RA in patients who respond inadequately to DMARDs. The combination of etanercept and methotrexate has been reported to be effective and promising in the treatment of RA.

DISPOSITION

- Remissions and exacerbations are common, but condition is chronically progressive in the majority of cases.

- Joint degeneration and deformity often lead to disability.
- Early diagnosis and treatment are important and can improve quality of life.

REFERRAL

Early referral to rheumatologist
Orthopedic consultation for corrective surgery

REFERENCES

Chen AL, Joseph TN, Zuckerman JD: Rheumatoid arthritis of the shoulder, *J Am Acad Orthop Surg* 11:12, 2003.

Choy EHS, Panayi GS: Cytokine pathways and joint inflammation in rheumatoid arthritis, *N Engl J Med* 344:907, 2001.

Cohen S et al: Treatment of rheumatoid arthritis with anakinra, a recombinant human interleukin-1 receptor antagonist, in combination with methotrexate: results of a twenty-four-week, multicenter, randomized, double-blind, placebo controlled trial, *Arthritis Rheum* 46:614, 2002.

Dayer J-M, Bresnihan B: Targeting interleukin-1 in the treatment of rheumatoid arthritis, *Arthritis Rheum* 46:574, 2002.

Gardner GC, Kadel MJ: Ordering and interpreting rheumatologic laboratory tests, *J Am Acad Orthop Surg* 11:60, 2003.

Genovese MC et al: Etanercept versus methotrexate in patients with early rheumatoid arthritis: two-year radiographic and clinical outcomes, *Arthritis Rheum* 46:1443, 2002.

Kremer JM: Rational use of new and existing disease-modifying agents in rheumatoid arthritis, *Ann Intern Med* 134:695, 2001.

Lipsky PE et al: Infliximab and methotrexate in the treatment of rheumatoid arthritis, *N Engl J Med* 343:1594, 2000.

Matteson FL: Current treatment strategies for rheumatoid arthritis, *Mayo Clin Proc* 75:69, 2000.

Pincus T et al: Combination therapy with multiple disease-modifying antirheumatic drugs in rheumatoid arthritis: a preventive strategy, *Ann Intern Med* 131:768, 1999.

Pisetsky DS, St. Clair EW: Progress in the treatment of rheumatoid arthritis, *JAMA* 286:2787, 2001.

Smith JB, Haynes MK: Rheumatoid arthritis: a molecular understanding, *Ann Intern Med* 136:908, 2002.

Van Everdingen AA et al: Low dose prednisone therapy for patients with early active rheumatoid arthritis: clinical efficacy, disease-modifying properties, and side effects, *Ann Intern Med* 136:1, 2002.

Weinblatt ME et al: A trial of etanercept, a recombinant tumor necrosis factor receptor: Fe fusion protein, in patients with rheumatoid arthritis receiving methotrexate, *N Engl J Med* 340:253, 1999.

Author: **Lonnie R. Mercier, M.D.**

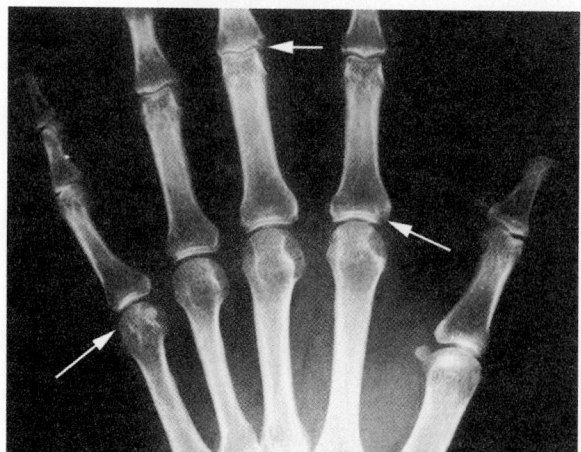
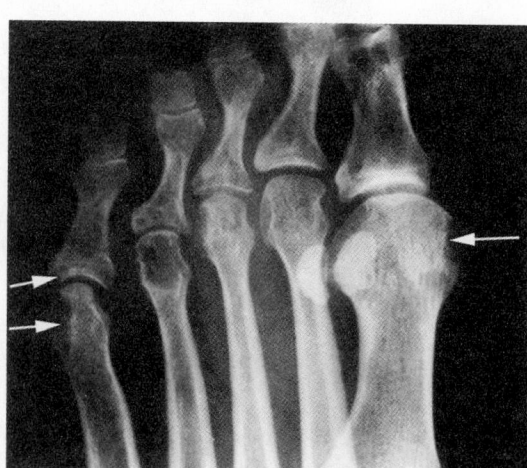

Fig. 1-31 **Rheumatoid arthritis. A,** Periarticular osteopenia and marginal erosions in MCPs and a PIP (*arrows*). **B,** In the same patient, marginal erosions at metatarsal heads. (From Canoso JJ [ed]: *Rheumatology in primary care,* Philadelphia, 1997, WB Saunders.)

TABLE 1-10   Selected Disease-Modifying Antirheumatic Drugs

TYPE/GENERIC (TRADE) NAME	RECOMMENDED DOSAGES	TOXIC EFFECTS	RECOMMENDED MONITORING
Gold compounds (Myochrysine)	IM: 10 mg followed by 25 mg 1 wk later, then 25-50 mg wkly until there is toxicity, major clinical improvement, or cumulative dose = 1 g. If effective, interval between doses is increased.	Pruritus, dermatitis (frequent—⅓ of pts), stomatitis, nephrotoxicity, blood dyscrasias, "nitritoid" reaction: flushing, weakness, nausea, dizziness 30 min after injection.	CBC, platelet count before every other injection. Urinalysis before each dose.
Aurothioglucose (Solganal)	IM: 10 mg; 2nd and 3rd doses 25 mg, 4th and subsequent 50 mg. Interval between doses: 1 wk. If improvement, no toxicity→decrease dose to 25 mg or increase interval between doses.	Dermatitis, stomatitis, nephrotoxicity, blood dyscrasias.	CBC, platelet count every 2 wk. Urinalysis before each dose.
Auranofin (Ridaura)	Oral: 3 mg bid or 6 mg qd. May increase to 3 mg tid after 6 months.	Loose stools, diarrhea (up to 50%), dermatitis.	Baseline CBC, platelet count, U/A, renal, liver function, at onset then CBC with platelet count, U/A 9 months.
Antimalarial Hydroxychloroquine (Plaquenil)	Oral: 400-600 mg qd with meals then 200-400 mg qd.	Retinopathy, dermatitis, muscle weakness, hypoactive DTRs, CNS.	Ophthalmologic examination every 3 months (visual acuity, slitlamp, funduscopic, visual field tests), neuromuscular examination.
Penicillamine (Cuprimine, Depen)	Oral: 125-250 mg qd, then increasing at monthly intervals doses to max 750-1000 mg by 125-250 mg.	Pruritus, rash/mouth ulcers, bone marrow depression, proteinuria, hematuria, hypogeusia, myesthenia, myositis, GI distress, pulmonary toxicity, teratogenic.	CBC every 2 weeks until dose stable, then every month. U/A weekly until dose stable, then every month. HCG as needed.
Methotrexate (Rheumatrex)	Oral: 7.5-15 mg weekly.	Pulmonary toxicity, ulcerative stomatitis, leukopenia, thrombocytopenia, GI distress, malaise, fatigue, chills, fever, CNS, elevated LFTs/liver disease, lymphoma, infection.	CBC with platelet count, LFTs weekly × 6 wk then monthly LFTs, U/A periodically, HCG as needed.
Azathioprine (Imuran)	Oral: 50-100 mg qd, increase at 4-wk intervals by 0.5 mg/kg/d up to 2.5 mg/kg/d.	Leukopenia, thrombocytopenia, GI, neoplastic if previous Rx with alkylating agents.	CBC with platelet count, wkly × 1 mo, 2×/mo. × 2 mo, then monthly, HCG as needed.
Sulfasalazine (Azulfidine)	Oral: 500 mg daily then increase up to 3 g daily.	GI, skin rash, pruritus, blood dyscrasias, oligospermia.	CBC, U/A q 2 wk × 3 mo, then monthly × 9 mo, then every 6 mo.
Alkylating agents Cyclophosphamide (Cytoxan)	Oral: 50-100 mg daily up to 2.5 mg/kg/d.	Leukopenia, thrombocytopenia, hematuria, GI, alopecia, rash, bladder cancer, non-Hodgkin's lymphoma, infection.	CBC with platelet count, regularly. HCG as needed.
Chlorambucil (Leukeran)	Oral: 0.1-0.2 mg/kg/d.	Bone marrow suppression, GI, CNS, infection.	CBC with platelet count every wk. WBCs 3-4 days after each CBC during 1st 3-6 wk at therapy. HCG as needed.
Cyclosporine (Sandimmune)	Oral 2.5-5 mg/kg/d.	Nephrotoxicity, tremor, hirsutism, hypertension, gum hyperplasia.	Renal function, liver function.
Pyrimidine, synthesis inhibitors Leflunomide (Arava)	Loading dose: 100 mg/d for 3 days. Maintenance therapy: 20 mg/d; if not tolerated, 10 mg/d.	Hepatotoxicity, carcinogenesis. Immunosuppression, long half-life.	LFTs every month, drug levels after discontinuation (after 1 month therapy, remains in blood for 2 years without use of cholestyramine).

From Rakel RE (ed): *Principles of family practice,* ed 6, Philadelphia, 2002, WB Saunders.
Bid, Twice a day; *CBC,* complete blood count; *CNS,* central nervous system; *DTR,* deep tendon reflex; *GI,* gastrointestinal; *HCG,* human chorionic gonadotropin; *IM,* intramuscular; *LFT,* liver function test; *qd,* every day; *tid,* three times a day; *U/A,* urinalysis; *WBC,* white blood cell count.

BASIC INFORMATION

■ **DEFINITION**
Asbestosis is a slowly progressive diffuse interstitial fibrosis resulting from dose-related inhalation exposure to fibers of asbestos.

ICD-9CM CODES
501 Asbestosis

■ **EPIDEMIOLOGY & DEMOGRAPHICS**
- In U.S.: 5 to 10 new cases/100,000 persons/yr
- Prolonged interval (20 to 30 yr) between exposures to inhaled fibers and clinical manifestations of disease
- Most common in workers involved in the primary extraction of asbestos from rock deposits and in those involved in the fabrication and installation of products containing asbestos (e.g., naval shipyards in World War II, installation of floor tiles, ceiling tiles, acoustic ceiling coverings, wall insulation, and pipe coverings in public buildings)

■ **PHYSICAL FINDINGS & CLINICAL PRESENTATION**
- Insidious onset of shortness of breath with exertion is usually the first sign of asbestosis.
- Dyspnea becomes more severe as the disease advances; with time, progressively less exertion is tolerated.
- Cough is frequent and usually paroxysmal, dry, and nonproductive.
- Scant mucoid sputum may accompany the cough in the later stages of the disease.

- Fine end respiratory crackles (rales, crepitations) are heard more predominantly in the lung bases.
- Digital clubbing, edema, jugular venous distention are present.

■ **ETIOLOGY**
Inhalation of asbestos fibers

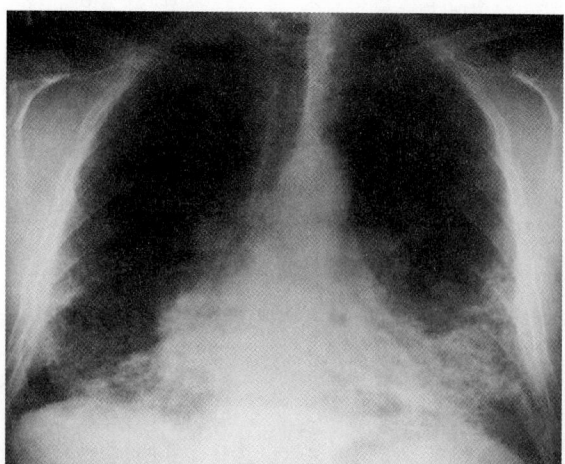 **DIAGNOSIS**

■ **DIFFERENTIAL DIAGNOSIS**
- Silicosis
- Siderosis, other pneumonoconioses
- Lung cancer
- Atelectasis

■ **WORKUP**
Documentation of exposure history, diagnostic imaging, pulmonary function testing

■ **LABORATORY TESTS**
- Generally not helpful
- Possible mild elevation of ESR, positive ANA and RF (These tests are nonspecific and do not correlate with disease severity or activity.)
- Pulmonary function testing: decreased vital capacity, decreased total lung capacity, decreased carbon monoxide gas transfer
- ABGs: hypoxemia, hypercarbia in advanced stages

■ **IMAGING STUDIES**
Chest x-ray examination (Fig. 1-32):
- Small, irregular shadows in lower lung zones
- Thickened pleural, calcified plaques (present under diaphragms and lateral chest wall)
CT scan of chest confirms the diagnosis.

TREATMENT

■ **NONPHARMACOLOGIC THERAPY**
- Smoking cessation, proper nutrition, exercise program to maximize available lung function
- Home oxygen therapy prn
- Removal of patient from further asbestos fiber exposure

■ **GENERAL Rx**
- Prompt identification and treatment of respiratory infections
- Supplemental oxygen on a prn basis
- Annual influenza vaccination, pneumococcal vaccination

■ **DISPOSITION**
- There is no specific treatment for asbestosis.
- Death is usually secondary to respiratory failure from cor pulmonale.
- Patients with asbestosis have increased risk for mesotheliomas, lung cancer, and TB. Recent reports indicate that the risk of asbestos-induced lung cancer may be overestimated.
- Survival in patients following development of mesothelioma is 4 to 6 yr.

■ **REFERRAL**
To pulmonologist initially

PEARLS & CONSIDERATIONS

■ **COMMENTS**
Patient information on asbestosis can be obtained from the American Lung Association, 1740 Broadway, New York, NY 10019.

REFERENCE
Camus M et al: Nonoccupational exposure to chrysotile asbestos and the risk of lung cancer, *N Engl J Med* 338:1565, 1998.
Author: **Fred F. Ferri, M.D.**

Fig. 1-32   Asbestosis. PA radiograph shows coarse linear opacities at both lung bases obscuring the cardiac borders. (From McLoud TC: *Thoracic radiology: the requisites,* St Louis, 1998, Mosby.)

BASIC INFORMATION

■ DEFINITION

Ascariasis is a parasitic infection caused by the nematode *Ascaris lumbricoides*. The majority of those infected are asymptomatic; however, clinical disease may arise from pulmonary hypersensitivity, intestinal obstruction, and secondary complications.

ICD-9CM CODES
127.0 Ascariasis

■ EPIDEMIOLOGY & DEMOGRAPHICS
INCIDENCE (IN U.S.):
• Unknown
• Three times the infection rates found in blacks as in whites
PREVALENCE (IN U.S.): Estimated at 4,000,000, the majority of which live in the rural southeastern part of the country
PREDOMINANT SEX: Both sexes probably equally affected, with a possible slight female preponderance
PREDOMINANT AGE: Most common in children, with estimated mean age of approximately 5 yr based on surveys in highly endemic areas
PEAK INCIDENCE: Unknown
NEONATAL INFECTION: Probable transmission, though not specifically studied

■ PHYSICAL FINDINGS & CLINICAL PRESENTATION
• Occurs approximately 9 to 12 days after ingestion of eggs (corresponding to the larva migration through the lungs)
• Nonproductive cough
• Substernal chest discomfort
• Fever
• In patients with large worm burdens, especially children, intestinal obstruction associated with perforation, volvulus, and intussusception
• Migration of worms into the biliary tree giving clinical appearance of biliary colic and pancreatitis as well as acute appendicitis with movement into that appendage
• Rarely, infection with *A. lumbricoides* producing interstitial nephritis and acute renal failure
• In endemic areas in Asia and Africa, malabsorption of dietary proteins and vitamins as a consequence of chronic worm intestinal carriage

■ ETIOLOGY
• Transmission is usually hand to mouth, but eggs may be ingested via transported vegetables grown in contaminated soil.
• Eggs are hatched in the small intestine, with larvae penetrating intestinal mucosa and migrating via the circulation to the lungs.
• Larval forms proceed through the alveoli, ascend the bronchial tree, and return to the intestines after swallowing, where they mature into adult worms.
• Estimated time until the female adult worm to begin producing eggs is 2 to 3 mo.
• Eggs are passed out of the intestines with feces.
• Within human host, adult worm lifespan is 1 to 2 yr.

DIAGNOSIS

■ DIFFERENTIAL DIAGNOSIS
• Radiologic manifestations and eosinophilia to be distinguished from drug hypersensitivity and Löffler's syndrome
• The differential diagnosis of intestinal helminths is described in Section II

■ LABORATORY TESTS
• Examination of the stool for *Ascaris* ova
• Expectoration or fecal passage of adult worm
• Eosinophilia: most prominent early in the infection and subsides as the adult worm infestation established in the intestines
• Anti-ascaris IgG4 blood levels by ELISA is a sensitive and specific marker of infection and may be useful in the evaluation of treatment
• Malondialdehyde levels clearly increase in patients infected with *A. lumbricoides*

■ IMAGING STUDIES
• Chest x-ray examination to reveal bilateral oval or round infiltrates of varying size (Löffler's syndrome); NOTE: infiltrates are transient and eventually resolve.
• Plain films of the abdomen and contrast studies to reveal worm masses in loops of bowel
• Ultrasonography and endoscopic retrograde cholangiopancreatography (ERCP) to identify worms in the pancreaticobiliary tract

TREATMENT

■ NONPHARMACOLOGIC THERAPY
Aggressive IV hydration, especially in children with fever, severe vomiting, and resultant dehydration

■ ACUTE GENERAL Rx
• Mebendazole (Vermox)
  1. Drug of choice for intestinal infection with *A. lumbricoides*
  2. 100 mg PO tid given for 3 days
• Albendazole, given as a single 400-mg dose PO
• Both mebendazole and albendazole are contraindicated in pregnancy.
• Pyrantel pamoate (Antiminth)
  1. Given at a dose of 11 mg/kg PO (maximum dose of 1 g/day)
  2. Considered safe for use in pregnant women
• Piperazine citrate
  1. Recommended in cases of intestinal or biliary obstruction
  2. Administered as a syrup, given via nasogastric tube, a 150 mg/kg loading dose, followed by six doses of 65 mg/kg q12h
  3. Considered safe in pregnancy, but cannot be given concurrently with chlorpromazine
• Complete obstruction should be managed surgically.

■ DISPOSITION
Overall prognosis is good.

■ REFERRAL
• To gastroenterologist in cases of visualized pancreaticobiliary tract or appendiceal obstruction
• To surgeon in cases of complete obstruction or suspected secondary complication (e.g., perforation or volvulus)

PEARLS & CONSIDERATIONS

■ COMMENTS
• Hepatic abscess, containing both viable and dead worms, complicating *Ascaris*-induced biliary duct disease has been documented.
• Given the known transmission of the parasite, routine hand washing and proper disposal of human waste would significantly decrease the prevalence of this disease.

REFERENCES

Amjad N et al: An unusual presentation of acute cholecystitis: biliary ascariasis *Hosp Med* 62(6):370, 2001.

Kilic E et al: Serum malondialdehyde level in patients infected with *Ascaris lumbricoides, World J Gastroenterol* 9(10):2332, 2003.

Rodriguez EJ et al: Ascariasis causing small bowel volvulus, *Radiographics* 23(5):1291, 2003.

Sangkhathat S et al: Massive gastrointestinal bleeding in infants with ascariasis, *J Pediatr Surg* 38(11):1696, 2003.

Santra A et al: Serodiagnosis of ascariasis with specific IgG4 antibody and its use in an epidemiological study, *Trans R Soc Trop Med Hyg* 95(3):289, 2001.

BASIC INFORMATION

■ DEFINITION
Cell death in components of bone: hematopoietic fat marrow and mineralized tissue.

■ SYNONYMS
Osteonecrosis, avascular necrosis

ICD-9CM CODES
733.40 Aseptic necrosis
733.43 Aseptic necrosis of femoral condyle
733.42 Aseptic necrosis of femoral head
733.41 Aseptic necrosis of humeral head
733.44 Aseptic necrosis of talus

■ EPIDEMIOLOGY & DEMOGRAPHICS
- 15,000 new cases per year in the U.S.
- Associated conditions:
  1. Corticosteroid treatment: 35%
  2. Alcohol abuse: 22%
  3. Idiopathic and other: 43%
- Common sites involved
  1. Femoral head
  2. Femoral condyle
  3. Humeral head
  4. Navicular and lunate wrist bones
  5. Talus

■ PHYSICAL FINDINGS & CLINICAL PRESENTATION
- May be asymptomatic
- Pain in the involved area exacerbated by movement or weight bearing

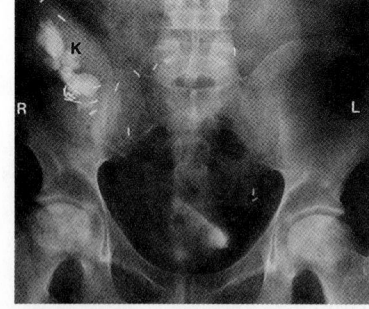

- Decreased range of motion as the disease progresses
- Functional limitation

■ ETIOLOGY
Final common pathway of conditions that lead to impairment of the blood supply to the involved bone.
Stages:
Stage 0
- Asymptomatic
- Normal imaging
- Histologic findings only (i.e., silent osteonecrosis)
Stage 1
- Asymptomatic or symptomatic
- Normal x-ray and CT scan
- Abnormal bone scan and/or MRI
Stage 2
- Abnormal x-rays and/or CT scan including linear sclerosis, focal bead mineralization, cysts; however, the overall architecture of the involved bone is normal
Stage 3
- Early evidence of mechanical bone failure (subchondral fracture), but the overall shape of the bone is still intact
Stage 4
- Flattening or collapse of the bone
Stage 5
- Joint space narrowing
Stage 6
- Extensive joint destruction

DIAGNOSIS

■ DIFFERENTIAL DIAGNOSIS
- None in late stages
- Early: any condition causing focal musculoskeletal pain including arthritis, bursitis, tendinitis, myopathy, neoplastic bone and joint diseases, traumatic injuries, pathologic fractures

■ IMAGING STUDIES See Fig. 1-33.
1. X-ray: insensitive early in the course. The earliest changes include diffuse osteopenia, areas of radiolucency with sclerotic border, and linear sclerosis. Later a subchondral lucency (crescent sign) indicates subchondral fracture. More advanced cases reveal flattening, collapsed bone and abnormal bone contour. In late disease, osteoarthritic changes are seen.
2. Bone scan:
- Early: "cold" area
- Later: increased radionuclide uptake as a result of remodeling
- Sensitivity in early disease is only 70% and specificity is poor
3. CT scan: may reveal central necrosis and area of collapse before those are visible in x-ray.
4. MRI: the most sensitive technology to diagnose early aseptic necrosis. The first sign is a margin of low signal. An inner border of high signal associated with a low-signal line is specific of aseptic necrosis ("double line sign"). Sensitivity is 75%-100%.

TREATMENT

■ PREVENTION
- Management of etiologic conditions
- Minimize corticosteroid use

■ MEDICAL TREATMENT
- Decrease weight bearing of affected area
- Pulsing electromagnetic fields applied externally (still experimental)
- Peripheral vasodilators (e.g., dihydrogotamine) (unproven)

■ SURGICAL TREATMENT
- Core decompression: effectiveness 35%-95% in early phases
- Bone grafting
- Osteotomies
- Joint replacement

■ PROGNOSIS
- When diagnosed at an early stage treatment is appropriate in all cases because 85%-90% can be expected to progress to a more advanced stage
- Contralateral joint involvement is common (30%-70%)

REFERENCE
Mazieres R: *Osteonecrosis:* In Klippel JH, Dieppe PA (eds): *Rhematology,* ed 2, St. Louis, 1998, Mosby.
Author: **Tom J. Wachtel**

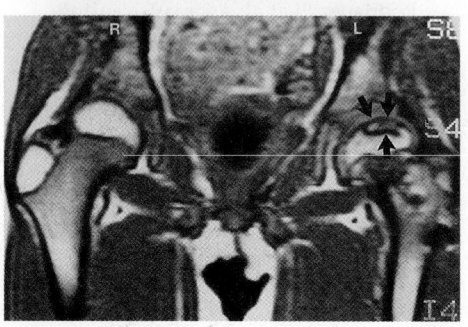

Fig. 1-33   Aseptic necrosis of the hips. A, Aseptic necrosis can occur from a number of causes, including trauma and steroid use. In this patient, an anteroposterior view of the pelvis shows a transplanted kidney (K) in the right iliac fossa. Use of steroids has caused this patient to have bilateral aseptic necrosis. The femoral heads are somewhat flattened, irregular, and increased in density. **B,** Aseptic necrosis in a different patient is demonstrated on a MRI scan as an area of decreased signal (*arrows*) in the left femoral head. This is the most sensitive method for detection of early aseptic necrosis. (From Mettler FA [ed]: *Primary care radiology,* Philadelphia, 2000, WB Saunders).

BASIC INFORMATION

■ DEFINITION

Aspergillosis refers to several forms of a broad range of illnesses caused by infection with *Aspergillus* species.

ICD-9CM CODES
117.3 Aspergillosis
117.3 Aspergillosis with pneumonia
117.3 *Aspergillus (flavus) (fumigatus)* (infection) *(terreus)*

■ EPIDEMIOLOGY & DEMOGRAPHICS

- *Aspergillus* species are ubiquitous in the environment internationally and occur as a mold found in soil
- Cause a variety of illness from hypersensitivity pneumonitis to disseminated overwhelming infection in immunosuppressed patients
- Incidence of invasive aspergillosis is increasing with advances in the treatment of life threatening diseases: aggressive chemotherapy; bone marrow and organ transplantation
- Frequently cultured from samples obtained in hospital wards from unfiltered outside air circulating through open windows
- Reaches the patient by airborne conidia (spores) that are small enough (2.5 to 3 μm) to reach the alveoli on inhalation
- Can also invade the nose and paranasal sinuses, external ear, or traumatized skin
- The clinical syndrome and pathologic spectrum of *Aspergillus* lung disease is dependent on the underlying lung architecture, the host's immune response, and the degree of inoculum.

■ ETIOLOGY

- *Aspergillus fumigatus* is the usual cause.
- *A. flavus* is the second most important species, particularly in invasive disease of immunosuppressed patients and in lesions beginning in the nose and paranasal sinuses.

ALLERGIC ASPERGILLOSIS:
- Represents a hypersensitivity pneumonitis
- Presents as cough, dyspnea, fever, chills, and malaise typically 4 to 8 hr after exposure
- Repeated attacks can lead to granulomatous disease and pulmonary fibrosis

ALLERGIC BRONCHOPULMONARY ASPERGILLOSIS (ABPA):
- Symptoms occur most commonly in atopic individuals during the third and fourth decades of life
- Hypersensitivity reaction of the airways to *Aspergillus* fungal antigens present in the bronchial tree
- Results from an initial type I (immediate hypersensitivity) and a type III reaction (immune complexes), which is most likely responsible for the roentgenographic features and more destructive changes of the bronchi
- Underdiagnosed pulmonary disorder in patients with asthma and cystic fibrosis

ASPERGILLOMAS ("FUNGUS BALLS"):
- In the absence of invasion or significant immune response, *Aspergillus* can colonize a preexisting cavity, causing pulmonary aspergilloma
- Forms masses of tangled hyphal elements, fibrin, and mucus
- Patients typically have a history of chronic lung disease, tuberculosis, sarcoidosis, or emphysema
- Manifests commonly as hemoptysis: blood-streaked sputum to active bleeding necessitating surgical reaction
- Many are asymptomatic

INVASIVE ASPERGILLOSIS:
- Patients with prolonged and profound granulocytopenia are predisposed to rapidly progressive *Aspergillus* pneumonia
- Lungs typically manifest a necrotizing bronchopneumonia, ranging from small areas of infiltrate to intensive bilateral hemorrhagic infarction
- Most common presentation is that of unremitting fever and a new pulmonary infiltrate despite broad-spectrum antibiotic therapy in an immunosuppressed patient
- Dyspnea and nonproductive cough are common; sudden pleuritic pain and tachycardia, sometimes with a pleural rub, may mimic pulmonary embolism; hemoptysis is uncommon

- Roentgenograms may reveal patchy bronchopneumonic, nodular densities, consolidation, or cavitation
- Immunocompromised patients: invasive pulmonary *Aspergillus* (IPA) generally is acute and evolves over days to weeks; less commonly, patients with normal or only mild abnormalities of their immune systems may develop a more chronic, slowly progressive form of IPA

EXTRAPULMONARY DISSEMINATION:
- Cerebral infarction from hematogenous dissemination may occur in immunosuppressed individuals
- Abscess formation may occur from direct extension of invasive disease in the sinuses
- Esophageal or gastrointestinal ulcerations caused by *Aspergillus* may occur in the immunosuppressed host
- Fatal perforation of the viscus or bowel infarction may occur
- Necrotizing skin ulcers involving the extremities (Fig. 1-34)
- Osteomyelitis
- Endocarditis

Patients with AIDS and a CD4 count of below 50 mm³ have increased susceptibility to invasive aspergillosis.

DIAGNOSIS

■ DIFFERENTIAL DIAGNOSIS
- Tuberculosis
- Cystic fibrosis
- Carcinoma of the lung
- Eosinophilic pneumonia
- Bronchiectasis
- Sarcoidosis
- Lung abscess

■ WORKUP
Physical examination and laboratory evaluation

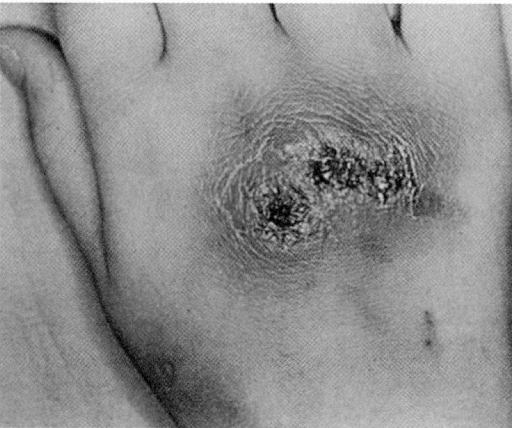

Fig. 1-34 Cutaneous aspergillosis in a patient with acute leukemia and marked neutropenia. The lesion developed at the site where a steel needle had been left for several days of intravenous infusion. (From Mandell GL [ed]: *Mandell, Douglas, and Bennett's principles and practice of infectious diseases*, ed 5, New York, 2000, Churchill Livingstone.)

■ LABORATORY TESTS
ALLERGIC BRONCHOPULMONARY ASPERGILLOSIS:
1. Peripheral blood eosinophilia and an elevated total serum IgE level
2. Skin test with *Aspergillus* antigenic extract usually is positive but is nonspecific
3. *Aspergillus* serum precipitating antibody is present in 70% to 100% of cases
4. Sputum cultures may be positive for *Aspergillus* spp. but are nonspecific

ASPERGILLOMAS:
1. Sputum culture
2. Serum precipitating antibody

INVASIVE ASPERGILLOSIS: Definitive diagnosis requires the demonstration of tissue invasion as seen on a biopsy specimen (i.e., septate, acute branching hyphae) or a positive culture from the tissue obtained by an invasive procedure such as transbronchial biopsy.
1. Sputum and nasal cultures: in high-risk patients a positive culture is strongly suggestive of invasive aspergillosis.
2. Serologic studies not helpful, rarely elevated in patients with invasive disease
3. Blood cultures: usually negative
4. Lung biopsy is necessary for definitive diagnosis
5. Biopsy and culture of extrapulmonary lesions

■ IMAGING STUDIES
ALLERGIC BRONCHOPULMONARY ASPERGILLOSIS:
- Chest roentgenograms show a variety of abnormalities from small, patchy, fleeting infiltrates (commonly in the upper lobes) to lobar consolidation and/or cavitation
- A majority of patients eventually develop central bronchiectasis

ASPERGILLOMAS: Chest roentgenograms or CT scans usually show the characteristic intracavity mass partially surrounded by a crescent of air (Fig. 1-35).

INVASIVE ASPERGILLOSIS: Chest roentgenograms and CT scanning may reveal cavity formation.

℞ TREATMENT

■ ACUTE GENERAL Rx
ALLERGIC BRONCHOPULMONARY ASPERGILLOSIS:
- Prednisone (0.5 to 1 mg/kg PO) until the chest roentgenogram has cleared, followed by alternate-day therapy at 0.5 mg/kg PO (3 to 6 mo)
- If a patient is corticosteroid dependent, prophylaxis for the prevention of *Pneumocystis carinii* infection and maintenance of bone mineralization should be considered

- Bronchodilators and physiotherapy
- Serial chest roentgenograms and serum IgE useful in guiding treatment
- Itraconazole 200 mg po bid for 4 to 6 mo, then taper over 4 to 6 mo; may be considered as a corticosteroid spanning agent or if corticosteroids are ineffective

ASPERGILLOMAS:
- Controversial and problematic
- Up to 10% of aspergillomas may resolve clinically without overt pharmacologic or surgical intervention
- Observation for asymptomatic patients
- Surgical resection/arterial embolization for those patients with severe hemoptysis or life-threatening hemorrhage
- For those patients at risk for marked hemoptysis with inadequate pulmonary reserve, consider itraconazole 200 to 400 mg/day PO

INVASIVE ASPERGILLOSIS:
- Amphotericin B deoxycholate 0.8 to 1.2 mg/kg IV qd to a total dose of 2 to 2.5 g; itraconazole 200 to 400 mg/d PO for 1 yr
- Amphotericin B lipid complex (ABLC) 5 mg/kg IV qd in those intolerant of or refractory to amphotericin B
- Amphotericin B colloidal dispersion (ABCD) 3 to 6 mg/kg IV qd; stepwise approach in those who have failed amphotericin B
- Liposomal amphotericin B (L-AMB) 3 to 5 mg/kg IV q day; stepwise approach is indicated as empiric therapy for presumed fungal infection in febrile neutropenic patients who are refractory to or intolerant of amphotericin B
- Itraconazole 200 mg IV bid × 4 doses followed by 200 mg IV qd or 200 mg tid for 4 days, then 200 mg bid PO—first-line therapy if not taking p450 inducers.

- Voriconazole 6 mg/kg IV bid followed by 6 mg/kg IV for up to 27 days, then 400 mg/day PO for up to 24 wk. Note that the optimal dose regimens have yet to be defined Posaconazole and Ravuconazole are two new azoles that are currently under investigation
- Caspofungins (Candigas) is the first of a new class of antifungals, the echinocandins approved by the FDA for the treatment of invasive aspergillosis in patients who fail to respond to or are unable to tolerate other antifungal drugs. The recommended dosage is 70 mg on the first day and 50 mg daily thereafter, given as a single dose IV over 1 hr. The two other echinocandins under investigation are micafungin and anidulafungin
Cytokine therapy may offer future treatment options in conjunction with the currently available antifungals

■ REFERRAL
Consultation with an infectious diseases specialist is highly recommended.

REFERENCES
Ferry TG, Yates RR: Aspergillomas: should we treat them all? *Infect Dis Clin Pract* 7:122, 1998.

Herbrecht R et al: Voriconazole versus amphotericin B for primary therapy of invasive aspergillosis, *N Engl J Med* 347:408, 2002.

Steinbach WJ, Stevens DA: Review of newer antifungal and immunomodulatory strategies for invasive aspergillosis, *Clin Infect Dis* 37(Supp 3):S 157, 2003.

Vlaharis N, Ausamit T: Diagnosis and treatment of allergic bronchopulmonary aspergillosis, *Mayo Clinic Proc* 76:30, 2001.

Author: **Sajeev Handa, M.D.**

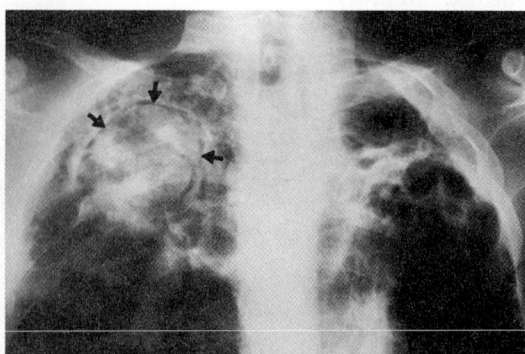

Fig. 1-35 Fungus ball or mycetoma caused by Aspergillus. Coned-down PA view of the chest of a patient with biapical fibrocavitary tuberculosis accompanied by volume loss. There is a mass in a large right upper-lobe cavity with air dissecting into the cavity producing "air crescents" (*arrows*). (From McLoud TC: *Thoracic radiology: the requisites,* St Louis, 1998, Mosby.)

BASIC INFORMATION

DEFINITION

The American Thoracic Society defines asthma as a "disease characterized by an increased responsiveness of the trachea and bronchi to various stimuli and manifested by a widespread narrowing of the airways that changes in severity either spontaneously or as a result of treatment." *Status asthmaticus* can be defined as a severe continuous bronchospasm.

SYNONYMS

Bronchospasm
Reactive airway disease
Bronchial asthma

ICD-9CM CODES

493.9 Asthma, unspecified
493.1 Intrinsic asthma
493.0 Extrinsic asthma

EPIDEMIOLOGY & DEMOGRAPHICS

- Asthma affects 5% of the population.
- It is more common in children (10% of children, 5% of adults).
- 50% to 80% of children with asthma develop symptoms before 5 yr of age.
- Overall asthma mortality in the U.S. is 20 per 1 million persons.

PHYSICAL FINDINGS & CLINICAL PRESENTATION

Physical examination varies with the stage and severity of asthma and may reveal only increased inspiratory and expiratory phases of respiration. Physical examination during status asthmaticus may reveal:
- Tachycardia and tachypnea
- Use of accessory respiratory muscles
- Pulsus paradoxus (inspiratory decline in systolic blood pressure >10 mm Hg)
- Wheezing: absence of wheezing (silent chest) or decreased wheezing can indicate worsening obstruction
- Mental status changes: generally secondary to hypoxia and hypercapnia and constitute an indication for urgent intubation
- Paradoxic abdominal and diaphragmatic movement on inspiration (detected by palpation over the upper part of the abdomen in a semirecumbent position): important sign of impending respiratory crisis, indicates diaphragmatic fatigue

- The following abnormalities in vital signs are indicative of severe asthma:
  1. Pulsus paradoxus >18 mm Hg
  2. Respiratory rate >30 breaths/min
  3. Tachycardia with heart rate >120 beats/min

ETIOLOGY

- Intrinsic asthma: occurs in patients who have no history of allergies; may be triggered by upper respiratory infections or psychologic stress
- Extrinsic asthma (allergic asthma): brought on by exposure to allergens (e.g., dust mites, cat allergen, industrial chemicals)
- Exercise-induced asthma: seen most frequently in adolescents; manifests with bronchospasm following initiation of exercise and improves with discontinuation of exercise
- Drug-induced asthma: often associated with use of NSAIDs, β-blockers, sulfites, certain foods and beverages
- There is a strong association of the ADAM 33 gene with asthma and bronchial hyperresponsiveness

DIAGNOSIS

DIFFERENTIAL DIAGNOSIS

- CHF
- COPD
- Pulmonary embolism (in adult and elderly patients)
- Foreign body aspiration (most frequent in younger patients)
- Pneumonia and other upper respiratory infections
- Rhinitis with postnasal drip
- TB
- Hypersensitivity pneumonitis
- Anxiety disorder
- Wegener's granulomatosis
- Diffuse interstitial lung disease

WORKUP

Medical history, physical examination, pulmonary function studies and peak flow meter determination, blood gas analysis and oximetry (during acute bronchospasm), chest radiography if infection is suspected

LABORATORY TESTS

Laboratory tests can be normal if obtained during a stable period. The following laboratory abnormalities may be present during an acute bronchospasm:
- ABGs can be used in staging the severity of an asthmatic attack:
Mild: decreased Pao_2 and $Paco_2$, increased pH
Moderate: decreased Pao_2, normal $Paco_2$, normal pH
Severe: marked decreased Pao_2, increased $Paco_2$, and decreased pH
- CBC, leukocytosis with "left shift" may indicate the existence of bacterial infection.
- Sputum: eosinophils, Charcot-Leyden crystals, PMNs, and bacteria may be found on Gram stain in patients with pneumonia.
- Useful diagnostic tests for asthma:
  1. Pulmonary function studies: during acute severe bronchospasm, FEV_1 is <1 L and peak expiratory flow rate (PEFR) <80 L/min
  2. Methacholine challenge test
  3. Skin test: to assess the role of atopy (when suspected)

IMAGING STUDIES

- Chest x-ray: usually normal, may show evidence of thoracic hyperinflation (e.g., flattening of the diaphragm, increased volume over the retrosternal air space)
- ECG: tachycardia, nonspecific ST-T wave changes are common during an asthmatic attack; may also show cor pulmonale, right bundle-branch block, right axial deviation, counterclockwise rotation

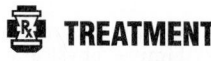 **TREATMENT**

NONPHARMACOLOGIC THERAPY

- Avoidance of triggering factors (e.g., salicylates, sulfites)
- Encouragement of regular exercise (e.g., swimming)
- Patient education regarding warning signs of an attack and proper use of medications (e.g., correct use of inhalers)

■ **ACUTE GENERAL Rx**

The Expert Panel of the National Asthma Education and Prevention Program (NAEPP) based on the classification of asthma severity (Table 1-11) recommends the following stepwise approach in the pharmacologic management of asthma in adults and children older than 5 yr:

STEP 1 (MILD INTERMITTENT ASTHMA): No daily medications are needed.

- Short-acting inhaled β_2-agonists as needed (e.g., albuterol [Ventolin, Proventil], terbutaline [Brethaire], bitolterol [Tornalate], pirbuterol [Maxair])

STEP 2 (MILD PERSISTENT ASTHMA): Daily treatment may be needed.

- Low-dose inhaled corticosteroid (e.g., beclomethasone [Beclovent, Vanceril], flunisolide [AeroBid], triamcinolone [Azmacort]) can be used.
- Cromolyn (Intal) or nedocromil (Tilade) can also be used.
- Additional considerations for long-term control are the use of the leukotriene receptor antagonist montelukast (Singulair).
- Quick relief of asthma can be achieved with short-acting inhaled β_2-agonists (see Step 1).

STEP 3 (MODERATE PERSISTENT ASTHMA): Daily medication is recommended.

- Low-dose or medium-dose inhaled corticosteroids (see Step 2) plus long-acting inhaled β_2-agonist (salmeterol [Serevent]), or long-acting oral β_2-agonists (e.g., albuterol, sustained-release tablets). Salmeterol is also available as a dry powder inhaler (Discus) that does not require a spacer device; the dosage is one puff bid. A salmeterol-fluticasone combination for the Discus inhaler (Advair) is now available and simplifies therapy for patients with asthma. It generally should be reserved for patients with at least moderately severe asthma not controlled by an inhaled corticosteroid alone.
- Use short-acting inhaled β-agonists on a prn basis for quick relief.

STEP 4 (SEVERE PERSISTENT ASTHMA):

- Daily treatment with high-dose inhaled corticosteroids plus long-acting inhaled β_2-agonists (e.g., long-acting oral β_2-agonist plus long-term systemic corticosteroids (e.g., methylprednisolone, prednisolone, prednisone) can be used.
- Short-acting β_2-agonists can be used on a prn basis for quick relief.

Treatment of *status asthmaticus* is as follows:

- Oxygen generally started at 2 to 4 L/min via nasal cannula or Venti-Mask at 40% Fio_2; further adjustments are made according to the ABGs.
- Bronchodilators: various agents and modalities are available. Inhaled bronchodilators are preferred when they can be administered quickly. Parenteral administration of sympathomimetics (e.g. SC epinephrine) when necessary should be accompanied by electrocardiographic monitoring.
- Albuterol (Proventil, Ventolin): 0.5 to 1 ml (2.5 to 5 mg) in 3 ml of saline solution tid or qid via nebulizer is effective.
- Corticosteroids
  1. Early administration is advised, particularly in patients using steroids at home.

TABLE 1-11   Classification of Asthma Severity

CLINICAL FEATURES BEFORE TREATMENT*	SYMPTOMS†	NIGHTTIME SYMPTOMS	LUNG FUNCTION
Step 4			
Severe Persistent	Continual symptoms Limited physical activity Frequent exacerbations	Frequent	■ FEV_1 or PEFR ≤60% predicted ■ PEFR variability >30%
Step 3			
Moderate Persistent	Daily symptoms Daily use of inhaled short-acting β_2-agonist Exacerbations affect activity Exacerbations ≥2 times a week; may last days	>1 time a week	■ FEV_1 or PEFR >60%-<80% predicted ■ PEFR variability >30%
Step 2			
Mild Persistent	Symptoms >2 times a week but <1 time a day Exacerbations may affect activity	>2 times a month	■ FEV_1 or PEFR ≥80% predicted ■ PEFR variability 20%-30%
Step 1			
Mild Intermittent	Symptoms ≤2 times a week Asymptomatic and normal PEFR between exacerbations Exacerbations brief (from a few hours to a few days); intensity may vary	≤2 times a month	■ FEV_1 or PEFR ≥80% predicted ■ PEFR variability <20%

Modified from National Asthma Education and Prevention Program, National Heart, Lung, and Blood Institute, Expert Panel Report 2: *Guidelines for the diagnosis and management of asthma.* Washington, DC, NIH Pub No 97-4051, July 1997.
*The presence of one of the features of severity is sufficient to place a patient in that category. An individual should be assigned to the most severe grade in which any feature occurs. The characteristics noted in this figure are general and may overlap because asthma is highly variable. Furthermore, an individual's classification may change over time.
†Patients at any level of severity can have mild, moderate, or severe exacerbations. Some patients with intermittent asthma experience severe and life-threatening exacerbations separated by long periods of normal lung function and no symptoms.
PEFR, Peak expiratory flow rate.

2. Patients may be started on hydro-cortisone (Solu-Cortef) 2.5 to 4 mg/kg or methylprednisolone (Solu-Medrol) 0.5 to 1 mg/kg IV loading dose, then q6h prn; higher doses may be necessary in selected patients (particularly those receiving steroids at home); steroids given by inhalation (e.g., beclomethasone 2 inhalations qid, maximum 20 inhalations/day) are also useful for controlling bronchospasm and tapering oral steroids and should be used in all patients with severe asthma.

3. Rapid but judicious tapering of corticosteroids will eliminate serious steroid toxicity; long-term low-dose methotrexate may be an effective means of reducing the systemic corticosteroid requirement in some patients with severe refractory asthma.

4. The most common errors regarding steroid therapy in acute bronchospasms are the use of "too little, too late" and too rapid tapering with return of bronchospasm.

- IV hydration: judicious use is necessary to avoid CHF in elderly patients.
- IV antibiotics are indicated when there is suspicion of bacterial infection (e.g., infiltrate on chest x-ray, fever, or leukocytosis).
- Intubation and mechanical ventilation are indicated when previous measures fail to produce significant improvement.
- General anesthesia: halothane may reverse bronchospasm in a severe asthmatic who cannot be ventilated adequately by mechanical means.
- IV magnesium sulfate supplementation in children with low or borderline-low magnesium levels may improve acute bronchospasm. Several reports in recent literature point to the beneficial effect on bronchospasm with a 20-min infusion of 40 mg/kg, up to a maximum of 2 g of magnesium sulfate in patients with acute asthma attack.

■ REFERRAL
Box 1-5 describes indications for referral to an asthma specialist.

REFERENCES
Braun-Fahrlander C et al: Environmental exposure to endotoxin and its relation to asthma in school-age children, *N Engl J Med* 347:869, 2002.

Ciarallo L et al: Higher dose IV magnesium therapy for children with moderate to severe acute asthma, *Arch Pediatr Adol Med* 154:979, 2000.

Diette GB et al: Asthma in older patients: factors associated with hospitalization, *Arch Intern Med* 162:1123, 2002.

Holgate ST: Therapeutic options for persistent asthma, *JAMA* 285:2637, 2001.

National Asthma Education and Prevention Program: *Expert panel report 2: guidelines for diagnosis and management of asthma*, Bethesda, Md, 1997, National Institutes of Health.

National Asthma Education and Prevention Program (NAEPP): Expert panel report: guidelines for the diagnosis and management of asthma—update on selected topics 2002, *J Allergy Clin Immunol* 110(suppl 5):5161, 2002.

Naureckas ET, Solway J: Mild asthma, *N Engl J Med* 345:1257, 2001.

Wood RA: Pediatric asthma, *JAMA* 288:745, 2002.

Author: **Fred F. Ferri, M.D.**

BOX 1-5   Possible Indications for Referral to an Asthma Specialist

Severe, acute asthma that has caused loss of consciousness, hypoxia, respiratory failure, convulsions, or near death

Poorly controlled asthma as indicated by admission to a hospital, frequent need for emergency care, need for oral corticosteroids, absence from school or work, disruption of sleep, interference with quality of life

Severe, persistent asthma requiring step 4 care (consider for patients who require step 3 care)

Patient less than 3 years old who requires step 3 or 4 care (consider for patient less than 3 years old who requires step 2 care)

Requirement for continuous oral corticosteroids or high-dose inhaled corticosteroids or more than two short courses of oral corticosteroids within 1 year

Need for additional diagnostic testing such as allergy skin testing, rhinoscopy, provocative challenge, complete pulmonary function testing, bronchoscopy

Consideration for immunotherapy

Need for additional education regarding asthma, complications of asthma and treatment of asthma, problems with adherence to management recommendations, or allergen avoidance

Uncertainty of diagnosis

Complications of asthma, including sinusitis, nasal polyposis, aspergillosis, severe rhinitis, vocal cord dysfunction, gastroesophageal reflux

Modified from National Asthma Education and Prevention Program, National Heart, Lung, and Blood Institute, Expert Panel Report 2: *Guidelines for the diagnosis and management of asthma.* Washington, DC, NIH Pub No 97-4051, July 1997.

BASIC INFORMATION

■ DEFINITION
Astrocytoma refers to a brain neoplasia arising from glial precursor cells (astrocytes).

■ SYNONYMS
Astroglial neoplasms

ICD-9CM CODES
191.9 Astrocytoma, unspecified site

■ EPIDEMIOLOGY & DEMOGRAPHICS
- Incidence of primary brain tumors is 6/100,000 persons.
- Approximately 18,000 primary brain tumors are diagnosed each year in the United States.
- In adults, glioblastoma is the most common brain tumor, followed by meningioma and astrocytoma. In children, astrocytomas are second only to medulloblastoma.
- Astrocytomas can be found at all ages, with an early peak between 0 to 4 years of age followed by a trough between the ages of 15 to 24 and then a steady rise in incidence occurs.
- Peak age incidence of low-grade astrocytoma is 34 yr.
- Peak age incidence of anaplastic astrocytoma is 41 yr.
- Peak age incidence of glioblastoma is 53 yr.

■ PHYSICAL FINDINGS & CLINICAL PRESENTATION
- Astrocytomas classically present with any one or more of the following features:
  1. Headache
  2. New-onset seizure
  3. Nausea and vomiting
  4. Focal neurologic deficit
  5. Change in mental status
  6. Papilledema

■ ETIOLOGY
- The specific etiology of astrocytoma is unknown.
- Genetic abnormalities leading to defective tumor-suppressing genes or activation of protooncogenes has been proposed.

DIAGNOSIS

A provisional diagnosis of astrocytoma is made on clinical grounds and radiographic imaging studies. Tissue pathology is needed to establish the diagnosis and to grade the astrocytoma.
- Two common grading systems used for astrocytomas are the World Health Organization (WHO) and the Saint Anne–Mayo grading system.
- WHO grades astrocytomas as follows:
  1. Grade I juvenile pilocytic astrocytoma, subependymal giant cell astrocytoma, and pleomorphic xanthoastrocytoma.
  2. Grade II astrocytoma
  3. Grade III anaplastic astrocytoma
  4. Grade IV glioblastoma multiforme
- The Saint Anne–Mayo system grades astrocytomas according to the presence or absence of four histologic features: nuclear atypia, mitoses, endothelial proliferation, and necrosis.
  1. Grade I tumors have none of the features.
  2. Grade II tumors have one feature.
  3. Grade III tumors have two features.
  4. Grade IV tumors have three or more features.
- Grades I and II astrocytomas are commonly called low-grade astrocytomas.
- Grades III and IV astrocytomas are called high-grade malignant astrocytomas.

■ DIFFERENTIAL DIAGNOSIS
The differential diagnosis is vast and includes any cause of headache, seizures, change in mental status, and focal neurologic deficits.

■ WORKUP
A CT scan or MRI of the head essentially makes the diagnosis of an intracranial brain tumor. However, tissue is needed to establish a diagnosis of astrocytoma.

■ LABORATORY TESTS
Blood tests are not very specific in the diagnosis of astrocytoma.

■ IMAGING STUDIES
MRI is the diagnostic imaging study of choice (Fig. 1-36). MRI and MRA are used to locate the margins of the tumor, distinguish vascular masses from tumors, detect low-grade astrocytomas not seen by CT scan, and provide clear views of the posterior fossa.

■ ACUTE GENERAL Rx
- Surgery is the initial treatment of almost all astrocytomas. Surgery helps in:
  1. Establishing a pathologic diagnosis
  2. Debulking the tumor
  3. Alleviating intracranial pressure
  4. Offering complete excision with hope for a cure
- Before surgery, dexamethasone 10 mg IV is given followed by 4 to 6 mg IV q6h.
- Phenytoin 300 mg qd is used for seizure control.

■ CHRONIC Rx
- Radiation therapy is used postoperatively in patients with low-grade astrocytoma (controversial) and in high-grade astrocytoma. Some authorities recommend waiting for symptoms to occur following surgery in patients with low-grade astrocytoma before using XRT.
- Chemotherapy has not been recommended in low-grade astrocytoma.
- Chemotherapeutic drugs carmustine and lomustine have been used with some effect in patients with high-grade astrocytoma.
- High-dose chemotherapy followed by autologous bone marrow transplantation is a consideration.

■ DISPOSITION

- Approximately 10% to 35% of astrocytomas (usually grade I pilocytic astrocytomas) are amenable to complete surgical excision and cure.
- The management of low-grade astrocytomas depends in part on the location of the tumor.
- In low-grade astrocytomas, the tumor is more infiltrative and therefore not amenable to complete excision. Nevertheless, most studies recommend surgery to remove as much of the tumor burden as possible.
- The prognosis of patients with low-grade astrocytoma is highly variable. A median of 7 yr is cited.
- Malignant astrocytomas, grades III and IV, usually require surgery for debulking. It is not known from prospective studies if surgery improves survival; however, retrospective studies suggest a survival benefit in the surgical treated group.
- Median survival for patients with high-grade astrocytomas is 2 yr for anaplastic type and 1 yr for glioblastoma multiforme.

■ REFERRAL

A team of specialty consultations is indicated in patients diagnosed with astrocytoma. A neurosurgeon, radiation oncologist, and neurooncologist are all needed to assist in establishing the diagnosis and to provide immediate and follow-up treatment.

☼ PEARLS & CONSIDERATIONS

■ COMMENTS

- Anaplastic astrocytomas and glioblastomas constitute more than 60% of all primary brain tumors.
- Other treatment modalities including stereotaxic radiosurgery using a gamma knife and interstitial brachytherapy are available.

REFERENCES

Black PM: Brain tumors. Part 1. *N Engl J Med* 324(21):1471, 1991.

Black PM: Brain tumors. Part 2. *N Engl J Med* 324(22):1555, 1991.

Burton EC, Prados MD: Malignant gliomas, *Curr Opin Oncol* 1(5):459, 2000.

Kaye AH, Walter DG: Low grade astrocytomas: controversies in management, *J Clin Neurosci* 7(6):475, 2000.

Author: **Peter Petropoulos, M.D.**

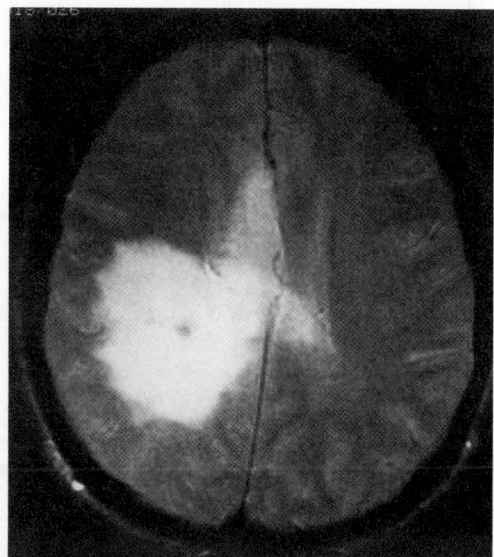 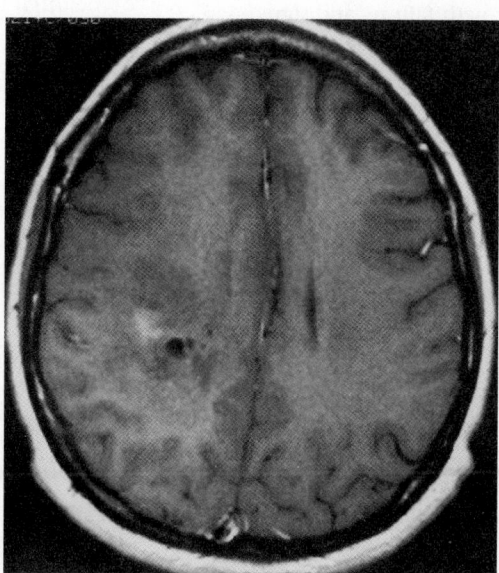

Fig. 1-36   Low-grade astrocytoma as imaged by MRI. On the left, T2-weighted image; on the right, T1-weighted image, gadolinium contrast with minimum enhancement. The images are typical of this tumor, which is being detected with increasing frequency in seizure patients by MRI. Many are invisible on CT scans. (From Goldman L, Bennett JC [eds]: *Cecil textbook of medicine,* ed 21, Philadelphia, 2000, WB Saunders.)

BASIC INFORMATION

■ DEFINITION
An autosomal recessive disorder of childhood characterized by progressive cerebellar ataxia, choreoathetosis, telangiectasias of the skin and conjunctiva (see Fig. 1-37), increased sensitivity to ionizing radiation, and a predisposition to malignancies.

ICD-9CM CODES
334.8 Ataxia telangiectasia

■ EPIDEMIOLOGY & DEMOGRAPHICS
INCIDENCE: 1/40,000 live births (most common of the degenerative ataxias)
PREDOMINANT SEX: Males = Females
PEAK INCIDENCE: Childhood
GENETICS: Autosomal recessive, chromosome 11q22-q23. The defective gene product is *ATM*, a protein kinase that is thought to be a regulator of cell cycle checkpoint in response to DNA damage.

■ PHYSICAL FINDINGS & CLINICAL PRESENTATION
- Children show normal early development until they start to walk, when gait and truncal ataxia become apparent.
- These findings are soon accompanied by polyneuropathy, cognitive dysfunction/arrested intellectual development, growth failure, and signs of premature aging (graying of the hair).
- Telangiectatic lesions occur in the outer parts of the bulbar conjunctivae, over the ears, on exposed parts of the neck, on the bridge of the nose, and in the flexor creases of the forearms.
- Recurrent sinopulmonary infections occur secondary to impaired humoral and cellular immunity
- Increased frequency of cancers is noted, particularly T-cell leukemia and lymphoma.

DIAGNOSIS

■ DIFFERENTIAL DIAGNOSIS (OF EARLY ONSET ATAXIAS)
- Friedreich's ataxia
- Abetalipoproteinemia (Bassen-Kornzweig Syndrome)
- Acquired Vitamin E deficiency
- Early onset cerebellar ataxia with retained reflexes (EOCA)
- Ataxia associated with biochemical abnormalities: associated with ceroid lipofuscinosis, xeroderma pigmentosa, Cockayne's syndrome, adrenoleukodystrophy, metachromatic leukodystrophy, mitochondrial disease, sialidosis, Niemann Pick

■ WORKUP
- Patients should be evaluated for IgA and IgE levels, which are decreased or absent
- Karyotype: high incidence of chromosomal breaks, especially on chromosome 14
- CT or MRI scans will show cerebellar atrophy
- Fibroblasts can be screened in vitro for x-ray sensitivity and radioresistant DNA synthesis
- Pathology shows cerebellar degeneration, loss of pigmented neurons, and posterior column degeneration in the spinal cord

TREATMENT

- Supportive, no effective treatment to date
- Surveillance for infections and neoplasms
- Minimize radiation as may induce further chromosomal damage and lead to neoplasms

■ PROGNOSIS
- 67% of children die by age 20, typically from infection or neoplasm

REFERENCES
Boutwood J: Ataxia telangiectasia gene mutations in leukemia and lymphoma, *J Clin Pathol* 54:512, 2001.
Meyn MS: Ataxia-telangiectasia, cancer and the pathobiology at the AMT gene, *Clin Genet* 55(5):289, 1999.
Authors: **Nicole J. Ullrich, M.D., Ph.D., and Maitreyi Mazumdar, M.D.**

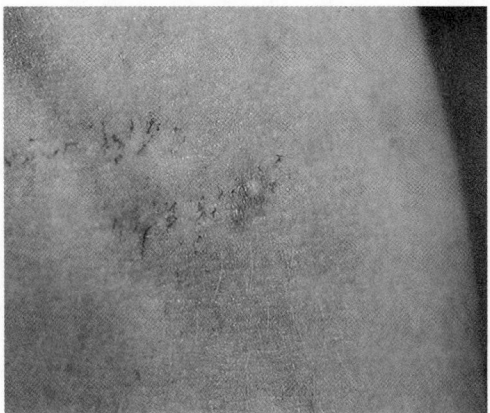
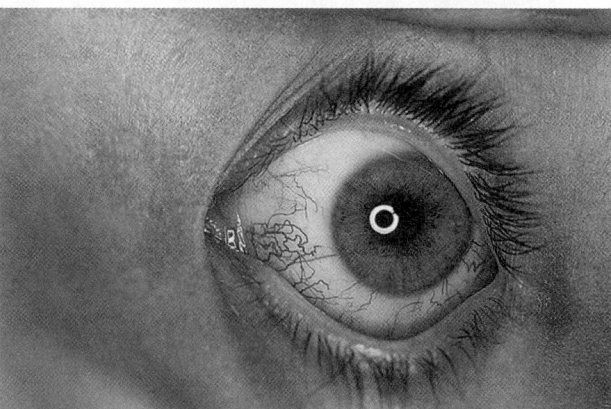

Fig. 1-37 **Ataxia telangiectasia.** (From Callen JP [ed]: *Color atlas of dermatology*, ed 2, Philadelphia, 2000, WB Saunders.)

BASIC INFORMATION

■ DEFINITION
Atelectasis is the collapse of lung volume.

ICD-9CM CODES
518.0 Atelectasis

■ EPIDEMIOLOGY & DEMOGRAPHICS
- Occurs frequently in patients receiving mechanical ventilation with higher Fio_2
- Dependent regions of the lung are more prone to atelectasis: they are partially compressed, they are not as well ventilated, and there is no spontaneous drainage of secretions with gravity

■ PHYSICAL FINDINGS & CLINICAL PRESENTATION
- Decreased or absent breath sounds
- Abnormal chest percussion
- Cough, dyspnea, decreased vocal fremitus and vocal resonance
- Diminished chest expansion, tachypnea, tachycardia

■ ETIOLOGY
- Mechanical ventilation with higher Fio_2
- Chronic bronchitis
- Cystic fibrosis
- Endobronchial neoplasms
- Foreign bodies
- Infections (e.g., TB, histoplasmosis)
- Extrinsic bronchial compression from neoplasms, aneurysms of ascending aorta, enlarged left atrium
- Sarcoidosis
- Silicosis
- Anterior chest wall injury, pneumothorax
- Alveolar injury (e.g., toxic fumes, aspiration of gastric contents)
- Pleural effusion, expanding bullae
- Chest wall deformity (e.g., scoliosis)
- Muscular weaknesses or abnormalities (e.g., neuromuscular disease)
- Mucus plugs from asthma, allergic bronchopulmonary aspergillosis, postoperative state

DIAGNOSIS

■ DIFFERENTIAL DIAGNOSIS
- Neoplasm
- Pneumonia
- Encapsulated pleural effusion
- Abnormalities of brachiocephalic vein and of the left pulmonary ligament

■ WORKUP
- Chest x-ray (Fig. 1-38)
- CT scan and fiberoptic bronchoscopy (selected patients)

■ IMAGING STUDIES
- Chest x-ray will confirm diagnosis.
- CT scan is useful in patients with suspected endobronchial neoplasm or extrinsic bronchial compression.
- Fiberoptic bronchoscopy (selected patients) is useful for removal of foreign body or evaluation of endobronchial and peribronchial lesions.

TREATMENT

■ NONPHARMACOLOGIC THERAPY
- Deep breathing, mobilization of the patient
- Incentive spirometry
- Tracheal suctioning
- Humidification
- Chest physiotherapy with percussion and postural drainage

■ ACUTE GENERAL Rx
- Positive-pressure breathing (CPAP by face mask, positive end-expiratory pressure [PEEP] for patients on mechanical ventilation)
- Use of mucolytic agents (e.g., acetylcysteine [Mucomyst])
- Recombinant human DNase (dornase alpha) in patients with cystic fibrosis
- Bronchodilator therapy in selected patients

■ CHRONIC Rx
Chest physiotherapy, humidification of inspired air, frequent nasotracheal suctioning

■ DISPOSITION
Prognosis varies with the underlying etiology.

■ REFERRAL
- Bronchoscopy for removal of foreign body or plugs unresponsive to conservative treatment
- Surgical referral for removal of obstructing neoplasms

PEARLS & CONSIDERATIONS

■ COMMENTS
Patients should be educated that frequent changes of position are helpful in clearing secretions. Sitting the patient upright in a chair is recommended to increase both volume and vital capacity relative to the supine position.

Author: **Fred F. Ferri, M.D.**

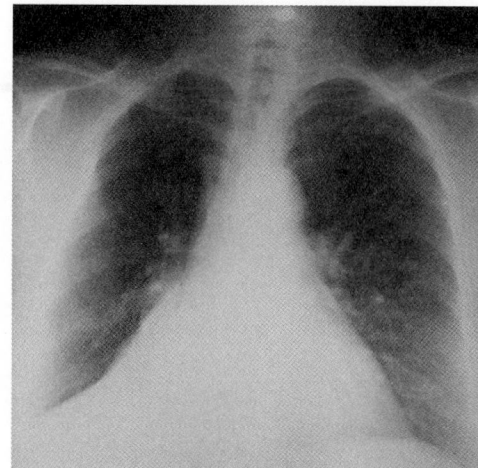

Fig. 1-38 Right middle and right lower lobe atelectasis that silhouettes the diaphram and the right heart border. (From Specht N [ed]: *Practical guide to diagnostic imaging,* St Louis, 1998, Mosby.)

BASIC INFORMATION

■ DEFINITION

Atrial fibrillation is totally chaotic atrial activity caused by simultaneous discharge of multiple atrial foci.

■ SYNONYMS

AF
A-fib

ICD-9CM CODES

427.31 Atrial fibrillation

■ EPIDEMIOLOGY & DEMOGRAPHICS

The prevalence of atrial fibrillation increases with age, from 2% in the general population, to 5% in patients older than 60 yr, to 9% of those aged 80 years or older

■ PHYSICAL FINDINGS & CLINICAL PRESENTATION

Clinical presentation is variable:
- Most common complaint: palpitations
- Fatigue, dizziness, light-headedness in some patients
- A few completely asymptomatic patients
- Cardiac auscultation revealing irregularly irregular rhythm

■ ETIOLOGY

- Coronary artery disease
- MS, MR, AS, AR
- Thyrotoxicosis
- Pulmonary embolism, COPD
- Pericarditis
- Myocarditis, cardiomyopathy
- Tachycardia-bradycardia syndrome
- Alcohol abuse
- MI
- WPW syndrome
- Other causes: left atrial myxoma, atrial septal defect, carbon monoxide poisoning, pheochromocytoma, idiopathic, hypoxia, hypokalemia, sepsis, pneumonia

DIAGNOSIS

■ DIFFERENTIAL DIAGNOSIS

- Multifocal atrial tachycardia
- Atrial flutter
- Frequent atrial premature beats

■ WORKUP

New-onset atrial fibrillation: ECG, echocardiogram, Holter monitor (selected patients), and laboratory evaluation

■ LABORATORY TESTS

- TSH, free T_4
- Serum electrolytes

■ IMAGING STUDIES

- ECG (see Fig. 1-39 for "Atrial flutter and atrial fibrillation")
  1. Irregular, nonperiodic wave forms (best seen in V1) reflecting continuous atrial reentry
  2. Absence of P waves
  3. Conducted QRS complexes showing no periodicity
- Echocardiography to evaluate left atrial size and detect valvular disorders
- Holter monitor: useful only in selected patients to evaluate paroxysmal atrial fibrillation

TREATMENT

■ NONPHARMACOLOGIC THERAPY

- Avoidance of alcohol in patients with suspected excessive alcohol use
- Avoidance of caffeine and nicotine

■ ACUTE GENERAL Rx

New-onset atrial fibrillation
- If the patient is hemodynamically unstable, perform synchronized cardioversion.
- Rate control with chronic anticoagulation is recommended for the majority of patients with atrial fibrillation.

- If the patient is hemodynamically stable, treatment options include the following:
  1. Diltiazem 0.25 mg/kg given over 2 min followed by a second dose of 0.35 mg/kg 15 min later if the rate is not slowed. May then follow with IV infusion 10 mg/hr (range 5-15 mg/hr). Onset of action following IV administration is usually within 3 min, with peak effect most often occurring within 10 min. After the ventricular rate is slowed, the patient can be changed to oral diltiazem 60 to 90 mg q 6 hr.
  2. Verapamil 2.5 to 5 mg IV initially, then 5 to 10 mg IV 10 min later if the rate is still not slowed. After the ventricular rate is slowed, the patient can be changed to oral verapamil 80 to 120 mg q 6-8 h.
  3. Digoxin, 0.5 mg IV loading dose (slow), then 0.25 mg IV 6 hr later. A third dose may be needed after 6 to 8 hr; daily dose varies from 0.125 to 0.25 mg (decrease dosage in patients with renal insufficiency and elderly patients). Digoxin is only effective for rate control at rest and should be used only as a second-line agent for rate control. Digoxin should be avoided in Wolff-Parkinson-White patients with atrial fibrillation. Procainamide is the preferred pharmacologic agent in these patients.
  4. Esmolol, metoprolol, atenolol are β-blockers that are available in IV preparations that can be used in atrial fibrillation.
  5. Other medications useful for converting atrial fibrillation to sinus rhythm are ibutilide, flecainide, propafenone, disopyramide, amiodarone, and quinidine.
- Anticoagulation with IV heparin or SC low-molecular-weight heparin and warfarin. Continue heparin until warfarin is therapeutic.

- Cardioversion is indicated if the ventricular rate is >140 bpm and the patient is symptomatic (particularly in acute MI, chest pain, dyspnea, CHF) or when there is no conversion to normal sinus rhythm after 3 days of pharmacologic therapy. The likelihood of cardioversion-related clinical thromboembolism is low in patients with atrial fibrillation lasting <48 hr. Patients with atrial fibrillation lasting >2 days have a 5% to 7% risk of clinical thromboembolism if cardioversion is not preceded by several weeks of warfarin therapy. However, if transesophageal echocardiography reveals no atrial thrombus, cardioversion may be performed safely after only a short period of anticoagulant therapy. Anticoagulant therapy should be continued for at least 1 mo after cardioversion to minimize the incidence of adverse thromboembolic events following conversion from atrial fibrillation to sinus rhythm.
- Most patients converted to sinus rhythm should not be placed on rhythm maintenance therapy because the risks outweigh the benefits.
- Long-term anticoagulation with warfarin (adjusted to maintain an INR of 2 to 3) is indicated in all patients with atrial fibrillation and associated cardiovascular disease, including the following:
  1. Rheumatic valvular disease (MS, MR, AI)
  2. Aortic stenosis
  3. Prostatic mitral valve
  4. History of previous embolism
  5. Known cardiac thrombus
  6. CHF
  7. Cardiomyopathy with poor left ventricular function
  8. Nonrheumatic heart disease (e.g., hypertensive cardiovascular disease, coronary artery disease, ASD)
- Anticoagulation is generally not recommended in young patients with lone atrial fibrillation (no associated cardiovascular disease).
- Aspirin 325 mg/day may be a suitable alternative to warfarin in patients >70 yr with increased risk of bleeding.
- Ximelagran is a promising new oral direct thrombin inhibitor that is also effective for stroke prevention in patients with nonvalvular atrial fibrillation. Its advantages over warfarin are no need to titrate dose and no routine coagulation monitoring.
- Medical cardioversion:
  1. Attempts at medical (pharmacologic) intervention should be considered only after proper anticoagulation because cardioversion can lead to systemic emboli. Following successful cardioversion, anticoagulation with warfarin should be continued for 4 wk.
  2. Useful agents for medical cardioversion are quinidine, flecainide, propafenone, amiodarone, ibutilide, sotalol, dofetilide, and procainamide.
  3. Amiodarone appears to be the most effective agent for converting to sinus rhythm in patients who do not respond to other agents.

■ **CHRONIC Rx**
- Anticoagulation with warfarin (see "Acute General Rx")
- Rate control with digoxin, verapamil, or diltiazem

■ **DISPOSITION**
Factors associated with maintenance of sinus rhythm following cardioversion:
- Left atrium diameter <60 mm
- Absence of mitral valve disease
- Short duration of atrial fibrillation

■ **REFERRAL**
Surgical treatment of atrial fibrillation:
- The maze procedure with its recent modifications creating electrical barriers to the macroreentrant circuits that are thought to underlie atrial fibrillation is being performed with good results in several medical centers (preservation of sinus rhythm in >95% of patients without the use of long-term antiarrhythmic medication). Clear indications for its use remain undefined. Generally surgery is reserved for patients with rapid heart rate refractory to pharmacologic therapy or who cannot tolerate pharmacologic therapy.
- Catheter-based radiofrequency ablation procedures designed to eliminate atrial fibrillation represent newer approaches to atrial fibrillation.
- Implantable pacemakers and defibrillators that combine pacing and cardioversion therapies to both prevent and treat atrial defibrillation are likely to have an increasing role in the future management of atrial fibrillation.

☼ PEARLS & CONSIDERATIONS

■ **COMMENTS**
- Amiodarone therapy should be considered for patients with recent atrial fibrillation and structural heart disease, particularly those with left ventricular dysfunction. Amiodarone should also be considered for patients with refractory conditions who do not have heart disease, before therapies with irreversible effects such as AV nodal ablation are attempted.
- In atrial fibrillation, rhythm control has not been shown to be superior to rate control in reducing morbidity and mortality in most patients. Rhythm control is preferred in patients who are symptomatic, have impaired exercise tolerance with rate control only, and in patients who desire rhythm control.

REFERENCES

Cooper JM et al: Implantable devices for the treatment of atrial fibrillation, *N Engl J Med* 346:2062, 2002.

Hart RG: Atrial fibrillation and stroke prevention, *N Engl J Med* 349:1015, 2003.

Hilek E et al: Effect of intensity of oral anticoagulation on stroke severity and mortality in atrial fibrillation. *N Engl J Med* 349:1019, 2003

Klein AL et al: Use of transesophageal echocardiography to guide cardioversions in patients with atrial fibrillation, *N Engl J Med* 344:1411, 2001.

Petersen P et al: Ximelagran versus warfarin for stroke prevention in patients with nonvalvular atrial fibrillation. SPORTIF II: A dose-guiding, tolerability, and safety study, *J Am Coll Cardiol* 41:1445, 2003.

Snow V et al: Management of newly detected atrial fibrillation: a clinical practice guideline from the Academy of Family Physicians and the American College of Physicians, *Ann Intern Med* 139:1009, 2003.

Author: **Fred F. Ferri, M.D.**

BASIC INFORMATION

■ DEFINITION
Atrial flutter is a rapid atrial rate of 280 to 340 bpm with varying degrees of intraventricular block.

■ ICD-9CM CODES
427.32 Atrial flutter

■ EPIDEMIOLOGY & DEMOGRAPHICS
Atrial flutter is common during the first week after open heart surgery.

■ PHYSICAL FINDINGS & CLINICAL PRESENTATION
- Fast pulse rate (approximately 150 bpm)
- Symptoms of cardiac failure, light-headedness, and angina pectoris

■ ETIOLOGY
- Atherosclerotic heart disease
- MI
- Thyrotoxicosis
- Pulmonary embolism
- Mitral valve disease
- Cardiac surgery
- COPD

DIAGNOSIS

■ DIFFERENTIAL DIAGNOSIS
- Atrial fibrillation
- Paroxysmal atrial tachycardia

■ WORKUP
- ECG
- Laboratory evaluation

■ LABORATORY TESTS
- Thyroid function studies
- Serum electrolytes

■ IMAGING STUDIES
ECG (Fig. 1-39)
- Regular, "sawtooth," or "F" wave pattern, best seen in II, III, and AVF and secondary to atrial depolarization
- AV conduction block (2:1, 3:1, or varying)

TREATMENT

■ NONPHARMACOLOGIC THERAPY
- Valsalva maneuver or carotid sinus massage usually slows the ventricular rate (increases grade of AV block) and may make flutter waves more evident.
- Electrical cardioversion is given at low energy levels (20 to 25 J).

■ ACUTE GENERAL Rx
- In absence of cardioversion, IV diltiazem or digitalization may be tried to slow the ventricular rate and convert flutter to fibrillation. Esmolol, verapamil, and adenosine may also be effective.
- Atrial pacing may also terminate atrial flutter.

- Atrial flutter is frequently associated with intermittent atrial fibrillation. It may be prudent to anticoagulate patients with atrial flutter and coexisting medical disorders (e.g., diabetes mellitus, hypertension, cardiac disease) before cardioversion. Anticoagulation should also be considered for all patients with atrial flutter who are older than 65 years of age.

■ CHRONIC Rx
- Chronic atrial flutter may respond to amiodarone.
- Radiofrequency ablation to interrupt the atrial flutter is also effective for patients with chronic or recurring atrial flutter.

■ DISPOSITION
- More than 85% of patients convert to regular sinus rhythm following cardioversion with as little as 25 to 50 J.
- Lone atrial flutter has a stroke risk at least as high as lone atrial fibrillation and carries a higher risk for subsequent development of atrial fibrillation than in the general population.

■ REFERRAL
For radiofrequency ablation in patients with chronic or recurring atrial flutter

REFERENCE
Halligan SC et al: The natural history of long atrial flutter, *Ann Int Med* 140:265, 2004.
Author: **Fred F. Ferri, M.D.**

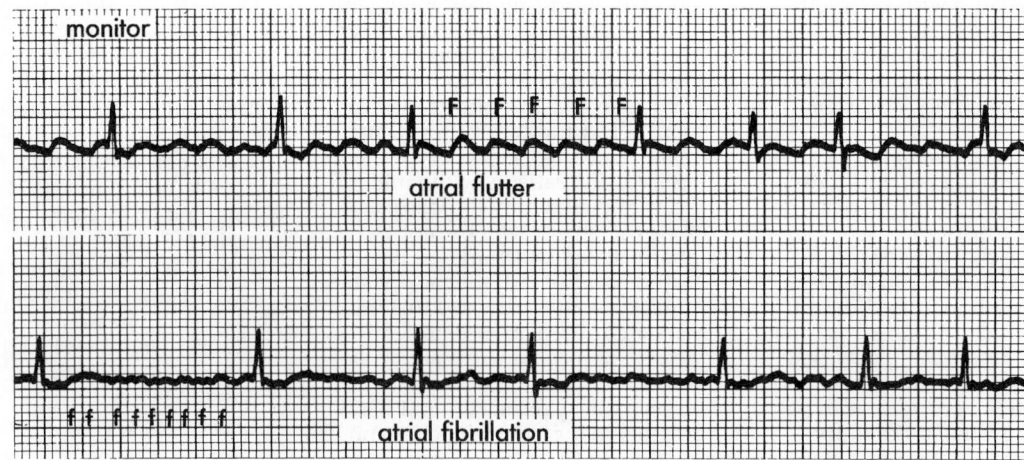

Fig. 1-39 Atrial flutter and fibrillation. Notice the sawtooth waves with atrial flutter (F) and the irregular fibrillatory waves with atrial fibrillation (f). (From Goldberger AL [ed]: *Clinical electrocardiography,* ed 5, St Louis, 1994, Mosby.)

BASIC INFORMATION

■ DEFINITION

- Atrial myxoma is a benign neoplasm of mesenchymal origin, and is the most common primary tumor of the heart

ICD-9CM CODES
212.7 Benign neoplasm, heart

■ EPIDEMIOLOGY & DEMOGRAPHICS

- Atrial myxomas account for 50% of all primary tumors of the heart.
- Approximately 75% of myxomas arise from the left atrium in close relationship to the fossa ovalis. Up to 15% of myxomas arise from the right atrium, with the remaining 10% arising from the left ventricle or from multiple sites.
- The prevalence of atrial myxoma is approximately 75 cases/1 million autopsies.
- Average age of sporadic cases is 56 yr.
- Average age of familial cases is 25 yr.
- 70% of sporadic cases occur in females.

■ PHYSICAL FINDINGS & CLINICAL PRESENTATION
Patients with atrial myxomas characteristically present in one of three ways:
- Mechanical valve obstruction (e.g., mitral or tricuspid valve)
  1. Dyspnea on exertion
  2. Orthopnea
  3. Paroxysmal nocturnal dyspnea
  4. Edema
  5. Dizziness, lightheadedness, or syncope
  6. Elevated jugular venous pressure
  7. Loud S1, increased intensity of the P2 component of S2 secondary to pulmonary hypertension
  8. Systolic murmurs of mitral regurgitation or tricuspid regurgitation and diastolic murmurs of mitral stenosis or tricuspid stenosis, depending on which chamber the myxoma arises from
  9. Third heart sound called a "tumor plop"
  10. Atrial fibrillation with an irregularly irregular pulse
- Systemic embolization may occur in up to 30% of cases leading to:
  1. Cerebrovascular accidents
  2. Pulmonary embolism
  3. Paradoxical embolism
- Constitutional symptoms
  1. Fever
  2. Weight loss
  3. Arthralgias
  4. Raynaud phenomenon

■ ETIOLOGY

- Most cases (90%) of atrial myxomas are sporadic with no known cause. In the remaining 10% of cases a familial pattern occurs having an autosomal dominant transmission. Some patients with familial cardiac myxomas have "Carney's syndrome," which consists of myxomas in other locations, skin pigmentation, and tumors of endocrine origin.

DIAGNOSIS

■ DIFFERENTIAL DIAGNOSIS

- Mitral stenosis
- Mitral regurgitaiton
- Tricuspid stenosis
- Tricuspid regurgitation
- Pulmonary hypertension
- Endocarditis
- Vasculitis
- Left atrial thrombus
- Pulmonary embolism
- Cerebrovascular accidents
- Collagen-vascular disease
- Carcinoid heart disease
- Ebstein's anomaly

■ WORKUP
A high index of suspicion is needed to make the diagnosis of atrial myxoma because the clinical manifestations are similar to many common cardiovascular and pulmonary diseases.

■ LABORATORY TESTS
Although not very specific, the following laboratory values may be abnormal in patients with atrial myxomas:
- CBC: anemia, polycythemia, thrombocytopenia may occur
- Erythrocyte sedimentation rate, C-reactive protein, and serum immunoglobulins are commonly elevated
- ECG: patients with atrial myxomas may have findings of left atrial enlargement, right atrial enlargement, atrial fibrillation, atrial flutter, premature ventricular contractions, ventricular tachycardia, and ventricular fibrillation

■ IMAGING STUDIES

- Echocardiography: initial imaging procedure of choice in suspected cases of atrial myxoma
- Chest x-ray examination: altered cardiac contour and chamber enlargement
- Transesophageal echocardiography: may pick up masses not visualized by transthoracic echocardiography
- MRI: Aids in delineating size, shape, and tumor characterizations
- Cardiac catheterization: usually not needed in diagnosing atrial myxoma; however, may be required in some circumstances to rule out coronary artery disease

TREATMENT

■ NONPHARMACOLOGIC THERAPY
None

■ ACUTE GENERAL THERAPY

- Surgical excision is the treatment of choice.
- Surgery should be done promptly because sudden death can occur while waiting for the procedure (see "Disposition").

■ CHRONIC Rx
Postoperative arrhythmias and conductions abnormalities were present in 26% of patients and can be treated according to standard convention.

■ DISPOSITION

- Surgical results have reported a 95% survival rate after a follow-up of 3 yr.
- Up to 5% of sporadic cases of atrial myxoma may recur within the first 6 yr after surgery.
- Up to 20% of familial cases of atrial myxoma may recur after surgery.
- Sudden death has been reported to occur in up to 15% of patients with atrial myxoma, with death resulting from coronary or systemic embolization or by obstruction of blood flow at the mitral or tricuspid valve.

■ REFERRAL

- Consultation with a cardiologist is recommended in the initial workup of a patient with signs and symptoms of valvular obstruction and/or systemic embolization thought to arise from the heart.
- Once the noninvasive workup has revealed a cardiac tumor, consultation with a cardiovascular surgeon is recommended for prompt surgical excision.

PEARLS & CONSIDERATIONS

■ COMMENTS
Although recurrence of atrial myxoma is rare following operative excision, yearly echocardiograms should be performed.

REFERENCES

Bhan A et al: Surgical experience with intracardiac myxomas: long-term follow-up, *Ann Thorac Surg* 66:810, 1998.

Centofanti P et al: Primary cardiac tumors: early and late results of surgical treatment in 91 patients, *Ann Thorac Surg* 68:1235, 1999.

Pérez de Isla L et al: Diagnosis and treatment of cardiac myxomas by transesophageal echocardiography, *Am J Cardiol* 90(12):1419, 2002.

Pinede L, Duhaut P, Loire R: Clinical presentation of left atrial cardiac myxoma. A series of 112 consecutive patients, *Medicine* 80:159, 2001.

Pucci A et al: Histopathologic and clinical characterization of cardiac myxoma: review of 53 cases from a single institution, *Am Heart J* 140:134, 2000.

Reymen K: Cardiac myxomas, *N Engl J Med* 333:1610, 1995.

BASIC INFORMATION

■ DEFINITION
Atrial septal defect (ASD) is an abnormal opening in the atrial septum that allows for blood flow between the atria. There are several forms (Fig. 1-40):
- Ostium primum: defect low in the septum
- Ostium secundum: occurs mainly in the region of the fossa ovalis
- Sinus venous defect: less common form, involves the upper part of the septum

■ SYNONYMS
ASD

ICD-9CM CODES
429.71 Atrial septal defect

■ EPIDEMIOLOGY & DEMOGRAPHICS
- 80% of cases of ASD involve persistence of ostium secundum.
- Incidence is higher in females.
- ASD accounts for 8% to 10% of congenital heart abnormalities.

■ PHYSICAL FINDINGS & CLINICAL PRESENTATION
- Pansystolic murmur best heard at apex secondary to mitral regurgitation (ostium primum defect)
- Widely split S_2
- Visible and palpable pulmonary artery pulsations
- Ejection systolic flow murmur
- Prominent right ventricular impulse
- Cyanosis and clubbing (severe cases)
- Exertional dyspnea
- Patients with small defects: generally asymptomatic

■ ETIOLOGY
Unknown

DIAGNOSIS

■ DIFFERENTIAL DIAGNOSIS
- Primary pulmonary hypertension
- Pulmonary stenosis
- Rheumatic heart disease
- Mitral valve prolapse
- Cor pulmonale

■ WORKUP
- ECG
- Chest x-ray examination
- Echocardiography
- Cardiac catheterization

■ IMAGING STUDIES
- ECG
  1. Ostium primum defect: left axis deviation, RBBB, prolongation of PR interval
  2. Sinus venous defect: leftward deviation of P axis
  3. Ostium secundum defect: right axis deviation, right bundle-branch block
- Chest x-ray: cardiomegaly, enlargement of right atrium and ventricle, increased pulmonary vascularity, small aortic knob
- Echocardiography with saline bubble contrast and Doppler flow studies: may demonstrate the defect and the presence of shunting. Transesophageal echocardiography is much more sensitive than transthoracic echocardiography in identifying sinus venous defects and is preferred by some for the initial diagnostic evaluation.
- Cardiac catheterization: confirms the diagnosis in patients who are candidates for surgery. It is useful if the patient has some anatomic finding on echocardiography that is not completely clear or has significant elevation of pulmonary artery pressures

TREATMENT

■ NONPHARMACOLOGIC THERAPY
Avoidance of strenuous activity in symptomatic patients

■ GENERAL Rx
- Children and infants: closure of ASD before age 10 yr is indicated if pulmonary:systemic flow ratio is >1.5:1.
- Adults: closure is indicated in symptomatic patients with shunts >2:1.
- Surgery should be avoided in patients with pulmonary hypertension with reversed shunting (Eisenmenger's syndrome) because of increased risk of right heart failure.
- Transcatheter closure is advocated in children when feasible.
- Prophylactic β-blocker therapy to prevent atrial arrhythmias should be considered in adults with ASD.
- Surgical closure is indicated in all patients with ostium primum defect and significant shunting unless patient has significant pulmonary vascular disease.

■ DISPOSITION
- Mortality is high in patients with significant ostium primum defect.
- Patients with small shunts have a normal life expectancy.
- Surgical mortality varies with the age of the patient and the presence of cardiac failure and systolic pulmonary artery hypertension; mortality ranges from <1% in young patients (<45 yr old) to >10% in elderly patients with presence of heart failure and systolic pulmonary hypertension.
- Preoperative atrial fibrillation is a risk factor for immediate postoperative and long-term atrial fibrillation.
- Thromboembolism after surgical repair of an ASD in an adult can occur in the early postoperative period. Giving early postoperative anticoagulation in patients >35 yr of age at the time of ASD repair and continuing it for at least 6 mo will decrease the risk.

REFERENCE
Moodie DS, Sterba R: Long-term outcomes excellent for ASD repair in adults, *Cleve Clin J Med* 67:591, 2000.
Author: **Fred F. Ferri, M.D.**

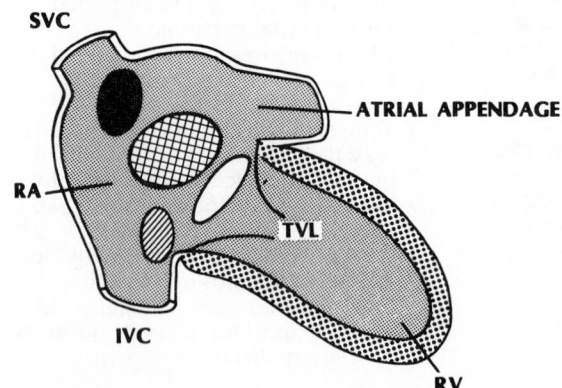

Fig. 1-40 Location of the four types of atrial septal defect. SVC, *Superior vena cava;* RA, *right atrium;* IVC, *inferior vena cava;* RV, *right ventricle;* TVL, *tricuspid valve leaflet.* (From Noble J [ed]: *Primary care medicine,* ed 2, St Louis, 1996, Mosby.)

■ Sinus venosus defect

⊠ Secundum defect

□ Primum defect

▨ Coronary sinus defect

BASIC INFORMATION

■ DEFINITION
Attention deficit hyperactivity disorder (ADHD) follows a persistent pattern (lasting at least 6 mo) of inattention *or* hyperactivity/impulsivity that is greater than expected for age and that begins before age 7 yr. The disorder is further defined by dysfunction in at least two settings (e.g., home, school, day care).

■ SYNONYMS
Hyperactivity
Attention deficit disorder (ADD)

ICD-9CM CODES
F90.X (DMS-IV 314.XX)

■ EPIDEMIOLOGY & DEMOGRAPHICS
PREVALENCE (IN U.S.): 35% of school-age children
PREDOMINANT SEX: Males > females, with rates ranging from 4:1 to 9:1
PREDOMINANT AGE:
- Onset must occur before age 7 yr.
- At least 20% experience spontaneous remissions by adolescence; however, the disorder may persist into adulthood.

PEAK INCIDENCE: Diagnosis is usually made after child begins school (ages 6 to 9 yr).
GENETICS:
- Familial pattern in many patients with ADHD
- Specific thyroid hormone abnormality in a very small fraction of familial ADHD

■ PHYSICAL FINDINGS & CLINICAL PRESENTATION
- Usually diagnosed in elementary school, where achievement is compromised and behavioral dyscontrol is less tolerated
- Wide array of symptoms, including difficulty sustaining attention, frequent careless mistakes, failure to follow instructions, difficulty organizing activities, distractibility, forgetfulness, fidgeting, inability to sit still or play quietly, excessive activity or speech, inability to await turn, or intrusiveness
- May exhibit bossiness, stubbornness, demoralization, mood lability, and poor self-esteem
- IQ scores slightly lower than the general population

■ ETIOLOGY
- Probability of multiple etiologies
- Associated and possibly etiologic factors: comorbid Tourette's, a history of abuse or neglect, lead poisoning, previous encephalitis, drug exposure in utero, low birth weight, and mental retardation. If possible, a specific diagnosis should be made
- Thyroid hormone metabolism abnormalities identified in a pedigree of familial ADHD

DIAGNOSIS

■ DIFFERENTIAL DIAGNOSIS
- In early childhood, may be difficult to distinguish from normal active children.
- ADHD may overlap symptoms in children with disruptive behavior such as conduct disorder or oppositional defiant disorders.
- School and behavioral problems are associated with a learning disability (these disorders often coexist).
- Bipolar disorder may be confused with ADHD, but it can be distinguished by the episodic nature of bipolar illness and the pervasive presence of ADHD.

■ WORKUP
- History with collateral information from parents and teachers is central to the diagnosis.
- Neurologic examination including imaging studies is used to uncover nonspecific, nonvocal, soft neurologic signs that frequently can be found in ADHD children.
- Questionnaires for parents and adolescents aid in the diagnosis.
- Psychologic testing is useful to diagnose a learning disability.

TREATMENT

■ NONPHARMACOLOGIC THERAPY
Children generally do better in special education settings with behavioral management of the disruptive behavior.

■ ACUTE GENERAL Rx
- Stimulants: mainstay of treating ADHD; include methylphenidate (Ritalin), dextroamphetamine (Dexedrine), and pemoline (Cylert; may cause rare, severe hepatotoxicity)

- The amphetamine-dextroamphetamine combination Adderall is also useful in children with ADHD. Once-daily Adderall is as effective as twice-daily methylphenidate and both are superior to once-daily methylphenidate
- Atomoxetine (strattera), a selective norepinephrine reuptake inhibitor was recently approved for treatment of ADHD
- Adjuncts: tricyclic antidepressants (rare cardiac deaths in children and adolescents warrant caution); serotonin reuptake–inhibiting antidepressants, bupropion (safer but efficacy not as well documented), clonidine, and neuroleptics

■ DISPOSITION
- Severity generally decreases with age.
- In late adolescence, the symptom severity is quite mild in many individuals.
- Full or partial aspects of the disorder are possibly persistent into mid-adulthood and require ongoing pharmacotherapy.

■ REFERRAL
- If diagnosis is complicated by coexisting conditions
- If treatment with stimulants is not adequately effective

REFERENCES
Chatfield J: AAP guideline on treatment of children with ADHD, *Am Fam Physician* 65:726, 2002.
Pecham WG et al: Once-a-day concerta methylphenidate versus three-times daily methylphenidate in laboratory and natural settings, *Pediatrics* 107:105, 2001.
Smucker WD et al: Evaluation and treatment of ADHD, *Am Fam Physician* 64:817, 2001.
Szymanski ML, Zolotor A: Attention-deficit/hyperactivity disorder: management, *Am Fam Physician* 64:1355, 2001.
Wender EH: Attention-deficit/hyperactivity disorder: Is it common? Is it overtreated? *Arch Pediatr Adolesc Med* 156:209, 2002.
Author: **Rif S. El-Mallakh, M.D.**

BASIC INFORMATION

■ DEFINITION

The term *autistic disorder* refers to impairment in the development of language, communication, and reciprocal social interaction along with a restricted behavioral repertoire, with onset before age 3 yr.

■ SYNONYMS

Autism
Early infantile autism
Childhood autism
Kanner's autism

ICD-9CM CODES

F84.0 Autistic disorder (DSM-IV coded 299.0 Autistic disorder)

■ EPIDEMIOLOGY & DEMOGRAPHICS

PREVALENCE (IN U.S.): 2 to 5 cases/10,000 persons (10 to 15 cases/10,000 persons when broader definitions are used)
PREDOMINANT SEX: Male:female ratio of 3-4:1
PREDOMINANT AGE: Lifelong illness
PEAK INCIDENCE: Before age 3 yr
GENETICS: Unknown genetic component; risk for sibling of affected individual: increases to 3%

■ PHYSICAL FINDINGS & CLINICAL PRESENTATION

- Marked impairment in the understanding and use of both verbal and nonverbal communication (probably underlies the profound impairment in social interaction)
- Stereotypic behavior or language

■ ETIOLOGY

- Majority of cases of autism are not associated with a medical condition.
- There is a significant increase in comorbid seizure disorder (25%) and mental retardation.
- Autism is sometimes associated with other neurologic conditions (e.g., encephalitis, phenylketonuria, fragile X, and others), suggesting that it may result from nonspecific neuronal injury.
- Specific abnormality that produces autistic symptoms has not been identified.

DIAGNOSIS

■ DIFFERENTIAL DIAGNOSIS

- Other pervasive developmental disorders
- Rett's syndrome: occurs in females, exhibits head growth deceleration, loss of previously acquired motor skills, and incoordination
- Childhood disintegration disorder: development normal until age 2 yr, followed by regression
- Childhood-onset schizophrenia: follows period of normal development
- Asperger's syndrome: lacks the language developmental abnormalities of autism
- Isolated symptoms of autism: when occurring in isolation, defined as disorders (i.e., selective mutism, expressive language disorder, mixed receptive-expressive language disorder, or stereotypic movement disorder)

■ WORKUP

A two-part process:
1. Establish the diagnosis.
2. Determine if there are any associated medical conditions.

■ LABORATORY TESTS

- PKU screen (usually done at birth in the U.S.)
- Chromosome analysis to rule out fragile X in both boys and girls (carrier girls may exhibit mild symptoms)

■ IMAGING STUDIES

- EEG to diagnose coexisting seizure disorder (a normal EEG does not rule out a seizure disorder.)
- Head CT scan or MRI to rule out tuberous sclerosis
- Possible BAER to rule out hearing deficit
- IQ testing to help determine functional level of the child

TREATMENT

■ NONPHARMACOLOGIC THERAPY

- A behavioral training program that is consistent in both the home and school environments is important.
- Educational needs should focus on language and social development.
- Most children need a highly structured environment.
- Educating the parents and teachers is of great value.

■ ACUTE GENERAL Rx

- Haloperidol or other high-potency neuroleptics are helpful in reducing aggression and stereotypy. Atypical neuroleptics, such as risperidone, also reduce aggression and irritability.
- Atypical neuroleptics, such as risperidone, also reduce aggression and irritability.
- Serotonin reuptake inhibitor antidepressants (fluoxetine, clomipramine, sertraline, paroxetine) are possibly useful in children with coexisting depression or with marked obsessive or ritualistic behaviors.
- Naltrexone is useful for children with self-injurious behaviors.
- Valproic acid and carbamazepine are preferred to phenytoin or phenobarbital for seizure control.

■ CHRONIC Rx

- Extended use of all medications used for acute management
- Potential for tardive dyskinesia with chronic use of neuroleptics
- Large doses of vitamin B_6 and magnesium supplementation (mild ameliorating effect)

■ DISPOSITION

- Most children (70%) will require some degree of assistance as adults, will not be able to work, and will not achieve proper social adjustment.
- Some 10% (particularly if IQ is in the normal range and speech is achieved by age 5 yr) may have a reasonable outcome.
- Children with Asperger's syndrome may have a very good outcome despite ongoing symptoms.

■ REFERRAL

Assistance may be needed in diagnosis, management, parental teaching, or intervention with the school system.

REFERENCE

Research Units on Pediatric Psychopharmacology Autism Network: Risperidone in children with autism and serious behavioral problems, *N Engl J Med* 347:314, 2002.

Authors: **Rif S. El-Mallakh, M.D., and Peter E. Tanguay, M.D.**

BASIC INFORMATION

■ DEFINITION
Babesiosis is a tick-transmitted protozoan disease of animals, caused by intraerythrocytic parasites of the genus *Babesia.* Humans are incidentally infected, resulting in a nonspecific febrile illness.

ICD-9CM CODES
088.82 Babesiosis

■ EPIDEMIOLOGY & DEMOGRAPHICS
INCIDENCE (IN U.S.): Unknown
PREVALENCE (IN U.S.):
- In areas of high endemicity, seropositivity ranging from 9% (Rhode Island) to 21% (Connecticut)
- Highest number of reported cases in New York

PREDOMINANT SEX: Males (most likely through increased exposure to vectors during recreational or occupational activities)
PREDOMINANT AGE: Severity apparently increasing with age >40 yr
PEAK INCIDENCE: Spring and summer months, May through September
GENETICS: None known
CONGENITAL INFECTION: At least one case of probable vertical transmission
NEONATAL INFECTION: At least two cases of perinatal transmission

■ PHYSICAL FINDINGS & CLINICAL PRESENTATION
- Incubation period 1 to 4 wk, or 6 to 9 wk in transfusion-associated disease
- Gradual onset of irregular fever, chills, diaphoresis, headache, myalgia, arthralgia, fatigue, and dark urine
- On physical examination: petechiae, frank or mild hepatosplenomegaly, and jaundice
- Infection with *B. divergens* producing a more severe illness with a rapid onset of symptoms and increasing parasitemia progressing to massive intravascular hemolysis and renal failure

■ ETIOLOGY
- Vector: Deer tick, *Ixodes scapularis* (also known as *I. dammini*)
  1. Feeds on rodents during the spring and summer while in its larval and nymphal stages and on deer as an adult
  2. During the warmer months in endemic areas, humans are readily infected while engaging in outdoor activities
- *B. microti,* along with *B. divergens* and *B. bovis,* account for most human infections.

- In the U.S., cases caused by *B. microti* are acquired on offshore islands of the northeastern coast, including Nantucket Island, Cape Cod, and Martha's Vineyard in Massachusetts; Block Island in Rhode Island; and Long Island, Fire Island, and Shelter Island in New York; as well as the nearby mainland including Connecticut and New Jersey.
- Sporadic cases reported from California, Georgia, Maryland, Minnesota, Virginia, Wisconsin, and most recently the WA-1 strain from Washington State and the MO-1 strain from Missouri.
- *B. divergens* and *B. bovis* are implicated in human disease in Europe, where the disease remains rare and predominantly associated with asplenia.
- Majority of cases are symptomatic.
- May be transmissible by transfusion, through platelets and erythrocytes.
- Mixed infections (*B. microti* and *Borrelia burgdorferi*) are estimated to occur in 10% (Rhode Island and Connecticut) to 60% (New York) of cases.

DIAGNOSIS

■ DIFFERENTIAL DIAGNOSIS
- Amebiasis
- Ehrlichiosis
- Hepatic abscess
- Leptospirosis
- Malaria
- Salmonellosis, including typhoid fever
- Acute viral hepatitis
- Hemorrhagic fevers

■ WORKUP
Should be suspected in any febrile patient living or traveling in an endemic area, irrespective of exposure history to ticks or tick bites, especially if asplenic

■ LABORATORY TESTS
- CBC to reveal mild to moderate pancytopenia
- Abnormally elevated serum chemistries, including creatinine, liver function profile, lactate dehydrogenase, and direct and total bilirubin levels
- Urinalysis to reveal proteinuria and hemoglobinuria
- Examination of Giemsa- or Wright-stained thick and thin blood films for intraerythrocytic parasites
  1. In its classic, though infrequently seen, form a "tetrad" or "Maltese Cross" composed of four daughter cells attached by cytoplasmic strands is observed (Fig. 1-41).
  2. More commonly, smaller forms composed of a single chromatin dot are eccentrically located within bluish cytoplasm.
  3. Parasitized erythrocytes may be multiply infected but not enlarged, or they may show evidence of pigment deposition, seen with *Plasmodium* species.
- Diagnosis achieved serologically by indirect immunofluorescence assay (IFA) is specific for *B. microti.*
  1. Titer of ≥1:64 is indicative of seropositivity, whereas one ≥1:256 is considered diagnostic of acute infection.
  2. Assay is hampered by the inability to distinguish between exposed patients and those who are actively infected.
  3. Immunoglobulin M indirect immunofluorescent-antibody test may be highly sensitive and specific for diagnosis.
  4. Babesial DNA by polymerase chain reaction (PCR) has comparable sensitivity and specificity to microscopic analysis of thin blood smears.

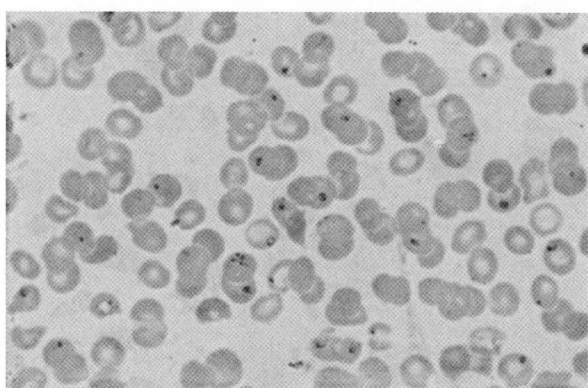

Fig. 1-41   Babesia microti-infected erythrocytes from a case of transfusion-induced babesiosis. Note ring and one tetrad form. (From Gorbach SL: *Infectious diseases,* ed 2, Philadelphia, 1998, WB Saunders.)

TREATMENT

■ NONPHARMACOLOGIC THERAPY
Supportive care with adequate hydration

■ ACUTE GENERAL Rx
- In patients with intact spleens: predominantly asymptomatic or if symptomatic, generally self-limited
- Therapy reserved for the severely ill patient, especially if asplenic or immunosuppressed
- Combination of quinine sulfate 650 mg PO tid plus clindamycin 600 mg PO tid (1.2 g parenterally bid) taken for 7 to 10 days: effective but may not eliminate parasites
- Combination of atovaquone 750 mg every 12 hr and azithromycin 500 mg on day 1 and 250 mg per day thereafter for 7 days appears to be as effective as a regimen of clindamycin and quinine with fewer adverse reactions
- Exchange transfusions in addition to antimicrobial therapy: successful treatment for severe infections in asplenic patients associated with high levels of *B. microti* or *B. divergens* parasitemia

■ DISPOSITION
Prognosis is usually good and fatal outcomes are rare.

■ REFERRAL
- For prompt consultation with an infectious disease specialist if the diagnosis is acutely suspected, especially in the asplenic, elderly, or immunocompromised patient
- For hospitalization for the severely ill patient who may require exchange transfusions in addition to antibiotic therapy

☼ PEARLS & CONSIDERATIONS

■ COMMENTS
- Prevention of babesiosis in asplenic or immunocompromised hosts is best achieved by avoidance of areas where the vector is endemic, especially during the months of May through September.
- If residence or travel in endemic areas is unavoidable, advise patients to perform daily cutaneous self-examination, wear light-colored clothing (to facilitate removal of ticks), and apply tick repellent (diethyltoluamide and dimethylphthalate) to skin or clothing.
- Advise a daily inspection for ticks in family pets (e.g., cats and dogs).

- Infection with *B. divergens*, especially in the asplenic patient, is often fatal.
- At least one case of concurrent babesiosis and Lyme disease has been documented.
- Clindamycin and quinine has been successfully used to treat Babesiosis during the third trimester of pregnancy without incurring apparent adverse effect on the fetus.

REFERENCES
Cable RG, Leiby DA: Risk and prevention of transfusion-transmitted babesiosis and other tick-borne diseases, *Curr Opin Hematol* 10(6):405, 2003.

Feder HM Jr et al: Babesiosis in pregnancy, *N Engl J Med* 349(2):195, 2003.

Herwaldt BL et al: Endemic babesiosis in another eastern state: New Jersey, *Emerg Infect Dis* 9(2):184, 2003.

Gelfand JA, Callahan MV: Babesiosis: an update on epidemiology and treatment, *Curr Infect Dis Rep* 5(1):53, 2003.

Gutman JD, Kotton CN, Kratz A: Case records of the Massachusetts General Hospital. Weekly clinicopathological exercises. Case 29-2003. A 60-year-old man with fever, rigors, and sweats. *N Engl J Med* 349(12):1168, 2003.

Krause PJ: Babesiosis diagnosis and treatment, *Vector Borne Zoonotic Dis* 3(1):45, 2003.

Author: **George O. Alonso, M.D.**

BASIC INFORMATION

■ DEFINITIONS
Baker's cyst refers to a fluid-filled popliteal bursa located along the medial border of the popliteal fossa.

■ SYNONYMS
Popliteal cyst

ICD-9CM CODES
727.51 Baker's cyst (knee)

■ EPIDEMIOLOGY & DEMOGRAPHICS
- Popliteal cysts occur at all ages.
- Incidence of Baker's cysts is unknown.
- Between 2% to 6% of all patients thought to have clinical DVT turn out to have symptomatic Baker's cysts.
- Approximately 5% of MRIs of the knees reveal popliteal cysts.

■ PHYSICAL FINDINGS & CLINICAL PRESENTATION
- Pain in the popliteal space
- Knee swelling
- Leg edema
- Prominence of the popliteal fossa
- Decreased range of motion of the knee
- Locking of the knee
- Foucher's sign: The cyst becomes hard with knee extension and soft with knee flexion.
- Neuropathic lancinating pains radiating from the knee down the back of the leg.
- Deep vein thrombosis (DVT)

■ ETIOLOGY
- Baker's cysts are believed to represent fluid distention of the bursal sac separating the semimembranous tendon from the medial head of the gastrocnemius.
- In children, Baker's cysts are thought to be secondary to trauma and irritation of the knee.
- In adults, Baker's cysts are usually associated with pathologic changes of the knee joint:
  1. Rheumatoid arthritis
  2. Osteoarthritis of the knee
  3. Meniscal tears
  4. Patellofemoral chondromalacia
  5. Fracture
  6. Gout
  7. Pseudogout
  8. Infection (tuberculosis)

DIAGNOSIS

Baker's cysts, like deep vein thrombosis, are very difficult to diagnose on clinical grounds alone. In fact, Baker's cyst frequently mimics a DVT and is sometimes called *pseudothrombophlebitis syndrome*.

■ DIFFERENTIAL DIAGNOSIS
- DVT
- Popliteal aneurysms
- Abscess
- Tumors
- Lymphadenopathy
- Varicosities
- Ganglion

■ WORKUP
Anyone suspected of having a popliteal cyst should undergo imaging studies to exclude other causes.

■ LABORATORY TESTS
Blood tests are not very specific in the diagnosis of Baker's cysts.

■ IMAGING STUDIES
- Plain x-ray (AP and lateral views) may show calcification in a solid tumor or in the posterior meniscal area.
- Ultrasound is easy, cost effective, and excludes other causes of popliteal fossa pathology.
- MRI of the knee identifies coexisting joint pathology (e.g., osteoarthritis, torn meniscus).
- Noninvasive venous studies to rule out DVT.

TREATMENT

Treatment is directed at the underlying pathology leading to the formation of the popliteal cyst.

■ NONPHARMACOLOGIC THERAPY
- Rest
- Strenuous activity avoidance
- Knee immobilization possibly necessary in some cases

■ ACUTE GENERAL Rx
- NSAIDs, ibuprofen 400 to 800 mg PO tid, or naproxen 250 to 500 mg PO bid can be used to treat Baker's cyst caused by RA, gout, and pseudogout.
- Intraarticular injection or injection of the cyst with corticosteroids, triamcinolone acetonide 40 mg is sometimes tried.

■ CHRONIC Rx
- Surgical procedures addressing the underlying cause or aimed at the cyst include:
  1. Arthroscopic surgery to remove loose cartilaginous fragment
  2. Partial or total meniscectomy
  3. Open excision of the cyst (Fig. 1-42)

■ DISPOSITION
- Baker's cyst may spontaneously resolve without treatment.
- Complications of Baker's cysts are:
  1. Rupture
  2. DVT
  3. Nerve impingement

■ REFERRAL
Because Baker's cysts are commonly the result of underlying rheumatologic causes, a consultation with rheumatology is often recommended.

☼ PEARLS & CONSIDERATIONS

■ COMMENTS
- Popliteal cysts was first described in 1877 by Baker in connection with disease of the knee joint.
- Baker's cyst and DVT can coexist. It is imperative to exclude the diagnosis of DVT before discharging the patient from the emergency room, hospital, or office.
- In the setting of meniscus injury, Baker's cysts commonly originate from the posterior horn of the medial meniscus with or without a tear.

REFERENCES
Drescher MJ, Smally AJ: Thrombophlebitis and pseudothrombophlebitis in the ED, *Am J Emerg Med* 15(7):683, 1997.

Handy JR: Popliteal cysts in adults: a review, *Semin Arthritis Rheum* 31(2):108, 2001.

Stone KR et al: The frequency of Baker's cysts associated with meniscal tears, *Am Sports Med* 24(5):670, 1996.

Torreggiani WC et al: The imaging spectrum of Baker's (Popliteal) cysts, *Clin Radiol* 57(8):681, 2002.

Author: **Peter Petropoulos, M.D.**

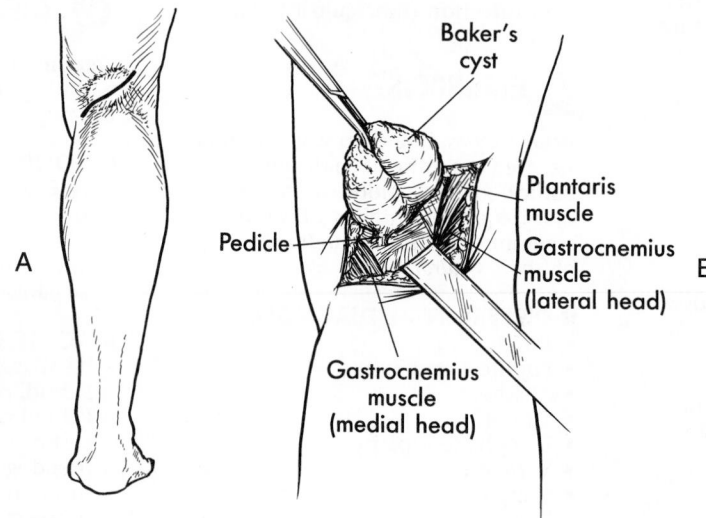

Fig. 1-42   **Removal of midline Baker's cyst. A,** Skin incision. **B,** After being exposed, pedicle is clamped, ligated, divided, and inverted. (Redrawn and modified from Meyerding HW, Van Demark GE: JAMA 122:858, 1943.)

BASIC INFORMATION

■ DEFINITIONS
Balanitis is an inflammation of the superficial tissues of the penile head (Fig. 1-43).

ICD-9CM CODES
112.2 Balanitis

■ EPIDEMIOLOGY & DEMOGRAPHICS
INCIDENCE (IN U.S.): Unknown
PREVALENCE (IN U.S.): Unknown
PREDOMINANT SEX: Exclusive to males
PEAK INCIDENCE: All ages, especially in sexually active men

■ PHYSICAL FINDINGS & CLINICAL PRESENTATION
- Itching and tenderness
- Pain, dysuria, and local edema
- Rarely, ulceration and lymph node enlargement
- Severe ulcerations leading to superimposed bacterial infections
- Inability to void: unusual, but a more distressing and serious complication

■ ETIOLOGY
- Poor hygiene, causing erosion of tissue with erythema and promoting growth of *Candida albicans*
- Sexual contact, urinary catheters, and trauma
- Allergic reactions to condoms or medications

DIAGNOSIS

■ DIFFERENTIAL DIAGNOSIS
- Leukoplakia
- Reiter's syndrome
- Lichen planus
- Balanitis xerotica obliterans
- Psoriasis
- Carcinoma of the penis
- Erythroplasia of Queyrat

■ WORKUP
- Sexually active males: assessment for evidence of other sexually transmitted diseases
- Biopsy if lesions do not heal

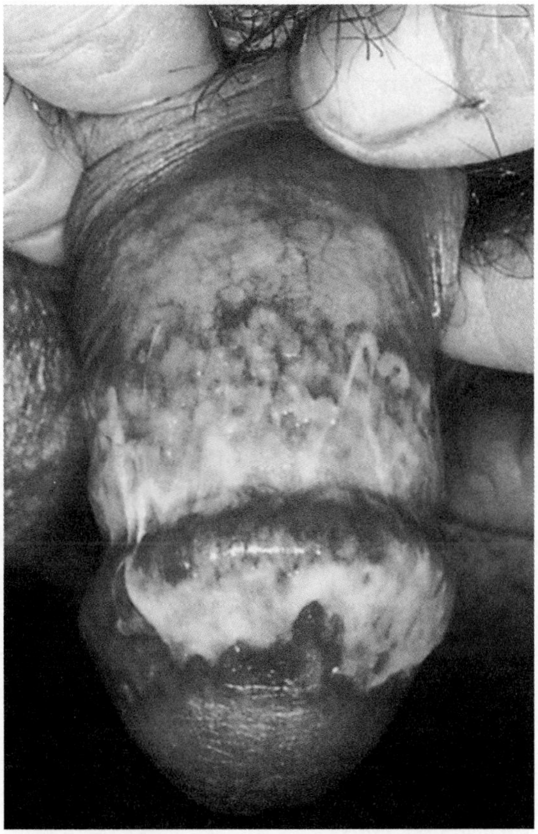

■ LABORATORY TESTS
- VDRL
- Serum glucose
- Wet mount
- KOH prep
- Microculture

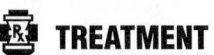 # TREATMENT

■ NONPHARMACOLOGIC THERAPY
- Maintenance of meticulous hygiene
- Retraction and bathing of prepuce several times a day
- Warm sitz baths to ease edema and erythema
- Consideration of circumcision, especially when symptoms are severe or recurrent
- With Foley catheters, strict catheter care strongly advised

■ MEDICATIONS
- Analgesics, such as acetaminophen and/or codeine
- Clotrimazole 1% cream applied topically twice daily to affected areas
- Bacitracin or Neosporin ointment applied topically 4 times daily
- With more severe bacterial superinfection: cephalexin 500 mg PO qid
- Topical corticosteroids added 4 times daily if dermatitis severe
- Patients with suspected urinary tract infections: trimethoprim-sulfa DS twice daily or ciprofloxacin 500 mg PO bid after obtaining appropriate cultures

■ REFERRAL
- For surgical evaluation for circumcision if symptoms are recurrent, especially if phimosis or meatitis occurs (NOTE: Severe phimosis with an inability to void may require prompt slit drainage.)
- For biopsy to rule out other diagnosis such as premalignant or malignant lesions if lesions are not healing

REFERENCES
Bielan B: What's your assessment? *Candida* balanitis, *Dermatol Nurs* 15(2):134, 2003.
Buechner SA: Common skin disorders of the penis, *BJU Int* 90(5):498, 2002.
Bunker CB: Topics in penile dermatology, *Clin Exp Dermatol* 26(6):469, 2001.
Huntley JS et al: Troubles with the foreskin: one hundred consecutive referrals to paediatric surgeons, *J R Soc Med* 96(9):449, 2003.
Author: **Joseph J. Lieber, M.D.**

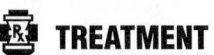

Fig. 1-43 *Candida* **balanitis.** The moist space between the skin surfaces of the uncircumcised penis is an ideal environment for *Candida* infection. This thick white exudates is typical of a severe acute infection. (From Habif TP: *Clinical dermatology: a color guide to diagnosis and therapy,* ed 3, St Louis, 1996, Mosby.)

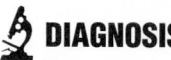
 BASIC INFORMATION

■ DEFINITION

Barrett's esophagus occurs when the squamous lining of the lower esophagus is replaced by columnar epithelium. The condition is associated with an increased risk of esophageal cancer.

■ SYNONYMS

Intestinal metaplasia of the lower esophagus

ICD-9CM CODES

530.2 Barrett's syndrome or ulcer

■ EPIDEMIOLOGY & DEMOGRAPHICS

- Male predominance with a 4:1 ratio of men to women
- Mean age of onset is 40 yr with a mean age of diagnosis of 55 to 60 yr
- Occurs more frequently in Caucasians and Hispanics than in African Americans with a ratio of 10-20:1
- Mean prevalence of 5% to 15% in patients undergoing endoscopy for symptoms of GERD

■ PHYSICAL FINDINGS & CLINICAL PRESENTATION

Symptoms:
- Typically, chronic (>5 yr) heartburn
- Less typical, asymptomatic, incidental finding
- Dysphagia for solid food
- Less frequent: chest pain, hematemesis, or melena

Physical findings:
- Nonspecific
- Ranges from epigastric tenderness on palpation to completely normal

■ ETIOLOGY

- Metaplasia is thought to be secondary to irritation of esophageal lining secondary to chronic gastroesophageal reflux (Fig. 1-44).

- Because not all individuals with GERD develop Barrett's esophagus, there is probably also a genetic propensity for the disease.

 DIAGNOSIS

■ DIFFERENTIAL DIAGNOSIS

- GERD, uncomplicated
- Erosive esophagitis
- Gastritis
- Hiatal hernia
- Peptic ulcer disease
- Angina
- Malignancy
- Stricture or Schatzki's ring

■ DIAGNOSTIC CRITERIA: CONTROVERSIAL

- Long segment (>3 cm, possible higher risk of dysplasia)
- Short segment (<3 cm)
- Junctional intestinal metaplasia

■ DIAGNOSTIC TESTS

- Endoscopy with biopsy necessary for diagnosis
- Histologic hallmark is intestinal metaplasia in esophagus (see Fig. 1-45)
- Upper GI with barium may reveal ulcer crater in esophagus (Fig. 1-46); however, UGI is nonspecific and insensitive for the diagnosis
- Screening for *H. pylori* infection in patients with GERD and Barrett's esophagus is not recommended

TREATMENT

■ NONPHARMACOLOGIC THERAPY

Same as treatment for GERD alone for symptoms of acid reflux (lifestyle modifications); however, chronic acid suppression is generally recommended to decrease inflammation effects on carcinogenesis

■ ACUTE GENERAL Rx

- Proton pump inhibitors (PPIs) are most effective.
- Adequate system control of GERD in patients with Barrett's esophagus may control symptoms and adequate acid suppression may impede the progression to dysplasia.
- If asymptomatic and incidentally found to have Barrett's esophagus, medication use is controversial, but thought to be helpful in impeding progression to dysplasia.

■ CHRONIC Rx

- Laser ablation, photodynamic therapy, endoscopic mucosal resection
- Surgery for: (1) management of GERD and associated sequelae or (2) cancer or precursor lesions

■ SCREENING

- GERD highly prevalent in general population
- Only 4% to 10% of patients with reflux symptoms develop Barrett's esophagus
- ACG recommends that patients with Barrett's undergo surveillance endoscopy and biopsy at intervals determined by the presence and grade of dysplasia, with a range of every 3 mo to 3 yr
- Patients should be treated aggressively for GERD before surveillance

■ DISPOSITION

- Overall, 30 to 50 times increased risk of adenocarcinoma of the esophagus in patients with Barrett's esophagus than in general population
- This risk corresponds to 500 cancers per yr per 100,000 persons with Barrett's esophagus
- Specifics of frequency of monitoring is controversial, no prospective controlled studies to prove that surveillance increases life expectancy
- Usual recommendation is periodic surveillance by endoscopy and multiple biopsies for detection of carcinoma or high-grade dysplasia
- Current generally accepted follow-up recommendations for patients with Barrett's esophagus (no dysplasia) include endoscopy every 2 to 3 yr and q6mo (×2), then once/yr for those with low-grade dysplasia

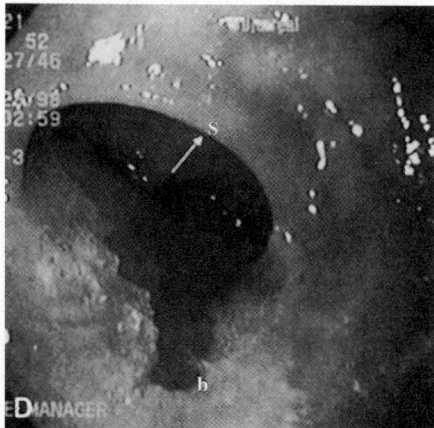

Fig. 1-44 Endoscopic view of the distal esophagus from a patient with gastroesophageal reflux disease showing a tongue of Barrett's mucosa (*b*) and a Schatzki's ring (*s*) (*arrow*). (From Goldman L, Bennett JC [eds]: *Cecil textbook of medicine,* ed 21, Philadelphia, 2000, WB Saunders.)

■ REFERRAL

- For endoscopy with biopsy in patients with chronic GERD symptomatology who have not had previous endoscopy
- For surveillance in those with a previous biopsy-proven diagnosis of Barrett's esophagus
- For those with high-grade dysplasia, biopsies should be confirmed by an expert pathologist, then esophageal resection or intensive surveillance should be offered

REFERENCES

Bammer T et al: Rationale for surgical therapy of Barrett esophagus, *Mayo Clin Proc* 76:335, 2001.

Cameron A: Management of Barrett's esophagus, *Mayo Clin Proc* 73:5, 1998.

Falk GW: Current challenges in Barrett's esophagus, *Cleve Clin J Med* 68:415, 2001.

Hirota WK: Specialized intestinal metaplasia, dysplasia, and cancer of the esophagus: prevalence and clinical date, *Gastroenterology* 116:277, 1999.

Morales TG, Sampliner RE: Barrett's esophagus, *Arch Intern Med* 159:1411, 1999.

Oatu-Lasear R, Fitzgerald RC, Triadafilopoulas G: Differentiation and proliferation in Barrett's esophagus and the effects of acid suppression, *Gastroenterology* 117:327, 1999.

Provenzale D, Schmitt C, Wong JB: Barrett's esophagus: a new look at surveillance based on emerging estimates of cancer risk, *Am J Gastroenterol* 94:2043, 1999.

Rajan E, Burgart LJ, Gostout CJ: Endoscopic and histologic diagnosis of Barrett esophagus, *Mayo Clin Proc* 76:217, 2001.

Samplinear RE: Practice guidelines on the diagnosis, surveillance, and therapy of Barrett's esophagus: the Practice Parameters Committee of the American College of Gastroenterology, *Am J Gastroenterol* 93:1028, 1998.

Shaheen N et al: Gastroesophageal reflux, Barrett esophagus, and esophageal cancer: clinical applications, *JAMA* 287(15):1982, 2002.

Sharma P: Short segment Barrett esophagus and specialized columnar mucosa at the gastroesophageal junction, *Mayo Clin Proc* 76:331, 2001.

Spechler SJ: Barrett's esophageus, *N Engl J Med* 346:836, 2002.

Wang KK, Samplinear RE: Mucosal ablation therapy of Barrett esophagus, *Mayo Clin Proc* 76:433, 2001.

Authors: **Laura Ofstead, M.D., and Rebecca Brienza, M.D., M.P.H.**

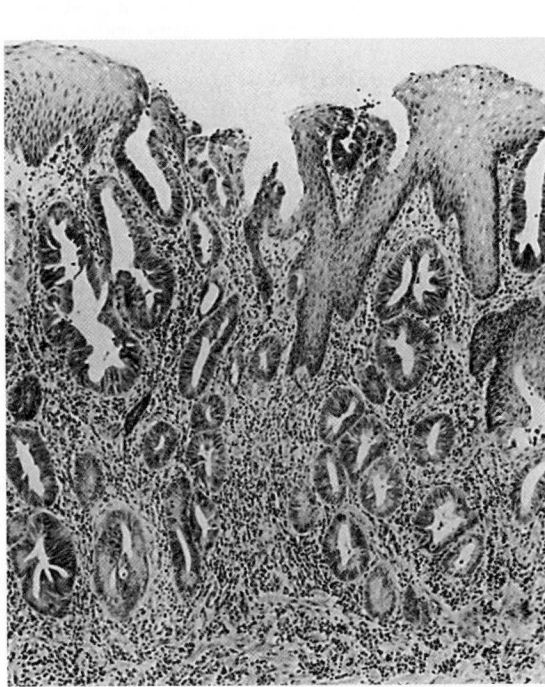

Fig. 1-45 Epithelial metaplasia (original magnification, x16). The esophageal mucosa consists of columnar epithelium (Barrett's esophagus) intermixed with squamous epithelium. (Photomicrograph courtesy Frank Mitros, M.D., Department of Pathology, University of Iowa. From Stein JH [ed]: *Internal medicine,* ed 5, St Louis, 1998, Mosby.)

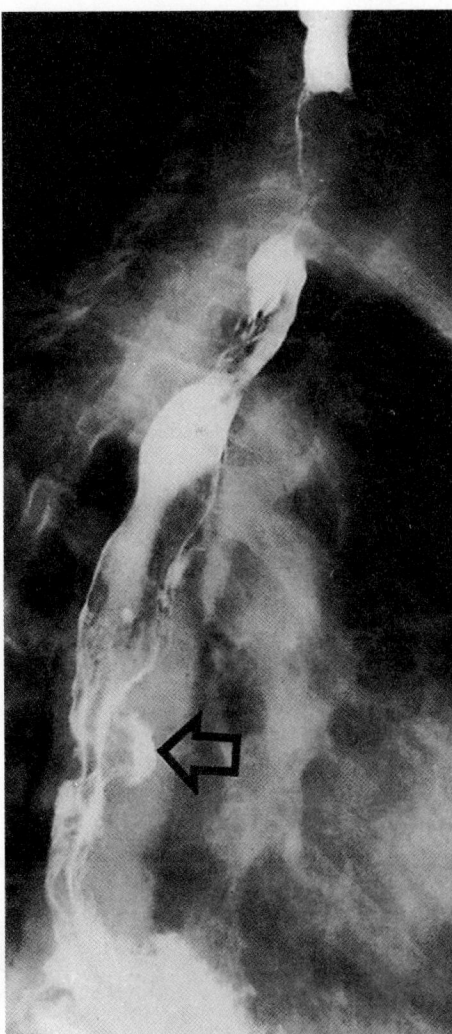

Fig. 1-46   Peptic esophageal ulcer. The occurrence of an ulcer crater (*arrow*) in the esophagus is indicative of Barrett's esophageal mucosal metaplasia. (Radiograph courtesy Charles C. Lu, M.D., Department of Radiology, University of Iowa. From Stein JH [ed]: *Internal medicine,* ed 5, St Louis, 1998, Mosby.)

BASIC INFORMATION

■ DEFINITION

Basal cell carcinoma is a malignant tumor of the skin arising from basal cells of the lower epidermis and adnexal structures. It may be classified as one of six types (nodular, superficial, pigmented, cystic, sclerosing or morpheaform, and nevoid). The most common type is nodular (21%); the least common is morpheaform (1%); a mixed pattern is present in approximately 40% of cases. Basal cell carcinoma advances by direct expansion and destroys normal tissue.

■ SYNONYMS

BCC

ICD-9CM CODES

179.9 Basal cell carcinoma, site unspecified
173.3 Basal cell carcinoma, face
173.4 Basal cell carcinoma, neck, scalp
173.5 Basal cell carcinoma, trunk
173.6 Basal cell carcinoma of the limb
173.7 Basal cell carcinoma, lower limb

■ EPIDEMIOLOGY & DEMOGRAPHICS

- Most common cutaneous neoplasm in humans (>400,000 cases/yr)
- 85% appear on the head and neck region
- Most common site: nose (30%)
- Increased incidence with age >40 yr
- Increased incidence in men
- Risk factors: fair skin, increased sun exposure, use of tanning salons with ultraviolet A or B radiation, history of irradiation (e.g., Hodgkin's disease), personal or family history of skin cancer, impaired immune system

■ PHYSICAL FINDINGS & CLINICAL PRESENTATION

Variable with the histologic type:
- Nodular: dome-shaped, painless lesion that may become multilobular and frequently ulcerates (rodent ulcer); prominent telangiectatic vessels

are noted on the surface; border is translucent, elevated, pearly white (Fig. 1-47); some nodular basal cell carcinomas may contain pigmentation, giving an appearance similar to a melanoma.
- Superficial: circumscribed scaling black appearance with a thin raised pearly white border; a crust and erosions may be present; occurs most frequently on the trunk and extremities.
- Morpheaform: flat or slightly raised yellowish or white appearance (similar to localized scleroderma); appearance similar to scars, surface has a waxy consistency.

■ ETIOLOGY

Sun exposure and use of tanning salons with equipment that emits ultraviolet A or B radiation

DIAGNOSIS

■ DIFFERENTIAL DIAGNOSIS

- Keratoacanthoma
- Melanoma (pigmented basal cell carcinoma)
- Xeroderma pigmentosa
- Basal cell nevus syndrome
- Molluscum contagiosum
- Sebaceous hyperplasia
- Psoriasis

■ WORKUP

Biopsy to confirm diagnosis

TREATMENT

■ NONPHARMACOLOGIC THERAPY

Avoidance of excessive tanning, use of sunscreens to prevent damage from excessive sun exposure

■ ACUTE GENERAL Rx

Variable with tumor size, location, and cell type:
- Excision surgery: preferred method for large tumors with well-defined borders on the legs, cheeks, forehead, and trunk
- Mohs' micrographic surgery: preferred for lesions in high-risk areas (e.g., nose, eyelid), very large primary tumors, recurrent basal cell carcinomas, and tumors with poorly defined clinical margins
- Electrodesiccation and curettage: useful for small (<6 mm) nodular basal cell carcinomas
- Cryosurgery with liquid nitrogen: useful in basal cell carcinomas of the superficial and nodular types with clearly definable margins; no clear advantages over the other forms of therapy; generally reserved for uncomplicated tumors
- Radiation therapy: generally used for basal cell carcinomas in areas requiring preservation of normal surround tissues for cosmetic reasons (e.g., around lips); also useful in patients who cannot tolerate surgical procedures or for large lesions and surgical failures

■ CHRONIC Rx

Periodic evaluation for at least 5 yr because of increased risk of recurrence of another basal cell carcinoma (>40% risk within 5 yr of treatment)

■ DISPOSITION

- More than 90% of patients are cured.
- A lesion is considered low risk if it is <1.5 cm in diameter, is nodular or cystic, is not in a difficult-to-treat area (H zone of face), and has not been previously treated.
- Nodular and superficial basal cell carcinomas are the least aggressive.
- Morpheaform lesions have the highest incidence of positive tumor margins (>30%) and the greatest recurrence rate.

Author: **Fred F. Ferri, M.D.**

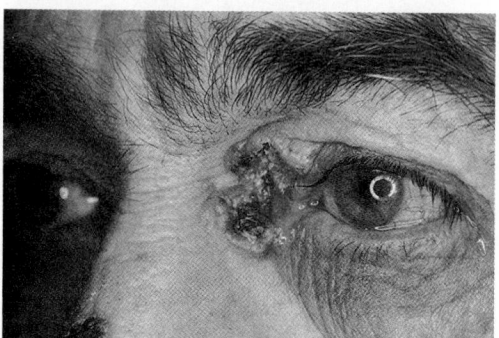

Fig. 1-47 **Basal cell carcinoma.** Note rolled translucent border and central ulceration in typical facial location. (From Noble J et al: *Textbook of primary care medicine,* ed 3, St Louis, 2001, Mosby.)

BASIC INFORMATION

■ DEFINITION

Behçet's disease is a chronic, relapsing, inflammatory disorder characterized by the presence of recurrent oral aphthous ulcers, genital ulcers, uveitis, and skin lesions (Figs. 1-48 and 1-49).

ICD-9CM CODES
136.1 Behçet's syndrome

■ EPIDEMIOLOGY & DEMOGRAPHICS

Behçet's disease is observed in two different geographic locations.
• One region consists of Japan, Korea, Turkey, and the Mediterranean basin.
  1. Prevalence ranges from 1:7000 to 1:10,000.
  2. Turkey has the highest prevalence at 80 to 370 cases per 100,000.
• The second region consists of North America and Northern Europe.
  1. Prevalence ranges from 1:20,000 to 1:100,000.
  2. Prevalence of Behçet's disease in the U.S. is 0.12 to 0.33 cases per 100,000.
• In these regions the prevalence of HLA-B51 is higher in patients with Behçet's disease
• Males = females

■ PHYSICAL FINDINGS & CLINICAL PRESENTATION

• Behçet's disease typically affects individuals in the third to fourth decade of life and primarily presents with painful aphthous oral ulcers. The ulcers occur in crops measuring 2 to 10 mm in size and are found on the mucous membrane of the cheek, gingiva, tongue, pharynx, and soft palate
• Genital ulcers are similar to the oral ulcers
• Decreased vision secondary to uveitis, keratitis, or vitreous hemorrhage, or occlusion of the retinal artery or vein may occur
• Skin findings include nodular lesions, which are histologically equally divided to erythema nodosum-like lesions superficial thrombophlebitis, and acne lesions, which are also presented at sites uncommon for ordinary acne (arms and legs)
• Arthritis and arthralgias
• CNS meningeal findings including headache, fever, and stiff neck can occur. Cerebellar ataxia and pseudobulbar palsy occur with involvement of the brainstem
• Vasculitis leading to both arterial and venous inflammation or occlusion can result in signs and symptoms of a myocardial infarction, intermittent claudication, deep vein thrombosis, hemoptysis, and aneurysm formation

■ ETIOLOGY

The etiology of Behçet's disease is unknown. An immune-related vasculitis is thought to lead to many of the manifestations of Behçet's disease. What triggers the immune response and activation is not yet known.

DIAGNOSIS

According to the International Study Group for Behçet's disease, the diagnosis of Behçet's disease is established when recurrent oral ulceration is present along with at least two of the following in the absence of other systemic diseases:
• Recurrent genital ulceration
• Eye lesions
• Skin lesions
• Positive pathergy test

■ DIFFERENTIAL DIAGNOSIS
• Ulcerative colitis
• Crohn's disease
• Lichen planus
• Pemphigoid
• Herpes simplex infection
• Benign aphthous stomatitis
• SLE
• Reiter's syndrome
• Ankylosing spondylitis
• AIDS
• Hypereosinophilic syndrome.
• Sweet's syndrome

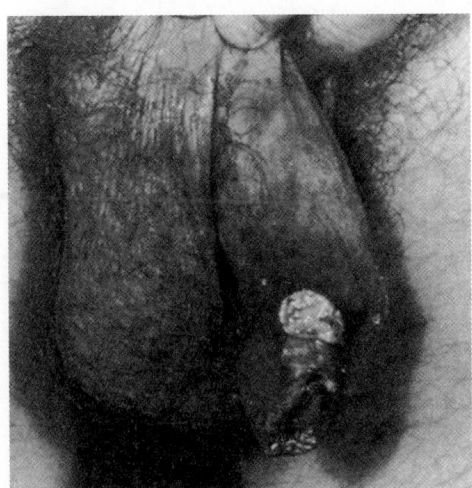

Fig. 1-48 Behçet's syndrome. Painful prepuceal ulcer in a male with superficial thrombophlebitis, oral ulcers, and bowel vasculitis. (From Canoso J: *Rheumatology in primary care,* Philadelphia, 1997, WB Saunders.)

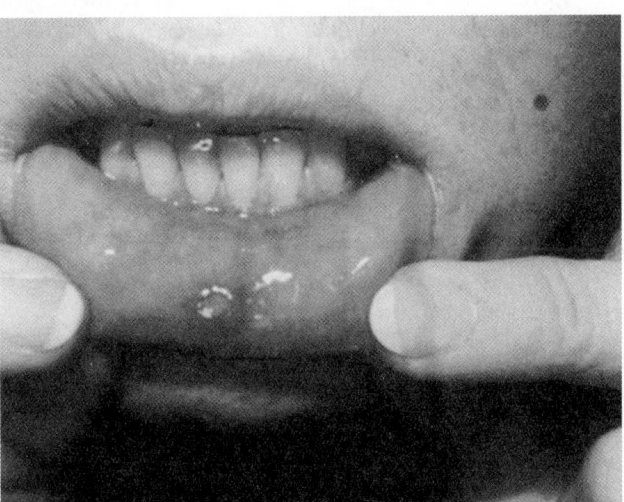

Fig. 1-49 Behçet's syndrome. Painful aphthous inner lower lip ulcer in a 30-year-old Chinese woman with relapsing oral and genital ulcers and uveitis. She did well on low-dose prednisone plus colchicines. (From Canoso J: *Rheumatology in primary care,* Philadelphia, 1997, WB Saunders.)

■ WORKUP

The diagnosis of Behçet's disease is a clinical diagnosis. Laboratory tests and x-ray imaging may be helpful in working up the complications of Behçet's disease or excluding other diseases in the differential.

■ LABORATORY TESTS

There are no diagnostic laboratory tests for Behçet's disease.

■ IMAGING STUDIES

CT scan, MRI, and angiography are useful for detecting CNS and vascular lesions

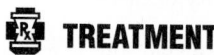 **TREATMENT**

Treatment is directed at the patient's clinical presentation (e.g., mucocutaneous lesions, ocular lesions, arthritis, GI, CNS, or vascular lesions).

■ NONPHARMACOLOGIC THERAPY

Supportive care

■ ACUTE GENERAL Rx

- Oral and genital ulcers
  1. Topical corticosteroids (e.g., triamcinolone acetonide ointment applied tid)
  2. Tetracycline tablets 250 mg dissolved in 5 cc water and applied to the ulcer for 2 to 3 min
  3. Colchicine 0.5 to 1.5 mg/kg/day PO
  4. Thalidomide 100 to 300 mg PO daily
  5. Dapsone 100 mg PO daily
  6. Pentoxifylline 300 mg/day PO
  7. Azathioprine 1-2.5 mg/kg/day PO
  8. Methotrexate 7.5-25 mg/wk PO or IV
- Ocular lesions
  1. Anterior uveitis is treated by an ophthalmologist with topical corticosteroids (e.g., betamethasone drops 1 to 2 drops tid). Topical injection with dexamethasone 1 to 1.5 mg has also been tried

  2. Infliximab 5 mg/kg single dose
- CNS disease
  1. Chlorambucil 0.1 mg/kg/day is used in the treatment of posterior uveitis, retinal vasculitis, or CNS disease. Patients not responding to chlorambucil can be tried on cyclosporine 5 to 7 mg/kg/day.
  2. In CNS vasculitis, cyclophosphamide 2 to 3 mg/kg/day is used. Prednisone can be used as an alternative.
- Arthritis
  1. NSAIDs (e.g., ibuprofen 400 to 800 mg tid PO or indomethacin 50 to 75 mg/day PO)
  2. Sulfasalazine 1 to 3 g/day PO is an alternative treatment
- GI lesions
  1. Sulfasalazine 1 to 3 g/day PO
  2. Prednisone 40 to 60 mg/day PO
- Vascular lesions
  1. Prednisone 40 to 60 mg/day PO
  2. Cytotoxic agents as mentioned previously
  3. Heparin 5000 to 20,000 U/day followed by oral warfarin

■ CHRONIC Rx

- Chronic therapy is usually continued for approximately 1 yr after remission.
- Surgery may be indicated in patients with complications of bowel perforation, vascular occlusive disease, and aneurysm formation.

■ DISPOSITION

- The aphthous oral ulcers last 1 to 2 wk, recurring more frequently than genital ulcers.
- Approximately 25% of patients with ocular lesions become blind.
- The disease course is unpredictable.
- Complications include:
  1. Meningitis
  2. Cerebrovascular accident (stroke)
  3. Aneurysm rupture
  4. Peripheral lower-extremity ischemia
  5. Mesenteric ischemia
  6. Myocardial infarction

■ REFERRAL

If the diagnosis of Behçet's disease is suspected, a referral to both rheumatology and ophthalmology is indicated because the disease is so rare.

☼ PEARLS & CONSIDERATIONS

■ COMMENTS

The pathergy test refers to the formation of a papule or pustule of 2 mm or more in size after oblique insertion of a sterile 20- or 25-gauge needle into the skin.

REFERENCES

International Study Group for Behçet's Disease: Criteria for diagnosis of Behçet's disease, *Lancet* 335:1078, 1990.

Meador R, Ehrlich E, Von Feldt JM: Behçet's disease: immunopathologic and therapeutic aspects, *Curr Rheumatol Rep* 4(1):47, 2002.

Saenz A et al: Pharmacotherapy for Behçet's syndrome, *Cochrane Database Syst Rev* 2:CD001084, 2000.

Sakane T et al: Behcet's disease, *N Engl J Med* 341(17):1284, 1999.

Sfikakis PP et al: Effect of infliximab on sight-threatening panuveitis in Behçet's disease, *Lancet* (358):295, 2001.

Yazici H: Behçet's syndrome: an update, *Curr Rheumatol Rep* (5):195, 2003.

Authors: **Mina Pantcheva, M.D., and Peter Petropoulos, M.D.**

BASIC INFORMATION

■ DEFINITION

Bell's palsy is an idiopathic, isolated, usually unilateral facial weakness in the distribution of the seventh cranial nerve (<1% of the facial palsies are bilateral)

■ SYNONYMS

Idiopathic facial paralysis

ICD-9CM CODES

351.0 Bell's palsy

■ EPIDEMIOLOGY & DEMOGRAPHICS

INCIDENCE: 13-34 cases/100,000 persons
RISK FACTORS:
- Pregnancy (especially third trimester/first postpartum week)
- Age >30
- Diabetes (present in 5%-10% of patients)
- Travel to area endemic for Lyme disease

■ PHYSICAL FINDINGS & CLINICAL PRESENTATION

- Unilateral paralysis of the upper and lower facial muscles (asymmetric eye closure, brow, and smile). Upward rolling of eye on attempted eye closure ("Bell's phenomenon")
- Ipsilateral loss of taste
- Ipsilateral ear pain, usually 2-3 days before presentation
- Increased or decreased unilateral eye tearing
- Hyperacusis
- Subjective (but not objective) ipsilateral facial numbness

■ ETIOLOGY

- Most cases are idiopathic.
- The cause is often viral (herpes simplex).
- Herpes zoster can cause Bell's palsy in association with herpetic blisters affecting the outer ear canal or the area behind the ear (Ramsay-Hunt Syndrome).
- Bell's palsy can also be one of the manifestations of Lyme disease.

DIAGNOSIS

■ DIFFERENTIAL DIAGNOSIS

- Neoplasms affecting the base of the skull or the parotid gland
- Bacterial infectious process (meningitis, otitis media, osteomyelitis of the base of the skull)
- Brainstem stroke
- Multiple sclerosis
- Sarcoidosis
- Head trauma with fracture of temporal bone
- Other: Guillain-Barré, carcinomatous or leukemic meningitis, leprosy, Melkersson-Rosenthal syndrome

■ WORKUP

Bell's palsy is a clinical diagnosis. A focused history and neurologic examination will confirm the diagnosis.

■ LABORATORY TESTS

- Fasting blood sugar to evaluate for diabetes
- Consider CBC, VDRL, ESR, ACE in selected patients
- Lyme titer in endemic areas

■ IMAGING STUDIES

- Contrast-enhanced MRI to exclude neoplasms is indicated only in patients with atypical features or course.
- Chest x-ray examination may be useful to exclude sarcoidosis or to rule out TB in selected patients before treating with steroids.

TREATMENT

■ NONPHARMACOLOGIC THERAPY

- Reassure patient that the disease is most likely a result of a virus attacking the nerve, not a stroke. It is also important to inform the patient that the prognosis is good.
- Avoid corneal drying by applying skin tape to the upper lid to keep the palpebral fissure narrowed. Lacri-Lube ophthalmic ointment at night and artificial tears during the day are also useful to prevent excessive drying.
- The patient should use dark glasses when going outside to minimize sun exposure.

■ ACUTE GENERAL Rx

- Although the benefits of corticosteroid therapy remain unproven, most practitioners use a brief course of prednisone therapy. Combination therapy with acyclovir and prednisone may possibly be effective in improvement of clinical recovery.
- If used, prednisone therapy should be started within 24-48 hr of symptom onset.
- Optimal steroid dose is unknown. Prednisone can be given as one 50-mg tablet qd for 7 days without tapering or can be started at 80 mg and tapered by 5 mg/day until finished. A Medrol dose-pack may also be given.

■ CHRONIC Rx

Patients should be monitored for evidence of corneal abrasion and ulceration or hemifacial spasm. Physical therapy including moist heat and massage may be beneficial.

■ DISPOSITION

- 71% of patients should recover completely. Prognosis is improved for those with clinical improvement within 3 wk and with less severity of symptoms at onset.
  Recovery begins within 3 wk in 85% of patients, with the remainder having some improvement within 3-6 mo.
- Recurrence is experienced in 5% of Bell's palsy cases.

■ REFERRAL

- Persistent redness or irritation of the eye requires referral to an ophthalmologist.
- Neurology referral is recommended if diagnosis is unclear or if the clinical course is atypical.

REFRENCES

Grogan PM: Practice parameter: steroids, acyclovir, and surgery for Bell's palsy (an evidence-based review): report of the Quality Standards Subcommittee of the American Academy of Neurology, *Neurology* 56(7):830, 2001.

Jabor, MA, Gianoli, G: Management of Bell's palsy, *J La State Med Soc* 148:279, 1996.

Mountain, RE, et al: The Edinburgh facial palsy clinic: a review of three years' activity, *J R Coll Surg Edinb* 39:275, 1994.

Peitersen, E: The natural history of Bell's palsy, *Am J Otol* 4:107, 1982.

Author: **Richard Isaacson, M.D.**

BASIC INFORMATION

■ DEFINITION

Bipolar disorder is an episodic, recurrent, and frequently progressive condition in which the afflicted individual suffers periods of mania and, possibly, depression. Depressive episodes are not essential for the diagnosis. However, the individual must experience at least one manic episode in which he or she experiences at least 1 wk of continuous symptoms of elevated, expansive, or irritable mood in association with three or four of the following:

- Decreased need for sleep
- Grandiosity
- Pressured speech
- Subjective or objective flight of ideas
- Distractibility
- Increased level of goal-directed activity
- Problematic behavior

■ SYNONYMS

Manic-depression
Cycloid psychosis

ICD-9CM CODES

296.4-6 Circular manic, circular depressed, circular type mixed

■ EPIDEMIOLOGY & DEMOGRAPHICS

INCIDENCE (IN U.S.): Approximately 1% of the population
PREVALENCE (IN U.S.): 0.4% to 1.6%
PREDOMINANT SEX: Equal distribution among male and female
PREDOMINANT AGE: Lifelong condition with age of onset 14 to 30 yr
PEAK INCIDENCE: Onset in 20s
GENETICS:

- Concordance rates for monozygotic twins: 0.7 to 0.9, for dizygotic twins: 0.2 to 0.4
- Risk of offspring with one affected parent: 0.2 to 0.4, with two affected parents: 0.4 to 0.7
- Displays the phenomenon of genetic anticipation (earlier onset with successive generations), which is a hallmark phenomenon of trinucleotide repeat diseases
- CAG trinucleotide repeats increased by approximately 30 repeats but location unknown
- Displays a parent of origin effect in which there is a higher frequency of the disease in maternal relatives
- Susceptibility locus mapped to chromosome 18p

■ PHYSICAL FINDINGS & CLINICAL PRESENTATION

- Mania associated with psychomotor activation that is usually goal directed but not necessarily productive
- Elevated and frequently labile mood
- Flight of ideas with rapid, loud, pressured speech
- Psychosis with delusions, hallucinations, and formal thought disorder possible
- Depressive episodes resembling major depression (see "Major Depression"); however, retardation usually extreme
- Catatonia possible in severe cases

■ ETIOLOGY

- Unknown
- Hypotheses:
  1. Abnormalities of membrane function
  2. Second messenger abnormalities
  3. Noradrenergic excess

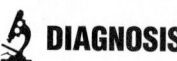

DIAGNOSIS

■ DIFFERENTIAL DIAGNOSIS

- Secondary manias caused by medical disorder (e.g., renal disease, AIDS, stroke, digoxin toxicity) are frequent.
- Onset of mania after age 40 yr is suggestive of secondary mania.
- Less severe, and probably distinct, conditions of bipolar type II and cyclothymia are possible.
- Cross-sectional examination of acutely manic patient can be confused with schizophreniform or a paranoid psychosis.

■ WORKUP

- History
- Physical examination
- Mental status examination

■ LABORATORY TESTS

- Because of high rate of secondary manias, initial presentation to confirm health of all major organ systems (routine chemistries, complete blood count, urinalysis, sedimentation rate)
- Low threshold for examination of CSF

■ IMAGING STUDIES

Imaging of anatomy (CT scan or MRI) as well as function (EEG) should be part of initial workup.

TREATMENT

■ NONPHARMACOLOGIC THERAPY

- Psychotherapy to help patients cope with consequences of the disease and improve compliance with medications
- Bright light therapy in the northern latitudes in individuals exhibiting a seasonal pattern of winter depression

■ ACUTE GENERAL Rx

- First-line agents for acute mania: lithium, valproate, carbamazepine lamotrigine, and olanzapine
- Useful adjuncts to acute treatment: antipsychotics and benzodiazepines
- Problematic because antidepressants can induce manic episodes

■ CHRONIC Rx

- Goal of long-term treatment: prevention
- Best agents for prophylaxis: lithium, valproate, and carbamazepine
- Useful second-line agents: antipsychotics (particularly the atypical agents such as clozapine)
- Long-term use of antidepressants: frequently destabilizes patient and leads to more frequent relapses

■ DISPOSITION

- Course is variable.
- More than 90% of patients having a single manic episode are likely to experience others.
- Uncontrolled manic or depressive episodes can lead to additional episodes ("illness begets illness").
- Untreated suicide rate approaches 20%; drops to only 8% to 10% with treatment.
- Psychosocioeconomic consequences of both mania and depression can be severe and disabling.

■ REFERRAL

- If use of antidepressant contemplated
- If patient is severely manic or suicidal

REFERENCES

Balderassini RJ, Tondo L: Suicide risk and treatment for patients with bipolar disorders, *JAMA* 290:1517, 2003.

El-Mallakh RS: *Lithium: actions and mechanisms,* Washington, DC, 1996, American Psychiatric Press.

El-Mallakh RS, Karippot A: Use of antidepressants to treat depression in bipolar disorder, *Psychiatr Serv* 53:580, 2002.

Author: **Rif S. El-Mallakh, M.D.**

BASIC INFORMATION

■ DEFINITION
A bite wound can be animal or human, accidental or intentional.

ICD-9CM CODES
879.8 Bite wound, unspecified site

■ EPIDEMIOLOGY & DEMOGRAPHICS
- Bite wounds account for 1% of emergency department visits.
- More than 1 million bites occur in humans annually in the U.S.
- Dog bites account for 85% to 90% of all bites and result in 10 to 20 fatalities yearly in the U.S.; cat bites, 10% to 20%. Typically the animal is owned by the victim.
- Infection rates are highest for cat bites (30% to 50%), followed by human bites (15% to 30%) and dog bites (5%).
- The extremities are involved in 75% of bites.

■ PHYSICAL FINDINGS & CLINICAL PRESENTATION
- The appearance of the bite wound is variable (e.g., puncture wound, tear, avulsion).
- Cellulitis, lymphangitis, and focal adenopathy may be present in infected bite wounds.
- Patient may experience fever and chills.

■ ETIOLOGY
- Increased risk of infection: human and cat bites, closed fist injuries, wounds involving joints, puncture wounds, face and lip bites, bites with skull penetration, bites in immunocompromised hosts
- Most frequent infecting organisms:
  1. *Pasteurella* spp.: responsible for majority of infections within 24 hr of dog (*P. canis*) and cat (*P. multocida, P. septica*) bites
  2. *Capnocytophaga canimorsus* (formerly DF-2 bacillus): a gram-negative organism responsible for late infection, usually following dog bites
  3. Gram-negative organisms (*Pseudomonas, Haemophilus*): often found in human bites
  4. *Streptococcus* spp., *Staphylococcus aureus*
  5. *Eikenella corrodens* in human bites

DIAGNOSIS

■ DIFFERENTIAL DIAGNOSIS
- Bite from a rabid animal (often the attack is unprovoked)
- Factitious injury

■ WORKUP
- Determination of the time elapsed since the patient was bitten, status of rabies immunization of the animal, and underlying medical conditions that might predispose the patient to infection (e.g., DM, immunodeficiency)
- Documentation of bite site, notification of appropriate authorities (e.g., police department, animal officer)

■ LABORATORY TESTS
- Generally not necessary
- Hct if there has been significant blood loss
- Wound cultures (aerobic and anaerobic) if there is evidence of sepsis or victim is immunocompromised patient; cultures should be obtained before irrigation of the wound but after superficial cleaning

■ IMAGING STUDIES
X-rays are indicated when bony penetration is suspected or if there is suspicion of fracture or significant trauma; x-rays are also useful for detecting presence of foreign bodies (when suspected).

TREATMENT

■ NONPHARMACOLOGIC THERAPY
- Local care with debridement, vigorous cleansing, and saline irrigation of the wound; debridement of devitalized tissue
- High-pressure irrigation to clean bite wound and ensure removal of contaminants (e.g., use saline solution with a 30- to 35-ml syringe equipped with a 20-gauge needle or catheter with tip of syringe placed 2 to 3 cm above the wound)
- Avoid blunt probing of wounds (increased risk of infection)

■ ACUTE GENERAL Rx
- Avoid suturing of hand wounds and any wounds that appear infected
- Puncture wounds should be left open
- Give antirabies therapy and tetanus immune globulin and toxoid as needed (Table 1-12)
- Use empiric antibiotic therapy in high-risk wounds (e.g., cat bite, hand bites, face bites, genital area bites, bites with joint or bone penetration, human bites, immunocompromised host): amoxicillin-clavulanate (Augmentin) 500 to 875 mg bid for 7 days or cefuroxime (Ceftin) 250 to 50 mg bid for 7 days
- In hospitalized patients, IV antibiotics of choice are cefoxitin 1 to 2 g q6h, ampicillin-sulbactam 1.5 to 3 g q6h, ticarcillin-clavulanate 3 g q6h, or ceftriaxone 1 to 2 g q24h
- Prophylactic therapy for persons bitten by others with HIV and hepatitis B (see Section V)

■ DISPOSITION
Prognosis is favorable with proper treatment. Box 1-6 describes risk factors for infection from animal bite.

■ REFERRAL
- Hospitalization and IV antibiotic therapy for infected human bites; bites with injury to joints, nerves, or tendons; or any animal bites unresponsive to oral therapy
- In the outpatient setting, bite wounds should be reevaluated within 48 hr to assess for signs of infection.

REFERENCE
Presutti RJ: Prevention and treatment of dog bites, *Am Fam Physician* 63:1567, 2001.
Author: **Fred F. Ferri, M.D.**

BOX 1-6   Risk Factors for Infection from Animal Bite

High Risk
Location

Hand, wrist, or foot
Scalp or face in patients with high risk of cranial perforation;
  CT or skull radiograph examination is mandatory
Over a major joint (possibility of perforation)
Through-and-through bite of cheek

Type of wound

Punctures that are difficult or impossible to irrigate adequately
Tissue crushing that cannot be debrided (typical of herbivores)
Carnivore bite over vital structure (artery, nerve, joint)

Patient

Older than 50 years
Asplenic
Chronic alcoholic
Altered immune status (chemotherapy, acquired immuno-
  deficiency syndrome [AIDS], immune defect)
Diabetic
Peripheral vascular insufficiency
Chronic corticosteroid therapy
Prosthetic or diseased cardiac valve (consider systemic pro-
  phylaxis)
Prosthetic or seriously diseased joint (consider systemic pro-
  phylaxis)

Species

Large cat (canine teeth produce deep punctures that can pene-
  trate joints, cranium)
Primates
Pigs (anecdotal evidence only)
Alligators, crocodiles

Low Risk
Location

Face, scalp, ears, and mouth (all facial wounds should be
  sutured)
Self-bite of buccal mucosa that does not go through to skin

Type of wound

Large, clean lacerations that can be thoroughly cleansed (the
  larger the laceration, the lower the infection rate)
Partial-thickness lacerations and abrasions

Species

Rodents
Quokkas
Bats (although high risk for rabies)

From Auerbach PS: *Wilderness medicine,* ed 4, St Louis, 2001, Mosby.
CT, Computed tomography.

TABLE 1-12   Tetanus Prophylaxis

HISTORY OF IMMUNIZATION (DOSES)	CLEAN MINOR WOUNDS		MAJOR DIRTY WOUNDS	
	TOXOID*	TIG†	TOXOID	TIG
Unknown	Yes	No	Yes	Yes
None to one	Yes	No	Yes	Yes
Two	Yes	No	Yes	No (unless wound older than 24 hr)
Three or more				
Last booster within 5 years	No	No	No	No
Last booster within 10 years	No	No	Yes	Yes
Last booster more than 10 years ago	Yes	No	Yes	Yes

From Auerbach PS: *Wilderness medicine,* ed 4, St Louis, 2001, Mosby.
*Toxoid: Adult: 0.5 ml DT intramuscularly (IM). Child less than 5 years old: 0.5 ml DPT IM. Child older than 5 years: 0.5 ml DT IM.
†Tetanus immune globulin (TIG): 250 to 500 units IM in limb contralateral to toxoid.

BASIC INFORMATION

■ DEFINITION
- Bees, wasps, and ants that sting
- Flies, mosquitoes, fleas, and lice that bite
- Two major classes of arthropods: insects, arachnida

ICD-9CM CODES
989.5 Anaphylactic shock or reaction
910-915 For bites/injury, superficial by site (0.4 if not infected, 0.5 if infected)

■ EPIDEMIOLOGY & DEMOGRAPHICS
- Occur during warm weather, near nests
- Bees attracted to bright clothing and perfumes
- Mosquitoes near standing water
- Flies near horses
- Fleas from pets
- Lice and scabies from person to person or clothing
- 0.4% to 4% of population allergic to venom of one or more stinging insects

■ PHYSICAL FINDINGS & CLINICAL PRESENTATION
BEE, WASP, AND ANT STINGS:
Local Reaction:
- Erythema
- Edema surrounding site; can be life threatening if involves mouth or throat and causes airway obstruction
- Stings around eye can lead to iris or lens damage
Toxic Reaction:
- Usually with more than 10 stings
- Vomiting, diarrhea, syncope or urticaria, or bronchospasm
Systemic or Anaphylactic Reaction:
- Rapid onset, symptoms intensify rapidly
- Urticaria, dry cough, progresses to chest constriction, wheezing, vertigo, vomiting, shock, within 30 min or less
Delayed Reaction:
- Serum sickness-like symptoms 10 to 14 days after sting
FLEA, LICE, AND SCABIES BITES:
- Similar lesions, small red spots or lines become erythematous
- Highly pruritic, thus usually see linear scratch marks
- Scabies concentrates on hands and feet, leaves zigzag red burrows

SPIDER AND SCORPION BITES:
- The class *Arachnida* contains the largest number of venomous species known and includes black widow spiders and brown recluse spiders.
- The classic symptomatology of the black widow spider is initially a pinprick sensation followed by swelling and redness; two small fang marks may be noticed.

■ ETIOLOGY
- Various insects
- Systemic reaction thought to be IgE-mediated, causing release of histamine and other anaphylactic mediators
- Venoms contain histamine and various antigens

DIAGNOSIS

■ DIFFERENTIAL DIAGNOSIS
History is crucial in attempting to correctly identify bees or hornets, which may be important if immunotherapy is a future consideration. Patients can usually identify fleas, flies, and mosquitoes. Body lice concentrate about waist, shoulder, neck, axillae. Head lice look like dandruff but can't be brushed out. Pubic lice appear as bluish spots on abdomen and thighs. Scabies causes burrows on hands and feet.

■ WORKUP
Physical examination: look for stingers and remove if possible. Scabies burrows can have mites that can be scraped with a blade and identified under a microscope.

TREATMENT

Stings:
- Remove stinger by scraping; do not use tweezers because this can squeeze venom into wound
- Local reactions: ice pack, oral antihistamines, analgesics, prednisone; elevate involved limbs
- Systemic reaction: epinephrine 1:1000, 0.3 to 0.5 ml SC; massage injection site to hasten absorption; second injection every 15 min as necessary; antihistamines IV

- Bronchospasm: β_2-agonist as necessary; intubate, if necessary, for airway obstruction
- Hypotension supportive care with isotonic fluids
- IV steroids: limit urticaria and edema
Fly, mosquito, and flea bites:
- Symptomatic treatment similar to stings, clean to prevent secondary infection
- Head lice: permethrin 5% (Elimite), repeat in 7 to 10 days; comb with fine comb to remove nits; safe in children over 2 mo
- Body lice: sterilization of clothing, disposal if possible
- Scabies: permethrin 5% cream, chin to toes; leave on 8 to 10 hr, repeat in 7 days
- Second-line agent for scabies is lindane 1%: not safe in children or pregnancy
Spider bite (black widow):
- Apply ice pack to bite area, immediate transport to ER
- Tetanus immunization should be instituted
- Symptomatic treatment (e.g., controlling muscle cramps with calcium gluconate, dantrolene sodium, diazepam)
- Cardiac monitoring, antivenin

■ DISPOSITION
- For patients with systemic reactions, send home with emergency epinephrine kit
- If severe or anaphylactic reaction, admit and observe for 48 hr for cardiac, renal, or neurologic problems

■ REFERRAL
For patients with systemic reactions, refer to allergist for immunotherapy; 95% to 98% effective in preventing anaphylaxis

REFERENCE
Blackman JR: Spider bites, *J Am Board Fam Pract* 8(4):288, 1995.
Author: **Gail M. O'Brien, M.D.**

BASIC INFORMATION

■ DEFINITION
Most stinging insects belong to the Hymenoptera order and include yellow jackets (most common cause of reactions), bumble bees, sweat bees, wasps, harvester ants, fire ants, and the Africanized honey bee "killer bee." Brown recluse spiders, although they are not insects, are another common cause of bites. The usual effect of a sting is to cause intense local pain, some immediate erythema, and often a small area of edema by injecting venom. Allergic reactions can be either local or generalized.

■ SYNONYMS
Venom allergy

ICD-9CM CODES
989.5 Stings (bees, wasps)
989.5 Bites (fire ant, brown recluse spider)

■ EPIDEMIOLOGY & DEMOGRAPHICS
PREVALENCE (OF BEE STINGS AND INSECT BITES):
- Unknown
- Between 0.4% and 4% of the population is allergic to the venom of one or more stinging insects
- Most anaphylactic reactions occur in those most likely to be exposed including children, males, outdoor workers
- Bites by fire ants and brown recluse spiders are less likely to cause systemic disease

INCIDENCE (IN U.S.): 50 to 150 people die each year from insect sting anaphylaxis; anaphylaxis occurs more often within 10 to 30 min of a sting. Delayed reactions are rare occurring only in <0.3% of stings.

■ PHYSICAL FINDINGS & CLINICAL PRESENTATION
Stings:
- Cutaneous: the skin is the most common site of an allergic reaction. Manifestations include flushing, urticaria, pruritus, and angioedema.
- Respiratory: hoarseness, difficulty speaking, choking, throat tightness or tingling may progress to stridor, laryngeal edema, laryngospasm, and bronchoconstriction. This is the leading cause of anaphylactic death.
- Cardiovascular: manifestations include tachycardia, hypotension, arrhythmia, in some cases progressing to profound hypovolemic shock. Myocardial infarction is rare. Cardiac manifestations are the second leading cause of death from anaphylaxis.

- Other symptoms: abdominal pain, nausea, vomiting, and diarrhea.
Bites:
Brown recluse spider:
- Erythematous, violaceous, or hemorrhagic discoloration at site within 8 hr
- Central necrosis: lesions <1 cm heal within weeks; lesions >1 cm take months to heal
- Mild hemolysis, mild coagulopathy
- Fevers, chills, vomiting, joint pain
Fire ant:
- Circularly arrayed pustules

■ ETIOLOGY
Stings:
- Most systemic reactions to insect stings are classic IgE-mediated allergic reactions.
- Reactions occur in previously sensitized patients who have produced high titers of IgE antibody to insect venom antigens.
- Sensitization to wasp venom requires only a few stings and can occur after a single sting.
- Sensitization to bee venom occurs mainly in people who have been stung frequently by bees.
Bites:
- Brown recluse spider venom contains enzymes that can cause tissue necrosis.
- Fire ant venom contains proteins toxic to the skin.

DIAGNOSIS

■ DIFFERENTIAL DIAGNOSIS
- Stings: cellulitis, bites
- Bites: stings, cellulitis

■ WORKUP
History is essential for accurate diagnosis including timing of sting or bite and type of insect (bee, wasp, spider, or ant) if known.

■ LABORATORY TESTS
- Skin test: either skin prick test or intradermal with bee and wasp venom.
- Measurement of serum bee-specific or wasp-specific IgE measured by radioallergosorbent tests (RAST) or other assays.

TREATMENT

■ ACUTE GENERAL Rx
Sting:
- Removal of the stinger, cleansing, and application of ice
- Treatment with oral antihistamines if limited reaction. Topical corticosteroids may provide some relief of inflammation

- Treatment for larger swellings and associated systemic symptoms is IM antihistamines, intravenous corticosteroids, adrenaline, IM epinephrine, and IV fluids
Bite:
- Supportive
- Application of ice
Brown recluse spider:
- Excision of lesion
- Dapsone
- IV corticosteroids

■ DISPOSITION
Sting:
Prognosis for a limited reaction is excellent. Anywhere from 20% to 80% of patients who have had generalized reaction to a sting will have no such reaction on subsequent sting and there is no evidence that the next sting will necessarily cause a more severe reaction. The reasons for the variable outcome include patient's immune status at the time of sting, dose of venom injected, and site of sting.
Bite:
- Prognosis for fire ant bite is excellent. Large lesions from brown recluse spider bites may take months to heal.

■ FURTHER MANAGEMENT
Patients with a history of sting allergies should carry syringes preloaded with epinephrine (EpiPen) and oral antihistamines to take if they are stung again. Consider a referral to an allergist for immunotherapy. Risk of subsequent anaphylaxis with immunotherapy falls to <3%. Venom immunotherapy for 3 to 5 yr induces long-term protection in most patients.

REFERENCES

Annila I: Bee venom allergy, *Clin Exp Allergy* 30(12):1682, 2000.
Ewan PW: ABC of allergies: venom allergy, *BMJ* 316(7141):1365, 1998.
Kemp ED: Bites and stings of the arthropod kind, *Postgrad Med* 103(6):88, 1998.
Koh WL: When to worry about spider bites: inaccurate diagnosis can have serious, even fatal, consequences, *Postgrad Med* 103(4):235, 1998.
Neugut Anaphylaxis in the United States: an investigation into its epidemiology, *Arch Intern Med* 161(1):15, 2001.
Youlton L: Insect sting reactions, *Clin Exp Dermatol* 24(4):338, 2000.
Author: **Jennifer Jeremiah, M.D.**

BASIC INFORMATION

■ DEFINITION
Injury resulting from snake biting a human.

ICD-9CM CODES
989.5 Venomous poisoning

■ EPIDEMIOLOGY & DEMOGRAPHICS
- 45,000 snake bites occur annually in the United States. Of the 8000 caused by poisonous snakes, approximately 9 to 15 result in fatality (i.e., ~1%-2%). Children, the elderly, and those in whom treatment has been delayed are at highest risk.
- In the United States at least one species of poisonous snake has been identified in every state except Alaska, Hawaii, and Maine. The majority of venomous snakes are members of the family Crotalidae, which includes rattlesnakes, copperheads, and cottonmouths. The Elapidae family, which includes the coral snake, accounts for the remainder.

■ PHYSICAL FINDINGS & CLINICAL PRESENTATION
In addition to local tissue injury, envenomation may affect the renal, neurologic, gastrointestinal, vascular, and coagulation systems. Species-specific signs and symptoms include:
CROTALIDAE (PIT VIPERS): Signs and symptoms:
- Fang punctures (see "Diagnosis")
- Pain within 5 min
- Edema within 30 min
- Erythema of site and adjacent tissues +/− lymphangitis

If no edema or erythema is manifested within 4 to 8 hr after a confirmed Crotalidae snakebite, it is safe to assume envenomation did not occur. Systemic manifestations may include:
- Perioral paresthesias, metallic taste, and tingling of fingers or toes (especially with rattlesnake bites)
- Fasciculations (local or generalized)
- Chills, fever, hypotension (due to increased vascular permeability), nausea, vomiting, headache, weakness

ELAPIDAE (CORAL SNAKES): Signs and symptoms:
- Local symptoms are far less pronounced (little or no pain/swelling immediately after the bite)

Systemic symptoms predominate, but onset may be delayed for 1 to 5 hr. Examples include:
- Ptosis
- Dysphagia
- Dysarthria
- Intense salivation
- Loss of DTRs and respiratory depression (late manifestations)

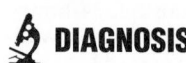 DIAGNOSIS

■ DIFFERENTIAL DIAGNOSIS
- Harmless snake bite
- Scorpion bite
- Insect bite
- Cellulitis
- Laceration or puncture wound

NOTE: Harmless snakebites are usually characterized by four rows of small scratches (teeth in upper jaw) separated from two rows of scratches (teeth in lower jaw). This is in distinction to venomous snake bites, which should have puncture wounds produced by the snake's fangs, whether other teeth marks are noted.

■ WORKUP
An estimated 25% of venomous snake bites do not result in envenomation, but observation is critical in all suspected cases:
- Clinical and laboratory evaluation are used to assess the severity of envenomation
- A nonstandardized classification system for grading envenomations was developed by Russell in 1964:
  Minimal: confined to the site of the bite, no significant systemic symptoms or signs, no laboratory abnormalities
  Moderate: manifestations extend beyond the site of the bite, but no life-threatening systemic symptoms
  Severe: extensive limb involvement, severe systemic symptoms and signs, or significant laboratory abnormalities (including abnormal coagulation studies)

Determination of severity is based on the most severe symptom, sign, or laboratory result. Continual reassessment is indicated throughout the observation period because grading may change.

■ LABORATORY TESTS
- For all suspected envenomations, obtain CBC, platelet count, coagulation profile (PT, PTT, fibrinogen), ECG, and urinalysis
- For more severe bites, consider: LFTs, sedimentation rate, serum electrolytes, BUN, Cr, creatine kinase (r/o rhabdomyolysis), and type and cross-match (see Box 1-7).

BOX 1-7 Diagnostic Studies in Evaluation of Venomous Snakebite Victims

Blood and Serum

Type and cross-match
Complete blood cell count
Peripheral smear
Coagulation studies (fibrinogen, fibrin degradation products, D-dimer, partial thromboplastin time, prothrombin time)
Electrolytes, glucose, creatinine, blood urea nitrogen, liver enzymes, bilirubin
Arterial blood gases
Myoglobin, creatine kinase

Urine

Bedside tests (glucose, blood, myoglobin [on each voided specimen])
Urinalysis

Stool

Test for blood

Radiographs

Chest (if over 40 yr old, history of underlying cardiopulmonary disease, or severe envenomation)
Bite site soft tissue films (if retained fangs possible; poor sensitivity)
Computed tomography of the brain (if presentation suggests intracranial hemorrhage)

Electrocardiogram

If patient is over 40 yr old, has a history of underlying cardiopulmonary disease, or has a severe envenomation

From Auerbach PS: *Wilderness medicine*, ed 4, St Louis, 2001, Mosby.

TREATMENT

■ ACUTE GENERAL Rx

IN THE FIELD: For a suspected snakebite

- Immobilize affected part below level of the heart.
- Remove any constricting items. Local pressure has been advocated for elapid bites, particularly in Australia, as a means of delaying absorption of neurotoxins. However, crotalid bites are far more common in the USA, and these frequently have tissue-necrosing venom, which will yield more damage with local pressure. Thus, as with incision and suction techniques, use by those without specialized training in snake-bite management is discouraged.
- DO NOT apply ice; keep victim warm.
- Avoid alcohol, stimulants (caffeine) or agents that can suppress mental status.
- Transport immediately to nearest medical facility and contact poison control center.

IN THE HOSPITAL:

- Establish intravenous access
- Obtain time of bite and description of snake if possible
- Obtain past medical history; ask about allergies to horse serum in those previously treated for snake bite
- Record vital signs: BP, HR, T, RR
- Inspect site of bite for fang marks, local symptoms
- Measure circumference of bitten part at two or more proximal sites and compare with unaffected limb; repeat every 15 to 20 min
- Neurologic examination
- Gauge the severity of the bite and decide whether administration of antivenom is necessary
- For minimal envenomation without progressive manifestations
  1. Clean and immobilize affected part
  2. Immunize against tetanus
  3. Observe patient for at least 8 to 12 hr. If, after this period, local and systemic sequelae are absent and lab values remain normal, the likelihood of significant envenomation is low, and the patient can be discharged from the acute setting
- Patients who have progressive symptoms (local or systemic) and/or moderate to severe envenomation should be considered for antivenom.

- Antivenom is most effective when given within 4 hr of the bite and least effective if delayed beyond 12 hr.

Once the decision is made to use antivenom:

- Most centers now have sheep immunoglobulin-based antivenom (Crofab) for crotalid bites. (A potent, safe, sheep-based antivenom for elapid bites exists but is not yet approved in the U.S.) Sheep-based antivenoms are very safe, but repeat administration may be necessary owing to a short half-life. An initial IV dose of 4 to 6 vials (depending on the size and age of the patient and the severity of the bite) is infused over 60 min. If the patient has not responded after 1 hr, a repeat dose of 4 to 6 vials is indicated. Additionally, patients with coagulopathic relapse (fibrinogen <50, platelets 3.0, or PTT >50 sec) require repeat doses of two vials q6hrs until resolution occurs. As many as ⅔ of patients with initial coagulopathy will require relapse dosing. 24-hour help in using the antivenom is available by calling 877-377-3784.
- Horse serum-based antivenoms are available for both crotalid and elapid (coral snake), but this runs a much higher risk of hypersensitivity reactions such as anaphylaxis and serum sickness. (Skin testing is available, but it is not recommended because it is not completely reliable and may delay time to administration beyond the most effective period.) For treatment considerations, see "Complications". Guidelines to dosage of horse serum-based antivenom are as follows:
- For pit viper bites
  Mild 5 vials
  Moderate 10 vials
  Severe 15 vials
  Shock 20 vials
- For coral snake bites (different formulation)
  3 vials, if symptoms evolve, repeat with 5 vials
- Zoos with exotic snakes are required to maintain a supply of snake-specific antivenom on their premises

Other considerations

- Initial dose of antivenom should be repeated until progression of symptoms has abated, but observation of bitten part should be continued for another 48 hr
- Children require more antivenom; increase dose by 50%
- Pregnancy is not a contraindication to antivenom

- Immunize against tetanus if no booster within past 5 yr; if never immunized, give immunoglobulin as well as toxoid
- Manage pain as needed (acetaminophen, codeine, meperidine)
- Avoid sedation in Mojave rattlesnake, eastern diamondback rattlesnake, and coral snake bites
- Antibiotics reserved for moderate to severe cases; use those with broad-spectrum coverage (which includes gram-negatives, i.e., quinolone derivatives)

■ DISPOSITION

Prognosis is good with prompt evaluation and treatment.

■ REFERRAL

To medical facility with ICU for administration of antivenin

PEARLS & CONSIDERATIONS

■ COMPLICATIONS

Most frequent complication of treated envenomations is serum sickness; occurs 7 to 14 days after antivenom administration and is characterized by fever, rash, arthralgias, and lymphadenopathy. It can be treated with PO prednisone 60 mg/day, tapered over 7 to 10 days. Acutely, there is the risk of anaphylaxis to antivenom as mentioned previously. This occurs within 30 min and is treated with

- IV epinephrine
- IV diphenhydramine
- IV hydrocortisone

Injuries also result from

- Tourniquet placement
- Cryotherapy

National poison-control hotline: (800)222-1222

REFERENCES

Gold BS et al: Bites of venomous snakes, *N Engl J Med* 347:347, 2002.

Juckett G, Honcox JG: Venomous snakebites in the United States: management review and update, *Am Fam Physician* 65:1367, 2002.

The Medical Letter: A new snake antivenom, *Med Lett Drugs Ther* 43:55, 2001.

Authors: **Jack Schwarzwald, M.D., and Rebecca A. Griffith, M.D.**

BASIC INFORMATION

■ DEFINITION

Bladder cancer is a heterogeneous spectrum of neoplasms ranging from non–life-threatening, low-grade, superficial papillary lesions to high-grade invasive tumors, which often have metastasized at the time of presentation. It is a field change disease in which the entire urothelium from the renal pelvis to the urethra may be susceptible to malignant transformation. *Types:* Transitional cell carcinoma (TCCa), squamous cell carcinoma, and adenocarcinoma.

ICD-9CM CODES
Primary: 188.9
Secondary: 198.1
CIS: 233.7
Benign: 223.3
Uncertain behavior: 236.7
Unspecified: 239.4

■ EPIDEMIOLOGY & DEMOGRAPHICS

Each year approximately 54,000 new cases are diagnosed and more than 12,000 deaths are attributed to bladder cancer.

Until 1990, the incidence of bladder cancer in the U.S. was rising. Since 1990, the incidence of bladder cancer is decreasing at a rate of 0.8% per year (1.2% among men and 0.4% among women).

PREDOMINANT SEX: In males, it is the fourth most common cancer; it accounts for 10% of all cancers. In females, it is the eighth most common cancer; it accounts for 4% of all cancers.

RISK: The lifetime risk of developing bladder cancer is 2.8% in white males, 0.9% in black males, 1% in white females, and 0.6% in black females.

Smoking:
- Users of "black" tobacco in place of "blond" tobacco have a twofold to threefold increase in developing bladder cancer.
- Smoking risk is based on consumption:

With a twofold to threefold increase for subjects smoking at least 10 cigarettes per day

The risk increases again when the daily consumption rises above 40-60 cigarettes per day

- Smokers of low-tar and nicotine cigarettes have a lower risk when compared with higher tar and nicotine cigarettes.
- Unfiltered cigarettes have a 50% increased risk of bladder cancer compared with those who smoke filtered cigarettes.

- Pipe smokers have a lower risk of bladder cancer compared with cigarette smokers.
- Cigar smoking, snuff, and chewing tobacco, although implicated in nonurologic cancers, are not believed to influence bladder cancer risk.

Diet:
- Diets rich in beef, pork, and animal fat consumption increase risk of bladder cancer.
- There is no indication that consumption of nonbeer alcoholic drinks contributes to bladder cancer development.
- Beer consumption has been linked to bladder cancer development as a result of the presence of nitrosamines in the beer. Similarly, these nitrosamines have been implicated in the development of rectal cancer.
- Drinking coffee is not believed to contribute to bladder cancer risk. There is additional evidence that coffee consumption is protective for colorectal cancers, possibly by diminishing fecal transit time.

PEAK INCIDENCE: Incidence increases with age, high >60 yr, uncommon <40 yr.

GENETICS: It is thought to be multifactorial in etiology, involving both genetic and environmental interactions. Overall, it is estimated that approximately 20% to 25% of the male population in the U.S. with bladder cancer has the disease as a result of occupational exposure.

DISTRIBUTION: In North America, transitional cell carcinomas comprise 93%, squamous cell carcinomas comprise 6%, and adenocarcinomas account for 1% of bladder cancers.

PATHOGENESIS: Two pathways exist for bladder cancer (TCCa):
1. Papillary superficial disease occasionally leading to invasive cancer (75%)
2. Carcinoma-in-situ (CIS) and solid invasive cancer with high risk of disease progression (25%)

Two distinct forms of "Superficial Cancer" exist:

T_a Papillary low-grade tumor High rate of recurrence Disease progression occurs 5%

T_1 Higher-grade papillary tumors that infiltrate the lamina propria Often associated with flat CIS that may involve the urothelium diffusely Disease progression occurs between 30% to 50%

Subdivided into:
T_{1a} Penetration of tumor up to the muscularis mucosae Disease progression 5.3%
T_{1b} Penetration of tumor through the muscularis mucosae Disease progression 53%

Flat CIS:
Entirely different and separate pathway of cancer development whose mechanism is manifested by dysplasia, which leads to the occurrence of poorly differentiated malignant cells that replace or undermine the normal urothelium and extend along the plane of the bladder wall. It penetrates the basement membrane and lamina propria in 20% to 30% of the cases and is associated with the development of solid tumor growth. A defect in chromosome 17p53 occurs in 50% of the cases.

At presentation, 72% of cancers are localized to the bladder, 20% of the cancers extend to the regional lymph nodes, and 3% present with distant metastases. 80% of superficial TCCa recur with up to 30% progressing to a higher stage or grade. Younger patients most commonly develop low-grade papillary noninvasive TCCa and are less likely to have recurrences when compared with older patients with similar lesions. Involvement of the upper tracts with tumor occurs in 25% to 50% of the cases.

STAGING (BASED ON THE TNM SYSTEM):

T_0 No tumor in specimen
T_{is} CIS
T_a Papillary TCCa noninvasive
T_1 Papillary TCCa into lamina propria
T_2 TCCa invasive of superficial ms
T_{3a} Invasive of deep ms
T_{3b} Invasive of perivesical fat
T_{4a} Invasive of adjacent pelvic organ
T_{4b} Invasive of pelvic wall with fixation

Invasive of nodal status:
N_0 No nodal involvement
N_{1-3} Pelvic nodes
N_4 Nodes above bifurcation
N_x Unknown

Invasive of metastatic status:
M_0 No distant metastases
M_1 Distant metastases
M_x Unknown

MOLECULAR EPIDEMIOLOGY: TCCa is usually a field change disease with tumors arising at different times and sites in the urothelium, suggesting a polyclonal etiology of bladder cancer. Bladder cancers have been associated with abnormalities on chromosomes 1, 4, 11, 5, 7, 3, 9, 21, 18, 13, 8; with alterations in suppressor genes P53, retinoblastoma gene, and P16; and with alterations in oncogenes H-ras and epidermal growth factor receptor.

■ PHYSICAL FINDINGS
- Gross painless hematuria
- Microhematuria
- Frequency, urgency, occasional dysuria

With locally invasive to distant metastatic disease, the presentation can include:
- Abdominal pain
- Flank pain
- Lymphedema
- Renal failure
- Anorexia
- Bone pain

■ ETIOLOGY
Bladder cancer is a potentially preventable disease associated with specific etiologic factors:
- Cigarette smoking is associated with 25% to 65% of the cases. The risk of developing a TCCa is 2 to 4 times higher in smokers than in nonsmokers, and that risk persists for many years, being equal to nonsmokers only after 12 to 15 yr of smoking abstinence. Smoking tobacco is associated with tumors that are characterized by higher histologic grade, increased tumor stage, increase in the numbers of tumor present, and increased tumor size.
- Occupational exposures: dye workers, textile workers, tire and rubber workers, petroleum workers
- Chemical exposure: O-toluidine, 2-naphthylamine, benzidine, 4-aminobiphenyl, and nitrosamines
- Exposure to HPV type 16

Squamous carcinomas are associated with:
- Schistosomiasis
- Urinary calculi
- Indwelling catheters
- Bladder diverticula

Miscellaneous causes:
- Phenacetin abuse
- Cyclophosphamide
- Pelvic irradiation
- Tuberculosis

Adenocarcinomas are associated with:
- Exstrophy
- Endometriosis
- Neurogenic bladder
- Urachal abnormalities
- As a secondary site for distant metastases from other organs (i.e., colon cancer)

■ DIAGNOSIS
- History and physical examination
- Urinalysis
- Cystoscopy with bladder barbotage and biopsy
- Transurethral resection of bladder tumor(s)
- There is insufficient evidence to determine whether a decrease in mortality from bladder cancer occurs with hematuria testing, urinary cytology, or a variety of other tests on exfoliated urinary cells or other substances.
- In addition to urinary cytologies and bladder barbotage, BTA, NMP22, and Fibrin Degradation Products (FDP) have been approved by the FDA as bladder cancer tumor markers. No marker has general, widespread acceptance because the results are affected by the presence of stents, recent urologic manipulation, stones, infection, bowel interposition, and prostatitis creating false-positive results.

■ DIFFERENTIAL DIAGNOSIS
- Urinary tract infection
- Frequency-urgency syndrome
- Interstitial cystitis
- Stone disease
- Endometriosis
- Neurogenic bladder

■ LABORATORY TESTS
RADIOLOGIC TESTS:
- IVP, renal ultrasound, retrograde pyelography, CT scan, and MRI.
- One or a combination of studies can be used. In the absence of skeletal symptoms, bone scan is not recommended.

■ TREATMENT
■ NONPHARMACOLOGIC THERAPY
- Initially, transurethral resection of bladder tumor (TURBT)
- Loop biopsy of the prostatic urethra if high-grade TCCa is suspected
- If superficial disease, follow-up protocol with repeat TURBT and/or the use of intravesical agents is recommended
- For advanced bladder cancer, radical cystectomy with urethrectomy (unless orthotopic diversion is planned) and either ileal loop conduit or orthotopic diversion

BLADDER PRESERVATION APPROACHES: Following cystectomy for muscle invasive disease, 50% or more of the patients will develop metastases. Most patients develop metastases at distant sites, a third relapse locally. Bladder preservation management is offered in those individuals who refuse surgery or who might not be suitable radical cystectomy patients. Bladder-sparing protocols include extensive TURBT or partial cystectomy with external beam or interstitial radiotherapy and systemic chemotherapy. Radiotherapy as a single treatment modality is not effective. The best predictor of successful bladder preservation is a complete response following the combination of initial TURBT and two cycles of CMV (cisplatin, methotrexate, vinblastine) chemotherapy seen with stages T2-T3a.

INDICATIONS FOR PARTIAL CYSTECTOMY:
- Tumor within a bladder diverticulum
- Solitary, primary, and muscle-invasive or high-grade lesion of a region of the bladder that allows complete excision with adequate surgical margins
- Inability to adequately resect tumor by TURBT alone because of size or location
- Tumor overlying a ureteral orifice requiring ureteral reimplantation
- Biopsy of a radiation-induced ulceration
- Palliation of severe local symptoms
- Patient refusal of urinary diversion
- Poor-risk patient who is not a diversion candidate

Contraindications:
- Multiple tumors
- CIS
- Cellular atypia on biopsy
- Prostatic invasion
- Invasion of the trigone
- Inability to achieve adequate surgical margins
- Prior radiotherapy
- Inability to maintain adequate bladder volume after resection
- Evidence of extravesical tumor extension
- Poor surgical risk

■ ACUTE GENERAL Rx
INDICATIONS FOR INTRAVESICAL CHEMOTHERAPY:
- High-grade tumor
- Tumor size >5 cm
- Tumor multiplicity

- Presence of CIS
- Positive urinary cytologies following a resection
- Incomplete tumor resection Intravesical agents: thiotepa, Adriamycin, mitomycin C, AD-32, BCG, interferon, bropirimine, Epodyl, interleukin-2, and keyhole-limpet hemocyanin. Photodynamic therapy with hematoporphyrin derivatives has also been used.

INDICATIONS FOR CYSTECTOMY:
- Large tumors not amenable to complete TURBT
- High-grade tumor
- Multiple tumors with frequent recurrences
- Diffuse CIS not responsive to intravesical chemotherapy
- Prostatic urethra involvement
- Irritative bladder symptoms with upper tract deterioration
- Muscle-invasive disease
- Disease outside of the bladder

SYSTEMIC CHEMOTHERAPY: Used as neoadjuvant and adjuvant therapy for systemic disease. The most effective agents are cisplatin, methotrexate, vinblastine, Adriamycin (MVAC). Other agents include mitoxantrone, vincristine, etoposide (VP16), 5FU, ifosfamide, Taxol, gemcitabine, Piritrexim, and gallium nitrate. Chemotherapy in combination can provide palliation and modest survival benefit.

RADIOTHERAPY: Conflicting reports suggest that superficial bladder cancer is more sensitive to radiotherapy. Squamous changes within the tumor and secretion of human chorionic gonadotropin by the lesion are associated with poor response to radiotherapy. Only 20% to 30% of patients with invasive bladder cancer can be cured by external beam radiation therapy alone. It is used in combination with surgery or with systemic agents to treat bladder cancer primarily in those patients who are not surgical candidates or who refuse surgery.

■ **CHRONIC Rx**
FOLLOW-UP RECOMMENDATIONS FOR SUPERFICIAL BLADDER CANCER:
- Cystoscopy, bladder barbotage, and bimanual examination every 3 mo for 2 yr, then every 6 mo for 2 yr, and annually thereafter.
- Upper tract studies are based on the risk of upper tract tumor development, generally every 2 to 5 yr.

FOLLOW-UP RECOMMENDATIONS FOR ADVANCED DISEASE:
Bladder Preservation:
- Cystoscopy, barbotage, bimanual examination, biopsy (when indicated), every 3 mo for 2 yr, then every 6 mo for 2 yr, yearly thereafter.
- CT scan of abdomen and pelvis every 6 mo for 2 yr in addition to chest x-ray examination, liver function testing, and serum creatinine.

Cystectomy with Ileal Loop/Orthotopic Bladder:
- Neobladder endoscopy and IVP yearly.
- CT scan of abdomen and pelvis every 6 mo for 2 yr in addition to chest x-ray examination, liver function tests, and serum creatinine.
- Loopogram every 6 mo for 2 yr, then yearly.

☼ **PEARLS & CONSIDERATIONS**

■ **COMMENTS**
- The most useful prognostic parameters for bladder tumor recurrence and subsequent cancer progression are tumor grade, depth of tumor penetration, multifocal tumors, frequency of recurrence, tumor size, CIS, lymphatic invasion, papillary or solid tumor configuration.
- Box 1-8 describes the American Urological Association Guideline Recommendations for bladder cancer.

REFERENCES
Lamm DL et al: Megadose vitamins in bladder cancer: a double-blind clinical trial, *J Urol* 151:21, 1994.
Messing EM: In Walsh PC et al. (eds): *Campbell's urology,* ed 8, Philadelphia, 2002, WB Saunders.
Author: **Philip J. Aliotta, M.D., M.S.H.A.**

BOX 1-8   American Urological Association Guideline Recommendations

1. Undiagnosed bladder tumor: obtain a histologic diagnosis of the tumor: Transurethral resection of the tumor is the most common method.
2. Stage Ta or T1 cancer: Complete surgical eradication of all visible tumors. The lesion can be treated with electrocautery resection, fulguration, or laser ablation. Adjuvant intravesical therapy is recommended for patients with carcinoma-in-situ, T1, or high-grade Ta tumors. The agent recommended is BCG or mitomycin C. Cystectomy is an option for this set of tumors because of risk of progression to muscle-invasive disease even after intravesical chemotherapy.
   An increased risk of disease progression is associated with large tumor, high-grade tumor, location of the tumor in a site that is poorly accessible to complete resection, diffuse disease, infiltration of lymphatic or vascular spaces, and prostatic urethral involvement.
3. Carcinoma-in-situ or high-grade T1 cancer and prior intravesical chemotherapy: Cystectomy is the recommendation based on the panel's expert opinion rather than evidence from outcomes data. The data show a substantial risk of progression to muscle-invasive cancer in patients with diffuse carcinoma-in-situ and high-grade T1 tumors. The response to intravesical chemotherapy in terms of altering this disease progression is unknown, and as a result of this, cystectomy is an option for the afflicted patient.

American Urological Association, Guideline Division, 1120 North Charles Street, Baltimore, MD 21201.

BASIC INFORMATION

■ DEFINITION
Blastomycosis is a systemic pyogranulomatous disease caused by a dimorphic fungus, *Blastomyces dermatitidis*.

ICD-9CM CODES
116.0 Blastomycosis
116.0 Primary pulmonary
116.1 Brazilian
116.1 South American
116.2 Keloidal
117.5 European

■ EPIDEMIOLOGY & DEMOGRAPHICS
Most patients reside in the southeastern and south central states, especially those bordering the Mississippi and Ohio River valleys, the Midwestern states, and Canadian provinces bordering the Great Lakes. Rare cases have been reported outside the United States. Widely disseminated disease is most common in immunocompromised hosts, especially those with acquired immunodeficiency syndrome (AIDS).

■ PHYSICAL FINDINGS & CLINICAL PRESENTATION
- Acute infection: 50% symptomatic, median incubation 30 to 45 days, symptoms are nonspecific: mimic influenza or bacterial infection with abrupt onset of myalgias, arthralgias, chills and fever; transient pleuritic pain, cough that is initially nonproductive; resolution within 4 wk is usual
- Chronic or recurrent infection: indolent and progressive; manifestations are diverse including pulmonary or extrapulmonary disease

Pulmonary manifestations:
Symptoms and signs of chronic pneumonia: productive cough, hemoptysis, pleuritic chest pain, weight loss, low-grade pyrexia

Extrapulmonary manifestations:
1. Cutaneous: most common; may occur with or without pulmonary disease. Two different lesions:
   Verrucous: beginning as a small papulopustular lesion on exposed body areas that may develop into an eschar with peripheral microabscesses
   Ulcerative
   Subcutaneous nodules (cold abscesses) may also occur.
2. Bone and joint: 10% to 50% of patients have osteolytic lesions; affects long bones, vertebrae, and ribs; lesions may present with a contiguous soft-tissue abscess or draining sinus that may spread to a joint, resulting in a pyarthrosis
3. Genitourinary: 10% to 30% of patients; prostatic involvement is most common and may manifest as obstruction; epididymis and testes may also be affected

4. Central nervous system: 5% normal host; 40% AIDS patients; meningitis and abscess formation

■ ETIOLOGY
B. dermatitidis exists in warm, moist soil that is rich in organic material. When these microfoci are disturbed, the aerosolized spores or conidia are inhaled into the lungs. Disease at other sites is a result of dissemination from the initial pulmonary infection; the latter may be acute or chronic.

DIAGNOSIS

■ DIFFERENTIAL DIAGNOSIS
PULMONARY INFECTION:
- Tuberculosis
- Bronchogenic carcinoma
- Histoplasmosis
- Bacterial pneumonia

CUTANEOUS INFECTION:
- Bromoderma
- Pyoderma gangrenosum
- *Mycobacterium marinum* infection
- Squamous cell carcinoma
- Giant keratoacanthoma

■ WORKUP
- Physical examination and laboratory evaluation
- Definitive diagnosis established by culture

■ LABORATORY TESTS
- Presumptive diagnosis can be made by visualizing the distinctive yeast forms in clinical specimens
- Culture: on Sabouraud's or more enriched media
  1. Aspirated material from abscesses
  2. Skin scrapings
  3. Prostatic secretions (urine culture with prostatic massage)
- Direct examination of clinical specimens
  1. Wet preparation with 10% KOH
  2. Histopathology: typically demonstrates pyogranulomas; yeast identification requires special stains
- Serologic tests: currently, a negative serologic test cannot be used to exclude blastomycosis, nor should a positive titer be an indication to start treatment

■ IMAGING STUDIES
In chronic disease, chest radiographic findings are nonspecific, but lobar or segmental alveolar infiltrates, especially of the upper lobes, are most common and may progress to cavitation.

TREATMENT

■ ACUTE BLASTOMYCOSIS
- Indication for chemotherapy remains controversial in patients with acute pulmonary blastomycosis.

- Because the acute form may be benign and self-limited, patients may be closely observed.
- Some patients progress to chronic infection with attendant significant morbidity and therefore may require treatment.
- Patients who are immunocompromised or have extrapulmonary disease or progressive pulmonary disease should be treated.

■ CHRONIC BLASTOMYCOSIS
- Itraconazole 200 mg IV bid × 4 doses followed by 200 mg IV qd or itraconazole 200 to 400 mg/day for 6 mo remains the drug of choice except for those patients with CNS disease or with fulminant illness who require amphotericin B.
- Ketoconazole 400 mg/day PO for 6 mo is an alternative in mild-moderate disease.
- Amphotericin B: total dose of 1.5 to 2.5 g IV is recommended in immunocompromised patients, those with life-threatening disease or CNS disease, or those for whom azole treatment has failed. In addition, amphotericin B is the only drug approved for treating blastomycosis in pregnant women.
- Amphotericin B lipid complex (ABLC) 5 mg/kg/day IV may be considered in patients who are intolerant of or refractory to amphotericin.
- Fluconazole 400 mg/day to 800 mg/day PO for 6 mo in those who cannot take itraconazole or who are unable to tolerate a full course of amphotericin B.
- Surgery may be indicated with antifungal therapy for drainage of large abscesses.

■ PROGNOSIS
- Before the development of antifungal chemotherapy, the disease had a progressive course with eventual extrapulmonary disease and a mortality exceeding 60%.
- Relapse rate for patients treated with amphotericin B is 5%; relapse is more common in AIDS patients.

■ REFERRAL
Consultation with an infectious diseases specialist is highly recommended, especially in chronic blastomycosis.

REFERENCE
Martynowicz MA et al: Pulmonary blastomycosis: an appraisal of diagnostic techniques, *Chest* 121(3):768, 2002.
Author: **Sajeev Handa, M.D.**

BASIC INFORMATION

■ DEFINITION
Blepharitis is an acute or, most often, chronic inflammation of the eyelid margins that is often refractory to treatment.

ICD-9 CM CODES
373.0 Blepharitis

■ PHYSICAL FINDINGS & CLINICAL PRESENTATION
- Chronically infected lids are usually diffusely erythematous, with collarettes (fibrin exudate) at the base of the lashes (Fig. 1-50).
- Lid margins thicken over time, with associated loss of eyelashes (madarosis), misdirected growth of lashes (trichiasis), and overflow or inspissation of the meibomian glands.
- Associated conjunctivitis with erythema and edema is frequent, but it is usually without discharge.
- Chalazia may develop.
- Superficial punctate erosions of the inferior corneal epithelium are common.
- More severe findings, such as corneal pannus, ulcerative keratitis, or lid ectropion, are less common.

■ ETIOLOGY
Multiple: bacterial and nonbacterial causes
- Staphylococcal infection
- Seborrheic dermatitis
- Rosacea
- Dry eye (keratoconjunctivitis sicca): includes a decrease in tear volume and/or increased rate of evaporation
- Meibomian gland dysfunction: normally there is keratinization of the meibomian gland duct; hyperkeratinization can plug up the duct.
- Two categories of blepharitis:
  1. Anterior blepharitis, most often associated with staphylococcal infection or seborrheic dermatitis
  2. Posterior blepharitis, associated with meibomian gland dysfunction

NOTE: most often bacteria isolated from blepharitis patients are normal skin microflora, but in greater amounts (mostly *S. epidermidis* and *P. acnes*). (*S. aureus* and coagulase-negative staphylococci can be cultured from the eyelid margins of 10%-35% and 90%-95% of healthy persons, respectively.)

DIAGNOSIS

■ DIFFERENTIAL DIAGNOSIS
- Keratoconjunctivitis sicca
- Eyelid malignancies
- Herpes simplex blepharitis
- Molluscum contagiosum
- Phthiriasis palpebrarum
- Phthirus pubis (pubic lice)
- Demodex folliculorum (transparent mites)
- Allergic blepharitis

■ WORKUP
Scrapings of the eyelids to show polymorphonuclear leukocytes and grampositive cocci

■ LABORATORY TESTS
Eyelid cultures and antibiotic sensitivity testing (usually not done unless patient fails to respond to initial treatment regimen)

TREATMENT

■ NONPHARMACOLOGIC THERAPY
- Lid scrubs are the oldest and most effective treatment.
- Alkaline soaps may be beneficial; alcohol and some detergents may be effective in removing surface lipids and microflora.
- Hot compresses applied to closed lids for 5 to 10 min: heat loosens debris from lid margins and increases meibomian gland fluidity.
- Firm massage of the lid margins to enhance the flow of secretions from glands, followed by cleansing of the lids with cotton-tipped applicators dipped in a 50:50 mixture of baby shampoo and water.
- Lashes and lid margins scrubbed vigorously while the eyelids are closed, followed by thorough rinsing.
- Following local massage and cleansing, the mainstay of treatment is application of topical antibiotic ointment to the eyelid margins.
- Antibiotics must be in ointment form for lids and drops or ointment for the ocular surface.
  1. Most effective topical antibiotics available are bacitracin and erythromycin opthalmic ointments; also effective are many aminoglycosides and fluoroquinolones.
  2. Ointment is applied 1 to 4 times daily, depending on the severity of inflammation, for 1 to 2 wk.
  3. Treatment is continued once daily, at bedtime, for another 4 to 8 wk.
  4. Treatment is continued for 1 mo after all signs of inflammation have disappeared.

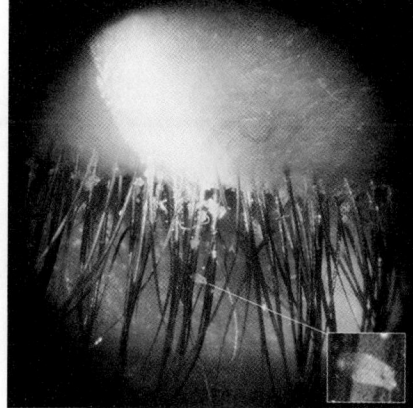
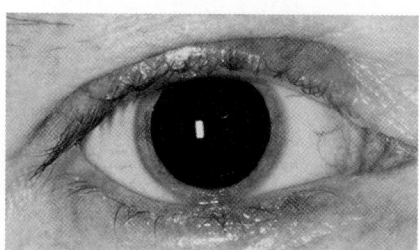

Fig. 1-50 A, Seborrheic blepharitis. The typical scales (scurf) are translucent and easily removed. **B,** Staphylococcal blepharitis showing the typical lid margin erythema and discharge. (From Palay D [ed]: *Ophthalmology for the primary care physician,* St Louis, 1997, Mosby.)

For patients with rosacea:
1. Tetracycline 250 mg orally 4 times daily or doxycycline 100 mg orally tid along with local treatment
2. Dosing reduced to once daily for several months, depending on the clinical situation

Recalcitrant cases with antibiotic resistance:
1. Vancomycin eye drops 1%
2. Ciprofloxacin or ofloxacin eyedrops

■ CHRONIC Rx

By definition, this is a chronic condition for which there is frequently no cure. This is complicated by the fact that long-term use of antibiotics results in development of resistance and cross-resistance.

Some newer agents being evaluated are flavonoid-type compounds (resveratrol, silymarin), which have antioxidant properties (may have a role in reducing the inflammatory response), azelaic acid, and glycolic acid (used to treat acne and have antikeratinizing effects).

Adapalene gel is also useful in treating acne; it has antiinflammatory properties and an antiproliferative effect on keratinocytes.

■ DISPOSITION

This condition is often refractory to treatment, and often requires prolonged courses of treatment. It is important that patients receive adequate education about treatment and compliance.

■ REFERRAL

To an ophthalmologist if patient fails to respond to local therapy.

REFERENCES

McCulley JP, Shine WE: Eyelid disorders, the meibomian gland, blepharitis and contact lenses. *Eye Contact Lens* 29(1 Suppl):S93, 2003.

McCulley JP, Shine WE: Changing concepts in the diagnosis and management of blepharitis: cornea 19(5):650, 2000.

Author: **Jane V. Eason, M.D.**

BASIC INFORMATION

DEFINITION

Primary malignant bone tumors are invasive, anaplastic, and have the ability to metastasize. Most arise from the marrow (myeloma), but tumors may develop from bone, cartilage, fat, and fibrous tissues. Leukemia and lymphoma are excluded from this discussion.
FIBROSARCOMA AND LIPOSARCOMA: Extremely rare. They are similar to those tumors arising in soft tissue.
OSTEOSARCOMA: A rare primary malignant tumor of bone characterized by malignant tumor cells that produce osteoid or bone. Several variants have been described: parosteal sarcoma, periosteal sarcoma, multicentric, and telangiectatic forms.
CHONDROSARCOMA: A malignant cartilage tumor that may develop primarily or secondarily from transformation of a benign osteocartilaginous exostosis or enchondroma.
EWING'S SARCOMA: A malignant tumor of unknown histogenesis.
MULTIPLE MYELOMA: A neoplastic proliferation of plasma cells.

SYNONYMS

Multiple myeloma:
1. Plasma cell myeloma
2. Plasmacytoma

ICD-9CM CODES

203.0 Multiple myeloma
170.9 Neoplasma, bone (periosteum), primary malignant
M9180/3 Osteosarcoma
N9220/3 Chondrosarcoma
M9260/3 Ewing's sarcoma

EPIDEMIOLOGY & DEMOGRAPHICS

MULTIPLE MYELOMA:
- The most common tumor in bone
- Age at onset: usually >40 yr
- Male:female ratio of 2:1
OSTEOGENIC SARCOMA:
- Average age at onset: 10 to 20 yr
- Males > females
- Parosteal sarcoma in older patients
CHONDROSARCOMA:
- Age at onset: 40 to 60 yr
- Male:female ratio of 2:1
EWING'S SARCOMA:
- Age at onset: 10 to 15 yr

PHYSICAL FINDINGS

MULTIPLE MYELOMA:
- May present as a systemic process or, less commonly, as a "solitary" lesion
- Early manifestations: anorexia, weight loss, and bone pain; majority of cases present initially with back pain that often leads to the detection of a destructive skeletal lesion
- Other organ systems eventually become involved, resulting in more bone pain, anemia, renal insufficiency, and/or bacterial infections, usually as a result of the dysproteinemia typical of this disorder

- Possible secondary amyloidosis, leading to cardiac failure or nephrotic syndrome
OSTEOSARCOMA:
- Most originating in the metaphysis
- 50% to 60% around the knee
- Possible pain and swelling, but otherwise healthy patient
- Osteosarcoma in conjunction with Paget's disease, manifested primarily as a sudden increase in bone pain
CHONDROSARCOMA:
- Tumor most commonly involving the pelvis, upper femur, and shoulder girdle
- Painful swelling
EWING'S SARCOMA:
- Painful soft tissue mass often present
- Possibly increased local heat
- Midshaft of a long bone usually affected (in contrast to other tumors)
- Weight loss, fever, and lethargy

DIAGNOSIS

DIFFERENTIAL DIAGNOSIS

- Osteomyelitis
- Metastatic bone disease
The age of the patient and the initial radiographic features often determine the next appropriate diagnostic steps.

LABORATORY TESTS

- Slightly elevated alkaline phosphatase in osteosarcoma
- In Ewing's sarcoma: reflective of systemic reaction; include anemia, an increase in WBC count, and an elevated sedimentation rate
- In multiple myeloma:
  1. Bence Jones protein in the urine
  2. Anemia and elevated sedimentation rate
  3. Characteristic dysproteinemia on serum protein electrophoresis
  4. Diagnostic feature: peak in the electrophoretic pattern suggestive of a monoclonal gammopathy
  5. Rouleaux formation in the peripheral blood smear
  6. Often, presence of hypercalcemia, but alkaline phosphatase levels usually normal

IMAGING STUDIES

- Classic osteogenic sarcoma penetrates the cortex early in many cases.
  1. A blastic (dense), lytic (lucent), or mixed response may be seen in the affected bone.
  2. An aggressive perpendicular sunburst pattern may be present as a result of periosteal reaction, and peripheral Codman's triangles are often noted.
  3. Margins of the tumor are poorly defined.
- Speckled calcifications in a destructive radiolucent lesion are usually suggestive of chondrosarcoma.

- Ewing's sarcoma is characterized radiographically by mottled, irregular destructive changes with periosteal new bone formation. The latter may be multilayered, producing the typical "onion skin" appearance.
- Typical roentgenographic finding in multiple myeloma is the "punched out" lesion with sharply demarcated edges.
  1. Multiple lesions are usual.
  2. Diffuse osteoporosis may be the only finding in many cases.
  3. Pathologic fractures are common.

TREATMENT

The evaluation and treatment of malignant bone tumors are complicated. Diagnostic studies and treatment should be supervised by an orthopedic cancer specialist and oncologist.

DISPOSITION

- In the past 20 yr, dramatic improvements have been made in the treatment protocols for osteosarcoma with the use of adjuvant multidrug regimens and limb-sparing surgery.
- Early diagnosis is important because most tumors have not metastasized at the time of the initial presentation.
- 70% 5-yr survival rates have been obtained in some series.
- Prognosis of multiple myeloma remains poor despite new therapies.
  1. Complete remissions are uncommon.
  2. Survival with a solitary lesion may be long, but most patients succumb after a median of 3 yr.
- Prognosis for Ewing's sarcoma has improved with a combination of chemotherapy, local resection, and radiation therapy.
- Chondrosarcomas are not sensitive to chemotherapy or radiation, and prognosis will depend on the grade of the tumor and the ability to obtain an adequate resection.

REFERENCES

Abe S et al: Long-term local intensive preoperative chemotherapy and joint-preserving conservative surgery for osteosarcoma around the knee, *Orthopedics* 24:671, 2001.

Bos GD: Foot tumors: diagnosis and treatment, *J Am Acad Orthop Surg* 10:259, 2002.

Papagelopoulos PJ et al: Current concepts in the evaluation and treatment of osteosarcoma, *Orthopedics* 23:858, 2000.

Scully, SP et al: Pathologic fracture in osteosarcoma. Prognostic importance and treatment implications, *J Bone Joint Surg* 84(A):49, 2002.

Wittig JC et al: Osteosarcoma: a multidisciplinary approach to diagnosis and treatment, *Am Fam Physician* 65:1123, 2002.

Author: **Lonnie R. Mercier, M.D.**

BASIC INFORMATION

■ DEFINITION

Botulism is an illness caused by a neurotoxin produced by *Clostridium botulinum*. Three types of disease can occur: foodborne botulism, wound botulism, and infant intestinal botulism. Recent concern has increased about a possible fourth type of disease: inhalational botulism. Does not occur naturally, but may occur as a result of bioterrorism.

ICD-9CM CODE
005.1 Botulism

■ EPIDEMIOLOGY & DEMOGRAPHICS
INCIDENCE (IN U.S.): Approximately 24 cases/yr of foodborne illness, 3 cases/yr of wound botulism, and 71 cases/yr of infant botulism

■ PHYSICAL FINDINGS & CLINICAL PRESENTATION
- Symptoms usually begin 12 to 36 hr following ingestion.
- Severity of illness is related to the quantity of toxin ingested.
- Significant findings:
  1. Cranial nerve palsies, with ocular and bulbar manifestations being most frequent (diplopia, ophthalmoplegia, ptosis, dysphagia, dysarthria, and dry mouth)
  2. Usually bilateral nerve involvement that may progress to a descending flaccid paralysis
  3. Typically, absence of sensory findings; sensorium intact
  4. GI symptoms (nausea, vomiting, diarrhea, or cramps)
  5. Usually no fever
- Wound botulism
  1. Occurs mostly in injecting drug users (subcutaneous heroin injection—"skin popping") or with traumatic injury.
  2. Presentation is similar to that of foodborne disease, except for a longer incubation period and the absence of GI symptoms.
  3. Wound infection is not always apparent, but injection sites frequently reveal cellulitis, draining pus, or abscess formation.

■ ETIOLOGY
- Cause is one of several types of neurotoxins (usually A, B, or E) produced by *C. botulinum*, an anaerobic, gram-positive bacillus. Spore production guarantees survival of the organism in extreme conditions. Botulinum toxin is the most powerful neurotoxin known.

- Disease results from absorption of toxin into the circulation from a mucosal surface or wound. Botulinum toxin does not penetrate intact skin.
- In foodborne variety, disease is caused by ingestion of preformed toxin. Although rapidly inactivated by heat, the toxin can survive the proteolytic environment of the stomach.
- In wound botulism, toxin is elaborated by organisms that contaminate a wound. Most cases reported are from California.
- In infant botulism, toxin is produced by organisms in the GI tract.
- Inhalational botulism has been demonstrated experimentally in primates. This manufactured form results from aerosolized toxin, and has been attempted by bioterrorists.

DIAGNOSIS

■ DIFFERENTIAL DIAGNOSIS
- Myasthenia gravis
- Guillain-Barré syndrome
- Tick paralysis
- CVA

■ WORKUP
- Search made for toxin and the organism (see "Laboratory Tests")
- Electrophysiologic studies (EMG) may aid in the diagnosis

■ LABORATORY TESTS
- Samples of food and stool are cultured for the organism.
- Food, serum, and stool are sent for toxin assay.

TREATMENT

■ NONPHARMACOLOGIC THERAPY
- Supportive care with intubation if respiratory failure occurs
- Debridement of the wound in wound botulism

■ ACUTE GENERAL Rx
- Give trivalent equine botulinum antitoxin as early as possible. Once a clinical diagnosis is made, antitoxin should be administered before laboratory confirmation.
  1. Give one vial by IM injection and one vial IV.
  2. The antitoxin is available from the Centers for Disease Control and Prevention [(404) 639-2206 or (404) 639-2888]; it is derived from horse serum, so there is a significant incidence of serum sickness.

  3. Skin testing, and possible desensitization, is recommended before treatment.
- Give wound botulism patients penicillin, 2 million U IV q4h.

■ CHRONIC Rx
- Supportive
- Rehabilitation/physical therapy

■ DISPOSITION
- Highest mortality in the first case in an outbreak, with subsequent cases receiving rapid treatment
- Complete recovery for most individuals

■ REFERRAL
Immediate for all cases to an ER and an infectious disease consultant

PEARLS & CONSIDERATIONS

■ COMMENTS
- Routine cooking inactivates the toxin, but spores are resistant to environmental factors. At room temperature, spores can germinate and produce toxin.
- Most outbreaks are associated with home-canned foods, especially vegetables.
- Patients must be closely monitored for progression to respiratory paralysis.
- There is increasing concern over the potential use of botulinum toxin as a biologic weapon, either by the enteric route or by aerosolization.
- Notify public health authorities.

REFERENCES

Amon SS et al: Botulinum toxin as a biological weapon, *Jama* 285(8):1059, 2001.

Bleck TP: *Clostridium botulinim* (botulism). In Mandell GL, Bennett JE, Dolin R (eds): *Principles and practice of infectious diseases*, ed 5, New York, 2000, Churchill Livingstone.

Maselli RA: Pathogenesis of human botulism, *Ann N Y Acad Sci* 841:122, 1998.

Shapiro RL et al: Botulism in the United States: a clinical and epidemiologic review, *Ann Intern Med* 129:221, 1998.

Werner SB et al: Wound botulism in California, 1951-1998: recent epidemic in heroin injectors, *Clin Infect Dis* 31:1018, 2000.

Author: **Maurice Policar, M.D.**

BASIC INFORMATION

DEFINITION

Brain neoplasms are primary (non-metastatic) tumors arising from one of many intracranial cellular substrates. Specific tumors subtypes and prognosis depend on the tumor cell of origin and pattern of growth.

SYNONYMS

Brain tumors
Primary tumors of the central nervous system

ICD-9CM CODES

225.0 Brain neoplasm (benign)
239.2 Brain neoplasm (unspecified)

EPIDEMIOLOGY & DEMOGRAPHICS

INCIDENCE (IN U.S.): 8 cases/100,000 persons/yr. Primary brain neoplasms account for ~2% of all cancers, ~20% of all cancers in children >15 yr. Most common cause of cancer death in children up to 15 yr.
PREVALENCE (IN U.S.): In 1990, there were >20,000 new cases of primary brain tumors
PREDOMINANT SEX: Male/female = 3/2, except for meningiomas: Female/male = 3/1
PREDOMINANT AGE: Male: 75+ yr; female: 65 to 74 yr

GENETICS

Most primary CNS neoplasms are sporadic; 5% are associated with hereditary syndromes that predispose to neoplasia. The most common of these include:
- Li Fraumeni syndrome → p53 mutation on chromosome 17q13 → gliomas
- Von Hippel-Lindau → VHL, chromosome 3p25 → hemangioblastoma
- Tuberous sclerosis → TSC1/TSC2 (chromosome 9q34/16p13) → subependymal giant cell astrocytoma
- Neurofibromatosis type 1 → NF1, chromosome 17q11 → neurofibroma, optic nerve glioma, Meningioma
- Neurofibromatosis type 2 → NF2, chromosome 22q12 → schwannoma, Meningioma, ependymoma
- Retinoblastoma → pRB, chromosome 13q → retinoblastoma
- Gorlin's syndrome → chromosome 9q31 → desmoplastic medulloblastoma

PHYSICAL FINDINGS & CLINICAL PRESENTATION

- In general, the location, size, and rate of growth will determine the symptoms and signs with development of progressive focal signs and symptoms
- Headache as presenting symptom is seen in 20% of patients and develops later in 60%
- Seizures in 33% of patients
- Symptoms and signs of hydrocephalus and raised intracranial pressure (headache, vomiting [particularly in children], clouding of consciousness, papilledema)

ETIOLOGY

- Most cases are idiopathic, though specific chromosomal abnormalities have been implicated in some tumor types.
- Exposure to ionizing radiation has been implicated in the genesis of meningiomas, gliomas, nerve sheath tumors. No convincing evidence has linked CNS tumors with trauma, occupation, diet, electromagnetic fields.

DIAGNOSIS

- Most common tumors in children → astrocytoma, medulloblastoma, ependymoma
- Most common adult tumors → Glioblastoma multiforma, anaplastic astrocytoma, meningioma

DIFFERENTIAL DIAGNOSIS

- Stroke
- Abscess/parasitic cyst
- Demyelinating disease
- Metastatic tumors
- Primary central nervous system lymphoma

LABORATORY TESTS

- CSF cytology may yield histologic diagnosis and test for tumor markers (for pineal tumors)
- NB: LP must never be performed if there is concern for increased ICP

IMAGING STUDIES (Fig. 1-51)

- A neuroradiologist is able to diagnose tumor type with considerable accuracy, but most tumors should be biopsied for 100% accuracy.
- MRI with contrast is highly sensitive, though CT scan is useful if calcification or hemorrhage suspected.
- PET scan is helpful to distinguish neoplastic lesions (with high rate of metabolism) from other lesions such as demyelination or radiation necrosis (with a much lower metabolic rate).

HISTOPATHOLOGY

- Ultimately, only a histologic examination can provide the exact diagnosis.
- There are several different classification schema. Typically, diagnosis is based on histopathology, although advances in molecular biology are facilitating genetic classification.

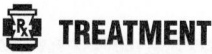 **TREATMENT**

NONPHARMACOLOGIC THERAPY

- Surgical removal or debulking is the treatment of choice.
- Biopsy alone is performed if the tumor is located in eloquent regions of brain or is inaccessible; this is essential for histopathologic diagnosis. Biopsy can be performed under CT or MRI guidance using stereotactic localization.
- If the tumor is of a benign nature (e.g., meningioma, acoustic neuroma), no further therapy is usually required.

ACUTE GENERAL Rx

Steroids (e.g., dexamethasone 4 mg PO q6h) may be used as a temporizing measure to reduce edema. In addition, steroids may be used following surgery or during radiation therapy.

■ **CHRONIC Rx**
- Depending on tumor type, chemotherapy may be necessary
- Chemotherapy → may be used before, during, or after surgery and radiation therapy (In children, chemotherapy is often used to delay radiation therapy.)
- Radiation is useful for certain types of tumors: Conventional radiation uses external beams over a period of weeks, whereas stereotactic radiosurgery delivers a single, high dose of radiation to a well-defined area (usually <1 cm)
- Long-term effects of radiation therapy include radiation necrosis (particularly of white matter), blood vessel hyalinization, secondary tumors (usually meningiomas, sarcomas and malignant astrocytomas)

■ **DISPOSITION/PROGNOSTIC FACTORS**
- Tumor histology/histologic diagnosis (WHO/grading system), including number of mitoses, capillary endothelial proliferation and necrosis (NB: there can be a high degree of morbidity based on tumor location, even with more benign histology)
- Age of the patient and Karnofsky performance score have predictive value for prognosis
- Terminal events typically result from raised intracranial pressure

■ **REFERRAL**
All cases warrant evaluation by an oncologist and neurosurgeon.

REFERENCE
Burton EC, Prados MD: Malignant gliomas, *Curr Opin Oncol* 1(5):459, 2000.
Author: **Nicole J. Ullrich, M.D., Ph.D.**

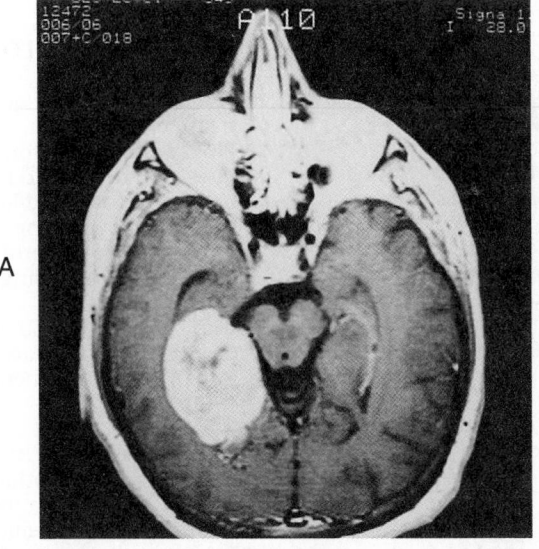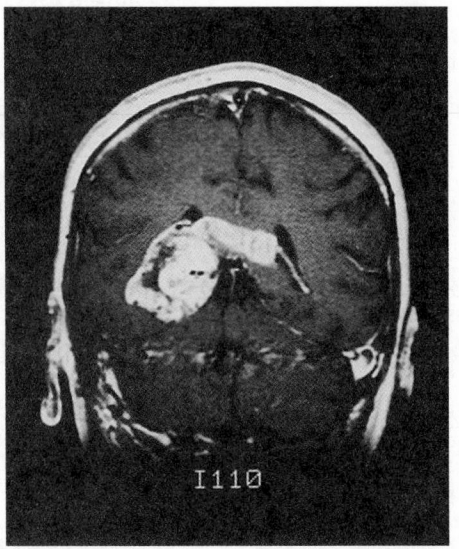

Fig. 1-51   Glioblastoma multiforme. Axial (**A**), and coronal (**B**), postcontrast enhanced T1-weighted image showing a large homogeneously contrast-enhancing mass in the right medial temporal lobe with extension across the midline. (From Specht N [ed]: *Practical guide to diagnostic imaging,* St Louis, 1998, Mosby.)

BASIC INFORMATION

■ DEFINITION

The term *breast cancer* refers to invasive carcinoma of the breast, whether ductal or lobular.

■ SYNONYMS

Carcinoma of the breast

ICD-9CM CODES

174.9 Malignant neoplasm female breast

■ EPIDEMIOLOGY & DEMOGRAPHICS

- Nearly exclusively the disease of women, with only 1% of breast cancers in males
- Steady increase in its incidence in the U.S., with 205,000 new patients annually
- Annual mortality of 40,000
- Risk steadily increases with age
- Genetically defined group of women with BRCA-1 or BRCA-2 identified to carry lifetime risk as high as 85%

■ PHYSICAL FINDINGS

- Increasing number of small breast cancers found by mammograms
- Patients usually completely free of physical findings
- Palpable tumors possibly as small as 1 cm or even smaller
- Size of the mass and its location measured and documented
- Skin and/or nipple retraction and skin edema/erythema/ulcer/satellite nodule
- Nodal enlargement in axilla and supraclavicular areas
- Advanced disease: clinical signs of pleural effusion and/or hepatomegaly
- Rare instances: clear, serous, or bloody discharge only symptom
- Nipple evaluation (see "Paget's disease of the breast")

■ ETIOLOGY

- Precise mechanism of carcinogenesis not understood
- Possibly interaction of ovarian estrogen, nonovarian estrogen, estrogens of exogenous origin with breast tissue of varied carcinogenic susceptibility to develop cancer
- Other known or suspected variables: childbearing, breast-feeding practice, diet, physical activities, body mass, alcoholic intake
- Have identified families with known high risk
- Women with BRCA-1 and BRCA-2 associated with high risk

DIAGNOSIS

■ DIFFERENTIAL DIAGNOSIS

The following nonmalignant breast lesions can simulate breast cancer on both physical and mammogram examinations:
1. Fibrocystic changes
2. Fibroadenoma
3. Hamartoma

■ IMAGING STUDIES

Mammograms: 30% to 50% of breast cancers detected by screening mammograms only as a spiculated mass, a mass with or without microcalcifications, or a cluster of microcalcifications (Fig. 1-52)

■ WORKUP

- Physical examination:
  1. Mass detected by patient or medical professional: workup required
  2. Negative mammogram: breast cancer not ruled out
  3. Sonogram: to demonstrate mass to be cyst, usually eliminating need for further workup
- To establish diagnosis:
  1. Positive aspiration cytology on a clinically and mammographically malignant mass—highly accurate but still requires open biopsy confirmation
  2. Stereotactic core needle biopsy diagnosis: reliable with invasive carcinoma identified, but negative or equivocal results require careful evaluation
  3. Atypical hyperplasia or in situ carcinoma found by core needle biopsy: open surgical biopsy confirmation still required
  4. Excisional or incisional biopsy: establishes diagnosis
- NOTE: Do not rely on negative mammogram or negative aspiration cytology to exclude malignancy. Make appropriate referral. Obtain imaging studies such as bone scan, chest x-ray examination, CT scan of abdomen, or CT scan of liver.
- Breast radiologic evaluation and an algorithm for breast cancer screening and evaluation are described in Section III. The differential diagnosis of breast lumps is described in Section II.

TREATMENT

■ NONPHARMACOLOGIC THERAPY

- Early breast cancer: primarily surgical or surgical and radiotherapeutic
- Choice in 60% to 70% of women between modified mastectomy and breast-conserving treatment, which consists of lumpectomy, axillary staging with sentinel node biopsy or axillary dissection, and breast irradiation

■ ACUTE GENERAL Rx

- May require adjuvant chemotherapy or endocrine therapy
- Evaluation and treatment by medical oncologist

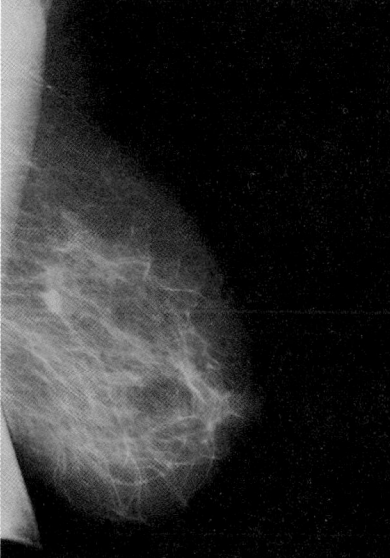
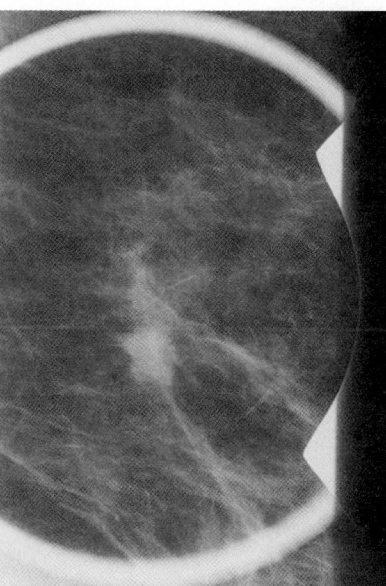

Fig. 1-52 **A,** Right mediolateral and, **B,** spot magnification view from routine screening mammography demonstrates a small, ill-defined mass with minimal spiculation. This was nonpalpable, and biopsy demonstrated infiltrating ductal carcinoma. (From Specht N [ed]: *Practical guide to diagnostic imaging,* St Louis, 1998, Mosby.)

■ CHRONIC Rx

Follow-up required after proper treatment of primary breast cancer includes:

1. Periodic clinical evaluations
2. Annual mammograms
3. Other tests as indicated
4. Patient instruction in monthly breast self-examination technique

■ DISPOSITION

- Prognosis after curative therapy: depends on size of tumor, extent of nodal metastasis, and pathologic grade of tumor
  1. Patient with 1-cm tumor with no axillary node metastasis: 10-yr disease-free survival rate of 90%
  2. Patient with 3-cm tumor with metastasis in four nodes: 10-yr disease-free survival rate of 15% if no systemic adjuvant therapy given
  3. Outlook for most patients is between these extremes
- Systemic adjuvant therapy: improves prognosis significantly

■ REFERRAL

Referral is necessary as soon as breast cancer is even remotely suspected.

☼ PEARLS & CONSIDERATIONS

Breast cancer in pregnancy and lactation:

1. Frequency in women 40 yr old or younger reported to be 15%
2. May carry worse prognosis because disease discovery delayed by engorged and nodular breast changes and/or because disease progression more rapid in pregnancy
3. Survival rates similar to those for nonpregnant early-stage breast cancer patients in same age group
4. Mass usually found by patient or obstetrician
5. Expedient workup recommended, including mammography and sonography
6. Diagnosis to be made without delay
7. Choice of mastectomy or lumpectomy with axillary dissection for treatment
8. Adjuvant chemotherapy delayed until third trimester or after delivery
9. Irradiation to breast after lumpectomy delayed until after delivery

Duct carcinoma in situ (DCIS, intraductal carcinoma):

1. "New" disease mostly found by mammogram as cluster of microcalcification and/or density
2. Less often, presents as palpable mass or nipple discharge
3. Before mammogram screening, DCIS accounted for 1% of all breast cancers
4. Now, 15% to 20% or even higher proportion present with DCIS
5. Formerly treated with mastectomy, now lumpectomy
6. Cure rates 98% to 99%
7. No axillary dissection required
8. With radiation, breast recurrences reduced
9. Mastectomy possibly required with extensive and/or high-grade DCIS
10. Systemic adjuvant treatment is not indicated

Inflammatory carcinoma:

1. Rare but rapidly progressive and often lethal form of breast cancer
2. Presents as erythematous and edematous breast resembling mastitis
3. Biopsy required, including skin
4. Treatment with combination chemotherapy followed by surgery and radiation therapy
5. Prognosis once dismal, now 5-yr disease-free survival in 50% of patients

■ COMMENTS

- Patient education material can be obtained from the following:
  1. SHARE: Self-Help for Women with Breast Cancer, 19 W 44th Street, No 415, New York, NY 10036-5902.
  2. Y-ME National Organization of Breast Cancer Information and Support, 18220 Harwood Avenue, Homewood, IL 80430.
- Breast radiologic evaluation, evaluation of nipple discharge, and evaluation of palpable mass are described in Section III.

REFERENCES

Boyd NF et al: Heritability of mammographic density, a risk factor for breast cancer, *N Engl J Med* 347:886, 2002.

Graham J et al: Stressful life experiences and risk of relapse of breast cancer: observational cohort study, *BMJ* 324:1420, 2002.

Hellekson KL: NIH statement on adjuvant therapy for breast cancer, *Am Fam Physician* 63:1857, 2001.

Humphrey LL et al: Breast cancer screening: a summary of the evidence for the U.S. Preventive Services Task Force, *Ann Intern Med* 137:347, 2002.

Kinsinger LS et al: Chemoprevention of breast cancer: a summary of the evidence for U.S. Preventive Services Task Force, *Ann Intern Med* 137:59, 2002.

Marchbanks PA et al: Oral contraceptives and the risk of breast cancer, *N Engl J Med* 346:2025, 2002.

Miller AB et al: The Canadian National Breast Screening Study—1: breast cancer mortality after 11 to 16 years of follow-up, *Ann Intern Med* 137:305, 2002.

Pruthi S: Detection and evaluation of palpable breast mass, *Mayo Clin Proc* 76:641, 2001.

Rebbeck TR et al: Prophylactic oophorectomy the risk of ovarian and breast cancer in carriers of BRCA1 or BRCA2 mutations, *N Engl J Med* 346:1616, 2002.

Slamon DJ et al: Use of chemotherapy plus a monoclonal antibody against HER2 for metastatic breast cancer that overexpresses HER2, *N Engl J Med* 344(11):783, 2001.

The ATAC Trialists' Group: Anastrozole alone or in combination with tamoxifen versus tamoxifen alone for adjuvant treatment of postmenopausal women with early breast cancer: first results of the ATAC randomized trial, *Lancet* 359:2131, 2002.

U.S. Preventive Services Task Force: Chemoprevention of breast cancer. Recommendations and rationale, *Ann Intern Med* 137:56, 2002.

Van 't Veer LJ et al: Gene expression profiling predicts clinical outcome of breast cancer, *Nature* 415:530, 2002.

Author: **Takuma Nemoto, M.D.**

BASIC INFORMATION

■ DEFINITION

Breech presentation exists when the fetal longitudinal axis is such that the cephalic pole occupies the uterine fundus. Three types exist, with respective percentages at term, frank (48% to 73%, flexed hips, extended thighs), complete (4.6% to 11.5%, flexed hips and knees), and footling (12% to 38%, hips extended).

ICD-9CM CODES
652.2 Breech presentation without mention of version

■ EPIDEMIOLOGY & DEMOGRAPHICS
INCIDENCE: Gestational age dependent: 3% to 4% overall, 14% at 29 to 32 wk, 33% at 21 to 24 wk
PERINATAL MORTALITY: 9% to 25%, or three to five times increase over vertex presentation at term. If one corrects for the associated increase in congenital anomalies and complications of prematurity, the morbidity and mortality approach that of the vertex presentation at term regardless of route of delivery.

■ PHYSICAL FINDINGS & CLINICAL PRESENTATION
- Maintain a high index of suspicion
- Lack of presenting part on vaginal examination
- Fetal heart tones heard above the umbilicus
- Leopold maneuvers revealing mobile fetal part in the uterine fundus

■ ETIOLOGY
- Abnormal placentation (fundal), uterine anomalies (fibroids, septa), pelvic or adnexal masses, alterations in fetal muscular tone, or fetal malformations
- Associated conditions: trisomy 13, 18, 21, Potter syndrome, myotonic dystrophy, prematurity

DIAGNOSIS

■ DIFFERENTIAL DIAGNOSIS
Vertex, oblique, or transverse lie

■ WORKUP
- If possible, determine reason for breech presentation, history of uterine anomalies, gestational age, or associated fetal congenital anomalies.
- Assess fetal status, by either continuous fetal heart rate monitoring or ultrasound.
- Assess pelvis to determine feasibility of vaginal delivery.

- Assess risk for safety of vaginal vs. abdominal delivery.

■ IMAGING STUDIES
Ultrasound to evaluate for:
- Fetal anomalies, such as hydrocephalus
- Placental location
- Position of fetal head relative to spine (check for hyperextension)
- Estimated fetal weight (2500 to 3800 g)
- Type of breech (frank, complete, footling)

■ CRITERIA FOR TRIAL OF LABOR
- Estimated fetal weight 2000 to 3800 g
- Frank breech
- Adequate pelvis
- Flexed fetal head
- Continuous fetal monitoring
- Normal progress of labor
- Bedside availability of anesthesia and capability for immediate C-section
- Informed consent
- Obstetrician trained in vaginal breech delivery

■ CRITERIA FOR C-SECTION
- Estimated fetal weight <1500 g or >4000 g
- Footling presentation (20% risk of cord prolapse, usually late in course of labor)
- Inadequate pelvis
- Hyperextended fetal head (21% risk of spinal cord injury)
- Nonreassuring fetal status
- Abnormal progress of labor
- Lack of trained obstetrician

TREATMENT

■ ACUTE GENERAL Rx
- Vaginal delivery in selected patient: allow maternal expulsive forces to deliver fetus until scapula visible (avoiding traction); with flexion and/or Piper forceps, deliver fetal head
- Perform C-section for the above-mentioned reasons
- External cephalic version, success 60% to 75%, after 37 wk, contraindicated with placental abruption, low-lying placenta, maternal hypertension, previous uterine incision, multiple gestation, nonreassuring fetal status
- Adequate pelvic/cervical relaxation essential for vaginal breech (i.e., need anesthesia in-room during birth [delivery] with uterine relaxants on hand [NTG, terbutaline])

■ COMPLICATIONS
- Head entrapment: leading cause of death (with the exception of anomalous fetuses), 88 cases/1000 deliveries, avoid by maintaining flexion of fetal head, use of Piper forceps or Dührssen's incisions. Before 36 wk, HC > AC, thus fetal predisposition. Tentorial tears secondary to hyperextended head. Association with trisomy 21 in 3% to 5% of cases. Avoid hyperextension of head during delivery.
- Cord prolapse: usually occurs late in the course of labor. Incidence depends on type of breech—frank (0.5%), complete (4% to 5%), footling (10%).
- Nuchal arm: arm extended above fetal head, occurs when there is undue traction before delivery of fetal scapulas. Treatment depends on bringing trapped arm across infant's face.

■ DISPOSITION
If confounding variables are corrected for, such as prematurity and associated congenital anomalies (6.3% of breeches vs. 2.4% in general population), route of delivery plays a less important role in fetal outcome than previously thought.

■ REFERRAL
An obstetrician trained in delivery of the vaginal breech is a prerequisite for attempting vaginal route, although it must be explained to the patient that with C-section certain risks (such as hyperextension of the fetal head with resultant spinal cord injury) may be minimized but not eliminated.

PEARLS & CONSIDERATIONS

■ COMMENTS
For breech presentation, in general, mortality is increased thirteenfold and morbidity sevenfold. The main reasons are an increase in congenital anomalies, perinatal hypoxia, birth injury, and prematurity.
There is no contraindication to induction of labor in the breech presentation, nor is labor prohibited in a primigravida.
Author: **Scott J. Zuccala, D.O.**

BASIC INFORMATION

■ **DEFINITION**
Bronchiectasis is the abnormal dilation and destruction of bronchial walls, which may be congenital or acquired.

ICD-9CM-CODES
494.0 Bronchiectasis

■ **EPIDEMIOLOGY & DEMOGRAPHICS**
• Cystic fibrosis is responsible for nearly 50% of all cases of bronchiectasis.
• Acquired primary bronchiectasis is uncommon because of rapid diagnosis of pulmonary infections and frequent use of antibiotics.
• Effective childhood immunizations have led to a significant decrease in the incidence of bronchiectasis resulting from pertussis.

■ **PHYSICAL FINDINGS & CLINICAL PRESENTATION**
• Moist crackles at lung bases
• Cough with expectoration of large amount of purulent sputum
• Fever, night sweats, generalized malaise, weight loss
• Hemoptysis
• Halitosis, skin pallor
• Clubbing (infrequent)

■ **ETIOLOGY**
• Cystic fibrosis
• Lung infections (pneumonia, lung abscess, TB, fungal infections, viral infections)
• Abnormal host defense (panhypogammaglobulinemia, Kartagener's syndrome, AIDS, chemotherapy)
• Localized airway obstruction (congenital structural defects, foreign bodies, neoplasms)
• Inflammation (inflammatory pneumonitis, granulomatous lung disease, allergic aspergillosis)

 DIAGNOSIS

■ **DIFFERENTIAL DIAGNOSIS**
• TB
• Asthma
• Chronic bronchitis or chronic sinusitis
• Interstitial fibrosis
• Chronic lung abscess
• Foreign body aspiration
• Cystic fibrosis
• Lung carcinoma

■ **WORKUP**
• Sputum for Gram stain and C&S, chest x-ray examination, bronchoscopy, spirometry
• Spirometry reveals reduced ration of FEV_1 to FVC, normal or slightly reduced FVC, and a reduced FEV_1

■ **LABORATORY TESTS**
• Sputum for Gram stain, C&S, and acid-fast bacteria (AFB)
• CBC with differential (leukocytosis with left shift, anemia)
• Serum protein electrophoresis to evaluate for hypogammaglobulinemia
• Antibody test for aspergillosis
• Sweat test in patients with suspected cystic fibrosis

■ **IMAGING STUDIES**
• Chest x-ray examination: hyperinflation, crowded lung markings, small cystic spaces at the base of the lungs
• High-resolution CT scan of the chest has become the best tool to detect cystic lesions and exclude underlying obstruction from neoplasm. The CT study should be a noncontrast study with the use of 1 to 1.5 mm window every 1 cm with acquisition time of 1 sec. Typical findings on CT include dilation of airway lumen, lack of tapering of an airway toward periphery, ballooned cysts at the end of bronchus, and varicose constrictions along airways.
• Bronchography is rarely used and may be considered only when surgery is contemplated.
• Pulmonary function tests generally reveal obstructive or mixed ventilatory defect.
• Bronchoscopy may be helpful to evaluate hemoptysis, rule out obstructive lesions, and remove mucus plugs.

TREATMENT

■ **NONPHARMACOLOGIC THERAPY**
• Postural drainage (reclining prone on a bed with the head down on the side) and chest percussion with use of inflatable vests or mechanical vibrators applied to the chest may enhance removal of respiratory secretions
• Adequate hydration
• Supplemental oxygen for hypoxemia

■ **ACUTE GENERAL Rx**
• Antibiotic therapy is based on the results of sputum, Gram stain, and C&S; in patients with inadequate or inconclusive results, empiric therapy with amoxicillin/clavulanate 500 mg to 875 mg q12h, TMP-SMX q12h, doxycycline 100 mg bid, or cefuroxime 250 mg bid for 10 to 14 days is recommended.
• Bronchodilators are useful in patients with demonstrable airflow obstruction.

■ **CHRONIC Rx**
• Avoidance of tobacco
• Maintenance of proper nutrition and hydration
• Prompt identification and treatment of infections
• Pneumococcal vaccination and annual influenza vaccination

■ **DISPOSITION**
Prognosis is variable with severity of the disease and underlying etiology of bronchiectasis.

■ **REFERRAL**
Surgical referral for partial lung resection in patients with localized severe disease unresponsive to medical therapy or in patients with massive hemoptysis

REFERENCE
Barker AF: Bronchiectasis, *N Engl J Med* 346:1383, 2002.
Author: **Fred F. Ferri, M.D.**

BASIC INFORMATION

■ DEFINITION
Acute bronchitis is the inflammation of trachea and bronchi.

ICD-9CM CODES
466.0 Acute bronchitis

■ EPIDEMIOLOGY & DEMOGRAPHICS
• Highest incidence in smokers, older adults, young children, and in winter months
• In the U.S. there are nearly 30 million ambulatory visits annually for cough, leading to more than 12 million diagnoses of "bronchitis"

■ PHYSICAL FINDINGS & CLINICAL PRESENTATION
• Cough, usually worse in the morning, often productive. Mainly caused by transient bronchial hyperresponsiveness
• Low-grade fever
• Substernal discomfort worsened by coughing
• Postnasal drip, pharyngeal injection
• Rhonchi that may clear after cough, occasional wheezing

■ ETIOLOGY
• Viral infections are the leading cause of bronchitis (rhinovirus, influenza virus, adenovirus, respiratory syncytial virus)
• Atypical organisms (*Mycoplasma, Chlamydia pneumoniae*)
• Bacterial infections (*Haemophilus influenzae, Moraxella, Streptococcus pneumoniae*)

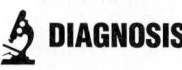

DIAGNOSIS

■ DIFFERENTIAL DIAGNOSIS
• Pneumonia
• Asthma
• Sinusitis
• Bronchiolitis
• Aspiration
• Cystic fibrosis
• Pharyngitis
• Cough secondary to medications
• Neoplasm (elderly patients)
• Influenza
• Allergic aspergillosis
• GERD
• CHF (in elderly patients)
• Bronchogenic neoplasm

■ WORKUP
Seldom necessary (e.g., to rule out pneumonia, neoplasm)

■ LABORATORY TESTS
• Tests are generally not necessary.
• CBC may reveal mild leukocytosis.
• Sputum culture, Gram stain, and blood cultures are generally not indicated.

■ IMAGING STUDIES
Chest x-ray examination is usually reserved for patients with suspected pneumonia, influenza, or underlying COPD and no improvement with therapy.

TREATMENT

■ NONPHARMACOLOGIC THERAPY
• Avoidance of tobacco and other pulmonary irritants
• Increased fluid intake
• Use of vaporizer to increase room humidity

■ ACUTE GENERAL Rx
• Inhaled bronchodilators (e.g., albuterol, metaproterenol) prn for 1 to 2 wk in patients with wheezing or troublesome cough. Inhaled albuterol has been proven effective in reducing the duration of cough in adults with uncomplicated acute bronchitis
• Cough suppression with guaifenesin; addition of codeine for cough suppression (e.g., Robitussin-AC) if cough is severe and is significantly interrupting patient's sleep pattern
• Use of antibiotics (TMP-SMX, amoxicillin, doxycycline, cefuroxime) for acute bronchitis is generally not indicated; should be considered only in patients with concomitant COPD and purulent sputum or in patients unresponsive to prolonged conservative treatment
• Antibiotics are overused in patients with acute bronchitis (70% to 90% of office visits for acute bronchitis result in treatment with antibiotics); this practice pattern is contributing to increases in resistant organisms

■ CHRONIC Rx
Avoidance of tobacco and other pulmonary irritants

■ DISPOSITION
• Complete recovery within 7 to 10 days in most patients
• Patients should be informed to expect to have a cough for 10 to 14 days after the visit

■ REFERRAL
For pulmonary function testing only in patients with recurrent bronchitis and suspected underlying asthma

☼ PEARLS & CONSIDERATIONS

■ COMMENTS
• Intervention studies reveal that patient and physician education are effective in reducing the use of antibiotic therapy.
• It is helpful to refer to acute bronchitis as a "chest cold." Patients should be informed that antibiotics are probably not going to be beneficial and may result in significant side effects.

REFERENCES

Evans AT et al: Azithromycin for acute bronchitis: a randomized, double-blind, controlled trial, *Lancet* 359:1648, 2002.

Knutson D, Braun C: Diagnosis and management of acute bronchitis, *Am Fam Physician* 65:2039, 2002.

Macfarlane J et al: Reducing antibiotic use for acute bronchitis in primary care: blinded, randomized controlled trial of patient information leaflet, *BMJ* 324:91, 2002.

Poole PJ, Black PN: Mucolytic agents for chronic bronchitis. *Cochrane Database Syst Rev* 2:CD001287, 2001.

Smucny JJ et al: Are beta-2 agonists effective treatment for acute bronchitis or acute cough in patients without underlying pulmonary disease? A systematic review, *J Fam Pract* 50:945, 2001.

Author: **Fred F. Ferri, M.D.**

BASIC INFORMATION

■ DEFINITION
Brucellosis is a zoonotic infection caused by one of four species of *Brucella*. It commonly presents as a nondescript febrile illness.

■ SYNONYMS
Malta fever
Bang's disease

ICD-9CM CODES
023.9 Brucellosis

■ EPIDEMIOLOGY & DEMOGRAPHICS
INCIDENCE (IN U.S.): About 100 cases/yr (may be underreported)
PREDOMINANT SEX: Male
PREDOMINANT AGE: Adult
CONGENITAL INFECTION: Recent evidence suggests a high rate of spontaneous abortions in untreated pregnant women during the first and second trimesters.
NEONATAL INFECTION: Can occur if mother is infected during pregnancy.

■ PHYSICAL FINDINGS
- Incubation period is 1 wk to 3 mo.
- Patients may be asymptomatic or have nonspecific symptoms such as fever, sweats, malaise, weight loss, and depression.
- Bacteremic patients may have arthralgias or arthritis. Patients may rarely present with abdominal pain.
- Fever is the most common finding.
- Hepatomegaly, splenomegaly, or lymphadenopathy is possible.
- Localized disease:
  1. Related to a single organ
  2. Includes endocarditis, meningitis, and osteomyelitis (especially vertebral)
Chronic hepatosplenic suppurative brucellosis (CHSB) presents with hepatic or splenic abscesses. This form is thought to be a reactivation and can occur years after the acute infection.

■ ETIOLOGY
- Caused by infection with *Brucella* species:
  1. Most commonly *melitensis*, but also *suis, abortus,* or *canis*
  2. A small, gram-negative coccobacillus
- Acquired through breaks in the skin or by inhalation or ingestion of organisms.

- Most cases occur after exposure to animals (sheep, goats, swine, cattle, or dogs), or animal products (i.e., milk, hides, tissue).
- Most cases (in U.S.) occur in men with occupational exposure to animals (farmers, ranchers, veterinarians, abattoir workers).
- Laboratory acquisition is possible.
- May occur in tourists to other countries who ingest goat milk or cheese.

DIAGNOSIS

■ DIFFERENTIAL DIAGNOSIS
Many febrile conditions without localizing manifestations (i.e., TB, endocarditis, typhoid fever, malaria, autoimmune diseases)

■ WORKUP
- Cultures of blood, bone marrow, or other tissue (lymph node, liver) should be sent and held for 4 wk, because *Brucella* grows slowly in vitro.
- Granulomas on biopsy are suggestive of diagnosis.

■ LABORATORY TESTS
- WBC count: normal or low
- Serology:
  1. Serum agglutination test (SAT) to detect antibodies to *B. abortus, melitensis,* and *suis*
  2. Specific antibody test to identify antibodies to *B. canis*
  3. False-negative SAT possibly resulting from a prozone effect
Serologic studies may be nondiagnostic in CHSB.

■ IMAGING STUDIES
- Radiographs to show splenic calcifications in chronic disease
- Bone scan and radiographs of the spine to suggest osteomyelitis
- Ultrasound or CT scan of the abdomen to show an enlarged liver or spleen
- Echocardiogram to reveal vegetations in endocarditis
In CHSB, abscesses and calcifications may be seen in the liver and spleen.

TREATMENT

■ NONPHARMACOLOGIC THERAPY
- Drainage of abscesses
- Valve replacement for endocarditis

■ ACUTE GENERAL Rx
Combination antibiotics required:
- Doxycycline 100 mg PO bid plus streptomycin 15 mg/kg IM qd for 6 wk
- Less effective: doxycycline 100 mg PO bid plus rifampin 600 mg PO qd or sulfamethoxazole 800 mg/ trimethoprim 160 mg one DS tablet PO qid
Courses <6 wk are associated with higher relapse rates; longer courses are recommended for complicated disease.

■ CHRONIC Rx
See "Acute General Rx."

■ DISPOSITION
Relapse is possible weeks to months after the completion of therapy, usually because of noncompliance with a prolonged medical regimen or a persistent focus of infection that requires surgical drainage.
Reactivation with CHSB has been reported up to 35 yr after initial illness.

■ REFERRAL
For all cases to an infectious disease specialist

PEARLS & CONSIDERATIONS

■ COMMENTS
- Alert the microbiology laboratory to the possibility of *Brucella*.
- Do not use doxycycline in children or pregnant women.
- Avoid aminoglycosides in pregnant women.

REFERENCES
Ariza J et al: Current understanding and management of chronic hepatosplenic suppurative brucellosis, *Clin Infect Dis* 32(7):995, 2001.
Fernandez MD et al: *Brucella* acute abdomen mimicking appendicitis, *Am J Med* 108:599, 2000.
Khan MY et al: Brucellosis in pregnant women, *Clin Infect Dis* 32(8):1172, 2001.
Memish Z et al: *Brucella* bacteremia: clinical and laboratory observations in 160 patients, *J Infect Dis* 40:59, 2000.
Author: **Maurice Policar, M.D.**

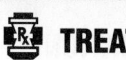
 BASIC INFORMATION

■ DEFINITION

Forcible clenching or grinding of the teeth during sleep or wakefulness, often leading to damage of the teeth.

ICD-9CM CODES
306.8 Bruxism

■ EPIDEMIOLOGY & DEMOGRAPHICS

Occurs in 15% of children and 75% of adults

■ PHYSICAL FINDINGS & CLINICAL PRESENTATION

Complaints of grinding of teeth from sleep partner or members of the family. In many cases, the masticatory system will adapt to the phenomenon, but in severe cases nearly every part of the masticatory system may be damaged. Excessive wearing of dentition is the most common physical finding. Tender or hypoatrophied masticatory muscles may also be observed.

■ ETIOLOGY

Cause is quite controversial. Possible causes in the literature include occlusal discrepancies, anatomy of the bony structures of the orofacial region, part of the sleep arousal response, disturbances of the central dopaminergic system, smoking, alcohol, drugs, stress, and personality.

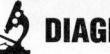 **DIAGNOSIS**

■ DIFFERENTIAL DIAGNOSIS
- Dental compression syndrome
- Temporomandibular joint disorders
- Chronic orofacial pain disorders
- Oral motor disorders
- Malocclusion

■ WORKUP

History should have an emphasis on sleep habits, including excessive snoring, pain in the temporal mandibular region, interview with close family members, health habits, personality quirks. Physical examination of the teeth and masticatory muscles is mandatory. Sleep studies in selected cases may be helpful.

■ LABORATORY TESTS

None indicated unless a systemic disease suspected (e.g., infection, autoimmune)

■ IMAGING STUDIES

X-ray studies of teeth and temporomandibular joints

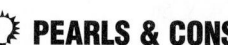 **TREATMENT**

■ NONPHARMACOLOGIC THERAPY

Biofeedback, psychological counseling, and elimination of harmful health habits have been used with limited success.

■ GENERAL Rx
- Oral splints; a nightguard to protect teeth may be useful
- Correction of malocclusion
- Pain management (e.g., gabapentin, ibuprofen)
- Medication to relieve anxiety and improve sleep (e.g., benzodiazepine or trazodone at hs)

■ DISPOSITION

Referral to dentist mandatory if damage to teeth evident.

☼ PEARLS & CONSIDERATIONS

Like any poorly understood disease, treatment is often unsatisfactory and subject to quackery.

REFERENCES

Attansio R: An overview of bruxism and its management, *Dent Clin North Am* 41(2):229, 1997.

Dae TT, Lavigne EJ: Oral splints: the crutches for temporomandibular disorders and bruxism, *Crit Rev Oral Biol Med* 9(3):345, 1998.

Lopbezoo F, Naeije M: Bruxism is mainly regulated centrally, not peripherally, *J Oral Rehabil* 28(12):1085, 2001.

Author: **Fred F. Ferri, M.D.**

BASIC INFORMATION

■ DEFINITION

Budd-Chiari syndrome (BCS) is the obstruction of hepatic venous blood flow. The site of obstruction may be anywhere from the small central lobar veins of the liver to the proximal inferior vena cava (IVC). Although BCS is frequently caused by thrombosis, extrinsic compression and venous malformations may also cause obstruction. BCS may result in portal hypertension, cirrhosis, and liver failure.

■ SYNONYMS

Hepatic vein thrombosis
Postsinusoidal obstruction
Hepatic venous outflow obstruction

ICD-9CM CODES
453.0 Budd-Chiari syndrome

■ EPIDEMIOLOGY & DEMOGRAPHICS

BCS is a rare disorder. Etiology varies with geography. Women are more commonly affected. Average age is 35 although the young and elderly can also be affected. In the U.S., BCS is more commonly associated with myeloproliferative disease, hypercoagulable states, IVC membranes, and tumors.

■ PHYSICAL FINDINGS & CLINICAL PRESENTATION

Variable according to the degree, location, and acuity of the obstruction
• Fulminant/Acute: Severe RUQ abdominal pain, jaundice, hepatomegaly, ascites, variceal bleeding, and encephalopathy. Early recognition and treatment are essential to survival. This presentation is more commonly seen in pregnant women
• Subacute/Chronic: Vague abdominal discomfort, gradual progression to hepatomegaly
• Portal hypertension with or without cirrhosis; ascites, lower extremity edema, esophageal varices, splenomegaly, coagulopathy, hepatopulmonary syndrome, and rarely, encephalopathy

■ ETIOLOGY

Myeloproliferative disease:
• Polycythemia vera
• Essential thrombocytosis
Hypercoagulable states:
• Protein C deficiency
• Antithrombin III deficiency
• Protein S deficiency
• Activated protein C resistance/factor V Leiden
• Antiphospholipid antibody
• Homocystinemia
• Pregnancy
• Oral contraceptive pills
• Sickle cell anemia

Infection:
• Liver abscess
• Filariasis
• Schistosomiasis
• Hydatid cyst
• Syphilis
• Tuberculosis
Malignancy:
• Adrenal
• Ovarian
• Bronchogenic
• Renal
• Hepatocellular
• Leiomyosarcoma
   Metastatic cancer
Other:
• Sarcoid
   Behçet's disease
   Paroxysmal nocturnal hemoglobinuria
• IVC membrane/congenital web
• Trauma

DIAGNOSIS

■ DIFFERENTIAL DIAGNOSIS
• Shock liver/ischemic hepatitis
• Viral hepatitis
• Toxic hepatitis
• Hepatic veno-occlusive disease
• Alcoholic hepatitis
• Pancreatitis
• Cholecystitis
• Perforated viscus
• Peptic ulcer disease
• Cardiac cirrhosis (i.e., chronic right-sided heart failure)
• Alcoholic cirrhosis
• Cirrhosis of other etiologies:
   Wilson's
   Hemochromatosis
   α-1-Antitrypsin deficiency
   Autoimmune

■ WORKUP
Physical examination, laboratory analysis, and imaging studies.

■ LABORATORY TESTS
Assessment of liver injury and function:
• Transaminases, prothrombin time, albumin, bilirubin
Diagnostic tests (directed by history):
• CBC, bone marrow biopsy, viral hepatitis panel, α-1-antitrypsin, serum iron, transferrin saturation, alkaline phosphatase, ceruloplasmin, toxicology screen, antismooth muscle antibody, antimitochondrial antibody, and double-stranded DNA antibody. Tests for hypercoagulable states may be difficult to interpret because many levels are abnormal due to liver dysfunction. Family studies may be the only way to identify a primary disorder

■ IMAGING STUDIES
• Color and pulsed Doppler U/S—most useful
• CT Scan with IV contrast
• MRI angiography
• Venography/arteriography—gold standard but invasive and mainly indicated if the abovementioned studies are negative despite a strong clinical suspicion and to guide surgical intervention

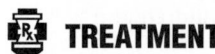

TREATMENT

■ ACUTE GENERAL Rx
• Supportive measures
• Liver transplant may be indicated for fulminant BCS
• Shunting, stenting, removal of IVC webs, or angioplasty to decompress the portal circulation may be indicated for acute BCS in patients in stable condition
• Thrombolytic therapy can be used to decompress the portal circulation

■ CHRONIC Rx
• Chronic anticoagulation may be needed to maintain shunt patency or in patients with thrombotic BCS
• ASA and hydroxyurea if underlying myeloproliferative disorder
• Treatment of underlying liver disease and complications related to portal hypertension
• Liver transplantation
• Shunt thrombosis is a common complication

■ DISPOSITION
Prognosis is dependent on multiple factors including time to recognition and treatment, etiology, acuity, the type of intervention, and the condition of the patient at the time of treatment.

■ REFERRAL
Prompt referral to a surgeon specializing in hepatobiliary disease is recommended.

REFERENCES

Granger DR et al: Transjugular intrahepatic portosystemic shunt (TIPS) for Budd Chiari syndrome or portal vein thrombosis, *Am J Gastroenterol* 94(3):559, 1999.
Slakey DP et al: Budd-Chiari syndrome: current management options, *Ann Surg* 233(4):522, 2001.
Valla, DC: The diagnosis and management of the Budd-Chiari syndrome: consensus and controversies, *Hepatology* 38(4): 793, 2003.
Authors: **James J. Ng, M.D., and Jennifer R. Hur, M.D.**

BASIC INFORMATION

■ DEFINITION
Bulimia nervosa is a prolonged illness characterized by a specific psychopathology (see below).

ICD-9CM CODES
783.6 Bulimia

■ EPIDEMIOLOGY & DEMOGRAPHICS
INCIDENCE/PREVALENCE: Affects 1% to 3% of female adolescents and young adults
PREDOMINANT SEX: Female:male ratio of 10:1
PREDOMINANT AGE: Adolescence to young adulthood; mean age of onset: 17 yr

■ PHYSICAL FINDINGS & CLINICAL PRESENTATION
- Parotid and salivary gland swelling
- Scars on the back of the hand and knuckles (Russell's sign) from rubbing against the upper incisors when inducing vomiting
- Eroded enamel, particularly on the lingual surface of the upper teeth; pyorrhea and other gum disorders possible
- Petechial hemorrhages of the cornea, soft palate, or face possibly noted after vomiting
- Loss of gag reflex, well-developed abdominal musculature
- Usually no emaciation; normal physical examination possible

■ ETIOLOGY
Etiology is unknown but likely multifactorial (sociocultural, psychologic, familial factors). Bulimia is much more common in Western societies where there is a strong cultural pressure to be slender. According to the American Psychiatric Association, patients with eating disorders display a broad range of symptoms that occur along a continuum between those of anorexia nervosa and bulimia.

DIAGNOSIS

■ DIFFERENTIAL DIAGNOSIS
- Schizophrenia
- GI disorders
- Neurologic disorders (seizures, Kleine-Levin syndrome, Klüver-Bucy syndrome)
- Brain neoplasms
- Psychogenic vomiting

■ WORKUP
- The following questions are useful to screen patients for bulimia:
  1. "Are you satisfied with your eating habits?"
  2. "Do you ever eat in secret?"
- Answering "no" to the first question and/or "yes" to the second question has 100% sensitivity and 90% specificity for bulimia. The SCOFF questionnaire can also be used as a screening tool for eating disorders (see "Anorexia Nervosa").
- A diagnosis can also be made using the following DSM-IV diagnostic criteria for bulimia nervosa:
  1. Recurrent episodes of binge eating (rapid consumption of a large amount of food in a discrete period)
  2. A feeling of lack of control over eating behavior during the eating binges
  3. Self-induced vomiting, use of laxatives or diuretics, strict dieting or fasting, or rigorous exercise to prevent weight gain
  4. A minimum of two binge-eating episodes a week for at least 3 mo
  5. Persistent overconcern with body shape and weight

■ LABORATORY TESTS
- Electrolyte abnormalities secondary to vomiting (hypokalemia and metabolic alkalosis) or to diarrhea from laxative abuse (hypokalemia and hyperchloremic metabolic acidosis)
- Hyponatremia, hypocalcemia, hypomagnesemia (caused by laxative abuse)
- Elevated cortisol, decreased LH, decreased FSH

TREATMENT

■ NONPHARMACOLOGIC THERAPY
- Cognitive behavioral therapy to control abnormal behaviors
- Use of food diaries, nutritional counseling, and planning meals at least a day in advance is useful to counter abnormal eating behaviors
- Correction of electrolyte abnormalities

■ ACUTE GENERAL Rx
- SSRIs are generally considered to be the safest medication option in these patients. They are useful in severely depressed patients and in those who fail to benefit from cognitive behavioral therapy.
- Prompt recognition and treatment of complications:
  1. Ipecac cardiotoxicity from laxative abuse

2. Electrolyte abnormalities (see Laboratory Tests)
3. Esophagitis and Mallory-Weiss tears; esophageal rupture from repeated vomiting
4. Aspiration pneumonia and pneumomediastinum
5. Menstrual irregularities (including amenorrhea)
6. GI abnormalities: acute gastric dilatation, pancreatitis, abdominal pain, constipation

■ CHRONIC Rx
- Psychotherapy continued for years and focused specifically on self-image and family and peer interactions is an integral part of successful recovery.
- Family therapy is also recommended, especially in younger patients.

■ DISPOSITION
Course is variable and marked by frequent recurrence of exacerbations.

■ REFERRAL
- In addition to the primary care physician, the multidisciplinary team should include a dietician, a psychiatrist, and a family therapist.
- Hospitalization should be considered for patients with severe electrolyte abnormalities or those with suicidal thoughts.

PEARLS & CONSIDERATIONS

■ COMMENTS
Bulimia has a close association with depression, bipolar disorder, obsessive-compulsive disorder, alcoholism, and substance abuse.

REFERENCES
American Psychiatric Association: Practice guideline for the treatment of patients with eating disorders, *Am J Psychiatry* 157(suppl):4, 2000.
Bacaltchuk J, Hay P, Trefiglio R: Antidepressants versus psychological treatments and their combination for bulimia nervosa, *Cochrane Database Syst Rev* (4):CD003385, 2001.
Mehler PS: Bulimia nervosa, *N Engl J Med* 349:875, 2003.
Prits SD, Susman J: Diagnosis of eating disorders in primary care, *Am Fam Physician* 67:297, 2003.
Author: **Fred F. Ferri, M.D.**

BASIC INFORMATION

■ DEFINITION
Bullous pemphigoid refers to an autoimmune, subepidermal blistering disease seen in the elderly.

■ SYNONYMS
Subepidermal autoimmune bullous dermatoses

ICD-9CM CODES
694.5 Pemphigoid

■ EPIDEMIOLOGY & DEMOGRAPHICS
- Commonly seen in the elderly older than 70 yr
- Incidence 10/1 million
- Equal prevalence between males and females
- No racial predilection
- Most common of the autoimmune bullous dermatoses

■ PHYSICAL FINDINGS & CLINICAL PRESENTATION
History
- Bullous pemphigoid typically starts as an eczematous or urticarial rash on the extremities.
- Blisters form between 1 wk to several months.

Physical findings
- Anatomic distribution
  1. Flexor surfaces of the arms, legs, groin, axilla, and lower abdomen
  2. Spares the head and neck
  3. Rare involvement of mucous membranes
- Lesion configuration
  1. May be localized to the extremities or generalized
  2. Lesions irregularly grouped but sometimes can be serpiginous (Fig. 1-53)
- Lesion morphology
  1. Blistering bullae characteristic findings measuring anywhere from 5 mm to 2 cm in diameter
  2. Contains clear or bloody fluid
  3. Arises from normal skin or from an erythematous base
  4. Heals without scarring if denuded

■ ETIOLOGY
Bullous pemphigoid is an autoimmune disease with IgG and/or C3 complement component reacting with antigens located in the basement membrane zone.

🔬 DIAGNOSIS

The diagnosis of bullous pemphigoid should be considered in any elderly individual with pruritic bullae.

■ DIFFERENTIAL DIAGNOSIS
- Cicatricial pemphigoid
- Herpes gestationis
- Epidermolysis bullosa acquisita
- Systemic lupus erythematosus
- Erythema multiforme
- Pemphigus
- Drug eruptions
- Pemphigoid nodularis

■ WORKUP
The clinical presentation and characteristic skin lesions assist in making the diagnosis of bullous pemphigoid. Specific laboratory tests, skin biopsy staining, and immunofluorescence studies confirm the diagnosis (Fig. 1-54).

■ LABORATORY TESTS
- Antibodies to the basement membrane zone are detected in the serum in 70% of patients with bullous pemphigoid.
- Skin biopsy staining with hematoxylineosin reveals subepidermal blisters.
- Direct and indirect immunofluorescence studies using salt-split skin detect the presence of IgG and C3 immune complexes on the basement membrane zone and can differentiate bullous pemphigus from other autoimmune blistering diseases.
- Immunoelectron microscopy also reveals immune deposits on the basement membrane zone.

■ IMAGING STUDIES
X-ray imaging studies are not very useful in the workup of patients with bullous pemphigoid.

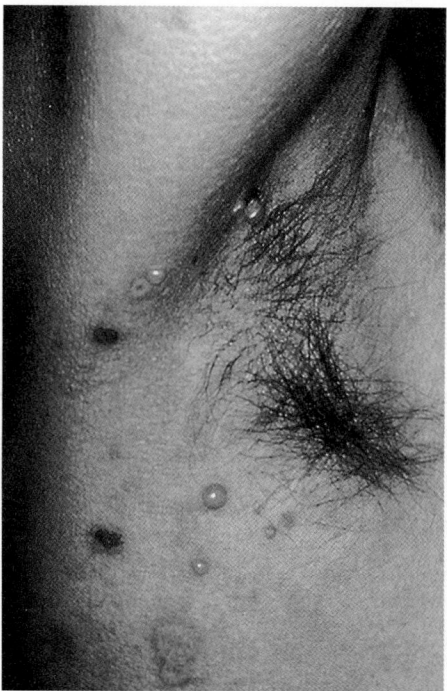

Fig. 1-53   Bullous pemphigoid. Note intact bullae with erosions in aflexural distribution. (From Goldstein BG, Goldstein AO: *Practical dermatology,* ed 2, St Louis, 1997, Mosby.)

TREATMENT

Treatment of bullous pemphigoid is based on the degree of involvement and rate of disease progression.

■ NONPHARMACOLOGIC THERAPY
- Avoid scratching.
- Use mild soaps and emollients after bathing to prevent dryness of the skin.

■ ACUTE GENERAL Rx
- Systemic corticosteroids are considered the standard treatment for more advanced bullous pemphigoid
  1. Prednisone 1 mg/kg/day is usually recommended and is continued until new blister formation ceases. The dose is tapered to 20 to 40 mg. Thereafter, the dose is gradually tapered according to the clinical findings.
- Topical steroids in general have been used in patients with localized bullous pemphigoid; however, recently topical corticosteroid therapy has been found to be effective for both moderate and severe bullous pemphigoid and superior to oral corticosteroid.
- If patients cannot take corticosteroids, dapsone, combination tetracycline and nicotinamide or azathioprine can be tried.

■ CHRONIC Rx
- Combination prednisone and azathioprine protocols are available in the treatment of bullous pemphigoid.
- Cyclophosphamide can be considered in attempt to reduce chronic long-term use of corticosteroids.

■ DISPOSITION
- Left untreated, patients with bullous pemphigoid run the risk of sepsis from infected bullae.
- Mortality rates are estimated at 19% at 1 yr, 6% at 2 yr, and 28% to 30% at 3 yr.

■ REFERRAL
If bullous pemphigoid is suspected, a dermatology consultation is recommended to assist with decisions regarding diagnosis, monitoring, and therapy.

PEARLS & CONSIDERATIONS

■ COMMENTS
- Bullous pemphigoid has been associated with diabetes, multiple sclerosis, pernicious anemia, rheumatoid arthritis, lichen planus, psoriasis, and vitiligo.
- Not known to transform into malignancies or represent a dermatologic manifestation of harboring malignancies.

REFERENCES

Joly P et al: A comparison of oral and topical corticosteroids in patients with bullous pemphigoid, *N Engl J Med* 346:321, 2002.

Korman NJ: Bullous pemphigoid: bullous diseases, *Dermatol Clin* 11:483, 1993.

Korman NJ: Bullous pemphigoid: the latest in diagnosis, prognosis and therapy, *Arch Dermatol* 134(9):1137, 1998.

Scott JE, Ahmed AR: The blistering diseases, *Med Clin North Am* 82(6):1239, 1998.

Vaillant L, et al: Evaluation of clinical criteria for diagnosis of bullous pemphigoid, *Arch Dermatol* 134(9):1075, 1998.

Author: **Peter Petropoulos, M.D.**

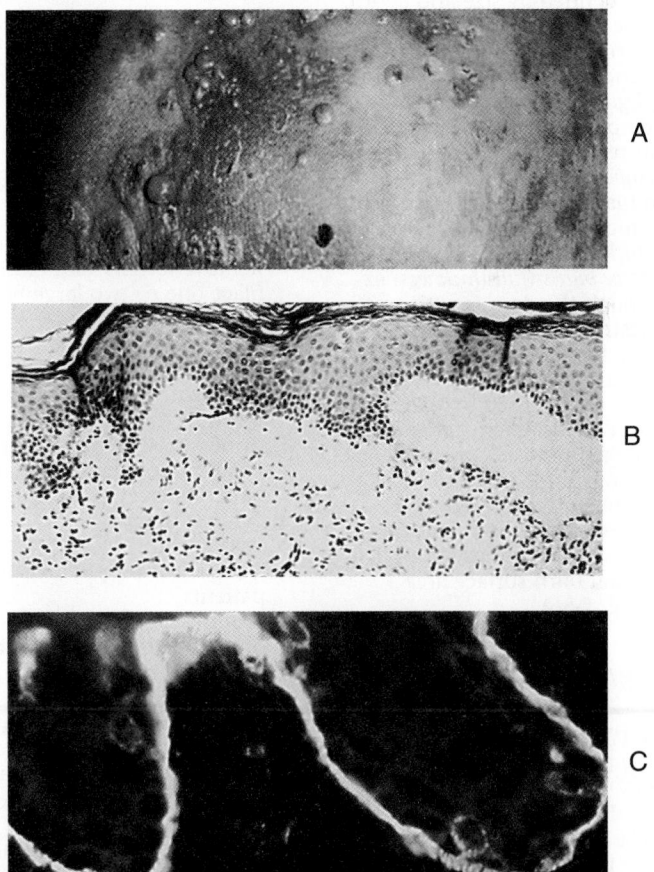

Fig. 1-54   Bullous pemphigoid. A, Clinical presentation with intact bullae and healing lesions. **B,** Hematoxylin and eosin stain of a blister reveals dermal-epidermal separation and a dermal inflammatory cell infiltrate. **C,** Indirect immunofluorescence performed on cryosections of rat tongue using serum from a patient with bullous pemphigoid, and fluorescein-labeled antihuman IgG. Note the binding of antibodies to the basement membrane zone in a linear and continuous pattern. (From Stein JH [ed]: *Internal medicine,* ed 5, St Louis, 1998, Mosby.)

BASIC INFORMATION

■ DEFINITION
Burn injuries consist of thermal injuries (flames, scalds, cigarettes), as well as chemical, electrical, and radiation burns.

■ SYNONYMS
Thermal injury

ICD-9CM CODES
942-949 (by region, % burn)

■ EPIDEMIOLOGY & DEMOGRAPHICS
PREVALENCE (IN U.S.): 2 million people/yr, 70-80 thousand require hospitalization.
PREDOMINANT SEX: Male:female ratio of 2:1
PREVALENT AGE: first few years of life and then 20-29 year olds

■ PHYSICAL FINDINGS & CLINICAL PRESENTATION
- Burns are defined by size and depth.
- *First-degree burns (superficial)* involve the epidermis only and appear painful and red.
- *Second-degree burns* involve the dermis and appear blistered, moist, and red with two-point discrimination intact (*superficial partial-thickness*) or red and blanched white with only sensation of pressure intact (*deep partial thickness*).
- *Third-degree burns (full-thickness)* extend through the dermis with associated destruction of hair follicles and sweat glands. The skin is charred, pale, *painless,* and leathery. These burns are caused by flames, immersion scalds, chemical and high voltage injuries.
- The "rule of nines" is useful for rapidly assessing the extent of a burn (see Fig. 1-55). Second- and third-degree burns are used to calculate the total burn surface area (TBSA) (Fig. 1-56).

DIAGNOSIS

■ CLASSIFICATION
Major burns: Partial-thickness burns >25% TBSA (or 20% if younger than 10 or older than 50 yr); full-thickness burns >10% TBSA; burns crossing major joints or involving the hands, face, feet, or perineum; electrical or chemical burns; those complicated by inhalation injury, or involving high-risk patients (extremes of age/comorbid diseases)
Moderate burns: Partial-thickness burns >15% to 25% TBSA (or 10% in children and older adults); full-thickness burns >2% to 10% TBSA and not in-volving the specific conditions of major burns
Minor burns: Partial-thickness burns <15% TBSA or full-thickness burns <2% TBSA

■ WORKUP
Diagnosis is based on clinical findings.

■ LABORATORY STUDIES
- CBC, electrolytes, BUN, creatinine, and glucose
- Serial ABG and carboxyhemoglobin if smoke inhalation suspected
- Urinalysis, urine myoglobin, and CPK levels if concern for rhabdomyolysis

■ IMAGING STUDIES
Chest x-ray and bronchoscopy if smoke inhalation suspected

TREATMENT

Minor burns are amenable to outpatient treatment, whereas moderate and major burns should be treated in specialized burn care facilities according to the principles described in Acute General Rx.

■ ACUTE GENERAL Rx
- Establish airway: inspect for inhalation injury and intubate for suspected airway edema (often seen 12 to 24 hr later); supplemental O₂
- Remove jewelry and clothing and place one or two large-bore peripheral IVs (if TBSA > 20%)
- Fluid resuscitation with Ringer's lactate at 2 to 4 ml/kg per %TBSA per 24 hr with half the calculated fluid given in the first 8 hr; may titrate to urine output of 0.5 to 1 ml/kg/hr
- Foley catheter and NG tube (20% of patients develop an ileus)
- Tetanus update
- Pain control
- Stress ulcer prophylaxis in high-risk patients
- Prophylactic antibiotics are not recommended; however, burn victims should be considered immunosuppressed
- High-voltage burn patients should have ECG monitoring because they are at increased risk for arrhythmia

■ BURN WOUND Rx
First-degree burns (e.g., sunburns) can be treated with cool compresses, antihistamines, emollients, and at times, a rapidly tapering dose of steroids.
Second-degree and third-degree burns:
- Wash burned skin with cool water or saline (1° to 5° C; immerse approximately 30 min if able) and cleanse with mild soap

- Sharp debridement of ruptured blisters (except palms and soles)
- There are several approaches to burn dressings after cleansing and debriding:
  1. Apply thin layer of antibiotic ointment (silver sulfadiazine can be used unless sulfa allergy or facial burn) and cover with a nonadherent dressing (e.g., Telfa or petroleum-soaked gauze) followed by a sterile gauze wrap. Wash wound and change dressing when dressing soaked.
  2. Apply saline-soaked gauze (Xeroform, Owen's), cover with 4 × 4 dressing and a bulky absorbent dressing such as Kerlex. Reevaluate in 5 to 7 days.
  3. Apply occlusive dressing (Duoderm, Tegaderm, Biobrane), remove in 7 to 10 days.
- Specialized care, such as excision and auto grafting is required for deep second-degree or third-degree burns.

■ DISPOSITION
- Respiratory injury, sepsis, and multi-organ failure may complicate severe burns.
- Scarring can be expected in many second-degree and all third-degree burns.

■ REFERRAL
Major and some moderate burns require referral to specialized burn centers for surgical debridement, grafting evaluation and rehabilitation

PEARLS & CONSIDERATIONS

Burn victims need to be reassessed frequently because the examination can change significantly in the first 24-72 hr.

■ COMMENTS

REFERENCES

Edlich R, Moghtader J: Thermal burns. In Rosen P (ed): *Emergency medicine: concepts and clinical practice,* ed 4, vol 1, St Louis, 1998, Mosby.

Schwartz L: Thermal burns. In Tintinalli J (ed): *Emergency medicine: a comprehensive study guide,* New York, 1996, McGraw-Hill.

Sheridan R: *Burn Care: Results of Technical and Organizational Progress,* JAMA 290(6):719, 2003.

Sheridan R: Burns. *Criti Care Med* 30(11)S;S500, 2002.

Authors: **Michael P. Johnson, M.D., and Michelle Stozek, M.D.**

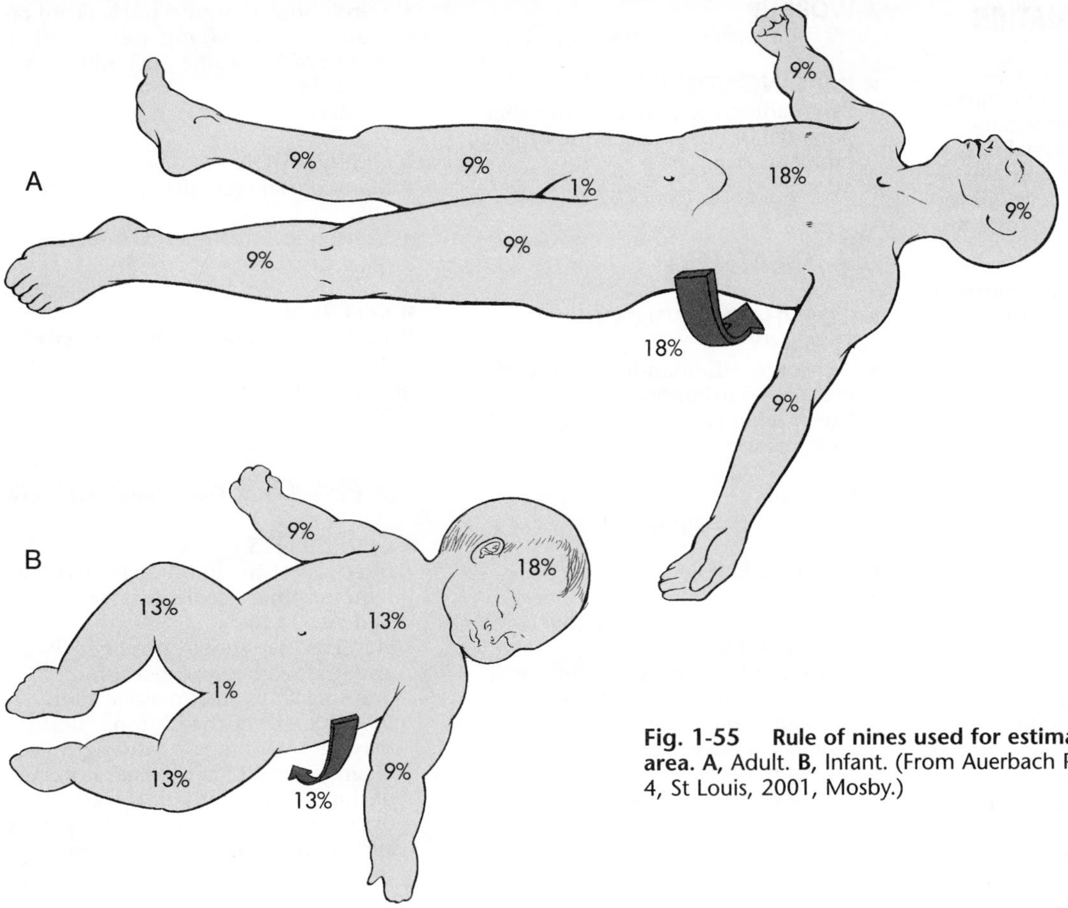

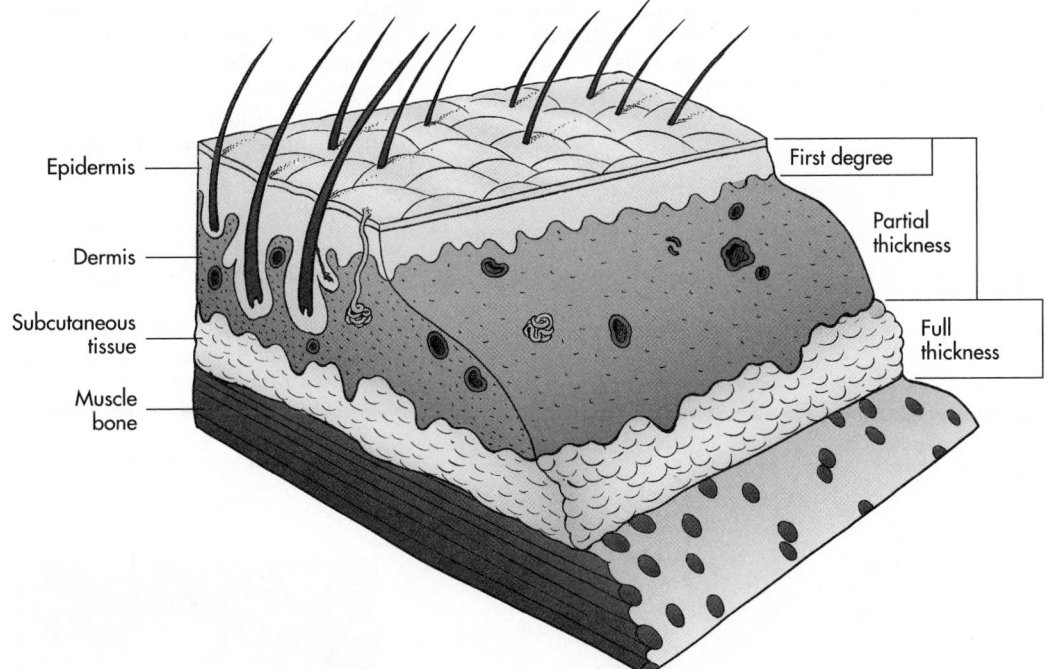

Fig. 1-55 **Rule of nines used for estimating burned surface area. A,** Adult. **B,** Infant. (From Auerbach PS: *Wilderness medicine,* ed 4, St Louis, 2001, Mosby.)

A

9%
9%
9%
1%
18%
9%
9%
18%
9%

B

9%
18%
13%
13%
1%
13%
9%
13%

Epidermis

Dermis

Subcutaneous tissue

Muscle bone

First degree

Partial thickness

Full thickness

Fig. 1-56 **Skin anatomy.** (From Auerbach PS: *Wilderness medicine,* ed 4, St Louis, 2001, Mosby.)

BASIC INFORMATION

■ DEFINITION
Bursitis is an inflammation of a bursa and is usually aseptic. A *bursa* is a closed sac lined with a synovial-like membrane that sometimes contains fluid that is found or that develops in an area subject to pressure or friction.

■ SYNONYMS
Housemaid's knee (prepatellar bursitis)
Weaver's bottom (ischial gluteal bursitis)
Baker's cyst (gastrocnemius-semimembranosus bursa)

ICD-9CM CODES
726.19 Subacromial bursitis
726.33 Olecranon bursitis
726.5 Ischiogluteal bursitis (hip)
726.5 Iliopsoas bursitis (hip)
726.61 Anserine bursitis
726.5 Trochanteric bursitis
726.65 Prepatellar bursitis
727.51 Baker's cyst
726.79 Retrocalcaneal bursitis

■ PHYSICAL FINDINGS & CLINICAL PRESENTATION
- Swelling, especially if bursa is superficial (olecranon, prepatellar)
- Local tenderness with pain on pressure against bursa
- Pain with joint movement
- Referred pain
- Palpable occasional fibrocartilaginous bodies (most common in olecranon and prepatellar bursae)

■ ETIOLOGY
- Acute trauma
- Repetitive trauma
- Sepsis
- Crystalline deposit disease
- Rheumatoid arthritis

DIAGNOSIS

DIFFERENTIAL DIAGNOSIS
- Degenerative joint disease
- Tendinitis (sometimes occurs in conjunction with bursitis)
- Cellulitis (if bursitis is septic)
- Infectious arthritis

■ WORKUP
Aspiration with Gram stain and C&S

■ IMAGING STUDIES
- Plain radiography to rule out other potential or coexisting bone or joint problems (Fig. 1-57)
- MRI

TREATMENT

■ NONPHARMACOLOGIC THERAPY
- If chronic, elimination of cause of pressure or irritation
- Use of relief pads, avoidance of direct pressure
- Rest
- Elevation
- Ice for acute trauma

■ ACUTE GENERAL Rx
- Septic:
  1. Appropriate antibiotic coverage and drainage
  2. Aspiration of purulent fluid with a large-bore needle (if there is no rapid clinical response, incision and drainage are indicated)
- Nonseptic:
  1. Aspiration of blood from acute trauma
  2. Application of compression dressing

■ CHRONIC Rx
- Aspiration if excessive fluid volume present, followed by application of compression dressing to prevent fluid reaccumulation (repeat aspiration may be required)

- Steroid injection into bursa (1 ml of triamcinolone, 40 mg, mixed with 1 to 3 cc of Xylocaine depending on size of bursa.)
- NSAIDs

■ DISPOSITION
- Many bursal sacs "dry up" eventually.
- Nonsurgical treatment is effective in most cases.

■ REFERRAL
For orthopedic consultation to assist in treatment of sepsis or for excision of chronic enlarged bursa when indicated

PEARLS & CONSIDERATIONS

■ COMMENTS
- Injection of trochanteric bursa may require spinal needle in large patient.
- Sterile bursae should not be incised and drained because a chronic draining sinus tract may develop.
- Involvement of the iliopsoas bursa may cause groin pain, although the diagnosis is difficult to make because of the inaccessibility of the area to direct examination. (This also makes steroid injection impossible even if the diagnosis could be established.)

REFERENCES
Bianchi S et al: Giant iliopsoas bursitis: sonographic findings with magnetic resonance correlations, *J Clin Ultrasound* 30:437, 2002.
Kim SM et al: Imaging features of ischial bursitis with an emphasis on ultrasonography, *Skeletal Radiol* 31:631, 2002.
Taira H et al: Localized cortical bone absorption induced by cubital bursitis in rheumatoid arthritis, *Orthopedics* 25:860, 2002.
Yamamoto T, Iwasaki Y, Kurosaka M: Tuberculosis of the greater trochanteric bursa occurring 51 years after tuberculous nephritis, *Clin Rheumatol* 21:397, 2002.
Author: **Lonnie R. Mercier, M.D.**

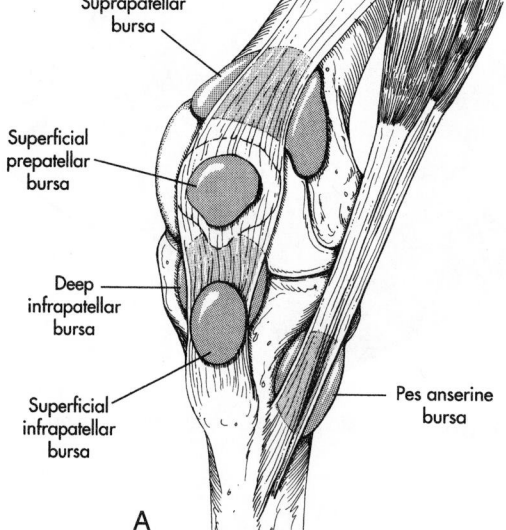
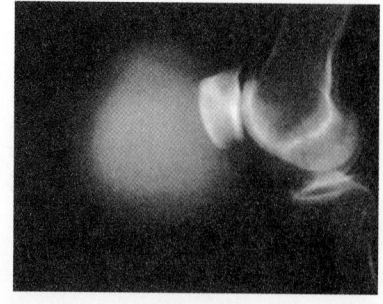

Fig. 1-57 A, Bursae around the knee. **B,** Markedly swollen prepatellar bursa. (From Scudieri G [ed]: *Sports medicine principles of primary care,* St Louis, 1997, Mosby.)

Suprapatellar bursa
Superficial prepatellar bursa
Deep infrapatellar bursa
Superficial infrapatellar bursa
Pes anserine bursa

A

B

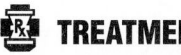

 BASIC INFORMATION

■ DEFINITION
Candidiasis is an inflammatory process involving the vulva and/or the vagina and is caused by superficial invasion of epithelial cells by *Candida* species.

■ SYNONYMS
Moniliasis
Thrush
Candidosis

ICD-9CM CODES
112.1 Moniliasis
112.0 Thrush
112 Candidosis

■ EPIDEMIOLOGY & DEMOGRAPHICS
- This is the second most common form of vaginitis in the U.S. It is estimated that up to 75% of women will have at least one episode of vulvovaginal candidiasis (VVC) during their childbearing years and about 45% will have a second attack. A small subpopulation of probably <5% of adult women has recurrent, often intractable episodes. *Candida* may be isolated in up to 20% of asymptomatic women of childbearing age.
- Factors that predispose to development of symptomatic VVC include pregnancy, antibiotic use, and diabetes. Antibiotic use disturbs normal vaginal flora and allows overgrowth of fungi; pregnancy and diabetes are associated with decrease in cell-mediated immunity.
- Factors associated with increased rates of asymptomatic vaginal colonization: pregnancy, high-estrogen oral contraceptives, uncontrolled diabetes mellitus, attendance at STD clinics.

UNCOMPLICATED VVC:
- Infrequent VVC
- Mild-to-moderate vaginitis and candida
- Likely to be *C. albicans*
- Nonimmunocompromised women

COMPLICATED VVC:
- Recurrent VVC
- Severe VVC
- Non-*albicans* candidiasis
- Women with uncontrolled diabetes, immunosuppression, or those who are pregnant

Rx OF COMPLICATED VVC:
- Recurrent VVS: 7 to 14 days of topical therapy
- 150 mg fluconazole PO, repeat in 3 days
- Maintenance regimen
  1. Clotrimazole: 500-mg vaginal suppositories once weekly
  2. Ketoconazole: 100 mg once daily
  3. Fluconazole: 100 to 150 mg PO once weekly
  4. Itraconazole 400 mg/mo or 100 mg/day
  5. Continue one of the above regimens for 6 mo

COMPROMISED HOST:
- Treat with traditional antimycotics for at least 7 to 14 days
- Pregnancy: topical azoles recommended for 7 days
- HIV-infected women: fluconazole 200 mg/wk
- Not usually an STD

■ PHYSICAL FINDINGS & CLINICAL PRESENTATION
Symptoms of VVC consist of:
- Vulvar pruritus with vaginal discharge that typically resembles cottage cheese
- Erythema and edema of labia and vulvar skin; possible discrete pustulopapular peripheral lesions (satellite lesions)
- Vagina may be erythematous with an adherent, whitish discharge
- Cervix may appear normal
- Symptoms characteristically exacerbated in the week preceding menses with some relief after onset of menstrual flow

■ ETIOLOGY
- *Candida* are dimorphic fungi (spores and mycelial forms).
- *C. albicans* is responsible for 85% to 90% of vaginal yeast infections.
- *C. glabrata, C. tropicalis* (non-*albicans* species) also cause vaginitis and may be more resistant to conventional therapy.

■ DIAGNOSIS

■ DIFFERENTIAL DIAGNOSIS
- Bacterial vaginosis
- Trichomoniasis

■ WORKUP
- Discharge may vary from watery to homogeneously thick. May have complaints of vaginal soreness, dyspareunia, vulvar burning, and irritation. External dysuria may be present
- Usually normal vaginal pH (<4.5)
- Budding yeast forms or mycelia will appear in as many as 80% of cases. Saline wet prep of vaginal secretions usually is normal; may be increased in inflammatory cells in severe cases
- Whiff test negative (KOH)
- 10% KCl useful and more sensitive than wet mount for microscopic identification
- Can make a presumptive diagnosis based on symptomatology in the absence of microscopy-proven fungal elements if the pH and wet prep are normal. Fungal culture is recommended to confirm diagnosis
- In chronic/recurrent, burning replaces itching as prominent symptom. Confirm diagnosis with direct microscopy and culture. Many may actually have chronic or atrophic dermatitis. Test for HIV

■ LABORATORY TESTS
If sending cultures, send on Nickerson's media or semiquantitative slide-stix cultures. There is no reliable serologic technique for diagnosis.

■ TREATMENT

■ ACUTE GENERAL Rx (UNCOMPLICATED)
TOPICAL BUTOCONAZOLE: 2% vaginal cream 5 g intravaginally for 3 days
- Butoconazole (sustained release)—5 gm intravaginally for 1 dose
TOPICAL CLOTRIMAZOLE:
- 1% cream 5 g intravaginally for 7 to 14 days
- 100-mg vaginal tablet for 7 days
- 100-mg vaginal tablets, two tablets for 3 days

- 500-mg vaginal tablet, single dose

TOPICAL MICONAZOLE:
- 2% cream 5 g intravaginally for 7 days
- 200-mg vaginal suppository for 3 days
- 100-mg vaginal suppository for 7 days

TOPICAL TIOCONAZOLE: 6.5% ointment 5 g intravaginally, single dose

TOPICAL TERCONAZOLE:
- 0.4% cream 5 g intravaginally for 7 days
- 0.8% cream 5 g intravaginally for 3 days
- 80-mg suppository for 3 days

ORAL FLUCONAZOLE: 150-mg single PO dose

■ CHRONIC Rx

Ketoconazole 400 mg PO qd or fluconazole 200 mg PO qd until symptoms resolve. Then maintenance on prophylactic doses of these agents for 6 mo (ketoconazole 100 mg/day, fluconazole 150 mg/wk).

■ DISPOSITION

Usually relatively limited in duration and occurrence. If chronic or recurrent, may consider screening for diabetes, HIV, or other immune deficiencies.

☼ PEARLS & CONSIDERATIONS

■ COMMENTS

- Azoles are more effective than nystatin. Symptoms usually take 2 to 3 days to resolve. Adjunctive treatment with weak topical steroid such as 1% hydrocortisone cream may help with relief of symptoms.
- Creams and suppositories are oil based and may weaken latex condoms and diaphragms

REFERENCES

Centers for Disease Control and Prevention: 2002 sexually transmitted diseases treatment guidelines, *MMWR Morb Mortal Wkly Rep* 51(RR-6), 2002.

Ostrosky-Zeichner L et al: Deeply invasive candidiasis, *Infect Dis Clin North Am.*

Watson MC et al: Oral versus intra-vaginal imidazole and triazole anti-fungal treatment of uncomplicated vulvovaginal candidiasis (thrush), *Cochrane Database Syst Rev* (4):CD002845, 2001.

Author: **Maria A. Corigliano, M.D.**

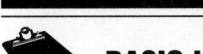 **BASIC INFORMATION**

■ **DEFINITION**
Carbon monoxide is a colorless, odorless, tasteless, nonirritating gas. When inhaled it produces toxicity by causing cellular hypoxia.

ICD-9CM CODES
986 Carbon monoxide poisoning

■ **EPIDEMIOLOGY & DEMOGRAPHICS**
• Carbon monoxide poisoning is seen more frequently during the winter months.
• Most common cause of lethal poisoning in the U.S.

■ **PHYSICAL FINDINGS & CLINICAL PRESENTATION**
• Symptoms of toxicity and prognosis do not correlate well with carboxyhemoglobin levels. See Table 1-13.
• Depend on the severity and duration of exposure. The brain and heart are most sensitive to carbon monoxide poisoning.

■ **ETIOLOGY**
Carbon monoxide causes tissue hypoxia by a number of mechanisms.
• Carbon monoxide binds to hemoglobin with an affinity 200 to 250 times greater than oxygen, thus displacing oxygen from hemoglobin and decreasing the oxygen-carrying capacity of blood.
• Carbon monoxide shifts the oxyhemoglobin curve to the left, thus decreasing oxygen release to tissue.
• Cellular respiration is depressed by inhibition of the mitochondrial cytochrome oxidase system.
• Cardiac function is depressed by direct binding to cardiac myoglobin.

• Neurologic toxicity is not explained by hypoxia alone and is thought to be related to the intracellular uptake of carbon monoxide, its role as a neural messenger, ischemic reperfusion injury of the brain, and delayed lipid peroxidation of brain tissue. Carbon monoxide poisoning occurs when individuals are exposed to smoke from fires; motor vehicle exhaust; or the burning of wood, charcoal, or natural gas for cooking or heating in poorly ventilated areas.
• Methylene chloride (paint stripper) fumes are converted to carbon monoxide by the liver.

DIAGNOSIS

■ **DIFFERENTIAL DIAGNOSIS**
• Viral syndromes
• Cyanide
• Hydrogen sulfide
• Methemoglobinemia
• Amphetamines and derivatives
• Cocaine
• Cyclic antidepressants
• Phencyclidine (PCP)
• Phenothiazines
• Theophylline

■ **WORKUP**
History of exposure to carbon monoxide, physical examination, laboratory tests

■ **LABORATORY TESTS**
• Carboxyhemoglobin level
NOTE: CoHgb level >5% in nonsmoker confirms exposure. Heavy smokers may have levels of 10%
• Direct measurement of arterial oxygen saturation

NOTE: Pulse oximetry and arterial blood gas may be falsely normal because neither measures oxygen saturation directly. Pulse oximetry is inaccurate because of the similar absorption characteristics of oxyhemoglobin and carboxyhemoglobin. An arterial blood gas is inaccurate because it measures oxygen dissolved in plasma (which is not affected by carbon monoxide) and then calculates oxygen saturation
• Electrolytes, glucose, BUN, creatinine, CPK, ABG (because lactic acidosis and rhabdomyolysis may develop)
• ECG (rule out ischemia)
• Pregnancy test (fetus at high risk)

TREATMENT

■ **ACUTE GENERAL Rx**
• Remove from site of carbon monoxide exposure
• Ensure adequate airway
• Continuous ECG monitor
• 100% oxygen by tight-fitting nonrebreather mask or endotracheal tube (this decreases the half-life of carboxyhemoglobin from 4 to 6 hr to 60 to 90 min)
• Measure carboxyhemoglobin level every 2 to 4 hr
• Continue oxygen until carboxyhemoglobin level is less than 10%
Hyperbaric oxygen (3 ATM) decreases half-life of carbon monoxide to 20 to 30 min
• Controversial if there is any beneficial effect over regular 100% oxygen
• Recent study suggests patients with acute (<24 hr), symptomatic carbon monoxide poisoning treated with 3 hyperbaric O2 sessions within 24 hr had lower rates of cognitive sequelae at 6 wk and 12 mo compared with those treated with normobaric O2

TABLE 1-13   Carboxyhemoglobin Poisoning and Signs and Symptoms

CARBOXYHEMOGLOBIN POISONING	SYMPTOMS	PHYSICAL FINDINGS
Mild	Mild headache, dyspnea on vigorous exertion	
Moderate	Nausea, vomiting, dizziness, fatigue, severe headache, blurred vision, confusion, dyspnea on exertion	Tachycardia, tachypnea, cognitive deficit, retinal hemorrhages
Severe	Dyspnea, chest pain	Lethargy, ataxia, arrhythmias, myocardial ischemia, pulmonary edema, syncope, seizures, coma, cherry-red skin, skin bullae

- Consider for individuals with:
  1. Severe intoxication (carboxyhemoglobin >25%, neurologic symptoms or signs, ischemic ECG changes, severe metabolic acidosis, rhabdomyolysis, pulmonary edema, shock)
  2. Those who remain symptomatic after 2 to 4 hr of oxygen at room air
  3. Pregnant women with carboxyhemoglobin >15% or signs of fetal distress: lower threshold for treatment suggested given the higher affinity of carbon monoxide for fetal hemoglobin
- Consult local poison control center
- Consider concomitant poisoning with other toxic/irritant gases that may be present in smoke and/or thermal injury to the airway

■ DISPOSITION
- Depends on severity of exposure
- Survivors of severe poisoning are at 14% to 40% risk for neurologic sequelae ranging from parkinsonism to neuropsychiatric symptoms (personality and memory disorders). Neurologic deficits are usually apparent within 3 wk of poisoning. Brain MRI may show changes in the white matter and basal ganglia
- High risk of fetal demise

■ REFERRAL
- Regional poison control center
- +/− Hyperbaric chamber

REFERENCES
Ahya SN, Flood K, Paranjothi S: *Washington manual of medical therapeutics,* ed 30, Philadelphia, 2001, Lippincott Williams and Wilkins.

Goldfrank LR et al: *Goldfrank's toxicologic emergencies,* ed 6, New York, 1998, McGraw-Hill.

Weaver LK et al: Hyperbaric oxygen for acute carbon monoxide poisoning, *N Engl J Med* 347:1057, 2002.

Author: **Sudeep K. Aulakh, M.D., F.R.C.P.C.**

BASIC INFORMATION

■ DEFINITION
Carcinoid syndrome is a symptom complex characterized by paroxysmal vasomotor disturbances, diarrhea, and bronchospasm. It is caused by the action of amines and peptides (serotonin, bradykinin, histamine) produced by tumors arising from neuroendocrine cells.

■ SYNONYMS
Flush syndrome
Argentaffinoma syndrome

ICD-9CM CODES
259.2 Carcinoid syndrome

■ EPIDEMIOLOGY & DEMOGRAPHICS
INCIDENCE: Carcinoid tumors are found incidentally in 0.5% to 0.75% of autopsies.

■ PHYSICAL FINDINGS & CLINICAL PRESENTATION
• Cutaneous flushing (75% to 90%)
   1. The patient usually has red-purple flushes starting in the face, then spreading to the neck and upper trunk.
   2. The flushing episodes last from a few minutes to hours (longer-lasting flushes may be associated with bronchial carcinoids).
   3. Flushing may be triggered by emotion, alcohol, or foods, or it may occur spontaneously.
   4. Dizziness, tachycardia, and hypotension may be associated with the cutaneous flushing.
• Diarrhea (>70%): often associated with abdominal bloating and audible peristaltic rushes
• Intermittent bronchospasm (25%): characterized by severe dyspnea and wheezing
• Facial telangiectasia
• Tricuspid regurgitation from carcinoid heart lesions

■ ETIOLOGY
• The carcinoid syndrome is caused by neoplasms originating from neuroendocrine cells.
• Carcinoid tumors are principally found in the following organs: appendix (40%); small bowel (20%; 15% in the ileum); rectum (15%); bronchi (12%); esophagus, stomach, colon (10%); ovary, biliary tract, pancreas (3%).
• Carcinoid tumors do not usually produce the syndrome unless liver metastases are present or the primary tumor does not involve the GI tract.

DIAGNOSIS

■ DIFFERENTIAL DIAGNOSIS
The carcinoid syndrome must be distinguished from idiopathic flushing (IF); patients with IF more often are females, younger, and with a longer duration of symptoms; palpitations, syncope, and hypotension occur primarily in patients with IF.

■ LABORATORY TESTS
• An algorithm for the diagnosis and treatment of carcinoid tumors is described in Section III, Fig. 3-40.
• The biochemical marker for carcinoid syndrome is increased 24-hr urinary 5-hydroxyindoleacetic acid (5-HIAA), a metabolite of serotonin (5-hydroxytryptamine).
• False elevations can be seen with ingestion of certain foods (bananas, pineapples, eggplant, avocados, walnuts) and certain medications (acetaminophen, caffeine, guaifenesin, reserpine); therefore patients should be on a restricted diet and should avoid these medications when the test is ordered.
• Liver function studies are an unreliable indicator of liver involvement.

■ IMAGING STUDIES
• Chest x-ray examination is useful to detect bronchial carcinoids.
• CT scans of abdomen or a liver and spleen radionuclide scan is useful to detect liver metastases (palpable in >50% of cases).
• Iodine-123 labeled somatostatin (123-ISS) can detect carcinoid endocrine tumors with somatostatin receptors.
• Scanning with radiolabeled octreotide can visualize previously undetected or metastatic lesions.

TREATMENT

■ NONPHARMACOLOGIC THERAPY
Avoidance of ethanol ingestion (may precipitate flushing)

■ GENERAL Rx
• Surgical resection of the tumor can be curative if the tumor is localized or palliative and result in prolonged asymptomatic periods if metastases are present. Surgical manipulation of the tumor can, however, cause severe vasomotor abnormalities and bronchospasm (carcinoid crisis).

• Percutaneous embolization and ligation of the hepatic artery can decrease the bulk of the tumor in the liver and provide palliative treatment of tumors with hepatic metastases.
• Cytotoxic chemotherapy: combination chemotherapy with 5-fluorouracil and streptozotocin can be used in patients with unresectable or recurrent carcinoid tumors; however, it has only limited success.
• Control of clinical manifestations:
   1. Diarrhea usually responds to diphenoxylate with atropine (Lomotil).
   2. Flushing can be controlled by the combination of H_1- and H_2-receptor antagonists (e.g., diphenhydramine 25 to 50 mg PO q6h and ranitidine 150 mg bid).
   3. Somatostatin analogue (SMS 201-995) is effective for both flushing and diarrhea in most patients.
   4. Bronchospasm can be treated with aminophylline and/or albuterol.
• Nutritional support: supplemental niacin therapy may be useful to prevent pellagra, because the tumor uses dietary tryptophan for serotonin synthesis, resulting in a nutritional deficiency in some patients.
• Subcutaneous somatostatin analogues (octreotide 150 μg SC tid) have been used successfully for long-term control of symptoms in patients with unresectable neoplasms.
• Echocardiography and monitoring for right-sided CHF are recommended for patients with unresectable disease because endocardial fibrosis, involving predominantly the endocardium, chordae, and valves of the right side of the heart, can occur and result in right-sided CHF.

■ DISPOSITION
• Prognosis varies with the stage and location of the tumor.
• Carcinoids of the appendix and rectum have a low malignancy potential and rarely produce the clinical syndrome; metastases are also uncommon if the size of the primary lesion is <2 cm in diameter.

Author: **Fred F. Ferri, M.D.**

I

BASIC INFORMATION

■ DEFINITION
Cardiac tamponade is compression of the heart by fluid within the pericardial sac that impairs dilation and filling of the ventricles during diastole.

ICD-9CM CODES
423.9 Unspecified diseases of the pericardium

■ PHYSICAL FINDINGS & CLINICAL PRESENTATION
Acute cardiac tamponade (e.g., penetrating wounds, iatrogenic, aortic dissection)
1. Beck's triad
   a. Decrease in systemic arterial pressure
   b. Elevated central venous pressure
   c. Small, quiet heart
Chronic accumulating pericardial effusion leading to tamponade
1. Pericardial friction rub may be present
2. Tachypnea and tachycardia
3. Raised jugular venous distention (prominent x descent with absent y descent) with peripheral venous distention in the forehead and scalp
4. Pulsus paradoxus defined as an inspiratory systolic fall in arterial pressure of 10 mm Hg or more during normal breathing
5. Soft heart sounds

■ ETIOLOGY
Acute
1. Penetrating trauma
2. Aortic dissection
3. Myocardial rupture after treatment of MI with thrombolytics and/or heparin
4. Iatrogenic (central line and pacemaker insertions, postcoronary bypass surgery)
Chronic accumulating pericardial effusion leading to tamponade
1. Malignancy (e.g., lung, breast, lymphoma)
2. Viral pericarditis (e.g., coxsackie, HIV)
3. Uremia
4. Bacterial, fungal, and tuberculosis
5. Myxedema (rare)
6. Collagen-vascular disease (e.g., SLE, RA, scleroderma)
7. Radiation

DIAGNOSIS

■ DIFFERENTIAL DIAGNOSIS
COPD, constrictive pericardial disease, restrictive cardiomyopathy, right ventricular infarction, and pulmonary embolism can all lead to elevated jugular venous pressure, decreased systemic pressure, and pulsus paradoxus.

■ WORKUP
Cardiac tamponade is a clinical diagnosis made at the bedside by noting the abovementioned physical findings. The echocardiogram will support the clinical diagnosis. Thereafter, one must pursue the etiology with specific laboratory work (see "Laboratory Tests").

■ LABORATORY TESTS
- Electrolytes, BUN, Cr, ESR, thyroid function tests, ANA, RF, PPD, blood cultures, viral titers, and pericardial fluid analysis and cultures will all help in identifying or excluding a possible etiology of the effusion leading to tamponade.
- 12-lead ECG findings are suggestive but not diagnostic.
  1. Low voltage (<5 mm QRS amplitude in the limb leads and <10 mm in the chest leads)
  2. PR depression
  3. Electrical alternans (alternating amplitude of the QRS complex in any or all leads)

■ IMAGING STUDIES
- The chest x-ray examination is not very specific. The heart size can be normal in acute tamponade or massive (water bottle configuration) in slow-forming effusions. At least 200 ml of fluid must accumulate before the cardiac silhouette is affected.
- The echocardiogram can detect effusions as small as 20 ml and can strongly suggest tamponade physiology (collapse of the right atrium and right ventricle during diastole).
- Right-sided cardiac catheterization and intrapericardial pressure measurements confirm the diagnosis.
- Typical findings are diastolic equalization of pressures usually between 15 to 30 mm Hg (pulmonary artery pressure = right ventricular diastolic pressure = right atrial pressure = intrapericardial pressure).

TREATMENT

■ NONPHARMACOLOGIC THERAPY
Cardiac tamponade should be treated urgently. Avoid drugs that will reduce preload and exacerbate tamponade (e.g., nitrates, diuretics).

■ ACUTE GENERAL Rx
- The acute forms of tamponade as mentioned earlier (see "Etiology") usually require emergency cardiothoracic surgery.
- Provide hemodynamic support with volume expansion and vasopressors along with emergency subxiphoid pericardiocentesis in the suspected tamponade code situation (e.g., electromechanical dissociation, patient in shock).

■ CHRONIC Rx
- Depends on etiology
- Semiacute treatment includes:
  1. Right-side heart catheter with echocardiographic-guided pericardiocentesis (can be done by cardiology). The catheter can be left in place for 48 hr to allow for continued drainage until a more definitive procedure is performed or the etiology is resolved (e.g., dialysis for uremia, levothyroxine for myxedema).
- Other surgical drainage procedures include:
  1. Subxiphoid pericardial drainage
  2. Limited pericardiectomy draining the pericardial fluid into the left hemithorax
  3. Complete pericardiectomy

■ DISPOSITION
The prognosis of cardiac tamponade depends on the underlying cause.

■ REFERRAL
- Cardiology consultation is made if the clinical suspicion of tamponade exists.
- Cardiothoracic surgeon consultation is made when tamponade is confirmed.

PEARLS & CONSIDERATIONS

■ COMMENTS
As little as 200 ml of fluid can lead to acute cardiac tamponade, whereas in the chronic formation, the pericardial sac can hold up to 5 L of fluid before tamponade occurs.

REFERENCES
Aikat S, Ghaffari S: A review of pericardial diseases: clinical, ECG and hemodynamic features and management, *Clev Clin J Med* 67(12):903, 2000.
Spodick DH: Acute cardiac tamponade, *N Engl J Med* 349(7):684, 2003.
Spodick DH: Pathophysiology of cardiac tamponade, *Chest* 113(5):1372, 1998.
Author: **Peter Petropoulos, M.D.**

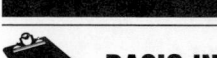

BASIC INFORMATION

■ DEFINITION
Cardiomyopathies are a group of diseases primarily involving the myocardium and characterized by myocardial dysfunction that is not the result of hypertension, coronary atherosclerosis, valvular dysfunction, or pericardial abnormalities. In dilated cardiomyopathy, the heart is enlarged, and both ventricles are dilated.

■ SYNONYMS
Congestive cardiomyopathy

ICD-9CM CODES
425.4 Other primary cardiomyopathies

■ EPIDEMIOLOGY & DEMOGRAPHICS
- The prevalence of dilated cardiomyopathy in the general adult population is approximately 1%.
- Incidence increases with age and approaches 10% at age 80 yr.

■ PHYSICAL FINDINGS & CLINICAL PRESENTATION
- Increased jugular venous pressure
- Small pulse pressure
- Pulmonary rales, hepatomegaly, peripheral edema
- S_3, S_4
- Mitral regurgitation, tricuspid regurgitation (less common)

■ ETIOLOGY
- Idiopathic
- Alcoholism (15% to 40% of all cases in Western countries)
- Collagen-vascular disease (SLE, RA, polyarteritis, dermatomyositis)
- Postmyocarditis
- Peripartum (last trimester of pregnancy or 6 mo postpartum)
- Heredofamilial neuromuscular disease
- Toxins (cobalt, lead, phosphorus, carbon monoxide, mercury, doxorubicin, daunorubicin)
- Nutritional (beriberi, selenium deficiency, carnitine deficiency, thiamine deficiency)
- Cocaine, heroin, organic solvents ("glue-sniffer's heart")
- Irradiation
- Acromegaly, osteogenesis imperfecta, myxedema, thyrotoxicosis, diabetes
- Hypocalcemia
- Antiretroviral agents (zidovudine, didanosine, zalcitabine)
- Phenothiazines
- Infections (viral [HIV], rickettsial, mycobacterial, toxoplasmosis, trichinosis, Chagas' disease)
- Hematologic (e.g., sickle cell anemia)

DIAGNOSIS

■ DIFFERENTIAL DIAGNOSIS
- Frank pulmonary disease
- Valvular dysfunction
- Pericardial abnormalities
- Coronary atherosclerosis
- Psychogenic dyspnea

■ WORKUP
- Chest x-ray examination, ECG, echocardiogram
- Medical history with emphasis on the following symptoms:
  1. Dyspnea on exertion, orthopnea, PND
  2. Palpitations
  3. Systemic and pulmonary embolism
- Cardiac troponin T levels: Persistently elevated troponin T levels are a marker of poor outcome in cardiomyopathy patients.

■ IMAGING STUDIES
CHEST X-RAY EXAMINATION:
- Massive cardiac enlargement
- Interstitial pulmonary edema

ECG:
- Left ventricular hypertrophy with ST-T wave changes
- RBBB or LBBB
- Arrhythmias (atrial fibrillation, PVC, PAC, ventricular tachycardia)

ECHOCARDIOGRAM:
- Low ejection fraction with global akinesia

TREATMENT

■ NONPHARMACOLOGIC THERAPY
- Limit activity when CHF is present
- Treatment of underlying disease (SLE, alcoholism)

■ ACUTE GENERAL Rx
- Treat CHF (cause of death in 70% of patients) with sodium restriction, diuretics, ACE inhibitors, β-blockers, spironolactone, and digitalis.
- Vasodilators (combined with nitrates and ACE inhibitors) are effective agents in all symptomatic patients with left ventricular dysfunction
- Prevent thromboembolism with oral anticoagulants in all patients with atrial fibrillation and in patients with moderate or severe failure
- Low-dose β-blockade with carvedilol or other β-blockers may improve ventricular function by interrupting the cycle of reflex sympathetic activity and controlling tachycardia.

- Diltiazem and ACE inhibitors have also been reported to have a long-term beneficial effect in idiopathic dilated cardiomyopathy.
- Use antiarrhythmic treatment as appropriate. Empiric pharmacologic suppression of asymptomatic ventricular ectopy does not reduce risk of sudden death or improve long-term survival. In patients with severe left ventricular dysfunction and/or symptomatic and sustained ventricular tachycardia, the use of an automatic implantable cardioverter-defibrillator should be considered.
- Preliminary studies have revealed that growth hormone administered for 3 mo to patients with idiopathic dilated cardiomyopathy increased myocardial mass and reduced the size of the left ventricular chamber, resulting in improvement in hemodynamics and clinical status.
- Patients with dilated cardiomyopathy (LVEF <25%) and associated coronary atherosclerosis (angina, ECG changes, reversible defects on thallium scan) may benefit from surgical revascularization.

■ DISPOSITION
Annual mortality is 20% in patients with moderate heart failure, and it exceeds 50% in patients with severe heart failure.

■ REFERRAL
Consider heart transplant for young patients (<60 yr old) who are no longer responsive to medical therapy.

PEARLS & CONSIDERATIONS

■ COMMENTS
- Patients should be encouraged to restrict or eliminate alcohol and decrease sodium intake.
- Vulnerability to cardiomyopathy among chronic alcohol abusers is partially genetic and is related to the presence of angiotensin-converting-enzyme (ACE) DD genotype.

REFERENCE
Lowes BD et al: Myocardial gene expression in dilated cardiomyopathy treated with beta-blocking agents, *N Engl J Med* 346:1357, 2002.
Author: **Fred F. Ferri, M.D.**

BASIC INFORMATION

DEFINITION
Cardiomyopathies are a group of diseases primarily involving the myocardium and characterized by myocardial dysfunction that is not the result of hypertension, coronary atherosclerosis, valvular dysfunction, or pericardial abnormalities. In hypertrophic cardiomyopathy (HCM) there is marked hypertrophy of the myocardium and disproportionally greater thickening of the intraventricular septum than that of the free wall of the left ventricle (asymmetric septal hypertrophy [ASH]).

SYNONYMS
Idiopathic hypertrophic subaortic stenosis (IHSS)
Hypertrophic obstructive cardiomyopathy (HOCM)
ASH
HCM

ICD-9CM CODES
425.4 Cardiomyopathy, hypertrophic nonobstructive
425.1 Cardiomyopathy, hypertrophic obstructive
746.84 Cardiomyopathy, hypertrophic congenital

EPIDEMIOLOGY & DEMOGRAPHICS
• The disease occurs in two major forms:
 1. A familial form, usually diagnosed in young patients and gene mapped to chromosome 14q
 2. A sporadic form, usually found in elderly patients
• The prevalence of phenotypically expressed HCM in the adult general population is 0.2% (most common genetic cardiovascular disease)

PHYSICAL FINDINGS & CLINICAL PRESENTATION
• Harsh, systolic, diamond-shaped murmur at the left sternal border or apex that increases with Valsalva maneuver and decreases with squatting
• Paradoxic splitting of S_2 (if left ventricular obstruction is present)
• S_4
• Double or triple apical impulse

• Increased obstruction
 1. Drugs: digitalis, β-adrenergic stimulators (isoproterenol, dopamine, epinephrine), nitroglycerin, vasodilators, diuretics, alcohol
 2. Hypovolemia
 3. Tachycardia
 4. Valsalva maneuver
 5. Standing position
• Decreased obstruction
 1. Drugs: β-adrenergic blockers, calcium channel blockers, disopyramide, α-adrenergic stimulators
 2. Volume expansion
 3. Bradycardia
 4. Hand grip exercise
 5. Squatting position

ETIOLOGY
• Autosomal dominant trait with variable penetrance caused by mutations in any of 1 to 10 genes, each encoding proteins of cardiac sarcomere
• Sporadic occurrence

DIAGNOSIS

DIFFERENTIAL DIAGNOSIS
• Coronary atherosclerosis
• Valvular dysfunction
• Pericardial abnormalities
• Chronic pulmonary disease
• Psychogenic dyspnea

WORKUP
• Chest x-ray examination, ECG, echocardiography
• Medical history with emphasis in the following manifestations:
 1. Dyspnea
 2. Syncope (usually seen with exercise)
 3. Angina (decreased angina in recumbent position)
 4. Palpitations
• 24-hr Holter monitor to screen for potential lethal arrhythmias (principal cause of syncope or sudden death in obstructive cardiomyopathy)

IMAGING STUDIES
• Chest x-ray examination: normal or cardiomegaly
• ECG is abnormal in 75% to 95% of patients: left ventricular hypertrophy, abnormal Q waves in anterolateral and inferior leads
• Two-dimensional echocardiography is used to establish the diagnosis. Findings include: ventricular hypertrophy, ratio of septum thickness to left ventricular wall thickness >1.3:1, increased ejection fraction.
• Magnetic resonance imaging may be of diagnostic value when echocardiographic studies are technically inadequate. MRI is also useful in identifying segmental LVH undetectable by echocardiography.

TREATMENT

NONPHARMACOLOGIC THERAPY
Advise avoidance of alcohol; alcohol use (even in small amounts) results in increased obstruction of the left ventricular outflow tract.

ACUTE GENERAL Rx
• Propranolol 160 to 240 mg/day. The beneficial effects of β-blockers on symptoms (principally dyspnea and chest pain) and exercise tolerance appear to be largely a result of a decrease in the heart rate with consequent prolongation of diastole and increased passive ventricular filling. By reducing the inotropic response, β-blockers may also lessen myocardial oxygen demand and decrease the outflow gradient during exercise, when sympathetic tone is increased.
• Verapamil also decreases left ventricular outflow obstruction by improving filling and probably reducing myocardial ischemia.
• IV saline infusion in addition to propranolol or verapamil is indicated in patients with CHF.
• Disopyramide is a useful antiarrhythmic because it is also a negative inotrope

- Use antibiotic prophylaxis for surgical procedures.
- Avoid use of digitalis, diuretics, nitrates, and vasodilators.
- Encouraging results have been reported on the use of DDD pacing for hemodynamic and symptomatic benefit in patients with drug-resistant hypertrophic obstructive cardiomyopathy.
- Implantable defibrillators are a safe and effective therapy in HCM patients prone to ventricular arrhythmias. Their use is strongly warranted for patients with prior cardiac arrest or sustained spontaneous ventricular tachycardia.

■ DISPOSITION

HCM is not a static disease. Some adults may experience subtle regression in wall thickness while others (approximately 5% to 10%) paradoxically evolve into an end stage resembling dilated cardiomyopathy and characterized by cavity enlargement, LV wall thinning, and diastolic dysfunction. Patients with HCM are at increased risk of sudden death, especially if there is onset of symptoms during childhood. Left ventricular outflow at rest is also a strong, independent predictor of severe symptoms of heart failure and of death. Adult patients can be considered low risk if they have no symptoms or mild symptoms and also if they have none of the following:

- A family history of premature death caused by hypertrophic cardiomyopathy
- Nonsustained ventricular tachycardia during Holter monitoring
- A marked outflow tract gradient
- Substantial hypertrophy (>20 mm)
- Marked left atrial enlargement
- Abnormal blood pressure response during exercise

■ REFERRAL

- Surgical treatment (myotomy-myectomy) is reserved for patients who have both a large outflow gradient (≥50 mm Hg) and severe symptoms of heart failure that are unresponsive to medical therapy. The risk of sudden death from arrhythmias is not altered by surgery.
- Nonsurgical reduction of interventricular septum represents a new, controversial, and unproven therapeutic approach that can be used in patients with HCM refractory to pharmacologic treatment. This technique involves the injection of ethanol in the septal perforator branch of the left anterior descending coronary artery, producing a controlled myocardial infarction of the interventricular septum and thereby reducing the left ventricular outflow tract gradient. This method may lead to improvement in both subjective and objective measures of exercise capacity but is associated with a high incidence of heart block, often requiring permanent pacing in about one fourth of patients.

☼ PEARLS & CONSIDERATIONS

■ COMMENTS

Screening of first-degree relatives with two-dimensional echocardiography is indicated, particularly if adverse HCM-related events have occurred in the family.

- Mortality rate in HCM is approximately 1% to 2%.
- It is important to remember that HCM is predominantly a non-obstructive disease (75% of patients do not have a sizable resting outflow tract gradient).

REFERENCES

Maron BJ: Hypertrophic cardiomyopathy, a systematic review, *JAMA* 287:1308, 2002.

Maron MS et al: Effect of left ventricular outflow tract obstruction on clinical outcome in hypertrophic cardiomyopathy, *N Engl J Med* 348:295, 2003.

Shamim W et al: Nonsurgical reduction of the interventricular septum in patients with hypertrophic cardiomyopathy, *N Engl J Med* 347:1326, 2002.

Author: **Fred F. Ferri, M.D.**

BASIC INFORMATION

■ DEFINITION

Cardiomyopathies are a group of diseases primarily involving the myocardium and characterized by myocardial dysfunction that is not the result of hypertension, coronary atherosclerosis, valvular dysfunction, or pericardial abnormalities. Restrictive cardiomyopathies are characterized by decreased ventricular compliance, usually secondary to infiltration of the myocardium.

ICD-9CM CODES
425.4 Other primary cardiomyopathies

■ EPIDEMIOLOGY & DEMOGRAPHICS

Relatively uncommon cardiomyopathy that is most frequently caused by amyloidosis (Fig. 1-58), myocardial fibrosis (after open heart surgery), and radiation

■ PHYSICAL FINDINGS & CLINICAL PRESENTATION

- Edema, ascites, hepatomegaly, distended neck veins
- Fatigue, weakness (secondary to low output)
- Kussmaul's sign: may be present
- Regurgitant murmurs
- Possible prominent apical impulse

■ ETIOLOGY

- Infiltrative and storage disorders (glycogen storage disease, amyloidosis, sarcoidosis, hemochromatosis)
- Scleroderma
- Radiation
- Endocardial fibroelastosis
- Endomyocardial fibrosis
- Idiopathic
- Toxic effects of anthracycline
- Carcinoid heart disease, metastatic cancers
- Diabetic cardiomyopathy
- Eosinophilic cardiomyopathy (Löffler's endocarditis)

DIAGNOSIS

■ DIFFERENTIAL DIAGNOSIS

- Coronary atherosclerosis
- Valvular dysfunction
- Pericardial abnormalities
- Chronic lung disease
- Psychogenic dyspnea

■ WORKUP

- Chest x-ray examination, ECG, echocardiogram
- Cardiac catheterization, MRI (selected cases)

■ IMAGING STUDIES

- Chest x-ray examination:
  1. Moderate cardiomegaly
  2. Possible evidence of CHF (pulmonary vascular congestion, pleural effusion)
- ECG:
  1. Low voltage with ST-T wave changes
  2. Possible frequent arrhythmias, left axis deviation, and atrial fibrillation
- Echocardiogram: increased wall thickness and thickened cardiac valves (especially in patients with amyloidosis)
- Cardiac catheterization to distinguish restrictive cardiomyopathy from constrictive pericarditis
  1. Constrictive pericarditis: usually involves both ventricles and produces a plateau of elevated filling pressures
  2. Restrictive cardiomyopathy: impairs the left ventricle more than the right (PCWP > RAP, PASP >50 mm Hg)
- MRI may also be useful to distinguish restrictive cardiomyopathy from constrictive pericarditis (thickness of the pericardium >5 mm in the latter)

TREATMENT

■ NONPHARMACOLOGIC THERAPY

Control CHF by restricting salt.

■ ACUTE GENERAL Rx

- Cardiomyopathy caused by hemochromatosis may respond to repeated phlebotomies to decrease iron deposition in the heart.
- Sarcoidosis may respond to corticosteroid therapy.
- Corticosteroid and cytotoxic drugs may improve survival in patients with eosinophilic cardiomyopathy.
- There is no effective therapy for other causes of restrictive cardiomyopathy.

■ CHRONIC Rx

Death usually results from CHF or arrhythmias; therefore therapy should be aimed at controlling CHF by restricting salt, administering diuretics, and treating potentially fatal arrhythmias.

■ DISPOSITION

Prognosis varies with the etiology of the cardiomyopathy.

■ REFERRAL

Cardiac transplantation can be considered in patients with refractory symptoms and idiopathic or familial restrictive cardiomyopathies.

Author: **Fred F. Ferri, M.D.**

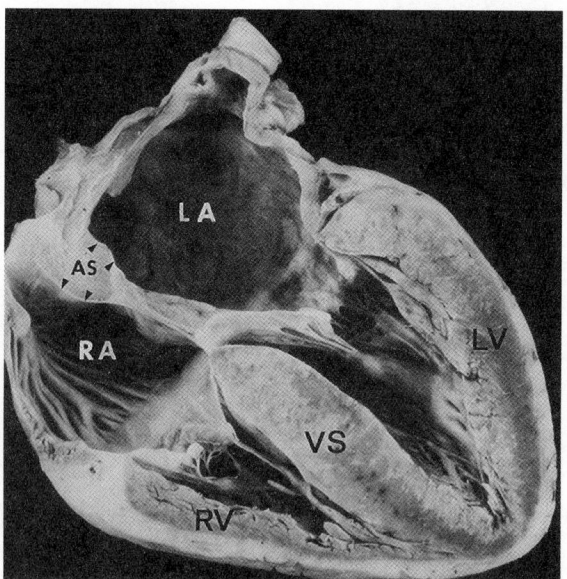

Fig. 1-58 A necropsy specimen of an amyloid heart demonstrating the thickened ventricular septum *(VS)*, atrial septum *(AS)*, and free wall of the left ventricle *(LV)* and right ventricle *(RV)*, and the dilated left atrium *(LA)*. RA, Right atrium. (Courtesy Dr. William Edwards, Mayo Clinic, Rochester, MN. In Goldman L, Bennett JC [eds]: *Cecil textbook of medicine*, ed 22, Philadelphia, 2004, WB Saunders.)

BASIC INFORMATION

■ DEFINITION

Dizziness, presyncope, or syncope in a patient with carotid sinus hypersensitivity is defined as *carotid sinus syndrome*. Carotid sinus hypersensitivity is the exaggerated response to carotid stimulation resulting in bradycardia, hypotension, or both.

■ SYNONYMS

Carotid sinus syncope
CSS

ICD-9CM CODES

337.0 Idiopathic peripheral autonomic neuropathy
Carotid sinus syncope or syndrome

■ EPIDEMIOLOGY & DEMOGRAPHICS

- The incidence of carotid sinus hypersensitivity is 10% in the adult population.
- The incidence increases with age.
- Men are affected more often than women (2:1).
- Carotid sinus syndrome is rarely found before the age of 50 yr.

■ PHYSICAL FINDINGS & CLINICAL PRESENTATION

Properly performed carotid sinus massage at the bedside is diagnostic. This maneuver can elicit three types of responses in the appropriate patient (see Diagnosis).
1. Carotid sinus massage (CSM) should be done in the supine position while monitoring the patient's blood pressure by cuff and heart rate by ECG.
2. CSM should not be performed on patients with carotid bruits or recent TIA/CVA.
3. CSM should be performed on only one artery at a time.
4. CSM should be applied for approximately 5 sec.

■ ETIOLOGY

- Idiopathic
- Head and neck tumors (e.g., thyroid)
- Significant lymphadenopathy
- Carotid body tumors
- Prior neck surgery

DIAGNOSIS

- The diagnosis of CSS is made when carotid sinus hypersensitivity is diagnosed by CSM and no other cause of syncope is identified.
- CSM can elicit three types of responses that are diagnostic of carotid sinus hypersensitivity:
  1. Cardioinhibitory type: CSM producing asystole for at least 3 sec

2. Vasodepressor type: CSM producing a decrease in systolic blood pressure of 50 mm Hg or 30 mm Hg in the presence of neurologic symptoms
3. Mixed type: CSM producing both types of responses
- It is not absolutely necessary to produce symptoms with CSM to diagnose CSS.

■ DIFFERENTIAL DIAGNOSIS

All causes of syncope, for example, cardiac tachyarrhythmias and bradyarrhythmias, cardiac valvular disease and obstructive cardiomyopathy, cerebrovascular events, seizures, drug-induced, autonomic dysfunction, orthostasis/hypovolemia, cough, micturition, hypoxemia, and hypoglycemia

■ WORKUP

The workup must exclude other causes of syncope as guided by the history and the physical examination. Blood tests, cardiac noninvasive studies (Holter, echocardiograms, ECG, tilt test, treadmill testing), cardiac invasive testing (electrophysiologic studies), EEG, and CT scan should be ordered in the appropriate clinical setting.

 TREATMENT

■ NONPHARMACOLOGIC THERAPY

Avoidance of triggering factors such as straining or applying neck pressure from tight collars, shaving, or rapid head turning.

■ ACUTE GENERAL Rx

Treatment will vary according to the type of carotid hypersensitivity response (e.g., cardioinhibitory, vasodepressor, or mixed) and symptoms present (see Chronic Rx). Acute treatment is usually not needed, because most patients at presentation are hemodynamically stable but present with either a fall resulting in an injury (e.g., hip fracture, laceration) or a complaint of true syncope with no injury.

■ CHRONIC Rx

For asymptomatic carotid sinus hypersensitivity of either the cardioinhibitory or vasodepressor type, it is generally agreed that pacemaker implantation is not necessary.
For patients with CSS with a cardioinhibitory response to CSM:
- Dual-chamber permanent pacemaker is indicated.
- Controversy exists as to whether to implant the pacemaker after the first syncopal episode or after a recurrent episode.

For patients with CSS with a vasodepressor response to CSM:
- Measures to maintain systolic blood pressure are tried:
  1. Sympathomimetics (ephedrine has been tried with success but has significant side effects, e.g., palpitations, tremors.)
  2. Fludrocortisone with its mineralocorticoid effect also has been tried with limited success.
  3. Dual-chamber pacemaker is *not* indicated in the patient with pure vasodepressor response.
  4. Elastic knee-high or thigh-high stockings help to maintain systolic blood pressure.
  5. Carotid sinus denervation is reserved for those patients refractory to the above mentioned treatment.
For patients with CSS with a mixed response to CSM:
- Dual-chamber permanent pacemaker and atropine can effectively treat the bradycardic response but have no major effect on the hypotensive response. The vasodepressor response should be treated as mentioned previously.

■ DISPOSITION

CSS occurs in the elderly population and presents with falls or syncope often resulting in injury. Up to 50% of the patients who present with symptoms will have recurrent symptoms. This is reduced in the group of patients for whom a pacemaker is indicated. There is no difference in survival in this group of patients when compared with the general population.

■ REFERRAL

Cardiology referral is indicated if a pacemaker is considered.

PEARLS & CONSIDERATIONS

■ COMMENTS

The most common type of response to CSM in this population is cardioinhibitory response followed by mixed and vasodepressor responses.

REFERENCES

Kapoor WN: Current evaluation and management of syncope, *Circulation* 106(13):1606, 2002.
Kenny RA, Richardson DA: Carotid sinus syndrome and falls in older adults, *Am J Geriatr Cardiol* 10(2):97, 2001.
Author: **Peter Petropoulos, M.D.**

BASIC INFORMATION

■ DEFINITION
Carpal tunnel syndrome is an entrapment neuropathy involving the median nerve at the wrist (Fig. 1-59). It is the most common entrapment neuropathy in the upper extremity.

■ ICD-9CM CODES
354.0 Carpal tunnel syndrome

■ EPIDEMIOLOGY & DEMOGRAPHICS
PREVALENT AGE: 30 to 60 yr (bilateral up to 50%)
PREVALENT SEX: Females are affected two to five times as often as males

■ PHYSICAL FINDINGS & CLINICAL PRESENTATION
- Nocturnal pain
- Occasional median nerve sensory impairment (often only index and long fingers)
- Positive Tinel's sign at wrist (tapping over the median nerve on the flexor surface of the wrist produces a tingling sensation radiating from the wrist to the hand)
- Positive Phalen's test (reproduction of symptoms after 1 min of gentle, unforced wrist flexion)
- Carpal compression test: Pressure with the examiner's thumb over the patient's carpal tunnel for 30 sec elicits symptoms
- Thenar atrophy in long-standing cases

■ ETIOLOGY
- Idiopathic in most cases
- Space-occupying lesions in carpal tunnel (tenosynovitis, ganglia, aberrant muscles)
- Often associated with hypothyroidism, hormonal changes of pregnancy
- Job-related mechanical overuse may be a risk factor
- Traumatic injuries to wrist

DIAGNOSIS

■ DIFFERENTIAL DIAGNOSIS
- Cervical radiculopathy
- Chronic tendinitis
- Vascular occlusion
- Reflex sympathetic dystrophy
- Osteoarthritis
- Other arthritides
- Other entrapment neuropathies

■ IMAGING STUDIES
Routine roentgenograms may be helpful in establishing cause or ruling out other conditions.

■ ELECTRODIAGNOSTIC STUDIES
Nerve conduction velocity tests and electromyography are useful in establishing the diagnosis and ruling out other syndromes.

TREATMENT

■ ACUTE GENERAL Rx
- Elimination of repetitive trauma
- Occupational splints or braces
- NSAIDs
- Injection of carpal canal on ulnar side of palmaris longus tendon at wrist flexor crease (avoiding median nerve)
- Low-dose oral corticosteroids (e.g., prednisolone 20 mg qd for 2 wk, followed by 10 mg qd for 2 more wk) are also effective for symptom relief in selected patients

■ DISPOSITION
Prognosis is variable. Some cases resolve spontaneously. Relief from local injection appears transient and symptoms recur in the majority of cases following injection.
Carpal tunnel syndrome is common in the third trimester of pregnancy, but symptoms subside after delivery in most cases, often dramatically. Symptoms may recur with subsequent pregnancies. Surgery is not recommended in pregnant patients because of the likelihood of spontaneous recovery.

■ REFERRAL
Surgical referral in cases of failed medical management or signs of motor weakness

REFERENCES
Bagatur AE, Zorer G: The carpal tunnel syndrome is a bilateral disorder, *J Bone Joint Surg Br* 83(5):655, 2001.

D'Arcy C, McGee S: Does this patient have carpal tunnel syndrome? *JAMA* 283:3110, 2000.

Gerritsen AM et al: Splinting vs surgery in the treatment of carpal tunnel syndrome, *JAMA* 288:1245, 2002.

Gonzalez MH, Bylak J: Steroid injection and splinting in the treatment of carpal tunnel syndrome, *Orthopedics* 24:479, 2001.

Katz JN, Simmons BP: Carpal tunnel syndrome, *N Engl J Med* 346:1807, 2002.

Nagle DJ: Evaluation of chronic wrist pain, *J Am Acad Orthop Surg* 8:45, 2000.

Robinson LR: Role of neurophysiologic evaluation in diagnoses, *J Am Acad Orthop Surg* 8:190, 2000.

Shum C et al: The role of flexor tenosynovectomy in the operative treatment of carpal tunnel syndrome, *J Bone Joint Surg* 84(A):221, 2002.

Vjera AJ: Management of carpal tunnel syndrome, *Am Fam Physician* 68:265, 2003.

Wong SM et al: Local vs. systemic caricosteroids in the treatment of carpal tunnel syndrome, *Neurology* 56:1565, 2001.
Author: **Lonnie R. Mercier, M.D.**

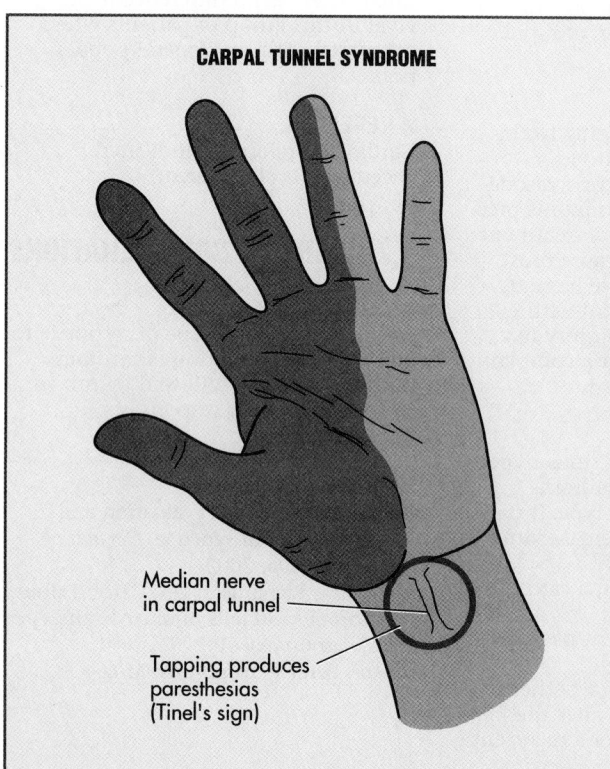

CARPAL TUNNEL SYNDROME

Median nerve in carpal tunnel

Tapping produces paresthesias (Tinel's sign)

Fig. 1-59 Distribution of pain and/or paresthesias (dark-shaded area) when the median nerve is compressed by swelling in the wrist (carpal tunnel). (From Arnett FC: Rheumatoid arthritis. In Andreoli TE [ed]: *Cecil essentials of medicine,* ed 4, Philadelphia, 1997, WB Saunders.)

BASIC INFORMATION

■ DEFINITION
Cataracts are the clouding and opacification of the crystalline lens of the eye. The opacity may occur in the cortex, the nucleus of the lens, or the posterior subcapsular region, but it is usually in a combination of areas.

■ SYNONYMS
Congenital cataracts (e.g., from rubella)
Metabolic cataracts (e.g., caused by diabetes)
Collagen-vascular disease cataracts (caused by lupus)
Hereditary cataracts
Age-related senile cataracts
Traumatic cataracts
Toxic or drug-induced cataracts (e.g., caused by steroids)

■ ICD-9CM CODES
366 Cataract

■ EPIDEMIOLOGY & DEMOGRAPHICS
INCIDENCE (IN U.S.): Highest cause of treatable blindness; cataract removal is the most frequent surgical procedure in patients >65 yr old (1.3 million operations/yr, with an annual cost of approximately $3 billion).
PREDOMINANT AGE: Elderly; some stage of cataract development is present in >50% of persons 65 to 74 yr old and 65% of those >75 yr old.
PEAK INCIDENCE:
• In early life: congenital and hereditary causes predominant
• In older age group: senile cataracts (after 40 yr of age)
GENETICS: Hereditary with such syndromes as galactosemia, homocystinuria, diabetes

■ PHYSICAL FINDINGS & CLINICAL PRESENTATION
Cloudiness and opacification of the crystalline lens of the eye (Fig. 1-60)

■ ETIOLOGY
• Heredity
• Trauma
• Toxins
• Age-related
• Drug-related
• Congenital
• Inflammatory

DIAGNOSIS

■ DIFFERENTIAL DIAGNOSIS
• Corneal lesions
• Retinal lesions

■ WORKUP
Complete eye examination, including slit lamp examination, funduscopic examination, and brightness acuity testing

■ LABORATORY TESTS
• Rarely, urinary amino acid screening and CNS imaging studies with congenital cataracts
• Fasting glucose in young adults with cataracts

TREATMENT

■ NONPHARMACOLOGIC THERAPY
• Wait until vision is compromised before doing surgery.
• Surgery is indicated when corrected visual acuity in the affected eye is >20/30 in the absence of other ocular disease; however, surgery may be justified when visual acuity is better in specific situations (especially disabling glare, monocular diplopia).

■ ACUTE GENERAL Rx
None necessary

■ CHRONIC Rx
• Change glasses as cataracts develop.
• Myopia is common, and glasses can be adjusted until surgery is contemplated.

■ DISPOSITION
Refer if sight compromised.

■ REFERRAL
Refer to ophthalmologist for extraction when vision is compromised (see Nonpharmacologic Therapy).

PEARLS & CONSIDERATIONS

■ COMMENTS
Success rate with surgery is 95% to 98%.

REFERENCES
Consultation section: Cataract surgical problem, *J Cataract Refract Surg* 28:577, 2002.
Solomon R, Donninfeld ED: Recent advances and future frontiers in treating age-related cataracts, *JAMA* 290:248, 2003.
Wong TY et al: Relation of ocular trauma to cortical, nuclear and posterior subcapsular cataracts, *Br J Ophthalmol* 86:152, 2002.
Author: **Melvyn Koby, M.D.**

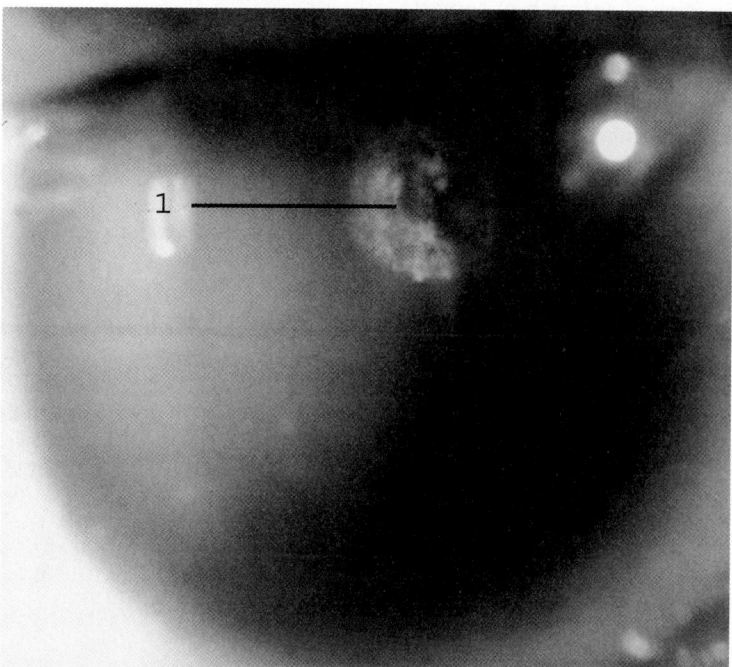

Fig. 1-60 The central location of a posterior subcapsular cataract *(1)*. (From Palay D [ed]: *Ophthalmology for the primary care physician*, St Louis, 1997, Mosby.)

BASIC INFORMATION

■ DEFINITION

Cat-scratch disease (CSD) is a syndrome consisting of gradually enlarging regional lymphadenopathy occurring after contact with a feline. Atypical presentations are characterized by a variety of neurologic manifestations as well as granulomatous involvement of the eye, liver, spleen, and bone. The disease is usually self-limiting, and recovery is complete; however, patients with atypical presentations, especially if immunocompromised, may suffer significant morbidity and mortality.

■ SYNONYMS

Cat-scratch fever
Benign inoculation lymphoreticulosis
Nonbacterial regional lymphadenitis

ICD-9CM CODES

078.3 Cat-scratch disease

■ EPIDEMIOLOGY & DEMOGRAPHICS

PREVALENCE: Unknown
INCIDENCE (IN U.S.):
• Unknown
• Majority of reported cases in children
PEAK INCIDENCE: August through January
GENETICS: Unknown

■ PHYSICAL FINDINGS & CLINICAL PRESENTATION

• Classic, most common finding: regional lymphadenopathy occurring within 2 wk of a scratch or contact with felines
• Tender, swollen lymph nodes most commonly found in the head and neck, followed by the axilla and the epitrochlear, inguinal, and femoral areas
• Erythematous overlying skin, showing signs of suppuration from involved lymph nodes
• On careful examination; evidence of cutaneous inoculation in the form of a nonpruritic, slightly tender pustule or papule (Fig. 1-61)
• Fever in most patients
• Malaise and headache in fewer than a third of patients

• Atypical presentations in fewer than 15% of cases
  1. Usually in association with lymph-adenopathy and a low-grade or frank fever (>101° F, >38.3° C)
  2. Include granulomatous involvement of the conjunctiva (Parinaud's oculoglandular syndrome) and focal masses in the liver, spleen, and mesenteric nodes
• CNS involvement: neuroretinitis, encephalopathy, encephalitis, transverse myelitis, seizure activity, and coma
• Osteomyelitis in adults and children

■ ETIOLOGY

• Major cause: *Bartonella (Rochalimaea) henselae*
• Mode of transmission: predominantly by direct inoculation through the scratch, bite, or lick of a cat, especially a kitten
• Limited evidence in support of an arthropod (flea) as an alternative vector of infection arising from bacteremic felines
• Rarely, associated with dogs, monkeys, and inanimate objects with which a feline has been in recent contact
• Approximately 2 wk after introduction of the bacteria into the host, regional lymphatic tissues displaying granulomatous infiltration associated with gradual hypertrophy
• Possible dissemination to distant sites (e.g., liver, spleen, and bone), usually characterized by focal masses or discrete parenchymal lesions

DIAGNOSIS

■ DIFFERENTIAL DIAGNOSIS

Granulomas of this syndrome must be differentiated from those associated with tularemia, tuberculosis, sarcoidosis, sporotrichosis, toxoplasmosis, lymphogranuloma venerum, fungal diseases, and benign and malignant tumors.

■ WORKUP

Diagnosis should be considered in patients who present with a predominant complaint of gradually enlarging regional (focal) lymphadenopathy, often with fever and a recent history of having contact with a cat.

■ LABORATORY TESTS

• Three of four of the following criteria are required:
  1. History of animal contact in the presence of a scratch, dermal, or eye lesion
  2. Culture of lymphatic aspirate that is negative for other causes
  3. Positive CSD skin test
  4. Biopsied lymph node histology consistent with CSD
• Enhanced culture techniques and serologies will augment establishment of the diagnosis.
• Histopathologically, Warthin-Starry silver stain has been used to identify the bacillus.
• Routine laboratory findings:
  1. Mild leukocytosis or leukopenia
  2. Infrequent eosinophilia
  3. Elevated ESR

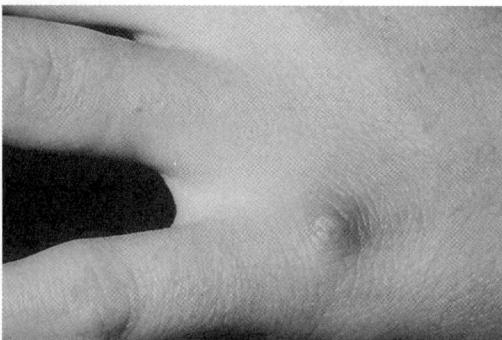

Fig. 1-61   Primary lesion of cat-scratch disease is a tender papule occurring 3 to 10 days after a scratch. (From Noble J [ed]: *Primary care medicine,* ed 2, St Louis, 1996, Mosby.)

- Abnormalities of bilirubin excretion and elevated hepatic transaminases are usually secondary to hepatic obstruction by granuloma, mass, or lymph node.
- In patients with neurologic manifestations, lumbar puncture usually reveals normal CSF, although there may be a mild pleocytosis and modest elevation in protein.
- The diagnosis may be confirmed by specific enzyme immunoassay (EIA) in association with a history of cat contact and a typical clinical presentation.

TREATMENT

■ NONPHARMACOLOGIC THERAPY
- Warm compresses to the affected nodes
- In cases of encephalitis or coma: supportive care

■ ACUTE GENERAL Rx
- There is no consensus over therapy, especially as the disease is self-limited in a majority of cases.
- It would be prudent to treat severely ill patients, especially if immuno-compromised, with antibiotic therapy, because these patients tend to suffer dissemination of infection and increased morbidity.
- *Bartonella* is usually sensitive to aminoglycosides, tetracycline, erythromycin, and the quinolones.
- When the isolate is proven by culture, the patient should receive antibiotic therapy as directed by the obtained sensitivities.
- Antipyretics and NSAIDs may also be used.

■ DISPOSITION
Overall prognosis is good.

■ REFERRAL
- To an appropriate subspecialist to evaluate specific lesions
- For diagnostic aspiration or excision in presence of regional lymph-adenopathy, bone lesions, and mesenteric lymph nodes and organs
- To ophthalmologist for ocular granulomas
  1. Usually diagnosed clinically
  2. Rarely require excision

✦ PEARLS & CONSIDERATIONS

■ COMMENTS
- A presentation of this syndrome, especially in patients with HIV infection or impaired cellular immunity, may be fever of unknown origin.
- Hepatic and splenic granulomas, coronary valve infections may offer few physical clues to diagnosis, emphasizing the need for a complete history.
- CSD should be considered in the differential diagnosis of school-aged children presenting with status epilepticus.
- Chronically immunocompromised patients considering the acquisition of a young feline should be made aware of the possible risk of infection.
- No signs of illness may be apparent in bacteremic kittens.

REFERENCES

Gonzalez BE et al: Cat-scratch disease occurring in three siblings simultaneously, *Pediatr Infect Dis J* 22(5):467, 2003.

Koehler JE et al: Prevalence of Bartonella infection among human immunodeficiency virus-infected patients with fever, *Clin Infect Dis* 37(4):559, 2003.

Metzkor-Cotter E et al: Long-term serological analysis and clinical follow-up of patients with cat scratch disease, *Clin Infect Dis* 37(9):1149, 2003.

Mirakhur B et al: Cat scratch disease presenting as orbital abscess and osteomyelitis, *J Clin Microbiol* 41(8):3991, 2003.

Resto-Ruiz S, Burgess A, Anderson BE: The role of the host immune response in pathogenesis of Bartonella henselae, *DNA Cell Biol* 22(6):431, 2003.

Rolain JM et al: Cat scratch disease with lymphadenitis, vertebral osteomyelitis, and spleen abscesses, *Ann N Y Acad Sci* 990:397, 2003.

Rolain JM et al: Detection by immunofluorescence assay of Bartonella henselae in lymph nodes from patients with cat scratch disease, *Clin Diagn Lab Immunol* 10(4):686, 2003.

Author: **George O. Alonso, M.D.**

BASIC INFORMATION

■ DEFINITION

Cavernous sinus thrombosis is an uncommon diagnosis usually stemming from infections of the face or paranasal sinuses resulting in thrombosis of the cavernous sinus and inflammation of its surrounding anatomic structures, including cranial nerves III, IV, V (ophthalmic and maxillary branch), and VI, and the internal carotid artery.

■ SYNONYMS

Intracranial venous sinus thrombosis or thrombophlebitis

ICD-9CM CODES

325 Phlebitis and thrombophlebitis of intracranial venous sinus

■ EPIDEMIOLOGY & DEMOGRAPHICS

- Cavernous sinus thrombosis is rare.
- Before antibiotics the mortality rate from cavernous sinus thrombosis was 80% to 100%.
- With antibiotics, the mortality rates range between 20% and 30%.
- Morbidity remains high (between 25% and 50%).

■ PHYSICAL FINDINGS & CLINICAL PRESENTATION

The classic findings include:
- Ptosis
- Proptosis
- Chemosis
- Cranial nerve palsies (III, IV, V, VI)
  1. Sixth nerve palsy is the most common.
  2. Sensory deficits of the ophthalmic and maxillary branch of the fifth nerve are common.

Other findings:
- Decreased visual acuity and blindness may occur.
- Venous engorgement and papilledema on funduscopic examination may be found.
- Fever, tachycardia, sepsis may be present.
- Headache with nuchal rigidity may occur.
- Pupil may be dilated and sluggishly reactive.

■ ETIOLOGY

- *Staphylococcus aureus* is the most common infectious microbe, found in 50% to 60% of the cases.
- *Streptococcus* is the second leading cause.
- Gram-negative rods and anaerobes may also lead to cavernous sinus thrombosis.
- The most common primary site of infection leading to cavernous sinus thrombosis is sphenoid sinusitis;

however, other sites of infection, including the middle ear, orbit, eye, eyelid, and face, can result in the same sequelae.

DIAGNOSIS

- The diagnosis of cavernous sinus thrombosis is made clinically.
- Proptosis, ptosis, chemosis, and cranial nerve palsy beginning in one eye and progressing to the other eye establish the diagnosis.

■ DIFFERENTIAL DIAGNOSIS

- Orbital cellulitis
- Internal carotid artery aneurysm
- CVA
- Migraine headache
- Allergic blepharitis
- Thyroid exophthalmos
- Brain tumor
- Meningitis
- Mucormycosis
- Trauma

■ WORKUP

Cavernous sinus thrombosis is a clinical diagnosis with laboratory tests and imaging studies confirming the clinical impression.

■ LABORATORY TESTS

- CBC, ESR, blood cultures, and sinus cultures help establish and identify an infectious primary source.
- Lumbar puncture is necessary to rule out meningitis.

■ IMAGING STUDIES

- Sinus films are helpful in the diagnosis of sphenoid sinusitis. Opacification, sclerosis, and air-fluid levels are typical findings.
- CT scan is the best study to diagnose sphenoid sinusitis; however, CT scan is not very sensitive in diagnosing cavernous sinus thrombosis.
- MRI is the imaging study of choice to diagnose cavernous sinus thrombosis.
- Cerebral angiography can be performed, but it is invasive and not very sensitive.
- Orbital venography is difficult to perform, but it is excellent in diagnosing occlusion of the cavernous sinus.

TREATMENT

■ NONPHARMACOLOGIC THERAPY

Recognizing the primary source of infection (i.e., facial cellulitis, middle ear, and sinus infections) and treating the primary source expeditiously is the best way to prevent cavernous sinus thrombosis.

■ ACUTE GENERAL Rx

- Broad-spectrum intravenous antibiotics are used until a definite pathogen is found.
  1. Nafcillin 1.5 g IV q4h
  2. Cefotaxime 1.5 to 2 g IV q4h
  3. Metronidazole 15 mg/kg load followed by 7.5 mg/kg IV q6h
- Anticoagulation with heparin is controversial. Retrospective studies show conflicting data. This decision should be made with subspecialty consultation.
- Steroid therapy is also controversial.

■ CHRONIC Rx

Surgical drainage with sphenoidotomy is indicated if the primary site of infection is thought to be the sphenoid sinus.

■ DISPOSITION

- Cavernous sinus thrombosis can be a life-threatening, rapidly progressive infectious disease with high morbidity and mortality rates despite antibiotic use.
- Complications in treated patients include oculomotor weakness, blindness, pituitary insufficiency, and hemiparesis.

■ REFERRAL

If the diagnosis is suspected, this should be considered a medical emergency. Depending on the primary site of infection, appropriate consultation should be made (i.e., ENT, ophthalmology, and infectious disease).

PEARLS & CONSIDERATIONS

■ COMMENTS

Realizing the cavernous sinus lies just above and lateral to the sphenoid sinus and drains the middle portion of the face via the superior and inferior ophthalmic veins and knowing that cranial nerves III, IV, V, and VI pass alongside or through the cavernous sinus make the clinical findings and diagnosis easier to understand.

REFERENCE

Ebright JR et al: Septic thrombosis of the cavernous sinuses, *Arch Intern Med* 161:2671, 2001.
Author: **Peter Petropoulos, M.D.**

BASIC INFORMATION

■ DEFINITION
Celiac disease is a chronic disease characterized by malabsorption and diarrhea precipitated by ingestion of food products containing gluten.

■ SYNONYMS
Gluten-sensitive enteropathy
Celiac sprue

■ ICD-9CM CODES
579.0 Celiac disease

■ EPIDEMIOLOGY & DEMOGRAPHICS
- Estimates of the incidence and prevalence of celiac sprue in the U.S. range from 50 to 500 cases/100,000 persons; it is highest in whites of northern European ancestry (1 in 300).
- Incidence is highest during infancy and the initial 36 mo (secondary to the introduction of foods containing gluten), in the third decade (frequently associated with pregnancy and severe anemia during pregnancy), and in the seventh decade.
- There is a slight female predominance.

■ PHYSICAL FINDINGS & CLINICAL PRESENTATION
- Physical examination may be entirely within normal limits.
- Weight loss, dyspepsia, short stature, and failure to thrive may be noted in children and infants.
- Weight loss, fatigue, and diarrhea are common in adults.
- Abdominal pain, nausea, and vomiting are unusual.
- Pallor as a result of iron deficiency anemia is common.
- Manifestations of calcium deficiency, such as tetany and seizures, are rare and can be exacerbated by coexistent magnesium deficiency.
- Angular cheilitis, aphthous ulcers, atopic dermatitis, and dermatitis herpetiformis are frequently associated with celiac disease.

■ ETIOLOGY
- Celiac sprue results from an inappropriate T-cell-mediated immune response against ingested gluten in genetically predisposed people. There is sensitivity to gliadin, a protein fraction of gluten found in wheat, rye, and barley.
- Recently a peptide that resists degradation by proteases in the small bowel was identified as the potential triggering molecule.

DIAGNOSIS

■ DIFFERENTIAL DIAGNOSIS
- IBD
- Laxative abuse

- Intestinal parasitic infestations
- Other: irritable bowel syndrome, tropical sprue, chronic pancreatitis, Zollinger-Ellison syndrome, cystic fibrosis (children), lymphoma, eosinophilic gastroenteritis, short bowel syndrome, Whipple's disease

■ WORKUP
Evaluation consists of laboratory tests followed by upper GI endoscopy with biopsy of duodenum or proximal jejunum.

■ LABORATORY TESTS
- Iron deficiency anemia (microcytic anemia, low ferritin level)
- Folic acid deficiency
- Vitamin B_{12} deficiency, hypomagnesemia, hypocalcemia
- Antigliadin IgA and IgG antibodies are elevated in >90% of patients; however, they are nonspecific. IgA endomysial antibodies are more specific for celiac sprue and are the best screening test for celiac disease, except in the case of patients with IgA deficiency. Tissue transglutinase autoantibody by ELISA is a newer serologic test for celiac sprue
- Biopsy of the small bowel is generally recommended to establish the diagnosis. It reveals absence or shortening of villi, intraepithelial lymphocytes, and crypt lengthening and hyperplasia. Several biopsy specimens should be obtained for proper diagnosis
- Tests for malabsorption are abnormal: fecal fat estimation for 72 hr is elevated (>7 g/day), D-xylose testing reveals malabsorption of sugar

■ IMAGING STUDIES
- Barium studies are usually unnecessary. Typical radiologic features include dilation of the small intestine with thickening or obliteration of the mucosal folds.
- Capsule endoscopy can also be used to evaluate the small intestinal mucosa, especially if future innovations will allow mucosal biopsy.

TREATMENT

■ NONPHARMACOLOGIC THERAPY
Patients should be instructed on gluten-free diet (avoidance of wheat, rye, and barley). Recent studies show that oats do not damage the mucosa in celiac disease.

■ GENERAL Rx
- Correct nutritional deficiencies with iron, folic acid, calcium, vitamin B_{12} as needed.

- Prednisone 20 to 60 mg qd gradually tapered is useful in refractory cases.
- Lifelong gluten-free diet is necessary.

■ DISPOSITION
- Prognosis is good with adherence to gluten-free diet. Rapid improvement is usually seen within a few days of treatment.
- Serial antigliadin or antiendomysial antibody tests can be used to monitor the patient's adherence to a gluten-free diet.
- Repeat small bowel biopsy following treatment generally reveals significant improvement. It is also useful to evaluate for increased risk of small bowel T-cell lymphoma in these patients (10%), especially in untreated patients.

■ REFERRAL
GI referral for small bowel biopsy.

PEARLS & CONSIDERATIONS

■ COMMENTS
- Some experts recommend a repeat biopsy only in selected patients who have an unsatisfactory response to a strict gluten-free diet.
- Celiac disease should be considered in patients with unexplained metabolic bone disease or hypocalcemia, especially because GI symptoms may be absent or mild. Clinicians should also consider testing children and young adults for celiac disease if unexplained weight loss, abdominal pain or distention, or chronic diarrhea is present.
- The prevalence of celiac disease in patients with dyspepsia is twice that of the general population. Screening for celiac disease should be considered in all patients with persistent dyspepsia.
- Celiac disease is associated with an increased risk for non-Hodgkin's lymphoma, especially of T-cell type and primarily localized in the gut.

REFERENCES
Farrell RJ, Kelly CP: Celiac sprue, *N Engl J Med* 346:180, 2002.
Fasano A: Celiac disease, how to handle a clinical chameleon, *N Eng J Med* 348:2568, 2003.
Hoffenberg EJ et al: A prospective study of the incidence of childhood celiac disease, *J Pediatr* 143:308, 2003.
Shan L et al: Structural basis for gluten intolerance in celiac sprue, *Science* 297:2275, 2002.
Author: **Fred F. Ferri, M.D.**

BASIC INFORMATION

■ DEFINITION
Cellulitis is a superficial inflammatory condition of the skin. It is characterized by erythema, warmth, and tenderness of the area involved.

■ SYNONYMS
Erysipelas (cellulitis generally secondary to group A β-hemolytic streptococci)

ICD-9CM CODES
682.9 Cellulitis

■ EPIDEMIOLOGY & DEMOGRAPHICS
- Occurs most frequently in diabetics, immunocompromised hosts, and patients with venous and lymphatic compromise
- Frequently found near skin breaks (trauma, surgical wounds, ulcerations, tinea infections)

■ PHYSICAL FINDINGS & CLINICAL PRESENTATION
Variable with the causative organism
- Erysipelas: superficial-spreading, warm, erythematous lesion distinguished by its indurated and elevated margin; lymphatic involvement and vesicle formation are common.
- Staphylococcal cellulitis: area involved is erythematous, hot, and swollen; differentiated from erysipelas by nonelevated, poorly demarcated margin; local tenderness and regional adenopathy are common; up to 85% of cases occur on the legs and feet.
- *H. influenzae* cellulitis: area involved is a blue-red/purple-red color; occurs mainly in children; generally involves the face in children and the neck or upper chest in adults.
- *Vibrio vulnificus:* larger hemorrhagic bullae, cellulitis, lymphadenitis, myositis; often found in critically ill patients in septic shock.

■ ETIOLOGY
- Group A β-hemolytic streptococci (may follow a streptococcal infection of the upper respiratory tract)
- Staphylococcal cellulitis
- *H. influenzae*
- *Vibrio vulnificus:* higher incidence in patients with liver disease (75%) and in immunocompromised hosts (corticosteroid use, diabetes mellitus, leukemia, renal failure)

- *Erysipelothrix rhusiopathiae:* common in people handling poultry, fish, or meat
- *Aeromonas hydrophila:* generally occurring in contaminated open wound in fresh water
- Fungi *(Cryptococcus neoformans):* immunocompromised granulopenic patients
- Gram-negative rods *(Serratia, Enterobacter, Proteus, Pseudomonas):* immunocompromised or granulopenic patients

DIAGNOSIS

■ DIFFERENTIAL DIAGNOSIS
- Necrotizing fasciitis
- DVT
- Peripheral vascular insufficiency
- Paget's disease of the breast
- Thrombophlebitis
- Acute gout
- Psoriasis
- Candida intertrigo
- Pseudogout
- Osteomyelitis

■ WORKUP
Physical examination and laboratory evaluation

■ LABORATORY TESTS
- Gram stain and culture (aerobic and anaerobic)
  1. Aspirated material from:
     a. Advancing edge of cellulitis
     b. Any vesicles
  2. Swab of any drainage material
  3. Punch biopsy (in selected patients)
- Blood cultures
- ALOS titer (in suspected streptococcal disease)

Despite the previous measures, the cause of cellulitis remains unidentified in most patients.

■ IMAGING STUDIES
CT or MRI in patients with suspected necrotizing fasciitis (deep-seated infection of the subcutaneous tissue that results in the progressive destruction of fascia and fat): patients present with diffuse swelling of an arm or leg followed by the appearance of bullae filled with clear fluid or maroon, violaceous fluid.

TREATMENT

■ NONPHARMACOLOGIC THERAPY
Immobilization and elevation of the involved limb

■ ACUTE GENERAL Rx
Erysipelas
- PO: dicloxacillin 500 mg PO q 6 h
- IV: nafcillin or oxacillin 2 g q 4 h or cefazolin 1 g q 8h
NOTE: Use erythromycin, cephalosporins, clindamycin, or vancomycin in patients allergic to penicillin.
Staphylococcus cellulitis
- PO: dicloxacillin 250 to 500 mg qid
- IV: nafcillin, 1 to 2 g q4-6h
- Cephalosporins (cephalothin, cephalexin, cephradine) also provide adequate antistaphylococcal coverage except for MRSA
- Use vancomycin in patients allergic to penicillin or cephalosporins and in patients with methicillin-resistant *S. aureus* (MRSA)
H. influenzae cellulitis
- PO: cefixime or cefuroxime
- IV: cefuroxime or ceftriaxone
Vibrio vulnificus
- Doxycycline 100 mg IV or PO bid +/− third-generation cephalosporin. Ciprofloxacin is an alternative antibiotic
- IV support and admission into ICU (mortality rate >50% in septic shock)
Erysipelothrix
- Penicillin
Aeromonas hydrophila
- Aminoglycosides
- Chloramphenicol
- Complicated skin and skin structure infections in hospitalized patients can be treated with daptomycin (cubicin) 4 mg/kg IV every 24 hr

■ DISPOSITION
Prognosis is good with prompt treatment.

■ REFERRAL
For surgical debridement in addition to antibiotics in patients with suspected necrotizing fasciitis

REFERENCE
Stulberg DL et al: Common bacterial skin infections, *Am Fam Physician* 66:119, 2002.
Author: **Fred F. Ferri, M.D.**

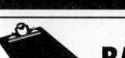

BASIC INFORMATION

■ DEFINITION
Cerebral palsy is a group of disorders of the central nervous system characterized by aberrant control of movement of posture, present since early in life and not the result of recognized progressive disease.

■ SYNONYMS
• Little's disease
• Congenital static encephalopathy
• Congenital spastic paralysis

ICD-9CM CODES
343 Infantile cerebral palsy
343.9 Infantile cerebral palsy, unspecified
EPDEMIOLOGY & DEMOGRAPHICS
INCIDENCE (IN U.S.): 1-2.4 per 1000 live births
PREDOMINANT SEX: Male = female
PREDOMINANT AGE: Diagnosis made at 3-5 yr

■ PHYSICAL FINDINGS & CLINICAL PRESENTATION
• Monoplegia, diplegia, quadriplegia, hemiplegia
• Often hypotonic in newborn period, followed by development of hypertonia
• Spasticity
• Athetosis
• Delay in motor milestones
• Hyperreflexia
• Seizures
• Mental retardation

■ ETIOLOGY
Mulitfactorial, including low birthweight, congenital malformation, asphyxia, multiple gestation, intrauterine exposure to infection, neonatal stroke, hyperbilirubinemia

 DIAGNOSIS

Mainly a clinical diagnosis, with exclusion of progressive disease

■ DIFFERENTIAL DIAGNOSIS
Other causes of neonatal hyptonia include muscular dystrophies, spinal muscular atrophy, Down syndrome, spinal cord injuries

■ LABORATORY TESTS
• Thyroid function tests
• Chromosomal analysis
• Urine organic acid screen

■ IMAGING STUDIES
Brain CT or MRI scan may show evidence of neonatal stroke or periventricular leukomalacia.

 TREATMENT

■ NONPHARMACOLOGIC THERAPY
• Physical therapy
• Special education

■ ACUTE GENERAL Rx
If present, treatment of seizures

■ CHRONIC Rx
• Physical therapy
• Treatment of seizures
• Baclofen
• Botulinum toxin

■ REFERRAL
If the child has difficulty with spasticity, physical medicine and rehabilitation referrals are especially helpful.

☼ PEARLS & CONSIDERATIONS

In full-term infants, history of traumatic delivery is usually not present.

REFERENCES
Kinsman SL: Predicting gross motor function in cerebral palsy, *JAMA* 288:1399, 2002.
Kuban KCK, Leviton A: Medical progress: cerebral palsy, *N Engl J Med* 330:188, 1994.
Nelson, KB: The epidemiology of cerebral palsy in term infants, *Ment Retard Dev Disabil Res Rev* 8(3):146, 2002.
Author: **Maitreyi Mazumdar, M.D.**

BASIC INFORMATION

■ DEFINITION
Cervical cancer is penetration of the basement membrane and infiltration of the stroma of the uterine cervix by malignant cells.

■ ICD-9CM CODES
180 Malignant neoplasm of cervix uteri

■ EPIDEMIOLOGY & DEMOGRAPHICS
INCIDENCE: There are approximately 15,000 new cases annually, with 4000 to 5000 associated deaths. The U.S. has an age-adjusted mortality of 2.6 cases/100,000 persons for cervical cancer.
PREDOMINANCE: Higher incidence rates occur in developing countries. Among the U.S. population, Hispanics have a higher incidence than African Americans, who likewise have a higher incidence than whites.
RISK FACTORS: Smoking, early age at first intercourse, multiple sexual partners, immunocompromised state, non-barrier methods of birth control, infection with high-risk HPV (types 16 and 18), multiparity.

■ PHYSICAL FINDINGS & CLINICAL PRESENTATION
- Unusual vaginal bleeding, particularly postcoital
- Vaginal discharge and/or odor
- Advanced cases may present with lower extremity edema or renal failure
- In early stages there may be little or no obvious cervical lesion, more advanced cases may present with large, bulky, friable lesions encompassing the majority of the vagina (Fig. 1-62)

■ ETIOLOGY
- Dysplastic cells progress to invasive carcinoma.
- Thought to be linked to the presence of HPV types 16, 18, 45, and 56 via interaction of E6 oncoproteins on p53 gene product.
- There may be an association between past infection with *Chlamydia trachomatis*.

DIAGNOSIS

■ DIFFERENTIAL DIAGNOSIS
- Cervical polyp or prolapsed uterine fibroid
- Preinvasive cervical lesions
- Neoplasia metastatic from a separate primary

■ WORKUP
- Thorough history and physical examination
- Pelvic examination with careful rectovaginal examination
- Colposcopy with directed biopsy and endocervical curettage
- Clinically staged, not surgically staged

■ LABORATORY TESTS
- CBC, chemistry profile
- Squamous cell carcinoma (SCC) antigen in research setting
- Carcinoembryonic antigen (CEA)

■ IMAGING STUDIES
- Chest x-ray examination
- IVP
- Depending on stage, may need cystoscopy, sigmoidoscopy or BE, CT scan or MRI, lymphangiography

TREATMENT

■ NONPHARMACOLOGIC THERAPY
- FIGO stage Ia: cone biopsy or simple hysterectomy

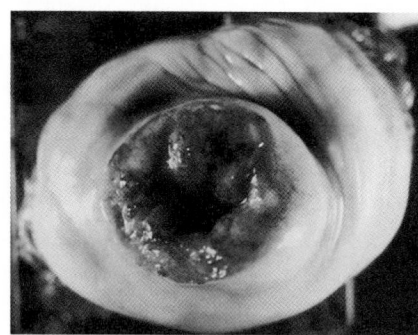

Fig. 1-62 Carcinoma of cervix (gross specimen). (From Mishell D [ed]: *Comprehensive gynecology*, ed 3, St Louis, 1997, Mosby.)

- FIGO stage Ib or IIa: type III radical hysterectomy and pelvic lymphadenectomy *or* pelvic radiation therapy
- Advanced or bulky disease: multi-modality therapy (radiation, chemotherapy, and/or surgery); platinum use before radiation therapy as a fertizer

■ ACUTE GENERAL Rx
Cervical cancer may present with massive and acute vaginal bleeding requiring volume and blood replacement, vaginal packing or other hemostatic modalities, and/or high-dose local radiotherapy.

■ CHRONIC Rx
- Physical examination with Pap smear every 3 mo for 2 yr, every 6 mo during the third to fifth year, and annually thereafter
- Chest x-ray examination annually

■ DISPOSITION
Five-year survival varies by stage:
- Stage I 60% to 90%
- Stage II 40% to 80%
- Stage III <60%
- Stage IV <15%

Early detection by Pap smear imperative to long-term improvements in survival.

■ REFERRAL
Gynecologic oncologist for all invasive disease

REFERENCES
Anttila T et al: Serotypes of *Chlamydia trachomatis* and risk for development of cervical squamous cell carcinoma, *JAMA* 285:47, 2001.

Morris M et al: Pelvic radiation with concurrent chemotherapy compared with pelvic and para-aortic radiation for high-risk cervical cancer, *N Engl J Med* 340:1137, 1999.

Nuono J et al: New tests for cervical cancer screening, *Am Fam Physician* 64:780, 2001.

Author: **Gil Farkash, M.D.**

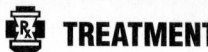
 BASIC INFORMATION

DEFINITION
Cervical disk syndromes refer to diseases of the cervical spine resulting from disk disorder, either herniation or degenerative change (spondylosis). When posterior osteophytes compress the anterior spinal cord, lower extremity symptoms may result, a condition termed *cervical spondylotic myelopathy.*

ICD-9CM CODES
722.4 Degenerative intervertebral cervical disk
722.71 Degenerative cervical disk with myelopathy

EPIDEMIOLOGY & DEMOGRAPHICS
PREVALENCE: 10% of general adult population (symptoms in 50% of population at some time in their life)
PREDOMINANT SEX: Male = female
PREDOMINANT AGE: 30 to 60 yr

PHYSICAL FINDINGS & CLINICAL PRESENTATION
- Neck pain, radicular symptoms, or myelopathy, either alone or in combination
- Limited neck movement
- Pain with neck motion, especially extension
- Referred unilateral interscapular pain, resulting in a local trigger point
- Radicular arm pain (usually unilateral), numbness, and tingling possible, most commonly involving the C6 (C5-C6 disk) or C7 (C6-C7 disk) nerve root
- Weakness and reflex changes (C6—biceps, C7—triceps)
- Myelopathy possibly resulting in gait disturbance, weakness, and even spasticity
- Sensory examination usually not helpful

ETIOLOGY
Unknown

🔬 **DIAGNOSIS**

DIFFERENTIAL DIAGNOSIS
- Rotator cuff tendinitis
- Carpal tunnel syndrome
- Thoracic outlet syndrome
- Brachial neuritis

A differential diagnosis for evaluation of neck pain is described in Section II.

WORKUP
In most cases, the diagnosis can be established on a clinical basis alone. Section III, Fig. 3-43 describes an algorithm for suspected cervical disc syndrome.

IMAGING STUDIES
- Plain roentgenograms within the first few weeks
  1. Usually normal in soft disk herniation
  2. With chronic degenerative disk disease, usually loss of height of the disk space, anterior and posterior osteophyte formation, and encroachment on the intervertebral foramen by osteophytes (see Fig. 1-63)
- Myelography, CT scanning, and MRI indicated in patients whose symptoms do not resolve or when other spinal pathology suspected
- Electrodiagnostic studies to confirm the diagnosis or rule out peripheral nerve disorders

💊 **TREATMENT**

NONPHARMACOLOGIC THERAPY
- Rest and cervical collar if needed
- Local modalities such as heat
- Physical therapy (Fig. 1-64)
- Avoid extreme range of motion exercises in degenerative disc disease

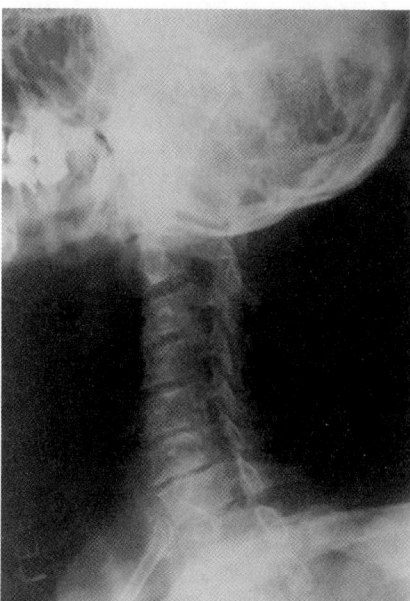

Fig. 1-63   Cervical spondylosis. Right anterior oblique x-ray of cervical spine demonstrates multilevel neural canal stenosis from C3-4 through C6-7 secondary to chronic degenerative spur formation arising from the uncinate processes. (From Goetz CG: *Textbook of clinical neurology,* Philadelphia, 1999, WB Saunders.)

■ **ACUTE GENERAL Rx**
- NSAIDs
- "Muscle relaxants" for their sedative effect
- Analgesics as needed
- Epidural steroid injection for radicular pain

■ **DISPOSITION**
- Usually improve with time
- Surgical intervention in <5%

■ **REFERRAL**
Orthopedic or neurosurgical consultation for intractable pain or neurologic deficit

☼ PEARLS & CONSIDERATIONS

■ **COMMENTS**
- Pain relief with physical therapy seems anecdotal and short-lived; any overall improvement usually parallels what would have probably occurred naturally.

- Sometimes carpal tunnel syndrome and cervical radiculopathy occur together; this is termed the *double-crush syndrome* and results from nerve compression at two separate levels. Proximal compression may decrease the ability of the nerve to tolerate a second, more distal compression.
- Surgical intervention is indicated primarily for relief of radicular pain caused by nerve root compression or for the treatment of myelopathy; it is generally not helpful when chief complaint is neck pain alone.
- In many cases of cervical spondylosis with myelopathy, the lower-extremity symptoms are much more disabling than the neck symptoms, a situation that can cause some difficulty in determining their etiology.

REFERENCES
Albert TJ, Murrell SE: Surgical management of cervical radiculopathy, *J Am Acad Orthop Surg* 7:368, 1999.
Emery SE: Cervical spondylotic myelopathy: diagnosis and treatment, *Am Acad Orthop Surg* 9:376, 2001.
Gorski JM, Schwartz LH: Shoulder impingement presenting as neck pain, *J Bone Joint Surg* 85A:635, 2003.
Linton SJ: A review of psychological risk factors in back and neck pain, *Spine* 25:1148, 2000.
Robinson LR: Role of neurophysiologic evaluation in diagnosis, *J Am Acad Orthop Surg* 8:190, 2000.
Author: **Lonnie R. Mercier, M.D.**

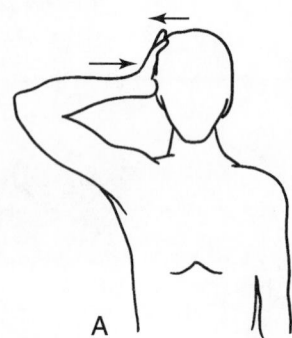 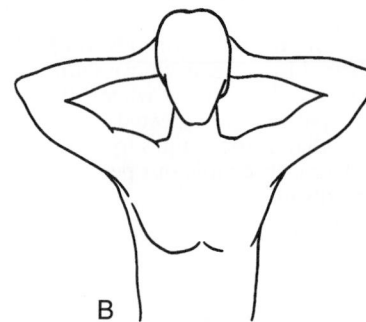 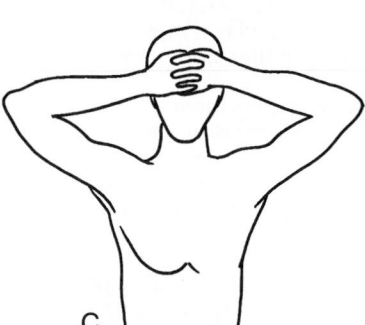

Fig. 1-64 Isometric neck exercises. A, The hand is placed against the side of the head slightly above the ear, and pressure is gradually increased while resisting with the neck muscles and keeping the head in the same position. The position is held 5 sec, relaxed, and repeated five times. **B,** The exercise is performed on the other side and then from the back and front (C). The exercise should be performed three to four times daily. (From Mercier LR [ed]: *Practical orthopedics,* ed 4, St Louis, 1995, Mosby.)

BASIC INFORMATION

■ DEFINITION

Cervical dysplasia refers to atypical development of immature squamous epithelium that does not penetrate the basement epithelial membrane. Characteristics include increased cellularity, nuclear abnormalities, and increased nuclear to cytoplasm ratio. A progressive polarized loss of squamous differentiation exists beginning adjacent to the basement membrane and progressing to the most advanced stage (severe dysplasia), which encompasses the complete squamous epithelial layer thickness (Fig. 1-65).
Classification systems:
Modified Papanicolaou: Class I, II, III, IV, and V
Dysplasia: Normal, atypia (mild, moderate, and severe), carcinoma in situ, and cancer
CIN: Normal, atypia (CIN I, II, or III), and cancer

BETHESDA 2001 UPDATED CLASSIFICATION:
Interpretation/result (including specimen adequacy)
- Negative for intraepithelial lesion or malignancy
- Organisms (i.e., *Trichomonas vaginalis, Candida* sp., bacterial vaginosis), reactive cellular changes (inflammation), atrophy
- Epithelial cell abnormalities: atypical squamous cells (ASC), of undetermined significance (ASC-US), cannot exclude HSIL (ASC-H), LSIL (CIN 1 and HPV), HSIL (CIN 2 & 3, CIS), squamous cell carcinoma
- Glandular cell abnormalities: atypical glandular cells (AGC): *(specify endocervical, endometrial, or NOS)*, atypical glandular cells, favor neoplastic *(specify endocervical, endometrial, or NOS)* endocervical adenocarcinoma in situ (AIS), adenocarcinoma
- Other: endometrial cells in a woman 40 yr of age

■ SYNONYMS

Class III or class IV Pap smear
Cervical intraepithelial neoplasia (CIN)
Low-grade or high-grade squamous intraepithelial lesion (LGSIL or HGSIL)

ICD-9CM CODES

622.1 Dysplasia of cervix (uteri)

■ EPIDEMIOLOGY & DEMOGRAPHICS

PEAK INCIDENCE:
- Age 35 yr
- Abnormal Pap smear rate revealing dysplasia approximates 2% to 5%, depending on population risk factors and false-negative rate variance
- False-negative rate approaching 40%
- Average age-adjusted incidence of severe dysplasia 35 cases/100,000 persons

PREVALENCE:
- Dysplasia: peak age, 26 yr (3600 cases/100,000 persons)
- CIS: peak age, 32 yr (1100 cases/100,000 persons)
- Invasive cancer: peak age, 77 yr (800 cases/100,000 persons)

■ PHYSICAL FINDINGS & CLINICAL PRESENTATION

- Cervical lesions associated with dysplasia usually are not visible to the naked eye; therefore physical findings are best viewed by colposcopy of a 3% acetic acid–prepared cervix.
- Patients evaluated by colposcopy are identified by abnormal cervical cytology screening from Pap smear screening
- Colposcopic findings:
  1. Leukoplakia (white lesion seen by the unaided eye that may represent condyloma, dysplasia, or cancer)
  2. Acetowhite epithelium with or without associated punctation, mosaicism, abnormal vessels
  3. Abnormal transformation zone (abnormal iodine uptake, "cuffed" gland openings)

■ ETIOLOGY

- Not clearly elucidated
- May be caused by abnormal reserve cell hyperplasia resulting in atypical metaplasia and dysplastic epithelium
- Strongly associated and initiated by oncogenic HPV infection (high-risk HPV types 16, 18, 31, 33, 35, 45, 51, 52, 56, and 58; low-risk HPV types 6, 11, 42, 43, and 44)

Risk factors:
1. Any heterosexual coitus
2. Coitus during puberty (T-zone metaplasia peak)
3. DES exposure
4. Multiple sexual partners
5. Lack of prior Pap smear screening
6. History of STD
7. Other genital tract neoplasia
8. HIV
9. TB
10. Substance abuse
11. "High-risk" male partner (HPV)
12. Low socioeconomic status
13. Early first pregnancy
14. Tobacco use
15. HPV

DIAGNOSIS

■ DIFFERENTIAL DIAGNOSIS

- Metaplasia
- Hyperkeratosis
- Condyloma
- Microinvasive carcinoma
- Glandular epithelial abnormalities
- Adenocarcinoma in situ
- VIN
- VAIN
- Metastatic tumor involvement of the cervix

■ WORKUP

Periodic history and physical examination (including cytologic screening), depending on age, risk factors, and history of preinvasive cervical lesions
- Consider screening for sexually transmitted disease (Gc, *Chlamydia,* VDRL, HIV, HPV)
- Abnormal cytology (HSIL/LSIL, initial ASC/ASC-US/ASC-H in high-risk patients, recurrent in low-risk/postmenopausal patients) and grossly evident suspicious lesions; refer for colposcopy and possible directed biopsy/ECC (examination should include cervix, vagina, vulva, and anus)
- For glandular cell abnormalities (AGC): refer for colposcopy and possible directed biopsy/ECC, and consider endometrial sampling
- In pregnancy: abnormal cytology followed by colposcopy in the first trimester and at 28 to 32 wk; only high-grade lesions suspect for cancer biopsied; ECC contraindicated

■ LABORATORY TESTS

- Gc, *Chlamydia* to rule out STD
- Pap cytology screening (requires appropriate sampling, preparation, cytologist interpretation and reporting)
- Colposcopy and directed biopsy, ECC for indications (see Workup)
- HPV-DNA typing if identified abnormal cytology

■ IMAGING STUDIES

- Cervicography
- Computer-enhanced Pap cytology screening (e.g., PAPNET)

TREATMENT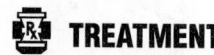

■ NONPHARMACOLOGIC THERAPY

- Superficial ablative techniques (cryosurgery, CO$_2$ laser, and electrocoagulation diathermy) considered for colposcopy-identified dysplasia (moderate to severe dysplasia or CIS) and negative ECC; mild dysplasia followed conservatively in a compliant patient

- Cone biopsy (LEEP, CO$_2$ laser, "cold knife" cone biopsy) considered for colposcopy-identified dysplasia (moderate to severe dysplasia or CIS) and positive ECC or if there is a two-grade or more discrepancy between the Pap smear, colposcopy, and biopsy or ECC findings
- Hysterectomy if patient has completed child bearing and has persistent or recurrent severe dysplasia or CIS
- In pregnancy: treatment for cervical dysplasia deferred until after delivery

■ ACUTE GENERAL Rx
Topical 5-fluorouracil (5-FU) is rarely used for recurrent cervicovaginal lesions.

■ CHRONIC Rx
- Because of the risk for persistent and recurrent dysplasia, long-term follow-up is individualized based on patient risk factors, Pap smear and colposcopy results, treatment history, and presence of high-risk HPV (e.g., Pap smear q3-4mo/yr, then q6mo/1 yr, then annually [if all normal], or repeat colposcopy examination and treat as indicated).
- Mild dysplasia with negative ECC should be followed conservatively in a compliant patient as a majority of these lesions persist or regress.

■ DISPOSITION
- Because of the large numbers of women in high-risk groups, the prevalence of HPV, and the high false-negative Pap smear rate, routine Pap smear screening should be reinforced for all women, especially those with a history of cervical dysplasia.
- Success rates for treatment approach 80% to 90%.
- Detection of persistence of recurrence requires careful follow-up.
- Cervical treatment possibly results in infertility (cervical stenosis or incompetence), which requires careful consideration and discretion for use of LEEP and cone biopsy.
- Appropriate counseling and informed consent needed when considering any form of management of cervical dysplasia.
- There has been no case of cervical dysplasia progressing to invasive cancer with appropriate screening, diagnosis, treatment, and follow-up.

■ REFERRAL
- Patients with abnormal Pap cytology should not be followed by repeat Pap smear screening.
- Patients with identified abnormal cytology should be evaluated by a skilled colposcopist (defined as documented didactic and preceptorship training including 50 cases of identified pathology, ongoing colposcopy activity with a minimum of 2 cases/wk, Q.A. log, and periodic CME).
- If treatment is required, patient should be referred to a gynecologist or gynecologic oncologist skilled in the diagnosis and treatment of preinvasive cervical disease.

☼ PEARLS & CONSIDERATIONS

■ COMMENTS
- Patient education material available from American College of Obstetricians and Gynecologists.

REFERENCES

Nuono J et al: New tests for cervical cancer screening, *Am Fam Physician* 64:780, 2001.

Schlecht NF et al: Persistent human papillomavirus infection as a predictor of cervical intraepithelial neoplasia, *JAMA* 286:3106, 2001.

Solomon D et al: Comparison of three management strategies for patients with atypical squamous cells of undetermined significance: baseline results from a randomized trial, *J Natl Cancer Inst* 93:293, 2001.

Solomon D et al: The 2001 Bethesda system terminology for reporting results of cervical cytology, *JAMA* 287:2114, 2002.

Stoler MH: New Bethesda terminology and evidence-based management guidelines for cervical cytology findings, *JAMA* 287:2140, 2002.

Wright TC et al: 2001 consensus guidelines for the management of women with cervical cytological abnormalities, *JAMA* 287:2120, 2002.

Author: **Dennis M. Weppner, M.D.**

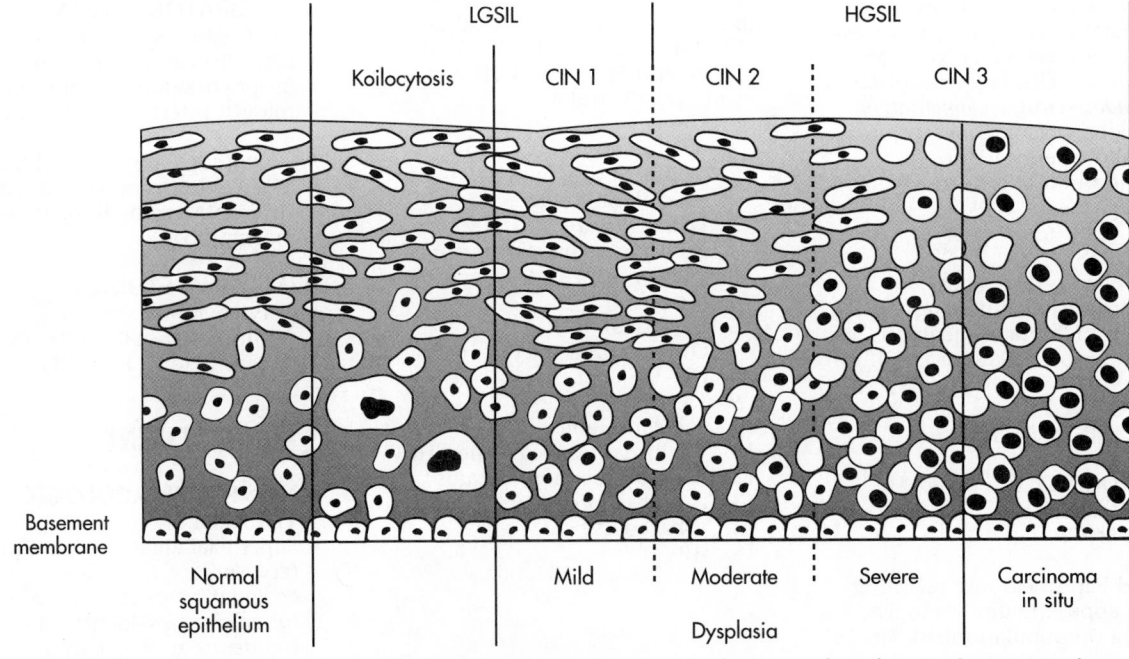

Fig. 1-65   Diagram of cervical epithelium showing various terminologies used to characterize progressive degrees of cervical epithelium. (From Mishell D [ed]: *Comprehensive gynecology,* ed 3, St Louis, 1997, Mosby.)

BASIC INFORMATION

■ DEFINITION

A cervical polyp is a growth protruding from the cervix or endocervical canal. Polyps that arise from the endocervical canal are called *endocervical polyps*. If they arise from the ectocervix, they are called *cervical polyps*.

ICD-9CM CODES
622.7 Mucous polyp of cervix

■ EPIDEMIOLOGY & DEMOGRAPHICS

Cervical polyps are common. Found in approximately 4% of all gynecologic patients. Most commonly present in perimenopausal and multigravid women between the ages of 30 and 50 yr. Endocervical polyps are more common than cervical polyps and are almost always benign (Fig. 1-66). Malignant degeneration is extremely rare.

■ PHYSICAL FINDINGS & CLINICAL PRESENTATION

Polyps may be single or multiple and vary in size from being extremely small (a few mm) to large (4 cm). They are soft, smooth, reddish-purple to cherry-red in color. They bleed easily when touched. Very large polyps can cause some cervical dilation. There may be vaginal discharge associated with cervical polyps if the polyp has become infected.

■ ETIOLOGY
• Most unknown
• Inflammatory
• Traumatic
• Pregnancy

DIAGNOSIS

■ DIFFERENTIAL DIAGNOSIS
• Endometrial polyp
• Prolapsed myoma
• Retained products of conception
• Squamous papilloma
• Sarcoma
• Cervical malignancy

■ WORKUP

Polyps are most commonly asymptomatic and are usually found at the time of annual gynecologic pelvic examination. Polyps are also found in women who present for evaluation of intermenstrual or postcoital bleeding and for profuse vaginal discharge. Polyps are painless. Unless a patient has a bleeding abnormality that necessitates her being evaluated by a physician, polyps would go undiagnosed until her next Pap smear was obtained.

TREATMENT

■ NONPHARMACOLOGIC THERAPY

Simple surgical excision can be done in the office. The physician should be prepared for bleeding, which can easily be controlled with silver nitrate or Monsel's solution. Most commonly, a polyp is excised by grasping it at the stalk and twisting it off. Polyps can also be excised by electrocautery or, in the case of very large polyps, in an outpatient surgical suite. Sexual intercourse and tampon usage are to be avoided until the patient's follow-up visit. Also, douching is not to be performed.

■ ACUTE GENERAL Rx
Generally, no medication is needed.

■ CHRONIC Rx
Patient is followed up in 2 wk for recheck of the surgical excision site unless there is active bleeding, in which case she would be seen immediately. The cervix should be checked at the patient's routine gynecologic visits.

■ DISPOSITION
Because these are almost always benign, usually no further treatment is needed. Annual gynecologic examinations should be performed to check for any regrowths.

■ REFERRAL
To a gynecologist for removal of polyps

PEARLS & CONSIDERATIONS

■ COMMENTS
A Pap smear should be obtained before removing the polyp. If an abnormal Pap smear is obtained, more than likely the cause will be secondary to the polyp. If a colposcopic evaluation is needed, this should also be performed. During pregnancy, the cervix is highly vascularized. If the polyps are stable and benign-appearing, they should just be observed during the pregnancy and removed only if they are causing bleeding.

REFERENCES

Copeland L: *Textbook of gynecology,* ed 2, Baltimore, 1999, Saunders.

Endo H et al: Cervical polyp with eccrine syringofibroadenoma-like features, *Histopathology* 42(3):301, 2003.

Rupke S: Family practice forum: clinical medicine. Evaluation and management of cervical polyps, *Hosp Pract* 33(6):81, 1998.

Scott PM: Procedures in family practice. Performing cervical polypectomy, *JAAPA* 12(6):81, 1999.

Author: **George T. Danakas, M.D.**

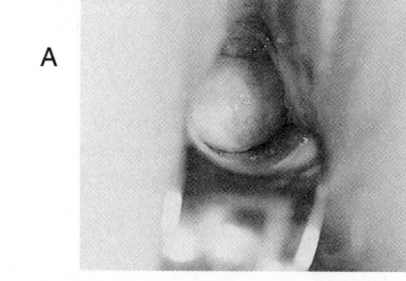
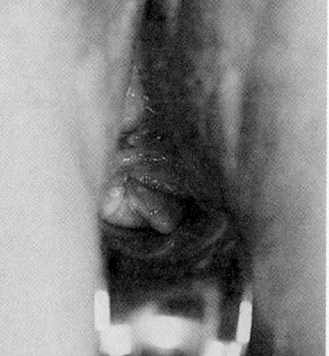

Fig. 1-66   A, Fibroid polyp protruding through the external cervical os. **B,** Small endocervical polyp. (From Symonds EM, Macpherson MBA: *Color atlas of obstetrics and gynecology,* St Louis, 1994, Mosby.)

BASIC INFORMATION

■ **DEFINITION**
Cervicitis is an infection of the cervix. It may result from direct infection of the cervix, or it may be secondary to uterine or vaginal infection.

■ **SYNONYMS**
Endocervicitis
Ectocervicitis
Mucopurulent cervicitis

ICD-9CM CODES
616.0 Cervicitis
098.15 Acute gonococcal cervicitis
079.8 Chlamydia infection

■ **EPIDEMIOLOGY & DEMOGRAPHICS**
Cervicitis accounts for 20% to 25% of patients presenting with abnormal vaginal discharge, and this affects women only. It is most common in adolescents, but it can be found in any sexually active woman. Practicing unsafe sex with multiple sexual partners increases the risk of developing cervicitis, as well as other sexually transmitted diseases.

■ **PHYSICAL FINDINGS**
Cervicitis is usually asymptomatic or associated with mild symptoms. Copious purulent or mucopurulent in vaginal discharge (Fig. 1-67), pelvic pain, and dyspareunia may be present if cervicitis is severe. The cervix can be erythematous and tender on palpation during bimanual examination. The cervix may also bleed easily when obtaining cultures or a Pap smear. May have postcoital bleeding.

■ **ETIOLOGY**
- *Chlamydia*
- *Trichomonas*
- *Neisseria gonorrhoeae*
- Herpes simplex
- *Trichomonas vaginalis*
- Human papillomavirus

🔬 **DIAGNOSIS**

■ **DIFFERENTIAL DIAGNOSIS**
- Carcinoma of the cervix
- Cervical erosion
- Cervical metaplasia

■ **WORKUP**
The patient usually presents with a vaginal discharge or history of postcoital bleeding. Otherwise the patient is diagnosed asymptomatically during routine examination. On examination there is gross visualization of yellow, mucopurulent material on the cotton swab.

■ **LABORATORY TESTS**
On a smear there will be ten or more polymorphonuclear leukocytes per microscopic field. Positive Gram stain is found. Cultures should be obtained for *Chlamydia* and *N. gonorrhoeae*. Use a wet mount to look for trichomonads. Obtain a Pap smear.

💊 **TREATMENT**

■ **NONPHARMACOLOGIC THERAPY**
Cervicitis is treated in an outpatient setting. Cryosurgery is an option for treatment of cervicitis with negative cultures and negative biopsies. Safe sex should be practiced with the use of condoms. Partners should be treated in all cases of infection proven by culture.

■ **ACUTE GENERAL Rx**
Because *Chlamydia* and *N. gonorrhoeae* make up >50% of the cause of infectious cervicitis, if it is suspected, treat without waiting for culture results. Administer ceftriaxone 125-mg IM single dose followed by doxycycline 100 mg PO bid for 7 days. If the patient is pregnant, treat with azithromycin (Zithromax) 1-g single dose instead of using doxycycline, which is contraindicated in pregnant or nursing mothers. Alternative treatments include: erythromycin base 500 mg PO qid for 7 days, erythromycin ethylsuccinate 800 mg PO qid for 7 days, ofloxacin 300 mg PO bid for 7 days, or levofloxacin 500 mg PO qd for 7 days. If *Trichomonas* is the etiologic agent, treat with metronidazole 2-g single dose. For herpes, treat with acyclovir 200 mg PO five times daily for 7 days.

■ **DISPOSITION**
Cervicitis responds well to antibiotics. Possible complications to watch for are a subsequent PID and infertility (found in 5% to 10% of patients). Repeat cultures should be performed after treatment. Sexual relations can be resumed after negative cultures.

■ **REFERRAL**
If subsequent PID develops, consider hospital admission for IV antibiotics.

🔆 **PEARLS & CONSIDERATIONS**

■ **COMMENTS**
Patient educational material can be obtained from local health clinics and clinics for sexually transmitted diseases.

REFERENCE
Centers for Disease Control and Prevention: 2002 sexually transmitted diseases treatment guidelines, *MMWR Morb Mortal Wkly Rep* 51(RR-6), 2002.
Author: **George T. Danakas, M.D.**

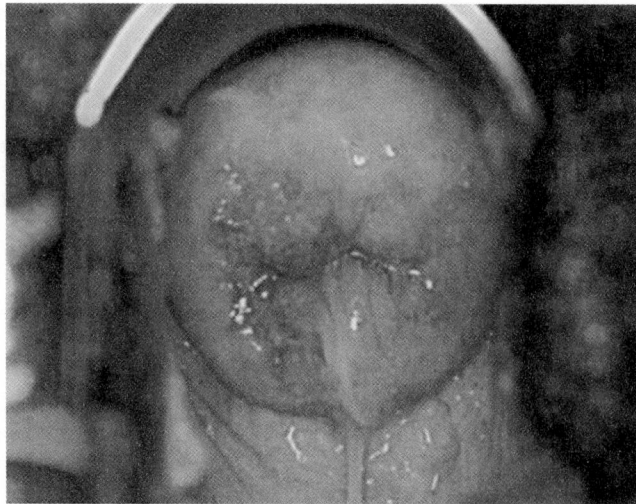

Fig. 1-67 Colposcopy of a woman with mucopurulent cervicitis and purulent discharge from endocervical os. (Courtesy Dr. David Soper, Richmond, VA. From Mandell GL [ed]: *Mandell, Douglas, and Bennett's principles and practice of infectious diseases,* ed 5, New York, 2000, Churchill Livingstone.)

BASIC INFORMATION

■ DEFINITION

Chagas' disease is an infection caused by the protozoan parasite *Trypanosoma cruzi*. The disease is characterized by an acute nonspecific febrile illness that may be followed, after a variable latency period, by chronic cardiac, GI, and neurologic sequelae.

■ SYNONYMS

American trypanosomiasis

ICD-9CM CODES

086.2 Chagas' disease

■ EPIDEMIOLOGY & DEMOGRAPHICS

INCIDENCE (IN U.S.):
- Four cases of autochthonous transmission in California and Texas
- In the last two decades, six cases of laboratory-acquired infection, three cases of transfusion-associated transmission, and nine cases of imported disease reported to the Centers for Disease Control and Prevention (none of the imported cases involving returning tourists)

PREVALENCE (IN U.S.): Based on regional seroprevalence studies in Hispanic blood donors, it is estimated that between 50,000 and 100,000 persons infected with *T. cruzi* are currently residing in the U.S.

PREDOMINANT SEX: Male = female

PREDOMINANT AGE:
- In highly endemic areas, mean age of acute infection: approximately 4 yr old
- Variable age distribution for both types of chronic disease, depending on geography
- Mean age of onset: usually between 35 and 45 yr

PEAK INCIDENCE: Unknown

GENETICS:

Congenital Infection: Congenital transmission has been documented with attendant high fetal mortality and morbidity in surviving infants.

Neonatal Infection: In rural areas, within substandard housing, transmission is likely to occur.

■ PHYSICAL FINDINGS & CLINICAL PRESENTATION

- Inflammatory lesion that develops about 1 wk after contamination of a break in the skin with infected insect feces (chagoma)
  1. Area of induration and erythema
  2. Usually accompanied by local lymphadenopathy
- Presence of Romaña's sign, which consists of unilateral painless palpebral and periocular edema, when conjunctiva is portal of entry

- Constitutional symptoms of fever, fatigue, and anorexia, along with edema of the face and lower extremities, generalized lymphadenopathy, and mild hepatosplenomegaly after the appearance of local signs of disease
- Myocarditis in a small portion of patients, sometimes with resultant CHF
- Uncommonly, CNS disease, such as meningoencephalitis, which carries a poor prognosis
- Symptoms and signs of disease persisting for weeks to months, followed by spontaneous resolution of the acute illness; patient then in the indeterminate phase of the disease (asymptomatic with attendant subpatent parasitemia and reactive antibodies to *T. cruzi* antigens)
- Chronic disease may become manifest years to decades after the initial infection:
  1. Most common organ involved: heart, followed by GI tract, and to a much lesser extent the CNS
     a. Cardiac involvement takes the form of arrhythmias or cardiomyopathy, but rarely both.
     b. Cardiomyopathy is bilateral but predominantly affects the right ventricle and is often accompanied by apical aneurysms and mural thrombi.
     c. Arrhythmias are a consequence of involvement of the bundle of His and have been implicated as the leading cause of sudden death in adults in highly endemic areas.
     d. Right-sided heart failure, thromboembolization, and rhythm disturbances associated with symptoms of dizziness and syncope are characteristic.
  2. Patients with megaesophagus: dysphasia, odynophagia, chronic cough, and regurgitation, frequently resulting in aspiration pneumonitis
  3. Megacolon: abdominal pain and chronic constipation, which, when severe, may lead to obstruction and perforation
  4. CNS symptoms: most often secondary to embolization from the heart or varying degrees of peripheral neuropathy

■ ETIOLOGY

- *T. cruzi*
  1. Found only in the Americas, ranging from the southern half of the U.S. to southern Argentina
  2. Transmitted to humans by various species of bloodsucking reduviid ("kissing") insects, primarily those of the genera *Triatoma, Panstrongylus,* and *Rhodnius*

  3. Usually found in burrows and trees where infected insects transmit the parasite to nonhuman mammals (e.g., opossums and armadillos), which constitute the natural reservoir
  4. Intrusion into enzootic areas for farmland, allowing insects to take up residence in rural dwellings, thus including humans and domestic animals in the cycle of transmission
  5. Initial infection of insects by ingesting blood from animals or humans that have circulating flagellated trypanosomes (trypomastigotes)
  6. Multiplication of ingested parasites in the insect midgut as epimastigotes, then differentiation into infective metacyclic trypomastigotes in the hindgut whereby the parasites are discharged with the feces during subsequent blood meals
  7. Transmission to the second mammalian host through contamination of mucous membranes, conjunctivae, or wounds with insect feces containing infected forms
- In the vertebrate host
  1. Movement of parasites into various cell types, intracellular transformation and multiplication in the cytoplasm as amastigotes, and thereafter differentiation into trypomastigotes
  2. Following rupture of the cell membrane, parasitic invasion of local tissues or hematogenous spread to distant sites, maintaining a parasitemia infective for vectors
- In addition to insect vectors, *T. cruzi* is transmitted through blood transfusions, transplacentally, and, occasionally, secondary to laboratory accidents

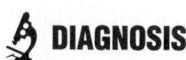

DIAGNOSIS

■ DIFFERENTIAL DIAGNOSIS

Acute disease
- Early African trypanosomiasis
- New World cutaneous and mucocutaneous leishmaniasis

Chronic disease
- Idiopathic cardiomyopathy
- Idiopathic achalasia
- Congenital or acquired megacolon

■ WORKUP

Principal considerations in diagnosis:
- A history of residence where transmission is known to occur
- Recent receipt of a blood product while in an endemic area
- Occupational exposure in a laboratory

■ LABORATORY TESTS

For acute diagnosis:
- Demonstration of *T. cruzi* in wet preparations of blood, buffy coat, or Giemsa-stained smears
- Xenodiagnosis, a technique involving laboratory-reared insect vectors fed on subjects with suspected infection thereafter examined for parasites, and culture of body fluids in liquid media to establish diagnosis
  1. Hampered by the length of time required for completion
  2. Of limited use in clinical decision making with regard to drug therapy
  3. Although xenodiagnosis and broth culture are considered to be more sensitive than microscopic examination of body fluids, sensitivities may not exceed 50%
- Recent advances in serologic testing include immunoblot assay, in situ indirect fluorescent antibody, PCR-based techniques, and an immunochromatographic assay (Chagas Stat Pak)

For chronic *T. cruzi* infection:
- Traditional serologic tests including: complement fixation (CF), indirect immunofluorescence (IIF), indirect hemagglutination, enzyme-linked immunosorbent assay (ELISA), and radioimmune precipitation assay
- Persistent problem with these tests: in addition to sensitivity and specificity, false-positive results
- Saliva ELISA may be useful as a screening diagnostic test in epidemiologic studies of chronic trypanosomiasis infection in endemic areas

℞ TREATMENT

■ NONPHARMACOLOGIC THERAPY

- Chronic chagasic heart disease: mainly supportive
- Megaesophagus: symptoms usually amenable to dietary measures or pneumonic dilation of the esophagogastric junction
- Chagasic megacolon: in its early stages responsive to a high-fiber diet, laxatives, and enemas

■ ACUTE GENERAL Rx

Nifurtimox (Lampit, Bayer 2502):
- Only drug available in the U.S. for the treatment of acute, congenital, or laboratory-acquired infection
- Recommended oral dosage for adults: 8 to 10 mg/kg/day given in four divided daily doses and continued for 90 to 120 days
- Parasitologic cure in approximately 50% of those treated; should be begun as early as possible

Benznidazole, a nitroimidazole derivative:
- Has demonstrated similar efficacy as nifurtimox in limited trials
- Recommended oral dosage: 5 mg/kg/day for 60 days

■ CHRONIC Rx

- In patients with indeterminate phase or chronic disease: no evidence of benefit with pharmacologic therapy
- In patients exhibiting bradyarrhythmias: pacemakers
- In individuals with congestive heart failure:
  1. Treat with modalities appropriate for dilated, especially right-sided, cardiomyopathic disease.
  2. Cardiac transplant is a controversial alternative for end-stage cardiomyopathy; however, reactivation rate found to be low and amenable to therapy without subsequent infection of the allograft in one study.
  3. Myotomy or esophageal resection is reserved for patients with advanced disease.
- In advanced chagasic megacolon associated with chronic fecal impaction, perforation, or, less commonly, volvulus: surgical resection

■ DISPOSITION

Based on few prospective studies, most patients infected with *T. cruzi* will not develop symptomatic Chagas' disease.

■ REFERRAL

- For consultation with an infectious disease specialist or communication with the Centers for Disease Control and Prevention when the disease is acutely suspected
- To a cardiologist for pacemaker implantation for patients with bradyarrhythmias
- To a surgeon for symptomatic disease in individuals with chagasic megaesophagus or megacolon

⚙ PEARLS & CONSIDERATIONS

■ COMMENTS

- In recipients of solid organ or bone marrow transplants, patients with AIDS, or those receiving chemotherapy, there may be reactivation of indeterminate phase disease.
- Mortality predictors associated with chagasic cardiomyopathy include CHF, QT-interval dispersion, left ventricular (LV) end-systolic dimension, the presence of pathological Q waves, frequent PVCs, and isolated LAFB on ECG.
- Patients with chagasic esophageal disease have an increased incidence of esophageal malignancy.
- The use of pyrethroid-impregnated curtains may represent an option for the reduction or elimination of Chagas' disease transmission in certain endemic areas.
- A recent study suggests that male gender and detection of *T. cruzi* DNA in serum by PCR may portend a higher risk of progression for chronic cardiomyopathy.

REFERENCES

Basquiera AL et al.: Risk progression to chronic Chagas cardiomyopathy: influence of male sex and of parasitemia detected by polymerase chain reaction, *Heart* 89(10):1186, 2003.

Herber O, Kroeger A: Pyrethroid-impregnated curtains for Chagas' disease control in Venezuela, *Acta Trop* 88(1):33, 2003.

Higuchi Mde L et al: Pathophysiology of the heart in Chagas' disease: current status and new developments, *Cardiovasc Res* 60(1):96, 2003.

Luquetti AO et al: Chagas' disease diagnosis: a multicentric evaluation of Chagas Stat-Pak, a rapid immunochromatographic assay with recombinant proteins of Trypanosoma cruzi, *Diagn Microbiol Infect Dis* 46(4):265, 2003.

Salles G et al: Prognostic value of QT interval parameters for mortality risk stratification in Chagas' disease: results of a long-term follow-up study, *Circulation* 108 (3):305, 2003.

Urbina JA, Docampo R: Specific chemotherapy of Chagas disease: controversies and advances, *Trends Parasitol* 19(11):495, 2003.

Author: **George O. Alonso, M.D.**

BASIC INFORMATION

■ DEFINITION
Chancroid is a sexually transmitted disease characterized by painful genital ulceration and inflammatory inguinal adenopathy.

■ SYNONYMS
Soft chancre
Ulcus molle

ICD-9CM CODES
099.0 Chancroid

■ EPIDEMIOLOGY & DEMOGRAPHICS
- Exact incidence is unknown.
- Occurs more frequently in men (male:female ratio of 10:1).
- Clinical infection is rare in women.
- There is a higher incidence in uncircumcised men and in tropical and subtropical regions.
- Incubation period is 4 to 7 days but may take up to 3 wk.
- High incidence of HIV infection associated with chancroid.

■ PHYSICAL FINDINGS & CLINICAL PRESENTATION
- One to three extremely painful ulcers (Fig. 1-68), accompanied by tender inguinal lymphadenopathy (especially if fluctuant)
- May present with inguinal bubo and several ulcers
- In women: initial lesion in the fourchette, labia minora, urethra, cervix, or anus; inflammatory pustule or papule that ruptures, leaving a shallow, nonindurated shallow ulceration, usually 1- to 2-cm diameter with ragged, undermined edges
- Unilateral lymphadenopathy develops 1 wk later in 50% of patients

■ ETIOLOGY
Haemophilus ducreyi, a bacillus

 DIAGNOSIS

■ DIFFERENTIAL DIAGNOSIS
- Other genitoulcerative diseases such as syphilis, herpes, LGV, granuloma inguinale
- A clinical algorithm for the initial management of genital ulcer disease is described in Section III

■ WORKUP
Diagnosis based on history and physical examination is often inadequate. Must rule out syphilis in women because of the consequences of inappropriate therapy in pregnant women. Base initial diagnosis and treatment recommendations on clinical impression of appearance of ulcer and most likely diagnosis for population. Definitive diagnosis is made by isolation of organism from ulcers by culture or Gram stain.

■ LABORATORY TESTS
Darkfield microscopy, RPR, HSV cultures, *H. ducreyi* culture, HIV testing recommended

 TREATMENT

■ NONPHARMACOLOGIC THERAPY
Fluctuant nodes should be aspirated through healthy adjacent skin to prevent formation of draining sinus. I&D not recommended, delays healing. Use warm compresses to remove necrotic material.

■ ACUTE GENERAL Rx
- Azithromycin 1 g PO (single dose) *or*
- Ceftriaxone 250 mg IM (single dose) *or*
- Ciprofloxacin 500 mg PO bid for 3 days *or*
- Erythromycin 500 mg PO qid for 7 days
NOTE: Ciprofloxacin is contraindicated in patients who are pregnant, lactating, or <18 yr.
- HIV-infected patients may need more prolonged therapy

■ DISPOSITION
- All sexual partners should be treated with a 10-day course of one of the previous regimens (see Acute General Rx).
- Patients should be reexamined 3 to 7 days after initiation of therapy. Ulcers should improve symptomatically within 3 days and objectively within 7 days after initiation of successful therapy.

☼ PEARLS & CONSIDERATIONS

■ COMMENTS
In the U.S. HSV-1 and syphilis are the most common causes of genital ulcers, followed by chancroid, LGV, and granuloma inguinale.

REFERENCE
Centers for Disease Control and Prevention: 2002 sexually transmitted diseases treatment guidelines, *MMWR Morb Mortal Wkly Rep* 51(RR-6), 2002.
Author: **Maria A. Corigliano, M.D.**

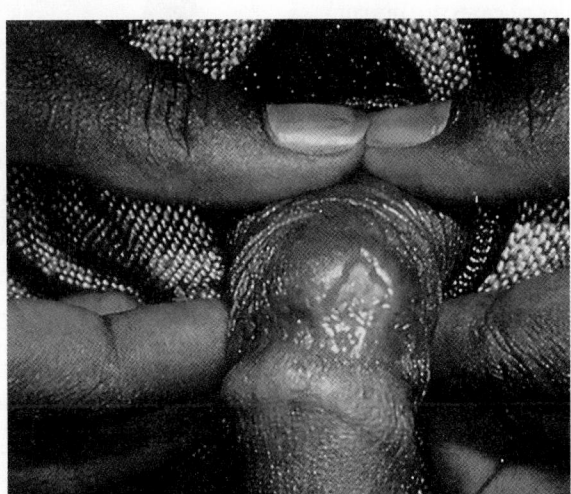

Fig. 1-68 Chancroid. Note shaggy, ragged-edged ulcer with edema and exudative base. (Courtesy Beverly Sanders, M.D. From Goldstein B [ed]: *Practical dermatology,* ed 2, St Louis, 1997, Mosby.)

BASIC INFORMATION

■ DEFINITION

Charcot-Marie-Tooth disease is a heterogeneous group of noninflammatory inherited peripheral neuropathies. It is the most common inherited neuromuscular disorder.

■ SYNONYMS

Peroneal muscular atrophy
Hereditary motor and sensory neuropathy (HMSN)
Idiopathic dominantly inherited hypertrophic polyneuropathy

ICD-9CM CODES

356.1 Charcot-Marie-Tooth disease, paralysis, or syndrome

■ EPIDEMIOLOGY & DEMOGRAPHICS

PREDOMINANT AGE: Onset usually 10 to 20 yr but can be delayed to 50 to 60 yr
PREDOMINANT SEX: Male:female ratio of 3:1

■ PHYSICAL FINDINGS & CLINICAL PRESENTATION

- Variable presentation from family to family, but affected individuals in a family tend to have similar symptomatology
- Usually, gradual onset, with slowly progressive disorder
- Foot deformity producing a high arch (cavus) and hammertoes
- Atrophy of the lower legs producing a stork-like appearance (muscle wasting does not involve the upper legs) (Fig. 1-69)
- Nerve enlargement
- Sensory loss or other neurologic signs, although the sensory involvement is usually mild
- Scoliosis
- Decreased proprioception that often interferes with balance and gait
- Painful paresthesias
- In late cases, possible involvement of hands
- Absence of DTRs in many cases
- Poorly healing foot ulcers in some patients

■ ETIOLOGY

Chronic segmental demyelination of peripheral nerves with hypertrophic changes caused by remyelination

DIAGNOSIS

■ DIFFERENTIAL DIAGNOSIS

- Other inherited neuropathies
- Toxic, metabolic, and nutritional polyneuropathies

■ WORKUP

- The early onset, slow progression, and familial nature of the disorder are usually sufficient to establish diagnosis.
- Electrophysiologic studies are often diagnostic and may also be helpful in defining various subtypes of this group of neuropathies.
- Occasionally, muscle and nerve (sural) biopsy may be required.

TREATMENT

■ ACUTE GENERAL Rx

- Genetic counseling
- Supportive physical therapy and occupational therapy
- Prevention of injury to limbs with diminished sensibility
- Bracing

■ CHRONIC Rx

Occasionally, surgery to add stability and restore a plantigrade foot

■ DISPOSITION

- Disability is usually mild and compatible with a long life.
- 10% to 20% of patients are asymptomatic.
- A small number of cases are nonambulators by the sixth or seventh decade.
- The condition is usually not life threatening.

■ REFERRAL

- For orthopedic consultation for bracing and treatment of deformity
- For genetic counseling

☼ PEARLS & CONSIDERATIONS

■ COMMENTS

Patient information on Charcot-Marie-Tooth disease is available from the Muscular Dystrophy Association, 3300 East Sunrise Drive, Tucson, Arizona 85718; phone: 1-800-572-1717.

REFERENCES

Gemiynani F, Marbini A: Charcot-Marie-Tooth disease (CMT) distinctive phenotypic and genotypic features in CMT type 2, *J Neurol Sci* 184:1, 2001.
Guyton GP, Mann RA: The pathogenesis and surgical management of foot deformity in Charcot-Marie-Tooth disease, *Foot Ankle Clin* 5:317, 2000.
Author: **Lonnie R. Mercier, M.D.**

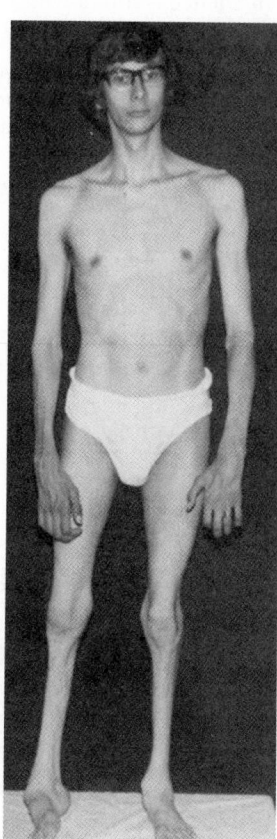

Fig. 1-69 Patient with Charcot-Marie-Tooth disease showing marked wasting of calf muscles and intrinsic foot muscles. (From Dubowitz V: *Muscle disorders in childhood,* London, 1995, WB Saunders. In Goetz CG: *Textbook of clinical neurology,* Philadelphia, 1999, WB Saunders.)

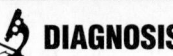 **BASIC INFORMATION**

■ DEFINITION

Charcot's joint is a chronic, progressive joint degeneration, often devastating, seen most commonly in peripheral weight-bearing joints and vertebrae, which develops as a result of the loss of normal sensory innervation of the joint. It was described by Charcot as a result of tabes dorsalis.

■ SYNONYMS

Neuropathic arthropathy

ICD-9CM CODES

094.0 Charcot's arthropathy

■ EPIDEMIOLOGY & DEMOGRAPHICS

PREVALENCE:
- 1 case/750 patients with diabetes mellitus; 5 cases/100 of those with peripheral neuropathy (foot is most commonly involved)
- 20% to 40% of patients with syringomyelia (shoulder most commonly involved)
- 5% to 10% of patients with tabes dorsalis; usually >60 yr (spine, hip, and knee most commonly involved)

■ PHYSICAL FINDINGS & CLINICAL PRESENTATION

Neuropathic joint disease is relatively painless, often in spite of considerable destruction
- Often, diffusely warm, swollen, and occasionally erythematous involved joint, the latter suggesting sepsis
- Possible progression of joint instability; palpable osseous debris; crepitus common
- Often, frank dislocation, leading to bony deformity, especially in more superficial joints

■ ETIOLOGY

The most widely accepted theory is the "neurotraumatic" theory:
- Impairment and loss of joint sensitivity decreases the protective mechanism about the joint.
- Rapid destruction occurs.
- Chronic inflammation and repetitive effusions develop, eventually contributing to joint instability and incongruity.

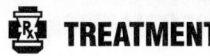 **DIAGNOSIS**

■ DIFFERENTIAL DIAGNOSIS

- Osteomyelitis, cellulitis, abscess
- Infectious arthritis
- Osteoarthritis
- Rheumatoid and other inflammatory arthritides

■ WORKUP

- An underlying neurologic disorder must always be present.
- Diabetes mellitus with peripheral neuropathy is the most common cause (Fig. 1-70).
- Syringomyelia, tabes dorsalis, Charcot-Marie-Tooth disease, congenital indifference to pain, alcoholism, and spinal dysraphism can all lead to the disorder.

■ LABORATORY TESTS

In questionable cases, aspiration, sometimes including biopsy, to rule out sepsis

■ IMAGING STUDIES

Plain roentgenography
- Sufficient to establish diagnosis in most cases, especially if etiology is known
- Findings: variable degrees of destruction and dislocation

TREATMENT

■ ACUTE GENERAL Rx

- Protection of effusions, sprains, and fractures until all hyperemic response has resolved
- Braces, special shoes with molded inserts, and elevation of the extremity
- Patient education with avoidance of weight bearing when lower extremity joints are involved
- Surgery: only limited value

■ DISPOSITION

Once the full-blown neuropathic joint has developed, treatment is difficult.

REFERENCES

Guyton GP, Saltzman CL: The diabetic foot: basic mechanisms of disease, *Instr Course Lect* 51:169, 2002.
Pakarinen TK et al: Charcot arthropathy of the diabetic foot: current concepts and review of 36 cases, *Scand J Surg* 91:195, 2002.
Pinzur MS et al: Current practice patterns in the treatment of Charcot foot, *Foot Ankle Int* 21:916, 2000.
Author: **Lonnie R. Mercier, M.D.**

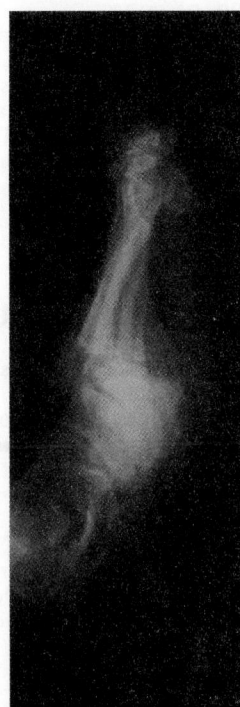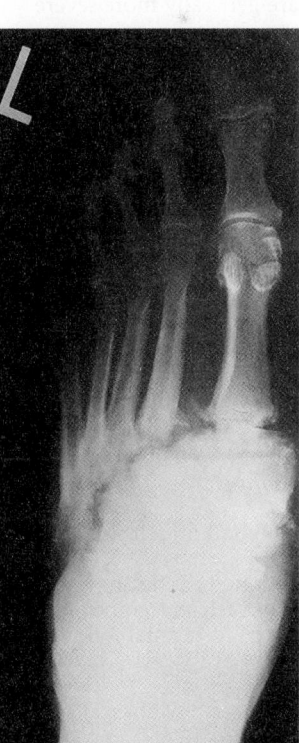

Fig. 1-70 Diabetes mellitus and neuropathic arthritis. Note lateral displacement of metatarsals (*left*) and fragmentation and osseous debris (*right*). (From Goldman L, Bennett JC [eds]: *Cecil textbook of medicine,* ed 21, Philadelphia, 2000, WB Saunders.)

BASIC INFORMATION

◾ DEFINITION

Chickenpox is a common viral illness characterized by acute onset of generalized vesicular rash and fever.

◾ SYNONYMS

Varicella

◾ ICD-9CM CODES

052.9 Varicella

◾ EPIDEMIOLOGY & DEMOGRAPHICS

- Chickenpox is extremely contagious. More than 90% of unvaccinated contacts become infected.
- The incubation period of chickenpox ranges from 9 to 21 days.
- Peak incidence is in the springtime.
- The predominant age is 5 to 10 yr.
- Infectious period begins 2 days before onset of clinical symptoms and lasts until all lesions have crusted.
- Most patients will have lifelong immunity following an attack of chickenpox; protection from chickenpox following varicella vaccine is approximately 6 yr.

◾ PHYSICAL FINDINGS & CLINICAL PRESENTATION

- Findings vary with the clinical course. Initial symptoms consist of fever, chills, backache, generalized malaise, and headache.
- Symptoms are generally more severe in adults.
- Initial lesions generally occur on the trunk (centripetal distribution) and occasionally on the face; these lesions consist primarily of 3- to 4-mm red papules with an irregular outline and a clear vesicle on the surface (dew drops on a rose petal appearance).
- Intense pruritus generally accompanies this stage.
- New lesion development generally ceases by the fourth day with subsequent crusting by the sixth day.
- Lesions generally spread to the face and the extremities (centrifugal spread).
- Patients generally present with lesions at different stages at the same time.
- Crusts generally fall off within 5 to 14 days.
- Fever is usually highest during the eruption of the vesicles; temperature generally returns to normal following disappearance of vesicles.

- Signs of potential complications (e.g., bacterial skin infections, neurologic complications, pneumonia, hepatitis) may be present on physical examination.
- Mild constitutional symptoms (e.g., anorexia, myalgias, headaches, restlessness) may be present (most common in adults).
- Excoriations may be present if scratching is prominent.

◾ ETIOLOGY

Varicella-zoster virus (VZV) is a human herpes virus III that can manifest with either varicella or herpes zoster (i.e., shingles, which is a reactivation of varicella).

DIAGNOSIS

◾ DIFFERENTIAL DIAGNOSIS

- Other viral infection
- Impetigo
- Scabies
- Drug rash
- Urticaria
- Dermatitis herpetiformis
- Smallpox

◾ WORKUP

Diagnosis is usually made based on patient's history and clinical presentation.

◾ LABORATORY TESTS

- Laboratory evaluation is generally not necessary.
- CBC may reveal leukopenia and thrombocytopenia.
- Serum varicella titers (significant rise in serum varicella IgG antibody level), skin biopsy, or Tzanck smear are used only when diagnosis is in question.

TREATMENT

◾ NONPHARMACOLOGIC THERAPY

- Use antipruritic lotions for symptomatic relief.
- Avoid scratching to prevent excoriations and superficial skin infections.
- Use a mild soap for bathing; hands should be washed often.

◾ ACUTE GENERAL Rx

- Use acetaminophen for fever and myalgias; aspirin should be avoided because of the increased risk of Reye's syndrome.

- Oral acyclovir (20 mg/kg qid for 5 days) initiated at the earliest sign (within 24 hr of illness) is useful in healthy, nonpregnant individuals 13 yr of age or older to decrease the duration and severity of signs and symptoms. Immunocompromised hosts should be treated with IV acyclovir 500 mg/m^2 or 10 mg/kg q8h IV for 7 to 10 days.
- Varicella-zoster immunoglobulin (VZIG) is effective in preventing chickenpox in susceptible individuals. Dose is 12.5 U/kg IM (up to a maximum of 625 U). May repeat dose 3 wk later if the exposure persists; VZIG must be administered as early as possible after presumed exposure.
- Varicella vaccine is available for children and adults; protection lasts at least 6 yr. Patients with HIV or other immunocompromised patients should not receive the live attenuated vaccine.
- Pruritus from chickenpox can be controlled with antihistamines (e.g., hydroxyzine 25 mg q6h) and oral antipruritic lotions (e.g., calamine).
- Oral antibiotics are not routinely indicated and should be used only in patients with secondary infection and infected lesions (most common infective organisms are *Streptococcus* sp. and *Staphylococcus* sp.).

◾ DISPOSITION

- The course is generally benign in immunocompetent adults and children.
- Infants who develop chickenpox are incapable of controlling the infection and should be given varicella-zoster immunoglobulin or γ-globulin if VZIG is not available.

◾ REFERRAL

Hospitalization and IV acyclovir are recommended for immunocompromised patients with chickenpox and for patients who develop neurologic complications or pneumonia.

PEARLS & CONSIDERATIONS

◾ COMMENTS

- VZIG can be obtained from the nearest regional Red Cross Blood Center or the Centers for Disease Control and Prevention in Atlanta, Georgia.
- Varicella immunization (Varivax) is recommended for all who have not had chickenpox; dosage for adults and adolescents (>13 yr old) is two 0.5-ml doses 4 to 8 wk apart.

Author: **Fred F. Ferri, M.D.**

BASIC INFORMATION

■ DEFINITION

Genital infection with *Chlamydia trachomatis* may result in urethritis, epididymitis, cervicitis, and acute salpingitis, but often it is asymptomatic in women (see "Pelvic Inflammatory Disease"). In men, urethritis, mucopurulent discharge, dysuria, urethral pruritus.

ICD-9CM CODES
597.80 Urethritis
604.0 Epididymitis
616.0 Cervicitis
381.51 Acute salpingitis

■ EPIDEMIOLOGY & DEMOGRAPHICS

• *Chlamydia trachomatis* is the most common cause of sexually transmitted disease in the U.S. More than 4 million infections occur annually, although the exact number is unknown because reporting is not required in all states. Occurrence is common worldwide, and recognition has been increasing steadily over the last two decades in the U.S., Canada, Australia, and Europe.
• Most women with endocervical or urethral infections are asymptomatic.
• Up to 45% of cases of gonococcal infection may have concomitant chlamydial infection.
• Infertility or ectopic pregnancy can result as a complication from symptomatic or asymptomatic chronic infections of the endometrium and fallopian tubes.
• Conjunctival and pneumonic infection of the newborn may result from infection in pregnancy.
• In men 15% to 55% of cases are of *C. trachomatis*. Complications of nongonococcal urethritis in men infected with *C. trachomatis* include epididymitis and Reiter's syndrome.

■ PHYSICAL FINDINGS & CLINICAL PRESENTATION

Clinical manifestations may be similar to those of gonorrhea: mucopurulent endocervical discharge, with edema, erythema, and easily induced endocervical bleeding caused by inflammation of endocervical columnar epithelium. Less frequent manifestations may include bartholinitis, urethral syndrome with dysuria and pyuria, perihepatitis (Fitz-Hugh–Curtis syndrome).

■ ETIOLOGY

• *Chlamydia trachomatis,* serotypes D through K
• Obligate, intracellular bacteria
• Trichomonal vaginalis
• Mycoplasma genitalium
• HSV

DIAGNOSIS

■ DIFFERENTIAL DIAGNOSIS

Gonorrhea, nongonococcal urethritis (nonchlamydial etiologies)

■ WORKUP

Diagnosis based on laboratory demonstration of evidence of infection in intraurethral or endocervical swab by various tests. The intracellular organism is less readily recovered from the discharge.

■ LABORATORY TESTS

• Cell culture is the reference method for diagnosis (single culture sensitivity 80% to 90%), but it is labor intensive and takes 48 to 96 hr; it is not suited for large screening programs.
• Nonculture methods:
  Direct fluorescent antibody (DFA) tests
  Enzyme immunoassay (EIA)
  DNA probes
  Polymerase chain reaction (PCR)
• With the exception of PCR, the other tests are probably less specific than cell culture and may yield false-positive results.
• Because this is an intracellular organism, purulent discharge is not an appropriate specimen. An adequate sample of infected cells must be obtained.
• 10 WBCs per high-power field.

TREATMENT

Nongonococcal urethritis, urethritis, cervicitis, conjunctivitis (except for LGV):
• Azithromycin 1 g PO × 1 *or*
• Doxycycline 100 mg PO bid for 7 days
• Alternatives
  1. Erythromycin base 500 mg PO qid for 7 days *or*
  2. Erythromycin ethylsuccinate 800 mg PO qid for 7 days *or*
  3. Ofloxacin 300 mg PO bid for 7 days *or*
  4. Levofloxacin 500 mg PO qd for 7 days

Infection in pregnancy:
• Erythromycin base 500 mg PO qid for 7 days *or*
• Amoxicillin 500 mg PO tid for 7 days
Alternatives:
1. Erythromycin base 250 mg PO qid for 7 days *or*
2. Erythromycin ethylsuccinate 800 mg PO qid for 7 days *or*
3. Erythromycin ethylsuccinate 400 mg PO qid for 14 days *or*
4. Azithromycin 1 g PO (single dose)
NOTE: Doxycycline and ofloxacin are contraindicated in pregnancy. Safety and efficacy of azithromycin are not established in pregnancy and lactation, although preliminary data indicate that it may be safe and effective. Erythromycin estolate is contraindicated in pregnancy because of drug-related hepatotoxicity.
FOLLOW UP:
Reculture after therapy completion and refer partners for evaluation and treatment.
RECURRENT AND PERSISTENT URETHRITIS:
Retreat noncompliant patients with the above regimens. If patient was initially complacent, recommended regimens: metronidazole 2 g PO in single dose plus erythromycin base 500 mg PO qid for 7 days or erythromycin ethylsuccinate 800 mg PO qid for 7 days.

■ DISPOSITION

See "Gonorrhea." In all patients being treated for chlamydia, presumptive treatment for concomitant infection with gonorrhea should be done. Also see Treatment in "Pelvic Inflammatory Disease."

REFERENCE

Centers for Disease Control and Prevention: 2002 sexually transmitted diseases treatment guidelines, *MMWR Morb Mortal Wkly Rep* 51(RR-6), 2002.
Author: **Maria A. Corigliano, M.D.**

BASIC INFORMATION

■ DEFINITION
Cholangitis refers to an inflammation and/or infection of the hepatic and common bile ducts associated with obstruction of the common bile duct.

■ SYNONYMS
Biliary sepsis
Ascending cholangitis
Suppurative cholangitis

ICD-9CM CODES
576.1 Cholangitis

■ EPIDEMIOLOGY & DEMOGRAPHICS
INCIDENCE (IN U.S.): Complicates approximately 1% of cases of cholelithiasis
PREVALENCE (IN U.S.): 2 cases/1000 hospital admissions
PREDOMINANT SEX:
- Females, for cholangitis secondary to gallstones
- Males, for cholangitis secondary to malignant obstruction and HIV infection

PREDOMINANT AGE: Seventh decade and older; unusual <50 yr of age
PEAK INCIDENCE: Seventh decade

■ PHYSICAL FINDINGS & CLINICAL PRESENTATION
- Usually acute onset of fever, chills, abdominal pain, tenderness over the RUQ of the abdomen, and jaundice (Charcot's triad)
- All signs and symptoms in only 50% to 85% of patients
- Often, dark coloration of the urine resulting from bilirubinuria
- Complications:
  1. Bacteremia (50%) and septic shock
  2. Hepatic abscess and pancreatitis

■ ETIOLOGY
Obstruction of the common bile duct causing rapid proliferation of bacteria in the biliary tree
- Most common cause of common bile duct obstruction: stones, usually migrated from the gallbladder
- Other causes: prior biliary tract surgery with secondary stenosis, tumor (usually arising from the pancreas or biliary tree), and parasitic infections from *Ascaris lumbricoides* or *Fasciola hepatica*
- Iatrogenic after contamination of an obstructed biliary tree by endoscopic retrograde cholangiopancreatoscopy (ERCP) or percutaneous transhepatic cholangiography (PTC)
- Primary sclerosing cholangitis (PSC)
- HIV-associated sclerosing cholangitis: associated with infection by CMV, *Cryptosporidium,* Microsporida, and *Mycobacterium avium* complex

DIAGNOSIS

■ DIFFERENTIAL DIAGNOSIS
- Biliary colic
- Acute cholecystitis
- Liver abscess
- PUD
- Pancreatitis
- Intestinal obstruction
- Right kidney stone
- Hepatitis
- Pyelonephritis

■ WORKUP
- Blood cultures
- CBC
- Liver function tests

■ LABORATORY TESTS
- Usually, elevated WBC count with a predominance of polynuclear forms
- Elevated alkaline phosphatase and bilirubin in chronic obstruction
- Elevated transaminases in acute obstruction
- Positive blood cultures in 50% of cases, typically with enteric gram-negative aerobes (e.g., *E. coli, Klebsiella pneumoniae*), enterococci, or anaerobes

■ IMAGING STUDIES
- Ultrasound:
  1. Allows visualization of the gallbladder and bile ducts to differentiate extrahepatic obstruction from intrahepatic cholestasis
  2. Insensitive but specific for visualization of common duct stones
- CT scan:
  1. Less accurate for gallstones
  2. More sensitive than ultrasound for visualization of the distal part of the common bile duct
  3. Also allows better definition of neoplasm
- ERCP:
  1. Confirms obstruction and its level
  2. Allows collection of specimens for culture and cytology
  3. Indicated for diagnosis if ultrasound and CT scan are inconclusive
  4. May be indicated in therapy (see Treatment)

TREATMENT

■ NONPHARMACOLOGIC THERAPY
Biliary decompression
- May be urgent in severely ill patients or those unresponsive to medical therapy within 12 to 24 hr
- May also be performed semielectively in patients who respond
- Options:
  1. ERCP with or without sphincterotomy or placement of a draining stent
  2. Percutaneous transhepatic biliary drainage for the acutely ill patient who is a poor surgical candidate
  3. Surgical exploration of the common bile duct

■ ACUTE GENERAL Rx
- Nothing by mouth
- Intravenous hydration
- Broad-spectrum antibiotics directed at gram-negative enteric organisms, anaerobes, and enterococcus: if infection is nosocomial, post-ERCP, or the patient is in shock, strong consideration of broader coverage to include hospital organisms such as *Pseudomonas aeruginosa,* resistant *Staphylococcus aureus,* and others

■ CHRONIC Rx
Repeated decompression may be necessary, particularly when obstruction is related to neoplasm.

■ DISPOSITION
Excellent prognosis if obstruction is amenable to definitive surgical therapy; otherwise relapses are common.

■ REFERRAL
- To biliary endoscopist if obstruction is from stones or a stent needs to be placed
- To interventional radiologist if external drainage is necessary
- To a general surgeon in all other cases
- To an infectious disease specialist if blood cultures are positive or the patient is in shock or otherwise severely ill

REFERENCES
Gouma DJ: Management of acute cholangitis, *Dig Dis* 21(1):25, 2003.
Lipsett PA, Hitt HA: Acute cholangitis, *Front Biosci* 8(s1229-39), 2003.
Author: **Michele Halpern, M.D.**

BASIC INFORMATION

■ DEFINITION

Cholecystitis is an acute or chronic inflammation of the gallbladder generally secondary to gallstones (>95% of cases).

■ SYNONYMS

Gallbladder attack

ICD-9CM CODES

575.0 Acute cholecystitis
574.0 Calculus of the gallbladder with acute cholecystitis
575.1 Cholecystitis without mention of calculus

■ EPIDEMIOLOGY & DEMOGRAPHICS

- Acute cholecystitis occurs most commonly in females during the fifth and sixth decades.
- The incidence of gallstones is 0.6% in the general population and much higher in certain ethnic groups (>75% of Native Americans by age 60 yr).

■ PHYSICAL FINDINGS & CLINICAL PRESENTATION

- Pain and tenderness in the right hypochondrium or epigastrium; pain possibly radiating to the infrascapular region
- Palpation of the RUQ eliciting marked tenderness and stoppage of inspired breath (Murphy's sign)
- Guarding
- Fever (33%)
- Jaundice (25% to 50% of patients)
- Palpable gallbladder (20% of cases)
- Nausea and vomiting (>70% of patients)
- Fever and chills (>25% of patients)
- Medical history often revealing ingestion of large, fatty meals before onset of pain in the epigastrium and RUQ

■ ETIOLOGY

- Gallstones (>95% of cases)
- Ischemic damage to the gallbladder, critically ill patient (acalculous cholecystitis)
- Infectious agents, especially in patients with AIDS (CMV, *Cryptosporidium*)
- Strictures of the bile duct
- Neoplasms, primary or metastatic

DIAGNOSIS

■ DIFFERENTIAL DIAGNOSIS

- Hepatic: hepatitis, abscess, hepatic congestion, neoplasm, trauma
- Biliary: neoplasm, stricture
- Gastric: PUD, neoplasm, alcoholic gastritis, hiatal hernia
- Pancreatic: pancreatitis, neoplasm, stone in the pancreatic duct or ampulla

- Renal: calculi, infection, inflammation, neoplasm, ruptured kidney
- Pulmonary: pneumonia, pulmonary infarction, right-sided pleurisy
- Intestinal: retrocecal appendicitis, intestinal obstruction, high fecal impaction
- Cardiac: myocardial ischemia (particularly involving the inferior wall), pericarditis
- Cutaneous: herpes zoster
- Trauma
- Fitz-Hugh–Curtis syndrome (perihepatitis)
- Subphrenic abscess
- Dissecting aneurysm
- Nerve root irritation caused by osteoarthritis of the spine

■ WORKUP

Workup consists of detailed history and physical examination coupled with laboratory evaluation and imaging studies. No single clinical finding or laboratory test is sufficient to establish or exclude cholecystitis without further testing.

■ LABORATORY TESTS

- Leukocytosis (12,000 to 20,000) is present in >70% of patients.
- Elevated alkaline phosphatase, ALT, AST, bilirubin; bilirubin elevation >4 mg/dl is unusual and suggests presence of choledocholithiasis.
- Elevated amylase may be present (consider pancreatitis if serum amylase elevation exceeds 500 U).

■ IMAGING STUDIES

- Ultrasound of the gallbladder is the preferred initial test; it will demonstrate the presence of stones and also dilated gallbladder with thickened wall and surrounding edema in patients with acute cholecystitis.
- Nuclear imaging (HIDA scan) is useful for diagnosis of cholecystitis: sensitivity and specificity exceed 90% for acute cholecystis. This test is only reliable when bilirubin is <5 mg/dl. A positive test will demonstrate obstruction of the cystic or common hepatic duct; the test will not demonstrate the presence of stones.
- CT scan of abdomen is useful in cases of suspected abscess, neoplasm, or pancreatitis.
- Plain film of the abdomen generally is not useful, because <25% of stones are radiopaque.

TREATMENT

■ NONPHARMACOLOGIC THERAPY

Provide IV hydration; withhold oral feedings.

■ ACUTE GENERAL Rx

- Cholecystectomy (laparoscopic is preferred, open cholecystectomy is acceptable); conservative management with IV fluids and antibiotics (ampicillin-sulbactam [Unasyn] 3 g IV q 6h *or* piperacillin-tazobactam [Zosyn] 4.5 g IV q 8 h) may be justified in some high-risk patients to convert an emergency procedure into an elective one with a lower mortality.
- ERCP with sphincterectomy and stone extraction can be performed in conjunction with laparoscopic cholecystectomy for patients with choledochal lithiasis; approximately 7% to 15% of patients with cholelithiasis also have stones in the common bile duct.
- IV fluids, broad-spectrum antibiotics, pain management (meperidine prn) should be used.

■ DISPOSITION

- Prognosis is good; elective laparoscopic cholecystectomy can be performed as outpatient procedure.
- Hospital stay (when necessary) varies from overnight with laparoscopic cholecystectomy to 4 to 7 days with open cholecystectomy.
- Complication rate is approximately 1% (hemorrhage and bile leak) for laparoscopic cholecystectomy and <0.5% (infection) with open cholecystectomy.

■ REFERRAL

Hospitalization and surgical referral in all patients with acute cholecystitis

PEARLS & CONSIDERATIONS

■ COMMENTS

- Patients should be instructed that stones may recur in bile ducts.
- Gallbladder aspiration in which all fluid visualized by ultrasound is aspirated represents a nonsurgical treatment when patients who are at high operative risk develop acute cholecystitis. Salvage cholecystectomy is reserved for nonresponders.

REFERENCES

Cuschieri A: Management of patients with gallstones and ductal calculi, *Lancet* 360:739, 2002.
Trowbridge RL et al: Does this patient have acute cholecystitis? *JAMA* 289:80, 2003.
Author: **Fred F. Ferri, M.D.**

BASIC INFORMATION

■ DEFINITION

Cholelithiasis is the presence of stones in the gallbladder.

■ SYNONYMS

Gallstones

ICD-9CM CODES

574.2 Calculus of the gallbladder without mention of cholecystitis
574.0 Calculus of the gallbladder with acute cholecystitis

■ EPIDEMIOLOGY & DEMOGRAPHICS

- Gallstone disease can be found in 20 million Americans. Of these, 2% to 3% (500,000 to 600,000) are treated with cholecystectomies each year.
- Annual medical expenditures for gallbladder surgeries in the U.S. exceed $5 billion.
- Incidence of gallbladder disease increases with age. Highest incidence is in the fifth and sixth decades. Predisposing factors for gallstones are female sex, pregnancy, age >40 yr, family history of gallstones, obesity, ileal disease, oral contraceptives, diabetes mellitus, rapid weight loss, estrogen replacement therapy.
- Patients with gallstones have a 20% chance of developing biliary colic or its complications at the end of a 20-yr period.

■ PHYSICAL FINDINGS & CLINICAL PRESENTATION

- Physical examination is entirely normal unless patient is having a biliary colic; 80% of gallstones are asymptomatic.
- Typical symptoms of obstruction of the cystic duct include intermittent, severe, cramping pain affecting the RUQ.
- Pain occurs mostly at night and may radiate to the back or right shoulder. It can last from a few minutes to several hours.

■ ETIOLOGY

- 75% of gallstones contain cholesterol and are usually associated with obesity, female sex, diabetes mellitus; mixed stones are most common (80%), pure cholesterol stones account for only 10% of stones.
- 25% of gallstones are pigment stones (bilirubin, calcium, and variable organic material) associated with hemolysis and cirrhosis. These tend to be black pigment stones that are refractory to medical therapy.
- 50% of mixed-type stones are radiopaque.

DIAGNOSIS

■ DIFFERENTIAL DIAGNOSIS

- PUD
- GERD
- IBD
- Pancreatitis
- Neoplasms
- Nonnuclear dyspepsia

■ LABORATORY TESTS

Generally normal unless patient has biliary obstruction (elevated alkaline phosphatase, bilirubin).

■ IMAGING STUDIES

- Ultrasound of the gallbladder will detect small stones and biliary sludge (sensitivity, 95%; specificity, 90%); the presence of dilated gallbladder with thickened wall is suggestive of acute cholecystitis.
- Nuclear imaging (HIDA scan) can confirm acute cholecystitis (>90% accuracy) if gallbladder does not visualize within 4 hr of injection and the radioisotope is excreted in the common bile duct.

TREATMENT

■ NONPHARMACOLOGIC THERAPY

Life-style changes (avoidance of diets high in polyunsaturated fats, weight loss in obese patients—however, avoid rapid weight loss)

■ ACUTE GENERAL Rx

- The management of gallstones is affected by the clinical presentation.
- Asymptomatic patients do not require therapeutic intervention.
- Surgical intervention is generally the ideal approach for symptomatic patients. Laparoscopic cholecystectomy is generally preferred over open cholecystectomy because of the shorter recovery period.
- Laparoscopic cholecystectomy after endoscopic sphincterectomy is recommended for patients with common bile duct stones and residual gallbladder stones. Where possible, single-stage laparoscopic treatments with removal of duct stones and cholecystectomy during the same procedure are preferable.

- Patients who are not appropriate candidates for surgery because of co-existing illness or patients who refuse surgery can be treated with oral bile salts: ursodiol (Actigall) 8 to 10 mg/kg/day in two to three divided doses for 16 to 20 mo, or chenodiol (Chenix) 250 mg bid initially, increasing gradually to a dose of 60 mg/kg/day. Candidates for oral bile salts are patients with cholesterol stones (radiolucent, noncalcified stones), with a diameter of ≤15 mm and having three or fewer stones. Candidates for medical therapy must have a functioning gallbladder and must have absence of calcifications on CT scans.
- Direct solvent dissolution with methyl *tert*-butyl ether (MTBE) can be used in patients with multiple stones with diameter ≥3 cm; this method should be used only by physicians experienced with contact dissolution. Administration of the solvent is either through percutaneous transhepatic placement of a catheter into the gallbladder or endoscopic retrograde catheter placement with subsequent continuous infusion and aspiration of the solvent either manually or by automatic pump system. MTBE is a powerful cholesterol solvent and can dissolve stones in a few hours (>90% dissolution over a 2-hr infusion).
- Extracorporeal shock wave lithotripsy (ESWL) is another form of medical therapy. It can be used in patients with stone diameter of ≤3 cm and having three or fewer stones.

■ DISPOSITION

- Recurrence rate after bile acid treatment is approximately 50% in 5 yr. Periodic ultrasound is necessary to assess the effectiveness of treatment.
- Gallstones recur after dissolution therapy with MTBE in >40% of patients within 5 yr.
- Following extracorporeal shock wave lithotripsy, stones recur in approximately 20% of patients after 4 yr.
- Patients with at least 1 gallstone <5 mm in diameter have a greater than fourfold increased risk of presenting with acute biliary pancreatitis. A policy of watchful waiting in such cases is generally unwarranted.
- A potential serious complication of gallstones is acute cholangitis. ERCP and endoscopic sphincterectomy (EC) followed by interval laparoscopic cholecystectomy is effective in acute cholangitis.

Author: **Fred F. Ferri, M.D.**

BASIC INFORMATION

■ **DEFINITION**

An acute diarrheal illness caused by *Vibrio cholerae*.

■ **SYNONYMS**

None

ICD-9CM CODES

001.0 Cholera

■ **EPIDEMIOLOGY & DEMOGRAPHICS**

INCIDENCE IN U.S. Previously, approximately 50 cases per year, mostly in travelers returning from endemic areas. From 1995 to 2000, 61 cases reported, 37 (61%) of which acquired outside the U.S.

PREDOMINANT SEX: None

PREDOMINANT AGE: In nonendemic areas, attack rates are equal in all age groups. In epidemic areas, children over the age of 2 yr are most commonly infected.

PEAK INCIDENCE:

None in the U.S.

Summer and fall in endemic areas

GENETICS: N/A

Familial disposition: N/A

Congenital infection: N/A

Neonatal infection: Illness is uncommon before the age of 2 yr, likely because of passive immunity.

■ **PHYSICAL FINDINGS**

Infection may result in asymptomatic illness or a mild diarrhea. The classic illness is described as the abrupt onset of voluminous watery diarrhea, which may lead to severe dehydration, acidosis, shock, and death. Vomiting may occur early in the illness, but fever and abdominal pain are usually absent. The typical "rice water" stools are pale with flecks of mucus and contain no blood. Muscle cramps may be prominent, and are the result of loss of fluid and electrolytes. Untreated illness results in hypovolemic shock, and death may occur in hours to days. With adequate fluid and electrolyte repletion, cholera is a self-limited illness that resolves in a few days. The use of antimicrobials can shorten the course of illness.

■ **ETIOLOGY**

The organism responsible for this illness is one of several strains of *V. cholerae*. Most infections result from the 01 serotype, the El Tor biotype. In the U.S., one outbreak occurred from the ingestion of illegally imported crab, and sporadic infection has been associated with the consumption of contaminated shellfish in Gulf Coast states. Most cases are seen in returning travelers. Transmission during epidemics is the result of the ingestion of contaminated water and, in some instances, contaminated food.

 DIAGNOSIS

■ **DIFFERENTIAL DIAGNOSIS**

• Mild illness may mimic gastroenteritis resulting from a variety of etiologies.
• Sudden, voluminous diarrhea causing marked dehydration is uncommon in other illnesses.

■ **WORKUP**

Stool should be sent for culture and microscopy. Treatment should not be delayed while awaiting culture results.

■ **LABORATORY TESTS**

• WBC may be elevated, and hemoglobin may be increased as a result of hemoconcentration.
• Elevated bun and creatinine suggests prerenal azotemia. Hypoglycemia may occur. Stool cultures on appropriate media may grow the organism. Wet mount of stool under dark field or phase contrast microscopy shows organisms with characteristic darting motility.

■ **IMAGING STUDIES**

None

TREATMENT

■ **NONPHARMACOLOGIC THERAPY**

The mainstay of therapy is adequate fluid and electrolyte replacement. This can usually be achieved using oral rehydration solutions containing salts and glucose. Some patients may require intravenous fluid and electrolyte replacement.

■ **ACUTE GENERAL Rx**

• Antimicrobial therapy can decrease shedding of fluid and organisms and can shorten the course of illness
  1. Doxycycline 100 mg PO bid for 5 days, *or*
  2. Septra, one DS tablet PO bid for 5 days
• Resistance to Septra is increasing in travel-associated infections

■ **CHRONIC Rx**

It is likely that asymptomatic chronic carriers exist, however, because they are difficult to identify, and their role in transmission of disease appears to be rather limited, there is no recommendation for treatment of these individuals.

■ **DISPOSITION**

The mortality of adequately hydrated patients is less than 1%.

■ **REFERRAL**

If more than mild illness occurs

PEARLS & CONSIDERATIONS

■ **COMMENTS**

• There is currently no indication for vaccination of travelers to endemic areas. The risk of infection is small, protection from available vaccines is limited, and side effects are prominent and frequent.
• Doxycycline should not be used to treat children or pregnant women.

REFERENCES

Ramakrishna BS et al: Amylase-resistant starch plus oral rehydration solution for cholera, *New Engl J Med* 342:308, 2000.

Steinberg EB et al: Cholera in the United States, 1995-2000: trends at the end of the twentieth century, *J Infect Dis* 184:799, 2001.

Author: **Maurice Policar, M.D.**

BASIC INFORMATION

■ DEFINITION

Chronic fatigue syndrome (CFS) is characterized by four or more of the following symptoms, present concurrently for at least 6 mo:
- Impaired memory or concentration
- Sore throat
- Tender cervical or axillary lymph nodes
- Muscle pain
- Multijoint pain
- New headaches
- Unrefreshing sleep
- Postexertion malaise

■ SYNONYMS

Yuppie flu
CFS
Chronic Epstein-Barr syndrome

ICD-9CM CODES

780.7 Chronic fatigue syndrome
300.8 Neurasthenia

■ EPIDEMIOLOGY & DEMOGRAPHICS

PREVALENCE IN U.S.: 100 to 300 cases/100,000 persons
PREDOMINANT AGE: Young adulthood and middle age
PREDOMINANT SEX: Female > male

■ PHYSICAL FINDINGS & CLINICAL PRESENTATION

- There are no physical findings specific for CFS.
- The physical examination may be useful to identify fibromyalgia and other rheumatologic conditions that may coexist with CFS.

■ ETIOLOGY

- The etiology of CFS is unknown.
- Many experts suspect that a viral illness may trigger certain immune responses leading to the various symptoms. Most patients often report the onset of their symptoms with a flu-like illness.
- Initial reports indicated a possible role of Epstein-Barr virus, but subsequent studies disproved this theory.

DIAGNOSIS

■ DIFFERENTIAL DIAGNOSIS

- Psychosocial depression, dysthymia, anxiety-related disorders, and other psychiatric diseases
- Infectious diseases (SBE, Lyme disease, fungal diseases, mononucleosis, HIV, chronic hepatitis B or C, TB, chronic parasitic infections)
- Autoimmune diseases: SLE, myasthenia gravis, multiple sclerosis, thyroiditis, RA
- Endocrine abnormalities: hypothyroidism, hypopituitarism, adrenal insufficiency, Cushing's syndrome, diabetes mellitus, hyperparathyroidism, pregnancy, reactive hypoglycemia
- Occult malignant disease
- Substance abuse
- Systemic disorders: chronic renal failure, COPD, cardiovascular disease, anemia, electrolyte abnormalities, liver disease
- Other: inadequate rest, sleep apnea, narcolepsy, fibromyalgia, sarcoidosis, medications, toxic agent exposure, Wegener's granulomatosis
- The differential diagnosis of fatigue is described in Section II

■ WORKUP

Because CFS is a clinical diagnosis and the symptoms are generally subjective, the history and physical examination are essential for excluding other causes of fatigue. A detailed mental status examination is necessary. Abnormalities should be further evaluated with appropriate psychiatric, psychologic, or neurologic examination. An algorithmic approach to the patient presenting with fatigue is described in Section III, Fig. 3-76.

■ LABORATORY TESTS

- No specific laboratory tests exist for diagnosing CFS. Initial laboratory tests are useful to exclude other conditions that may mimic or may be associated with CFS.
  1. Screening laboratory tests: CBC, ESR, ALT, total protein, albumin, globulin, alkaline phosphatase, calcium, phosphorus, glucose, BUN, creatinine, electrolytes, TSH, and urinalysis are useful.
  2. Serologic tests for Epstein-Barr virus, *Candida albicans,* human herpesvirus 6, and other studies for immune cellular abnormalities are not useful; these tests are expensive and generally not recommended.
- Other tests may be indicated depending on the history and physical examination (e.g., ANA, RF in patients presenting with joint complaints or abnormalities on physical examination, Lyme titer in areas where Lyme disease is endemic).

■ IMAGING STUDIES

Generally not recommended unless history and physical examination indicate specific abnormalities (e.g., chest x-ray examination in any patient suspected of TB or sarcoidosis)

TREATMENT

■ NONPHARMACOLOGIC THERAPY

- Education and counseling help to develop realistic goals and expectations.
- Support groups (see Chronic Rx) are useful.
- Patients should be reassured that the illness is not fatal and that most patients improve over time.
- An initially supervised exercise program to preserve and increase strength is beneficial for most patients and can improve symptoms.

■ ACUTE GENERAL Rx

Therapy is generally palliative. The following medications may be helpful:
- Antidepressants: The choice of antidepressant varies with the desired side effects. Patients with difficulty sleeping or fibromyalgia-like symptoms may benefit from low-dose tricyclics (doxepin 10 mg hs or amitriptyline 25 mg qhs). When sedation is not desirable, low-dose SSRIs (paroxetine 20 mg qd) often help alleviate fatigue and associated symptoms.
- NSAIDs can be used to relieve muscle and joint pain and headaches.
- Fludrocortisone as monotherapy for neurally mediated hypotension is no more efficacious than placebo.
- Low-dose hydrocortisone therapy provides a few benefits in quality of life; however, it is associated with frequent side effects and is not recommended.
"Alternative" medications (herbs, multivitamins, nutritional supplements) are very popular with many CFS patients but are generally not very helpful.

■ CHRONIC Rx

Psychiatric referral and treatment are helpful in coping with the disease in the majority of patients.

■ DISPOSITION

Moderate to complete recovery at 1 yr occurs in 22% to 60% of patients with CFS.

PEARLS & CONSIDERATIONS

■ COMMENTS

In CFS the symptoms are serious enough to reduce daily activities by >50% and in absence of any other medically identifiable disorders.

REFERENCE

Koelle DM et al: Markers of viral infection in monozygotic twins discordant for chronic fatigue syndrome, *Clin Infect Dis* 35:518, 2002.
Author: **Fred F. Ferri, M.D.**

BASIC INFORMATION

■ DEFINITION

Chronic obstructive pulmonary disease (COPD) is a disorder characterized by the presence of airflow limitation that is not fully reversible. COPD encompasses *emphysema,* characterized by loss of lung elasticity and destruction of lung parenchyma with enlargement of air spaces, and *chronic bronchitis,* characterized by obstruction of small airways and productive cough greater than 3 months' duration for more than 2 successive years. Patients with COPD are classically subdivided in two major groups based on their appearance:

1. *"Blue bloaters"* are patients with chronic bronchitis; the name is derived from the bluish tinge of the skin (secondary to chronic hypoxemia and hypercapnia) and from the frequent presence of peripheral edema (secondary to cor pulmonale); chronic cough with production of large amounts of sputum is characteristic.
2. *"Pink puffers"* are patients with emphysema; they have a cachectic appearance but pink skin color (adequate oxygen saturation); shortness of breath is manifested by pursed-lip breathing and use of accessory muscles of respiration.

■ SYNONYMS

COPD
Emphysema
Chronic bronchitis

ICD-9CM CODES

496 COPD
492.8 Emphysema

■ EPIDEMIOLOGY & DEMOGRAPHICS

- COPD affects 16 million Americans and is responsible for >80,000 deaths/yr.
- Highest incidence is in males >40 yr.
- 16 million office visits, 500,000 hospitalizations, and >$18 billion in direct health care costs annually can be attributed to COPD.

■ PHYSICAL FINDINGS & CLINICAL PRESENTATION

- Blue bloaters (chronic bronchitis): peripheral cyanosis, productive cough, tachypnea, tachycardia
- Pink puffers (emphysema): dyspnea, pursed-lip breathing with use of accessory muscles for respiration, decreased breath sounds
- Possible wheezing in both patients with chronic bronchitis and emphysema
- Features of both chronic bronchitis and emphysema in many patients with COPD
- Acute exacerbation of COPD is mainly a clinical diagnosis and generally manifests with worsening dyspnea, increase in sputum purulence, and increase in sputum volume

■ ETIOLOGY

- Tobacco exposure
- Occupational exposure to pulmonary toxins (e.g., cadmium)
- Atmospheric pollution
- α-1 antitrypsin deficiency (rare; <1% of COPD patients)

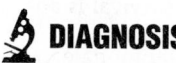

DIAGNOSIS

■ DIFFERENTIAL DIAGNOSIS

- CHF
- Asthma
- Respiratory infections
- Bronchiectasis
- Cystic fibrosis
- Neoplasm
- Pulmonary embolism
- Sleep apnea, obstructive
- Hypothyroidism

■ WORKUP

Chest x-ray examination, pulmonary function testing, blood gases (in patients with acute exacerbation)

■ LABORATORY TESTS

- CBC may reveal leukocytosis with "shift to the left" during acute exacerbation.
- Sputum may be purulent with bacterial respiratory tract infections. Sputum staining and cultures are usually reserved for cases that are refractory to antibiotic therapy.
- ABGs: normocapnia, mild to moderate hypoxemia may be present.

- Pulmonary function testing: abnormal diffusing capacity, increased total lung capacity and/or residual volume, fixed reduction in FEV_1 are present with emphysema; normal diffusing capacity, reduced FEV_1 are present with chronic bronchitis. Generally, acute spirometry should not be used to diagnose an exacerbation or assess its severity.

■ IMAGING STUDIES

Chest x-ray examination:
- Hyperinflation with flattened diaphragm, tending of the diaphragm at the rib, and increased retrosternal chest space
- Decreased vascular markings and bullae in patients with emphysema
- Thickened bronchial markings and enlarged right side of the heart in patients with chronic bronchitis

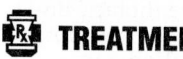

TREATMENT

■ NONPHARMACOLOGIC THERAPY

- Weight loss in patients with chronic bronchitis.
- Avoidance of tobacco use and elimination of air pollutants.
- Supplemental oxygen, usually through a face mask to ensure oxygen saturation >90% measured by pulse oximetry.
- Pulmonary toilet: careful nasotracheal suction is indicated in patients with excessive secretions and inability to expectorate. Mechanical percussion of the chest as applied by a physical or respiratory therapist is ineffective with acute exacerbations of COPD.

■ ACUTE GENERAL Rx

- Acute exacerbation of COPD can be treated with:
  1. Aerosolized β-agonists (e.g., metaproterenol nebulizer solution 5% 0.3 mL or albuterol nebulized 5% solution 2.5-5 mg).
  2. Anticholinergic agents, which have equivalent efficacy to inhaled β-adrenergic agonists. Inhalant solution of ipratropium bromide 0.5 mg can be administered every 4 to 8 hr.

3. Short courses of systemic corticosteroids, which have been shown to improve spirometric and clinical outcomes. In the hospital setting give IV methyl-prednisolone 50- to 100-mg bolus, then q6-8h; taper as soon as possible. In the outpatient setting, oral prednisone 40 mg/day initially, decreasing the dose by 10 mg every other day is generally effective.

4. Judicious oxygen administration (hypercapnia and further respiratory compromise may occur after high-flow oxygen therapy); use of a Venturi-type mask delivering an inspired oxygen fraction of 24% to 28% is preferred to nasal cannula.

5. Noninvasive positive pressure ventilation delivered by a facial or nasal mask in the treatment of chronic restrictive thoracic disease may obviate the need for intratracheal intubation.

6. IV aminophylline administration is controversial and generally not recommended. When used, serum levels should be closely monitored to minimize risks of tachyarrhythmias.

- Antibiotics are indicated in suspected respiratory infection (e.g., increased purulence and volume of phlegm).
  1. *Haemophilus influenzae, Streptococcus pneumoniae* are frequent causes of acute bronchitis.
  2. Oral antibiotics of choice are azithromycin, levofloxacin, amoxicillin-clavulanate, and cefuroxime.
  3. The use of antibiotics is beneficial in exacerbations of COPD presenting with increased dyspnea and sputum purulence (especially if the patient is febrile).
- Guaifenesin may improve cough symptoms and mucus clearance; however, mucolytic medications are generally ineffective. Their benefits may be greatest in patients with more advanced disease.
- Intubation and mechanical ventilation may be necessary if previous measures fail to provide improvement.

■ **DISPOSITION**
- Following the initial episode of respiratory failure, 5-yr survival is approximately 25%.
- Development of cor pulmonale or hypercapnia and persistent tachycardia are poor prognostic indicators.

✧ PEARLS & CONSIDERATIONS

■ **COMMENTS**
- All patients with COPD should receive pneumococcal vaccine and yearly influenza vaccine.
- Correction of resting arterial hypoxemia with oxygen therapy for more than 15 hr/day prolongs survival of COPD patients if resting P_{AO_2} is <55 mm Hg.

REFERENCES

Aaron SD et al: Outpatient oral prednisone after emergency treatment of chronic obstructive pulmonary disease, *N Engl J Med* 348:2618, 2003.

Man PS et al: Contemporary management of chronic obstructive pulmonary disease, clinical applications, *JAMA* 290:2313, 2003.

Sethi S et al: New strains of bacteria and exacerbations of chronic obstructive pulmonary disease, *N Engl J Med* 347:465, 2002.

Sin DD et al: Contemporary management of chronic obstructive pulmonary disease, a scientific review, *JAMA* 290:2301, 2003.

Stoller JK: Acute exacerbations of chronic obstructive pulmonary disease, *N Engl J Med* 346:988, 2002.

Author: **Fred F. Ferri**, M.D.

BASIC INFORMATION

■ DEFINITION
Churg-Strauss syndrome refers to a systemic vasculitis accompanied by severe asthma, hypereosinophilia, and necrotizing vasculitis with extravascular eosinophil granulomas.

■ SYNONYMS
Allergic angiitis and granulomatosis

ICD-9CM CODES
446.4 Angiitis, allergic granulomatous

■ EPIDEMIOLOGY & DEMOGRAPHICS
- Churg-Strauss syndrome is a rare disease
- At the Mayo Clinic, 90 cases were observed over a 19-yr period from 1976-1995
- Affects males > females (2:1)
- Can occur at any age but usually affects young to middle-aged adults (~40 yr of age)

■ PHYSICAL FINDINGS & CLINICAL PRESENTATION
Churg-Strauss syndrome can be described as occurring in three distinct phases:
1. The prodromal phase or allergic phase characterized by severe asthma, either with or without allergic rhinitis, sinusitis, headache, cough, and wheezing
2. The eosinophilic phase characterized by peripheral eosinophilia and eosinophilic tissue infiltration producing signs and symptoms of cough, fever, anorexia, weight loss, sweats, malaise, abdominal pain, and diarrhea
3. The vasculitic phase, which may involve any organ, including the heart (most frequent), lung, CNS, kidney, lymph nodes, muscle, and skin, and manifesting in chest pain, dyspnea, hemophysis, arthralgia, myalgias, peripheral neuropathy (mononeuritis multiplex), joint swelling, skin rash, and signs of CHF

■ ETIOLOGY
- The cause of Churg-Strauss syndrome is unknown—a hypersensitivity immunological etiology has been proposed.
- Although similar and at times grouped with patients with polyarteritis nodosa (PAN), Churg-Strauss syndrome differs in that:
  1. Churg-Strauss syndrome vasculitis involves not only small-sized arteries but also veins and venules.
  2. Churg-Strauss syndrome, unlike PAN, predominantly involves the lung. Other organs affected include heart, GI, CNS, kidney, and skin.
  3. Churg-Strauss biopsy shows necrotizing vasculitis along with a granulomatous extravascular reaction infiltrated by eosinophils.

DIAGNOSIS

The American College of Rheumatology has established criteria for the diagnosis of Churg-Strauss syndrome. For the diagnosis to be made at least 4 of the following 6 criteria must be met:
- Asthma
- Eosinophilia >10%
- Mononeuropathy or polyneuropathy
- Pulmonary infiltrates
- Paranasal sinus abnormalities
- Extravascular eosinophils

The presence of any 4 or more of the 6 criteria yields a sensitivity of 85% and a specificity of 99.7%.

■ DIFFERENTIAL DIAGNOSIS
- Polyarteritis nodosa
- Wegener's granulomatosis
- Sarcoidosis
- Loeffler syndrome
- Henoch-Schönlein purpura
- Allergic bronchopulmonary aspergillosis
- Rheumatoid arthritis
- Leukocytoclastic vasculitis

■ WORKUP
If the clinical suspicion of Churg-Strauss is raised, further workup including blood tests, x-rays, and tissue biopsy help establish the diagnosis.

■ LABORATORY TESTS
- CBC with differential may reveal one diagnostic criterion: eosinophilia with counts ranging from 5000 to 10,000 eosinophils/mm³.
- ESR is usually elevated and a marker of inflammation.
- BUN/creatinine may be elevated, suggesting renal involvement.
- Urinalysis may show hematuria and proteinuria.
- 24-hour urine for protein if greater than 1 g/day is a poor prognostic factor.
- Antineutrophil cytoplasmic antibodies (ANCA), although not diagnostic of Churg-Strauss syndrome, are found in up to 70% of patients.
- AST, ALT, and CPK may indicate liver or muscle (skeletal or cardiac) involvement.
- RA and ANA may be positive.
- Biopsy substantiates the diagnosis if the characteristic findings as previously described are seen.

■ IMAGING STUDIES
- Chest x-ray is abnormal in >50% of the cases and can show patchy migratory infiltrates, interstitial lung disease, or nodular infiltrates (Fig. 1-71).
- Paranasal sinus films may reveal sinus opacification.
- Angiography is sometimes done in patients with mesenteric ischemia or renal involvement.

TREATMENT

■ NONPHARMACOLOGIC THERAPY
Oxygen therapy in severe asthmatic exacerbations

■ ACUTE GENERAL Rx
- Corticosteroids are the treatment of choice. Prednisone 1 mg/kg/day is the starting dose and is continued for the first month. Thereafter, prednisone is tapered progressively to 10 mg/day at 1 yr.
- A drop in the eosinophil count and the ESR documents a response. Antineutrophil cytoplasmic antibodies do not reliably correspond with disease activity.

■ **CHRONIC Rx**
- Cyclophosphamide plus corticosteroids are used in patients with multiorgan involvement and poor prognostic factors.
- Many with persistent symptoms of asthma will require long-term corticosteroids even if vasculitis is no longer present.

■ **DISPOSITION**
- Clinical remissions are obtained in more than 90% of patients.
- With treatment, long-term prognosis is good, with a 5-yr survival rate of 80%. Despite successful treatment of Churg-Strauss syndrome, asthma generally remains persistent.
- The 5-yr survival of untreated Churg-Strauss is 25%.
- Death usually occurs from progressive refractory vasculitis, myocardial involvement, or severe GI involvement (mesenteric ischemia, pancreatitis, etc.).

■ **REFERRAL**
If a patient is suspected of having Churg-Strauss syndrome, a pulmonary referral for diagnosis and management is appropriate.

☼ PEARLS & CONSIDERATIONS

■ **COMMENTS**
- The diagnosis of Churg-Strauss is many times missed initially, because asthma and rhinitis or sinusitis are very common and these symptoms can precede the onset of vasculitis by many years (mean 8 yr).
- Churg-Strauss syndrome is distinguished from other vasculitides by the nearly universal presence of asthma that typically precedes all other symptoms.
- Poor prognostic factors include:
  1. Renal insufficiency
  2. Proteinuria >1 g/day
  3. GI involvement
  4. Cardiac involvement
  5. CNS involvement

- Churg-Strauss syndrome was first described by Churg and Strauss in 1951 after reviewing a number of autopsy cases previously classified as polyarteritis nodosa.

REFERENCES

Conron M, Beynon HL: Churg-Strauss syndrome, *Thorax* 55(10):870, 2000.

Masi AT et al: American College of Rheumatology 1990 criteria for the classification of Churg-Strauss syndrome, *Arthritis Rheumatol* 33:1094, 1990.

Noth I, Strek ME, Leff AL: Churg-Strauss Syndrome, *Lancet* 361(9357):587, 2003.

Vogel P, Schissel D: Churg-Strauss syndrome (allergic granulomatosis), e *Medicine Journal* 2(10), 2001. (www.emedicine.com).

Watts RA, Scott DG, Lane SE: Epidemiology of Wegener's granulomatosis, microscopic polyangiitis, and Churg-Strauss syndrome, *Cleve Clin J Med* 69(Suppl 2):SII84, 2002.

Author: **Peter Petropoulos, M.D.**

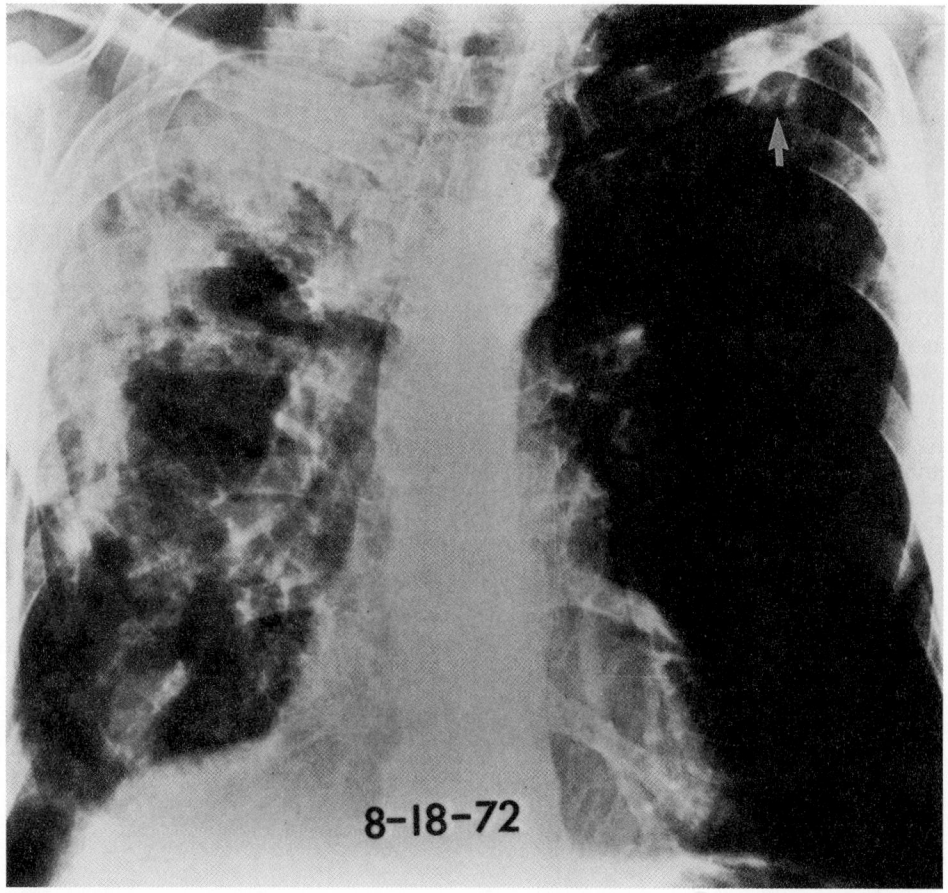

Fig. 1-71 **Allergic angitis and granulomatosis.** PA chest radiograph demonstrates peripheral air-space consolidation in the right lung and a nodule (*arrow*) in the left upper lobe in this asthmatic patient. (From McLoud TC [ed]: *Thoracic radiology, the requisites,* St Louis, 1998, Mosby.)

BASIC INFORMATION

■ DEFINITION
Cirrhosis is defined histologically as the presence of fibrosis and regenerative nodules in the liver. It can be classified as micronodular, macronodular, and mixed; however, each form may be seen in the same patient at different stages of the disease. Cirrhosis manifests clinically with portal hypertension, hepatic encephalopathy, and variceal bleeding.

ICD-9CM CODES
571.5 Cirrhosis of the liver
571.2 Cirrhosis of the liver secondary to alcohol

■ EPIDEMIOLOGY & DEMOGRAPHICS
- Cirrhosis is the eleventh leading cause of death in the U.S. (death rate 9 deaths/100,000 persons/yr).
- Alcohol abuse and viral hepatitis are the major causes of cirrhosis in the U.S.

■ PHYSICAL FINDINGS & CLINICAL PRESENTATION
SKIN: Jaundice, palmar erythema (alcohol abuse), spider angiomata, ecchymosis (thrombocytopenia or coagulation factor deficiency), dilated superficial periumbilical vein (caput medusae), increased pigmentation (hemochromatosis), xanthomas (primary biliary cirrhosis), needle tracks (viral hepatitis)
EYES: Kayser-Fleischer rings (corneal copper deposition seen in Wilson's disease; best diagnosed with slit lamp examination), scleral icterus
BREATH: Fetor hepaticus (musty odor of breath and urine found in cirrhosis with hepatic failure)
CHEST: Possible gynecomastia in men
ABDOMEN: Tender hepatomegaly (congestive hepatomegaly), small, nodular liver (cirrhosis), palpable, nontender gallbladder (neoplastic extrahepatic biliary obstruction), palpable spleen (portal hypertension), venous hum auscultated over periumbilical veins (portal hypertension), ascites (portal hypertension, hypoalbuminemia)
RECTAL EXAMINATION: Hemorrhoids (portal hypertension), guaiac-positive stools (alcoholic gastritis, bleeding esophageal varices, PUD, bleeding hemorrhoids)
GENITALIA: Testicular atrophy in males (chronic liver disease, hemochromatosis)

EXTREMITIES: Pedal edema (hypoalbuminemia, failure of right side of the heart), arthropathy (hemochromatosis)
NEUROLOGIC: Flapping tremor, asterixis (hepatic encephalopathy), choreoathetosis, dysarthria (Wilson's disease)

■ ETIOLOGY
- Alcohol abuse
- Secondary biliary cirrhosis, obstruction of the common bile duct (stone, stricture, pancreatitis, neoplasm, sclerosing cholangitis)
- Drugs (e.g., acetaminophen, isoniazid, methotrexate, methyldopa)
- Hepatic congestion (e.g., CHF, constrictive pericarditis, tricuspid insufficiency, thrombosis of the hepatic vein, obstruction of the vena cava)
- Primary biliary cirrhosis
- Hemochromatosis
- Chronic hepatitis B or C
- Wilson's disease
- α-1 antitrypsin deficiency
- Infiltrative diseases (amyloidosis, glycogen storage diseases, hemochromatosis)
- Nutritional: jejunoileal bypass
- Others: parasitic infections (schistosomiasis), idiopathic portal hypertension, congenital hepatic fibrosis, systemic mastocytosis, autoimmune hepatitis, hepatic steatosis, IBD

DIAGNOSIS

■ WORKUP
Diagnostic workup is aimed at identifying the most likely cause of cirrhosis. The history is extremely important:
- Alcohol abuse: alcoholic liver disease
- History of hepatitis B (chronic active hepatitis, primary hepatic neoplasm, or hepatitis C)
- History of IBD (primary sclerosing cholangitis)
- History of pruritus, hyperlipoproteinemia, and xanthomas in a middle-aged or elderly female (primary biliary cirrhosis)
- Impotence, diabetes mellitus, hyperpigmentation, arthritis (hemochromatosis)
- Neurologic disturbances (Wilson's disease, hepatolenticular degeneration)
- Family history of "liver disease" (hemochromatosis [positive family history in 25% of patients], α-1 antitrypsin deficiency)
- History of recurrent episodes of RUQ pain (biliary tract disease)
- History of blood transfusions, IV drug abuse (hepatitis C)

- History of hepatotoxic drug exposure
- Coexistence of other diseases with immune or autoimmune features (ITP, myasthenia gravis, thyroiditis, autoimmune hepatitis)

■ LABORATORY TESTS
- Decreased Hgb and Hct, elevated MCV, increased BUN and creatinine (the BUN may also be "normal" or low if the patient has severely diminished liver function), decreased sodium (dilutional hyponatremia), decreased potassium (as a result of secondary aldosteronism or urinary losses)
- Decreased glucose in a patient with liver disease indicating severe liver damage
- Other laboratory abnormalities:
  1. Alcoholic hepatitis and cirrhosis: there may be mild elevation of ALT and AST, usually <500 IU; AST > ALT (ratio >2:3).
  2. Extrahepatic obstruction: there may be moderate elevations of ALT and AST to levels <500 IU.
  3. Viral, toxic, or ischemic hepatitis: there are extreme elevations (>500 IU) of ALT and AST.
  4. Transaminases may be normal despite significant liver disease in patients with jejunoileal bypass operations or hemochromatosis or after methotrexate administration.
  5. Alkaline phosphatase elevation can occur with extrahepatic obstruction, primary biliary cirrhosis, and primary sclerosing cholangitis.
  6. Serum LDH is significantly elevated in metastatic disease of the liver; lesser elevations are seen with hepatitis, cirrhosis, extrahepatic obstruction, and congestive hepatomegaly.
  7. Serum γ-glutamyl transpeptidase (GGTP) is elevated in alcoholic liver disease and may also be elevated with cholestatic disease (primary biliary cirrhosis, primary sclerosing cholangitis).
  8. Serum bilirubin may be elevated; urinary bilirubin can be present in hepatitis, hepatocellular jaundice, and biliary obstruction.
  9. Serum albumin: significant liver disease results in hypoalbuminemia.
  10. Prothrombin time: an elevated PT in patients with liver disease indicates severe liver damage and poor prognosis.

11. Presence of hepatitis B surface antigen implies acute or chronic hepatitis B.
12. Presence of antimitochondrial antibody suggests primary biliary cirrhosis, chronic hepatitis.
13. Elevated serum copper, decreased serum ceruloplasmin, and elevated 24-hr urine may be diagnostic of Wilson's disease.
14. Protein immunoelectrophoresis may reveal decreased α-1 globulins (α-1 antitrypsin deficiency), increased IgA (alcoholic cirrhosis), increased IgM (primary biliary cirrhosis), increased IgG (chronic hepatitis, cryptogenic cirrhosis).
15 An elevated serum ferritin and increased transferrin saturation are suggestive of hemochromatosis.
16. An elevated blood ammonia suggests hepatocellular dysfunction; serial values are not useful in following patients with hepatic encephalopathy because there is poor correlation between blood ammonia level and degree of hepatic encephalopathy.
17. Serum cholesterol is elevated in cholestatic disorders.
18. Antinuclear antibodies (ANA) may be found in autoimmune hepatitis.
19. Alpha fetoprotein: levels >1000 pg/ml are highly suggestive of primary liver cell carcinoma.
20. Hepatitis C viral testing identifies patients with chronic hepatitis C infection.
21. Elevated level of serum globulin (especially γ-globulins), positive ANA test may occur with autoimmune hepatitis.

■ IMAGING STUDIES
- Ultrasonography is the procedure of choice for detection of gallstones and dilation of common bile ducts.
- CT scan is useful for detecting mass lesions in liver and pancreas, assessing hepatic fat content, identifying idiopathic hemochromatosis, early diagnosing of Budd-Chiari syndrome, dilation of intrahepatic bile ducts, and detection of varices and splenomegaly.

- Technetium-99m sulfur colloid scanning is useful for diagnosing cirrhosis (there is a shift of colloid uptake to the spleen, bone marrow), identifying hepatic adenomas (cold defect is noted), diagnosing Budd-Chiari syndrome (there is increased uptake by the caudate lobe).
- ERCP is the procedure of choice for diagnosing periampullary carcinoma, common duct stones; it is also useful in diagnosing primary sclerosing cholangitis.
- Percutaneous transhepatic cholangiography (PTC) is useful when evaluating patients with cholestatic jaundice and dilated intrahepatic ducts by ultrasonography; presence of intrahepatic strictures and focal dilation is suggestive of PSC.
- Percutaneous liver biopsy is useful in evaluating hepatic filling defects, diagnosing hepatocellular disease or hepatomegaly, evaluating persistently abnormal liver function tests, and diagnosing hemachromatosis, primary biliary cirrhosis, Wilson's disease, glycogen storage diseases, chronic hepatitis, autoimmune hepatitis, infiltrative diseases, alcoholic liver disease, drug-induced liver disease, and primary or secondary carcinoma.

℞ TREATMENT

■ NONPHARMACOLOGIC THERAPY
Avoid any hepatotoxins (e.g., ethanol, acetaminophen); improve nutritional status.

■ GENERAL Rx
- Correct any mechanical obstruction to bile flow (e.g., calculi, strictures).
- Provide therapy for underlying cardiovascular disorders in patients with cardiac cirrhosis.
- Remove excess body iron with phlebotomy and deferoxamine in patients with hemochromatosis.
- Remove copper deposits with D-penicillamine in patients with Wilson's disease.
- Long-term ursodiol therapy will slow the progression of primary biliary cirrhosis. It is, however, ineffective in primary sclerosing cholangitis.

- Glucocorticoids (prednisone 20 to 30 mg/day initially or combination therapy or prednisone and azathioprine) is useful in autoimmune hepatitis.
- Liver transplantation may be indicated in otherwise healthy patients (age <65 yr) with sclerosing cholangitis, chronic hepatitis cirrhosis, or primary biliary cirrhosis with prognostic information suggesting <20% chance of survival without transplantation; contraindications to liver transplantation are AIDS, most metastatic malignancies, active substance abuse, uncontrolled sepsis, uncontrolled cardiac or pulmonary disease.
- Treatment of complications of portal hypertension (ascites, esophagogastric varices, hepatic encephalopathy, and hepatorenal syndrome).

■ DISPOSITION
- Prognosis varies with the etiology of the patient's cirrhosis and whether there is ongoing hepatic injury. Mortality rate exceeds 80% in patients with hepatorenal syndrome.
- Two markers of portal hypertension, thrombocytopenia and splenomegaly, moderately increase the likelihood of large esophageal varices.
- If advanced cirrhosis is present and transplantation is not feasible, survival is 1 to 2 yr.

■ REFERRAL
- Hospital admission for bleeding varices, hepatic encephalopathy, or onset of hepatorenal syndrome
- Liver transplantation in suitable candidates is the only effective long-term treatment of complications resulting from cirrhosis

☼ PEARLS & CONSIDERATIONS

■ COMMENTS
Thrombocytopenia and advanced Child-Pugh cases are associated with the presence of varices. These factors are useful to identify cirrhotic patients who benefit most from referral for endoscopic screening for varices.
Author: Fred F. Ferri, M.D.

BASIC INFORMATION

■ DEFINITION

Primary biliary cirrhosis (PBC) is a chronic progressive disease, most often affecting women, characterized by progressive destruction of the small intrahepatic bile ducts with portal inflammation leading to fibrosis, cirrhosis, liver failure, and the need for liver transplantation.

ICD-9CM CODES
571.6 Biliary cirrhosis

■ EPIDEMIOLOGY & DEMOGRAPHICS
- PBC affects all races and accounts for 0.6% to 2% of deaths from cirrhosis worldwide.
- Approximately 95% of patients are female.
- PBC is reported only rarely in Africa and the Indian subcontinent.
- Prevalence estimates range from 19 to 151 cases per million population; incidence estimates range from 3.9 to 15 cases per million population per year.
- Genetic factors are important in the development of PBC; however, there is no clear dominant or recessive pattern of inheritance. Prevalence in families with one affected member is estimated to be 100 times higher than the general population. There is a weak association between PBC and HLA-DR8, and recent data suggest that infection with Chlamydia pneumoniae may be a triggering or causative event in PBC.
- Onset typically occurs between the ages of 30 and 65 yr.
- Up to 84% patients with PBC have at least one other autoimmune disorder, such as Sjögren's syndrome, rheumatoid arthritis, Raynaud's phenomenon, scleroderma, or thyroiditis.

■ PHYSICAL FINDINGS & CLINICAL PRESENTATION
SYMPTOMS:
- Variable dependent on stage of diagnosis. Fatigue and pruritus are the usual presenting symptoms. However, as many as 48% to 60% may be asymptomatic
- Pruritus may first occur during pregnancy but is distinguished from pruritus of pregnancy because it persists into the postpartum period
- Pruritus is worse at night, under constricting, coarse garments; in association with dry skin; and in hot, humid weather
- Musculoskeletal complaints caused by inflammatory arthropathy in 40% to 70% of patients: 5% to 10% develop chronic RA; 10% develop "arthritis of PBC"
- Unexplained RUQ pain
PHYSICAL:
- Variable: dependent on stage of disease at time of presentation. Early may be completely normal.

- 25% to 50% have hypopigmentation of skin.
- Excoriations may be present.
- Hepatomegaly and splenomegaly may be present in more advanced disease.
- Xanthomas, jaundice, and features of chronic liver disease/cirrhosis are all features of advanced disease.

■ ETIOLOGY
- Cause remains unknown.
- Most data point to inherited abnormality of immunoregulation.

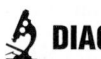

DIAGNOSIS

■ DIFFERENTIAL DIAGNOSIS
Drug-induced cholestasis
Other etiologies of chronic liver disease and cirrhosis:
- Alcoholic cirrhosis
- Viral hepatitis (chronic)
- Primary sclerosing cholangitis
- Autoimmune chronic active hepatitis
- Chemical/toxin-induced cirrhosis
- Other hereditary or familial disorders (e.g., CF, α1-antitrypsin deficiency)

■ WORKUP
History, physical examination, laboratory evaluation, and liver biopsy

■ LABORATORY TESTS
- Antimitochondrial antibodies (found in 95% of patients with PBC and are 98% specific)
- Markedly elevated alkaline phosphatase (of hepatic origin)
- Elevated GGTP
- Normal or slightly elevated aminotransferases
- Bilirubin normal early; increases with disease progression (direct and indirect)
- Markedly elevated serum lipids (total cholesterol, LDL, and especially HDL) Elevated ceruloplasmin
- Eosinophilia
- Percutaneous liver biopsy is the confirmatory test

■ IMAGING STUDIES
If history, physical examination, blood tests, and liver biopsy are all consistent with PBC, neither imaging nor cholangiography is necessary.

■ PROGNOSIS
- Progressive but variable
- Median survival asymptomatic: 10 to 16 yr; symptomatic: 7 yr
- Neither presence nor titer of antimitochondrial antibodies predicts survival
- Prognostic laboratory measures: serum bilirubin, albumin, prothrombin time
- At risk for both osteoporosis and osteomalacia
- Presence of cirrhosis, increased risk for hepatocellular carcinoma
- May develop deficiencies of fat-soluble vitamins, especially vitamin A

TREATMENT

- Management decisions vary depending on clinical status of patient.
- No generally accepted treatment of underlying disease process.
- Treatment focuses on management of complications (pruritus, metabolic bone diseases, hyperlipidemia) because liver transplantation is the only definitive treatment for this disease.

■ ACUTE GENERAL Rx
- Ursodiol, colchicine, and methotrexate have shown encouraging results.
- Ursodiol extends survival and lengthens the time before liver transplantation; normalizes bilirubin, may mask need for transplantation.
- Colchicine and methotrexate yield less impressive results but are still modestly effective.
- Prednisone, azathioprine, penicillamine, and cyclosporine have limited efficacy and predictable toxicity.

■ CHRONIC Rx
- Diet low in neutral triglycerides and high in medium chain triglycerides decreases steatorrhea and improves nutritional status
- Treatment for acute bacterial cystitis, which occurs with greater frequency in these patients
- Treatment for osteoporosis
- Vitamin A, K, E deficiencies can be clinically important in advanced cases and respond to oral replacement
- Pruritus: use cholestyramine resin, antihistamines, colestipol, rifampin, ursodiol, or naloxone
- Monitoring antimitochondrial antibody titer is not useful in assessing response to therapy
- Liver transplantation definitive
- 85% to 90% survival at 1 yr; survival rates thereafter resemble age/sex-matched healthy persons
- PBC does not recur in the new liver if appropriate immunosuppression is used

■ DISPOSITION
Definitive treatment requires liver transplantation; survival is 7 to 16 yr, dependent on symptoms.

■ REFERRAL
Evaluation for liver transplantation or treatment of refractory variceal bleeding

REFERENCES
Kaplan, MM: Primary biliary cirrhosis: past, present, and future, *Gastroenterology* 123(4): 1392, 2002.
Kaplan, MM: Primary biliary cirrhosis (review), *N Engl J Med* 335:1570, 1996.
Phillips JR et al: Fat-soluble vitamin levels in patients with primary biliary cirrhosis, *Am J Gastroenterol* 96:2745, 2001.
Authors: **Rebecca S. Brienza, M.D., M.P.H., and Jennifer R. Hur, M.D.**

BASIC INFORMATION

DEFINITION
Claudication refers to leg pain brought on by exertion and relieved with rest.

SYNONYMS
Intermittent claudication

ICD-9CM CODES
443.9 Peripheral vascular disease, unspecified
440.21 Intermittent claudication due to atherosclerosis

EPIDEMIOLOGY & DEMOGRAPHICS
INCIDENCE: 3 to 8 cases/1000 persons
PREVALENCE: 2% to 4% in the general population
RISK: Major risk factors of tobacco, hypertension, diabetes, and hypercholesterolemia increase the chance of developing claudication. Cigarette smoking is the major determinant of disease progression.

PHYSICAL FINDINGS & CLINICAL PRESENTATION
- Diminished pulses
- Bruits over the distal aorta, iliac or femoral arteries
- Pallor of the distal extremities on elevation
- Rubor with prolonged capillary refill on dependency
- Cool skin temperature
- Trophic changes of hair loss and muscle atrophy noted
- Nonhealing ulcers, necrotic tissue, and gangrene possible

ETIOLOGY
Primary cause of claudication is atherosclerosis with subsequent stenosis of peripheral vessels and ischemia to working muscle.

DIAGNOSIS

The history of buttock, thigh, or calf pain or fatigue brought on by exertion and relieved by rest along with the above mentioned physical findings makes the diagnosis of claudication fairly certain. Noninvasive studies help confirm the diagnosis.

DIFFERENTIAL DIAGNOSIS
Spinal stenosis (neurogenic claudication), muscle cramps, degenerative osteoarthritic joint disease particularly of the lumbar spine and hips, and compartment syndrome may all resemble claudication.

WORKUP
- Noninvasive vascular testing confirms the clinical impression of claudication and aids in locating the major occlusive site. Noninvasive testing uses continuous-wave Doppler to measure systolic arterial pressures and reports the ankle-brachial index (ABI) and segmental systolic pressures as well as Doppler waveforms.
- Ankle-brachial index (ABI): The ratio of ankle pressure to brachial pressure is usually about 1.
  1. In claudication, the ABI ranges from 0.5 to 0.8.
  2. In patients with rest pain or impending limb loss, ABI ≤0.3.
- Segmental systolic pressures usually are measured from the high thigh, above the knee, below the knee, and the ankle. Normally there should not be >20 mm Hg difference in pressures between adjacent segments. If the gradient is >20 mm Hg, significant narrowing is suspected in the intervening segment.
- Both ABI and segmental pressures can be done before and after exercise.

IMAGING STUDIES
- Duplex ultrasound can be used to locate the occluded areas and assess the patency of the distal arterial system or prior vein grafts.
- MRA and spiral CT angiography are newer imaging techniques available.
- Angiography remains the gold standard for imaging peripheral arterial occlusion. Complications can occur, and the study should be done only if surgical reconstruction is being considered.

TREATMENT

NONPHARMACOLOGIC THERAPY
- Tobacco cessation is vital.
- Diet to control diabetes and blood pressure, as well as to reduce cholesterol, should be followed.
- Daily exercise must be emphasized. Exercise will increase walking distances before symptoms occur and improve functional status. Walking 30 to 60 min/day for 5 days at about 2 mi/hr is recommended.

ACUTE GENERAL Rx
Most patients with claudication respond to conservative management mentioned above. If this fails, medication can be tried (see Chronic Rx). Surgical reconstruction has its specific indications reserved for patients with impending limb loss (see Chronic Rx).

CHRONIC Rx
- Pentoxifylline (Trental) and cilostazol (Pletal) have been approved for use in patients with intermittent claudication who have not responded well to conservative measures. Pentoxifylline 400 mg tid or cilostazol 100 mg bid for 3 mo should be tried. If there is no improvement in symptoms, the medicine can be discontinued.
- Surgical reconstruction is indicated in patients with refractory rest pain, limb ischemia, nonhealing ulcers, or gangrene and in a select group of patients with functional disability. Common surgical procedures:
  1. Aortoiliofemoral reconstruction: perioperative mortality <3%
  2. Infrainguinal bypass (e.g., femoropopliteal, femorotibial): perioperative mortality, 2% to 5%
  3. Extraanatomic bypass (e.g., axillofemoral or femorofemoral bypass)
  4. Angioplasty is used on short, discrete stenotic lesions in the iliac or femoropopliteal artery
  5. Atherectomy, stents, and lasers are newer techniques

DISPOSITION
- Intermittent claudication progressing to an ischemic leg or limb loss is an unusual course, especially if maintaining the conservative treatment of exercise and abstaining from tobacco.
- The 5-yr risk for developing ischemic ulceration in patients treated for diabetes and with ABI <0.5 was 30% compared with only 5% in patients with neither characteristic.

REFERRAL
Consultation with the vascular surgeon is recommended in the patient with threatened limb loss, rest pain, nonhealing ulcers, functional disability from pain, and gangrene.

❂ PEARLS & CONSIDERATIONS

- About 70% of patients with peripheral vascular disease will have concomitant coronary artery disease.

■ COMMENTS

- Claudication is a marker for generalized atherosclerosis. This group of patients has a higher risk of death from cardiovascular events than from limb loss. This should be kept in mind when deciding to proceed with surgical evaluation. Every effort should be made toward conservative measures.

- The ABI is more closely associated with leg function in persons with peripheral arterial disease than is intermittent claudication or other leg symptoms.

REFERENCES

Aquino R et al: Natural history of claudication: long-term serial follow-up study of 1244 claudicants, *J Vasc Surg* 34:962, 2002.

Dormandy JA, Rutherford RB: Management of peripheral arterial disease (PAD): TASC Working Group, *J Vasc Surg* 31(1Pt2):S1, 2000.

Hiatt WR: Drug therapy: medical treatment of peripheral arterial disease and claudication, *N Engl J Med* 344:1608, 2001.

McDermott MM et al: The ankle brachial index is associated with leg function and physical activity: the walking and leg circulation study, *Ann Intern Med* 136:873, 2002.

Stewart KJ, Hiatt WR, et al: Medical progress: exercise training for claudication, *N Engl J Med* 347:1941, 2002.

Authors: **Peter Petropoulos, M.D., and Mel Anderson, M.D.**

BASIC INFORMATION

■ DEFINITION

Cocaine is an alkaloid derived from the coca plant *Erythroxylon coca*, native to South America, which contains approximately 0.5% to 1% cocaine. The drug produces physiologic and behavioral effects when administered orally, intranasally, intravenously, or via inhalation following smoking. Cocaine has potent pharmacologic effects on dopamine, norepinephrine, and serotonin neurons in the central nervous system (CNS) involving alteration and blockade of cellular membrane transport and prevention of reputake.

■ SYNONYMS

Cocaine hydrochloride: topical solution (FDA approved as a topical anesthetic)

Free base: aqueous solution of cocaine hydrochloride converted to a more volatile base state by the addition of alkali, thereby extracting the cocaine base in a residue or precipitate

Crack: potent, purified smokable form; produces effects similar to those of intravenous administration

Street names include Bernice, Bernies, C, Cadillac or Champagne of drugs, Carrie, Cecil, Charlie, Coke, Dust, Dynamite, Flake, Gin, Girl, Gold dust, Green gold, Jet, Powder, Star dust, Paradise, Pimp's drug, Snowflake, Stardust, White girl

Liquid lady = alcohol + cocaine

Speedball = heroin + cocaine

Street measures: Hit (2-200 mg), snort, line, dose, spoon (approximately 1 g)

ICD-9CM CODES

304.2 Cocainism

■ EPIDEMIOLOGY & DEMOGRAPHICS

The 1993 National Household Survey on Drug Abuse estimated that 4.5 million Americans used cocaine in 1992, with 1.3 million reporting use at least monthly. By 1998 this had not significantly changed.

Between 1993 and 1994, intravenous cocaine and heroin abusers accounted for a major new group of persons with human immunodeficiency virus (HIV) in several metropolitan areas.

In 1999 an estimated 25 million Americans admitted that they used cocaine at least once, 3.7 million the previous year, and 1.5 million were current users. It is the most frequent cause of drug-related deaths reported by medical examiners.

■ PHYSICAL FINDINGS & CLINICAL PRESENTATION

PHASE I:
- CNS: euphoria, agitation, headache, vertigo, twitching, bruxism, nonintentional tremor
- Nausea, vomiting, fever, hypertension, tachycardia

PHASE II:
- CNS: lethargy, hyperreactive deep tendon reflexes, seizures (status epilepticus)
- Sympathetic overdrive: tachycardia, hypertension, hyperthermia
- Incontinence

PHASE III:
- CNS: flaccid paralysis, coma, fixed dilated pupils, loss of reflexes
- Pulmonary edema
- Cardiopulmonary arrest

Psychologic dependence manifests with habituation, paranoia, hallucinations (cocaine "bugs").

Central nervous system: cerebral ischemia and infarction, cerebral arterial spasm, cerebral vasculitis, cerebral vascular thrombosis, subarachnoid hemorrhage, intraparenchymal hemorrhage, seizures, cerebral atrophy, movement disorders

Cardiac: acute myocardial ischemia and infarction, arrhythmias and sudden death, dilated cardiomyopathy and myocarditis, infective endocarditis, aortic rupture

Pulmonary: (secondary to smoking crack cocaine) inhalation injuries: cartilage and nasal septal perforation, oropharyngeal ulcers; immunologically mediated diseases: hypersensitivity pneumonitis, bronchiolitis obliterans; pulmonary vascular lesions and hemorrhage, pulmonary infarction, pulmonary edema secondary to left ventricular failure, pneumomediastinum, and pneumothorax

Gastrointestinal: gastroduodenal ulceration and perforation; intestinal infarction and/or perforation, colitis

Renal: acute renal failure secondary to rhabdomyolysis and myoglobinuria; renal infarction; focal segmental glomerulosclerosis

Obstetric: placental abruption, low infant weight, prematurity, and microcephaly

Psychiatric: anxiety, depression, paranoia, delirium, psychosis, and suicide

■ ETIOLOGY

Cocaine may be absorbed through different routes with varying degrees of speed
- Nasal insufflation/snorting: 2.5 min
- Smoking: <30 sec
- Oral: 2 to 5 min
- Mucosal: <20 min
- Intravenous injection: <30 sec

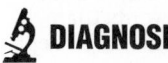 DIAGNOSIS

■ DIFFERENTIAL DIAGNOSIS
- Methamphetamine ("speed") abuse
- Methylenedioxyamphetamine ("ecstasy") abuse
- Cathione ("khat") abuse
- Lysergic acid diethylamide (LSD) abuse

■ WORKUP

Physical examination and laboratory evaluation

■ LABORATORY TESTS
- Toxicology screen (urine): Cocaine is metabolized within 2 hr by the liver to major metabolites, benzoylecogonine and ecgonine methylester, which are excreted in the urine. Metabolites can be identified in urine within 5 min of IV use and up to 48 hr after oral ingestion
- Blood: CBC, electrolytes, glucose, BUN, creatinine, calcium
- ABG analysis
- ECG
- Serum creatinine kinase and troponin concentration

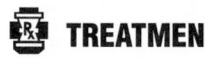 TREATMENT

There is no specific antidote and, at present, no drug therapy is uniquely effective in treating cocaine abuse and dependence. In addition, adulterants, contaminants, and other drugs may be admixed with street cocaine. Amantadine may provide effective treatment for cocaine-dependent patients with severe cocaine withdrawal symptoms, as well as the other dopamine agonist bromocriptine (1.5 mg PO tid), which may alleviate some of the symptoms of craving associated with acute cocaine withdrawal.

■ ACUTE GENERAL Rx

Acute cocaine toxicity requires following advanced poisoning treatment and life support. A suspected "body-packer" should have an abdominal radiograph to detect the continued presence of cocaine-containing condoms in the intestinal tract. If present, gentle catharsis with charcoal and mineral oil should be performed with ICU admission and monitoring. Management of cocaine-related toxicity is also outlined in Table 1-14.

■ SPECIFIC TREATMENT

For an outline of treatment, see Table 1-14

INHALATION: Wash nasal passages
ANXIETY: Diazepam 15 to 20 mg PO IV for severe agitation
SEIZURE MANAGEMENT (STATUS EPILEPTICUS):
- Diazepam 5 to 10 mg IV over 2 to 3 min, may be repeated every 10 to 15 min
- Lorazepam 2 to 3 mg IV over 2 to 3 min, may be repeated

- Phenytoin loading dose 15 to 18 mg/kg IV at a rate not to exceed 25 to 50 mg/min under cardiac monitoring
- Phenobarbital loading dose 10 to 15 mg/kg IV at a rate of 25 mg/min; an additional 5 mg/kg may be given in 30 to 45 min if seizures are not controlled.
- Refractory seizures, consider:
  Pancuronium 0.1 mg/kg IV
  Halothane general anesthesia
  Both require EEG monitoring to determine brain seizure activity.

HYPERTENSION:
- Nifedipine 10 mg SL
- Labetalol 10 to 80 mg IV
- Propranolol 1 mg IV/q min, up to 6 mg
- Phentolamine may be required (unopposed adrenergic effects)
- If diastolic pressure >120 mm Hg: hydralazine hydrochloride 25 mg IM or IV; may repeat q1h
- If hypertension uncontrolled or hypertensive encephalopathy is present: sodium nitroprusside initially at 0.5 μg/kg/min not to exceed 10 μg/kg/min

VENTRICULAR ARRHYTHMIAS:
- Antiarrhythmia agents should be used in caution during the early period after cocaine exposure as a result of their proarrhythmic and proconvulsant effects
- Propranolol 1 mg/min IV for up to 6 mg
- Lidocaine 1.5 mg/kg IV bolus followed by IV infusion (controversial: may cause seizures)
- Termination of ventricular arrhythmias may be resistant to lidocaine and even cardioversion
- $NaHCO_3^-$ is under investigation in cocaine-mediated conduction abnormalities and rhythm disturbances.

■ REFERRAL

Consider psychotherapy and/or behavioral therapy once stable.

REFERENCE

Lange RA, Hillis LD: Cardiovascular complications of cocaine use, *N Engl J Med* 345:351, 2001.
Author: **Sajeev Handa, M.D.**

TABLE 1-14 **Management of Cocaine-Related Toxicity**

CONDITION	DIAGNOSIS	MANAGEMENT
Rhabdomyolysis	CK <5-10 times normal Muscle tenderness Urine dip insensitive	Vigorous hydration, urine output at least 2 ml/kg Mannitol or bicarb for rhabdomyolysis resistant to hydration
Hyperthemia	Rectal temperature CK Electrolytes	Continuous rectal probe. Bring temperature down to 101° F within 30-45 min
Hyptertension	Continuous blood pressure monitoring; consider arterial line	Nitroprusside, phentolamine, labetalol
Chest pain	Chest x-ray film, ECG, cardiac enzymes for patients with abnormal ECGs or persistant cardiac-sounding chest pain	Benzodiazepines for agitation; aspirin and nitroglycerin drip for ischemic pain; see text for discussion of indications for admission; PCTA possibly better than thrombolysis for presumed cocaine-associated MI
Agitation	Clinical evaluation; stat glucose	Benzodiazepines

From Rosen P (ed): *Emergency medicine,* ed 4, St Louis, 1998, Mosby.

BASIC INFORMATION

■ DEFINITION
Coccidioidomycosis is an infectious disease caused by the fungus *Coccidioides immitis*. It is usually asymptomatic and characterized by a primary pulmonary focus with infrequent progression to chronic pulmonary disease and dissemination to other organs.

■ SYNONYMS
San Joaquin Valley fever

ICD-9CM CODES
114.0 Coccidioidax pneumonia
114.1 Cutaneous or extrapulmonary (primary) coccidioidomycosis
114.3 Disseminated or prostate coccidioidomycosis
114.5 Pulmonary coccidioidomycosis
114.2 Meninges coccidioidomycosis
114.4 Chronic coccidioidomycosis

■ EPIDEMIOLOGY & DEMOGRAPHICS
PREVALENCE: Unknown
INCIDENCE (IN U.S.): Estimated annual infection rate 100,000 persons, predominantly in southwest U.S.
PREDOMINANT SEX: Males, between the ages of 25 to 55 yr
PEAK INCIDENCE: Unknown
GENETICS:
Familial Disposition: Unknown
Congenital Infection: Documented, but considered to occur rarely
Neonatal Infection:
- Occurs equally between the sexes
- Clinical disease more severe than in older children and adults

■ PHYSICAL FINDINGS & CLINICAL PRESENTATION
- Asymptomatic infections or illness consistent with a nonspecific upper respiratory tract infection in at least 60%
- Symptoms of primary infection—cough, malaise, fever, chills, night sweats, anorexia, weakness, and arthralgias (desert rheumatism)—in remaining 40% within 3 wk of exposure
- Skin rashes, such as erythema nodosum and erythema multiforme, usually with a significant female preponderance
- Scattered rales and areas that are dull on percussion with auscultation
- Spontaneous improvement within 2 wk of illness, with complete recovery usual

- Subsequent pulmonary residua in the form of pulmonary nodules and cavities in <10% of those patients with primary infection; half of these patients asymptomatic
- In a small portion of these patients: a progressive pneumonitis, often with a fatal outcome
- Some, especially if immunocompromised and/or diabetic, progressing to chronic pulmonary disease
- Over many years, granulomas rupture, leading to new cavity formation and continued fibrosis, often accompanied by hemoptysis
- Possible bronchiectasis with acute or chronic disease
- Disseminated or extrapulmonary disease in approximately 0.5% of acutely infected patients
  1. Early signs of probable dissemination: fever, malaise, hilar adenopathy, and elevated ESR persisting in the setting of primary infection
  2. Most organs are susceptible to dissemination, with heart and GI tract generally spared
- Musculoskeletal involvement
  1. Occurs one third of the time in disseminated disease
  2. Usually presents with local pain, swelling of a joint, bone, or muscle
  3. Majority of bone lesions unifocal and usually involve the skull, metacarpals, metatarsals, and tibia
  4. Vertebral column possibly affected with usually multiple lesions involving the arch and contiguous ribs and sparing the intravertebral disk
  5. Joint lesions predominantly unifocal, most commonly involving the ankle and knee, and often accompanying adjacent sites of osteomyelitis
- Meningeal involvement
  1. Occurs approximately one third of the time with dissemination
  2. Usually presents within 6 mo of primary infection or may appear concurrently
  3. Mass lesions rare, with approximately 40 cases reported this century
  4. Usually, absence of classic signs of meningeal irritation, but possible focal deficits, seizure activity, and stiff neck
  5. Most common complaint: headache
  6. Presenting symptoms: fever, weakness, confusion, lethargy, vomiting

- Cutaneous involvement, excluding rash
  1. Variable in appearance, taking the form of pustules, papules, plaques, nodules, ulcers, abscesses, or proliferative lesions
  2. Lesions most characteristically verrucous
  3. Dissemination and fatal outcomes most common in men, pregnant women, neonates, immunocompromised hosts, and individuals of dark-skinned races, especially those of African, Filipino, Mexican, and Native American ancestry

■ ETIOLOGY
- *Coccidioides immitis* is endemic to the American continent, including northern, central, and southern parts.
- In the U.S., most cases are acquired in Arizona, California, New Mexico, and Texas.
- Endemic areas coincide with the Lower Sonoran Life Zone, with semi-arid climate, sparse flora, and alkaline soil.
- Fungus exists in the mycelial phase in soil, having barrel-shaped hyphae (arthroconidia).
- Windswept spores from easily fragmented arthroconidia are dispersed to infect other soil (saprophytic cycle) or are inhaled by animals, including rodents and humans.
- Arthrospore deposits in the alveoli, then fungus converts to thick-walled spherule.
- Internal spherical spores (endospores) are released through spherule rupture and mature into new spherules (parasitic cycle).
- Fungus incites a granulomatous reaction in host tissue, usually with caseation necrosis.

DIAGNOSIS

■ DIFFERENTIAL DIAGNOSIS
- Acute pulmonary coccidioidomycoses:
  1. Community-acquired pneumonias caused by *Mycoplasma* and *Chlamydia*
  2. Granulomatous diseases, such as *Mycobacterium tuberculosis* and sarcoidosis
  3. Other fungal diseases, such as *Blastomyces dermatitidis* and *Histoplasma capsulatum*
- Coccidioidomas: true neoplasms

■ WORKUP
- Suspected in patients with a history of residence or travel in an endemic area, especially during periods favorable to spore dispersion (e.g., dust storms and drought followed by heavy rains)
- Suspected with a patient history of handling fomites from endemic areas (e.g., fruit and cotton), as in textile workers or fruit handlers

■ LABORATORY TESTS
- CBC to reveal eosinophilia, especially with erythema nodosum
- Routine chemistries: usually normal but may reveal hyponatremia
- Elevated serum levels of IgE; associated with progressive disease
- CSF cell counts and chemistry: pleocytosis with mononuclear cell predominance associated with hypoglycorrhachia and elevated protein level
- Definitive diagnosis based on demonstration of the organism by culture from body fluids or tissues (Fig. 1-72)
  1. Greatest yield with pus, sputum, synovial fluid, and soft tissue aspirations, varying with the degree of dissemination
  2. Possible positive cultures of blood, gastric aspirate, pleural effusion, peritoneal fluid, and CSF, but less frequently obtained
  3. In patients with AIDS: failure of sputum cultures to grow the fungus, so pulmonary biopsy is needed
- Serologic evaluations
  1. Latex agglutination and complement fixation
  2. Elevated serum complement-fixing antibody (CFA) titers ≥1:32 (Smith and Saito) strongly correlated with disseminated disease, except with meningitis where lower titers seen
  3. Variable discriminating titers depending on method, so must be based on reference ranges provided
  4. In meningeal disease: CFA detected in CSF except with high serum CFA titers secondary to concurrent extraneural disease
  5. Enzyme-linked immunosorbent assay (ELISA) against a 33-kDa spherule antigen to detect and monitor CNS disease
- Coccidioidin, the mycelial phase antigen, and spherulin, the parasitic phase antigen
  1. Positive (>5 mm) 1 mo following onset of symptomatic primary infection
  2. Useful in assessing prior infection
  3. Negative skin test with primary infection: latent or future dissemination

■ IMAGING STUDIES
Chest x-ray examination:
- Reveals unilateral infiltrates, hilar adenopathy, or pleural effusion in primary infection
- Shows areas of fibrosis containing usually solitary, thin-walled cavities that persist as residua of primary infection
- Possible coccidioidoma, a coin-like lesion representing a healed area of previous pneumonitis

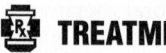 TREATMENT

■ NONPHARMACOLOGIC THERAPY
- Supportive care in mild symptomatic disease
- In patients with extrapulmonary manifestations involving draining skin, joint, and soft tissue infection: local wound care to avoid possible bacterial superinfection

■ ACUTE GENERAL Rx
- In general, drug therapy is not required for patients with asymptomatic pulmonary disease and most patients with mild symptomatic primary infection.
- Chemotherapy is indicated under the following circumstances:
  1. Severe symptomatic primary infection
  2. High serum CFA titers
  3. Persistent symptoms >6 wk
  4. Prostration
  5. Progressive pulmonary involvement
  6. Pregnancy
  7. Infancy
  8. Debilitation
  9. Concurrent illness (e.g., diabetes, asthma, COPD, malignancy)
  10. Acquired or induced immunosuppression

A   B   C

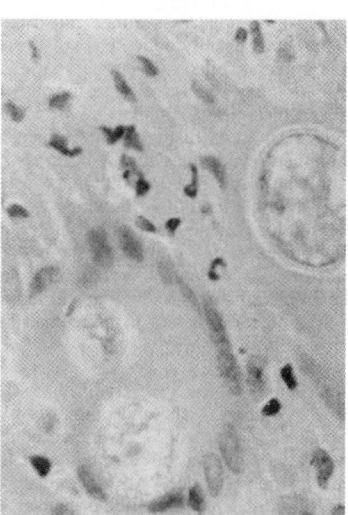 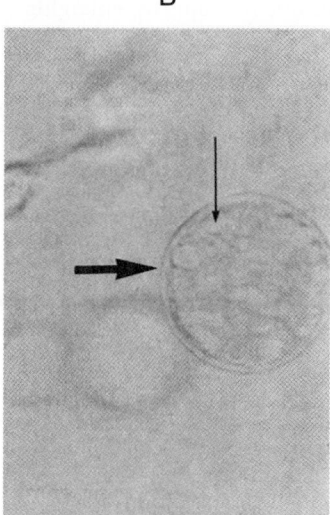 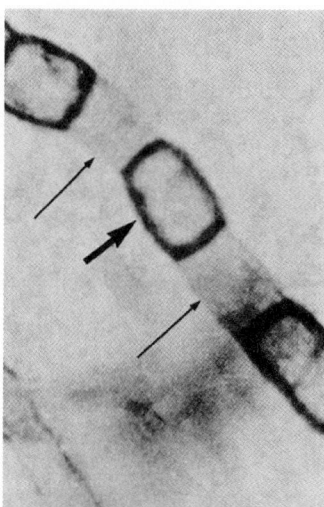

Fig. 1-72 Morphologic appearance of *Coccidioides immitis*. A, Spherules within Langerhans' giant cells, shown by hematoxylin and eosin stain. **B,** Spherule in unstained potassium hydroxide preparation. The endospores within spherule *(small arrow)* and the clearly defined double wall of spherule *(large arrow)* are evident. **C,** Mycelial form with barrel-shaped arthroconidia *(large arrow)* spaced between intercalating "ghost cells" *(small arrows).* (From Stein JH [ed]: *Internal medicine,* ed 5, St Louis, 1998, Mosby.)

11. Racial group with known predisposition for disseminated disease
- Fluconazole
  1. Most commonly, oral therapy with 400 mg/day up to 1.2 g/day appears to be the drug of choice for meningeal and deep-seated mycotic infections.
  2. In patients with AIDS, fluconazole may be considered the drug of choice for initial and maintenance therapy.
  3. All patients with coccidioidal meningitis should continue azole therapy indefinitely.
- Itraconazole
  1. 400 to 600 mg/day achieves 90% response rate in bone, joint, soft tissue, lymphatic, and genitourinary infections.
  2. Itraconazole may be more efficacious than fluconazole in the treatment of skeletal (bone) infections.
- For pulmonary infections, treatment with either fluconazole or itraconazole, given for 6 to 12 wk, appears to be equal in efficacy.
- Amphotericin B is the classic therapy for disseminated extraneural disease, dose 1 to 1.5 mg/kg/day, qd for the first week and qid thereafter, for a total dose of 1 to 2.5 g or until clinical and serologic remission is accomplished.
  1. Local instillation into body cavities such as sinuses, fistulae, and abscesses has been adjunct to therapy.
  2. Liposomal amphotericin B is probably equally effective, but further studies are needed.
  3. Duration of therapy for extraneural disease is undefined but probably about 1 yr.
- With meningeal disease:
  1. Intrathecal amphotericin B remains the traditional treatment modality, given alone or preceding the use of oral agents.
  2. Begin in doses of 0.01 to 0.025 mg/day, gradually increasing the dose as tolerated, to 0.5 mg/day with the patient in Trendelenburg's position.

3. If given via Ommaya reservoir, as in ventriculitis, dose may be increased to 1.5 mg/day if tolerated.
4. Concomitant parenteral therapy with amphotericin B is used for simultaneous extraneural disease as standard doses and with purely meningeal disease in smaller doses, although not strictly indicated.
5. Intrathecal therapy is usually given three times a week for at least 3 mo, then discontinued or gradually tapered until once every 6 wk through 1 yr of therapy.
6. Patients need routine monitoring of CSF, CFA, cell count, and chemistries for at least 2 yr following cessation of therapy.
- For osteomyelitis, soft-tissue closed space infections, and pulmonary fibrocavitary disease: surgical debridement, drainage, or resection, respectively, in addition to oral azole therapy or parenteral administration of amphotericin B

■ CHRONIC Rx
For chronically immunocompromised patients, lifelong therapy with oral azoles or amphotericin B

■ DISPOSITION
- Prognosis for primary symptomatic infection is good.
- Immunocompromised patients are most likely to have disseminated disease and higher morbidity and mortality.

■ REFERRAL
- To surgeon for the evaluation of chronic hemoptysis, enlarging cavitary lesions despite chemotherapy and intrapleural rupture, osteomyelitis, and other synovial or soft tissue closed space infections
- For neurosurgical consultation in patients with meningeal disease to establish the delivery route of intrathecal drug therapy

⚙ PEARLS & CONSIDERATIONS

■ COMMENTS
- Infected body fluids contained within a closed moist environment (e.g., sputum in a specimen cup) provide the opportunity for the fungus to revert to its hyphal form whereby spores may be made airborne on opening of the container. Purulent drainage into a cast, allowing conversion of fungus to the saprophytic phase, has been responsible for acute disease when the cast was opened and the spores were unintentionally made airborne.
- Patients with a remote history of exposure, especially if immunosuppressed by medication or disease, may reactivate primary disease and suffer rapid dissemination.
- Although cardiac disease is rare, constrictive pericarditis in the setting of disseminated coccidioidomycosis has been documented and is potentially fatal.
- Organ transplant recipients may develop disease if the transplant donor has unrecognized active coccidioidomycosis at the time of death.

REFERENCES
Blair JE et al: Incidence and prevalence of coccidioidomycosis in patients with end-stage liver disease, *Liver Transpl* 9(8):843, 2003.

Caraway NP et al: Coccidioidomycosis osteomyelitis masquerading as a bone tumor. A report of 2 cases, *Acta Cytol* 47(5):777, 2003.

Chiller TM et al: Coccidioidomycosis, *Infect Dis Clin North Am* 17(1):41, 2003.

Copeland B, White D, Buenting J: Coccidioidomycosis of the head and neck, *Ann Otol Rhinol Laryngol* 112(1):98, 2003.

Crum NF et al: A cluster of disseminated coccidioidomycosis cases at a US military hospital, *Mil Med* 168(6):460, 2003.

Komotar RJ et al: Coccidioidomycosis of the brain, mimicking en plaque meningioma, *J Neurol Neurosurg Psychiatry* 74(6):806, 2003.

Visbal AL et al: Coccidioidal pericarditis: implications of surgical treatment in the elderly, *Ann Thorac Surg* 75(4):1328, 2003.

Wright PW et al: Donor-related coccidioidomycosis in organ transplant recipients, *Clin Infect Dis* 37(9):1265, 2003.
Author: **George O. Alonso, M.D.**

BASIC INFORMATION

■ DEFINITION
Acute self-limited febrile illness caused by infection with a Coltivirus

ICD-9CM CODES
066.1 Colorado Tick Fever

■ EPIDEMIOLOGY & DEMOGRAPHICS
- Incidence: approximately 330 cases reported per year in the U.S.
- Demographics: children and adults of both genders
- Geography: Rocky Mountains at elevations of 4000 to 10,000 feet.
- Colorado has the highest incidence (see Fig. 1-73)

■ PHYSICAL FINDINGS & CLINICAL PRESENTATION
- Incubation: 3 to 4 days is usual, but can be up to 14 days
- First symptoms: fever, chills, severe headache, severe myalgias, and hyperesthetic skin
- Initial signs and symptoms
  1. Tick bite
  2. Fever and chills
  3. Headache
  4. Myalgias
  5. Weakness
  6. Prostration and indifference
  7. Injected conjunctivae
  8. Erythematous pharyngitis
  9. Lymphadenopathy
  10. Maculopapular or petechial rash

These first symptoms last for 1 wk or less but 50% of the cases experience a febrile relapse 2 to 3 days following an initial remission. Weakness and fatigue may persist for several months after the acute phase(s). This chronic phase is more likely in older patients.
In children, 5% to 10% of cases are complicated by aseptic meningitis. In adults, rare complications include pneumonia, hepatitis, myocarditis, and epididymoorchitis. Vertically transmitted fetal infection is possible.

■ ETIOLOGY & PATHOGENESIS
- Infectious agent: Coltiviruses; 7 species, including 3 in the U.S.
- Vector: wood tick, *Dermacentor andersoni*
- Pathogenesis: human transmission occurs via tick bite. Tick season spans from March to September. The virus infects marrow erythrocytic precursors, explaining the protracted disease course as viremia lasts for the lifespan of the infected RBC

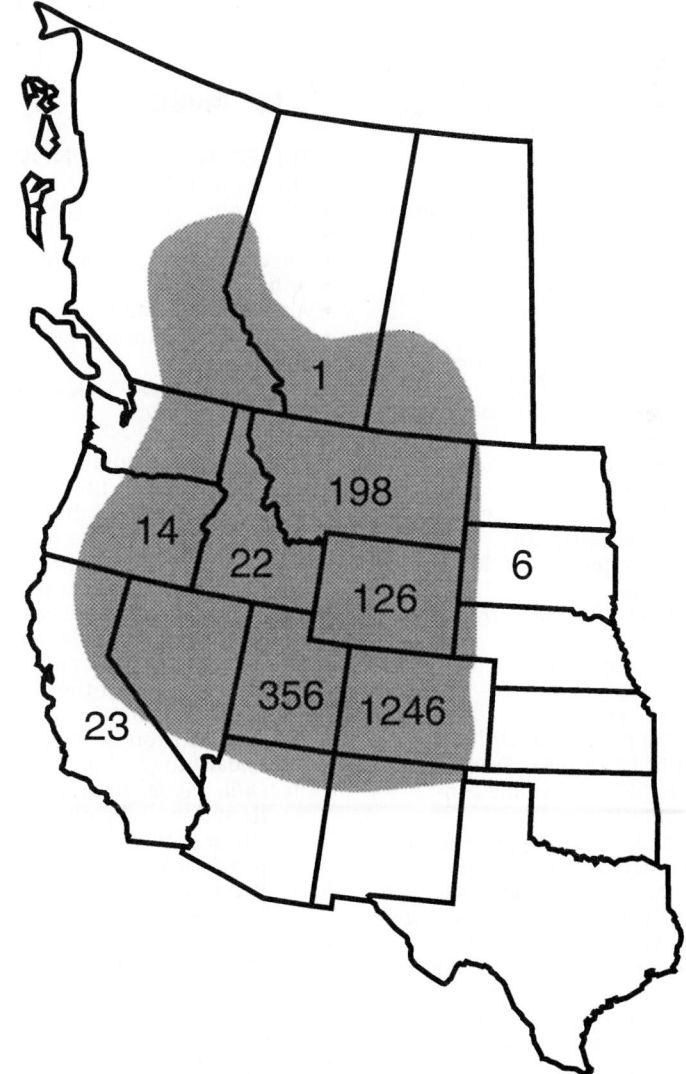 **DIAGNOSIS**

■ DIFFERENTIAL DIAGNOSIS
Rocky Mountain spotted fever, influenza, leptospirosis, infectious mononucleosis, CMV infection, pneumonia, hepatitis, meningitis, endocarditis, scarlet fever, measles, rubella, typhus, Lyme disease, ITP, TTP, Kawasaki disease, toxic shock syndrome, vasculitis

■ WORKUP
Consider Colorado tick fever in the presence of the above symptoms associated with travel to an endemic area coupled with a history of tick exposure

■ LABORATORY TESTS
- CBC
  1. Leukopenia
  2. Atypical lymphocytes
  3. Moderate thrombocytopenia
- Virus identification in RBCs by indirect immunofluorescence
- Serology using ELISA, neutralization, or complement fixation

 TREATMENT

- No specific therapy although Coltiviruses are sensitive to ribavirin
- Bedrest, fluids, acetaminophen
- Avoid aspirin because of thrombocytopenia
- Prevention: tick avoidance measures

REFERENCE
Tsai TF: Coltiviruses (Colorado tick fever). In Mandell GL, Bennett JF, Dolin R (eds): *Principles and practice of infectious diseases*, ed 5, Philadelphia, 2000, Churchill Livingstone.
Author: **Tom J. Wachtel, M.D.**

Fig. 1-73 Geographic distribution of *Dermacentor andersoni* (wood ticks) and reported cases of Colorado tick fever, 1990-1996, United States and Canada. (From Mandell GL: *Mandell, Douglas, and Bennett's principles and practice of infectious diseases*, ed 5, New York, 2000, Churchill Livingstone.)

BASIC INFORMATION

■ DEFINITION
Colorectal cancer is a neoplasm arising from the luminal surface of the large bowel: descending colon (40% to 42%), rectosigmoid and rectum (30% to 33%), cecum and ascending colon (25% to 30%), transverse colon (10% to 13%).

ICD-9CM CODES
154.0 Colorectal cancer

■ EPIDEMIOLOGY & DEMOGRAPHICS
- Colorectal cancer is the second leading cause of cancer deaths in the U.S. (>135,000 new cases and >50,000 deaths/yr).
- Peak incidence is in the seventh decade of life.
- 50% of rectal cancers are within reach of the examiner's finger, 50% of colon cancers are within reach of the flexible sigmoidoscope.
- Colorectal cancer accounts for 14% of all cases of cancer (excluding skin malignancies) and 14% of all yearly cancer deaths.
- Risk factors:
  1. Hereditary polyposis syndromes
     a. Familial polyposis (high risk)
     b. Gardner's syndrome (high risk)
     c. Turcot's syndrome (high risk)
     d. Peutz-Jeghers syndrome (low to moderate risk)
  2. IBD, both ulcerative colitis and Crohn's disease
  3. Family history of "cancer family syndrome"
  4. Heredofamilial breast cancer and colon carcinoma
  5. History of previous colorectal carcinoma
  6. Women undergoing irradiation for gynecologic cancer
  7. First-degree relatives with colorectal carcinoma
  8. Age >40 yr
  9. Possible dietary factors (diet high in fat or meat, beer drinking, reduced vegetable consumption)
  10. Hereditary nonpolyposis colon cancer (HNPCC): autosomal-dominant disorder characterized by early age of onset (mean age of 44 yr) and right-sided or proximal colon cancers, synchronous and metachronous colon cancers, mucinous and poorly differentiated colon cancers; it accounts for 1% to 5% of all cases of colorectal cancer
  11. Previous endometrial or ovarian cancer, particularly when diagnosed at an early age

■ PHYSICAL FINDINGS & CLINICAL PRESENTATION
- Physical examination may be completely unremarkable.
- Digital rectal examination can detect approximately 50% of rectal cancers.
- Palpable abdominal masses may indicate metastasis or complications of colorectal carcinoma (abscess, intussusception, volvulus).
- Abdominal distention and tenderness are suggestive of colonic obstruction.
- Hepatomegaly may be indicative of hepatic metastasis.

■ ETIOLOGY
Colorectal cancer can arise through two mutational pathways: microsatellite instability or chromosomal instability. Germline genetic mutations are the basis of inherited colon cancer syndromes; an accumulation of somatic mutations in a cell is the basis of sporadic colon cancer.

DIAGNOSIS

■ DIFFERENTIAL DIAGNOSIS
- Diverticular disease
- Strictures
- IBD
- Infectious or inflammatory lesions
- Adhesions
- Arteriovenous malformations
- Metastatic carcinoma (prostate, sarcoma)
- Extrinsic masses (cysts, abscesses)

■ WORKUP
- The clinical presentation of colorectal malignancies is initially vague and nonspecific (weight loss, anorexia, malaise). It is useful to divide colon cancer symptoms into those usually associated with right side of colon and those commonly associated with left side of colon, because the clinical presentation varies with the location of the carcinoma.
  1. Right side of colon
     a. Anemia (iron deficiency secondary to chronic blood loss)
     b. Dull, vague, and uncharacteristic abdominal pain may be present or patient may be completely asymptomatic
     c. Rectal bleeding is often missed because blood is mixed with feces
     d. Obstruction and constipation are unusual because of large lumen and more liquid stools
  2. Left side of colon
     a. Change in bowel habits (constipation, diarrhea, tenesmus, pencil-thin stools)
     b. Rectal bleeding (bright red blood coating the surface of the stool)
     c. Intestinal obstruction is frequent because of small lumen
- Early diagnosis of patients with surgically curable disease (Dukes' A, B) is necessary, because survival time is directly related to the stage of the carcinoma at the time of diagnosis. Appropriate screening recommendations are discussed in Section V.

■ CLASSIFICATION
Dukes' and UICC classification for colorectal cancer:
  A Confined to the mucosa-submucosa (I)
  B Invasion of muscularis propria (II)
  C Local node involvement (III)
  D Distant metastasis (IV)

■ LABORATORY TESTS
- Positive fecal occult blood test.
- Newer modalities for early detection of colorectal neoplasms include the detection of mutations in the adenomatous polyposis coli (APC) gene from stool samples
- Microcytic anemia
- Elevated plasma carcinoembryonic antigen (CEA). CEA should not be used as a screening test for colorectal cancer because it can be elevated in patients with many other conditions (smoking, IBD, alcoholic liver disease). A normal CEA does not exclude the diagnosis of colorectal cancer
- Liver function tests

■ IMAGING STUDIES
- Colonoscopy with biopsy (primary assessment tool)
- CT scan of abdomen to assist in preoperative staging
- Chest x-ray examination to look for evidence of metastatic disease
- Air-contrast barium enema only in patients refusing colonoscopy or unable to tolerate colonoscopy

TREATMENT

■ GENERAL Rx
- Surgical resection: 70% of colorectal cancers are resectable for cure at presentation; 45% of patients are cured by primary resection.
- Radiation therapy is a useful adjunct to fluorouracil and levamisole therapy for stage II or III rectal cancers.
- Adjuvant chemotherapy with combination of 5-fluorouracil (5-FU) and levamisole substantially increases cure rates for patients with stage III colon cancer and should be considered standard treatment for all such patients and selected patients with high-risk stage II colon cancer.

- Weekly treatment with irinotecan plus fluorouracil and leucovorin is superior to a widely used regimen of fluorouracil and leucovorin for metastatic colorectal cancer in terms of progression-free survival and overall survival.
- In patients who undergo resection of liver metastases from colorectal cancer, postoperative treatment with a combination of hepatic arterial infusion of floxuridine and IV fluorouracil improves the outcome at 2 yr.
- Irinotecan (Camptosar), a potent inhibitor of topoisomerase I, a nuclear enzyme involved in the unwinding of DNA during replication, can be used to treat metastatic colorectal cancer refractory to other drugs, including 5-FU; it may offer a few months of palliation but is expensive and associated with significant toxicity.
- Oxiliplatin (Eloxatin), an inhibitor of DNA synthesis, has been approved by the FDA for chemotherapy of advanced colorectal cancer for use in combination with fluorouracil and leucovorin for patients with metastatic colorectal cancer whose disease has recurred or progressed despite treatment with fluorouracil/leucovorin plus irinotecan.

■ CHRONIC Rx
Follow-up is indicated with:
- Fecal occult blood testing every 6 mo for 4 yr, then yearly
- Colonoscopy yearly for the initial 2 yr, then every 3 yr
- CEA level should be obtained baseline; if elevated, it can be used postoperatively as a measure of completeness of tumor resection or to monitor tumor recurrence; if used to monitor tumor recurrence, CEA should be obtained every 2 mo for 2 yr, then every 4 mo for 2 yr, and then yearly. The role of CEA for monitoring patients with resected colon cancer has been questioned because of the small number of cures attributed to CEA monitoring despite the substantial cost in dollars and physical and emotional stress associated with monitoring

■ DISPOSITION
- The 5-yr survival varies with the stage of the carcinoma:
  1. Dukes' A 5-yr survival, >80%
  2. Dukes' B 5-yr survival, 60%
  3. Dukes' C 5-yr survival, 20%
  4. Dukes' D 5-yr survival, 3%
- Overall 5-yr disease-free survival is approximately 50% for colon cancer.
- High-frequency microsatellite instability in colorectal cancer is independently predictive of a relatively

favorable outcome and, in addition, reduces the likelihood of metastases.
- In patients with Dukes' C (stage III) colorectal cancer there is improved 5-year survival among women treated with adjuvant chemotherapy (53% with chemotherapy vs. 33% without) and among patients with right-sided tumors treated with adjuvant chemotherapy.
- Retention of 18q alleles in microsatellite-stable cancers and mutation of the gene for the type I receptor for TGF-B1 in cancers with high levels of microsatellite instability point to a favorable outcome after adjuvant chemotherapy with fluorouracil-based regimens for stage II colon cancer.

■ REFERRAL
- Surgical referral for resection
- Oncology referral for adjuvant chemotherapy in selected patients
- Radiation oncology referral for patients with stage II or III rectal cancers

✺ PEARLS & CONSIDERATIONS

■ COMMENTS
- Decreased fat intake to 30% of total energy intake, increased fiber, and fruit and vegetable consumption may lower colorectal cancer risk. Recent literature reports, however, do not support a protective effect from dietary fiber against colorectal cancer in women.
- Chemoprophylaxis with aspirin (81 mg/day) reduces the incidence of colorectal adenomas in persons at risk.
- The National Cancer Institute has published consensus guidelines for universal screening for hereditary nonpolyposis colon cancer (HNPCC) in patients with newly diagnosed colorectal cancer. Tumors in mutation carriers of HNPCC typically exhibit microsatellite instability, a characteristic phenotype that is caused by expansions or contractions of short nucleotide repeat sequences. These guidelines (Bethesda Guidelines) are useful for selective patients for microsatellite instability testing. Screening patients with newly diagnosed colorectal cancer for HNPCC is cost effective, especially if the benefits to their immediate relatives are considered.
- Expression of guanylyl cyclase C mRNA in lymph nodes is associated with recurrence of colorectal cancer in patients with stage II disease. Analysis of guanylyl cyclase mRNA expression by RT-PCR may be useful for colorectal cancer staging.

- The use of either annual or biennial fecal occult-blood testing significantly reduces the incidence of colorectal cancer.
- The detection of mutations in the adenomatous polyposis coli (APC) gene from stool samples is a promising new modality for early detection of colorectal neoplasms.

REFERENCES
Baron JA et al: A randomized trial of aspirin to prevent colorectal adenomas, *N Engl J Med* 348:891, 2003.

Calvert P, Frucht H: The genetics of colorectal cancer, *Ann Intern Med* 137:603, 2002.

Elsaleh H et al: Association of tumor site and sex with survival benefit from adjuvant chemotherapy in colorectal cancer, *Lancet* 355:1745, 2000.

Green RJ et al: Surveillance for second primary colorectal cancer after adjuvant chemotherapy: an analysis of Intergroup 0089, *Ann Intern Med* 136:261, 2002.

Gryfe R et al: Tumor microsatellite instability and clinical outcome in young patients with colorectal cancer, *N Engl J Med* 342:69, 2000.

Imperiale TF et al: Results of screening colonoscopy among persons 40-49 years of age, *N Engl J Med* 346:1781, 2002.

Raedle J et al: Bethesda guidelines: relation to microsatellite instability and MLH1 promoter methylation in patients with colorectal cancer, *Ann Intern Med* 135:566, 2001.

Ransohoff DF, Sandler RS: Screening for colorectal cancer, *N Engl J Med* 346:40, 2002.

Saltz LB et al: Irinotecan plus fluorouracil and leucovorin for metastatic colorectal cancer, *N Engl J Med* 343:905, 2000.

Swaroop V, Larson MV: Colonoscopy as a screening test for colorectal cancer in average-risk individuals, *Mayo Clin Proc* 77:951, 2002.

Traverso G et al: Detection of APC mutations in fecal DNA from patients with colorectal tumors, *N Engl J Med* 346:311, 2002.

U.S. Preventive Services Strike Force: Screening for colorectal cancer: recommendations and rationale, *Ann Intern Med* 137:129, 2002.

Watanabe T et al: Molecular predictors of survival after adjustment chemotherapy for colon cancer, *N Engl J Med* 344:1186, 2001.

Author: **Fred F. Ferri, M.D.**

BASIC INFORMATION

■ **DEFINITION**
Condyloma acuminatum is a sexually transmitted viral disease of the vulva, vagina, and cervix that is caused by the human papillomavirus (HPV).

■ **SYNONYMS**
Genital warts
Venereal warts
Anogenital warts

ICD-9CM CODES
078.11 Condyloma acuminatum

■ **EPIDEMIOLOGY & DEMOGRAPHICS**
• Seen mostly in young adults with a mean age of onset of 16 to 25 yr
• A sexually transmitted disease spread by skin-to-skin contact
• Highly contagious, with 25% to 65% of sexual partners developing it
• Virus shed from both macroscopic and microscopic lesions
• Average incubation time 2 mo (range: 1 to 8 mo)
• Predisposing conditions: diabetes, pregnancy, local trauma, and immunosuppression (e.g., transplant patients, those with HIV infection)

■ **PHYSICAL FINDINGS & CLINICAL PRESENTATION (FIG. 1-74)**
• Usually found in genital area, but can be present elsewhere
• Lesions usually in similar positions on both sides of perineum
• Initial lesions pedunculated, soft papules about 2 to 3 mm in diameter, 10 to 20 mm long; may occur as single papule or in clusters
• Size of lesions varies from pinhead to large cauliflower-like masses
• Usually asymptomatic, but if infected, can cause pain, odor, or bleeding
• Vulvar condyloma more common than vaginal and cervical
• There are four morphologic types: condylomatous, keratotic, papular, and flat warts

■ **ETIOLOGY**
• HPV DNA types 6 and 11 usually found in exophytic warts and have no malignant potential
• HPV types 16 and 18 usually found in flat warts and are associated with increased risk of malignancy
• Recurrence associated with persisting viral infection of adjacent normal skin in 25% to 50% of cases

■ **DIAGNOSIS**

■ **DIFFERENTIAL DIAGNOSIS**
• Abnormal anatomic variants or skin tags around labia minora and introitus
• Dysplastic warts

■ **WORKUP**
• Colposcopic examination of lower genital tract from cervix to perianal skin with 3% to 5% acetic acid
• Biopsy of vulvar lesions that lack the classic appearance of warts and that become ulcerated or fail to respond to treatment
• Biopsy of flat white or ulcerated cervical lesions

■ **LABORATORY TESTS**
• Pap smear
• Cervical cultures for *N. gonorrhoeae* and *Chlamydia*
• Serologic test for syphilis
• HIV testing offered
• Wet mount for trichomoniasis, *Candida albicans,* and *Gardnerella vaginalis*
• Testing for diabetes (blood glucose)

■ **TREATMENT**

■ **NONPHARMACOLOGIC THERAPY**
• Keep genital area dry and clean.
• Keep diabetes, if present, well controlled.
• Advise use of condoms to prevent spread of infection to sexual partner.

■ **ACUTE GENERAL Rx**
Keratolytic agents:
• Podophyllin
  1. Acts by poisoning mitotic spindle and causing intense vasospasm
  2. Applied directly to lesion weekly and washed off in 6 hr
  3. Used in minimal vulvar or anal disease
  4. Applied cautiously to nonkeratinized epithelial surfaces
  5. Contraindicated in pregnancy
  6. Discontinued if lesions do not disappear in 6 wk; switch to other treatment
• Trichloroacetic acid (30% to 80% solution)
  1. Acts by precipitation of surface proteins
  2. Applied twice monthly to lesion
  3. Indicated for vulvar, anal, and vaginal lesions; can be used for cervical lesions
  4. Less painful and irritating to normal tissue than podophyllin
• Fluorouracil
  1. Causes necrosis and sloughing of growing tissue
  2. Can be used intravaginally or for vulvar, anal, or urethral lesions
  3. Better tolerated; 3 g (two thirds of vaginal applicator) applied weekly for 12 wk
  4. Possible vaginal ulceration and erythema
  5. Patient's vagina examined after four to six applications
  6. 80% cure rate

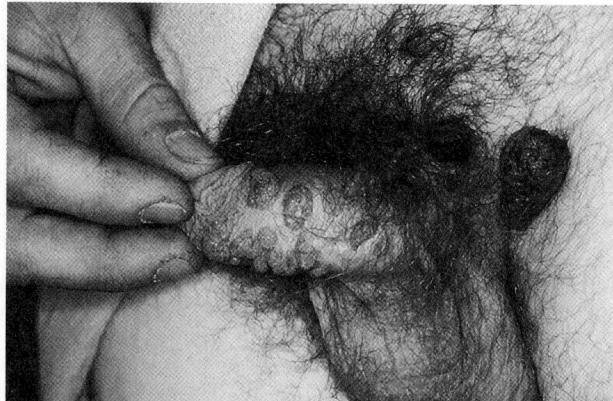

Fig. 1-74   Condylomata. Verrucoid pigmented lesions on the penis. (From Noble J: *Primary care medicine,* ed 3, St Louis, 2001, Mosby.)

Physical agents:
- Cryotherapy
  1. Can be used weekly for 3 to 6 wk
  2. 62% to 79% success rate
  3. Not suitable for large warts
- Laser therapy
  1. Done by physician with necessary expertise and equipment
  2. Painful; requires anesthesia
- Electrocautery or excision
  1. For recurrent, very large lesions
  2. Local anesthesia needed

Immunotherapy
- Interferon
  1. Injected intralesionally at a dose of 3 million U/m² three times weekly for 8 wk
  2. Side effects: fever, chills, malaise, headache
- Autologous vaccine
  1. Made from host's own condyloma acuminatum; not very effective

- Imiquimod 5% cream: increases wart clearance after 3 mo
- Interferon, topical: increases wart clearance at 4 wk

■ DISPOSITION
Follow closely with pelvic examinations and Pap smears every 3 mo for 6 mo, every 6 mo for 12 mo, and then yearly if no evidence of recurrence.

■ REFERRAL
Consult gynecologist in case of extensive lesions or lesions resistant to treatment with keratolytic agents (podophyllin and trichloroacetic acid).

REFERENCES
Czegledy J: Sexual and non-sexual transmission of human papillomavirus, *Acta Microbiol Immunol Hung* 48(3-4):511, 2001.

Moore RA et al: Imiquimod for the treatment of genital warts: a quantitative systematic review, *BMC Infect Dis* 1(1):3, 2001.

Pearson GW, Langley RG: Topical imiquimod, *J Dermatolog Treat* 12(1):37, 2001.

Author: **George T. Danakas, M.D.**

BASIC INFORMATION

■ DEFINITION
Congestive heart failure is a pathophysiologic state characterized by congestion in the pulmonary and/or systemic circulation. It is caused by the heart's inability to pump sufficient oxygenated blood to meet the metabolic needs of the tissues.

■ CLASSIFICATION
The American College of Cardiology and the American Heart Association describe the following four stages of heart failure:

A. At high risk for heart failure, but without structural heart disease or symptoms of heart failure (e.g., CAD, hypertension)

B. Structural heart disease but without symptoms of heart failure

C. Structural heart disease with prior or current symptoms of heart failure

D. Refractory heart failure requiring specialized interventions

The New York Heart Association (NYHA) defines the following functional classes:

I. Asymptomatic
II. Symptomatic with moderate exertion
III. Symptomatic with minimal exertion
IV. Symptomatic at rest

■ SYNONYMS
CHF
Cardiac failure
Heart failure

ICD-9CM CODES
428.0 Congestive heart failure

■ EPIDEMIOLOGY & DEMOGRAPHICS
• CHF is the most common admission diagnosis (20%) in elderly patients.
• Heart failure occurs in 4.7 million persons in the U.S. and is the discharge diagnosis in 3.5 million hospitalizations annually.

■ PHYSICAL FINDINGS & CLINICAL PRESENTATION
The findings on physical examination in patients with CHF vary depending on the severity and whether the failure is right-sided or left-sided.
• Common clinical manifestations are:
1. Dyspnea on exertion initially, then with progressively less strenuous activity, and eventually manifesting when patient is at rest; caused by increasing pulmonary congestion
2. Orthopnea caused by increased venous return in the recumbent position

3. Paroxysmal nocturnal dyspnea (PND) resulting from multiple factors (increased venous return in the recumbent position, decreased Pao_2, decreased adrenergic stimulation of myocardial function)
4. Nocturnal angina resulting from increased cardiac work (secondary to increased venous return)
5. Cheyne-Stokes respiration: alternating phases of apnea and hyperventilation caused by prolonged circulation time from lungs to brain
6. Fatigue, lethargy resulting from low cardiac output
• Patients with failure of the left side of the heart will have the following abnormalities on physical examination: pulmonary rales, tachypnea, S_3 gallop, cardiac murmurs (AS, AR, MR), paradoxic splitting of S_2.
• Patients with failure of right side of the heart manifest with jugular venous distention, peripheral edema, perioral and peripheral cyanosis, congestive hepatomegaly, ascites, hepatojugular reflux.
• In patients with heart failure, elevated jugular venous pressure and a third heart sound are each independently associated with adverse outcomes.
• Acute precipitants of CHF exacerbations are: noncompliance with salt restriction, pulmonary infections, arrhythmias, medications (e.g., calcium channel blockers/antiarrhythmic agents), and inappropriate reductions in CHF therapy.

■ ETIOLOGY
LEFT VENTRICULAR FAILURE:
• Systemic hypertension
• Valvular heart disease (AS, AR, MR)
• Cardiomyopathy, myocarditis
• Bacterial endocarditis
• Myocardial infarction
• IHSS
Left ventricular failure is further differentiated according to systolic dysfunction (low ejection fraction) and diastolic dysfunction (normal or high ejection fraction), or "stiff ventricle." It is important to make this distinction because treatment is significantly different (see Treatment).
• Common causes of systolic dysfunction are post-MI, cardiomyopathy, myocarditis.
• Causes of diastolic dysfunction are hypertensive cardiovascular disease, valvular heart disease (AS, AR, MR, IHSS), restrictive cardiomyopathy.

RIGHT VENTRICULAR FAILURE:
• Valvular heart disease (mitral stenosis)
• Pulmonary hypertension
• Bacterial endocarditis (right-sided)
• Right ventricular infarction

BIVENTRICULAR FAILURE:
• Left ventricular failure
• Cardiomyopathy
• Myocarditis
• Arrhythmias
• Anemia
• Thyrotoxicosis
• AV fistula
• Paget's disease
• Beriberi

DIAGNOSIS

■ DIFFERENTIAL DIAGNOSIS
• Cirrhosis
• Nephrotic syndrome
• Venous occlusive disease
• COPD, asthma
• Pulmonary embolism
• ARDS
• Heroin overdose
• Pneumonia

■ WORKUP
• Chest x-ray examination, electrocardiography, echocardiography, cardiac catheterization (selected patients)
• Standard 12-lead ECG is useful to diagnose ischemic heart disease and obtain information about rhythm abnormalities

■ LABORATORY TESTS
• CBC (to rule out anemia, infections), BUN, creatinine, liver enzymes, TSH
• β-type natriuretic peptide is a cardiac neurohormone specifically secreted from the ventricles in response to volume expansion and pressure overload. Elevated levels are indicative of left ventricular dysfunction. Bedside measurement of β-type natriuretic peptide is useful in establishing or excluding the diagnosis of CHF in patients with acute dyspnea

■ IMAGING STUDIES
• Chest x-ray examination:
1. Pulmonary venous congestion
2. Cardiomegaly with dilation of the involved heart chamber
3. Pleural effusions
• Two-dimensional echocardiography is useful to assess global and regional left ventricular function and estimate ejection fraction.

- Exercise stress testing may be useful for evaluating concomitant coronary disease and assess degree of disability. The decision to perform exercise stress testing should be individualized.
- Cardiac catheterization remains an excellent method to evaluate ventricular diastolic properties, significant coronary artery disease, or valvular heart disease; however, it is invasive. The decision to perform cardiac catheterization should be individualized.

℞ TREATMENT

■ NONPHARMACOLOGIC THERAPY

- Determine if CHF is secondary to systolic or diastolic dysfunction and treat accordingly.
- Identify and correct precipitating factors (i.e., anemia, thyrotoxicosis, infections, increased sodium load, medical noncompliance).
- Decrease cardiac workload in patients with systolic dysfunction: restrict patients' activity only during periods of acute decompensation; the risk of thromboembolism during this period can be minimized by using heparin 5000 U SC q12h in hospitalized patients. In patients with mild to moderate symptoms aerobic training may improve symptoms and exercise capacity.
- Restrict sodium intake to ≤3 g/day.
- Restricting fluid intake to 2 L or less may be useful in patients with hyponatremia.

■ ACUTE GENERAL Rx
TREATMENT OF CHF SECONDARY TO SYSTOLIC DYSFUNCTION:

1. Diuretics: indicated in patients with systolic dysfunction and volume overload. The most useful approach to selecting the dose of, and monitoring the response to, diuretic therapy is by measuring body weight, preferably daily.
   a. Furosemide: 20 to 80 mg/day produces prompt venodilation and diuresis. IV therapy may produce diuresis when oral therapy has failed; when changing from IV to oral furosemide, doubling the dose is usually necessary to achieve an equal effect.
   b. Thiazides are not as powerful as furosemide but are useful in mild to moderate CHF.
   c. The addition of metolazone to furosemide enhances diuresis.
   d. Blockade of aldosterone receptors by spironolactone (12.5 to 25 mg qd) used in conjunction with ACE inhibitors reduces both mortality and morbidity in patients with severe CHF and is generally not associated with hyperkalemia. It should be considered in patients with recent or recurrent class IV (NYHA) symptoms.
   e. Frequent monitoring of renal function and electrolytes is recommended in all patients receiving diuretics.
2. ACE inhibitors:
   a. They cause dilation of the arteriolar resistance vessels and venous capacity vessels, thereby reducing both preload and afterload.
   b. They are associated with decreased mortality and improved clinical status when used in patients with CHF caused by systolic dysfunction. They are also indicated in patients with ejection fraction <40%.
   c. They can be used as first-line therapy or they can be added to diuretics in patients with CHF poorly controlled with only diuretic therapy.
   d. Therapy with ACE inhibitors should be initiated at low dose (e.g., captopril 6.25 mg tid or enalapril 2.5 mg bid) to prevent hypotension and rapidly titrated up to high doses if tolerated.
   e. Contraindications to use of ACE inhibitors are renal insufficiency (creatinine >3.0 or creatinine clearance <30 ml/min), renal artery stenosis, persistent hyperkalemia (K+ >5.5 mEQ/L), symptomatic hypotension, and history of adverse reactions (e.g., angioedema).
3. β-blockers: All patients with stable NYHA class II or III heart failure caused by left ventricular systolic dysfunction should receive a β-blocker unless they have a contraindication to its use or are intolerant to it. β-blockers are especially useful in patients who remain symptomatic despite therapy with ACE inhibitors and diuretics. Effective agents are carvedilol (Coreg) 3.125 mg bid, bisoprolol 1.25 mg qd, or metoprolol 12.5 mg bid initially, titrated upward as tolerated.
4. Angiotensin II receptor blockers (ARBS) block the A-II type 1 (AT) receptor, which is responsible for many of the deleterious effects of angiotensin II. These receptors are potent vasoconstrictors that may contribute to the impairment of LV function. ARBS are useful in patients unable to tolerate ACE inhibitors because of angioedema or intractable cough. They can also be used in combination with a β-blocker.
5. Digitalis may be useful because of its positive inotropic and vagotonic effects in patients with CHF secondary to systolic dysfunction; it is of limited value in patients with mild CHF and normal sinus rhythm. It is more beneficial in patients with rapid atrial fibrillation, severe CHF, or ejection fraction of <30%; it can be added to diuretics and ACE inhibitors in patients with severe CHF. In patients with chronic heart failure and normal sinus rhythm, digoxin does not reduce mortality, but it does reduce the rate of hospitalization both overall and for worsening heart failure. Digoxin has a narrow therapeutic window. Its beneficial effects are found with a low dose that results in a serum concentration of approximately 0.7 ng/ml. Higher doses may be detrimental.
6. Direct vasodilating drugs (nesiritide, hydralazine, isosorbide) are useful in the therapy of systolic dysfunction with CHF because they can reduce the systemic vascular resistance and pulmonary venous pressure, especially when used in combination. Nesiritide (Natrecor), a recombinant human brain, or B-type, natriuretic peptide has venous, arterial, and coronary vasodilatory properties that decrease preload and afterload and increase cardiac output without direct inotropic effects. In hospitalized patients with acutely decompensated CHF, the addition of IV nesiritide to standard care improves hemodynamic function (decreased PCWP) and self-reported symptoms more effectively than IV nitroglycerin. Usual nesiritide dosage is 2 mcg/kg IV bolus, then 0.01 mcg/kg/min.
7. Anticoagulants:
   a. Anticoagulation is not recommended for patients in sinus rhythm and no prior history of stroke, left ventricular thrombi, or arteriolar emboli.
   b. Anticoagulation therapy is appropriate for patients with heart failure and atrial fibrillation or a history of embolism.

8. Surgical revascularization should be considered in patients with both heart failure and severe limiting angina.

9. Antiarrhythmic therapy with amiodarone has a modest effect in reducing mortality in patients with CHF; however, it is not recommended for general use in CHF. Its benefits must be weighed against the risk for adverse effects, especially potentially fatal pulmonary toxicity.

10. Atrioventricular pacing significantly improves exercise tolerance and quality of life in patients with chronic heart failure and intraventricular conduction delay.

11. Obstructive sleep apnea has an adverse effect on heart failure. Recognition and treatment of coexisting obstructive sleep apnea by continuous positive airway pressure reduces systolic blood pressure and improves left ventricular systolic function.

TREATMENT OF CHF SECONDARY TO DIASTOLIC DYSFUNCTION: THERAPEUTIC OPTIONS ARE DETERMINED BY THE CAUSE

1. Hypertension
   a. Calcium channel blockers (verapamil)
   b. ACE inhibitors
   c. β-blockers or verapamil to control heart rate and prolong diastolic filling
   d. Diuretics: vigorous diuresis should be avoided, because a higher filling pressure may be needed to maintain cardiac output in patients with diastolic dysfunction
   e. ARBs
2. Aortic stenosis
   a. Diuretics
   b. Contraindicated medications: ACE inhibitors, nitrates, digitalis (except to control rate of atrial fibrillation)
   c. Aortic valve replacement in patients with critical stenosis

3. Aortic insufficiency and mitral regurgitation
   a. ACE inhibitors increase cardiac output and decrease pulmonary wedge pressure. They are agents of choice along with diuretics.
   b. Hydralazine combined with nitrates can be used if ACE inhibitors are not tolerated.
   c. Surgery
4. IHSS
   a. β-blockers or verapamil
   b. Contraindicated medications (they increase outlet obstruction by decreasing the size of the left ventricle in end systole): diuretics, digitalis, ACE inhibitors, hydralazine
   c. Restoration of intravascular volume with IV saline solution if necessary in acute pulmonary edema
   d. Septal myotomy and DDD pacing are useful in selected patients

TREATMENT OF CHF SECONDARY TO MITRAL STENOSIS:

1. Diuretics
2. Control of the heart rate and atrial fibrillation with digitalis, verapamil, and/or β-blockers is critical to allow emptying of left atrium and relief of pulmonary congestion
3. Repairing or replacing the mitral valve is indicated if CHF is not readily controlled by the above measures
4. Balloon valvuloplasty is useful in selected patients

■ **DISPOSITION**
- Annual mortality ranges from 10% in stable patients with mild symptoms to >50% in symptomatic patients with advanced disease.
- Sudden death secondary to ventricular arrhythmias occurs in >40% of patients with heart failure.
- Cardiac transplantation has a 5-yr survival rate of >70% in many centers and represents a viable option in selected patients.

- The use of a left ventricular assist device in patients with advanced heart failure can result in a clinically meaningful survival benefit and improve quality of life. It is an acceptable alternative therapy in selected patients who are not candidates for cardiac transplantation.

REFERENCES

Cardioselective beta-blockers in patients with reactive airway disease: a meta-analysis, *Ann Intern Med* 137:715, 2002.

Cuffe MS et al: Short-term intravenous milrinone for acute exacerbation of chronic heart failure, *JAMA* 287:1541, 2002.

Goldstein S: Benefits of beta-blocker therapy in heart failure, *Arch Intern Med* 162:641, 2002.

Jessup M, Brozena S: Heart failure, *N Engl J Med* 348:2007, 2003.

King DE et al: Acute management of heart failure, *Am Fam Physician* 66:249, 2002.

Kukin ML: Beta blockers in chronic heart failure, *Mayo Clin Proc* 77:1199, 2002.

Maisel AS et al: Rapid measurement of B-type natriuretic peptide in the emergency diagnosis of heart failure, *N Engl J Med* 347:161, 2002.

Nesiritide for decompensated congestive heart failure, *Med Lett Drugs Ther* 43:100, 2001.

Nohria A et al: Medical management of advanced heart failure, *JAMA* 287:628, 2002.

Pfeffer MA et al: Valsartan, captopril, or both in myocardial infarction complicated by heart failure, left ventricular dysfunction, or both, *N Engl J Med* 349:1893, 2003.

Publications Committee for the VMAC Investigators: Intravenous nesiritide vs nitroglycerin for the treatment of decompensated congestive heart failure, *JAMA* 287:1531, 2002.

Author: **Fred F. Ferri, M.D.**

BASIC INFORMATION

■ DEFINITION
The term *conjunctivitis* refers to an inflammation of the conjunctiva resulting from a variety of causes, including allergies and bacterial, viral, and chlamydial infections.

■ SYNONYMS
"Red eye"
Acute conjunctivitis
Subacute conjunctivitis
Chronic conjunctivitis
Purulent conjunctivitis
Pseudomembranous conjunctivitis
Papillary conjunctivitis
Follicular conjunctivitis
Newborn conjunctivitis

ICD-9CM CODES
372.30 Conjunctivitis, unspecified

■ EPIDEMIOLOGY & DEMOGRAPHICS
INCIDENCE (IN U.S.): Newborn 1.6% to 12%
PREVALENCE (IN U.S.):
• Very common
• Often seasonal and can be extremely contagious
PREDOMINANT AGE: Occurs at any age
PEAK INCIDENCE: More common in the fall when viral infections and pollens increase

■ PHYSICAL FINDINGS & CLINICAL PRESENTATION
• Injection and chemosis of conjunctivae with discharge (Fig. 1-75)
• Cornea clear
• Vision usually normal

■ ETIOLOGY
• Bacterial
• Viral
• Chlamydial
• Allergic

DIAGNOSIS

■ DIFFERENTIAL DIAGNOSIS
• Acute glaucoma
• Corneal lesions
• Acute iritis
• Episcleritis
• Scleritis
• Uveitis
• Canalicular obstruction
• The differential diagnosis of red eye is described in Section II

■ WORKUP
• History and physical examination
• Reports of itching, pain, visual changes

■ LABORATORY TESTS
Cultures are useful if not successfully treated with antibiotic medications; initial culture is usually not necessary.

TREATMENT

■ NONPHARMACOLOGIC THERAPY
• Warm compresses if infective conjunctivitis
• Cold compresses in irritative or allergic conjunctivitis

■ ACUTE GENERAL Rx
• Antibiotic drops (e.g., levofloxacin, ofloxin, ciprofloxacin, tobramycin, gentamicin ophthalmic solution one or two drops q2-4h)
• Caution: be careful with corticosteroid treatment and avoid unless sure of diagnosis; corticosteroids can exacerbate infections

■ CHRONIC Rx
• Depends on cause
• If allergic, nonsteroidals such as Voltaren ophthalmic solution, mast cell stabilizers such as Alocril, Patanol, Zaditor are useful
• If infections, antibiotic drops (see Acute General Rx)

■ DISPOSITION
Follow carefully for the first 2 wk to make sure secondary complications do not occur.

■ REFERRAL
To ophthalmologist if symptoms refractory to initial treatment

PEARLS & CONSIDERATIONS

■ COMMENTS
Do not use steroids indiscriminately; use only when the diagnosis is certain.

REFERENCES
Nichols GR: The red eye, *N Engl J Med* 343(21):1577, 2000.
Sheikh A, Hurwitz B: Topical antibiotics for acute bacterial conjunctivitis: a systematic review, *Br J Gen Pract* 51:473, 2001.
Snyder-Perlmutter LS, Katz HR, Melia M: Effect of topical ciprofloxacin and ofloxacin on the reduction of bacterial flora on the human conjunctiva, *J Cataract Refract Surg* 26(11):1620, 2000.
Author: **Melvyn Koby, M.D.**

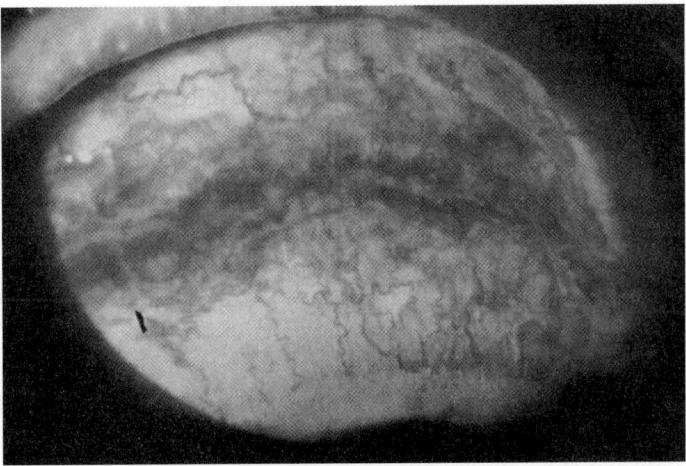

Fig. 1-75   Conjunctival infection from viral conjunctivitis. (From Marx JA [ed]: *Rosen's emergency medicine*, ed 5, St Louis, 2002, Mosby.)

BASIC INFORMATION

■ DEFINITION

Contraception refers to the various options that a sexually active couple have to prevent pregnancy. These options can be either medical or non-medical and used by men or women or both. The options are as follows:

- No contraception: failure rate 85% both typical and perfect
- Abstinence
  1. 12.4% of unmarried men
  2. 13.2% of unmarried women
  3. More frequently practiced before age 17 yr
  4. No intercourse experienced by 13% of women ages 30 to 34 yr old
  5. Failure rate 0%
- Withdrawal
  1. Used in only 2% of sexually active women
  2. Failure rate with perfect use, 4%; with typical use, 19%
- Rhythm method (natural family planning)
  1. Failure rate with perfect use, 1% to 9%; with typical use, 20%
  2. Symptothermal type: mucus method and ovulation pain combined with basal body temperature
  3. Ovulation (Billings' method): takes into account mucus quality
  4. Basal body temperature method: uses biphasic temperature chart
  5. Lactation amenorrhea method: effective in fully breast-feeding women, especially 70 to 100 days after delivery; depends on number of feedings per day
- Barriers
  1. Diaphragm and cervical cap: failure rate 5% to 9% in nulliparous women, 20% in multiparous women
  2. Female condom: failure rate with perfect use, 5.1%; with typical use, 12.4%; FDA labeling states 25% failure rate
  3. Male condom: failure rate with perfect use, 3%, with typical use, 12%
  4. Spermicides (aerosols, foam, jellies, creams, tabs): failure rate with perfect use, 3%; with typical use, 21%
- Oral contraceptives
  1. Failure rate with perfect use, <1%; with typical use, 3%
  2. Come in combinations of estrogen/progestin or as progestin only
- Hormonal implants and injectables
  1. Norplant
     a. Most typically used in U.S.
     b. Failure rate in first 5 yr: 1%
     c. Failure rate after 6 yr: 2%
     d. May be extended to 7 yr use

  2. Depo-Provera: failure rate 0.3% in first year of use
  3. Lunelle (approved October 2000): failure rate 0.2% in first year
  4. Etonogestrel implant: 2-yr cumulative pregnancy rate 0%
  5. Nestorone-releasing single implant: not yet available
  6. Jadelle implant
- Mini pill (progesterone only pill)
  1. Failure rate with typical use, 1.1% to 13.2%
  2. With perfect use, 5 pregnancies/1000 women
- Emergency postcoital contraception
  1. Decreases pregnancy rate by 75% with women treated immediately postcoitally
  2. Involves hormonal use or IUD insertion
- IUD (available OTC in some states)
  1. Progestasert: failure rate with perfect use, 2%; with typical use, 3%
  2. Copper T (380-A): failure rate with perfect use, 0.8%; with typical use, 3%
  3. Levonorgestrel Intrauterine System (Mirena)
     a. 1-yr failure rate, 1%
     b. 5-yr cumulative failure rate, 0.71/100 women
- Female sterilization (tubal ligation): failure rate with perfect use, 0.2%; with typical use, 3%
- Male sterilization (vasectomy): failure rate of 0.1% in first year
- Vaginal ring (Nuva ring): failure rate pearl index 0.77
- Contraceptive patch (Orthoevra): failure rate 0.4% to 0.7%

■ SYNONYMS

Birth control
Family planning

ICD-9CM CODES

V25.01 Oral contraceptives
V25.02 Other contraceptive measures
V25.09 Family planning
V25.1 IUD
V25.2 Sterilization

■ EPIDEMIOLOGY & DEMOGRAPHICS

For women at risk for pregnancy, ranges for use of most commonly used birth control are dependent, as follows:

- Oral contraceptives: 3% (40 to 44 yr old) to 60% (20 to 24 yr old)
- Condoms: 9% (40 to 44 yr old) to 26% (15 to 19 yr old)
- Diaphragm: 0.8% (15 to 19 yr old) to 8% (30 to 34 yr old)
- Periodic abstinence: 0.7% (15 to 19 yr old) to 3% (35 to 39 yr old)
- Withdrawal: 1.1% (40 to 44 yr old) to 3% (20 to 30 yr old)
- IUD: 0% (15 to 19 yr old) to 3% (30 to 34 yr old)

- Spermicides: 0.8% (15 to 19 yr old) to 2.7% (35 to 39 yr old)
- No method: 6.3% (35 to 39 yr old) to 19.8% (15 to 19 yr old)
- Sterilization
  Female: 0.2% (15 to 19 yr old) to 47% (40 to 44 yr old)
  Male: 0.2% (15 to 19 yr old) to 21% (40 to 44 yr old)

Women are more likely to use contraception. The only two male forms available are condoms and vasectomy (sterilization).

DIAGNOSIS

■ WORKUP

- Thorough medical history
- Thorough surgical history
- Obstetric history (fertility desired?)
- Gynecologic history, including:
  1. History of previous sexually transmitted diseases
  2. Number of partners
  3. Previous difficulties with contraception
  4. Frequency of intercourse
- Family history

■ LABORATORY TESTS

- Pap smear
- Cultures, aerobic and *Chlamydia*
- Pregnancy test if suspected pregnancy
- Lipid profile if family history of premature vascular event

TREATMENT

■ NONPHARMACOLOGIC THERAPY

- Male condoms
  1. 95% latex (rubber), 5% skin or natural membrane
  2. Proper use: place on an erect penis and leave one-half-inch empty space at the tip of the condom; use with non–oil-based lubricants
  3. Effectiveness increased when used with spermicides
- Female condoms
  1. Composed of polyurethane, with one end open and one end closed
  2. Proper use: place closed end over cervix, open end hanging out of vagina to cover penis and scrotum
  3. Highly effective against HIV
- Spermicides
  1. Types: nonoxynol, octoxynol
  2. Forms: jellies, creams, foams, suppositories, tablets, soluble films
  3. Proper use: put in immediately before intercourse; may be used with other barrier methods

- Diaphragm and cervical cap
  1. Must be fitted by practitioner, used with contraceptive gels, and refitted with weight gain or loss
  2. Diaphragm sizes: 50 to 95 mm; cervical cap sizes: 22, 25, 28, and 31 mm
  3. Proper use of diaphragm: put in immediately before intercourse and keep in for 6 hr after intercourse; must not remain in the vagina for longer than 24 hr
  4. Proper use of cervical cap: fit over the cervix exactly; must not remain in place for longer than 48 hr
- Lactation amenorrhea method
  1. Depends on number of breastfeedings per day; effective as birth control for 6 mo if 15 or more feedings, lasting 10 min each, are accomplished daily
  2. Not a common practice in the U.S
- Withdrawal
  1. Withdrawal of the penis from the vagina before ejaculation
  2. Dependent on self-control
- Rhythm method
  1. Dependent on awareness of physiology of male and female reproductive tracts
  2. Sperm viable in vagina for 2 to 7 days
  3. Ovum life span 24 hr
- Sterilization
  1. Male:
     a. Vasectomy to interrupt vas deferens and block passage of sperm to seminal ejaculate
     b. Scalpel and nonscalpel techniques available
     c. More easily performed procedure than female sterilization and does not require general anesthesia
  2. Female:
     a. Leading method of birth control in U.S. in women older than 30 yr
     b. Interrupts fallopian tubes, blocking passage of ovum proximally and sperm distally through tube
     c. Several types; modified Pomeroy done during cesarean section or laparoscopic done in nonpregnant females most common
     d. Essure-tubal occlusion through hysteroscopic placement of micro-inserts into the fallopian tubes.

■ **ACUTE GENERAL Rx**
- Combination oral contraceptives
  1. Taken daily for 21 days, pill-free interval of 7 days
  2. Less than 50 μg ethynyl estradiol in most common combination oral contraceptives; progestins most commonly used in combination pills are norethindrone, levonorgestrel, norgestrel, norethindrone acetate, ethynodiol diacetate, norgestimate, or desogestrel; triphasic combination oral contraceptives (give varying doses of progestin and estrogens throughout cycle); monophasic oral contraceptives: offer same dose of progestin and estrogen throughout cycle, taken daily at same time; estrophasic pill (constant progesterone with variation of estrogen throughout the cycle)
  3. If pill taken with antibiotics, efficacy affected by inadequate gastrointestinal absorption in most cases; only rifampin truly reduces pill's effectiveness
  4. Increased body weight decreases effectiveness
- Mini pill
  1. Progestin only; taken without a break
  2. Causes much irregular bleeding because of the lack of estrogen effect on the lining of the uterus
- Hormonal implants and injectables
  1. Norplant
     a. Progestin only; inserted under the skin
     b. Six levonorgestrel implants placed subcutaneously in upper inner arm effective for 5 yr
  2. Depo-Provera
     a. Medroxyprogesterone acetate given every 3 mo in IM injection form
     b. Major side effect: irregular bleeding
     c. Fertility return possibly delayed up to 18 mo after discontinuation
  3. Lunelle: monthly injectable administered intramuscularly. Contains 0.5 ml aqueous, 5 mg estradiol cypionate and 25 mg medroxyprogesterone acetate
  4. Etonogestrel implant: single-rod release etonogestrel for 3 yr placed subdermally

- Postcoital contraception
  1. Done on emergency basis, usually secondary to noncompliance with birth control or failure of birth control (e.g., condom breakage) at the time of ovulation
  2. Methods:
     a. IUD insertion within 7 days of coitus
     b. Hormonal methods (combination pills and danazol) given within 48 hr of coitus
- IUD
  1. Device inserted into uterus to prevent sperm and ovum from uniting in fallopian tube
  2. Types available in the U.S.:
     a. Progestasert: a T-shaped device that is an ethylene vinyl acetate copolymer T; vertical stem contains 38 mg progesterone and must be changed yearly
     b. ParaGard (Copper T/380-A): a polyethylene T wrapped with a fine copper wire that is effective for 10 yr of use
     c. Mirena Levonorgestrel Intrauterine System (LNGIUS): a T-shaped system with a chamber that contains LNG. Releases 20 μg per day; is effective for 5 yr
- Vaginal ring (brand name Nuvaring)
  1. Provides daily dose of 120 μg of etonogestrel and 15 μg ethinyl estradiol
  2. Stays in vagina 3 wk and removed the fourth
  3. Increased body weight decreases effectiveness
- Contraceptive patch (brand name Evra)
  1. Provides low daily dose of steroids
  2. Releases a progestin and estrogen (ethinyl estradiol)
  3. Patch size 20 cm²
  4. Each patch contains 6 mg norelgestromin and delivers an estimated continuous systemic dose of 150 μg norelgestromin and 20 μg of ethinyl estradiol; common dose 250 μg/day progestin and 25 μg/day estrogen
  5. Worn 3 of 4 wk
  6. Increased body weight decreases effectiveness

I

■ CHRONIC Rx

- With all of the previously mentioned types of birth control, patient is followed at least yearly, or as necessary, if problems arise.
- Full history, physical examination, and Pap smear, including cultures when needed, are performed yearly.
- Patients with medical problems are followed about every 6 mo when taking hormonal therapy.

■ DISPOSITION

- Follow yearly or more frequently according to patient's side effects.
- Tailor birth control to patient according to different needs or side effects present at different times in life.

■ REFERRAL

With hormonal contraception, if neurologic or cardiac symptoms arise, stop method immediately, evaluate, and refer to internist when appropriate.

☼ PEARLS & CONSIDERATIONS

■ COMMENTS

- Patient education information available through American College of Obstetricians and Gynecologists (ACOG) at 1-800-673-8444 and through various drug companies representing and supplying the particular type of contraception.
- A clinical algorithm on the use of oral contraceptives is described in Section III, Fig. 3-47.

REFERENCES

Clinical proceedings: *Association of Reproductive Health Professionals,* February 2001.

Dieben T: Efficacy cycle control and user acceptability of a novel combined contraceptive vaginal ring, *Obstet Gynecol* 100(3):585, 2002.

Gordon J: Transdermal contraception: a new technology for women, *The Female Patient* (Suppl):1, 2002.

Grimes DA: Switching emergency contraception to over-the-counter status, *N Engl J Med* 347:846, 2002.

Holt VL et al: Body weight and risk of oral contraceptive failure, *Obstet Gynecol* 99:820, 2002.

Sivin I, Moo-Young A: Recent developments in contraceptive implants at the population council contraception, 65(1):113, 2002.

Author: **Maria A. Corigliano, M.D.**

BASIC INFORMATION

■ **DEFINITION**
Conversion disorder is an alteration or loss of voluntary motor or sensory function suggestive of a physical disorder but without demonstrable physical cause and related to a psychologic stress or a conflict.

■ **SYNONYMS**
Hysteria
Hysterical conversion
Pseudoneurologic illness
Nondisease
Psychosomatic illness
Persistent somatization
Function illness

ICD-9CM CODES
300.11 Conversion disorder

■ **EPIDEMIOLOGY & DEMOGRAPHICS**
INCIDENCE (IN U.S.): 22 cases/100,000 persons/yr (in Iceland, 11 cases/100,000 persons/yr)
PREVALENCE (IN U.S.): 11 to 300 cases/100,000 persons
PREDOMINANT SEX: More common in women (2-10:1)
PREDOMINANT AGE: Generally a disease of adults
PEAK INCIDENCE: Older than 10 yr and younger than 35 yr
GENETICS: Monozygotic twins have increased risk, but dizygotic twins do not.

■ **PHYSICAL FINDINGS & CLINICAL PRESENTATION**
• Dysfunction of voluntary activity or sensation
• Most common symptoms: amnesia, difficulty swallowing, speech dysfunction, deafness, visual problems, loss of sensation, fainting, pseudoseizures, gait abnormalities, paresis, and paralysis
• In women: left side of the body more commonly affected
• Other presentations, such as hyperemesis
• In children <10 yr old: gait difficulties or pseudoseizures
• Physical abnormalities (if present) insufficient to explain the presentation
• Proximal psychologic issue identifiable

■ **ETIOLOGY**
The term *conversion* was coined by Freud and Breuer, who proposed that psychic energy of a conflict is converted into physical symptoms; this remains one of the best theoretical formulations.

DIAGNOSIS

■ **DIFFERENTIAL DIAGNOSIS**
• Malingering: dysfunction is consciously created for the purpose of secondary gain or avoidance of noxious duties
• Factitious disorder (e.g., Munchausen's syndrome): dysfunction is consciously created for the purpose of assuming the patient role
• Somatization: a related disorder in which psychologic difficulties present with a wide range of somatic complaints that affect several organ systems

■ **WORKUP**
Physical examination and laboratory evaluation must be sufficient to rule out a physical cause for the dysfunction.

■ **LABORATORY TESTS**
• No specific laboratory tests
• Goal of tests: to exclude physical cause for the dysfunction

■ **IMAGING STUDIES**
Goal of tests: to exclude physical cause for the dysfunction

TREATMENT

■ **NONPHARMACOLOGIC THERAPY**
• Psychotherapy that attempts to address the underlying psychologic conflicts is generally recommended.
• Affected individuals generally are not ideal psychotherapy candidates; supportive psychotherapy is possibly the only reasonable intervention.
• Patients are frequently suggestible, so interventions such as suggestion and hypnosis can be useful.

■ **ACUTE GENERAL Rx**
Amobarbital (sodium amytal) interviews are sometimes used both diagnostically and therapeutically; conversion may disappear under the influence of Amytal.

■ **CHRONIC Rx**
Conversion has a high recurrence rate, so ongoing psychotherapy may be cost effective.

■ **DISPOSITION**
• Among hospitalized patients with conversion disorder, remission typically occurs within 2 wk. However, recurrence may occur in 20% to 25% of patients within 1 yr. Recurrences foretell future recurrences.
• Symptoms of pseudoseizures and tremor are less likely to remit than symptoms of paralysis, aphonia, or blindness.

■ **REFERRAL**
If supportive interventions are not helpful, disability is extreme, or there is no improvement in 2 wk

PEARLS & CONSIDERATIONS

■ **COMMENTS**
Many patients "elaborate" on symptoms to convince the physician they are ill; this may considerably complicate appropriate diagnosis and therapy.

REFERENCES
Moene FC et al: Organic syndromes diagnosed as conversion disorder: identification and frequency in a study of 85 patients, *J Psychosom Res* 49:7, 2000.
Zeharia A et al: Conversion reaction: management by the paediatrician, *Eur J Ped* 158:160, 1999.
Author: **Rif S. El-Mallakh, M.D.**

BASIC INFORMATION

■ **DEFINITION**
Cor pulmonale refers to the enlargement of the right ventricle caused by pulmonary hypertension. Cor pulmonale may be acute or chronic.

■ **SYNONYMS**
• Acute cor pulmonale
• Chronic cor pulmonale

ICD-9CM CODES
415.0 Cor pulmonale, acute
416.9 Cor pulmonale, chronic

■ **EPIDEMIOLOGY & DEMOGRAPHICS**
• Cor pulmonale is the third most common cardiac disorder after the age of 50.
• More common in men than in women.

■ **PHYSICAL FINDINGS & CLINICAL PRESENTATION**
No symptoms are specific for cor pulmonale. Typically cor pulmonale presents according to the underlying disease process such as pulmonary embolism or COPD.
• Dyspnea, pleuritic chest pain, and cough
• Leg swelling
• Hemoptysis
• Wheezing and rales
• Tachypnea and tachycardia
• Cyanosis
• Jugular venous distention with large V waves
• Holosystolic murmur heard best along the left parasternal line, fourth intercostal space and is augmented during inspiration
• Pulsatile hepatomegaly

■ **ETIOLOGY**
• Cor pulmonale is caused by pulmonary hypertension.
• Mechanisms leading to pulmonary hypertension include:
 1. Pulmonary vasoconstriction resulting from any condition causing alveolar hypoxia and/or acidosis
 2. Lung parenchymal disorders (e.g., emphysema, interstitial lung disease, pulmonary emboli)
 3. Conditions leading to increased bloom viscosity (e.g., polycythemia vera, Waldenstrom's macroglobulinemia)
 4. Idiopathic primary pulmonary hypertension

🔬 **DIAGNOSIS**

The diagnosis of cor pulmonale is made in any patient with underlying evidence of pulmonary hypertension and findings of right-sided heart failure.

■ **DIFFERENTIAL DIAGNOSIS**
• Pulmonary thromboembolic disease
• Chronic obstructive pulmonary disease (COPD)
• Interstitial lung disease
• Neuromuscular diseases causing hypoventilation (e.g., ALS)
• Collagen-vascular disease (e.g., SLE, CREST, systemic sclerosis)
• Pulmonary venous disease
• Primary pulmonary hypertension

■ **WORKUP**
Any patient suspected of cor pulmonale should undergo a workup consisting of blood tests, chest x-ray, echocardiogram, MRI, and occasionally, right-side heart catheterization.
LABORATORY TESTS
• CBC may show erythrocytosis secondary to hypoxia
• Arterial blood gas (ABGs) confirming hypoxemia and acidosis or hypercapnia
IMAGING STUDIES
• Chest x-ray may show evidence of COPD and pulmonary hypertension.
• Echocardiogram with continuous, pulse, and color Doppler can estimate pulmonary artery pressure. M-mode and two-dimensional measures chamber size and wall thickness.
• Radionuclide ventriculography reveals depressed right ventricular ejection fraction.
• MRI is a sensitive test to measure right ventricular dimensions and detect hypertrophy.
• Right-side catheterization measures pulmonary artery pressures and vascular resistance. It also helps determine response to various therapies (e.g., oxygen, calcium blockers, angiotensin-converting enzyme inhibitors, etc.).

℞ **TREATMENT**

The treatment of cor pulmonale is directed at the underlying etiology while at the same time reversing hypoxemia, hypercapnia, and acidosis.

■ **NONPHARMACOLOGIC THERAPY**
• Chest physiotherapy is beneficial in patients with COPD and infectious exacerbations.
• Continuous positive airway pressure (CPAP) is used in patients with obstructive sleep apnea.
• Long-term oxygen supplementation has improved survival in hypoxemic patients with COPD.

■ **ACUTE GENERAL Rx**
• Pulmonary embolism is the most common cause of acute cor pulmonale. Treatment includes:
 1. Thrombolytic therapy (urokinase, tPA, streptokinase) in the hemodynamically unstable patient

 2. Heparin IV followed by warfarin therapy maintaining an INR between 2 and 3 is the standard therapy for pulmonary embolism (see "Pulmonary Embolism")

■ **CHRONIC Rx**
• Treatment of chronic cor pulmonale is directed at:
 1. The underlying cause (e.g., COPD, the most common cause of chronic cor pulmonale)
 2. The underlying pathologic process (e.g., pulmonary hypertension)
 3. The underlying pathologic sequelae (e.g., right ventricular [RV] failure)
• Cause
 1. COPD is treated in the standard fashion with metered dose inhalers (see "Chronic Obstructive Pulmonary Disease")
• Rx of pulmonary hypertension
 1. Oxygen supplementation
 2. Vasodilators including nitroglycerine, calcium channel blockers, and angiotensin-converting enzyme inhibitors can be tried
• Rx of RV failure with diuretics (e.g., furosemide 40 to 80 mg PO qd and digoxin 0.25 mg PO qd)

■ **DISPOSITION**
• Nearly 50,000 people die each year from acute pulmonary embolism.
• The prognosis of patients with severe COPD and cor pulmonale is poor (survival <2 yr).

💡 **PEARLS & CONSIDERATIONS**

■ **COMMENTS**
• Acute elevation of pulmonary artery pressures (30 to 40 mm Hg) results in:
 1. RV dilatation
 2. LV compression
 3. Decreased LV end-diastolic volume
 4. Decreased cardiac output
 5. Hypotension
 6. Mean pulmonary artery pressures >40 mm Hg usually signify a chronic underlying process.

REFERENCES
MacNee W: Pathophysiology of cor pulmonale in chronic obstructive pulmonary disease, *Am J Respir Crit Care Med* 150:833, 1994.
Romano PM, Peterson S: The management of cor pulmonale, *Heart Dis* 2(6):431, 2000.
Author: **Peter Petropoulos, M.D.**

BASIC INFORMATION

■ DEFINITION

A corneal abrasion is a loss of surface epithelial tissue of the cornea caused by trauma.

■ SYNONYMS

Corneal erosion
Corneal contusion

■ ICD-9CM CODES

918.1 Corneal abrasion

■ EPIDEMIOLOGY & DEMOGRAPHICS

INCIDENCE (IN U.S.): A universal problem
PREDOMINANT AGE: Any age
PEAK INCIDENCE: Childhood through active adulthood

■ PHYSICAL FINDINGS & CLINICAL PRESENTATION

• Haziness of the cornea
• Disruption of the corneal surface (Fig. 1-76)
• Redness and infection of the conjunctiva
• Pain
• Sensation of a foreign body

■ ETIOLOGY

Trauma (direct mechanical event)

DIAGNOSIS

■ DIFFERENTIAL DIAGNOSIS

• Acute angle glaucoma
• Herpes ulcers and other corneal ulcers
• Foreign body in the cornea (be certain it is not a keratitis)

■ WORKUP

• Fluorescein staining, slit lamp evaluation
• Assessment of visual acuity
• Intraocular pressure

TREATMENT

■ NONPHARMACOLOGIC THERAPY

• Warm compresses
• Pressure dressing (controversial)
• Removal of any foreign particles if present

■ ACUTE GENERAL Rx

• Topical antibiotics such as 10% sulfacetamide or Ocuflox qid
• Pressure patching of eye with eyelid closed
• Cycloplegics such as 5% homatropine

■ CHRONIC Rx

Topical antibiotics to prevent secondary infection

■ DISPOSITION

Follow-up in 24 hr and then every 3 days until abrasion has cleared and vision has returned to normal

■ REFERRAL

To ophthalmologist if patient experiences no relief within 24 hr

PEARLS & CONSIDERATIONS

■ COMMENTS

Never give patient topical anesthetic to use at home because these can cause decomposition of the cornea and permanent damage.

REFERENCES

Le Sage N et al: Efficiency of eye patching for traumatic corneal abrasions: a controlled clinical trial, *Ann Emerg Med* 78:129, 2001.
Michael JG et al: Management of corneal abrasion in children, *Ann Emerg Med* 40(1):67, 2002.
Author: **Melvyn Koby, M.D.**

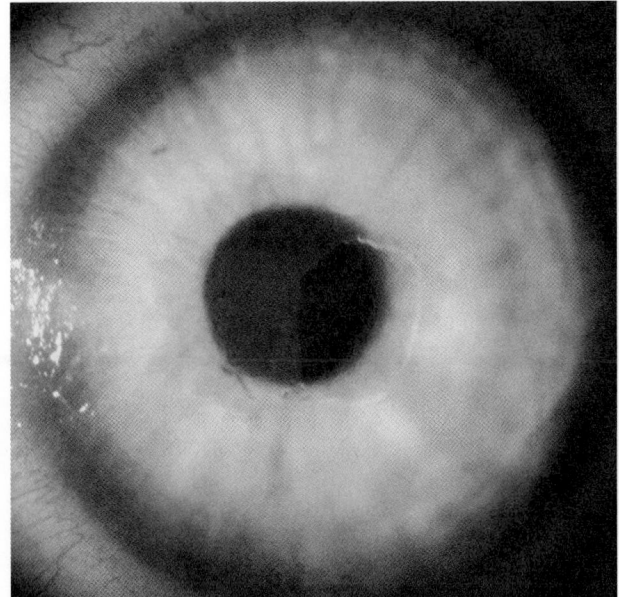
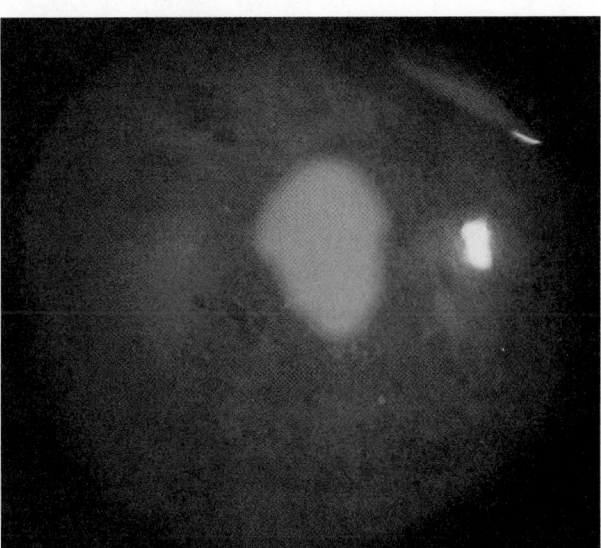

Fig. 1-76   Corneal epithelial abrasion. A, Epithelial defect without fluorescein highlighting the defect. An irregularity in the otherwise smooth corneal surface is the key to identifying the defect if no fluorescein is available. **B,** Classic fluorescein staining of an epithelial defect. (From Palay D [ed]: *Ophthalmology for the primary care physician,* St Louis, 1997, Mosby.)

BASIC INFORMATION

■ DEFINITION

Corneal ulceration refers to the disruption of the corneal surface and/or deeper layers caused by trauma or infection.

■ SYNONYMS

Infectious keratitis
Bacterial keratitis
Viral keratitis
Fungal keratitis

ICD-9CM CODES

370.0 Corneal ulcer NOS

■ EPIDEMIOLOGY & DEMOGRAPHICS

INCIDENCE (IN U.S.): 4 to 6 cases/mo seen by average general ophthalmologist
PREVALENCE (IN U.S.): Common
PREDOMINANT SEX: Either
PREDOMINANT AGE: All ages

■ PHYSICAL FINDINGS

- Localized, well-demarcated, infiltrative lesion with corresponding focal ulcer (Fig. 1-77) or oval, yellow-white stromal suppuration with thick mucopurulent exudate and edema
- Eye possibly painful, with conjunctival edema and infection

■ ETIOLOGY

- Complication of contact lens wear, trauma, or diseases such as herpes simplex keratitis, keratoconjunctivitis sicca
- Viral causes often contagious

 ## DIAGNOSIS

■ DIFFERENTIAL DIAGNOSIS

- *Pseudomonas* and pneumococcus infection—virulent
- *Moraxella, Staphylococcus, α-Streptococcus* infection—less virulent
- Herpes simplex infection or disease caused by other viruses

■ WORKUP

- Fluorescein staining, slit lamp
- Appearance often typical

■ LABORATORY TESTS

Microscopic examination and culture of scrapings

TREATMENT

■ NONPHARMACOLOGIC THERAPY

- Warm compresses
- Remove eyelid crusting

■ ACUTE GENERAL Rx

- An ophthalmic emergency
- Bacterial infection: subconjunctival cefazolin or gentamicin
- Fungal infection: hospitalization and topical application of antifungal agents

■ DISPOSITION

Ideally treated by an ophthalmologist if the patient does not rapidly respond to antibiotics (within 24 hr)

PEARLS & CONSIDERATIONS

■ COMMENTS

Do not use topical steroids because herpes, fungal, or other ulcers may be aggravated, leading to perforation of the cornea.

REFERENCES

Price FW: New pieces for the puzzle: nonsteroidal anti-inflammatory drugs and corneal ulcers, *J Cataract Refract Surg* 26(9):1263, 2000.
Schaefer F et al: Bacterial keratitis: a prospective clinical and microbiological study, *Br J Ophthalmol,* 85(7):42, 2001.

Author: **Melvyn Koby, M.D.**

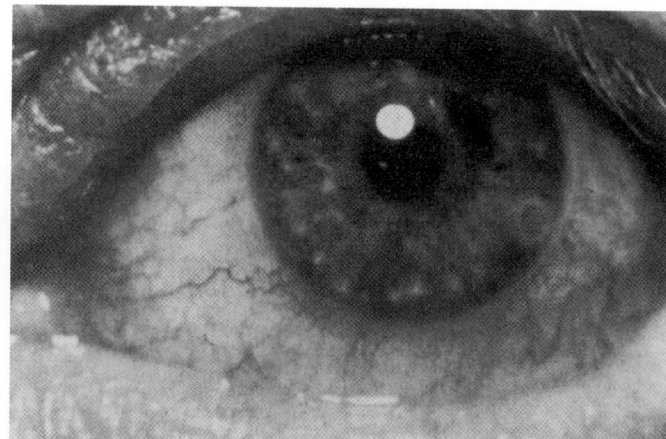

Fig. 1-77 **Peripherally located corneal ulcer.** (From Marx JA [ed]: *Rosen's emergency medicine,* ed 5, St Louis, 2002, Mosby.)

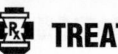

BASIC INFORMATION

■ DEFINITION
Costochondritis is a poorly defined chest wall pain of uncertain cause.

■ SYNONYMS
• Benign chest wall pain syndrome
• Costosternal syndrome
• Costosternal chondrodynia

ICD-9CM CODES
733.6 Costochondritis

■ EPIDEMIOLOGY & DEMOGRAPHICS
PREVALENCE: Unknown
PREVALENT SEX: Women > men
PREVALENT AGE: Over age 40 yr

■ PHYSICAL FINDINGS & CLINICAL PRESENTATION
• Tenderness of costochondral junctions (second through fifth) and/or sternum
• Pain with coughing and deep breathing
• Both sides of chest equal in frequency of involvement

■ ETIOLOGY
• Unknown
• May be a form of regional fibrositis
• May be referred pain from cervical or thoracic spine

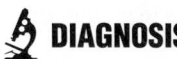

DIAGNOSIS

■ DIFFERENTIAL DIAGNOSIS
• Tietze's syndrome
• Cardiovascular disease
• GI disease
• Pulmonary disease
• Osteoarthritis (see Table 1-15)
• Cervical disc syndrome

■ WORKUP
There are no laboratory or radiographic abnormalities.

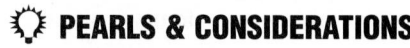

TREATMENT

■ ACUTE GENERAL Rx
• Explanation, reassurance
• Tricyclic antidepressants for sleep disturbance
• Aerobic exercise program

■ DISPOSITION
• The duration of the disorder is variable.
• Spontaneous remission is the rule.

PEARLS & CONSIDERATIONS

■ COMMENTS
In spite of the name, no inflammation is present. After other, more serious conditions are ruled out, the treatment is strictly symptomatic and supportive.

REFERENCES
Gregory PL, Biswas AC, Batt ME: Musculoskeletal problems of the chest wall in athletes, *Sports Med* 32:325, 2002.
Jenson S: Musculoskeletal causes of chest pain, *Am Fam Physician* 30:834, 2001.
Author: **Lonnie R. Mercier, M.D.**

TABLE 1-15   Musculoskeletal Chest Pain

DISORDER	CLINICAL FEATURES	COMMENTS
Tietze's syndrome	Pain and swelling of sternoclavicular joint or second or third costochondral junctions (usually left). Worse with cough and deep breathing. Local tenderness.	Traumatic cause? Rare.
Costochondritis	Pain and tenderness but no swelling. Costochondral junctions of ribs 2-5. Increased pain with cough and sneeze.	Sometimes associated with headache and hyperventilation.
Seronegative spondyloarthropathy (ankylosing spondylitis)	Sternoclavicular or manubriosternal joint. Worse in AM. Relieved by activity. May be associated with swelling.	Local chest findings usually associated with other symptoms of ankylosing spondylitis such as sacroilitis. May need HLA-B27 antigen testing.
Cervical, thoracic disc disease	Referred regional pain from affected area. No local swelling. Often aggravated by spine motion and may be accompanied by radicular pain into arm if cervical or along intercostal nerve if thoracic.	May mimic chest disease if spinal complaints are minimal and referred or radicular symptoms predominate.
Fibromyalgia	Widespread pain with other sites involved. Symptoms often change in location. Local "tender points" but no swelling or objective findings.	Female:male ratio of 9:1. Prevalent age 30-50 yr
Osteoarthritis, sternoclavicular or manubriosternal joint	Dull, aching local pain with tenderness. Occasional bony joint enlargement with soft-tissue swelling.	Crepitus may rarely be present.

BASIC INFORMATION

■ DEFINITION

Craniopharyngiomas are tumors arising from squamous cell remnants of Rathke's pouch, located in the infundibulum or upper anterior hypophysis.

■ SYNONYMS

Subset of nonadenomatous pituitary tumors

ICD-9CM CODES

237.0 Craniopharyngioma

■ EPIDEMIOLOGY & DEMOGRAPHICS

PEAK INCIDENCE: Occurs at all ages; peak during the first two decades of life, with a second small peak occurring in the sixth decade.
PREDOMINANT SEX: Both sexes are usually equally affected. Craniopharyngiomas represent 2% to 4% of intracranial neoplasms and 10% of central nervous system tumors in childhood.

■ PHYSICAL FINDINGS & CLINICAL PRESENTATION

- Presenting symptoms are usually related to the effects of a sella turcica mass. Approximately 75% of patients complain of headache and have visual disturbances.
- The usual visual defect is bitemporal hemianopsia. Optic nerve involvement with decreased visual acuity and scotomas and homonymous hemianopsia from optic tract involvement may also occur.
- Other symptoms include mental changes, nausea, vomiting, somnolence, or symptoms of pituitary failure. In adults, sexual dysfunction is the most common endocrine complaint, with impotence in males and primary or secondary amenorrhea in females. Diabetes insipidus is found in 25% of cases. In children, craniopharyngiomas may present with dwarfism.

■ ETIOLOGY

Craniopharyngiomas are believed to arise from nests of squamous epithelial cells that are commonly found in the suprasellar area surrounding the pars tuberalis of the adult pituitary.

DIAGNOSIS

■ DIFFERENTIAL DIAGNOSIS

- Pituitary adenoma
- Empty sella syndrome
- Pituitary failure of any cause
- Primary brain tumors (e.g., meningiomas, astrocytomas)
- Metastatic brain tumors
- Other brain tumors
- Cerebral aneurysm

■ LABORATORY TESTS

- Hypothyroidism (low TT_4, TT_3, T_3RU, FT_4, FT_3) with low TSH
- Hypercortisolism (low cortisol) with low ACTH
- Low sex hormones (testosterone, estriol) with low FSH and LH
- Diabetes insipidus (see "Diabetes insipidus")
- Prolactin may be normal or slightly elevated
- Pituitary stimulation tests may be required in some cases

■ IMAGING STUDIES

- Visual field testing for bitemporal hemianopsia
- Skull film
  Enlarged or eroded sella turcica (50%)
  Suprasellar calcification (50%)
- Head CT scan or MRI (Fig. 1-78)

TREATMENT

- Surgical resection (curative or palliative)
  Transsphenoidal surgery for small intrasellar tumors
  Subfrontal craniotomy for most patients
- Postoperative radiation
- Intralesional ^{32}P irradiation or bleomycin for unresectable tumors

■ PROGNOSIS

- Operative mortality: 3% to 16% (higher with large tumors)
- Postoperative recurrence rate: 10% to 40%
- 5-yr and 10-yr survival: 88% and 76%, respectively, with surgery and radiation

REFERENCES

Asa SL, Horvath E, Kovacs K: Craniopharyngiomas. In Mazzaferri EL, Samaan NA (eds): *Endocrine tumors*, Boston, 1993, Blackwell Scientific.

Leavens ME et al: Nonadenomatous intrasellar and parasellar neoplasms. In Mazzaferri EL, Samaan NA (eds): *Endocrine tumors*, Boston, 1993, Blackwell Scientific.

Melmed S: Evaluation of pituitary masses. In DeGroot LJ, Jameson JL (eds): *Endocrinology*, ed 4, Philadelphia 2001, WB Saunders.
Author: **Tom J. Wachtel, M.D.**

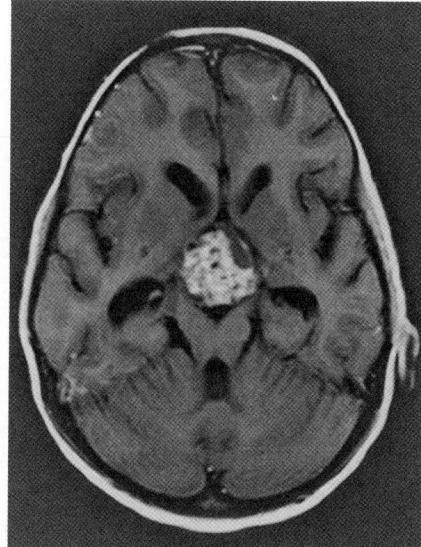

Fig. 1-78 MRI scan of a craniopharyngioma, demonstrating a cystic contrast-enhancing mass in the suprasellar area extending upward and compressing the hypothalamus. (From Goetz CG: *Textbook of clinical neurology*, Philadelphia, 1999, WB Saunders.)

BASIC INFORMATION

■ DEFINITION

Creutzfeldt-Jakob disease is a progressive, fatal, dementing illness caused by an infectious agent known as a *prion*.

■ SYNONYMS

Transmissible spongiform encephalopathy
Prion disease

ICD-9CM CODES

046.1 Creutzfeldt-Jakob disease

■ EPIDEMIOLOGY & DEMOGRAPHICS

- Incidence of 1 per 1,000,000 population per yr
- Peak age 60 yr (range 16-82 yr)
- 5%-10% familial, remaining cases are sporadic; iatrogenic cases (corneal transplants, dura mater allograft, human pituitary extract) very rare
- Normal prion protein gene found on human chromosome 20

■ PHYSICAL FINDINGS & CLINICAL PRESENTATION

- All patients present with cognitive deficits (dementing illness—memory loss, behavioral abnormalities, higher cortical function impairment).
- More than 80% will have myoclonus.
- Pyramidal tract signs (weakness), cerebellar signs (clumsiness), and extrapyramidal signs (parkinsonian features) are seen in more than 50% of the cases.
- Less common features include cortical visual abnormalities, abnormal eye movements, vestibular dysfunction, sensory disturbances, autonomic dysfunction, lower motor neuron signs, and seizures.

■ ETIOLOGY

Small proteinaceous infections particle (prion). Noninfectious prion protein (PrP) is a cellular protein found on the surfaces of neurons. Normal function is not known. Protein is converted to protease resistant and infectious agent (PrP^{sc}) by infectious prion protein (PrP^{sc}).

DIAGNOSIS

- Definite CJD: Neuropathologically confirmed spongiform encephalopathy in a case of progressive dementia.
- Probable CJD: History of rapidly progressive dementia (less than 2 yr) with typical EEG with at least two of the following clinical features: myoclonus, visual or cerebellar dysfunction, pyramidal or extrapyramidal features, akinetic mutism.
- Possible CJD: Same as probable CJD without EEG findings.

■ DIFFERENTIAL DIAGNOSIS

- Alzheimer's disease
- Frontotemporal dementia
- Lewy Body disease
- Vascular dementia
- Others (hydrocephalus, infectious, vitamin deficiency, endocrine)

A clinical algorithm for the evaluation of dementia is described in Section III, Fig. 3-56.

■ WORKUP

- Evaluate for treatable causes of dementia (see "Alzheimer's disease").
- Brain biopsy can be diagnostic, but it is usually not performed because there is no treatment or cure.

■ LABORATORY TESTS

- Presence of periodic sharp wave complexes on EEG (Fig. 1-79) in cases of rapidly progressive dementia has a sensitivity of 67% and a specificity of 86%.
- Presence of the 14,3,3 protein in CSF has a 95% positive predictive value with its absence having a 92% negative predictive value in cases of probable or possible CJD.

■ IMAGING STUDIES

MRI scan can show areas of increased signal in basal ganglia and areas of restricted diffusion in the cerebral cortex.

TREATMENT

■ NONPHARMACOLOGIC THERAPY

Full time caregiver and/or nursing home

■ ACUTE GENERAL Rx

No known therapy

■ CHRONIC Rx

No known therapy

■ DISPOSITION

The disease is fatal. Mean duration of illness is 8 mo (range 1-130 mo).

■ REFERRAL

Neurology for evaluation of any rapidly progressive dementia
Social work

PEARLS & CONSIDERATIONS

■ COMMENTS

- Related diseases in humans: Kuru, Fatal Familial Insomnia, Gerstmann-Sträussler-Scheinker syndrome, new-variant Creutzfeldt-Jacob disease.
- Related diseases in animals: Scrapie, bovine spongiform encephalopathy (Mad cow disease).

REFERENCES

Brown P et al: Human spongiform encephalopathy: The National Institutes of Health series of 300 cases of experimentally transmitted disease, *Ann Neurol* 35:513, 1994.

Hsich G et al: The 14-3-3 brain protein in cerebrospinal fluid as a marker for transmissible spongiform encephalopathies, *N Engl J Med* 335:924, 1996.

Johnson RT, Gibbs CJ: Creutzfeldt-Jakob disease and related transmissible spongiform encephalopathies, *N Engl J Med* 339:1994, 1998.

Masters CL et al: Creutzfeldt-Jakob disease: patterns of worldwide occurrence and the significance of familial and sporadic clustering, *Ann Neurol* 5:177, 1979.

Steinhoff BJ et al: Accuracy and reliability of periodic sharp wave complexes in Creutzfeldt-Jakob disease, *Arch Neurol* 53:162, 1996.
Author: **Chun Lim, M.D., Ph.D.**

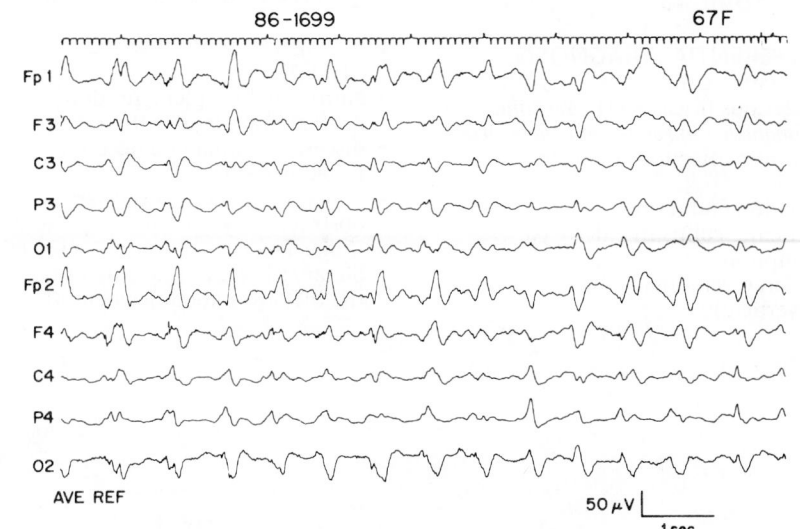

Fig. 1-79 Periodic sharp wave pattern in a woman with Creutzfeldt-Jakob disease. Generalized bisynchronous diphasic sharp waves occur approximately 1.5–2.0 per second. (From Bradley WG et al: *Neurology in Clinical Practice,* 3rd ed, Newton, MA, 2000, Butterworth Heinemann.)

BASIC INFORMATION

■ DEFINITION

Crohn's disease is an inflammatory disease of the bowel of unknown etiology, most commonly involving the terminal ileum and manifesting primarily with diarrhea, abdominal pain, fatigue, and weight loss.

■ SYNONYMS

Regional enteritis
Inflammatory bowel disease (IBD)

ICD-9CM CODES

555.9 Crohn's disease, unspecified site
555.0 Crohn's disease, small intestine
555.1 Crohn's disease involving large intestine

■ EPIDEMIOLOGY & DEMOGRAPHICS

PREVALENCE: 1 case/1000 persons; most common in Caucasians and Jews

■ PHYSICAL FINDINGS & CLINICAL PRESENTATION

- Abdominal tenderness, mass, or distention
- Hyperactive bowel sounds in patients with partial obstruction, bloody diarrhea
- Delayed growth and failure of normal development in children
- Perianal and rectal abscesses, mouth ulcers, and atrophic glossitis
- Extraintestinal manifestations: joint swelling and tenderness, hepatosplenomegaly, erythema nodosum, clubbing, tenderness to palpation of the sacroiliac joints

■ ETIOLOGY

Unknown

DIAGNOSIS

■ DIFFERENTIAL DIAGNOSIS

- Ulcerative colitis
- Infectious diseases (TB, *Yersinia, Salmonella, Shigella, Campylobacter*)
- Parasitic infections (amebic infection)
- Pseudomembranous colitis
- Ischemic colitis in elderly patients
- Lymphoma
- Colon carcinoma
- Diverticulitis

- Radiation enteritis
- Collagenous colitis
- Fungal infections (*Histoplasma, Actinomyces*)
- Gay bowel syndrome (in homosexual patient)
- Carcinoid tumors
- Celiac sprue
- Mesenteric adenitis

■ LABORATORY TESTS

- Decreased Hgb and Hct from chronic blood loss
- Hypokalemia, hypomagnesemia, hypocalcemia, and low albumin in patients with chronic diarrhea
- Vitamin B_{12} and folate deficiency
- Endoscopic features of Crohn's disease include asymmetric and discontinued disease, deep longitudinal fissures, cobblestone appearance, presence of strictures. Crypt distortion and inflammation are also present. Granulomas may be present

■ IMAGING STUDIES

- Barium imaging studies reveal deep ulcerations (often longitudinal and transverse) and segmental lesions (skip lesions, strictures, fistulas, cobblestone appearance of mucosa caused by submucosal inflammation); "thumbprinting" is common, "string sign" in terminal ileum may be noted.
- In 5% to 10% of patients with IBD, a clear distinction between ulcerative colitis and Crohn's disease cannot be made. Generally, Crohn's disease can be distinguished from ulcerative colitis by presence of transmural involvement and the frequent presence of noncaseating granulomas and lymphoid aggregates.

TREATMENT

■ NONPHARMACOLOGIC THERAPY

- Nutritional supplementation is needed in patients with advanced disease. TPN may be necessary in selected patients.
- Low-residue diet is necessary when obstructive symptoms are present.
- If diarrhea is prominent, increased dietary fiber and lowering of fat in the diet are sometimes helpful.

- Psychotherapy is useful for situational adjustment crises. A trusting and mutually understanding relationship and referral to self-help groups are very important because of the chronicity of the disease and the relatively young age of the patients.
- Avoid oral feedings during acute exacerbation to decrease colonic activity: a low-roughage diet may be helpful in early relapse.

■ ACUTE GENERAL Rx

- Sulfasalazine, 500 mg PO qid initially, increased qd or qod by 1 g until therapeutic dosages of 4 to 6 g/day are achieved. The oral salicylates, mesalamine (Asacol, Rowasa) are as effective as sulfasalazine and better tolerated but more expensive; they may be useful in patients allergic to the sulfa moiety of sulfasalazine molecule. Individuals with sulfa allergies should avoid sulfasalazine. Folate supplementation is recommended because sulfasalazine inhibits folate absorption.
- Corticosteroids (prednisone) 40 to 60 mg/day are useful for acute exacerbation. Steroids are usually tapered over approximately 2 to 3 mo. Some patients require a low dose for prolonged period of maintenance.
- Steroid analogues are locally active corticosteroids that target specific areas of inflammation in the GI tract. Budesonide (Entocort EC) is available as a controlled-release formulation and is approved for mild to moderate active Crohn's disease involving the ileum and/or ascending colon. The adult dose is 9 mg qd for a maximum of 8 wk.
- Immunosuppressants such as azathioprine (Imuran) 150 mg/day, methotrexate, or cyclosporine can be used for severe, progressive disease. In patients with Crohn's disease who enter remission after treatment with methotrexate, a low dose of methotrexate maintains remission.
- Metronidazole (Flagyl) 50 mg qid is useful for colonic fistulas.

- Infliximab (Remicade), a chimeric monoclonal antibody targeting tumor necrosis factor-α, is effective in the treatment of enterocutaneous fistulas. This medication can induce clinical improvement in 80% of patients with Crohn's disease refractory to other agents. Its mechanism of action is incompletely understood. It is very costly. A PPD test should be done before using this medication.
- Natalizumab, a selective adhesion-molecule inhibitor, has been reported effective in increasing the rate of remission and response in patients with active Crohn's disease.
- Hydrocortisone (Cortenema) enema bid or tid is useful for proctitis.
- Most patients who have anemia associated with Crohn's disease respond to iron supplementation.

Erythropoietin is useful in patients with anemia refractory to treatment with iron and vitamins.

■ CHRONIC Rx
- Monitor disease activity with symptom review and laboratory evaluation (CBC and sedimentation rate)
- Liver tests and vitamin B_{12} levels monitored on a yearly basis

■ DISPOSITION
- One tenth of patients have prolonged remission, three quarters have a chronic intermittent disease course, and one eighth have an unremitting course.

■ REFERRAL
- Surgical referral is needed for complications such as abscess formation, obstruction, fistulas, toxic mega-colon, refractory disease, or severe hemorrhage. A conservative surgical approach is necessary, because surgery is not curative. Multiple surgeries may also result in short bowel syndrome.

REFERENCES
Ghosh S et al: Natalizumab for active Crohn's disease, *N Engl J Med* 348:24, 2003.

Knutson D et al: Management of Crohn's disease: a practical approach, *Am Fam Physician* 68:707, 2003.

Podolsky DK: Inflammatory bowel disease, *N Engl J Med* 347:417, 2002.

Author: **Fred F. Ferri, M.D.**

BASIC INFORMATION

■ DEFINITION
Cryptococcosis is an infection caused by the fungal organism *Cryptococcus neoformans*.

ICD-9CM CODES
117.5 Cryptococcosis

■ EPIDEMIOLOGY & DEMOGRAPHICS
INCIDENCE (IN U.S.)
- 1 to 2 cases/1 million (non–HIV-infected) persons annually
- 6% to 7% in HIV-infected persons

PREDOMINANT SEX: Equal sex distribution when corrected for HIV status

PREDOMINANT AGE: Less than 2 yr of age; 20 to 40 yr of age

PEAK INCIDENCE: 20 to 40 yr (parallel to AIDS epidemic)

NEONATAL INFECTION: Very uncommon

■ PHYSICAL FINDINGS & CLINICAL PRESENTATION
- More than 90% present with meningitis; almost all have fever and headache.
- Meningismus, photophobia, mental status changes are seen in approximately 25%.
- Focal intracranial infection occurs in rare cases with focal deficit, increased intracranial pressure.
- Most common infections outside the CNS:
  1. In the lungs (fever, cough, dyspnea)
  2. In the skin (cellulitis, papular eruption)
  3. In the lymph nodes (lymphadenitis)
  4. Potential involvement of virtually any organ

■ ETIOLOGY
- Caused by the fungal organism *C. neoformans*
- Transmission by the respiratory route
- Disseminates to the CNS in most cases, usually without recognizable lung involvement
- Almost always in the setting of AIDS or other disorders of cellular immune function (hematologic malignancies, long-term corticosteroid therapy, immunosuppressive therapy following organ transplantation), or pregnancy

DIAGNOSIS

■ DIFFERENTIAL DIAGNOSIS
- Acute or subacute meningitis (caused by *Neisseria meningitidis*, *Streptococcus pneumoniae*, *Haemophilus influenzae*, *Listeria monocytogenes*, *Mycobacterium tuberculosis*, *Histoplasma capsulatum*, viruses)
- Intracranial mass lesion (neoplasms, toxoplasmosis, TB)
- Pulmonary involvement confused with *Pneumocystis carinii* pneumonia when diffuse or confused with TB or bacterial pneumonia when focal or involving the pleura
- Skin lesions confused with bacterial cellulitis or molluscum contagiosum

■ WORKUP
- Lumbar puncture to exclude cryptococcal meningitis.
- CT scan of the head when focal lesion or increased intracranial pressure is suspected.
- Biopsy of enlarged lymph nodes and skin lesions if feasible.

■ LABORATORY TESTS
- Culture and India ink stain (60% to 80% sensitive in culture-proven cases [Fig. 1-80]), examination of the CSF in all cases when CNS involvement is suspected
- Blood and serum cryptococcal antigen assay (>90% sensitivity and specificity)
- Culture and histologic examination of biopsy material

■ IMAGING STUDIES
- CT scan or MRI of the head if focal neurologic involvement is suspected
- Chest x-ray examination to exclude pulmonary involvement

TREATMENT

■ ACUTE GENERAL Rx
- Therapy is initiated with IV amphotericin B (0.5 mg/kg/day) with or without flucytosine.
- After stabilization (usually several weeks), consider fluconazole (200 to 400 mg qd PO) for additional 6 to 8 wk.
- Alternative: IV fluconazole for initial therapy in patients unable to tolerate amphotericin B.
- If symptomatic increased intracranial pressure, consider therapeutic lumbar taps or intraventricular shunt.

■ CHRONIC Rx
Fluconazole (200 mg PO qd) is highly effective in preventing a relapse in HIV-infected patients.

■ DISPOSITION
Without maintenance therapy, relapse rate is >50% among AIDS patients.

■ REFERRAL
- For consultation with infectious diseases specialist in all cases
- For neurologic consultation if level of consciousness is depressed or focal lesion is present

PEARLS & CONSIDERATIONS

■ COMMENTS
Cryptococcosis is considered an AIDS-defining infection when it occurs in the absence of other known causes of immunodeficiency; thus all patients should be advised to be HIV tested and, if positive, referred for evaluation and follow-up by a physician experienced in the management of HIV infection.

REFERENCES
Powderly WG: Current approach to the acute management of cryptococcal infections, *J Infect Dis* 41:18, 2000.

Vilchez RA et al: Cryptococcosis in organ transplant recipients: an overview, *A J Transplant* 2(7):575, 2002.

Author: **Joseph R. Masci, M.D.**

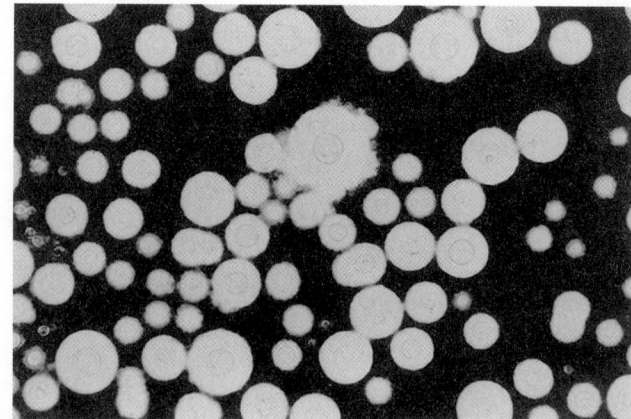

Fig. 1-80 India ink preparation of cerebrospinal fluid revealing encapsulated cryptococci. Note the large capsules surrounding the smaller organisms. (From Andreoli TE [ed]: *Cecil essentials of medicine*, ed 4, Philadelphia, 1997, WB Saunders.)

BASIC INFORMATION

■ DEFINITION

Cryptorchidism is the failure of descent of the testes into the scrotum during fetal development. Cryptorchid testes neither reside in nor can be manipulated into the scrotum. Testes that can be manually manipulated into the scrotum are called retractile.

■ SYNONYMS

Undescended testis

ICD-9CM CODES

752.51 Cryptorchidism

■ EPIDEMIOLOGY & DEMOGRAPHICS

Cryptorchidism is the most common genitourinary disorder of male children. Approximately 30% of premature and 5% of full-term males will have an undescended testicle. Within the first year of life, most cryptorchid testes descend into the scrotum so that the incidence of cryptorchidism becomes approximately 1% in boys. Increased rates are associated with premature birth, low birth weight, and twinning. Associations have been seen with Kallmann's and Prader-Willi syndromes, pituitary hypoplasia, testicular feminization, and Reifenstein syndrome.

■ PHYSICAL FINDINGS & CLINICAL PRESENTATION

- Typically asymptomatic and is noted incidentally on screening examination
- The testis may be impalpable or palpable in a location other than the scrotum but usually along the path of normal descent (Fig. 1-81)
- Associated with infertility and a 10- to 20-fold increase in risk of testicular cancer, which can occur in the contralateral descended testis. Testes that remain in an intraabdominal location are associated with a 40-fold increased risk of developing testicular carcinoma

■ ETIOLOGY

Normal testicular descent is a complex interplay between differential growth and endocrine, gubernaculum, and genitofemoral nerve function. Developmental problems among some or all of these are postulated in causing cryptorchidism.

DIAGNOSIS

■ DIFFERENTIAL DIAGNOSIS

- Retractile testis
- Ascended testis
- Dislocated testis
- Anorchia

■ WORKUP

Physical examination, hormonal challenge, imaging studies

■ PHYSICAL EXAMINATION

When properly done in a warm room, an examination identifies presence or absence of palpable testes and location of palpable testes. An examination should be done in both the supine and standing positions with adequate cremasteric relaxation to differentiate true cryptorchidism from retractile testes. Cryptorchid testes are often associated with an indirect inguinal hernia as the tunica vaginalis fails to close above the testis.

■ HORMONAL CHALLENGE

Administration of human chorionic gonadotropin (hCG) will confirm the presence of functioning testicular tissue. If the follicular stimulating hormone (FSH) level is 3× normal and there is no elevation of testosterone in response to hCG, functional testes are absent.

■ IMAGING

Ultrasound, CT scan, or MRI can be used to identify impalpable testes, but the sensitivity is inadequate. Inguinal exploration is not reliable. Laparoscopy is preferred and can be used therapeutically.

TREATMENT

Treatment of the undescended testicle can be hormonal, surgical, or both. Treatment is recommended as early as 6 mo of age and should be completed before age 2 yr because early treatment offers protection of fertility. Early referral to a pediatric urologist is recommended. There is no proof that placement of the undescended testicle into the scrotum reduces the risk of testicular cancer, but placement of both testes in the scrotum facilitates testicular examination.

■ FOLLOW-UP

- Repeat examination at 3 mo of age, because many testes will descend spontaneously. Spontaneous descent of true undescended testes is rare after 3 mo of age
- Lifelong testicular examination after puberty to screen for malignancy

■ HORMONAL Rx

Administration of hCG can cause testicular descent and is often tried before surgical intervention. hCG will cause retractile testes to remain in the scrotum.

■ SURGICAL Rx

Although the risk of testicular cancer is higher in men with cryptorchidism, the removal of all intraabdominal testes is not warranted. Orchiopexy, which is the surgical placement of an undescended testis into the scrotum, is a well-established operation for the palpable undescended testicle. For the nonpalpable testis, laparoscopic surgery is indicated to identify and locate the testis.

■ DISPOSITION

Prognosis is fair. Fertility and malignancy risks not greatly affected by treatment.

REFERENCES

Docimo S, Silver R, Cromie W: The undescended testicle: diagnosis and management, *Am Fam Physician* 62:2037, 2000.
Gill B, Kogan S: Cryptorchidism: current concepts, *Pediatr Clin North Am* 44(5):1211, 1997.
Rozanski TA, Bloom DA: The undescended testis: theory and management, *Urol Clin North Am* 22(1):107, 1995.

Authors: **Iris Tong, M.D., and Michael Picchioni, M.D.**

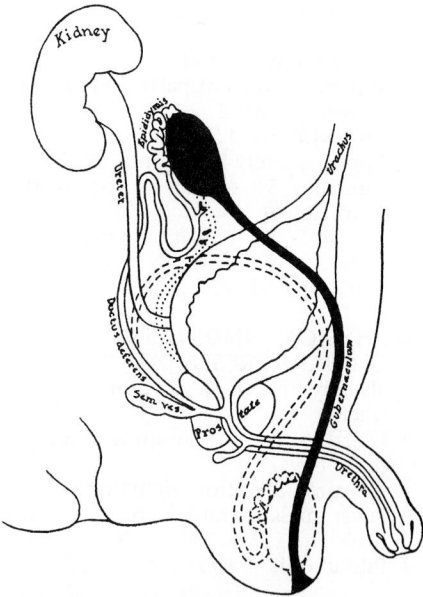

Fig. 1-81 Undescended testes are common in male neonates with neuromuscular disease already symptomatic at birth, regardless of the etiology. The gubernaculums is a cylinder of striated muscle surrounding a core of smooth muscle that actively pulls the testicle into the scrotum in late gestation. Weakness of the gubernaculums in a generalized myopathy of fetal life prevents or delays the descent of the testis. (Reproduced with permission from Sarnat HB, Sarnat MS: Disorders of muscle in the newborn. In Moss AJ, Stern L [eds]: *Pediatrics update*, ed 4, New York, 1983, Elsevier-North Holland.)

BASIC INFORMATION

■ DEFINITION

The intracellular protozoan parasite *Cryptosporidium parvum* is associated with gastrointestinal disease and diarrhea, especially in AIDS patients or immunocompromised hosts. It is also associated with waterborne outbreak in immunocompetent hosts.

Other species, including *C. felis, C. muris,* and *C. meleagridis,* are now described to be pathogens as well.

■ SYNONYMS

Cryptosporidiosis

ICD-9CM CODES

00.7.4 Cryptosporidia infection

■ EPIDEMIOLOGY & DEMOGRAPHICS

PREVALENCE: Worldwide, especially third world countries; associated with poor hygiene as a waterborne pathogen

TRANSMISSION:
- Person to person (daycare, family members)
- Animal to person (pets, farm animals)
- Environmental (water-associated outbreaks, including travel associated with swimming in or drinking contaminated water)
- May be significant pathogen causing diarrhea in AIDS

INCIDENCE (IN U.S.):
- Approximately 2% in industrial countries, 5% to 10% in third world countries
- 10% to 20% HIV patients may excrete cyst in U.S.

PREDOMINANT SEX: Male = female

■ PHYSICAL FINDINGS & CLINICAL PRESENTATION

- Usually limited to gastrointestinal tract
- Diarrhea, severe abdominal pain (2 to 28 days)
- Impaired digestion, dehydration
- Fever, malaise, fatigue, nausea, vomiting
- Pneumonia if aspirated

■ ETIOLOGY

Cryptosporidium parvum, C. felis, C. muris, C. meleagridis

DIAGNOSIS

Clinical presentation of acute gastrointestinal illness, especially associated with HIV or with travel and waterborne outbreaks.

■ DIFFERENTIAL DIAGNOSIS

- *Campylobacter*
- *Clostridium difficile*
- *Entamoeba histolytica*
- *Giardia lamblia*
- *Salmonella*
- *Shigella*
- *Microsporida*
- *Cytomegalovirus*
- *Mycobacterium avium*

Disease may cause cholecystitis, reactive arthritis, hepatitis, pancreatitis, pneumonia in immunocompromised or HIV-infected patients.

■ WORKUP

- Stool evaluation looking for characteristic oocyst by modified acid-fast stain (Fig. 1-82)
- Serologic testing investigational
- May be seen in mucosal surfaces of GI lumen by biopsy

TREATMENT

- May be self-limited in normal host—often requiring hydration. Antidiarrhea agents Pepto-Bismol, Kaopectate, or loperamide may give symptomatic relief.

- Pharmacologic treatment with antibiotics has to date varying and usually poor response. Oocyst excretion reduction has been shown with paromomycin (1 g bid)/azithromycin and nitazoxanide therapy along with decreasing stool frequency. If treatment failure, consider metronidazole or Bactrim.
- Nitazoxanide elixir has been approved for the treatment of cryptosporidiosis in children ages 1 to 11 yr.
- Biliary cryptosporidiosis can be treated with antiretroviral therapy in the HIV setting.

REFERENCES

Chen XM et al: Cryptosporidiosis, *N Engl J Med* 346:1723, 2002.

Rossignol JF, Ayoub A, Ayers, MS: Treatment of diarrhea caused by Cryptosporidium parvum. A prospective randomized, double-blind, placebo-controlled study of nitazoxanide, *J Infect Dis* 184:103, 2001.

Smith NH et al: Combination drug therapy for cryptosporidiosis in AIDS, *J Infect Dis* 178:900, 1998.

Tzipori S: Cryptosporidiosis: laboratory investigations and chemotherapy, *Adv Parasitol* 40:187, 1998.

Authors: **Glenn G. Fort M.D., and Dennis J. Mikolich, M.D.**

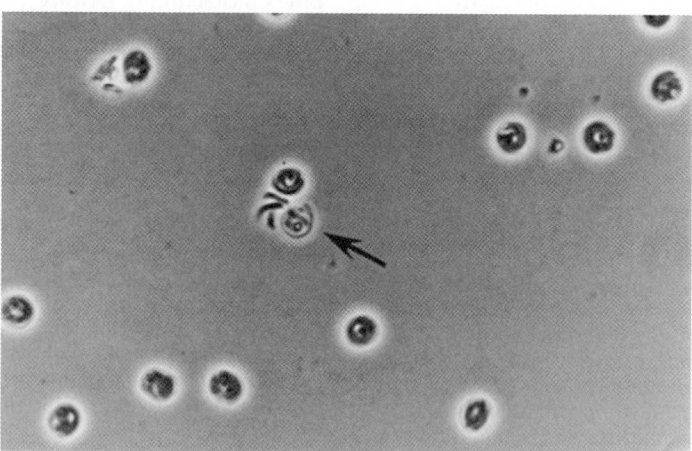

Fig. 1-82 **Human stool-derived *Cryptosporidium* oocysts.** Excysting oocyst *(arrow)* is releasing three of its four sporozoites. (Phase-control microscopy x630.) (From Gorbach SL: *Infectious diseases,* ed 2, Philadelphia, 1998, WB Saunders.)

BASIC INFORMATION

■ **DEFINITION**
Compression of the ulnar nerve behind the elbow (cubitus)

■ **SYNONYMS**
Tardy ulnar palsy

ICD-9CM CODES
354.2 Cubital tunnel syndrome

■ **EPIDEMIOLOGY & DEMOGRAPHICS**
Prevalent sex: Males = females

■ **PHYSICAL FINDINGS & CLINICAL PRESENTATION**
• Paresthesias and numbness along distribution of ulnar nerve (ulnar one and one-half fingers)
• Positive Tinel's sign at elbow
• Positive elbow flexion test (flexion of elbow with wrist extended for 30 sec may reproduce symptoms)
• May be diminished sensation to tip of small finger
• Ulnar nerve may be subluxable with elbow motion or by manipulation
• Cubitus valgus may be present if prior bony injury
• Interosseous weakness in long-standing cases with atrophy (Fig. 1-83)

■ **ETIOLOGY**
• Direct pressure
• Cubitus valgus deformity
• Subluxation of ulnar nerve
• Repeated stretching during throwing motion
• Elbow synovitis
• Local muscular hypertrophy

 DIAGNOSIS

■ **DIFFERENTIAL DIAGNOSIS**
• Medial epicondylitis
• Medial elbow instability
• Carpal tunnel syndrome
• Cervical disc syndrome with radicular arm symptoms
• Ulnar nerve compression at wrist (Guyon's canal)

■ **WORKUP**
Diagnosis can usually be established clinically

■ **IMAGING STUDIES**
• Routine roentgenograms may be helpful in establishing cause or ruling out other conditions
• Electrodiagnostic studies: nerve conduction tests and electromyography are useful in establishing diagnosis and ruling out other syndromes

TREATMENT

■ **GENERAL THERAPY**
• Protect nerve from pressure
• Elbow pads
• Avoid prolonged elbow flexion (talking on phone with elbow bent)

■ **DISPOSITION**
• Prognosis is variable
• Mild to moderate cases recover well if offending activity can be eliminated. If muscle atrophy has developed, recovery of strength may be incomplete in spite of treatment

■ **REFERRAL**
Surgical referral in cases of failed medical management or if signs of motor impairment are present

REFERENCES

Grana W: Medial epicondylitis and cubital tunnel syndrome in the throwing athlete, *Clin Sports Med* 20(3):541, 2001.
Kato H et al: Cubital tunnel syndrome associated with medial elbow ganglia and osteoarthritis of the elbow, *J Bone Joint Surg* 84(A):1413, 2002.
Sasaki J et al: Ultrasonographic assessment of ulnar collateral ligament and medial elbow laxity in college baseball players, *J Bone Joint Surg* 84(A):525, 2002.
Author: **Lonnie R. Mercier, M.D.**

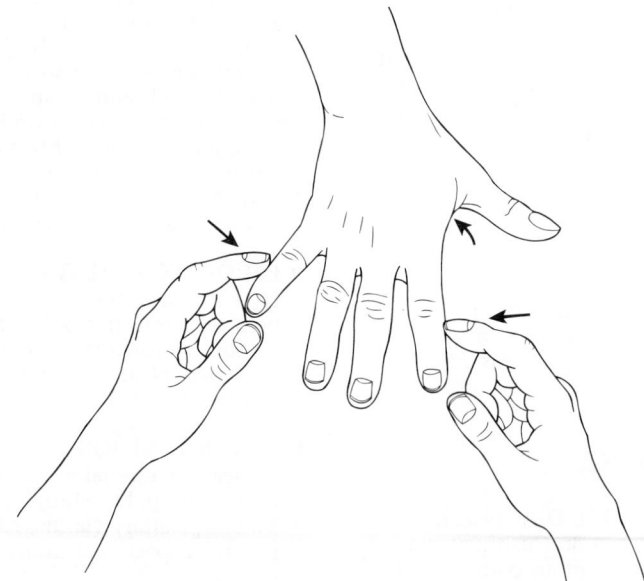

Fig. 1-83 Testing for intrinsic (ulnar) motor weakness (fanning the fingers against resistance). Always look for atrophy of the first dorsal interosseus *(curved arrow)* when ulnar nerve lesions are suspected. (From Mercier LR: *Practical orthopedics*, ed 5, St Louis, 2000, Mosby.)

BASIC INFORMATION

■ DEFINITION

- Cushing's syndrome is the occurrence of clinical abnormalities associated with glucocorticoid excess secondary to exaggerated adrenal cortisol production or chronic glucocorticoid therapy.
- Cushing's disease is Cushing's syndrome caused by pituitary ACTH excess.

ICD-9CM CODES
255.0 Cushing's disease or syndrome

■ PHYSICAL FINDINGS & CLINICAL PRESENTATION

- Hypertension
- Central obesity with rounding of the facies (moon facies); thin extremities
- Hirsutism, menstrual irregularities, hypogonadism
- Skin fragility, ecchymoses, red-purple abdominal striae, acne, poor wound healing, hair loss, facial plethora, hyperpigmentation (when there is ACTH excess)
- Psychosis, emotional lability, paranoia
- Muscle wasting with proximal myopathy

NOTE: The previous characteristics are not commonly present in Cushing's syndrome secondary to ectopic ACTH production. Many of these tumors secrete a biologically inactive ACTH that does not activate adrenal steroid synthesis. These patients may have only weight loss and weakness.

■ ETIOLOGY

- Iatrogenic from chronic glucocorticoid therapy (common)
- Pituitary ACTH excess (Cushing's disease; 60%)
- Adrenal neoplasms (30%)
- Ectopic ACTH production (neoplasms of lung, pancreas, kidney, thyroid, thymus; 10%)

DIAGNOSIS

■ DIFFERENTIAL DIAGNOSIS

- Alcoholic pseudo-Cushing's syndrome (endogenous cortisol overproduction)
- Obesity associated with diabetes mellitus
- Adrenogenital syndrome

■ WORKUP

- In patients with a clinical diagnosis of Cushing's syndrome the initial screening test is the overnight dexamethasone suppression test:
  1. Dexamethasone 1 mg PO given at 11 pm
  2. Plasma cortisol level measured 9 hr later (8 am)
  3. Plasma cortisol level <5 μg/100 ml excludes Cushing's syndrome
- Serial measurements (two or three consecutive measurements) of 24-hr urinary free cortisol and creatinine (to ensure adequacy of collection) are undertaken if overnight dexamethasone test is suggestive of Cushing's syndrome. Persistent elevated cortisol excretion (>300 μg/24 hr) indicates Cushing's syndrome.
- The low-dose (2 mg) dexamethasone suppression test is useful to exclude pseudo-Cushing's syndrome if the previous results are equivocal. CRH stimulation after low-dose dexamethasone administration (dexamethasone-CRH test) is also used to distinguish patients with suspected Cushing's syndrome from those who have mildly elevated urinary free cortisol level and equivocal findings.
- The high-dose (8 mg) dexamethasone test and measurement of ACTH by RIA are useful to determine the etiology of Cushing's syndrome.
  1. ACTH undetectable or decreased and lack of suppression indicates adrenal etiology of Cushing's syndrome.
  2. ACTH normal or increased and lack of suppression indicate ectopic ACTH production.
  3. ACTH normal or increased and partial suppression suggest pituitary excess (Cushing's disease).
- A single midnight serum cortisol (normal diurnal variation leads to a nadir around midnight) >7.5 μg/dl has been reported as 96% sensitive and 100% specific for the diagnosis of Cushing's syndrome.

■ LABORATORY TESTS

- Hypokalemia, hypochloremia, metabolic alkalosis, hyperglycemia, hypercholesterolemia
- Increased 24-hr urinary free cortisol (>100 μg/24 hr)

■ IMAGING STUDIES

- CT scan of adrenal glands in suspected adrenal Cushing's syndrome
- MRI of pituitary gland with gadolinium in suspected pituitary Cushing's syndrome
- Additional imaging studies to localize neoplasms of the lung, pancreas, kidney, thyroid, or thymus in patients with ectopic ACTH production

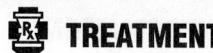 TREATMENT

■ GENERAL Rx
The treatment of Cushing's syndrome varies with its cause:
- Pituitary adenoma: transsphenoidal microadenomectomy is the therapy of choice in adults. Pituitary irradiation is reserved for patients not cured by transsphenoidal surgery. In children, pituitary irradiation may be considered as initial therapy, because 85% of children are cured by radiation. Stereotactic radiotherapy (photon knife or gamma knife) is effective and exposes the surrounding neuronal tissues to less irradiation than conventional radiotherapy. Total bilateral adrenalectomy is reserved for patients not cured by transsphenoidal surgery or pituitary irradiation.
- Adrenal neoplasm:
  1. Surgical resection of the affected adrenal
  2. Glucocorticoid replacement for approximately 9 to 12 mo after the surgery to allow time for the contralateral adrenal to recover from its prolonged suppression
- Bilateral micronodular or macronodular adrenal hyperplasia: bilateral total adrenalectomy
- Ectopic ACTH:
  1. Surgical resection of the ACTH-secreting neoplasm
  2. Control of cortisol excess with metyrapone, aminoglutethimide, mifepristone, or ketoconazole
  3. Control of the mineralocorticoid effects of cortisol and 11-deoxycorticosteroid with spironolactone
  4. Bilateral adrenalectomy: a rational approach to patients with indolent, unresectable tumors

■ DISPOSITION
Prognosis is favorable in patients with surgically amenable disease.

PEARLS & CONSIDERATIONS

■ COMMENTS
- Screening for MEN I should be considered in patients with Cushing's disease.
- An algorithm for the diagnosis of Cushing's syndrome is described in Section III

REFERENCE
Boscaro M et al: The diagnosis of Cushing's syndrome, *Arch Intern Med* 160:3045, 2000.
Author: **Fred F. Ferri, M.D.**

BASIC INFORMATION

■ DEFINITION
Cystic fibrosis (CF) is an autosomal recessive disorder characterized by dysfunction of exocrine glands.

ICD-9CM CODES
277.0 Cystic fibrosis

■ EPIDEMIOLOGY & DEMOGRAPHICS
- It is the most common fatal hereditary disorder of caucasians in the U.S. (1 case/2500 caucasians).
- Median survival is 30 yr.

■ PHYSICAL FINDINGS & CLINICAL PRESENTATION
- Failure to thrive in children
- Increased anterior/posterior chest diameter
- Basilar crackles and hyperresonance to percussion
- Digital clubbing
- Chronic cough
- Abdominal distention
- Greasy, smelly feces

■ ETIOLOGY
Chromosome 7 gene mutation (CFTR gene) resulting in abnormalities in chloride transport and water flux across the surface of epithelial cells; the abnormal secretions cause obstruction of glands and ducts in various organs and subsequent damage to exocrine tissue (recurrent pneumonia, atelectasis, bronchiectasis, diabetes mellitus, biliary cirrhosis, cholelithiasis, intestinal obstruction, increased risk of GI malignancies)

DIAGNOSIS

■ DIFFERENTIAL DIAGNOSIS
- Immunodeficiency states
- Celiac disease
- Asthma
- Recurrent pneumonia

■ WORKUP
A diagnosis of CF requires a positive quantitative pilocarpine iontophoresis test with one or more phenotypic features consistent with CF (e.g., chronic suppurative obstructive lung disease, pancreatic insufficiency) or documented CF in a sibling or first cousin.

■ LABORATORY TESTS
- Pilocarpine iontophoresis ("sweat test"): diagnostic of cystic fibrosis in children if sweat chloride is >60 mmol/L (>80 mmol/L in adults) on two separate tests on consecutive days
- DNA testing may be useful for confirming the diagnosis and providing genetic information for family members.

- Sputum C&S and Gram stain (frequent bacterial infections with *Staphylococcus aureus, Pseudomonas, Haemophilus influenzae*)
- Low albumin level, increased 72-hr fecal fat excretion
- Pulse oxymetry or ABGs: hypoxemia
- Pulmonary function studies: decreased TLC, forced vital capacity, pulmonary diffusing capacity

■ IMAGING STUDIES
- Chest x-ray examination: may reveal focal atelectasis, peribronchial cuffing, bronchiectasis, increased interstitial markings, hyperinflation
- High-resolution chest CT scan: bronchial wall thickening, cystic lesions, ring shadows (bronchiectasis)

TREATMENT

■ NONPHARMACOLOGIC THERAPY
- Postural drainage and chest percussion
- Encouragement of regular exercise and proper nutrition
- Psychosocial evaluation and counseling of patient and family members

■ ACUTE GENERAL Rx
- Antibiotic therapy based on results of Gram stain and C&S of sputum (PO ciprofloxacin or floxacillin for *Pseudomonas*, cephalosporins for *S. aureus*, IV aminoglycosides plus ceftazidime for life-threatening *Pseudomonas* infections. Macrolides are also active against *pseudomona aeruginosa*. A recent study using azithromycin maintenance in children with CF for 6 mo found less use of additional antibiotics and improvement in some aspects of pulmonary function. Additional studies may be necessary to determine if azithromycin should be used as a primary therapy or rescue treatment
- Bronchodilators for patients with air flow obstruction
- Chronic pancreatic enzyme replacement
- Alternate-day prednisone (2 mg/kg) possibly beneficial in children with cystic fibrosis (decreased hospitalization rate, improved pulmonary function); routine use of corticosteroids not recommended in adults; among children with cystic fibrosis who have received alternate-day treatment with prednisone, boys, but not girls, have persistent growth impairment after treatment is discontinued
- Proper nutrition and vitamin supplementation
- Recombinant human deoxyribonuclease (DNase [Dornase alpha]) 2.5 mg qd or bid given by aerosol for patients with viscid sputum. It is

useful to improve mucociliary clearance by liquefying difficult-to-clear pulmonary secretions. It is, however, very expensive (annual cost to the pharmacist is >$10,000); most beneficial in patients with FVC values >40% of predicted. Its cost can be decreased by using alternate-day rhDnase therapy
- Intermittent administration of inhaled tobramycin has been reported beneficial in CF
- Treatment of glucose intolerance and diabetes mellitus

■ CHRONIC Rx
Pneumococcal vaccination, yearly influenza vaccination

■ DISPOSITION
- More than 50% of children with cystic fibrosis live beyond age 20 yr.
- Lung transplantation is the only definitive treatment; 3-yr survival following transplantation exceeds 50%.
- Obstructive azoospermia is present in >98% of postpubertal males.

■ REFERRAL
- To regional ambulatory care cystic fibrosis center
- For lung transplantation in selected patients
- For screening of family members with DNA analysis

PEARLS & CONSIDERATIONS

■ COMMENTS
- Genetic testing for CF should be offered to adults with a positive family history of CF, to couples currently planning a pregnancy, and to couples seeking prenatal care.

REFERENCES

Equi A et al: Long-term azithromycin in children with cystic fibrosis: a randomized, placebo-controlled crossover trial, *Lancet* 360:978, 2002.

Groman JD et al: Variant cystic fibrosis phenotypes in the absence of CFTR mutations, *N Engl J Med* 347:401, 2002.

Kulich M et al: Improved survival among young patients with cystic fibrosis, *J Pediatr* 142:631, 2003.

West SE et al: Respiratory infections with *Pseudomonas aeruginosa* in children with cystic fibrosis, *JAMA* 287:2958, 2002.

Wilschanski M et al: Gentamicin-induced correction of CFTR function in patients with cystic fibrosis and CFTR stop mutations, *N Engl J Med* 349:1433, 2003.

Author: **Fred F. Ferri, M.D.**

BASIC INFORMATION

■ DEFINITION

Neurocysticercosis is present when cysts from the eggs of *Taenia solium* are deposited in the central nervous system. Cysticercosis represents a tissue infection with the cysts of *T. solium*. Cysticerci are the larval form of the pork tapeworm *T. solium* enclosed in bladderlike cysts. The mature tapeworm resides in the host intestine, but egg ingestion can lead to cysts being deposited in both soft tissue and the central nervous system.

ICD-9CM CODES
123.1 Cysticercosis

■ EPIDEMIOLOGY & DEMOGRAPHICS

Neurocysticercosis is the most common parasitic disease of the CNS. It affects thousands of people in Latin America, Asia, and Africa. Increasing numbers of immigrants from developing countries and improved diagnostic procedures have led to increased recognition of the entity in the United States. Neurocysticercosis is no longer an exotic disease in the United States, and it accounts for up to 2% of neurologic and neurosurgical admissions in southern California and more than 1000 cases per year nationally.

■ PHYSICAL FINDINGS & CLINICAL PRESENTATION

- Soft tissue deposition of cysts can cause local inflammation, which results in only minor morbidity compared with the damage possible in neurocysticercosis.
- Epilepsy caused by intracerebral cysts is most common manifestation of neurocysticercosis (70% to 90% of cases). The patient with a seizure history often has no unusual physical findings.
- Less common: headache, nausea and vomiting resulting from increased intracranial pressure, and altered mental status, including psychosis.
- Inflammation around degenerating cysts can cause focal encephalitis, vasculitis, chronic meningitis, and cranial nerve palsies.
- Cysts can occur in the ventricles and cause hydrocephalus; more rarely, they can be found in the spinal cord and eye.

■ ETIOLOGY

Ingestion of the *T. solium* cysticerci in infected, undercooked pork results in human intestinal tapeworms, and excretion of eggs in the feces follows. Eggs can be ingested by the source patient or transmitted via food handlers. Ingestion of the *T. solium* eggs leads to release of an oncosphere, which tra-

verses the intestinal wall and enters the circulation. Oncospheres mature into cysticerci; these can be deposited in the soft tissue or the CNS. The presence of viable cysts in the CNS is usually asymptomatic. With time, inflammation around degenerating cysts causes symptoms dependent on the cysts' location, number, and size. Neurocysticercosis has been reported in AIDS patients; immunosuppression does not seem to increase the incidence of the infection.

DIAGNOSIS

■ DIFFERENTIAL DIAGNOSIS
- Idiopathic epilepsy
- Migraine
- Vasculitides
- Primary neoplasia of CNS
- Toxoplasmosis
- Brain abscess
- Granulomatous disease such as sarcoidosis

■ WORKUP
- Comprehensive clinical history
- Stool examination for ova if intestinal tapeworms also suspected
- Imaging studies (precedes laboratory tests if CNS involvement suspected)
- CSF examination
- Laboratory tests (serology)

■ LABORATORY TESTS
- CSF examination: may show pleocytosis, with lymphocytic or eosinophilic predominance, low glucose, elevated protein with neurocysticercosis
- Immunotest: both serum and CSF can be studied for antibodies. ELISA sensitivity and specificity >90% when done in inflammatory CSF

■ IMAGING STUDIES
Head CT scan can show living cysticerci (hypodense lesions) and degenerating cysts (isodense or hyperdense lesions). Typically, there are multiple lesions. CT scan is the best method for detecting calcification associated with prior infection. Brain MRI provides detailed images of living and degenerating cysts, but it may not detect destroyed lesions. MRI is the best means to diagnose intraventricular cysticerci noninvasively.

TREATMENT

A plan for treatment should follow a clear definition of the characteristics of the cysts and the degree of the immune response to the parasite.

- Inactive infection: patients with seizures and calcifications alone on neuroimaging studies are not

thought to have viable parasites. Cysticidal therapy is usually not undertaken. Anticonvulsants can control seizures. For patients with hydrocephalus, ventriculoperitoneal shunting can resolve symptoms.

- Active parenchymal infection (most common form presentation): eradication of cysts is less controversial for active disease. Anticonvulsants should be given to control seizures. Some argue that only treatment of seizures, not antiparasitic therapy, is needed.
- Extraparenchymal neurocysticercosis: refer to a neurosurgeon.
- Ventricular: usually presents with obstructive hydrocephalus. The mainstay of therapy is the rapid correction of hydrocephalus.
- Subarachnoid: is associated with arachnoiditis. Diversion of CSF and steroid therapy may be needed.
- Cysticidal therapy: praziquantel has been the mainstay of therapy and is effective; albendazole is now being used more frequently, and it may have greater efficacy at a lesser cost than praziquantel.
- Dosage: PO praziquantel 50 mg/kg/day divided into three doses for 14 days. NOTE: Praziquantel is metabolized via P-450 and levels may be reduced when given in combination with anticonvulsants. Levels can increase with cimetidine.
- PO albendazole 15 mg/kg/day divided into three doses for 8 days. May add to steroid therapy, especially if treatment causes worsening of inflammation.

■ REFERRAL
Neurosurgical consultation if extraparenchymal neurocysticercosis or obstructive hydrocephalus suspected

PEARLS & CONSIDERATIONS

■ PREVENTION
Eradication of taeniasis/cysticercosis is possible, as demonstrated in countries that were endemic earlier in this century. The disease disappears with implementation of meat inspection, improvement of pig husbandry, and betterment of sociocultural conditions.

REFERENCE
Pal KD et al: Neurocysticercosis and epilepsy in developing countries, *J Neurol Neurosurg Psychiatry* 68:137, 2000.
Authors: **Gail O'Brien, M.D., and Karoll Cortez, M.D.**

Note: Dr. Cortez wrote this monograph while employed by the U.S. government; therefore it is public domain.

BASIC INFORMATION

■ DEFINITION

Infection with cytomegalovirus (CMV), a herpes virus, is common in the general population, with multiple mechanisms for transmission, often during childhood and adolescence. CMV is associated with pregnancy and can be a congenital disease. CMV is also associated with immunocompromised states and may be life threatening.

■ SYNONYMS

CMV
Heterophil-negative mononucleosis
Cytomegalic inclusion disease virus

ICD-9CM CODES

078.5 CMV infection
771.1 Congenital or perinatal CMV infection
V01.7 Exposure to CMV

■ EPIDEMIOLOGY & DEMOGRAPHICS

- Seroprevalence is widespread: 40% to 100% antibody positivity in adults.
- Increased infection develops perinatally, in day care exposure, and then during reproductive age, related to sexual activity.

■ ROUTES OF TRANSMISSION

- Blood transfusions
- Sexually (STDs) via uterus, cervix, and semen
- Perinatally via breast milk
- Transplant of organs—bone marrow, kidneys, liver, heart, or lung

■ PHYSICAL FINDINGS & CLINICAL PRESENTATION

Children: Congenital—25% of infected children with symptoms if congenital:
- Jaundice
- Petechial rash
- Hepatosplenomegaly
- Lethargy
- Respiratory distress
- CNS involvement
- Seizures
Postnatal acquisition:
- CMV mononucleosis
- Pharyngitis
- Bronchitis
- Pneumonia
- Croup
Healthy adults:
Common
- May be asymptomatic
- CMV mononucleosis similar to EBV mononucleosis
- Fever—lasting 9 to 30 days—mean of 19 days
Less common
- Exudative pharyngitis
- Rare lymphadenopathy—splenomegaly

- Interstitial pneumonia (rare)
- Cervical adenopathy
- Nonspecific rash
- Thrombocytopenia/hemolytic anemia
Rare
- Hepatitis
- Guillain-Barré syndrome
- Meningoencephalitis
- Myocarditis
- Granulomatous hepatitis
Immunosuppressed patients:
- Febrile mononucleosis
- GI ulcerations, hepatitis, pneumonitis, retinitis, encephalopathy, meningoencephalopathy
- HIV associated—dementia, demyelination, retinitis (Fig. 1-84), acalculous cholecystitis, adrenalitis, diarrhea, enterocolitis, esophagitis
- Diabetes associated with pancreatitis
- Adrenalitis associated with HIV

■ ETIOLOGY

Cytomegalovirus infection can remain latent, reactive with immunosuppression.

DIAGNOSIS

■ DIFFERENTIAL DIAGNOSIS

Congenital:
- Acute viral, bacterial, parasitic infections including other congenitally transmitted agents (toxoplasmosis, rubella, syphilis, pertussis, croup, bronchitis)
Acquired:
- EBV mononucleosis
- Viral hepatitis—A, B, C
- Cryptosporidiosis
- Toxoplasmosis
- *Mycobacterium avium* infections
- Human herpesvirus 6

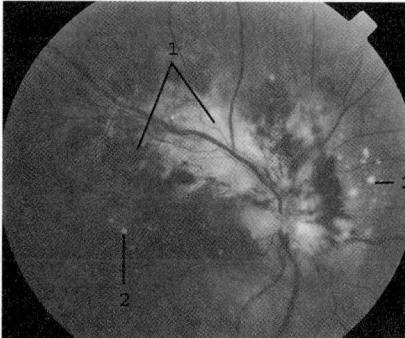

Fig. 1-84 Sight-threatening CMV retinitis involves the macula and optic nerve of this HIV-positive young man. White, infected retina with intraretinal hemorrhage is present in the arcuate distribution of the nerve fiber layer *(1)*. A small amount of lipid exudation near the fovea and nasal to the optic nerve is also seen *(2)*. (From Palay D [ed]: *Ophthalmology for the primary care physician,* St Louis, 1997, Mosby.)

- Drug reaction
- Acute HIV infection

■ WORKUP

- Laboratory confirmation combined with clinical findings often with leukopenia, thrombocytopenia, lymphocytosis
- Demonstration of virus in tissue or serologic testing including CMV IgM antibodies, rising titers of complement fixation (CF) and indirect fluorescent antibody (IFA) or anticomplement IFA
- Funduscopic—necrotic patches with white granular component of retina
- Cultures—(viral) human fibroblast from urine, cervical swab, tissue buffy coat
- Biopsy—"owl's eye" inclusion bodies on tissue sample

■ IMAGING STUDIES

- Chest x-ray—if pneumonitis suspected, consider bronchoscopy
- Endoscopy—if GI involvement
- Funduscopy—retinitis
- CT scan/MRI—if CNS involvement

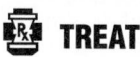

TREATMENT

■ NONPHARMACOLOGIC THERAPY

- Strict handwashing and education about standard precautions can control CMV transmission in health care facilities
- Highly active antiretroviral therapy (HAART) in patients with CD4 count <50/mm³ for the goal of CD4 >100/mm³ for a 3-6 mo period

■ ACUTE GENERAL Rx

For compromised hosts with CMV retinitis or pneumonitis:
- Ganciclovir 5 mg/kg bid IV × 21 days, then 5 mg/kg/day IV, or 1 g po tid or occular implant
- Foscarnet 60 mg/kg tid × 3 wk, then 90 mg/kg/day
- Cidofovir 5 mg/kg IV, repeat 1 wk later, then q2 wk IV
- Fomivirsen-salvage therapy for CMV retinitis 300 μg injected into vitreous

REFERENCES

MacDonald JC et al: High active antiretroviral therapy-related immune recovery in AIDS patients with cytomegalovirus retinitis, *Ophthalmology* 107:877, 2000.

Taylor GH: Cytomegalovirus, *Am Fam Physician* 67:3, 2003.

Whitcup SM: Cytomegalovirus retinitis in the era of highly active antiretroviral therapy, *JAMA* 283:653, 2000.

Authors: **Mina Pantcheva, M.D., and Dennis J. Mikolich, M.D.**

BASIC INFORMATION

DEFINITION
Decubitus ulcers (pressure ulcers) are any damage to the skin and the underlying tissue or both that results from pressure, friction, or shearing forces that usually occur over bony prominences such as the sacrum or heels.

SYNONYMS
Pressure ulcers
Pressure sores
Bed sores
Sacral decubitus
Decubiti

ICD-9CM CODES
707.0 Decubitus ulcers

EPIDEMIOLOGY & DEMOGRAPHICS
Pressure ulcers are present in 5% to 10% of patients in all health care settings: hospitals, nursing homes, and home-confined. Pressure ulcers are associated with significant morbidity and mortality. Pain occurs in two thirds of patients with stage II or greater pressure ulcers. Cellulitis, osteomyelitis, abscesses, and sepsis are all associated with pressure ulcers. One-year mortality approaches 40%.

PHYSICAL FINDINGS & CLINICAL PRESENTATION
All pressure ulcers should be staged according to the depth and type of tissue damage.

Stage I	Nonblanchable erythema of intact skin or boggy mushy feeling of skin
Stage II	Partial-thickness skin loss involving the epidermis, dermis, or both
Stage III	Full-thickness skin loss involving damage or necrosis of subcutaneous tissue that may extend down to, but not through, underlying fascia or muscle
Stage IV	Full-thickness skin loss with extensive destruction and tissue damage to muscle, bone, or supporting structures (e.g., tendons, joint capsule)

ETIOLOGY
- Prolonged unrelieved pressure often associated with impaired or restricted mobility
- Friction or shearing forces on skin

DIAGNOSIS

DIFFERENTIAL DIAGNOSIS
- Venous stasis ulcers
- Arterial ulcers
- Diabetic ulcers
- Skin cancer
- Cellulitis

WORKUP
All ulcers should have a description of the ulcer (i.e., stage, location, size); the wound bed (i.e., epithelialization, granulation tissue, necrotic tissue, eschar); the presence of any exudates, which includes type and amount; the wound edges (i.e., undermining, sinus tracts, tunneling, or fistulas); signs of infection; and pain. In addition, pressure ulcer risk factors and their causes should be reassessed.

LABORATORY TESTS
Directed at identifying the cause of risk factors or any complications arising from the pressure ulcer (e.g., abscess or osteomyelitis); wound cultures of the wound bed are not helpful and should not be performed.

IMAGING STUDIES
MRI or bone scans may help identify osteomyelitis when clinically suspected.

TREATMENT

PREVENTION STRATEGIES
- Identify high-risk patients using standardized risk assessment scales (e.g., Bradon scale)
- Routine skin inspection and good skin care for high-risk patients
- Minimize prolonged skin exposure to moisture, including urine and stool
- Avoid excessive drying and cracking of skin
- Reduce skin pressure through repositioning and pressure-reducing devices (e.g., foam mattresses, low air loss beds, pillows, or foam wedges when in bed and chair)
- Use adequate support surfaces while in bed and chair to prevent "bottoming out" (defined as less than 1 inch between patient and support surface measured by putting hand under support surface and feeling thickness to patient)
- Shear and friction reduction

MANAGEMENT STRATEGIES FOR PRESSURE ULCERS
- Pressure ulcers should be cleaned at each dressing change, and necrotic tissue should be debrided.
- Wound irrigation should not exceed 15 psi and is best done with an 18-gauge angiocatheter.

- No one dressing or product is superior but should be used to keep ulcer bed moist and protect it from urine and stool.
- Avoid agents that are cytotoxic to epithelial cells (e.g., iodine, iodophor, sodium hypochlorite, hydrogen peroxide, acetic acid, and alcohol).
- Reduce pressure by using foam mattress, dynamic support surface (e.g., low-air-loss bed), and frequent repositioning (e.g., q2h).
- Hyperbaric oxygen, ultrasound, ultraviolet and low-energy radiation, and growth factors either are ineffective or have not been extensively evaluated to conclude their efficacy.
- Correct poor nutrition.
- Minimize urinary and fecal incontinence.
- Use standardize assessment tool (e.g., PUSH tool) to monitor wound healing on weekly basis.

DISPOSITION
When systematic risk assessments are done and preventive measures are followed, most pressure ulcers can be prevented. Most pressure ulcers heal when appropriate management strategies are followed.

REFERRAL
- To physical and occupational therapists to improve bed and chair mobility
- Wounds with necrotic tissue to physicians, nurses, or physical therapists trained in sharp debridement
- To plastic surgeons for operative repair for large stage III or IV ulcers that do not respond to optimal care

REFERENCES
Bergstrom A: prospective study on pressure sore risk among institutionalized elderly, *JAGS*747, 1992.
Lyder C: Pressure ulcer prevention and management, *JAMA* 289(2):223, 2003.
National Pressure Ulcer Advisory Panel 9 (NPUAP): Pressure Ulcer Scale for Healing (PUSH), PUSH tool version 3.0 http://www.npuap.org/push3-0.htm
Pressure ulcers in adults: prediction and prevention, Clinical practice guideline No 3; Treatment of pressure ulcers, Clinical practice guideline No 4, AHCPR Publication No 92-0047 & 95-0652, Rockville, Md, 1994, US Department of Health and Human Services, Public Health Service, Agency for Health Care Policy and Research.
Author: **David R. Gifford, M.D., M.P.H.**

I

BASIC INFORMATION

■ DEFINITION

Delirium tremens refers to overactivity of the central nervous system after cessation of alcohol intake. The time interval is variable; it usually occurs within 1 wk after reduction or cessation of heavy alcohol intake and persists for 1 to 3 days.

■ SYNONYMS

Alcohol withdrawal syndrome
DTs
Alcoholic delirium

ICD-9CM CODES

291.00 Alcohol withdrawal delirium

■ EPIDEMIOLOGY & DEMOGRAPHICS

INCIDENCE (IN U.S.): Up to 500,000 cases annually
PREDOMINANT SEX: Male
PEAK INCIDENCE: 30 yr and older
PEAK AGE: Teenage years and older
GENETICS: More common with patients who have relatives who are alcoholics

■ PHYSICAL FINDINGS & CLINICAL PRESENTATION

- Initially: anxiety, insomnia, tremulousness
- Early: tachycardia, sweating, anorexia, agitation, headache, GI distress
- Late: seizures, visual hallucinations, delirium

■ ETIOLOGY

Alcoholism

DIAGNOSIS

■ DIFFERENTIAL DIAGNOSIS

Be alert for coexisting illness, trauma, and drug usage.

■ WORKUP

- Frequent rating of symptoms (hallucinations, tremor, sweating, agitation, orientation).
- The Clinical Institute Withdrawal Assessment-Alcohol (CIWA-A) scale can be used to measure the severity of alcohol withdrawal. It consists of the 10 following items: nausea; tremor; autonomic hyperactivity; anxiety; agitation; tactile, visual, and auditory disturbances; headache; and disorientation. The maximum score is 67. When the CIWA-A score is ≥8, patients are usually given 2 to 4 mg of lorazepam hourly.

■ LABORATORY TESTS

- Electrolytes
- Close monitoring of glucose levels
- Drug screen

■ IMAGING STUDIES

CT scan of head if there is a history of head trauma

TREATMENT

■ NONPHARMACOLOGIC THERAPY

Refer to drug rehabilitation program after patient recovers.

■ ACUTE GENERAL Rx

1. Admission to a detoxification unit where patient can be observed closely
2. Vital signs q30min (neurologic signs, if necessary)
3. Use of lateral decubitus or prone position if restraints are necessary
4. NPO: NG tube for abdominal distention may be necessary but should not be routinely used
5. Vigorous hydration (4-6 L/day): IV with glucose (Na^+, K^+, PO_4^{-3}, and Mg^{2+} replacement)
6. Vitamins: thiamine, 100 mg IV qd. The initial dose of thiamine should precede the administration of IV dextrose; multivitamins (may be added to the hydrating solution)
7. Sedation
   a. Initially: lorazepam 2 to 5 mg IM/IV repeated prn
   b. Maintenance (individualized dosage): chlordiazepoxide, 50 to 100 mg PO q4-6h, lorazepam 2 mg PO q4h, or diazepam 5 to 10 mg PO tid; withhold doses or decrease subsequent doses if signs of oversedation are apparent
   c. Midazolam is also effective for managing DTs. Its rapid onset (sedation within 2 to 4 min of IV injection) and short duration of action (approximately 30 min) make it an ideal agent for titration in continuous infusion
8. Treatment of seizures: Diazepam 2.5 mg/min IV until seizure is controlled (check for respiratory depression or hypotension) may be beneficial for prolonged seizure activity; IV lorazepam 1 to 2 mg every 2 hr can be used in place of diazepam; generally, withdrawal seizures are self-limited and treatment is not required; the use of phenytoin or other anticonvulsants for short-term treatment of alcohol withdrawal seizures is not recommended
9. Diagnosis and treatment of concomitant medical, surgical, or psychiatric conditions

■ CHRONIC Rx

Alcoholics Anonymous has the best record in breaking addiction, but the results are still disappointing.

■ DISPOSITION

Refer to drug rehabilitation program.

■ REFERRAL

If cardiac arrhythmias are prominent or respiratory distress develops

PEARLS & CONSIDERATIONS

■ COMMENTS

This is a potentially lethal disease if not carefully treated. Mortality is 15% in untreated patients.

REFERENCE

Kosten TR, O'Connor PG: Management of drug and alcohol withdrawal, *N Engl J Med* 348:1786, 2003.
Author: **Fred F. Ferri, M.D.**

BASIC INFORMATION

■ DEFINITION

Major depression is an episodic, frequently recurrent syndrome lasting at least 2 wk with five of the following symptoms: depressed mood, diminished interest, pleasure, energy, self-worth, ability to think and concentrate, altered sleep pattern, appetite, and level of psychomotor activity.

■ SYNONYMS

Unipolar depression
Depressive episode

ICD-9CM CODES

296.2 Major depressive disorder, single episode

■ EPIDEMIOLOGY & DEMOGRAPHICS

INCIDENCE (IN U.S.): 10% of men; 20% of women
PREVALENCE (IN U.S.): 2.5% of men; 8% of women; 1% of children
PREDOMINANT SEX: Female > male; equal before puberty
PREDOMINANT AGE: 25 to 44 yr; 5% of adolescents
PEAK INCIDENCE: 30 to 40 yr; 13% of postpartum women
GENETICS:
- Clear evidence of familial predominance
- No established pattern of inheritance

■ PHYSICAL FINDINGS & CLINICAL PRESENTATION

- Psychomotor retardation with slowed thinking, slowed responses, slowed physical movements, depressed affect and mood, sleep disturbance, appetite disturbance
- May be associated with mood-congruent delusional thinking (paranoid and melancholic themes)
- May be associated with active or passive suicidal ideation

■ ETIOLOGY

- Unknown
- Several factors possible: neuroendocrine response to unremitting stress, hormones, social/developmental factors

DIAGNOSIS

■ DIFFERENTIAL DIAGNOSIS

- Hypothyroidism
- Neurosyphilis
- Major organ system disease (e.g., cardiovascular, liver, renal, neuronal diseases, and others) with depressive symptoms

- Elderly patients: frequently coexists with dementia
- Bipolar patients will frequently present with depression, but routine treatment with antidepressant medications may be detrimental in this group.

■ WORKUP

- History
- Physical examination
- Mental status examination
- Screening questionnaires may enhance recognition of depression
- A clinical approach to the treatment of depression in primary care is described in Section III, Fig. 3-57

■ LABORATORY TESTS

All done to rule out other major organ system disease:
- Routine chemistries
- CBC with differential
- Sedimentation rate
- Thyroid function studies

■ IMAGING STUDIES

With unusual presentations (e.g., associated with new-onset severe headache, focal neurologic signs, a cognitive or sensory disturbance), the following may be performed:
- EEG (diffuse slowing indicates metabolic encephalopathy)
- Anatomic brain imaging (CT scan or MRI)

TREATMENT

■ NONPHARMACOLOGIC THERAPY

- Many forms of psychotherapy are helpful.
- Behavioral, cognitive, and interpersonal psychotherapies have efficacy rates of 40% to 50%.

■ ACUTE GENERAL Rx

- Many antidepressants are available, all with efficacy rates of 60% to 65%.
- Serotonin reuptake inhibitors generally are first-line agents.
- Therapy should be continued for 6 to 12 mo.
- Several treatment-refractory strategies are available.

■ CHRONIC Rx

The risk of recurrence exceeds 90% in individuals having experienced three or more depressive episodes; for these individuals continuous prophylactic therapy is recommended.

■ DISPOSITION

- Course is variable.

- Additional episodes are experienced by >60% of individuals having one depressive episode.
- There can be increasing or decreasing numbers of episodes into old age.
- Without treatment, episodes last an average of 8 mo.
- Depression associated with physical disorders generally does not resolve until physical disorder improves.
- No evidence that antidepressants improve medical outcome unless major depression can be diagnosed.

■ REFERRAL

- If treatment refractory
- If patient imminently suicidal

PEARLS & CONSIDERATIONS

■ CAUTION

All threats of suicide should be taken very seriously.

REFERENCES

Brent DA, Birmaher B: Adolescent depression, *N Engl J Med* 347:667, 2002.
Bull SA et al: Discontinuation of use and switching of antidepressants, influence of patient-physician communication, *JAMA* 288:1403, 2002.
El-Mallakh RS et al: Clues to depression in primary care practice, *Postgrad Med* 100:85, 1996.
Lapid M, Rummans TA: Evaluation and management of geriatric depression in primary care. Mayo Clin Proc 78:1423, 2003.
Miller LJ: Postpartum depression, *JAMA* 287:762, 2002.
Pignone MP et al: Screening for depression in adults: a summary of the evidence for the U.S. Preventive Services Task Force, *Ann Intern Med* 136:765, 2002.
Sharp LK, Lipsky MS: Screening for depression across the lifespan: a review of measures for use in primary care settings, *Am Fam Physician* 66:1001, 2002.
Sullivan M et al: Depression-related costs in heart failure care, *Arch Intern Med* 162:1860, 2002.
U.S. Preventive Services Task Force: Screening for depression: recommendations and rationale, *Ann Intern Med* 136:760, 2002.
Whooler MA, Simon GE: Managing depression in medical outpatients, *N Engl J Med* 343:1842, 2000.
Wisner KL et al: Postpartum depression, *N Engl J Med* 347:194, 2002.

Author: **Rif S. El-Mallakh, M.D.**

BASIC INFORMATION

■ DEFINITION
De Quervain's tenosynovitis refers to a stenosing inflammatory process of the first dorsal retinacular compartment containing the tendons of the abductor pollicis longus (APL) and extensor pollicis brevis (EPB).

■ SYNONYMS
Stenosing tenosynovitis of the radial styloid
Stenosing tenovaginitis of the first dorsal compartment

ICD-9CM CODES
727.04 Tenosynovitis radial styloid

■ EPIDEMIOLOGY & DEMOGRAPHICS
- More common in women than in men (10:1)
- Usually occurs between the ages of 30 to 50
- Associated with rheumatoid arthritis
- Seen in occupations (e.g., clerical, assembly, and manual labor)

■ PHYSICAL FINDINGS & CLINICAL PRESENTATION
- Pain over the styloid process of the radius
- Swelling
- Positive Finkelstein's test (Fig. 1-85): stretching the tendons of the APL and EPB by clasping the thumb with the fingers and passive deviation of the wrist to the ulnar side. Provocation of pain is a positive sign
- Crepitance

■ ETIOLOGY
- The cause is usually repetitive use or overuse of the hands.

DIAGNOSIS

- The diagnosis of de Quervain's tenosynovitis is based on the clinical triad of:
  1. Tenderness over the radial styloid
  2. Swelling over the first dorsal retinacular compartment
  3. Positive Finkelstein's test (Fig. 1-85)
- Sometimes 1.5 cc of 1% Xylocaine can be injected into the tenosynovial sac, and if all three physical signs resolve, the diagnosis is confirmed.

■ DIFFERENTIAL DIAGNOSIS
- Carpal tunnel syndrome
- Ostearthritis
- Gout
- Infiltrative tenosynovitis
- Radiculopathy
- Compression neuropathy (e.g., superficial branch of the radial nerve "bracelet syndrome")

- Infection (e.g., tuberculosis, bacterial)

■ WORKUP
The workup of suspected de Quervain's tenosynovitis requires laboratory testing and x-rays to exclude other causes of wrist and hand pain.

■ LABORATORY TESTS
- ESR is usually normal in patients with de Quervain's tenosynovitis. If elevated, a search for an infectious or infiltrative cause should be pursued
- Aspiration with examination of the specimen under polarized microscope to rule out gout
- Gram stain and culture of aspirate to rule out infectious etiology

■ IMAGING STUDIES
- X-ray studies of the hand may show findings of osteoarthritis of the first carpometacarpal joint that can mimic de Quervain's tenosynovitis.

TREATMENT

■ NONPHARMACOLOGIC THERAPY
- Rest
- Splinting
- Physiotherapy

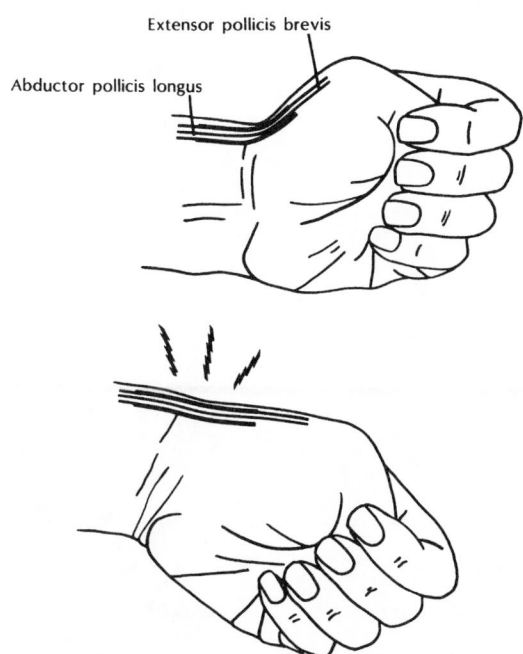

Extensor pollicis brevis

Abductor pollicis longus

Fig. 1-85 Finkelstein's test is positive in de Quervain's stenosing synovitis. Ulnar flexion of the wrist produces pain over the dorsal compartment containing the extensor policis brevis and abductor pollicis longus. (From Noble J [ed]: *Textbook of primary care medicine,* ed 2, St Louis, 1996, Mosby.)

■ **ACUTE GENERAL Rx**
- Corticosteroid injection using 20 to 40 mg triamcinolone acetonide and 1% Xylocaine is effective in relieving pain.
- NSAIDs ibuprofen 800 mg tid or naproxen 500 mg bid can be tried in patients refusing steroid injection therapy.

■ **CHRONIC Rx**
- Surgical release is generally reserved for patients not responding to NSAIDs and corticosteroid injection therapy.

■ **DISPOSITION**
- Approximately 90% of patients have relief of symptoms with either single or multiple steroid injections.
- Complications of steroid injections include:
  1. Infection
  2. Tendon rupture

- Surgical control of symptoms occurs in 90% of cases.
- Complications of surgery include:
  1. Radial nerve damage
  2. Paresthesia (~10%)
  3. Neuroma

■ **REFERRAL**
Consultation with either a rheumatologist or an orthopedist is recommended in patients with de Quervain's tenosynovitis requiring injection therapy.

☼ **PEARLS & CONSIDERATIONS**

■ **COMMENTS**
- Dr. Fritz de Quervain published the original article on stenosing tenovaginitis in 1895.
- Finkelstein's description of stenosing tenosynovitis was originally published in *J Bone Joint Surg* in 1930.

REFERENCES
Anderson BC, Manthey R, Brounds MC: Treatment of de Quervain's tenosynovitis with corticosteroids: a prospective study of the response to local injection, *Arthr Rheum* 34(7):793, 1991.

Chin DH, Jones NF: Repetitive motion hand disorder, *J Calif Dent Assoc* 30(2):149, 2002.

Conoso JJ: *Rheumatology in primary care*, Baltimore, 1997, Saunders.

Moore JS: De Quervain's tenosynovitis: stenosing tenosynovitis of the first dorsal compartment, *J Occup Environ Med* 39(10):990, 1997.

Saldana TS: Trigger digit: diagnosis and treatment, *J Am Acad Orthop Surg* 9(4):246, 2001.
Author: **Peter Petropoulos, M.D.**

BASIC INFORMATION

■ DEFINITION

Atopic dermatitis is a genetically determined eczematous eruption that is pruritic, symmetric, and associated with personal family history of allergic manifestations (atopy).

■ SYNONYMS

Eczema
Atopic neurodermatitis
Atopic eczema

ICD-9CM CODES
691.8 Atopic dermatitis

■ EPIDEMIOLOGY & DEMOGRAPHICS

- Incidence is between 5 and 25 cases/1000 persons.
- Highest incidence is among children (5%-10 %). It accounts for 4% of acute care pediatric visits.
- Onset of disease before age 5 yr in 85% of patients.
- More than 50% of children with generalized atopic dermatitis develop asthma and allergic rhinitis by age 13 yr.
- Concordance in monozygotic twins is 86%.

■ PHYSICAL FINDINGS & CLINICAL PRESENTATION

- There are no specific cutaneous signs for atopic dermatitis, and there is a wide spectrum of presentations ranging from minimal flexural eczema to erythroderma.
- The primary lesions are a result of itching caused by severe and chronic pruritus. The repeated scratching modifies the skin surface, producing lichenification, dry and scaly skin, and redness.
- The lesions are typically on the neck, face, upper trunk, and bends of elbows and knees (symmetric on flexural surfaces of extremities).
- There is dryness, thickening of the involved areas, discoloration, blistering, and oozing.
- Papular lesions are frequently found in the antecubital and popliteal fossae.
- In children, red scaling plaques are often confined to the cheeks and the perioral and perinasal areas.
- Inflammation in the flexural areas and lichenified skin is a very common presentation in children.
- Constant scratching may result in areas of hypopigmentation or hyperpigmentation (more common in blacks).
- In adults, redness and scaling in the dorsal aspect of the hands or about the fingers are the most common expression of atopic dermatitis; oozing and crusting may be present.
- Secondary skin infections may be present (*Staphylococcus aureus*, dermatophytosis, herpes simplex).

■ ETIOLOGY

Unknown; elevated T-lymphocyte activation, defective cell immunity, and B cell IgE overproduction may play a significant role.

DIAGNOSIS

■ DIFFERENTIAL DIAGNOSIS

- Scabies
- Psoriasis
- Dermatitis herpetiform
- Contact dermatitis
- Photosensitivity
- Seborrheic dermatitis
- Candidiasis
- Lichen simplex chronicus
- Other: Wiskott-Aldrich syndrome, PKU, mycosis fungoides, ichthyosis, HIV dermatitis, nonnummular eczema, histiocytosis X

■ WORKUP

Diagnosis is based on the presence of three of the following major features and three minor features.

MAJOR FEATURES:
- Pruritus
- Personal or family history of atopy: asthma, allergic rhinitis, atopic dermatitis
- Facial and extensor involvement in infants and children
- Flexural lichenification in adults

MINOR FEATURES:
- Elevated IgE
- Eczema-perifollicular accentuation
- Recurrent conjunctivitis
- Ichthyosis
- Nipple dermatitis
- Wool intolerance
- Cutaneous *S. aureus* infections or herpes simplex infections
- Food intolerance
- Hand dermatitis (nonallergic irritant)
- Facial pallor, facial erythema
- Cheilitis
- White dermographism
- Early age of onset (after 2 mo of age)

■ LABORATORY TESTS

- Tests are generally not helpful.
- Elevated IgE levels are found in 80% to 90% of atopic dermatitis.
- Blood eosinophilia correlates with disease severity.

TREATMENT

■ NONPHARMACOLOGIC THERAPY

Avoidance of triggering factors:
- Sudden temperature changes, sweating, low humidity in the winter
- Contact with irritating substance (e.g., wool, cosmetics, some soaps and detergents, tobacco)
- Foods that provoke exacerbations (e.g., eggs, peanuts, fish, soy, wheat, milk)
- Stressful situations
- Allergens and dust
- Excessive hand washing
- Clip nails to decrease abrasion of skin

■ GENERAL Rx

- Emollients can be used to prevent dryness. Severely affected skin can be optimally hydrated by occlusion in addition to application of emollients.
- Topical corticosteroids (e.g., 1% to 2.5% hydrocortisone) may be helpful. Consider intermediate-potency steroids (e.g., triamcinolone, fluocinolone) for more severe cases and limit potent corticosteroids (e.g., betamethasone, desoximetasone, clobetasol) to severe cases.
- Pimecrolimus cream (Elidel) 1% applied bid is a steroid-free compound with antiinflammatory effects secondary to blockage of activated T-cell cytokine production. It is highly effective in atopic dermatitis without having the adverse effects associated with topical corticosteroids.
- Tacrolimus (Protopic) ointment (0.03% or 0.1%) applied bid represents an effective alternative to topical corticosteroids. It does not cause skin atrophy and may be particularly useful on the face and neck. It is a macrolide that decreases activation of T-lymphocytes, inhibits release of inflammatory mediators from cutaneous mast cells and basophils, and suppresses humoral and cell-mediated immune responses.
- Oral antihistamines (e.g., hydroxyzine, diphenhydramine) are effective in controlling pruritus and inducing sedation, restful sleep, and prevention of scratching during sleep. Doxepin and other tricyclic antidepressants also have antihistamine effect, induce sleep, and reduce pruritus.
- Oral prednisone, IM triamcinolone, Goeckerman regimen, PUVA are generally reserved for severe cases.
- Methotrexate, cyclosporine azathioprine, and systemic corticosteroids are sometimes tried for recalcitrant disease.

■ DISPOSITION

- Resolution occurs in approximately 40% of patients by adulthood.
- Most patients have a course characterized by remissions and intermittent flares.

REFERENCES

Barnetson RC, Rogers M: Childhood atopic eczema, *BMJ* 324(7350):1376, 2002.
Ong et al: Endogenous antimicrobial peptides and skin infections in atopic dermatitis, *N Engl J Med* 347:1151, 2002.
Author: **Fred F. Ferri, M.D.**

BASIC INFORMATION

■ DEFINITION
Contact dermatitis is an acute or chronic skin inflammation, usually eczematous dermatitis resulting from exposure to substances in the environment. It can be subdivided into "irritant" contact dermatitis (nonimmunologic physical and chemical alteration of the epidermis) and "allergic" contact dermatitis (delayed hypersensitivity reaction).

■ SYNONYMS
Irritant contact dermatitis
Allergic contact dermatitis

ICD-9CM CODES
692 Contact dermatitis and other eczema

■ EPIDEMIOLOGY & DEMOGRAPHICS
- 20% of all cases of dermatitis in children are caused by allergic contact dermatitis.
- Rhus dermatitis (poison ivy, poison oak, and poison sumac) is responsible for most cases of contact dermatitis.
- Frequent causes of irritant contact dermatitis are soaps, detergents, and organic solvents.

■ PHYSICAL FINDINGS & CLINICAL PRESENTATION
IRRITANT CONTACT DERMATITIS:
- Mild exposure may result in dryness, erythema, and fissuring of the affected area (e.g., hand involvement in irritant dermatitis caused by exposure to soap, genital area involvement in irritant dermatitis caused by prolonged exposure to wet diapers).
- Eczematous inflammation may result from chronic exposure.
ALLERGIC CONTACT DERMATITIS:
- Poison ivy dermatitis can present with vesicles and blisters; linear lesions (as a result of dragging of the resins over the surface of the skin by scratching) are a classic presentation.
- The pattern of lesions is asymmetric; itching, burning, and stinging may be present.
- The involved areas are erythematous, warm to touch, swollen, and may be confused with cellulitis.

■ ETIOLOGY
- Irritant contact dermatitis: cement (construction workers), rubber, ragweed, malathion (farmers), orange and lemon peels (chefs, bartenders), hair tints, shampoos (beauticians), rubber gloves (medical, surgical personnel)
- Allergic contact dermatitis: poison ivy, poison oak, poison sumac, rubber (shoe dermatitis), nickel (jewelry), balsam of Peru (hand and face dermatitis), neomycin, formaldehyde (cosmetics)

DIAGNOSIS

■ DIFFERENTIAL DIAGNOSIS
- Impetigo
- Lichen simplex chronicus
- Atopic dermatitis
- Nummular eczema
- Seborrheic dermatitis
- Psoriasis
- Scabies

■ WORKUP
- Medical history: gradual onset vs. rapid onset, number of exposures, clinical presentation, occupational history
- Physical examination: contact dermatitis in the neck may be caused by necklaces, perfumes, after-shave lotion; involvement of the axillae is often secondary to deodorants, clothing; face involvement can occur with cosmetics, airborne allergens, aftershave lotion

■ LABORATORY TESTS
- Patch testing is useful to confirm the diagnosis of contact dermatitis; it is indicated particularly when inflammation persists despite appropriate topical therapy and avoidance of suspected causative agent; patch testing should not be used for irritant contact dermatitis because this is a nonimmunologic-mediated inflammatory reaction.
- Gram stain and cultures are indicated only in cases of suspected secondary infection or impetigo.

TREATMENT

■ NONPHARMACOLOGIC THERAPY
Avoidance of suspected allergens

■ ACUTE GENERAL Rx
- Removal of the irritant substance by washing the skin with plain water or mild soap within 15 min of exposure is helpful in patients with poison ivy, poison oak, or poison sumac dermatitis.
- Cold or cool water compresses for 20 to 30 min five to six times a day for the initial 72 hr are effective during the acute blistering stage.
- Oral corticosteroids (e.g., prednisone 20 mg bid for 6 to 10 days) are generally reserved for severe, widespread dermatitis.
- IM steroids (e.g., Kenalog) are used for severe reactions and in patients requiring oral corticosteroids but unable to tolerate PO.
- Oral antihistamines (e.g., hydroxyzine 25 mg q6h) will control pruritus, especially at night; calamine lotion is also useful for pruritus; however, it can lead to excessive drying.
- Colloidal oatmeal (Aveeno) baths can also provide symptomatic relief.
- Patients with mild to moderate erythema may respond to topical steroid gels or creams.
- Patients with shoe allergy should change their socks at least once a day; use of aluminum chloride hexahydrate in a 20% solution (Drysol) qhs will also help control perspiration.
- Use hypoallergenic surgical gloves in patients with rubber and surgical glove allergy.

■ DISPOSITION
Allergic contact dermatitis generally resolves within 2 to 4 wk if reexposure to allergen is prevented.

■ REFERRAL
For patch testing in selected patients (see Laboratory Tests)

PEARLS & CONSIDERATIONS

■ COMMENTS
- Commercially available corticosteroid dose packs should be avoided, because they generally provide an inadequate amount of medication.
Author: **Fred F. Ferri, M.D.**

BASIC INFORMATION

■ DEFINITION
Dermatitis herpetiformis is a rare, chronic skin disorder characterized by an intensely burning, pruritic, vesicular rash. It is strongly associated with gluten-sensitive enteropathy. From 20% to 70% of patients with dermatitis herpetiformis will have gastrointestinal symptoms, whereas approximately 10% of patients with celiac sprue will have dermatitis herpetiformis.

ICD-9CM CODES
694.0 Dermatitis herpetiformis

■ EPIDEMIOLOGY & DEMOGRAPHICS
PREVALENCE: 1.2 to 39.2 cases/100,000 persons in northern Europe. Reported prevalence in Utah in 1987 was 11.2 cases/100,000 persons
PREDOMINANT AGE: Third and fourth decades
PREDOMINANT SEX: Slight male predominance
PREDOMINANT RACE: Rarely seen in Blacks/African Americans or Asians

■ PHYSICAL FINDINGS & CLINICAL PRESENTATION
- Pruritic, burning vesicles initially, frequently grouped (hence the name "herpetiform") (see Fig. 1-86)
- Symmetrically distributed on extensor surfaces: elbows, knees, scalp, nuchal area, shoulder, and buttocks; rarely found in mouth
- May evolve in time to intensely burning urticarial papules, vesicles, and rarely bullae

- Celiac-type permanent-tooth enamel defects found in 53% of patients

DIAGNOSIS

Diagnosis is confirmed histologically by the demonstration of IgA deposits found along the subepidermal basement membrane.

■ DIFFERENTIAL DIAGNOSIS
- Linear IgA bullous dermatosis (not associated with gluten-sensitive enteropathy)
- Herpes simplex infection
- Herpes zoster infection
- Bullous erythema multiforme
- Bullous pemphigoid

■ WORKUP
History of chronic diarrhea and pruritic, vesicular rash highly suggestive of diagnosis

■ LABORATORY TESTS
- Skin biopsy for immunofluorescence studies. Diagnosis is confirmed by IgA deposits along the subepidermal basement membrane. >90% will have granular or fibrillar IgA deposits in the dermal papillae. Multiple specimens may be needed to obtain positive findings because of the focal nature of deposits. Biopsies are taken from adjacent normal skin because the diagnostic Ig deposits are usually destroyed by the blistering process.
- Circulating antibody levels
  1. IgA antiendomysial antibody: found in 70% of patients with rash and who are not on gluten-free diet and in 100% of patients

with rash and grade 3 to 4 flattening of intestinal mucosa, and in all patients with untreated celiac disease. Levels decrease to 0% when gluten is avoided for 3 mo.
  2. IgA antigliadin antibodies: found in 66% of patients; also present in patients with pemphigus and pemphigoid.
  3. IgA reticulin antibody: found in 36% of patients with dermatitis herpetiformis.
  4. IgA antitissue transglutaminase: elevated levels in patients with DH as compared with patients with skin or intestinal diseases unrelated to DH.

TREATMENT

Patients may be given a trial of pharmacologic therapy if they are extremely uncomfortable. Symptoms are often dramatically relieved within hours or days of initiation of medical therapy.

■ PHARMACOLOGIC
- Dapsone: Initial dose of 100 to 150 mg PO qd. Itching and burning are controlled in 12 to 48 hr and new lesions stop appearing. The dosage is adjusted to the lowest level that provides adequate relief, usually in the range of 50 to 200 mg/day; although some patients may require 25 mg/day, others may require 400 mg/day. Peripheral motor neuropathy can occur in the first few months of therapy. Paresthesias and weakness of the distal upper and lower extremities and footdrop are

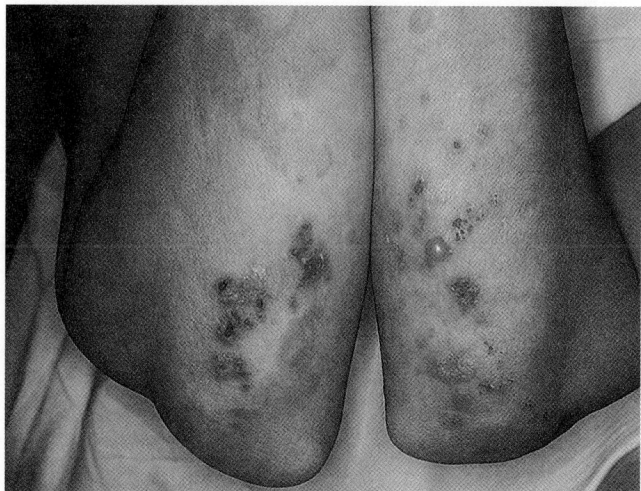

Fig. 1-86   Dermatitis herpetiformis is an immunologically mediated blistering disease. There is a strong association of dermatitis herpetiformis with HLA-B8, DR3. Gluten-sensitive enteropathy is a common associated finding. The lesions are grouped (herpetiform) and extremely pruritic. (From Callen JP [ed]: *Color atlas of dermatology,* ed 2, Philadelphia, 2000, WB Saunders.)

the most common manifestations. Symptoms slowly improve over months to years after dapsone is discontinued. Hemolysis, anemia, and methemoglobinemia occur to some degree in all patients receiving dapsone therapy. Patients at risk for having G6PD should have levels drawn before therapy because dapsone may cause severe hemolytic anemia in these patients. Probenecid blocks the renal excretion of dapsone, and rifampin increases the rate of its clearance.

- Sulfapyridine: Initial dosage 500 to 1500 mg/day. Sulfapyridine does not cause neuropathy, but it is associated with agranulocytosis and aplastic anemia. It also may cause severe hemolysis in patients with G6PD.
- Tetracycline: Successful treatment has been reported with tetracycline 500 mg PO qd-tid and minocycline 100 mg PO bid. Cessation resulted in a flare of the rash.
- Nicotinamide: Successful treatment has been reported with nicotinamide 500 mg PO bid-tid. Cessation resulted in a flare of the rash.

■ NONPHARMACOLOGIC

- Gluten-free diet: for at least 6 mo, which will allow most patients to begin to decrease or discontinue sulfone therapy. The diet usually needs

to be followed for 2 yr before medications can be discontinued. Although intestinal villous architecture improves, symptoms and lesions recur in 1 to 3 wk if a normal diet is resumed. Most patients need to follow diet indefinitely. Gluten is found in all grains except rice and corn.

- Elemental diet: Other dietary factors may also be important in dermatitis herpetiformis. Antigens stimulate the production of antibodies, leading to the formation of immune complexes. Most antigens that elicit a humoral immune response are proteins. Thus, a diet without full proteins, an elemental diet, is not likely to contain major antigens. A diet of amino acids, fat, and carbohydrates can produce a rapid benefit and allow a decrease in the dosage of dapsone within 2 wk.

■ ACUTE GENERAL Rx

Initiation of sulfone therapy to relieve symptoms

■ CHRONIC Rx

Gluten-free diet

■ REFERRAL

To dermatologist for skin biopsy

✪ PEARLS & CONSIDERATIONS

- There is an increased incidence of other autoimmune disorders, including thyroid disease, type 1 diabetes mellitus, systemic lupus erythematosus, vitiligo, and Sjögren's syndrome in patients with dermatitis herpetiformis.
- Small bowel lymphoma and nonintestinal lymphoma have been reported in patients with dermatitis herpetiformis and celiac disease.
- Linear IgA bullous dermatosis is not associated with gluten-sensitive enteropathy or with IgA antiendomysial Ab.

REFERENCES

Cotran RS: *Robbins pathologic basis of disease,* ed 6, Philadelphia, 1999. WB Saunders.

Dieterich W et al: Antibodies to tissue Transglutaminase as serologic markers in patients with dermatitis herpetiformis, *J Invest Dermatol* 113(1):133, 1999.

Habif TP: *Clinical dermatology.* ed 3, St Louis, 1996, Mosby.

Author: **Iris L. Tong, M.D.**

BASIC INFORMATION

■ DEFINITION
Dermatomyositis (DM) refers to a chronic idiopathic inflammatory myopathy characterized by a skin rash and proximal muscle weakness.

■ SYNONYMS
Idiopathic inflammatory myopathy
ICD-9CM CODES710.3
Dermatomyositis

■ EPIDEMIOLOGY & DEMOGRAPHICS
- Dermatomyositis (DM) occurs in children and in adults
- Incidence 1:100,000
- Prevalence 1 to 10 cases per million in adults and 1 to 3.2 cases per million in children
- More common in females than males (2:1)
- Average age at diagnosis is 40. The average age of onset in children is between 5 and 14 yr
- DM usually occurs alone but sometimes can be associated with systemic sclerosis and mixed connective tissue disease
- Approximately 15% to 20% of patients with DM over the age of 50 have associated malignancies

■ PHYSICAL FINDINGS & CLINICAL PRESENTATION
- Most patients with DM have a subacute onset, over weeks to months
- Symmetrical proximal muscle weakness involving the shoulder and pelvic girdle
- Difficulty getting up from a chair, climbing stairs, or combing hair
- Distal muscle and ocular involvement is uncommon
- Dysphagia and dysphonia resulting from proximal pharyngeal muscle involvement
- Rales, dyspnea, and respiratory failure
- Skin findings
  1. Heliotrope rash on the upper eyelids (Fig. 1-87)
  2. Erythematous rash on the face (see Fig. 1-87)
  3. Can also involve the back and shoulders (shawl sign), neck and chest (V-shape), knees and elbows
  4. Photosensitive
  5. Gottron's papules (violaceous papules overlying dorsal interphalangeal or metacarpophalangeal areas, elbow or knee joints)
  6. Nail cracking, thickening, and irregularity with periungual telangiectasia (Fig. 1-88)
  7. Mechanic's hand: fissured, hyperpigmented, scaly and hyperkeratotic also associated with in-

creased risk of interstitial lung disease

■ ETIOLOGY
The cause of DM is not known but is believed to be an immune-related phenomenon.

DIAGNOSIS

The diagnosis of DM requires at least one skin lesion and four findings from the following items 2 through 9.
1. Skin lesions (e.g., heliotrope, Groton's sign, or erythema on the extensor surface of extremity joints)
2. Proximal muscle weakness
3. Elevated muscle enzymes
4. EMG abnormalities suggesting a myopathic process
5. Muscle biopsy confirmation
6. Muscle pain on grasping
7. Positive anti-Jo-1 antibody test
8. Systemic inflammatory signs (e.g., temperature >98.6 F, elevated C-reactive protein or ESR >20 mm)

■ DIFFERENTIAL DIAGNOSIS
- Polymyositis
- Inclusion body myositis
- Muscular dystrophies
- Amyotrophic lateral sclerosis
- Myasthenia gravis
- Eaton-Lambert syndrome
- Drug-induced myopathies
- Diabetic amyotrophy
- Guillain-Barré syndrome
- Hyperthyroidism or hypothyroidism

- Lichen planus
- SLE
- Contact dermatitis
- Atopic dermatitis
- Psoriasis
- Seborrheic dermatitis

■ WORKUP
Patients suspected of having DM by clinical presentation should have an EMG, muscle biopsy, and specific blood tests to confirm the diagnosis.

■ LABORATORY TESTS
- ESR, although not specific, is elevated in the majority of cases.
- Creatine kinase is the most sensitive muscle enzyme test and can be elevated as much as 50 times above normal.
- Aldolase, AST, ALT, alkaline phosphatase, and LDH can be elevated.
- Anti-Jo-1 antibodies are more common in polymyositis than DM.
- Electrolytes, TSH, Ca, and Mg should be requested to exclude other causes.
- Electromyography (EMG) is abnormal in 90% of patients and distinguishes a myopathic from neuropathic process.
- Muscle biopsy is the definitive test. Characteristic findings separate DM from polymyositis, inclusion body myositis, and neuromuscular disorders mimicking DM.

■ IMAGING STUDIES
- A chest x-ray to rule out pulmonary involvement. If suspicious for pulmonary interstitial disease, a high-resolution CT scan of the chest may be helpful.

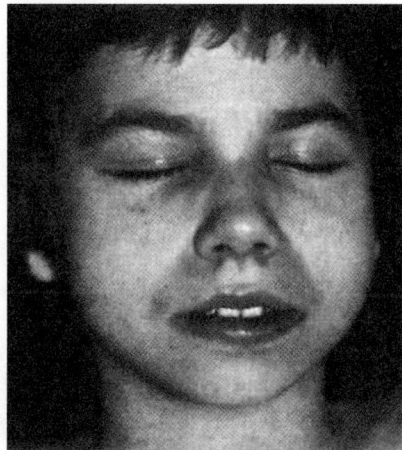

Fig. 1-87 The facial rash of juvenile dermatomyositis. There is erythema over the bridge of the nose and malar areas, with violaceous (heliotropic) discoloration of the upper eyelids. (From Behrman RE: *Nelson textbook of pediatrics,* ed 16, Philadelphia, 2000, WB Saunders.)

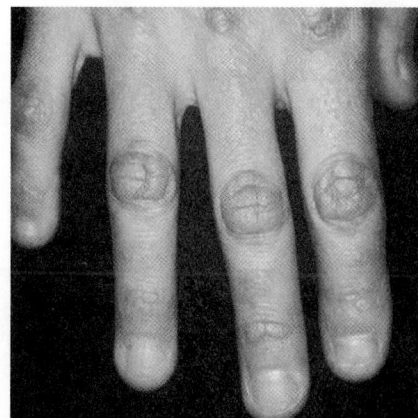

Fig. 1-88 Dermatomyositis (Gottron's papules). Note erythematous papules over joints and periungual telangiectasias. (From Nobel J [ed]: *Textbook of primary care medicine,* ed 2, St Louis, 1996, Mosby.)

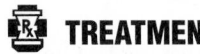
- A barium swallow to look for upper esophageal dysfunction in patients with dysphagia and DM.
- MRI can help to locate sites of muscle involvement.

TREATMENT

The therapeutic goal is to maintain function and prevent or minimize sequelae.

■ NONPHARMACOLOGIC THERAPY
- Sun-blocking agents with SPF 15 or greater for skin lesions
- Physical therapy is beneficial in increasing muscle tone and strength
- Occupational therapy to assist with activities of daily living
- Speech therapy for dysphagia and swallowing problems

■ ACUTE GENERAL Rx
- Prednisone 1 to 2 mg/kg/day is the treatment of choice in patients with DM. The dose is continued until muscle strength improves and/or muscle enzymes have returned to normal for 4 wk. Thereafter, taper by 10 mg/mo until off prednisone.
- Immunosuppressive agents (azathioprine, cyclophosphamide, or methotrexate) should be used if the patient fails to improve on prednisone or muscle enzymes begin rising when tapering off prednisone. See Chronic Rx for specific dosage.
- Hydroxychloroquine is used to treat the cutaneous lesions of DM.

■ CHRONIC Rx
- Chronic prednisone therapy may be needed for years.

- Azathioprine (2.5 to 3.5 mg/kg/day) or methotrexate (0.5 mg/kg/wk) can be added as stated previously.
- Azathioprine 2 to 3 mg/kg/day tapered to 1 mg/kg/day once steroid is tapered to 15 mg/day. Reduce dosage monthly by 25 mg intervals. Maintenance dosage is 50 mg/day.
- Methotrexate 7.5 to 10 mg PO/wk, increased by 2.5 mg/wk to total of 25 mg/wk.
- Cyclophosphamide 1 to 3 mg/kg/day PO or 2 to 4 mg/kg/day in conjunction with prednisone.
- Other drugs considered in the chronic treatment of DM include mycophenolate, cyclosporine, hydroxychloroquine, and IV immunoglobulins.

■ DISPOSITION
- As treatment is initiated, the muscle enzymes should return to normal before symptoms improve.
- During exacerbations, enzymes will rise first before symptoms appear.
- Approximately 50% of the patients will go into remission and stop therapy within 5 yr. The remaining will either have active disease requiring ongoing treatment or inactive disease with permanent muscle atrophy and contractures.
- Poor prognostic indicators include:
  1. Delay in diagnosis
  2. Older age
  3. Recalcitrant disease
  4. Malignancy
  5. Interstitial pulmonary fibrosis
  6. Dysphagia
  7. Leukocytosis
  8. Fever
  9. Anorexia

- Infection, malignancy, and cardiac and pulmonary dysfunction are the most common causes of death.
- With early treatment 5- and 8-yr survival rates of 80% and 73% have been reported.

■ REFERRAL
For any suspected cases of DM a rheumatology referral should be made to help establish the diagnosis and implement treatment.

PEARLS & CONSIDERATIONS

■ COMMENTS
- When assessing response to treatment, it is best to follow clinical muscle strength over muscle enzyme tests.
- The concern of malignancies (ovary, lung, breast, GI) associated with myositis is legitimate and merits screening in patients over the age of 40.
- Malignancies can occur before, during, or after the diagnosis of dermatomyositis.
- There does not appear to be any association between juvenile dermatomyositis and malignancy.
- Overlap syndrome are patients with dermatomyositis who also meet criteria for other connective tissue disorder (e.g., rheumatoid arthritis, scleroderma, SLE).

REFERENCES
Callen JP: Dermatomyositis, *Lancet* 355(9197):53, 2000.
Koler RA, Montemarano A: Dermatomyositis, *Am Fam Physician* 64(156):5, 2001.
Author: **Peter Petropoulos, M.D.**

BASIC INFORMATION

■ DEFINITION

Diabetes insipidus is a polyuric disorder resulting from insufficient production of antidiuretic hormone (ADH) (pituitary [neurogenic] diabetes insipidus) or unresponsiveness of the renal tubules to ADH (nephrogenic diabetes insipidus).

ICD-9CM CODES
253.5 Diabetes insipidus

■ EPIDEMIOLOGY & DEMOGRAPHICS
GENETICS:
- Nephrogenic diabetes insipidus can be inherited as sex-linked recessive.
- There is also a rare autosomal dominant form of neurogenic diabetes insipidus.

■ PHYSICAL FINDINGS & CLINICAL PRESENTATION
- Polyuria: urinary volumes ranging from 2.5 to 6 L/day
- Polydipsia (predilection for cold or iced drinks)
- Neurologic manifestations (seizures, headaches, visual field defects)
- Evidence of volume contractions

NOTE: The previous physical findings and clinical manifestations are generally not evident until vasopressin secretory capacity is reduced <20% of normal.

■ ETIOLOGY
NEUROGENIC DIABETES INSIPIDUS:
- Idiopathic
- Neoplasms of brain or pituitary fossa (craniopharyngiomas, metastatic neoplasms from breast or lung)
- Posttherapeutic neurosurgical procedures (e.g., hypophysectomy)
- Head trauma (e.g., basal skull fracture)
- Granulomatous disorders (sarcoidosis or TB)
- Histiocytosis (Hand-Schüller-Christian disease, eosinophilic granuloma)
- Familial (autosomal dominant)
- Other: interventricular hemorrhage, aneurysms, meningitis, postencephalitis, multiple sclerosis

NEPHROGENIC DIABETES INSIPIDUS:
- Drugs: lithium, amphotericin B, demeclocycline, methoxyflurane anesthesia
- Familial: X-linked
- Metabolic: hypercalcemia or hypokalemia
- Other: sarcoidosis, amyloidosis, pyelonephritis, polycystic disease, sickle cell disease, postobstructive

DIAGNOSIS

■ DIFFERENTIAL DIAGNOSIS
- Diabetes mellitus, nephropathies
- Primary polydipsia, medications (e.g., chlorpromazine)
- Osmotic diuresis (glucose, mannitol, anticholinergics)
- Psychogenic polydipsia, electrolyte disturbances

■ WORKUP
- The diagnostic workup is aimed at showing that the polyuria is caused by the inability to concentrate urine and determining whether the problem is secondary to decreased ADH or insensitivity to ADH. This is done with the water deprivation test:
  1. Following baseline measurement of weight, ADH, plasma sodium, and urine and plasma osmolarity, the patient is deprived of fluids under strict medical supervision.
  2. Frequent (q2h) monitoring of plasma and urine osmolarity follows.
  3. The test is generally terminated when plasma osmolarity is >295 or the patient loses ≥3.5% of initial body weight.
  4. Diabetes insipidus is confirmed if the plasma osmolarity is >295 and the urine osmolarity is <500.
  5. To distinguish nephrogenic from neurogenic diabetes insipidus, the patient is given 5 U of vasopressin (ADH) and the change in urine osmolarity is measured. A significant increase (>50%) in urine osmolarity following administration of ADH is indicative of neurogenic diabetes insipidus.
- A diagnostic algorithm for diabetes insipidus is described in Section III.

■ LABORATORY TESTS
- Decreased urinary specific gravity (≤1.005)
- Decreased urinary osmolarity (usually <200 mOsm/kg) even in the presence of high serum osmolality
- Hypernatremia, increased plasma osmolarity, hypercalcemia, hypokalemia

■ IMAGING STUDIES
MRI of the brain if neurogenic diabetes insipidus is confirmed

TREATMENT

■ NONPHARMACOLOGIC THERAPY
- Patient education regarding control of fluid balance and prevention of dehydration with adequate fluid intake
- Daily weight

■ ACUTE GENERAL Rx
Therapy varies with the degree and type of diabetes insipidus:
NEUROGENIC DIABETES INSIPIDUS:
1. Desmopressin acetate (DDAVP) 10 to 40 µg qd intranasally in one to three divided doses or in tablet form 0.1 or 0.2 mg. Usual oral dose is 0.1 to 1.2 mg/day in two to three divided doses Desmopressin is also available in injectable form given as 2 to 4 µg/day SC or IV in two divided doses
2. Vasopressin tannate in oil: 2.5 to 5 U IM q24-72h; useful for long-term management because of its long life
3. In mild cases of neurogenic diabetes insipidus, the polyuria may be controlled with HCTZ 50 mg qd (decreases urine volume by increasing proximal tubular reabsorption of glomerular infiltrate) or chlorpropamide (Diabinese) 100-250 mg qd; enhances the effect of vasopressin at the renal tubule

NEPHROGENIC DIABETES INSIPIDUS:
1. Adequate hydration
2. Low-sodium diet and chlorothiazide to induce mild sodium depletion
3. Polyuria of diabetes insipidus secondary to lithium can be ameliorated by using amiloride (5 mg PO bid initially, increased to 10 mg bid after 2 wk)

■ CHRONIC Rx
Patients should be aware of the danger of dehydration and the need for liberal water intake.

■ REFERRAL
Endocrinology evaluation for diagnostic testing

PEARLS & CONSIDERATIONS

■ COMMENTS
Patients should be instructed to wear a medical identification tag or bracelet identifying their medical illness.

REFERENCE
Maghnie M et al: Central diabetes insipidus in children and young adults, *N Engl J Med* 343:998, 2000.
Author: **Fred F. Ferri, M.D.**

■ BASIC INFORMATION

■ DEFINITION

- Diabetes mellitus (DM) refers to a syndrome of hyperglycemia resulting from many different causes (see Etiology). It can be classified into type 1 insulin-dependent (formerly IDDM) and type 2 non–insulin-dependent (formerly NIDDM) DM. Because "insulin-dependent" and "non–insulin-dependent" refer to stage at diagnosis, when a type 2 diabetic needs insulin, he or she remains classified as type 2 and does not revert to type 1. Table 1-16 provides a general comparison of the two types of diabetes mellitus.
- The American Diabetes Association (ADA) defines DM as (1) a fasting plasma glucose ≥126 mg/dl or (2) a nonfasting plasma glucose ≥200 mg/dl or (3) an oral glucose tolerance test (OGTT) ≥200 mg/dl in the 2-hr sample. Furthermore, the ADA also defines a value of 110 mg/dl on fasting blood sugar as the upper limit of normal for glucose. A fasting glucose between 110 mg/dl and 126 mg/dl is classified as "Impaired Fasting Glucose" (IFG). When results of the oral glucose test are between 110 mg/dl and 200 mg/dl, the patient is also classified as having IFG.

■ SYNONYMS

IDDM (insulin-dependent diabetes mellitus)
NIDDM (non–insulin-dependent diabetes mellitus)
Type 1 diabetes mellitus (insulin-dependent diabetes mellitus)
Type 2 diabetes mellitus (non-insulin-dependent diabetes mellitus)

ICD-9CM CODES

250.0 Diabetes mellitus (NIDDM)
250.1 Insulin-dependent diabetes mellitus without complication (IDDM)

■ EPIDEMIOLOGY & DEMOGRAPHICS

- DM affects 5% to 7% of the U.S. population. Prevalence in Pima Indians is 35%.
- Incidence increases with age, with 2% in persons ages 20 to 44 yr to 18% in persons 65 to 74 yr of age.
- Diabetes accounts for 8% of all legal blindness and is the leading cause of end-stage renal disease in the U.S.
- Patients with diabetes are twice as likely as nondiabetic patients to develop cardiovascular disease.

■ PHYSICAL FINDINGS & CLINICAL PRESENTATION

1. Physical examination varies with the presence of complications and may be normal in early stages.
2. Diabetic retinopathy:
   a. Nonproliferative (background diabetic retinopathy):
      (1) Initially: microaneurysms, capillary dilation, waxy or hard exudates, dot and flame hemorrhages, AV shunts
      (2) Advanced stage: microinfarcts with cotton wool exudates, macular edema
   b. Proliferative retinopathy: characterized by formation of new vessels, vitreal hemorrhages, fibrous scarring, and retinal detachment
3. Cataracts and glaucoma occur with increased frequency in diabetics.
4. Peripheral neuropathy: patients often complain of paresthesias of extremities (feet more than hands); the symptoms are symmetric, bilateral, and associated with intense burning pain (particularly during the night).

TABLE 1-16 General Comparison of the Two Most Common Types of Diabetes Mellitus

	TYPE 1	TYPE 2
Previous terminology	Insulin-dependent diabetes mellitus (IDDM), type I, juvenile-onset diabetes	Non-insulin-dependent diabetes mellitus, type II, adult-onset diabetes
Age of onset	Usually <30 yr, particularly childhood and adolescence, but any age	Usually >40 yr, but any age
Genetic predisposition	Moderate; environmental factors required for expression; 35%-50% concordance in monozygotic twins; several candidate genes proposed	Strong; 60%-90% concordance in monozygotic twins; many candidate genes proposed; some genes identified in maturity-onset diabetes of the young
Human leukocyte antigen associations	Linkage to DQA and DQB, influenced by DRB(3 and 4) [DR2 protective]	None known
Other associations	Autoimmune; Graves' disease, Hashimoto's thyroiditis, vitiligo, Addison's disease, pernicious anemia	Heterogenous group, ongoing subclassification based on identification of specific pathogenic processes and genetic defects
Precipitating and risk factors	Largely unknown; microbial, chemical, dietary, other	Age, obesity (central), sedentary lifestyle, previous gestational diabetes
Findings at diagnosis	85%-90% of patients have one and usually more autoantibodies to ICA512/IA-2/IA-2β, GAD$_{65}$, insulin (IAA)	Possibly complications (microvascular and macrovascular) caused by significant preceeding asymptomatic period
Endogenous insulin levels	Low or absent	Usually present (relative deficiency), early hyperinsulinemia
Insulin resistance	Only with hyperglycemia	Mostly present
Prolonged fast	Hyperglycemia, ketoacidosis	Euglycemia
Stress, withdrawal of insulin	Ketoacidosis	Nonketotic hyperglycemia, occasionally ketoacidosis

From Andreoli TE (ed): *Cecil essentials of medicine*, ed 5, Philadelphia, 2001, WB Saunders.
GAD, Glutamic acid decarboxylase; *IA-2/IA-2β*, tyrosine phosphatases; *IAA*, insulin autoantibodies; *ICA*, islet cell antibody; *ICA512*, islet cell autoantigen 512 (fragment of IA-2).

a. Mononeuropathies involving cranial nerves III, IV, and VI, intercostal nerves, and femoral nerves are also common.
b. Physical examination may reveal:
   (1) Decreased pinprick sensation, sensation to light touch, and pain sensation
   (2) Decreased vibration sense
   (3) Loss of proprioception (leading to ataxia)
   (4) Motor disturbances (decreased DTR, weakness and atrophy of interossei muscles); when the hands are affected, the patient has trouble picking up small objects, dressing, and turning pages in a book
   (5) Diplopia, abnormalities of visual fields
5. Autonomic neuropathy:
   a. GI disturbances: esophageal motility abnormalities, gastroparesis, diarrhea (usually nocturnal)
   b. GU disturbances: neurogenic bladder (hesitancy, weak stream, and dribbling), impotence
   c. Orthostatic hypotension: postural syncope, dizziness, lightheadedness
6. Nephropathy: pedal edema, pallor, weakness, uremic appearance.
7. Foot ulcers: occur frequently and are usually secondary to peripheral vascular insufficiency, repeated trauma (unrecognized because of sensory loss), and superimposed infections.
8. Neuropathic arthropathy (Charcot's joints): bone or joint deformities from repeated trauma (secondary to peripheral neuropathy).
9. Necrobiosis lipoidica diabeticorum: plaquelike reddened areas with a central area that fades to white-yellow found on the anterior surfaces of the legs; in these areas the skin becomes very thin and can ulcerate readily.

■ ETIOLOGY
IDIOPATHIC DIABETES:
Type 1 DM
• Hereditary factors:
   1. Islet cell antibodies (found in 90% of patients within the first year of diagnosis)
   2. Higher incidence of HLA types DR3, DR4
   3. 50% concordance in identical twins
• Environmental factors: viral infection (possibly coxsackie virus, mumps virus)

Type 2 DM
• Hereditary factors: 90% concordance in identical twins
• Environmental factor: obesity
DIABETES SECONDARY TO OTHER FACTORS:
• Hormonal excess: Cushing's syndrome, acromegaly, glucagonoma, pheochromocytoma
• Drugs: glucocorticoids, diuretics, oral contraceptives
• Insulin receptor unavailability (with or without circulating antibodies)
• Pancreatic disease: pancreatitis, pancreatectomy, hemochromatosis
• Genetic syndromes: hyperlipidemias, myotonic dystrophy, lipoatrophy
• Gestational diabetes

🔬 DIAGNOSIS

Diagnosis is made on the basis of the following tests and should be confirmed by repeated testing on a different day:
1. Fasting glucose ≥126 mg/dl (ADA criteria)
2. Nonfasting plasma glucose ≥200 mg/dl

Use of glycosylated hemoglobin (Hb A1c) level is not recommended for diagnosis at this time by the ADA because of lack of standardization of hemoglobin Alc values and the imperfect correlation between HbAlc and fasting plasma glucose levels. However, some physicians use this test to make the diagnosis of diabetes mellitus if the random plasma glucose is >200 mg/dl and the hemoglobin Alc level is ≥2 standard deviations above the laboratory mean.

■ DIFFERENTIAL DIAGNOSIS
• Diabetes insipidus
• Stress hyperglycemia
• Diabetes secondary to hormonal excess, drugs, pancreatic disease

💊 TREATMENT

■ NONPHARMACOLOGIC THERAPY
1. Diet
   a. Calories
      (1) The diabetic patient can be started on 15 calories/lb of ideal body weight; this number can be increased to 20 calories/lb for an active person and 25 calories/lb if the patient does heavy physical labor.

   (2) The calories should be distributed as 55% to 60% carbohydrates, 25% to 35% fat, and 15% to 20% protein.
   (3) The emphasis should be on complex carbohydrates rather than simple and refined starches and on polyunsaturated instead of saturated fats in a ratio of 2:1.
   b. Seven food groups
      (1) The exchange diet of the ADA includes protein, bread, fruit, milk, and low- and intermediate-carbohydrate vegetables.
      (2) The name of each exchange is meant to be all-inclusive (e.g., cereal, muffins, spaghetti, potatoes, rice are in the bread group; meats, fish, eggs, cheese, peanut butter are in the protein group).
      (3) The *glycemic index* compares the rise in blood sugar after the ingestion of simple sugars and complex carbohydrates with the rise that occurs after the absorption of glucose; equal amounts of starches do not give the same rise in plasma glucose (pasta equal in calories to a baked potato causes less of a rise than the potato): thus it is helpful to know the glycemic index of a particular food product.
      (4) Fiber: insoluble fiber (bran, celery) and soluble globular fiber (pectin in fruit) delay glucose absorption and attenuate the postprandial serum glucose peak; they also appear to lower the elevated triglyceride level often present in uncontrolled diabetics.
2. Exercise increases the cellular glucose uptake by increasing the number of cell receptors. The following points must be considered:
   a. Exercise program must be individualized and built up slowly.
   b. Insulin is more rapidly absorbed when injected into a limb that is then exercised, and this can result in hypoglycemia.
3. Weight loss: to ideal body weight if the patient is overweight

■ PHARMACOLOGIC THERAPY

- When the previous measures fail to normalize the serum glucose, oral hypoglycemic agents (e.g., metformin, glitazones, or a sulfonylurea) should be added to the regimen in type 2 DM. Table 1-17 describes commonly used oral hypoglycemic agents. The sulfonamides and the biguanide metformin are the oldest and most commonly used classes of hypoglycemic drugs.
- Metformin's primary mechanism is to decrease hepatic glucose output. Because metformin does not produce hypoglycemia when used as a monotherapy, it is preferred for most patients. It is contraindicated in patients with renal insufficiency.
- Sulfonylureas and repaglinide work best when given before meals because they increase the postprandial output of insulin from the pancreas. All sulfonylureas are contraindicated in patients allergic to sulfa.
- Acarbose and miglitol work by competitively inhibiting pancreatic amylase and small intestinal glucosidases delay gastrointestinal absorption of carbohydrates, thereby reducing alimentary hyperglycemia. The major side effects are flatulence, diarrhea, and abdominal cramps.
- Pioglitazone and rosiglitazone increase insulin sensitivity and are useful in addition to other agents in type 2 diabetics whose hyperglycemia is inadequately controlled. Serum transaminase levels should be obtained before starting therapy and monitored periodically.
- Insulin is indicated for the treatment of all type 1 DM and type 2 DM patients who cannot be adequately controlled with diet and oral agents. Table 1-18 describes commonly used types of insulin. The risks of insulin therapy include weight gain, hypoglycemia, and, in

TABLE 1-17 Oral Antidiabetic Agents as Monotherapy

	SULFONYLUREAS	BIGUANIDES	α-GLUCOSIDASE INHIBITORS	THIAZOLIDINEDIONES	MEGLITINIDES
Generic name	Glimepiride, glyburide, glipizide, chlorpropamide, tolbutamide	Metformin	Acarbose, miglitol	Troglitazone, rosiglitazone, pioglitazone	Repaglinide, nateglinide
Mode of action	↑↑ Pancreatic insulin secretion chronically	↓↓ HGP; ↓ peripheral IR; ↓ intestinal glucose absorption	Delays PP digestion of carbohydrates and absorption of glucose	↓↓ Peripheral IR; ↑↑ glucose disposal; ↓ HGP	↑↑ Pancreatic insulin secretion acutely
Preferred patient type	Diagnosis age >30 yr, lean, diabetes <5 yr, insulinopenic	Overweight, IR, fasting hyperglycemia, dyslipidemia	PP hyperglycemia	Overweight, IR, dyslipidemia, renal dysfunction	PP hyperglycemia, insulinopenic
Therapeutic effects					
↓ HBA_{1c}* (%)	1-2	1-2	0.5-1	0.8-1	1-2
↓ FPG* (mg/dl)	50-70	50-80	15-30	25-50	40-80
↓ PPG* (mg/dl)	~90	80	40-50	—	30
Insulin levels	↑	—	—	—	↑
Weight	↑	–/↓	—	–/↑	↑
Lipids	—	↓ LDL / ↓↓ TG	—	↑ Large "fluffy" LDL / ↓↓ TG / ↑ HDL	—
Side effects	Hypoglycemia	Diarrhea, lactic acidosis	Abdominal pain, flatulence, diarrhea	Idiosyncratic hepatotoxicity with troglitazone; edema	Hypoglycemia (low-risk)
Dose(s)/day	1-3	2-3	1-3	1	1-4+
Maximum daily dose (mg)	Depends on agent	2550	150 (<60-kg bw) / 300 (>60-kg bw)	Depends on agent	16 (repaglinide), 360 (nateglinide)
Range/dose (mg)	Depends on agent	500-1000	25-50 (<60-kg bw) / 25-100 (>60-kg bw)	Depends on agent	0.5-4 (repaglinide), 60, 120 (nateglinide)
Optimal administration time	~30 min premeal (some with food, others on empty stomach)	With meal	With first bite of meal	With meal (breakfast)	Preferably <15 (0-30 min) premeals (omit if no meal)
Main site of metabolism/ excretion	Hepatic/renal, fecal	Not metabolized/ renal	Only 2% absorbed/fecal	Hepatic/fecal	Hepatic/fecal

Modified from Andreloi TE (ed): *Cecil essentials of medicine,* ed 5, Philadelphia, 2001, WB Saunders.
↑, Increased; ↓, decreased; —, unchanged; *bw,* body weight; *FPG,* fasting plasma glucose; *HDL,* high-density lipoprotein; *HGP,* hepatic glucose production; *IR,* insulin resistance; *LDL,* low-density lipoprotein; *PP,* postprandial; *PPG,* postprandial plasma glucose; *TG,* triglyceride.
*Values combined from numerous studies; values are also dose dependent.

TABLE 1-18   Types of Insulin

INSULIN TYPE	GENERIC NAME	PREPRANDIAL INJECTION TIMING* (HR)	ONSET* (HR)	PEAK* (HR)	DURATION* (HR)	BLOOD GLUCOSE (BG) NADIR* (HR)
Rapid acting	Lispro†	0-0.2	0.2-0.5	0.5-2	<5	2-4
Short acting	Regular	0.5-(1)	0.3-1	2-6	4-8 (≤16)	3-7 (Pre-next meal)
	Lente		1-2	4-12		
Intermediate acting	NPH	0.5-(1)	1-3	6-15	16-26	6-13
Long acting‡	Ultralente	0.5-(1)	4-6	8-30	24-36	10-28
Mixed, short/intermediate acting	70/30					
	50/50	0.5-(1)	0.5-1	3-12	16-24	3-12

From Andreoli TE (ed): *Cecil essentials of medicine,* ed 5, Philadelphia, 2001, WB Saunders.
70/30, 70% NPH, 30% regular; *50/50,* 50% NPH, 50% regular; *NPH,* neutral protamine Hagedorn.
*Times depend on several factors including dose, anatomic site of injection, method (SQ, IM, IV), duration of diabetes, degree of insulin resistance, level of activity, and body temperature. Some time ranges are wide to include data from several separate studies. Preprandial injection depends on premeal BG values as well as insulin type. If BG is low, may need to inject insulin and eat immediately (carbohydrate portion of meal first). If BG is high, may delay meal after insulin injection and eat carbohydrate portion last.
†Insulin analogue with reversal of lysine and proline at positions 28 and 29 on the β chain.
‡Insulin glargine [rDNA origin] is a newer, once-daily insulin analog (Lantus) that provides 24-hour basal glucose-lowering with once-a-day bedtime dosing. Onset of action is 2-3 hr, duration of action is 24+ hr.

rare cases, allergic or cutaneous reactions.
- Combination therapy of various hypoglycemic agents is commonly used when monotherapy results in inadequate glycemic control.
- Continuous subcutaneous insulin infusion (CSII, or insulin pump) provides better glycemic control than does conventional therapy and comparable to or slightly better control than multiple daily injections. It should be considered for diabetes presenting in childhood or adolescence and during pregnancy.
- Low-dose ASA to decrease the risk of cerebrovascular disease is beneficial for diabetics over age 30 with other risk factors (hypertension, dyslipidemia, smoking, obesity).
- A fasting serum lipid panel should be obtained yearly on all adult diabetic patients. Strict lipid control (LDL <100 mg/dl) is indicated in all diabetics. Use of statins is often necessary to achieve therapeutic goals.

■ DISPOSITION
The Diabetes Control and Complications Trial (DCCT) proved that intensive treatment decreases the development and progression of complications of DM. In this trial, the risks of retinopathy, nephropathy, and neuropathy were decreased by 35% to 90%. Each patient should be made aware of these findings.

- Retinopathy occurs in approximately 15% of diabetic patients after 15 yr and increases 1%/yr after diagnosis.
- The frequency of neuropathy in type 2 diabetics approaches 70% to 80%. Gabapentin (900-3600 mg/day) is effective for the symptomatic treatment of peripheral neuropathic pain. Amitriptyline or carbamazepine is also modestly effective.
- Nephropathy occurs in 35% to 45% of patients with type 1 DM and in 20% of type 2 DM. The first sign of renal involvement in patients with DM is most often microalbuminuria, which is classified as incipient nephropathy. ACE inhibitors are effective in slowing the progression of renal disease in both type I and type II DM, independently of their reduction in blood pressure. ARBs and nondihydropyridine calcium channel blockers are also effective in protecting against the progression of nephropathy in diabetics, especially in type 2 DM.
- Infections are generally more common in diabetics because of multiple factors, such as impaired leukocyte function, decreased tissue perfusion secondary to vascular disease, repeated trauma because of loss of sensation, and urinary retention secondary to neuropathy.
- Diabetic ketoacidosis and hyperosmolar coma are described in detail in Section I.

■ REFERRAL
- Diabetic patients should be advised to have annual ophthalmologic examination. In type 1 DM, ophthalmologic visits should begin within 3 to 5 yr, whereas type 2 DM patients should be seen from disease onset.
- Podiatric care can significantly reduce the rate of foot infections and amputations in patients with DM.

◯ PEARLS & CONSIDERATIONS

■ COMMENTS
- Because normalization of serum glucose level is the ultimate goal, every patient should measure his or her blood glucose unless contraindicated by senility or blindness.
- For blood glucose monitoring, glucose oxidase strips are used in conjunction with a meter to give a digital reading. The testing can be done once day, but the time should be varied each day so that over time the serum glucose level before meals and at bedtime can be assessed frequently without pricking the patient's fingers four times daily.
- Glycosylated hemoglobin should be measured at least twice yearly; measurement of microalbumin in the urine on a yearly basis is also recommended.
- Underinsured children and those with psychiatric illness are at higher risk for acute complications in type 1 DM.

REFERENCES

American Diabetes Association Position Statement: Standards of medical care for patients with diabetes mellitus, *Diabetes Care* 25:S33, 2002.

Barr RG et al: Tests of glycemia for the diagnosis of type 2 diabetes mellitus, *Ann Intern Med* 137:263, 2002.

Beckman JA et al: Diabetes and atherosclerosis, *JAMA* 287:2570, 2002.

DeWitt DE, Hirsch IB: Outpatient insulin therapy in type 1 and type 2 DM, *JAMA* 289:2254, 2003.

Diabetes Control and Complications Trial (DCCT)/Epidemiology of Diabetes Interventions and Complications (EDIC) Research Group: Beneficial effects of intensive therapy of diabetes during adolescence: outcomes after the conclusion of the Diabetes Control and Complications Trial (DCCT), *J Pediatr* 139:804, 2001.

Diabetes Control and Complications Trial/Epidemiology of Diabetes Interventions and Complications Research Group: Effect of intensive therapy on the microvascular complications of type 1 diabetes mellitus, *JAMA* 287:2563, 2002.

Holmboe ES: Oral antihyperglycemic therapy for type 2 diabetes, *JAMA* 287:373, 2002.

Nathan DM: Initial management of glycemia in type 2 diabetes mellitus, *N Engl J Med* 347:1342, 2002.

Pickup J et al: Glycemic control with continuous subcutaneous insulin infusion compared with intensive insulin injections with type 1 diabetes: meta-analysis of randomized controlled trials, *BMJ* 324:705, 2002.

Remuzzi G et al: Nephropathy in patients with type 2 diabetes, *N Engl J Med* 346:1145, 2002.

Stern MP et al: Identification of persons at high risk for type 2 diabetes mellitus: do we need the oral glucose tolerance test? *Ann Intern Med* 136:575, 2002.

U.S. Preventive Services Task Force: Screening for type 2 DM in adults: recommendations and rationale, *Ann Intern Med* 138:212, 2003.

Zandbergen AM et al: Effect of losartan on microalbuminuria in normotensive patients with type 2 DM, *Ann Intern Med* 139:90, 2003.

Author: **Fred F. Ferri, M.D.**

BASIC INFORMATION

■ DEFINITION

Diabetic ketoacidosis (DKA) is a life-threatening complication of diabetes mellitus resulting from severe insulin deficiency and manifested clinically by severe dehydration and alterations in the sensorium.

■ SYNONYMS

DKA

ICD-9CM CODES

250.1 Diabetic ketoacidosis

■ EPIDEMIOLOGY & DEMOGRAPHICS

INCIDENCE/PREVALENCE: 46 episodes/10,000 diabetics; cause of 14% of all hospital admissions of diabetic patients
PREDOMINANT AGE: 1 to 25 yr

■ PHYSICAL FINDINGS & CLINICAL PRESENTATION

- Evidence of dehydration (tachycardia, hypotension, dry mucous membranes, sunken eyeballs, poor skin turgor)
- Clouding of mental status
- Tachypnea with air hunger (Kussmaul's respiration)
- Fruity breath odor (caused by acetone)
- Lipemia retinalis in some patients
- Possible evidence of precipitating factors (infected wound, pneumonia)
- Abdominal or CVA tenderness in some patients

■ ETIOLOGY

Metabolic decompensation in diabetics usually precipitated by an infectious process (up to 40% of cases). Poor compliance with insulin therapy and severe medical illness (e.g., CVA, MI) are other common causes. Cocaine abuse has been reported as a risk factor for DKA, particularly in patients with multiple admissions.

DIAGNOSIS

■ DIFFERENTIAL DIAGNOSIS

- Hyperosmolar nonketotic state (Table 1-19)
- Alcoholic ketoacidosis
- Uremic acidosis
- Metabolic acidosis secondary to methyl alcohol, ethylene glycol
- Salicylate poisoning

■ WORKUP

- Laboratory evaluation (see Laboratory Tests) to confirm diagnosis and evaluate precipitating factors
- Admission ECG to evaluate electrolyte abnormalities and rule out myocardial ischemia/infarction as a contributing factor

■ LABORATORY TESTS

- Glucose level reveals severe hyperglycemia (serum glucose generally >300 mg/dl).
- ABGs reveal acidosis: arterial pH usually <7.3 with Pco_2 <40 mm Hg.

- Serum electrolytes:
  1. Serum bicarbonate is usually <15 mEq/L.
  2. Serum potassium may be low, normal, or high. There is always significant total body potassium depletion regardless of the initial potassium level.
  3. Serum sodium is usually decreased as a result of hyperglycemia, dehydration, and lipemia. Assume 1.6 mEq/L decrease in extracellular sodium for each 100 mg/dl increase in glucose concentration.
  4. Calculate the anion gap (AG):

$$AG = Na^+ - (Cl^- + HCO^{-3})$$

In DKA the anion gap is increased; hyperchloremic metabolic acidosis may be present in unusual circumstances when both the glomerular filtration rate and the plasma volume are well maintained.

- CBC with differential, urinalysis, urine and blood cultures to rule out infectious precipitating factor.
- Serum calcium, magnesium, and phosphorus; the plasma phosphate and magnesium levels may be significantly depressed and should be rechecked within 24 hr because they may decrease further with correction of DKA.
- BUN and creatinine generally reveal significant dehydration.
- Amylase, liver enzymes should be checked in patients with abdominal pain.

TABLE 1-19 A Comparison of Diabetic Ketoacidosis (DKA) and Hyperosmolar Nonketotic Syndrome (HNKS)

FEATURE	DKA	HNKS
Age of patient	Usually <40 yr	Usually >60 yr
Duration of symptoms	Usually <2 days	Usually >5 days
Serum glucose concentration	Usually <800 mg/dl	Usually >800 mg/dl
Serum sodium concentration (Na+)	More likely to be normal or low	More likely to be normal or high
Serum bicarbonate concentration (HCO₃)	Low	Normal
Ketone bodies	At least 4 + in 1:1 dilution	<2 + in 1:1 dilution
pH	Low	Normal
Serum osmolality	Usually <350 mOsm/kg	Usually >350 mOsm/kg
Cerebral edema	Occasionally clinical symptoms	Rarely (never?) clinical
Prognosis	3% to 10% mortality	10% to 20% mortality
Subsequent course	Insulin therapy required in almost all cases	Insulin therapy not required in most cases

From Andreoli TE (ed): *Cecil essentials of medicine,* ed 5, Philadelphia, 2001, WB Saunders.

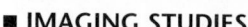
■ IMAGING STUDIES

Chest x-ray examination is helpful to rule out infectious process. The initial chest x-ray may be negative if the patient has significant dehydration. Repeat chest x-ray examination after 24 hr if pulmonary infection is strongly suspected.

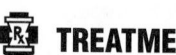 **TREATMENT**

■ NONPHARMACOLOGIC THERAPY

- Monitor mental status, vital signs, and urine output qh until improved, then monitor q2-4h.
- Monitor electrolytes, renal function, and glucose level (see Acute General Rx).

■ ACUTE GENERAL Rx
FLUID REPLACEMENT (THE USUAL DEFICIT IS 6 TO 8 L)

1. Do not delay fluid replacement until laboratory results have been received.
2. The initial fluid replacement should be with 0.9% NS until blood pressure and organ perfusion are restored (usually 1 L or more). In patients with severe hypernatremia (serum sodium > 160 mEq/L), 0.45 % saline infusion can be used. Careful monitoring for fluid overload is necessary in elderly patients and those with a history of CHF.
3. The rate of fluid replacement varies with the age of the patient and the presence of significant cardiac or renal disease.
   - The usual rate of infusion is 500 ml to 1 L over the first hour; 300 to 500 ml/hr for the next 12 hr.
   - Continue the infusion at a rate of 200 to 300 ml/hr, using 0.45% NS until the serum glucose level is <300 ml/dl, then change the hydrating solution to D_5W to prevent hypoglycemia, replenish free water, and introduce additional glucose substrate (necessary to suppress lipolysis and ketogenesis).

INSULIN ADMINISTRATION

1. The patient should be given an initial loading IV bolus of 0.15 to 0.2 U/kg of regular insulin followed by a constant infusion at a rate of 0.1 U/kg/hr (e.g., 25 U of regular insulin in 250 ml of 0.9% saline solution at 70 ml/hr equals 7 U/hr for a 70-kg patient).
2. Monitor serum glucose qh for the first 2 hr, then monitor q2-4h.
3. The goal is to decrease serum glucose level by 80 mg/dl/hr (follow-ing an initial drop because of rehydration); if the serum glucose level is not decreasing at the expected rate, double the rate of insulin infusion.
4. When the serum glucose level approaches 250 mg/dl, decrease the rate of insulin infusion to 2 to 3 U/hr and continue this rate until the patient has received adequate fluid replacement, HCO^-_3 is close to normal, and ketones have cleared.
5. Approximately 30 to 60 min before stopping the IV insulin infusion, administer an SC dose of regular insulin (dose varies with the patient's demonstrated insulin sensitivity); this SC dose of regular insulin is necessary because of the extremely short life of the insulin in the IV infusion.
6. When the patient is able to eat, NPH insulin 10-15 U is given in the morning and regular insulin is administered before each meal and at bedtime by using a sliding scale. In newly diagnosed diabetics, the total daily dose to maintain metabolic control ranges from 0.5 to 0.8 U/kg/day. Split dose therapy with regular and NPH insulin may be given, with two thirds of the total daily dose administered in the morning and one third in the evening.

ELECTROLYTE REPLACEMENT

Potassium Replacement: The average total potassium loss in DKA is 300 to 500 mEq.

- The rate of replacement varies with the patient's serum potassium level, degree of acidosis (decreased pH, increased potassium level), and renal function (potassium replacement should be used with caution in patients with renal failure).
- As a rule of thumb, potassium replacement may be started when there is no ECG evidence of hyperkalemia (tall, narrow, or tent-shaped T waves, decreased or absent P waves, short QT intervals, widening of QRS complex).
- In patients with normal renal function, potassium replacement can be started by adding 20 to 40 mEq KCl/L of IV hydrating solution if serum potassium is 4 to 5 mEq/L, more if serum potassium level is lower than 4 mEq/L.
- Monitor serum potassium level qh for the first 2 hr, then monitor q2-4h.

Phosphate Replacement: If the serum PO_4 is <1.5 mEq/L, give 2.5 mg/kg IV over 6 hr of elemental phosphate.

Routine replacement of phosphate (in absence of laboratory evidence of significant hypophosphatemia) is not indicated. Rapid IV phosphate administration can cause hypocalcemia.

Magnesium Replacement: Replacement indicated only in the presence of significant hypomagnesemia or refractory hypokalemia.

BICARBONATE THERAPY: Routine use of bicarbonate in DKA is contraindicated, because it can worsen hypokalemia and intracellular acidosis and cause cerebral edema. Bicarbonate therapy should be used only if the arterial pH is <7. In these patients 44 to 88 mEq of sodium bicarbonate can be added to a liter of 0.45% NS q2-4h until pH increases >7. Use of bicarbonate therapy is particularly dangerous in the pediatric population. Children with DKA who have low partial pressures of arterial carbon dioxide and high serum urea nitrogen concentration at presentation and who are treated with bicarbonate are at increased risk for cerebral edema. Bicarbonate therapy in children with DKA should be limited to those with severe circulatory failure and a high risk of cardiac decompensation resulting from profound acidosis.

■ DISPOSITION

- Average mortality in DKA is 5% to 10%.
- In children <10 yr of age, DKA causes 70% of diabetes-related deaths.
- Cerebral edema occurs in 1% of episodes of DKA in children and is associated with a mortality rate of 40% to 90%.

■ REFERRAL

Patients with DKA should be admitted to the ICU.

☼ PEARLS & CONSIDERATIONS

■ COMMENTS

- Potential complications of DKA therapy include hypoglycemia, cerebral edema, cardiac arrhythmias, shock, MI, and acute pancreatitis.
- Underinsured children and those with psychiatric illness are at higher risk for DKA.

REFERENCE

Glaser N et al: Risk factor for cerebral edema in children with diabetic ketoacidosis, *N Engl J Med* 344:264, 2001.
Author: **Fred F. Ferri, M.D.**

BASIC INFORMATION

DEFINITION

Diffuse interstitial lung disease is a group of blood disorders involving the lung interstitium and characterized by inflammation of the alveolar structures and progressive parenchymal fibrosis.

SYNONYMS

Interstitial lung disease
ILD

ICD-9CM CODES

136.3 Acute interstitial lung disease
515 Chronic interstitial lung disease

EPIDEMIOLOGY & DEMOGRAPHICS

• The incidence of interstitial lung disease is 5 cases/100,000 persons
• There are >100 known disorders that can cause interstitial lung disease (see Etiology).

PHYSICAL FINDINGS & CLINICAL PRESENTATION

• The patient generally presents with progressive dyspnea and nonproductive cough; other clinical manifestations vary with the underlying disease process.
• Physical examination typically shows end respiratory dry rales (Velcro rales), cyanosis, clubbing, and right-sided heart failure.

ETIOLOGY

• Occupational and environmental exposure: pneumoconiosis, asbestosis, organic dust, gases, fumes, berylliosis, silicosis
• Granulomatous lung disease: sarcoidosis, infections (e.g., fungal, mycobacterial)
• Drug-induced: bleomycin, busulfan, methotrexate, chlorambucil, cyclophosphamide, BCNU (carmustine), gold salts, tetrazolium chloride, amiodarone, tocainide, penicillin, zidovudine, sulfonamide
• Radiation pneumonitis
• Connective tissue diseases: SLE, rheumatoid arthritis, dermatomyositis
• Idiopathic pulmonary fibrosis: bronchiolitis obliterans, interstitial pneumonitis, DIP
• Infections: viral pneumonia, *Pneumocystis* pneumonia
• Others: Wegener's granulomatosis, Goodpasture's syndrome, eosinophilic granuloma, lymphangitic carcinomatosis, chronic uremia, chronic gastric aspiration, hypersensitivity pneumonitis, lipoid pneumonia, lymphoma, lymphoid granulomatosis

DIAGNOSIS

DIFFERENTIAL DIAGNOSIS

• CHF
• Chronic renal failure
• Lymphangitic carcinomatosis
• Sarcoidosis
• Allergic alveolitis

WORKUP

Chest x-ray, ABGs, PFTs, bronchoscopy with bronchioloalveolar lavage, biopsy, laboratory evaluation
• Pulmonary function testing: findings are generally consistent with restrictive disease (decreased VC, TLC, and diffusing capacity).
• Bronchoscopy with bronchioloalveolar lavage may be useful to characterize the pulmonary inflammatory response; the effector cell population in patients with interstitial lung disease consists of two major cell types:
  1. Lymphocytes (e.g., sarcoidosis, berylliosis, silicosis, hypersensitive pneumonitis)
  2. Neutrophils (e.g., asbestosis, collagen-vascular disease, idiopathic pulmonary fibrosis)
• Open lung biopsy or transbronchial biopsy is useful to identify the underlying disease process and exclude neoplastic involvement; transbronchial biopsy is less invasive but provides less tissue for analysis (this factor may be important in patients with irregular pulmonary involvement).

LABORATORY TESTS

• ABGs provide only limited information; initially ABGs may be normal but with progression of the disease, hypoxemia may be present.
• Antineutrophil cytoplasmic antibody (c-ANCA) is frequently positive in Wegener's granulomatosis.
• Antiglomerular basement membrane (anti-GBM) and antipulmonary basement membrane antibody are often present in Goodpasture's syndrome.
• Pulmonary function testing: findings are generally consistent with restrictive disease (decreased VC, TLC, and diffusing capacity).
• Bronchoscopy with bronchioloalveolar lavage is useful to characterize the pulmonary inflammatory response; the effector cell population in patients with interstitial lung disease consists of two major cell types:
  1. Lymphocytes (e.g., sarcoidosis, berylliosis, silicosis, hypersensitive pneumonitis)
  2. Neutrophils (e.g., asbestosis, collagen-vascular disease, idiopathic pulmonary fibrosis)

IMAGING STUDIES

Chest x-ray may be normal in 10% of patients.
• Ground-glass appearance is often an early finding.
• A coarse reticular pattern is usually a late finding.
• CHF causing interstitial changes on chest x-ray must always be ruled out.
• Differential diagnosis of interstitial patterns include the following: pulmonary fibrosis, pulmonary edema, PCP, TB, sarcoidosis, eosinophilic granuloma, pneumoconiosis, and lymphangitic spread of carcinoma.
• Gallium-67 scanning plays a limited role in the evaluation of interstitial lung disease because it is not specific and a negative result does not exclude the disease (e.g., patients with end-stage fibrosis may have a negative scan).

TREATMENT

NONPHARMACOLOGIC THERAPY

Avoidance of tobacco and removal of any other offending agent (e.g., environmental exposure)

ACUTE GENERAL Rx

• Treatment of infectious process with appropriate antibiotic therapy
• Supplemental oxygen in patients with significant hypoxemia
• Corticosteroids in symptomatic patients with sarcoidosis
• Immunosuppressive therapy in selected cases (e.g., cyclophosphamide in patients with Wegener's granulomatosis)
• Treatment of any complications (e.g., pneumothorax, pulmonary embolism)

DISPOSITION

Overall mortality is 50% within 5 yr of diagnosis.

REFERRAL

• Surgical referral for biopsy
• Pulmonary referral for bronchoscopy and bronchoalveolar lavage (selected patients)
• Consider lung transplantation in selected patients with intractable end-stage ILD

PEARLS & CONSIDERATIONS

COMMENTS

Although open lung biopsy is the gold standard for diagnosis, it may be inappropriate in elderly patients; therefore individual consideration is advisable.
Author: **Fred F. Ferri, M.D.**

BASIC INFORMATION

■ DEFINITION
Acute or chronic consumption of digitalis leading to signs and symptoms of toxicity. May occur when serum levels are within the therapeutic range.

■ SYNONYMS
Cardiac glycosides: clinically available forms are digoxin and digitoxin

ICD-9CM CODES
972.1 Digitalis overdose

■ PHARMACOKINETICS
• Steady state levels (not peak levels) correlate with toxicity; digoxin reaches steady state 6 hr after ingestion

BIOAVAILABILITY: (1) digoxin about 80%, (2) digitoxin about 100%
VOLUME OF DISTRIBUTION: (1) digoxin 5 to 7 L/kg, (2) digitoxin 0.6 L/kg
HALF-LIFE: (1) digoxin 36 hr, (2) digitoxin 5 to 7 days
EXCRETION: (1) digoxin predominantly renal, (2) digitoxin predominantly hepatic
THERAPEUTIC LEVEL: (1) digoxin 0.8 to 2 ng/ml, (2) digitoxin 10 to 30 ng/ml

■ EPIDEMIOLOGY & DEMOGRAPHICS
• Digitalis toxicity occurs in up to 5% of individuals on therapy.

• Factors that potentiate toxicity: advanced age, renal insufficiency, cardiac disease, drugs that affect elimination (amiodarone, quinidine, verapamil, diltiazem, captopril, spironolactone, cyclosporine, erythromycin, clarithromycin, tetracyclines, indomethacin), coingestion of cardiotoxic drugs (β-blockers, calcium channel blockers, tricyclic antidepressants), hypokalemia, hypomagnesemia, hypercalcemia, hypoxemia, hypothyroidism, and volume depletion.

■ PHYSICAL FINDINGS & CLINICAL PRESENTATION
Cardiac, gastrointestinal, and central nervous systems are affected. Fatigue and weakness are common complaints.
CARDIAC
Any dysrhythmia; most frequent are AV junctional block and increased ventricular automaticity
GI
Anorexia, nausea, vomiting, diarrhea, abdominal pain
CNS
Headache, dizziness, visual disturbance (scotoma, blurred vision, change in color perception, decreased visual acuity), confusion, hallucinations, delirium.

■ ETIOLOGY
Cardiac glycosides reversibly inhibit the function of the sodium-potassium ATPase pump that increases myocardial contractility. Toxicity causes:

• **AV Block** by the following effects on the AV node:
1. Decreased conduction velocity
2. Increased refractory period
• **Extrasystoles and tachyarrhythmias** by the following effects on the atria and ventricles:
1. Increased automaticity
2. Increased excitability
3. Decreased conduction velocity
4. Decreased refractoriness

DIAGNOSIS

■ DIFFERENTIAL DIAGNOSIS
• β-Blockers
• Calcium channel blockers
• Clonidine
• Cyclic antidepressants
• Encainide and flecainide
• Procainamide
• Propoxyphene
• Quinidine
• Plants producing glycosides similar to digitalis (foxglove, oleander, lily of the valley)

■ WORKUP
History, physical examination, laboratory tests

■ LABORATORY TESTS
• Stat digoxin or digitoxin levels (may not correlate with severity of intoxication in acute ingestion)
• Electrolytes, BUN, creatinine, magnesium
• ECG (Figs. 1-89 and 1-90)

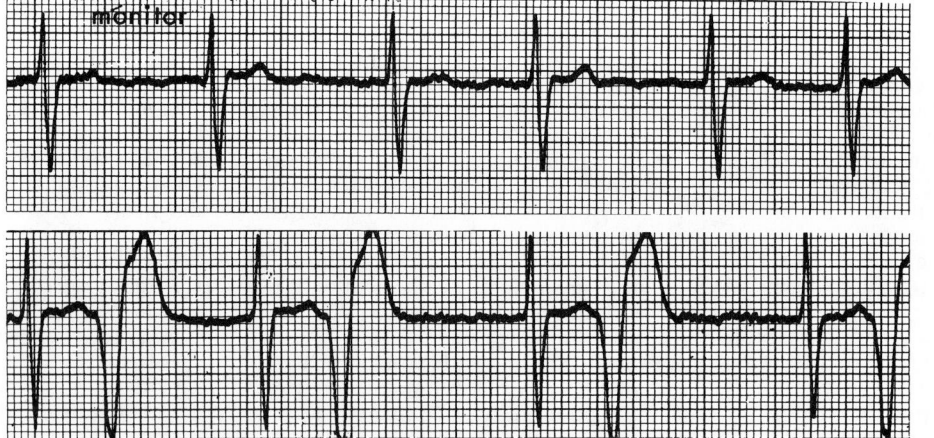

Fig. 1-89   Ventricular bigeminy caused by digitalis toxicity. Ventricular ectopy is one of the most common signs of digitalis toxicity. The underlying rhythm in **(A)** is atrial fibrillation. In **(B)** each normal QRS is followed by a VPB. (From Goldberger AL [ed]: *Clinical electrocardiography,* ed 5, St Louis, 1994, Mosby.)

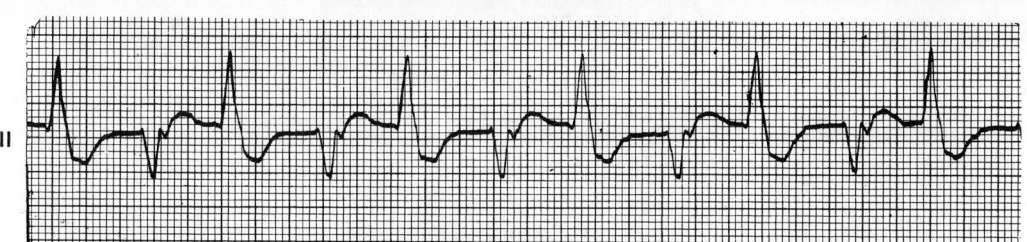

Fig. 1-90   This digitalis-toxic arrhythmia is a special type of ventricular tachycardia (bidirectional tachycardia) with QRS complexes that alternate in direction from beat to beat. No P waves are present. (From Goldberger AL [ed]: *Clinical electrocardiography,* ed 5, St Louis, 1994, Mosby.)

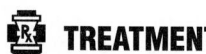 **TREATMENT**

■ **NONPHARMACOLOGIC THERAPY**
- Ensure adequate airway
- ECG monitor for 12 to 24 hr after ingestion

■ **ACUTE GENERAL Rx**
DECREASE TOXICITY:
- Acute toxicity: Activated charcoal if within 1 hr of ingestion, multiple doses may be indicated for digitoxin intoxication (because of significant enterohepatic circulation). Gastric emptying considered for massive acute overdose presenting <1 hr after ingestion.
- Treat hypokalemia and hypomagnesemia. Follow potassium level closely; hyperkalemia can increase AV block, and in acute intoxication, patients may develop hyperkalemia.
- Fab fragments of digoxin-specific antibodies (Digibind):
  1. Specific antibodies that bind to digoxin and to a lesser extent digitoxin and other cardiac glycosides
  2. Initial response usually seen in 30 min, and complete reversal usually occurs within 4 hr
  3. Indications: hyperkalemia (≥5 mEq/L), life-threatening arrhythmia, massive overdose (acute ingestion of ≥10 mg digoxin or digoxin serum level ≥10 ng/ml 6 hr postingestion), coingestion of cardiotoxic drugs or plants containing cardiac glycosides
  4. Dosing: 1 vial (38 mg) of Fab fragments binds 0.5 mg of digoxin or digitoxin

   a. Digoxin **Acute ingestion:** number of vials = [(ingested digoxin mg × 0.8]/ 0.5 **Chronic ingestion:** number of vials = [(serum digoxin level ng/ml) × weight kg]/100

   b. Digitoxin **Acute ingestion:** number of vials = (ingested digitoxin mg)/ 0.5 **Chronic ingestion:** number of vials = [(serum digitoxin level ng/ml) × weight kg]/1000

   c. If neither the amount ingested nor serum level are known, treat empirically:
- acute intoxication—10 vials and repeat if needed
- chronic toxicity—6 vials

5. After use of Fab fragments the digoxin level is falsely elevated; accurate measurement of free digoxin level can be obtained by fluorescence polarization assay of protein-free ultrafiltrate
6. Inactive complex excreted in urine, half-life of complex is 15 to 20 hr. In renal failure, consider plasma exchange (within 3 hr) to remove Fab-digoxin complex; theoretically, complexes may dissociate before excretion
7. Class C for pregnancy
8. Adverse effects of treatment: May undo desirable action of drug and exacerbate heart failure and increase ventricular response in previously controlled atrial fibrillation, hypokalemia, hypersensitivity reaction, and serum sickness
9. Hemodialysis and hemoperfusion: not useful because of extensive tissue binding and large volume of distribution

COMPLICATIONS:
Hyperkalemia:
- Sodium bicarbonate
- Glucose and insulin
- Sodium polystyrene sulfonate (Kayexalate)
- Do not use calcium because it may worsen ventricular arrhythmias
Bradycardia and heart block:
- Atropine
- Temporary pacemaker if symptomatic
Supraventricular and ventricular tachycardia:
- Lidocaine or phenytoin: decrease ventricular automaticity without significantly slowing AV node conduction
- Avoid quinidine, bretylium, procainamide, and verapamil; may increase ventricular arrhythmias/AV node block
- Elective cardioversion is contraindicated, because it may precipitate ventricular fibrillation.

■ **DISPOSITION**
- Good with prompt treatment
- Chronic poisoning is associated with higher mortality than acute poisoning

REFERENCE

Marx JA: *Rosen's emergency medicine: concepts and clinical practice,* ed 5, St Louis, 2002, Mosby.
Author: **Sudeep K. Aulakh, M.D., F.R.C.P.C**

BASIC INFORMATION

■ DEFINITION
Diphtheria is an infection of the mucous membranes or skin caused by *Corynebacterium diphtheriae*.

■ ICD-9CM CODES
032.9 Diphtheria

■ EPIDEMIOLOGY & DEMOGRAPHICS
INCIDENCE (IN U.S.):
- Fewer than 5 cases/yr since 1980 (<0.002 cases/100,000 persons)
- Last culture-confirmed indigenous case in 1988

PREDOMINANT AGE: Adult years

■ PHYSICAL FINDINGS & CLINICAL PRESENTATION
RESPIRATORY DIPHTHERIA:
- Commonly presenting as pharyngitis, but any part of the respiratory tract may be involved, including the nasopharynx, larynx, trachea, or bronchi
- Areas of gray or white exudate coalescing to form a "pseudomembrane" that bleeds when removed
- Possible fever and dysphagia
- Complications: respiratory tract obstruction and pneumonia
- Systemic effects of the toxin: myocarditis and polyneuritis (frequently involving a bulbar distribution)
- Occurs mostly in nonimmune individuals; usually milder and less likely to be complicated in those adequately immunized

CUTANEOUS DIPHTHERIA:
- Usually complicates existing skin lesion (i.e., impetigo or scabies)
- Resembles the underlying condition

■ ETIOLOGY
- Caused by *C. diphtheriae,* an aerobic, gram-positive rod
- Transmitted by close contact through droplets of nasopharyngeal secretions
- Symptomatic disease of the respiratory system caused by toxin-producing strains (tox⁺)
- Systemic effects of toxin: ranging from nausea and vomiting to polyneuropathy, myocarditis, and vascular collapse
- Presence of strains not producing toxin (tox⁻) in the respiratory tract of asymptomatic carriers and in skin lesions of cutaneous diphtheria

DIAGNOSIS

■ DIFFERENTIAL DIAGNOSIS
- *Streptococcus* pharyngitis
- Viral pharyngitis
- Mononucleosis

■ WORKUP
- Presence of a pseudomembrane in the oropharynx suggestive of diagnosis (not always present)
- Gram stains of secretions to show club-shaped organisms, which appear as "Chinese letters"
- Nasolaryngoscopy to identify lesions in the nares, nasopharynx, larynx, or tracheobronchial tree
- Electrocardiogram
- Possible ICU monitoring

■ LABORATORY TESTS
- Cultures of mucosal lesions or of nasal discharge
  1. Positive culture for *C. diphtheriae* confirms the diagnosis.
  2. Laboratory is notified of the suspected diagnosis so that appropriate culture medium (Tinsdale agar) is used.
- Testing of all isolated organisms for toxin production

■ IMAGING STUDIES
- Chest x-ray examination to rule out pneumonia
- Bronchopneumonia has been described in fatal cases

TREATMENT

■ NONPHARMACOLOGIC THERAPY
- Intubation or tracheostomy if signs of respiratory distress occur
- Nasogastric or parenteral nutrition in those with bulbar signs
- ICU monitoring for patients with signs of systemic toxicity
- Cardiac pacing in patients with heart block
- Respiratory isolation

■ ACUTE GENERAL Rx
- Administration of diphtheria antitoxin once a clinical diagnosis is made
- If tests for hypersensitivity to horse serum are negative: 50,000 U given for mild to moderate disease or 60,000 to 120,000 U for critically ill patients
- IV infusion of antitoxin over 60 min

- Serum sickness in 10% of treated individuals; those with hypersensitivity to horse serum should be desensitized before administration of antitoxin
- Antibiotics to eradicate the organism in carriers or patients
- For respiratory diphtheria:
  1. Erythromycin 500 mg qid PO or IV or IM penicillin 600,000 U bid for 14 days
  2. Carriers or patients with cutaneous disease: erythromycin 500 mg PO qid or rifampin 600 mg PO qd for 7 days

■ CHRONIC Rx
Antibiotics to limit toxin production and eradicate carrier state, thereby preventing transmission

■ DISPOSITION
Complete recovery with adequate supportive measures and antitoxin

■ REFERRAL
- Hospitalization and referral to an infectious disease specialist for all suspected patients
- To an otolaryngologist for evaluation in cases of respiratory diphtheria
- All cases reported to the public health authorities

☼ PEARLS & CONSIDERATIONS

■ COMMENTS
- Most cases are imported by travelers in epidemic areas, so recent epidemics in Europe are a cause for concern. A widespread epidemic of diphtheria began in 1990 in the former Soviet Union.
- Vaccination with diphtheria toxoid (attenuated toxin) is safe and effective in the form of DPT or Td; Td boosters should be given to adults every 10 yr.
- According to serologic studies, 20% to 60% of U.S. adults >20 yr of age are susceptible to diphtheria.

REFERENCES
Bisgard KM et al: Respiratory diphtheria in the United States: 1980 through 1995, *Am J Pub Health* 88:787, 1998.
Hadfield TL et al: The pathology of diphtheria, *J Infect Dis* 181:s116, 2000.
Markina SS et al: Diphtheria in the Russian Federation in the 1990s, *J Infect Dis* 181 (Suppl 1):S27, 2000.
Author: **Maurice Policar, M.D.**

BASIC INFORMATION

■ DEFINITION
Discoid lupus erythematosus (DLE) refers to a chronic cutaneous usually localized skin disorder sometimes associated with systemic lupus erythematosus (SLE). Erythematous plaque lesions with scaling, follicular plugging, atrophy, and scarring characterize DLE.

■ SYNONYMS
Chronic cutaneous lupus erythematosus

ICD-9CM CODES
695.4 Lupus erythematosus (local discoid)

■ EPIDEMIOLOGY & DEMOGRAPHICS
- Discoid lupus is more common in African Americans.
- DLE is more common in females, with peak incidence in the fourth decade of life.
- Less than 5% of patients with DLE progress to SLE.
- Approximately 10% to 20% of patients with SLE will also have discoid lupus skin lesions.

■ PHYSICAL FINDINGS & CLINICAL PRESENTATION
History
- Appearance of single or multiple asymptomatic plaque lesions (Fig. 1-91)
Physical findings
- Anatomic distribution
  1. DLE commonly involves the scalp, face, and ears but is not limited to these areas.
- Lesion configuration
  1. Irregularly grouped

- Lesion morphology
  1. Plaque lesions with scales
  2. Follicular plugging
  3. Atrophy
  4. Scarring
  5. Telangiectasia
- Color
  1. Erythematous
  2. Red to violaceous
  3. Hyperpigmentation or hypopigmentation
- Alopecia can occur and is permanent
- Urticaria (5%)
- May be associated with other criteria for SLE (e.g., oral ulcers, arthritis, pleuritis, pericarditis)

■ ETIOLOGY
The exact cause of DLE is not known, although an immune complex mediated mechanism is thought to be responsible.

🔬 DIAGNOSIS

Clinical inspection and skin biopsy usually establish the diagnosis of DLE.

■ DIFFERENTIAL DIAGNOSIS
- Psoriasis
- Lichen planus
- Secondary syphilis
- Superficial fungal infections
- Photosensitivity eruption
- Sarcoidosis
- Subacute cutaneous lupus erythematosus
- Rosacea
- Keratoacanthoma
- Actinic keratosis
- Dermatomyositis

■ WORKUP
The workup for isolated DLE includes laboratory tests and x-rays looking for diagnostic criteria for SLE.

■ LABORATORY TESTS
Laboratory tests are done to exclude criteria for SLE. The following statements refer to patients having SLE with DLE.
- CBC is usually normal in isolated DLE.
- BUN/creatinine is normal.
- ESR is elevated in active disease associated with SLE.
- Urinalysis looking for proteinuria and hematuria.
- ANA may be positive in 20% of patients with isolated DLE.
- Anti-Ro (SS-A) autoantibodies are present in approximately 1% to 3% of patients.
- dsDNA and antiSm antibodies are rarely present.
- Complement levels may be low in patients with SLE but not in DLE.
- Skin biopsy shows degeneration of the basal cell layer with follicular plugging and atrophy of the epidermis.

■ IMAGING STUDIES
Chest x-ray examination is not specific in the diagnosis of DLE; however, it is helpful when assessing for SLE.

℞ TREATMENT

■ NONPHARMACOLOGIC THERAPY
- The goals of management are to control existing lesions and limit scarring, and to prevent development of further lesions.
- Avoid sun exposure from 10 AM to 4 PM.
- Use sunscreens with sun protective factor (SPF) of at least 15.

■ ACUTE GENERAL Rx
- Topical steroid is first-line therapy for DLE.
- Intradermal steroid triamcinolone acetonide, 3 mg/ml with 1% Xylocaine is injected into the lesion.
- Hydroxychloroquine 400 mg PO qd for 1 mo, then decrease the dose to 200 mg qd. Treatment is continued for 3 to 6 mo.

■ CHRONIC Rx
- Dapsone 100 mg/day can be used in patients who fail to respond to topical steroid or hydroxychloroquine.
- Other alternatives include
  1. Chloroquine 250-500 mg PO qd
  2. Auranofin 6 mg/day PO qd or divided bid; after 3 mo, may increase to 9 mg/day divided tid
  3. Thalidomide 100-300 mg PO hs, aq, and >1 hr pc
  4. Azathioprine 1 mg/kg/day PO for 6-8 wk, increase by 5 mg/kg q4wk until response is seen or dose reaches 2.5 mg/kg/day

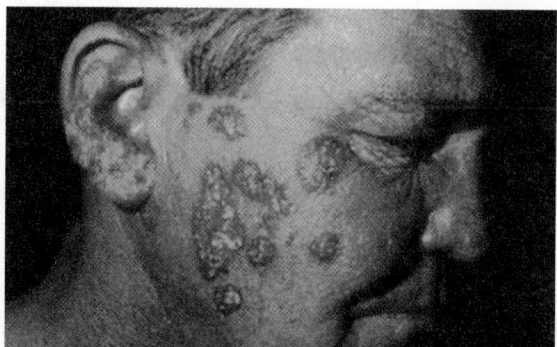

Fig. 1-91 Scaling plaques with thick scales on the ear and face of a patient who has discoid lupus. (Courtesy Department of Dermatology, University of North Carolina at Chapel Hill. In Goldstein BG, Goldstein AO [eds]: *Practical dermatology*, ed 2, St Louis, 1977, Mosby.)

5. If all of the previous treatments fail, mycophenolate 1 g PO bid or interferon ∝-2b (2 million units/m² SQ 3 times/wk for 30 days) have been tried

DISPOSITION
- If left untreated, DLE is a chronic disorder that can lead to atrophy and scarring of the skin.
- A minority of patients with isolated cutaneous DLE progress to systemic lupus erythematosus. Prognosis is better in this group than unselected SLE patients.

REFERRAL
Patients with isolated DLE involving the face and scalp should be referred to a dermatologist. If associated with SLE, a rheumatology consultation is recommended.

☼ PEARLS & CONSIDERATIONS

COMMENTS
- Cutaneous lesions account for 4 of the 11 criteria in the diagnosis of SLE (e.g., malar rash, discoid rash, photosensitivity, and oral ulcers).
- Cutaneous lupus erythematosus is classified as:
  1. Chronic cutaneous lupus erythematosus (discoid lupus is included in this category)
  2. Subacute cutaneous lupus erythematosus
  3. Acute cutaneous lupus erythematosus
- DLE lesions are not as photosensitive as the subacute cutaneous lesions.
- Rarely does DLE degenerate into a malignant nonmelanotic skin cancer.

REFERENCES
Callen JP: Collagen vascular diseases, *Med Clin North Am* 82(6):1217, 1998.
Callen JP: Lupus erythematosus, discoid *e* Medicine Journal, 2(11) 2001 (www.emedicine.com).
Jessop S, Whitelaw D, Jordaan F: Drugs for discoid lupus erythematosus, *Cochrane Database Syst Rev* (1):C0002954, 2001.
Werth V: Current treatment of cutaneous lupus erythematosus, *Dermatology Online Journal* 7(1):2, 2001.
Author: **Peter Petropoulos, M.D.**

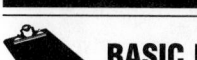

BASIC INFORMATION

■ DEFINITION
Disseminated intravascular coagulation (DIC) is an acquired thromboembolic disorder characterized by generalized activation of the clotting mechanism, which results in the intravascular formation of fibrin and ultimately thrombotic occlusion of small and midsize vessels.

■ SYNONYMS
Consumptive coagulopathy
DIC
Defibrination syndrome

ICD-9CM CODES
286.6 Disseminated intravascular coagulation

■ EPIDEMIOLOGY & DEMOGRAPHICS
Greater than 50% of cases are associated with gram-negative sepsis or other septicemic infections.

■ PHYSICAL FINDINGS & CLINICAL PRESENTATION
• Wound site bleeding, epistaxis, gingival bleeding, hemorrhagic bullae
• Petechiae, ecchymosis, purpura
• Dyspnea, localized rales, delirium
• Oliguria, anuria, GI bleeding, metrorrhagia

■ ETIOLOGY
• Infections (e.g., gram-negative sepsis, Rocky Mountain spotted fever, malaria, viral or fungal infection)
• Obstetric complications (e.g., dead fetus, amniotic fluid embolism, toxemia, abruptio placentae, septic abortion, eclampsia)
• Tissue trauma (e.g., burns, hypothermia-rewarming)
• Neoplasms (e.g., adenocarcinomas [GI, prostate, lung, breast], acute promyelocytic leukemia)
• Quinine, cocaine-induced rhabdomyolysis
• Liver failure
• Acute pancreatitis
• Transfusion reactions
• Respiratory distress syndrome
• Other: SLE, vasculitis, aneurysms, polyarteritis, cavernous hemangiomas

DIAGNOSIS

■ DIFFERENTIAL DIAGNOSIS
• Hepatic necrosis: normal or elevated Factor VIII concentrations
• Vitamin K deficiency: normal platelet count
• Hemolytic uremic syndrome
• Thrombocytopenic purpura
• Renal failure, SLE, sickle cell crisis, dysfibrinogenemias

■ WORKUP
Diagnostic workup includes laboratory screening to confirm the diagnosis and exclude conditions noted in the differential diagnosis.

■ LABORATORY TESTS
• Peripheral blood smear generally shows RBC fragments and low platelet count.
• Coagulation factors are consumed at a rate in excess of the capacity of the liver to synthesize them, and platelets are consumed in excess of the capacity of the bone marrow megakaryocytes to release them. Diagnostic characteristics of DIC are increased PT, PTT, TT, fibrin split products, d-dimer; decreased fibrinogen level, thrombocytopenia.
• Coagulopathy secondary to DIC must be differentiated from that secondary to liver disease or vitamin K deficiency.
  1. Vitamin K deficiency manifests with prolonged PT and normal PTT, TT, platelet, and fibrinogen level; PTT may be elevated in severe cases.
  2. Patients with liver disease have abnormal PT and PTT; TT and fibrinogen are usually normal unless severe disease is present; platelets are usually normal unless splenomegaly is present.
  3. Factors V and VIII are low in DIC, but they are normal in liver disease with coagulopathy.

■ IMAGING STUDIES
Imaging studies are generally not useful. Chest x-ray examination may be helpful to exclude infectious processes in patients presenting with pulmonary symptoms such as dyspnea, cough, or hemoptysis.

TREATMENT

■ NONPHARMACOLOGIC THERAPY
No specific precautions regarding activity level are necessary unless thrombocytopenia is severe.

■ ACUTE GENERAL Rx
• Correct and eliminate underlying cause (e.g., antimicrobial therapy for infection).
• Give replacement therapy with FFP and platelets in patients with significant hemorrhage:
  1. FFP 10 to 15 ml/kg can be given with a goal of normalizing INR.
  2. Platelet transfusions are given when platelet count is <10,000 (or higher if major bleeding is present).
  3. Cryoprecipitate 1 U/5 kg is reserved for hypofibrinogen states.
  4. Antithrombin III treatment may be considered as a supportive therapeutic option in patients with severe DIC. Its modest results and substantial cost are limiting factors.
• Heparin therapy at a dose lower than that used in venous thrombosis (300 to 500 U/hr) may be useful in selected cases to increase neutralization of thrombin (e.g., DIC associated with acute promyelocytic leukemia, purpura fulminans, acral ischemia).

■ CHRONIC Rx
Follow-up management includes coagulation screening to assess factor replacement therapy. Laboratory abnormalities generally correct with treatment of the underlying disorder. Chronic laboratory monitoring is not required.

■ DISPOSITION
Mortality in severe DIC exceeds 75%. Death generally results from progression of the underlying disease and complications such as acute renal failure, intracerebral hematoma, shock, or cardiac tamponade.

■ REFERRAL
Hematology consultation is recommended in all cases of DIC.

PEARLS & CONSIDERATIONS

■ COMMENTS
The treatment of chronic DIC is controversial. Low-dose SC heparin and/or combination antiplatelet agents such as aspirin and dipyridamole may be useful.
Author: **Fred F. Ferri, M.D.**

BASIC INFORMATION

■ DEFINITION
- Colonic diverticula are herniations of mucosa and submucosa through the muscularis. They are generally found along the colon's mesenteric border at the site where the vasa recta penetrates the muscle wall (anatomic weak point).
- *Diverticulosis* is the asymptomatic presence of multiple colonic diverticula.
- *Diverticulitis* is an inflammatory process or localized perforation of diverticulum.

ICD-9CM CODES
562.10 Diverticulosis of colon
562.11 Diverticulitis of colon

■ EPIDEMIOLOGY & DEMOGRAPHICS
- Incidence of diverticulosis in the general population is 35% to 50%.
- Diverticulosis is more common in Western countries, affecting >30% of people >40 yr and >50% of people >70 yr.

■ PHYSICAL FINDINGS & CLINICAL PRESENTATION
- Physical examination in patients with diverticulosis is generally normal.
- Painful diverticular disease can present with LLQ pain, often relieved by defecation; location of pain may be anywhere in the lower abdomen because of the redundancy of the sigmoid colon.
- Diverticulitis can cause muscle spasm, guarding, and rebound tenderness predominantly affecting the LLQ.

■ ETIOLOGY
- Diverticular disease is believed to be secondary to low intake of dietary fiber.

DIAGNOSIS

■ DIFFERENTIAL DIAGNOSIS
- Irritable bowel syndrome
- IBD
- Carcinoma of colon
- Endometriosis
- Ischemic colitis
- Infections (pseudomembranous colitis, appendicitis, pyelonephritis, PID)
- Lactose intolerance

■ LABORATORY TESTS
- WBC count in diverticulitis reveals leukocytosis with left shift.
- Microcytic anemia can be present in patients with chronic bleeding from diverticular disease. MCV may be elevated in acute bleeding secondary to reticulocytosis.

■ IMAGING STUDIES
- Barium enema will demonstrate multiple diverticula and muscle spasm ("sawtooth" appearance of the lumen) in patients with painful diverticular disease. Barium enema can be hazardous and should not be performed in the acute stage of diverticulitis because it may produce free perforation.
- A CT scan of the abdomen can be used to diagnose acute diverticulitis; typical findings are thickening of the bowel wall, fistulas, or abscess formation.
- Evaluation of suspected diverticular bleeding:
  1. Arteriography if the bleeding is faster than 1 ml/min (advantage: the possible infusion of vasopressin directly into the arteries supplying the bleeding, as well as selective arterial embolization; disadvantages: its cost and invasive nature)
  2. Technetium-99m sulfa colloid
  3. Technetium-99m labeled RBC (can detect bleeding rates as low as 0.12 to 5 ml/min)

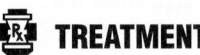

TREATMENT

■ NONPHARMACOLOGIC THERAPY
- Increase in dietary fiber intake and regular exercise to improve bowel function
- NPO and IV hydration in severe diverticulitis; NG suction if ileus or small bowel obstruction is present

■ ACUTE GENERAL Rx
TREATMENT OF DIVERTICULITIS:
- Mild case: broad-spectrum PO antibiotics (e.g., Ciprofloxacin 500 mg bid to cover aerobic component of colonic flora and metronidazole 500 mg q6h for anaerobes) and liquid diet for 7 to 10 days
- Severe case: NPO and aggressive IV antibiotic therapy
  a. Ampicillin-sulbactam (Unasyn) 3 g IV q6h *or*
  b. Piperacillin-tazobactam (Zosyn) 4.5 g IV q8h *or*
  c. Ciprofloxacin 400 mg IV q12h plus metronidazole 500 mg IV q6h *or*
  d. Cefoxitin 2 g IV q8h plus metronidazole 500 mg IV q6h
- Life-threatening case: Imipenem 500 mg IV q6h *or* meropenem 1 g IV q8h
- Surgical treatment consisting of resection of involved areas and reanastomosis (if feasible); otherwise a diverting colostomy with reanastomosis performed when infection has been controlled; surgery should be considered in patients with:
  1. Repeated episodes of diverticulitis (two or more)
  2. Poor response to appropriate medical therapy (failure of conservative management)
  3. Abscess or fistula formation
  4. Obstruction
  5. Peritonitis
  6. Immunocompromised patients, first episode in young patient (<40 yr old)
  7. Inability to exclude carcinoma (10% to 20% of patients diagnosed with diverticulosis on clinical grounds are subsequently found to have carcinoma of the colon)

DIVERTICULAR HEMORRHAGE: 70% of diverticular bleeding occurs in the right colon.
1. Bleeding is painless and stops spontaneously in the majority of patients (60%); it is usually caused by erosion of a blood vessel by a fecalith present within the diverticular sac.
2. Medical therapy consists of blood replacement and correction of volume and any clotting abnormalities.
3. Colonoscopic treatment with epinephrine injections, bipolar coagulation, or both may prevent recurrent bleeding and decrease the need for surgery.
4. Surgical resection is necessary if bleeding does not stop spontaneously after administration of 4 to 5 U of PRBCs or recurs with severity within a few days; if attempts at localization are unsuccessful, total abdominal colectomy with ileoproctostomy may be indicated (high incidence of rebleeding if segmental resection is performed without adequate localization).

■ CHRONIC Rx
Asymptomatic patients with diverticulosis can be treated with a high-fiber diet or fiber supplements.

■ DISPOSITION
- Most patients with diverticulitis respond well to antibiotic management and bowel rest. Up to 30% of patients with diverticulitis will eventually require surgical management.
- Diverticular bleeding can recur in 15% to 20% of patients within 5 yr.

■ REFERRAL
Surgical referral when considering resection (see Acute General Rx)
Author: **Fred F. Ferri, M.D.**

BASIC INFORMATION

■ DEFINITION
Down syndrome is a chromosomal abnormality causing mental retardation and multiple organ defects.

■ SYNONYMS
Trisomy 21

ICD-9CM CODES
758.0 Down Syndrome

■ EPIDEMIOLOGY & DEMOGRAPHICS
INCIDENCE (IN U.S.): 1 in 800 births
PREVALENCE (IN U.S.): 300,000 persons
PREDOMINANT SEX: Male:female ratio of 1.3:1.0
PREDOMINANT AGE: Newborn to early adulthood
PEAK INCIDENCE: Newborn
GENETICS: Nondisjunction causing trisomy 21
PHYSICAL FINDINGS: (SEE FIG. 1-92)
- Microcephaly
- Flattening of occiput and face
- Upward slant to eyes with epicanthal folds
- Brushfield spots in iris
- Broad stocky neck
- Small feet, hands, digits
- Single palmar crease

- Associated with congenital heart disease, malformations of the GI tract, cataracts, hypothyroidism, hip dysplasia

■ ETIOLOGY
Nondisjunction of chromosome 21

DIAGNOSIS

- Prenatal cytogenic diagnosis by amniocentesis or chorionic villus sampling
- Combined use of serum screening and fetal ultrasound testing for thickened nuchal fold has 80% detection rate with 5% false positives
- Postnatal chromosomal karyotype

TREATMENT

- Treatment consists of vigilant monitoring for comorbid states, such as obesity, hypothyroidism, leukemia, hearing loss, and valvular heart disease
- Thyroid screen at birth, at age 6 mo, and yearly thereafter
- Prevention of obesity with low-calorie, high-fiber diet
- Monitoring for hematologic problems

- Auditory brainstem responses in all newborns and aggressive testing for hearing loss in children with chronic otitis media
- Echocardiogram in all newborns and cardiac assessment of adolescents for development of mitral valve prolapse
- Ophthalmologic assessment by age 6 mo for congenital cataracts and annual exams for monitoring of refractive errors and strabismus
- Regular dental care

■ REFERRAL
Down syndrome clinics use a preventive checklist to anticipate many clinical challenges.

■ COMMENTS
- Screening for atlantoaxial subluxation is controversial.
- Most patients develop neuropathologic changes typical of Alzheimer's disease. If suspected, screen for treatable diseases such as depression or hypothyroidism.
- This disease accounts for approximately one third of moderate to severe cases of mental retardation.
- Though increased maternal age is a risk factor, most children with Down syndrome are born to women under the age of 35 yr.

REFERENCES
Racial disparities in median age at death of persons with Down syndrome–United States, 1968-97, *MMWR* 50:463, 2001.
Roizen NJ, Patterson D: Down syndrome, *Lancet* 361:1281, 2003.
Author: **Maitreyi Mazumdar, M.D.**

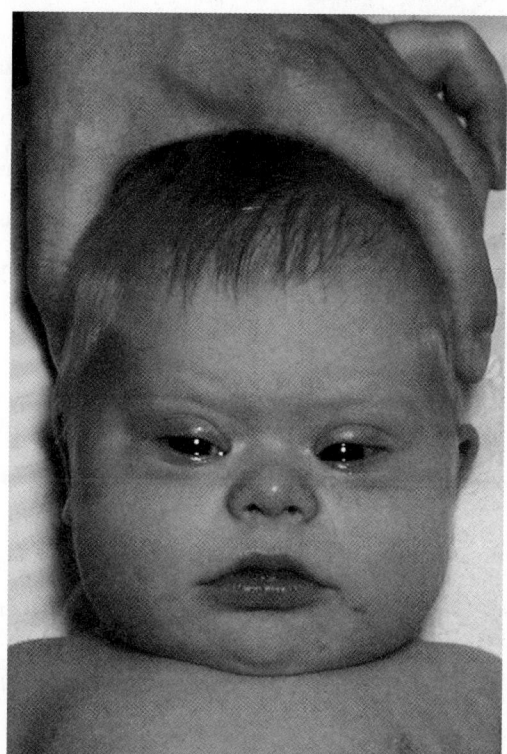

Fig. 1-92 **Down syndrome.** Note depressed nasal bridge, epicanthal folds, mongoloid slant of eyes, low-set ears, and large tongue. (From Zitelli BJ, Davis HW: *Atlas of pediatric physical diagnosis,* ed 3, St Louis, 1997, Mosby.)

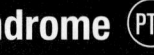
 BASIC INFORMATION

■ **DEFINITION**

Dumping syndrome refers to the constellation of postprandial symptoms as a result of rapid delivery of stomach contents into the small bowel seen after definitive surgery for peptic ulcer disease.

■ **SYNONYMS**

Early postgastrectomy syndrome

ICD-9CM CODES

564.2 Postgastric surgery syndromes

■ **EPIDEMIOLOGY & DEMOGRAPHICS**

Incidence is 10% of all patients having gastric surgery.
• Vagotomy and pyloroplasty (8.5% to 20%)
• Vagotomy and antrectomy (4% to 27%)
• Subtotal gastrectomy (10% to 40%)
• Parietal cell vagotomy (3% to 5%)
• Affects males and females equally

■ **PHYSICAL FINDINGS & CLINICAL PRESENTATION**

Early dumping
• Symptoms start within 1 hr after eating food
• No symptoms in fasting state
• Nausea, vomiting, and belching
• Epigastric fullness, cramping, and diarrhea
• Dizziness, flushing, diaphoresis, and syncope
• Palpitations and tachycardia
Late dumping
• Symptoms occurring 1 to 3 hr after eating
• Diaphoresis
• Irritability
• Difficulty concentrating
• Tremulous

■ **ETIOLOGY**

Dumping syndrome occurs almost exclusively in patients having gastric surgery.
• Systemic symptoms are thought to be due to hypovolemia caused by rapid shifts of fluid from the intravascular space into the lumen of the bowel.
• Increase in vasoactive substances is thought to play a role in dumping syndrome.
• Late dumping symptoms are thought to be due to reactive hypoglycemia.

 DIAGNOSIS

A detailed clinical history and evidence of prior gastric surgery usually makes the diagnosis of dumping syndrome. Oral glucose challenge test and radiographic imaging studies aid in establishing the diagnosis.

■ **DIFFERENTIAL DIAGNOSIS**

• Pancreatic insufficiency
• Inflammatory bowel disease
• Afferent loop syndromes
• Bile acid reflux after surgery
• Bowel obstruction
• Gastroenteric fistula

■ **WORKUP**

Typically the diagnosis is made on clinical grounds. In certain clinical settings (e.g., symptoms in patients with no prior history of gastric surgery), a workup, including oral glucose challenge and imaging studies, may be pursued.

■ **LABORATORY TESTS**

Oral glucose challenge test:
• Oral intake of 50 g of glucose is followed by serial measurements of heart rate, serum glucose, and hydrogen breath test every 15 min for 6 hr.
• An increase in the heart rate >12 beats/min and a rise in hydrogen breath excretion had a sensitivity of 94% and specificity >92%. A nadir blood glucose <3.3 mmol/L was present in 75% of late dumpers.

■ **IMAGING STUDIES**

• Upper GI series properly defines anatomy.
• Scintigraphic imaging documents rapid gastric emptying and may be useful in patients with dumping syndrome and no prior history of gastric surgery.

 TREATMENT

■ **NONPHARMACOLOGIC THERAPY**

• Diet modification
1. Divide calorie intake over six small meals
2. Limit fluid intake with meals (try to avoid 30 min before meals)
3. Decrease carbohydrate intake and avoid simple sugars
4. Increase/supplement dietary fibers
5. Avoid milk/milk products

■ **ACUTE GENERAL Rx**

• Acarbose 50 mg PO qd can be tried if dietary modification does not help.
• Octreotide 25 to 50 μg SC 30 min before meals is effective in relieving symptoms of dumping syndrome.

■ **CHRONIC Rx**

• Surgery is considered in patients with severe symptoms refractory to the above mentioned dietary and acute general treatment.
• Surgical procedures include: reconstruction of the pylorus, converting Billroth II to a Billroth I anastomosis, and a Roux-en-Y reconstruction.

■ **DISPOSITION**

• Dumping syndrome improves with time. Approximately 1% to 2% of patients will continue to have significant symptoms several months after surgery.
• Dietary modification effectively treats the majority of patients.

■ **REFERRAL**

• A GI consult is recommended in patients suspected of having dumping syndrome.
• If medical management is unsuccessful, a general surgical consultation is warranted.

PEARLS & CONSIDERATIONS

■ **COMMENTS**

• The majority of patients usually manifest with early dumping symptoms or combination of early and late symptoms. Few have late dumping symptoms alone.
• Octreotide has an inhibitory effect on the release of insulin and other vasoactive substances released by the gut. It also works by decreasing gastric emptying.

REFERENCES

Li-Ling J, Irving M: Therapeutic value of octreotide for patients with severe dumping syndrome: a review of randomized controlled trials, *Postgrad Med J* 77(909):441, 2001.
Vecht J, Masclee AAM, Lamers CBHW: The dumping syndrome: current insights into pathophysiology, diagnosis and treatment, *Scand J Gastroenterol* 32 (223):21, 1997.
Authors: **Hemchand Ramberan, M.D., and Peter Petropoulos, M.D.**

BASIC INFORMATION

■ DEFINITION
Dupuytren's contracture is a disease of the palmar fascia characterized by nodular fibroblastic proliferation that often results in progressive contractures of the fascia and flexion deformity of the fingers.

ICD-9CM CODES
728.6 Dupuytren's contracture

■ EPIDEMIOLOGY & DEMOGRAPHICS
PREVALENCE: Varies depending on nationality
PREVALENT AGE: 40 to 60 yr
PREVALENT SEX: Male:female ratio of 10:1

■ PHYSICAL FINDINGS & CLINICAL PRESENTATION
- Usually asymptomatic
- Most common complaints: deformity and interference with the use of the hand by the flexed, contracted fingers (Fig. 1-93)
- Process usually begins in the ulnar side of the hand, often starting at the ring finger
- Isolated painless nodules that eventually harden and mature into a longitudinal cord that extends into the finger
- Lesion often begins in the distal palmar crease
- Overlying skin adherent to the fascia
- Later stages: fibrous cord begins to contract and pull the finger into flexion
- Possible involvement of other fingers, particularly small finger

■ ETIOLOGY
Unknown

DIAGNOSIS

■ DIFFERENTIAL DIAGNOSIS
Soft tissue tumor, tendon cyst

TREATMENT

■ NONPHARMACOLOGIC THERAPY
- Stretching exercises
- Local heat

■ DISPOSITION
Rate of development is variable.

■ REFERRAL
- If joint contracture begins to develop
- For excision of rare nodule that is painful (at any stage)

PEARLS & CONSIDERATIONS

■ COMMENTS
- Dupuytren's contracture develops earlier and more often in certain families.
- The disorder is more common in Scandinavians, and some Northern Europeans have a 25% prevalence over age 60 yr.
- About 5% of patients develop a similar condition elsewhere, such as Peyronie's disease or Ledderhose disease (involvement of the plantar fascia).
- Soft tissue "pads" in the knuckles may also be present.
- Individuals with these additional findings are considered to have Dupuytren's diathesis, and their disease is generally more severe and recurrent.

REFERENCES
Frank PL: An update on Dupuytren's contracture, *Hosp Med* 62:678, 2001.
McFarlane RM: On the origin and spread of Dupuytren's disease, *J Hand Surg* 27:385, 2002.
Ragsowansi RH, Britto JA: Genetic and epigenetic influence on the pathogenesis of Dupuytren's disease, *J Hand Surg* 26:1157, 2001.
Author: **Lonnie R. Mercier, M.D.**

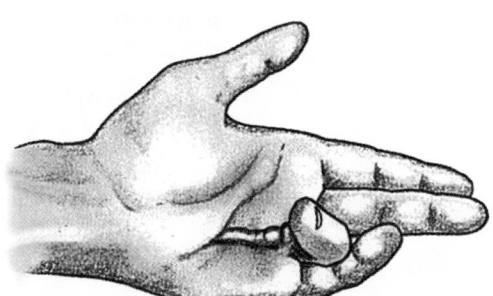

Fig. 1-93 Dupuytren's contracture. A flexion deformity of the finger is present, with nodular thickening of the fascia to the ring finger.

BASIC INFORMATION

■ DEFINITION

Dysfunctional uterine bleeding (DUB) describes abnormal uterine bleeding in the absence of disease in the pelvis, pregnancy, or medical illness. Specific types of abnormal bleeding include the following:

- Hypermenorrhea: excessive bleeding in amount during normal duration of regular menstrual cycles.
- Hypomenorrhea: decreased bleeding in amount in regular menstrual cycles.
- Menorrhagia: regular normal intervals, excessive flow and duration.
- Metrorrhagia: irregular intervals, excessive flow and duration.
- Menometrorrhagia: irregular or excessive bleeding during menstruation and between periods.
- Oligomenorrhea: intervals greater than 35 days.
- Polymenorrhea: intervals less than 21 days.

■ SYNONYMS

DUB

ICD-9CM CODES

626 Disorders of menstruation and other abnormal bleeding from female genital tract
626.2 Hypermenorrhea
626.1 Hypomenorrhea
626.2 Menorrhagia
626.6 Metrorrhagia
626.2 Menometrorrhagia
626.1 Oligomenorrhea
626.2 Polymenorrhea

■ EPIDEMIOLOGY & DEMOGRAPHICS

- Most cases of DUB occur in post-menarchal and perimenopausal age groups.
- During reproductive age, <20% of abnormal bleeding results from anovulatory DUB.

■ PHYSICAL FINDINGS & CLINICAL PRESENTATION

- A clinical diagnosis of exclusion
- Thorough physical and pelvic examination to exclude the other causes of abnormal bleeding
  1. Includes thyroid, breasts, liver, presence or absence of ecchymotic lesions
  2. Patient possibly obese and hirsute (polycystic ovarian disease)
  3. No evidence of any vulvar, vaginal, cervical lesions, uterine (fibroid) or ovarian tumor, urethral caruncle, urethral diverticula, hemorrhoids, anal fissure, colorectal lesions
  4. Bimanual pelvic examination: normal-sized or slightly enlarged uterus

■ ETIOLOGY & PATHOGENESIS

- 90% is caused by anovulation.
- 10% is ovulatory in origin; can be caused by dysfunction of corpus luteum or midcycle bleeding.
- Section II describes the various causes of abnormal uterine bleeding.

DIAGNOSIS

■ DIFFERENTIAL DIAGNOSIS

- Pregnancy-related cause
- Anatomic uterine causes:
  1. Leiomyomas
  2. Adenomyosis
  3. Polyps
  4. Endometrial hyperplasia
  5. Cancer
  6. Sexually transmitted diseases
  7. Intrauterine contraceptive devices
- Anatomic nonuterine causes:
  1. Cervical neoplasia, cervicitis
  2. Vaginal neoplasia, adhesions, trauma, foreign body, atrophic vaginitis, infections, condyloma
  3. Vulvar trauma, infections, neoplasia, condyloma, dystrophy, varices
  4. Urinary tract: urethral caruncle, diverticulum, hematuria
  5. GI tract: hemorrhoids, anal fissure, colorectal lesions
- Systemic diseases:
  1. Exogenous hormone intake
  2. Coagulopathies: von Willebrand's disease, thrombocytopenia, hepatic failure
  3. Endocrinopathies: thyroid disorder, hypo- and hyperthyroidism, diabetes mellitus
  4. Renal diseases
- Table 2-206 describes a differential diagnosis of vaginal bleeding abnormalities.

■ WORKUP

- A detailed history and thorough physical examination, including a pelvic examination to exclude above mentioned causes.
- Clinical algorithms for the evaluation of vaginal bleeding are described in Section III, Fig. 3-32.

■ LABORATORY TESTS
- CBC with platelets; possible iron deficiency anemia or thrombocytopenia
- Prothrombin (PT); partial thromboplastin and bleeding time if coagulopathy is suspected
- Serum human chorionic gonadotropin (hCG)
- Chemistry profile, including liver function tests
- Thyroid profile
- Stool testing for occult blood
- Urinalysis for hematuria
- Pap smear
- Cultures for gonorrhea and *Chlamydia*
- Serum gonadotropins and prolactin
- Serum androgens
- Endometrial biopsy in women >35 yr old, or earlier, if longstanding history of anovulatory bleeding
- Hysterogram and hysteroscopy

■ IMAGING STUDIES
- Pelvic ultrasound, including measurement of endometrial thickness
- Hydrosonogram

 TREATMENT

■ NONPHARMACOLOGIC THERAPY
Increase iron intake in the form of pills and in a diet rich in iron.

■ ACUTE GENERAL Rx
- Progestational agents
  1. Progesterone in oil, 100 to 200 mg
  2. Medroxyprogesterone acetate, 20 to 40 mg qd for 15 days
  3. Megestrol acetate, 40 to 120 mg daily in divided doses × 15 days
  4. Oral contraceptives: any oral contraceptive pill, one tablet qid for 5 to 7 days, followed by one tablet low-dose estrogen qd for 21 days; causes one heavy withdrawal bleeding, should then be on cyclical Provera or continue on oral contraceptives
- Estrogens
  1. Conjugated estrogen (Premarin) 25 mg IV q4h until bleeding is under control (in cases of severe or life-threatening bleeding); maximum three doses
  2. For prolonged bleeding that is not life-threatening: Premarin 1.25 mg (Estrace 2 mg) q4h for 24 hr, followed by Provera to bring on withdrawal bleeding; then sequential regimen of estrogen and progestin (Premarin 1.25 mg qd for 24 days; Provera 10 mg for last 10 days) or oral contraceptives
- Surgical treatment
  1. Dilation and curettage (D&C) and hysteroscopy
  2. Endometrial ablation
  3. Hysterectomy

■ CHRONIC Rx
- Progestational agents
  1. Medroxyprogesterone acetate 10 mg qd for 12 days, then cyclically to induce monthly withdrawal bleeding
  2. Norethindrone 1 mg qd for 12 days
  3. Depo-Provera 150 mg IM and then 150 mg q3mo
  4. Oral contraceptives one tablet qd
- Clomiphene citrate: patients with anovulatory bleeding who want to become pregnant
- Others
  1. Antiprostaglandins
  2. Danazol
  3. Gonadotropin-releasing hormone analogs (GNRH)
  4. Human menopausal gonadotropin (HMG)
- Surgical treatment
  1. D&C and hysteroscopy
  2. Endometrial ablation
  3. Hysterectomy

■ DISPOSITION
Cyclical treatment on birth control pills or Provera for several cycles, then discontinue pill and watch patient for onset of regular menses

■ REFERRAL
To gynecologist in case of failure of treatment

☼ PEARLS & CONSIDERATIONS

■ COMMENTS
Patient education material may be obtained from the American College of Obstetricians and Gynecologists, 409 12th Street SW, Washington, DC 20024-2188; phone (202) 638-5577.

REFERENCES
Gallinat A, Nugent W: NovaSure impedance-controlled system for endometrial ablation, *J Am Assoc Gynecol Laparosc* 9(3):283, 2002.

Mihm LM et al: The accuracy of endometrial biopsy and saline sonohysterography in the determination of the cause of abnormal uterine bleeding, *Am J Obstet Gynecol* 186:858, 2002.

Mishell DR, Stenchever MA, Drogemuller W: *Comprehensive gynecology,* ed 3, St Louis, 1997, Mosby.

Speroff L: *Clinical gynecologic endocrinology and infertility,* ed 6, Baltimore, 1999, Williams & Wilkins.

Author: **Mandeep K. Brar, M.D.**

BASIC INFORMATION

■ DEFINITION
Dysmenorrhea is pain with menstruation, usually as cramping and usually centered in the lower abdomen. It is defined as *primary dysmenorrhea* when there is no associated organic pathology and *secondary dysmenorrhea* when there is demonstrable organic pathology.

■ SYNONYMS
Menstrual cramps
Painful periods

ICD-9CM CODES
625.3 Dysmenorrhea

■ EPIDEMIOLOGY & DEMOGRAPHICS
Approximately 50% of menstruating women are affected by dysmenorrhea, with approximately 10% of them having severe dysmenorrhea with incapacitation for 1 to 3 days/mo. Dysmenorrhea is most common in the age group from 20 to 24 yr, and primary dysmenorrhea usually appears within 6 to 12 mo after menarche.

■ PHYSICAL FINDINGS & CLINICAL PRESENTATION
- Sharp, crampy, midline, lower abdomen pain without a lower quadrant or adnexal component but possible radiation to the lower back and upper thighs
- Unremarkable pelvic examination in nonmenstruating patient
- Accompanying symptoms: nausea, vomiting, headaches, anxiety, fatigue, diarrhea, fainting, and abdominal bloating
- Cramps usually lasting <24 hr and seldom lasting >2 to 3 days
- Secondary dysmenorrhea: dyspareunia is a common complaint, and bimanual pelvic-abdominal examination may demonstrate uterine or adnexal tenderness, fixed uterine retroflexion, uterosacral nodularity, a pelvic mass, or an enlarged, irregular uterus

■ ETIOLOGY
Prostaglandin $F_2\alpha$ (PG $F_2\alpha$) is the agent responsible for dysmenorrhea. It stimulates uterine contractions, cervical stenosis or narrowing, and increased vasopressin release. Behavior and psychologic factors have also been implicated in the etiology of primary dysmenorrhea. Primary dysmenorrhea only occurs in ovulatory cycles. Secondary dysmenorrhea is usually caused by endometriosis, adenomyosis, leiomyomas and, less commonly, chronic salpingitis, IUD use, or congenital or acquired outflow tract obstruction, including cervical stenosis.

DIAGNOSIS

■ DIFFERENTIAL DIAGNOSIS
- Adenomyosis
- Adhesions
- Allen-Masters syndrome
- Cervical structures or stenosis
- Congenital malformation of müllerian system
- Ectopic pregnancy
- Endometriosis, endometritis
- Imperforate hymen
- IUD use
- Leiomyomas
- Ovarian cysts
- Pelvic congestion syndrome, PID
- Polyps
- Transverse vaginal septum

■ WORKUP
- Primary dysmenorrhea: characteristic history, physical examination normal with the absence of an identifiable cause of pelvic pain
- Secondary dysmenorrhea: history of onset generally >2 yr after menarche, physical examination may reveal uterine irregularity, cul-de-sac tenderness, or nodularity or pelvic masses

■ LABORATORY TESTS
- No specific tests diagnostic for dysmenorrhea
- Elevated WBC count in the presence of infection
- hCG to rule out ectopic pregnancy

■ IMAGING STUDIES
- Ultrasound scan of the pelvis to evaluate the presence of leiomyomas, ovarian cysts, or ectopic pregnancy
- Hysterosalpingogram to assess the uterine cavity to rule out endometrial polyps, submucosal or intraluminal leiomyomas

TREATMENT

■ NONPHARMACOLOGIC THERAPY
- Applying heat to the lower abdomen with hot compresses, heating pads, or hot water bottles seems to offer some relief.
- Other reassurance that this is a treatable condition.

■ ACUTE GENERAL Rx
- Nonsteroidal antiinflammatory drugs such as ibuprofen 400 to 600 mg q4-6h or naproxen sodium 550 mg q12h, mefenamic acid 500 mg initial dose followed by 250 mg q6h prn, aspirin 650 mg q4-6h, or oral contraceptives
- Nifedipine 30 mg qd in difficult cases of dysmenorrhea
- Magnesium supplements have been found likely to be beneficial
- Thiamine supplements may reduce pain
- Secondary dysmenorrhea: treatment directed to the specific underlying condition; surgery plays a greater role
- Endometriosis: use of nonsurgical approaches, such as using danazol, gonadotropin-releasing hormone agonists, and oral contraceptives

■ CHRONIC Rx
Acupuncture and transcutaneous electrical nerve stimulation (TENS) may be tried. In cases in which medical therapy has not worked, laparoscopy should be considered, as well as other surgical treatments depending on the secondary cause of the dysmenorrhea.

■ DISPOSITION
The majority of patients are satisfactorily treated with good outcomes. It is thought that primary dysmenorrhea generally improves with age and parity and that secondary dysmenorrhea usually has good results with adequate treatment. Possible chronic complications with primary dysmenorrhea that has not been adequately treated can lead to anxiety and depression. With certain causes of secondary dysmenorrhea infertility can become a problem.

■ REFERRAL
If a secondary cause of dysmenorrhea is revealed, refer to the appropriate specialist for further medical or surgical treatment (gynecologist, pain management center).

PEARLS & CONSIDERATIONS

■ COMMENTS
Patient education materials can be obtained through various pharmaceutical companies (e.g., booklet "Painful periods" from Warner Lambert, Inc.)
Author: **George T. Danakas, M.D.**

BASIC INFORMATION

■ DEFINITION
Persistent and/or recurrent sexual intercourse associated pain

ICD-9CM CODES
625.0 Pain associated with female genital organs
302.76 Sexual deviations and disorders with functional dyspareunia, psychogenic dyspareunia

■ EPIDEMIOLOGY & DEMOGRAPHICS
PREVALENCE: 7% to 60% depending on definition
PREDOMINANT SEX: Female
AT RISK POPULATION
No consistent findings regarding:
- Age
- Parity
- Educational status
- Race
- Income
- Marital status

RISK FACTORS
Lower:
- Frequency of intercourse
- Levels of desire and arousal
- Orgasmic response
- Physical and emotional satisfaction
- General happiness

HISTORICAL FACTORS
- Pain parameters
  1. Character
  2. Location (Introital/middle/deep)
  3. Onset
  4. Duration
  5. Timing
  6. Chronicity
  7. Cyclicity
  8. Recurrence
- Gynecologic history
  1. History of STD
  2. History of HSV or HPV
  3. Other sexual dysfunctions
  4. Prior abdominal or gynecologic surgery
  5. Prior pelvic or abdominal radiation
  6. History of endometriosis, fibroids
  7. History of genital/uterine prolapse
  8. History of gynecologic infection
  9. History of pelvic pain
  10. History of menopausal symptoms
  11. Sexual misinformation
- OB history
  1. Lacerations
  2. Episiotomy
- General medical causes
  1. History of chronic diseases
  2. GI or GU symptoms
  3. Medications
  4. History of psychological disorders
  5. History of dermatologic condition
  6. Religious beliefs
  7. Generalized anxiety

■ PHYSICAL FINDINGS & CLINICAL PRESENTATION
- Primary vs. secondary dyspareunia
  1. Latter with history of pain-free coitus
- Visual inspection
  1. Discoloration
  2. Ulcerations
  3. Discharge
  4. Prolapse
  5. Dysplastic changes
  6. Infestations
- Physical examination
  1. Sensitivity to light touch
  2. Tenderness to palpation
  3. Genital prolapse
     a. Uterus
     b. Bladder
     c. Cervix
     d. Vagina
     e. Adnexa
     f. Rectum
     g. Bowel
  4. Ridges/septum
  5. Levator muscle tone
  6. Evidence of previous surgery
  7. Vaginal length/depth/caliber constrictions

■ ETIOLOGY
- Pathology or alteration/reduction of genital-associated tissue
- Psychosocial factors
- Marital/relationship discord
- History of sexual abuse

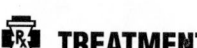

DIAGNOSIS

■ DIFFERENTIAL DIAGNOSIS
(Not an exhaustive list)
- Congenital deformities (septa/agenesis)
- Imperforate hymen
- Menopausal changes
- Atrophic tissue
- Impaired lubrication
- Psychogenic
- Vaginismus
- Inadequate foreplay
- Endometriosis
- Levator ani myalgia
- Chronic pelvic pain
- Previous surgery (posterior colporrhaphy/perineorrhaphy)
  1. Alteration in vaginal length/depth/caliber
  2. Adhesions
- Infectious
  1. Human papilloma
  2. Herpes simplex
  3. Candidiasis
  4. Tinea cruris
  5. Acute/chronic salpingitis/endometritis
- Pelvic carcinoma
- Previous radiation
- Adnexal attachment or tubal prolapse
- Pelvic tumor

- Uterine prolapse/malpositions/enlargement/retroversion
- Genital prolapse
- Cystocele/rectocele/enterocele
- Urethral/bladder pathology
- Pelvic congestion
- Vulvar vestibulitis
- Postcoital cystitis
- Broad ligament pathology
- Neuroma at the site of previous episiotomy
- Previous sexual abuse
- Vulvodynia
- Contact or allergic dermatitis
- Vitamin A, B, or C deficiency
- Equestrian dyspareunia
- Interstitial cystitis
- Pudendal neuralgia
- Myofacial pain syndrome
- Rectal pathology
- Structural abnormalities/alterations
  1. Muscle
  2. Bone
  3. Ligament

■ WORKUP
- History and physical examination are key
- If needed
  1. Colposcopy
  2. Cystoscopy
  3. Consider laparoscopy for unexplained deep dyspareunia

■ LABORATORY TESTS
- ESR
- WBC
- Wet mount
- Cultures
  1. Cervical
     a. Gonorrhea
     b. Chlamydia
  2. Vaginal
  3. Lesions
  4. Urine
- Vulva/vaginal/cervical biopsy
- Pap smear
- Herpes simplex virus antibodies
- Gonadotropin levels

■ IMAGING STUDIES
Pelvic/abdominal ultrasonography

TREATMENT

■ NONPHARMACOLOGIC THERAPY
- Patient education
- Discontinue exacerbating activity and irritants
- Lubrication with colitis
- Coital position changes: female superior position
- Warm or cool soaks
- Reassurance to patient of nonmalignant condition
- Psychosocial interventions
  1. Systemic desensitization techniques

2. Behavior modification
- Vaginal dilators
- Vaginal muscle exercises and relaxation techniques
- Excision of pathologic tissue
- Surgical correction of altered/reduced/deformed tissues

■ ACUTE GENERAL THERAPY
- Topical lidocaine
- Corticosteroids
- Antiinfective agents
- Trigger point injections
- Massage
- Acupuncture
- TENS
- Stress reduction techniques
- Safe sexual practices
- Hormonal replacement therapy
- Antiviral agents
- Intralesional interferon
- Mild analgesics
- Antidepressants

■ CHRONIC Rx
All the previous plus:
- Set supportive visits, as needed
- Oral contraceptives
- Regular sexual activity
- Balanced diet
- Vitamin supplementation
- Proper hygiene

■ DISPOSITION
Most patients will have a reduction and/or resolution of their symptoms by using the appropriate therapeutic approaches.

■ REFERRAL
A multidisciplinary approach using the expertise of psychologists, dermatologists, gynecologic surgeons, infectious disease specialists, or urologists is helpful.

☼ PEARLS & CONSIDERATIONS

- Dyspareunia is a symptom complex resulting from a multitude of etiologies, some of which are acting simultaneously.
- Uncovering the etiology of dyspareunia is predominately based on a comprehensive history and physical examination.
- The differential diagnoses can be sorted into superficial, intermediate, and deep dyspareunia categories.
- As with the physical evaluation of any painful condition, attempt, by precise touching (moistened cotton swab), palpation, or applied pressure, to reproduce the patient's chief complaint.
- Performing a one-finger pelvic exam, without concurrent abdominal palpation, allows for a more precise assessment of the source of genital pain.
- Individualize therapy.
- Initiate and maintain an honest diagnosis and compassionate demeanor with the patient and her mate.
- Be open-minded, approachable, nonjudgmental, and diligent in your search for a solution to help these often silently suffering patients.

REFERENCES
Helm LJ: Evaluation and differential diagnosis of dyspareunia, *Am Fam Physician* 63:1535, 2001.
Nichols D: *Reoperative gynecologic and obstetric surgery,* ed 2, St Louis, 1997, Mosby.
Author: **David I. Kurss, M.D.**

BASIC INFORMATION

DEFINITION
Dystonia is characterized by involuntary muscle contractions (sustained or spasmodic) that lead to abnormal body movements or postures. Dystonia can be generalized or focal.

SYNONYMS
Blepharospasm
Oromandibular dystonia
Torticollis
Writer's cramp

ICD-9CM CODES
333.6 Dystonia musculorum deformans
335.7 Dystonia caused by drugs
333.7 Dystonia, torsion, symptomatic

EPIDEMIOLOGY & DEMOGRAPHICS
PREVALENCE: Estimated at 1 in 3000 persons.
PREDOMINANT SEX: Cervical dystonia has a 3:2 female preponderance.
PREDOMINANT AGE:
- Focal cervical dystonia usually has its onset in the fifth decade.
- Hereditary forms may have an onset in childhood or adulthood.
GENETICS: Autosomal dominant, autosomal recessive, and X-linked forms of dystonia have been identified.

PHYSICAL FINDINGS & CLINICAL PRESENTATION
Focal dystonias produce abnormal sustained muscle contractions in an area of the body:
- Neck (torticollis): most commonly affected site with a tendency for the head to turn to one side
- Eyelids (blepharospasm): involuntary closure of the eyelids
- Mouth (oromandibular dystonia): involuntary contraction of muscles of the mouth, tongue, or face
- Hand (writer's cramp) (Fig. 1-94)
Generalized dystonia affects multiple areas of the body and can lead to marked joint deformities.

ETIOLOGY
- Exact pathophysiology is unknown, thought to involve abnormalities of basal ganglia.
- Hereditary forms have been described, including the severe progressive form, dystonia musculorum deformans.
- Sporadic or idiopathic forms occur.
- Dystonia can occur secondary to other diseases such as CNS disease, hypoxia, kernicterus, Huntington's disease, Wilson's disease, Parkinson syndrome, lysosomal storage diseases.

- Acute dystonia can occur following treatment with drugs that block dopamine receptors, such as phenothiazines or butyrophenones.
- Tardive dyskinesia or dystonia can result from long-term treatment with antipsychotic drugs such as phenothiazines or butyrophenones.

DIAGNOSIS

DIFFERENTIAL DIAGNOSIS
- Parkinson's disease
- Progressive supranuclear palsy
- Wilson's disease
- Huntington's disease
- Drug effects

WORKUP
History (including family history, birth history, medication use) and physical examination

LABORATORY TESTS
- Usually not helpful for establishing diagnosis
- Serum ceruloplasmin if Wilson's disease is suspected

IMAGING STUDIES
CT scan or MRI of brain if a CNS lesion is suspected

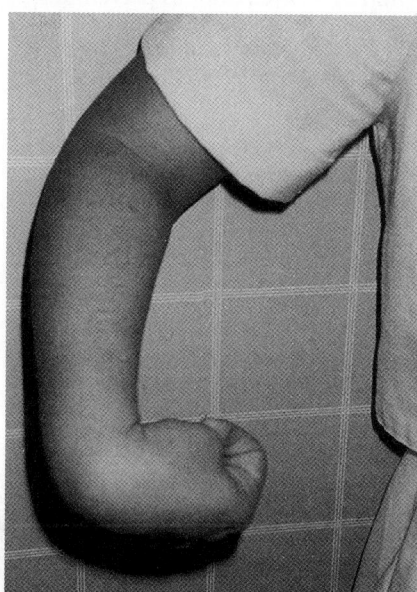

Fig. 1-94 Focal dystonia of the distal right arm. (From Goldman L, Bennett JC [eds]: *Cecil textbook of medicine,* ed 21, Philadelphia, 2000, WB Saunders.)

TREATMENT

NONPHARMACOLOGIC THERAPY
- Heat, massage, physical therapy to relieve pain
- Splints to prevent contractures

ACUTE Rx
For acute dystonic reactions to phenothiazines or butyrophenones: use diphenhydramine 50 mg IV or benztropine 2 mg IV

CHRONIC Rx
- Treatment is often ineffective.
- Slowly withdraw potentially offending agents.
- Diazepam, baclofen, or carbamazepine may be helpful.
- Trihexyphenidyl may be helpful in tardive dyskinesia or dystonia.
- Injections of botulinum toxin into the affected muscles can be used for refractory cases of focal dystonias.
- Surgical procedures including myectomy, rhizotomy, or thalamotomy may be helpful for severe, refractory cases.

DISPOSITION
Spontaneous remission of focal cervical dystonia can occur, but dystonia is generally progressive and pharmacologic therapy is often ineffective.

REFERRAL
To neurologist for severe or refractory cases

REFERENCE
Tan N-C et al: Hemifacial spasm and involuntary facial movements, *QJM* 95(8):493, 2002.
Author: **Mark J. Fagan, M.D.**

BASIC INFORMATION

■ DEFINITION
Echinococcosis is a chronic infection caused by the larval stage of several animal cestodes (flat worms) of the genus *Echinococcus*.

■ SYNONYMS
Hydatid disease

ICD-9-CM CODES
122.9 *Echinococcus* infection

■ EPIDEMIOLOGY & DEMOGRAPHICS
INCIDENCE (IN U.S.): Seen primarily in immigrants; varies widely depending on areas of origin.
PREVALENCE (IN U.S.): See Incidence
PREDOMINANT SEX: Male = female
PREDOMINANT AGE: 20 to 50 yr of age
PEAK INCIDENCE: Presumed to be acquired in childhood or early adulthood in most cases.

■ PHYSICAL FINDINGS & CLINICAL PRESENTATION
- Signs of an enlarging mass lesion in a visceral site such as the liver, lungs, kidneys, bone, or CNS
- Occasional cyst rupture causing allergic manifestations such as urticaria, angioedema, or anaphylaxis that bring the patient to medical attention
- Incidental discovery of cysts by abdominal or thoracic imaging studies performed for other reasons

■ ETIOLOGY
- Four species of *Echinococcus*: *E. granulosus*, *E. multilocularis*, *E. oligarthrus*, and *E. vogeli*.
  1. *E. granulosus* is the cause of cystic hydatid disease.
  2. *E. multilocularis* and *E. vogeli* are the causes of alveolar and polycystic disease.
- The disease is transmitted to humans by infected canines (domestic or wild dogs, wolves, foxes) and seen most commonly in livestock-producing areas of the Middle East, Africa, Australia, New Zealand, Europe, and the Americas, including the southwestern U.S.
- Eggs are present in the feces of infected canines; human infection occurs by ingestion of viable eggs in contaminated food.
- It is common in many areas of the world, especially the Middle East.

DIAGNOSIS

■ DIFFERENTIAL DIAGNOSIS
- Cystic neoplasms
- Abscess (amebic or bacterial)
- Congenital polycystic disease

■ WORKUP
- Antibody assay
- Imaging study (CT scan, ultrasonography)
- Histologic examination of cyst or contents obtained by aspiration or resection (if possible) to confirm diagnosis

■ LABORATORY TESTS
Antibody assays (ELISA and Western blot): >90% sensitive and specific for liver cysts, but less accurate for cysts in other sites

■ IMAGING STUDIES
Ultrasonography and/or CT scan:
- Both are extremely sensitive for the detection of cysts, especially in the liver (Fig. 1-95).
- Both lack specificity and are inadequate to establish the diagnosis of echinococcosis with certainty.

TREATMENT

■ NONPHARMACOLOGIC THERAPY
- Treatment of choice for echinococcal cysts is surgical resection, when feasible.
- If resection is not feasible, perform percutaneous drainage with instillation of 95% ethanol to prevent dissemination of viable larvae.
- Surgical therapy is followed by medical therapy with albendazole (see Acute General Rx).

■ ACUTE GENERAL Rx
For echinococcosis confined to the liver:
- Albendazole (400 mg bid for 28 days followed by 14 days of rest for at least three cycles)
- Mebendazole (50 to 70 mg/kg qd) if albendazole not available

■ CHRONIC Rx
See Acute General Rx.

■ DISPOSITION
- Long-term follow-up is necessary following surgical or medical therapy because of the high incidence of late relapse.
- Antibody assays and imaging studies are repeated every 6 to 12 mo for several years following successful surgical or medical therapy.

■ REFERRAL
- All patients for evaluation for possible surgical resection of cysts
- For consultation with a physician experienced in the medical and surgical management of echinococcosis

PEARLS & CONSIDERATIONS

■ COMMENTS
Surgical resection, if indicated, should be performed by surgeons experienced in the management of echinococcal cysts.

REFERENCES
Anadol D et al: Treatment of hydatid disease, *Paediatr Drugs* 3(2):123, 2001.
Chrieki M: Echinococcosis, an emerging parasite in the immigrant population, *Am Fam Physician* 66:817, 2002.
Eckert J, Conraths FJ, Tackman K: Echinococcosis: an emerging or reemerging zoonosis? *Int J Parasitol* 30(12-13):1283, 2000.
Pedrosa I et al: Hydatid disease: radiologic and pathologic features and complications, *Radiographics* 20(30):795, 2000.
Siles-Lucas MM, Gottstein BB: Molecular tools for the diagnosis of cystic and alveolar echinococcosis, *Trop Med Int Health* 6(6):463, 2001.
Author: **Joseph R. Masci, M.D.**

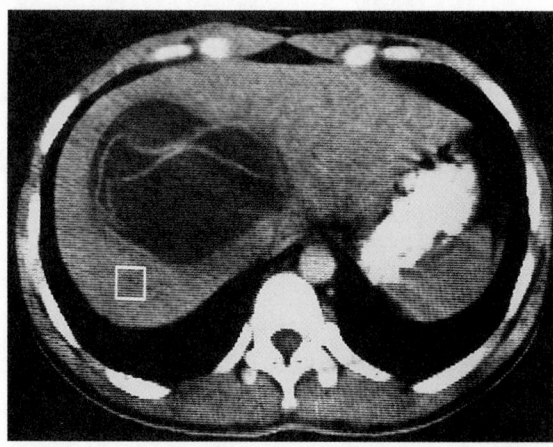

Fig. 1-95 Computed tomography scan of an echinococcal cyst in a 25-year-old man, demonstrating the complex structure of the wall and the interior. (From Goldman L, Bennett JC [eds]: *Cecil textbook of medicine*, ed 21, Philadelphia, 2000, WB Saunders.)

BASIC INFORMATION

■ **DEFINITION**

Eclampsia is the occurrence of seizures or coma in a woman with preeclampsia, occurring at >20 wk gestation or <48 hr postpartum. Atypical eclampsia occurs at <20 wk gestation or as much as 14 days postpartum.

■ **SYNONYMS**

Toxemia
Seizures of pregnancy

ICD-9CM CODES
642.6 Eclampsia

■ **EPIDEMIOLOGY &
DEMOGRAPHICS**

INCIDENCE: 1 case/150 to 3000 pregnancies; 2% to 4% of those with preeclampsia
RISK FACTORS: Multifetal gestation (3.6% in twin gestation), molar pregnancy, nonimmune hydrops fetalis, uncontrolled hypertension, preexisting hypertension or renal disease
GENETICS: Increased incidence with first-degree relatives (sister or mother) having had eclampsia

■ **PHYSICAL FINDINGS &
CLINICAL PRESENTATION**

- Seizure begins as facial twitching then spreads to generalized clonicotonic state, with cessation of respiration, followed by a postictal period of amnesia, agitation, and confusion.
- 40% have severe hypertension, 40% have mild to moderate hypertension, and 20% are normotensive.
- Generalized edema with rapid weight gain (>2 lb/wk) may be one of the earliest signs of eclampsia.
- Persistent occipital headache and hyperreflexia with clonus occur in 80% of patients with eclampsia; epigastric pain exists in 20% of these patients.

■ **ETIOLOGY**

Although the exact etiology is unknown, the common pathway relates to abnormalities in autoregulation of cerebral blood flow. This may involve transient vasospasm, ischemia, cerebral hemorrhage, and edema, occurring by a mechanism involving hypertensive encephalopathy, decreased colloid osmotic pressure, and prostaglandin imbalance.

■ **DIAGNOSIS**

■ **DIFFERENTIAL DIAGNOSIS**

- Preexisting seizure disorder
- Metabolic abnormalities (hypoglycemia, hyponatremia, hypocalcemia)
- Substance abuse
- Head trauma, infection (meningitis, encephalitis)
- Intracerebral bleeding or thrombosis
- Amniotic fluid embolism
- Space-occupying brain lesions or neoplasms
- Pseudoseizure

■ **WORKUP**

- Rule out other causes of seizures during pregnancy.
- Atypical presentations such as prolonged postictal state, status epilepticus, gestational age <20 wk or >48 hr postpartum, or signs of meningitis, substance abuse, or severe uncontrolled hypertension should prompt a search for other seizure etiologies.

■ **LABORATORY TESTS**

- Proteinuria: severe (49%), mild to moderate (29%), absent (22%)
- Hct: elevated secondary to hemoconcentration
- Platelet count: decreased; LFTs elevated in HELLP syndrome
- BUN and creatinine: elevated with renal involvement
- Serum electrolytes, glucose, calcium, toxicology profile: to rule out other causes of seizures
- Hyperuricemia: >6.9 mg/dl found in 70% of eclamptics
- ABG: maternal acidemia and hypoxia

■ **IMAGING STUDIES**

- CT scan or MRI indicated in atypical presentation, suspected intracerebral bleeding, focal neurologic deficit.
- There are abnormal findings, including cerebral edema, hemorrhage, and infarction, in 50% of patients.

■ **TREATMENT**

■ **NONPHARMACOLOGIC
THERAPY**

- Airway protection (risk of aspiration)
- Supportive care during acute event

■ **ACUTE GENERAL Rx**

- Maintain airway, adequate oxygenation, and IV access.
- Fetal resuscitation, involving maternal oxygenation, left lateral positioning, and continuous fetal heart rate monitoring, is needed.
- Magnesium sulfate is drug of choice. Give magnesium sulfate 6 g IV load over 20 min, then 3 g/hr maintenance, for recurrent seizure prophylaxis. If repeated convulsion, may give an additional 2 g IV over 3 to 5 min. About 10% to 15% of patients will have a second seizure after initial loading dose. Check magnesium level 1 hr after loading dose, then q6h (therapeutic range 4 to 6 mg/dl). Antidote for toxicity is calcium gluconate 10 ml of 10% solution. Phenytoin has been used as an alternative in patients in whom magnesium sulfate is contraindicated (renal insufficiency, heart block, myasthenia gravis, hypoparathyroidism).
- Give sodium amobarbital 250 mg IV over 3 min for persistent seizures.
- Treat blood pressure if >160 mm Hg/110 mm Hg, with labetalol 20- to 40-mg IV bolus, hydralazine 10 mg IV, or nifedipine 10 to 20 mg sublingual q20min.
- Evaluate patient for delivery.

■ **CHRONIC Rx**

- The first priority is stabilization of the mother in terms of adequate oxygenation, hemodynamics, and laboratory abnormalities, such as associated coagulopathies.
- Cervical status and gestational age should be assessed. If unfavorable cervix and <30 wk consider C-section, otherwise consider induction.
- Controlled epidural is the anesthesia of choice for labor or C-section.
- Avoid general anesthesia in uncontrolled hypertension to minimize risk of catastrophic cerebral events.

■ **DISPOSITION**

The maternal mortality rate for eclampsia averages 5% to 6%. Morbidity is 25%, including placental abruption (10%), maternal apnea with fetal asphyxia, aspiration pneumonia, pulmonary edema (4%), renal failure, cardiopulmonary arrest, and coma.

■ **REFERRAL**

Because of the potential for serious permanent maternal and fetal sequelae, all cases should be managed by a team approach of obstetrician, neonatologist, and intensivist.

PEARLS & CONSIDERATIONS

■ **COMMENTS**

- Eclampsia antepartum, 50%; intrapartum, 20%; and postpartum, 30%
- Postseizure there is an associated period of fetal bradycardia from 1 to 9 min; if there is evidence of fetal compromise beyond that time, consider alternative etiologies such as placental abruption (23% incidence).

REFERENCE

Schroeder BM: ACOG practice bulletin on diagnosing and managing preeclampsia and eclampsia, *Am Fam Physician* 66:330, 2002.
Author: **Scott J. Zuccala, D.O.**

BASIC INFORMATION

■ DEFINITION

An ectopic pregnancy (EP) is one in which a fertilized ovum implants outside the endometrial lining of the uterus.

■ SYNONYMS

Abdominal pregnancy (1% to 2%)
Cervical pregnancy (0.5%)
Interstitial pregnancy (2% to 3%)
Ovarian pregnancy (1%)
Tubal pregnancy (97%)

ICD-9CM CODES

633 Ectopic pregnancy

■ EPIDEMIOLOGY & DEMOGRAPHICS

• 1% to 2% of pregnancies
• 13% of maternal deaths
PREVALENCE (IN U.S.): Increasing number of EPs; 17,800 reported cases in 1970 and 108,000 reported cases in 1992.
RISK FACTORS: Previous salpingitis, previous EP, previous tubal ligation, previous tuboplasty, IUD use, progestin-only pill, and assisted reproductive techniques

■ PHYSICAL FINDINGS & CLINICAL PRESENTATION

• Abdominal tenderness: 95%
• Adnexal tenderness: 87% to 99%
• Peritoneal signs: 71% to 76%
• Adnexal mass: 33% to 53%
• Enlarged uterus: 6% to 30%
• Shock: 2% to 17%
• Amenorrhea or abnormal vaginal bleeding: 75%
• Shoulder pain: 10%
• Tissue passage: 6% to 7%

■ ETIOLOGY

• Anatomic obstruction to zygote passage
• Abnormalities in tubal motility
• Transperitoneal migration of the zygote

DIAGNOSIS

■ DIFFERENTIAL DIAGNOSIS

• Corpus luteum cyst
• Rupture or torsion of ovarian cyst
• Threatened or incomplete abortion
• PID
• Appendicitis
• Gastroenteritis
• Dysfunctional uterine bleeding
• Degenerating uterine fibroids
• Endometriosis

■ WORKUP

1. The classic presentation of EP includes the triad of abnormal vaginal bleeding, pelvic pain, and an adnexal mass. Consider in all women with abdominal-pelvic pain and a positive pregnancy test
2. Culdocentesis is clinically useful when other diagnostic modalities are not readily available
   • Positive tap means nonclotting blood with Hct >12%.
   • Negative tap means clear or blood-tinged fluid.
   • Nondiagnostic tap means clotted blood or no fluid.
3. Laparoscopy

■ LABORATORY TESTS

• hCG: if normal IUP, 85% have doubling time of 2 days. If abnormal gestation, will show <66% increase of QhCG within 2 days. However, 13% of ectopic pregnancies have a normal doubling time (Section III, Fig. 3-69)
• Progesterone: decreased production in EP, <5 ng/ml strongly predictive of abnormal pregnancy. If >25 ng/ml, strongly predictive of normal IUP
• Dropping Hct associated with tubal rupture
• Leukocytosis

■ IMAGING STUDIES

• Ultrasound: presence of an IUP rules out EP.
• If QhCG >6000 mIU/ml, should see IUP on abdominal scan, and QhCG >1500 mIU/ml for transvaginal scan.
• Findings on ultrasound in EP include:
  1. Empty uterus
  2. Adnexal mass
  3. Cul-de-sac fluid
  4. Fetal sac in tube
  5. Fetal cardiac activity in adnexa

TREATMENT

■ NONPHARMACOLOGIC THERAPY

Surgery: can be performed by laparoscopy if patient is stable or by laparotomy if patient is unstable. Salpingiosis: direct injection of chemotherapy into ectopic via laparoscopy, transvaginal ultrasound, or hysteroscopy.
• Conservative surgery-salpingostomy or segmental resection depends on tubal location and size of ectopic.
• Salpingectomy should be considered in the following circumstances:
  1. Ruptured tube
  2. Future fertility not desired
  3. Recurrent ectopic in the same tube
  4. Uncontrolled hemorrhage

■ ACUTE GENERAL Rx

• If the patient is stable and compliant may consider medical management with methotrexate. Patient should not have contraindications to methotrexate such as hepatic or renal disease, thrombocytopenia, leukopenia, or significant anemia. There should be no evidence of hemoperitoneum on transvaginal ultrasound. Ectopic should be <4 cm mass with QhCG <30,000 mIU/ml.
• Most common regimen is methotrexate 50 mg/m² body surface area. May require second dose or surgical intervention if QhCG increases or plateaus after 7 days.

■ CHRONIC Rx

Persistent EP results from residual trophoblastic tissue or secondary implantation after conservative surgery. There is a 5% incidence of persistent ectopic with conservative treatment.

■ DISPOSITION

If diagnosed and treated early (before rupture) prognosis is excellent for good recovery. Follow QhCG weekly until negative. Use reliable contraception until hCG negative. With subsequent pregnancies, follow QhCG and perform early ultrasound to confirm IUP. There is a 12% recurrence rate for EP.

■ REFERRAL

Should obtain gynecologic consultation if EP is suspected.

PEARLS & CONSIDERATIONS

■ COMMENTS

Patient information can be obtained through American College of Obstetricians and Gynecologists, 409 12th St SW, Washington, DC 20024-2188.

REFERENCES

Della-Giustina D, Denny M: Ectopic pregnancy, *Emerg Med Clin North Am* 21(3):565, 2003.
Gracia CR, Barnhart KT: Diagnosing ectopic pregnancy: decision analysis comparing six strategies, *Obstet Gynecol* 97(3):464, 2001.
Lipscomb GH, Stovall TG, Ling FW: Nonsurgical treatment of ectopic pregnancy, *N Engl J Med* 343:1325, 2000.
Author: **George T. Danakas, M.D.**

BASIC INFORMATION

■ DEFINITION

Ehlers-Danlos syndrome (EDS) refers to a group of inherited, clinically variable, and genetically heterogeneous connective tissue disorders. EDS is characterized by skin hyperextensibility, skin fragility, and joint laxity and hyperextensibility. The revised classification scheme and diagnostic criteria (1998) are listed below.

■ ICD-9CM CODES
756.83 Ehlers-Danlos syndrome

■ EPIDEMIOLOGY & DEMOGRAPHICS
The prevalence of EDS is estimated to be about 1 in 5000 births, although it is somewhat higher in African Americans. Types I, II, and III are most prevalent. Types I and II account for approximately 80% of reported cases. In most cases, transmission is autosomal dominant except for V and IX (X-linked) and X and VIIC (autosomal recessive).

■ PHYSICAL FINDINGS & CLINICAL PRESENTATION
See Fig. 1-96.
- Classic: (EDS I and II) hyperextensibility ("Gorlin's sign": ability to touch tip of tongue to nose), easy scarring and bruising ("cigarette-paper scars"), smooth, velvety skin, subcutaneous spheroids (small, firm cyst-like nodules) along shins or forearms
- Hypermobility (EDS III): Joint hypermobility and some skin hypermobility with or without very smooth skin.
- Vascular (EDS IV): Thin, translucent skin with visible veins; marked bruising; pinched nose; acrogeria; spontaneous rupture of medium and large arteries and hollow organs, especially large intestine and uterus.
- Kyphoscoliotic (EDS VI): Characterized by joint hypermobility, progressive scoliosis; ocular fragility and possible globe rupture, mitral valve prolapse and aortic dilation.
- Arthrochalasia (EDS VII A and B): Prominent joint hypermobility with subluxations, congenital hip dislocation, skin hyperextensibility, and tissue fragility.
- Dermatosparaxis (EDS VIIC): Severe skin fragility with decreased elasticity, bruising, hernias.
- Unclassified type:
  1. EDS V: Classic characteristics
  2. EDS VIII: Classic characteristics and periodontal disease
  3. EDS IX: Classic characteristics
  4. EDS X: Mild classic characteristics, mitral valve prolapse
  5. EDS XI: Joint instability

■ ETIOLOGY
Defects of collagen in extracellular matrices of multiple tissues (skin, tendons, blood vessels, and viscera) underlie all forms of EDS. EDS I and II are associated with defects in type V collagen, corresponding to mutations of the COL5A genes. EDS IV involves a deficiency in type III collagen, and several studies suggest that mutations of gene COL3A1 lead to this deficiency. EDS VIIA and VIIB result from a defect in type I collagen, caused by mutations in the COL1A1 and COL1A2 genes.

 DIAGNOSIS

Diagnosis is based solely on clinical criteria. It is important to identify patients with EDS type IV because of the grave consequences of the disease.

■ DIFFERENTIAL DIAGNOSIS
Generally limited to types of EDSs. Some individuals with Marfan's syndrome have joint laxity. Some patients with osteogenesis imperfecta have joint laxity and easy bruising. Patients with joint hypermobility without skin changes are more likely to have familial joint hypermobility. Patients with autosomal dominant cutis laxa have skin redundancy and loss of elasticity but do not have easy bruising or tissue fragility.

■ WORKUP
Diagnosis is based solely on clinical criteria.

■ LABORATORY TESTS
- Limited biochemical assays and gene analyses are performed for known molecular defects.
- Plain radiographs may reveal calcified nodules along the shin or forearms, corresponding to the subcutaneous spheroids.
- Echocardiogram can identify MVP and aortic dilation.

 TREATMENT

- All patients should receive genetic counseling about the mode of inheritance of their EDS and the risk of having children with EDS.
- Management of most skin and joint problems should be conservative and preventive. Joint hypermobility and pain in EDS usually does not require surgical intervention. Physical therapy to strengthen muscles is helpful. Surgical repair and tightening of joint ligaments require careful evaluation of individual patients because ligaments frequently will not hold sutures.
- Vascular type requires special surgical care because of increased friability of tissues. Women with EDS type IV should be counseled to avoid pregnancy.
- Patients should be advised to avoid contact sports, and elevated blood pressure should be aggressively treated.

■ DISPOSITION
Prognosis varies according to type of EDSs.

■ REFERRAL
Referral to cardiology, orthopedic, and general surgery, and physical therapy as needed.

REFERENCES
Pepin M et al: Clinical and genetic features of Ehlers-Danlos syndrome type IV, the vascular type, *N Engl J Med* 342:673, 2000.
Pyeritz R: Ehlers-Danlos syndrome, *N Engl J Med* 342(10):730, 2000
Pyeritz RE: Ehlers-Danlos syndromes. In Goldman L, Bennett JC (eds): *Cecil textbook of medicine*, ed 21, vol 1, Philadelphia, 2000, WB Saunders.
Shapiro, JR: Heritable disorders of structural proteins, *Kelley's textbook of rheumatology*, ed 6, Philadelphia, 2001, WB Saunders.
Author: **Iris Tong, M.D.**

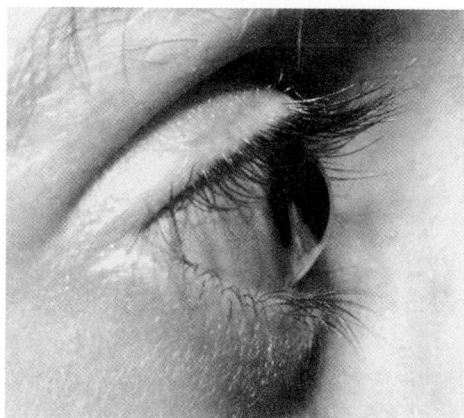

Fig. 1-96 Ehlers-Danlos syndrome is characterized by poor cross-linking of collagen. This results in joint hypermobility, skin hyperextensibility, easy bruising, and a propensity toward tissue rupture. A blue sclera (as seen here) results from thinning of the sclera. (From Palay D [ed]: *Ophthalmology for the primary care physician*, St Louis, 1997, Mosby.)

BASIC INFORMATION

■ DEFINITION
The three clinically significant disorders of ejaculation are ejaculatory failure, retrograde ejaculation, and premature ejaculation. Ejaculatory failure is the lack of production of seminal emission. Retrograde ejaculation is a backward flow of the emission into the bladder. Premature ejaculation is the inability to control ejaculation for sufficient time to allow adequate penetration and intercourse.

ICD-9CM CODES
606.9 Male infertility unspecified
608.9 Unspecified disorder of male genital organs
302.75 Premature ejaculation (psychosexual)
302.74 Orgasm inhibited male psychosexual

■ EPIDEMIOLOGY & DEMOGRAPHICS
Ejaculatory failure and retrograde ejaculation are uncommon disorders seen predominantly with diseases affecting the autonomic nervous system. Premature ejaculation is a common functional problem seen mostly in younger men.

■ PHYSICAL FINDINGS & CLINICAL PRESENTATION
Varies with disorder:
Ejaculatory failure: no ejaculate is expelled; physical findings may be normal or may show autonomic or central nervous system dysfunction (e.g., spinal cord injury); results in infertility.
Retrograde ejaculation: no ejaculate is expelled at orgasm and subsequent bladder void reveals cloudy urine; physical examination is often normal but may reveal autonomic nervous system dysfunction; results in infertility.

Premature ejaculation: ejaculation occurs quickly following excitation; physical examination is normal.

■ ETIOLOGY
Ejaculatory failure: lumbar sympathectomy, spinal cord injury, duct obstruction, sympatholytic drugs, substance abuse, psychologic factors, aging
Retrograde ejaculation: open or transurethral prostatectomy, urethral or bladder procedures, congenital urethral anomalies, lumbar sympathectomy, sympatholytic drugs (antihypertensives, psychotropics), diabetes
Premature ejaculation: fears, sexual ignorance

DIAGNOSIS

■ WORKUP
History, physical examination, and laboratory analysis
Imaging occasionally

■ HISTORY
Psychosexual history, medication and substance use, history of genitourinary surgeries or infections, and past medical and trauma history

■ PHYSICAL EXAMINATION
Neurologic and genitourinary examinations

■ LABORATORY TESTS
Postorgasmic urine should be evaluated for spermatozoa, viscosity, and fructose to differentiate ejaculatory failure from retrograde ejaculation.

■ IMAGING STUDIES
Transrectal ultrasound or vasography can show dilated seminal vesicles or ejaculatory ducts if obstruction is present.

TREATMENT

■ NONPHARMACOLOGIC THERAPY
Ejaculatory failure: vibratory or electrical stimulation of emission
Retrograde ejaculation: viable sperm can be recovered from the bladder
Premature ejaculation: sex therapy

■ GENERAL Rx
Offending drugs should be eliminated if possible. Alpha-adrenergic sympathomimetics such as pseudoephedrine, ephedrine, or phenylpropanolamine may convert retrograde to antegrade ejaculation. Psychotropic medications such as sertraline, fluoxetine, and clomipramine have shown success in delaying premature ejaculation. Topical anesthetics such as lidocaine cream have also been used.

■ SURGICAL Rx
Correction of anatomic abnormalities, such as relieving obstruction or improving the competence of the internal urethral sphincter apparatus

■ REFERRAL
All fertility issues and suspected anatomic problems should be referred to a urologist.

REFERENCES
Master VA, Turek PJ: Ejaculation physiology and dysfunction, *Urol Clin North Am* 28(2):363, 2001.
Murphy JB, Lipshultz LI: Abnormalities of ejaculation, *Urol Clin North Am*, 14(3):583, 1987.
Levine SB: Marital sexual dysfunction: ejaculation disturbance, *Ann Intern Med* 84(5):575, 1976.

Author: **Michael Picchioni, M.D.**

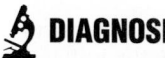

 BASIC INFORMATION

■ DEFINITION

Premature ejaculation is a persistent and recurrent problem in which a male experiences orgasm or ejaculation in the early phases of sexual contact and before he wishes it. Other definitions have emphasized elapsed time after intromission (with durations of 30 sec to several min), number of thrusts, or rate of partner satisfaction.

■ SYNONYMS

Rapid ejaculation
Early ejaculation
Inadequate ejaculatory control

ICD-9CM CODES
F52.4 Premature ejaculation (DSM-IV Code 302.75)

■ EPIDEMIOLOGY & DEMOGRAPHICS
INCIDENCE (IN U.S.): Reported as 21% in 1988; 46% in 1970
PREVALENCE (IN U.S.): 7% to 38%
PREDOMINANT SEX: Only males affected
PREDOMINANT AGE: None defined
PEAK INCIDENCE: Adolescence and young adulthood
GENETICS: No identifiable genetic factors

■ PHYSICAL FINDINGS & CLINICAL PRESENTATION
- Complaint of ejaculation before, upon, or shortly after penetration
- Frequently associated anxiety related to either sexual activity or more generalized anxiety disorder
- Premature ejaculation secondary to a medical condition frequently associated with low anxiety, low desire, and/or erectile insufficiency

■ ETIOLOGY
- Unclear etiology; different theoretical frameworks emphasizing anxiety related to performance or personal interactions, behavioral concepts of learned expectations related to early experience, or heightened penile sensitivity

- Organic factors in a small fraction of individuals (e.g., abdominal or pelvic trauma or surgery, neuropathies, or urologic pathology such as prostatic urethritis)

 DIAGNOSIS

■ DIFFERENTIAL DIAGNOSIS
- In as many as 25% of men with complaints of premature ejaculation, partner is anorgasmic.
- In young adolescents, premature ejaculation is normally experienced as a consequence of heightened excitation.

■ WORKUP
- History with a specific emphasis on sexual activities, beliefs, orientation, and gender identity
- History of relationships
- Collateral information from sexual partner when possible
- Additional history regarding surgery, trauma, and mycologic symptoms
- History of prescribed and recreational drugs revealing contributory factors (e.g., tricyclic antidepressants, alcohol, opiates)

■ LABORATORY TESTS
Urinalysis and urine culture after prostatic massage may uncover a urinary or prostatic infection (prostatitis found in 47.8% of men with premature ejaculation).

■ IMAGING STUDIES
None indicated

TREATMENT

■ NONPHARMACOLOGIC THERAPY
- Behavioral and psychotherapeutic interventions: strongly guided by a specific theoretical framework; often inadequate data to suggest the superiority of any particular approach

- Use of condoms frequently recommended to reduce penile sensitivity
- Use of pause-squeeze technique, in which 4 sec of moderate pressure is applied to the frenulum to reduce ejaculatory urge

■ GENERAL Rx
- Topical anesthetics increase ejaculatory latency.
- Anxiolytics (benzodiazepines) may be useful in individuals with anxiety.
- Serotonin reuptake inhibiting antidepressants, which frequently delay orgasm in both men and women, are a common intervention but have not been extensively studied.
- Sildenafil may be superior to antidepressants in delaying ejaculation.

■ DISPOSITION
- Premature ejaculation is frequently a chronic, lifelong problem.
- There is gradual improvement with age but few spontaneous remissions.
- Impact of successful therapy may be prolonged.

■ REFERRAL
If behavioral sex therapy or psychotherapy is indicated or if significant urologic abnormalities are discovered

REFERENCES
Abdel-Hamid IA et al: Assessment of as needed use of pharmacotherapy and the pause-squeeze technique in premature ejaculation, *Int J Impot Res* 13:41, 2001.
Screponi E et al: Prevalence of chronic prostatitis in men with premature ejaculation, *Urology* 58:198, 2001.
Author: **Rif S. El-Mallakh, M.D.**

BASIC INFORMATION

■ DEFINITION
Electrical injuries are wounds occurring as a result of contact with an electrical current (Fig. 1-97).

■ SYNONYMS
None

ICD-9CM CODES
994.8 Electrical shock, nonfatal

■ EPIDEMIOLOGY & DEMOGRAPHICS
- Electrical injuries cause approximately 1000 deaths annually, with two thirds occurring in persons between 15 and 40 yr of age.
- Electrical injury ranks fifth as the cause of occupational fatalities.
- Electrical injuries account for 4% to 6.5% of all admissions to burn units.
- Deaths typically occur in the young.
- Most electrical burns in adults are occupationally related.
- Children commonly experience oral burns from electrical appliances.

■ PHYSICAL FINDINGS & CLINICAL PRESENTATION
- Depending on the extent of injury, the patient may be unconscious, seizing, or confused and unable to present a history
- Extensive burns (~10% to 25% of the body surface)
  1. Located over the entry and exit sites
  2. Most common entry sites are the hands and skull
  3. Most common exit sites are the heels
  4. "Kissing burns" over the flexor creases
  5. Superficial partial thickness
  6. Oral burns in children
  7. Bleeding from the labial artery may present 7 to 10 days after the injury
- Cardiac arrest (asystole or ventricular fibrillation) may be the initial presenting rhythm
- Pulseless extremities
- Fractures
- Compartment syndrome from severe muscle tissue damage
- Headaches
- Weakness and paresthesias
- Motor and sensory deficits

■ ETIOLOGY
- Electricity causes tissue injury by converting electrical energy into heat.
- The higher the electrical voltage, the greater the tissue destruction.
- The longer the duration of contact with the electrical source, the greater the damage.
  1. Direct current (DC) contact causes a single muscle contraction throwing the patient away from the source.
  2. Alternating current (AC) contact precipitates a tetanic contraction, not allowing the patient to withdraw from the source and prolonging the duration of contact.
  3. Therefore AC contact is more ominous than DC contact.
- Electrical injuries are arbitrarily divided into high voltage (1000 volts) and low voltage (500 volts).
- The entry and exit path the electrical current travels in the body determines which tissues are affected.

DIAGNOSIS

The diagnosis of electrical injury is based on history and physical examination.

■ WORKUP
A detailed workup is indicated in patients with electrical injuries because the physical examination may not reveal the extent of damage that has occurred.

■ LABORATORY TESTS
- CBC
- Electrolytes
- BUN/creatinine
- Arterial blood gases
- Myoglobin
- Creatinine kinase CPK with isoenzyme fractionation
- Urinalysis including screening for myoglobinuria
- LFTs
- Type and cross-match
- EKG

■ IMAGING STUDIES
- C-spine films in patients with suspected spinal injury
- X-ray any suspicious area for bone fractures
- CT scan of the head and skull in patients with major head injury
- Technetium pyrophosphate scanning may locate areas of myonecrosis

TREATMENT

■ NONPHARMACOLOGIC THERAPY
- If at the scene of the injury, make sure the power source is turned off before approaching the victim
- Maintain urine output of at least 50 cc/hr with IV fluids
- Cardiac monitoring
- Oxygen
- Tetanus prophylaxis

■ ACUTE GENERAL Rx
- Alkalinization of the urine (sodium bicarbonate 50 mEq in 1 L of normal saline) is indicated in patients who are suspected of having myoglobinuria.
- Furosemide 20 to 40 mg PO or IV may be used to force diuresis.
- Mannitol 12.5 g/kg/hr assists in maintaining diuresis.
- Seizures are treated in the standard fashion.
- Treat burns with sulfadiazine silver dressings.

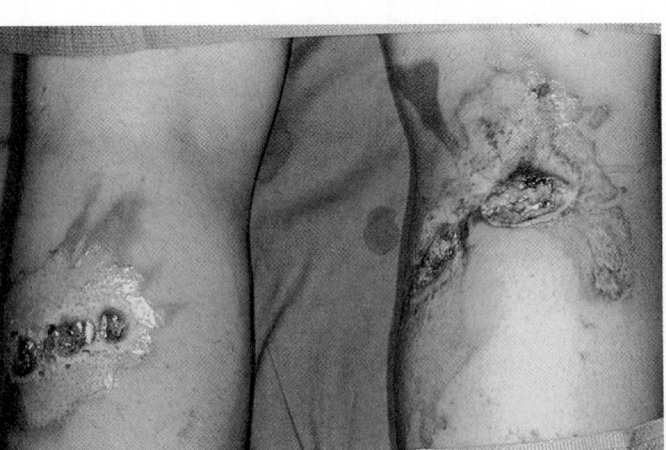

Fig. 1-97 Charring of the skin of both calves indicates points of contact with a high-voltage electrical current. These contact points are surrounded by full-thickness cutaneous burns caused by arcing of current. The extent of deep tissue destruction is often not related to the size of the cutaneous manifestations of the injury. (From Goldman L, Bennett JC [eds]: *Cecil textbook of medicine*, ed 21, Philadelphia, 2000, WB Saunders.)

■ CHRONIC Rx
- Asymptomatic patients with a normal physical examination, negative urinalysis, and normal ECG findings may be discharged home with close follow-up.

■ DISPOSITION
- Patients with severe burns should be transferred to the regional burn center.
- Complications of electrical injuries include:
  1. Infection
  2. Renal failure from rhabdomyolysis
  3. Seizure disorder
  4. Fasciotomies
  5. Amputation
- Delayed neurologic damage may present as ascending paralysis, amyotrophic lateral sclerosis, or transverse myelitis weeks to years after the injury.
- Vascular damage may also present in a delayed fashion.

■ REFERRAL
A general surgery consultation is recommended in any patient with significant electrical injuries and tissue damage. Plastic surgery is recommended in children with oral burns. Ophthalmology consultation is also recommended screening for cataract formation.

☼ PEARLS & CONSIDERATIONS

■ COMMENTS
- Electrical injuries are caused by:
  1. Direct contact with the electrical source.
  2. Conversion of electrical energy to heat.
  3. Blunt trauma after being thrown from the electrical source or from continuous muscle contraction (tetany).
- Electrical burns are the most frequent cause of amputation in burn units.

- Cataract formation has been shown to occur within 1 to 24 mo following a high-voltage electrical injury in approximately 5% to 20% of patients.
- The absence of physical findings on the initial examination does not exclude extensive underlying tissue damage.

REFERENCES
Cooper MA: Electrical and lightning injuries. In Rosen P, Barkin R: *Emergency medicine: concepts and clinical practice,* ed 4, St Louis, 1998, Mosby.

Fish RM: Electrical injury, part III: cardiac monitoring indications, the pregnant patient, and lightning, *J Emerg Med* 18(2):181, 2000.

Jeschke RJ, Herndon RE: Electrical injuries: a 30-year review, *J Trauma* 46(5):933, 1999.

Martinez JA, Nguyen T: Electrical injuries, *South Med J* 93(12):1165, 2000.
Author: **Peter Petropoulos, M.D.**

BASIC INFORMATION

■ DEFINITION
Electromechanical dissociation (EMD) is the absence of effective cardiac output in the presence of organized electrical activity.

■ SYNONYMS
Pulseless electrical activity (PEA)

ICD-9CM CODES
426.89 Electromechanical dissociation

■ EPIDEMIOLOGY & DEMOGRAPHICS
• Less frequent than VT/VF, asystole
• May be last electrical activity of dying myocardium

■ PHYSICAL FINDINGS & CLINICAL PRESENTATION
PRIMARY EMD:
• Organized electrical activity (not VT/VF)
• No palpable pulse
SECONDARY EMD:
Primary EMD and may also have:
• Bradycardia: drug overdose
• Tachycardia: hypovolemia, massive PE
• Decreased JVP: hypovolemia
• Elevated JVP and no pulse with CPR: cardiac tamponade, massive PE, tension pneumothorax
• Absent unilateral breath sounds with mechanical ventilation and tracheal deviation: tension pneumothorax
• Cyanosis: hypoxia

■ ETIOLOGY
PRIMARY EMD: Myocardial excitation and contraction uncoupling secondary to advanced heart muscle disease
SECONDARY EMD: Because of changes in the loading conditions of the heart, ischemia, myocardial depressants
• Massive MI
• Massive PE

• Hypovolemia
• Cardiac tamponade
• Tension pneumothorax
• Hypothermia
• Hyperkalemia/hypokalemia
• Hypomagnesemia
• Hypoxia
• Acidosis
• Drug overdose: β-blockers, calcium channel blockers, digoxin, tricyclic antidepressants

DIAGNOSIS

■ DIFFERENTIAL DIAGNOSIS
• Pseudo-EMD
• Idioventricular rhythm
• Postdefibrillation idioventricular rhythm
• Ventricular escape rhythm
• Bradyasystolic rhythm

■ WORKUP
• Stabilizing patient and workup to establish etiology of EMD should proceed simultaneously
• History, physical examination, laboratory tests, imaging studies

■ LABORATORY TESTS
• Potassium, magnesium
• Arterial blood gas
• ECG (Fig. 1-98):
Low voltage: tamponade
Right heart strain: PE, pneumothorax
Arrhythmias: MI, metabolic abnormalities, drug effects
ST changes, Q waves: MI

■ IMAGING STUDIES
Guided by clinical suspicion of reversible causes and what can be performed without compromising patient safety:
• Chest x-ray: rule out pneumothorax
• Pulmonary arteriogram: rule out PE

• Echocardiogram: rule out pseudo-EMD, tamponade, valve dysfunction, and atrial myxoma
• Abdominal x-ray: rule out rupture of abdominal aortic aneurysm

TREATMENT

■ NONPHARMACOLOGIC THERAPY
• Activate emergency medical service system
• Begin CPR
• Intubate and ventilate
• Obtain IV access
• Continuous cardiac monitor
• Confirm absence of blood flow with Doppler ultrasound, arterial line, or bedside echocardiogram

■ ACUTE GENERAL Rx
NOTE: Epinephrine and atropine can be given via tracheal tube. Give 2 to 2.5 times the IV dose in 10 ml of normal saline or distilled water.
• Epinephrine 1 mg IV push, repeat q3-5min
• If bradycardic (<60 beats/min): atropine 1 mg IV q3-5min to a maximum of 3 mg
• If preexisting hyperkalemia: sodium bicarbonate 1 mEq/kg
• Treat specific cause if known
PROBABLY HELPFUL:
Sodium bicarbonate 1 mEq/kg if:
• Preexisting bicarbonate responsive acidosis
• Tricyclic antidepressant overdose
• Drug overdoses that respond to alkalization of urine
POSSIBLY HELPFUL:
Sodium bicarbonate 1 mEq/kg if:
• Intubated and prolonged arrest
• Successful resuscitation after prolonged arrest
Epinephrine at higher doses:
• 2 to 5 mg IV push q3-5min
• 1 mg, 3 mg, 5 mg IV push, 3 min apart
• 0.1 mg/kg IV push q3-5min

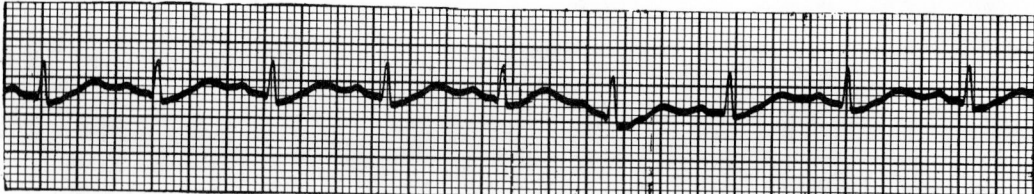

Fig. 1-98 Sinus rhythm with electromechanical dissociation (EMD). Although the ECG showed sinus rhythm, the patient had no pulse or blood pressure. In this case the EMD was a result of depressed myocardial function after a cardiac arrest. (From Goldberg AL: *Clinical electrocardiography*, ed 5, St Louis, 1994, Mosby.)

■ DISPOSITION

- Poor overall. Of hospitalized patients who develop EMD, 4% to 15% survival to discharge reported. Survival rates much lower in patients with prehospital EMD.
- Prompt treatment may be successful in secondary EMD.

REFERENCES

ECG Guidelines: Part 6: advanced cardiovascular life support: section 7: algorithm approach to ACLS emergencies, *Circulation* 102(suppl I):I136, 2000.

Eisenberg MS, Mengert TJ: Cardiac resuscitation, *N Engl J Med* 344(17):1304, 2001.

Emergency Cardiac Care Committee and Subcommittees, American Heart Association: Guidelines for cardiopulmonary resuscitation and emergency cardiac care, part III: adult advanced cardiac life support, *JAMA* 268(16):2199, 1992.

Parish DC, Dane FC, Montgomery M: Resuscitation in the hospital: differential relationship between age and survival across rhythms, *Crit Care Med* 27(10):2137, 1999.

Saklayen M, Liss H, Markert R: In-hospital cardiopulmonary resuscitation: survival in one hospital and literature review, *Medicine* 74(4):163, 1995.

Author: **Sudeep K. Aulakh, M.D., F.R.C.P.C.**

BASIC INFORMATION

■ DEFINITION

An accumulation of pus in the pleural space, most often caused by bacterial infection.

■ ICD-CM CODES

511.9

■ EPIDEMIOLOGY & DEMOGRAPHICS

Empyema occurs in a variety of clinical settings. Most often it is seen as a complication of bacterial pneumonia, especially in association with pneumococcal or anaerobic infection. Empyema may also occur as a complication of thoracic surgery, penetrating chest trauma, or bronchopleural fistulae resulting from malignancy or lung biopsy. Although pleural effusions occur in many other disease states, most notably congestive heart failure, end-stage liver disease, collagen-vascular, and malignancy, the term *empyema* refers to the presence of pus in the pleural space and does not encompass most pleural effusions.

■ PHYSICAL FINDINGS & CLINICAL PRESENTATION

The clinical presentation of empyema may be abrupt and dramatic or chronic and insidious depending on the etiologic agent and host factors. Empyema complicating pneumococcal pneumonia typically presents as progressive pleuritic chest pain, persistent fever, and other sustained signs and symptoms of infection. In the case of anaerobic empyema, particularly that caused by the actinomycetes, the clinical picture may be dominated by non-respiratory symptoms and signs, such as weight loss, malaise, and a slowly enlarging chest wall mass. As a complication of thoracic trauma or surgery, empyema typically results from superinfection of blood or other material in the pleural space several days following the event.

The physical findings of empyema are those of pleural effusion. Decreased breath sounds and dullness to percussion over the involved part of the thorax is typical. Systemic signs of infection include fever, tachycardia, leukocytosis and, occasionally, warmth and erythema over the involved area.

■ ETIOLOGY

Empyema results from the accumulation of infected material within the pleural space. Infection of the lung parenchyma with *Streptococcosis pneumoniae, Hemophilus influenzae, Staphylococcus aureus, Legionella species,* or a variety of oral anaerobic bacteria.

 DIAGNOSIS

■ DIFFERENTIAL DIAGNOSIS

- Uninfected parapneumonic effusion
- Congestive heart failure
- Malignancy involving the pleura
- Tuberculous pleurisy
- Collagen vascular disease (particularly rheumatoid lung and systemic lupus erythematosus)

■ LABORATORY TESTS

- Complete blood count; arterial blood gas
- Blood cultures

■ Pleural fluid analysis including cell count and differential, LDH and protein levels, pH, Gram stain and culture. Empyema fluid is expected to have the characteristics of pleural exudates with a ratio of pleural fluid protein to serum protein of >0.5 or a ratio of pleural fluid LDH to serum LDH of >0.6. In addition, the presence of gross pus; visible organisms on Gram stain of the pleural fluid; pleural fluid glucose <50 mg/dL or pleural fluid pH below 7 are characteristic of empyema. Any of these latter findings justify immediate drainage by chest tube or surgery because of the high risk of loculation and progressive systemic infection.

■ IMAGING STUDIES

- Chest roentgenogram
- Lateral decubitus view to establish the presence of free fluid in the pleural space
- Computed tomography to establish the presence of fluid loculation, underlying mass lesions, and other intrathoracic pathology

TREATMENT

■ NONPHARMACOLOGIC THERAPY

Prompt drainage by thoracostomy (chest tube) or open thoracotomy

■ ACUTE GENERAL THERAPY

- Maintenance of drainage until infection controlled
- Antibiotics directed at suspected or proven bacterial or fungal pathogens
- Thoracoscopy or instillation of thrombolytic agents (streptokinase or urokinase) may be considered in refractory, loculated empyema.

■ CHRONIC THERAPY

- If thorough drainage cannot be accomplished, open thoracotomy with pleural decortication may be required.
- Lung function should be monitored following completion of therapy.

■ DISPOSITION

- Hospitalization
- Supplemental oxygen with ventilatory support if necessary

■ REFERRAL

Consultation by infectious diseases, pulmonary or thoracic surgical specialists may be appropriate.

PEARLS & CONSIDERATIONS

■ COMMENTS

- Empyema caused by actinomycetes may present with erosion through the chest wall and formation of a fistulous tract.
- Nosocomial infection caused by relatively resistant bacterial or fungal pathogens may result in empyema in patients with indwelling thoracostomy tubes.

REFERENCES

De Hoyos A, Sundaresan S: Thoracic empyema, *Surg Clin North Am* 82(3):643, 2002.

Pierrepoint MJ et al: Pigtail catheter drain in the treatment of empyema thoracis, *Arch Dis Child* 87(4):331, 2002.

Jaffe A, Cohen G: Thoracic empyema, *Arch Dis Child* 88(10):839, 2003.

Author: **Joseph R. Masci, M.D.**

BASIC INFORMATION

■ DEFINITION

Acute viral encephalitis is an acute febrile syndrome with evidence of meningeal involvement and of derangement of the function of the cerebrum, cerebellum, or brainstem.

■ SYNONYMS

Arboviral encephalitis
Brainstem encephalitis
Acute necrotizing encephalitis
Rasmussen encephalitis
Encephalitis lethargica

ICD-9CM CODES

049.9 Viral encephalitis NOS

■ EPIDEMIOLOGY & DEMOGRAPHICS

INCIDENCE (IN U.S.): About 20,000 cases/yr are reported to the CDC.
PREVALENCE (IN U.S.): Unknown
PREDOMINANT SEX: Male = female
PREDOMINANT AGE: Any age
PEAK INCIDENCE: Any age
GENETICS: No specific genetic or congenital predisposition

■ ETIOLOGY

- Can be caused by a host of viruses, with herpes simplex the most common virus identified
- Arboviruses: agents causing Eastern equine encephalitis, Western equine encephalitis, St. Louis encephalitis, Venezuelan equine encephalitis, California virus encephalitis, Japanese B encephalitis, Murray Valley and West Nile encephalitis, Russian spring-summer encephalitis, as well as other lesser known agents
- Also implicated: rabies-causing agents, CMV, Epstein-Barr, varicella-zoster, echo virus, mumps, adenovirus, coxsackie, rubeola, and herpes viruses
- Meningoencephalitis: acute retroviral infection

■ PHYSICAL FINDINGS & CLINICAL PRESENTATION

- Initially, fever and evidence of meningeal irritation
- Headache and stiff neck
- Later, development of signs of cortical dysfunction: lethargy, coma, stupor, weakness, seizures, facial weakness, as well as brainstem findings
- Cerebellar findings: ataxia, nystagmus, hypotonia; myoclonus, cranial nerve palsies, and abnormal tendon reflexes
- Patients with rabies: hydrophobia, anxiety, facial numbness, psychosis, coma, or dysarthria
- Rarely, movement disorders, such as chorea, hemiballismus, or dystonia
- Recall of a prodromal viral-like illness (this finding is not at all uniform)

🔬 DIAGNOSIS

■ DIFFERENTIAL DIAGNOSIS

- Bacterial infections: brain abscess, toxic encephalopathies, TB
- Protozoal infections
- Behçet's disease
- Lupus encephalitis
- Sjögren's syndrome
- Multiple sclerosis
- Syphilis
- Cryptococcus
- Toxoplasmosis
- Brucellosis
- Leukemic or lymphomatous meningitis
- Other metastatic tumors
- Lyme disease
- Cat-scratch disease
- Vogt-Koyanagi-Harada syndrome
- Mollaret's meningitis

■ WORKUP

- Lumbar puncture to reveal pleocytosis, usually lymphocytic although neutrophils may be seen early on
- Usually, elevated CSF protein
- Normal or low CSF glucose
- In herpes simplex encephalitis: RBCs and xanthochromia
- EEG changes showing periodic high-voltage sharp waves in the temporal regions and slow wave complexes suggestive of herpes encephalitis
- CT scan and MRI to reveal edema and hemorrhage in the frontal and temporal lobes
- Arboviral infections suspected during outbreaks in specific areas
- Rising titers of neutralizing antibodies from the acute to the convalescent stage demonstrated but often not helpful in the acutely ill patient
- Polymerase chain reaction that amplifies DNA from the CSF for herpes simplex encephalitis
- Rarely, brain biopsy to assist in the diagnosis; viral culture of cerebral tissue obtained if biopsy done
- Classic herpetic skin lesions suggestive of herpes encephalitis
- In diagnosing arboviral encephalitis:
  1. Presence of antiviral IgM within the first few days of symptomatic disease; detected and quantified by ELISA
  2. Unusual to recover an arbovirus from the blood or CSF

■ LABORATORY TESTS

- Aside from the lumbar puncture, most other laboratory studies are nonspecific.
- Skin lesions and urine may be cultured for herpes simplex and CMV.

🔬 TREATMENT

■ ACUTE GENERAL Rx

- Supportive care, frequent evaluation, and neurologic examination
- Ventilatory assistance for patients who are moribund or at risk for aspiration
- Avoidance of infusion of hypotonic fluids to minimize the risk of hyponatremia
- For patients who develop seizures: anticonvulsant therapy and follow-up in a critical care setting
- For comatose patients:
  1. Aggressive care to avoid decubiti, contractures, and DVT
  2. Close attention to weights, input/output, and serum electrolytes
- Acyclovir 30 mg/kg/day IV for 14 days for herpes simplex encephalitis
- Short courses of corticosteroids to control brain edema and prevent herniation
- In patients with suspected rabies:
  1. Human rabies immune globulin (HRIG) should be given at a dose of 20 U/kg.
  2. Active immunization may be stimulated by recently developed rabies vaccine, which is grown on a human diploid cell line (HDCV) and has reduced the number of doses needed to five.
  3. If suspect animal can be found, observe closely for 10 days to detect rabid behavior.
  4. If signs are seen, animal should be euthanized and its brain examined for signs of rabies.
- No specific pharmacologic therapy for most other viral pathogens

■ CHRONIC Rx

Some patients may develop permanent neurologic sequelae; these patients will gain benefit from intensive rehabilitation programs, including physical, occupational, and speech therapy.

REFERENCES

Beckwith WH et al: Isolation of eastern equine encephalitis virus and West Nile virus from crows during increased arbovirus surveillance in Connecticut, 2000, *Am J Trop Med Hyg* 66(4):422, 2002.

Centers for Disease Control and Prevention: Provisional surveillance summary of the West Nile virus epidemic—United States, January-November, 2002, *MMWR Morb Mortal Wkly Rep* 51(50):1129, 2002.

Miravalle A, Roos KL: Encephalitis complicating smallpox vaccination, *Arch Neurol* 60(7):925, 2003.

Romero JR, Newland JG: Viral meningitis and encephalitis: traditional and emerging viral agents, *Semin Pediatr Infect Dis* 14(2):72, 2003.

Srey VH et al: Etiology of encephalitis syndrome among hospitalized children and adults in Takeo, Cambodia, 1999-2000, *Am J Trop Med Hyg* 66(2):200, 2002.

Author: **Joseph J. Lieber, M.D.**

BASIC INFORMATION

■ DEFINITION
Encopresis is the voluntary or involuntary passage of stool into inappropriate places, in children over the developmental age of 4 yr, with the absence of direct physiologic causes.

■ SYNONYMS
Functional incontinence of stool

ICD-9CM CODES
787.6 Incontinence of feces
307.7 Encopresis

■ EPIDEMIOLOGY & DEMOGRAPHICS
INCIDENCE (IN U.S.): 1% of 5 yr olds
PREVALANCE (IN U.S.): 3% of the pediatric population
PREDOMINANT SEX: Male > female
PREDOMINANT AGE: 4 to 9 yr of age
PEAK INCIDENCE: 4 to 5 yr of age
GENETICS: Factors that contribute to slow gut motility may predispose to encopresis

■ PHYSICAL FINDINGS & CLINICAL PRESENTATION
- When constipation and overflow incontinence are causative, defecation is usually uncomfortable or painful, so patient avoids defecation with consequent stool retention.
- Stool is usually poorly formed and leakage is continuous (occurring during sleep and wakefulness).
- Encopresis resolves when the constipation is resolved.
- When there is no constipation with overflow incontinence, stool is more likely to be normal in character.
- Soiling is intermittent and usually in a prominent location.
- Coexisting oppositional-defiant or conduct disorders are frequent.

■ ETIOLOGY
- Approximately 96% of children will have bowel movements between three times daily to once every other day. When bowel movements are less frequent, stool becomes drier and harder and much more uncomfortable to pass. Children may avoid the discomfort by avoiding elimination, but this only results in worsening constipation.
- Soiling results from more liquid stool that leaks around the main stool mass.
- Constipation may begin gradually as a result of a slow decrease in elimination frequency or more acutely after an illness, dehydration, or prolonged bed rest.
- In encopresis without constipation and overflow incontinence, soiling is usually intentional. This frequently occurs in the setting of comorbid oppositional-defiant disorder or conduct disorder.
- Incontinence can also result from anal masturbation.

DIAGNOSIS

■ DIFFERENTIAL DIAGNOSIS
- Hirschsprung's disease
- Cerebral palsy
- Myelomeningocele
- Pseudoobstruction
- Anorectal lesions
- Malformations
- Trauma
- Rectal prolapse
- Hypothyroidism
- Medications

■ WORKUP
- History: pay particular attention to frequency of elimination, character of the stool, associated pain, and presence of enuresis (with which it is frequently associated)
- Physical examination: pay particular attention to the abdomen, anus, rectum, and saddle sensation.

■ LABORATORY TESTS
- Thyroid profile
- Electrolytes (including calcium)
- Adrenal function
- Urinalysis and urine culture

■ IMAGING STUDIES
- Abdominal x-rays to determine extent of obstruction or megacolon
- Anorectal manometric studies to determine sphincter function if Hirschsprung's disease is suspected; if abnormal, followed up with a barium enema and rectal biopsy

TREATMENT

■ NONPHARMACOLOGIC THERAPY
- Psychotherapy or family therapy in chronic encopresis
- Biofeedback to improve sphincter function

■ ACUTE GENERAL Rx
- Disimpaction with hypertonic phosphate (30 ml/5 kg body weight) or isotonic saline enemas
- Resistant cases: repeated instillation of 200 to 600 ml of milk of magnesia enemas
- If child does not permit enemas: oral disimpaction with large doses of mineral oil or lactulose until stool mass is cleared (NOTE: this is frequently more painful and more uncomfortable than an enema)

■ CHRONIC Rx
- Prevention of recurrence of constipation by increased dietary fiber and the use of laxatives
- In immediate postdisimpaction period (3 mo following acute treatment) laxatives needed because bowel tone remains low
- Laxatives possibly required for several years or indefinitely

■ DISPOSITION
In most cases encopresis is self-limited and of relatively brief duration; it is rarely chronic.

■ REFERRAL
If patient is resistant to treatment, complicated family factors are involved, or encopresis is purposeful

REFERENCE
Mikkelsen EJ: Enuresis and encopresis: ten years of progress, *J Am Acad Child Adolesc Psychiatry* 40:1146, 2001.
Author: **Rif S. El-Mallakh, M.D.**

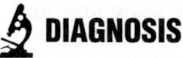

BASIC INFORMATION

■ DEFINITION

Infective endocarditis is an infection of the endocardial surface of the heart or mural endocardium.

ACUTE ENDOCARDITIS: Usually caused by *Staphylococcus aureus, Streptococcus pyogenes,* pneumococcus, and *Neisseria* organisms; classic clinical presentation of fever, positive blood cultures, vascular and immunologic phenomenon

SUBACUTE ENDOCARDITIS: Usually caused by viridans streptococci in the presence of valvular pathology; less toxic, often indolent presentation with lower fevers, night sweats, fatigue

INFECTIVE ENDOCARDITIS IN INJECTION DRUG USERS: Often involving *S. aureus* or *Pseudomonas aeruginosa* with variation that may be geographically influenced; tricuspid or multiple valvular involvement; high mortality rate of 50% to 60%

EARLY PROSTHETIC VALVE ENDOCARDITIS: Usually caused by *S. epidermidis* within 2 mo of valve replacement; other organisms include *S. aureus,* gram-negative bacilli, diphtheroids, *Candida* organisms

LATE PROSTHETIC VALVE ENDOCARDITIS: Typically develops >60 days after valvular replacement; involved organisms similar to early prosthetic valve endocarditis, including viridans streptococci, enterococci, and group D streptococci

NOSOCOMIAL ENDOCARDITIS: Secondary to intravenous catheters, TPN lines, pacemakers; coagulase negative staphylococci, *S. aureus,* and streptococci most common

■ SYNONYMS

Bacterial endocarditis

ICD-9CM CODES

421.0 Infective endocarditis
996.61 Prosthetic valve endocarditis

■ EPIDEMIOLOGY & DEMOGRAPHICS

INCIDENCE (IN U.S.): 1.7 to 3.8 cases/100,000 persons/yr
NOSOCOMIAL ENDOCARDITIS: 14% to 28% of cases
PREVALENCE (IN U.S.): 0.3 to 3 cases/1000 hospital admissions
PREDOMINANT SEX: Male > female
PREDOMINANT AGE: 45 to 65 yr
PEAK INCIDENCE: Females: often <35 yr old; males: 45 to 65 yr old

■ PHYSICAL FINDINGS & CLINICAL PRESENTATION

- Fever may be variable in presentation; may be high, hectic, or absent.
- Fever, chills, fatigue, and rigors occur in 25% to 80% of patients.
- Heart murmur may be absent in right-sided endocarditis.
- Embolic phenomenon with peripheral manifestations is found in 50% of patients.
- Skin manifestations include petechiae, Osler nodes, splinter hemorrhages, Janeway lesions.
- Splenomegaly is more common with subacute course.

■ ETIOLOGY

Streptococcal and staphylococcal infections are the most common causes of infective endocarditis. Variation in incidence may occur that is influenced by the patient's risk for developing infection.

ACUTE ENDOCARDITIS:
- *S. aureus*
- *Streptococcus pneumoniae*
- Streptococcal species and groups A through G
- *Haemophilus influenzae*

SUBACUTE ENDOCARDITIS:
- Viridans streptococci (α-hemolytic)
- *S. bovis*
- Enterococci
- *S. aureus*

ENDOCARDITIS IN IV DRUG ADDICTS:
- *S. aureus*
- *P. aeruginosa*
- *Candida* species
- Enterococci

PROSTHETIC VALVE (EARLY):
- *S. epidermidis*
- *S. aureus*
- Gram-negative bacilli
- Group D streptococci

PROSTHETIC VALVE (LATE):
- *S. epidermidis*
- Viridans streptococci
- *S. aureus*
- Enterococci and group D streptococci

NOSOCOMIAL ENDOCARDITIS:
- Coagulase negative *Staphylococcus*
- *S. aureus*
- Streptococci: viridans, group B, enterococcus

HACEK ORGANISMS:
- Fastidious gram-negative bacilli
- *Haemophilus parainfluenzae*
- *Haemophilus aphrophilus*
- *Actinobacillus actinomycetemcomitans*
- *Cardiobacterium hominis*
- *Eikenella corrodens*
- *Kingella kingae*

RISK FACTORS
- Poor dental hygiene
- Long-term hemodialysis
- Diabetes mellitus
- HIV infection
- Mitral valve prolapse

DIAGNOSIS

■ DIFFERENTIAL DIAGNOSIS
- Brain abscess
- FUO
- Pericarditis
- Meningitis
- Rheumatic fever
- Osteomyelitis
- Salmonella
- TB
- Bacteremia
- Pericarditis
- Glomerulonephritis

■ WORKUP
Physical examination to evaluate for the previous physical findings followed by laboratory testing (see Laboratory Tests)

■ LABORATORY TESTS
- Blood cultures: three sets in first 24 hr
- More culturing if patient has received prior antibiotic
- CBC (anemia possibly present, subacute)
- WBC (leukocytosis is higher in acute endocarditis)
- ESR (elevated)
- Positive rheumatoid factor (subacute endocarditis)
- False-positive VDRL
- Proteinuria, hematuria, RBC casts

■ IMAGING STUDIES
- Echocardiogram: two-dimensional
- Transesophageal echocardiography: more sensitive in detecting vegations if two-dimensional is negative, especially helpful with prosthetic valves or in detecting perivalvular disease

TREATMENT

Initial IV antibiotic therapy (before culture results) is aimed at the most likely organism:

- In patients with prosthetic valves or patients with native valves who are allergic to penicillin: vancomycin plus rifampin and gentamicin
- In IV drug users: nafcillin or oxacillin plus gentamicin; if MRSA, vancomycin plus gentamicin
- In native valve endocarditis: combination of penicillin and gentamicin; a penicillase-resistant penicillin (oxacillin or nafcillin) can be used if acute bacterial endocarditis is present or if *S. aureus* is suspected as one of the possible causative organisms; for Hacek organisms, treat with third-generation cephalosporin
- Ceftriaxone and an aminoglycoside for 2 wk can be used in streptococcus viridans endocarditis

Antibiotic therapy after identification of the organism should be guided by susceptibility testing.

⚙ PEARLS & CONSIDERATIONS

■ COMMENTS

For endocarditis prophylaxis refer to Section II and Tables 5-25 and 5-26.

REFERENCES

DiSalvo G, Habib G, Pergola V: Echocardiography predicts embolic events in infective endocarditis, *J Am Coll Cardiol* 37:1069, 2001.

Heiro M et al: Diagnosis of infective endocarditis, *Arch Intern Med* 158:18, 1998.

Mylonakis E, Calderwood SB: Infective endocarditis in adults, *N Engl J Med* 345:1318, 2001.

Authors: **Glenn G. Fort, M.D., and Dennis J. Mikolich, M.D.**

BASIC INFORMATION

■ DEFINITION
Endometrial cancer is a malignant transformation of endometrial stroma and/or glands typified by irregular nuclear membranes, nuclear atypia, mitotic activity, loss of glandular pattern, irregular cell size (Fig. 1-99).

■ SYNONYMS
Uterine cancer (some forms)

ICD-9CM CODES
182 Malignant neoplasm of body of uterus

■ EPIDEMIOLOGY & DEMOGRAPHICS
INCIDENCE: 21.2 cases/100,000 persons; approximately 30,000 new cases annually
PREDOMINANCE: Median age at onset: 60 yr; only 5% occur in women <40 yr
RISK FACTORS: Obesity, diabetes, nulliparity, early menarche and late menopause, unopposed estrogen therapy, tamoxifen use, endometrial atypical hyperplasia

■ PHYSICAL FINDINGS & CLINICAL PRESENTATION
- Abnormal uterine bleeding or post-menopausal bleeding in 90%
- Pyometra or hematometra
- Abnormal Pap smear

■ ETIOLOGY
Endogenous or exogenous chronic unopposed estrogen stimulation of the endometrium

DIAGNOSIS

■ DIFFERENTIAL DIAGNOSIS
- Atypical hyperplasia
- Other genital tract malignancy
- Polyps
- Atrophic vaginitis
- Granuloma cell tumor
- Fibroid uterus

■ WORKUP
- Complete history and physical examination
- Endometrial biopsy or dilation and curettage
- Assessment of operative risk

■ LABORATORY TESTS
- CBC
- Chemistry profile including liver function tests
- Consider CA-125 level

■ IMAGING STUDIES
- Chest x-ray examination
- Possible CT scan, BE, and/or pelvic ultrasound
- Endovaginal ultrasound in postmenopausal women with vaginal bleeding

TREATMENT

■ NONPHARMACOLOGIC THERAPY
- Surgery is the mainstay of treatment, with or without radiation, depending on tumor stage and grade.

- Surgery consists of pelvic washings, total abdominal hysterectomy and bilateral salpingo-oophorectomy, omental biopsy, and selective pelvic and periaortic lymphadenectomy, depending on stage and grade.
- Brachytherapy and/or teletherapy are added in an advanced stage.
- Chemotherapy (cisplatin, Adriamycin) or tamoxifen may also be used.

■ ACUTE GENERAL Rx
- A thorough workup should be completed before any therapy for endometrial cancer.
- Surgery is the treatment of choice.

■ CHRONIC Rx
- Physical and pelvic examination every 3 mo for 2 yr, then every 6 mo for 2 yr, annually thereafter
- Yearly Pap smear
- Hormone replacement (combination) a consideration in low-risk patients (stage I or early stage II)

■ DISPOSITION
The majority of cases present early, where the 5-yr survival is generally good:
Stage I   75% to 100%
Stage II   60%
Stage III 50%
Stage IV   20%
Some histologic types (clear cell, serous papillary) have poorer survival rates.

■ REFERRAL
A gynecologist may manage early-stage disease, otherwise refer to a gynecologic oncologist.

☼ PEARLS & CONSIDERATIONS

■ COMMENTS
Estrogen replacement therapy (ERT) after surgery for endometrial cancer remains controversial. Recent data suggest that ERT does not increase endometrial cancer recurrence rates.

REFERENCES
Smith-Bindman R et al: Endovaginal ultrasound to exclude endometrial cancer and other endometrial abnormalities, *JAMA* 280:1510, 1998.
Suriano KA et al: Estrogen replacement therapy in endometrial cancer patients, *Obstet Gynecol* 97:555, 2001.
Tabor A et al: Endometrial thickness as a test for endometrial cancer in women with postmenopausal vaginal bleeding, *Obstet Gynecol* 99:529, 2002.
Author: **Gil Farkash, M.D.**

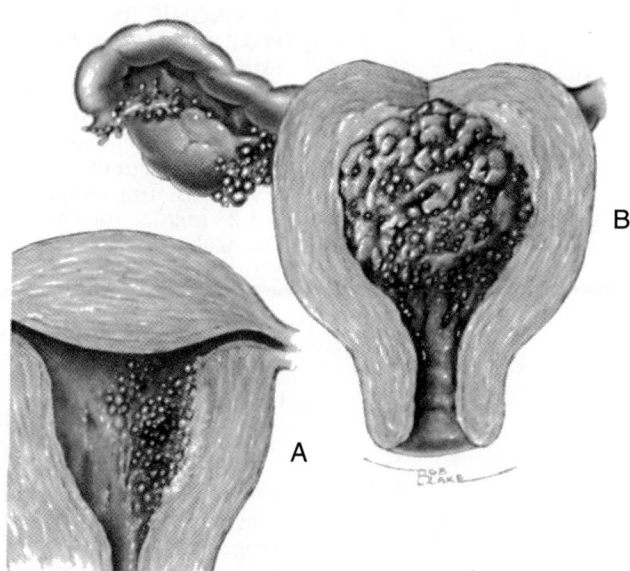

Fig. 1-99   Carcinoma of the endometrium. A, Stage I. **B,** Stage III, myometrial invasion. (From Sabiston D: *Textbook of surgery,* ed 15, Philadelphia, 1997, WB Saunders.)

BASIC INFORMATION

■ DEFINITION
Endometriosis is defined as the presence of functioning endometrial glands and stroma outside the uterine cavity (Fig. 1-100).

ICD-9CM CODES
617.9 Endometriosis

■ EPIDEMIOLOGY & DEMOGRAPHICS
PREVALENCE:
- In asymptomatic woman: 2%-22%
- Women with dysmenorrhea: 40%-60%
- Subfertile women: 20%-30%
- Incidence peaks at about age 40

MOST COMMON AGE AT DIAGNOSIS:
25 to 29 yr

GENETICS:
- Multifactorial inheritance pattern
- 6.9% occurrence rate in first-degree female relatives

■ PHYSICAL FINDINGS & CLINICAL PRESENTATION
- Classic triad is dysmenorrhea, dyspareunia, and infertility.
- Presence of pelvic pain *not correlated* with the total area of endometriosis, type of lesion, or volume of disease, but it *is correlated* with the depth of infiltration.
- Most severe discomfort is associated with lesions >1 cm in depth.
- Bimanual examination may reveal tender uterosacral ligaments, cul-de-sac nodularity, induration of the rectovaginal septum, fixed retroversion of the uterus, adnexal mass, and generalized or localized tenderness.

■ ETIOLOGY
- Reflux and direct implantation theory: retrograde menstruation with implantation of viable endometrial cells to surrounding pelvic structures
- Coelomic metaplasia theory: transformation of multipotential cells of the coelomic epithelium into endometrium-like cells
- Vascular dissemination theory: transport of endometrial cells to distant sites via the uterine vascular and lymphatic systems
- Autoimmune disease theory: disorder of immune surveillance allows growth of endometrial implants

DIAGNOSIS

■ DIFFERENTIAL DIAGNOSIS
- Ectopic pregnancy
- Acute appendicitis
- Chronic appendicitis
- PID
- Pelvic adhesions
- Hemorrhagic cyst
- Hernia
- Psychologic disorder
- Irritable bowel syndrome
- Uterine leiomyomata
- Adenomyosis
- Nerve entrapment syndrome
- Scoliosis
- Muscular/skeletal strain
- Interstitial cystitis

■ WORKUP
- Thorough history and physical examination, including inquiry about physical and emotional abuse
- Colonoscopy if rectal bleeding present

- Laparoscopy for definitive diagnosis
- Revised American Fertility Society (RAFS) scale to classify endometriosis (since 1985):

Stage I   minimal
Stage II   mild
Stage III moderate
Stage IV severe

■ LABORATORY TESTS
Cancer antigen 125 (CA125)
- Also elevated in ovarian epithelial neoplasm, myomas, adenomyosis, acute PID, ovarian cysts, pancreatitis, chronic liver disease, menstruation, and pregnancy
- CA 125 value >35 U/ml: positive predictive value of 0.58 and a negative predictive value of 0.96 for the presence of endometriosis

■ IMAGING STUDIES
- Ultrasound: for evaluating adnexal mass; cannot reliably distinguish endometriomas from other benign or malignant ovarian conditions
- MRI:
  1. Highly accurate in detecting endometriomas
  2. Limited sensitivity in detecting diffuse pelvic endometriosis

TREATMENT

■ NONPHARMACOLOGIC THERAPY
Expectant management (observation for 5 to 12 mo) for stage I or stage II endometriosis-associated infertility

■ ACUTE GENERAL Rx
NSAIDs for symptomatic relief of dysmenorrhea

■ CHRONIC Rx
PHARMACOLOGIC MANAGEMENT:
Estrogen-progesterone:
- State of "pseudopregnancy" created by continuous use of combination oral contraceptives for 6 to 12 mo
- Breakthrough bleeding treated by administering conjugated estrogens 1.25 mg/day for 2 wk

Danazol:
- Initial dose 200 mg PO bid
- If no improvement within 6 wk, dosage increased to 300 or 400 mg PO bid
- Treatment generally continued for 6 mo, after which up to 90% of patients with mild to moderate endometriosis experience alleviation of pelvic pain
- Treatment begun after menses to avoid fetal exposure

Progestins:
- Medroxyprogesterone acetate 10 to 30 mg PO qd and occasionally up to 100 mg PO qd

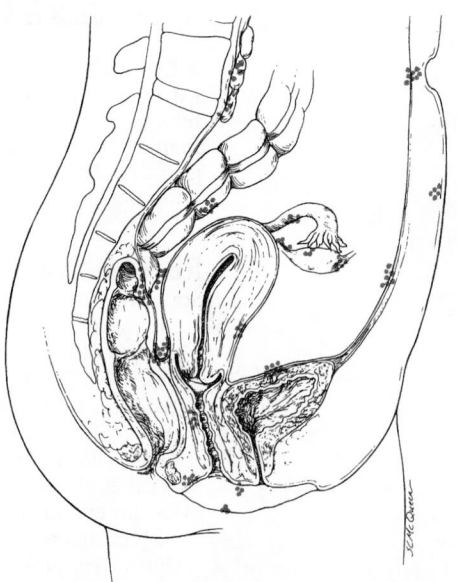

Fig. 1-100   Common pelvic sites of endometriosis. (From Mishell D [ed]: *Comprehensive gynecology*, ed 3, St Louis, 1997, Mosby.)

- Alternatively, 100 mg IM q2wk for four doses, followed by 200 mg IM monthly for 4 mo
- Breakthrough bleeding treated with ethinyl estradiol (20 µg/day) or conjugated estrogens (1.25 mg/day) for 1 to 2 wk
- Comparison with danazol: progestins cost less, have a more tolerable side-effect profile, and have comparable efficacy with regard to pain relief, so are often the first-line drug

Gonadotropin-releasing hormone (GnRH) agonists:
- Use usually limited to 6 mo
- Leuprolide acetate depot 3.75 mg IM monthly *or* 11.25 mg IM q3mo
- *or* nafarelin 200 µg nasal puffs bid
- *or* goserelin 3.6 mg SC monthly
- As effective as danazol for relief of pelvic pain
- Add-back therapy for protection against vasomotor symptoms and bone loss: norethindrone acetate 5 mg PO qd alone *or* in combination with conjugated estrogen 0.625 mg PO qd
- Add-back therapy allows GnRH agonist use to be extended to 1 yr

SURGICAL MANAGEMENT:
Conservative:
- Directed at enhancing fertility or treating pain unresponsive to first-line medical treatment
- Usually accomplished through laparoscopy
- Removal or destruction of endometriotic implants by excision, electrocautery, or laser
- Cystectomy
- Unless pregnancy is desired, patient is usually started on GnRH agonist therapy immediately after surgery

- For those desiring pregnancy, surgery alone results in significant increase in fertility

Definitive:
- Directed at relieving endometriosis-associated pain
- Total abdominal hysterectomy with bilateral salpingo-oophorectomy and complete excision or ablation of endometriosis
- Thorough abdominal exploration to ensure removal of all disease
- Must be prepared to manage possible GI and urinary tract endometriosis
- 90% effective in pain relief
- Estrogen replacement therapy (ERT) to be considered in all women undergoing definitive surgical management; after ERT, recurrence rate of 0% to 5% in women with endometriosis confined to the pelvis but 18% in women with bowel involvement

MANAGEMENT OF ENDOMETRIOSIS-ASSOCIATED INFERTILITY:
Conservative Surgery:
- Yields significantly increased pregnancy rate than does expectant management, in part because of correction of mechanical factors such as adhesions

Assisted Reproductive Technologies:
- Can be used to circumvent unknown mechanism of endometriosis-associated infertility
- Superovulation with clomiphene citrate or human menopausal gonadotropins; clomiphene citrate results in threefold pregnancy rate over either danazol or expectant management
- Further improvement with intrauterine insemination combined with superovulation

- In vitro fertilization if above mentioned unsuccessful

■ DISPOSITION
Tends to recur unless definitive surgery is performed

■ REFERRAL
To a reproductive endocrinologist for advanced surgical management or infertility management

☼ PEARLS & CONSIDERATIONS

■ COMMENTS
Patient information can be obtained through the following organizations: Endometriosis Association, 8585 North 76th Place, Milwaukee, WI 53223, 414-355-2200 or 800-992-ENDO; Women's Reproductive Health Network, P.O. Box 30167, Portland, OR 97230-9067; phone: 503-667-7757.

REFERENCES
Hornstein MD et al for the Lupron Addback Study Group: Leuprolide acetate depot and hormonal add-back in endometriosis: a 12-month study, *Obstet Gynecol* 91:16, 1998.
Johnson KM: Endometriosis: the immunoendocrine factor, *Female Patient* 21:15, 1996.
Olive DL, Pritts EA: Treatment of endometriosis, *N Engl J Med* 345:266, 2001.
Winkel CA: Evaluation and management of women with endometriosis, Obstetrics and gynecology, 102(2):397, 2003.
Author: **Wan J. Kim, M.D.**

BASIC INFORMATION

■ DEFINITION
Endometritis is defined as a uterine infection following delivery or abortion.

■ SYNONYMS
Endomyometritis
Endoperimetritis
Metritis

ICD-9CM CODES
615.9 Endometritis

■ EPIDEMIOLOGY & DEMOGRAPHICS
• Overall rate of postpartum infection: estimated between 1% and 8%
• Most common genital tract infection following delivery
• Usually presents early in postpartum period; more commonly seen following C-section than vaginal delivery; also seen with an incomplete abortion (spontaneous abortion, legal abortion, or illegal abortion)
• More common in preterm deliveries
• Possible following any uterine manipulation in the presence of an undiagnosed cervicitis or vaginitis

■ PHYSICAL FINDINGS & CLINICAL PRESENTATION
• Postpartum oral temperature >37.8° C
• Localized uterine tenderness, purulent or foul lochia; physical examination revealing uterine or parametrial tenderness
• Nonspecific signs and symptoms such as malaise, abdominal pain, chills, and tachycardia

■ ETIOLOGY
Endometritis is usually associated with multiple organisms: group A or B streptococci, *Staphylococcus aureus* and *Bacteroides* species, *Neisseria gonorrhoeae, Chlamydia trachomatis,* enterococci, *Gardnerella vaginalis, E. coli,* and *Mycoplasma.*

DIAGNOSIS

■ DIFFERENTIAL DIAGNOSIS
Causes of postoperative or postprocedural infections

■ WORKUP
Diagnosis based on symptoms of fever, malaise, abdominal pain, uterine tenderness, and purulent, foul vaginal discharge

■ LABORATORY TESTS
CBC, blood cultures, and uterine culture

■ IMAGING STUDIES
Ultrasound may be useful if retained products are considered a possible source of infection.

TREATMENT

■ ACUTE GENERAL Rx
• In treating endometritis after a vaginal delivery, ampicillin 2 g IV q6h plus gentamicin loading dose IV or IM (2 mg/kg of body weight), followed by a maintenance dose (1.5 mg/kg of body weight) q8h are used.
• Regimen should be continued for at least 48 hr after substantial clinical improvement. If response is not adequate, check cultures and treat with appropriate antibiotics (Table 1-20).
• Endometritis following C-section should be treated with ampicillin 2 g IV q6h plus gentamicin loading dose IV or IM (2 mg/kg of body weight), followed by a maintenance dose (1.5 mg/kg of body weight) q8h and clindamycin 900 mg IV q8h. If *Chlamydia* is one of the etiologic agents, add doxycycline 100 mg PO bid for completion of a 14-day course of therapy (if breast feeding, use erythromycin).

■ CHRONIC Rx
Watch for recurrent infection.

■ DISPOSITION
With appropriate antibiotic therapy, 95% to 98% cure rate

■ REFERRAL
For patients who do not respond within 48 to 72 hr of appropriate antibiotic therapy, obtain an infectious disease consult or gynecologic consultation.

REFERENCES

Centers for Disease Control and Prevention: Sexually transmitted disease treatment guideline, *MMWR* 47(RR-1), 1998.
French LM, Smaill FM: Antibiotic regimens for endometritis after delivery, *Cochrane Database of Sysstematic Reviews* (1):CD001067, 2002.
Smaill F, Hofmeyr GJ: Antibiotic prophylaxis for cesarean section, *Cochrane Database of Systematic Reviews* (3):CD000933, 2002.
Author: **George T. Danakas, M.D.**

TABLE 1-27 **Identified Causes of Poor Response to Antibiotic Therapy in Patients with Endometritis**

CAUSE	APPROXIMATE PREVALENCE (%)
Infected mass, including abscess, hematoma, septic pelvic thrombophlebitis, pelvic cellulitis, retained placenta	40-50
Resistant organisms, commonly enterococci, in a patient receiving clindamycin-aminoglycoside or a cephalosporin	20
Additional cause, including catheter phlebitis, inadequate dose of antibiotics	10
No cause evident but response to empirical change in antibiotic therapy	20-30

From Gorbach SL: *Infectious diseases,* ed 2, Philadelphia, 1998, WB Saunders.

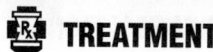
 BASIC INFORMATION

■ DEFINITION
Enuresis refers to the voiding of urine into clothes or in bed that is usually involuntary but occasionally intentional in individuals who are expected to be continent (i.e., >5 yr of age). The diagnosis is made if voiding occurs at least twice a week for 3 mo.

■ SYNONYMS
Urinary incontinence
Bed-wetting
Self-wetting

ICD-9CM CODES
F98.0
DMS-IV Code 307.6

■ EPIDEMIOLOGY & DEMOGRAPHICS
PREVALENCE (IN U.S.):
- Age 5: 7% of males and 3% of females
- Age 10: 3% of males and 2% of females
- Age 18: 1% of males and even fewer females

PREDOMINANT SEX: Twice as many males as females
PREDOMINANT AGE: By definition, enuresis does not begin before age 5 yr, at which time the prevalence is highest, and decreases steadily through life.
PEAK INCIDENCE: Early childhood, ages 5 to 10 yr
GENETICS:
- Approximately 75% of children with enuresis have a first-degree relative with enuresis.
- Concordance rate may be higher in monozygotic twins than dizygotic twins.

■ PHYSICAL FINDINGS & CLINICAL PRESENTATION
Three subtypes are defined:
- Nocturnal only: usually occurs in first third of sleep, frequently during REM sleep; child may recall a dream with voiding
- Diurnal only: more frequent in girls and rarely after age 9 yr; voiding occurs in early afternoon on school days
- Combined nocturnal and diurnal enuresis

■ ETIOLOGY
- No clear etiology
- Hypotheses: lax toilet training, stress, inability to concentrate urine, and altered smooth muscle physiology
- Diurnal enuresis associated with a higher rate of urinary tract infections

🔬 DIAGNOSIS

■ DIFFERENTIAL DIAGNOSIS
- May be associated with encopresis and sleep disorders such as sleep terrors
- Must rule out organic causes associated with polyuria or urgency but may coexist if enuresis was present before or after treatment of the associated medical condition

■ WORKUP
History and physical examination to rule out anatomic abnormalities
NOTE: Because children frequently experience shame, gentleness and care must be exercised when questioning or examining the child.

■ LABORATORY TESTS
- Urinalysis to determine specific gravity
- Urine culture to rule out urinary tract infection
- Serum studies to rule out diabetes and fluid balance abnormalities

■ IMAGING STUDIES
- In complicated cases: sleep studies possibly useful
- If an anatomic abnormality suspected: renal ultrasound or IVP possibly indicated

℞ TREATMENT

■ NONPHARMACOLOGIC THERAPY
- Scheduled voiding to reduce the frequency of enuretic episodes
- Conditioning, psychotherapy, and bed alarms: all reported as useful but not found to be adequate by the children's caregivers

■ ACUTE GENERAL Rx
- Desmopressin (DDAVP) administered intranasally at bedtime significantly reduces the incidence of bed-wetting.
- Imipramine: used with mixed results; the use of tricyclic antidepressants in children is problematic because of the risk of sudden death.
- Serotonin reuptake inhibitors: lack of adequate trials is notable.

■ DISPOSITION
- After age 5 yr, the rate of spontaneous remissions is 5% to 10%/yr.
- Usually the disorder resolves by adolescence.
- Fewer than 1% will experience enuresis as adults.

■ REFERRAL
If coexisting psychiatric condition complicates the course of treatment

REFERENCES
Glazener CM, Evans JH: Desmopressin for nocternal enuresis in children, *Cochrane Database of Systematic Reviews* (3):CD002112, 2002.
Mikkelsen EJ: Enuresis and encopresis: ten years of progress, *J Am Acad Child Adolesc Psychiatry* 40:1146, 2001.
Author: **Rif S. El-Mallakh, M.D.**

BASIC INFORMATION

■ DEFINITION

Eosinophilic fasciitis is a rare inflammatory disease of the skin and subcutaneous tissue that is initially characterized by pain, swelling, and peripheral eosinophilia. This condition may progress to sclerosis and contractures.

■ SYNONYMS

Shulman's syndrome

ICD-9CM CODES

728.89 Eosinophilic fasciitis

■ EPIDEMIOLOGY & DEMOGRAPHICS

• Males and females are affected equally.
• The disease most commonly presents in the fourth and fifth decades.

■ PHYSICAL FINDINGS & CLINICAL PRESENTATION

• Initial presentation consists of swelling and pain with or without erythema.
• The extremities are usually symmetrically involved.
• Upper extremities are more commonly affected than lower extremities.
• The face, fingers, and toes tend to be spared.
• The skin may appear deeply rippled with an orange-peel texture.
• Sunken veins may be seen when the extremity is elevated (Fig. 1-101).
• The groove sign marks the borders of different muscle groups.
• Arthritis is found in 40% of cases.
• Chronic complications are carpal tunnel syndrome and flexion contractures.
• Spontaneous resolution or improvement has been reported after 2 to 5 yr.

■ ETIOLOGY

• The etiology is unclear. A defect in humoral immunity has been hypothesized to cause the disease.
• Elevated polyclonal IgG levels and immune complexes have been associated with the disease.
• Eosinophilic fasciitis has been seen in association with myelodysplastic syndromes, aplastic anemia, thrombocytopenia, monoclonal gammopathy, and Hodgkin's disease.

DIAGNOSIS

■ DIFFERENTIAL DIAGNOSIS

• Systemic sclerosis
• Chemical induced sclerosis
• Generalized lichen sclerosus et atrophicus
• Graft-versus-host disease
• Porphyria cutanea tarda
• Chronic Lyme borreliosis

■ WORKUP

• Physical examination to confirm characteristic distribution
• Some authorities suggest bone marrow biopsy to rule out hematological malignancy
• Ultrasound sonography and MRI might be useful to detect the thickened fascia

■ LABORATORY TESTS

• Peripheral eosinophilia in up to 70%
• Elevated erythrocyte sedimentation rate
• Hypergammaglobulinemia
• Occasionally thrombocytopenia and anemia

■ DEEP TISSUE BIOPSY

Skin biopsy that penetrates to muscle is optimal for diagnosis:
• Epidermis is usually normal.
• Dermis may demonstrate mild inflammation with lymphocytes, histiocytes, plasma cells, and eosinophils with some fibrosis.

• Subcutaneous tissue shows moderate inflammation and sclerosis of fat septa.
• Muscle demonstrates perivascular mixed inflammatory cell infiltrate.

TREATMENT

• Oral steroids are effective in most patients, but the duration and extent of symptom reduction are variable.
• Methotrexate and cimetidine have also been used.
• Surgery is sometimes required to reduce contractures and maintain function.

■ DISPOSITION

Prognosis is generally good with frequent spontaneous regression and response to steroids. However, 10% may develop blood dyscrasias, and contractures are common.

■ REFERRAL

Dermatology referral may be needed for definitive diagnosis (biopsy). Functional impairment requires surgical evaluation.

REFERENCE

Costenbader KH et al: Eosinophilic fasciitis presenting as pitting edema of the extremities, *Am J Med* 111(4):318, 2001.

Author: **James J. Ng, M.D.**

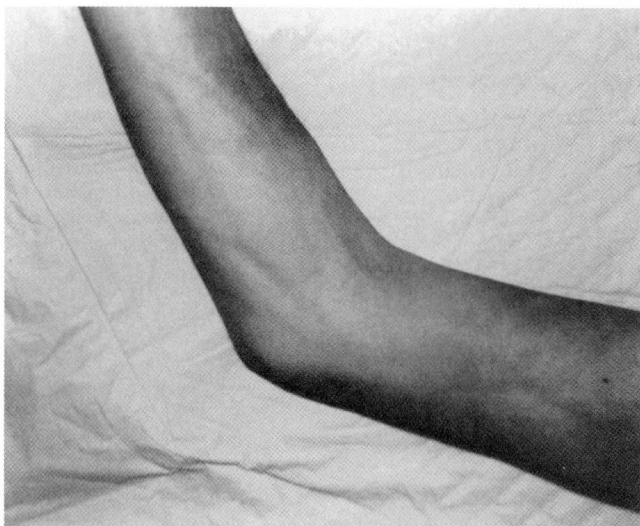

Fig. 1-101   Eosinophilic fasciitis. This 29-year-old butcher had to stop working because of a generalized painful induration of his skin. Fingers were spared. As he raised his forearms, the collapsed veins appeared as grooves (the "groove sign"), which is pathognomonic of eosinophilic fasciitis. Four years later his condition subsided, leaving joint contractures. (From Canoso J: *Rheumatology in primary care*, Philadelphia, 1997, WB Saunders.)

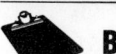

BASIC INFORMATION

■ DEFINITION
Eosinophilic pneumonias are a group of disorders characterized by infiltrates on chest radiographs (x-rays), pulmonary parenchymal eosinophilia, and peripheral blood eosinophilia.

ICD-9CM CODES
518.3 Eosinophilic pneumonia

■ EPIDEMIOLOGY & DEMOGRAPHICS
Varies depending on the specific cause of the pneumonia

■ PHYSICAL FINDINGS & CLINICAL PRESENTATION
- Usually a combination of fever, cough, and shortness of breath
- Varies depending on the specific cause

■ ETIOLOGY
SIMPLE PULMONARY EOSINOPHILIA (LÖFFLER'S SYNDROME):
- Transient infiltrates
- Symptoms range from asymptomatic to dyspnea and dry cough
- Usually idiopathic
- May be secondary to parasitic infection or drugs such as nitrofurantoin or penicillin
- Therapy consists of removing the offending agent
- If idiopathic and severe symptoms, then give glucocorticoid therapy

CHRONIC EOSINOPHILIC PNEUMONIA:
- Idiopathic disease
- Presents with productive cough, dyspnea, malaise, weight loss, night sweats, and fever
- Progressive peripheral pulmonary infiltrates
- Blood eosinophilia is not always present
- Diagnose by bronchoalveolar lavage (BAL) or lung biopsy
- Spontaneous remission in 10% of cases
- Treatment with glucocorticoids is rapidly effective
- Relapses are common

ALLERGIC BRONCHOPULMONARY ASPERGILLOSIS:
- Hypersensitivity reaction to *Aspergillus*
- Occurs most often in patients with asthma and atopy

- Fever, flulike symptoms, myalgias, and lassitude
- Chest x-ray: infiltrates (sometimes migratory) and atelectasis
- Blood and sputum eosinophilia
- Diagnosis by:
  1. *Aspergillus* isolation from multiple sputum samples
  2. Positive skin test to *Aspergillus* antigen
  3. Elevated serum IgE
  4. *Aspergillus*-specific IgE and IgG antibodies
- Treatment: systemic corticosteroids

TROPICAL PULMONARY EOSINOPHILIA:
- Onset of asthma, fever, marked blood eosinophilia
- Basilar reticulonodular and alveolar infiltrates
- Presumed etiology: filariasis

PULMONARY VASCULITIS (ALLERGIC GRANULOMATOSIS AND ANGIITIS):
- Vasculitis and necrotizing granulomatous inflammation that involves many organ systems
- Blood eosinophilia and elevated IgE levels

HYPEREOSINOPHILIC SYNDROME:
- A disease of elevated eosinophils with no known cause
- Cardiac problems are the prominent clinical feature
- Pulmonary involvement results in fever, cough, weight loss, and wheezing
- Diagnosis of exclusion
- Check echocardiogram
- Treat with steroids if symptoms or cardiac abnormalities

ACUTE EOSINOPHILIC PNEUMONIA:
- Acute onset of cough, dyspnea, fever, tachypnea, and rales
- Patients often require mechanical ventilation
- Tends to affect the young
- Often blood eosinophilia
- Chest radiographs show alveolar infiltrates
- BAL eosinophils often >20%
- Glucocorticoid therapy often leads to rapid improvement
- Relapses are rare
- May be secondary to drugs or cigarette smoking

DIAGNOSIS

- Diagnosis varies depending on the specific cause of the eosinophilic pneumonia.
- Usually involves a combination of chest radiograph, peripheral eosinophil count, and BAL.

■ DIFFERENTIAL DIAGNOSIS
- Tuberculosis
- Brucellosis
- Fungal diseases
- Bronchogenic carcinoma
- Hodgkin's disease
- Immunoblastic lymphadenopathy
- Rheumatoid lung disease
- Sarcoidosis

■ WORKUP
Physical examination, laboratory tests, and bronchoscopy

■ LABORATORY TESTS
- WBC counts are often normal
- Often there is an increase in blood eosinophils
- BAL will often reveal an elevation in the eosinophil count

■ IMAGING STUDIES
Chest radiograph may show a variety of infiltrates depending on the cause of the eosinophilic pneumonia.

TREATMENT

- Varies depending on the cause of the pneumonia
- Remove or treat any offending agent
- Steroids may be helpful
- Supportive respiratory care

■ REFERRAL
Consultation with a pulmonologist may be necessary if a BAL is needed to establish the diagnosis.

REFERENCE
Allen JN et al: The eosinophilic pneumonias, *Sem Resp Crit Care Med* 23(2):127, 2002.

Author: **Jennifer Clarke, M.D.**

BASIC INFORMATION

■ DEFINITION
Epicondylitis is an inflammation of the musculotendinous origin of the common extensors at the lateral elbow or the flexor pronator group at the medial elbow.

■ SYNONYMS
Tennis elbow (lateral epicondylitis)
Golfer's elbow (medial epicondylitis)

ICD-9CM CODES
726.31 Medial epicondylitis
726.32 Lateral epicondylitis
723.4 Radial nerve neuralgia

■ EPIDEMIOLOGY & DEMOGRAPHICS
PREVALENCE: 10% to 15% of regular (2 hr/wk) tennis players
PREVALENT AGE: 20 to 40 yr
The lateral side is involved 5 times more often than the medial.

■ PHYSICAL FINDINGS & CLINICAL PRESENTATION
• Local tenderness over affected epicondyle
• Reproduction of pain by resistance against wrist extension (lateral) (Fig. 1-102) or flexion (medial)

■ ETIOLOGY
• Unknown
• Overuse probably causing minor tendinous tears resulting in inflammation
• Posterior interosseous nerve syndrome: compression of this nerve has occasionally been cited as a possible etiology, especially in cases that have failed traditional medical and surgical treatment. In this disorder, the site of tenderness is 2-3 cm distal to the epicondyle

DIAGNOSIS

■ DIFFERENTIAL DIAGNOSIS
• Cervical radiculopathy
• Intraarticular elbow pathology (osteoarthritis, osteochondritis dissecans, loose body)
• Radial nerve compression
• Ulnar neuropathy
• Medial collateral ligament instability

■ IMAGING STUDIES
Traction spur or minor soft tissue calcification may be present on plain radiography. Other studies are not usually needed.

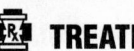 ## TREATMENT

• Rest, restricted activities
• Ice after exercise
• Stretching exercise program
• NSAIDs
• Local steroid/lidocaine injection (Table 1-21), (Fig. 1-103)
• Counterforce brace
• Proper technique in sports activities
• Intermittent immobilization

■ DISPOSITION
Disorder is self-limited in most cases. Resolution of symptoms may take months to years.

■ REFERRAL
• If symptoms fail to respond to medical management
• For surgical consideration

REFERENCES

Chen FS, Rokito AS, Jobe FW: Medial elbow problems in the overhead-throwing athlete, *J Am Acad Orthop Surg* 9:99, 2001.
Cicotti MG, Charlton WP: Epicondylitis in the athlete, *Clin Sports Med* 20:77, 2001.
David TS: Medial elbow pain in the throwing athlete, *Orthopedics* 26:94, 2003.
Haake M et al: Extracorporeal shock wave therapy in the treatment of lateral epicondylitis, *J Bone Joint Surg* 84(A):1982, 2002.
Hay EM et al: Pragmatic randomized controlled trial of local corticosteroid injection and naproxen for treatment of lateral epicondylitis of elbow in primary care, *BMJ* 319:964, 1999.
Smidt N et al: Corticosteroid injections, physiotherapy, or wait-and-see policy for lateral epicondylitis: a randomized controlled trial, *Lancet* 359:657, 2002.
Wang AA et al: Pain levels after injection of corticosteroid to hand and elbow, *Am J Orthop* 32:383, 2003.
Wang CJ, Chen HS: Shock wave therapy for patients with lateral epicondylitis of the elbow: a one- to two-year follow-up study, *Am J Sports Med* 30:422, 2002.
Author: **Lonnie R. Mercier, M.D.**

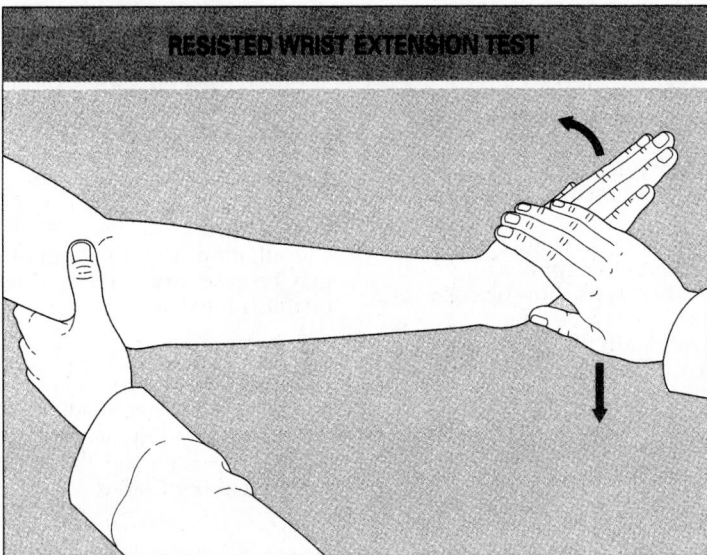

Fig. 1-102   Resisted wrist extension to test for lateral epicondylitis. The examiner asks the patient to try to extend the wrist, but prevent movement by fixing the wrist; this puts tension on the lateral epicondyle without moving the elbow and reproduces the pain of lateral epicondylitis. (From Klippel J, Dieppe P, Ferri F [eds]: *Primary care rheumatology*, London, 1999, Mosby.)

TABLE 1-21 **Guidelines for Common Steroid Injections**

Using 1 ml of the appropriate steroid, the volume is increased by the addition of local anesthetic. Injecting a "space" should not cause pain during the injection. If it does, the needle tip may be in the synovium, capsule, or fat pad, and the needle should be redirected or the shot may not be as effective. Injecting soft tissue should be performed slowly so as not to cause pain from the sudden volume pressure.

SITE	DIAGNOSIS	NEEDLE SIZE (GAUGE, INCHES)	ANESTHETIC VOLUME (ml)
Subacromial bursa	Rotator cuff tendinitis	22,1½	4 to 5
Bicipital groove	Biceps tendinitis	22,1½	2 to 3
A-C joint	Arthritis	25,1½	1 to 2
L, M epicondyle	Epicondylitis	25,⅝	1.5
First extensor sheath	De Quervain's disease	25,⅝	1.5
Trochanteric bursa	Tendinitis	22, spinal	4 to 5
Knee joint	Arthritis	22,1½	5 to 10
Knee, soft tissue	Tendinitis	25,1½	3 to 4
Plantar fascia	Fasciitis	25,1½	1.0
Toe MPJ	Arthritis	25,⅝	1.5

From Mercier LR: *Practical orthopedics,* ed 5, St Louis, 2000, Mosby.

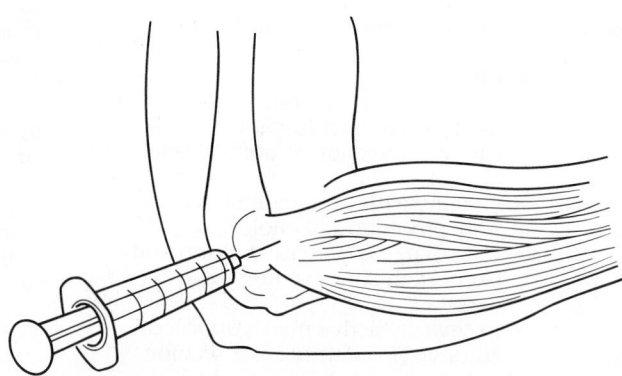

Fig. 1-103 **Soft-tissue injection for lateral epicondylitis.** The patient is supine, and the elbow is flexed 90 degrees. A 25-gauge needle is used to inject the tender spot, which is usually about 1 cm distal to the bony epicondyle. (From Mercier L: *Practical orthopedics,* ed 5, St Louis, 2000, Mosby.)

BASIC INFORMATION

■ **DEFINITION**
Epididymitis is an inflammatory reaction of the epididymis caused by either an infectious agent or local trauma.

■ **SYNONYMS**
Nonspecific bacterial epididymitis
Sexually transmitted epididymitis

ICD-9CM CODES
604.90 Nonvenereal epididymitis
098.0 Gonococcal epididymitis

■ **EPIDEMIOLOGY & DEMOGRAPHICS**
INCIDENCE (IN U.S.): Cause of >600,000 visits to physicians per year
PREDOMINANT SEX: Exclusive to males
PREDOMINANT AGE: All ages affected but usually in sexually active men or older males
PEAK INCIDENCE: Sexually active years
CONGENITAL: Congenital urologic structural disorders possibly predisposing to infections

■ **PHYSICAL FINDINGS & CLINICAL PRESENTATION**
• Tender swelling of the scrotum with erythema, usually unilateral testicular pain and tenderness
• Dysuria and/or urethral discharge
• Fever and signs of systemic illness (less common)
• Pain and redness on scrotal examination
• Hydrocele or even epididymoorchitis, especially late
• Chronic draining scrotal sinuses with a "beadlike" enlargement of the vas deferens in tuberculous disease

■ **ETIOLOGY**
• In young, sexually active men, the most common infectious agents isolated are *N. gonorrhoeae* and *Chlamydia trachomatis.*
• In men >35 yr or with underlying urologic disease:
   1. Gram-negative aerobic rods are predominant.
   2. Similar organisms are found in men following invasive urologic procedures.
   3. Gram-positive cocci are rarely seen in these groups.
   4. Mycobacteria are also a cause of epididymitis.

• Young, prepubertal boys may present with epididymitis caused by coliform bacteria; almost always a complication of underlying urologic disease such as reflux.
• Recently, in AIDS patients, CMV and *Salmonella* epididymitis have been described. CMV may have a negative urine culture. Toxoplasmosis should also be considered as a cause of epididymitis in AIDS patients.

 DIAGNOSIS

■ **DIFFERENTIAL DIAGNOSIS**
• Orchitis
• Testicular torsion, trauma, or tumor
• Epididymal cyst
• Hydrocele
• Varicocele
• Spermatocele
• Testicular torsion should be considered in all cases but is more common in adolescents and men without evidence of inflammation. If a diagnosis is in question, a specialist should be consulted immediately.

■ **WORKUP**
• Consideration of a full assessment of the urologic tract in patients with bacterial infection, especially if recurrent
• Imaging with sonogram or IVP (possibly procedures of choice)
• If discharge is present: cultures and Gram stain smear of urethral exudate
• In sexually active men: gonococcal cultures of the throat and rectum possibly of value
• If testicular torsion a consideration: radionuclear imaging
• Examination of first void uncentrifugal urine for leukocytes if the urethral Gram stain is negative. A culture and Gram-stained smear of this urine specimen should be obtained

■ **LABORATORY TESTS**
• Urinalysis and urine culture if dysuria is present or if urinary tract infection is suspected
• VDRL in sexually active men
• PPD placed and chest x-ray viewed if TB suspected
• Rarely, biopsy to assure the diagnosis of tuberculous epididymitis
• HIV testing and counseling

 TREATMENT

■ **ACUTE GENERAL Rx**
• Ice packs and scrotal elevation for relief of pain
• Analgesia with acetaminophen with or without codeine or NSAIDs (such as ibuprofen or Naprosyn)
• Antibiotics to cover suspected pathogens
• In sexually active men, doxycycline 100 mg PO bid or tetracycline 500 mg PO qid for 10 days to cover both gonococci and chlamydiae; ceftriaxone 250 mg IM is a single dose may be adequate for gonococci alone
• Best treatment for older men with gram-negative bacteria and leukocyturia: ofloxacin 300 mg PO bid for 10 days or levofloxacin 500 mg PO qd for 10 days
• *Pseudomonas* covered by ciprofloxacin or ceftazidime (1 g IV q6-8h)
• Gentamicin in toxic-appearing patients (1 mg/kg IV q8h following a loading dose of 2 mg/kg): doses must be adjusted for renal function and these agents may be more toxic
• Vancomycin (1 g IV q12h) to cover suspected gram-positive infections
• Surgical aspiration of local abscesses or even open surgical drainage
• Diabetics: especially prone to develop more extensive scrotal infections, including Fournier's gangrene
• Reinforcement of compliance with antibiotics to avoid partial treatment

■ **CHRONIC Rx**
• Repair of underlying structural defects is considered especially if infections are severe or recur.
• Surgical repair of reflux in young boys should be undertaken promptly and at a young age when possible.
• Sex partners of patient should be referred for evaluation and treatment.

■ **DISPOSITION**
Usually self-limited

■ **REFERRAL**
• If abscess or chronic structural problems suspected
• If other diagnosis, such as testicular torsion, strongly considered

REFERENCE
Centers for Disease Control and Prevention: 2002 Sexually transmitted diseases treatment guidelines. *MMWR* 51(RR-6), 2002.
Author: **Joseph J. Lieber, M.D.**

BASIC INFORMATION

■ DEFINITION
Epiglottitis is a rapidly progressive cellulitis of the epiglottis and adjacent soft tissue structures with the potential to cause abrupt airway obstruction.

■ SYNONYMS
Supraglottitis
Cherry-red epiglottitis

ICD-9CM CODES
464.30 Epiglottitis

■ EPIDEMIOLOGY
INCIDENCE (IN U.S.): Highest in young children, 2 to 4 yr old
INCIDENCE (IN U.S.): Unknown
PREDOMINANT SEX: Males
PEAK INCIDENCE: Peaks in young boys ages 2 to 4 yr, but it is reported in adults as well

■ PHYSICAL FINDINGS & CLINICAL PRESENTATION
- Irritability, fever, dysphonia, and dysphagia
- Respiratory distress, with child tending to lean up and forward
- Often, drooling or oral secretions
- Often, presence of tachycardia and tachypnea
- On visualization, edematous and cherry-red epiglottis
- Often, no classic barking cough as seen in croup
- Possibly fulminant course (especially in children), leading to complete airway obstruction

■ ETIOLOGY
- In children, *Haemophilus influenzae* type b is usual.
- In adults, *H. influenzae* can be isolated from blood and/or epiglottis (about 26% of cases).
- Pneumococci, streptococci, and staphylococci are also implicated.
- Role of viruses in epiglottitis unclear.

DIAGNOSIS

■ DIFFERENTIAL DIAGNOSIS
- Croup
- Angioedema
- Peritonsillar abscess
- Retropharyngeal abscess
- Diphtheria
- Foreign body aspiration
- Lingual tonsillitis

■ WORKUP
- Cultures of blood and urine
- Lateral neck radiograph to show an enlarged epiglottis, ballooning of the hypopharynx, and normal subglottic structures (Fig. 1-104)

1. Radiographs are of only moderate sensitivity and specificity and take time to perform.
2. Epiglottis should be visualized directly to secure diagnosis and only when prepared to urgently secure the airway.
3. Visualization of the epiglottis may be safer in adults than in children.
- Cultures of the epiglottis

■ LABORATORY TESTS
- CBC: may reveal a leukocytosis with a shift to the left
- Chest x-ray examination: may reveal evidence of pneumonia in close to 25% of cases
- Cultures of blood, urine, and the epiglottis, as noted previously

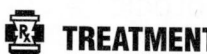 TREATMENT

■ ACUTE GENERAL Rx
- Maintenance of adequate airway is critical.
- Early placement of an endotracheal or nasotracheal tube in a child is advised.
- Closely follow adult patient and defer intubation, provided the airway reveals no signs of obstruction.
- In children, visualization and intubation are best done in the most controlled environment, such as an operating room; pay close attention to vital signs, oxygen saturation, respiratory rate, input, and output, because abrupt deterioration can occur.
- *H. influenzae* in children may be less common thanks to the HIB vaccine.

- Use antibiotics such as ceftriaxone (80 to 100 mg/kg/day in two divided doses), cefotaxime (50 to 180 mg/kg/day in four divided doses), or ampicillin (200 mg/kg/day in four divided doses) with chloramphenicol (75 to 100 mg/kg/day in four divided doses).
- If possible, obtain cultures before initiating antibiotics, but do not delay antibiotic therapy if cultures cannot be obtained quickly.
- Treat adult patients with similar antibiotic regimens.
- Give close family contacts of the patient who are <4 yr old rifampin 20 mg/kg/day for 4 days (up to 600 mg/day) for prophylaxis.
- Role of epinephrine or corticosteroids in the management of epiglottitis is not firmly established.

■ REFERRAL
For effective management:
- Close cooperation between the pediatrician or internist, anesthesiologist, and otorhinolaryngologist, especially when epiglottis is visualized and when the patient requires endotracheal intubation
- Best managed in a critical care setting or ICU

REFERENCES
Nakamura H et al: Acute epiglottitis: a review of 80 patients, *J Laryngol Otol* 115(1):31, 2001.
Sack JL, Brock CD: Identifying acute epiglottitis in adults: high degree of awareness, close monitoring are key, *Postgrad Med* 112(1):81, 2002.
Author: **Joseph J. Lieber, M.D.**

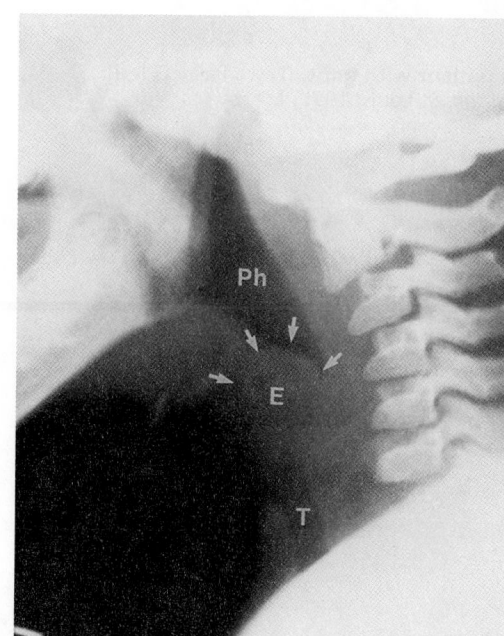

Fig. 1-104   Epiglottitis. A lateral soft tissue view of the neck shows a ballooned pharynx *(Ph)* with swollen epiglottis *(E)* in the shape of a large thumbprint *(arrows)*. *T,* Trachea. (From Mettler FA [ed]: *Primary care radiology,* Philadelphia, 2000, WB Saunders.)

BASIC INFORMATION

■ DEFINITION

Episcleritis is an inflammation of the episclera, or thin layer of vascular elastic tissue between the sclera and conjunctiva.

ICD-9CM CODES

379.0 Scleritis and episcleritis

■ EPIDEMIOLOGY & DEMOGRAPHICS

INCIDENCE (IN U.S.): Relatively rare in an ophthalmologic practice
PREDOMINANT SEX: None
PREDOMINANT AGE: 43 yr
PEAK INCIDENCE: Most common in middle and old age

■ PHYSICAL FINDINGS & CLINICAL PRESENTATION

• Red, vascular injection of conjunctiva with engorged and enlarged blood vessels beneath the conjunctions (Fig. 1-105)
• Pain in area of inflammation

■ ETIOLOGY

Associated with collagen-vascular diseases

DIAGNOSIS

■ DIFFERENTIAL DIAGNOSIS

• Acute glaucoma
• Conjunctivitis
• Scleritis
• Subconjunctival hemorrhage
• Congenital or lymphoid masses
• The differential diagnosis of "red eye" is described in Section II.

■ WORKUP

Eye examination

■ LABORATORY TESTS

Studies for collagen-vascular disease

TREATMENT

■ NONPHARMACOLOGIC THERAPY

Warm compresses

■ ACUTE GENERAL Rx

Topical steroids, 1% prednisolone if no glaucoma; nonsteroidals if there is a tendency for glaucoma

■ CHRONIC Rx

NSAIDs such as Voltaren or Acular qid

■ DISPOSITION

Close follow-up needed

■ REFERRAL

To ophthalmologist if patient unresponsive to treatment after a few days

PEARLS & CONSIDERATIONS

■ COMMENTS

Usually related to systemic disease

REFERENCES

Jabs DA et al: Episcleritis and scleritis: clinical features and treatment results, *Am J Ophthalmol* 130(4):469, 2000.
Paresio CE, Meier FM: Systemic disorders associated with episcleritis and scleritis, *Curr Opin Ophthalmology* 12(6):471, 2002.
Author: **Melvyn Koby, M.D.**

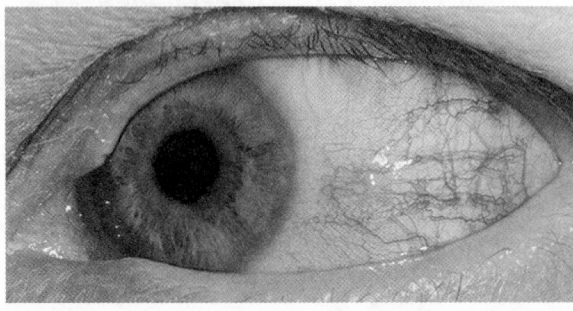

Fig. 1-105   Nodular episcleritis in a patient with gout. (From Palay D [ed]: *Ophthalmology for the primary care physician,* St Louis, 1997, Mosby.)

BASIC INFORMATION

■ DEFINITION
Epistaxis is defined as bleeding from the nose or nasal hemorrhage and is classified as either anterior or posterior.

■ SYNONYMS
Nosebleed

■ ICD-9CM CODES
784.7 Epistaxis

■ EPIDEMIOLOGY & DEMOGRAPHICS
- Epistaxis is usually anterior and occurs from Kiesselbach's plexus (Fig. 1-106).
- Only 5% of patients with epistaxis have posterior bleeds.

■ PHYSICAL FINDINGS & CLINICAL PRESENTATION
- Nosebleed
- Hypotension and hemodynamic instability with acute severe epistaxis

■ ETIOLOGY
- The cause of epistaxis is multifactorial including:
  1. Cold, dry environment
  2. Trauma (nose picking, accidents, and physical altercations)
  3. Infection (sinusitis)
  4. Allergies
  5. Foreign bodies in the nasal cavity
  6. Tumors
  7. Irritants
  8. Hypertension
  9. Coagulopathy (hemophilia, von Willebrand's disease, thrombocytopenia)
  10. Osler-Weber-Rendu disease
  11. Renal failure
  12. Drugs: aspirin, NSAIDs, warfarin, and alcohol

DIAGNOSIS

■ DIFFERENTIAL DIAGNOSIS
The differential diagnosis is as described under Etiology.

■ WORKUP
The diagnosis of epistaxis is self-evident. The workup should include laboratory blood testing to exclude obvious causes and to prepare in case the bleeding cannot be stopped.

■ LABORATORY TESTS
- Hemoglobin and hematocrit
- Platelet count
- BUN/creatinine
- Coagulation studies (PT and PTT)
- Type and crossmatching of blood products

■ IMAGING STUDIES
X-ray studies are usually not helpful in the assessment of patients with epistaxis.

TREATMENT

■ NONPHARMACOLOGIC THERAPY
- Digital compression or pinching the nose for 4 to 5 min
- Cotton or tissue plug
- Bend forward at the waist allowing blood to flow out of the nostrils as opposed to bending backward, which would allow the blood to flow down the throat
- Application of cold compresses to the bridge of the nose, causing a vasoconstrictive effect

■ ACUTE GENERAL Rx
Anterior Epistaxis
- Local vasoconstriction is performed by moistening a cotton pledget with either:
  1. 4% lidocaine with 1:1000 epinephrine
  2. 4% lidocaine with 1% phenylephrine (Neo-Synephrine)
  3. 4% lidocaine with 0.05% oxymetazoline (Afrin)
  4. 4% cocaine

Then insert the pledget into the nasal cavity with bayonet forceps.
- Cauterization with silver nitrate is performed once hemostasis is achieved.
- Anterior nasal packing is needed when local measures are unsuccessful in controlling hemostasis. Nasal packing is done by inserting Vaseline gauze strips in layers from the floor of the nasal cavity to the front entrance of the nasal orifice. Enough pressure is placed to tamponade the epistaxis (Fig. 1-107).
- Other commercially available nasal packing using sponge packs that expand when exposed to blood or moisture can be used for anterior epistaxis.

Posterior Epistaxis
- Posterior nasal packing
  1. Commercially available nasal sponge packing can be applied
  2. Rolled gauze technique (see reference)
- Foley catheter balloon insertion into the nasopharynx can be tried in patients with posterior epistaxis (for the proper technique, please refer to the reference).

■ CHRONIC Rx
- If acute treatment fails to stop the bleeding or the site of bleeding cannot be located, endoscopic cauterization can be used.

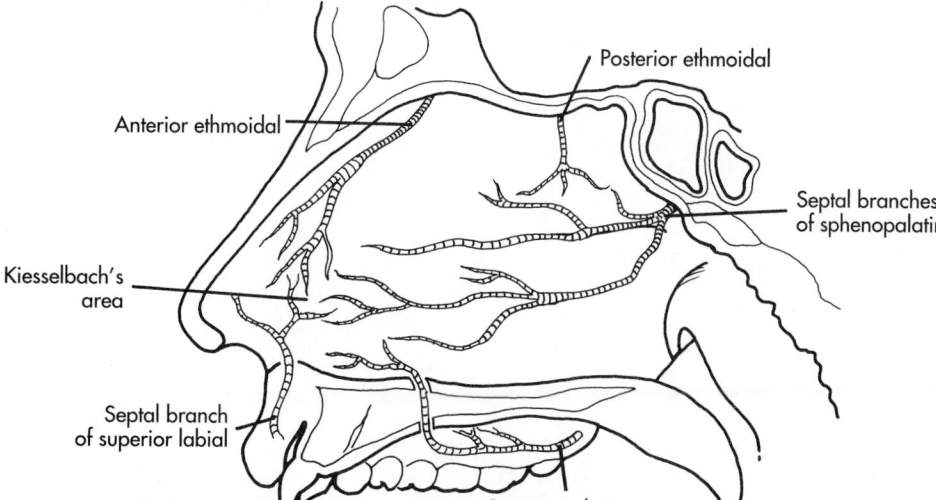

Fig. 1-106 Kiesselbach's plexus on the anterior septum derives blood supply from the superior labial, descending palatine, and sphenopalatine arteries. (From Noble J: *Primary care medicine,* ed 3, St Louis, 2001, Mosby.)

Labels in figure:
- Posterior ethmoidal
- Anterior ethmoidal
- Septal branches of sphenopalatine
- Kiesselbach's area
- Septal branch of superior labial
- Greater palatine

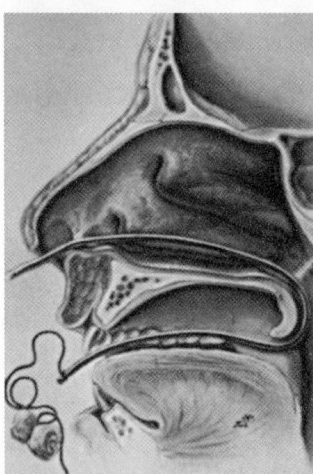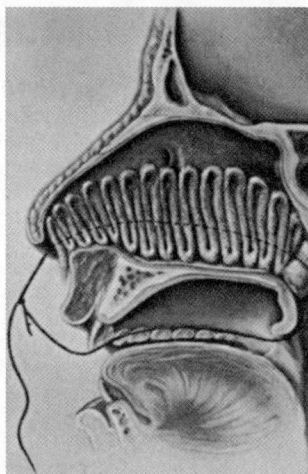

Fig. 1-107 Packing of the nose for epistaxis with a postnasal pack and an anterior nose pack. (From Boies LR et al: *Fundamentals of otolaryngology: a textbook of ear, nose, and throat diseases,* ed 4, Philadelphia, 1964, WB Saunders.)

- Arterial ligation or embolization has been used in refractory posterior epistaxis.

■ DISPOSITION
- Most cases of anterior epistaxis from Kiesselbach's plexus can be stopped by nasal compression and local vasoconstriction or cauterization.
- Nasal packing with gauze or sponge can control 90% of anterior epistaxis.
- Anterior and posterior packs are removed in 2 to 3 days.

- Although rare, epistaxis can lead to death by aspiration of blood, hemodynamic compromise from rapid excessive blood loss, or toxic shock syndrome.

■ REFERRAL
- If epistaxis cannot be controlled in the acute setting by the above mentioned nonpharmacologic and pharmacologic measures, ENT specialist should be called for assistance.
- ENT specialist should be consulted in any patient with posterior epistaxis requiring posterior packing.

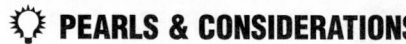

PEARLS & CONSIDERATIONS

■ COMMENTS
- Silver nitrate cauterization, if done on both sides of the nasal septum, can lead to septal perforation and should be discouraged.
- If anterior nasal packing is done, broad-spectrum antibiotics (e.g., amoxicillin-clavulanate 250 mg PO tid or trimethoprim-sulfamethoxazole 1 tab PO bid) are used until the anterior packs are removed.
- Complications of nasal packing include
  1. Aspiration
  2. Dislodged packing
  3. Infection
  4. Nasal trauma

REFERENCES
Bentley B: Nasal emergencies. In Cline DM et al (eds): *Emergency medicine: a comprehensive study guide,* ed 4, American College of Emergency Physicians, New York, 1996, McGraw-Hill.

Kotecha B et al: Management of epistaxis: a national survey, *Ann R Coll Surg Engl* 78:444, 1996.

Parshen D, Stevens M: Management of epistaxis in general practice, *Aust Fam Physician* 31(8):717, 2002.

Pond F, Sizeland A: Epistaxis: strategies for management, *Aust Fam Physician* 29(10):933, 2000.

Tan LKS, Calhoun KH: Epistaxis, *Med Clin North Am* 83(1):43, 1999.

Author: **Peter Petropoulos, M.D.**

BASIC INFORMATION

DEFINITION
Epstein-Barr virus infection refers to a disease caused by Epstein-Barr virus (EBV), a human herpesvirus.

SYNONYMS
Infectious mononucleosis

ICD-9CM CODES
075 Mononucleosis

EPIDEMIOLOGY & DEMOGRAPHICS
INCIDENCE (IN U.S.): 45 cases/100,000 persons/yr of infectious mononucleosis (IM)
PREDOMINANT SEX: Neither, although peak incidence occurs about 2 years earlier in women
PREDOMINANT AGE:
- Infectious mononucleosis: occurs most commonly between the ages of 15 and 24 yr.
- EBV infection: occurs earlier in life in lower socioeconomic groups.

PHYSICAL FINDINGS
- Most EBV infections either are asymptomatic or cause a nonspecific illness.
- Incubation period is 1 to 2 mo, possibly followed by a prodrome of anorexia, malaise, headache, and chills; after several days, clinical triad of pharyngitis, fever, and adenopathy may appear, accompanied by fatigue and malaise.
- Pharyngitis is usually the most severe symptom; exudates are common.
- Lymphadenopathy is most prominent in the cervical region but may be diffuse.
- Splenomegaly is possible, most commonly during the second week of illness.
- Rash is uncommon, but will occur in nearly all patients who receive ampicillin.
- Possible IM presentation: fever and adenopathy without pharyngitis.
- Although complications may be severe, they are also uncommon and tend to resolve completely.
- Involvement of the hematologic, pulmonary, cardiac, or nervous systems possible; splenic rupture is rare.
- IM is usually a self-limited illness, but symptoms of malaise and fatigue may last months before resolving.
- Besides IM, EBV is also related to lymphoproliferative syndromes in transplant recipients and in AIDS patients.
- Increasing evidence showing an association between EBV infection and both African Burkitt's lymphoma and nasopharyngeal carcinoma.

ETIOLOGY
- Ubiquitous virus
- Prevalence is higher in lower socioeconomic groups than in age-matched controls in more affluent groups
- Infection during childhood is much less likely to cause significant illness
- Frequency of IM in late adolescence is attributed to the onset of social contact between the sexes
- Close personal contact is usually necessary for transmission, although EBV is occasionally transmitted by blood transfusion; transfer via saliva while kissing may be responsible for many cases

DIAGNOSIS

DIFFERENTIAL DIAGNOSIS
- Heterophile-negative infectious mononucleosis caused by CMV
- Although clinical presentation similar, CMV more frequently follows transfusion
- Bacterial and viral causes of pharyngitis
- Toxoplasmosis
- Acute retroviral syndrome of HIV
- Lymphoma

WORKUP
Heterophile antibody and CBC

LABORATORY TESTS
- Increased WBC common, with a relative lymphocytosis and neutropenia
- Hallmark of IM: atypical lymphocytes (not pathognomonic)
- Mild thrombocytopenia
- Falling Hct signaling splenic rupture
- Elevated hepatocellular enzymes and cryoglobulins in most cases
- Heterophile antibody
  1. As measured by the Monospot test, may be positive at presentation or may appear later in the course of illness.
  2. Negative test is repeated if clinical suspicion is high.
  3. A positive test has been reported with primary HIV infection.
- Virus-specific antibodies possibly responding to IM: determination of these EBV-specific antibodies is rarely necessary to diagnose IM

IMAGING STUDIES
Chest x-ray examination
- May rarely show infiltrates
- Possible elevated left hemidiaphragm with splenic rupture

TREATMENT

NONPHARMACOLOGIC THERAPY
- Supportive
- Rest advocated by some; impact on outcome not clear
- Splenectomy if rupture occurs
- Transfusions for severe anemia or thrombocytopenia

ACUTE GENERAL Rx
- Pharmacologic therapy is not indicated in uncomplicated illness
- Use of steroids
  1. Suggested in patients who have severe thrombocytopenia or hemolytic anemia, or impending airway obstruction resulting from enlarged tonsils
  2. Prednisone 60 to 80 mg PO qd for 3 days, then tapered over 1 to 2 wk
- There is no role for antiviral agents such as acyclovir in the management of IM.

CHRONIC Rx
An extremely rare, chronic form of IM with persistent fevers and other objective findings has been described and should be differentiated from chronic fatigue syndrome, which is not related to EBV.

DISPOSITION
Eventual resolution of all symptoms

REFERRAL
If more than mild illness

PEARLS & CONSIDERATIONS

COMMENTS
Avoidance of contact sports during the first month of illness, because splenic rupture can occur even in the absence of clinically detectable splenomegaly.

REFERENCES
Auwaerter PG: Infectious mononucleosis in middle age, *JAMA* 281:454, 1999.
Cohen JI: Epstein-Barr virus infection, *N Engl J Med* 343:481, 2000.
Vidrih JA et al: Positive Epstein-Barr virus heterophile antibody tests in patients with primary human immunodeficiency virus infection, *Am J Med* 111(3):237, 2001.

Author: **Maurice Policar, M.D.**

BASIC INFORMATION

■ DEFINITION
Erectile dysfunction is the inability to achieve or sustain an erection of adequate rigidity to make intercourse possible.

■ SYNONYMS
Impotence
Male erectile disorder
Sexual dysfunction (a nonspecific term)

ICD-9CM CODES
F52.2 Male erectile disorder (DSM-IV Code: 302.72 Male erectile disorder)

■ EPIDEMIOLOGY & DEMOGRAPHICS
INCIDENCE (IN U.S.): Unknown
PREVALENCE (IN U.S.):
- Increases with age
- About 7% for men between 18 and 29 yr, 18% for men in their 50s, 25% for men in their 60s, 80% for men in their 80s
PREDOMINANT SEX: By definition, only in males
PREDOMINANT AGE: Increases with age

■ PHYSICAL FINDINGS & CLINICAL PRESENTATION
- Psychogenic impotence: inability to obtain erection, inability to obtain or maintain an adequate erection, or the loss of erection before completion of sexual intercourse; nocturnal penile tumescence usually normal
- Organic impotence: inability to obtain an erection or inability to obtain an adequate erection; nocturnal penile tumescence usually abnormal

■ ETIOLOGY
- Psychogenic erectile dysfunction resulting from a wide range of experiential, historical, or even psychotic processes
- Organic impotence resulting from a wide variety of insults to neurologic, hormonal, or vascular structures
- Medications (antihypertensives, antidepressants, antipsychotics, histamine blockers, nicotine, alcohol, and others) commonly causative
- Endocrinopathies such as diabetes, hypogonadism, hypo- or hyperthyroidism, and hyperprolactinemia
- Neurogenic causes including spinal cord lesions, cortical lesions, and peripheral neuropathies

DIAGNOSIS

■ DIFFERENTIAL DIAGNOSIS
- Treatment dependent on the etiology
- Psychogenic dysfunction distinguished from organic
- Etiology of organic dysfunction to be determined
- Erectile dysfunction possible in the setting of another psychiatric condition (e.g., depression or obsessive-compulsive disorder)

■ WORKUP
- History (often including partner report) with a focus on risk factors (e.g., smoking, alcohol)
- Report of nocturnal erections
- Physical examination to rule out neuronal damage, direct penile damage (e.g., fibrosis), or testicular atrophy

■ LABORATORY TESTS
Screen for endocrinopathy with AM testosterone levels, fasting glucose, and thyroid profile.

■ IMAGING STUDIES
- Nocturnal penile tumescence very specific for distinguishing psychogenic and organic causes
- Vascular etiologies screened by the penile-brachial pressure index (measures the loss of systolic blood pressure between the arm and penis) or with Doppler studies
- Neurogenic etiologies examined by the bulbocavernosus reflex or the pudendal-evoked response
- Intracorporeal injection of prostaglandin E_1 to distinguish vascular and nonvascular etiologies (erection is achieved in patients with nonvascular etiologies)

TREATMENT

■ NONPHARMACOLOGIC THERAPY
- Various psychotherapeutic approaches: cognitive behavioral therapy preferred because it is the most focused; success rates decrease with advancing age and duration of symptoms.
- Sex therapy and couples' therapy are used to address technical or social issues that contribute to impotence.
- Vacuum devices (70% to 90% effective) work for many men, but they are difficult to use and cumbersome.

■ ACUTE GENERAL Rx
- Sildenafil (Viagra) 50 mg or vardenafil (Levitra) 10 mg PO 1 hr before sexual activity; avoid concomitant use of nitrates
- Intracavernosal injections of vasodilators (e.g., papaverine, alprostadil, or prostaglandin E_1 pellet)
- Oral medications such as pentoxifylline and yohimbine (limited success)

■ CHRONIC Rx
- Psychogenic impotence: open-ended, insight psychotherapies possibly curative but time-consuming and require extraordinary motivation
- Successful acute approaches maintained over time, but intracavernosal injections of papaverine associated with penile scarring
- For men failing other approaches: penile prosthesis (does not address issues of sexual drive or orgasm)
- Testosterone therapy in elderly hypogonadal males

■ DISPOSITION
- When erectile dysfunction is secondary to an organic cause, it does not remit unless the organic cause is corrected; therefore, it is usually a chronic condition.
- Psychogenic acquired erectile dysfunction will remit spontaneously in 15% to 30% of the cases.
- Lifelong erectile dysfunction is usually a chronic and unremitting condition.
- Situational erectile dysfunction may remit with changes in social environment, but it usually recurs.

■ REFERRAL
If psychotherapy, sex therapy, or invasive organic treatment required

REFERENCES
Fink HA et al: Sildenafil for male erectile dysfunction, *Arch Intern Med* 162:1349, 2002.
Miller TA: Diagnostic evaluation of erectile dysfunction, *Am Fam Physician* 61:95, 2000.
Author: **Rif S. El-Mallakh, M.D.**

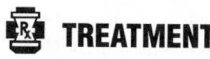

 BASIC INFORMATION

■ **DEFINITION**
Erysipelas is a type of cellulitis caused by infection of the superficial layers of the skin and cutaneous lymphatics. Erysipelas is characterized by redness, induration, and a sharply demarcated, raised border.

■ **SYNONYMS**
St. Anthony's fire

ICD-9CM CODES
035 Erysipelas

■ **EPIDEMIOLOGY & DEMOGRAPHICS**
Erysipelas occurs most often in the young or old, in patients with impaired lymphatic or venous drainage (mastectomy, saphenous vein harvesting), and in immunocompromised patients. Recurrence is relatively common.

■ **PHYSICAL FINDINGS & CLINICAL PRESENTATION**
- Distinctive red, warm, tender skin lesion with induration and a sharply defined, advancing, raised border is present (Fig. 1-108).
- Most common sites are lower extremities or face.

- Systemic signs of infection (fever) are often present.
- Vesicles or bullae may develop.
- After several days, lesions may appear ecchymotic.
- After 7 to 10 days desquamation of affected area may occur.

■ **ETIOLOGY**
- Usually group A β-hemolytic streptococci
- Less often group B, C, or G streptococci
- Rarely *Staphylococcus aureus*

■ **COMPLICATIONS**
- Abscess
- Necrotizing fasciitis
- Thrombophlebitis
- Gangrene
- Metastatic infection

🔬 **DIAGNOSIS**

■ **DIFFERENTIAL DIAGNOSIS**
- Other types of cellulitis
- Necrotizing fasciitis
- DVT
- Contact dermatitis
- Erythema migrans (Lyme disease)
- Insect bite
- Herpes zoster
- Erysipeloid

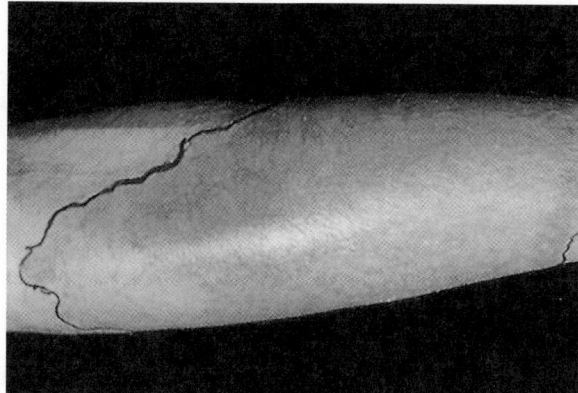

Fig. 1-108   Erysipelas. Note well-demarcated erythematous plaque on arm. (From Goldstein B [ed]: *Practical dermatology,* ed 2,, St Louis, 1997, Mosby. Courtesy Department of Dermatology, University of North Carolina at Chapel Hill.)

- Acute gout
- Pseudogout

■ **WORKUP**
History, physical examination, and laboratory evaluation

■ **LABORATORY TESTS**
Diagnosis is usually made by characteristic clinical setting and appearance.
- CBC and WBC often elevated
- Blood cultures positive in 5% of patients
- Gram stain and culture of any drainage from skin lesions
- Culture of aspirated fluid from leading edge of skin lesion has low yield

■ **IMAGING STUDIES**
- Duplex ultrasound for patients suspected of having DVT
- CT scan or MRI for patients with suspected necrotizing fasciitis

℞ **TREATMENT**

■ **NONPHARMACOLOGIC THERAPY**
- Elevation of the affected limb
- Warm compresses

■ **ACUTE GENERAL Rx**
Typical erysipelas of extremity in non-diabetic patient:
- PO: penicillin V 250 mg to 500 mg qid
- IV: penicillin G (aqueous) 1 to 2 million units q6h
NOTE: Use erythromycin or cephalosporin in patients allergic to penicillin.
Facial erysipelas (include coverage for *Staphylococcus aureus*):
- PO dicloxacillin 500 mg q6h
- IV nafcillin or oxacillin 2 g q4h

■ **DISPOSITION**
Prognosis is good with antibiotic treatment, but recurrence is common.

■ **REFERRAL**
For surgical debridement for patients with necrotizing fasciitis or for drainage of abscess
Author: **Mark J. Fagan, M.D.**

BASIC INFORMATION

■ DEFINITION
Erythema multiforme is an inflammatory disease believed to be secondary to immune complex formation and subsequent deposition in the skin and mucous membranes.

■ SYNONYMS
EM

ICD-9CM CODES
695.1 Erythema multiforme

■ EPIDEMIOLOGY & DEMOGRAPHICS
- Predominant age: 20 to 40 yr
- Often associated with herpes simplex and other infectious agents, drugs, and connective tissue diseases

■ PHYSICAL FINDINGS & CLINICAL PRESENTATION
- Symmetric skin lesions with a classic "target" appearance (caused by the centrifugal spread of red maculopapules to circumference of 1 to 3 cm with a purpuric, cyanotic, or vesicular center) are present (Fig. 1-109).
- Lesions are most common in the back of the hands and feet and extensor aspect of the forearms and legs. Trunk involvement can occur in severe cases.

- Urticarial papules, vesicles, and bullae may also be present and generally indicate a more severe form of the disease.
- Individual lesions heal in 1 or 2 wk without scarring.
- Bullae and erosions may also be present in the oral cavity.

■ ETIOLOGY
- Immune complex formation and subsequent deposition in the cutaneous microvasculature may play a role in the pathogenesis of erythema multiforme.
- The majority of EM cases follow outbreaks of herpes simplex.
- In >50% of patients, no specific cause is identified.
- Erythema multiforme associated with bupropion use has been recently reported.

DIAGNOSIS

■ DIFFERENTIAL DIAGNOSIS
- Chronic urticaria
- Secondary syphilis
- Pityriasis rosea
- Contact dermatitis
- Pemphigus vulgaris
- Lichen planus
- Serum sickness
- Drug eruption
- Granuloma annulare

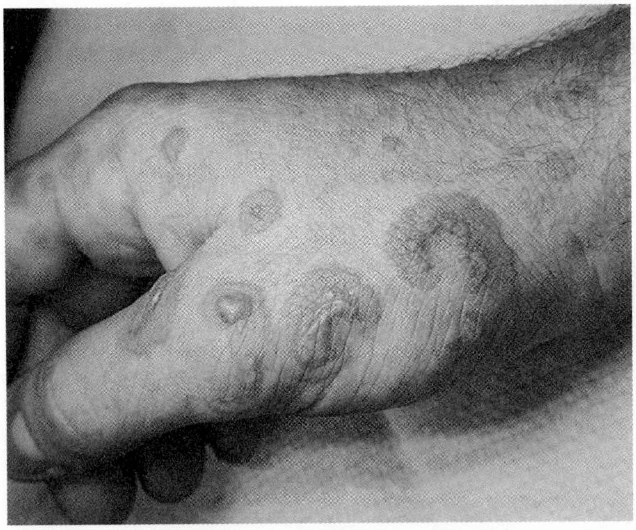

Fig. 1-109 Iris and arcuate lesions of erythema multiforme. Note erythematous lesions with multiform configurations—target, arcuate, and vesicles. (From Noble J et al: *Textbook of primary care medicine,* ed 2, St Louis, 1995, Mosby.)

■ WORKUP
- Medical history with emphasis on drug ingestion
- Laboratory evaluation in patients with suspected collagen-vascular diseases
- Skin biopsy when diagnosis is unclear

■ LABORATORY TESTS
- CBC with differential
- ANA
- Serology for *Mycoplasma pneumoniae*
- Urinalysis

TREATMENT

■ NONPHARMACOLOGIC THERAPY
- Mild cases generally do not require treatment; lesions resolve spontaneously within 1 mo.
- Potential drug precipitants should be removed.

■ ACUTE GENERAL Rx
- Treatment of associated diseases (e.g., acyclovir for herpes simplex, erythromycin for *Mycoplasma* infection).
- Prednisone 40 to 80 mg/day for 1 to 3 wk may be tried in patients with many target lesions; however, the role of systemic steroids remains controversial.
- Levamisole, an immunomodulator, may be effective in treatment of patients with chronic or recurrent oral lesions (dose is 150 mg/day for 3 consecutive days used alone or in combination with prednisone).

■ DISPOSITION
The rash of EM generally evolves over a 2-wk period and resolves within 3 to 4 wk without scarring. A severe bullous form can occur (see "Stevens-Johnson syndrome").

■ REFERRAL
Hospital admission in patients with Stevens-Johnson syndrome

PEARLS & CONSIDERATIONS

■ COMMENTS
The risk of recurrence of erythema multiforme exceeds 30%.

REFERENCE
Lineberry TW et al: Bupropion-induced erythema multiforme, *Mayo Clin Proc* 76:664, 2001.
Author: **Fred F. Ferri, M.D.**

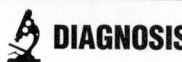

BASIC INFORMATION

■ DEFINITION

Erythema nodosum is an acute, tender, erythematous, nodular skin eruption resulting from inflammation of subcutaneous fat, often associated with bruising.

■ ICD-9CM CODES

695.2 Erythema nodosum
017.10 Erythema nodosum, tuberculous, NOS

■ EPIDEMIOLOGY & DEMOGRAPHICS

INCIDENCE: 2 to 3 cases per 100,000 persons per year
PEAK AGE: 25 to 40 yr
SEX DISTRIBUTION: Ratio of 3-4:1 (female:male)

■ PHYSICAL FINDINGS & CLINICAL PRESENTATION

- Acute onset of tender nodules typically located on shins (Fig. 1-110), occasionally seen on thighs and forearms

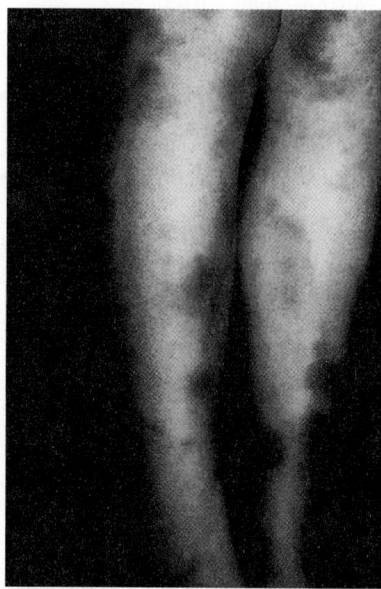

Fig. 1-110   Erythema nodosum.
(From Arndt KA et al: *Cutaneous medicine and surgery,* vol 1, Philadelphia, 1997, WB Saunders.)

- The nodules are usually one eighth to 1 inch in diameter, but can be as large as 4 inches; they begin as light red lesions, then become darker and often ecchymotic. The nodules heal within 8 wk without ulceration
- Associated findings
  Fever
  Lymphadenopathy
  Arthralgia
  Signs of the underlying illness

■ ETIOLOGY

Cell-mediated hypersensitivity reaction seen more frequently in persons with HLA antigen B8. The lesion results from an exaggerated interaction between an antigen and cell-mediated immune mechanisms leading to granuloma formation.
Infections:
- Bacteria
  Streptococcal pharyngitis
  Salmonella enteritis
  Yersinia enteritis
  Psittacosis
  Chlamydia pneumoniae infection
  Mycoplasma pneumonia
  Meningococcal infection
  Gonorrhea
  Syphilis
  Lymphogranuloma venereum
  Tularemia
  Cat-scratch disease
  Leprosy
  Tuberculosis
- Fungi
  Histoplasmosis
  Coccidioidomycosis
  Blastomycosis
  Trichophyton verrucosum
- Viruses
  Cytomegalovirus
  Hepatitis B
  Epstein-Barr virus
- Drugs
  Sulfonamides
  Penicillins
  Oral contraceptives
  Gold salts
  Prazosin
  Aspirin
  Bromides
- Sarcoidosis
- Cancer, usually lymphoma
- Ankylosing spondylosis and reactive arthropathies (e.g., associated with inflammatory bowel disease)

DIAGNOSIS

■ DIFFERENTIAL DIAGNOSIS

- Insect bites
- Posttraumatic ecchymoses
- Vasculitis
- Weber-Christian disease
- Fat necrosis associated with pancreatitis

■ WORKUP

- Physical examination
- Diagnosis of underlying illness by history, physical examination, and laboratory tests as indicated

■ LABORATORY TESTS

- Erythrocyte sedimentation rate (ESR)
- Throat culture and antistreptolysin O titer
- PPD
- Others depending on index of suspicion

■ IMAGING STUDIES

- Chest x-ray for sarcoidosis and TB
- Skin biopsy in doubtful cases
Early lesion: inflammation and hemorrhage in subcutaneous tissue
Late lesion: giant cells and granulomata

TREATMENT

The disease is self-limited and treatment is symptomatic
- NSAIDs for pain
- Systemic steroids in severe cases

■ PROGNOSIS

Typical case:
- Pain for 2 wk
- Resolution within 8 wk

REFERENCE

Dixey J: Erythema nodosum. In Klippel JH et al (eds): *Rheumatology,* St Louis, 1998, Mosby.
Author: **Tom J. Wachtel, M.D.**

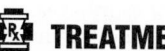

BASIC INFORMATION

■ DEFINITION

Esophageal tumors are defined as benign and malignant tumors arising from the esophagus. Approximately 15% of esophageal cancers arise in the cervical esophagus, 50% in the middle third of the esophagus, and 35% in the lower third. Eighty-five percent of esophageal tumors are squamous cell carcinoma (arising from squamous epithelium). Adenocarcinomas arise from columnar epithelium in the distal esophagus, which have become dysplastic secondary to chronic gastric reflux.

ICD-9CM CODES
150.8 Esophageal cancer, NEC
150.9 Esophageal cancer, NOS
230.1 Carcinoma of esophagus, in situ

■ EPIDEMIOLOGY & DEMOGRAPHICS

Carcinomas of the esophageal epithelium, both squamous cell and adenocarcinoma, are by far the most common and important tumors of the esophagus. Benign neoplasms are much less common and include leiomyoma, papilloma, and fibrovascular polyps. Prevalence of esophageal carcinoma varies widely in different parts of world, from 7.6 cases per 100,000 persons in the U.S. to 130 cases per 100,000 persons in China. It occurs frequently within the so-called Asian "esophageal cancer belt," extending from the southern shore of the Caspian Sea to northern China, with certain high-incidence pockets in Finland, Ireland, SE Africa, and NW France. In the U.S., it is more common among blacks than whites and is more predominant in men (male:female ratio of 3:1). It usually develops in the seventh and eighth decades of life and is an illness associated with lower socioeconomic status.

■ PHYSICAL FINDINGS & CLINICAL PRESENTATION

Symptoms and signs:
- Dysphagia: initially occurs with solid foods and gradually progresses to include semisolids and liquids; latter signs usually indicate incurable disease with tumor involving more than 60% of the esophageal circumference
- Weight loss: usually of short duration
- Hoarseness: suggests recurrent laryngeal nerve involvement
- Odynophagia: an unusual symptom
- Cervical adenopathy: usually involving supraclavicular lymph nodes
- Dry cough: suggests tracheal involvement
- Aspiration pneumonia: caused by development of a fistula between the esophagus and trachea
- Massive hemoptysis or hematemesis: results from the invasion of vascular structures
- Advanced disease spreads to liver, lungs, and pleura
- Hypercalcemia: usually associated with squamous cell carcinoma because of the secretion of a tumor peptide similar to the parathyroid hormone

■ ETIOLOGY

- Excess alcohol consumption: accounts for 80% to 90% of esophageal cancer in the U.S., with whiskey being associated with a higher incidence than wine or beer
- Cigarette smoking: alcohol and tobacco use combined increase the risk substantially
- Other ingested carcinogens:
  Nitrates (converted to nitrites): South Asia, China
  Smoked opiates: Northern Iran
  Fungal toxins in pickled vegetables
- Mucosal damage:
  Long-term exposure to extremely hot tea
  Lye ingestion
- Radiation-induced strictures
- Chronic achalasia: incidence is seven times higher
- Host susceptibility secondary to precancerous lesions:
  Plummer-Vinson syndrome (Paterson-Kelly): glossitis with iron deficiency
  Congenital hyperkeratosis and pitting of palms and soles
- Chronic GERD leading to Barrett's esophagus (whites are affected more than blacks)
- Possible association with celiac sprue or dietary deficiencies of molybdenum, zinc, vitamin A

DIAGNOSIS

■ DIFFERENTIAL DIAGNOSIS
- Achalasia of the esophagus
- Scleroderma of the esophagus
- Diffuse esophageal spasm
- Esophageal rings and webs

■ PHYSICAL EXAMINATION
- Monitor weight
- Findings are limited to cervical and supraclavicular lymph nodes
- Signs of lung consolidation from aspiration pneumonia

■ LABORATORY TESTS
Complete blood cell count, chemistries, liver enzymes

■ IMAGING STUDIES
- Double contrast esophagogram effectively identifies large esophageal lesions (Fig. 1-111).

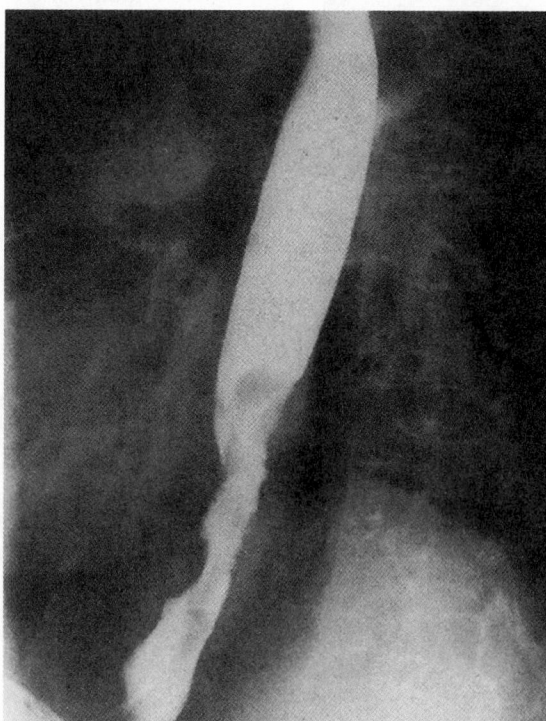

Fig. 1-111 Barium swallow demonstrating the classic findings in cancer of the distal third of the espophagus. (From Nobel J [ed]: *Primary care medicine,* ed 2, St Louis, 1996, Mosby.)

- In contrast to benign esophageal leiomyomata, which cause esophageal narrowing with preservation of normal mucosal pattern, esophageal carcinomas cause ragged ulcerating changes in the mucosa in association with deeper infiltration.
- Smaller tumors can be missed by esophagogram, therefore esophagoscopy is recommended.
- Esophagoscopy is performed to visualize tumor and obtain histopathologic confirmation.
- This population is also at risk for cancers of head, neck, and lung; therefore endoscopic inspection of larynx, trachea, and bronchi should also be performed.
- Endoscopic biopsies fail to recover malignant tissue one third of the time, thus cytologic examination of tumor brushings should be routinely performed.
- Examination of the fundus of the stomach via retroflexion of the endoscope is also imperative.
- Chest and abdominal CT scan should be performed to determine the extent of tumor spread to mediastinum, paraaortic lymph nodes, and liver.

 TREATMENT

■ ACUTE GENERAL Rx
SURGICAL RESECTION:
- Surgical resection of squamous cell and adenocarcinoma of the lower third of the esophagus is done in most centers if there is no widespread metastasis.

- Less than 20% of patients who survive a total resection can be expected to survive after 5 yr. Usually stomach or colon is used for esophageal replacement.

POSSIBLE COMPLICATIONS OF SURGERY: Anatomic fistula (usually with colon interposition, subphrenic abscesses); respiratory complications are less common as a result of advances in surgical techniques, respiratory therapy, hyperalimentation, and anesthetic support during surgery. Cardiovascular complications are by far the most common including MI, CVA, and PE.

RADIATION THERAPY:
- Squamous cell carcinomas are more radiosensitive than adenocarcinoma, and radiation achieves good local control and is an excellent palliative modality for obstructive symptoms. Usually employed for tumors in upper third of esophagus, often for middle third tumors as well.
- About 40% of tumors cannot be destroyed even after 6000 rads.
- Palliative radiation therapy for bone metastasis is also effective.
- Single agent resulted in significant tumor regression in 15% to 25% of patients and combination chemotherapy including cisplatin achieved significant tumor reduction in 30% to 60% of patients.

COMPLICATIONS OF RADIATION THERAPY:
- Esophageal stricture, radiation-induced pulmonary fibrosis, transverse myelitis are the most feared complications.
- Radiation-induced cardiomyopathy and skin changes occur less frequently given modern techniques.

- Mucositis, GI toxicity, and myelosuppression occur frequently.
- Nephrotoxicity, ototoxicity and neurotoxicity can develop with cisplatin.

COMBINATION CHEMOTHERAPY, RADIATION Rx, AND SURGICAL Rx:
- Combination therapy has been found to be associated with increased mortality rate and does not confer a survival advantage.
- Palliative procedures such as repeated endoscopic dilation, surgical placement of feeding tube, or polyvinyl prosthesis to bypass tumors have been used for surgically unresectable patients.

■ DISPOSITION
- Surgery: 5-yr survival rate is 48% in stages I and II, 20% in advanced stages.
- Radiation therapy: 5-yr survival rate is between 6% and 20%.
- Chemotherapy: Simple agent response rate 15% to 38%; combination response rate 80%.
- Combined modality: 18% response rate.

REFERENCES
Enzinger PC, Mayer RJ: Esophageal cancer, *N Engl J Med* 349:2241, 2003.

Shaheen N et al: Gastroesophageal reflux, Barrett esophagus, and esophageal cancer: clinical applications, *JAMA* 287(15):1982, 2002.

Authors: **Lynn McNicoll, M.D., and Madhavi Yerneni, M.D.**

BASIC INFORMATION

■ **DEFINITION**

A predominantly postural and action tremor that is bilateral and tends to progress slowly over the years in the absence of other neurological abnormalities.

ICD-CM CODES

333.1 Essential tremor

■ **EPIDEMIOLOGY & DEMOGRAPHICS**

About 415/100,000 in persons over 40 yr. No gender or racial predominance.

■ **PHYSICAL FINDINGS & CLINICAL PRESENTATION**

- Patients complain of tremor, especially when under emotional duress and drinking liquids
- Tremor, 4 to 12 Hz, bilateral postural and action tremor of the upper extremities. May also affect the head, voice, trunk, and legs. Typically is the same amplitude throughout the action, such as bringing a cup to the mouth. No other neurologic abnormalities on examination. Patients often note improvement with small amount of alcohol.

■ **ETIOLOGY**

Often an inherited disease, autosomal dominant; sporadic cases without a family history are frequently encountered

DIAGNOSIS

■ **DIFFERENTIAL DIAGNOSIS**

- Parkinson's disease—tremor is usually asymmetric, especially early on in the disease, and is predominantly a resting tremor. Patients with Parkinson's disease will also have increased tone, decreased facial expression, slowness of movement, and shuffling gait.
- Cerebellar tremor—an intention tremor that increases at the end of a goal-directed movement (such as finger to nose testing). Other associated neurologic abnormalities include ataxia, dysarthria, and difficulty with tandem gait.
- Drug-induced—there are many drugs that enhance normal, physiologic tremor. These include caffeine, nicotine, lithium, levothyroxine, B-adrenergic bronchodilators, valproate, and SSRIs.
- Wilson's Disease—wing-beating tremor that is most pronounced with shoulders abducted, elbows flexed, and fingers pointing towards each other. Usually there are other neurologic abnormalities including dysarthria, dystonia, and Keyser Fleischer rings on ophthalmologic examination.

■ **WORKUP**

- All imaging studies normal (MRI, CT) and are usually unnecessary unless there are other associated neurologic abnormalities
- Check TSH
- In patients younger than 40 yr with other neurologic abnormalities, send ceruloplasmin, Cu, 24-hr Cu to rule out Wilson's disease

TREATMENT

Do not need to treat essential tremor unless it is functionally impairing. Patients need to understand that treatments are only 40%-70% effective.

■ **NONPHARMACOLOGIC THERAPY**

Reduction of stress. Minimize use of caffeine. Small quantities of alcohol at social functions tend to be beneficial.

■ **ACUTE GENERAL Rx**

Can take a dose of propranolol (20-40 mg) in preparation for specific event.

■ **CHRONIC Rx**

First-line agents
- Propranolol: Usual starting dose is 30 mg. Usual therapeutic dose is 160-320 mg. Must be used with caution in those with asthma, depression, cardiac disease, and diabetes.
- Primidone: Usual starting dose is 12.5 to 25 mg hs. Usual therapeutic dose is between 62.5 and 750 mg daily. Sedation and nausea when first begin medication are biggest side effects.

Other agents
- Neurontin: 400 mg qhs, usual therapeutic dose is 1200-3600 mg
- Topamax: 25 mg qhs, may titrate up to about 400 mg
- Alprazolam: 0.75-2.75 mg

■ **SURGICAL Rx**

Thalamic deep brain stimulation contralateral to side of tremor

■ **DISPOSITION**

Patients should be reassured that the condition is not associated with other neurologic disabilities; however, it can become quite functionally disabling over time.

■ **REFERRAL**

This is a condition that usually can be treated by the primary care physician; however, if patient fails first-line therapies then patient should be referred to specialists for other drug trials and other possible surgical options.

PEARLS & CONSIDERATIONS

Essential tremor is the most common of all movement disorders. The newer anticonvulsants are found to be the most effective therapy with the fewest side effects.

REFERENCES

Deuschel G, Volkmann J: Tremors: Differential diagnosis, pathophysiology, and therapy. In Jankovic J, Tolosa E (eds): *Parkinson's disease and movement disorders*, ed 4, 2002, pp. 270-291.

Louis ED: Essential tremor, *N Engl J Med* 345(12):887, 2001.

Zesiewicz TA et al: Phenomenology and treatment of tremor disorders. In Hurtig H, Stern M (eds): *Neurologic clinics: Movement disorders* 19:3, 2001, pp. 651-680.

Author: **Cindy Zadikoff, M.D.**

BASIC INFORMATION

■ DEFINITION
Acute fatty liver of pregnancy (AFLP) is characterized histologically by microvesicular fatty cytoplasmic infiltration of hepatocytes with minimal hepatocellular necrosis.

■ SYNONYMS
Acute fatty metamorphosis
Acute yellow atrophy

ICD-9CM CODES
646.7 Liver disorders in pregnancy

■ EPIDEMIOLOGY & DEMOGRAPHICS
INCIDENCE:
- Approximately 1 in 10,000 pregnancies
- Equal frequencies in all races and at all maternal ages

AVERAGE GESTATIONAL AGE: 37 wk (range 28 to 42 wk)

RISK FACTORS:
- Primiparity
- Multiple gestation
- Male fetus

GENETICS: Some with a familial deficiency of long-chain 3-hydroxyacyl-CoA dehydrogenase (LCHAD)

■ PHYSICAL FINDINGS & CLINICAL PRESENTATION
- Initial manifestations
  1. Nausea and vomiting (70%)
  2. Pain in RUQ or epigastrium (50% to 80%)
  3. Malaise and anorexia
- Jaundice often in 1 to 2 wk
- Late manifestations
  1. Fulminant hepatic failure
  2. Encephalopathy
  3. Renal failure
  4. Pancreatitis
  5. GI and uterine bleeding
  6. Disseminated intravascular coagulation
  7. Seizures
  8. Coma
- Liver
  1. Usually small
  2. Normal or enlarged in preeclampsia, eclampsia, HELLP (hemolysis, elevated liver enzymes, and low platelets) syndrome, and acute hepatitis
  3. Coexistent preeclampsia in up to 46% of patients

■ ETIOLOGY
- Postulated that inhibition of mitochondrial oxidation of fatty acids may lead to microvesicular fatty infiltration of liver
- Fatty metamorphosis of preeclamptic liver disease thought to be of different etiology

DIAGNOSIS

■ DIFFERENTIAL DIAGNOSIS
- Acute gastroenteritis
- Preeclampsia or eclampsia with liver involvement
- HELLP syndrome
- Acute viral hepatitis
- Fulminant hepatitis
- Drug-induced hepatitis caused by halothane, phenytoin, methyldopa, isoniazid, hydrochlorothiazide, or tetracycline
- Intrahepatic cholestasis of pregnancy
- Gallbladder disease
- Reye's syndrome
- Hemolytic-uremic syndrome
- Budd-Chiari syndrome
- SLE

■ WORKUP
- A clinical diagnosis is based predominantly on physical and laboratory findings.
- Most definitive diagnosis is through liver biopsy with oil red O staining and electron microscopy.
- Liver biopsy is reserved for atypical cases only and only after any existing coagulopathy corrected with FFP.

■ LABORATORY TESTS
Tests to determine the following:
- Hypoglycemia (often profound)
- Hyperammonemia
- Elevated aminotransferases (usually <500 U/ml)
- WBC count >15,000
- Hyperbilirubinemia (usually <10 mg/dl)
- Low albumin
- DIC (in 75%)

■ IMAGING STUDIES
- Ultrasound: best used to rule out other diseases in the differential diagnosis such as gallbladder disease
- CT scan: plays minimal role because of a high false-negative rate

TREATMENT

■ NONPHARMACOLOGIC THERAPY
- Patient is admitted to intensive care unit for stabilization.
- Fetus is delivered; spontaneous resolution usually follows delivery.
- Mode of delivery is based on obstetric indications and clinical assessment of disease severity.

■ ACUTE GENERAL Rx
- Decrease in endogenous ammonia through dietary protein restriction; neomycin 6 to 12 g/day PO to decrease presence of ammonia-producing bacteria; magnesium citrate 30 to 50 ml PO or enema to evacuate nitrogenous wastes from colon
- Administration of intravenous fluids with glucose to keep glucose levels >60 mg/dl
- Coagulopathy corrected with FFP
- Avoidance of drugs metabolized by liver
- Aggressive avoidance and treatment for nosocomial infections; consideration of prophylactic antibiotics

■ CHRONIC Rx
Orthotopic liver transplantation is the only treatment for irreversible liver failure.

■ DISPOSITION
- Before 1980, both maternal and fetal mortalities: approximately 85%
- After 1980, both maternal and fetal mortalities: below 20%
- Usually rapid return of liver function to normal after delivery
- Minimal risk of recurrence with future pregnancies

■ REFERRAL
To tertiary health care facility as soon as diagnosis is suspected

REFERENCES
Cunningham FG et al: Gastrointestinal disorders. In Cunningham FG et al (eds): *Williams' obstetrics*, ed 20, Stamford, Conn, 1997, Appleton & Lange.
Davidson KM: Acute fatty liver of pregnancy, *Postgrad Obstet Gynecol* 15:1, 1995.
Knox TA, Olans LB: Liver disease in pregnancy, *N Engl J Med* 335:569, 1996.
Sawai SK: Acute fatty liver of pregnancy. In Foley MR, Strong TH Jr: *Obstetric intensive care: a practical manual*, Philadelphia, 1997, WB Saunders.
Toro Ortiz JC et al: Acute fatty liver of pregnancy. *J Matern Fetal Neonatl Med* 12(4):277, 2003.
Author: **Wan J. Kim, M.D.**

BASIC INFORMATION

■ DEFINITION

Felty's syndrome (FS) is defined as the triad of rheumatoid arthritis (RA), splenomegaly, and granulocytopenia. It is an extraarticular manifestation of seropositive RA in which recurrent local and systemic infections are the major source of morbidity and mortality.

ICD-9CM CODES
714.1 Felty's syndrome

■ EPIDEMIOLOGY & DEMOGRAPHICS
• FS occurs in less than 1% of patients with RA
• 60% to 80% are women
• Recognized in the fifth through seventh decades in patients who have had RA for 10 yr or more
• FS patients are more likely to have a family history of RA and HLA-DR4
• Rare in African Americans (low frequency of HLA-DR4)

■ PHYSICAL FINDINGS & CLINICAL PRESENTATION
• Rarely, splenomegaly and granulocytopenia are present before the arthritis.
• Articular involvement is usually more severe in patients with FS as compared with other patients with RA; however, one third may have relatively inactive synovitis with elevated ESR.
• Degree of splenomegaly varies and may be detectable only by imaging studies.
• The degree of splenomegaly has no correlation with the degree of granulocytopenia.
• FS patients have a greater frequency of extraarticular manifestations (nodules, weight loss, Sjögren's syndrome, etc.) than other patients with RA.
• Approximately 25% of patients have refractory leg ulcers, often associated with hyperpigmentation of the anterior tibia.
• Mild hepatomegaly is common (up to 68%).
• Patients with FS have a 20 times increased frequency of infections as compared with other RA patients.
• There is usually an adequate response to appropriate antibiotic therapy.

■ ETIOLOGY
The pathogenesis of FS is probably multifactorial and no clear explanation has been elucidated.

Proposed mechanisms of the granulocytopenia:
• Splenic sequestration and peripheral destruction of granulocytes secondary to immune complexes and antineutrophil antibodies
• Impaired granulopoiesis in bone marrow as a result of decreased cytokine production, presence of inhibitors, or humoral and cell-mediated immune suppression
• Excessive margination

DIAGNOSIS

■ DIFFERENTIAL DIAGNOSIS
• Drug reaction
• Myeloproliferative disorders
• Lymphoma/reticuloendothelial malignancies
• Hepatic cirrhosis with portal hypertension
• Sarcoidosis
• Tuberculosis
• Amyloidosis
• Chronic infections

■ WORKUP
Physical examination and laboratory evaluation

■ LABORATORY TESTS
• Complete blood count with differential, looking for:
  1. Granulocytopenia
  2. Mild to moderate anemia
  3. Mild thrombocytopenia
• ESR
• Bone marrow biopsy in most patients will show myeloid hyperplasia with an excess of immature granulocyte precursors ("maturation arrest")
• Rheumatoid factor: positive in 98%, usually high titer
• ANA: positive in 67%
• Antihistone antibody: positive in 83%
• HLA-DR4: positive in 95%
• Antineutrophil cytoplasmic antibodies
• Immunoglobulins: level may be higher than in RA patients
• Complement: level may be lower than in RA patients

■ IMAGING STUDIES
Ultrasonography or CT scan may be useful in diagnosing splenomegaly

TREATMENT

There is no uniformly effective therapy for FS.

■ ACUTE GENERAL Rx
Splenectomy
• Standard therapy since 1932
• Acutely reverses hematologic abnormalities
• Ongoing infections may resolve after operation as the granulocyte count rises
• 25% to 30% will have recurrent granulocytopenia, but the granulocyte count usually remains above the presplenectomy level
• Improvement in frequency of recurrent infection variable and not correlated with hematologic improvement
• Usually reserved for patients with profound granulocytopenia ($<1000/mm^3$) and severe recurrent infections
Lithium
• Stimulates granulopoiesis
• Little evidence of long-term benefit or conclusive reduction in rate of infection
• Used as short-term therapy while awaiting response to other measures
Parenteral testosterone: Efficacy limited by toxicity, especially in women
Corticosteroids
• Pulse dosing is a potential alternative for short-term elevation of neutrophils
• Overwhelming infection is the main barrier to the use of corticosteroids
Antirheumatic drugs: Second-line drugs, may improve the granulocytopenia in FS
Gold salt injections: Good hematologic response—60%, partial response—20%
Penicillamine: Controversial, should never be the first choice for FS
Methotrexate: The frequency of infection may decrease, but still not well proven
Recombinant G-CSF
• Improves neutrophil count but not arthritis and anemia of FS
• May be useful as adjunctive therapy during serious infection or in preparation for surgery
Other immunosuppressants: Cyclophosphamide, cyclosporine, azathioprine, leflunomide, TNF-α: limited experience

■ REFERRAL
• To rheumatologist for treatment of RA
• To hematologist for treatment of granulocytopenia

Authors: Etsuko Aoki, M.D., and Rebecca A. Griffith, M.D.

BASIC INFORMATION

■ DEFINITION

A femoral neck fracture occurs within the capsule of the hip joint between the base of the head and the intertrochanteric line.

■ SYNONYMS

Intracapsular fracture
Subcapital fracture
ICD-9CM CODES
820.8 Femoral neck fracture

■ EPIDEMIOLOGY & DEMOGRAPHICS

PREVALENCE: Lifetime risk in women approximately 16%
PREVALENT SEX: Female:male ratio of 3:1
PREVALENT AGE: 90% over age 60

■ PHYSICAL FINDINGS & CLINICAL PRESENTATION

• A hip or groin pain
• Affected limb usually shortened and externally rotated in displaced fractures
• Impacted fractures: possibly no deformity and only mild pain with hip motion
• Mild external bruising

■ ETIOLOGY

• Trauma
• Age-related bone weakness, usually caused by osteoporosis
• Increased risk of fractures in elderly (decline in muscle function, use of psychotropic medication, etc.)

DIAGNOSIS

■ DIFFERENTIAL DIAGNOSIS

Osteoarthritis of hip
Pathologic fracture
Lumbar disc syndrome with radicular pain
Insufficiency fracture of pelvis

■ WORKUP

Diagnosis usually obvious based on clinical and radiographic findings

■ IMAGING STUDIES

• Standard roentgenograms consisting of an AP of the pelvis and a cross-table lateral of the hip to confirm the diagnosis (Fig. 1-112)
• If initial roentgenograms negative and diagnosis of an occult femoral neck fracture suspected, hospital admission and further radiographic assessment with either bone scanning or MRI
• Bone scanning most sensitive after 48 to 72 hr.

TREATMENT

• Orthopedic consultation
• Surgery indicated in most cases, usually within 24 hr
• DVT prophylaxis

■ DISPOSITION

• Mortality rate within 1 yr in elderly patients is 25% to 30%.
• Dementia is a particularly poor prognostic sign.

PEARLS & CONSIDERATIONS

■ COMMENTS

• Complications: nonunion and avascular necrosis
• Intracapsular fractures: occasionally occur in nonambulatory patients
  1. Usually treated nonsurgically, especially in the patient with dementia and limited pain perception
  2. Early bed-to-chair mobilization and vigilant nursing care to avoid skin breakdown
  3. Fracture usually pain free in a short time even if solid bony healing does not occur
• As a result of the increasing life span of the female population, femoral neck fractures are becoming more common. The initial physical examination and roentgenographic studies may be completely negative. Groin pain, sometimes quite severe, may be the only early clue to the diagnosis.

• The rate of hip fracture could be reduced by:
  1. Elimination of environmental hazards (poor lighting, loose rugs)
  2. Regular exercise for balance and strength
  3. Patient education about fall prevention
  4. Medication review to minimize side effects
  5. Prevention and treatment of osteoporosis

REFERENCES

Bettelli G et al: Relationship between mortality and proximal femur fractures in the elderly, *Orthopedics* 26:1045, 2003.
Jain R et al: Comparison of early and delayed fixation of subcapital hip fractures in patients sixty years of age or less, *Bone Joint Surg* 84(A):1605, 2002.
Lawrence VA et al: Medical complications and outcomes after hip fracture repair, *Ann Intern Med* 162:2053, 2003.
McClung MR et al: Effect of risedronate on the risk of hip fracture in elderly women. Hip Intervention Program Study Group, *N Engl J Med* 344(5):333, 2001.
McKinley JC, Robinson CM: Treatment of displaced intracapsular fractures with total hip arthroplasty, *J Bone Joint Surg* 84(A):2010, 2002.
Schoofs MW et al: Thiazide diuretics and the risk for hip fractures, *Ann Intern Med* 139:476, 2003.
Stevens JA, Olson S: Reducing falls and resulting hip fractures among older women, *Home Care Prov* 5(4):134, 2000.

Author: **Lonnie R. Mercier, M.D.**

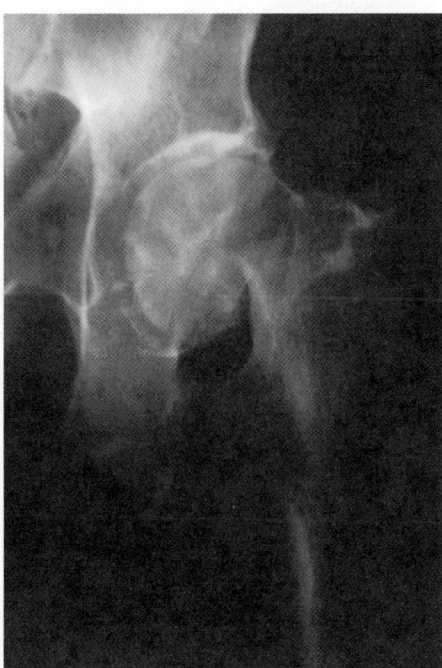

Fig. 1-112　Femoral neck fracture. (From Scudieri G [ed]: *Sports medicine: principles of primary care,* St Louis, 1997, Mosby.)

BASIC INFORMATION

■ DEFINITION

Fever of undetermined origin (FUO) was defined by Petersdorf in 1961 as an illness characterized by temperatures surpassing 101° F for more than 3 wk with no known cause despite extensive workup.

- Persistence for greater than 2 wk separates a FUO from an insignificant viral illness.
- Traditionally, diagnosis made only after at least a 1-wk inpatient workup.
- In contemporary practice, much of the workup is performed outpatient; taking time for a complete history and physical examination is still essential.
- Different settings—community vs. hospital vs. oncology ward—dictate duration needed for FUO designation.

ICD-9CM CODES

780.6 Pyrexia of undetermined origin

■ EPIDEMIOLOGY & DEMOGRAPHICS

Incidence is difficult to calculate because of inconsistent designation of febrile illnesses as FUO. The incidence of undiagnosed FUO has dropped to less than 10% in most recent studies.

■ ETIOLOGY

Classic (1 wk workup after 2 wk persistently febrile): Divided among infection, malignancy, collagen-vascular, and other etiology; proportion for each dependent on age, geography, host and microbial factors, hospital and health services. Etiology has also changed over time. A partial list of eventual etiologies, with most common diagnoses in *italics*:

- *Factitious fever, Munchausen syndrome*
- *Abscess: dental, abdominal, pelvic*
- *Lymphoma and leukemia*
- Endocarditis (especially caused by difficult-to-isolate organisms)
- Biliary tract infection
- Osteomyelitis
- Tuberculosis
- Whipple's disease
- Psittacosis
- Fungal: histoplasmosis, cryptomycosis
- Leishmaniasis
- Renal cell carcinoma, other solid malignancies
- Systemic lupus erythematosus
- Still's disease
- Hypersensitivity vasculitis
- Temporal arteritis
- Drug-induced fever
- Inflammatory bowel disease
- Sarcoidosis
- Granulomatous hepatitis
- Central fever (rare)

Neutropenic (PMN <500 and febrile >3 days): With blood cultures from onset negative, ruling out *Pseudomonas* and other gram-negative bacteremia, staphylococcal bacteremia from line infection; urinalysis and chest x-ray negative. Possible etiologies:

- Perianal infection
- Occult fungal infection
- Drug fever
- Cytomegalovirus infection in post-transplant patients or patients who are on immunosuppressants

HIV-associated: Etiology depends on CD4 count. HIV itself may be the cause. With low CD4 count—MAI bacteremia, non-Hodgkin's lymphoma

Nosocomial (febrile for 3 days in hospital): UTI, pneumonia, line-related bacteremia, *Clostridium difficile* diarrhea, or sinusitis secondary to intubation

- Noninfectious etiology: deep venous thrombosis, hematoma, drug fever

DIAGNOSIS

■ DIFFERENTIAL DIAGNOSIS

Factitious fever: body temperature not elevated when accurately measured.

■ WORKUP

- Accurate history and careful physical examination is essential
- Laboratory tests and radiologic examinations dependent on historical clues, physical findings
- "Shotgun" approach, ordering every test for every possibility, is rarely helpful
- Tests and procedures should be thoughtful, directed toward localizing signs and symptoms (Section III, Fig. 3-77).
- When in doubt, perform another complete history and physical examination

■ HISTORICAL CLUES

- Fever duration, tempo; inciting factors
- Associated symptoms: rash, myalgia, weight loss, pain
- Sick contacts
- Past medical history: HIV, malignancies, surgeries
- Medications
- Family history: tuberculosis in a relative, malignancies, familial Mediterranean fever
- Social history: daily routine, rural vs. urban, pets and animal contacts, arthropod bites, travel—recent and remote, socioeconomic status, occupation, military service, sexual history

■ PHYSICAL FINDINGS

- HEENT: rule out sinusitis, dental abscesses; examine eyes carefully
- Neck: check adenopathy
- Lungs: auscultate for rales

- Heart: listen for murmur
- Abdomen: check for organomegaly
- Rectal: examine for prostate tenderness
- Pelvic: rule out cervical motion tenderness, check for inguinal adenopathy
- Extremities: look for clubbing, splinter hemorrhages; examine IV access site
- Musculoskeletal: examine for joint effusions
- Skin: note any rashes, wounds

■ LABORATORY TESTS

- Base on historical clues and physical findings.
- Blood cultures, CBC, urinalysis, transaminases, PPD testing is important in most FUO workups.
- Base on leads from history, examination—whether need for serum antibody testing, lumbar puncture, thyroid function testing, stool culture and *C. difficile* assay, bone marrow biopsy, skin biopsy, ANA.
- May need to repeat laboratory examinations at regular intervals until diagnosis is established.

■ IMAGING STUDIES

- Base on historical clues and physical findings.
- Chest x-ray, abdominal CT scan are important eventually in most workups in which diagnosis is elusive.

TREATMENT

■ PHARMACOTHERAPY

Antibiotics and other treatment are indicated only after definitive or highly probable diagnosis is established, unless patient appears severely ill or septic.

■ DISPOSITION

Diagnoses are found in majority of fevers with initially undetermined origin. Some will continue to defy diagnosis for years.

■ REFERRAL

To an infectious disease specialist if no diagnosis after thoughtful workup

REFERENCES

Mackowiak PA, Durack DT: Fever of unknown origin. In Mandel G, Bennett J, Dolin R (eds): *Principles and practice of infectious disease,* ed 5, Philadelphia, 2000, Churchill Livingstone.

Petersdorf R, Beeson P: Fever of unexplained origin: report of 100 cases, *Medicine* 40:1, 1961.

Roth AR, Basello GM: Approach to the adult patient with fever of unknown origin, *Am Fam Physician* 68:2223, 2003.

Authors: **Etsuko Aoki, M.D., and Anne Spaulding, M.D.**

BASIC INFORMATION

■ DEFINITION

Fibrocystic breast disease (FCD) is a "nondisease" that includes nonmalignant breast lesions such as microcystic and macrocystic changes, fibrosis, ductal or lobular hyperplasia, adenosis, apocrine metaplasia, fibroadenoma, papilloma, papillomatosis, and other changes. Atypical ductal or lobular hyperplasia is associated with a moderate increase in breast cancer risk.

■ SYNONYMS

Cystic changes
Chronic cystic mastitis
Mammary dysplasia

ICD-9CM CODES

610.0 Solitary cyst of the breast
610.1 Fibrocystic disease of the breast

■ EPIDEMIOLOGY & DEMOGRAPHICS

- Ubiquitous in premenopausal women after 20 yr of age
- Palpable nodular changes in the breast termed *FCD* clinically; such changes observable in more than half of adult women 20 to 50 yr of age

■ PHYSICAL FINDINGS & CLINICAL PRESENTATION

- Tender breasts
- Nodular areas
- Dominant mass
- Thickening
- Nipple discharge
- Can vary with menstrual cycle

■ ETIOLOGY

- Although frequently seen and diagnosed, mechanism of development not understood.
- Because found in majority of healthy breasts, regarded as non-pathologic process.
- With hormone replacement therapy, may be carried into menopausal age.

 # DIAGNOSIS

■ DIFFERENTIAL DIAGNOSIS

- If presenting as dominant mass or masses: exclude possible carcinoma.
- Carcinoma: detection is difficult with FCD, particularly among premenopausal women.
- If presenting with nipple discharge: differentiate from discharge of possible malignant origin.

■ WORKUP

- Exclude breast carcinoma if breast mass, thickening, discharge, and pain present.
- Perform biopsy of suspected area for histologic confirmation.

■ IMAGING STUDIES

Mammography and ultrasound studies required:
- For mammographic changes (suspicious densities, microcalcifications, architectural distortion): careful evaluation, including possibly biopsy to exclude breast cancer
- Ultrasound study: to establish cystic nature of clinical or mammographic mass lesion

TREATMENT

■ NONPHARMACOLOGIC THERAPY

- Not considered a "disease" and does not require treatment
- Surgical intervention diagnostic to eliminate possibility of breast cancer
- Periodic physician examination to follow patients with FCD who have pronounced nodular features
- Aspiration for palpable cysts (NOTE: Cysts often recur; repeat aspiration is not always required unless pain is a problem.)

■ ACUTE GENERAL Rx

Majority of women require no treatment.

■ CHRONIC Rx

For breast pain:
- Danocrine (Danazol): limited success reported
- Bromocriptine or tamoxifen: used less frequently
- Limited caffeine intake: not as successful in controlling pain or nodularity as originally suggested

■ DISPOSITION

- Careful evaluation to exclude suspicious changes for breast cancer, then reassurance and periodic reevaluation as required
- Regular self-examination, annual physician examination, and annual mammograms for women with atypical ductal or lobular hyperplasia

■ REFERRAL

- For further evaluation and/or biopsy if there are suspicious changes that may be associated with FCD (including changing of dominant mass or thickening, persistent or spontaneous discharge, suspicious mammographic changes or lesions)
- To alleviate anxiety associated with breast symptoms or changes

PEARLS & CONSIDERATIONS

■ COMMENTS

Patient education material is available from American College of Obstetricians and Gynecologists, 408 12th Street SW, Washington, DC 20024-2188.

REFERENCE

Zera RT et al: Atypical hyperplasia, proliferative fibrocystic change, and exogenous hormone use, *Surgery* 130(4):732, 2001.
Author: **Takuma Nemoto, M.D.**

BASIC INFORMATION

■ DEFINITION

Fibromyalgia is a poorly defined disorder characterized by multiple trigger points and referred pain.

■ SYNONYMS

Myofascial pain syndrome
Fibrositis
Psychogenic rheumatism
Nonarticular rheumatism
Fibromyalgia syndrome (FS)

ICD-9CM CODES

729.0 Rheumatism, unspecified and fibrositis
729.1 Myalgia and myositis, unspecified

■ EPIDEMIOLOGY & DEMOGRAPHICS

PREVALENCE: 1% to 2% of the general population
PREVALENT SEX: Female:male ratio of 9:1
PREVALENT AGE: 30 to 50 yr

■ PHYSICAL FINDINGS

Tender "nodules" and tender points (Fig. 1-113)

■ ETIOLOGY

- Unknown
- Pain magnification may play a role

DIAGNOSIS

■ DIFFERENTIAL DIAGNOSIS

- Polymyalgia rheumatica
- Referred discogenic spine pain
- Rheumatoid arthritis
- Localized tendinitis
- Connective tissue disease
- Osteoarthritis
- Thyroid disease
- Spondyloarthropathies

■ WORKUP

- Subsets of this disorder are often described:
  1. If symptoms develop in conjunction with other conditions (rheumatoid disease or acute stress)
  2. If findings are more regionally distributed, such as those in the neck following motor vehicle accidents
- The primary condition is often suggested by the following criteria from the American College of Rheumatology:
  1. History of widespread pain
  2. Pain in 11 of 18 selected tender spots on digital palpation (mainly in the spine, elbows, and knees)

■ LABORATORY TESTS

There are no abnormalities in fibromyalgia, but laboratory assessment may be required to rule out other conditions and may include:

- CBC, ESR, rheumatoid factor, ANA
- CPK, T_4

TREATMENT

■ ACUTE GENERAL Rx

- Self-management
- Explanation, reassurance
- Tricyclic antidepressants for sleep disturbance
- Aerobic and stretching exercise, particularly swimming
- Mild analgesics; avoidance of chronic narcotic use
- Trigger point injections
- Physical therapy

■ DISPOSITION

- Prognosis is uncertain.
- Symptoms come and go for years in spite of an aggressive multifaceted approach to treatment.

PEARLS & CONSIDERATIONS

■ COMMENTS

- Before making this diagnosis, all other more likely disorders should be ruled out.
- The term "fibrositis" is often used, but no inflammation has ever been found.
- The number of trigger points needed to establish the diagnosis is debated.

REFERENCES

Clauw DJ: Elusive syndromes: treating the biologic basis of fibromyalgia and related syndromes, *Cleve Clin J Med* 68:830, 2001.

Goldenberg DL: Fibromyalgia syndrome a decade later: what have we learned? *Arch Intern Med* 159:777, 1999.

Gracely RH et al: Functional magnetic resonance imaging evidence of augmented pain processing in fibromyalgia, *Arthritis Rheum* 46:1333, 2002.

Hakkinen A et al: Strength training induced adaptations in neuromuscular function of premenopausal women with fibromyalgia: comparison with healthy women, *Ann Rheum Dis* 60:21, 2001.

Leventhal LJ: Management of fibromyalgia, *Ann Intern Med* 131:850, 1999.

O'Malley PG et al: Treatment of fibromyalgia with antidepressants: a meta-analysis, *J Gen Intern Med* 15:659, 2000.

Richards SCM, Scott DL: Prescribed exercise in people with fibromyalgia: parallel group randomized controlled trial, *BMJ* 325:185, 2002.

Worrel LM et al: Treating fibromyalgia with a brief interdisciplinary program: initial outcomes and predictors of response, *Mayo Clin Proc* 76:381, 2001.

Author: **Lonnie R. Mercier, M.D.**

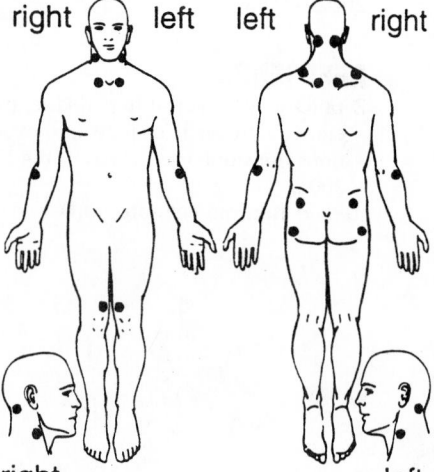

1. Occiput
2. Low cervical
3. Trapezius
4. Supraspinatus
5. Second rib
6. Lateral epicondyle
7. Gluteal
8. Greater trochanter
9. Knees

Fig. 1-113 The sites of the 18 tender points of the 1990 ACR criteria for the classification of fibromyalgia. (From Conn R: *Current Diagnosis,* ed 9, Philadelphia, 1997, WB Saunders.)

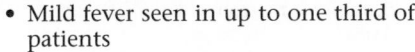

BASIC INFORMATION

■ DEFINITION

Fifth disease is a viral exanthem of childhood affecting primarily school-age children, which is caused by parvovirus B-19. Erythema infectiosum was the "fifth" in a series of described viral exanthems of childhood and is the most common clinical syndrome associated with parvovirus B-19.

■ SYNONYMS

Erythema infectiosum

ICD-9CM CODES

057.0 Fifth disease (eruptive)

■ EPIDEMIOLOGY & DEMOGRAPHICS

- Peak age range 5 to 18 yr old
- Peak incidence in late winter and spring, especially April and May
- Fifty to sixty percent of adults have demonstrated protective antibodies to parvovirus B-19

■ PHYSICAL FINDINGS & CLINICAL PRESENTATION

- Typical bright red nontender maxillary rash with circumoral pallor over cheeks, producing the classic "slapped cheek" appearance (Fig. 1-114)
- Reticular nonpruritic lacy, erythematous maculopapular rash over trunk and extremities lasting for up to several weeks after the acute episode. May be worsened by heat or sunlight
- Polyarthritis and arthralgias are commonly seen in older patients; less common in children. Arthritis involves small joints of extremities in symmetric fashion

- Mild fever seen in up to one third of patients

■ ETIOLOGY

- Syndrome caused by parvovirus B-19, a single-stranded DNA virus, which has been reclassified in a new genus "erythrovirus." It remains the only accepted member of this genus, although new variants have recently been described. Designation as "parvovirus" is still common in recent literature

DIAGNOSIS

■ DIFFERENTIAL DIAGNOSIS

- Juvenile rheumatoid arthritis (Still's disease)
- Rubella, measles (rubeola), and other childhood viral exanthems
- Mononucleosis
- Lyme disease
- Acute HIV infection
- Drug eruption

■ WORKUP

- Diagnosis made by typical clinical picture
- Parvovirus B-19 IgM antibody seen in 90% of patients with acute illness

■ LABORATORY TESTS

- Complete blood count. Transient aplastic crisis is a syndrome distinct from fifth disease, which may be seen in patients with chronic hematologic illness (described with sickle cell disease, spherocytosis, and other hemolytic processes) or AIDS, who are infected with parvovirus B-19. It is usually self-limited and associated with prodrome of fever and malaise. Lasts for 1 to 2 wk followed by marrow recovery. Rash usually absent. These patients are highly infective.

- hCG in women of childbearing age. Infection during early pregnancy may result in fetal death (10%) or severe anemia but is usually asymptomatic and not associated with congenital malformations.
- Antibody testing usually not necessary. IgM levels may be elevated early in the course of the illness.
- Lyme titers, monospot performed.
- Testing for other viral diseases as indicated by clinical picture.

TREATMENT

■ ACUTE GENERAL Rx

- Treatment is supportive only
- NSAIDs for arthralgias/arthritis
- Intravenous immunoglobulin and transfusion support may be used in patients with immunocompromised state with red cell aplasia
- Consider immunoglobulin treatment or prophylaxis in pregnancy

■ DISPOSITION & PROGNOSIS

- Self-limited illness lasting 1 to 2 wk
- Arthritis lasts for weeks. In some patients it may be chronic and develop into rheumatoid arthritis as adult
- Pregnant women should avoid contact with patients who have marrow suppression
- Patients with transient aplastic crisis or chronic parvovirus B-19 infection pose a risk for nosocomial spread and, when hospitalized, should be isolated with contact and respiratory precautions
- Children with fifth disease are not contagious and may attend school and day care
- Vaccine is under development

■ REFERRAL

- For signs of marrow suppression
- For signs of severe or erosive arthritis

REFERENCES

Katta, R: Parvovirus B19: a review, *Dermatol Clin* 20(2):333, 2002.
Sabella C, Goldfarls J: Parvovirus B19 infections, *Am Fam Physician* 60(5):1455, 1999.
Author: **Dominick Tammaro, M.D.**

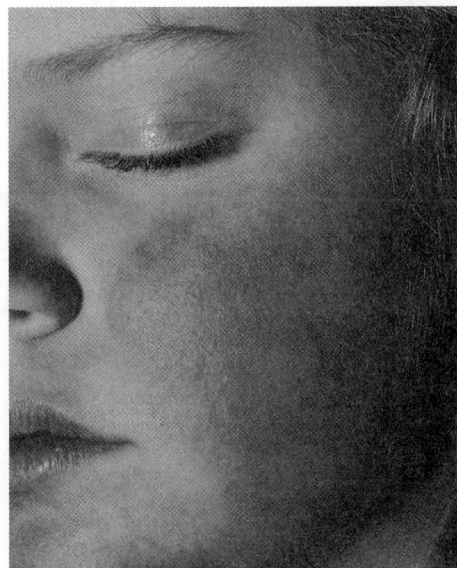

Fig. 1-114 Fifth disease (erythema infectiosum). Facial erythema "slapped cheek." The red plaque covers the cheek and spares the nasolabial and the circumoral region. (From Habif TP: *Clinical dermatology: a color guide to diagnosis and therapy,* ed 3, St Louis, 1996, Mosby.)

BASIC INFORMATION

■ DEFINITION
Filariasis is a general term for an infection caused by nematodes (round-worms) of the genera *Wuchereria* and *Brugia,* found in the tropical and subtropical regions of the world. The disease is variably characterized by acute lymphatic inflammation or chronic lymphatic obstruction associated with intermittent fevers or recurrent episodes of dyspnea and bronchospasm.

■ SYNONYMS
Lymphatic filariasis

ICD-9CM CODES
125.0 Bancroftian
125.1 Brugian
125.9 Filariasis

■ EPIDEMIOLOGY & DEMOGRAPHICS
INCIDENCE (IN U.S.): Unknown
PREDOMINANT SEX: Male
PREDOMINANT AGE: For both males and females, risk is greatest between the ages of 15 to 35 yr.
PEAK INCIDENCE: Unknown

■ PHYSICAL FINDINGS & CLINICAL PRESENTATION
- Clinical manifestations result from acute lymphatic inflammation or chronic lymphatic obstruction.
- Many patients are asymptomatic despite the presence of microfilaremia.
- Episodes of lymphangitis and lymphadenitis are associated with fever, headache, and back pain.
- Acute funiculitis and epididymitis or orchitis may also be present; all usually resolve within days to weeks but tend to recur.
- Chronic infections may be associated with lymphedema, most commonly manifested by hydrocele.
- It is a progressive disease, leading to nonpitting edema and brawny changes that may involve a whole limb (Fig. 1-115).
- Elephantiasis occurs in about 10% of patients, with skin of the scrotum or leg becoming thickened and fissured; patient is thereafter plagued by recurrent ulceration and infection.
- Chyluria, a condition that develops when lymphatic vessels rupture into the urinary tract, may occur.

■ ETIOLOGY
Caused by one of three types of nematode parasites, all of which are transmitted to humans by mosquitoes.
- *W. bancrofti:* distributed in Africa, areas of Central and South America, the Pacific Islands, and the Caribbean Basin

- *B. malayi:* restricted to Southeast Asia
- *B. timori:* confined to the Indonesian archipelago

After bite of an infected mosquito:
- Filarial larvae move into lymphatic vessels and nodes, settling and maturing over 3 to 15 mo into adult male and female worms.
- After fertilization, the female nematode produces large numbers of larvae or microfilariae that enter into the blood stream via the lymphatics.
- Nocturnal periodicity, characteristic of *B. malayi,* is an increased presence of microfilariae in the circulation during the night.
- Microfilariae of *W. bancrofti* are maximal during late afternoon.
- Most microfilariae remain in the body as immature forms for 6 mo to 2 yr.
- Infected larvae are ingested by mosquitoes, then transmitted to humans where the microfilariae mature into new adult worms.

Acute and chronic inflammatory and granulomatous changes in the lymphatic channels:
- Result from complex interaction of adult worms and host's immune systems
- Eventually lead to fibrosis and obstruction
- Most likely to develop into obstructive lymphatic disease with recurrent exposure over many years

DIAGNOSIS

■ DIFFERENTIAL DIAGNOSIS
- Elephantiasis is distinguished from other causes of chronic lymphedema, including Milroy's disease, postoperative scarring, and lymphedema of malignancy.

■ WORKUP
Diagnosis is suspected in individuals who have resided in endemic areas for at least 3 to 6 mo or more and complain of recurrent episodes of lymphangitis, lymphadenitis, scrotal edema, or thrombophlebitis, with or without fever.

■ LABORATORY TESTS
- Demonstration of microfilariae on a blood smear for definitive diagnosis
- For patients from southeastern Asia: blood sample drawn at night, especially between midnight and 2 AM
- Occasionally, microfilaremia in chylous urine or hydrocele fluid
- Prominent eosinophilia only during periods of acute lymphangitis or lymphadenitis
- Serologic tests for antibody, including enzyme-linked immunosorbent assay and indirect fluorescent antibody (often unable to distinguish among the various forms of filariasis or between acute and remote infection)

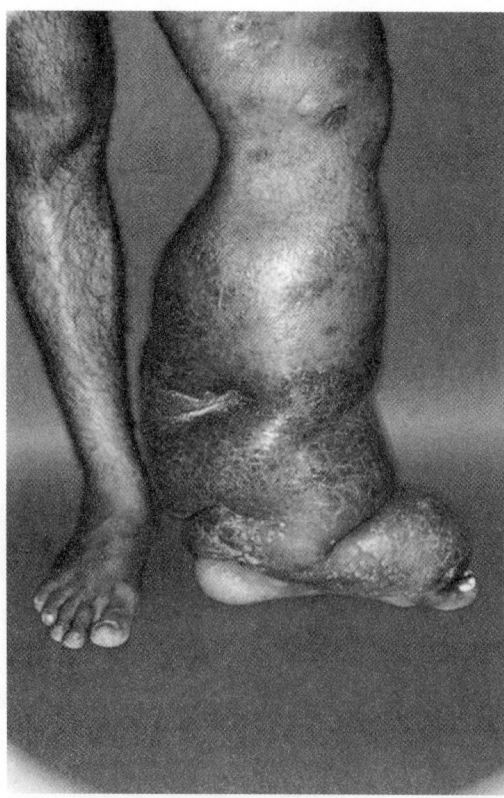

Fig. 1-115 Filariasis that eventually leads to elephantiasis. Note massive swelling of the extremity. (From Goldstein B [ed]: *Practical dermatology,* ed 2, St Louis, 1997, Mosby.)

- Immunoassays (such as circulating filaria antigen [CFA]): more successful in antigen detection in patients who are microfilaremic than in those who are amicrofilaremic

■ IMAGING STUDIES
- Chest x-ray examination: reticular nodular infiltrates (tropical pulmonary eosinophilia syndrome)
- In men proven to be microfilaremic, scrotal ultrasonography to aid in the detection of adult worms
- Compared with adults, children with FS have more sleep disturbances, fewer tender points, and a better prognosis

 TREATMENT

■ NONPHARMACOLOGIC THERAPY
- Standard of care for elephantiasis:
  1. Elevation of the affected limb
  2. Use of elastic stockings
  3. Local foot care
- General wound care for chronic ulcers and prevention of secondary infection

■ ACUTE GENERAL Rx
- Diethylcarbamazine citrate (DEC) to reduce microfilaremia by 90%
  1. Effect on adult worms, especially those of the *Wuchereria* species, less certain
  2. Given in an oral dose of 6 mg/kg qd for 12 to 14 days

- Ivermectin alone or in combination with diethylcarbamazine citrate to decrease microfilaremia
- Both drugs are similar in efficacy and tolerability; advantage of ivermectin: administration in a single oral dose of 200 μg/kg
- World Health Organization (WHO) recommendation: DEC given as a single dose, alone or (preferably) in combination with ivermectin as treatment in endemic areas

■ CHRONIC Rx
- Surgical drainage of hydroceles
- No satisfactory therapy for those patients with chyluria

■ DISPOSITION
Rarely fatal, but the psychologic impact of limb and scrotal deformities associated with elephantiasis are substantial.

■ REFERRAL
To a surgeon for management of hydrocele

☼ PEARLS & CONSIDERATIONS

- Studies in endemic areas suggest that filarial-specific IgG1 is associated with amicrofilaremic states highest in children, regardless of sex.
- Levels of IgE and IgG4 increase with age and are associated with increased levels of microfilaremia.

■ COMMENTS
Individuals who intend to travel or reside in endemic areas should be advised to institute preventive measures such as the use of netting and insect repellents, especially at night.

REFERENCES
Malhotra I et al: Influence of maternal filariasis on childhood infection and immunity to Wuchereria bancrofti in Kenya, *Infect Immun* 71(9):5231, 2003.

Rahmah N et al: Multicentre laboratory evaluation of Brugia Rapid dipstick test for detection of brugian filariasis, *Trop Med Int Health* 8(10):895, 2003.

Ramaiah KD et al: The prevalences of Wuchereria bancrofti antigenemia in communities given six rounds of treatment with diethylcarbamazine, ivermectin or placebo tablets, *Ann Trop Med Parasitol* 97(7):737, 2003.

Walther M, Muller R: Diagnosis of human filariases (except onchocerciasis), *Adv Parasitol* 53:149, 2003.

Watanabe K et al: Bancroftian filariasis in Nepal: a survey for circulating antigenemia of Wuchereria bancrofti and urinary IgG4 antibody in two rural areas of Nepal, *Acta Trop* 88(1):11, 2003.
Author: **George O. Alonso, M.D.**

BASIC INFORMATION

■ DEFINITION
Folliculitis is the inflammation of the hair follicle as a result of infection, physical injury, or chemical irritation.

■ SYNONYMS
Sycosis barbae

ICD-9CM CODES
704.8 Other specified diseases of hair and hair follicles

■ EPIDEMIOLOGY & DEMOGRAPHICS
• Staphylococcal folliculitis is the most common form of infectious folliculitis; it occurs most commonly in persons with diabetes.
• Sycosis barbae occurs most frequently in men who have commenced shaving.

■ PHYSICAL FINDINGS & CLINICAL PRESENTATION
• The lesions generally consist of painful yellow pustules surrounded by erythema; a central hair is present in the pustules.
• Patients with sycosis barbae may initially present with small follicular papules or pustules that increase in size with continued shaving; deep follicular pustules may occur surrounded by erythema and swelling; the upper lip is frequently involved (Fig. 1-116).

• "Hot tub" folliculitis occurs within 1 to 4 days following use of hot tub with poor chlorination, and it is characterized by pustules with surrounding erythema generally affecting torso, buttocks, and limbs.

■ ETIOLOGY
• *Staphylococcus* infection (e.g., sycosis barbae), *Pseudomonas aeruginosa* ("hot tub" folliculitis)
• Gram-negative folliculitis (*Klebsiella, Enterobacter, Proteus*) associated with antibiotic treatment of acne
• Chronic irritation of the hair follicle (use of cocoa butter or coconut oil, chronic irritation from workplace)
• Initial use of systemic corticosteroid therapy (steroid acne), eosinophilic folliculitis (AIDS patients), *Candida albicans* (immunocompromised patients)
• *Pityrosporum orbiculare*

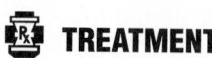

DIAGNOSIS

■ DIFFERENTIAL DIAGNOSIS
• Pseudofolliculitis barbae (ingrown hairs)
• Acne vulgaris
• Dermatophyte fungal infections
• Keratosis biliaris
• Cutaneous candidiasis
• Superficial fungal infections
• Miliaris

■ WORKUP
Physical examination and medical history (e.g., use of hot tub: "hot tub" folliculitis; adolescent patients who have started shaving: sycosis barbae; use of occlusive topical steroid therapy: *Staphylococcus* folliculitis).

■ LABORATORY TESTS
Gram stain is useful to identify the infective organisms in infectious folliculitis and to differentiate infectious folliculitis from noninfectious.

TREATMENT

■ NONPHARMACOLOGIC THERAPY
• Prevention of chemical or mechanical skin irritation
• Glycemic control in diabetics
• Proper chlorination of hot tubs and spas
• Shaving with a clean razor

■ ACUTE GENERAL Rx
• Cleansing of the area with chlorhexidine and application of saline compresses to involved area
• Application of 2% mupirocin ointment (Bactroban) for bacterial folliculitis affecting a limited area (e.g., sycosis barbae)
• Treatment of severe cases of *Pseudomonas* folliculitis with ciprofloxacin
• Treatment of *S. aureus* folliculitis with dicloxacillin 250 mg qid for 10 days

■ CHRONIC Rx
• Chronic nasal or perineal *S. aureus* carriers with frequent folliculitis can be treated with rifampin 300 mg bid for 5 days.
• Mupirocin (Bactroban ointment 2%) applied to nares bid is also effective for nasal carriers.

■ DISPOSITION
• Most cases of bacterial folliculitis resolve completely with proper treatment.
• Steroid folliculitis responds to discontinuation of steroids.

PEARLS & CONSIDERATIONS

■ COMMENTS
Patients should be instructed in good personal hygiene and avoidance of sharing razors, towels, and washcloths.
Author: **Fred F. Ferri, M.D.**

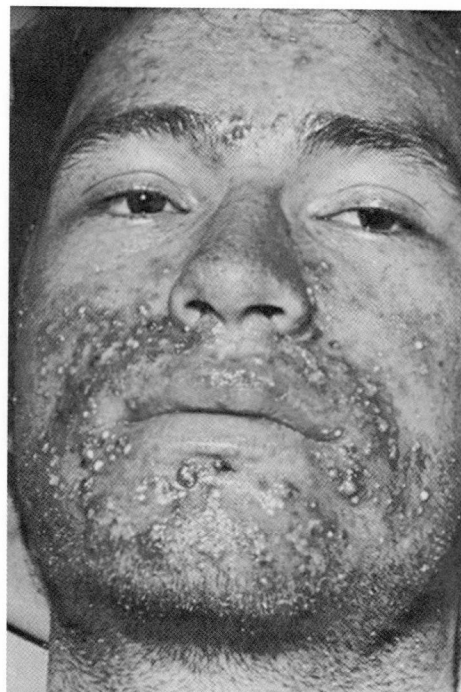

Fig. 1-116 Folliculitis. Note the pustular eruption with small abscess formation in the hair-bearing areas of the face. General symptoms are usually absent. (From Mandell GL: *Mandell, Douglas, and Bennett's principles and practice of infectious diseases,* ed 5, New York, 2000, Churchill Livingstone.)

BASIC INFORMATION

■ DEFINITION
Food poisoning is an illness caused by ingestion of food contaminated by bacteria and/or bacterial toxins.

ICD-9CM CODES
See specific illness.

■ EPIDEMIOLOGY & DEMOGRAPHICS
INCIDENCE (IN U.S.):
- Estimated range of 6 to 80 million cases/yr
- Majority of identifiable causes are bacterial

PREDOMINANT AGE: Varies with specific agent

PEAK INCIDENCE: Varies with specific organism
- Summer: *Staphylococcus aureus, Salmonella, Shigella*
- Summer and fall: *Clostridium botulinum, Vibrio parahaemolyticus*
- Spring and fall: *Campylobacter jejuni*
- Winter: *Clostridium perfringens, Yersinia*

NEONATAL INFECTION: Rare but severe with *Shigella*

■ PHYSICAL FINDINGS & CLINICAL PRESENTATION
- Any combination of GI symptoms and fever
- Specific organisms suspected on the basis of the incubation period and predominant symptoms, although a great deal of overlap exists
  1. Short incubation period (1 to 6 hr): involve the ingestion of pre-formed toxin; noninvasive
     a. *S. aureus:* nausea, profuse vomiting, and abdominal cramps common; diarrhea possible, but fever uncommon; usually resolves within 24 hr; foods implicated in outbreaks include meats, mayonnaise, and cream pastries
     b. *B. cereus:* two forms, a short incubation (emetic) form (characterized by vomiting and abdominal cramps in virtually all patients, diarrhea in one third of patients, fever uncommon) and a long incubation *(diarrheal)* form; illness usually mild, resolves within 12 hr; unrefrigerated rice most often implicated as vehicle
  2. Moderate incubation period (8 to 16 hr): involves the in vivo production of toxin; noninvasive
     a. *C. perfringens:* severe crampy abdominal pain and watery diarrhea common; fever and vomiting unlikely; symptoms usually resolving within 24 hr; outbreaks invariably related to cooked meat or poultry that is allowed to cool without refrigeration; most cases in the fall and winter months
     b. *B. cereus:* diarrheal (or long incubation) form most commonly beginning with diarrhea, abdominal cramps, and occasionally vomiting; fever uncommon; usually resolves within 24 hr; the responsible food is usually fried rice
  3. Long incubation period (>16 hr): some toxin-mediated, some invasive
     a. Toxin-producing organisms include:
        (1) *C. botulinum:* should be considered when a diarrheal illness coincides with or precedes paralysis; severity of illness related to the quantity of toxin ingested; characteristic cranial nerve palsies progressing to a descending paralysis; fever usually absent; usually associated with home-canned foods
        (2) Enterotoxigenic *E. coli* (ETEC): most common cause of travelers' diarrhea; after 1- to 2-day incubation period, abdominal cramps and copious diarrhea occur; vomiting and fever uncommon; usually resolves after 3 to 4 days; vehicle usually unbottled water or contaminated salad or ice
        (3) Enterohemorrhagic *E. coli* (EHEC): can cause severe abdominal cramps and watery diarrhea, which may eventually become bloody; bacteria (strain O157:H7) are noninvasive; no fever; illness may be complicated by hemolytic-uremic syndrome; associated with contaminated beef
        (4) *V. cholerae:* varies from a mild, self-limited illness to life-threatening cholera; diarrhea, nausea and vomiting, abdominal cramps, and muscle cramps; no fever; severe cases may progress to shock and death within hours of onset; survivors usually have resolution of symptoms in 1 wk; U.S. cases are either imported or result from ingestion of imported food
     b. Invasive organisms include:
        (1) *Salmonella:* associated most often with nonty-phoidal strains; incubation period generally 12 to 48 hr; nausea, vomiting, diarrhea, and abdominal cramps typical; fever possible; outbreaks of gastroenteritis related to contaminated poultry, meat, and dairy products
        (2) *Shigella:* asymptomatic infection possible, but some with fever and watery diarrhea that may progress to bloody diarrhea and dysentery; with mild illness, usually self-limited, resolves in a few days; with severe illness, may develop complications; transmission usually from person to person but can occur via contaminated food or water
        (3) *C. jejuni:* the most common food-borne bacterial pathogen; incubation period is about 1 day, then a prodrome of fever, headache, and myalgias; intestinal phase marked by diarrhea associated with fever, malaise, and abdominal pain; diarrhea mild to profuse and bloody; usually resolves in about 7 days, but relapse is possible; associated with undercooked meats and poultry, unpasteurized dairy products, and drinking from freshwater streams
        (4) *Y. enterocolitica* and *Y. pseudotuberculosis:* infrequent causes of enteritis in U.S.; children affected more often than adults; fever, diarrhea, and abdominal pain lasting 1 to 3 wk; some with mesenteric adenitis that mimics acute appendicitis; contaminated food or water is usually responsible
        (5) *V. parahaemolyticus:* In U.S., most outbreaks in coastal states or on cruise ships during the summer months; incubation period usually <1 day, followed by explosive watery diarrhea in the majority of cases; nausea, vomiting, abdominal cramps, and headache also common; fever less common; usually resolves by 1 wk; related to ingestion of seafood

(6) Enteroinvasive *E. coli* (EIEC): a rare cause of disease in the U.S.; high incidence of fever and bloody diarrhea; may resemble bacillary dysentery

(7) *V. vulnificus:* may cause serious, often fatal illness in persons with chronic liver disease; GI symptoms usually absent, but fever, chills, hypotension, and hemorrhagic skin lesions possible; patients with liver disease or at increased risk of developing liver disease should avoid eating raw oysters

■ ETIOLOGY
Classically categorized as either inflammatory (invasive) or noninflammatory:

- Noninflammatory: *B. cereus, S. aureus, C. botulinum, C. perfringens, V. cholerae,* enterotoxigenic *E. coli* (ETEC), and enterohemorrhagic *E. coli* (EHEC); toxin-producing organisms that are noninvasive; fecal leukocytes are not seen.
- Inflammatory: *Campylobacter,* enteroinvasive *E. coli* (EIEC), *Salmonella, Shigella, V. parahaemolyticus,* and *Yersinia;* cause disease by invasion of intestinal tissue; fecal leukocytes are seen.

🔬 DIAGNOSIS

■ DIFFERENTIAL DIAGNOSIS
Gastroenteritis caused by viruses (Norwalk or rotavirus), parasites *(Amoeba histolytica, Giardia lamblia),* or toxins (ciguatoxins, mushrooms, heavy metals)

■ LABORATORY TESTS
- Test stool for fecal leukocytes to help narrow the differential diagnosis:
  1. Send stool for culture and for ova and parasites.
  2. Send stool for *C. difficile* toxin in patients with current or recent antibiotic use.

3. NOTE: Some pathogens are not identified on routine stool culture; laboratory should be advised if *Yersinia, C. botulinum, Vibrio,* or enterohemorrhagic *E. coli* (O157:H7) are suspected.
4. Finding *B. cereus, C. perfringens,* or *E. coli* in stool is of little value, because these may be part of the normal bowel flora.
- If botulism suspected, send food, serum, and stool for toxin assay.
- Blood cultures are needed for all febrile patients.

💊 TREATMENT

■ NONPHARMACOLOGIC THERAPY
Adequate rehydration is the mainstay of therapy.

■ ACUTE GENERAL Rx
- Gastroenteritis caused by the following organisms requires no antimicrobial treatment: *B. cereus, S. aureus, C. perfringens, V. parahaemolyticus, Yersinia,* and enterohemorrhagic and enteroinvasive *E. coli.*
- The usual cause of traveler's diarrhea is enterotoxigenic *E. coli.* Although usually a self-limited illness, antibiotics can shorten the course.
  1. SMX/TMP one DS tab bid for 3 days
  2. Ciprofloxacin 500 mg PO bid for 3 days
- The mainstay of therapy for cholera is fluid replacement. Antibiotics should be given to decrease shedding and duration of illness.
  1. Doxycycline 100 mg PO bid for 3 days
  2. SMX/TMP one DS tab bid for 3 days
- Treatment is not indicated for *Salmonella* gastroenteritis. Patients who are at high risk of developing bacteremia may be treated for 48 to 72 hr (see "Salmonellosis").
- Although shigellosis tends to be a self-limited illness, antibiotics shorten the course of illness and may limit transmission of the illness (see "Shigellosis").

- Those with moderate or severe *Campylobacter* diarrhea may benefit from treatment.
  1. Erythromycin 500 mg PO qid for 5 days
  2. Ciprofloxacin 500 mg PO bid for 5 days
- *V. vulnificus* sepsis should be treated with:
  1. Doxycycline 100 mg IV bid for 2 wk
  2. Ceftazidime 2 g IV q8h for 2 wk
- For suspected botulism, antitoxin should be administered early (see "Botulism").

■ CHRONIC Rx
Patients with *Salmonella* infections may become carriers and may require treatment (see "Salmonellosis").

■ DISPOSITION
- Most infections are self-limited and do not require therapy.
- In immunocompromised host or patient with underlying disease, serious complications are possible.
- Postinfectious syndromes are important with some infections:
  1. Reiter's syndrome: *Salmonella, Shigella, Campylobacter, Yersinia;* more common in genetically susceptible host (HLA-B27+)
  2. Guillain-Barré syndrome: *Campylobacter*

■ REFERRAL
If more than a mild illness

🔆 PEARLS & CONSIDERATIONS

■ COMMENTS
- Grossly underreported and undiagnosed
- All cases to be reported to the local health department
- Table 2-74 compares incubation period, symptoms, and common vehicles for microbial causes of food poisoning.

REFERENCE
Centers for Disease Control and Prevention: Diagnosis and management of foodborne illnesses: a primer for physicians, *MMWR Recomm Rep* 50(RR-2):1, 2001.
Author: **Maurice Policar, M.D.**

BASIC INFORMATION

■ DEFINITION

Friedreich's ataxia is the most common neurodegenerative hereditary ataxic disorder, caused by degeneration of dorsal root ganglions, posterior columns, spinocerebellar and corticospinal tracts and large sensory peripheral neurons.

ICD-9CM CODES

334.0 Friedreich's ataxia

■ EPIDEMIOLOGY & DEMOGRAPHICS

INCIDENCE (IN U.S.): Not reported
PREVALENCE (IN U.S.): 2-4/100,000. Carrier rate 1:120-1:160. Lower prevalence in Asians and people of African descent.
PREDOMINANT SEX: Male = Female
PEAK INCIDENCE: 8 to 15 yr
GENETICS: Autosomal recessive; 96% of affected patients are homozygous, 4% compound heterozygous (2 different mutations)

■ PHYSICAL FINDINGS

- Onset of progressive appendicular and gait ataxia, with absent muscle stretch reflexes in the lower extremities
- With disease progression (within 5 yr): dysarthria, distal loss of position and vibration sense, pyramidal leg weakness, areflexia in all 4 limbs, extensor plantar responses
- Common findings: progressive scoliosis, distal atrophy, pes cavus, and cardiomyopathy (symmetric concentric hypertrophic form in most cases)
- Insulin-requiring diabetes mellitus may occur in 10% of patients, with glucose intolerance occurring in an additional 10%-20%

■ ETIOLOGY

- Genetic: Frataxin gene is localized to the centromeric region of chromosome 9q13.
- Normal sequence has 6-27 repeats; abnormal sequence has 120-1700 GAA repeats.
- Frataxin deficiency leads to impaired mitochondrial iron homeostasis.

DIAGNOSIS

■ DIFFERENTIAL DIAGNOSIS

- Charcot-Marie-Tooth disease type (in early cases)
- Abetalipoproteinemia (Bassen-Kornzweig syndrome)
- Severe vitamin E deficiency with malabsorption

- Early-onset cerebellar ataxia with retained reflexes
- Autosomal dominant cerebellar ataxia (Spinocerebellar ataxia)

■ WORKUP

- Diagnostic criteria include electrophysiological evidence for a generalized axonal sensory neuropathy
- Electrocardiogram (ECG) shows widespread T-wave inversion and evidence of left ventricular hypertrophy in 65% of patients
- Sural nerve biopsy shows major loss of large myelinated fibers
- Specific gene testing for the expanded GAA trinucleotide repeat

■ LABORATORY TESTS

- EMG/NCS
- ECG and echocardiogram.
- Peripheral blood smear for acanthocytes
- Lipid profile
- Glucose levels (fasting or 2 hr postprandial; consider glucose tolerance test if necessary)
- Vitamin E levels (if necessary)

■ IMAGING STUDIES

MRI of the spinal cord may demonstrate spinal cord atrophy with essentially normal cerebrum, brainstem, and cerebellum (Fig. 1-117).

TREATMENT

■ NONPHARMACOLOGIC THERAPY

- Surgical correction of scoliosis and foot deformities in selected patients
- Prosthetic devices as required (e.g., ankle-foot orthosis for foot drop)
- Physical therapy
- Communication devices for patients with severe dysarthria

■ ACUTE GENERAL Rx

None established.
An antioxidant, idebenone (short-chain analogue of coenzyme Q10) administered orally at 5mg/kg/day with or without vitamin E may improve outcomes in patients with cardiomyopathy without clinical deterioration. This is treatment is experimental and research may be reviewed on www.idebenone.org.

■ CHRONIC Rx

Chronic management of congestive heart failure required. Cardiac arrhythmias will warrant pacemaker implantation.

■ DISPOSITION

- Loss of ambulation typically occurs within 15 yr of symptom onset, and 95% are wheelchair bound by age 45 yr.
- Life expectancy is reduced, particularly if heart disease with/without diabetes mellitus is present.

■ REFERRAL

- If uncertain about diagnosis
- For genetic counseling (recommended if available)

REFERENCE

Alper G, Narayanan V: Friedreich's ataxia, *Pediatr Neurol* 28:335, 2003.
Author: **Eroboghene E. Ubogu, M.D.**

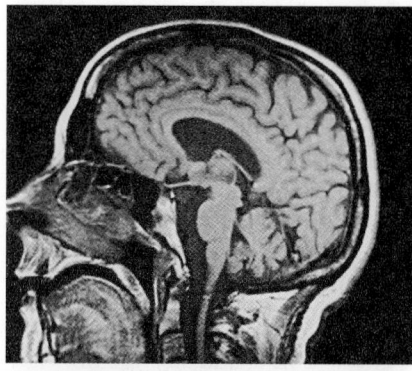

A

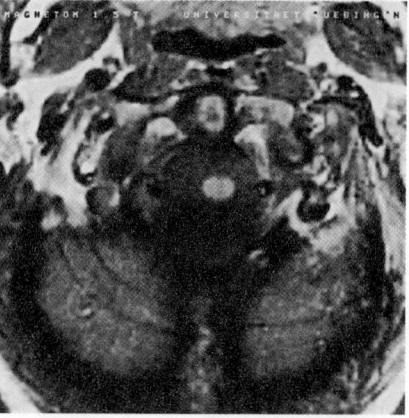

B

Fig. 1-117 T1-weighted MRIs of the brain and cervical spinal cord in Friedreich's ataxia. The images are, **A,** midsagittal plane of the head and, **B,** an axial slice at the level of the dens axis. There is severe shrinkage of the cervical spinal cord. In contrast, the cerebellum and brainstem are of normal size. (From Goetz CG: *Textbook of clinical neurology,* Philadelphia, 1999, WB Saunders.)

BASIC INFORMATION

■ DEFINITION

Frostbite represents tissue injury (or death) from freezing and vasoconstriction induced by severe environmental cold exposure.

■ SYNONYMS

Cold-induced tissue injury

ICD-9CM CODES

991.3 Frostbite

■ EPIDEMIOLOGY & DEMOGRAPHICS

- Environmental factors include wind chill factor, temperature, duration of exposure, altitude, and degree of wetness.
- Host factors include immobility, history of cold injuries, lack of acclimatization, skin damage, psychiatric illness, preexisting CNS or cardiovascular disease, diabetes, malnutrition, tobacco use, sedative drugs (especially alcohol), fatigue, hypothyroidism, anemia, and perhaps race (African Americans may be more susceptible).

■ PHYSICAL FINDINGS & CLINICAL PRESENTATION

- Frostbite may be classified into degrees of injury or, more practically, into *superficial* and *deep* groups.
- *Superficial* frostbite involves the skin and subcutaneous tissue. The frozen part is waxy, white, and firm but soft and resilient below the surface when gently depressed. After rewarming, the frostbitten area may appear mottled and swollen, and superficial blisters with clear or milky fluid may form within 6 to 24 hr (Fig.1-118). There is no ultimate tissue loss.
- *Deep* frostbite extends into subcutaneous tissues and may involve muscles, nerves, tendons, or bones. The skin may be hard or wooden, without tissue resilience. Edema, cyanosis, hemorrhagic bullae (after 3 to 7 days), tissue necrosis, and gangrene may develop. Affected tissue has a poor prognosis.
- Patients initially experience numbness, prickling, and itching. More severe injury can produce paresthesias, stiffness, and burning or throbbing pain on thawing.
- Severity of frostbite injury appears to correlate with duration of exposure, rather than with ambient temperature.

DIAGNOSIS

- Diagnosis is clinically based on the appropriate environmental conditions.
- Other locally induced cold injuries include:
  Pernio (chilblains): cold-induced vasculitis of dermal vessels often affecting dorsum of hands and feet and seen with repeated cold exposure.
  Cold immersion (trench) foot: caused by ischemic injury resulting from sustained severe vasoconstriction in cold-immersed appendage.

■ WORKUP

- CBC
- Wound and blood cultures in more severe cases
- Technetium scintigraphy, MRI, and MRA appear to be the most promising modalities for assessment of tissue viability, but a delay of 2 to 3 wk is generally required to reliably distinguish a level of debridement or amputation

TREATMENT

■ NONPHARMACOLOGIC THERAPY

- Remove constricting or wet clothing and gently insulate and immobilize the affected area.
- Avoid thawing if there is any risk of refreezing.
- Never rub or massage the affected area, and avoid dry heat.
- If there is associated hypothermia, core temperature must first be stabilized with warmed, humidified oxy-

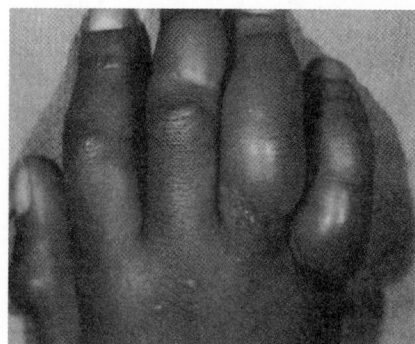

Fig. 1-118 Large, clear frostbite blisters on the right hand. (From Rosen P [ed]: *Emergency medicine,* ed 4, St Louis, 1998, Mosby.)

gen, heated IV saline (45° to 65° C), and warming blankets.

■ ACUTE GENERAL Rx

- Immerse affected area in circulating warm water that is 40° to 42° C for 15 to 30 min
- Parenteral narcotics are often required for pain control
- Topical aloe vera (Dermaide) q6h (thromboxane inhibitor)
- Td prophylaxis
- Streptococcal prophylaxis for 48 to 72 hr with IV penicillin for severe cases
- Limb elevation to minimize edema
- Sterile dressing

■ POST-THAW Rx

- Ibuprofen 400 mg bid to tid (inhibits coagulation cascade and produces fibrinolysis)
- Blister management is controversial. Debride broken clear vesicles and leave hemorrhagic vesicles intact
- Whirlpool hydrotherapy with an antiseptic for 20 to 30 min bid to tid for several weeks
- Gentle, progressive physical therapy after edema resolves
- Avoid all vasoconstrictors, including nicotine

■ DISPOSITION

Long-term residual symptoms including neuropathic pain, sensory deficits, hyperhidrosis, secondary Raynaud's disease, edema, hair or nail deformities, and arthritis occur in 65% of patients.

■ REFERRAL

- Hospitalize if patient has systemic hypothermia or more than superficial frostbite.
- Surgical decisions regarding amputation should be deferred until there is clear demarcation of viable tissue (may take months) unless refractory pain, sepsis, or supervening gangrene occurs.

REFERENCES

Danzl D: Frostbite. In Rosen P (ed): *Emergency medicine: concepts and clinical practice,* vol 1, ed 5, St Louis, 2002, Mosby.

Kare JA, Shneiderman A: Hyperthermia and hypothermia in the older population, *Top Emerg Med* 23(3):39, 2001.

Murphy JV et al: Frostbite: pathogenesis and treatment, *J Trauma Inj Infect & Crit Care,* 48(1):171, 2000.

Reamy B: Frostbite: review and current concepts, *J Am Board Fam Pract* 11(1):341, 1998.

Author: **Michael P. Johnson, M.D.**

I

BASIC INFORMATION

■ DEFINITION
Frozen shoulder is a condition unique to the shoulder and characterized by pain and restricted passive and active range of motion (Fig. 1-119).

■ SYNONYMS
Adhesive capsulitis
Periarthritis
Pericapsulitis
Check-rein shoulder

ICD-9CM CODES
726.0 Adhesive shoulder capsulitis

■ EPIDEMIOLOGY & DEMOGRAPHICS
PREVALENT AGE: Over 40 yr
PREVALENT SEX: Females > males

■ PHYSICAL FINDINGS & CLINICAL PRESENTATION
- Arm held protectively at the side with apprehension caused by pain
- Varying degrees of deltoid and spinatus atrophy
- Generalized shoulder tenderness
- Restricted active and passive shoulder motion of varying degrees

■ ETIOLOGY
- Unknown
- Fig. 1-119 illustrates the sequence of events terminating in frozen shoulder

DIAGNOSIS

■ DIFFERENTIAL DIAGNOSIS
- Secondary causes of shoulder stiffness (prolonged immobilization following trauma or surgery)
- Posterior shoulder dislocation
- Ruptured rotator cuff
- Glenohumeral osteoarthritis
- Rotator cuff inflammation
- Superior sulcus tumor
- Cervical disk disease
- Brachial neuritis

■ WORKUP
Laboratory and radiographic studies are generally normal.

TREATMENT

■ NONPHARMACOLOGIC THERAPY
Prevention is important. Shoulder motion should be maintained during those periods when the patient may be inactive as a result of illness or injury.

■ ACUTE GENERAL Rx
- Moist heat, sedation, and analgesics as needed
- A local steroid/lidocaine mixture injected into the subacromial space and joint (Table 1-21)
- Home exercise program
- Manipulation of shoulder under anesthesia (rarely needed)

■ DISPOSITION
- The initial stage of pain followed by stiffness may last several months; recovery phase may also last several months; complete recovery is usually the case.
- Recurrence in the same shoulder is rare, although the opposite limb may develop the same symptoms.
- Some patients have mild residual loss of movement but without any significant functional impairment.

■ REFERRAL
Orthopedic consultation in patients with resistant disease

PEARLS & CONSIDERATIONS

■ COMMENTS
- "Capsulitis" with an inflammatory infiltrate is not consistently found pathologically.
- Frozen shoulder is increased in patients with diabetes, thyroid disease, and recent cardiopulmonary conditions.
- Some cases present with findings of reflex sympathetic dystrophy.

REFERENCES
Griggs SM, Ahn A, Green A: Idiopathic adhesive capsulitis: a prospective functional outcome study of nonoperative treatment, *J Bone Joint Surg* 82A:1398, 2000.
Kivimaki J, Pohjolainen T: Manipulation for frozen shoulder with and without steroid injection, *Arch Phys Med Rehabil* 82:1188, 2001.
Tuten HR, Young DC et al: Adhesive capsulitis of the shoulder in male cardiac surgery patients, *Orthopedics* 23:693, 2000.
Wolf JM, Green A: Influence of comorbidity on self-assessment instrument scores of patients with idiopathic adhesive capsulitis, *J Bone Joint Surg* 84(A):1167, 2002.
Author: **Lonnie R. Mercier, M.D.**

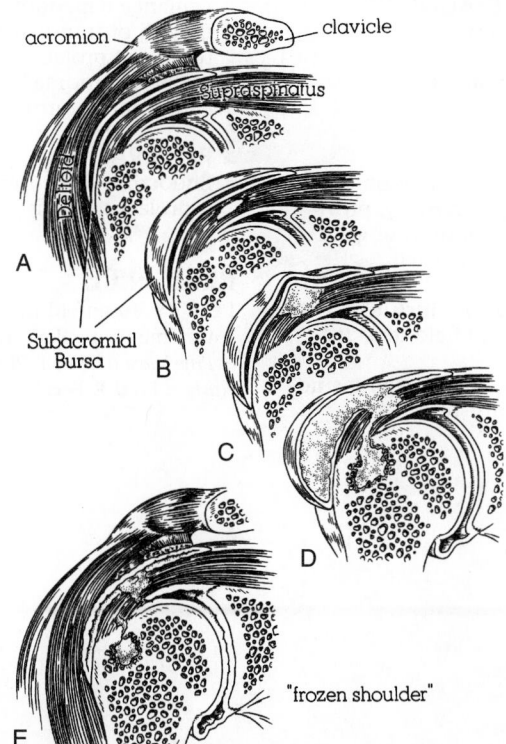

Fig. 1-119   **Sequence of events terminating in frozen shoulder. A,** Normal structures of the shoulder. **B,** Supraspinatus tendonitis, sometimes calcific, in the "critical zone." **C,** Spread of inflammation to the tendon sheath and a bulge into the floor of the subacromial bursa. **D,** Rupture into the subacromial bursa and extension of the inflammatory process as an osteitis into the humeral head and greater tuberosity. **E,** Frozen shoulder with involvement of tendons, bursa, capsule, synovium, and muscle with fibrous contracture and markedly diminished volume of the shoulder joint space. (From Noble J [ed]: *Primary care medicine,* ed 2, St Louis, 1996, Mosby.)

BASIC INFORMATION

■ DEFINITION

Galactorrhea can be defined as inappropriate lactation (in absence of pregnancy and postpartum state) secondary to nonphysiologic augmentation of prolactin release.

ICD-CM CODES

611.6 Galactorrhea

■ PHYSICAL FINDINGS AND CLINICAL PRESENTATION

- Milky discharge from nipples usually occurring bilaterally
- Evidence of chest wall irritation from ill-fitting clothing, herpes zoster, or atopic dermatitis may be present
- Visual field defects may be present with prolactinomas
- Evidence of acromegaly, Cushing's disease, or hypothyroidism when galactorrhea is secondary to these disorders

■ ETIOLOGY

- Medications (phenothiazines, metoclopramide, SSRIs, anxiolytics, buspirone, atenolol, valproic acid, conjugated estrogen and medroxyprogesterone, methyldopa, verapamil, H2 receptor blockers, octreotide, danazol, tricyclics, isoniazid, amphetamine, reserpine, opiates, sumatriptan, rimantadine, oral contraceptive formulations)
- Breast stimulation (prolonged suckling), sexual intercourse
- Pituitary tumors (prolactinomas, craniopharyngiomas
- Chest wall irritation from ill-fitting clothing, herpes zoster, atopic dermatitis, burns
- Hypothyroidism (elevated TSH increases TRH, which increases prolactin)
- Increased stress, major trauma

- Chronic renal failure (decreased prolactin clearance)
- Cushing's disease
- Herbs (e.g. fennel, red clover, anise, red raspberry, marshmallow)
- Cannabis
- Spinal cord surgery or injury, or tumors
- Severe GERD, esophagitis (stimulation of thoracic nerves via cervical and thoracic ganglia)
- Breast surgery
- Idiopathic
- Neonatal ("witch's milk" produced by 2%-5% of neonates because of precipitous drop in maternal estrogen and progesterone postdelivery)
- Lymphomas, Hodgkin's disease, bronchogenic carcinoma, renal adenocarcinomas
- Sarcoidosis and other infiltrative disorders
- Tuberculosis affecting pituitary gland
- Pituitary stalk resection
- Multiple sclerosis
- Empty sella syndrome
- Acromegaly

DIAGNOSIS

■ DIFFERENTIAL DIAGNOSIS

- Intraductal papilloma
- Breast cancer
- Paget's disease of breast
- Breast abscess

■ WORKUP

- Complete history focusing on menstrual irregularity, infertility, previous pregnancies, duration of galactorrhea, medications, visual complaints, fatigue
- Physical examination: hirsutism, acne, obesity, visual field defects, goiter
- Laboratory testing and imaging studies (see "Laboratory Tests")

■ LABORATORY TESTS

- Prolactin level (elevated, usually >200 ng/ml in prolactinoma)
- Human chorionic gonadotropin level (positive in pregnancy)
- TSH, TRH (both elevated in hypothyroidism)
- BUN, creatinine (elevated in renal failure), glucose (elevated in Cushing's syndrome)
- Urinalysis (hematuria in renal cell carcinoma)
- Microscopic examination of nipple discharge (scant cellular material, numerous fat globules)

■ IMAGING STUDIES

- MRI of brain if prolactin level is elevated, amenorrhea is present or visual fields defects are detected on physical examination

 TREATMENT

- Discontinuation of potential offending agents
- Avoidance of excessive breast stimulation
- Galactorrhea resulting from prolactinoma can be managed medically, surgically, or with careful surveillance depending on size and growth of tumor, associated symptoms and prolactin level. Please refer to "Prolactinoma" in Section I for additional information

■ REFERRAL

- Endocrine and surgical consultation if prolactinoma is detected

REFERENCE

Pena KS, Rosenfeld JA: Evaluation and treatment of galactorrhea, *Am Fam Physician* 63:1763, 2001.
Author: **Fred F. Ferri, M.D.**

BASIC INFORMATION

■ DEFINITION
Ganglia are cystic structures thought to derive from a tendon sheath or joint capsule.

■ ICD-9CM CODES
727.43 Ganglion

■ EPIDEMIOLOGY & DEMOGRAPHICS
- Ganglia are more common in women than men (3:1)
- Can occur at any age but usually occurs between second and fourth decades of life
- Most common soft tissue tumor of the hand and wrist

■ PHYSICAL FINDINGS & CLINICAL PRESENTATION
- Most ganglia occur on the dorsum of the wrist (50% to 70%) (Fig. 1-120).
- Volar wrist (18% to 20%) is the next most common site.
- Ganglia can also involve the proximal digital flexor tendons and the distal interphalangeal joints.
- Left and right hands are equally affected.
- Ganglia are usually solitary, firm, smooth, round, and fluctuant.
- Pain from mass effect or compression up against nearby structure may be present (e.g., median nerve and radial nerve).
- Hand numbness may be present.
- Patient may experience hand muscle weakness.
- Ganglia usually develop over a period of months but may arise suddenly.

■ ETIOLOGY
- Ganglia are thought to derive from synovial herniation or expansion from the joint capsule or tendon sheath.

DIAGNOSIS

Direct inspection and localization of the cyst often is enough to make the diagnosis of ganglia.

■ DIFFERENTIAL DIAGNOSIS
- Lipoma
- Fibroma
- Epidermoid inclusion cyst
- Osteochondroma
- Hemangioma
- Infection (tuberculosis, fungi, and secondary syphilis)
- Gout
- Rheumatoid nodule
- Radial artery aneurysm

■ WORKUP
The workup of ganglia usually consists of history, physical examination, and x-ray imaging.

■ LABORATORY TESTS
Blood tests are not specific in the diagnosis of ganglia.

■ IMAGING STUDIES
- X-ray of the hand and wrist is done to rule out other bone or joint abnormalities.
- Ultrasound studies are helpful in the diagnosis of ganglia, demonstrating smooth cystic walls that may be septated.
- CT scan can be done if the ultrasound is equivocal.
- MRI although not done often for the diagnosis of ganglia aids in differentiating malignant bone lesions from cystic structures.
- Arthrography may demonstrate a communication between the joint and ganglia (not commonly done).

TREATMENT

Treatment is indicated for pain, muscle weakness, and cosmetic purposes.

■ NONPHARMACOLOGIC THERAPY
- Attempts to rupture the cyst by sharp blows with a book or with finger compression.
- Aspiration, heat, and sclerotherapy have been tried but met with high recurrence rates (60%).

■ ACUTE GENERAL Rx
- Aspiration with a large-bore needle (18-gauge) followed by injection of 20 to 40 mg of triamcinolone acetonide can be tried.
- This may be repeated if the ganglia recurs (35% to 40%).

■ CHRONIC Rx
Total ganglionectomy is the surgical procedure of choice.

■ DISPOSITION
- Ganglia spontaneously resolve in approximately 40% to 50% of cases.
- Aspiration with steroid injection is successful in approximately 65% of cases.
- Surgery provides cure in 85% to 95% of the cases.
- Complications of ganglia include:
  1. Carpal tunnel syndrome with pain and muscle atrophy
  2. Radial nerve impingement
  3. Radial artery compression
- Complications of ganglion surgery include:
  1. Infection
  2. Recurrence (5% to 15%) usually secondary to inadequate excision
  3. Reflex sympathetic dystrophy
  4. Scar formation

■ REFERRAL
It is best to refer patients with symptomatic ganglia to a hand surgeon.

PEARLS & CONSIDERATIONS

■ COMMENTS
- Ganglia synovial membrane maintains its secretory function. Aspiration of ganglia often demonstrates a viscous, mucinous clear fluid containing albumin, globulin, and hyaluronic acid.
- Dorsal ganglia usually originate from the scapholunate ligament.
- Volar ganglia typically originate between the tendons of the flexor carpi radialis and brachioradialis.

REFERENCES
Ho PC et al: Current treatment of ganglion of the wrist, *Hand Surg* 6(1):49, 2001.

Thornburg LE: Ganglions of the hand and wrist, *J Am Acad Orthop Surg* 7(4):231, 1999.

Wang AA, Hutchinson DT: Longitudinal observation of pediatric hand and wrist ganglia, *J Hand Surg* 26(4):599, 2001.

Author: **Peter Petropoulos, M.D.**

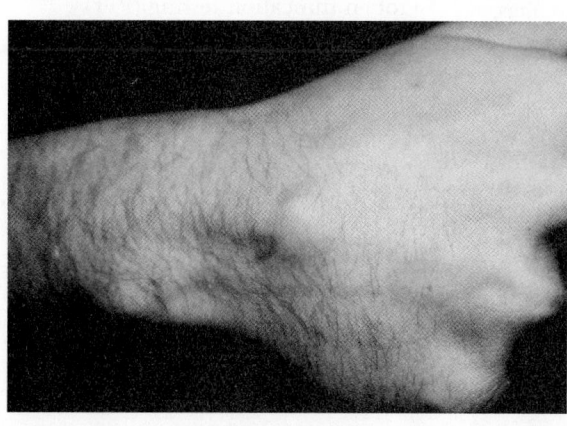

Fig. 1-120 Round and firm ganglion cyst bulging from the dorsal aspect of the hand. (From Kelly WN: *Textbook of rheumatology,* ed 5, Philadelphia, 1997, WB Saunders.)

BASIC INFORMATION

■ DEFINITION
Gardner's syndrome is a variant of familial adenomatous polyposis (FAP), with prominent extraintestinal manifestations. It is an autosomal dominant condition characterized by:
- Adenomatous intestinal polyps
- Soft-tissue tumors
- Osteomas

ICD-9CM CODES
211.3 Gardner's syndrome

■ EPIDEMIOLOGY & DEMOGRAPHICS
- FAP accounts for less than 1% of all colorectal cancers.
- The entire GI tract may have polyps, but the malignant potential is highest in the colon. Individuals with Gardner's syndrome develop hundreds to thousands of colorectal adenomatous polyps.
- Polyps occur at a mean age of 16 yr.
- Cancer develops in 7% of individuals by age 21 yr, 50% by age 39 yr, and 90% by age 45 yr. There is 100% chance of developing colorectal cancer.
- Individuals with Gardner's syndrome are at increased risk for other cancers: about 10% develop desmoid tumors and 10% develop duodenal periampullary cancer. Risk for brain (medulloblastoma), thyroid, childhood hepatoblastoma, and pancreatic cancer is also increased.

■ CLINICAL PRESENTATION
There is phenotypic variability even in individuals and families with the same mutation.
Soft tissue and bone abnormalities may precede intestinal disease.
- Congenital hypertrophy of the retinal pigment epithelium (often the first sign of the syndrome) is diagnosed by ophthalmologic examination
- Dental abnormalities: supernumerary teeth, unerupted teeth
- Soft tissue lesions: epidermoid cysts, sebaceous cysts, fibromas, lipomas, desmoid tumors
- Bony abnormalities of skull, mandible and long bones
- Abdominal mass, occult blood in stool

■ ETIOLOGY
- Gardner's syndrome is caused by mutations of the adenomatous polyposis coli (APC) gene on chromosome 5q21. More than 300 mutations of the APC gene have been identified that result in FAP. The site of the mutation may explain the prominent extraintestinal lesions that differentiate Gardner's syndrome from other variants of FAP.
- Spontaneous mutations are responsible for 20%-30% of FAP cases.

DIAGNOSIS
In individuals with a family history, diagnosis is confirmed by >100 adenomatous polyps in the colon, >3 pigmented ocular lesions on fundoscopic examination, or genetic testing.

■ DIFFERENTIAL DIAGNOSIS
- FAP
- Turcot's syndrome
- Attenuated adenomatous polyposis coli
- Peutz-Jeghers syndrome
- Juvenile polyposis
- MYH polyposis

■ WORKUP
History, physical examination, laboratory tests, imaging studies

■ LABORATORY TESTS
Genetic tests for APC gene mutations:
- Protein truncation testing (an in vitro synthesized protein assay on patient's blood)
NOTE: Genetic counseling should be performed and written informed consent obtained before genetic testing.

■ IMAGING STUDIES
Sigmoidoscopy, upper endoscopy

■ SCREENING
Screening should be offered to first-degree relatives of affected individuals >10 yr of age and individuals with >100 colorectal adenomas.
GENETIC TESTS:
Protein truncation testing (PTT)
- Able to identify a mutation in 80% of families with FAP. To ensure that the mutation affecting the family is identifiable, a family member known to have FAP should be tested first.

- If the test is positive in the affected individual, other family members can be screened and the test can differentiate with 100% accuracy affected and unaffected family members. If the family member with disease tests negative, screening family members will not be useful in determining disease status (because the pedigree represents the 20% of families whose mutation is not detected with PTT).
- If there is no known family member with the disorder, screening the individual in question is reasonable. A positive test rules in the condition, but a negative test does not rule it out.
- Other genetic tests (sequencing, linkage, single-strand conformation polymorphism testing) can be considered if PTT is not informative.
CONGENITAL HYPERTROPHY OF THE RETINAL PIGMENT EPITHELIUM (CHRPE): CHRPE lesions occur in some families and are a reliable indicator of affected status in these families.
SIGMOIDOSCOPY
- Sigmoidoscopy surveillance is sufficient to determine if the patient is expressing the syndrome.
- Pedigrees with an identified APC mutation: positive genetic tests: annual sigmoidoscopy beginning at age 12 yr; negative genetic test: sigmoidoscopy at age 25 yr.
- Pedigrees with an unidentified APC mutation: family members should have annual sigmoidoscopy starting at age 12 yr; every 2 yr starting at age 25 yr; every 3 yr starting at age 35 yr; and then per age-appropriate guidelines starting at age 50.
UPPER GASTROINTESTINAL ENDOSCOPY (INCLUDING VISUALIZATION OF THE AMPULLA OF VATER): Screening for gastric and duodenal polyps should begin once colonic polyps are detected and continue every 2 to 4 yr. If polyps are present in the UGI track, screening should occur yearly.
HEPATOBLASTOMA: It is suggested that children of affected parents be screened annually (from infancy to 7 yr of age) with alpha-fetoprotein levels and ultrasound imaging of the liver.
ANNUAL PHYSICAL EXAM: Examine for extraintestinal lesions (thyroid nodule, abdominal mass, etc.)

TREATMENT

- Colectomy is recommended once polyps are seen on sigmoidoscopy.
- Regular screening of remaining GI tract and extraintestinal manifestations must continue after colectomy.
- Treat other complications and cancers.

■ **DISPOSITION**

There is a 100% chance of colorectal cancer in untreated individuals. Many other neoplasms occur at higher rates.

■ **REFERRAL**

- GI for sigmoidoscopy
- Surgery for prophylactic colectomy at detection of polyps
- Genetic counseling

PEARLS & CONSIDERATIONS

- Sulindac (nonselective NSAID) and celecoxib (cox-2 inhibitor) have been found to cause polyp regression in individuals with FAP. Celecoxib is FDA approved for this indication. Whether cancer risk is changed is not clear. Neither replaces colon resection for cancer prevention.
- Desmoid tumors have been induced and promoted by surgical procedures and OCP use.

REFERENCES

Cruz-Correa M, Giardiello FM: Diagnosis and management of hereditary colon cancer, *Gastroenterol Clin North Am* 31(2):537, 2002.

Giardiello FM, Brensinger JD, Petersen GM: American Gastroenterologic Association Practice Guidelines: AGA technical review on hereditary colorectal cancer and genetic testing, *Gastroenterology* 121(1):198, 2001.

Author: **Sudeep K. Aulakh, M.D., F.R.C.P.C.**

BASIC INFORMATION

■ DEFINITION
Gastric cancer is an adenocarcinoma arising from the stomach.

■ SYNONYMS
Stomach cancer
Linitis plastica

ICD-9CM CODES
451 Malignant neoplasm of stomach

■ EPIDEMIOLOGY & DEMOGRAPHICS
- Annual incidence of gastric cancer in the U.S. is 7 cases/100,000 persons. The incidence is much higher in Japan, with rates as high as 80 cases/100,000 persons.
- Most gastric cancers arise in the antrum (35%).
- The incidence of proximal tumors of the cardia and fundus is on the rise.
- Gastric cancer occurs most commonly in male patients >65 yr (70% of patients are >50 yr).
- Incidence of gastric cancer has been declining over the past 30 yr.
- Male:female ratio is 3:2.
- Familiar diffuse gastric cancer is a disease with autosomal dominant inheritance in which gastric cancer develops at a young age. Germ-line truncating mutations in the E-cadherin gene (CDH1) is found in these families.

■ PHYSICAL FINDINGS & CLINICAL PRESENTATION
- Medical history may reveal complaints of postprandial fullness with significant weight loss (70% to 80%), nausea/emesis (20% to 40%), dysphagia (20%), and dyspepsia, usually unrelieved by antacids; epigastric discomfort, usually lessened by fasting and exacerbated by food intake, is also common.
- Epigastric or abdominal mass (30% to 50%), epigastric pain.
- Skin pallor secondary to anemia.
- Hard, nodular liver: generally indicates metastatic disease to the liver.
- Hemoccult-positive stools.
- Ascites, lymphadenopathy, or pleural effusions: may indicate metastasis.

■ ETIOLOGY
Risk factors:
- Chronic *H. pylori* gastritis. Gastric cancer develops in persons infected with *H. pylori* but not in uninfected persons. Those with histologic find-

ings of severe gastric atrophy, corpus-predominant gastritis, or intestinal metaplasia are at increased risk. Persons with *H. pylori* infection and duodenal ulcer are not at risk, whereas those with gastric ulcers, nonulcer dyspepsia, and gastric hyperplastic polyps are.
- Tobacco abuse, alcohol consumption
- Food additives (nitrosamines), smoked foods, occupational exposure to heavy metals, rubber, asbestos
- Chronic atrophic gastritis with intestinal metaplasia, hypertrophic gastritis, and pernicious anemia

DIAGNOSIS

■ DIFFERENTIAL DIAGNOSIS
- Gastric lymphoma (5% of gastric malignancies)
- Hypertrophic gastritis
- Peptic ulcer
- Reflux esophagitis

■ WORKUP
Upper endoscopy with biopsy will confirm diagnosis.

■ LABORATORY TESTS
- Microcytic anemia
- Hemoccult-positive stools
- Hypoalbuminemia
- Abnormal liver enzymes in patients with metastasis to the liver
- Mutation-specific predictive genetic testing by PCR amplification followed by restriction—enzyme digestion and DNA sequencing for truncating mutations in the E-cadherin gene (CDH1) is recommended in families of patients with familiar diffuse cancer because gastric cancer develops in three of every four carriers of a mutant CDH1 gene.

■ IMAGING STUDIES
- Upper GI series with air contrast (90% accurate) if endoscopy is not readily available
- Abdominal CT scan to evaluate for metastasis (70% accurate for regional node metastases)

TREATMENT

■ ACUTE GENERAL Rx
- Gastrectomy is performed in patients with curative potential (<30% of patients at time of diagnosis).
- Palliative resection may prolong duration and quality of life.

- Chemotherapy (FAM: 5-fluorouracil, Adriamycin, and mitomycin C) may provide some palliation; however, it generally does not prolong survival.
- Postoperative chemoradiotherapy should be considered for all patients at high risk for recurrence of adenocarcinoma of the stomach or gastroesophageal junction who have undergone curative resection.
- Postoperative chemotherapy and radiotherapy, compared with surgical resection alone, can extend the survival of patients with gastric cancer in those who are able to complete adjuvant therapy.

■ DISPOSITION
- 5-yr survival rate of gastric carcinoma is 12% overall.
- 5-yr survival for early gastric cancers (usually detected incidentally with endoscopy in populations where screening is recommended) is >35%.

■ REFERRAL
Surgical referral for resection

PEARLS & CONSIDERATIONS

■ COMMENTS
- Gastrectomy patients will need vitamin B_{12} replacement. They are also at risk for dumping syndrome and should be advised to ingest frequent, small meals.
- Prophylactic gastrectomy should be considered in young asymptomatic carriers of germ-line truncating CDH1 mutations who belong to families with highly penetrant heredity diffuse gastric cancer.

REFERENCES
Huntsman DE et al: Early gastric cancer in young, asymptomatic carriers of germ-line E-cadherin mutations, *N Engl J Med* 344:1906, 2001.
Macdonald JS et al: Chemoradiotherapy after surgery compared with surgery alone for adenocarcinoma of the stomach or gastroesophageal junction, *N Engl J Med* 345:725, 2001.
Vemura N et al: *Helicobacter pylori* infection and the development of gastric cancer, *N Engl J Med* 345:784, 2001.
Wong BC et al: H. pylori eradication to prevent gastric cancer in a high-risk region of China, *JAMA* 291:187, 2004.
Author: **Fred F. Ferri, M.D.**

BASIC INFORMATION

■ DEFINITION

Histologically, gastritis refers to inflammation in the stomach.
Endoscopically, "gastritis" refers to a number of abnormal features such as erythema, erosions, and subepithelial hemorrhages. Gastritis can also be subdivided into erosive, nonerosive, and specific types of gastritis with distinctive features both endoscopically and histologically.

■ SYNONYMS

Erosive gastritis
Hemorrhagic gastritis
Helicobacter pylori gastritis

ICD-9CM CODES

535.5 Gastritis (unless otherwise specified)
535.0 Gastritis, acute
535.3 Alcoholic gastritis
535.1 Atrophic (chronic) gastritis
535.4 Erosive gastritis
535.2 Hypertrophic gastritis

■ EPIDEMIOLOGY & DEMOGRAPHICS

- Erosive and hemorrhagic gastritis are most commonly seen in patients taking NSAIDs, alcoholics, and critically ill patients (usually on ventilator support).
- *H. pylori* infection with gastritis is believed to be present in 30% to 50% of the population; however, the majority are asymptomatic.
- The prevalence of *H. pylori* infection increases with age from <10% in Caucasians <40 yr old to >50% in patients >50 yr.

■ PHYSICAL FINDINGS & CLINICAL PRESENTATION

- Patients with gastritis generally present with nonspecific clinical signs and symptoms (e.g., epigastric pain, abdominal tenderness, bloating, anorexia, nausea [with or without vomiting]). Symptoms may be aggravated by eating.
- Epigastric tenderness in acute alcoholic gastritis (may be absent in chronic gastritis).
- Foul-smelling breath.
- Hematemesis ("coffee-ground" emesis).

■ ETIOLOGY

- Alcohol, NSAIDs, stress (critically ill patients usually on mechanical respiration), hepatic or renal failure, multiorgan failure
- Infection (bacterial, viral)
- Bile reflux, pancreatic enzyme reflux
- Gastric mucosal atrophy, portal hypertension gastropathy
- Irradiation

DIAGNOSIS

■ DIFFERENTIAL DIAGNOSIS

- Peptic ulcer disease
- GERD
- Nonulcer dyspepsia
- Gastric lymphoma or carcinoma
- Pancreatitis
- Gastroparesis

■ WORKUP

Diagnostic workup includes a comprehensive history and endoscopy with biopsy.

■ LABORATORY TESTS

- Serologic (IgG antibody to *H. pylori*) or breath test (^{13}C urea breath tests) for *H. pylori*; patients should not receive proton pump inhibitors for 2 wk before undergoing urea breath test for *H. pylori* infection. Serum antibody tests are not reliable because of a high rate of false-positive results and the fact that antibodies persist even after treatment. The urea breath test is more sensitive and specific; however, it is not readily available. Histologic evaluation of endoscopic biopsy samples is currently the gold standard for accurate diagnosis of *H. pylori* infection.
- Stool antigen test for *H. pylori* is useful to confirm successful eradication of *H. pylori* following treatment.
- Vitamin B_{12} level in patients with atrophic gastritis.
- Hct (low if significant bleeding has occurred).

■ IMAGING STUDIES

Upper GI series is generally insensitive for the detection of gastritis. Gastroscopy with biopsy is the gold standard diagnostic test and will also detect *H. pylori*.

TREATMENT

■ NONPHARMACOLOGIC THERAPY

- Avoidance of mucosal irritants such as alcohol and NSAIDs
- Lifestyle modifications with avoidance of tobacco and foods that trigger symptoms

■ ACUTE GENERAL Rx

- Eradication of infectious agents: *H. pylori* therapy with
  1. Proton pump inhibitors (PPI) bid (e.g., omeprazole 20 mg bid or lansoprazole 30 mg bid) *plus* clarithromycin 500 mg bid *and* amoxicillin 1000 mg bid for 7 to 10 days
  2. PPI bid *plus* amoxicillin 500 mg bid *plus* metronidazole 500 mg for 7 to 10 days
  3. PPI bid *plus* clarithromycin 500 mg bid *and* metronidazole 500 mg bid for 7 days
  4. Recent trials indicate that a 1-day quadruple therapy may be as effective as a 7-day triple therapy regimen. The 1-day quadruple therapy regimen consists of two tablets of 262 mg bismouth subsalicylate qid, one 500-mg metronidazole tablet qid, 2 grams of amoxicillin suspension qid, and two capsules of 30 mg of lansoprazole.
  5. Bismouth compound qid *plus* tetracycline 500 mg qid *and* metronidazole 500 mg qid for 14 days
- Prophylaxis and treatment of stress gastritis with sucralfate suspension 1 g orally q4-6h, H_2-receptor antagonists, or PPIs in patients on ventilator support
- Misoprostol (Cytotec) in patients on chronic NSAIDs therapy

■ CHRONIC Rx

- Misoprostol 100 µg qid in patients receiving chronic NSAIDs
- Avoidance of alcohol, tobacco, and prolonged NSAID use
- Surveillance gastroscopy in patients with atrophic gastritis (increased risk of gastric cancer)

■ DISPOSITION

- Prognosis is good with most cases resolving with treatment. Successful eradication of *H. pylori* infection can be achieved in >80% of patients with appropriate therapy.
- Undetectable stool antigen 4 wk after therapy accurately confirm cure of *H. pylori* infection in initially seropositive healthy subjects with reasonable sensitivity.
- Most patients with atrophic gastritis and intestinal metaplasia improve within 12 mo following successful *H. pylori* eradication.

REFERENCES

Lara LF et al: One day quadruple therapy compared with 7-day triple therapy for helicobacter pylori infection, *Arch Intern Med* 163:2079, 2003.

Meurer L et al: Management of *helicobacter pylori* infection, *Am Fam Physician* 65:1327, 2002.

Suerbaum S, Michetti P: *Helicobacter pylori* infection, *N Engl J Med* 347:1175, 2002.

Vaira D et al: The stool antigen test for detection of *Helicobacter pylori* after eradication therapy, *Ann Intern Med* 136:280, 2002.

Author: **Fred F. Ferri, M.D.**

BASIC INFORMATION

■ **DEFINITION**

Gastroesophageal reflux disease (GERD) is a motility disorder characterized primarily by heartburn and caused by the reflux of gastric contents into the esophagus.

■ **SYNONYMS**

Peptic esophagitis
Reflux esophagitis
GERD

ICD-9CM CODES

530.81 Gastroesophageal reflux disease
530.1 Esophagitis
787.1 Heartburn

■ **EPIDEMIOLOGY & DEMOGRAPHICS**

GERD is one of the most prevalent GI disorders. Nearly 7% of persons in the United States experience heartburn daily, 20% experience it monthly, and 60% experience it intermittently. Incidence in pregnant women exceeds 80%. Nearly 20% of adults use antacids or OTC H_2-blockers at least once a week for relief of heartburn.

■ **PHYSICAL FINDINGS & CLINICAL PRESENTATION**

• Physical examination: generally unremarkable
• Clinical signs and symptoms: heartburn, dysphagia, sour taste, regurgitation of gastric contents into the mouth
• Chronic cough and bronchospasm
• Chest pain, laryngitis, early satiety, abdominal fullness, and bloating with belching
• Dental erosions in children

■ **ETIOLOGY**

• Incompetent LES
• Medications that lower LES pressure (calcium channel blockers, β-adrenergic blockers, theophylline, anticholinergics)
• Foods that lower LES pressure (chocolate, yellow onions, peppermint)
• Tobacco abuse, alcohol, coffee
• Pregnancy
• Gastric acid hypersecretion
• Hiatal hernia (controversial) present in >70% of patients with GERD; however, most patients with hiatal hernia are asymptomatic

DIAGNOSIS

■ **DIFFERENTIAL DIAGNOSIS**

• Peptic ulcer disease
• Unstable angina
• Esophagitis (from infections such as herpes, *Candida*), medication induced (doxycycline, potassium chloride)
• Esophageal spasm (nutcracker esophagus)
• Cancer of esophagus

■ **WORKUP**

Aimed at eliminating the conditions noted in the differential diagnosis and documenting the type and extent of tissue damage with upper endoscopy

■ **LABORATORY TESTS**

• 24-hr esophageal pH monitoring and Bernstein test are sensitive diagnostic tests; however, they are not very practical and generally not done. They are useful in patients with atypical manifestations of GERD, such as chest pain or chronic cough.
• Esophageal manometry is indicated in patients with refractory reflux in whom surgical therapy is planned.

■ **IMAGING STUDIES**

• Upper GI series can identify ulcerations and strictures; however, it may miss mucosal abnormalities. Only one third of patients with GERD have radiographic signs of esophagitis.
• Upper GI endoscopy is useful to document the type and extent of tissue damage in GERD and to exclude potentially malignant conditions such as Barrett's esophagus. The American College of Gastroenterology recommends endoscopy to screen for Barrett's esophagus in patients who have chronic GERD symptoms. The data demonstrating the cost-effectiveness of endoscopic screening remain controversial.

TREATMENT

■ **NONPHARMACOLOGIC THERAPY**

• Lifestyle modifications with avoidance of foods (e.g., citrus- and tomato-based products) and drugs that exacerbate reflux (e.g., caffeine, β-blockers, calcium channel blockers, α-adrenergic agonists, theophylline)
• Avoidance of tobacco and alcohol use
• Elevation of head of bed (4 to 8 in) using blocks
• Avoidance of lying down directly after late or large evening meals
• Weight reduction, decreased fat intake
• Avoidance of clothing that is tight around the waist

■ **GENERAL Rx**

• Proton pump inhibitors (PPIs) (esomeprazole 40 mg qd, omeprazole 20 mg qd, lansoprazole 30 mg qd, rabeprazole 20 mg qd, or pantoprazole 40 mg qd) are safe, tolerated, and very effective in most patients.
• H_2-Blockers (nizatidine 300 mg qhs, famotidine 40 mg qhs, ranitidine 300 mg qhs, or cimetidine 800 mg qhs) can be used but are generally much less effective than PPIs.
• Antacids (may be useful for relief of mild symptoms; however, they are generally ineffective in severe cases of reflux).
• Prokinetic agents (metoclopramide) are indicated only when PPIs are not fully effective. They can be used in combination therapy; however, side effects limit their use.
• For refractory cases: surgery with Nissen fundoplication. Potential surgical candidates should have reflux esophagitis documented by EGD and normal esophageal motility as evaluated by manometry. Surgery generally consists of reduction of hiatal hernia when present and placement of a gastric wrap around the GE junction (fundoplication). Although laparoscopic fundoplication is now widely used, surgery should not be advised with the expectation that patients with GERD will no longer need to take antisecretory medications or that the procedure will prevent esophageal cancer among those with GERD and Barrett's esophagus.

- Endoscopic radiofrequency heating of the GE junction (Stretta procedure) is a newer treatment modality for GERD patients unresponsive to traditional therapy. Its mechanism of action remains unclear. Endoscopy gastroplasty (EndoCinch procedure) also aims at treating GERD. Initial results appear encouraging; however, long-term studies are needed before recommending these procedures.
- Lifestyle modification must be followed lifelong, because this is generally an irreversible condition.

■ DISPOSITION
- The majority of the patients respond well to therapy.
- Recurrence of reflux is common if treatment is discontinued.

- Postsurgical complications occur in nearly 20% of patients (dysphagia, gas, bloating, diarrhea, nausea). Long-term follow-up studies also reveal that within 3 to 5 yr 52% of patients who had undergone antireflux surgery are taking antireflux medications again.

■ REFERRAL
- There is a strong and probably causal relation between symptomatic prolonged and untreated GERD, Barrett's esophagus, and esophageal adenocarcinoma. GI referral for upper endoscopy is needed when there are concerns about associated PUD, Barrett's esophagus, or esophageal cancer.
- Patients with Barrett's esophagus should undergo surveillance endoscopy with mucosal biopsy every 2 yr or less because the risk of developing adenocarcinoma of esophagus is at least 30 times greater than that of the general population.
- All children with dental erosions should be evaluated for GERD.

REFERENCES
Heidelbaugh JL et al: Management of gastroesophageal reflux disease, *Am Fam Physician* 68:1311, 2003.

Kabrilas PJ: Radiofrequency energy treatment of GERD, *Gastroenterology* 125:970, 2003.

Shaheen N, Ransohoff DF: Gastroesophageal reflux, Barret esophagus, and esophageal cancer, *JAMA* 287:1972, 2002.

Author: **Fred F. Ferri, M.D.**

BASIC INFORMATION

■ DEFINITION
Giant cell arteritis (GCA) is a segmental systemic granulomatous arteritis affecting medium- and large-sized arteries in individuals >50 years. Inflammation primarily targets extracranial blood vessels, and although the carotid system is usually affected, pathology in posterior cerebral artery has been reported.

■ SYNONYMS
Temporal arteritis
Cranial arteritis
Horton's disease

ICD-9CM CODES
446.5 Temporal arteritis

■ EPIDEMIOLOGY & DEMOGRAPHICS
PREVALENCE: 200 cases/100,000 persons; female-to-male predominance of two- to four-fold
INCIDENCE: 17 to 23.3 new cases/100,000 persons >50 yr

■ CLINICAL PRESENTATION & PHYSICAL FINDINGS
GCA can present with the following clinical manifestations:
- Headache, often associated with marked scalp tenderness
- Constitutional symptoms (fever, weight loss, anorexia, fatigue)
- Polymyalgia syndrome (aching and stiffness of the trunk and proximal muscle groups)
- Visual disturbances (transient or permanent monocular visual loss)
- Intermittent claudication of jaw and tongue on mastication
Important physical findings in GCA:
- Vascular examination: Tenderness, decreased pulsation, and nodulation of temporal arteries; diminished or absent pulses in upper extremities

■ ETIOLOGY
Vasculitis of unknown etiology

DIAGNOSIS

Clinical history and vascular examination are cornerstones of diagnosis.
The presence of any three of the following five items allows the diagnosis of GCA with a sensitivity of 94% and a specificity of 91%:
- Age of onset >50 yr
- New-onset or new type of headache
- Temporal artery tenderness or decreased pulsation on physical examination
- Westergren ESR >50 mm/hr
- Temporal artery biopsy with vasculitis and mononuclear cell infiltrate or granulomatous changes

■ DIFFERENTIAL DIAGNOSIS
- Other vasculitic syndromes
- Nonarteritic Anterior Ischemic Optic Neuropathy (AION)
- Primary amyloidosis
- TIA, stroke
- Infections
- Occult neoplasm, multiple myeloma

■ WORKUP

■ LABORATORY TESTS
- ESR >50 mm/hr; however, up to 22.5% patients with GCA have normal ESR before treatment
- C-reactive protein is typically included in lab investigation; it has greater sensitivity than ESR
- Mild-to-moderate normochromic normocytic anemia, elevated platelet count
- IL-6 levels hold promise for a more sensitive modality, but at this stage remains experimental

■ IMAGING STUDIES
- Reliability of color duplex ultrasonography of temporal artery is controversial as it is thought that it does not improve diagnostic accuracy over careful physical examination
- Fluorescein angiogram of ophthalmic vessels may be warranted to differentiate between arteritic AION (i.e., GCA) and nonarteritic AION

TREATMENT

■ ACUTE GENERAL Rx
- Intravenous methylprednisolone (500-1000 mg qd for 3-5 days) is indicated in those with significant clinical manifestations (e.g., visual loss).
- Oral prednisone (1 mg/kg/day) may be used under less urgent circumstances or following the initial period of treatment with intravenous methylprednisolone. High-dose oral regimen should be continued at least until symptoms resolve and ESR returns to normal.
- Prednisone should be tapered gradually (~5 mg every other wk) initially and subsequently even more slowly (2.5 mg every 2-4 wk). Steroid treatment is usually required for at least 6 mo, and sometimes as much as 2 yr.
- Methotrexate or azathioprine may be added to the steroid regimen for their steroid-sparing effect, but efficacy is unproven.

■ DISPOSITION
If steroid therapy is initiated early, GCA has excellent prognosis; however, 20% of patients have permanent partial or complete loss of vision. Once there is visual loss, improvement is dismal: in one study, only 4% of eyes improved in both visual acuity and central visual field.

■ REFERRAL
- Surgical referral for biopsy of temporal artery
- Ophthalmology referral in patients with visual disturbances and following initiation of corticosteroid therapy
- Rheumatology referral for difficult cases

PEARLS & CONSIDERATIONS

■ COMMENTS
- The relationship between polymyalgia rheumatica and GCA is unclear, but the two may frequently coexist.
- Clinical picture rather than ESR should be the prime yardstick for continuing prednisone therapy.
- A rising ESR in a clinically asymptomatic patient with normal hematocrit should raise suspicion for alternate explanations (e.g., infections, neoplasms).
- Although pathologic findings on temporal artery biopsy are the gold standard for the diagnosis of GCA, the false-negative rate is around 9% (the false-negative rate may be lower in the hands of an experienced surgeon); in some cases, a second biopsy from the contralateral side may be required.
- GCA is associated with a markedly increased risk for the development of aortic aneurysm, which is often a late complication and may cause death. Annual chest radiograph in chronic CGA patients has been suggested, as well as emergent chest CT or MRI for clinical suspicion.

REFERENCES
Please refer to references within these papers as well as associated 'Letters to the Editor' for further details.
Gold R et al: Therapy of neurological disorders in systemic vasculitis, *Sem Neurol* 23(2):207, 2003.
Hayreh SR et al: Visual improvement with corticosteroid therapy in giant cell arteritis. Report of large study and review of the literature, *Acta Opththalmol Scand* 80:355, 2002.
Hoffman GS et al: A multicenter, randomized, double-blind, placebo-controlled trial of adjuvant methotrexate for giant-cell arteritis, *Arthritis and Rheum* 46(5):1309, 2002.
Norborg E, Norborg C: Giant cell arteritis: epidemiological clues to its pathogenesis and an update on its treatment, *Rheumatol* 42:413, 2003.
Salvarani C et al: Polymyalgia rheumatica and giant-cell arteritis, *N Engl J Med* 347(4):261, 2002.
Smetana GW, Shmerling RH: Does this patient have temporal arteritis? *JAMA* 287:92, 2002.
Author: U. Shivraj Sohur, M.D, Ph.D.

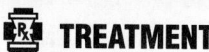

 BASIC INFORMATION

■ DEFINITION

Giardiasis is an intestinal and/or biliary tract infection caused by the protozoal parasite *Giardia lamblia*.

■ ICD-9CM CODES

007.1 Giardiasis

■ EPIDEMIOLOGY & DEMOGRAPHICS

INCIDENCE (IN U.S.):
- Exact incidence unknown
- Frequently occurs in outbreaks

PREVALENCE (IN U.S.): 4%

PREDOMINANT SEX: Male = female

PREDOMINANT AGE:
- Preschool children, especially if in day care
- 20 to 40 yr old, especially among sexually active homosexual men

PEAK INCIDENCE:
- Varies with risk factors, outbreaks
- All age groups affected

GENETICS:

Familial Disposition: Patients with common variable immunodeficiency or X-linked agammaglobulinemia are at increased risk of infection.

Neonatal Infection: Rare; infection is common among preschool children in day care.

■ PHYSICAL FINDINGS & CLINICAL PRESENTATION

- More than 70% with one or more intestinal symptoms (diarrhea, flatulence, cramps, bloating, nausea)
- Fever in <20%
- Malaise, anorexia
- Chronic diarrhea, malabsorption, and weight loss

- GI bleeding is unusual
- Continuous or intermittent symptoms, lasting for weeks
- Of infected patients, 20% to 25% are asymptomatic

■ ETIOLOGY

Infection is acquired by ingestion of viable cysts of the organism, typically in contaminated water or by fecal-oral contact.

🔬 DIAGNOSIS

■ DIFFERENTIAL DIAGNOSIS

- Other agents of infective diarrhea (amebae, *Salmonella* sp., *Shigella* sp., *Staphylococcus aureus*, *Cryptosporidium*, etc.)
- Noninfectious causes of malabsorption

■ WORKUP

Stool specimen (three specimens yield 90% sensitivity) or duodenal aspirate for microscopic examination to establish diagnosis and exclude other pathogens (Fig. 1-121)

■ LABORATORY TESTS

- Serum albumin, vitamin B_{12} levels, and stool fat test to exclude malabsorption
- Serum antibody test if desired for epidemiologic purposes

■ IMAGING STUDIES

- Not necessary unless biliary obstruction is suspected
- In detection of organism, possible interference by barium in stool from radiographic studies

🔬 TREATMENT

■ NONPHARMACOLOGIC THERAPY

Avoidance of milk products to reduce symptoms of transient lactase deficiency that occur in many patients

■ ACUTE GENERAL Rx

Adults:
- Metronidazole 250 mg PO three times daily for 7 days (metronidazole avoided in pregnancy) *or*
- Paromomycin 25 to 30 mg/kg/day in three doses for 5 to 10 days

■ CHRONIC Rx

May require retreatment

■ DISPOSITION

Reinfection is possible.

■ REFERRAL

For evaluation by gastroenterologist if malabsorption and weight loss do not resolve with therapy

⚙ PEARLS & CONSIDERATIONS

■ COMMENTS

Travelers to endemic areas (developing world, wilderness areas) should be cautioned to boil drinking water, or if this is impossible, use halogenated water purification tablets.

REFERENCES

Grant J et al: Wheat germ supplement reduces cyst and trophozoite passage in people with giardiasis, *Am J Trop Med Hyg* 65(6):705, 2001.

Hoque ME et al: Nappy handling and risk of giardiasis, *Lancet* 357(9261): 1017, 2001.

Lane S, Loyd D: Current trends in research into the waterborne parasite *Giardia, Crit Rev Microbiol* 28(2):123, 2002.

Minenoa T, Avery MA: Giardiasis: recent progress in chemotherapy and drug development, *Curr Pharm Des* 9(11):841, 2003.

Newman RD et al: A longitudinal study of *Giardia lamblia* infection in northeast Brazilian children, *Trop Med Int Health* 6(8):624, 2001.

Author: **Joseph R. Masci, M.D.**

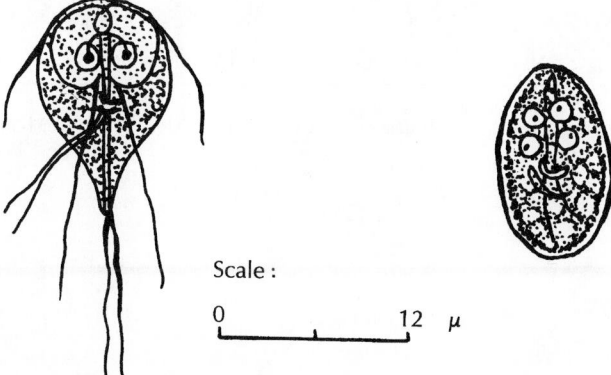

Scale:

0 ————— 12 μ

Fig. 1-121 *Giardia* organisms. The trophozoite (*left*) is 12 to 15 μm long and has four pairs of flagella. This form is not commonly seen in stools. Cysts (*right*) are 9 to 19 μm long and may have two to four nuclei. (From Hoekelman R [ed]: *Primary pediatric care,* ed 3, St Louis, 1997, Mosby.)

BASIC INFORMATION

■ DEFINITION
Gilbert's disease is an autosomal dominant disease characterized by indirect hyperbilirubinemia caused by impaired glucuronyl transferase activity.

■ SYNONYMS
Gilbert's syndrome

ICD-9CM CODES
277.4 Gilbert's syndrome

■ EPIDEMIOLOGY & DEMOGRAPHICS
- Probable autosomal dominant disease affecting >5% of the U.S. population
- Male:female ratio of 3:1
- Most common hereditary hyperbilirubinemia (genotypic prevalence 12%)

■ PHYSICAL FINDINGS & CLINICAL PRESENTATION
- No abnormalities on physical examination other than mild jaundice when bilirubin exceeds 3 mg/dl.
- A family history of unconjugated hyperbilirubinemia may be present.

■ ETIOLOGY
Decreased elimination of bilirubin in bile is caused by inadequate conjugation of bilirubin. Alcohol consumption and starvation diet can increase the bilirubin level. The pathogenesis of Gilbert's syndrome has been linked to a reduction in bilirubin UGT-1 gene (HUG-Brl) transcription resulting from a mutation in the promoter region.

DIAGNOSIS

■ DIFFERENTIAL DIAGNOSIS
- Hemolytic anemia
- Liver disease (chronic hepatitis, cirrhosis)
- Crigler-Najjar syndrome

■ WORKUP
- Most patients are diagnosed during or after adolescence, when isolated hyperbilirubinemia is detected as an incidental finding on routine biochemical testing
- Laboratory evaluation to exclude hemolysis and liver diseases as a cause of the elevated bilirubin level (Table 1-22)

■ LABORATORY TESTS
Elevated indirect (unconjugated) bilirubin (rarely exceeds 5 mg/dl)

TREATMENT

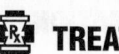

■ ACUTE GENERAL Rx
Treatment is generally unnecessary. Phenobarbital (if clinical jaundice is present) can rapidly decrease serum indirect bilirubin level.

■ DISPOSITION
Prognosis is excellent. Treatment is generally unnecessary.

■ REFERRAL
Referral is generally not necessary.

PEARLS & CONSIDERATIONS

■ COMMENTS
- Patients should be reassured about the benign nature of their condition.
- Fasting for 2 days or significant dehydration may raise the bilirubin level and result in the clinical recognition of jaundice.

Author: **Fred F. Ferri, M.D.**

TABLE 1-22 Characteristic Patterns of Liver Function Tests

DISORDER	BILIRUBIN	ALKALINE PHOSPHATASE	AST	ALT	PROTHROMBIN TIME	ALBUMIN
Gilbert's syndrome (abnormal bilirubin metabolism)	↑	NL	NL	NL	NL	NL
Bile duct obstruction (pancreatic cancer)	↑↑↑	↑↑↑	↑	↑	↑-↑↑	NL
Acute hepatocellular damage (toxic, viral hepatitis)	↑-↑↑↑	↑-↑↑	↑↑↑	↑↑↑	NL-↑↑↑	NL-↓↓
Cirrhosis	NL-↑	NL-↑	NL-↑	NL-↑	NL-↑↑	NL-↓↓

From Andreoli TE (ed): *Cecil essentials of medicine*, ed 4, Philadelphia, 1997, WB Saunders.
ALT, Alanine aminotransferase; *AST*, aspartate aminotransferase; *NL*, normal; ↑, increase; ↓, decrease (arrows indicate extent of change: ↑-↑↑↑, slight to large).

BASIC INFORMATION

DEFINITION
Inflammation of the gums covering the maxilla and mandible

SYNONYMS
None

ICD-9-CM CODE
523.1

EPIDEMIOLOGY & DEMOGRAPHICS
INCIDENCE IN US: N/A
PREVALENCE IN US: N/A
PREDOMINANT SEX: None
PREDOMINANT AGE: Adults
PEAK INCIDENCE: None
GENETICS: N/A
    Familial Disposition: N/A
    Congenital Infection: N/A
    Neonatal Infection: N/A

PHYSICAL FINDINGS
Inflammation is usually painless. Bleeding may occur with minor trauma such as brushing teeth. A bluish discoloration of the gums and halitosis are sometimes present. Subgingival plaque may be seen on close examination, and in time, there is detachment of soft tissue from the tooth surface. Long-standing infection may lead to destructive periodontal disease, which may involve teeth and bones.

A dramatic form of gingivitis called *acute ulcerative necrotizing gingivitis* (ANUG or "trench mouth") can occur. This is manifested by acute, painful, inflammation of the gingivae, with bleeding, ulceration, and halitosis. At times this is accompanied by fever and lymphadenopathy.

Linear gingival erythema ("HIV Gingivitis") presents as a brightly inflamed band of marginal gingiva. It may be painful, with easy bleeding and rapid destruction.

Severe periodontitis can occur in patients with diabetes mellitus or HIV infection and in primary HIV infection (acute retroviral syndrome).

Pregnancy may be associated with an acute form of gingivitis. Gingivae become inflamed and hypertrophic; this is likely due to hormonal shifts.

ETIOLOGY
- A variety of organisms may be found in the environment of plaque. Anaerobes play a predominant role in periodontal disease.
- Improper hygiene and poorly fitting dentures may contribute to development of gingivitis.
- Excessive use of tobacco and alcohol may predispose individuals to gingival disease.
- In patients with HIV infection, gram-negative anaerobes, enteric organisms, and yeast predominate.
- Appropriate oral hygiene, such as flossing and tooth brushing, can prevent the accumulation of bacterial plaque.
- Once plaque is present, adequate hygiene becomes more difficult.

DIAGNOSIS

DIFFERENTIAL DIAGNOSIS
Gingival hyperplasia, which may be caused by phenytoin or nifedipine

WORKUP
Oral examination

LABORATORY TESTS
Elevated serum glucose in diabetics

IMAGING STUDIES
Radiographs of the teeth and facial bones may reveal extension of infection to these structures.

TREATMENT

NONPHARMACOLOGIC THERAPY
Removal of plaque, and at times, debridement of soft tissue

ACUTE GENERAL Rx
Penicillin VK, 500 mg po qid for 1 to 2 wk, *or*
Clindamycin, 300 mg po qid for 1 to 2 wk
For *linear gingival erythema,* clorhexidene rinses and nystatin rinses or troches may be used.

CHRONIC Rx
Extensive or recurrent infection may require periodic evaluation and debridement.

DISPOSITION
Continued inflammation can eventually lead to destruction of teeth and bone.

REFERRAL
Patients should be referred to a dentist or oral surgeon.

PEARLS & CONSIDERATIONS

COMMENTS
- Presence of periodontal disease is associated with an increased incidence of anaerobic pleuropulmonary infections.
- Existing data support the recommendation to change a toothbrush every 3 mo. Worn brushes seem to be less effective in plaque reduction.

REFERENCES
Obernesser MS: Gingivitis and periodontitis syndromes, In *Up To Date,* Clinical reference CD, vol 8.1, 2000.
Sharma NC et al: Antiplaque and antigingivitis effectiveness of a hexetidine mouthwash, *J Clin Periodontol* 30(7):590, 2003.
Warren PR et al: A clinical investigation into the effect of toothbrush wear on efficacy, *J Clin Dent* 13:119, 2002.
Author: **Maurice Policar, M.D**

BASIC INFORMATION

■ DEFINITION
Chronic open-angle glaucoma refers to optic nerve damage often associated with elevated intraocular pressure; it is a chronic, slowly progressive, usually bilateral disorder associated with visual loss, eye pain, and optic nerve damage. High pressure is a definite risk factor for glaucoma.

■ SYNONYM
Chronic simple glaucoma

ICD-9CM CODES
365.1 Open-angle glaucoma

■ EPIDEMIOLOGY & DEMOGRAPHICS
INCIDENCE (IN U.S.): Third most common cause of visual loss (75% to 95% of all glaucomas are open angle.)
PREVALENCE (IN U.S.):
- 15,000,000 Americans may have glaucoma and 1,600,000 have visual field loss.
- 150,000 patients suffer bilateral blindness.
- Disease occurs in 2% of people >40 yr old.
- Prevalence is higher in diabetics, with high myopia, and among older persons.

PREDOMINANT AGE:
- Persons >50 yr old
- Can occur in 30s and 40s

PEAK INCIDENCE: Increases after 40 yr
GENETICS:
- Four to six times higher incidence in blacks than whites
- No clear-cut hereditary patterns but a strong hereditary tendency

■ PHYSICAL FINDINGS
- High intraocular pressures and large optic nerve cup
- Abnormal visual fields
- Open-angle gonioscopy

■ ETIOLOGY
- Uncertain hereditary tendency
- Topical steroids
- Trauma
- Inflammatory
- High-dose oral corticosteroids taken for prolonged periods

DIAGNOSIS

■ DIFFERENTIAL DIAGNOSIS
- Other optic neuropathies
- Secondary glaucoma from inflammation and steroid therapy

■ WORKUP
- Intraocular pressure
- Slit lamp examination
- Visual fields
- Gonioscopy
- Nerve fiber analysis
- Corneal thickness

■ LABORATORY TESTS
Blood sugar

■ IMAGING STUDIES
- Optic nerve photography
- Visual field testing
- GDx (laser scan of nerve fiber layer)

TREATMENT

■ ACUTE GENERAL Rx
- β-Blockers (Timolol)
- Diamox or pilocarpine
- Hyperosmotic agents (mannitol)
- Prostaglandins
- Laser trabeculoplasty (SLT)

■ CHRONIC Rx
At least biannual checks of intraocular pressure and adjustment of medication

■ DISPOSITION
Usually followed by ophthalmologist

■ REFERRAL
Immediately to ophthalmologist

PEARLS & CONSIDERATIONS

■ COMMENTS
- Early diagnosis and treatment may minimize visual loss.
- Glaucoma is not solely caused by increased intraocular pressure, because approximately 20% of patients with glaucoma have normal intraocular pressure, but high pressure is definitely a risk factor to be considered.

REFERENCES
Gordon MO et al: Baseline factors that predict the onset of primary open-angle glaucoma, *Arch Ophthalmol* 120:714, 2002.

Heijl A et al: Reduction of intraocular pressure and glaucoma progression: Results from the early manifest glaucoma trial, *Arch Ophthalmol* 120:1268, 2002.

Rezaie T et al: Adult-onset primary open-angle glaucoma caused by mutations in optineurin, *Science* 295:1077, 2002.
Author: **Melvyn Koby, M.D.**

BASIC INFORMATION

■ DEFINITION
Primary closed-angle glaucoma occurs when elevated intraocular pressure is associated with closure of the filtration angle.

■ SYNONYMS
Glaucoma
Pupillary block glaucoma
Narrow-angle glaucoma

ICD-9CM CODES
365.2 Primary angle-closure glaucoma

■ EPIDEMIOLOGY & DEMOGRAPHICS
INCIDENCE (IN U.S.):
- In 2% to 8% of all patients with glaucoma
- Higher incidence among those with hyperopia

PREDOMINANT SEX: Females > males
PREDOMINANT AGE: 50 to 60 yr
PEAK INCIDENCE: Greater after 50 yr of age
GENETICS: High family history

■ PHYSICAL FINDINGS & CLINICAL FINDINGS
- Hazy cornea (Fig. 1-122)
- Narrow angle
- Red eyes
- Pain
- Injection of conjunctiva

■ ETIOLOGY
- Narrow angles with acute closure

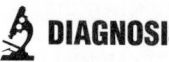

DIAGNOSIS

■ DIFFERENTIAL DIAGNOSIS
- Open-angle glaucoma
- Conjunctivitis
- Corneal disease-keratitis

■ WORKUP
- Intraocular pressure
- Gonioscopy
- Slit lamp examination
- Visual field examination
- GDx examination (laser scan of nerve fiber layer)

■ LABORATORY TESTS
Blood sugar and CBC (if diabetes or inflammatory disease is suspected)

■ IMAGING STUDIES
- Fundus photography
- Fluorescein angiography for neurovascular disease

TREATMENT

The goal of treatment is to acutely lower pressure on eye and keep it down.

■ NONPHARMACOLOGIC THERAPY
Laser iridotomy early in disease process

■ ACUTE GENERAL Rx
- IV mannitol
- Pilocarpine
- β-Blockers
- Diamox
- Laser iridotomy

■ CHRONIC Rx
- Iridotomy
- Trabeculectomy

■ DISPOSITION
Refer to ophthalmologist immediately.

■ REFERRAL
This is an emergency—refer immediately to an ophthalmologist.

PEARLS & CONSIDERATIONS

■ COMMENTS
- After iridotomy, the majority of patients will be totally cured and will need no further medication and have no visual loss.
- Lower socioeconomic status and higher levels of social deprivation are risk factors for delayed detection and probable worse outcomes in glaucoma.

REFERENCES
Fraser S et al: Deprivation and late presentation of glaucoma: case control study, *BMJ* 322:638, 2001.
Kapur SB: The lens and angle-closure glaucoma, *J Cataract Refract Surg* 27(2):176, 2001.
Lam DS et al: Angle-closure glaucoma, *Opthalmology* 109:1, 2002.
Author: **Melvyn Koby, M.D.**

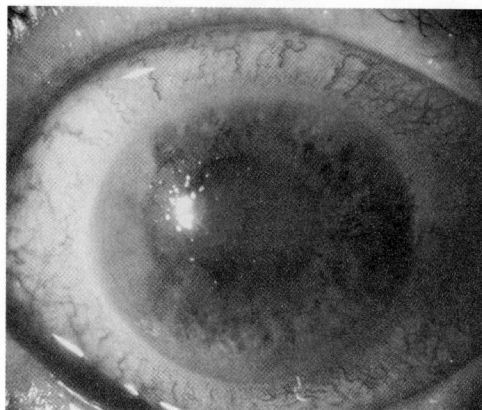

A

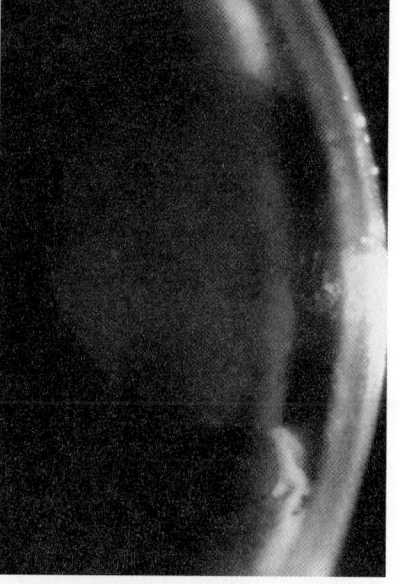

B

Fig. 1-122 Acute angle-closure glaucoma. A, Acutely elevated pressure produces an inflamed eye with corneal edema (note fragmented light reflex) and a middilated pupil. **B,** Slit lamp examination shows a very shallow central anterior chamber (space between cornea and iris) and no peripheral chamber. (From Palay D [ed]: *Ophthalmology for the primary care physician,* St Louis, 1997, Mosby.)

BASIC INFORMATION

■ DEFINITION

Complete separation or displacement of the humeral head from the glenoid surface. (Partial separation is termed *subluxation*.) Most often the cause is traumatic, and the humeral head dislocates anterior and inferior. This may cause a tear of the glenoid labrum (the Bankart lesion). Less commonly, the head dislocates posteriorly.
Rarely, multidirectional instability may be present in which dislocation or subluxation, often bilateral, may occur in multiple directions, usually the result of excessive joint laxity and generally without trauma.

ICD-9CM CODES
831.01 Anterior
831.02 Posterior
831.03 Inferior
718.31 Recurrent
718.81 Instability

■ PHYSICAL FINDINGS & CLINICAL PRESENTATION

Traumatic
- The arm is held in external rotation with anterior dislocation, internal rotation with posterior dislocation.
- Little movement is possible without pain.
- The acromion may appear more prominent and there is absence of the normal "fullness" beneath the acromion.
- The status of the axillary nerve must always be checked (sensation to the middeltoid should be assessed).

- The apprehension test may become positive if anterior instability persists (pain and apprehension that the shoulder will dislocate when the relaxed arm is manually placed in the "throwing position" of external rotation and abduction).
- Recurrent episodes of anterior dislocation may occur with minor movement such as putting on a coat or turning a light off at night.
Multidirectional
- Often difficult to diagnose, especially if only subluxation occurs
- Recurrent episodes of giving out, weakness, often bilateral without trauma
- Sulcus sign often positive (the arms are pulled downward with the patient standing; a sulcus [indentation] will form between the acromion and humeral head, indicating excessive inferior movement of the head)
- Other signs of generalized joint laxity may be present, such as joint hyperextensibility and the ability of the patient to touch the thumb against the flexor aspect of the forearm

■ ETIOLOGY
- Trauma
- Generalized joint laxity (multidirectional)
- Seizures (posterior dislocations)

DIAGNOSIS

■ DIFFERENTIAL DIAGNOSIS
- Rotator cuff rupture
- Frozen shoulder (posterior dislocation)
- Suprascapular nerve paralysis
- Anterior instability

■ IMAGING STUDIES
- Acute shoulder injury: True AP roentgenogram plus lateral view of the glenohumeral joint, either transaxillary or transcapular (Fig. 1-123)
- MRI: To determine soft tissue status, especially the presence of Bankart lesion or rotator cuff tear; may be indicated following a second episode of dislocation
- Arthrogram: To determine if concurrent rotator cuff tear has occurred, especially in older patient

TREATMENT

- Reduction of the acute dislocation by gentle straight traction in the relaxed patient followed by light immobilization
- Gentle limited range of motion exercises as pain subsides followed by strengthening exercises at 2 wk

■ DISPOSITION
- Recurrence of anterior dislocation is common in the young; this patient may have to avoid the arm position associated with dislocation (external rotation with abduction)

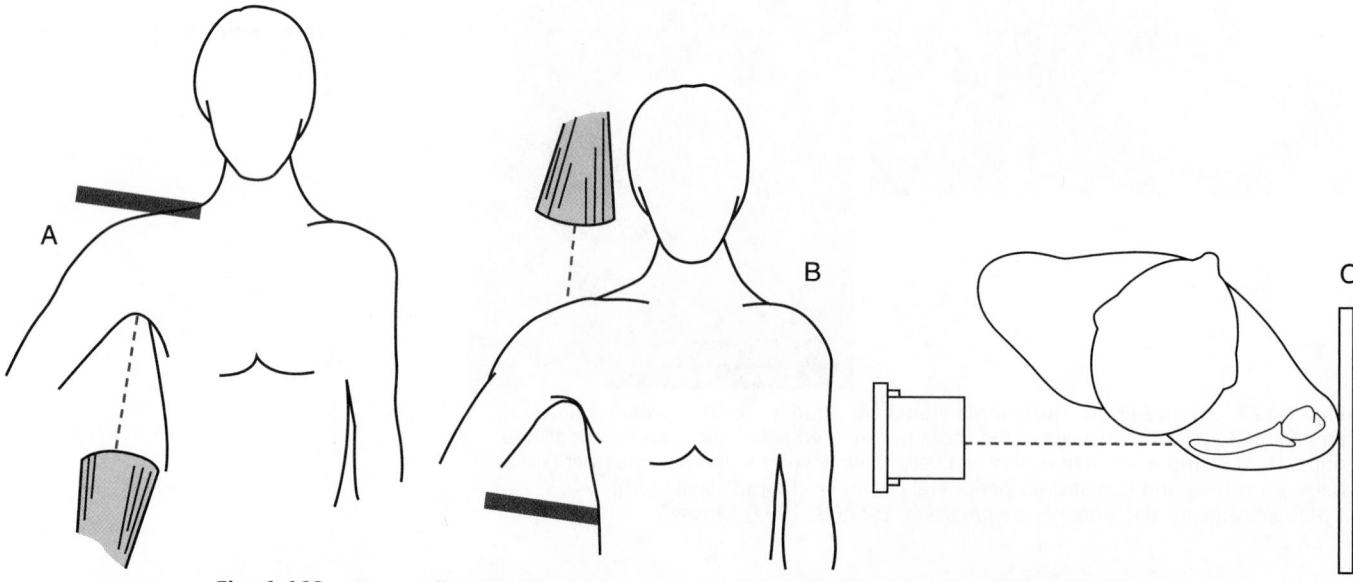

Fig. 1-123   Transaxillary (**A, B**) and transscapular "Y" views (**C**) of the glenohumeral joint.

- Primary dislocations in patients over 40 yr are not generally complicated by recurrence, but may result in shoulder stiffness and may have associated rotator cuff injuries
- There is an almost 100% recurrence after the third dislocation

■ REFERRAL
- Surgical reconstruction may be required in the recurrent dislocator

◌ PEARLS & CONSIDERATIONS

■ COMMENTS
- It is important to know if there was an injury involved in the first episode and if a radiograph was taken to determine direction.

- Up to 50% of posterior dislocations are missed by the first examiner, usually the result of an inadequate lateral radiograph of the glenohumeral joint.
- "Voluntary" posterior dislocators should always be treated nonsurgically.
- Sports activities may be resumed when there is pain-free full flexibility and normal strength.
- Multidirectional instabilities are usually treated nonsurgically with strengthening exercises.

REFERENCES

Orlinski I et al: Comparative study of intra-articular lidocaine and intravenous meperidine/diazepam for shoulder dislocation, *J Emerg Med* 22:241, 2001.

Pagnini N, Dome DC: Surgical treatment of traumatic anterior shoulder instability in the American football players, *J Bone Joint Surg* 84(A):711, 2002.

Robinson CN, Kelly M, Wakefield AE: Redislocation of the shoulder during the first 6 weeks after a primary anterior dislocation: risk factor and results of treatment, *J Bone Joint Surg* 84:1552, 2002.

Sugaya H, Moriishi J, et al: Glenoid rim morphology in recurrent anterior glenohumeral instability, *J Bone Joint Surg* 85:878, 2003.

Author: **Lonnie R. Mercier, M.D.**

BASIC INFORMATION

■ DEFINITION
Acute glomerulonephritis is an immunologically mediated inflammation primarily involving the glomerulus that can result in damage to the basement membrane, mesangium, or capillary endothelium. Table 1-23 summarizes primary renal diseases that present as acute glomerulonephritis.

■ SYNONYMS
Postinfectious glomerulonephritis
Acute nephritic syndrome

ICD-9CM CODES
583.9 Glomerulonephritis, acute

■ EPIDEMIOLOGY & DEMOGRAPHICS
- Over 50% of cases involve children <13 yr old.
- Glomerulonephritis is the most common cause of chronic renal failure (25%).
- IgA nephropathy glomerulonephritis (Berger's disease) is the most common glomerulonephritis worldwide.

■ PHYSICAL FINDINGS & CLINICAL FINDINGS
- Edema (peripheral, periorbital, or pulmonary)
- Joint pains, oral ulcers, malar rash (frequently seen with lupus nephritis)
- Dark urine
- Hypertension
- Findings of palpable purpura in patients with Henoch-Schönlein purpura
- Heart murmurs may indicate endocarditis
- Impetigo, skin pallor, tenderness in the abdomen and/or back, pharyngeal erythema may be present

■ ETIOLOGY
Acute glomerulonephritis may be due to primary renal disease or a systemic disease. A number of pathogenic processes (e.g., antibody deposition, cell-mediated immune mechanisms, complement activation, hemodynamic alterations) have been implicated in the pathogenesis of glomerular inflammation. Medical disorders generally associated with glomerulonephritis are:
- Post group A β-hemolytic *Streptococcus* infection (other infectious etiologies including endocarditis and visceral abscess)
- Collagen-vascular diseases (SLE)
- Vasculitis (Wegener's granulomatosis, polyarteritis nodosa)
- Idiopathic glomerulonephritis (membranoproliferative, idiopathic, crescentic, IgA nephropathy)
- Goodpasture's syndrome
- Other cryoglobulinemia (Henoch-Schönlein purpura)
- Drug-induced (gold, penicillamine)
- Table 1-23 is a summary of primary renal diseases that present as acute glomerulonephritis

🔬 DIAGNOSIS

■ DIFFERENTIAL DIAGNOSIS
- Cirrhosis with edema and ascites
- CHF
- Acute interstitial nephritis
- Severe hypertension
- Hemolytic-uremic syndrome
- SLE, diabetes mellitus, amyloidosis, preeclampsia, sclerodermal renal crisis

■ WORKUP
Initial evaluation of suspected glomerulonephritis consists of laboratory testing.

■ LABORATORY TESTS
- Urinalysis (hematuria [dysmorphic erythrocytes and red cell casts], proteinuria)
- Serum creatinine (to estimate GFR), BUN
- 24-hr urine for protein excretion and creatinine clearance (to document degree of renal dysfunction and amount of proteinuria). Proteinuria in acute glomerulonephritis typically ranges from 500 mg/day to 3 g/day but nephrotic-range proteinuria (>3.5 g/day) may be present
- Streptococcal tests (Streptozyme), antistreptolysin O (ASO) quantitative titer (highest in 3 to 5 wk); ASO titer, however, is not related to severity of renal disease, duration, or prognosis
- Additional useful tests depending on the history: Anti-DNA antibodies (rule out SLE), CH_{50} level (if elevated, obtain C_3, C_4 levels), triglycerides, cryoglobulins, hepatitis B and C serologies, ANCA (antineutrophil cytoplasmic antibody), c-ANCA (in suspected cases of Wegener's granulomatosis), p-ANCA found in pauci-immune (lack of immune deposits) idiopathic rapidly progressive glomerulonephritis with or without systemic vasculitis, anti-glomerular basement membrane (type alpha[3] IV collagen) antibodies
- Hct (decrease in glomerulonephritis), platelet count (thrombocytopenia in cases of lupus nephritis)
- Anti-GBM antibody (in Goodpasture's syndrome)
- Blood cultures are indicated in all febrile patients

■ IMAGING STUDIES
- Chest x-ray examination: pulmonary congestion, Wegener's granulomatosis, and Goodpasture's syndrome
- Renal ultrasound if GFR is depressed to evaluate renal size and determine extent of fibrosis. A kidney size of <9 cm is suggestive of extensive scarring and low likelihood of reversibility
- Echocardiogram in patients with new cardiac murmurs or positive blood cultures to rule out endocarditis and pericardial effusion
- Renal biopsy and light, electron, and immunofluorescent microscopy to confirm diagnosis
- Kidney biopsy: generally reveals a granular pattern in poststreptococcal glomerulonephritis, linear pattern in Goodpasture's syndrome; absence of immune deposits suggests vasculitis; renal biopsy: although helpful to define the etiology of glomerulonephritis, is not usually essential. It is useful to determine the degree of inflammation and fibrosis. It is also especially important for patients with RPGN where prompt diagnosis and treatment is essential
- Immunofluorescence: generally reveals C_3; negative immunofluorescence suggests Wegener's granulomatosis, idiopathic crescentic glomerulonephritis, or polyarteritis nodosa
- Angiography or biopsy of other affected organs if systemic vasculitis is suspected

💊 TREATMENT

■ NONPHARMACOLOGIC THERAPY
- Avoidance of salt if edema or hypertension is present
- Low-protein intake (approximately 0.5 g/kg/day) in patients with renal failure
- Fluid restriction in patients with significant edema
- Avoidance of high-potassium foods

■ ACUTE GENERAL Rx
- Correction of electrolyte abnormalities (hypocalcemia, hyperkalemia) and acidosis (if present)
- Treatment of streptococcal infection with penicillin (or erythromycin in penicillin-allergic patients)
- Furosemide in patients with significant hypertension and/or edema; hydralazine or nifedipine in patients with hypertension

TABLE 1-23 Summary of Primary Renal Diseases That Present as Acute Glomerulonephritis

DISEASES	POSTSTREPTOCOCCAL GLOMERULONEPHRITIS (PSGN)	IgA NEPHROPATHY	MEMBRANOPROLIFERATIVE GLOMERULONEPHRITIS	IDIOPATHIC RAPIDLY PROGRESSIVE GLOMERULONEPHRITIS (RPGN)
Clinical manifestations				
Age and sex	All ages, mean 7 yr, 2:1 male	15-35 yr, 2:1 male	15-30 yr, 6:1 male	Mean 58 yr, 2:1 male
Acute nephritic syndrome	90%	50%	90%	90%
Asymptomatic hematuria	Occasionally	50%	Rare	Rare
Nephrotic syndrome	10%-20%	Rare	Rare	10%-20%
Hypertension	70%	30%-50%	Rare	25%
Acute renal failure	50% (transient)	Very rare	50%	60%
Other	Latent period of 1-3 wk	Follows viral syndromes	Pulmonary hemorrhage; iron-deficiency anemia	None
Laboratory findings	↑ ASO titers (70%) Positive streptozyme (95%) ↓ C3-C9 Normal C1, C4	↑ Serum IgA (50%) IgA in dermal capillaries	Positive anti-GBM antibody	Positive ANCA
Immunogenetics	HLA-B12, D "EN" (9)*	HLA-Bw 35, DR4 (4)*	HLA-DR2 (16)*	None established
Renal pathology				
Light microscopy	Diffuse proliferation	Focal proliferation	Focal → diffuse proliferation with crescents	Crescentic GN
Immunofluorescence	Granular IgG, C3	Diffuse mesangial IgA	Linear IgG, C3	No immune deposits
Electron microscopy	Subepithelial humps	Mesangial deposits	No deposits	No deposits
Prognosis	95% resolve spontaneously 5% RPGN or slowly progressive	Slow progression in 25%-50%	75% stabilize or improve if treated early	75% stabilize or improve if treated early
Treatment	Supportive	None established	Plasma exchange, steroids, cyclophosphamide	Steroid pulse therapy

Modified from Goldman L, Ausiello D (eds): *Cecil textbook of medicine*, ed 22, Philadelphia, 2004, WB Saunders.
ANCA, Antineutrophil cytoplasm antibody; *GBM*, glomerular basement membrane; *GN*, glomerulonephritis; *Ig*, immunoglobulin.
*Relative risk.

- Immunosuppressive treatment in patients with heavy proteinuria or rapidly decreasing glomerular filtration rate (high-dose steroids, cyclosporin A, cyclophosphamide); corticosteroids generally not useful in poststreptococcal glomerulonephritis
- Fish oil (n-3 fatty acids) 12 g/day: may prevent or slow down loss of renal function in patients with IgA nephropathy
- Plasma exchange therapy and immunosuppressive drugs (prednisone and cyclophosphamide): effective in Goodpasture's syndrome
- Short-term therapy with IV cyclophosphamide followed by maintenance therapy with mycophenolate mofetil or azathioprine is more efficacious and safer than long-term therapy with IV cyclophosphamide in patients with proliferative lupus nephritis

■ CHRONIC Rx

- Frequent monitoring of urinalysis, serum creatinine, and blood pressure in the initial 12 mo
- Monitoring for onset of hypertensive retinopathy, encephalopathy
- Aggressive treatment of infections, particularly streptococcal infections
- Dosage adjustment of all renally excreted medications

■ DISPOSITION

- Prognosis is generally related to histology with excellent prognosis in patients with minimal change glomerulonephritis and focal segmental proliferative glomerulonephritis; 25% to 30% of patients with mesangial IgA disease and membranous glomerulonephritis generally progress to chronic renal failure; >70% of patients with mesangial capillary glomerulonephritis will develop chronic renal failure.
- Generally prognosis is worse in patients with heavy proteinuria, severe hypertension, and significant elevations of creatinine.
- Recovery of renal function occurs within 8 to 12 wk in 95% of patients with poststreptococcal glomerulonephritis.

■ REFERRAL

- Nephrology consultation. The urgency for referral depends on the GFR. Urgent consultation is recommended if GFR is significantly abnormal, rapidly deteriorating, or if there are systemic symptoms
- Surgical referral for biopsy in selected cases

☼ PEARLS & CONSIDERATIONS

■ COMMENTS

- Anticoagulation to prevent DVT should be considered in patients with a low level of physical activity.
- Monitoring of lipids and aggressive treatment of hyperlipidemias is recommended.
- Close monitoring of side effects of immunosuppressive drugs and complications of corticosteroids is necessary.

REFERENCES

Contreras G et al: Sequential therapies for proliferative lupus nephritis, *N Engl J Med* 350:971, 2004.

Hricik D et al: Glomerulonephritis, *N Engl J Med* 339:888, 1998.

Madaio MP, Harrington JT: The diagnosis of glomerular diseases, *Arch Intern Med* 161:25, 2001.

Author: **Fred F. Ferri, M.D.**

📋 BASIC INFORMATION

■ DEFINITION

Glossitis is an inflammation of the tongue that can lead to loss of filiform papillae.

ICD-9CM CODES

529.0 Glossitis

■ EPIDEMIOLOGY & DEMOGRAPHICS

Glossitis is seen more frequently in patients of lower socioeconomic status, malnourished patients, alcoholics, smokers, elderly patients, immunocompromised patients, and patients with dentures.

■ PHYSICAL FINDINGS & CLINICAL PRESENTATION

- The appearance of the tongue is variable depending on the etiology of the glossitis. Loss of filiform papillae results in red, smooth-surfaced tongue (Fig. 1-124).

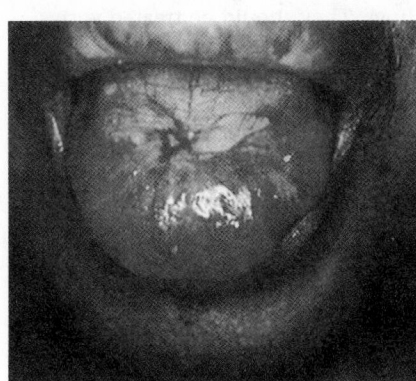

Fig. 1-124   Glossitis. (From Seidel HM [ed]: *Mosby's guide to physical examination,* ed 4, St Louis, 1999, Mosby.)

- The tongue may appear pale in patients with significant anemia.
- Pain and swelling of the tongue may be present when glossitis is associated with infections, trauma, or lichen planus.
- Ulcerations may be present in patients with herpetic glossitis, pemphigus, or streptococcal infection.
- Excessive use of mouthwash may result in a "hairy" appearance of the tongue.

■ ETIOLOGY

- Nutritional deficiencies (vitamin E, riboflavin, niacin, vitamin B_{12}, iron deficiency)
- Infections (viral, candidiasis, TB, syphilis)
- Trauma (generally caused by poorly fitting dentures)
- Irritation of the tongue secondary to toothpaste, medications, alcohol, tobacco, citrus
- Lichen planus, pemphigus vulgaris, erythema multiforme
- Neoplasms

🔬 DIAGNOSIS

■ DIFFERENTIAL DIAGNOSIS

- Infections
- Use of chemical irritants
- Neoplasms
- Skin disorders (e.g., Behçet's syndrome, erythema multiforme)

■ WORKUP

- Laboratory evaluation to exclude infectious processes, vitamin deficiencies, and systemic disorders
- Biopsy of lesion only when there is no response to treatment

■ LABORATORY TESTS

- CBC: Decreased Hgb and Hct, low MCV (iron deficiency anemia), elevated MCV (vitamin B_{12} deficiency)
- Vitamin B_{12} level
- 10% KOH scrapings in patients with white patches suspect for candidiasis

💊 TREATMENT

■ NONPHARMACOLOGIC THERAPY

Avoidance of primary irritants such as hot foods, spices, tobacco, and alcohol

■ ACUTE GENERAL Rx

Treatment varies with the etiology of the glossitis.
- Malnutrition with avitaminosis: multivitamins
- Candidiasis: fluconazole 200 mg on day 1, then 100 mg/day for at least 2 wk or nystatin 400,000 U suspension qid for 10 days or 200,000 pastilles dissolved slowly in the mouth four to five times qd for 10 to 14 days
- Painful oral lesions: rinsing of the mouth with 2% lidocaine viscous, 1 to 2 tablespoons q4h prn; triamcinolone 0.1% applied to painful ulcers prn for symptomatic relief

■ CHRONIC Rx

- Lifestyle changes with elimination of tobacco, alcohol, and other primary irritants
- Dental evaluation for correction of ill-fitting dentures
- Correction of associated metabolic abnormalities such as hyperglycemia from diabetes mellitus

■ DISPOSITION

Most patients experience prompt improvement with identification and treatment of the cause of the glossitis.

■ REFERRAL

Surgical referral for biopsy of solitary lesions unresponsive to treatment to rule out neoplasm

⚙ PEARLS & CONSIDERATIONS

■ COMMENTS

If the primary cause of glossitis is not identified or cannot be corrected, enteric nutritional replacement therapy should be considered in malnourished patients.

Author: **Fred F. Ferri, M.D.**

BASIC INFORMATION

■ DEFINITION
Gonorrhea is a sexually transmitted bacterial infection with a predilection for columnar and transitional epithelial cells. It commonly manifests as urethritis, cervicitis, or salpingitis. Infection may be asymptomatic. It differs in males and females in course, severity, and ease of recognition.

■ SYNONYMS
Gonococcal urethritis
Gonococcal vulvovaginitis
Gonococcal cervicitis
Gonococcal bartholinitis
Clap
GC

ICD-9CM CODES
098 Gonococcal infections

■ EPIDEMIOLOGY & DEMOGRAPHICS
- The disease is common worldwide, affects both sexes, all ages, especially younger adults; highest incidence is in inner-city areas, with an estimated 3 million new cases annually.
- Asymptomatic anterior urethral carriage may occur in 12% to 50% of cases in men.
- Asymptomatic in 50% to 80% of cases in women. Most common dissemination by mucosal passage to fallopian tubes, resulting in PID in 10% to 15% of infected women. Hematogenous spread may result in septic arthritis and skin lesions. Conjunctivitis rarely occurs but may result in blindness if not rapidly treated. Infection can occur in both men and women in oropharynx and anorectally.
- 600,000 new infections/yr.

■ PHYSICAL FINDINGS & CLINICAL PRESENTATION
- Males: purulent discharge from anterior urethra with dysuria appearing 2 to 7 days after infecting exposure. May have rectal infection causing pruritus, tenesmus, and discharge or may be asymptomatic.
- Females: initial urethritis, cervicitis may occur a few days after exposure, frequently mild. In about 20% of cases, uterine invasion occurs after menstrual period with signs and symptoms of endometritis, salpingitis, or pelvic peritonitis. The patient may have purulent discharge, inflamed Skene's or Bartholin's glands.

- Classic presentation of acute gonococcal PID is fever, abdominal and adnexal tenderness, often absence of purulent discharge. Physical examination may be normal if asymptomatic.

■ ETIOLOGY
Neisseria gonorrhoeae is the gonococcus. Plasmids coding for β-lactamase render some strains resistant to penicillin or tetracycline (PPNG, TRNG). There is an increasing frequency of chromosomally mediated resistance to penicillin, tetracycline, and cefoxitin. In the Far East, high-level resistance to spectinomycin is endemic.

There is a rising number of cases of quinolone-resistant *N. gonorrhoeae* (QRNG) worldwide, with the expected number to rise in the U.S. from importation. As long as the total number of QNRG strains remains less than 1% of strains isolated, fluoroquinolones may still be used with confidence.

🔬 DIAGNOSIS

■ DIFFERENTIAL DIAGNOSIS
- Nongonococcal urethritis (NGU)
- Nongonococcal mucopurulent cervicitis
- *Chlamydia trachomatis*

■ WORKUP
- Diagnosis is dependent on bacteriologic investigation.
- Gram-negative intracellular diplococci are diagnostic in male urethral smears. There is a false-negative rate of 60% to 70% in female cervical or urethral smears. Culture is essential in women.

■ LABORATORY TESTS
- Gonorrhea culture on Thayer-Martin medium (Organism is fastidious, requires aerobic conditions with increased carbon dioxide atmosphere. Incubate ASAP.)
- Serologic testing for syphilis on all patients
- *Chlamydia* testing on all patients
- Offer of HIV counseling and testing

💊 TREATMENT

■ ACUTE GENERAL Rx
Uncomplicated infections of the cervix, urethra, and rectum:
- Cefixime 400 mg PO × 1 dose *or*
- Ceftriaxone 125 mg IM × 1 dose *or*

- Ciprofloxacin 500 mg PO × 1 dose *or*
- Ofloxacin 400 mg PO × 1 dose *plus* azithromycin 1 g PO × 1 dose *or*
- Doxycycline 100 mg PO bid × 7 days
- Dual treatment with azithromax and doxycycline may prevent the development of antimicrobial resistant *N. gonorrhoeae.*

Alternatives: Spectinomycin 2 g IM × 1 dose
Quinolones:
- Gatifloxacin 400 mg PO × 1 dose
- Norfloxacin 800 mg PO × 1 dose
- Lomefloxacin 400 mg PO × 1 dose
- Not recommended for person <18 yr

Uncomplicated pharyngeal infection:
- Ceftriaxone 125 mg IM × 1 dose *or*
- Ciprofloxacin 500 mg PO × 1 dose *or*
- Ofloxacin 400 mg PO × 1 dose *plus* azithromycin 1 g PO × 1 dose *or*
- Doxycycline 100 mg PO bid × 7 days

Pregnancy: patients should not be treated with quinolones or tetracyclines. They should be treated with one of the previous recommended or alternative cephalosporins.

■ DISPOSITION
- Pregnant patients require test of cure (as do those treated with regimens other than ceftriaxone/doxycycline); reculture 4 to 7 days after treatment.
- Treatment failure in nonpregnant patients is rare, and test of cure is not required. Rescreening in 1 to 2 mo detects treatment failures and reinfections.
- Sexual partners should all be identified, examined, cultured, and receive presumptive treatment.

■ REFERRAL
PID requiring hospitalization, disseminated gonococcal infection

☼ PEARLS & CONSIDERATIONS

■ COMMENTS
- This is a reportable disease.

REFERENCE
Centers for Disease Control and Prevention: 2002 sexually transmitted diseases treatment guidelines, *MMWR Morb Mortal Wkly Rep* 51(RR-6), 2002.
Author: **Maria A. Corigliano, M.D.**

BASIC INFORMATION

■ DEFINITION
Goodpasture's syndrome is characterized by idiopathic recurrence of alveolar hemorrhage and rapidly progressive glomerulonephritis. It can also be defined by the triad of glomerulonephritis, pulmonary hemorrhage, and antibody to basement membrane antigens.

ICD-9CM CODES
446.2 Goodpasture's syndrome

■ EPIDEMIOLOGY & DEMOGRAPHICS
- Goodpasture's syndrome affects predominantly young white male smokers.
- Male:female ratio is 6:1.
- Goodpasture's syndrome accounts for 5% of all cases of rapidly progressive glomerulonephritis.
- 80% of patients are HLA-BR2 positive.

■ PHYSICAL FINDINGS & CLINICAL PRESENTATION
- Dyspnea, cough, hemoptysis
- Skin pallor, fever, arthralgias (may be mild or absent at the time of initial presentation)

■ ETIOLOGY
Presence of glomerular basement membranes (GBM) antibody deposition in kidneys and lungs with subsequent pulmonary hemorrhage and glomerulonephritis.

DIAGNOSIS

■ DIFFERENTIAL DIAGNOSIS
- Wegener's granulomatosis
- SLE
- Systemic necrotizing vasculitis
- Idiopathic rapidly progressive glomerulonephritis
- Drug-induced renal pulmonary disease (e.g., penicillamine)

■ WORKUP
Laboratory evaluation, diagnostic imaging, immunofluorescence studies of renal biopsy

■ LABORATORY TESTS
- Presence of circulating serum anti-GBM antibodies
- Absence of circulating immunocomplexes, antineutrophils, cytoplasmic antibodies, and cryoglobulins
- Urinalysis revealing microscopic hematuria and proteinuria
- Elevated BUN and creatinine from rapidly progressive glomerulonephritis
- Immunofluorescence studies of renal biopsy material: linear deposits of anti-GBM antibody, often accompanied by C3 deposition
- Anemia from iron deficiency (secondary to blood loss and iron sequestration in the lungs)

■ IMAGING STUDIES
Chest x-ray examination: fluffy alveolar infiltrates, evidence of pulmonary hemorrhage (Fig. 1-125)

TREATMENT

■ ACUTE GENERAL Rx
- Plasma exchange therapy
- Immunosuppressive therapy with prednisone (1 mg/kg/day) and cyclophosphamide (2 mg/kg/day)
- Dialysis support in patients with renal failure

■ DISPOSITION
Life-threatening pulmonary hemorrhage and irreversible glomerular damage are the major causes of death.

■ REFERRAL
- Surgical referral for renal biopsy to guide the management
- Referral of patients with renal failure to dialysis center
- Consideration for renal transplantation in patients with end-stage renal failure

Author: **Fred F. Ferri, M.D.**

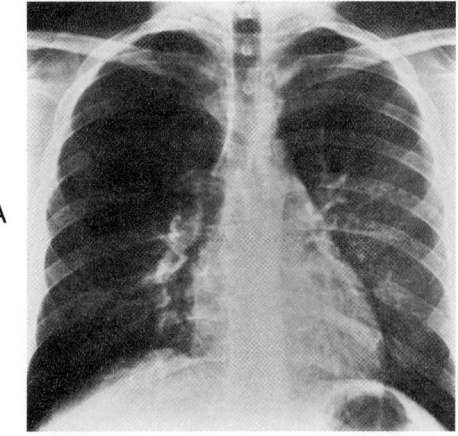
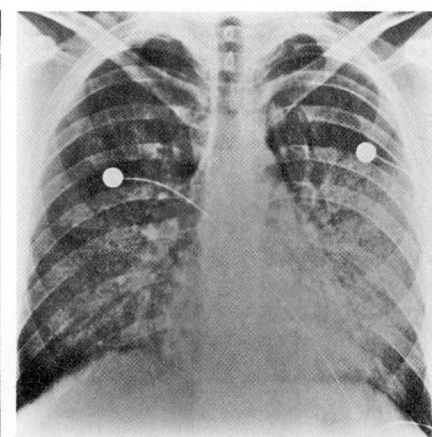

Fig. 1-125   Goodpasture's syndrome. PA chest radiographs several days apart demonstrate consolidation in the left lung, **A,** which progressed to diffuse alveolar disease (consolidation), **B.** (From McLoud TC [ed]: *Thoracic radiology: the requisites,* St Louis, 1998, Mosby.)

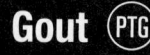 **BASIC INFORMATION**

■ **DEFINITION**

Gout is a clinical disorder in which crystals of monosodium urate become deposited in tissue as a result of hyperuricemia. Gout and hyperuricemia can be classified as either primary or secondary if resulting from another disorder.

ICD-9CM CODES
274.9 Gout

■ **EPIDEMIOLOGY & DEMOGRAPHICS**
PREVALENCE: 3 cases/1000 persons
PREDOMINANT SEX: 95% males, rare in females before menopause
PREDOMINANT AGE: 30 to 50 yr

■ **PHYSICAL FINDINGS & CLINICAL PRESENTATION**
• Usually, initial attack in a single joint or an area of tenosynovium
• Mainly a disease of the lower extremities
• First site of involvement: classically, MP joint of the great toe
• Another common site of acute attack: extensor tenosynovium on the dorsum of the midfoot
• Severe pain and inflammation, which may be precipitated by exercise, dietary indiscretions, and physical or emotional stress
• Attacks following illness or surgery
• Presence of swelling, heat, redness, and other signs of inflammation (the physical findings simulating cellulitis)
• Exquisite soft tissue tenderness
• Fever, tachycardia, and other constitutional symptoms
• Eventually, deposits of urate crystals (tophi) in the subcutaneous tissue

■ **ETIOLOGY**
• Hyperuricemia and gout develop from excessive uric acid production, a decrease in the renal excretion of uric acid, or both.
• Primary gout results from an inborn error of metabolism and may be attributed to several biochemical defects.

• Secondary hyperuricemia may develop as a complication of acquired disorders (e.g., leukemia) or as a result of the use of certain drugs (e.g., diuretics).

🔬 **DIAGNOSIS**

■ **DIFFERENTIAL DIAGNOSIS**
• Pseudogout
• Rheumatoid arthritis
• Osteoarthritis
• Cellulitis
• Infectious arthritis
Section II describes the differential diagnosis of acute monoarticular and oligoarticular arthritis.

■ **WORKUP**
Hyperuricemia accompanying a typical history of monoarticular acute arthritis is usually sufficient to establish the diagnosis.

■ **LABORATORY TESTS**
• Mild leukocytosis
• Elevated ESR
• Hyperuricemia
• Synovial aspirate: usually cloudy and markedly inflammatory in nature; urate crystals in fluid: needle-shaped and birefringent under polarized light

■ **IMAGING STUDIES**
• Plain radiography to rule out other disorders
• No typical findings in early gouty arthritis but late disease possibly associated with characteristic punched-out lesions and joint destruction

℞ **TREATMENT**

■ **NONPHARMACOLOGIC THERAPY**
• Modification of diet (avoidance of foods high in purines [e.g., anchovies, organ meat, liver, spinach, mushrooms, asparagus, oatmeal, cocoa, sweetbreads]) and lifestyle
• Treatment for obesity

• Moderation in alcohol intake, no more than two drinks per day
• Hypertension and its management requiring careful assessment and possibly nondiuretic drugs

■ **ACUTE GENERAL Rx**
• Quick-acting NSAIDs such as ibuprofen
• Colchicine (given PO or IV)
• Corticosteroids or ACTH for those who are intolerant of NSAIDs or colchicine
• Intraarticular cortisone when oral medication cannot be given
• General measures, such as rest, elevation, and analgesics as needed
• Table 1-24 describes treatment options for gout

■ **CHRONIC Rx**
• Prevention is achieved through normalization of serum urate concentration.
• Uricosuric agents (e.g., probenecid) or xanthine oxidase inhibitors (allopurinol) are used in patients with recurrent attacks despite adequate dietary restrictions.
• A 24-hr urine collection is useful in deciding which antihyperuricemic agent is indicated. Allopurinol is generally used if the uric acid output is >900 mg/day on a regular diet. However, hyperuricemic therapy should not be started for at least 2 wk after the acute attack has resolved because it may prolong the acute attack and it can also precipitate new attacks by rapidly lowering the serum uric acid level.
• Urinary uric acid hypoexcretors (<700 mg/day) can be given probenecid (250 mg bid for 1 wk, then increased to 500 mg bid) to block absorption of uric acid. Probenecid should be started only after the acute attack of gout has completely subsided.
• Colchicine 0.6 mg bid is indicated for acute gout prophylaxis before starting hyperuricemic therapy. It is generally discontinued 6 to 8 wk after normalization of serum urate levels. Long-term colchicine therapy (0.6 mg qd or bid) may be necessary in patients with frequent gout attacks despite the use of uricosuric agents.

- Surgery usually limited to excision of large tophi and, occasionally, arthroplasty.

■ DISPOSITION

- Musculoskeletal complications are usually limited to joint disease.
- Surgical intervention may occasionally be indicated.
- Renal disease is the most frequent complication of gout after arthritis; most gouty patients develop renal disease as a result of parenchymal urate deposition but the involvement is only slowly progressive and often has no effect on life expectancy.
- Incidence of urolithiasis is increased, with 80% of calculi being uric acid stones.

■ REFERRAL

For orthopedic consultation when joint destruction has occurred

☼ PEARLS & CONSIDERATIONS

■ COMMENTS

- No significant correlation between coronary artery disease and gout
- No indication to treat asymptomatic hyperuricemia
- Acute attacks of gout occasionally associated with normal levels of uric acid

REFERENCES

Agudelo CA, Wise CM: Crystal-associated arthritis in the elderly, *Rheum Dis Clin North Am* 26:527, 2000.

Agudelo CA, Wise CM: Gout: diagnosis, pathogenesis, and clinical manifestations, *Curr Opin Rheumatol* 13:234, 2001.

Schlesinger N, Schumacher HR: Gout: can management be improved? *Curr Opin Rheumatol* 13:240, 2001.

Schlesinger N et al: Local ice therapy during bouts of acute gouty arthritis, *J Rheumatol* 29:331, 2002.

Snaith ML: Gout: diet and uric acid revisited, *Lancet* 358:521, 2001.

Wortmann RL: Effective management of gout: an analogy, *Am J Med* 105:513, 1998.

Author: **Lonnie R. Mercier, M.D.**

TABLE 1-24 Treatment of Gout

ACUTE GOUT	INTERVAL GOUT	LONG-TERM TREATMENT
Therapeutic goal: Terminate acute inflammatory attack.	**Therapeutic goal:** Prevent recurrent attacks.	**Therapeutic goals:** Prevent attacks, resolve tophi, maintain serum urate at ≤6 mg/dl.
NSAIDs *(preferred):* Indomethacin, 50 mg qid, or ibuprofen, 800 mg tid (or other NSAIDs in full doses) *(lower dose in renal insufficiency; contraindicated with peptic ulcer disease).* *OR*	**Colchicine, oral:** 0.6-1.2 mg daily as prophylaxis against recurrent attacks.	**Colchicine, oral:** 0.6-1.2 mg daily for 1-2 wk before initiating hypouricemic therapy and for several months afterward to prevent recurrent attacks during initial period of hypouricemic therapy.
Colchicine, oral *(used infrequently):* 0.6–1.2 mg (1-2 tablets), then 0.6 mg (1 tablet) q1-2h until attack subsides or until nausea, diarrhea, or GI cramping develops. Maximum total dose, 4-6 mg. If ineffective in 48 hr, do not repeat.	**Hypouricemic agent:** Start only if indicated by frequent attacks, severe hyperuricemia, presence of tophi, urolithiasis, or urate overexcretion.	**Allopurinol:** Dose variable; usually 300 mg once daily, but up to 900 mg may be needed in occasional patient; dose should be reduced to 100 mg daily or every other day in patients with renal insufficiency. *OR*
Colchicine, IV *(only if oral medication is precluded):* 1-2 mg in 20 ml 0.9% saline infused slowly *(extravasation causes tissue necrosis);* dose may be repeated once in 6 hr. Few GI symptoms with IV use. Maximum total dose, 4 mg per attack. Monitor blood counts	**Other:** Diet—moderate protein, low fat; avoid excessive alcohol. Treat hypertension if present. High fluid intake to promote uric acid excretion in a dilute urine (for uric acid overexcretors).	**Uricosuric agent** *(reduced efficacy if creatinine clearance <80 ml; ineffective if <30 mL):* Probenecid, 0.5-1 g bid, or sulfinpyrazone, 100 mg tid or qid; usually well tolerated, but may cause headache, GI upset, rash.
Steroids *(if NSAIDs or colchicines are contraindicated or if oral medication is precluded, e.g., postoperatively):* Triamcinolone acetonide, 60 mg IM, *or* ACTH, 40 U IM *or* 25 U by slow IV infusion, *or* prednisone, 20-40 mg daily. Intra-articular steroids may be used to treat a single inflamed joint: triamcinolone hexacetonide, 5-20 mg, or dexamethasone phosphate, 1-6 mg.		**Other:** Diet—moderate protein, low fat; avoid excessive alcohol. Treat hypertension if present. For uric acid overexcretors or when initiating uricosuric agent: high fluid intake, particularly at night, to promote uric acid excretion in a dilute urine. Acetazolamide, 250 mg at bedtime, may be used to keep urine pH >6.
Hypouricemic agents: Of no benefit for inflammatory attack and may initiate recurrent attack. Should not be started until attack has resolved, but *ongoing use should not be interrupted during an attack.*		

From Goldman L, Ausiello D (eds): *Cecil textbook of medicine,* ed 22, Philadelphia, 2004, WB Saunders.
ACTH, Adrenocorticotropic hormone; *bid,* twice daily; *GI,* gastrointestinal; *IM,* intramuscularly; *IV,* intravenously; *NSAIDs,* nonsteroidal antiinflammatory drugs; *q1-2h,* every 1 to 2 hours; *qid,* four times daily; *tid,* three times daily.

BASIC INFORMATION

■ DEFINITION
A chronic, inflammatory disorder of the dermis.

ICD-9CM CODES
695.89 Granuloma annulare

■ EPIDEMIOLOGY & DEMOGRAPHICS
- Most common in children and young adults
- Female predominance (2:1)
- Disseminated form associated with diabetes mellitus
- Recurrent in 40% of affected individuals

■ PHYSICAL FINDINGS & CLINICAL PRESENTATION
- Start as small ring of colored skin or pale erythematous papules
- Coalesce and evolve into annular plaques over several weeks
- Plaques undergo central involution and increase in diameter over several months (0.5 to 5 cm) (Fig. 1-126)
- Most frequently found on the lateral and dorsal surfaces of the hands and feet
- Most lesions resolve spontaneously after several months

■ ETIOLOGY
Unknown, but may be related to vasculitis, trauma, monocyte activation, or delayed hypersensitivity.

DIAGNOSIS

■ DIFFERENTIAL DIAGNOSIS
- Tinea corporis
- Lichen planus
- Necrobiosis lipoidica diabeticorum
- Sarcoidosis
- Rheumatoid nodules
- Late secondary or tertiary syphilis

■ WORKUP
Diagnosis is based on clinical appearance and presentation.

■ LABORATORY TESTS
Biopsy shows collagen degeneration.

TREATMENT

■ NONPHARMACOLOGIC THERAPY
Reassurance

■ CHRONIC Rx
Intralesional steroid injection into elevated border with triamcinolone 2.5 to 10 mg/ml

■ DISPOSITION
Most lesions will resolve spontaneously within 2 yr.

■ REFERRAL
Dermatology referral recommended for symptomatic, disseminated disease

REFERENCE
Hsu S et al: Differential diagnosis of annular lesions, *Am Fam Physician* 64:284, 2001.
Author: **Jennifer R. Souther, M.D.**

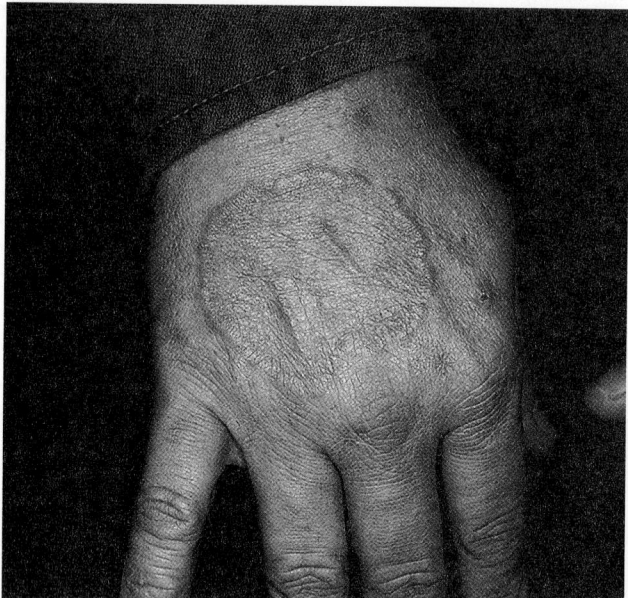
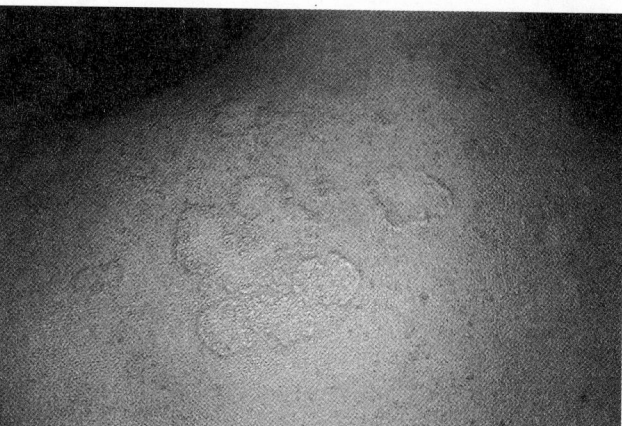

Fig. 1-126   Granuloma annulare. (From Callen JP [ed]: *Color atlas of dermatology,* ed 2, Philadelphia, 2000, WB Saunders.)

BASIC INFORMATION

■ DEFINITION
Granuloma inguinale is caused by a gram-negative bacterium, *Calymmatobacterium granulomatis,* that may be sexually transmitted, possibly by anal intercourse. It can also be spread through close, chronic nonsexual contact.

■ SYNONYMS
Donovanosis

ICD-9CM CODES
099.2 Granuloma inguinale

■ EPIDEMIOLOGY & DEMOGRAPHICS
- Rare in the U.S. (<100 cases reported annually) and other developed countries
- Endemic in Australia, India, Caribbean, and Africa
- Can affect both males and females
- Incubation period is variable: 1 to 2 wk

■ PHYSICAL FINDINGS & CLINICAL PRESENTATION
- Indurated nodule is the primary lesion and is usually painless.
- Lesion erodes to granulomatous heaped ulcer (Fig. 1-127); progresses slowly.

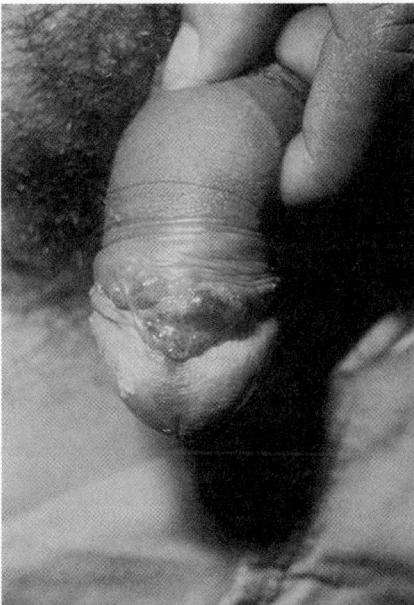

Fig. 1-127 Involvement of the penis, with a beefy red, granulomatous ulceration in a patient with granuloma inguinale. (From Goldstein B [ed]: *Practical dermatology,* ed 2, St Louis, 1997, Mosby.)

- Pathogenic features are as follows:
  1. Large infected mononuclear cell containing many Donovan bodies
  2. Intracytoplasmic location

■ ETIOLOGY
Calymmatobacterium granulomatis is a gram-negative bacillus that reproduces within PMNs, plasma cells, and histiocytes, causing the infected cells to rupture 20 to 30 organisms.

DIAGNOSIS

■ DIFFERENTIAL DIAGNOSIS
- Carcinoma
- Secondary syphilis: condylomata lata
- Amebiasis: necrotic ulceration
- Concurrent infections
- Lymphogranuloma venereum
- Chancroid
- Genital herpes

■ WORKUP
- Check for clinical manifestations.
  1. Lesions bleed easily.
  2. Lesions sharply defined and painless.
  3. Secondary infection may ensue.
  4. Inguinal involvement may cause pseudobuboes.
  5. Elephantiasis can result from obstruction of lymphatics.
  6. Suppuration and sinus formation are rare in female patients.
- Screen for other sexually transmitted diseases.
- Exclude other causes of lesions.
- Obtain stained, crushed prep from lesion.
- A clinical algorithm for evaluation of genital ulcer disease is described in Section III, Fig. 3-79.
Section II describes the differential diagnosis of genital sores.

■ LABORATORY TESTS
Wright stain: observation of Donovan bodies (intracellular bacteria); organisms in vacuoles within macrophages

TREATMENT

■ ACUTE GENERAL Rx
Recommended regimens:
- Doxycycline 100 mg orally bid × 3 wk minimum
- Trimethoprim/sulfamethoxazole, one double-strength tablet orally bid × 3 wk minimum

Alternative regimens:
- Ciprofloxacin 750 mg PO bid × 3 wk
- Erythromycin base 500 mg PO od × 3 wk
- Azithromycin 1 g PO/wk × 3 wk
- All gentamycin 1 mg/kg IV q8h if no improvement within the first few days of therapy

■ CHRONIC Rx
If there is a poor initial response, extend treatment. Treatment of relapses is often necessary. Patients should be counseled to avoid risky sex practices and not resume having sex until infection is cleared.

■ DISPOSITION
Follow clinically until signs and symptoms have resolved, then routine annual or semiannual visits

■ REFERRAL
If response is poor, consider referral to infectious disease specialist.

☿ PEARLS & CONSIDERATIONS

■ COMMENTS
- Sexual partners should be examined and offered therapy.
- Pregnant women should be treated with erythromycin regimen.
- Patient education material can be obtained from local and state health clinics and also from ACOG.

REFERENCES
Centers for Disease Control and Prevention: 2002 sexually transmitted diseases treatment guidelines, *MMWR Morb Mortal Wkly Rep* 51(RR-6), 2002.
Mead PB et al: *Protocols for infectious diseases in obstetrics and gynecology,* ed 2, Cambridge, Mass, 2000, Blackwell Science.
Author: **George T. Danakas, M.D.**

BASIC INFORMATION

■ DEFINITION
Graves' disease is a hypermetabolic state characterized by thyrotoxicosis, diffuse goiter, and infiltrative ophthalmopathy (edema and inflammation of the extraocular muscles and an increase in orbital connective tissue and fat); infiltrative dermopathy characterized by lymphocytic infiltration of the dermis, accumulation of glycosaminoglycans, and edema is occasionally present.

■ SYNONYMS
Thyrotoxicosis

ICD-9CM CODES
242.0 Toxic diffuse goiter

■ EPIDEMIOLOGY & DEMOGRAPHICS
INCIDENCE/PREVALENCE:
Hyperthyroidism affects 2% of women and 0.2% of men in their lifetimes. More than 80% of these cases are caused by Graves' disease.
PREDOMINANT AGE: Most common before age 50 yr
GENETICS: Increased prevalence of HLA-B8 and HLA-DR3 in whites with Graves' disease. Concordance rate is 20% among monozygotic twins.

■ PHYSICAL FINDINGS & CLINICAL FINDINGS
- Tachycardia, palpitations, tremor, hyperreflexia
- Goiter, exophthalmos (50% of patients), lid retraction, lid lag
- Nervousness, weight loss, heat intolerance, atrial fibrillation
- Increased sweating, brittle nails, clubbing of fingers
- Nervousness, weight loss, heat intolerance, and atrial fibrillation
- Localized dermopathy (1% to 2% of patients) is most frequent over the anterolateral aspects of the skin but can be found at other sites (especially after trauma)

■ ETIOLOGY
Autoimmune etiology: the activity of the thyroid gland is stimulated by the action of T cells, which induce specific B cells to synthesize antibodies against TSH receptors in the follicular cell membrane.

DIAGNOSIS

■ DIFFERENTIAL DIAGNOSIS
- Anxiety disorder
- Premenopausal state
- Thyroiditis
- Other causes of hyperthyroidism (e.g., toxic multinodular goiter, toxic adenoma)
- Other: metastatic neoplasm, diabetes mellitus, pheochromocytoma

■ WORKUP
The diagnostic workup includes a detailed medical history followed by laboratory and imaging studies. Patients often present with anxiety, heat intolerance, menstrual dysfunction, increased appetite, and weight loss. Elderly patients can have an atypical presentation (apathetic hyperparathyroidism). For additional information, refer to the topic "Hyperthyroidism."

■ LABORATORY TESTS
- Increased free thyroxine (T_4) and free triiodothyronine (T_3)
- Decreased TSH
- Presence of thyroid autoantibodies (useful in selected patients to differentiate Graves' disease from toxic nodular goiter)

■ IMAGING STUDIES
- 24-hr radioactive iodine uptake (RAIU): increased homogeneous uptake
- CT or MRI of the orbits is useful if there is uncertainty about the cause of ophthalmopathy

TREATMENT

■ NONPHARMACOLOGIC THERAPY
Patient education and discussion of therapeutic options

■ ACUTE GENERAL Rx
- Antithyroid drugs (ATDs) to inhibit thyroid hormone synthesis or peripheral conversion of T_4 to T_3
  1. Propylthiouracil (PTU) 50 to 100 mg q8h or methimazole (Tapazole) 10 to 20 mg q8h for 6 to 24 mo
  2. Side effects: skin rash (3% to 5%), arthralgias, myalgias, granulocytopenia (0.5%); rare side effects: aplastic anemia, hepatic necrosis (PTU), cholestatic jaundice (methimazole)
- Radioactive iodine (RAI)
  1. Treatment of choice for patients >21 yr of age and younger patients who have not achieved remission after 1 yr of ATD therapy
  2. Contraindicated during pregnancy and lactation
- Surgery: near-total thyroidectomy is rarely performed; indications: obstructing goiters despite RAI and ATD therapy, patients who refuse RAI and cannot be adequately managed with ATDs, and pregnant women inadequately managed with ATDs
- Adjunctive therapy: propranolol (20 to 40 mg q6h) to alleviate the β-adrenergic symptoms of hyperthyroidism (tachycardia, tremor); contraindicated in patients with CHF and bronchospasm
- Graves' ophthalmopathy: methylcellulose eye drops to protect against excessive dryness, sunglasses to decrease photophobia, systemic high-dose corticosteroids for severe exophthalmos; worsening of ophthalmopathy after RAI therapy often transient and can be prevented by the administration of prednisone

■ CHRONIC Rx
Patients undergoing treatment with ATDs should be seen every 1 to 3 mo until euthyroidism is achieved and every 3 to 4 mo while they are receiving ATDs.

■ DISPOSITION
- ATDs induce sustained remission in <60% of cases.
- The incidence of hypothyroidism post RAI is >50% within first year and 2%/yr thereafter.
- Complications of surgery include hypothyroidism (28% to 43% after 10 yr), hypoparathyroidism, and vocal cord paralysis (1%).
- Successful treatment of hyperthyroidism requires lifelong monitoring for the onset of hypothyroidism or the recurrence of thyrotoxicosis.
- RAI therapy is followed by the appearance or worsening of ophthalmopathy more often than is therapy with methimazole, particularly in patients who are cigarette smokers. It can be prevented with the administration of prednisone 0.5 mg/kg of body weight per day starting 2 to 3 days post RAI, continued for 1 mo, then tapered off over 2 mo.
- Mild to moderate ophthalmopathy often improves spontaneously. Severe cases can be treated with high-dose glucocorticoids, orbital irradiation, or both. Orbital decompression may be used in patients with optic neuropathy and exophthalmos.

REFERENCE
Weetman AP: Graves' disease, *N Engl J Med* 343:1236, 2000.
Author: **Fred F. Ferri, M.D.**

BASIC INFORMATION

■ DEFINITION

Guillain-Barré syndrome (GBS) is an acute immune-mediated polyradiculoneuropathy (affects nerve roots and peripheral nerves), with predominant motor involvement. Maximal clinical weakness occurs within 4 wk of disease onset.

■ SYNONYMS

Acute polyneuropathy
Ascending paralysis
Postinfectious polyneuritis

ICD-9CM CODES

357.0 Guillain-Barré

■ EPIDEMIOLOGY & DEMOGRAPHICS

INCIDENCE: 0.6-1.9 cases/100,000 persons annually. Incidence increases with age.
PREDISPOSING FACTORS: Viral (HIV, CMV, EBV, influenza) and bacterial (*Campylobacter jejuni, Mycoplasma pneumonia*) infections; systemic illness (Hodgkin's lymphoma, immunizations)

■ PHYSICAL FINDINGS & CLINICAL PRESENTATION

- Symmetric weakness, initially involving proximal muscles, subsequently involving both proximal and distal muscles; difficulty in ambulating, getting up from a chair, or climbing stairs
- Depressed or absent reflexes bilaterally
- Minimal to moderate glove and stocking paresthesias/dysesthesia/anesthesia and/or back pain
- Pain (caused by involvement of posterior nerve roots) may be prominent
- Autonomic abnormalities (brady- or tachyarrhythmias, hypo- or hypertension)
- Respiratory insufficiency (caused by weakness of bulbar/intercostal muscles)
- Facial paresis, ophthalmoparesis, dysphagia (secondary to cranial nerve involvement)

■ ETIOLOGY

Unknown. Preceding infectious illness 1-4 wk before disease onset in 66% of patients. Humoral and cell-mediated immune attack of peripheral nerve myelin, Schwann cells; sometimes with axonal involvement

DIAGNOSIS

■ DIFFERENTIAL DIAGNOSIS

- Toxic peripheral neuropathies: heavy metal poisoning (lead, thallium, arsenic), medications (vincristine, disulfiram), organophosphate poisoning, hexacarbon (glue sniffer's neuropathy)
- Nontoxic peripheral neuropathies: acute intermittent porphyria, vasculitic polyneuropathy, infectious (poliomyelitis, diphtheria, Lyme disease); tick paralysis
- Neuromuscular junction disorders: myasthenia gravis, botulism, snake envenomations
- Myopathies; such as polymyositis, acute necrotizing myopathies caused by drugs
- Metabolic derangements such as hypermagnesemia, hypokalemia, hypophosphatemia
- Acute central nervous system disorders such as basilar artery thrombosis with brainstem infarction, brainstem encephalomyelitis, transverse myelitis, or spinal cord compression
- Hysterical paralysis or malingering

■ WORKUP

1. Exclude other causes based on clinical history, examination, and laboratory tests.
2. Lumbar puncture (may be normal in the first 1-2 wk of the illness)
- Typical findings include elevated CSF protein with few mononuclear leukocytes (albuminocytologic dissociation) in 80%-90% of patients. Elevated CSF cell counts is an expected feature in cases associated with HIV seroconversion.
3. EMG/NCS: May be normal in the first 10-14 days of the disease. The earliest electrodiagnostic abnormality is prolongation or absence of H-reflexes.

■ LABORATORY TESTS

- CBC may reveal early leukocytosis with left shift. Electrolytes to exclude metabolic causes
- Heavy metal testing, urine porphyria screen, creatine kinase, HIV titers, neuroimaging of the brain and spinal cord if diagnosis uncertain

TREATMENT

■ NONPHARMACOLOGIC THERAPY

- Close monitoring of respiratory function (frequent measurements of vital capacity, negative inspiratory force and pulmonary toilet), because respiratory failure is the major complication in GBS
- Frequent repositioning of patient to minimize formation of pressure sores
- Prevention of thromboembolism with antithrombotic stockings and SC heparin (5000 U q12h) in nonambulatory patients
- Emotional support and social counseling

■ ACUTE GENERAL Rx

- Infusion of IV immunoglobulins (IVIg; 0.4 g/kg/day for 5 days). Always check serum IgA levels before infusion to prevent anaphylaxis in deficient patients.
- Early therapeutic plasma exchange (TPE or plasmapheresis: 200-250mL/kg over 5 sessions qod), started within 7 days of onset of symptoms, is beneficial in preventing paralytic complications in patients with rapidly progressive disease. It is contraindicated in patients with cardiovascular disease (recent MI, unstable angina), active sepsis, and autonomic dysfunction.
- Mechanical ventilation may be needed if FVC is <12 to 15 ml/kg, vital capacity is rapidly decreasing or is <1000 ml, negative inspiratory force < -20 cm H_2O, Pao_2 is <70, the patient is having significant difficulty clearing secretions or is aspirating.

■ CHRONIC Rx

- Ventilatory support: may be necessary in 10% to 20% of patients. Adequate fluid/electrolyte support and nutrition necessary, especially in patients with dysautonomia or bulbar dysfunction
- Aggressive nursing care to prevent decubiti, infections, fecal impactions, and pressure nerve palsies
- Monitoring and treatment of autonomic dysfunction (bradyarrhythmias or tachyarrhythmias, orthostatic hypotension, systemic hypertension, altered sweating)
- Treatment of back pain and dysesthesia with low-dose tricyclics, gabapentin, etc.
- Stress ulcer prevention in patients receiving ventilator support
- Physical and occupational therapy rehabilitation, including supportive devices

■ DISPOSITION

- Mortality is approximately 5%-10%. A recent study showed 62% complete recovery, 14% mild weakness, 9% moderate weakness, 4% bedbound or ventilated, and 8% dead at 1 yr.
- Predictors for poor recovery (inability to walk independently at 1 yr): age >60 yr, preceding diarrheal illness, recent CMV infection, fulminant or rapidly progressing course, ventilatory dependence, reduced motor amplitudes (<20% normal), or inexcitable nerves on NCS.

■ REFERRAL

Tracheostomy may be necessary in patients with prolonged ventilatory support. Percutaneous endoscopic gastrostomy may be temporarily required.

⚙ PEARLS & CONSIDERATIONS

■ COMMENTS

Patient education information may be obtained from the Guillain-Barré Foundation International, Box 262, Wynnewood, PA 19096; phone: (610) 667-0131.

REFERENCE

Gorson KC, Ropper AH: Guillain-Barré syndrome (acute inflammatory demyelinating neuropathy) and related disorders. In: Katirji B et al. (eds): *Neuromuscular disorders in clinical practice.* Boston, 2002, Butterworth-Heinemann.

Author: **Eroboghene E. Ubogu, M.D.**

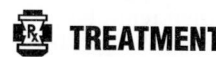

 BASIC INFORMATION

■ DEFINITION

Hand-foot-mouth (HFM) disease is a viral illness that is characterized by superficial lesions of the oral mucosa and of the skin of the extremities. HFM is highly contagious. Although children are predominantly affected, adults are also at risk. This disease is usually self-limited and benign.

■ SYNONYMS

Vesicular stomatitis with exanthem
Coxsackievirus infection

ICD-9CM CODES

074.0 Hand-foot-mouth disease

■ EPIDEMIOLOGY & DEMOGRAPHICS

- Children under the age of 5 yr are at the highest risk and have the most severe cases
- HFM is usually found in children below the age of 10 yr.
- Close contacts of affected children, including family members and health care workers, are the most commonly affected adults.
- Outbreaks tend to occur during the summer.
- Infection leads to immunity, but a second episode may occur after infection with a different agent.

■ PHYSICAL FINDINGS & CLINICAL PRESENTATION

Symptoms:
- After a 3-day incubation period, patients may complain of odynophagia, sore throat, malaise, and fever (38.3-40° C) and anorexia.
- One to 2 days later the characteristic oral lesions appear.
- In 75% of cases, skin lesions on the extremities accompany these oral manifestations.
- 11% of adults have cutaneous findings.
- Lesions appear over the course of 1 or 2 days.
Physical findings:
- Oral lesions, usually between five and ten, are commonly found on the tongue, buccal mucosa, gingivae, and hard palate.
- Oral lesions initially start as 1- to 3-mm erythematous macules and evolve into gray vesicles on an erythematous base.
- Vesicles are frequently broken by the time of presentation and appear as superficial gray ulcers with surrounding erythema.

- Skin lesions of the hands and feet start as linear erythematous papules (3 to 10 mm in diameter) that evolve into gray vesicles that may be mildly painful (Fig. 1-128). These vesicles are usually intact at presentation and remain so until they desquamate within 2 wk.
- Involvement of the buttocks and perineum is present in 31% of cases.
- In rare cases, encephalitis, meningitis, myocarditis, and pulmonary edema may develop.
- Spontaneous abortion may occur if the infection takes place early in pregnancy.

■ ETIOLOGY

Coxsackievirus group A, type 16, was the first and is the most common viral agent isolated. Coxsackieviruses A5, A7, A9, A10, B1, B2, B3, B5, and enterovirus 71 have also been implicated.

🔬 DIAGNOSIS

■ DIFFERENTIAL DIAGNOSIS

- Aphthous stomatitis
- Herpes simplex infection
- Herpangina
- Behçet's disease
- Erythema multiforme
- Pemphigus
- Gonorrhea
- Acute leukemia
- Lymphoma
- Allergic contact dermatitis

■ WORKUP

The diagnosis is usually made on the basis of history and characteristic physical examination.

■ LABORATORY TESTS

Not indicated unless the diagnosis is in doubt
Throat culture or stool specimen may be obtained for viral testing

💊 TREATMENT

■ ACUTE GENERAL Rx

- Palliative therapy is given for this usually self-limited disease.
- One small, uncontrolled case series reported a decrease in duration of symptoms in response to acyclovir.

■ DISPOSITION

Prognosis is excellent except in rare cases of CNS or cardiac involvement. Most are managed as outpatients.

■ REFERRAL

Not usually needed

REFERENCE

Chang LY et al: Clinical features and risk of pulmonary edema after enterovirus-related hand, foot, and mouth disease, *Lancet* 354(9191):1682, 1999.

Authors: **James J. Ng, M.D., and Jennifer Jeremiah, M.D.**

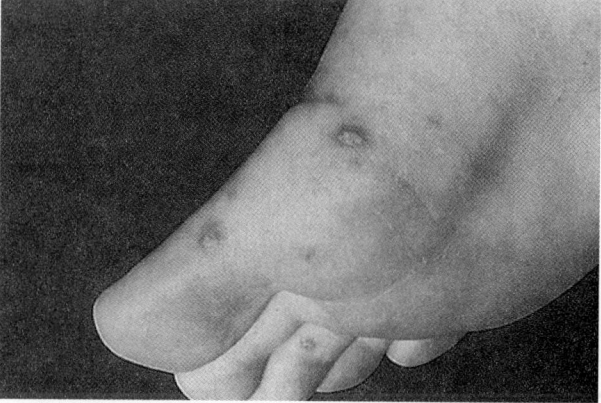

Fig. 1-128   Hand-foot-mouth disease. Note oval lesions on an erythematous base. (From Goldstein B [ed]: *Practical dermatology,* ed 2, St Louis, 1997, Mosby.)

BASIC INFORMATION

■ DEFINITION
The term *cluster headache* refers to recurrent episodes of intense, unilateral, orbitotemporal headache lasting 30 to 120 min with associated autonomic dysfunction. Headaches occur in clusters lasting up to 1 yr, during which one to three episodes occur per day at predictable times, typically during sleep. The episodes then remit for months to years. See Box 1-9 for the IHS classification for cluster headache.

ICD-9CM CODES
346.2 Variants of migraine

■ EPIDEMIOLOGY & DEMOGRAPHICS
- Estimated to occur in 0.05% to 1% of the population with males at least five times more common than females
- Peak age of onset between 25 and 50 yr.

■ PHYSICAL FINDINGS & CLINICAL PRESENTATION
- During attack: ipsilateral conjunctival injection, lacrimation, nasal congestion, rhinorrhea, facial sweating, Horner's syndrome.
- In contrast to migraine sufferers, patients are agitated and active during an attack.
- Permanent partial Horner's syndrome in 5% of patients; otherwise examination normal.

■ ETIOLOGY
Unknown

DIAGNOSIS

■ DIFFERENTIAL DIAGNOSIS
- Migraine
- Trigeminal neuralgia
- Temporal arteritis
- Postherpetic neuralgia
- Pheochromocytoma
- Glaucoma
- Section II describes the differential diagnosis of headaches

■ WORKUP
Diagnosis is usually established by characteristic history.

■ IMAGING STUDIES
None, unless history or examination suggests focal neurological deficit

TREATMENT

■ NONPHARMACOLOGIC THERAPY
Avoidance of ethanol and tobacco during clusters

■ ABORTIVE Rx
- Inhalation of 100% oxygen by face mask at 8 to 10 L/min for 15 min often aborts an attack.

- Triptans Cafergot or dihydroergotamine may abort an attack or prevent one if given just before a predictable episode. Acute episode is typically resolved before oral analgesics become effective, although idomethacin and other NSAIDS may also be effective in prolonged attacks.

■ PROPHYLAXIS Rx
Various medications have been tried without great success, although good responses may be obtained in up to 50% of cases. Examples include:
- Verapamil: up to 480 mg/day as tolerated (the drug of choice)
- Lithium: 200 mg tid with frequent monitoring and adjustment to maintain therapeutic serum level of 0.4 to 1 mEq/L. Equally effective as verapamil, but more side effects
- Methysergide: 1 to 2 mg tid; requires familiarity with the potential adverse effects and use of "drug holidays" to decrease risk of fibrosis
- Ergotamine tartrate: 3-4 mg/day during clusters
- Prednisone: 60 mg po qd x 1 wk followed by taper. Headaches can return during taper

■ DISPOSITION
Headache-free periods tend to increase with increasing age.

■ REFERRAL
- Refractory cluster headaches
- If surgical opinion is desired for medication failure

REFERENCES
Ekbom K, Hardebo JE: Cluster headache: aetiology, diagnosis and management, *Drugs* 62(1):61, 2002.
Weiss HD: The treatment of migraine and cluster headaches. In Johnson RT et al. (eds): *Current therapy in neurologic disease.* Philadelphia, 2002, Mosby.
Author: **Chun Lim, M.D., Ph.D.**

BOX 1-9 International Headache Criteria for Cluster Headache

Severe unilateral orbital, supraorbital, or temporal pain peaking in 10 to 15 min and lasting 30 to 45 min (occasionally up to 180 min). Pain rapidly resolves. Cluster headaches have a propensity to occur at night and may lead to sleep deprivation. Cycles generally last for a few weeks or months but may last for more than 1 yr.

Headache is associated with at least one of the following on the painful side:
- Conjunctival injection
- Rhinorrhea
- Lacrimation
- Miosis
- Nasal congestion
- Ptosis
- Forehead and facial sweating
- Eyelid edema

Additionally:
- Frequency of attacks ranges from one to eight daily.
- There have been at least five episodes of headache.

From Graber MA: *The family practice handbook,* ed 4, St Louis, 2001, Mosby.

BASIC INFORMATION

■ DEFINITION
Migraine headaches are recurrent headaches that are preceded by an aura (migraine with aura), occur independently (migraine without aura), or have atypical presentations (migraine variants). Migraine with aura typically has a visual aura that develops or marches gradually over more than 5 min. Migraine without aura is often unilateral, pulsatile, and associated with nausea and vomiting and photophobia and phonophobia. See Boxes 1-10 and 1-11 for IHS classification of migraine.

ICD-9CM CODES
346 Migraine

■ EPIDEMIOLOGY & DEMOGRAPHICS
PREVALENCE (IN U.S.): Females: 18%; males: 6%
PREDOMINANT SEX: Female:male ratio of 3:1
INCIDENCE: Increases from infancy, peaks during the third decade of life then decreases
GENETICS:
- Familial predisposition, with over 50% of migraine sufferers having an affected family member
- Autosomal dominant transmission for some rare migraine variants

(Familial hemiplegic migraine, CADASIL)

■ PHYSICAL FINDINGS & CLINICAL PRESENTATION
- Normal between episodes
- Normal for migraine without aura. Focal motor or sensory abnormalities possible with migraine with aura or migraine variants
- Common aura types include scintillating scotomata, bright zigzags, homonymous visual disturbance, hemisensory disturbance, speech disturbances, and hemiparesis

■ ETIOLOGY
A primary neuronal event resulting in a trigeminovascular reflex causing neurogenic inflammation. Serotonin also plays a role but exact mechanism is unknown.

DIAGNOSIS

■ DIFFERENTIAL DIAGNOSIS
- Subarachnoid hemorrhage
- Cluster headache
- Chronic daily headaches (drug rebound headaches)
- Arteriovenous malformation
- Vasculitis
- Tumor
- Section II describes the differential diagnosis of headaches

■ WORKUP
- Generally no additional investigation is needed with recurrent, typical attacks with usual age of onset, family history, and a normal physical examination.
- If there is an unusual presentation and/or unexpected findings on examination, investigation for other causes is required.

■ LABORATORY TESTS
Lumbar puncture for history of abrupt onset headaches and uncertain diagnosis of migraine

■ IMAGING STUDIES
- Imaging should be done in patients with headaches and an unexplained abnormal finding on the neurological examination.
- Imaging should be considered in patients with rapidly increasing headache frequency, history of dizziness or incoordination, subjective numbness or tingling, headache causing wakening from sleep, or headaches worsening with Valsalva maneuver.

BOX 1-10 International Headache Society Criteria for Migraine without Aura

Migraine without aura must have at least five attacks meeting the following criteria:
Headache attacks last 4 to 72 hr
Headache has at least two of the following:
- Unilateral location
- Pulsating quality
- Moderate or severe intensity (inhibits daily activity)
- Aggravation by routine physical activity
During the headache, at least one of the following:
- Nausea or vomiting
- Photophobia and phonophobia
No organic etiology found by history, physical, or neurologic examination

From Graber MA: *The family practice handbook,* ed 4, St Louis, 2001, Mosby.

BOX 1-11 International Headache Society Criteria for Migraine with Aura

Migraine with aura must have at least two attacks fulfilling the following criteria:
At least three of the following are present:
- One or more fully reversible aura symptoms indicating focal cerebral cortical or brainstem dysfunction
- At least one aura symptom develops gradually over more than 4 min
- No aura symptom lasts more than 60 min (duration proportionally increases if more than one aura symptom present)
- HA follows the aura within 60 min (but HA may begin before or with the aura); HA usually lasts 4 to 72 hr but may have only the aura
- No organic etiology found by history, physical, or neurologic examination
Note: Common aura types include scintillating scotomata, multiple small dots, homonymous visual disturbance, hemisensory disturbance, difficulty communicating, and occasionally vertigo.

From Graber MA: *The family practice handbook,* ed 4, St Louis, 2001, Mosby.
HA, Headache.

TREATMENT

Consider the use of a headache log/diary to identify triggers of headaches, to record efficacy of treatments, and to track history of the headaches.

■ NONPHARMACOLOGIC THERAPY

- Avoid any identifiable provoking factors: caffeine, tobacco, and alcohol may trigger attacks, as may dietary or other environmental precipitants (less common)
- Avoid stressors in life and minimize variations in daily routine with regular sleep, meals, and exercise
- Relaxation training and biofeedback

■ ACUTE ANALGESIC Rx

- Many oral agents are ineffective because of poor absorption secondary to migraine-induced gastric stasis. Nonoral route of administration should be selected in patients with severe nausea or vomiting
- Nonspecific treatment for pain.
- Acetaminophen, NSAIDS, combination analgesics, benzodiazepines, opioids, barbiturates

■ ACUTE ABORTIVE Rx

- Intravenous antiemetics (prochlorperazine, metoclopramide, domperidone). Acute dystonic reactions and akathisia are rare side effects. Generally not used as monotherapy
- Triptans (SC, PO, and Intranasal), ergotamine and ergotamine combinations (PO/PR), and dihydroergotamine (DHE 45) (SC, IV, IM, Nasal) all have well-documented efficacy against migraines (less so with ergotamines). DHE 45 usually administered in combination with an antiemetic drug (Table 1-25)
- Early administration improves effectiveness

■ PROPHYLAXIS Rx

- Prophylactic treatment is generally indicated when headaches occur more than once a week or when symptomatic treatments are contraindicated or not effective. They are most effective when initiated during headache-free period. All prophylaxis should be maintained for at least 3 mo before deeming the medication a failure.
- Well-established options for prophylactic treatment include β-blockers (propanolol, timolol, atenolol, metoprolol), tricyclic antidepressants (amitriptyline), and the antiepileptic drug valproic acid.
- Less established options include Ca-channel blockers, SSRI, the antiepileptic drugs gabapentin and topiramate.

■ DISPOSITION

After age 30 yr, 40% of patients are migraine free.

■ REFERRAL

If uncertain about diagnosis or treatment not effective

⚙ PEARLS & CONSIDERATIONS

- Avoid overuse of narcotics, barbiturates, caffeine, and benzodiazepines, as they are habit-forming.
- Chronic use of analgesic medications can result in drug-induced or rebound headaches.

REFERENCES

Ferrari MD et al: Migraine—current understanding and treatment, *N Engl J Med* 346:257, 2002.
Silberstein SD, for the US Headache Consortium: Practice parameter: Evidence-based guidelines for migraine headache (an evidence based review), *Neurology* 55:754, 2000.
Author: **Chun Lim, M.D., Ph.D.**

TABLE 1-25 Abortive and Analgesic Therapy for Migraine*

DRUG	DOSE	ROUTE
Triptans (serotonin agonists)		
Sumatriptan	6 mg, repeat in 2 hr (max 2 doses/day)	Subcutaneous
Sumatriptan	25 mg, 50 mg, 100 mg, repeat in 2 hr (max 200 mg/day)	Oral
Sumatriptan	5 mg and 20 mg, repeat in 2 hr (max 200 mg/day)	Nasal spray
Zolmitriptan	2.5 mg, 5 mg, repeat in 2 hr (max 10 mg/day)	Oral
Naratriptan	1 mg, 2.5 mg, repeat in 2 hr (max 5 mg/day)	Oral
Rizatriptan	5 mg, 10 mg, repeat in 2 hr (max 30 mg/day)	Oral
Almotriptan	6.25 mg, 12.5 mg, may repeat in 1 hr (max 25 mg/day)	Oral
Eletriptan	20 mg, 40 mg, may repeat in 2 hr (max 80 mg/day)	Oral
Frovatriptan	2.5 mg, may repeat in 2 hr (max 7.5 mg/day)	Oral
Ergotamine preparations		
Ergotamine and caffeine	2 tablets, repeat in 1 hr; max 4/day	Oral
Ergotamine and caffeine	1 suppository, repeat in 1 hr; max 2/day	Rectal
Ergotaminel	1 tablet, repeat in 1 hr; max 2/day	Sublingual
Dihydroergotamine	0.5-1.0 mg, repeat twice at 1-hr intervals (max 3 mg/attack)	Intramuscular
		Subcutaneous
		Intravenous
Sympathomimetics (with or without barbiturates or codeine)		
Isometheptene	2 capules, repeat in 1 hr, max 2/day	Oral
Acetaminophen	2 capsules, repeat in 1 hr, max 2/day	Oral
Dichloralphenazone	2 capsules, repeat in 1 hr, max 2/day	Oral
Nonsteroidal antiinflammatory drugs		
Naproxen	550-750 mg, repeat in 1 hr; max 3 times/wk	Oral
Meclofenamate	100-200 mg, repeat in 1 hr; max 3 times/wk	Oral
Flurbiprofen	50-100 mg, repeat in 1 hr; max 3 times/wk	Oral
Ibuprofen	200-300 mg, repeat in 1 hr; max 3 times/wk	Oral
Antiemetics		
Promethazine	50-125 mg	Oral
		Intramuscular
Prochlorperazine	1-25 mg	Oral
	2.5-25 mg (suppository)	Rectal
	5-10 mg	Intramuscular
Chlorpromazine	10-25 mg	Oral
	50-100 mg (suppository)	Rectal
	Up to 35 mg	Intravenous
Trimetobenzamide	250 mg	Oral
	200 mg	Rectal
Metoclopramide	5-10 mg	Oral
	10 mg	Intramuscular
	5-10 mg	Intravenous
Dimenhydrinate	50 mg	Oral

Modified from Wiederholt WC: *Neurology for non-neurologists*, ed 4, Philadelphia, 2000, WB Saunders.
*For side effects and contraindications consult the manufacturer's drug insert before prescribing any of these drugs.

BASIC INFORMATION

■ DEFINITION

Tension-type headaches are recurrent headaches lasting 30 min to 7 days without nausea or vomiting and with at least two of the following characteristics: pressing or tightening quality, mild or moderate intensity, bilateral, and not aggravated by routine physical activity.

■ SYNONYMS

Muscle contraction headache
Tension headache
Stress headache
Essential headache

ICD-9CM CODES

307.81 Tension headache

■ EPIDEMIOLOGY & DEMOGRAPHICS

INCIDENCE (IN U.S.):
- Undetermined
- Believed to be the most common type of headache; as high as 70% of all headaches presenting to primary care physician

PREVALENCE (IN U.S.): Males: 63%/yr; females: 86%/yr
PREDOMINANT SEX: Females > males
PEAK INCIDENCE: Occurs at all ages
GENETICS: Not established

■ PHYSICAL FINDINGS & CLINICAL PRESENTATION

Pressure or "band-like" tightness all around the head, may be worse at the vertex. Cervical, paracervical and trapezius muscle spasm and/or percussion tenderness may be present. Scalp tenderness or hypersensitivity to pain also occurs. Symptoms suggestive of migraine are usually not present (e.g., throbbing pain, nausea/vomiting, photo/phonophobia, visual complaints, aura).

■ ETIOLOGY

- Unclear; little data to support postulated muscle contraction component. More recently has been thought of as a multifactorial disorder with several possible concurrent pathophysiological mechanisms
- No recent data to support the long-standing belief that these headaches arise from stress or other psychologic factors. However, components of stress, sleep deprivation, hunger, and eyestrain may exacerbate symptoms
- These headaches respond poorly to standard migraine therapy

DIAGNOSIS

■ DIFFERENTIAL DIAGNOSIS

- Migraine (would expect associated symptoms see "Headache, Migraine")
- Cervical spine disease
- Intracranial mass (may present with focal neurologic signs, seizures, or headache awakening patient from sleep)
- Idiopathic intracranial hypertension (found more often in obese women of child-bearing age, may have papilledema, visual loss, or diplopia)
- Rebound headache from overuse of analgesics
- Secondary headache (e.g., temporomandibular joint syndrome, thyrotoxicosis, polycythemia, drug side-effects)
- Migraine and tension-type headache may often coexist and may be difficult to differentiate (suggest headache calendar)
- Section II describes the differential diagnosis of headaches

■ WORKUP

- Thorough history and physical examination for any new-onset headache
- Neuroimaging should be performed when unexplained neurologic findings are present on exam or in cases of atypical new-onset sudden and severe headaches. Although data are insufficient, imaging studies may be considered if there is a change in the pattern, frequency, or severity of headaches but may be of lower yield

■ LABORATORY TESTS

- No routine tests
- ESR in elderly patients suspected of having cranial arteritis

■ IMAGING STUDIES

CT scan and/or MRI may be used to exclude intracranial pathology. MRI is better for imaging the posterior fossa. Contrast should be used if mass lesion is suspected.

TREATMENT

■ NONPHARMACOLOGIC THERAPY

- Relaxation training
- Biofeedback
- Heat
- Transcutaneous electrical nerve stimulation (TENS)
- Physical therapy including stretching exercises, massage, and ultrasound

■ ACUTE GENERAL Rx

Nonnarcotic analgesics with limited frequency to prevent drug-induced headache

■ CHRONIC Rx

- Tricyclic antidepressants (e.g., amitriptyline 10 to 150 mg hs) and SSRIs
- Avoid narcotics, limit NSAIDs, consider indomethacin; if related to cervical muscle spasm, may consider trial of muscle relaxants

■ DISPOSITION

May not respond fully to treatment

■ REFERRAL

If uncertain about diagnosis or unexplained focal neurologic findings on examination

PEARLS & CONSIDERATIONS

It is imperative to avoid overuse of caffeine- and barbiturate-containing medications because of the risk of rebound headaches

REFERENCES

Bendtsen L: Central sensitization in tension-type headache—possible pathophysiological mechanisms, *Cephalalgia* 20(5):486, 2000.

Headache Classification Committee of the International Headache Society: Classification and diagnostic criteria for headache disorders, cranial neuralgias and facial pain, *Cephalalgia,* 8(suppl 7):19, 1988.

Holroyd KA et al: Management of chronic tension-type headache with tricyclic anti-depressant medication, stress management therapy, and their combination: a randomized controlled trial, *JAMA* 285(17):2208, 2001.

Jensen R: Pathophysiological mechanisms of tension-type headache: a review of epidemiological and experimental studies, *Cephalalgia* 19(6):602, 1999.

Millea P, Brodie J: Tension-type headache, *Am Fam Physician* 66:797, 2002.

Rollnik, JD, et al: Botulinum toxin type A and EMG: A key to the understanding of chronic tension-type headaches? *Headache* 41:985, 2001.

Silberstein, SD, Rosenberg, J: Multispecialty consensus on diagnosis and treatment of headache, *Neurology* 54:1553, 2000.

Author: **Richard S. Isaacson, M.D.**

BASIC INFORMATION

■ DEFINITION
In complete heart block, there is complete blockage of all AV conduction. The atria and ventricles have separate, independent rhythms.

■ SYNONYMS
Third-degree AV block

ICD-9CM CODES
426.0 Complete heart block

■ EPIDEMIOLOGY & DEMOGRAPHICS
Over 100,000 permanent pacemakers are implanted worldwide each year for complete heart block.

■ PHYSICAL FINDINGS & CLINICAL PRESENTATION
Physical examination may be normal. Patients may present with the following clinical manifestations:
- Dizziness, palpitations
- Stokes-Adams syncopal attacks
- CHF
- Angina

■ ETIOLOGY
- Degenerative changes in His-Purkinje system
- Acute anterior wall MI
- Calcific aortic stenosis
- Cardiomyopathy
- Trauma
- Cardiovascular surgery
- Congenital

DIAGNOSIS

■ DIFFERENTIAL DIAGNOSIS
The differential diagnosis involves only the etiology. ECG will confirm diagnosis.

■ WORKUP
ECG:
- P waves constantly change their relationship to the QRS complexes (Fig. 1-129).
- Ventricular rate is usually <50 bpm (may be higher in congenital forms).
- Ventricular rate is generally lower than the atrial rate.
- QRS complex is wide.

TREATMENT

■ ACUTE GENERAL Rx
- Immediate pacemaker insertion unless the patient has congenital third-degree AV block and is completely asymptomatic
- Therapy of underlying etiology

■ CHRONIC Rx
Patients with permanent pacemakers need regular follow-up and pacemaker monitoring to ensure proper sensing.

■ DISPOSITION
Prognosis is favorable following insertion of pacemaker and related to the underlying etiology of complete AV block (e.g., MI, cardiomyopathy).

■ REFERRAL
Referral for implantation of permanent pacemaker

PEARLS & CONSIDERATIONS

■ COMMENTS
- Patients should be instructed on avoidance of activities that may damage the pacemaker (e.g., contact sports).
- Common environmental causes of pacemaker malformation are electrocautery, transthoracic defibrillation, MRI, extracorporeal shock wave lithotripsy, transcutaneous electrical nerve stimulation, therapeutic radiation, ECT, diathermy, radiofrequency ablation for treatment of tachyarrhythmias.

REFERENCE
Bayce M et al: Evolving indications for permanent pacemakers, *Ann Intern Med* 134:1130, 2001.
Author: **Fred F. Ferri, M.D.**

THIRD-DEGREE (COMPLETE) AV BLOCK

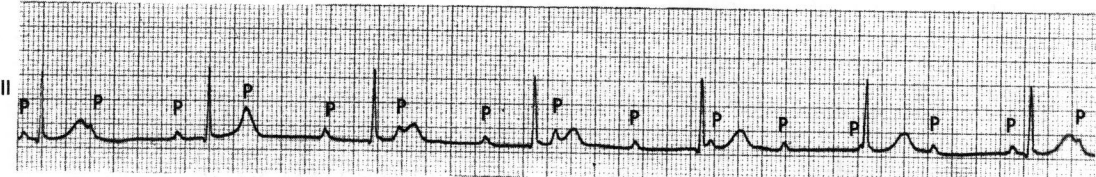

Fig. 1-129 Third-degree complete AV heart block is characterized by independent atrial (*P*) and ventricular (QRS) activity. The atrial rate is always faster than the ventricular rate. The PR intervals are completely variable. Some P waves fall on the T wave, distorting its shape. Others may fall in the QRS complex and be "lost." Notice that the QRS complexes are of normal width, indicating that the ventricles are being paced from the AV junction. (From Goldberger AL [ed]: *Clinical electrocardiography*, ed 5, St Louis, 1994, Mosby.)

BASIC INFORMATION

■ DEFINITION
Second-degree heart block is the blockage of some (but not all) impulses from the atria to the ventricles. There are two types of second-degree AV block:

MOBITZ TYPE I (WENCKEBACH):
- There is a progressive prolongation of the PR interval before an impulse is completely blocked; the cycle repeats periodically.
- Cycle with dropped beat is less than two times the previous cycle.
- Site of block is usually AV node (proximal to the bundle of His).

MOBITZ TYPE II:
- There is a sudden interruption of AV conduction without prior prolongation of the PR interval.
- Site of block is infranodal.

■ SYNONYMS
Wenckebach block (Mobitz type I block)
Mobitz type II block

ICD-9CM CODES
426.13 Mobitz type I
426.12 Mobitz type II

■ EPIDEMIOLOGY & DEMOGRAPHICS
Mobitz type I block is more common and may occur in individuals with heightened vagal tone or secondary to some medications such as β-blockers or calcium channel blockers.

■ PHYSICAL FINDINGS & CLINICAL PRESENTATION
- Patients with Mobitz type I are usually asymptomatic.
- Sudden loss of consciousness without warning (Adams-Stokes attack) can occur in patients with Mobitz type II; however, it is much more common in patients with complete heart block.
- Irregular pulse with dropped beats is present (Mobitz type I).
- Irregular pulse with occasional dropped beats is present (Mobitz type II).

■ ETIOLOGY
MOBITZ TYPE I:
- Vagal stimulation
- Degenerative changes in the AV conduction system
- Ischemia at the AV nodes (particularly in inferior wall MI)
- Drugs (digitalis, quinidine, procainamide, adenosine, calcium channel blockers, β-blockers)
- Cardiomyopathies
- Aortic regurgitation
- Lyme carditis

MOBITZ TYPE II:
- Degenerative changes in the His-Purkinje system
- Acute anterior wall MI
- Calcific aortic stenosis

DIAGNOSIS

■ DIFFERENTIAL DIAGNOSIS
The ECG will distinguish between Mobitz type I and Mobitz type II block and other conduction abnormalities.

■ WORKUP
ECG, 24-hr Holter monitor (selected patients)
MOBITZ TYPE I (Fig. 1-130): ECG shows:
- Gradual prolongation of PR interval leading to a blocked beat
- Shortened PR interval after dropped beat

MOBITZ TYPE II: ECG shows:
- Fixed duration of PR interval
- Sudden appearance of blocked beats

TREATMENT

■ NONPHARMACOLOGIC THERAPY
Elimination of drugs that may induce AV block

■ ACUTE GENERAL Rx
MOBITZ TYPE I:
- Treatment generally is not necessary. This type of block is usually transient.
- If symptomatic (e.g., dizziness), atropine 1 mg (may repeat once after 5 min) may be tried to increase AV conduction; if no response, insert temporary pacemaker.
- If block is secondary to drugs (e.g., digitalis), discontinue the drug.
- If associated with anterior wall MI and wide QRS escape rhythm, consider insertion of temporary pacemaker.
- Significant AV block post-MI may be caused by adenosine produced by the ischemic myocardium. These arrhythmias (which may be resistant to conventional therapy such as atropine) may respond to theophylline (adenosine antagonist).

MOBITZ TYPE II:
- Pacemaker insertion is needed, because this type of block is usually permanent and often progresses to complete AV block.

■ DISPOSITION
Prognosis is good with insertion of pacemaker in patients with Mobitz type II.

■ REFERRAL
Referral for pacemaker insertion (see Acute General Rx)

PEARLS & CONSIDERATIONS

■ COMMENTS
Patients with Mobitz type I should be followed routinely for potential development of high-grade AV block.

REFERENCE
Barold S, Hayes D: Second-degree atrioventricular block: a reappraisal, *Mayo Clin Proc* 76:44, 2001.
Author: **Fred F. Ferri, M.D.**

WENCKEBACH (MOBITZ TYPE I) SECOND-DEGREE AV BLOCK

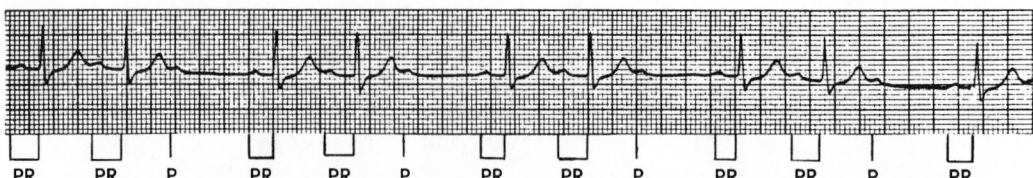

PR PR P PR PR P PR PR P PR PR P PR

Fig. 1-130   Wenckebach (Mobitz type I) second-degree AV block. Notice the progressive increase in PR intervals, with the third P wave in each sequence not followed by a QRS. Wenckebach block produces a characteristically syncopated rhythm with grouping of the QRS complexes (group beating). (From Goldberger AL [ed]: *Clinical electrocardiography*, ed 5, St Louis, 1994, Mosby.)

BASIC INFORMATION

■ DEFINITION

HEAT EXHAUSTION: An illness resulting from prolonged heavy activity in a hot environment with subsequent dehydration, electrolyte depletion, and rectal temperature >37.8° C but <40° C.

HEAT STROKE: A life-threatening heat illness characterized by extreme hyperthermia, dehydration, and neurologic manifestations (core temperature >40° C).

■ SYNONYMS

Heat illness
Hyperthermia

ICD-9CM CODES

992.0 Heat stroke
992.5 Heat exhaustion

■ EPIDEMIOLOGY & DEMOGRAPHICS

- Heat exhaustion and stroke occur more frequently in elderly patients, especially those taking diuretics or medications that impair heat dissipation (e.g., phenothiazines, anticholinergics, antihistamines, β-blockers).
- Incidence of heat stroke in United States is approximately 20 cases/100,000 population.

■ PHYSICAL FINDINGS & CLINICAL PRESENTATION

HEAT EXHAUSTION:
- Generalized malaise, weakness, headache, muscle and abdominal cramps, nausea, vomiting, hypotension, and tachycardia
- Rectal temperature is usually normal
- Sweating is usually present

HEAT STROKE:
- Neurologic manifestations (seizures, tremor, hemiplegia, coma, psychosis, and other bizarre behavior)
- Evidence of dehydration (poor skin turgor, sunken eyeballs)
- Tachycardia, hyperventilation
- Skin is hot, red, and flushed
- Sweating is often (not always) absent, particularly in elderly patients

■ ETIOLOGY

- Exogenous heat gain (increased ambient temperature)
- Increased heat production (exercise, infection, hyperthyroidism, drugs)
- Impaired heat dissipation (high humidity, heavy clothing, neonatal or elderly patients, drugs [phenothiazines, anticholinergics, antihistamines, butyrophenones, amphetamines, cocaine, alcohol, β-blockers])

DIAGNOSIS

■ DIFFERENTIAL DIAGNOSIS

- Infections (meningitis, encephalitis, sepsis)
- Head trauma
- Epilepsy
- Thyroid storm
- Acute cocaine intoxication
- Malignant hyperthermia
- Heat exhaustion can be differentiated from heat stroke by the following:
  1. Essentially intact mental function and lack of significant fever in heat exhaustion
  2. Mild or absent increases in CPK, AST, LDH, ALT in heat exhaustion

■ WORKUP

- Heat stroke: comprehensive history, physical examination, and laboratory evaluation
- Heat exhaustion: in most cases, laboratory tests are not necessary for diagnosis

■ LABORATORY TESTS

Laboratory abnormalities may include the following:
- Elevated BUN, creatinine, Hct
- Hyponatremia or hypernatremia, hyperkalemia or hypokalemia
- Elevated LDH, AST, ALT, CPK, bilirubin
- Lactic acidosis, respiratory alkalosis (secondary to hyperventilation)
- Myoglobinuria, hypofibrinogenemia, fibrinolysis, hypocalcemia

TREATMENT

- Treatment of **heat exhaustion** consists primarily of placing the patient in a cool, shaded area and providing rapid hydration and salt replacement.
  1. Fluid intake should be at least 2 L q4h in patients without history of CHF.
  2. Salt replacement can be accomplished by using one-quarter teaspoon of salt or two 10-grain salt tablets dissolved in 1 L of water.
  3. If IV fluid replacement is necessary, young athletes can be given normal saline IV (3 to 4 L over 6 to 8 hr); in elderly patients, consider using $D_5\frac{1}{2}NS$ IV with rate titrated to cardiovascular status.
- Patients with **heat stroke** should undergo rapid cooling.
  1. Remove the patient's clothes and place the patient in a cool and well-ventilated room.
  2. If unconscious, position patient on his or her side and clear the airway. Protect airway and augment oxygenation (e.g, nasal O_2 at 4 L/min to keep oxygen saturation >90%).
  3. Monitor body temperature every 5 min. Measurement of the patient's core temperature with a rectal probe is recommended.

The goal is to reduce the body temperature to 39° C (102.2° F) in 30 to 60 min.
  4. Spray the patient with a cool mist and use fans to enhance airflow over the body (rapid evaporation method).
  5. Immersion of the patient in ice water, stomach lavage with iced saline solution, intravenous administration of cooled fluids, and inhalation of cold air are advisable only when the means for rapid evaporation are not available. Immersion in tepid water (15° C 59° F]) is preferred over ice water immersion to minimize risk of shivering.
  6. Use of ice packs on axillae, neck, and groin is controversial because they increase peripheral vasoconstriction and may induce shivering.
  7. Antipyretics are ineffective because the hypothalamic set point during heat stroke is normal despite the increased body temperature.
  8. Intubate a comatose patient, insert a Foley catheter, and start nasal O_2. Continuous ECG monitoring is recommended.
  9. Insert at least two large-bore IV lines and begin IV hydration with NS or Ringer's lactate.
  10. Draw initial lab studies: electrolytes, CBC, BUN, creatinine, AST, ALT, CPK, LDH, glucose, INR, PTT, platelet count, Ca^{2+}, lactic acid, ABGs.
  11. Treat complications as follows:
      a. Hypotension: vigorous hydration with normal saline or Ringer's lactate.
      b. Convulsions: diazepam 5 to 10 mg IV (slowly).
      c. Shivering: chlorpromazine 10 to 50 mg IV.
      d. Acidosis: use bicarbonate judiciously (only in severe acidosis).
  12. Observe for evidence of rhabdomyolysis, hepatic, renal, or cardiac failure and treat accordingly.

■ DISPOSITION

Most patients recover completely within 48 hr. Mortality can exceed 30% in patients with prolonged and severe hyperthermia.

REFERENCES

Bouchama A, Knochel JP: Heat stroke, *N Engl J Med* 346:1978, 2002.
Wexler RK: Evaluation and treatment of heat-related illness, *Am Fam Physician* 65:230, 2002.
Author: **Fred F. Ferri, M.D.**

BASIC INFORMATION

■ DEFINITION

The HELLP syndrome is a serious variant of preeclampsia. HELLP is an acronym for *H*emolysis, *E*levated *L*iver function, and *L*ow *P*latelet count. It is the most frequently encountered microangiopathy of pregnancy. There are three classes of the syndrome based on the degree of maternal thrombocytopenia as a primary indicator of disease severity.
Class 1: platelets 50,000/mm³
Class 2: platelets >50,000/mm³ to 100,000/mm³
Class 3: platelets >100,000/mm³

ICD-9CM CODES
642.50 HELLP, episode of care
642.51 HELLP, delivered
642.52 HELLP, delivered with postpartum complications
642.53 HELLP, antepartum complications
642.54 HELLP, postpartum complications

■ EPIDEMIOLOGY & DEMOGRAPHICS
- Among women with severe preeclampsia, 6% will manifest with one abnormality suggestive of HELLP syndrome, 12% will develop two abnormalities, and approximately 10% will develop all three.
- The HELLP Syndrome, like preeclampsia, is rare before 20 wk gestation.
- One third of all cases occur postpartum; of these, only 80% were diagnosed with preeclampsia before delivery.
RISK FACTORS: Women older than 35 yr, Caucasian, multiparity
RECURRENCE RATE: 3% to 25%

■ PHYSICAL FINDINGS & CLINICAL PRESENTATION
- Definitive laboratory criteria remain to be validated prospectively.
- Most commonly used criteria include hemolysis defined by the presence of an abnormal peripheral smear with schistocytes, lactate dehydrogenase (LDH) >600 U/L, and total bilirubin >1.2 mg/dl; elevated liver enzymes as serum aspartate aminotransferase (AST) >70 U/L and LDH >600 U/L; low platelet count as less than 100,000/mm³.
- Although many women with HELLP syndrome will be asymptomatic, 80% report right upper quadrant pain and 50% to 60% present with excessive weight gain and worsening edema.

■ ETIOLOGY
As with other microangiopathies, endothelial dysfunction, with resultant activation of the intravascular coagulation cascade, has been proposed as the central pathogenesis of HELLP syndrome.

DIAGNOSIS

■ DIFFERENTIAL DIAGNOSIS
Appendicitis, gallbladder disease, peptic ulcer, enteritis, hepatitis, pyelonephritis, systemic lupus erythematosus, thrombotic thrombocytopenic purpura/hemolytic uremic syndrome, acute fatty liver of pregnancy. See Table 1-26.

■ WORKUP
Because the HELLP syndrome is a disease entity based on laboratory values, initial assessment is detailed as follows.

■ LABORATORY TESTS
- Initial assessment of suspected HELLP syndrome should include a complete blood count (CBC) to evaluate platelets, urinalysis, serum creatinine, LDH, uric acid, indirect and total bilirubin levels, and AST/ALT.
- Tests of prothrombin time, partial thromboplastin time, fibrinogen and fibrin split products are reserved for those women with a platelet count well below 100,000/mm³.

■ IMAGING STUDIES
There are none to aid in diagnosis.

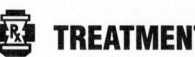 TREATMENT

Treatment is dependent on gestational age of the fetus, severity of HELLP, and maternal status. Stabilization of the mother is the first priority.

■ ACUTE GENERAL Rx
- Assess gestational age thoroughly. Fetal status should be monitored with nonstress tests, contraction stress tests, and/or biophysical profile
- Maternal status should be evaluated by history, physical examination, and laboratory testing
- Magnesium sulfate is administered for seizure prophylaxis regardless of blood pressure
- Blood pressure control is achieved with agents such as hydralazine or labetalol
- Indwelling Foley catheter to monitor maternal volume status and urine output

TABLE 1-26   Liver Diseases Unique to Pregnancy

	TRIMESTER OF ONSET	SYMPTOMS	LABORATORY ABNORMALITIES	RECURRENCE WITH FUTURE PREGNANCIES
Hyperemesis gravidarum	1	Nausea, vomiting	Elevated AST/ALT (60-1000 U/L), occasionally hyperbilirubinemia	
Cholestasis	2, 3	Pruritus	Bile acids >8 μM, elevated AST/ALT and bilirubin in more severe cases	Common
Acute fatty liver	3	Nausea, vomiting, abdominal pain	Elevated AST/ALT (100-1000 U/L), bilirubin >5 mg/dl, prolonged prothrombin time*	Rare
HELLP syndrome	2, 3, or postpartum	Abdominal pain, nausea, vomiting	Elevated AST/ALT (60-15000 U/L), platelets <100,000/mm³, LDH >600 U/L, microangiopathic anemia	3-25%

From Goldman L, Ausiello D (eds): *Cecil textbook of medicine*, ed 22, Philadelphia, 2004, WB Saunders.
ALT, Alanine aminotransferase; *AST*, aspartate aminotransferase.
*Useful diagnostic distinction from HELLP syndrome, in which prothrombin time, partial thromboplastin time, and fibrinogen are usually normal.

■ CHRONIC Rx

- In those pregnancies 34 wk or Class 1 HELLP syndrome, delivery, either vaginal or abdominal, within 24 hr is the goal.
- In the preterm fetus, corticosteroid therapy to enhance fetal lung maturation is indicated.
- Some reports have shown temporary amelioration of HELLP severity with the administration of high dose of steroids measured by increased urine output, improvement in platelet count and LFTs.
- Judicious use of blood products, especially in those requiring surgery.
- The patient requires intensive observation for 48 hr postpartum; laboratory levels should begin to improve during this time.

■ DISPOSITION

The natural history of this disorder is a rapidly deteriorating condition requiring close monitoring of maternal and fetal well-being.

■ REFERRAL

Preterm patients with the HELLP syndrome should be stabilized hemodynamically and transferred to a tertiary care center. Term patients can be treated at a local hospital depending on the availability of obstetric, neonatal, and blood banking services.

☼ PEARLS & CONSIDERATIONS

Not all women with HELLP have hypertension or proteinuria.

REFERENCES

Egerman RS, Sibai BM: HELLP syndrome, *Clin Obstet Gynecol* 42(2):381, 1999.

Gabbe SG, et al: *Obstetrics: normal and problem pregnancies,* ed 3, Philadelphia, 1996, Churchill Livingstone.

Magann EF, Martin JN: Twelve steps to optimal management of HELLP syndrome, *Clin Obstet Gynecol* 42(3):532, 1999.

Martin JN et al: Pregnancy complicated by preeclampsia-eclampsia with the syndrome of hemolysis, elevated liver enzymes, and low platelet count. How rapid is recovery? *Obstet Gynecol* 76:737, 1990.

Norwitz ER, Hsu CD, Repke JT: Acute complications of preeclampsia, *Clin Obstet Gynecol* 45(2):308, 2002.

Author: **Sonya S. Abdel-Razeq, M.D.**

BASIC INFORMATION

■ DEFINITION
Hemochromatosis is an autosomal recessive disorder characterized by increased accumulation of iron in various organs (adrenals, liver, pancreas, heart, testes, kidneys, pituitary) and eventual dysfunction of these organs if not treated appropriately.

■ SYNONYMS
Bronze diabetes

ICD-9CM CODES
275.0 Hemochromatosis

■ EPIDEMIOLOGY & DEMOGRAPHICS
- Hemochromatosis is generally diagnosed in males in their fifth decade.
- Diagnosis in females is generally not made until 10 to 20 yr after menopause.
- Incidence in whites is approximately 1 in 300 persons.
- Most common genetic disorder in North European ancestry.

■ PHYSICAL FINDINGS & CLINICAL PRESENTATION
Examination may be normal; patient with advanced case may present with the following:
- Increased skin pigmentation
- Hepatomegaly, splenomegaly, hepatic tenderness, testicular atrophy
- Loss of body hair, peripheral edema, gynecomastia, ascites
- Amenorrhea (25% of females)
- Loss of libido (50% of males)
- Arthropathy
- Joint pain (44%)
- Fatigue (45%)

■ ETIOLOGY
Autosomal recessive disease; the gene HFE, which contains two missense mutations (C 282Y and H 63D), was recently identified.

DIAGNOSIS

■ DIFFERENTIAL DIAGNOSIS
- Hereditary anemias with defect of erythropoiesis
- Cirrhosis
- Repeated blood transfusions

■ WORKUP
Medical history, physical examination, and laboratory evaluation should be focused on affected organ systems (see Physical Findings). Liver biopsy is the gold standard for diagnosis; it reveals iron deposition in hepatocytes, bile ducts, and supporting tissues.

■ LABORATORY TESTS
- Transferrin saturation is the best screening test. Plasma ferritin is also a good indicator of total body iron stores but may be elevated in many other conditions (inflammation, malignancy). Some authors recommend measurement of both fasting transferrin saturation and serum ferritin level as initial tests for population-based screening to detect and treat hemochromatosis before iron loading occurs.
- Elevated AST, ALT, alkaline phosphatase.
- Hyperglycemia.
- Endocrine abnormalities (decreased testosterone, LH, FSH).
- Measurement of hepatic iron index (hepatic iron concentration [HIC] divided by age) in liver biopsy specimen can confirm diagnosis.
- Genetic testing (HFE genotyping for the C 282 Y and H63 D mutations) may be useful in selected patients with liver disease and suspected iron overload (e.g., patients with transferrin saturation >40%). Genetic testing should not be performed as part of initial routine evaluation for hereditary hemochromatosis. Once a patient has been identified, first-degree relatives of the index patient should also be screened. The HFE gene test is a PCR-based test usually performed on whole blood sample. Cost is approximately $150 to $200.

■ IMAGING STUDIES
CT scan or MRI of the liver is useful to exclude other etiologies and may in some cases show iron overload in the liver.

TREATMENT

■ NONPHARMACOLOGIC THERAPY
Weekly phlebotomies of 500 ml of blood should be continued for several weeks until depletion of iron stores is achieved. Subsequent phlebotomies can be performed on a prn basis to maintain a normal transferrin saturation and a ferritin level <50 µg/L.

■ ACUTE GENERAL Rx
Deferoxamine (iron chelating agent) is generally reserved for patients with severe hemochromatosis with diffuse organ involvement (e.g., liver disease, heart disease) and when phlebotomy is not possible. It is administered in a dose of 0.5 to 1 g IM qd or 20 mg SC over a 12- to 24-hr period with a constant infusion pump.

■ CHRONIC Rx
Phlebotomy on a prn basis depending on the Hct level; generally, Hct should not exceed 40%.

■ DISPOSITION
Prognosis is good if phlebotomy is started early (before onset of cirrhosis or diabetes mellitus); women can have the full phenotypic expression of the disease, including cirrhosis, and should also be aggressively treated.

■ REFERRAL
For liver biopsy if diagnosis is uncertain

☼ PEARLS & CONSIDERATIONS

■ COMMENTS
- Recent data reveal that patients with hemochromatosis and serum ferritin levels <1000 mcg/L are unlikely to have cirrhosis. Liver biopsy to screen for cirrhosis may be unnecessary in such patients.
- Cirrhotic patients must be periodically monitored (ultrasound or CT scan) because of their increased risk of hepatocellular carcinoma.
- HFE gene testing for C282Y mutation is a cost-effective method of screening relatives of patients with hereditary hemochromatosis.

REFERENCES
Brandhagen DJ et al: Recognition and management of hereditary hemochromatosis, *Am Fam Physician*, 65:853, 2002.

Morrison ED et al: Serum ferritin level predicts advanced hepatic fibrosis among US patients with phenotypic hemochromatosis, *Ann Intern Med* 138:627, 2003.

Waalen J et al: Prevalence of hemochromatosis-related symptoms among individuals with mutations in the HFE gene, *Mayo Clin Proc* 77:522, 2002.

Author: **Fred F. Ferri, M.D.**

BASIC INFORMATION

■ DEFINITION
Hemolytic-uremic syndrome refers to an acute syndrome characterized by hemolytic anemia, thrombocytopenia, and severe renal failure.

■ SYNONYMS
HUS

ICD-9CM CODES
283.11 Hemolytic-uremic syndrome

■ EPIDEMIOLOGY & DEMOGRAPHICS
- HUS affects mainly children younger than 10 yr old
- Incidence is 2.6 cases/100,000 in people younger than 5 yr of age
- Incidence is 0.97 cases/100,000 in people over the age of 18
- May be epidemic, most commonly occurring during the summer months
- Most common cause of acute renal failure in children
- In the United States 300 to 700 new cases occur each year

■ PHYSICAL FINDINGS & CLINICAL PRESENTATION
- HUS usually preceded by diarrhea in 90% of cases
- Bloody diarrhea (75%)
- Abdominal pain
- Vomiting
- Fever
- Irritability, lethargy, and seizures (10%)
- Hypertension
- Pallor
- Anuria or oliguria

■ ETIOLOGY
Pathologically, it is thought that thrombin generation (probably the result of accelerated thrombogenesis) and inhibition of fibrinolysis leads to renal arteriolar and capillary microthrombi preceding renal injury.
In children:
- *E. coli* serotype O157:H7 is the leading cause of HUS.
- The infection is acquired by eating undercooked red meat, especially hamburgers.

Other causes of HUS in children and adults are:
- Drugs (cyclosporine, mitomycin, tacrolimus, ticlopidine, clopidogrel, cisplatin, quinine, penicillin, penicillamine, oral contraceptives, and quinine used to treat muscle cramps)
- Infection (*Salmonella, Shigella, Yersinia, Campylobacter,* coxsackievirus, rubella, influenza virus, Epstein-Barr virus)
- Toxins

- Pregnancy (usually postpartum) and oral contraceptives
- HIV-associated thrombotic microangiopathy
- Pneumococcal infection

DIAGNOSIS

The triad of thrombocytopenia, acute renal failure, and microangiopathic hemolytic anemia establishes the diagnosis of HUS.

■ DIFFERENTIAL DIAGNOSIS
- The differential is vast, including all causes of bloody and nonbloody diarrhea because the GI symptoms usually precede the triad of HUS
- Thrombotic thrombocytopenic purpura
- Disseminated intravascular coagulation
- Prosthetic valve hemolysis
- Malignant hypertension
- Vasculitis

■ WORKUP
The workup for suspected HUS patients includes blood tests and stool cultures.

■ LABORATORY TESTS
- CBC with hemoglobin <10 g/dl
- Peripheral smear shows the hallmark microangiopathic hemolytic anemia with schistocytes, burr cells, and helmet cells
- Thrombocytopenia (platelet counts usually <60,000/mm³)
- Reticulocyte count is high
- LDH level is elevated
- Haptoglobin is low
- Indirect bilirubin is elevated
- BUN and creatinine are elevated
- Urinalysis reveals proteinuria, microscopic hematuria, and pyuria
- Stool cultures for *E. coli* O157:H7 are positive in over 90% of cases if obtained during the first week of illness. After the first week only one third are positive

■ IMAGING STUDIES
Imaging studies are not very helpful in the diagnosis of HUS.

TREATMENT

The treatment of HUS is primarily supportive.

■ NONPHARMACOLOGIC THERAPY
- Blood transfusions for severe anemia
- Antibiotics should be avoided and are not indicated for the treatment of *E. coli* O157:H7

- Correction of electrolyte abnormalities

■ ACUTE GENERAL Rx
Hypertension control

■ CHRONIC Rx
For anuric or oliguric renal failure, dialysis may be required.

■ DISPOSITION
- Adults presenting with HUS have a worse prognosis than children do with HUS.
- Mortality rate is 5%.
- Morbidity includes:
  1. Proteinuria (31%)
  2. Renal insufficiency (31%)
  3. Hypertension (6%)

■ REFERRAL
- The local health department should be notified if the bacteria *E. coli* O157:H7 has been isolated.
- Consultation with hematology and nephrology specialist is recommended in patients with HUS.

☼ PEARLS & CONSIDERATIONS

■ COMMENTS
- Hemolytic-uremic syndrome was first described by Gasser and colleagues in 1955.
- Children testing positive for the *E. coli* O157:H7 serotype should not return to school or day care facilities until two consecutive stools test negative for the microorganism.
- *E. coli* O157:H7 can be transmitted from person to person, therefore universal precautions and hand washing are recommended in preventing the spread of the infection.

REFERENCES
Begue RE, Mehta D, Blecker U: *Escherichia coli* and the hemolytic-uremic syndrome, *South Med J* 91(9):798, 1998.

Boyce TG, Swerdlow DL, Griffin PM: *Escherichia coli* O157:H7 and the hemolytic-uremic syndrome, *N Engl J Med* 333(6):364, 1995.

Chandler WL et al: Prothrombotic coagulation abnormalities preceding the hemolytic-uremic syndrome, *N Engl J Med* 346:23, 2002.

Gordjani N et al: Hemolytic uremic syndromes in childhood, *Semin Thromb Hem* 23(3):281, 1997.

Medina PJ, Sipolis JM, George JN: Drug-associated thrombotic thrombocytopenic purpura-hemolytic uremic syndrome, *Curr Opin Hematol* 8:286, 2001.
Authors: **Peter Petropoulos, M.D., and Dennis J. Mikolich, M.D.**

BASIC INFORMATION

DEFINITION
Hemophilia is a hereditary bleeding disorder caused by low factor VIII coagulant activity (hemophilia A) or low levels of Factor IX coagulant activity (hemophilia B).

SYNONYMS
Hemophilia A: Classic hemophilia, factor VIII deficiency hemophilia
Hemophilia B: Christmas disease, factor IX hemophilia

ICD-9CM CODES
286.0 Hemophilia A
286.1 Hemophilia B

EPIDEMIOLOGY & DEMOGRAPHICS
INCIDENCE/PREVALENCE (IN U.S.):
Hemophilia A: 100 cases/1 million males, hemophilia B: 20 cases/1 million males
GENETIC FACTORS: Both hemophilias have an X-linked recessive pattern of inheritance with only males affected.

PHYSICAL FINDINGS & CLINICAL PRESENTATION
- The clinical features of hemophilia A and B are generally indistinguishable from each other.
- Bleeding is most commonly seen in joints (knees, ankles, elbows) resulting in hot, swollen, painful joints and subsequent crippling joint deformity.
- Bleeding can also occur into the muscles and the GI tract.
- Compartment syndromes can occur from large hematomas.
- Hematuria may be present.

ETIOLOGY
- Hemophilia A: low factor VIII coagulant (VIII:C) activity; can be classified as mild if factor VIII:C levels are >5%, moderate: levels are 1% to 5%, severe: levels are <1%.
- Hemophilia B: low levels of factor IX coagulant activity.
- Both disorders are congenital.
- Spontaneous acquisition of factor VIII inhibitors (acquired hemophilia) is rare.

DIAGNOSIS

DIFFERENTIAL DIAGNOSIS
- Other clotting factor deficiencies
- Platelet function disorders
- Vitamin K deficiency

WORKUP
Patients with mild hemophilia bleed only in response to major trauma or surgery and may not be diagnosed until young adulthood. Diagnostic workup includes laboratory evaluation (see Laboratory Tests).

LABORATORY TESTS
- Partial thromboplastin time (PTT) is prolonged.
- Reduced factor VIII:C level distinguishes hemophilia A from other causes of prolonged PTT.
- Factor VIII antigen, PT, fibrinogen level, and bleeding time are normal.
- Factor IX coagulant activity levels are reduced in patients with hemophilia B.
- Coagulation factor activity measurement is useful to correlate with disease severity: normal range is 50 to 150 U/dl; 5 to 20 U/dl indicates mild disease, 2 to 5 U/dl indicates moderate disease, and <2 U/dl indicates severe disease with spontaneous bleeding episodes.

TREATMENT

NONPHARMACOLOGIC THERAPY
- Avoidance of contact sports
- Patient education regarding their disease; promotion of exercises such as swimming
- Avoidance of aspirin or other NSAIDs
- Orthopedic evaluation and physical therapy evaluation in patients with joint involvement
- Hepatitis vaccination

ACUTE GENERAL Rx
HEMOPHILIA A:
- Reversal and prevention of acute bleeding in hemophilia A and B are based on adequate replacement of deficient or missing factor protein.
- The choice of the product for replacement therapy is guided by availability, capacity, concerns, and cost. Recombinant factors cost two to three times as much as plasma-derived factors, and the limited capacity to produce recombinant factors often results in periods of shortage. In the U.S., 60% of patients with severe hemophilia use recombinant products.
- Factor VIII concentrates are effective in controlling spontaneous and traumatic hemorrhage in severe hemophilia. The new recombinant factor VIII is stable without added human serum albumin (decreased risk of transmission of infectious agents).

- Recombinant activated factor VII is useful to stop spontaneous hemorrhages and prevent excessive bleeding during surgery in 75% of patients with inhibitors. Recommended dose is 90 µg/mg of body weight every 2-3 hr for treatment of life-threatening hemorrhage. It is, however, very expensive ($1 per µg).
- Desmopressin acetate 0.3 µg/kg q24h (causes release of factor VIII:C) may be used in preparation for minor surgical procedures in mild hemophiliacs.
- Aminocaproic acid (EACA, Amicar) 4 g PO q4h can be given for persistent bleeding that is unresponsive to factor VIII concentrate or desmopressin.

HEMOPHILIA B:
- Infuse factor IX concentrates. It is important to remember that factor IX concentrates contain other proteins that may increase the risk of thrombosis with recurrent use. Therefore factor IX concentrates must be used only when clearly indicated.
- Daily administration of oral cyclophosphamide and prednisone without empirical factor VIII therapy is an effective and well-tolerated treatment for acquired hemophilia.

CHRONIC Rx
- The aim of chronic treatment is to prevent spontaneous bleeding and to prevent excessive bleeding during any surgical intervention.
- Implantation of genetically altered fibroblasts that produce factor VIII is safe and well tolerated. This form is feasible in patients with severe hemophilia. Hemophilia will likely be the first common, severe genetic disease to be cured by gene therapy.

DISPOSITION
- Despite the advent of virally safe blood products and blood treatment programs, nearly 70% of hemophiliacs are HIV-seropositive. Survival is of normal expectancy in HIV-negative patients with mild disease.
- Intracranial bleeds are the second most common cause of death in hemophiliacs after AIDS. They are fatal in 30% of patients, occur in 10% of patients, and are generally secondary to trauma.

REFERENCE
Mannucci PM, Tuddenham E: The hemophilias, from royal genes to gene therapy, *N Engl J Med* 344:1773, 2001.
Author: **Fred F. Ferri, M.D.**

BASIC INFORMATION

■ DEFINITION
A hemorrhoid is a varicose dilation of a vein of the superior or inferior hemorrhoidal plexus, resulting from a persistent increase in venous pressure. External hemorrhoids are below the pectinate line (inferior plexus). Internal hemorrhoids are above the pectinate line (superior plexus) (Fig. 1-131).

■ SYNONYMS
Piles

ICD-9CM CODES
455.6 Hemorrhoids

■ EPIDEMIOLOGY & DEMOGRAPHICS
Potential for development of symptomatic hemorrhoids in all adults
PREVALENCE: Estimated 50% of the adult population in the U.S.
PREDOMINANT SEX: Males = females

■ PHYSICAL FINDINGS & CLINICAL PRESENTATION
- Painless bleeding with defecation; bleeding is bright red and staining on toilet paper
- Perianal irritation
- Mucofecal staining of underclothes
- Acute external hemorrhoids: painful, swollen, and often thrombosed
- Pain on sitting, standing, or defecating (thrombosed hemorrhoid)
- Prolapse
- Constipation

■ ETIOLOGY
- Low-fiber, high-fat diet
- Chronic constipation and straining with defecation
- High resting anal sphincter pressures
- Pregnancy
- Obesity
- Rectal surgery (i.e., episiotomy)
- Prolonged sitting
- Anal intercourse

DIAGNOSIS

■ DIFFERENTIAL DIAGNOSIS
- Fissure
- Abscess
- Anal fistula
- Condylomata acuminata
- Hypertrophied anal papillae
- Rectal prolapse
- Rectal polyp
- Neoplasm

■ WORKUP
- Inspection
- Digital rectal examination
- Anoscopy
- Sigmoidoscopy

TREATMENT

■ NONPHARMACOLOGIC THERAPY
- Avoidance of constipation and straining with defecation
- Avoidance of prolonged sitting on toilet
- High-fiber diet (20 to 30 g/day)

- Increased fluid intake (six to eight glasses of water per day)
- Cleaning with mild soap and water after defecation
- Warm soaks or ice to soothe
- Sitz baths

■ ACUTE GENERAL Rx
- Fiber supplements to provide bulk (psyllium extracts or mucilloids)
- Medicated compresses with witch hazel
- Topical hydrocortisone (1% to 3% cream or ointment)
- Topical anesthetic spray
- Glycerin suppositories
- Stool softeners
- Surgically remove during first 72 hr after onset

■ CHRONIC Rx
- Rubber-band ligation
- Injection sclerotherapy
- Photocoagulation
- Cryodestruction
- Hemorrhoidectomy
- Anal dilation
- Laser or cautery hemorrhoidectomy
- Observance for complications: thrombosis, bleeding, infection, anal stenosis or weakness

■ DISPOSITION
Should resolve, but there is a high rate of recurrence

■ REFERRAL
To colorectal or general surgeon for any hemorrhoid that does not respond to conservative therapy

☼ PEARLS & CONSIDERATIONS

■ COMMENTS
- Patients need to understand the importance of a healthy diet, regular exercise, and rectal hygiene.
- Stress the importance of avoiding prolonged sitting and straining on the toilet.
- Stress the need not to defer the urge to defecate.

REFERENCE
Zuber TJ: Hemorrhoidectomy for thrombosed external hemorrhoids, *Am Fam Physician* 65:1629, 2002.
Author: **Maria A. Corigliano, M.D.**

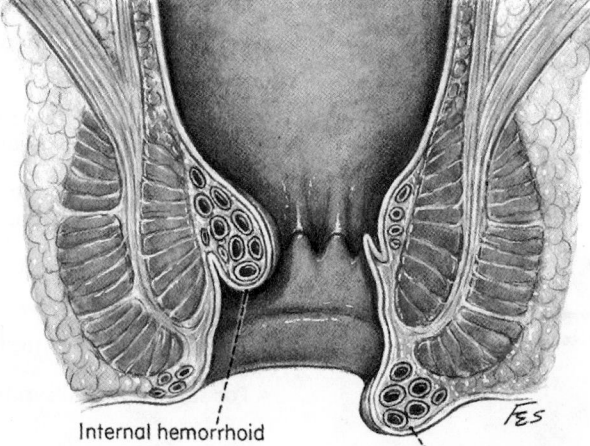

Internal hemorrhoid

External hemorrhoid

Fig. 1-131   Anatomy of internal and external hemorrhoids. (From Noble J [ed]: *Textbook of primary care medicine,* ed 2, St Louis, 1996, Mosby.)

BASIC INFORMATION

■ DEFINITION
Henoch-Schönlein purpura (HSP) is a systemic small vessel vasculitis characterized by palpable purpura in dependent areas (buttocks, legs), gastrointestinal bleeding and other symptoms, arthralgias, arthritis, and renal involvement.

■ SYNONYMS
Anaphylactoid purpura
Allergic purpura

ICD-9CM CODES
287.0 Henoch-Schönlein purpura

■ EPIDEMIOLOGY & DEMOGRAPHICS
HSP is the most common vasculitis seen in children and younger age groups. It has an annual incidence of 14 cases/100,000 population. It is seen mostly from 4 to 15 yr of age, although it can also be seen in older adolescents and young adults. A 2:1 male to female ratio exists. Peak incidence is seen in spring, although cases are seen throughout the year.

■ PHYSICAL FINDINGS & CLINICAL PRESENTATION
- Palpable purpura of dependent areas, especially lower extremities (Fig. 1-132), and areas subjected to pressure such as the beltline
- Subcutaneous edema
- Arthralgias and arthritis in 80% of patients
- GI symptoms are seen in approximately one third of patients. Common findings are nausea, vomiting, diarrhea, cramping, abdominal pain, hematochezia, and melena
- Anecdotally may follow upper respiratory infection
- Renal involvement is seen in up to 80% of older children, usually

within the first month of illness. Less than 5% of cases progress to end-stage renal failure

■ ETIOLOGY
The presumptive etiology is exposure to a trigger antigen that causes antibody formation. Antigen-antibody (immune) complex deposition then occurs in arteriole and capillary walls of skin, renal mesangium, and GI tract. IgA deposition is most common. Antigen triggers postulated include drugs, foods, immunization, and upper respiratory and other viral illnesses. Serologic and pathologic evidence exists, suggesting an association between Parvovirus B19 and HSP. This association may explain observed cases of HSP, which does not respond to corticosteroids or other immunosuppressive therapy.

DIAGNOSIS

Diagnosis is made on clinical grounds. Skin manifestations are most common. Palpable purpura is seen in 70% of adult patients and is less pronounced in children, in whom GI complaints are more common. Skin biopsy will show leukocytoclastic vasculitis.

■ DIFFERENTIAL DIAGNOSIS
Other forms of cutaneous or leukocytoclastic vasculitis:
- Polyarteritis nodosa
- Meningococcemia
- Thrombocytopenic purpura

■ WORKUP
History, physical examination, laboratory testing to rule out other diagnostic considerations, and skin biopsy

■ LABORATORY TESTS
- Electrolytes, BUN, and creatinine

- Urinalysis
- CBC
- Prothrombin time, fibrinogen, and fibrin degradation products
- Blood cultures

Laboratory abnormalities are not specific for HSP. Leukocytosis and eosinophilia may be seen. IgA levels are elevated in approximately 50% of patients. Glomerulonephritis may be present and result in microscopic hematuria, proteinuria, and RBC casts.

■ IMAGING STUDIES
Imaging studies are not useful in diagnosis of HSP. Arteriography or magnetic resonance angiography may be helpful in distinguishing from polyarteritis nodosa.

TREATMENT

- Prednisone 1 mg/kg PO is given if renal or severe GI disease, although benefits are not clear
- Corticosteroids and azathioprine may be beneficial if rapidly progressive glomerulonephritis present. Pulse methylprednisolone therapy has also been proposed in patients with glomerulonephritis, mesenteric vasculitis, or pulmonary involvement
- NSAIDs for arthritis and arthralgias

■ NONPHARMACOLOGIC THERAPY
Supportive care with pain management, adequate hydration, and nutrition

■ DISPOSITION & PROGNOSIS
- Prognosis excellent with spontaneous recovery of most patients within 4 wk.
- End-stage renal disease occurs in 5% of patients. Chronic renal insufficiency is the most common long-term morbidity.
- GI complications include mesenteric infarction, perforation, and intussusception.
- Recurrences can occur.

■ REFERRAL
- For renal or gastrointestinal complications
- For severe clinical syndrome

REFERENCE
Dillon MJ: Henoch-Schönlein purpura (treatment and outcome), *Cleve Clin J Med* 69(Suppl 2):SII 121, 2002.
Author: **Dominick Tammaro, M.D.**

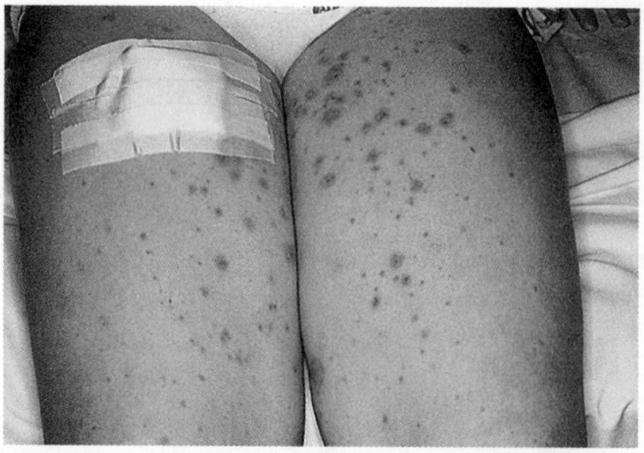

Fig. 1-132   Henoch-Schönlein purpura on the lower extremities of a child. (Courtesy Medical College of Georgia, Division of Dermatology. From Goldstein B [ed]: *Practical dermatology*, ed 2, St Louis, 1997, Mosby.)

BASIC INFORMATION

DEFINITION
Hepatic encephalopathy is an abnormal mental status occurring in patients with severe impairment of liver function and consequent accumulation of toxic products not metabolized by the liver.

SYNONYMS
Hepatic coma

ICD-9CM CODES
572.2 Hepatic encephalopathy

EPIDEMIOLOGY & DEMOGRAPHICS
INCIDENCE/PREVALENCE: Hepatic encephalopathy occurs in >50% of all cases of cirrhosis.

PHYSICAL FINDINGS & CLINICAL PRESENTATION
Hepatic encephalopathy can be classified in stages or grades 1 to 4:
- Grades 1 and 2: mild obtundation
- Grades 3 and 4: stupor to deep coma, with or without decerebrate posturing

The physical examination in hepatic encephalopathy varies with the stage and may reveal the following abnormalities:
- Skin: jaundice, palmar erythema, spider angiomata, ecchymosis, dilated superficial periumbilical veins (caput medusae) in patients with cirrhosis
- Eyes: scleral icterus, Kayser-Fleischer rings (Wilson's disease)
- Breath: fetor hepaticus
- Chest: gynecomastia in men with chronic liver disease
- Abdomen: ascites, small nodular liver (cirrhosis), tender hepatomegaly (congestive hepatomegaly)
- Rectal examination: hemorrhoids (portal hypertension), guaiac-positive stool (alcoholic gastritis, bleeding esophageal varices, PUD, bleeding hemorrhoids)
- Genitalia: testicular atrophy in males with chronic liver disease
- Extremities: pedal edema from hypoalbuminemia
- Neurologic: flapping tremor (asterixis), obtundation, coma with or without decerebrate posturing

ETIOLOGY
- Precipitating factors in patients with underlying cirrhosis (UGI bleeding, hypokalemia, hypomagnesemia, analgesic and sedative drugs, sepsis, alkalosis, increased dietary protein)
- Acute fulminant viral hepatitis
- Drugs and toxins (e.g., isoniazid, acetaminophen, diclofenac and other NSAIDs, statins, methyldopa, loratadine, PTU, lisinopril, labetalol, halothane, carbon tetrachloride, erythromycin, nitrofurantoin, troglitazone)
- Reye's syndrome
- Shock and/or sepsis
- Fatty liver of pregnancy
- Metastatic carcinoma, hepatocellular carcinoma
- Other: autoimmune hepatitis, ischemic venooclusive disease, sclerosing cholangitis, heat stroke, amebic abscesses

DIAGNOSIS

DIFFERENTIAL DIAGNOSIS
- Delirium secondary to medications or illicit drugs
- CVA, subdural hematoma
- Meningitis, encephalitis
- Hypoglycemia
- Uremia
- Cerebral anoxia
- Hypercalcemia
- Metastatic neoplasm to brain
- Alcohol withdrawal syndrome

WORKUP
Exclude other etiologies with comprehensive history (obtained from patient, relatives, and others), physical examination, laboratory and imaging studies. A pertinent history should include exposure to hepatitis, ethanol intake, drug history, exposure to toxins, IV drug abuse, measles or influenza with aspirin use (Reye's syndrome), history of carcinoma (primary or metastatic).

LABORATORY TESTS
- ALT, AST, bilirubin, alkaline phosphatase glucose, calcium, electrolytes, BUN, creatinine, albumin
- CBC, platelet count, PT, PTT
- Serum and urine toxicology screen in suspected medication or illegal drug use
- Blood and urine cultures, urinalysis
- Venous ammonia level
- ABGs

IMAGING STUDIES
CT scan of head may be useful in selected patients to exclude other etiologies.

TREATMENT

NONPHARMACOLOGIC THERAPY
- Identification and treatment of precipitating factors
- Restriction of protein intake (30 to 40 g/day) to reduce toxic protein metabolites

ACUTE GENERAL Rx
REDUCTION OF COLONIC AMMONIA PRODUCTION:
- Lactulose 30 ml of 50% solution qid initially, dose is subsequently adjusted depending on clinical response. Ornithine aspartate 9 g tid is also effective.
- Neomycin 1 g PO q4-6h or given as a 1% retention enema solution (1 g in 100 ml of isotonic saline solution); neomycin should be used with caution in patients with renal insufficiency; metronidazole 250 mg qid may be as effective as neomycin and is not nephrotoxic; however, long-term use can be associated with neurotoxicity. Rifaximin 1200 mg/day is a viable alternative to metronidazole.
- A combination of lactulose and neomycin can be used when either agent is ineffective alone.

TREATMENT OF CEREBRAL EDEMA:
Cerebral edema is often present in patients with acute liver failure, and it accounts for nearly 50% of deaths. Monitoring intracranial pressure by epidural, intraparenchymal, or subdural transducers and treatment of cerebral edema with mannitol (100 to 200 ml of 20% solution [0.3 to 0.4 g/kg of body weight]) given by rapid IV infusion is helpful in selected patients (e.g., potential transplantation patients); dexamethasone and hyperventilation (useful in head injury) are of little value in treating cerebral edema from liver failure

CHRONIC Rx
- Avoidance of any precipitating factors (e.g., high-protein diet, medications)
- Consideration of liver transplantation in selected patients with progressive or recurrent encephalopathy

DISPOSITION
Prognosis varies with the underlying etiology of the liver failure and the grade of encephalopathy (generally good for grades 1, 2; poor for grades 3, 4).

REFERRAL
The early stages of hepatic encephalopathy can be managed in the outpatient setting, whereas stages 3 or 4 require hospital admission.

PEARLS & CONSIDERATIONS

COMMENTS
Patients not responding to supportive therapy should be evaluated for liver transplantation.
Author: **Fred F. Ferri, M.D.**

BASIC INFORMATION

■ DEFINITION
Hepatitis A is generally an acute self-limiting infection of the liver by an enterically transmitted picorna virus, hepatitis A virus (HAV). Infection may range from asymptomatic to fulminant hepatitis.

ICD-9CM CODES
070.1 Hepatitis A

■ EPIDIMIOLOGY & DEMOGRAPHICS
INCIDENCE:
- It occurs worldwide, affecting 1.4 million people annually and accounting for 20%-40% of cases of viral hepatitis in U.S.
- The seroprevalence increases with age, ranging from 10% in individuals <5 yr to 74% in those >50 yr.
- In the U.S. average disease rate is approximately 15 cases/100,000 persons/yr.
- The incidence is relatively higher in some regions in the U.S., including Arizona, Alaska, California, Idaho, Nevada, New Mexico, Okalahoma, Oregon, South Dakota, and Washington.
- At-risk groups include:
  1. Residents and staff of group homes
  2. Children, employees of day care centers
  3. Persons who engage in oral-anal contact, regardless of sexual orientation
  4. Intravenous drug abusers
  5. Travel to endemic areas
  6. Areas of overcrowding, poor sanitation, inadequate sewage treatment

PREVALENCE
- Approximately three fourths of U.S. population has serologic evidence of prior infection
- Anti-HAV prevalence has inverse relation to income and household size

PREDOMINANT SEX: None, except higher infection rates seen in homosexual males who engage in oral-anal contact.

PREDOMINANT AGE/PEAK INCIDENCE
- In areas of high rates of hepatitis A, virtually all children are infected while younger than 10 yr, but disease is rare.
- In areas of moderate rates of hepatitis A, disease occurs in late childhood and young adults.
- In areas of low rates of hepatitis A, most cases occur in young adults.

INCUBATION PERIOD: Averages 30 days (15 to 50)

■ PHYSICAL FINDINGS & CLINICAL PRESENTATION
- Infection with HAV may have acute or subacute presentation, icteric or anicteric. Severity of illness seems to increase with age (90% of infection in children <5 yr may be subclinical)
- A preicteric, prodromal phase of approximately 1-14 days. 15% no apparent prodrome. Symptoms are usually abrupt in onset and may include anorexia, malaise, nausea, vomiting, fever, headache, abdominal pain
- Less common symptoms are chills, myalgias, arthralgias, upper respiratory symptoms, constipation, diarrhea, pruritis, urticaria
- Jaundice occurs in >70% of patients
- The icteric phase is preceded by dark urine
- Bilirubinuria is typically followed a few days later by clay-colored stools and icterus

■ PHYSICAL EXAM
- Jaundice
- Hepatomegaly
- Splenomegaly
- Cervical lymphadenopathy
- Evanescent rash
- Petechiae
- Cardiac arrhythmias

■ COMPLICATION
- Cholestasis
- Fulminant hepatitis
- Arthritis
- Myocarditis
- Optic neuritis
- Transverse myelitis
- Thrombocytopenic purpura
- Aplastic anemia
- Red cell aplasia

■ ETIOLOGY
- Caused by HAV, a 27nm, nonenveloped, icosahedra, positive-stranded RNA virus
- Transmission is fecal-oral route, from person to person. Transmission requires close contact
- Parenteral transmission is considered rare
- Vertical transmission also reported

DIAGNOSIS

■ DIFFERENTIAL DIAGNOSIS
- Other hepatitis virus (B, C, D, E)
- Infectious mononucleosis
- Cytomegalovirus infection
- Herpes simplex virus infection
- Leptospirosis
- Brucellosis
- Drug-induced liver disease
- Ischemic hepatitis
- Autoimmune hepatitis

■ WORKUP
- IgM antibody specific for HAV
- Liver function tests; ALT and AST elevations are sensitive for liver damage but not specific for HAV
- Elevated ESR
- CBC; may find mild lymphocytosis

■ LABORATORY TESTS
- Diagnosis confirmed by IgM anti HAV; it is detectable in almost all infected patients at presentation and remains positive for 3 to 6 mo
- A fourfold rise in titer of total antibody (IgM and IgG) to HAV confirms acute infection
- HAV detection in stool and body fluids by electron microscopy
- HAV RNA detection in stool, body fluids, serum, and liver tissue
- ALT and AST usually more than eight times normal in acute infection
- Bilirubin usually five to 15 times normal
- Alkaline phosphatase minimally elevated but higher level in cholestasis
- Albumin and prothrombin time are generally normal, if elevated may herald hepatic necrosis

■ IMAGING STUDIES
- Rarely useful
- Sonogram (fulminant hepatitis)

TREATMENT

- Usually self-limited
- Supportive care
- Those with fulminant hepatitis may require hospitalization and treatment of associated complications
- Activity as tolerated
- Advise to avoid alcohol and hepatoxic drugs
- Patients with fulminant hepatitis should be assessed for liver transplantation

■ CHRONIC Rx
No chronic HAV and no chronic carrier state

■ DISPOSITION
Follow-up as outpatient

■ PREVENTION
- Improvement in hygiene and sanitation
- Heating food
- Avoidance of water and foods from endemic area

■ PASSIVE IMMUNIZATION
- Immunoglobulin provides protection against HAV through passive transfer of antibody

- Preexposure prophylaxis indicated for person traveling to endemic areas (0.6 ml protects for <5 mo)
- Postexposure prophylaxis indicated for persons with recent exposure (within 2 wk) to HAV and who have not been previously vaccinated. In high-risk patients vaccine may administered with immunoglobulin

■ ACTIVE IMMUNIZATION

- There are several inactivated and attenuated hepatitis vaccines; only the inactivated vaccines are currently available for use and they have been found to be safe and highly immunogenic
- Protective antibody levels were reached in 94% to 100% of adults 1 mo after the first dose, similar results have been found for children and adolescents
- Theoretic analyses of antibody levels estimate duration of immunity to be 10 to 20 yr
- Vaccine should be considered for persons who are at risk: those traveling to or working in endemic areas, homosexual men, illegal drug users, persons with chronic liver disease, children in areas with high rates of hepatitis A infection

REFERENCES

Craig A, Schaffner W: Prevention of hepatitis A with the hepatitis A vaccine, *N Engl J Med* 350:476, 2004.

Rezende G. et al: Viral and clinical factors associated with the fulminant course of hepatitis A infection, *Hepatology* 38:613, 2003.

Vento S. et al: Fulminant hepatitis associated with hepatitis A virus superinfection in patients with chronic hepatitis C, *N Engl J Med* 338:286, 1998.

Author: **Vasanthi Arumugam, M.D.**

BASIC INFORMATION

■ DEFINITION

Hepatitis B is an acute infection of the liver parenchymal cells caused by the hepatitis B virus (HBV).

■ SYNONYMS

Serum hepatitis
Long incubation (30 to 180 days)
Hepatitis

ICD-9CM CODES

070.3 Hepatitis B

■ EPIDEMIOLOGY & DEMOGRAPHICS

INCIDENCE (IN U.S.):
- Approximately 200,000 to 300,000 infections annually in U.S.
- Much higher incidence in Europe (approximately 1 million new cases annually) and in areas of high endemicity
- In U.S., transmission is mainly horizontal (percutaneous and mucous membrane exposure to infectious blood and other body fluids, [e.g., sexual transmission, either homosexual or heterosexual]); also from needle sharing amongst drug abusers; occupational exposure to contaminated blood and blood products; persons receiving transfusions of blood and blood products; hemodialysis patients

NOTE: improved screening of blood and blood products has greatly reduced, although not eliminated, the risk of posttransfusion HBV infection.
- In areas of high endemicity, transmission is largely vertical (perinatal): HBV exists in the blood and body fluids. Perinatal transmission from HBsAg-positive mothers is as high as 90%

PREVALENCE (IN U.S.):
- North America, Western Europe, and Australia are areas of low prevalence, <2%.
- Africa, Asia, and the Western Pacific region are areas of high prevalence, ≥8%.
- Southern and Eastern Europe have intermediate rates, 2% to 7%.
- Chronically infected persons, those with positive HBsAg for >6 mo, represent the major source of infection.
- Up to 95% of infants and children <5 yr of age, who typically have subclinical acute infection, will become chronic HBV carriers.
- Adults are more likely to have clinically evident acute infection, but only 1% to 5% will develop chronic infection.
- Approximately 0.1% with acute infection will develop fulminant acute hepatitis resulting in death.

PREDOMINANT SEX:
- Predominant in males because of increased intravenous drug abuse, homosexuality
- Females more commonly terminate in chronic carrier state

PREDOMINANT AGE: 20 to 45 yr
PEAK INCIDENCE: 30 to 45 yr of age, at rates of 5% to 20%
GENETICS:
Neonatal infection:
- Rare in U.S.
- High (up to 90%) in areas of high endemicity (only 5% to 10% of perinatal infections occur in utero)

■ PHYSICAL FINDINGS & CLINICAL PRESENTATION (FIG. 1-133)

- Often nonspecific symptoms
- Profound malaise
- Many asymptomatic cases
- Prodrome:
  1. 15% to 20% serum sickness (urticaria, rash, arthralgia) during early HBsAg
  2. HBsAg-Ab complex disease (arthritis, arteritis, glomerulonephritis)
- Hepatomegaly (87%) with RUQ tenderness
  1. Hepatic punch tenderness
  2. Splenomegaly: rare (10% to 15%)

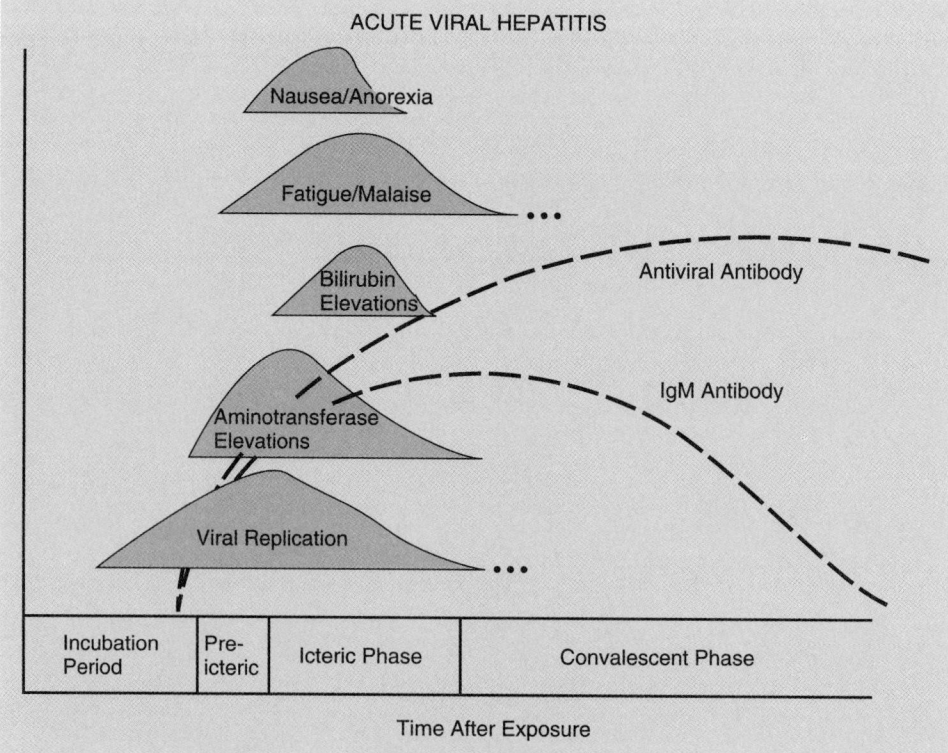

Fig. 1-133   The typical course of acute viral hepatitis. (From Goldman L, Ausiello D [eds]: *Cecil textbook of medicine,* ed 22, Philadelphia, 2004, WB Saunders.)

- Jaundice, dark urine, with occasional pruritus
- Variable fever (when present, generally precedes jaundice and rapidly declines following onset of icteric phase)
- Spider angiomata: rare; resolves during recovery
- Rare polyarteritis nodosa, cryoglobulinemia

■ ETIOLOGY
- Caused by hepatitis B virus (42-nm hepadnavirus with an outer surface coat [HBsAg], inner nucleocapsid core [HBcAg; HBeAg]; DNA polymerase; and partially double-stranded DNA genome)
- Transmission by parenteral route (needle use, tattooing, ear piercing, acupuncture, transfusion of blood and blood products, hemodialysis, sexual contact), perinatal transmission
- Infection may result from contact of infectious material with mucous membranes and open skin breaks (e.g., HBV is stable and can be transmitted from toothbrushes, utensils, razors, baby toys, various medical equipment [respirators, endoscopes])
- Oral intake of infectious material may result in infection through breaks in the oral mucosa
- Food or water virtually never found to be sources of HBV infection
- Infection occurring primarily in liver, where necrosis probably results from cytotoxic T-cell response, direct cytopathic effect of HBcAg (core antigen), high-level HBsAg (surface antigen) expression, or co-infection with delta (D) hepatitis virus (RNA delta core within HBsAg envelope)
- Recovery (>90%):
  1. Fulminant hepatitis occurring in <1% (especially if coinfected with hepatitis D); 80% fatal
  2. Unusual (5%) prolonged acute disease for 4 to 12 mo, with recovery
  3. Overall fatality increases with age and viral inoculation (e.g., transfusions)
- Chronic infection (1% to 2%):
  1. Persistent carrier state without hepatitis (HBsAg positive)
  2. Chronic persistent hepatitis (CPH) (clinically well), or chronic active hepatitis (CAH) (HBsAg positive and HBeAg positive)
  3. Cirrhosis
  4. Hepatocellular carcinoma (especially after neonatal infection)
  5. Chronic infection: more common following low-dose exposure and mild acute hepatitis, with earlier age of infection, in males, or if immunosuppressed

6. One third to one quarter of chronically infected will develop progressive liver disease (cirrhosis, hepatocellular carcinoma)

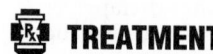 **DIAGNOSIS**

■ DIFFERENTIAL DIAGNOSIS
- Acute disease confused with other viral hepatitis infections (A, C, D, E)
- Any viral illness producing systemic disease and hepatitis (e.g., yellow fever, EBV, CMV, HIV, rubella, rubeola, coxsackie B, adenovirus, herpes simplex or zoster)
- Nonviral etiologies of hepatitis (e.g., leptospirosis, toxoplasmosis, alcoholic hepatitis, drug-induced [e.g., acetaminophen, INH], toxic hepatitis [carbon tetrachloride, benzene])

■ WORKUP
- Acute serum specimen for hepatitis B serology (HBsAg, HBsAb, HBcAb, HBeAg, HBeAb)
- LFTs
- CBC
- Liver biopsy: rarely indicated for diagnosis of fulminant viral hepatitis, chronic hepatitis, cirrhosis, carcinoma

■ LABORATORY TESTS
- Diagnosis of acute HBV infection is best confirmed by IgM HBcAb in acute or early convalescent serum.
  1. Generally, IgM present during onset of jaundice
  2. Coexisting HBsAg
- HBsAg and IgG-HBcAb during acute jaundice are strongly suggestive of remote HBV infection and another etiology for current illness.
- HBsAb alone is suggestive of immunization response.
- With recovery, HBeAg is rapidly replaced by HBeAb in 2 to 3 mo, and HBsAg is replaced by HBsAb in 5 to 6 mo.
- In chronic HBV hepatitis, HBsAg and HBeAg are persistent without corresponding Ab.
- In chronic carrier state, HBsAg is persistent, but HBeAg is replaced by HBe AB.
- HBcAb develops in all outcomes.
- HBeAg correlation with highest infectivity; appearance of HBeAb heralds recovery.
- LFTs:
  1. ALT and AST: usually more than eight times normal (often 1000 U/L) at onset of jaundice (minimal acute ALT/AST rises often followed by chronic hepatitis or hepatocellular carcinoma)
  2. Bilirubin: variably elevated in icteric viral hepatitis

3. Alkaline phosphatase: minimally elevated (one to three times normal) acutely
- Albumin and prothrombin time:
  1. Generally normal
  2. If abnormal, possible harbinger of impending hepatic necrosis (fulminant hepatitis)
- WBC and ESR: generally normal

■ IMAGING STUDIES
- Rarely useful
- Sonogram to document rapid reduction in liver size during fulminant hepatitis or mass in hepatocellular carcinoma

Rx **TREATMENT**

■ NONPHARMACOLOGIC THERAPY
- Symptomatic treatment as necessary
- Activity as tolerated
- High-calorie diet preferred; often best tolerated in morning

■ ACUTE GENERAL Rx
- In most cases of acute HBV infection no treatment necessary; >90% of adults will spontaneously clear infection
- Hospitalization advisable for any patient in danger from dehydration caused by poor oral intake, whose PT is prolonged, who has rising bilirubin level >15 to 20 μg/dl, or who has any clinical evidence of hepatic failure
- IV therapy needed (rarely) for hydration during severe vomiting
- Avoid hepatically metabolized drugs
- No therapeutic measures are beneficial
- Steroids not shown helpful

■ CHRONIC Rx
The aim of therapy in chronic HBV infection is to eradicate the virus.
The two modalities of therapy available to achieve this goal have been: immune modulators (interferon alpha) and antiviral agents in the form of nucleoside analogues (e.g., lamivudine, famciclovir).
- Until recently, IFN-α has been the mainstay of therapy. Its mechanism of action is to stimulate the immune system to attack HBV-infected hepatocytes, thus inhibiting viral protein synthesis.
- A 4-month course of treatment results in a 30% to 40% response with significant reduction of serum HBV DNA, normalization of ALT, and loss of HBeAg. Seroconversion from HBeAg to HBeAb occurs in 15% to 20%.

- Factors that increase the likelihood of response to IFN-α therapy include:
  1. Adult onset of infection
  2. High baseline ALT
  3. Low baseline HBV DNA
  4. Absence of cirrhosis
  5. Female
  6. HBeAg positive
- Infrequent relapse after successful completion of therapy
- 80% of patients who lose HBeAg during therapy lose HBsAg in the decade after therapy
- >50% of patients who do not seroconvert after initial therapy develop a delayed HBeAg seroconversion months to years after therapy
- Overall incidence of cirrhosis and hepatocellular carcinoma is decreased in those treated with IFN-α
- IFN-α is successful only in patients with an active immune response; therefore it is not effective in patients with HIV infection and organ transplant patients
- Asians respond poorly to IFN-α
- Treatment with IFN-α in general is also poorly tolerated: side effects include flulike symptoms, injection-site reactions, rash, weight loss, anxiety, depression, alopecia, thrombocytopenia, granulocytopenia, thyroid dysfunction
- Nucleoside analogues block viral replication by inhibiting HBV polymerase
- Lamivudine is, to date, the only one of these agents approved for treatment of chronic HBV infection; it has been shown to rapidly reduce HBV replication and suppress HBV DNA to undetectable levels after a few weeks of treatment, and treatment for 1 yr is as effective as IFN-α with respect to loss of HBeAg seroconversion to HBeAb and loss of HBV DNA
  1. It is better tolerated than IFN-α
  2. Easier administration: given orally

---

3. Suppression of HBV replication regardless of sex, ethnicity, disease severity
- Other nucleoside agents under evaluation include famciclovir (found less effective than lamivudine), adefovir and adefovir dipivoxil, ganciclovir, lobucavir, entecavir, emtricitabine
- A problem with the antiviral therapies is emergence of resistant HBV strains (YMDD variants [tyrosine-methionine-aspartate-aspartate])
- Combination therapy with two or three nucleoside analogues or combination therapy with IFN-α currently under investigation
- Liver transplantation (consider for fulminant hepatitis)

■ DISPOSITION
- Follow-up as outpatient
- Acute disease: usually <6 wk
- Rare fatalities (fulminant hepatitis)
- Possible chronic carrier state, cirrhosis, hepatocellular carcinoma

■ REFERRAL
To infectious disease specialist and gastroenterologist for consultation regarding fulminant hepatitis or prolonged cholestasis, for cases of uncertain etiology, or for treatment of chronic active hepatitis

☼ PEARLS & CONSIDERATIONS

■ COMMENTS
- Virus and HBsAg in high titers in blood for 1 to 7 wk before jaundice and for a variable time thereafter.
- Transmission is possible during entire period of HBsAg (and especially during HBeAg) in serum.
- Universal precautions should be followed for all contacts with blood or secretions/excretions contaminated with blood.

- Preventing before exposure:
  1. Lifestyle changes
  2. Meticulous testing of blood supply (although some chronically infected, infectious donors are HBsAg negative)
  3. Sterilization via steam or hypochlorite
  4. Hepatitis B vaccine for high-risk groups given IM in deltoid to induce HBsAb (response should be confirmed) is protective (>90% effective)
  5. Recommendation for universal childhood immunization with doses at birth, 1 mo, and 6 mo
- Prevention after exposure:
  1. HBV hyperimmune globulin (HBIG) given immediately after needlestick, within 14 days of sexual exposure, or at birth, followed by HBV vaccination
  2. Standard immune globulin: nearly as effective as HBIG

Section V, Tables 5-15 and 5-17 describe hepatitis B prophylaxis.

REFERENCES

Jonas MM et al: Clinical trial of lamivudine in children with chronic hepatitis B, *N Engl J Med* 346(22):1706, 2002.

Lin KW, Kirchner JT: Hepatitis B, *Am Fam Physician* 69:75, 2004.

Maddrey WC: Hepatitis B: an important public health issue, *J Med Virol* 61:362, 2000.

Torresi J, Locarnini S: Antiviral chemotherapy for the treatment of hepatitis B virus infections, *Gastroenterol* 118:S83, 2000.

Weinberg MS et al: Preventing transmission of hepatitis B virus from people with chronic infection, *Am J Prev Med* 20(4):272, 2001.

Author: **Jane V. Eason, M.D.**

BASIC INFORMATION

■ DEFINITION

Hepatitis C is an acute liver parenchymal infection caused by hepatitis C virus (HCV).

■ SYNONYMS

Transfusion-related non-A, non-B hepatitis (incubation period averages 6 wk, intermediate between hepatitis A and B)

ICD-9CM CODES
070.51 Other viral hepatitis

■ EPIDEMIOLOGY & DEMOGRAPHICS

Hepatitis C infection is the most common chronic blood-borne infection in the U.S.

INCIDENCE (IN U.S.):
- 150,000 new cases/yr (37,500, symptomatic; 93,000, later chronic liver disease; 30,700, cirrhosis)
- Approximately 9000 of these ultimately die of HCV infection; most common (40%) cause of nonalcoholic liver disease in U.S.

PREVALENCE (IN U.S.):
- Overall prevalence of anti-HCV is 1.8% (an estimated 3.9 million persons nationwide)
- Highest prevalence in hemophiliacs transfused before 1987 and injecting-drug users, 72% to 90%
- Among low-risk groups, prevalence 0.6%

PREDOMINANT SEX: Slight male predominance

PREDOMINANT AGE: Highest prevalence in 30 to 49 yr age group (65%)

PEAK INCIDENCE:
- 20 to 39 yr old
- African Americans and whites have similar incidence of acute disease; Hispanics have higher rates
- Prevalence substantially higher among non-Hispanic blacks than among non-Hispanic whites

GENETICS: Neonatal infection: Rare. Increased risk with maternal HIV-1 coinfection

PHYSICAL FINDINGS & CLINICAL PRESENTATION
- Symptoms usually develop 7 to 8 wk after infection (2 to 26 wk), but 70% to 80% of cases are subclinical.
- 10% to 20% report acute illness with jaundice and nonspecific symptoms (abdominal pain, anorexia, malaise).
- Fulminant hepatitis may rarely occur during this period.
- After acute infection, 15% to 25% have complete resolution (absence of HCV RNA in serum, normal ALT).
- Progression to chronic infection is common, 50% to 84%. 74% to 86% have persistent viremia; spontaneous clearance of viremia in chronic infection is rare. 60% to 70% of patients will have persistent or fluctuating ALT levels, 30% to 40% with chronic infection have normal ALT levels.
- 15% to 20% of those with chronic HCV will develop cirrhosis over a period of 20 to 30 yr; in most others chronic infection leads to hepatitis and varying degrees of fibrosis.
- 0.4% to 2.5% of patients with chronic infection develop hepatocellular carcinoma.
- 25% of patients with chronic infection continue to have an asymptomatic course with normal LFTs and benign histology.
- In chronic HCV infection, extrahepatic sequelae include a variety of immunologic and lymphoproliferative disorders (e.g., cryoglobulinemia, membranoproliferative glomerulonephritis, and possibly Sjögren syndrome, autoimmune thyroiditis, polyarteritis nodosa, aplastic anemia, lichen planus, porphyria cutanea tarda, B-cell lymphoma, others).

■ ETIOLOGY
- Caused by HCV (single-stranded RNA flavivirus)
- Most HCV transmission is parenteral
- In the U.S., advances in screening of blood and blood products in 1990 and 1992 have made transfusion-related HCV infection rare (the risk is estimated to be 0.001%/unit transfused)
- Injecting-drug use accounts for most HCV transmission in the U.S. (60% of newly acquired cases, 20% to 50% of chronically infected persons)
- Occupational needlestick exposure from an HCV-positive source has a seroconversion rate of 1.8% (range 0% to 7%)
- Nosocomial transmission rates (from surgery and procedures such as colonoscopy, hemodialysis) are extremely low
- Sexual transmission and maternal-fetal transmission are infrequent (estimated at 5%)
- No identifiable risk in 40% to 50% of community-acquired HIV infection
- HCV infection may stimulate production of cytotoxic T lymphocytes and cytokines (inf-γ), which likely mediate hepatic necrosis

DIAGNOSIS

■ DIFFERENTIAL DIAGNOSIS
- Other hepatitis viruses (A, B, D, E)
- Other viral illnesses producing systemic disease (e.g., yellow fever, EBV, CMV, HIV, rubella, rubeolae, coxsackie B, adenovirus, HSV, HZV)
- Nonviral hepatitis (e.g., leptospirosis, toxoplasmosis, alcoholic hepatitis, drug-induced hepatitis [acetaminophen, INH], toxic hepatitis)

■ WORKUP
- Acute hepatitis C antibody (Table 1-27)
- LFTs; CBC

NOTE: ALT is an easy and inexpensive test to monitor infection and efficacy of therapy. However, ALT levels may fluctuate or even be normal in active or chronic infection and even with cirrhosis, and ALT may remain elevated even after clearance of viremia.
- Liver biopsy with histologic staging is the gold standard for assessing the degree of disease activity and the likelihood of disease progression, and also help rule out other causes of liver disease.

■ LABORATORY TESTS
Diagnosis is often by exclusion, because it takes 6 wk to 12 mo to develop anti-HCV antibody (70% positive by 6 wk, 90% positive by 6 mo). Diagnostic tests include serologic assays for antibodies and molecular tests for viral particles.
1. Enzyme immunoassay is the test for anti-HCV antibody:
   - The current version can detect antibody within 4 to 10 wk after infection
   - False-negative rate in low-risk populations is 0.5% to 1%
   - False-negatives also in immune-compromised persons, HIV-1, renal failure, HCV-associated essential mixed cryoglobulinemia
   - False positives in autoimmune hepatitis, paraproteinemia, and persons with no risk factors
2. Recombinant immunoblot is used to confirm positive enzyme immunoassays:
   - Recommended only in low-risk settings
3. Qualitative and quantitative HCV RNA tests using PCR:
   - Lower limit of detection is <100 copies HCV RNA/ml
   - Used to confirm viremia and to assess response to treatment
   - Qualitative PCR useful in patients with negative enzyme immunoassay in whom infection is suspected
   - Quantitative tests use either branched-chain DNA or reverse transcription PCR; the latter is more sensitive
4. Viral genotyping can distinguish among genotypes 1, 2, and 3, which is helpful in choosing therapy; most of these tests use PCR

TABLE 1-27 Tests for Hepatitis C Virus (HCV) Infection

TEST/TYPE	APPLICATION	COMMENTS
Hepatitis C Virus Antibody (anti-HCV)		
EIA (enzyme immunoassay) Supplemental assay (i.e., recombinant immunoblot assay [RIBA])	Indicates past or present infection but does not differentiate among acute, chronic, or resolved infection All positive EIA results should be verified with a supplemental assay	Sensitivity ≥97% EIA alone has low-positive predictive value in low-prevalence populations
HCV RNA (Hepatitis C Virus Ribonucleic Acid) *Qualitative Tests*†*		
Reverse transcriptase polymerase chain reaction (RT-PCR) amplification of HCV RNA by in-house or commercial assays (e.g., Amplicor HCV)	Detect presence of circulating HCV RNA Monitor patients on antiviral therapy	Detect virus as early as 1-2 wk after exposure Detection of HCV RNA during course of infection might be intermittent; a single negative RT-PCR is not conclusive False-positive and false-negative results might occur
Quantitative Tests*†		
RT-PCR amplification of HCV RNA by in-house or commercial assays (e.g., Amplicor HCV Monitor) Branched chain DNA‡ (bDNA) assays (e.g., Quantiplex HCV RNA Assay)	Determine concentration of HCV RNA Might be useful for assessing the likelihood of response to antiviral therapy	Less sensitive than qualitative RT-PCR Should not be used to exclude the diagnosis of HCV infection or to determine treatment end point
Genotype*†		
Several methodologies available (e.g., hybridization, sequencing)	Group isolates of HCV based on genetic differences, into 6 genotypes and >90 subtypes With new therapies, length of treatment might vary based on genotype	Genotype 1 (subtypes 1a and 1b) most common in U.S. and associated with lower response to antiviral therapy
Serotype*		
EIA based on immunoreactivity to synthetic peptides (e.g., Murex HCV Serotyping 1-6 Assay)	No clinical utility	Cannot distinguish among subtypes Dual infections often observed

From *MMWR Morb Mortal Rep Wkly* 47(RR-19) 1998.
*Currently not U.S. Food and Drug Administration approved; lack standardization.
†Samples require special handling (e.g., serum must be separated within 2-4 hours of collection and stored frozen [−20° C or −70° C]; frozen samples should be shipped on dry ice).
‡Deoxyribonucleic acid.

(NOTE: genotypes 1, 2, and 3 predominate in the U.S. and Europe [1 is especially common in North America])
5. LFTs:
   - ALT and AST may be elevated to more than eight times normal in acute infection; in chronic infection ALT may be normal or fluctuate
   - Bilirubin may be 5 to 10 times normal
   - Albumin and prothrombin time generally normal; if abnormal, may be harbinger of impending hepatic necrosis
6. WBC and ESR are generally normal

■ IMAGING STUDIES
- Rarely useful
- Sonogram: rapid liver size reduction during fulminant hepatitis or mass in hepatocellular carcinoma

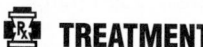 **TREATMENT**

■ NONPHARMACOLOGIC THERAPY
Activity and diet as tolerated

■ ACUTE GENERAL Rx
- Supportive care
- Avoid hepatically metabolized drugs
- Specific Rx for acute HCV infection
- Recent studies demonstrate that *early* treatment with IFN-α-2b during acute HCV infection prevents chronic infection. The aim is to decrease viral load early in infection and allow the patient's immune system to control viral replication, thus preventing progression to chronic infection. The primary end point was sustained virologic response, with absence of HCV RNA in serum 24 wk after completion of therapy.
- Further investigations are in progress.

■ CHRONIC Rx
- Response to therapy is influenced by HCV genotype. Patients with genotype 1 rarely respond to interferon alone, and response to combination therapy with interferon and ribavirin is less than for genotypes 2 and 3.
- IFN-α alone or combined with ribavirin have been the mainstays of therapy.
- IFN-α monotherapy for 12 to 18 mo achieves initial response (normalization of transaminases and undetectable HCV RNA) in 40%, but most have relapse after therapy; sustained response in only 6% to 21%; those with genotype 1 and those with cirrhosis at time of therapy have even lower response rates.
- Combination INF-α and ribavirin given thrice weekly has been shown to achieve sustained virologic response in up to 40% of patients. Those with genotype 1 and those

with high viral loads required 48 wk of therapy to achieve optimal response (versus 24 wk for those with genotypes 2 and 3 and those with low viral loads).

- 49% of patients who relapse after IFN-α monotherapy have a sustained virologic response to IFN-α and ribavirin combination therapy. In those with contraindications to ribavirin, a more prolonged course of treatment with higher dose IFN-α or PEG-interferon may be an option.
- Both IFN-α and ribavirin have numerous contraindications (absolute and relative) to use and may cause a variety of side effects. IFN-α can cause flulike symptoms, thrombocytopenia, granulocytopenia, rash, alopecia, anorexia, psychiatric disturbances, others. Ribavirin can cause hemolysis, nausea, anemia, nasal congestion, pruritus.
- In patients who fail to respond to IFN-α or combination therapy with ribavirin, <10% will respond to retreatment.
- Pegylated interferons are IFN-α with an attached polyethylene glycol molecule. The PEG molecule confers a longer half-life and extended therapeutic activity compared with IFN-α, and reduced dosing, once a week.
- Recent treatment trials have shown that pegylated interferon alone achieves higher response rates than does IFN-α alone in patients with chronic hepatitis C without cirrhosis, and in patients with chronic hepatitis C with cirrhosis or bridging fibrosis. Their enhanced efficacy over INF-α may be the result of a more vigorous immune response

(e.g., increased hepatitis C-specific T-helper-1 response).
- Pegylated interferons can be used in the treatment of persons who cannot be treated with ribavirin.
- Optimal regimens with pegylated interferons have yet to be determined; currently trials are underway using pegylated interferon in combination with ribavirin.

Liver transplantation:
- Hepatitis C is the main indication for liver transplantation in the U.S.
- It is the only option for patients with deteriorating HCV-related cirrhosis and for some patients with hepatocellular carcinoma.
- Recurrent infection occurs in almost all patients with progressive fibrosis and cirrhosis; up to 20% progress to cirrhosis within 5 yr posttransplant.

Coinfection with HIV:
- These patients have a poor response to IFN-α alone.
- Consider initiating therapy for HCV before starting antiretrovirals, because immune reconstitution syndrome occurring with initiation of antiretrovirals may exacerbate HCV-related hepatitis.

■ DISPOSITION

- Follow-up as outpatient
- Monitor ALT levels as a clue for chronic disease
- Chronic carrier state, cirrhosis, hepatic carcinoma more common than with hepatitis A and B

☼ PEARLS & CONSIDERATIONS

- More rapid progression of disease in persons who drink alcohol regularly, persons of advanced age at time of infection, and those coinfected with other viruses (HIV, hepatitis B).
- No preventive vaccine available; postexposure immune globulin may provide minimal protection.
- Preventive measures include use of universal precautions, careful screening of blood and blood products, lifestyle changes.

REFERENCES

Centers for Disease Control: Hepatitis C, *MMWR Morb Mortal Wkly Rep* 51(RR-6), 2002.

Germer HH, Zein NN: Advances in the molecular diagnosis of hepatitis C and their implications, *Mayo Clin Proc* 76:911, 2001.

Hadziyannis JJ et al: Peginterferon α-2a and ribavirin combination therapy in chronic hepatitis C, *Ann Intern Med* 140:346, 2004.

Herrine SK: Approach to the patient with chronic hepatitis C virus infection, *Ann Intern Med* 136:747, 2002.

Jaeckel E et al: Treatment of acute hepatitis C with interferon alfa-2b, *N Engl J Med* 345(20):1452, 2001.

Lauer GM, Walker BD: Hepatitis C virus infection, *N Engl J Med* 345(1):41, 2001.

Sulkowski MS, Ray SC, Thomas DL: Needlestick transmission of hepatitis C, *JAMA* 287(18):2406, 2002.

Author: **Jane V. Eason, M.D.**

BASIC INFORMATION

■ DEFINITION
Autoimmune hepatitis is a chronic inflammatory condition of the liver, characterized by the presence of circulating autoantibodies. Two types have been described: type 1 or "classic" autoimmune hepatitis and type 2, characterized by the presence of antibodies to liver/kidney microsomes.

■ SYNONYMS
Autoimmune chronic active hepatitis
Chronic active hepatitis
Lupoid hepatitis

ICD-9CM CODES
571.49 Chronic hepatitis

■ EPIDEMIOLOGY & DEMOGRAPHICS
- Type 1 can occur at any age
- Type 2 is more common in children
- More common in women
- Estimated 100,000 to 200,000 cases in U.S.
- Accounts for 5.9% of liver transplants in U.S.

■ PHYSICAL FINDINGS & CLINICAL PRESENTATION
- Varies from asymptomatic elevations of liver enzymes to advanced cirrhosis
- Symptoms may include fatigue, anorexia, nausea, abdominal pain, pruritus, and arthralgia
- Jaundice
- Hepatomegaly/splenomegaly
- Autoimmune findings may include arthritis, xerostomia, keratoconjunctivitis, cutaneous vasculitis, and erythema nodosum
- For patients presenting with advanced disease: ascites, edema, abnormal bleeding, jaundice

■ ETIOLOGY
- Exact etiology unknown; liver histology demonstrates cell-mediated immune attack against hepatocytes
- Presence of a variety of autoantibodies suggests an autoimmune mechanism
- Strong genetic predisposition

■ DIAGNOSIS

■ DIFFERENTIAL DIAGNOSIS
Acute Disease:
- Acute viral hepatitis (A, B, C, D, E, cytomegalovirus, Epstein-Barr, herpes)
- Chronic viral hepatitis (B, C)
- Toxic hepatitis (alcohol, drugs)
- Primary biliary cirrhosis
- Primary sclerosing cholangitis
- Hemochromatosis
- Nonalcoholic steatohepatitis
- SLE
- Wilson's disease
- Alpha-1-antitrypsin deficiency

■ WORKUP
- History and physical examination with attention to the presence of autoimmune abnormalities such as arthritis, vasculitis, or sicca syndrome
- LFTs
- Tests for autoantibodies
- Liver biopsy for establishing diagnosis and disease severity

■ LABORATORY TESTS
- Aminotransferases generally elevated, may fluctuate
- Bilirubin and alkaline phosphatase moderately elevated or normal
- Hypergammaglobulinemia usually present
- Circulating autoantibodies often present
  1. Rheumatoid factor
  2. Antinuclear antibodies
  3. Anti-smooth muscle antibodies
  4. Antibodies to liver/kidney microsomes
- Hypoalbuminemia and prolonged prothrombin time with advanced disease

■ IMAGING STUDIES
Ultrasound of liver and biliary tree to rule out obstruction or hepatic mass

■ TREATMENT

■ NONPHARMACOLOGIC THERAPY
Avoid alcohol and hepatotoxic drugs

■ CHRONIC Rx
- Indications for treatment:
  1. Serum aminotransferase >10 times the upper limit of normal
  2. Serum aminotransferase >5 times the upper limit of normal, with serum gammaglobulin level twice the upper limit of normal
  3. Young age
  4. Histologic features of bridging necrosis or multiacinar necrosis
- Treatment may not be indicated in patients with inactive cirrhosis
- Initial treatment: prednisone 60 mg PO/day or combination treatment with prednisone 30 mg PO/day plus azathioprine 50 mg PO/day
- Combination therapy allows for lower prednisone doses and less steroid side effects
- Goal of therapy is remission (normalization of gammaglobulin and bilirubin, reduction of aminotransferases to <2 times the upper limit of normal)
- Patients who develop end-stage liver disease are candidates for liver transplantation

■ DISPOSITION
- Follow-up as outpatient
- Long-term treatment may be necessary for sustained remission
- 65% of patients achieve remission by 18 mo; 80% achieve remission by 3 yr
- Approximately 10% of patients fail to improve with therapy
- Patients who develop end-stage liver disease are candidates for liver transplantation

■ REFERRAL
To gastroenterologist for long-term management

⚇ PEARLS & CONSIDERATIONS

A variety of autoimmune conditions can be seen in association with autoimmune hepatitis, including thyroiditis, Graves' disease, ulcerative colitis, rheumatoid arthritis, uveitis, pernicious anemia, Sjögren's syndrome, mixed connective tissue disease, CREST syndrome, and vitiligo.

REFERENCE
Al-Khalidi JA, Czaja AJ: Current concepts in the diagnosis, pathogenesis, and treatment of autoimmune hepatitis, *Mayo Clin Proc* 76:1237, 2001.
Author: **Mark J Fagan, M.D.**

BASIC INFORMATION

■ **DEFINITION**

Hepatocellular carcinoma is a malignant tumor of the liver, arising from hepatocytes.

■ **ICD-9CM CODES**

155.0 Hepatocellular carcinoma

■ **SYNONYMS**

Hepatoma

■ **EPIDEMIOLOGY & DEMOGRAPHICS**

Incidence of hepatocellular carcinoma varies widely in parts of the world:

- Areas with high rates of hepatitis B and hepatitis C (Asia, sub-Saharan Africa) have correspondingly high rates of hepatocellular carcinoma.
- Males are affected more commonly than females.
- Peak incidence is in fifth and sixth decades in Western countries, earlier in areas with perinatal transmission of hepatitis B.

■ **RISK FACTORS**

- Chronic liver disease
- Cirrhosis
- Chronic hepatitis B or C infection, especially in the presence of HBeAg
- Hepatotoxins including alcohol, mycotoxins (aflatoxin B_1), high-dose anabolic steroids, vinyl chloride, possibly estrogen

- Systemic diseases affecting the liver such as alpha-1 antitrypsin deficiency, hemochromatosis, tyrosinemia

■ **PHYSICAL FINDINGS & CLINICAL PRESENTATION**

- One third of patients are asymptomatic.
- Signs of underlying cirrhosis are often present (e.g., weight loss, ascites).
- Previously compensated cirrhosis with new ascites, encephalopathy, jaundice or bleeding

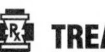 **DIAGNOSIS**

■ **DIFFERENTIAL DIAGNOSIS**

- Metastatic tumor to liver
- Benign liver tumors such as adenomas, focal nodular hyperplasia, hemangiomas
- Focal fatty infiltration

■ **WORKUP**

- History with regard to risk factors (see Risk Factors)
- Physical examination with attention to signs of chronic liver disease
- Laboratory evaluation and imaging

■ **LABORATORY TESTS**

- LFTs
- Elevated alpha-fetoprotein in 70% of patients (sensitivity 40%-65%; specificity 80%-94%)

- Paraneoplastic syndromes associated with hepatocellular carcinoma may cause abnormalities such as hypercalcemia, hypoglycemia, and polycythemia

■ **IMAGING STUDIES**

Ultrasound, CT scan, or MRI (Fig. 1-134)

■ **BIOPSY**

Percutaneous biopsy under ultrasound or CT scan usually is diagnostic.

■ **SCREENING**

Screening high-risk patients with ultrasound and α-fetoprotein may identify hepatocellular carcinoma at an early stage.

TREATMENT

- Depends on size of lesion and severity of underlying liver disease
- For patients with small solitary lesions <5 cm, good liver function, and no portal hypertension, surgical resection is the best option
- For patients who are not candidates for surgical resection, percutaneous ethanol injection, transcatheter arterial chemotherapy with or without embolization of the tumor, or ultrasound-guided cryoablation can be used for local tumor control. Chemotherapy not used routinely for advanced disease

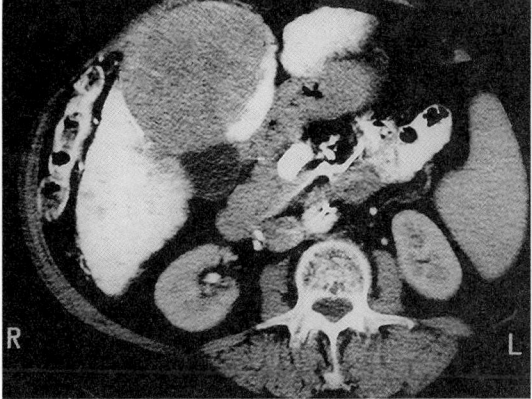 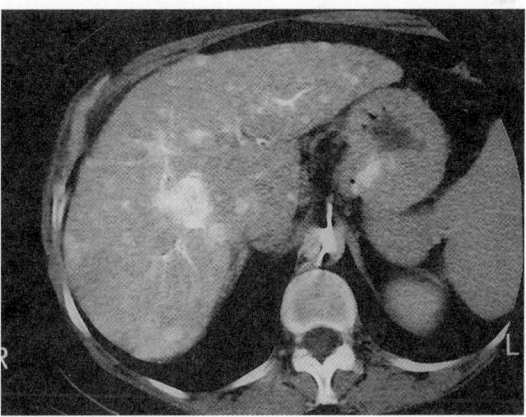

Fig. 1-134 **A,** CT scan through the lower portion of the liver obtained during the portal venous phase shows a single large hypodense lesion. Percutaneous biopsy confirmed a hepatoma. **B,** CT scan through the cranial portion of the liver during the arterial phase demonstrates multiple additional hypervascular lesions, suggesting an unresectable, multicentric hepatoma. (From Goldman L, Ausiello D [eds]: *Cecil textbook of medicine,* ed 22, Philadelphia, 2004, WB Saunders.)

- Patients with advanced cirrhosis and small tumors should be considered for liver transplantation
- For patients with hepatitis C virus, associated hepatocellular carcinoma, postoperative treatment with interferon-alpha decreases the rate of tumor recurrence

■ DISPOSITION
- For unresectable tumors, prognosis is poor.
- Five-year survival following surgical resection ranges from 30%-50%.

■ REFERRAL
For treatment planning

⚙ PEARLS & CONSIDERATIONS

Prevention:
- Hepatitis B vaccination
- Eliminate aflatoxin contamination of food
- Decrease alcohol consumption
- Identify and treat hemochromatosis
- Interferon therapy in patients with hepatitis C reduces the risk of hepatocellular carcinoma

REFERENCES

Gupta S et al: Test characteristics of α-fetoprotein for detecting hepatocellular carcinome in patients with Hepatitis C: a systematic review and critical analysis, *Ann Intern Med* 139:46, 2003.

Hwai-Yang et al: Hepatitis B antigen and the risk of hepatocellular carcinoma, *N Engl J Med* 347:168, 2002.

Kubo S et al: Effects of long-term postoperative interferon–alpha therapy on intrahepatic recurrence after resection of hepatitis C virus-related hepatocellular carcinoma: a randomized controlled trial, *Ann Intern Med* 134:963, 2001.

Authors: **Christine Duffy, M.D., and Mark J. Fagan, M.D.**

BASIC INFORMATION

■ DEFINITION
Hepatorenal syndrome (HRS) is a condition of intense renal vasoconstriction resulting from loss of renal autoregulation occurring as a complication of severe liver disease.

■ SYNONYMS
Hepatic nephropathy
Oliguric renal failure of cirrhosis
HRS

■ ICD-9CM CODES
572.4 Hepatorenal syndrome

■ EPIDEMIOLOGY & DEMOGRAPHICS
The probability of HRS in patients with cirrhosis is 18% at 1 yr and 39% at 5 yr.

■ PHYSICAL FINDINGS & CLINICAL PRESENTATION
- Evidence of cirrhosis is usually present: jaundice, spider angiomas, splenomegaly, ascites, fetor hepaticus, pedal edema
- Hepatic encephalopathy: flapping tremor (asterixis), coma
- Tachycardia and bounding pulse
- Oliguria

■ ETIOLOGY
An exacerbation of end-stage liver disease, HRS may occur after significant reduction of effective blood volume (e.g., paracentesis, GI bleeding, diuretics) or in the absence of any precipitating factors.

 DIAGNOSIS

■ DIFFERENTIAL DIAGNOSIS
- Prerenal azotemia: response to sustained plasma expansion is good (prompt diuresis with volume expansion).
- Acute tubular necrosis: urinary sodium >30, FENa >1.5%, urinary/plasma creatinine ratio <30, urine/plasma osmolality ratio = 1,

urine sediment reveals casts and cellular debris, there is no significant response to sustained plasma expansion.

■ WORKUP
Patients with acute azotemia and oliguria in the setting of liver disease should undergo laboratory evaluation to differentiate HRS from acute tubular necrosis and volume challenge to differentiate HRS from prerenal azotemia if FENa <1%.

■ LABORATORY TESTS
- Obtain serum electrolytes, BUN, creatinine, osmolality, urinalysis, urinary sodium, urinary creatinine, urine osmolality.
- Calculate fractional excretion of sodium (FENa).
- In HRS: urinary sodium <10 mEq/L, FENa <1%, urinary plasma creatinine ratio >30, urinary-plasma osmolality ratio >1.5, urine sediment is unremarkable.

■ IMAGING STUDIES
Renal ultrasound may be indicated if renal obstruction is suspected.

 TREATMENT

■ NONPHARMACOLOGIC THERAPY
Avoidance of precipitating factors

■ ACUTE GENERAL Rx
- Volume challenge (to increase mean arterial pressure) followed by large-volume paracentesis (to increase cardiac output and decrease renal venous pressure) may be useful to distinguish HRS from prerenal azotemia in patients with FENa <1%. In patients with prerenal azotemia, the increase in renal perfusion pressure and renal blood flow will result in prompt diuresis; the volume challenge can be accomplished by giving a solution of 100 g of albumin in 500 ml of isotonic saline.

- The only effective treatment of HRS is liver transplantation; low-dose dopamine or ornipressin is used in some liver units to avoid further deterioration of renal function in patients awaiting liver transplantation.
- Vasopressin analogues may improve renal perfusion by reversing splanchnic vasodilation, which is the hallmark of HRS. Encouraging results were found in a recent study using continuous IV noradrenalin in combination with albumin and furosemide. In this study, reversal of HRS was achieved in 10 out of 12 patients.

■ DISPOSITION
Mortality rate exceeds 80%; liver transplantation is the only curative treatment.

■ REFERRAL
Referral for liver transplantation when indicated (see Comments)

✷ PEARLS & CONSIDERATIONS

■ COMMENTS
Liver transplantation may be indicated in otherwise healthy patients (age preferably <65 yr) with sclerosing cholangitis, chronic hepatitis with cirrhosis, or primary biliary cirrhosis; contraindications to liver transplantation are AIDS, most metastatic malignancies, active substance abuse, uncontrolled sepsis, uncontrolled cardiac or pulmonary disease.

REFERENCE
Duvoux C et al: Effects of noradrenalin and albumin in patients with type 1 hepatorenal syndrome: a pilot study, *Hepatology* 36:374, 2002.
Author: **Fred F. Ferri, M.D.**

BASIC INFORMATION

■ DEFINITION
Herpangina is a self-limited upper respiratory tract infection associated with a characteristic vesicular rash on the soft palate.

ICD-9CM CODES
074.0 Herpangina

■ EPIDEMIOLOGY & DEMOGRAPHICS
INCIDENCE (IN U.S.): Unknown
PREVALENCE (IN U.S.): Unknown
PREDOMINANT SEX: Male = female
PREDOMINANT AGE: 3 to 10 yr
PEAK INCIDENCE: Summer outbreaks common

■ PHYSICAL FINDINGS & CLINICAL PRESENTATION
- Characterized by ulcerating lesions typically located on the soft palate (Fig. 1-135)
- Usually fewer than six lesions that evolve rapidly from a diffuse pharyngitis to erythematous macules and subsequently to vesicles that are moderately painful
- Fever, vomiting, and headache in the first few days of illness but subsiding spontaneously
- Pharyngeal lesions typical for several more days

■ ETIOLOGY
- Most caused by coxsackie A viruses (A2, A4, A5, A6, A10)
- Occasional cases caused by other viruses

DIAGNOSIS

■ DIFFERENTIAL DIAGNOSIS
- Herpes simplex
- Bacterial pharyngitis
- Tonsillitis
- Aphthous stomatitis
- Hand-foot-mouth disease

■ WORKUP
Diagnosis is typically based on characteristic lesions on the soft palate.

■ LABORATORY TESTS
Viral and bacterial cultures of the pharynx to exclude herpes simplex infection and streptococcal pharyngitis if the diagnosis is in doubt

TREATMENT

- Symptomatic treatment for sore throat
- No antiviral therapy indicated

■ NONPHARMACOLOGIC THERAPY
Analgesic throat lozenges are helpful in some cases.

■ ACUTE GENERAL Rx
Antipyretics when indicated

■ CHRONIC Rx
Self-limited infection

■ DISPOSITION
- Generally, resolution of symptoms within 1 wk
- Persistence of fever or mouth lesions beyond 1 wk suggestive of an alternative diagnosis (see Differential Diagnosis)

■ REFERRAL
For consultation with otolaryngologist or infectious disease specialist if the diagnosis is in doubt

PEARLS & CONSIDERATIONS

■ COMMENTS
Household outbreaks may occur, especially during the summer months.

REFERENCES
Chang LY et al: Risk factors of enterovirus 71 infection and associated hand, foot, and mouth disease/herpangina in children during an epidemic in Taiwan, *Pediatrics* 109(6):e88, 2002.
Stone MS: Viral exanthems, *Dermatol Online J* 9(3):4, 2003.
Author: **Joseph R. Masci, M.D.**

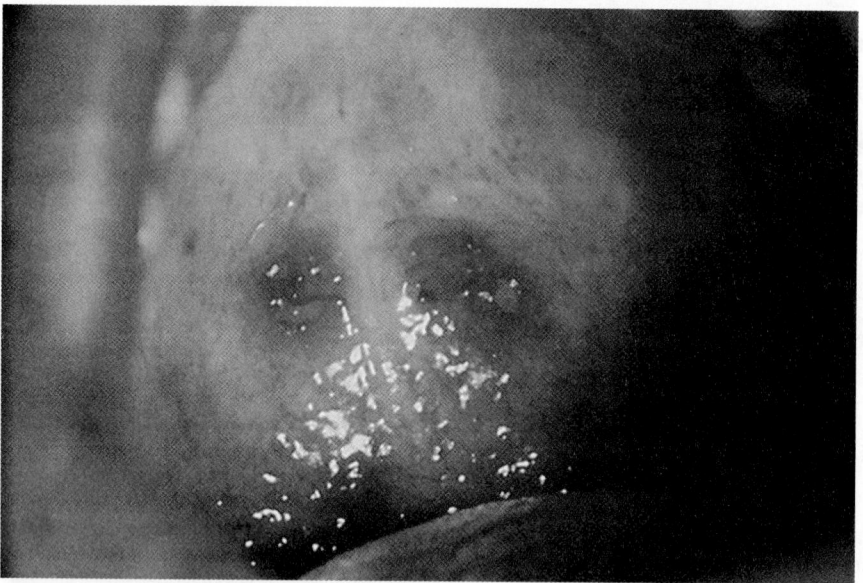

Fig. 1-135   Herpangina with shallow ulcers in the roof of the mouth. (Courtesy Marshall Guill, M.D. From Goldstein B [ed]: *Practical dermatology,* ed 2, St Louis, 1997, Mosby.)

BASIC INFORMATION

■ DEFINITION
Herpes simplex is a viral infection caused by the herpes simplex virus (HSV); HSV-1 is associated primarily with oral infections, whereas HSV-2 causes mainly genital infections; however, each type can infect any site; following the primary infection, the virus enters the nerve endings in the skin directly below the lesions and ascends to the dorsal root ganglia where it remains in a latent stage until it is reactivated.

■ SYNONYMS
Genital herpes
Herpes labialis
Herpes gladiatorum
Herpes digitalis

ICD-9CM CODES
054.10 Genital herpes
054.9 Herpes labialis

■ EPIDEMIOLOGY & DEMOGRAPHICS
- More than 85% of adults have serologic evidence of HSV-1 infection. The seroprevalence of adults with HSV-2 in the United States is 25%; however, only about 20% of these persons recall having symptoms of HSV infection.
- Most cases of eye or digital herpetic infections are caused by HSV-1.
- Frequency of recurrence of HSV-2 genital herpes is higher than HSV-1 oral labial infection.
- The frequency of recurrence is lowest for oral labial HSV-2 infections.

- The incidence of complications from herpes simplex (e.g., herpes encephalitis) is highest in immunocompromised hosts.

■ PHYSICAL FINDINGS
PRIMARY INFECTION:
- Symptoms occur from 3 to 7 days after contact (respiratory droplets, direct contact).
- Constitutional symptoms include low-grade fever, headache and myalgias, regional lymphadenopathy, and localized pain.
- Pain, burning, itching, and tingling last several hours.
- Grouped vesicles (Fig. 1-136) usually with surrounding erythema appear and generally ulcerate or crust within 48 hr.
- The vesicles are uniform in size (differentiating it from herpes zoster vesicles, which vary in size).
- During the acute eruption the patient is uncomfortable; involvement of lips and inside of mouth may make it unpleasant for the patient to eat; urinary retention may complicate involvement of the genital area.
- Lesions generally last from 2 to 6 wk and heal without scarring.

RECURRENT INFECTION:
- Generally caused by alteration in the immune system; fatigue, stress, menses, local skin trauma, and exposure to sunlight are contributing factors.
- The prodromal symptoms (fatigue, burning and tingling of the affected area) last 12 to 24 hr.

- A cluster of lesions generally evolve within 24 hr from a macule to a papule and then vesicles surrounded by erythema; the vesicles coalesce and subsequently rupture within 4 days, revealing erosions covered by crusts.
- The crusts are generally shed within 7 to 10 days, revealing a pink surface.
- The most frequent location of the lesions is on the vermilion border of the lips (HSV-1), the penile shaft or glans penis and the labia (HSV-2), buttocks (seen more frequently in women), fingertips (herpetic whitlow), and trunk (may be confused with herpes zoster).
- Rapid onset of diffuse cutaneous herpes simplex (eczema herpeticum) may occur in certain atopic infants and adults. It is a medical emergency, especially in young infants, and should be promptly treated with acyclovir.
- Herpes encephalitis, meningitis, and ocular herpes can occur in patients with immunocompromised status and occasionally in normal hosts.

■ ETIOLOGY
HSV-1 and HSV-2 are both DNA viruses.

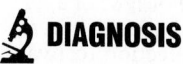 DIAGNOSIS

■ DIFFERENTIAL DIAGNOSIS
- Impetigo
- Behçet's syndrome
- Coxsackie virus infection
- Syphilis
- Stevens-Johnson syndrome

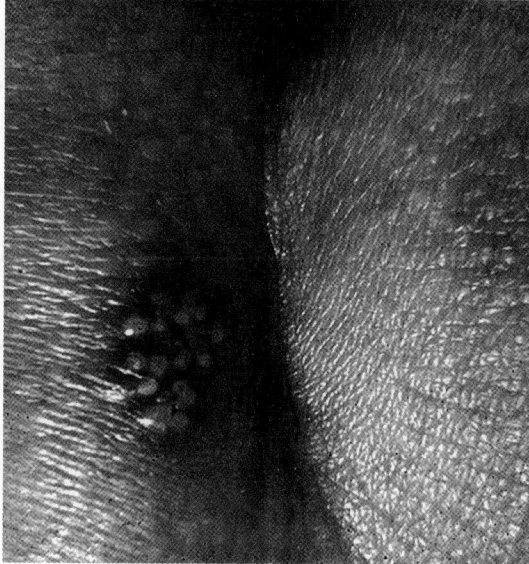
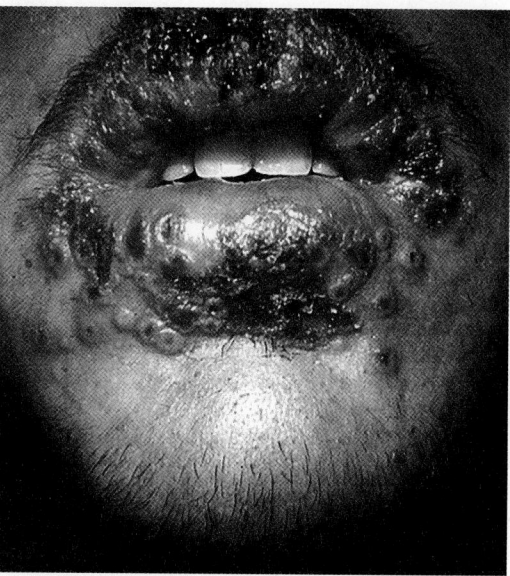

Fig. 1-136 Herpes simplex. (From Scuderi G [ed]: *Sports medicine: principles of primary care,* St Louis, 1997, Mosby.)

- Herpangina
- Aphthous stomatitis
- Varicella
- Herpes zoster

■ WORKUP

Diagnosis is based on clinical presentation. Laboratory evaluation will confirm diagnosis.

■ LABORATORY TESTS

- Direct immunofluorescent antibody slide tests will provide a rapid diagnosis.
- Viral culture is the most definitive method for diagnosis; results are generally available in 1 or 2 days; the lesions should be sampled during the vesicular or early ulcerative stage; cervical samples should be taken from the endocervix with a swab.
- Tzanck smear is a readily available test; it will demonstrate multinucleated giant cells. However, it is not a very sensitive test.
- Pap smear will detect HSV-infected cells in cervical tissue from women without symptoms.
- Serologic tests for HSV: IgG and IgM serum antibodies. Antibodies to HSV occur in 50% to 90% of adults. Routine tests do not discriminate between antibodies that are HSV-1 and HSV-2; the presence of IgM or a fourfold or greater rise in IgG titers indicates a recent infection (convalescent sample should be drawn 2 to 3 wk after the acute specimen is drawn).

℞ TREATMENT

■ NONPHARMACOLOGIC THERAPY

Application of topical cool compresses with Burow's solution for 15 min four to six times daily may be soothing in patients with extensive erosions on the vulva and penis (decrease edema and inflammation, debridement of crusts and purulent material).

■ ACUTE GENERAL Rx

- Acyclovir ointment or cream (Zovirax) applied using finger-cot or rubber glove q3-6h (six times daily) for 7 days may be useful for the first clinical episode of genital herpes. Severe primary genital infections may be treated with IV acyclovir (5 mg/kg infused at a constant rate over 1 hr q8h for 7 days in patients with normal renal function) or oral acyclovir 200 mg five times daily for 7 to 10 days. Topical acyclovir 5% cream can also be used for herpes labialis; when started at the prodrome or papule stage, it decreases the duration of an episode by about one-half day.
- Valacyclovir caplets (Valtrex) can also be used for the initial episode of genital herpes (1 g bid for 10 days).
- Valacyclovir 2 g PO q12h for 1 day begun within the first symptoms of herpes labialis can modestly shorten its duration.
- Penciclovir 1% cream (Denavir) can be used for recurrent herpes labialis on the lips and face. It should be applied q2h while awake for 4 days. Treatment should be started at the earliest sign or symptom. Its use decreases healing time of orolabial herpes by about one day.
- Docosanol 10% cream (Abbreva), a long-chain saturated alcohol, inhibits fusion between the plasma membrane and the viral envelope, blocking viral entry and subsequent replication. It is available over the counter and, when applied at the first sign of recurrence of herpes labialis, may shorten the durations of the episode by about 12 hr.

■ CHRONIC Rx

- Recurrent episodes of genital herpes can be treated with acyclovir. A short course (800 mg tid for 2 days) is effective. Other treatment options include 800 mg PO bid for 5 days, generally started during the prodrome or within 2 days of onset of lesions; famciclovir (Famvir) is also useful for treatment of recurrent genital herpes (dose is 125 mg q12h for 5 days in patients with normal renal function) started at the first sign of symptoms, or valacyclovir (Valtrex) (dose is 500 mg q12h for 5 days in patients with normal renal function).
- Acyclovir-resistant mucocutaneous lesions in patients with HIV can be treated with foscarnet (40 to 60 mg/kg IV q8h in patients with normal renal function); HPMPC has also been reported to be effective in HSV infections resistant to acyclovir or foscarnet.
- Patients with 6 recurrences of genital herpes/year can be treated with valacyclovir 1 g qd, acyclovir 400 mg bid, or famciclovir 250 mg bid.

■ DISPOSITION

Most patients recover from the initial episode or recurrences without complications; immunocompromised hosts are at risk for complications (e.g., disseminated herpes simplex infection, herpes encephalitis).

■ REFERRAL

Hospital admission in patients with herpes encephalitis, herpes meningitis, and in immunocompromised hosts with diffuse herpes simplex infection Ophthalmology referral in patients with suspected ocular herpes

⚙ PEARLS & CONSIDERATIONS

■ COMMENTS

- Provide patient education regarding transmission of HSV.
- Condom use offers significant protection against HSV-1 infection in susceptive women.
- Patients should be instructed on the use of condoms for sexual intercourse and on avoiding kissing or sexual intercourse until lesions are crusted.
- Patients should also avoid contact with immunocompromised hosts or neonates while lesions are present.
- Proper hand-washing techniques should be explained.
- Patients with herpes gladiatorum (cutaneous herpes in athletes involved in contact sports) should be excluded from participation in active sports until lesions have resolved.
- For additional information on genital herpes simplex, refer to "Herpes Simplex, Genital" in Section I.
- Many new HSV-2 infections are asymptomatic, but new symptoms may result from old infections.

REFERENCES

Centers for Disease Control and Prevention: 2002 sexually transmitted diseases treatment guidelines, *MMWR Morb Mortal Wkly Rep* 51(RR-6), 2002.
Corey L et al: Once-daily valacyclovir to reduce the risk of transmission of genital herpes, *N Engl J Med* 350:11, 2004.
Author: **Fred F. Ferri, M.D.**

BASIC INFORMATION

■ DEFINITION

Herpes simplex infection is a sexually transmitted disease caused by a double-stranded DNA virus. Two forms of infection exist: HSV-1, or oral herpes (15% of genital cases), and HSV-2, or genital herpes.

ICD-9CM CODES

054.10 Genital herpes

■ EPIDEMIOLOGY & DEMOGRAPHICS

INCIDENCE:
- 1% to 2%, with 500,000 new cases/yr
- Antibodies to HSV-1 or HSV-2 in up to 80% of adults

RISK FACTORS:
- Promiscuity
- Highest frequency in 15- to 29-yr-old population
- Associated with other sexually transmitted diseases, such as syphilis, gonorrhea, or chlamydia

GENETICS: No associated genetic predisposition

■ PHYSICAL FINDINGS & CLINICAL PRESENTATION

Three separate syndromes, as follows:
- First episode primary:
  1. No antibodies to HSV-1 or HSV-2
  2. Severe local symptoms such as painful bilateral genital ulcers or vesicles, inguinal adenopathy
  3. Constitutional findings of fever, malaise, myalgia
  4. Lesions persisting >16 days, with extragenital symptoms on fingers, buttock, or mouth
- First episode nonprimary:
  1. Presence of antibodies to HSV-1 and HSV-2
  2. Milder clinical course with symptoms similar to those of recurrent disease
- Recurrent herpes:
  1. Shorter duration (5 to 10 days)
  2. Mild symptoms
  3. Unilateral distribution
  4. Few systemic symptoms
  5. Prodrome of itching or burning before lesions appear

■ ETIOLOGY

Double-stranded DNA virus with a lytic as well as a latent phase

DIAGNOSIS

- Classic appearance of vesicles or ulcers in various stages of development

- Clinical history of recurrent prodromal symptoms and recurrences

■ DIFFERENTIAL DIAGNOSIS

- Human papillomavirus
- Molluscum contagiosum
- HIV infection
- Fungal infections (*Candida*)
- Bacterial infections (syphilis, chancroid, granuloma inguinale)
- Follicular abscess
- Hidradenitis suppurativa
- Vulvar dystrophies
- Cancer of the vulva

Section II describes the differential diagnosis of genital sores.

■ WORKUP

- Clinical history, including a thorough search for other sexually transmitted diseases
- Complete physical examination, including culture of suspected sites
- Possibly antibody screening

■ LABORATORY TESTS

- Viral culture
  1. Gold standard
  2. Requires 48 to 72 hr in most cases, with a higher chance of a positive culture with more viral load (first episode or early vesicular lesions)
  3. Disease not excluded by a negative culture result
- Tzanck smear
  1. Low sensitivity
  2. Tests for presence of intranuclear inclusions or giant cells
- Monoclonal antibody, ELISA
- HSV type I/type II antibody is the best test

TREATMENT

■ NONPHARMACOLOGIC THERAPY

- Exposure of affected areas to dry environment, avoiding contact of early vesicles with noninfected tissue
- Avoidance of intercourse during outbreak or with prodromal symptoms, with consideration of condom use if there are frequent recurrent episodes

■ ACUTE GENERAL Rx

- First clinical episode: acyclovir 200 mg PO × 5 for 7 to 10 days or until resolution of symptoms or valacyclovir 1 g PO bid × 7 to 10 days
- Recurrent disease:
  1. Course of recurrence shortened if treatment begun during prodromal phase or within initial phase of disease
  2. Acyclovir 200 mg PO × 5 for 5 days, 400 mg × 3 for 5 days, or 800 mg PO × 2 for 5 days

  3. Valacyclovir 500 mg PO bid × 5 days or 1 g PO bid × 7 days initially
- Severe disease (encephalitis, pneumonia, or hepatitis):
  1. Requires intravenous treatment
  2. Acyclovir 5 to 10 mg/kg q8h for 7 days

■ CHRONIC Rx

Suppressive therapy:
- Indicated for patients with >6 recurrences per year
- Acyclovir 400 mg PO bid, valacyclovir 500 mg qd, or famciclovir 250 mg bid
- Reevaluation after 1 yr of therapy to assess for continued suppression
- May reduce frequency of recurrences by 75%

■ DISPOSITION

Most cases responsive to initial therapy with acyclovir, but for those with recurrences, suppressive treatment (noted in Chronic Rx) is indicated.

■ REFERRAL

To infectious disease specialist or obstetrician for patients with life-threatening diseases or who are pregnant, especially in third trimester

PEARLS & CONSIDERATIONS

■ COMMENTS

HSV infection during pregnancy requires consideration of fetus as well as mother:
- Culture of any lesion suspicious for herpes should be performed.
- If active disease is suspected at the time of delivery, C-section may be indicated to decrease chance of neonatal infection.

REFERENCES

Centers for Disease Control and Prevention: 2002 sexually transmitted diseases treatment guidelines, *MMWR Morb Mortal Wkly Rep* 51(RR-6), 2002.

Corey L et al: Once-daily valacyclovir to reduce the risk of transmission of genital herpes, *N Engl J Med* 350:11, 2004.

Leone PA et al: Valacyclovir for episodic treatment of genital herpes: a shorter 3-day treatment course compared with 5 day treatment, *Clin Infect Dis* 34:958, 2002.

Wald A et al: Two-day regimen of acyclovir for treatment of recurrent genital herpes simplex virus type 2 infection, *Clin Infect Dis* 34:944, 2002.

Author: **Scott J. Zuccala, D.O.**

BASIC INFORMATION

■ DEFINITION

Herpes zoster is a disease caused by reactivation of the varicella-zoster virus. Following the primary infection (chickenpox) the virus becomes latent in the dorsal root ganglia and reemerges when there is a weakening of the immune system (secondary to disease or advanced age).

■ SYNONYMS

Shingles

ICD-9CM CODES

053.9 Herpes zoster

■ EPIDEMIOLOGY & DEMOGRAPHICS

- Herpes zoster occurs during lifetime in 10% to 20% of the population.
- There is an increased incidence in immunocompromised patients (AIDS, malignancy), the elderly, and children who acquired chickenpox when younger than 2 mo.

■ PHYSICAL FINDINGS & CLINICAL PRESENTATION

- Pain generally precedes skin manifestation by 3 to 5 days and is generally localized to the dermatome that will be affected by the skin lesions.
- Constitutional symptoms are often present (malaise, fever, headache).
- The initial rash consists of erythematous maculopapules generally affecting one dermatome (thoracic region in majority of cases); some patients (<50%) may have scattered vesicles outside of the affected dermatome.
- The initial maculopapules evolve into vesicles and pustules by the third or the fourth day.
- The vesicles have an erythematous base, are cloudy, and have various sizes (a distinguishing characteristic from herpes simplex in which the vesicles are of uniform size).
- The vesicles subsequently become umbilicated and then form crusts that generally fall off within 3 wk; scarring may occur.
- Pain during and after the rash is generally significant.
- Secondary bacterial infection with *Staphylococcus aureus* or *Streptococcus pyogenes* may occur.
- Regional lymphadenopathy may occur.
- Herpes zoster may involve the trigeminal nerve (most frequent cranial nerve involved); involvement of the geniculate ganglion can cause facial palsy and a painful ear, with the presence of vesicles on the pinna and external auditory canal (*Ramsay Hunt syndrome*).

■ ETIOLOGY

Reactivation of varicella virus (human herpesvirus III)

DIAGNOSIS

■ DIFFERENTIAL DIAGNOSIS

- Rash: herpes simplex and other viral infections
- Pain from herpes zoster: may be confused with acute myocardial infarction, pulmonary embolism, pleuritis, pericarditis, renal colic

■ LABORATORY TESTS

Laboratory tests are generally not necessary (viral cultures and Tzanck smear will confirm diagnosis in patients with atypical presentation).

TREATMENT

■ NONPHARMACOLOGIC THERAPY

- Wet compresses (using Burow's solution or cool tap water) applied for 15 to 30 min 5 to 10 times a day are useful to break vesicles and remove serum and crust.
- Care must be taken to prevent any secondary bacterial infection.

■ ACUTE GENERAL Rx

- Gabapentin 300 to 1800 mg qd is effective in the treatment of pain and sleep interference associated with postherpetic neuralgia.
- Lidocaine patch 5% (Lidoderm) is also effective in relieving postherpetic neuralgia. Patches are applied to intact skin to cover the most painful area for up to 12 hr within a 24-hr period.
- Oral antiviral agents can decrease acute pain, inflammation, and vesicle formation when treatment is begun within 48 hr of onset of rash. Treatment options are:
  1. Acyclovir (Zovirax) 800 mg 5 times daily for 7 to 10 days
  2. Valacyclovir (Valtrex) 1000 mg tid for 7 days
  3. Famciclovir (Famvir) 500 mg tid for 7 days
- Immunocompromised patients should be treated with IV acyclovir 500 mg/m² or 10 mg/kg q8h in 1-hr infusions for 7 days, with close monitoring of renal function and adequate hydration; vidarabine (continuous 12-hr infusion of 10 mg/kg/day for 7 days) is also effective for treatment of disseminated herpes zoster in immunocompromised hosts.
- Patients with AIDS and transplant patients may develop acyclovir-resistant varicella-zoster; these patients can be treated with foscarnet (40 mg/kg IV q8h) continued for at least 10 days or until lesions are completely healed.
- Capsaicin cream (Zostrix) can be useful for treatment of postherpetic neuralgia. It is generally applied three to five times daily for several weeks after the crusts have fallen off.
- Sympathetic blocks (stellate ganglion or epidural) with 0.25% bupivacaine and rhizotomy are reserved for severe cases unresponsive to conservative treatment.
- Corticosteroids should be considered in older patients if there are no contraindications. Initial dose is prednisone 60 mg/day tapered over a period of 21 days. When used there is a decrease in the use of analgesics and time to resumption of usual activities, but there is no effect on the incidence and duration of postherpetic neuralgia.

■ DISPOSITION

- The incidence of postherpetic neuralgia (defined as pain that persists more than 30 days after onset of rash) increases with age (30% by age 40 yr, >70% by age 70 yr); antivirals reduce the risk of postherpetic neuralgia.
- Incidence of disseminated herpes zoster is increased in immunocompromised hosts (e.g., 15% to 50% of patients with active Hodgkin's disease).
- Immunocompromised hosts are also more prone to neurologic complications (encephalitis, myelitis, cranial and peripheral nerve palsies, acute retinal necrosis). The mortality rate is 10% to 20% in immunocompromised hosts with disseminated zoster.
- Motor neuropathies occur in 5% of all cases of zoster; complete recovery occurs in >70% of patients.

■ REFERRAL

- Hospitalization for IV acyclovir in patients with disseminated herpes zoster
- Patients with herpes zoster ophthalmicus should be referred to an ophthalmologist
- Surgical referral for rhizotomy in patients with severe pain unresponsive to conventional treatment
- Sympathetic blocks in selected patients

REFERENCE

Gnann JW, Whitley RJ: Herpes zoster, *N Engl J Med* 347:340, 2002.

Author: **Fred F. Ferri, M.D.**

BASIC INFORMATION

■ DEFINITION

A hiatal hernia is the herniation of a portion of the stomach into the thoracic cavity through the diaphragmatic esophageal hiatus.

■ SYNONYMS

Diaphragmatic hernias

ICD-9CM CODES

750.6 Hiatal hernia

■ EPIDEMIOLOGY & DEMOGRAPHICS

- Found in 50% of patients over the age of 50
- Increases with age

- More prevalent in Western countries than in Africa and Asia
- Sliding hiatal hernias are more common in women than men (4:1)
- Associated with diverticulosis (25%), esophagitis (25%), duodenal ulcers (20%), and gallstones (18%)
- More than 90% of patients with documented endoscopic esophagitis have hiatal hernias

■ PHYSICAL FINDINGS & CLINICAL PRESENTATION

Most patients with hiatal hernias are asymptomatic. Symptomatic patients present similar to patients with GERD.
- Heartburn
- Dysphagia
- Regurgitation

- Chest pain
- Postprandial fullness
- GI bleed
- Dyspnea
- Hoarseness
- Wheezing with bowel sounds heard over the left lung base

■ ETIOLOGY

- Hiatal hernias are classified as:
  1. Sliding (Fig. 1-137 and 1-138, *A*), axial, or concentric hiatal hernia (most common type, 99%). The GE junction protrudes through the hiatus into the thoracic cavity
  2. Paraesophageal hernia (Fig. 1-138, *B*) (1%). The GE junction stays at the level of the diaphragm, but part of the stomach

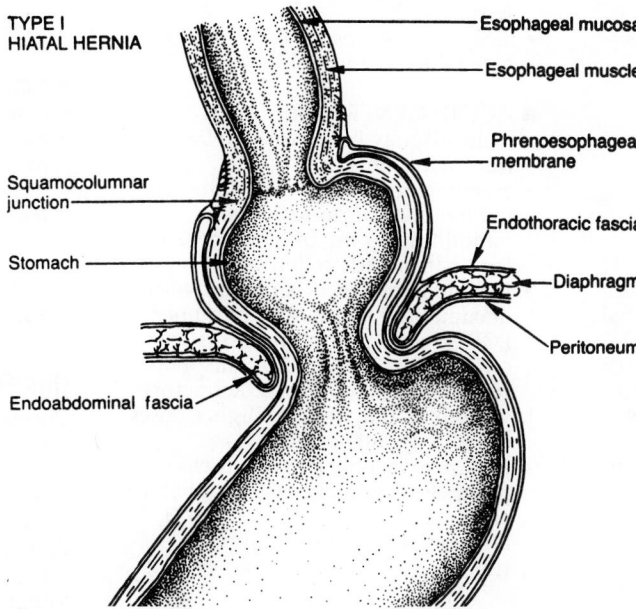

Fig. 1-137   Schematic diagram of a type I sliding hiatal hernia. (From Sabiston DC, Jr [ed]: *Textbook of surgery*, ed 13, Philadelphia, 1986, WB Saunders.)

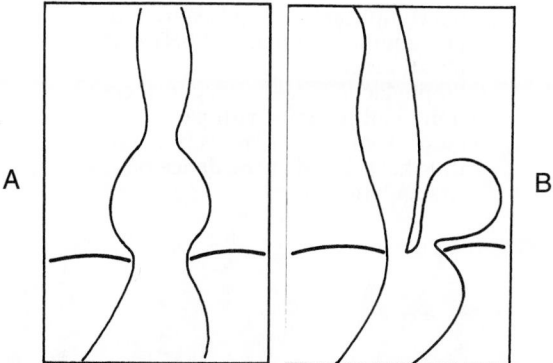

Fig. 1-138   Types of esophageal hiatal hernia. A, Sliding hiatal hernia, the most common type. **B,** Paraesophageal hiatal hernia. (From Behrman RE: *Nelson textbook of pediatrics*, ed 16, Philadelphia, 2000, WB Saunders.)

bulges into the thoracic cavity and stays there at all times, not being affected by swallowing
3. Mixed (rare)
- Hiatal hernias are thought to develop from an imbalance between normal pulling forces of the esophagus through the diaphragmatic hiatus during swallowing and the supporting structures maintaining normal esophagogastric junction positioning in association with repetitive stretching that results in rupture of the phrenoesophageal membrane.

DIAGNOSIS

The diagnosis of hiatal hernia relies on history and imaging studies.

■ DIFFERENTIAL DIAGNOSIS
- Peptic ulcer disease
- Unstable angina
- Esophagitis (e.g., *Candida*, herpes, NSAIDs, etc.)
- Esophageal spasm
- Barrett's esophagus
- Schatzki's ring
- Achalasia
- Zenker's diverticulum
- Esophageal cancer

■ WORKUP
- The workup is directed at excluding conditions noted in the differential diagnosis and documenting the presence of a hiatal hernia. Upper endoscopy may also be needed to exclude abnormal metaplasia, dysplasia, or neoplasia.
- A clinical algorithm for evaluation of heartburn is described in Section III, Fig. 3-83.

■ LABORATORY TESTS
- Blood tests are not very specific in diagnosing hiatal hernias.
- Esophageal manometry, although not commonly done, can be used in establishing a diagnosis.

■ IMAGING STUDIES
- Barium contrast UGI series best defines the anatomic abnormality. A hiatal hernia is considered to be present if the gastric cardia is herniated 2 cm above the hiatus. UGI may reveal a tortuous esophagus.

- Upper GI endoscopy is useful to document the presence of a hiatal hernia and also to exclude common associated findings of esophagitis and Barrett's esophagus. A hiatal hernia can be found incidentally and is diagnosed if >2 cm of gastric rugal fold is seen above the margins of the diaphragmatic crura.

℞ TREATMENT

■ NONPHARMACOLOGIC THERAPY
- Lifestyle modifications with avoidance of foods and drugs that decrease lower esophageal pressure (e.g. caffeine, chocolate, mint, calcium channel blockers, and anticholinergics)
- Weight loss
- Avoid large quantities of food with meals
- Sleep with the head of the bed elevated 4 to 6 in with blocks

■ ACUTE GENERAL Rx
- Antacids may be useful to relieve mild symptoms.
- H_2 antagonists (e.g., cimetidine 400 mg bid, ranitidine 150 mg bid, or famotidine 20 mg bid) can be used for symptomatic relief.
- If significant GERD is present with documented esophagitis by upper EGD, proton pump inhibitors (e.g., omeprazole 20 mg qd or lansoprazole 30 mg qd) are used. Refractory symptoms may require higher doses of PPI (e.g., BID dosing).
- Prokinetic agents (e.g., metoclopramide 10 mg taken 30 min before each meal) can be added to an H_2 antagonist or proton pump inhibitor.

■ CHRONIC Rx
- Although rarely indicated, surgery can be done in patients with refractory symptoms impairing quality of life and causing both intestinal (e.g., recurrent GI bleeds) and extraintestinal complications (e.g., aspiration pneumonia, asthma, and ENT complications).
- Prophylactic surgery is a consideration in all patients with paraesophageal hiatal hernias because they have a higher incidence of strangulation.

■ DISPOSITION
- More than 90% of patients with a hiatal hernia having GERD symptoms respond well to medical therapy.
- Complications of hiatal hernias are similar to complications occurring in patients with GERD:
  1. Erosive esophagitis
  2. Ulcerative esophagitis
  3. Barrett's esophagus
  4. Peptic stricture
  5. GI hemorrhage
  6. Extraintestinal complications

■ REFERRAL
All patients with documented hiatal hernia refractory to conventional H_2 antagonists, antacids, and proton pump inhibitors or having complications as mentioned previously should be referred to a gastroenterologist.

✣ PEARLS & CONSIDERATIONS

■ COMMENTS
- Once in a lifetime upper endoscopy has been proposed in the literature to exclude Barrett's esophagus.
- Approximately 5% of patients with Barrett's esophagus go on to develop esophageal cancer.
- Yearly surveillance by upper EGD is recommended in patients with Barrett's esophagus.

REFERENCES

Christensen J, Miftakhnr R: Hiatus hernia: a review of evidence for its origin in esophageal longitudinal muscle dysfunction, *Am J Med* 108(Suppl 4a):35, 2000.

Epstein FH: The esophagogastric junction, *N Engl J Med* 336(13):924, 1997.

Mittal RK: Hiatal hernia: myth or reality? *Am J Med* 103(5A):33S, 1997.

Sloan S, Rademaker AW, Kahrilas PJ: Determinants of gastroesophageal junction incompetence: hiatal hernia, lower esophageal sphincter or both? *Ann Intern Med* 117:977, 1992.

Authors: **Hemchand Ramberan, M.D., and Peter Petropoulos, M.D.**

BASIC INFORMATION

■ DEFINITION
Histiocytosis X is a rare disorder characterized by the abnormal proliferation of pathologic Langerhans cells.

■ SYNONYMS
- Eosinophilic granuloma
- Hand-Schüller-Christian disease
- Letterer-Siwe disease
- Langerhans cell histiocytosis
- Langerhans cell granulomatosis

ICD-9CM CODES
277.8 Histiocytosis X

■ EPIDEMIOLOGY & DEMOGRAPHICS
- Histiocytosis X is a rare disease in adults
- Peak incidence is from 1 to 3 yr
- Incidence 4 per 1 million
- Affects males more often than females—2:1
- Disseminated histiocytosis X usually occurs before 2 yr of age
- Approximately 50% of isolated eosinophilic granuloma cases occur before the age of 5

■ PHYSICAL FINDINGS & CLINICAL PRESENTATION
- A characteristic feature of histiocytosis X is its variable clinical presentation. The clinical spectrum ranges from:
  1. A benign isolated bony lesion (eosinophilic granuloma)
  2. Multiple bone lesions with soft tissue gingival and oral mucosal involvement (Hand-Schüller-Christian disease)
  3. An aggressive disseminated disease infiltrating organs and causing organ dysfunction (Letterer-Siwe disease)
- Bone lesions (80% to 100%)
  1. May be isolated or multiple
  2. Painful
  3. Skull most frequently involved, followed by long bones; lesions rarely seen in small bones of hands and feet
  4. Proptosis
  5. Mastoiditis
  6. Loose teeth
  7. Gingival hypertrophy
- Skin is involved in more than 80% of patients with disseminated disease and in 30% of patients with less extensive disease.
  1. Seborrhea-like scaling of scalp, petechial and purpuric lesions, ulcers, and bronzing of the skin may occur
  2. Common sites: scalp, neck, trunk, groin, and extremities
- Lymphadenopathy (10%): cervical and inguinal

- Lung involvement may manifest with cough, tachypnea, cyanosis, inspiratory crackles, pleural effusions, or pneumothorax.
- Liver involvement manifesting with jaundice and hepatomegaly
- Splenomegaly (5%)
- CNS involvement occurs in 1% to 4% of patients primarily manifesting as diabetes insipidus with insatiable thirst and urination

■ ETIOLOGY
- The etiology of histiocytosis is unknown.
- Initially, histiocytosis was thought to represent an abnormal immune response to a virus or other stimulant resulting in the proliferation of pathologic Langerhans cells. More recent evidence suggests histiocytosis X as a monoclonal proliferative neoplastic disorder.

DIAGNOSIS

Tissue biopsy revealing pathologic Langerhans cells characterized by the presence of surface nucleoprotein, CD1a antigen, and "Birbeck granules" noted on electron microscopy establishes the diagnosis of histiocytosis X.

■ DIFFERENTIAL DIAGNOSIS
The differential diagnosis is extensive, including all causes of diabetes insipidus, lytic bone lesions, dermatitis, hepatomegaly, and lymphadenopathy.

■ WORKUP
The workup of patients suspected of having histiocytosis X includes blood tests and imaging studies to assess the extent of disease involvement.

■ LABORATORY TESTS
- CBC is not specific in the diagnosis of histiocytosis X but may reveal cytopenias in patients with bone marrow involvement.
- Electrolytes, BUN, creatinine, urinalysis, and urine and serum osmolality are helpful in the diagnosis of diabetes insipidus during fluid deprivation testing.
- LFTs may be elevated in patients with liver involvement.
- Bronchoalveolar lavage (BAL) may show increased numbers of CD1a-positive histiocytes or Langerhans cells in patients with pulmonary histiocytosis X.

■ IMAGING STUDIES
- X-ray studies of affected areas show lytic lesions with or without sclerotic margins
- X-ray bone survey is done searching for other lesions

- Bone scan complements the bone survey studies
- Panoramic dental view of the mandible and maxilla for children with oral involvement
- Chest x-ray can show interstitial reticulonodular infiltrates (Fig. 1-139)
- High-resolution CT scan of the chest confirms interstitial lung scarring
- CT scans of the temporal bone looking at the mastoid, and inner and middle ear
- Ultrasound of the abdomen may show hepatosplenomegaly
- MRI of the brain visualizing the hypothalamic-hypophyseal region in patients suspected of having diabetes insipidus

TREATMENT

Treatment is based on the extent of involvement:
- Single-system disease:
  1. Single site: single bone lesion, isolated skin disease, or solitary lymph node
  2. Multiple site: multiple bone lesions, multiple lymph nodes
- Multiple disease: Multiple organ involvement, with or without dysfunction

■ ACUTE GENERAL Rx
Isolated bone lesions can be treated by:
- Curettage at the time of diagnosis
- Intralesional steroid injection
- Radiation therapy
Single skin lesions are treated with:
- Topical steroid (e.g., triamcinolone acetonide) applied bid
- Nitrogen mustard in 20% solution
Solitary lymph node
- Excision at the time of diagnosis
- Systemic oral prednisone
Multisystem disease treatment includes:
- Vinblastine 6 mg/m² IV bolus qwk × 6 mo or etoposide 150 mg/m² IV for 3 days q3wk for 6 mo plus
- Methylprednisolone 30 mg/kg/day for 3 days

■ CHRONIC Rx
- High-risk patients not responding to initial treatment should be considered for salvage therapy, including either bone marrow transplantation or combination cyclosporin A, antithymocyte globulin, and prednisolone.
- Diabetes insipidus is treated with DDAVP 0.1 mg to 0.8 mg PO or 1 spray bid to tid.

■ **DISPOSITION**

- A poor prognostic feature in the multisystem treatment group is the failure to respond to therapy in the first 6 wk.
- Multisystem disease patients categorized as low-risk group were patients >2 yr of age with no evidence of organ involvement (e.g., bone marrow, liver, lung, or spleen).
- Age of onset (<2 yr) with organ involvement is considered a high-risk group.
- In patients with disseminated histiocytosis X and <2 yr of age, the mortality rate is 30%.
- The association of histiocytosis X with other malignancies (e.g., ALL, acute nonlymphoblastic leukemia, and solid tumors) has been cited. It remains unclear if the associated malignancies result from the treatment of histiocytosis X or chance events.

■ **REFERRAL**

Histiocytosis X patients require a multidisciplinary approach including pediatric oncologist, radiation oncologists, oral maxillary surgeons, ENT specialists, audiology, dermatology, endocrinology, and family counseling.

☼ **PEARLS & CONSIDERATIONS**

■ **COMMENTS**

- Dr. Alfred Hand, Jr. described the first case of histiocytosis X in 1893. Drs. Letterer, Siwe, Schüller, and Christian also described similar cases between 1915 and 1933.
- Dr. Louis Lichtenstein noted the similarities of the cases and coined the term name *histiocytosis X*.
- In 1987, the Histiocyte Society was formed and the disease was officially termed *Langerhans cell histiocytosis*.

REFERENCES

Arico M, Egeler RM: Clinical aspects of Langerhans cell histiocytosis, *Hematol/Oncol Clin North Am* 12(2):247, 1998.

Broadbent V, Gadner H: Current therapy for Langerhans cell histiocytosis, *Hematol/Oncol Clin North Am* 12(2):327, 1998.

Coppes-Zantinga A, Egeler RM: The Langerhans cell histiocytosis X files revealed, *Br J Haematol* 116:3, 2002.

Lamper F: Langerhans cell histiocytosis: historical perspectives, *Hematol/Oncol Clin North Am* 12(2):213, 1998.

Nicholson HS, Egeler RM, Nesbit ME: The epidemiology of Langerhans cell histiocytosis, *Hematol/Oncol Clin North Am* 12(2):379, 1998.

Schmitz L, Favara BE: Nosology and pathology of Langerhans cell histiocytosis, *Hematol/Oncol Clin North Am* 12(2):221, 1998.

Author: **Peter Petropoulos, M.D.**

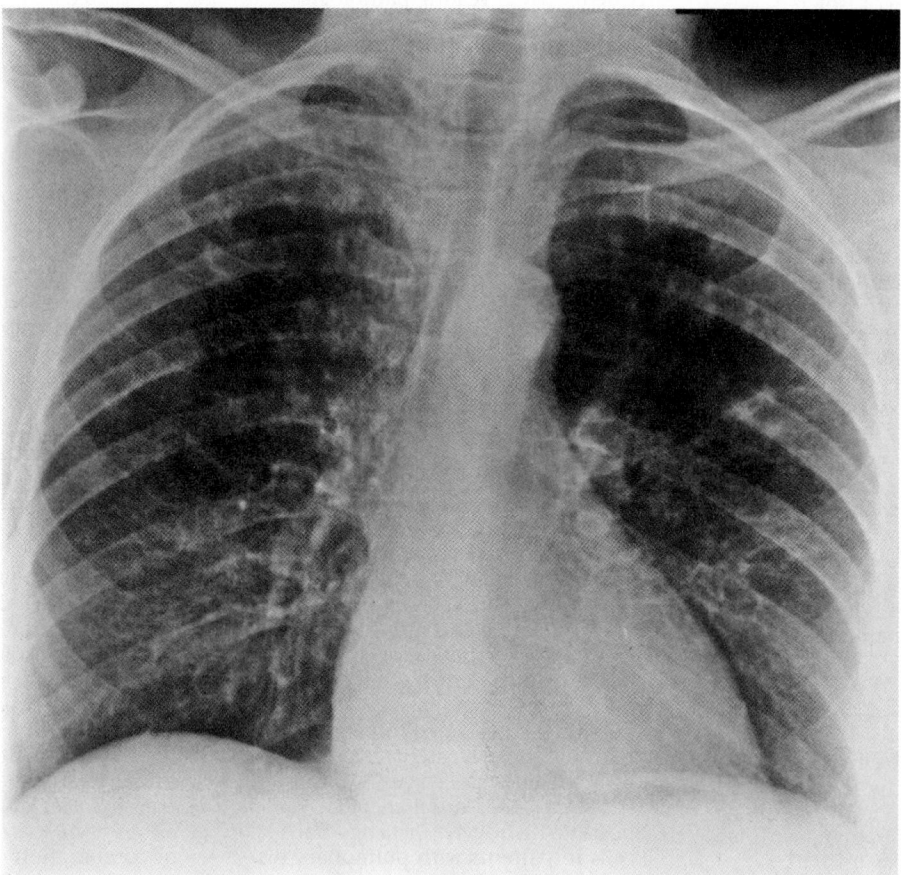

Fig. 1-139   Histiocytosis X. There is a reticular nodular pattern in the upper lobes. The lung volumes are preserved. (From McLoud TC [ed]: *Thoracic radiology, the requisites,* St Louis, 1998, Mosby.)

BASIC INFORMATION

■ DEFINITION

Histoplasmosis is an infectious disease caused by the fungus *Histoplasma capsulatum,* which is usually asymptomatic and characterized by a primary pulmonary focus with occasional progression to chronic pulmonary histoplasmosis (CPH) or various forms of dissemination. Progressive disseminated histoplasmosis (PDH) may present with a diverse clinical spectrum, including adrenal necrosis, pulmonary and mediastinal fibrosis, and ulcerations of the oropharynx and GI tract. In those patients who are concurrently infected with the human immunodeficiency virus (HIV), it is a defining disease for acquired immunodeficiency syndrome (AIDS).

ICD-9CM CODES
115.90 Histoplasmosis
115.94 Histoplasmosis with endocarditis
115.91 Histoplasmosis with meningitis
115.93 Histoplasmosis with pericarditis
115.95 Histoplasmosis with pneumonia
115.92 Histoplasmosis with retinitis

■ EPIDEMIOLOGY & DEMOGRAPHICS
INCIDENCE (IN U.S.):
- Unknown for acute pulmonary disease
- For CPH, estimated at 1/100,000 cases in endemic areas
- For PDH in immunocompetent adults, estimated at 1/2000 cases of histoplasmosis

PREVALENCE: Unknown
PREDOMINANT SEX: Clinically evident disease is most common in males; male:female ratio of 4:1
PREDOMINANT AGE:
- CPH is most often seen in males >50 yr old with an associated history of COPD.
- Presumed ocular histoplasmosis syndrome (POHS) is most commonly diagnosed between ages of 20 and 40 yr.

PEAK INCIDENCE: Unknown

■ PHYSICAL FINDINGS & CLINICAL PRESENTATION
- Conidia are deposited in alveoli, then fungus is converted to a yeast in the initial focus of bronchopneumonia and spreads to regional lymph nodes and other organs, especially liver and spleen, via lymphatics.
- From 7 to 18 days after onset, granulomatous inflammatory response marking host's cellular immunity begins to contain the yeast in the form of discrete granulomas.
- In normal host, fungistasis is achieved slowly as granulomas undergo contraction and, later, fibrosis with frequent calcification.
- With maturation of specific cellular immunity, there is development of delayed-type cutaneous hypersensitivity to *Histoplasma* antigens, usually 3 to 6 wk after exposure.
- Clinical disease manifests in various forms, depending on host cellular immunity and inoculum size:
  1. Acute primary pulmonary histoplasmosis
     a. Overwhelming number of patients are asymptomatic.
     b. Most clinically apparent infections manifest by complaints of fever, headache, malaise, pleuritic chest pain, nonproductive cough, and weight loss.
     c. Less than 10%, mainly women, complain of arthralgias, myalgias, and skin manifestations such as erythema multiforme or erythema nodosum.
     d. Acute pericarditis presents in smaller percentage of patients.
     e. On auscultation findings are minimal; hepatosplenomegaly, seen sometimes in adults, is most commonly observed in children.
     f. With particularly heavy exposure, there is severe dyspnea, marked hypoxemia, impending respiratory failure.
     g. Most patients are asymptomatic within 6 wk.
  2. CPH
     a. Presents insidiously with low-grade fever, malaise, weight loss, cough, sometimes with blood-streaked sputum or frank hemoptysis.
     b. Most patients with cavitary lesions present with associated COPD or chronic bronchitis, masking underlying fungal disease.
     c. Tends to worsen preexisting pulmonary disease and further contribute to eventual respiratory insufficiency.
  3. PDH
     a. In both acute and subacute forms, constitutional symptoms of fever, fatigue, malaise, and weight loss are common.
     b. Acute form (seen most commonly in infants and children) is distinguished by predominance of respiratory symptoms, fevers consistently >101° F (38.3° C), generalized lymphadenopathy, marked hepatosplenomegaly, and fulminant course resembling septic shock associated with a high fatality rate.
     c. Subacute form is more common in adults and associated with lower temperatures, hepatosplenomegaly, oropharyngeal ulceration, focal organ involvement (including Addison's disease secondary to adrenal destruction, endocarditis, chronic meningitis, and intracerebral mass lesions).
     d. Course of subacute form is relentless, with untreated patient dying within 2 yr.
     e. Chronic PDH is found in adults and marked by gradual, often intermittent, symptoms of weight loss, weakness, easy fatigability; fever only uncommonly and usually of low grade when present; oropharyngeal ulcerations and hepatomegaly and/or splenomegaly in one third of patients.
     f. Less clinical evidence of focal organ involvement in chronic form than in subacute form.
     g. Natural history of chronic form protracted and intermittent, spanning months to years.
- Histoplasmoma
  1. A healed area of caseation necrosis surrounded by a fibrous capsule
  2. Usually asymptomatic
- Mediastinal fibrosis
  1. A rare consequence of a fibroblastic process that encases caseating mediastinal lymph nodes after primary histoplasma bronchopneumonia
  2. Progressive fibrosis producing severe retraction, compression, and distortion of mediastinal structures
  3. Constriction of the bronchi resulting in bronchiectasis, also esophageal stenosis associated with dysphagia, and superior vena cava syndrome
- POHS
  1. Diagnosis characterized by distinct clinical features, including atrophic choroidal scars and maculopathy in patient with a history suggestive of exposure to the fungus (e.g., residence in an endemic area)
  2. Patient complains of distortion or loss of central vision without pain, redness, or photophobia
  3. Usually no evidence of systemic infection except for a positive skin reaction to histoplasmin

- In patients with AIDS
  1. Possible presentation as overwhelming infection similar to acute PDH seen in children
  2. Constitutional symptoms: fever, weight loss, malaise, cough, dyspnea
  3. About 10% with cutaneous maculopapular, erythematous eruptions or purpuric lesions on face, trunk, and extremities
  4. Up to 20% with CNS involvement, manifesting as intracerebral mass lesions, chronic meningitis, or encephalopathy
  5. Infrequent oropharyngeal ulceration

■ ETIOLOGY

- *H. capsulatum* is a dimorphic fungus present in temperate zones and river valleys around the world.
- In the U.S., it is highly endemic in southeastern, mid-Atlantic, and central states.
- Exists as mold at ambient temperature and favors surface soil enriched with bird or bat droppings.
- In endemic areas, contaminated dusty soil containing spores (microconidia) may be windswept or otherwise made airborne by sweeping, raking, or bulldozing, and then be inhaled.

🔬 DIAGNOSIS

■ DIFFERENTIAL DIAGNOSIS

- Acute pulmonary histoplasmosis
  1. *Mycobacterium tuberculosis*
  2. Community-acquired pneumonias caused by *Mycoplasma* and *Chlamydia*
  3. Other fungal diseases, such as *Blastomyces dermatitidis* and *Coccidioides immitis*
- Chronic cavitary pulmonary histoplasmosis: *M. tuberculosis*
- Yeast forms of histoplasmosis on tissue section: cysts of *Pneumocystis carinii*, which tend to be larger, extracellular, and do not display budding
- Intracellular parasites of *Leishmania* and *Toxoplasma* species: distinguishable by inability to take up methenamine silver
- Histoplasmomas: true neoplasms

■ WORKUP

- Suspect diagnosis in patients who present with an influenza-like illness and a history of residence or travel in an endemic area, especially if engaged in occupations (e.g., outside construction or street cleaning) or hobbies (e.g., cave exploring and aviary keeper) that increase the likelihood of exposure to fungal spores.

- Suspect diagnosis in immunosuppressed patients with remote history of exposure, especially if associated with characteristic calcifications on chest x-ray examination.

■ LABORATORY TESTS

- Demonstration of organism on culture from body fluid or tissues to make definitive diagnosis
  1. Especially high yield in patients with AIDS
  2. Characteristic oval yeast cells in neutrophils stained with Wright-Giemsa on peripheral smear
  3. Preparations of infected tissue with Gomori's silver methenamine for revealing yeast forms, especially in areas of caseation necrosis
- Serologic tests, including complement-fixing (CF) antibodies and immunodiffusion assays
  1. To establish previous infection and suggest active disease
  2. Possibly limited by inability to distinguish acute disease from remote infection and cross-reactivity with other fungi
- Detection of *Histoplasma* antigen in urine: may be influenced by infections with *Blastomyces* and *Coccidioides*
- Skin testing with histoplasmin: useful epidemiologically but essentially useless for diagnosis of acute disease
- In PDH
  1. Pancytopenia
  2. Marked elevations in alkaline phosphatase and alanine aminotransferase (ALT) common
  3. Most evident in acute and subacute forms and to a lesser extent in chronic form
- In chronic meningitis (majority of cases)
  1. CSF pleocytosis with either lymphocytes or neutrophils predominating
  2. Elevated CSF protein levels
  3. Hypoglycorrhachia

■ IMAGING STUDIES

- Chest x-ray examination in acute pulmonary histoplasmosis
  1. Singular or multiple patchy infiltrates, especially in the lower lung fields
  2. Hilar or mediastinal lymphadenopathy with or without pneumonitis
  3. Diffuse nodular or confluent bilateral miliary infiltrates characteristic of heavier exposure
  4. Infrequent pleural effusions, except when associated with pericarditis
- Chest x-ray examination in histoplasmoma: coin lesion displaying central calcification, ranging from 1

to 4 cm in diameter, predominantly located in the subpleural regions
- Chest x-ray examination in CPH:
  1. Upper lobe disease frequently associated with cavities (thick-walled, secondarily infected with an *Aspergillus* fungus ball)
  2. Preexisting calcifications in the hilum associated with peribronchial streaking extending to the parenchyma
- Chest x-ray examination in acute PDH: hilar adenopathy and/or diffuse nodular infiltrates
- CT scan of adrenals to reveal bilateral enlargement and low-attenuation centers

℞ TREATMENT

■ NONPHARMACOLOGIC THERAPY

For life-threatening disease seen in acute disseminated disease or infection in patients with AIDS: supportive therapy with IV fluids

■ ACUTE GENERAL Rx

- No drug therapy is required for patients with asymptomatic pulmonary disease and most patients with mild symptomatic pulmonary disease.
- Brief course of therapy with ketoconazole 400 mg/day or itraconazole 200 mg/day PO for 3 to 6 wk may be beneficial in some patients with acute pulmonary distress.
- Same therapy appropriate for immunocompetent, mild to moderately symptomatic patients with CPH and subacute and chronic forms of PDH, but duration of therapy is longer, ranging for 6 to 12 mo.
- Use amphotericin B 0.7 to 1 mg/kg IV for 6 to 12 mo in patients hypersensitive to or intolerant of azole therapy.
- Do not give immunocompromised patients, especially those with AIDS, ketoconazole as primary therapy for disseminated histoplasmosis.
- Give amphotericin B for life-threatening disease or continued illness as a result of primary failure or relapse of adequate azole therapy.
  1. For acute pulmonary histoplasmosis associated with acute respiratory distress syndrome (ARDS), acute PDH, and histoplasma meningitis: dose of 0.7 to 1 mg/kg IV >4 hr
  2. End point of therapy for patient with complicated acute pulmonary disease: total dose of 500 mg
  3. End point for patient with acute PDH: total dose 35 mg/kg or 2.5 g total

4. Concomitant administration of prednisone 60 to 80 mg/day beneficial for severe fungal hypersensitivity complicating acute pulmonary disease
- Endocarditis: surgical treatment is preferable, with excision of infected valve or graft combined with amphotericin for a total dose of 35 mg/kg or 2.5 g
- For pericardial disease:
  1. Antifungal therapy: no apparent benefit
  2. Best managed with NSAIDs
- For POHS:
  1. Antifungal therapy: no apparent benefit
  2. May respond to laser therapy

■ CHRONIC Rx
In patients with AIDS: lifelong suppressive therapy with either itraconazole, given 200 mg PO qd, or IV amphotericin B at a dose of 50 mg once weekly

■ DISPOSITION
- Most immunocompetent patients with acute histoplasmosis are asymptomatic.
- For those with chronic or progressive disease, especially if immunocompromised by virtue of disease or medication, outcome and favorable prognosis are dependent on prompt recognition of varied forms of disease and timely administration of appropriate antifungal drugs.

■ REFERRAL
- For consultation with infectious disease specialist in suspected cases of disseminated disease, especially if immunocompromised
- To a pulmonologist for patients with CPH form because progressive respiratory compromise usually results from chronic infection and underlying COPD
- For consultation with a thoracic surgeon for decompression procedures in patients symptomatic as a consequence of progressive mediastinal fibrosis

☼ PEARLS & CONSIDERATIONS

- *H. capsulatum,* variety *duboisii,* also known as African histoplasmosis, is restricted to Senegal, Nigeria, Zaire, and Uganda.
- Unlike *H. capsulatum,* pulmonary forms of *duboisii* are not seen, and the disease is limited to the skin, soft tissues, and bone.

■ COMMENTS
- Patients living in endemic areas, especially if immunocompromised, should be advised to take appropriate respiratory precautions when sweeping or disposing of bird waste from rooftop or home aviaries.

- Appropriate respiratory precautions should also be taken when leisure traveling to areas that act as a natural haven for the fungus, such as bat caves.
- Immunocompetent hosts are generally unaware of fungal infection, but the immunocompromised suffer devastating consequences.

REFERENCES
Ball SC: Histoplasmosis in a patient with AIDS, *AIDS Read* 13(3):112, 2003.

Kumar N et al: Adrenal histoplasmosis: clinical presentation and imaging features in nine cases, *Abdom Imaging* 28(5):703, 2003.

Quraishi NA et al: Histoplasmosis as the cause of a pathological fracture, *J Bone Joint Surg Br* 85(5):732, 2003.

Saccente M et al: Cerebral histoplasmosis in the azole era: report of four cases and review, *South Med J* 96(4):410, 2003.

Spencer WH et al: Detection of histoplasma capsulatum DNA in lesions of chronic ocular histoplasmosis syndrome, *Arch Ophthalmol* 121(11):1551, 2003.

Weinberg M et al: Severe histoplasmosis in travelers to Nicaragua, *Emerg Infect Dis* 9 (10):1322, 2003.

Wheat LJ, Kauffman CA: Histoplasmosis, *Infect Dis Clin North Am* 17(1):1, 2003.
Author: **George O. Alonso, M.D.**

BASIC INFORMATION

■ DEFINITION

Hodgkin's disease is a malignant disorder of lymphoreticular origin, characterized histologically by the presence of multinucleated giant cells (Reed-Sternberg cells) usually originating from B lymphocytes in germinal centers of lymphoid tissue.

ICD-9CM CODES

201.9 Hodgkin's disease, unspecified
201.4 Hodgkin's disease, lymphocyte predominance
201.5 Hodgkin's disease, nodular sclerosis
201.6 Hodgkin's disease, mixed cellularity
201.7 Hodgkin's disease, lymphocyte depletion

■ EPIDEMIOLOGY & DEMOGRAPHICS

- There is a bimodal age distribution (15 to 34 yr and >50 yr).
- Concordance for Hodgkin's disease in identical twins suggests that a genetic susceptibility underlies Hodgkin's disease in young adulthood.
- The disease is more common in males (in childhood Hodgkin's disease, >80% occurs in males), in Caucasians, and in higher socioeconomic groups.
- Overall incidence of Hodgkin's disease in the U.S. is approximately 4:100,000.

■ PHYSICAL FINDINGS & CLINICAL PRESENTATION

- Palpable lymphadenopathy, generally painless
- Most common site of involvement: neck region
- See Workup for description of common symptoms

■ ETIOLOGY

Unknown; evidence implicating Epstein-Barr virus remains controversial.

DIAGNOSIS

■ DIFFERENTIAL DIAGNOSIS

- Non-Hodgkin's lymphoma
- Sarcoidosis
- Infections (e.g., CMV, Epstein-Barr virus, toxoplasma, HIV)
- Drug reaction

■ WORKUP

Symptomatic patients with Hodgkin's disease usually present with the following manifestations:

- Fever and night sweats: fever in a cyclical pattern (days or weeks of fever alternating with afebrile periods) is known as Pel-Epstein fever
- Weight loss, generalized malaise
- Persistent, nonproductive cough
- Pain associated with alcohol ingestion, often secondary to heavy eosinophil infiltration of the tumor sites
- Pruritus
- Others: superior vena cava syndrome and spinal cord compression (rare)

Diagnosis can be made with lymph node biopsy. There are four main **histologic subtypes,** based on the number of lymphocytes, Reed-Sternberg cells, and the presence of fibrous tissue:

1. Lymphocyte predominance
2. Mixed cellularity
3. Nodular sclerosis
4. Lymphocyte depletion

Nodular sclerosis is the most common type and occurs mainly in young adulthood, whereas the mixed cellularity type is more prevalent after age 50 yr.

Staging for Hodgkin's disease follows the **Ann Arbor staging classification.**

Stage I: Involvement of a single lymph node region
Stage II: Two or more lymph node regions on the same side of the diaphragm
Stage III: Lymph node involvement on both sides of diaphragm, including spleen
Stage IV: Diffuse involvement of external sites

Suffix A: No systemic symptoms
Suffix B: Presence of fever, night sweats, or unexplained weight loss of 10% or more body weight over 6 mo
Suffix X: Indicates bulky disease >1/3 widening of mediastinum or >10 cm maximum dimension of nodal mass on a chest film.

Proper staging requires the following:

- Detailed history (with documentation of "B symptoms" and physical examination)
- Surgical biopsy
- Laboratory evaluation (CBC, sedimentation rate, BUN, creatinine, alkaline phosphatase, LFTs, albumin, LDH, uric acid)
- Chest x-ray studies (PA and lateral)
- Bilateral bone marrow biopsy
- CT scan of the chest (when abnormal findings are noted on chest x-ray examination) and of the abdomen and pelvis to visualize the mesenteric, hepatic, portal and splenic hilar nodes
- Bipedal lymphangiography in selected patients to define periaortic and iliac lymph node involvement
- Exploratory laparotomy and splenectomy (selected patients):
  1. Decision to perform staging laparotomy depends on the therapeutic plan; it is generally not indicated in patients who have a large mediastinal mass (these patients will generally be treated with combined chemotherapy and radiation). Staging laparotomy may also not be required in patients with clinical stage I or unlikely to have abdominal disease (e.g., females with supradiaphragmatic disease).
  2. Exploratory laparotomy and splenectomy may be used for patients with clinical stage I-IIA or IIB.
  3. It is useful in identifying patients who can be treated with irradiation alone with curative intent.
  4. Polyvalent pneumococcal vaccine should be given prophylactically to all patients before splenectomy (increased risk of sepsis from encapsulated organisms in splenectomized patients).
- Gallium scan

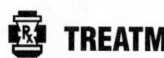
■ LABORATORY TESTS
See Workup.

■ IMAGING STUDIES
See Workup.

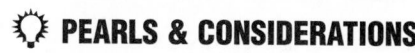

TREATMENT

■ ACUTE GENERAL Rx
The main therapeutic modalities are radiotherapy and chemotherapy; the indication for each vary with pathologic stage and other factors.
- Stage I and II: radiation therapy alone unless a large mediastinal mass is present (mediastinal to thoracic ratio ≥1.3); in the latter case, a combination of chemotherapy and radiation therapy is indicated.
- Stage IB or IIB: total nodal irradiation is often used, although chemotherapy is performed in many centers.
- Stage IIIA: treatment is controversial. It varies with the anatomic substage after splenectomy.
  1. III_1A and minimum splenic involvement: radiation therapy alone may be adequate.
  2. III_2 or III_1A with extensive splenic involvement: there is disagreement whether chemotherapy alone or a combination of chemotherapy and radiation therapy is the preferred treatment modality.
  3. IIIB and IVB: the treatment of choice is chemotherapy with or without adjuvant radiotherapy.

Various regimens can be used for combination of chemotherapy. Most oncologists prefer the combination of doxorubicin plus bleomycin plus vincristine plus dacarbazine (ABVD). Other commonly used regimens are MOPP, MOPP-ABV, MOPP-ABVD, MOPP-BAP.
- In patients with advanced Hodgkin's disease, increased-dose bleomycin, etoposide, doxorubicin, cyclophosphamide, vincristine, procarbazine, and prednisone (BEACOPP) offers better tumor control and overall survival than COPP-ABVD.

■ DISPOSITION
- The overall survival at 10 yr is approximately 60%.
- Cure rates as high as 75% to 80% are now possible with appropriate initial therapy.
- Poor prognostic features include presence of "B symptoms," advanced age, advanced stage at initial presentation, mixed-cellularity, and lymphocyte depletion histology.
- Chemotherapy significantly increases the risk of leukemia.
- The peak in risk of leukemia is seen approximately 5 yr after the initiation of chemotherapy.
- The risk of leukemia is greater for those who undergo splenectomy and for patients with advanced stages of Hodgkin's disease; the risk is unaffected by concomitant radiotherapy.
- Involved-field radiotherapy does not improve the outcome in patients with advanced-stage Hodgkin's lymphoma who have a complete remission after MOPP-ABV chemotherapy.

Radiotherapy may benefit patients with a partial response after chemotherapy.
- Mediastinal irradiation increases the risk of subsequent death from heart disease caused by sclerosis of coronary artery secondary to irradiation. Risk increases with high mediastinal doses, minimal protective cardiac blocking, young age at irradiation, and increased duration of follow-up.
- Both chemotherapy and radiation therapy increase the risk of developing secondary solid tumors (e.g., carcinoma of the lung, breast, and stomach).

■ REFERRAL
- Surgical referral for lymph node biopsy
- Hematology/oncology referral

PEARLS & CONSIDERATIONS

■ COMMENTS
Young male patients should consider sperm banking before the initiation of therapy.

REFERENCES
Aleman B et al: Involved-field radiotherapy for advanced Hodgkin's lymphoma, *N Engl J Med* 348:2396, 2003.

Diehl V et al: Standard and increased-dose BEACOPP chemotherapy compared with COPP-ABVD for advanced Hodgkin's disease, *N Engl J Med* 348:2386, 2003.

Author: **Fred F. Ferri, M.D.**

BASIC INFORMATION

■ DEFINITION
Hookworm is a parasitic infection of the intestine caused by helminths.

ICD-9CM CODES
126.35 Hookworm

■ EPIDEMIOLOGY & DEMOGRAPHICS
INCIDENCE (IN U.S.):
- Varies greatly in different areas of the U.S.
- Most common in rural areas of southeastern U.S.
- Poor sanitation and increased rainfall increase likelihood

PREVALENCE (IN U.S.): Varies from 10% to 90% in regions where it is found

PREDOMINANT AGE: Schoolchildren

■ PHYSICAL FINDINGS & CLINICAL PRESENTATION
- Nonspecific abdominal complaints
- Because these organisms consume host RBCs, symptoms related to iron-deficiency anemia, depending on the amount of iron in the diet and the worm burden
- Fatigue, tachycardia, dyspnea, and high-output failure
- Hypoproteinemia and edema from loss of proteins into the intestinal tract
- Unusual for pulmonary manifestations to occur when the larvae migrate through the lungs
- Skin rash at sites of larval penetration in some individuals without prior exposure

■ ETIOLOGY
Two species can cause this disease: *Necator americanus* and *Ancylostoma duodenale*. *N. americanus* is the predominant cause of hookworm in the U.S.
- Infection occurs via penetration of the skin by the larval form, with subsequent migration via the blood stream to the alveoli, up the respiratory tract, then into the GI tract
- Sharp mouth parts allow for attachment to intestinal mucosa

DIAGNOSIS

■ DIFFERENTIAL DIAGNOSIS
- Strongyloidiasis
- Ascariasis

■ WORKUP
Examine stool for hookworm eggs.

■ LABORATORY TESTS
CBC to show hypochromic, microcytic anemia; possible mild eosinophilia and hypoalbuminemia

■ IMAGING STUDIES
Chest x-ray examination: occasionally shows opacities

TREATMENT

■ NONPHARMACOLOGIC THERAPY
Prevention of disease by not walking barefoot and by improving sanitary conditions

■ ACUTE GENERAL Rx
- Mebendazole 100 mg PO bid for 3 days
- Iron supplementation may be helpful

■ DISPOSITION
Easily treated

■ REFERRAL
If diagnosis uncertain

☼ PEARLS & CONSIDERATIONS

■ COMMENTS
Appropriate disposal of human wastes is important in controlling the disease in areas with a high prevalence of hookworm infestation.

REFERENCES
Biegel Y et al: Clinical problem-solving: letting the patient off the hook, *N Engl J Med* 342:1658, 2000.

Grover JK et al: Antihelminthics: a review, *Trop Gastroenterol* 22:180, 2001.
Author: **Maurice Policar, M.D.**

BASIC INFORMATION

DEFINITION
A hordeolum is an acute inflammatory process affecting the eyelid and arising from the meibomian (posterior) or Zeis (anterior) glands. It is most often infectious and usually caused by *Staphylococcus aureus.*

SYNONYMS
Stye

ICD-9CM CODES
373.11 External hordeolum
373.12 Internal hordeolum

EPIDEMIOLOGY & DEMOGRAPHICS
INCIDENCE (IN U.S.): Unknown
PREVALENCE (IN U.S.): Unknown
PREDOMINANT SEX: No gender predilection
PREDOMINANT AGE: May occur at any age
PEAK INCIDENCE: May occur at any age
NEONATAL INFECTION: Rare in the neonatal period

PHYSICAL FINDINGS & CLINICAL PRESENTATION
- Abrupt onset with pain and erythema of the eyelid
- Localized, tender mass in the eyelid (Fig. 1-140)
- May be associated with blepharitis
- External hordeolum: points toward the skin surface of the lid and may spontaneously drain
- Internal hordeolum: can point toward the conjunctival side of the lid and may cause conjunctival inflammation

ETIOLOGY
- 75% to 95% of cases are caused by *S. aureus.*
- Occasional cases are caused by *Streptococcus pneumoniae,* other streptococci, gram-negative enteric organisms, or mixed bacterial flora.

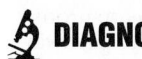 **DIAGNOSIS**

DIFFERENTIAL DIAGNOSIS
- Eyelid abscess
- Chalazion
- Allergy or contact dermatitis with conjunctival edema
- Acute dacryocystitis
- Herpes simplex infection
- Cellulitis of the eyelid

LABORATORY TESTS
- Generally, none are necessary.
- If incision and drainage are performed, specimens should be sent for bacterial culture.

IMAGING STUDIES
None necessary

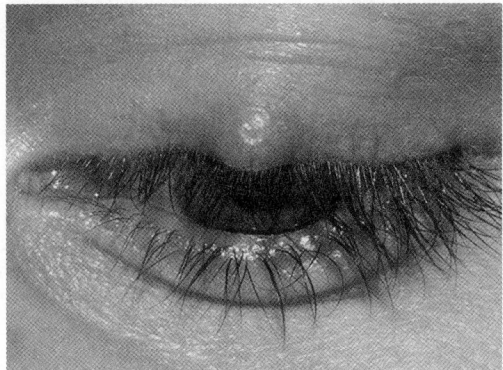

Fig. 1-140 External stye. (From Palay D [ed]: *Ophthalmology for the primary care physician,* St Louis, 1997, Mosby.)

 TREATMENT

NONPHARMACOLOGIC THERAPY
Usually responds to warm compresses

ACUTE GENERAL Rx
- Systemic antibiotics generally not necessary
- In refractory cases, an oral anti-staphylococcal agent (e.g., dicloxacillin 500 mg PO qid) possibly helpful
- Topical erythromycin ophthalmic ointment applied to the lid margins two to four times daily until resolution
- Incision and drainage: rarely needed but should be considered for progressive infections

CHRONIC Rx
None necessary

DISPOSITION
- Usually sporadic occurrence
- Possible relapse if resolution is not complete

REFERRAL
- For evaluation by an ophthalmologist if visual acuity or ocular movement is affected or if the diagnosis is in doubt
- For surgical drainage if necessary

PEARLS & CONSIDERATIONS

COMMENTS
Seborrheic dermatitis may coexist with hordeolum.

REFERENCES
Kiratli HK, Akar Y: Multiple recurrent hordeola associated with selective IgM deficiency, *J AAPOS* 5(1):60, 2001.
Maldonado M, Juberias J, Moreno-Montanes J: Extensive corneal epithelial defect associated with internal hordeolum after uneventful laser in situ keratomileusis, *J Cataract Refract Surg* 28(9):1700, 2002.
Author: **Joseph R. Masci, M.D.**

BASIC INFORMATION

■ DEFINITION

Horner's syndrome is the clinical triad of ipsilateral ptosis, miosis, and sometimes anhidrosis of the face. These physical findings are the result of disruption of the cervical sympathetic pathway along its course from the hypothalamus to the eye. Disruption of any of the three neurons involved in the pathway (central, preganglionic, or postganglionic) can cause Horner's syndrome.

■ SYNONYMS

Oculosympathetic paresis

ICD-9CM CODES

337.9 Horner's syndrome

■ EPIDEMIOLOGY & DEMOGRAPHICS

- May occur congenitally
- Associated with vascular disease and neoplasms

■ PHYSICAL FINDINGS & CLINICAL PRESENTATION

- Miosis results from loss of sympathetic pupillodilator activity (Fig. 1-141).
- Affected pupil reacts normally to light and accommodation. Anisocoria is greater in darkness.
- Ptosis results from loss of sympathetic tone to eyelid muscles.

- The presence of anhidrosis is variable, and depends on the site of injury in the sympathetic pathway. Anhidrosis may occur with lesions affecting the central or preganglionic neurons.
- Conjunctival or facial hyperemia may occur on the affected side because of loss of sympathetic vasoconstrictor activity.
- In congenital Horner's syndrome, the iris on the affected side may fail to become pigmented, resulting in heterochromia of the iris, with the affected iris remaining blue-gray.

■ ETIOLOGY

Lesions affecting any of the neurons involved in the sympathetic pathway can cause Horner's syndrome.
Mechanical:
- Syringomyelia
- Trauma
- Benign tumors
- Malignant tumors (especially Pancoast tumor)
- Metastatic tumor
- Lymphadenopathy
- Neurofibromatosis
- Cervical rib
- Cervical spondylosis
Vascular (ischemia, hemorrhage or AVM):
- Brainstem lesion: commonly occlusion of the posterior inferior cerebellar artery but almost any of the vessels may be responsible (vertebral; superior, middle or inferior lateral medullary arteries; superior or anterior inferior cerebellar arteries)

- Internal carotid artery aneurysm or dissection. Injury of other major vessels (carotid artery, subclavian artery, ascending aorta) can also cause Horner's syndrome
- Cluster headache, migraine
Miscellaneous:
- Congenital
- Demyelination (multiple sclerosis)
- Infection (apical TB, herpes zoster)
- Pneumothorax
- Iatrogenic (angiography, internal jugular/subclavian catheter, chest tube, surgery)
- Radiation

DIAGNOSIS

■ DIFFERENTIAL DIAGNOSIS

Causes of anisocoria (unequal pupils):
- Normal variant
- Mydriatic use
- Prosthetic eye
- Unilateral cataract
- Iritis
Disorders causing ptosis are described in Section II.

■ WORKUP

History, physical examination, and imaging

■ IMAGING STUDIES

- Chest x-ray for patients with suspected apical lung (Pancoast) tumor
- CT scan or MRI of the head and neck to identify lesions affecting the cervical sympathetic pathway

TREATMENT

Treatment depends on underlying cause.

■ DISPOSITION

Prognosis depends on underlying cause. Horner's syndrome is an uncommon presentation for malignancy. In one study, 60% of cases were idiopathic.

■ REFERRAL

- Vascular surgeon for carotid disease
- Oncologist for Pancoast tumor

Authors: **Mark J. Fagan, M.D., and Sudeep K. Aulakh, M.D., F.R.C.P.C.**

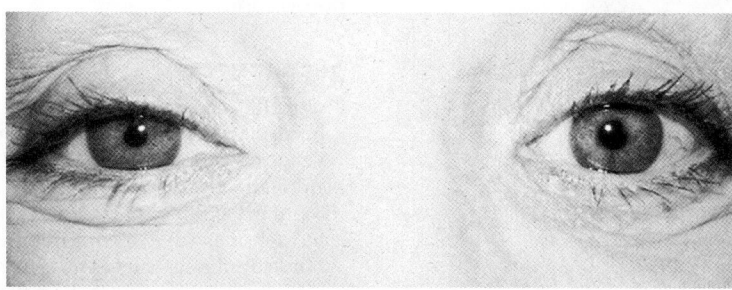

Fig. 1-141   Horner's syndrome. The mild ptosis (1 to 2 mm) and the smaller pupil (in room light) can be seen on the affected right side. (From Palay D [ed]: *Ophthalmology for the primary care physician,* St Louis, 1997, Mosby.)

BASIC INFORMATION

■ **DEFINITION**
Sudden onset of intense warmth that begins in the neck or face or in the chest and progresses to the neck and face, often associated with profuse sweating, anxiety, and palpitations

ICD-CM CODES
627.2 Hot flashes

■ **EPIDEMIOLOGY & DEMOGRAPHICS**
• Hot flashes affect 75% of post-menopausal women.
• Most hot flashes begin 1 to 2 yr before menopause and resolve after 2 yr.
• 15% of women report duration of hot flashes longer than 15 yr.

■ **PHYSICAL FINDINGS & CLINICAL PRESENTATION**
• Profuse sweating and red blotching of skin may be noted during the vasomotor event.
• Palpitations and hyperreflexia may be present during the hot flash.
• Hot flushes typically last 1-5 min.
• Each hot flush is associated with increase in temperature, increased pulse rate, and increased blood flow into the hands and face.
• Episodes of hot flush during sleep are common and are referred to as "night sweats."
• There is considerable variation in the frequency of hot flashes. One third of women report more than 10 flushes per day.

■ **ETIOLOGY**
• Dysfunction of central thermoregulatory centers caused by changes in estrogen level at the time of menopause
• Tamoxifen use
• Chemotherapy-induced ovarian failure
• Androgen ablation therapy for prostate carcinoma

 DIAGNOSIS

■ **DIFFERENTIAL DIAGNOSIS**
• Carcinoid syndrome
• Anxiety disorder
• Idiopathic flushing
• Lymphoma (night sweats)
• Hyperthyroidism

■ **WORKUP**
Evaluation of hot flashes is aimed at excluding conditions listed in the differential diagnosis

■ **LABORATORY TESTS**
• FSH, LH
• TSH

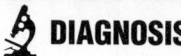 **TREATMENT**

■ **NONPHARMACOLOGIC THERAPY**
• Behavioral interventions such as relaxation training and paced respiration have been reported effective in reducing symptoms in some women.
• Avoidance of caffeine, alcohol, and tobacco, and spicy foods may be beneficial.

■ **GENERAL THERAPY**
• Estrogen replacement therapy reduces hot flashes by 80%-90%. Estrogen therapy, however, is contraindicated in many women and others are fearful of its use. Potential risks and side effects should be considered before using estrogen in any patient.
• Megestrol acetate, a progestational agent, is a safer alternative to estrogen in women with a history of breast or uterine cancer and in men receiving androgen ablation therapy for prostate cancer. Usual dose is 20 mg bid.
• The antidepressant venlaxefine has been reported to be 60% effective in reducing hot flashes and represents an alternative treatment modality in women unable or unwilling to use estrogens. Starting dose is 37.5 mg qd, increased as tolerated up to a maximum of 300 mg/day. Other antidepressants such as the SSRIs fluoxetine and paroxetine are also used by clinicians for hot flashes; however, they appear to be less effective than venlafaxine.
• The anticonvulsant gabapentin (300-1200 mg/day) represents another nonhormonal alternative in the treatment of hot flashes and can be used alone or in combination with venlafaxine.
• Vitamin E (800 IU/day) may be effective in patients with mild symptoms that do not interfere with sleep or daily function.
• Soy protein (use of soy extracts which contain plant-derived estrogens [phytoestrogens]) is often used; however, clinical trials have not shown clear efficacy.
• Several classes of herbal remedies are available to patients and commonly used without significant benefit. Frequently used agents are *Cimicifuga racemosa* (black cohosh, snakeroot, bugbane), *angelica sinensis,* and evening primrose (evening star).

REFERENCES
Fitzpatrick LA, Santen RJ: Hot flashes: the old and the new, what is really true? *Mayo Clin Proc* 77:1155, 2002.
Loprinzi CL et al: Pilot evaluation of Gabapentin for treating hot flashes, *Mayo Clin Proc* 77:1159, 2002.
Shanafelt TD et al: Pathophysiology and treatment of hot flashes, *Mayo Clin Proc* 77:1207, 2002.
Women's Health Initiative Investigators: Risks and benefits of estrogen plus progestin in healthy postmenopausal women: principal results from the Women's Health initiative randomized controlled trial, *JAMA* 288:321, 2002.
Author: **Fred F. Ferri, M.D.**

BASIC INFORMATION

■ DEFINITION

Human granulocytic ehrlichiosis (HGE) is a zoonotic infection of granulocytes, caused by an *Ehrlichia* species closely related to *E. phagocytophila*, *E. equi*, and *E. ewingii*, with multisystem manifestations.

ICD-9CM CODES
082-8 Other tick-borne rickettsiosis

■ EPIDEMIOLOGY & DEMOGRAPHICS

INCIDENCE (IN U.S.): Highest overall incidence in New York, New Jersey, Connecticut, Wisconsin, Minnesota, and northern California. >600 cases identified in the U.S. since 1990
PREDOMINANT SEX: Males outnumber females by 2 to 1
PREDOMINANT AGE: Most severe disease 50 to 70 yr
PEAK INCIDENCE: Occurs throughout the year, with peak incidence between May and July and again in November

■ PHYSICAL FINDINGS & CLINICAL PRESENTATION

- Most common initial symptoms
  1. Fever
  2. Chills, rigor
  3. Headache
  4. Myalgia
- Subsequent symptoms
  1. Anorexia, nausea
  2. Arthralgia
  3. Cough
  4. Confusion
  5. Abdominal pain
  6. Rash (erythematous to pustular) rare (<11%)
- Complications
  1. Hepatitis
  2. Interstitial pneumonitis
  3. Noncardiogenic pulmonary edema
  4. Renal insufficiency
  5. Bilateral facial palsy
  6. Meningitis

■ ETIOLOGY

- Obligate intracellular gram-negative bacterium (family *Rickettsiaceae*, genus *Ehrlichia*), closely related to *E. phagocytophila*, *E. equi* and *E. ewingii*
- Vector
  1. Almost certainly tick-borne, recently transmitted by infected blood
  2. Transmitted by *Ixodes scapularis* in the northeastern and upper midwestern states and *Ixodes pacificus* in the Pacific western states
  3. Tick exposure reported in >90% of patients, with approximately 60% reporting tick bite

- Mammalian host: deer, horses, dogs, white-footed mice, cattle, sheep, goats, bison
- Precise pathogenesis is unclear, although host inflammatory and immune responses may define final spectrum of disease beyond granulocytes, including hepatitis, interstitial pneumonitis, and nephritis with mild azotemia
- Between 6% and 21% of patients with HGE also have serologic evidence of other infection, both transmitted by *Ixodes* spp. tick bites
- Recovery is usual outcome; fatality rate of HGE is <1%

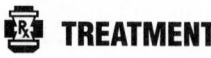

DIAGNOSIS

■ DIFFERENTIAL DIAGNOSIS

- Human monocytic ehrlichiosis (HME)
  1. Caused by *E. chaffeensis* (vector: tick *Amblyomma americanum*, possibly *Dermocenter variabilis*)
  2. Rash more common, sometimes petechial
  3. Morulae in monocytes
- Rocky Mountain spotted fever, Colorado tick fever, Q fever, relapsing fever
- Babesiosis
- Leptospirosis
- Typhus
- Lyme disease
- Legionnaire's disease
- Tularemia
- Typhoid fever, paratyphoid fever
- Brucellosis
- Viral hepatitis
- Enteroviral infections
- Meningococcemia
- Influenza
- Adenovirus pneumonia

■ WORKUP

- Acute blood samples for Giemsa-stained smears
- CBC
- Prothrombin time
- Acute serum samples for serology
- Chest x-ray examination
- Liver function and renal function tests
- MRI
- CSF analysis
- Bone marrow rarely needed

■ LABORATORY TESTS

- Giemsa-stained smear demonstrating morulae of *Ehrlichia* within granulocytes
- CBC progressive leukopenia and thrombocytopenia with nadir near day 7
- C reactive protein concentration is generally elevated

- LFT—twofold to fourfold increase in concentration of hepatic transaminases
- Serologic titer (IFA) >80 or fourfold increase in titer to *E. equi* antigen
- Polymerase chain reaction (PCR) to facilitate early diagnosis
- Culture on the first 7 days of illness
- Spinal tap for PCR analysis

■ IMAGING STUDIES

- Chest x-ray examination to show interstitial pneumonitis (unusual)
- MRI of the brain

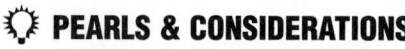

TREATMENT

■ ACUTE GENERAL Rx

- Immediate therapy to limit extent of acute illness and complication
- Tetracycline and doxycycline have demonstrated marked activity against the HGE, although doxycycline has been preferred because of a better pharmacokinetic profile and better toleration by patient
- Rifampin is an alternative drug of choice

■ CHRONIC Rx
Probably unnecessary; undefined

■ PROGNOSIS
Poor prognostic indicators include:
1. Advanced age
2. Concomitant chronic illness (such as diabetes mellitus, collagen-vascular disease)
3. Lack of diagnosis recognition
4. Delayed onset of specific antibiotic therapy

■ DISPOSITION
- Follow-up as outpatient
- Repeat CBC every 2 to 4 wk until normal

■ REFERRAL
- For consultation with infectious diseases specialist and hematologist in suspected cases
- For coagulopathy

PEARLS & CONSIDERATIONS

■ COMMENTS
Duration of time tick must be attached to produce illness is at least 24 hr.

REFERENCES
Olano JP, Walker DH: Human ehrlichiosis, *Med Clin North Am* 86(2):375,2002.
Singh-Behl D et al: Tick-borne infections, *Dermatol Clin* 21(2):237, 2003.
Author: **Vasanthi Arumugam, M.D.**

BASIC INFORMATION

■ DEFINITION
The human immunodeficiency virus, type 1 (HIV) causes a chronic infection that culminates, usually after several years, in acquired immunodeficiency syndrome (AIDS).

■ SYNONYMS
Acquired immunodeficiency syndrome (AIDS) when a patient with HIV infection meets specific diagnostic criteria (see "Acquired Immunodeficiency Syndrome" in Section I)

ICD-9CM CODES
044.9 HIV, unspecified

■ EPIDEMIOLOGY & DEMOGRAPHICS
INCIDENCE (IN U.S.):
- No complete incidence data available.
- Greatest incidence is in metropolitan areas with population >500,000.

PREVALENCE (IN U.S.): Estimated at 1 to 2 million cases

PREDOMINANT SEX:
- Adults: Most recently, estimated to be 74% males, 24% females, but is changing toward more women
- Children: male = female

PREDOMINANT AGE: 80% of cases occur between ages 20 and 40 yr

PEAK INCIDENCE: Age 30 to 35 yr

GENETICS:
Familial Disposition: Although there is no proven genetic predisposition, individuals with deletions in the CCR5 gene are immune from infection with macrophage tropic virus (the predominant virus in sexual transmission).

Congenital Infection:
- 80% of childhood cases are caused by peripartum infection, which may occur in utero, during delivery, or after delivery via breast-feeding.
- No specific congenital abnormalities are associated with HIV infection, although risk of spontaneous abortion and low birth weight is greater.

Neonatal Infection:
- May occur during delivery or via breast-feeding
- Typically asymptomatic

■ PHYSICAL FINDINGS & CLINICAL PRESENTATION
- Signs and symptoms variable with stage of disease
- In acute infection:
  1. May cause a self-limited mononucleosis-like illness characterized by fever, sore throat, lymphadenopathy, headache, and a rash resembling roseola
  2. In a minority of acute cases: frank aseptic meningitis, Bell's palsy, or peripheral neuropathy

- Later in the course of infection, after a prolonged asymptomatic phase: nonspecific symptoms of lymphadenopathy, weight loss, diarrhea, and skin changes including seborrheic dermatitis, localized herpes zoster, or fungal infection
- Advanced disease: characterized by the infections and malignancies associated with acquired immunodeficiency syndrome (see specific disorders)
- Section II describes rheumatic syndromes in HIV infection
- Some studies suggest that HIV infection in women is associated with lower levels of viral load at comparable degrees of immunosuppression when compared with men. Further, women may, on average have higher CD4 lymphocyte counts at the time of AIDS diagnosis
- Another special consideration in women infected with HIV is the high incidence of human papillomavirus (HPV) coinfection and the risk for cervical neoplasm that this presents. Even women with normal Pap smears should have this test repeated after 6 mo and annually thereafter

■ ETIOLOGY
- RNA retrovirus (Fig. 1-142)
- Transmitted by sexual contact, shared needles, blood transfusion, or from mother to child during pregnancy, delivery, or breast-feeding
- Primary target of infection: CD4 lymphocyte
- Direct CNS involvement: manifested as encephalopathy, myelopathy, or neuropathy in advanced cases

- Renal failure, rheumatologic disorders, thrombocytopenia, or cardiac abnormalities

DIAGNOSIS

■ DIFFERENTIAL DIAGNOSIS
- Acute infection: mononucleosis or other respiratory viral infections
- Late symptoms: similar to those produced by other wasting illnesses such as neoplasms, TB, disseminated fungal infection, malabsorption, or depression
- HIV-related encephalopathy: confused with Alzheimer's disease or other causes of chronic dementia (cognitive impairment in HIV infection is described in Section II); myelopathy and neuropathy possibly resembling other demyelinating diseases such as multiple sclerosis

■ WORKUP
Diagnosis is established by voluntary testing for antibody to the virus, available through public health laboratories or private facilities.

■ LABORATORY TESTS
HIV antibody detected by a two-step technique:
- ELISA as a sensitive screening test
- Confirmation of positive ELISA tests with the more specific Western blot technique
- The CD4 count and HIV RNA PCR should be measured in all patients
- The CD4 count is a marker of current immune status
- The HIV RNA PCR (viral load) is predictive of disease progression

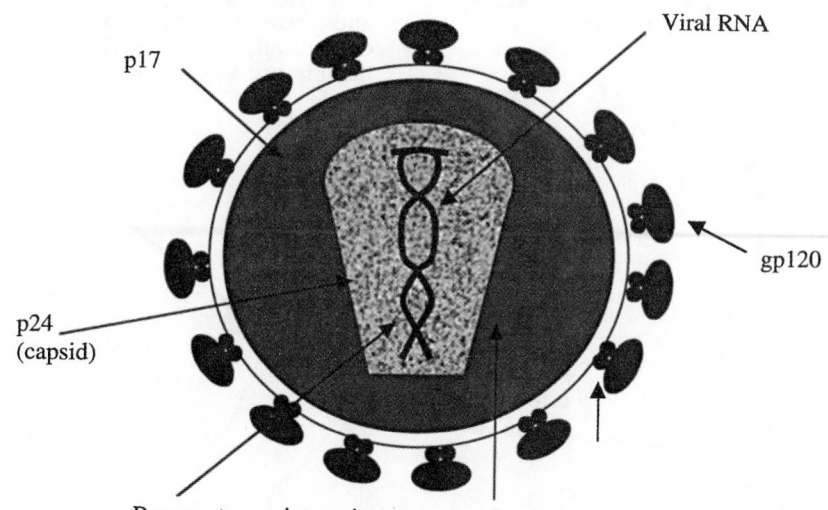

Fig. 1-142 **Locations of viral proteins and nucleic acids in the HIV-1 virion.** (From Mandell GL [ed]: *Mandell, Douglas, and Bennett's principles and practice of infectious diseases,* ed 5, New York, Churchill Livingstone.)

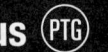
Fig. 1-143 describes the immunologic response to HIV infection

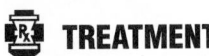 **TREATMENT**

■ **NONPHARMACOLOGIC THERAPY**
Maintenance of adequate nutrition

■ **ACUTE GENERAL Rx**
• Acute management of opportunistic infections and malignancies (see AIDS-associated disorders, "*Pneumocystis carinii* pneumonia," "Cryptococcosis," "Tuberculosis," "Toxoplasmosis" elsewhere in this text)
• Acute HIV syndrome:
  1. Early therapy during acute infection may reset viral set point and lead to attenuated disease progression.
  2. Given the need to further study the best way to approach patients with acute HIV infection, an attempt should always be made to refer these patients into clinical trials. If clinical trials are not available, therapy with combination antiretroviral therapy is recommended.

■ **CHRONIC Rx**
• Naïve chronically infected patients should be considered for therapy based on their current CD4 counts, likelihood for disease progression (viral loads), and ability to remain adherent with combination antiretroviral therapy. Please see current HIV treatment guidelines of the Department of Health and Human Services (http://www.aidsinfo.nih.gov/guidelines/).
  1. Patients with CD4 counts <200 cells/mm³ should be treated regardless of viral load.

2. Those with CD4 counts >350 cells/mm3 should generally be observed without therapy; however, in cases of extremely elevated viral loads therapy should be considered.
3. The benefits of therapy for patients with CD4 counts between 200-350 cells/mm3 remains controversial, although most authorities recommend treatment.
4. The current guidelines recommend the use of lamivudine (Epivir) 1 zidovudine (Retrovir) or tenofovir (Viread) or stavudine (Zerit) 1 lopinavir/ritonavir (Kaletra) or efavirenz (Sustiva) as the preferred initial antiretroviral regimen. Many alternative regimens and drugs are available.
• All patients should have genotypic resistance testing upon entry into medical care.
• Later antiretroviral regimen should be constructed based on past antiretroviral experience and the results of genotypic testing.
• Patients with CD4 lymphocyte count <200/mm³ should be given preventive therapy for *Pneumocystis carinii* pneumonia (PCP) (see "*Pneumocystis carinii* pneumonia").
• Evaluation of chronic diarrhea in patients with HIV is described in Section III, Fig. 3-62.
• Table 1-5 describes primary prophylaxis of opportunistic infections in adults and adolescents with HIV infection. Criteria for discontinuing and restarting opportunistic prophylaxis for adults with HIV infection is described in Section I, "Acquired Immunodeficiency Syndrome."
• HIV infection in a pregnant woman poses special challenges and considerations. Appropriate and timely antiretroviral therapy given to mother and newborn has been shown to dramatically reduce the risk of perinatal transmission of HIV. All preg-

nant women with newly diagnosed HIV infection should be offered antiretroviral therapy. Antiretroviral therapy should be initiated at the end of the first trimester, include zidovudine when possible, and continue through the baby's birth. The goal of therapy is to achieve an undetectable viral load. In women with viral loads persistently >1000 copies/ml despite appropriate ARV, C-section may further lower risk of transmission. Zidovudine (AZT) should also be given to the newborn for the first 6 wk of life, and mothers should completely avoid nursing. Efavirenz (Sustiva) should be avoided because of its potential teratogenic effects.

■ **DISPOSITION**
• Ongoing care consisting of frequent medical evaluations and T-lymphocyte subset analysis
• Long-term care focused on providing up-to-date antiretroviral therapy and prophylaxis of PCP and other opportunistic infections, as well as early detection of complications (see Section III, Figs. 3-90 to 3-92)

■ **REFERRAL**
To a physician knowledgeable and experienced in the management of HIV infection and its complications

PEARLS & CONSIDERATIONS

■ **COMMENTS**
HIV chemoprophylaxis after occupational exposure is described in Section V, Tables 5-29 and 5-30.

REFERENCES
Carpenter C et al: Antiretroviral therapy in adults, updated recommendations of the International AIDS Society-USA Panel, *JAMA* 283:381, 2000.
Kasten MJ: Human immunodeficiency virus: the initial physician-patient encounter, *Mayo Clin Proc* 77:957, 2002.
Levine AM: Evaluation and management of HIV-infected women, *Ann Intern Med* 136:228, 2002.
Schacker TW et al: Biological and virologic characteristics of primary HIV infection, *Ann Intern Med* 128:613, 1998.
Watts DH: Management of human immunodeficiency virus infection in pregnancy, *N Engl J Med* 346(24):1879, 2002.
Yeni PG: Antiretroviral treatment for adult HIV infection in 2002: updated recommendations of the International AIDS Society–USA panel, *JAMA* 288:222, 2002.
Author: **Joseph R. Masci, M.D.**

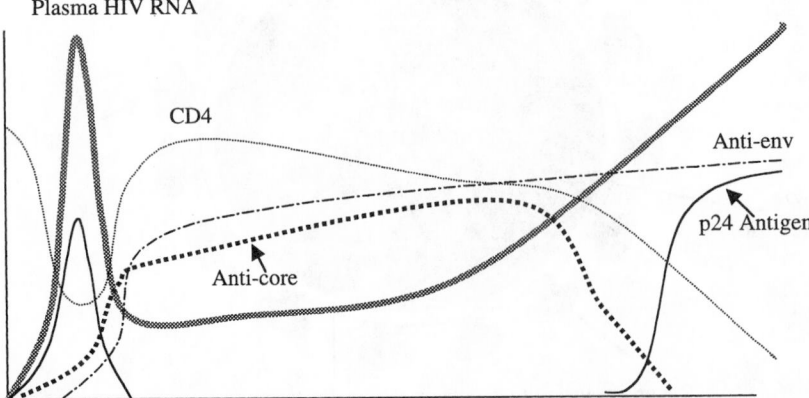
Fig. 1-143 Course of human immunodeficiency virus infection. (From Mandell GL [ed]: *Mandell, Douglas, and Bennett's principles and practice of infectious diseases,* ed 5, New York, Churchill Livingstone.)

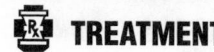

BASIC INFORMATION

■ DEFINITION
Huntington's chorea is an inherited neurodegenerative disorder characterized by involuntary movements, psychiatric disturbance, and cognitive decline.

■ SYNONYMS
Huntington's disease

ICD-9CM CODES
333.4 Huntington's chorea

■ EPIDEMIOLOGY & DEMOGRAPHICS
PREVALENCE (IN U.S.): 4.1 to 5.4 cases/100,000 persons
PREDOMINANT SEX: Female = male
PREDOMINANT AGE: Adulthood
PEAK INCIDENCE: Late 30s and 40s, with onsets from age 2 to 70 yr
GENETICS: Autosomal dominant

■ PHYSICAL FINDINGS & CLINICAL PRESENTATION
- Chorea (irregular rapid, flowing, nonstereotyped involuntary movements). When there is a writhing quality, it is referred to as choreoathetosis. 90% of affected patients have chorea, but virtually any expression of basal ganglia dysfunction, including rigidity and dystonia, can be seen. Chorea is present early on and tends to decrease in end stages of disease.
- Dance-like, lurching gait, often caused by chorea.
- Westphal variant: cognitive dysfunction, bradykinesia, and rigidity. This variant is more commonly seen in juvenile onset HD.
- Oculomotor abnormalities are common early on and include increased latency of response and insuppressible eye blinking.
- Psychiatric disorders (can be present early on): depression is commonly seen. Also, obsessive-compulsive behaviors and aggression associated with impaired impulse control.

■ ETIOLOGY
- Trinucleotide repeat disorder.
- Unstable repeat results in CAG expansion.
- The responsible gene is the Huntington gene located on chromosome 4. Its function is not known.

DIAGNOSIS

■ DIFFERENTIAL DIAGNOSIS
- Drug-induced chorea—dopamine, stimulants, anticonvulsants, antidepressants, and oral contraceptives have all been known to cause chorea.
- Sydenham's chorea—decreased incidence with decline of rheumatic fever.
- Benign hereditary chorea—autosomal dominant with onset in childhood. There is no progression of symptoms and no associated dementia or behavioral problems.
- Senile chorea.
- Wilson's disease—autosomal recessive; tremor, dysarthria, and dystonia are more common presentations than chorea. 95% of patients with neurologic manifestations will have Keyser-Fleischer rings.
- Neuroacanthocytosis—autosomal recessive. Chorea, dystonia, tics, and orolingual dyskinesias that can result in self-mutilation. Must look for acanthocytes in peripheral smear.
- Dentatorubropallidoluysian atrophy—autosomal dominant, triplet repeat disease. Presentation is variable and includes chorea, myoclonus, dementia, and ataxia. More common in Japan. Can be confirmed by genetic testing.
- Postinfectious.
- Systemic lupus erythematosus—can be the presenting feature of lupus. Only occurs in about 1% of individuals with lupus. Pathophysiology unknown.
- Chorea gravidarum—presents during first 4-5 mo of pregnancy and resolves after delivery.
- Paraneoplastic—seen most commonly in small cell lung cancer and lymphoma.

■ WORKUP
Onset of symptoms in an individual with an established family history requires no additional investigation.

■ LABORATORY TESTS
- Confirm diagnosis by chromosome analysis.
- If normal, obtain CBC with smear, ESR, electrolytes, serum ceruloplasmin, 24-hr urinary copper excretion, TFTs, ANA, LFTs, HIV, and ASO titer. Consider paraneoplastic markers.

■ IMAGING STUDIES
CT scan or MRI scan will show atrophy most notably in the caudate and putamen. Cortex is involved to a lesser extent. A normal scan does not exclude the diagnosis.

TREATMENT

■ NONPHARMACOLOGIC THERAPY
- Supportive counseling
- Physical and occupational therapy
- Home health care
- Genetic counseling

■ CHRONIC Rx
- Chorea does not need to be treated unless disabling
- Chorea may be diminished by low doses of neuroleptics (e.g., haloperidol 1 to 10 mg/day)
- Can also try clozapine or other atypical antipsychotics such as quetiapine, which decreases chorea with fewer extrapyramidal side effects
- Amantadine (up to 300-400 mg divided tid)
- Tetrabenazine. This is a dopamine depletor that is not currently available in the United States. Side effects include parkinsonism and depression
- Depression with suicidal ideation is common; may improve with tricyclic or SSRI antidepressants

■ DISPOSITION
Relentless course of variable duration leading to progressive disability and death

■ REFERRAL
- Should refer to psychiatry and neurology for treatment of mood disorders and movement disorders
- Genetic counselors

☼ PEARLS AND CONSIDERATIONS

- Suicide rate is fivefold that of the general population.
- The number of repeats does correlate with age of onset but does not clearly correlate with disease severity. Interpretation of number of repeats is still difficult at this time and therefore it is debatable whether to disclose this information to patients.

REFERENCES
Biglan K, Shoulson I: Huntington's disease. In Jankovic J, Tolosa E (eds): *Parkinson's disease and movement disorders.* Philadelphia, 2002, Lippincott Williams & Wilkins.
Higgins D: Chorea and its disorders, *Neuro Clin* 19(3):707, 2001.
Author: **Cindy Zadikoff M.D.**

BASIC INFORMATION

■ DEFINITION
A hydrocele is a fluid collection in a serous scrotal space usually between the layers of the tunica vaginalis (Figs. 1-144 and 1-145).

ICD-9CM CODES
603.9 Hydrocele

■ PHYSICAL FINDINGS & CLINICAL PRESENTATION
Symptoms:
- Scrotal enlargement
- Scrotal heaviness or discomfort radiating to the inguinal area
- Back pain

Physical findings:
- Scrotal distention (testicle may be impossible to palpate)
- Transillumination

■ ETIOLOGY & PATHOGENESIS
Hydroceles may occur as a congenital abnormality where the processus vaginalis fails to close. In this case, an inguinal hernia is virtually always associated with the malformation. Congenital hydroceles are most common in infants and children. In adults, hydroceles are more frequently caused by infection, tumor, or trauma. Infection of the epididymis often results in the development of a secondary hydrocele. Tropical infections such as filariasis may produce hydroceles.

DIAGNOSIS

■ DIFFERENTIAL DIAGNOSIS
- Spermatocele
- Inguinoscrotal hernia
- Testicular tumor
- Varicocele
- Epididymitis

■ IMAGING
Scrotal ultrasound (useful to rule out a testicular tumor as the cause of the hydrocele)

TREATMENT

- No treatment if asymptomatic and testicle is thought to be normal
- Surgical repair

REFERENCE
Rowland RG, Foster RS, Donohue JP: Scrotum and testis. In Gillenwater JY et al. (eds): *Adult and pediatric urology,* ed 3, St Louis, 1996, Mosby.

Author: **Tom J. Wachtel, M.D.**

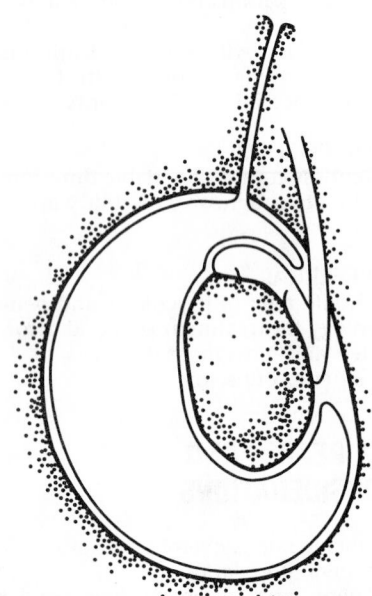

Fig. 1-144 A hydrocele is a fluid collection in the serous space between the layers of the tunica vaginalis. The tunica vaginalis may or may not remain patent, allowing the hydrocele to communicate with the peritoneum.

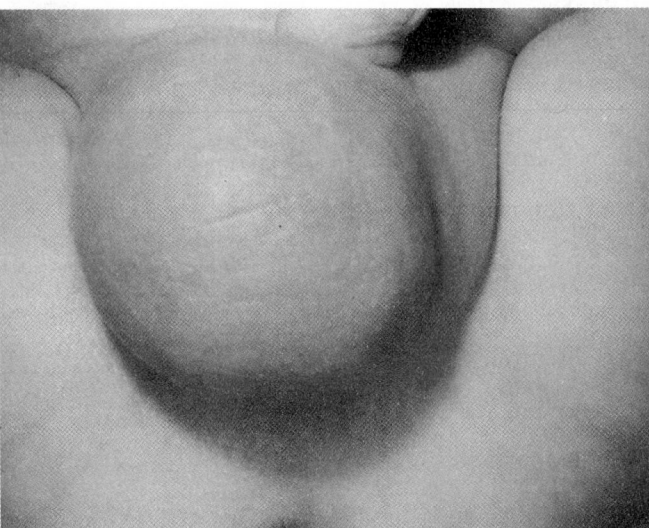

Fig. 1-145 **Newborn with large right hydrocele.** (From Behrman RE: *Nelson textbook of pediatrics,* ed 16, Philadelphia, 2000, WB Saunders.)

BASIC INFORMATION

■ DEFINITION

Normal pressure hydrocephalus (NPH) is a syndrome of symptomatic hydrocephalus in the setting of normal CSF pressure. The classic clinical triad of NPH includes gait disturbance, cognitive decline, and incontinence.

■ ICD-9CM CODES

331.3 Communicating hydrocephalus

■ EPIDEMIOLOGY & DEMOGRAPHICS

PREDOMINANT SEX: Males = females
PREDOMINANT AGE: Fourth to sixth decades, but can occur at any age
INCIDENCE: 1 per 100,0000

■ PHYSICAL FINDINGS & CLINICAL PRESENTATION

- **Gait difficulty:** patients often have difficulty initiating ambulation, and the gait may be broad-based and shuffling, with the appearance that the feet are stuck to the floor (i.e., "magnetic gait" or "frontal gait disorder")
- **Cognitive decline:** mental slowing, forgetfulness and inattention without agnosia, aphasia, or other "cortical" disturbances
- **Incontinence:** initially may have urinary urgency; later incontinence develops. Occasionally fecal incontinence also occurs

- On physical examination, look for signs of disease that may mimic NPH

■ ETIOLOGY

- Approximately 50% of cases are idiopathic; remaining cases are from secondary causes, including prior subarachnoid hemorrhage, meningitis, trauma, or intracranial surgery.
- Symptoms are presumed to result from stretching of sacral motor and limbic fibers that lie near the ventricles, as dilation occurs.

DIAGNOSIS

■ DIFFERENTIAL DIAGNOSIS

- Alzheimer's disease with extrapyramidal features
- Cognitive impairment in the setting of Parkinson's disease or Parkinson's Plus syndromes
- Diffuse Lewy Body disease
- Frontotemporal dementia
- Cervical spondylosis with cord compromise in setting of degenerative dementia
- Multifactorial gait disorder
- Multiinfarct dementia

■ WORKUP

- **Large volume lumbar puncture:**
  1. Mental status testing and time to walk a prespecified distance (usu-
     ally 25 feet) are measured, followed by removal of 30-50 ml of CSF.
  2. Retest of mental status and timed walking are done at 1 and 4 hr. Patients who have significant improvement in gait or mental status tend to have better surgical outcome; those with mild or negative response can have variable outcomes.
  3. Opening and closing pressure are measured; if pressure is elevated, alternative etiologies must be considered.
- Occasionally, continuous lumbar CSF drainage may be performed.
- CSF infusion and CSF pressure monitoring are sometimes used to help predict surgical outcome.

■ LABORATORY TESTS

CSF should be sent for routine fluid analyses to exclude other pathology.

■ IMAGING STUDIES

- CT scan (Fig. 1-146) or MRI can be used to document ventriculomegaly. The distinguishing feature of NPH is ventricular enlargement out of proportion to sulcal atrophy.
- MRI has advantages over CT, including better ability to visualize structures in the posterior fossa, visualize transependymal CSF flow, and to document extent of white matter lesions.

A
B

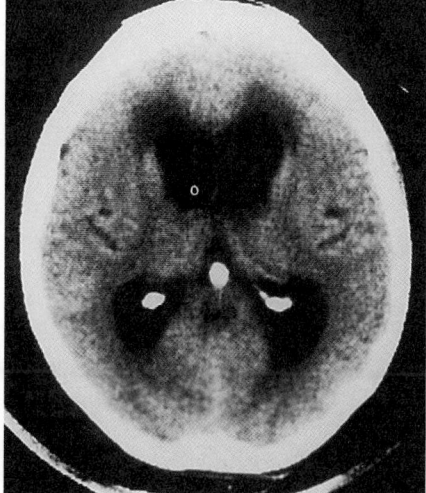
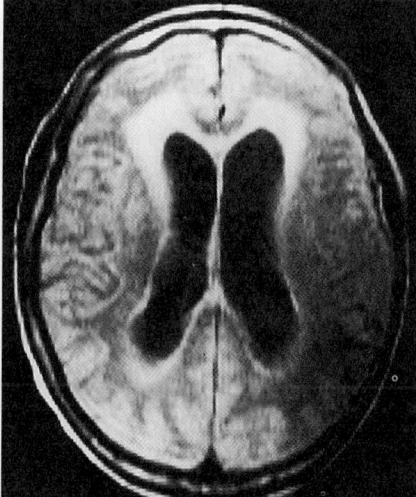

Fig. 1-146 **(A)** CT scan showing enlarged ventricles in the absence of cortical sulcal atrophy and **(B)** MRI scan showing enlarged ventricles with transependymal CSF flow into the brain parenchyma surrounding the ventricles. (From Andreoli TE [ed]: *Cecil essentials of medicine,* ed 4, Philadelphia, 1997, WB Saunders.)

- Isotope cisternography and dynamic MRI studies have not been shown to be superior in predicting shunt outcome.

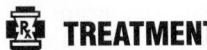

TREATMENT

■ NONPHARMACOLOGIC THERAPY

Some patients (30% of those with idiopathic NPH and 60% of patients with a known etiology) show significant improvement from shunting.

Factors that may predict positive outcome with surgery:

- NPH secondary to prior trauma, subarachnoid hemorrhage, or meningitis
- History of mild impairment in cognition <2 yr
- Onset of gait abnormality before cognitive decline

- Imaging demonstrates hydrocephalus without sulcal enlargement
- Transependymal CSF flow visualized on MRI

Factors that may predict negative outcome with surgery

- Extensive white matter lesions or diffuse cerebral atrophy on MRI
- Moderate to severe cognitive impairment
- Onset of cognitive impairment before gait disorder
- History of alcohol abuse

■ ACUTE GENERAL Rx

Shunting in selected patients

■ REFERRAL

Neurosurgical referral for shunting in appropriate patients

PEARLS & CONSIDERATIONS

Each of the cardinal symptoms of NPH are commonly seen in the elderly and can be seen in multiple disease processes, therefore keep possible differential diagnosis in mind.

■ CAUTION

Shunt complications occur in 30%-40% of patients.

REFERENCE

Vanneste JA: Diagnosis and management of normal-pressure hydrocephalus, *J Neurol* 247(1):5, 2000.

Author: **Tamara G. Fong, M.D., Ph.D.**

BASIC INFORMATION

■ DEFINITION
Hydronephrosis is dilation of the renal pyelocalyceal system, most often as a result of impairment of urinary flow.

■ SYNONYMS
Hydroureter (dilation of ureter, often seen with hydronephrosis when obstruction is in lower urinary tract)
Urinary tract obstruction

ICD-9CM CODES
591 Acquired hydronephrosis
753.2 Congenital hydronephrosis

■ EPIDEMIOLOGY & DEMOGRAPHICS
Children usually have congenital malformations, whereas adults tend to have acquired defects as etiologies.

■ PHYSICAL FINDINGS & CLINICAL PRESENTATION
HISTORY:
- Pain is caused by distention of collecting system or renal capsule and is more related to the rate of onset than the degree of obstruction. It can vary in location from flank to lower abdomen to testes/labia. Pain in flank occurring only on micturition is highly suggestive of vesicoureteral reflux.
- Anuria can occur with total obstruction of urinary flow (bilateral hydronephrosis or unilateral if only one kidney is present).
- Polyuria or nocturia can occur with chronic (incomplete) obstruction because of deleterious effects on renal concentrating ability (nephrogenic diabetes insipidus).
- Urinary frequency, hesitancy, postvoid dribbling, and difficulty initiating stream are all symptoms that can occur with obstruction at or below the bladder (e.g., prostatic hyperplasia).
- Chronic urinary infections can either result from chronic urinary obstruction (organisms favoring growth with stasis of urine) or lead to conditions (e.g., urine pH changes) that favor stone formation and subsequent obstruction.

PHYSICAL EXAMINATION:
- Hypertension can be caused by increased renin release in acute or subacute obstruction
- Fever or CVA tenderness can suggest urinary tract infection
- Distended bladder or kidneys present
- Rectal examination should be done to evaluate prostate for size and nodularity and also to check rectal sphincter tone

- Pelvic examination is done to assess for vaginal anatomy, pelvic mass, or pelvic inflammatory disease (PID)
- Penile examination performed to rule out meatal stenosis or phimosis
- Bladder catheterization is needed to assess postvoid residual volume if urinary tract obstruction is considered. Should rule out postrenal obstruction in unexplained acute renal failure

■ ETIOLOGY
MECHANICAL IMPAIRMENTS:
- Congenital: ureteropelvic junction narrowing, ureterovesical junction narrowing, ureterocele, retrocaval ureter, bladder neck obstruction, urethral valves, urethral stricture, meatal stenosis
- Acquired:
  1. Intrinsic to urinary tract: calculi, inflammation, trauma, sloughed papillae, ureteral tumor, blood clots, prostatic hypertrophy or cancer, bladder cancer, urethral stricture, phimosis
  2. Extrinsic to urinary tract: gravid uterus, retroperitoneal fibrosis or tumor (e.g., lymphoma), aortic aneurysm, uterine fibroids, trauma (surgical or nonsurgical), PID, pelvic malignancies (e.g., prostate, colorectal, cervical, uterine, bladder)

FUNCTIONAL IMPAIRMENTS:
- Neurogenic bladder (often with adynamic ureter) can occur with spinal cord disease or diabetic neuropathy.
- Pharmacologic agents such as α-adrenergic antagonists and anticholinergic drugs can inhibit bladder emptying.
- Vesicoureteral reflux may occur.
- Pregnancy can cause hydroureter and hydronephrosis (right more often than left) as early as the second month. Hormonal effects on ureteral tone combine with mechanical factors.

DIAGNOSIS

■ DIFFERENTIAL DIAGNOSIS
- Urinary stones
- Neoplastic disease
- Prostatic hypertrophy
- Neurologic disease
- Urinary reflux
- Urinary tract infection
- Medication effects
- Trauma
- Congenital abnormality of urinary tract

■ LABORATORY TESTS
- Serum BUN and creatinine to assess for renal insufficiency (usually im-

plies bilateral obstruction or unilateral obstruction of a solitary kidney)
- Electrolytes may reveal hypernatremia (if nephrogenic DI), hyperkalemia (from renal failure and effects on tubular function), or distal renal tubular acidosis
- Urinalysis and examination of sediment may reveal WBCs, RBCs, or bacteria in the appropriate setting (e.g., infection, stones), but often the sediment is normal in obstructive renal disease

■ IMAGING STUDIES
- Abdominal plain film of kidneys, ureters, and bladder is used to look for nephrocalcinosis or a radiopaque stone.
- Assess kidney and bladder size with ultrasound; contour of pyelocalyces and ureters (Fig. 1-147). Ultrasound is about 90% sensitive and specific for hydronephrosis and is noninvasive, so it will not worsen preexisting renal insufficiency.
- Intravenous pyelogram (IVP) helps localize the site of obstruction (Fig. 1-148) when hydronephrosis is seen on ultrasound, but the contrast may have deleterious effects on the kidneys if there is renal insufficiency.
- Antegrade or retrograde urograms can be performed if renal failure is a concern with IVP and either of these two procedures could be extended to provide relief of the obstruction.
- Abdominal CT scan without IV contrast provides excellent localization of the site of obstruction.
- Voiding cystourethrogram is helpful in diagnosing vesicoureteral reflux and obstructions of the bladder neck or urethra.

TREATMENT

- Urgent treatment is required if urinary tract obstruction is associated with urinary tract infection, acute renal failure, or uncontrollable pain.
- Conservative management of calculi with IV fluid, IV antibiotics (if evidence of infection), and aggressive analgesia may be enough to treat acute unilateral urinary tract obstruction depending on the size (90% of stones <5 mm will pass spontaneously).
- Urethral catheter is adequate to relieve most obstructions at or distal to the bladder, but occasionally a suprapubic catheter will be required (e.g., impassable urethral stricture or urethral injury). Neurogenic bladder may require intermittent clean catheterization if frequent voiding and pharmacologic treatments are ineffective.

- Nephrostomy tube can be placed percutaneously to facilitate urinary drainage.
- Extracorporeal shock wave lithotripsy (ESWL) is used to fragment large stones to facilitate spontaneous passage or subsequent extraction (NOTE: ESWL is contraindicated in pregnancy).
- Nephroscopy is performed for extraction of proximal stones under direct vision.
- Cystoscopy with ureteroscopy is used for removal of distal ureteral stones using a loop or basket with or without fragmentation by ultrasonic or laser lithotripsy.
- Ureteral stents can be used for extrinsic and some intrinsic ureteral obstructions.

- Urethral dilation or internal urethrotomy can be used for urethral strictures.
- Nephrectomy or ureteral diversion may be required in severe cases (e.g., malignancy).
- Ureterovesical reimplantation can be used for reflux disease.
- Transurethral retrograde prostatectomy (TURP) is used for severe obstruction from benign prostatic hypertrophy (BPH).
- IV fluid and electrolyte replacement is needed; the patient must be monitored closely during the postobstructive diuresis (usually lasting several days to a week).

■ DISPOSITION

Aggressive treatment of infections and early relief of obstruction can usually prevent progressive loss of renal function; however, chronic bilateral obstruction (often from BPH) can lead to chronic renal failure.

■ REFERRAL

- Urologist consultation early for diagnostic and/or therapeutic procedures
- Oncologist if a neoplasm is diagnosed
- Gynecologist if pregnancy or female pelvic anatomy is involved

Author: **William F. Boyd, M.D.**

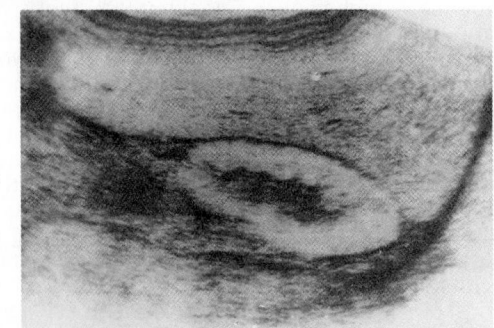 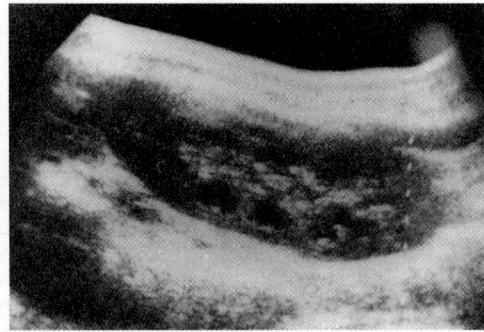

A   B

Fig. 1-147   Renal ultrasound. A, Normal features include peripheral homogeneous thick cortex (*white*) and central heterogeneous fluid-filed calyces (*black*). Note that individual calyces cannot be visualized. **B,** In acute hydronephrosis, features include normal cortex (*gray*) and dilated calyces (gray areas within central white). (From Harrington J [ed]: *Consultation in internal medicine,* ed 2, St Louis, 1997, Mosby.)

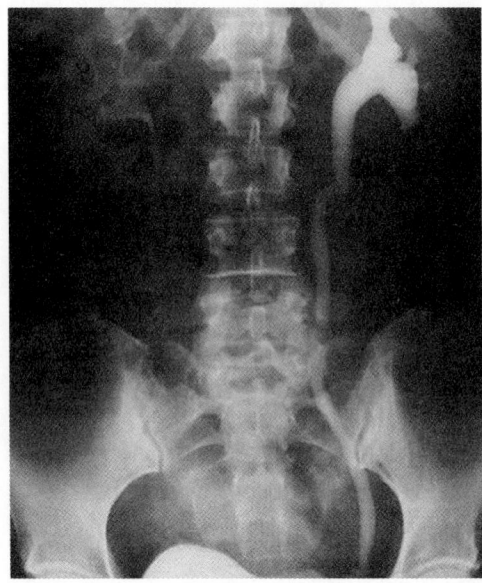

Fig. 1-148   Left-side obstruction demonstrating dense nephrogram-dilated collecting system and ureter. Calculus of the ureterovesicle junction is responsible for the obstruction. (From Stein JH [ed]: *Internal medicine,* ed 5, St Louis, 1998, Mosby.)

■ BASIC INFORMATION

■ DEFINITION

Hypercholesterolemia refers to a blood cholesterol measurement >200 mg/dl. A cholesterol level of 200 to 239 mg/dl is considered borderline high, and a level of ≥240 mg/dl is considered to be a high cholesterol measurement.

■ SYNONYMS

Hypercholesteremia
Hypercholesterinemia
Type II familial hyperlipoproteinemia

ICD-9CM CODES

272.0 Hypercholesterolemia

■ EPIDEMIOLOGY & DEMOGRAPHICS

INCIDENCE/PREVALENCE:
- There are well over 100 million Americans with a total serum cholesterol >200 mg/dl.
- Elevated cholesterol requires drug therapy in about 60 million Americans.
- Incidence of heterozygous familial hypercholesterolemia: about 1:500.
- Incidence of homozygous familial hypercholesterolemia: about 1:1 million.
- Prevalence of hypercholesterolemia increases with increasing age.

GENETICS:
- Familial hypercholesterolemia: autosomal dominant disorder
- Familial combined hyperlipidemia: possibly an autosomal dominant disorder
- Multifactorial predilection: apparent in majority of affected individuals

RISK FACTORS:
- Dietary intake
- Genetic predisposition
- Sedentary lifestyle
- Associated secondary causes

■ PHYSICAL FINDINGS & CLINICAL PRESENTATION

- Most patients: no physical findings
- Possible findings particularly in the familial forms
  1. Tendon xanthomas
  2. Xanthelasma
  3. Arcus corneae
  4. Arterial bruits (young adulthood)

■ ETIOLOGY

Primary
1. Genetics
2. Obesity
3. Dietary intake

Secondary
1. Diabetes mellitus
2. Alcohol
3. Oral contraceptives
4. Hypothyroidism
5. Glucocorticoid use
6. Most diuretics
7. Nephrotic syndrome
8. Hepatoma
9. Extrahepatic biliary obstruction
10. Primary biliary cirrhosis

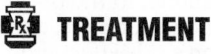 DIAGNOSIS

■ DIFFERENTIAL DIAGNOSIS

No real differential diagnosis; however, consider underlying secondary causes/etiologies for the elevated cholesterol.

■ LABORATORY TESTS

PRIMARY PREVENTION WITHOUT ATHEROSCLEROSIS:
1. Total cholesterol <200 mg/dl, and the HDL >40: repeat in 5 yr.
2. Cholesterol 200 to 239 mg/dl and the HDL >40: discuss dietary modification, repeat in 1 to 2 yr.
3. Total cholesterol >240 mg/dl or the HDL <40 mg/dl: need a fasting lipid profile (cholesterol, HDL, triglycerides, from which an LDL can be calculated).

4. Fasting lipid profile with LDL <130 mg/dl and 1 or no risk factors: dietary guidance and repeat in 5 yr.
5. Fasting lipid profile with LDL 130 to 159 mg/dl (borderline high risk), and less than two risk factors for CAD: diet and exercise modification, with repeat profile in 12 wk.
6. Fasting lipid profile with LDL >160 mg/dl or borderline LDL and two or more risk factors for CAD: need drug therapy.

SECONDARY PREVENTION WITHOUT ATHEROSCLEROSIS OR DIABETES MELLITUS:
1. All patients: fasting lipid profile
2. If LDL <100 mg/dl: instruction on diet and exercise, and repeat annually
3. If LDL >100 mg/dl: drug therapy required

■ TREATMENT

■ NONPHARMACOLOGIC THERAPY

- First line of treatment: dietary therapy (see "Hyperlipoproteinemia")
- Dietary modifications
  1. Low-cholesterol, low-fat diet (fat intake to 30% or less of the total caloric intake)
  2. Saturated fats <7% of total calories
  3. No more than 200 mg/day of cholesterol
- Increased activity with aerobic exercise: encourage 20 to 30 min of aerobic exercise three to four times a week
- Smoking cessation encouraged
- Counseling on CAD risk factors

■ ACUTE GENERAL Rx

No acute treatment needed

■ **CHRONIC Rx**
- In primary prevention: needed for patients with LDL >160 mg/dl or LDL 130 to 159 mg/dl with two or more risk factors for CAD
- In secondary prevention: needed for patients with known CAD, vascular disease or diabetes mellitus, and LDL >100 mg/dl
- In primary prevention: considered in patients on dietary therapy with LDL >190 mg/dl with no risk factors, LDL >160 mg/dl with two or more risk factors, or HDL <30 mg/dl
- Medications that can be used (see Table 1-28):
  1. Bile acid sequestrants (poorly tolerated)
  2. Niacin (poorly tolerated)
  3. HMG-CoA reductase inhibitors ("statins")
  4. Fibric acids
  5. Medication tailored to the patient's lipid profile, lifestyle, and the medication's side-effect profile

- Cholesterol absorption inhibitors (ezetimibe)
- Bile acid sequestrants to lower LDL
- Niacin to lower LDL and triglycerides and raise HDL
- HMG-CoA reductase inhibitors to lower LDL
- Fibric acids work to lower triglycerides more than LDL

■ **DISPOSITION**
- After initiation of therapy, repeat laboratory tests in 4 to 6 wk, with modifications as necessary.
- Once goal is achieved, lifelong medication and monitoring are needed at least three to four times a year.
- Dietary modification is needed to continue with drug therapy.
- Repeat review for additional CAD risk factors.

💡 **PEARLS & CONSIDERATIONS**

■ **COMMENTS**
See "Hyperlipoproteinemia."

REFERENCES

Cleeman JI: Detection and evaluation of dyslipoproteinemia, *Endocrinol Metab Clin North Am* 27(3):597, 1998.

Illingworth DR: Management of hypercholesterolemia, *Med Clin North Am* 84(1):23, 2000.

National Cholesterol Education Program: Second Report on the Expert Panel on Detection, Evaluation, and Treatment of High Cholesterol in Adults (adult treatment panel III), *JAMA* 285:2486, 2001.

Safeer R, Ugalat P: Cholesterol treatment guidelines update, *Am Fam Physician* 65:871, 2002.
Author: **Beth J. Wutz, M.D.**

TABLE 1-28 Drugs Affecting Lipoprotein Metabolism

DRUG CLASS	AGENTS AND DAILY DOSES	LIPID/LIPOPROTEIN EFFECTS		SIDE EFFECTS	CONTRAINDICATIONS
HMG-CoA reductase inhibitors (statins)	Lovastatin (20-80 mg) Pravastatin (20-80 mg) Simvastatin (20-80 mg) Fluvastatin (20-80 mg) Atorvastatin (10-80 mg)	LDL HDL TG	↓18%-55% ↑5%-15% ↓7%-30%	Myopathy Increased liver enzymes	Absolute: • Active or chronic liver disease Relative: • Concomitant use of certain drugs*
Bile acid sequestrants	Cholestyramine (4-16 g) Colestipol (5-20 g) Colesevelam (2.6-3.8 g)	LDL HDL TG	↓1.5%-30% ↑3%-5% No change or increase	Gastrointestinal distress Constipation Decreased absorption of other drugs	Absolute: • Dysbetalipoproteinemia • TG >400 mg/dl Relative: • TG >200 mg/dl
Nicotinic acid	Immediate release (crystalline) nicotinic acid (1.5-3 g), extended-release nicotinic acid (Niaspan) 1-2 g), sustained release nicotinic acid (1-2 g)	LDL HDL TG	↓5%-25% ↑15%-35% ↓20%-50%	Flushing Hyperglycemia Hyperuricemia (or gout) Upper GI distress Hepatotoxicity	Absolute: • Chronic liver disease • Severe gout Relative: • Diabetes • Hyperuricemia • Peptic ulcer disease
Fibric acids	Gemfibrozil (600 mg bid) Fenofibrate (160 mg qd) Clofibrate (1000 mg bid)	LDL *(may be increased in patients with high TG)* HDL TG	↓5%-20% ↑10%-20% ↓20%-50%	Dyspepsia Gallstones Myopathy	Absolute: • Severe renal disease • Severe hepatic disease
Cholesterol absorption inhibitors	Ezetimibe (10 mg QD)	LDL HDL TG	↓18% ↑1% ↓7%-8%	Abdominal pain myalgias	• Severe renal disease • Severe hepatic disease

Modified from The National Cholestrol Education Program, *JAMA* 285:2486, 2001.
CoA, Coenzyme A; *GI,* gastrointestinal; *HDL,* high-density lipoprotein; *HMG,* 3-hydroxy-3 methylglutanyl; *LDL,* low-density lipoprotein; *TG,* triglyceride.
*Cyclosporine, macrolide antibiotics, various antifungal agents, and cytochrome P-450 inhibitors (fibrates and niacin should be used with appropriate caution).

BASIC INFORMATION

■ DEFINITION
A hypercoagulable state is an inherited or acquired condition associated with an increased risk of thrombosis.

ICD-9CM CODES
289.8 Hypercoagulable state
795.79 Antiphospholipid antibody syndrome

■ EPIDEMIOLOGY & DEMOGRAPHICS (Table 1-29)
- Risk of thrombosis increases with age.
- Most people with a genetic defect or laboratory abnormality will not suffer thrombotic disease.
- About half of patients with thrombosis have a predisposing hereditary or acquired blood protein defect.
- Annual risk of thrombosis is <1%.

■ HISTORY
A hypercoagulable state is strongly suggested by:
- Spontaneous thrombosis: absence of other medical conditions associated with increased risk of thrombosis
- Less than 45 yr old at first episode of thrombosis
- Family history of thrombosis
- Recurrent thrombotic events
- Thrombosis in unusual anatomic location
- Thrombosis in pregnancy, postpartum, or associated with oral contraceptive use
- Fetal loss associated with placental infarction, recurrent or severe placental abruption, severe intrauterine growth restriction, severe preeclampsia in second or early third trimester
- Warfarin-induced skin necrosis

■ PHYSICAL FINDINGS & CLINICAL PRESENTATION
- Thrombosis
- Medical conditions associated with increased risk of thrombosis

■ ETIOLOGY (Table 1-29)
- Often a multifactorial process with genetic, environmental, and acquired factors
- Multiple genetic factor defects are not uncommon, often strong synergistic effect with multiple risk factors

COMMON INHERITED:
Factor V Leiden (FVL)
- Mutation causing activated protein C resistance (APCR); 80% to 90% of APCR is caused by FVL mutation
- Most common genetic risk factor for venous thrombosis; accounts for 40% to 50% of inherited thrombophilia cases
- Important cause of thrombosis in the elderly
- Heterozygous carrier has seven-fold increased risk and homozygous carrier has eighty-fold increased risk of thrombosis
- OCP use and pregnancy induce APCR. Carriers have a four- to eight-fold increased risk of thrombosis with OCP use and pregnancy. OCP use in heterozygous carriers is associated with a thirty-five-fold increased risk of thrombosis compared with noncarriers not using OCP
- Accounts for about 40% of thrombotic events in pregnancy.

Associated with late first-, second-, and third-trimester fetal loss; severe intrauterine growth retardation; severe preeclampsia; and placental abruption
- Risk of recurrent thrombotic event not well defined

Prothrombin G20210A Mutation
- Second most common inherited thrombophilia
- Responsible for 17% of thrombosis in pregnancy. Associated with increased risk of fetal loss, severe intrauterine growth retardation, severe preeclampsia, and placental abruption

Hyperhomocysteinemia
- Can be inherited (most commonly a mutation in methylene tetrahydrofolate reductase gene) but more frequently secondary to poor dietary intake. Deficiency of folate, vitamin B_6 or vitamin B_{12} account for two thirds of cases
- Associated with fetal neural tube defects, fetal loss, severe intrauterine growth retardation, severe preeclampsia, and placental abruption

Factor VIII
Levels >150% found to be associated with increased risk of venous thrombosis

UNCOMMON INHERITED:
Protein C, Protein S, Antithrombin Deficiency:
- Autosomal dominant inheritance
- Decreased level or abnormal function
- First episode of thrombosis usually in young adults

TABLE 1-29 Hypercoagulable Conditions

	PREVALENCE IN GENERAL POPULATION	PREVALENCE IN POPULATION WITH THROMBOSIS	ARTERIAL (A)/ VENOUS (V) EVENTS	FETAL LOSS	RELATIVE RISK OF THROMBOSIS
FVL	• 6% of whites	12-20%	V	yes	7
Prothrombin G20210A	• Rare in nonwhites	6%	V	yes	3
AT	• 2% of whites	0.5-1%	V	yes	25-50
PC	• Rare in nonwhites	3%	V	yes	10-15
PS	0.02%	3%	V	yes	2
Factor VIII (activity level >150%)	0.2-0.3%	25%	V	yes	5 (activity level >150% compared with those of activity level <100%)
Hyperhomocysteinemia	1-2%	10%	V+A		2.5 (if homocysteine level >95 percentile of control population)
Antiphospholipid Antibody syndrome	11%	10%	V+A		

NOTE: There is significant variation in the prevalence rates and thrombotic risks reported in different studies. This may reflect variations in the genetic defects, the presence of other unknown or unmeasured coagulation defects or different populations.

- Increased risk of recurrent thrombosis
- Associated with an eightfold increased risk of venous thrombosis in pregnancy/postpartum in carriers versus noncarriers

Protein C:

- By age 45 yr, about half of all carriers have had venous thrombosis
- Homozygous condition very rare, usually associated with lethal thrombosis in infancy
- Risk of thrombosis in pregnancy/postpartum: 5% to 20%. Associated with increased risk of fetal loss, severe intrauterine growth retardation, severe preeclampsia; and placental abruption
- Associated with warfarin-induced skin necrosis, which occurs secondary to depletion of vitamin K dependent anticoagulant factors sooner than procoagulant factors in the first few days of therapy

Protein S:

- Risk of hypercoagulable potential unclear: one large case-control study found no increased thrombotic risk in individuals with PS deficiency
- Risk of thrombosis in pregnancy/postpartum 5% to 20%. Associated with increased risk of fetal loss, severe intrauterine growth retardation, severe preeclampsia, and placental abruption
- Associated with warfarin-induced skin necrosis

Antithrombin (AT) Deficiency:

- Common in young people presenting with thrombosis; by age 25 yr about half of all carriers have venous thrombosis
- Most thrombogenic of the identified inherited factors
- Homozygous condition very rare, probably not compatible with normal fetal development
- Risk of thrombosis in pregnancy 12% to 60% and postpartum 11% to 33%. Increases risk of pregnancy loss twofold to fivefold. Because of low prevalence, it is rarely the cause of fetal loss, intrauterine growth retardation, preeclampsia, or placental abruption
- Associated with high recurrence risk of thrombosis, about 60% of individuals have recurrent thrombosis
- Can cause heparin resistance

Other causes: dysfibrinogenemia, heparin cofactor II, Factor XII or plasminogen deficiency

ACQUIRED:

Antiphospholipid Antibody Syndrome:

- Defined as the presence of
  1. Thrombosis or morbidity with pregnancy (fetal loss after 10 wk of anatomically normal fetus; premature birth [≤34 wk] of anatomically normal fetus as a result of preeclampsia or placental

insufficiency; ≥3 fetal losses before 10 wk gestation in the absence of chromosomal abnormalities, or abnormal maternal hormones/anatomy)
  2. Persistence of lupus anticoagulant or anticardiolipin antibodies (tested at least 6 wk apart)
- About two thirds of patients will have a venous thrombosis and one third will have an arterial thrombosis. An initial venous event is usually followed by venous events, and an initial arterial event is usually followed by arterial events
- Increased risk of fetal loss (late first trimester and second trimester), preeclampsia, preterm delivery, placental abruption, and intrauterine growth retardation. Live birth rates of 70% to 80% can be achieved with treatment
- Associated with high recurrence risk of thrombosis (50% to 70%). Thrombosis recurs in 30% of patients/yr if not anticoagulated
- Associated with thrombocytopenia

Medical Conditions Associated with Increased Risk of Thrombosis:

- Trauma
- Chronic medical illness: CHF, DM, obesity, nephrotic syndrome, inflammatory bowel disease, paroxysmal nocturnal hemoglobinuria, sickle cell anemia
- Pregnancy, postpartum, OCP (fourfold increased risk of thrombosis with OCP use; risk about two times higher with third-generation vs. second-generation OCP), HRT, tamoxifen
- Immobilization, surgery (especially orthopedic)
- Myeloproliferative disorders
- Cancer: disease or treatment related
- Heparin-induced thrombocytopenia and thrombosis
- Cigarette smoking

🔬 DIAGNOSIS

■ WORKUP

- History, physical examination, laboratory tests
- Varying recommendations on extent of workup. Little cost-effectiveness and outcomes data. It is currently not recommended that individuals with medical conditions associated with increased risk of thrombosis be screened for the inherited or acquired defects. A notable exception is made for thrombosis associated with pregnancy, postpartum, or OCP use.
- Currently screening for Factor VIII is not suggested.

VENOUS THROMBOSIS

Among individuals without medical conditions associated with increased thrombotic risk:

- Screen individuals for protein C, protein S, antithrombin deficiency, FVL, prothrombin G20210A mutation, hyperhomocysteinemia, and antiphospholipid antibodies if any of the following are present: <45 yr old at first episode of thrombosis, family history of thrombosis, recurrent thrombotic events, thrombosis in unusual anatomic location, warfarin-induced skin necrosis, thrombosis in pregnancy/postpartum, characteristic pregnancy complications or associated with OCP use.
- Screen all caucasians and all women on HRT for FVL, prothrombin G20210A mutation, hyperhomocysteinemia, and antiphospholipid antibodies.
- Screen all others for hyperhomocysteinemia and antiphospholipid antibodies.

ARTERIAL THROMBOSIS

Screen for antiphospholipid antibody syndromes and hyperhomocysteinemia.

TIMING OF WORKUP

Ideally 2 wk after discontinuation of anticoagulation (except for antiphospholipid antibodies because this will influence duration of anticoagulation)

■ LABORATORY TESTS

- CBC, electrolytes, renal function, liver function tests, PT/PTT, PSA

NOTE: Acute thrombosis, anticoagulation and many medical conditions can affect the results and must be considered in the interpretation of the workup.

- APCR: clotting assay (using factor V-deficient plasma) and genetic test for FVL mutation. Increased factor VIII level or lupus anticoagulant can cause APCR
- Prothrombin G20210A mutation: genetic test (PCR)
- Antithrombin deficiency: functional assay (AT heparin cofactor assay) and immunologic assay
- Protein C deficiency: functional assay (level and activity) and immunologic assay. Functional assay may be false positive if have APCR or elevated factor VIII level. Results may be unreliable if lupus anticoagulant is present
- Protein S deficiency: functional assay (level and activity) and immunologic assay of free and total level. Results affected by the presence of APCR and lupus anticoagulant
- Antiphospholipid antibody syndrome: either of the following found on two occasions at least 6 wk apart
  1. Lupus anticoagulant: clotting assay
  2. Anticardiolipin antibody: enzyme-linked immunosorbent assay

- Hyperhomocysteinemia: fasting plasma homocysteine level (if normal but suspicion is high, can proceed with methionine loading test and genotyping for methylene tetrahydrofolate reductase)
- Factor VIII: clotting factor level

■ IMAGING STUDIES

As appropriate to diagnose thrombosis and to rule out medical conditions associated with increased thrombotic risk

 TREATMENT

■ NONPHARMACOLOGIC THERAPY

OCP use and smoking should be avoided.

■ PROPHYLAXIS

- Symptomatic and asymptomatic carriers (identified by family screening) should receive prophylactic anticoagulation in high-risk situations.
- Patients with antithrombin deficiency may benefit from antithrombin concentrates in the perioperative and postoperative periods.
- Patients with hyperhomocysteinemia should receive folic acid supplement (and vitamin B_6 and B_{12} if deficient); this may decrease risk of thrombosis by decreasing plasma homocysteine levels.

PREGNANCY PROPHYLAXIS
- Asymptomatic women with AT deficiency, homozygous FVL mutation or homozygous prothrombin G20210A mutation should receive full heparin anticoagulation throughout pregnancy. LMWH is preferred because of less need for monitoring, and lower risk of osteopenia, thrombocytopenia and hemorrhage. If LMWH is used, it should be changed to unfractionated heparin at 36 wk to decrease the risk of hematomas associated with epidural anesthesia during labor. Postpartum anticoagulation should be resumed with heparin or warfarin for at least 6 wk. AT concentrates may be used during labor, delivery, and obstetric complications if deficiency is present.
- Women with a history of both FVL mutation and prothrombin G20210A mutation, thrombophilia and thrombosis or a spontaneous thrombosis should receive prophylaxis during pregnancy and for 6 wk postpartum.
- Women with a history of thrombosis associated with a nonrecurring risk factor and without inherited or acquired thrombophilia do not need prophylaxis in pregnancy. They should receive prophylactic anticoagulation postpartum.

- Asymptomatic carriers of thrombophilia should receive prophylactic anticoagulation postpartum if they have a cesarean section or if a first-degree relative has a history of thrombosis.
- Women with antiphospholipid antibody syndrome and a history of thrombosis should replace warfarin with full heparin anticoagulation preconception. Once pregnant, add ASA 81 mg/day. Postpartum resume warfarin anticoagulation.
- Women with antiphospholipid antibody syndrome but no history of venous thrombosis should be treated with ASA 81 mg/day preconception and add unfractionated heparin 10,000 U s/c bid postconception. Adjust heparin to get mid-interval PTT level similar to baseline (or use LMWH). Continue both until term. Anticoagulate with heparin or warfarin for 6 wk postpartum.

■ ACUTE GENERAL Rx
VENOUS THROMBOSIS
- Unfractionated heparin or LMWH followed by warfarin. Continue heparin for at least 5 days or until INR is therapeutic for 48 hr, continue warfarin for 6 mo. Aim for INR of 2 to 3, unless antiphospholipid antibodies are present, in which case an INR of 3 to 3.5 is more protective.
- In pregnancy, full heparin anticoagulation for at least 4 mo, followed by prophylactic heparin for the remainder of the pregnancy. Prophylaxis with heparin or warfarin should be continued for at least 6 wk postpartum.

ARTERIAL THROMBOSIS
Anticoagulation and surgical consult for definitive procedure
PROTEIN C DEFICIENCY
- Warfarin-induced skin necrosis: after full heparin or LMWH anticoagulation, begin gradual warfarin loading (2 mg qd for 3 days and increase by 2 to 3 mg qd until target INR is reached). Continue heparin for 5 to 7 days until warfarin-induced anticoagulation is achieved.
- Protein C concentrates may be used for deficiency states.

AT DEFICIENCY
Heparin resistance, severe thrombosis, or recurrent thrombosis despite anticoagulation can be treated with AT concentrates.
LUPUS ANTICOAGULANT
Low molecular weight heparin or unfractionated heparin (check heparin levels or anti-factor Xa activity) followed by warfarin (INR 3 to 3.5)
Duration of Therapy: Must consider risk and benefit, risk of major bleeding 2% to 3%/yr in general population on anticoagulation but as high as 7% to 9%/yr in the elderly.

Indefinite anticoagulation suggested if
- One spontaneous thrombosis associated with one of the following
  1. Life-threatening thrombosis
  2. More than one genetic defect
  3. Presence of antithrombin deficiency or antiphospholipid antibodies
- Two or more spontaneous thrombosis

■ DISPOSITION
Depends on underlying condition

■ REFERRAL
Hematology, high-risk obstetrics

☼ PEARLS & CONSIDERATIONS

Consider screening family members: may be able to decrease risk with lifestyle modification
Interpreting workup: Many medical conditions cause acquired abnormalities.
- Heparin therapy: antithrombin levels decrease.
- Warfarin therapy: protein C, protein S levels and function decrease, antithrombin levels may increase.
- Antithrombin and protein S levels decrease with acute thrombosis (<10 days), surgery liver disease, DIC, nephrotic syndrome, pregnancy, estrogen therapy (HRT, OCP).
- Protein C decreases with acute thrombosis (10 days), surgery, liver disease, severe infection, and DIC. Levels increase with age and hyperlipidemia.
- APCR is increased with pregnancy and estrogen therapy (HRT, OCP).
- Factor VIII levels increase with acute thrombosis.

REFERENCES

Bauer KA: The thrombophilias: well-defined risk factors with uncertain therapeutic implications, *Ann Intern Med* 135:367, 2001.

Guideline: investigation and management of heritable thrombophilia, *Br J Haematol* 114:512, 2001.

Lockwood CJ: Inherited thrombophilias in pregnancy patients: detection and treatment paradigm, *Obstet Gynecol* 99(2):333, 2002.

Marques MB, Triplett DA: When to suspect hypercoagulability and how to investigate it, *Ann Diagn Pathol* 5(3):177, 2001.

Shehata HA, Nelson-Piercy C, Khamashta MA: Antiphospholipid syndrome: management of pregnancy in antiphospholipid syndrome, *Rheum Dis Clin North Am* 27:643, 2001.

Author: **Sudeep K. Aulakh, M.D., F.R.C.P.C.**

BASIC INFORMATION

■ DEFINITION
Hyperemesis gravidarum is the persistent nausea and vomiting with onset in the first trimester of pregnancy, resulting in weight loss and fluid and electrolyte and acid-base imbalances.

ICD-9CM CODES
643.1 Hyperemesis gravidarum

■ EPIDEMIOLOGY & DEMOGRAPHICS
INCIDENCE: 0.5 to 10 cases/1000 pregnancies
GENETICS: No genetic disposition
RISK FACTORS:
- Multiple pregnancy
- Molar pregnancy
- Previous history of unsuccessful pregnancy
- Nulliparity
- Hyperemesis gravidarum in a prior pregnancy
- No correlation with race, socioeconomic status, or marital status
PEAK ONSET: 8 to 12 wk of gestation

■ PHYSICAL FINDINGS & CLINICAL PRESENTATION
- Weight loss
- Rapid heart rate
- Fall in blood pressure
- Dry mucous membranes
- Loss of skin elasticity
- Ketotic odor
- In severe cases, Wernicke's encephalopathy as a result of thiamine deficiency

■ ETIOLOGY
Specific etiology is unknown.

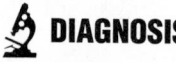 **DIAGNOSIS**

■ DIFFERENTIAL DIAGNOSIS
Pancreatitis, cholecystitis, hepatitis, pyelonephritis

■ WORKUP
Hyperemesis gravidarum is a diagnosis of exclusion. A detailed history and physical examination along with laboratory tests to rule out other causes of vomiting in early pregnancy are indicated.

■ LABORATORY TESTS
- Urinalysis to document ketonuria and proteinuria
- Urine C&S to rule out pyelonephritis
- Serum electrolytes to rule out electrolyte and acid-base imbalance
- Serum concentration of aminotransferases and bilirubin to rule out hepatitis
- Serum amylase to rule out pancreatitis
- Free T_4 and TSH (Elevated T_4 with suppressed TSH levels present in up to 60% of patients with hyperemesis gravidarum. This biochemical hyperthyroidism usually spontaneously resolves after 18 wk.)

■ IMAGING STUDIES
- Pelvic ultrasound examination to rule out multiple gestation and molar pregnancy
- Ultrasound of the gallbladder to rule out cholecystitis

 TREATMENT

■ NONPHARMACOLOGIC THERAPY
- Reassurance
- Psychologic support
- Avoidance of foods that trigger nausea
- Frequent small meals once oral intake has resumed
- Accupressure with the use of a wrist band
- Ginger has been studied as a promising herbal remedy, but data are relatively sparse

■ ACUTE GENERAL Rx
- NPO
- Fluid and electrolyte replacement
- Parenteral vitamin supplementation
- Daily supplementation of thiamine 100 mg IM or IV to prevent Wernicke's encephalopathy

- Pyridoxine (vitamin B_6) 30 mg daily may reduce nausea. It should not exceed 25 mg/day.
- Antiemetics, such as promethazine (Phenergan) or droperidol (Inapsine), have not been found to be associated with fetal malformations when given in early pregnancy. Promethazine given as a low-dose continuous infusion of 25 mg in each liter of IV fluid has been shown to be very effective in controlling nausea and vomiting.
- Restart oral intake gradually no less than 48 hr after vomiting has ceased.

■ CHRONIC Rx
If the previous acute therapy does not resolve vomiting and oral intake is not feasible, parenteral hyperalimentation may be necessary.

■ DISPOSITION
- Untreated hyperemesis gravidarum can result in maternal renal and hepatic damage or death from fluid and electrolyte imbalance.
- Hyperemesis gravidarum with severe weight loss has been associated with lower average birth weight and with CNS malformations in neonates.

■ REFERRAL
For parenteral hyperalimentation if required

☼ PEARLS & CONSIDERATIONS

■ COMMENTS
Although the specific etiology of hyperemesis gravidarum is not known, psychogenic causes proposed in older literature have been largely discredited. "Behavioral therapies" for hyperemesis gravidarum are inappropriate.

REFERENCE
Strong T: Alternative therapies of morning sickness, *Clin Obstet Gynecol* 44:653, 2001.
Author: **Laurel White, M.D.**

BASIC INFORMATION

■ DEFINITION
Hypereosinophilic syndrome (HES) refers to a group of disorders of unknown cause characterized by sustained overproduction of eosinophils and organ dysfunction.

■ SYNONYMS
Idiopathic hypereosinophilic syndrome

■ ICD-9CM CODES
288.3 Hypereosinophilic syndrome

■ EPIDEMIOLOGY & DEMOGRAPHICS
- HES usually occurs between the ages of 20 and 50 yr
- Occurs in men more often than women (9:1)

■ PHYSICAL FINDINGS & CLINICAL PRESENTATION
- Clinical presentation of patients with HES may vary from an incidental finding of eosinophilia on peripheral blood smear to sudden onset of cardiac or neurologic symptoms.
- *Cardiac manifestations* (58%) include dyspnea, orthopnea, signs and symptoms of congestive heart failure, murmurs of mitral regurgitation or tricuspid regurgitation.
  1. Symptoms are the result of endocardial infiltration of eosinophils leading to tissue necrosis. Thrombosis of the damaged tissue ensues and ultimately results in scarring and fibrosis.
  2. The pathologic process may result in a restrictive cardiomyopathy, dilated cardiomyopathy, and valvular heart disease.
- *Neurologic manifestations* (54%) may be of three types:
  1. Thromboembolic (e.g., cardiac emboli or local vascular thrombosis)
  2. CNS dysfunction—confusion, loss of memory, ataxia, upper motor neuron signs, Babinski's sign, seizures, and behavior changes. The cause is unknown
  3. Peripheral neuropathy may be symmetric or asymmetric, sensory or mixed sensory and motor deficits

- *Pulmonary manifestations* (40%) include a chronic persistent nonproductive cough, shortness of breath, and dyspnea on exertion.
- *Cutaneous manifestations* (56%) usually include urticaria, angioedema, or erythematous pruritic papules and nodules.
- *GI manifestations* (23%) include diarrhea but findings of gastritis, colitis, pancreatitis, and hepatitis can occur.
- *Ocular manifestations* (23%) are thought to be due to microemboli causing visual disturbances (e.g., blurring).

■ ETIOLOGY
- The etiology of HES is unknown.
- HES is thought to be a composite of many diseases.

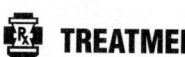

DIAGNOSIS

Criteria for the diagnosis of idiopathic HES include:
- Persistent eosinophilia of >1500 eosinophils/mm³ for more than 6 mo
- Exclusion of other conditions causing eosinophilia (e.g., parasites, allergies)
- Signs and symptoms of organ system dysfunction (e.g., heart, liver, lung)

■ DIFFERENTIAL DIAGNOSIS
The differential includes all causes of peripheral blood eosinophilia. Parasitic infections (filariasis, schistosomiasis, ascariasis, trichinosis, etc.), coccidioidomycosis, cat-scratch disease, asthma, Churg-Strauss syndrome, allergic rhinitis, atopic dermatitis, drug reactions, aspergillosis, eosinophilic pneumonia, hypersensitivity pneumonitis, HIV, eosinophilic gastroenteritis, inflammatory bowel disease.

■ WORKUP
The workup of a patient who is suspected of having HES should exclude other causes mentioned in the Differential Diagnosis leading to peripheral eosinophilia.

■ LABORATORY TESTS
- CBC with total eosinophil count; often the total white cell count ranges from 10,000 to 30,000/mm³ with eosinophilia of 30% to 70%
- Erythrocyte sedimentation rate (ESR)
- Electrolytes, BUN, and creatinine
- LFTs
- Urinalysis
- HIV assay
- Stools for ova and parasites × 3
- Serologic blood tests for parasitic infections (e.g., *Strongyloides*)
- Total IgE level
- Rheumatoid factor
- Bone marrow aspirate and biopsy
- Duodenal aspirate
- ECG

■ IMAGING STUDIES
- Chest x-ray may be clear or show infiltrates, effusions, or fibrotic scarring
- CT scan of chest, abdomen, and pelvis
- Echocardiogram can assess for ventricular function, valvular pathology including regurgitation and thrombi formation

TREATMENT

Treatment is usually not initiated unless there is evidence of organ involvement and therapy is designed at controlling organ damage.

■ NONPHARMACOLOGIC THERAPY
In patients with hypereosinophilia without organ involvement, serial echocardiograms are recommended at 6-mo intervals.

■ ACUTE GENERAL Rx
- In patients with organ involvement, initial therapy is with prednisone 1 mg/kg/day or 60 mg/day in adults.
- Patient's symptoms and peripheral eosinophil counts are monitored as a means of assessing response.
- Doses may be tapered to alternate day prednisone use in patients whose eosinophil counts have been suppressed.

■ **CHRONIC Rx**
- Patients not responding to corticosteroids, hydroxyurea 1 to 2 g/day may be tried.
- Hydroxyurea is aimed at reducing the total WBC count to <10,000/mm³.
- If the disease continues to progress, vincristine, etoposide, interferon-α, cyclosporine, and leukapheresis are alternative choices.
- Anticoagulation with warfarin and/or antiplatelet agents is often used in patients with HES.
- If all else fails, bone marrow transplantation may be considered.

■ **DISPOSITION**
- Before the use of cardiac imaging (echo) and cardiac surgeries (valve replacement), patients with HES had a poor prognosis with a mean survival of 9 mo and a 3-yr survival of 12%.

- Deaths usually resulted from congestive heart failure, valvular endocarditis, and systemic embolization.
- Patients responding to corticosteroids (reduction of eosinophil counts to normal range) have a better prognosis than patients who do not respond to corticosteroids.
- There are now reports of 5-, 10-, and 15-yr survival rates.

■ **REFERRAL**
HES is a rare and complicated disorder requiring a multidisciplinary approach. Cardiology, neurology, pulmonary, ophthalmology, and hematology consultations should be requested in the appropriate clinical setting.

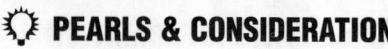 **PEARLS & CONSIDERATIONS**

■ **COMMENTS**
There is still much to be learned about HES. The etiology and exact mechanism of organ damage caused by eosinophils remains unknown, and research is ongoing to attempt to answer these and other questions.

REFERENCES
Ackerman SJ: *Hematology basic principles and practice*, ed 3, New York, 2000, Churchill Livingstone.
Brito-Babapulle F: The eosinophilias, including the idiopathic hypereosinophilic syndrome, *Br J Haematol* 121:203, 2003.
Weller PF, Bubley GJ: The idiopathic hypereosinophilic syndrome, *Blood* 83(10):2749, 1994.
Weller PF, Dvorak AM: The idiopathic hypereosinophilic syndrome, *Arch Dermatol* 132(5):583, 1996.
Author: **Dennis Mikolich, M.D.**

BASIC INFORMATION

■ DEFINITION

Primary hyperlipoproteinemia refers to a group of genetic disorders of the lipid transport proteins in the blood, which manifests as abnormally elevated levels of cholesterol, triglycerides, or both in the serum of affected patients (Table 1-30).

■ SYNONYMS

Hyperlipidemia

ICD-9CM CODES

272.4 Hyperlipoproteinemia
272.3 Fredrickson type I
272.0 Fredrickson type IIa
272.2 Fredrickson type IIb, III
272.1 Fredrickson type IV
272.3 Fredrickson type V

■ EPIDEMIOLOGY & DEMOGRAPHICS

INCIDENCE:
- Variable depending on the genetic defect
- Spectrum spans the common familial hypercholesterolemia, with an incidence of 1:500, to the rare familial lipoprotein lipase deficiency

PREDOMINANT SEX: None
GENETICS:
- Familial lipoprotein lipase deficiency: autosomal recessive, resulting in an elevation in the plasma chylomicrons and triglycerides
- Familial apoprotein CII deficiency: autosomal recessive, resulting in increased serum chylomicrons, VLDL, and hypertriglyceridemia
- Familial type 3 hyperlipoproteinemia: single-gene defect requiring contributory factors to manifest
- Familial hypercholesterolemia: autosomal dominant defect of the LDL receptor resulting in an elevated serum cholesterol level and normal triglycerides
- Familial hypertriglyceridemia: common, autosomal dominant defect resulting in elevated VLDL and triglycerides
- Multiple lipoprotein–type hyperlipidemia: autosomal dominant, manifesting as isolated hypercholesterolemia, isolated hypertriglyceridemia, or hyperlipidemia
- Polygenic hypercholesterolemia: multifactorial
- Polygenic hyperalphalipoproteinemia: autosomal dominant or polygenic, causing an elevated HDL

■ PHYSICAL FINDINGS & CLINICAL PRESENTATION

- Familial lipoprotein lipase deficiency: recurrent bouts of abdominal pain in infancy, eruptive xanthomas, hepatomegaly, splenomegaly, lipemia retinalis
- Familial apoprotein CII deficiency: occasional eruptive xanthomas
- Familial type 3 hyperlipoproteinemia: after age 20 yr see xanthoma striata palmaris or tuberoeruptive xanthomas, xanthelasmas, arterial bruits at a young age, gangrene of the lower extremities at a young age
- Familial hypercholesterolemia: tendon xanthomas, arcus corneae, xanthelasma
- Familial hypertriglyceridemia: associated obesity; with exacerbations eruptive xanthomas can develop
- Multiple lipoprotein type hyperlipidemia: no discerning physical findings
- Polygenic hypercholesterolemia: no discerning physical findings
- Polygenic hyperalphalipoproteinemia: no discerning physical findings

■ ETIOLOGY

Genetic defects causing lipid abnormalities

TABLE 1-30 Classification of Lipoprotein Disorders by Phenotypes, Genotypes, and Corresponding Clinical Manifestations

| PHENOTYPE | PLASMA LIPID LEVELS | | GENOTYPE | XANTHOMAS | OTHER CLINICAL MANIFESTATIONS |
	CHOLESTEROL	TRIGLYCERIDE			
I	Normal or elevated	Elevated lipemia	Familial lipoprotein lipase deficiency, Apo C-II deficiency	Eruptive, tuberoeruptive	Recurrent abdominal pain, other gastrointestinal symptoms, hepatosplenomegaly
IIA	Normal	Elevated	FHC, familial combined hyperlipidemia—polygenic and sporadic hypercholesterolemia	Tendinous, xanthelasma, tuberous; planar (homozygous)	Premature CAD, arcus corneae, aortic stenosis (homozygous FHC), arthritic symptoms
IIB	Elevated	Elevated	Familial combined hyperlipidemia, FHC		
III	Elevated	Elevated	Familial dysbetalipoproteinemia	Planar (especially palmar), tuberous	Premature CAD and peripheral vascular disease, male > female, obesity, abnormal glucose tolerance, hyperuricemia, aggravated by hypothyroidism, good response to therapy
IV	Normal or elevated	Elevated	Familial hypertriglyceridemia, familial combined hyperlipidemia, sporadic hypertriglyceridemia	Usually none; rarely eruptive or tuberoeruptive	CAD and peripheral vascular disease, obesity, abnormal glucose tolerance, hyperuricemia, arthritic symptoms, gallbladder disease
V	Normal or elevated	Elevated	Homozygous FHC	Eruptive, tuberoeruptive	Recurrent abdominal pain, other gastrointestinal symptoms, hepatosplenomegaly, peripheral paresthesia

From Graber MA: *The family practice handbook*, ed 4, St Louis, 2001, Mosby.
CAD, Coronary artery disease; *FHC,* familial hypercholesterolemia.

DIAGNOSIS

■ **DIFFERENTIAL DIAGNOSIS**
Secondary causes of hyperlipopro-
teinemias:
• Diabetes mellitus
• Glycogen storage diseases
• Lipodystrophies
• Glucocorticoid use/excess
• Alcohol
• Oral contraceptives
• Renal disease
• Hepatic dysfunction

■ **WORKUP**
• Detailed family history for prema-
ture cardiac disease
• Recurrent pancreatitis
• Thorough physical examination

■ **LABORATORY TESTS**
• Lipoprotein analysis
• Lipoprotein electrophoresis

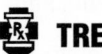 **TREATMENT**

■ **NONPHARMACOLOGIC
THERAPY**
• Cornerstone of treatment: dietary
therapy
• Familial lipoprotein lipase deficiency
and familial apoprotein CII deficiency: fat-free diet

• Remainder of cases, except those
with polygenic hyperalphalipoproteinemia: fat- and cholesterol-
restricted diets

■ **ACUTE GENERAL Rx**
No acute treatment needed

■ **CHRONIC Rx**
• Familial lipoprotein lipase deficiency, polygenic hyperalphalipoproteinemia, or familial apoprotein CII deficiency: no chronic drug
therapy
• Familial type 3 hyperlipoproteinemia: usually responds well to secondary causes being treated and diet
therapy; if not, fibric acids may be
tried
• Familial hypercholesterolemia: bile
acid sequestrants, HMG-CoA reductase inhibitors, or niacin
• Familial hypertriglyceridemia: fibric
acids
• Multiple lipoprotein type hyperlipidemia: drug therapy aimed at the
predominant lipid abnormality
noted
• Recent data suggest in patients with
lipoprotein abnormalities that treatment goals should be based on non-
HDLC rather than LDL-C

■ **DISPOSITION**
• Those with polygenic hyperalphalipoproteinemia: excellent prognosis
for longevity
• Those with familial hypercholesterolemia, familial type 3 hypercholesterolemia, and multiple lipoprotein type hyperlipidemia: even with
aggressive treatment, at high risk for
accelerated atherosclerosis and CAD

✿ **PEARLS & CONSIDERATIONS**

■ **COMMENTS**
Patient information is available
through the American Heart
Association.
See Tables 1-31 and 1-32 and Boxes
1-12 through 1-16.

REFERENCES
Cleeman JI: Detection and evaluation of
dyslipoproteinemia, *Endocrinol Metab
Clin North Am* 27(3):597, 1998.
Davignon J, Genesh J, Jr: Genetics of
lipoprotein disorders, *Endocrinol Metab
Clin North Am* 27(3):521, 1998.
National Cholesterol Education Program:
Second report on the Expert Panel on
Detection, evaluation and treatment of
high cholesterol in adults (adult treat-
ment panel III), *JAMA* 285:2486, 2001.
Author: **Beth J. Wutz, M.D.**

TABLE 1-31 **LDL Cholesterol Goals and Cutpoints for Therapeutic Lifestyle Changes (TLC)
and Drug Therapy in Different Risk Categories**

RISK CATEGORY	LDL GOAL (mg/dl)	LDL LEVEL AT WHICH TO INITIATE THERAPEUTIC LIFESTYLE CHANGES (mg/dl)	LDLD LEVEL AT WHICH TO CONSIDER DRUG THERAPY (mg/dl)
CHD or CHD risk equivalents (10-yr risk >20%)	<100	≥100	≥130 (100-129: drug optional)*
2+ Risk factors (10-yr risk ≤20%)	<130	≥130	10-yr risk 10%-20%: ≥130 10-yr risk <10%: ≥160
0-1 Risk factor†	<160	≥160	≥190 (160-189: LDL-lowering drug optional)

From National Cholesterol Education Program Expert Panel on Detection, Evaluation, and Treatment of High Blood Cholesterol in Adults (Adult Treatment
Panel III), National Institutes of Health, *JAMA* 285:2486, 2001.
CHD, Coronary heart disease; *LDL,* low-density lipoprotein.
*Some authorities recommend use of LDL-lowering drugs in this category if an LDL cholesterol level of <100 mg/dl cannot be achieved by therapeutic
lifestyle changes. Others prefer use of drugs that primarily modify triglycerides and HDL (e.g., nicotinic acid or fibrate). Clinical judgment also may call for
deferring drug therapy in this subcategory.
†Almost all people with 0-1 risk factor have a 10-year risk <10%; thus 10-year risk assessment in people with 0-1 risk factor is not necessary.

TABLE 1-32 **Comparison of LDL Cholesterol and Non-HDL Cholesterol Goals
for Three Risk Categories**

RISK CATEGORY	LDL GOAL (mg/dl)	NON-HDL GOAL (mg/dl)
CHD and CHD risk equivalent (10-yr risk for CHD >20%)	<100	<130
Multiple (2+) risk factors and 10-yr risk ≤20%	<130	<160
0-1 Risk factor	<160	<190

From National Cholesterol Education Program Expert Panel on Detection, Evaluation, and Treatment of High Blood Cholesterol in Adults (Adult Treatment
Panel III), National Institutes of Health, *JAMA* 285:2486, 2001.
CHD, Coronary heart disease; *HDL,* high-density lipoprotein; *LDL,* low-density lipoprotein.

BOX 1-12   Nutrient Composition of the Therapeutic Lifestyle Changes (TLC) Diet

Nutrient	Recommended Intake
Saturated fat*	<7% of total calories
Polyunsaturated fat	Up to 10% of total calories
Monounsaturated fat	Up to 20% of total calories
Total fat	25%-35% of total calories
Carbohydrate†	50%-60% of total calories
Fiber	20-30 g/day
Protein	Approximately 15% of total calories
Cholesterol	<200 mg/day
Total calories‡	Balance energy intake and expenditure to maintain desirable body weight/prevent weight gain

From National Cholesterol Education Program Expert Panel on Detection, Evaluation, and Treatment of High Blood Cholesterol in Adults (Adult Treatment Panel III), National Institutes of Health, *JAMA* 285:2486, 2001.
*Trans fatty acids are another LDL-raising fat that should be kept at a low intake.
†Carbohydrates should be derived predominantly from foods rich in complex carbohydrates, including grains, especially whole grains, fruits, and vegetables.
‡Daily energy expenditure should include at least moderate physical activity (contributing approximately 200 kcal/day).

BOX 1-13   ATP III Classification of LDL, Total, and HDL Cholesterol (mg/dl)

LDL cholesterol

<100	Optimal
100-129	Near or above optimal
130-159	Borderline high
160-189	High
≥190	Very high

Total cholesterol

<200	Desirable
200-239	Borderline high
≥240	High

HDL cholesterol

<40	Low
≥60	High

From National Cholesterol Education Program Expert Panel on Detection, Evaluation, and Treatment of High Blood Cholesterol in Adults (Adult Treatment Panel III), National Institutes of Health, *JAMA* 285:2486, 2001.
ATP, Adult treatment panel; *HDL,* high-density lipoprotein, *LDL,* low-density lipoprotein.

BOX 1-14   Major Risk Factors (Exclusive of LDL Cholesterol) That Modify LDL Goals*

Cigarette smoking
Hypertension (blood pressure ≥140/90 mm Hg or on antihypertensive medication)
Low HDL cholesterol (<40 mg/dl)†
Family history of premature CHD (CHD in male first-degree relative (<55 yr; CHD in female first-degree relative <65 yr)
Age (men ≥45 yr; women ≥55 yr)

From National Cholesterol Education Program Expert Panel on Detection, Evaluation, and Treatment of High Blood Cholesterol in Adults (Adult Treatment Panel III), National Institutes of Health, *JAMA* 285:2486, 2001.
HDL, High-density lipoprotein; *LDL,* low-density lipoprotein.
*Diabetes is regarded as a coronary heart disese (CHD) risk equivalent.
†HDL cholesterol ≥60 mg/dl counts as a "negative" risk factor; its presence removes 1 risk factor from the total count.

BOX 1-15   **Interventions to Improve Adherence**

Focus on the Patient

Simplify medication regimens
Provide explicit patient instruction and use good counseling techniques to teach the
    patient how to follow the prescribed treatment
Encourage the use of prompts to help patients remember treatment regimens
Use systems to reinforce adherence and maintain contact with the patient
Encourage the support of family and friends
Reinforce and reward adherence
Increase visits for patients unable to achieve treatment goal
Increase the convenience and access to care
Involve patients in their care through self-monitoring

Focus on the Physician and Medical Office

Teach physicians to implement lipid treatment guidelines
Use reminders to prompt physicians to attend to lipid management
Identify a patient advocate in the office to help deliver or prompt care
Use patients to prompt preventive care
Develop a standardized treatment plan to structure care
Use feedback from past performance to foster change in future care
Remind patients of appointments and follow up missed appointments

Focus on the Health Delivery System

Provide lipid management through a lipid clinic
Utilize case management by nurses
Deploy telemedicine
Utilize the collaborative care of pharmacists
Execute critical care pathways in hospitals

From National Cholesterol Education Program Expert Panel on Detection, Evaluation, and Treatment of High
Blood Cholesterol in Adults (Adult Treatment Panel III), National Institutes of Health, *JAMA* 285:2486, 2001.

BOX 1-16   **Clinical Identification of the Metabolic Syndrome**

RISK FACTOR	DEFINING LEVEL
Abdominal obesity* (waist circumference)†	
Men	>102 cm (>40 in)
Women	>88 cm (>35 in)
Triglycerides	≥150 mg/dl
High-density lipoprotein cholesterol	
Men	<40 mg/dl
Women	<50 mg/dl
Blood pressure	≥130/≥85 mm Hg
Fasting glucose	≥110 mg/dl

From National Cholesterol Education Program Expert Panel on Detection, Evaluation, and Treatment of High
Blood Cholesterol in Adults (Adult Treatment Panel III), National Institutes of Health, *JAMA* 285:2486, 2001.
*Overweight and obesity are associated with insulin resistance and the metabolic syndrome. However, the pres-
ence of abdominal obesity is more highly correlated with the metabolic risk factors than is an elevated body
mass index (BMI). Therefore, the simple measure of waist circumference is recommended to identify the body
weight component of the metabolic syndrome.
†Some male patients can develop multiple metabolic risk factors when the waist circumference is only margin-
ally increased, for example, 94-102 cm (37-40 in). Such patients may have strong genetic contribution to
insulin resistance, and they should benefit from changes in life habits, similarly to men with categorical increases in waist circumference.

BASIC INFORMATION

■ DEFINITION

Hyperosmolar coma (nonketotic hyperosmolar syndrome) is a state of extreme hyperglycemia, marked dehydration, serum hyperosmolarity, altered mental status, and absence of ketoacidosis.

■ SYNONYMS

Nonketotic hyperosmolar syndrome
Hyperosmolar nonketotic state

ICD-9CM CODES

250.2 Hyperosmolar coma

■ PHYSICAL FINDINGS & CLINICAL PRESENTATION

- Evidence of extreme dehydration (poor skin turgor, sunken eyeballs, dry mucous membranes)
- Neurologic defects (reversible hemiplegia, focal seizures)
- Orthostatic hypotension, tachycardia
- Evidence of precipitating factors (pneumonia, infected skin ulcer)
- Coma (25% of patients), delirium

■ ETIOLOGY

- Infections, 20% to 25% (e.g., pneumonia, UTI, sepsis)
- New or previously unrecognized diabetes (30% to 50%)
- Reduction or omission of diabetic medication
- Stress (MI, CVA)
- Drugs: diuretics (dehydration), phenytoin, diazoxide (impaired insulin secretion)

DIAGNOSIS

■ DIFFERENTIAL DIAGNOSIS

- Diabetic ketoacidosis
- The differential diagnosis of coma is described in Section II.

■ LABORATORY TESTS

- Hyperglycemia: serum glucose usually >600 mg/dl.
- Hyperosmolarity: serum osmolarity usually >340 mOsm/L.
- Serum sodium: may be low, normal, or high; if normal or high, the patient is severely dehydrated, because an elevated glucose draws fluid from intracellular space decreasing the serum sodium; the corrected sodium can be obtained by increasing the serum sodium concentration by 1.6 mEq/dl for every 100 mg/dl increase in the serum glucose level over normal.
- Serum potassium: may be low, normal, or high; regardless of the initial serum level, the total body deficit is approximately 5 to 15 mEq/kg.
- Serum bicarbonate: usually >12 mEq/L (average is 17 mEq/L).
- Arterial pH: usually >7.2 (average is 7.26); both serum bicarbonate and arterial pH may be lower if lactic acidosis is present.
- BUN: azotemia (prerenal) is usually present (BUN generally ranges from 60 to 90 mg/dl).
- Phosphorus: hypophosphatemia (average deficit is 70 to 140 mm).
- Calcium: hypocalcemia (average deficit is 50 to 100 mEq).
- Magnesium: hypomagnesemia (average deficit is 50 to 100 mEq).
- CBC with differential, urinalysis, blood and urine cultures should be performed to rule out infectious etiology.

■ IMAGING STUDIES

- Chest x-ray examination is useful to rule out infectious process. The initial chest x-ray may be negative if the patient has significant dehydration. Repeat chest x-ray examination after 24 hr of hydration if pulmonary infection is suspected.
- CT scan of head should be performed in patients with suspected CVA.

TREATMENT

■ NONPHARMACOLOGIC THERAPY

- Monitor mental status, vital signs, urine output qh until improved, then monitor q2-4h.
- Monitor electrolytes, renal function, and glucose level (see Acute General Rx).

■ ACUTE GENERAL Rx

- Vigorous fluid replacement: the volume and rate of fluid replacement are determined by renal and cardiac function. Typically, infuse 1000 to 1500 ml/hr for the initial 1 to 2 L; then decrease the rate of infusion to 500 ml/hr and monitor urinary output, blood chemistries, and blood pressure; use 0.9% NS (isotonic solution) if the patient is hypotensive or serum osmolarity is <320 mOsm/L; otherwise use 0.45% NS solution. Slower infusion rate may be used initially in patients with compromised cardiovascular or renal status.

- Replace electrolytes and monitor serum levels frequently (e.g., serum sodium and potassium q2h for the first 12 hr). Serum KCl replacement in patients with normal renal function and adequate urinary output is started when the serum potassium level is <5.2 mEq/L (e.g., 10 mEq KCl/hr if potassium level is 4 to 5.2 mEq/L). Continuous ECG monitoring and hourly measurement of urinary output are recommended.
- Correct hyperglycemia. The goal is for plasma glucose to decline by at least 75 to 100 mg/dl/hr.
  1. Vigorous IV hydration will decrease the serum glucose level in most patients by 80 mg/dl/hr; a regular insulin IV bolus (10 U) is often not necessary.
  2. Low-dose insulin infusion at 1 to 2 U/hr (e.g., 25 U of regular insulin in 250 ml of 0.9% saline solution at 20 ml/hr) until the serum glucose level approaches 300 mg/dl; then the patient is started on regular SC insulin with sliding scale coverage. If the plasma glucose does not decrease over 2 to 4 hr despite adequate fluid administration and urine output, consider doubling the hourly insulin dose.
  3. Glucose should be monitored q1-2h in the initial 12 hr.
- In the absence of renal failure, phosphate can be administered at a rate of 0.1 mmol/kg/hr (5 to 10 mmol/hr) to a maximum of 80 to 120 mmol in 24 hr. Magnesium replacement, in absence of renal failure, can be administered IM (0.05 to 0.10 ml/kg of 20% magnesium sulfate) or as IV infusion (4 to 8 ml of 20% magnesium sulfate [0.08 to 0.16 mEq/kg]). Repeat magnesium, phosphate, and calcium levels should be obtained after 12 to 24 hr.

■ DISPOSITION

Mortality in nonketotic hyperosmolar coma ranges from 20% to 50%.

PEARLS & CONSIDERATIONS

■ COMMENTS

The typical patient presenting with hyperosmolar coma is an elderly or bed-confined diabetic with impaired ability to communicate thirst who is evaluated after an interval of 1 to 2 wk of prolonged osmotic diuresis.
Author: **Fred F. Ferri, M.D.**

BASIC INFORMATION

■ **DEFINITION**

Primary hyperparathyroidism is an endocrine disorder caused by the excessive secretion of parathyroid hormone (PTH) from the parathyroid glands.

ICD-9CM CODES

252.0 Primary hyperparathyroidism
253.9 Ectopic hyperparathyroidism
588.8 Secondary hyperparathyroidism in chronic renal disease

■ **EPIDEMIOLOGY & DEMOGRAPHICS**

PREVALENCE: 1 case/1000 persons
PREDOMINANT AGE AND SEX:
- Primary hyperparathyroidism occurs most frequently in postmenopausal women; prevalence in this group may be as high as 3%. The condition is asymptomatic in >50% of patients
- Incidence: 1 case/1000 men and 2 to 3 cases/1000 women

GENETICS: Hyperparathyroidism can occur in conjunction with MEN I or II.

■ **PHYSICAL FINDINGS & CLINICAL PRESENTATION**

Physical examination may be entirely normal. The presence of signs and symptoms varies with the rapidity of development and degree of hypercalcemia. The following abnormalities may be present:
- GI: constipation, anorexia, nausea, vomiting, pancreatitis, ulcers
- CNS: confusion, obtundation, psychosis, lassitude, depression, coma
- GU: nephrolithiasis, renal insufficiency, polyuria, decreased urine-concentrating ability, nocturia, nephrocalcinosis
- Musculoskeletal: myopathy, weakness, osteoporosis, pseudogout, bone pain
- Other: hypertension, metastatic calcifications, band keratopathy (found in medial and lateral margin of the cornea), pruritus

■ **ETIOLOGY**

- A single adenoma is found in 80% of patients; 90% of the adenomas are found within one of the parathyroid glands, the other 10% are in ectopic sites (lateral neck, thyroid, mediastinum, retroesophagus).
- Parathyroid gland hyperplasia occurs in 20% of patients.

🔬 **DIAGNOSIS**

■ **DIFFERENTIAL DIAGNOSIS**

Other causes of hypercalcemia:
- Malignancy: neoplasms of breast, lung, kidney, ovary, pancreas; myeloma, lymphoma
- Granulomatous disorders (e.g., sarcoidosis)
- Paget's disease
- Vitamin D intoxication, milk-alkali syndrome
- Thiazide diuretics
- Other: familial hypocalciuric hypercalcemia, thyrotoxicosis, adrenal insufficiency, prolonged immobilization, vitamin A intoxication, recovery from acute renal failure, lithium administration, pheochromocytoma, disseminated SLE

■ **WORKUP**

- The serum PTH level is the single best test for initial evaluation of confirmed hypercalcemia. The "intact" PTH (iPTH) is the best assay. The iPTH distinguishes primary hyperparathyroidism from hypercalcemia caused by malignancy when the serum calcium level is >12 mg/dl.
- A high level of urinary cyclic AMP is also suggestive of primary hyperparathyroidism.
- Parathyroid hormone–like protein (PLP) is increased in hypercalcemia associated with solid malignancies.
- ECG may reveal shortening of the QT interval secondary to hypercalcemia.

■ **LABORATORY TESTS**

- Elevated serum ionized calcium level, low serum phosphorus, and normal or elevated alkaline phosphatase
- Elevated urine calcium level (in contrast with very low urinary calcium levels seen in patients with familial hypocalciuric hypercalcemia)
- Possibly elevated serum chloride levels, decreased serum CO_2, hyperchloremic metabolic acidosis
- The differential diagnosis of hypercalcemia is described in Sections II and IV

■ **IMAGING STUDIES**

- A bone survey may show evidence of subperiosteal bone resorption (suggesting PTH excess). The classic bone disease of primary hyperparathyroidism is *osteitis fibrosa cystica*.

- Parathyroid localization with technetium-99m sestamibi has been shown to have a high sensitivity and specificity for single adenomas.
- Screen for osteopenia with measurement of bone mineral density in all postmenopausal women.

℞ **TREATMENT**

■ **NONPHARMACOLOGIC THERAPY**

- Unless contraindicated, patients should maintain a high intake of fluids (3 to 5 L/day) and sodium chloride (>400 mEq/day) to increase renal calcium excretion. Calcium intake should be 1000 mg/day.
- Potential hypercalcemic agents (e.g., thiazide diuretics) should be discontinued.
- Surgery is the only effective treatment for primary hyperparathyroidism. It is generally indicated in all patients under age 50 and patients with complications from hyperthyroidism, such as nephrolithiasis and osteopenia. The conventional surgical approach is bilateral neck exploration under general anesthesia. Minimally invasive adenomectomy guided by preoperative technetium-99-m sestamibi scanning or ultrasound plus spiral CT is an alternative to conventional neck exploration. With the minimally invasive approach, the solitary adenoma is excised through a small unilateral incision with the patient under local cervical block anesthesia.
- Percutaneous ethanol injection into the parathyroid gland should be considered in selected patients who have undergone a subtotal parathyroidectomy for multigland disease and have recurrent hyperparathyroidism as a result of remnant gland.
- Asymptomatic elderly patients can be followed conservatively with periodic monitoring of serum calcium level and review of symptoms. Serum creatinine and PTH levels should also be obtained at 6- to 12-mo intervals, bone density (cortical and trabecular) yearly.

■ ACUTE GENERAL Rx

Acute severe hypercalcemia (serum calcium >13 mg/dl) or symptomatic patients can be treated with the following:

- Vigorous IV hydration with NS followed by IV furosemide. Use NS with caution in patients with cardiac or renal insufficiency to avoid fluid overload.
- Calcitonin 4 IU/kg q12h is indicated when saline hydration and furosemide are ineffective or contraindicated.
- Biphosphonates (pamidronate, etidronate), mithramycin, and gallium nitrate are also effective for severe hypercalcemia.

✷ PEARLS & CONSIDERATIONS

■ COMMENTS

- Patients with hyperparathyroidism should undergo further evaluation for the presence of MEN I or II.
- Decreased bone mineral density and nephrolithiasis are the major sequelae of untreated hyperparathyroidism.
- An experienced endocrine surgeon cures more than 95% of patients undergoing bilateral neck exploration and incurs <1% perioperative mortality.

REFERENCES

Monchik JM et al: Minimally invasive parathyroid surgery in 103 patients with local/regional anesthesia, without exclusion criteria, *Surgery* 131:502, 2002.

Udelsman R: Six hundred fifty-six consecutive explorations for primary hyperparathyroidism, *Ann Surg* 235:665, 2002.

Author: **Fred F. Ferri, M.D.**

BASIC INFORMATION

■ DEFINITION

Hypersensitivity pneumonitis (HP) is a group of pulmonary diseases. It is characterized by an immunologically induced inflammation of the lung parenchyma, which is due to intense or repeated inhalation of an organic agent or inorganic chemicals.

■ SYNONYMS

Extrinsic allergic alveolitis (EAA)
Some specific examples:
- Bird fancier's lung
- Farmer's lung
- Chemical worker's lung
- Humidifier lung
- Hot tub lung
- Sauna taker's lung

ICD-9CM CODES

495.9 Pneumonitis, hypersensitivity

■ EPIDEMIOLOGY & DEMOGRAPHICS

Anyone with exposure to an offending antigen is susceptible. The list of identified agents is extensive and can essentially be caused by microbes, animal or plant proteins, organic and inorganic chemicals. Most causative agents have been recognized in a wide variety of occupations. Therefore the disease is less common than 20 years ago. Now, the important exposures occur at home (birds, humidifiers, mold), and residential exposure is more difficult to diagnose.

■ PHYSICAL FINDINGS & CLINICAL PRESENTATION

Vary depending on frequency and intensity of antigen exposure.
- *Acute:* Fever, cough, and dyspnea 4 to 6 hr after an intense exposure, lasting 18 to 24 hr
- *Subacute:* Insidious onset of productive cough, dyspnea on exertion, anorexia, and weight loss, usually from a heavy, sustained exposure
- *Chronic:* Gradually progressive cough, dyspnea, malaise, and weight loss, usually from low-grade or recurrent exposure

Physical examination: cyanosis and "crepitant rales," possible fever

■ ETIOLOGY

- Numerous environmental agents, often encountered in occupational settings
- Common sources of antigens: "moldy" hay, silage, grain, or vegetables; bird droppings or feathers; low-molecular-weight chemicals (i.e., isocyanates), pharmaceutical products

DIAGNOSIS

■ DIFFERENTIAL DIAGNOSIS

Acute stages:
Acute bronchopulmonary aspergillosis
Pulmonary embolism
Asthma
Aspiration pneumonia
Recurrent pneumonia
BOOP
Sarcoidosis
Churg-Strauss syndrome
Wegener's granulomatosis

Chronic stages:
IPF
Bronchiectasis
Chronic bronchitis

■ WORKUP

There is no single radiologic, physiologic, or immunologic test specific for the diagnosis of HP. HP must be suspect in any patient presenting with cough, dyspnea, fever, and malaise. A thorough history focusing on potential exposures is essential. See Box 1-17 for diagnostic criteria.

■ LABORATORY TESTS

- Routine lab tests do not make the diagnosis, but typically the ESR, CRP, and leukocyte count are increased; the total IgG is elevated and RF is often positive; peripheral eosinophil count and serum IgE are generally normal
- Pulmonary function tests: Restrictive ventilatory patterns are typically seen. Decreased FEV1, decreased VC, decreased diffusing capacity, and decreased static compliance
- ABG: Mild hypoxemia
- Serum precipitin test: Sensitive but not specific for HP (asymptomatic patients may have IgG antibodies in serum)
- Skin testing: Unclear if helpful. However, some feel it to be a safe, effective, and rapid procedure in the diagnosis and follow-up of patients with HP. Sensitivity is similar to that of the precipitin test but the specificity is higher

---

BOX 1-17 Diagnostic Criteria for Hypersensitivity Pneumonitis

Major criteria:
1. History of symptoms compatible with HP that appear to worsen within hours after antigen exposure.
2. Confirmation of exposure to the offending agent by history, investigation of the environment, serum precipitin test, and/or BAL antibody.
3. Compatible changes on cxr or HRCT of the chest.
4. BAL fluid lymphocytosis (if performed).
5. Compatible histologic changes by lung bx (if performed).
6. Positive natural challenge (reproduction of symptoms and laboratory abnormalities after exposure to the suspected environment) or by controlled inhalation challenge.

Minor criteria:
1. Basilar crackles
2. Decreased diffusion capacity
3. Arterial hypoxemia (either at rest or with exercise)

■ IMAGING STUDIES

Chest x-ray: Nonspecific; may be normal in early stage.
- *Acute/subacute:* Bilateral interstitial and alveolar nodular infiltrates (Fig. 1-149) in a patchy or homogeneous distribution. Apices are often spared.
- *Chronic:* Diffuse reticulonodular infiltrates and fibrosis. Honeycombing may develop.

High-resolution chest CT scan: No pathognomonic features but demonstrates airspace and interstitial patterns in the acute and subacute stage. The chronic stage reveals honeycombing and bronchiectasis.

℞ TREATMENT

■ NONPHARMACOLOGIC THERAPY

Early recognition and avoidance of the causative antigen

■ ACUTE GENERAL Rx

- Glucocorticoids accelerate initial lung recovery but may have no effect long term
- Prednisone 0.5-1mg/Kg usually over 1-2 wk then tapered over 4 wk

■ DISPOSITION/PROGNOSIS

See Table 1-33.

■ REFERRAL

- Bronchoscopy: BAL provides useful supportive data in the diagnosis of HP. Usually reveals intense lymphocytosis of predominantly CD 8+ suppressor cells. In acute stages neutrophils predominate but as the disease progresses to chronic form the ratio of CD 4+ to CD 8+ cells increase. When fibrosis is present the number of neutrophils increase.
- Lung biopsy: The histopathologic features of HP are distinctive but not pathognomonic. Typically bronchiolitis and interstitial pneumonitis with granuloma formation is seen.
- Laboratory inhalation challenge: Testing to prove a direct relationship between a suspected antigen and disease; extract of antigen is inhaled via a nebulizer.

REFERENCES

Ferran M, Roger A, Cruz MJ: Correspondence: usefulness of specific skin tests in the diagnosis of hypersensitivity pneumonitis,

Fraser et al: *Synopsis of diseases of the chest*, ed 2, 1994.

Patel AM, Ryu JH, Reed CE: Hypersensitivity pneumonitis: current concepts and further questions, *J Allergy Clin Immunol* 108:661, 2001.

Schuyler M, Cormier Y: The diagnosis of hypersensitivity pneumonitis, *Chest* 111:534, 1997.

Authors: **Carolyn J. O'Connor, M.D., and Jeanne M. Oliva, M.D.**

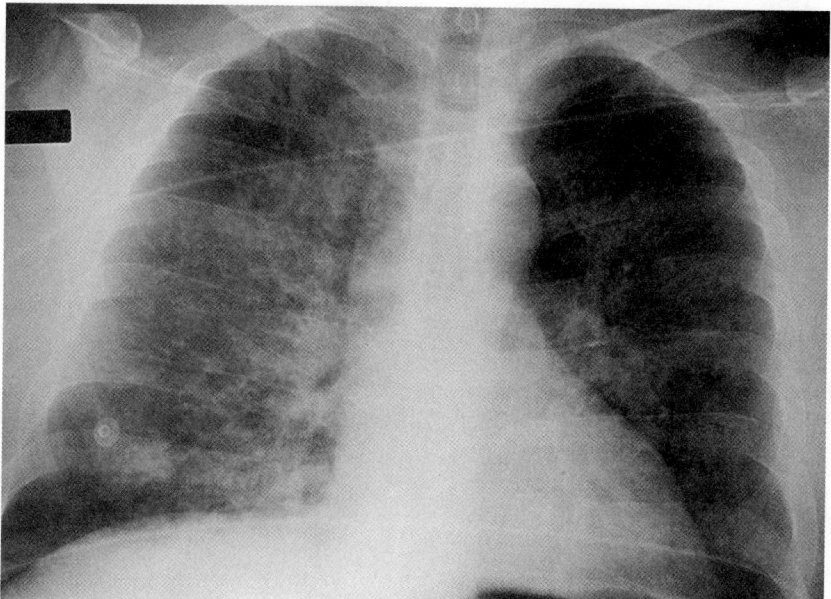

Fig. 1-149 Chest radiograph of a patient with acute hypersensitivity pneumonitis. Bilateral interstitial infiltrates are evident, more on the right side than the left. Note the absence of pleural effusion, hilar adenopathy, and hyperinflation. (From Altman LV [ed]: *Allergy in primary care*, Philadelphia, 2000, WB Saunders.)

TABLE 1-33 Key Features of the Stages of Hypersensitivity Pneumonitis

	TIME FRAME	CLINICAL FEATURES	HRCT FINDINGS	IMMUNOPATH	PROGNOSIS
Acute	4-48 hr	Fever, chills, cough, hypoxia, malaise	Ground-glass infiltrates	Alveolitis, immune complex	Good
Subacute	Weeks-4 mo	Dyspnea, cough, episodic flares	Micronodules, air trapping	Granulomas, bronchiolitis	Good
Chronic	4 mo-years	Dyspnea, cough, fatigue, weight loss	Fibrosis +/-, honeycombing, emphysema	Lymphocytic infiltration and fibrosis, neutrophil-mediated air space destruction	Poor

BASIC INFORMATION

■ DEFINITION

Hypersplenism is a syndrome characterized by splenomegaly, cytopenia (decrease of one or more of the peripheral cell lines), and compensatory hyperplastic bone marrow.

ICD-9CM CODES

289.4 Hypersplenism

■ EPIDEMIOLOGY & DEMOGRAPHICS

Most often seen in patients with liver disease, hematologic malignancy, or infection.

■ PHYSICAL FINDINGS & CLINICAL PRESENTATION

- History: early satiety, abdominal discomfort/fullness, left upper quadrant pleuritic pain (abscess, infarction), episodes of acute left upper quadrant pain (sequestration crisis), referred pain to left shoulder
- Physical examination: splenomegaly, presence of a rub in left upper quadrant (suggestive of a splenic infarct), stigmata of cytopenias

■ ETIOLOGY

The spleen's normal activities are augmented when it is enlarged.

- Splenomegaly increases the proportion of blood channeled through the red pulp, causing inappropriate splenic pooling of both normal and abnormal blood cells. The size of the spleen determines the amount of cell sequestration. Up to 90% of platelets may be pooled in an enlarged spleen.
- Splenomegaly leads to increased destruction of RBCs. Platelets and WBCs have about normal survival time even when sequestered and may be available if needed.
- Splenomegaly causes plasma volume expansion and thus exacerbates cytopenias by dilution.

■ DIAGNOSIS

■ DIFFERENTIAL DIAGNOSIS

Hypersplenism can be caused by splenomegaly of almost any cause.

- Splenic congestion: cirrhosis, CHF, portal, splenic or hepatic vein thrombosis
- Hematologic causes: hemolytic anemia, sickle cell anemia, thalassemia, spherocytosis, elliptocytosis
- Infections: viral (hepatitis, infectious mononucleosis, CMV, HIV), bacterial (endocarditis, tuberculosis, brucellosis, lyme), parasitic (malaria, leishmaniasis, schistosomiasis, toxoplasmosis), fungal
- Malignancy: leukemia, lymphoma, polycythemia vera, myeloproliferative diseases, metastatic tumors
- Inflammatory diseases: Felty syndrome, SLE, sarcoidosis
- Infiltrative diseases: amyloidosis, Gaucher's disease, Niemann-Pick disease, glycogen storage disease

■ WORKUP

History (including travel), physical examination, laboratory tests, imaging studies

■ LABORATORY TESTS

- CBC with differential
- Peripheral smear
- Bone marrow biopsy: hyperplasia of corresponding cellular element
- Tests to diagnose suspected cause of splenomegaly
- NOTE: Red cell mass may be used to assess severity of anemia. It remains normal when low Hgb/Hct are secondary to hemodilution

■ IMAGING STUDIES

- Ultrasound to determine splenic size
- CT scan/MRI to obtain structural information; rule out cysts, tumors, infarcts
- Consider other studies as suggested by history and exam: CXR, cardiac echo, and so forth

■ TREATMENT

■ ACUTE GENERAL Rx

- Treat underlying disease
- Splenectomy is considered if
  1. Cannot treat underlying cause
  2. Have persistent symptomatic disease
  3. Necessary for diagnosis

Risks:

- Increase infections: can be decreased with pneumococcal vaccine
- Rapid increase in platelet count may cause thromboembolic complications

■ DISPOSITION

- Thrombocytopenia is rarely of clinical consequence because of the ability to slowly mobilize platelets from the spleen if needed.
- Cytopenias are usually correctable with splenectomy, cell counts return to normal within a few weeks.
- Splenectomy may alleviate portal hypertension.
- Prognosis depends on the underlying disease.

■ REFERRAL

Hematology for bone marrow biopsy

REFERENCE

Beutler E et al: *Williams hematology*, ed 6, New York, 2001, McGraw-Hill.
Author: **Sudeep K. Aulakh, M.D., F.R.C.P.C.**

BASIC INFORMATION

■ DEFINITION

The Joint National Committee on Prevention, Detection, Evaluation, and Treatment of High Blood Pressure (JNC 7) classifies normal blood pressure in adults as <120 mm Hg systolic and <80 mm Hg diastolic. "Prehypertension" is defined as systolic pressure 120-139 mm Hg or diastolic pressure 80-89 mm Hg. "Stage 1 hypertension" is systolic BP 140-159 mm Hg or diastolic BP 90-99 mm HG. "Stage 2 hypertension" is systolic BP ≥160 mm Hg or diastolic BP ≥100 mm Hg.

■ SYNONYMS

Essential hypertension
Idiopathic hypertension
High blood pressure

ICD-9CM CODES

401.1 Essential hypertension
401.0 Malignant hypertension caused by renal artery stenosis
642 Hypertension complicating pregnancy
405.01 Malignant hypertension secondary to renal artery stenosis
437.2 Hypertensive encephalopathy

■ EPIDEMIOLOGY & DEMOGRAPHICS

- Incidence of hypertension in adult population: 10% to 15%
- Increased incidence in males and in the elderly
- 50 million individuals in the U.S. and approximately 1 billion individuals worldwide meet the criteria for diagnosis of hypertension

■ PHYSICAL FINDINGS & CLINICAL PRESENTATION

Physical examination may be entirely within normal limits except for the presence of hypertension. A proper initial physical examination on a hypertensive patient should include the following:
- Measure height and weight.
- Evaluate skin for the presence of café-au-lait spots (neurofibromatosis), uremic appearance (CRF), striae (Cushing's syndrome).
- Perform careful funduscopic examination: check for papilledema, retinal exudates, hemorrhages, arterial narrowing, AV compression.
- Examine the neck for carotid bruits, distended neck veins, or enlarged thyroid gland.

- Perform extensive cardiopulmonary examination: check for loud aortic component of S_2, S_4, ventricular lift, murmurs, arrhythmias.
- Check abdomen for masses (pheochromocytoma, polycystic kidneys), presence of bruits over the renal artery (renal artery stenosis), dilation of the aorta.
- Obtain two or more BP measurements separated by 2 min with the patient either supine or seated and after standing for at least 2 min. Measure BP in both upper extremities (if values are discrepant, use the higher value).
- Examine arterial pulses (dilated or absent femoral pulses and BP greater in upper extremities than lower extremities suggest aortic coarctation).
- Note the presence of truncal obesity (Cushing's syndrome) and pedal edema (CHF, nephrosis).
- Perform full neurologic assessment.
- The clinical evaluation should help determine if the patient has primary or secondary (possibly reversible) hypertension, if there is target organ disease present, and if there are cardiovascular risk factors in addition to hypertension.

■ ETIOLOGY

- Essential (primary) hypertension (85%)
- Drug-induced or drug-related (5%)
- Renal hypertension (5%)
  1. Renal parenchymal disease (3%)
  2. Renovascular hypertension (<2%)
- Endocrine (4% to 5%)
  1. Oral contraceptives (4%)
  2. Primary aldosteronism (0.5%)
  3. Pheochromocytoma (0.2%)
  4. Cushing's syndrome and chronic steroid therapy (0.2%)
  5. Hyperparathyroidism or thyroid disease (0.2%)
- Coarctation of the aorta (0.2%)

DIAGNOSIS

■ WORKUP

Pertinent history:
- Age of onset of hypertension, previous antihypertensive therapy
- Family history of hypertension, stroke, cardiovascular disease
- Diet, salt intake, alcohol, drugs (e.g., oral contraceptives, NSAIDs, decongestants, steroids)
- Occupation, lifestyle, socioeconomic status, psychologic factors

- Other cardiovascular risk factors: hyperlipidemia, obesity, diabetes mellitus, carbohydrate intolerance
- Symptoms of secondary hypertension:
  1. Headache, palpitations, excessive perspiration (possible pheochromocytoma)
  2. Weakness, polyuria (consider hyperaldosteronism)
  3. Claudication of lower extremities (seen with coarctation of aorta)

■ LABORATORY TESTS

- Urinalysis: for evidence of renal disease.
- BUN, creatinine: to rule out renal disease. High-serum creatinine is a predictor of cardiovascular risk in essential hypertension.
- Serum electrolyte levels: low potassium is suggestive of primary aldosteronism, diuretic use.
- Screening for coexisting diseases that may adversely affect prognosis:
  1. Fasting serum glucose
  2. Serum lipid panel, uric acid, calcium
  3. If pheochromocytoma is suspected: 24-hr urine for VMA and metanephrines

■ IMAGING STUDIES

- ECG: check for presence of left ventricular hypertrophy (LVH) with strain pattern.
- MRA of the renal arteries: in suspected renovascular hypertension (renal artery stenosis).

TREATMENT

■ NONPHARMACOLOGIC THERAPY

Life-style modifications:
- Lose weight if overweight.
- Limit alcohol intake to ≤1 oz of ethanol per day in men or ≤0.5 oz in women.
- Exercise (aerobic) regularly (at least 30 min/day, most days).
- Reduce sodium intake to <100 mmol/day (<2.3 g of sodium).
- Maintain adequate dietary potassium (>3500 mg/day) intake.
- Stop smoking and reduce dietary saturated fat and cholesterol intake for overall cardiovascular health.
Consume diet rich in fruits and vegetables.

■ ACUTE GENERAL Rx

According to the Seventh Report of the Joint National Committee on Detection, Evaluation, and Treatment of High Blood Pressure:

- Antihypertensive drug therapy should be initiated in patients with stage 1 hypertension. Diuretics or β-blockers are preferred for initial therapy because a reduction in morbidity and mortality has been demonstrated and because of their lower cost.
- ACE inhibitors, calcium antagonists, α-1 receptor blockers, and α-β blockers are also effective.
- Two-drug combination is necessary for most patients with stage 2 hypertension.
- When selecting drugs, also consider the cost of the medication, metabolic and subjective side effects, and drug-drug interactions.
- The major advantages and limitations of each class of drugs are described as follows:
  1. Diuretics
     a. Advantages: inexpensive, once per day dosing. Useful in edema states, CHF, chronic renal disease, elderly patients (decreased incidence of hip fractures in elderly patients)
     b. Disadvantages: significant adverse metabolic effects, increased risk of cardiac arrhythmias, sexual dysfunction, possible adverse effects on lipids and glucose levels
  2. β-Blockers
     a. Advantages: ideal in hypertensive patients with ischemic heart disease or post-MI. Favored in hyperkinetic, young patients (resting tachycardia, wide pulse pressure, hyperdynamic heart) and stable (Class II-III) CHF patients.
     b. Disadvantages: adverse effect on quality of life (increased incidence of fatigue, depression, impotence, bronchospasm, hypoglycemia, peripheral vascular disease, adverse effects on lipids, masking of signs and symptoms of hypoglycemia in diabetics.
  3. Calcium antagonists
     a. Advantages: helpful in hypertensive patients with ischemic heart disease. Generally favorable effect on quality of life; can be used in patients with bronchospastic disorders, renal disease, peripheral avascular disease, metabolic disorders, and salt sensitivity. Nondihydropyridine calcium channel blockers (verapamil, diltiazem) are useful in reducing proteinuria.
     b. Disadvantages: diltiazem and verapamil should be avoided in patients with CHF because of their chronotropic and inotropic effects; pedal edema may occur with nifedipine and amlodipine; constipation can be severe in elderly patients receiving verapamil.
  4. ACE inhibitors
     a. Advantages: well tolerated, favorable impact on quality of life; useful in hypertension complicated by CHF; helpful in prevention of diabetic renal disease; effective in decreasing LVH.
     b. Disadvantages: cough is a frequent side effect (5% to 20% of patients); hyperkalemia may occur in patients with diabetes or severe renal insufficiency; hypotension may occur in volume-depleted patients.
  5. Angiotensin II receptor blockers (ARB)
     a. Advantages: well tolerated, favorable impact on quality of life; useful in patients unable to tolerate ACE inhibitors because of persistent cough and in CHF and diabetic patients; single daily dose.
     b. Disadvantages: excessive cost; hypotension may occur in volume-depleted patients; contraindicated in pregnancy.
  6. α-Adrenergic blockers
     a. Advantages: no adverse effect on blood lipids or insulin sensitivity; helpful in BPH.
     b. Disadvantages: frequent postural hypotension; syncope can be avoided by giving an initial low dose at bedtime.

TREATMENT OF RENOVASCULAR HYPERTENSION (RVH): The therapeutic approach varies with the cause of the RVH.
1. Young patients with fibromuscular dysplasia can be treated with percutaneous transluminal renal angioplasty (PTRA).
2. Medical therapy is advisable in elderly patients with atheromatous renal vascular hypertension; useful agents are:
   a. β-Blockers: very effective in patients with elevated plasma renin.
   b. ACE inhibitors: very effective; however, should be avoided in patients with bilateral renal artery stenosis or in patients with solitary kidney and renal stenosis.
   c. Diuretics: often used in combination with ACE inhibitors.
3. Surgical revascularization is generally reserved for atheromatous RVH in patients responding poorly to medical therapy (uncontrolled hypertension, deteriorating renal function).

HYPERTENSION DURING PREGNANCY:
1. Hypertension complicates 5% to 12% of all pregnancies.
2. The American Obstetrical Committee defines blood pressure of 130/80 mm Hg as the upper limit of normal at any time during pregnancy.
3. A rise of 30 mm Hg systolic or 15 mm Hg diastolic is also considered abnormal regardless of the absolute values obtained.
4. Chronic hypertension (occurring before pregnancy) must be distinguished from preeclampsia, because the risk to mother and fetus is much greater in the latter.
5. Treatment of chronic hypertension during pregnancy is as follows:
   a. Initial treatment with conservative measures (proper nutrition, limited physical activity)
   b. When drug therapy is necessary, initiation of one of the following agents—methyldopa, hydralazine, labetalol, or atenolol—is preferred.
   c. ACE inhibitors can cause fetal and neonatal complications; their use should be avoided in pregnancy
   d. The safety of calcium channel blockers remains unclear
   e. Diuretics should be used only if there is a specific reason for initiating and maintaining their use (e.g., hypertension associated with severe fluid overload or left ventricular dysfunction)

MALIGNANT HYPERTENSION, HYPERTENSIVE EMERGENCIES, AND HYPERTENSIVE URGENCIES:
- Definitions:
1. **Malignant hypertension** is a potentially life-threatening situation that is secondary to elevated BP.
   a. The rate of BP rise is a critical factor.
   b. The clinical manifestations are grade IV hypertensive retinopathy (exudates, hemorrhages, and papilledema), cardiovascular and/or renal compromise, and encephalopathy.
   c. It requires immediate BP reduction (not necessarily into normal ranges) to prevent or limit target organ disease.
2. **Hypertensive emergencies** are situations that require rapid (within 1 hr) lowering of BP to prevent end-organ damage.

3. **Hypertensive urgencies** are significant BP elevations that should be corrected within 24 hr of presentation.

• Therapy:

The choice of therapeutic agents in malignant hypertension varies with the cause.

1. Nitroprusside is the drug of choice in hypertensive encephalopathy, hypertension and intracranial bleeding, malignant hypertension, hypertension and heart failure, dissecting aortic aneurysm (used in combination with the propranolol); its onset of action is immediate. Fenoldopam is a newer vasodilator agent useful for the short-term (up to 48 hr) management of severe hypertension when rapid but quickly reversible reduction of blood pressure is required.

2. The following are important points to remember when treating hypertensive emergencies:

   a. Introduce a plan for long-term therapy at the time of the initial emergency treatment.

   b. Agents that reduce arterial pressure can cause the kidney to retain sodium and water; therefore the judicious administration of diuretics should accompany their use.

   c. The initial goal of antihypertensive therapy is not to achieve a normal BP, but rather to gradually reduce the BP; cerebral hyperperfusion may occur if the mean BP is lowered >40% in the initial 24 hr.

3. Hypertensive urgencies can be effectively treated with oral clonidine 0.1 mg q20min (to a maximum of 0.8 mg); sedation is common.

⚙ PEARLS & CONSIDERATIONS

■ COMMENTS

In patients with hypertension and chronic renal insufficiency, it is not uncommon to see a small rise in serum creatinine as the blood pressure is lowered. Most physicians will respond by decreasing the dose of the antihypertensive medication. This approach should be discouraged because it is not optimal for the long-term preservation of renal function because a small, nonprogressive increase in serum creatinine in the context of improved blood pressure control is indicative of successful reduction of the intraglomerular pressure.

REFERENCES

Magill MK et al: New developments in the management of hypertension, *Am Fam Physician* 68:853, 2003.

Murphy MB et al: Fenoldopam, a selective peripheral dopamine-receptor agonist for the treatment of severe hypertension, *N Engl J Med* 345:1548, 2001.

Oparil S et al: Pathogenesis of hypertension, *Ann Intern Med* 139:761, 2003.

Seventh Report of the Joint National Committee on Prevention, Detection, Evaluation, and Treatment of High Blood Pressure, *JAMA* 289:2560, 2003.

Author: **Fred F. Ferri, M.D.**

BASIC INFORMATION

■ DEFINITION
Hyperthyroidism is a hypermetabolic state resulting from excess thyroid hormone.

■ SYNONYMS
Thyrotoxicosis

ICD-9CM CODES
242.9 Hyperthyroidism
242.0 Hyperthyroidism with goiter
242.2 Hyperthyroidism, multinodular
242.3 Hyperthyroidism, uninodular

■ EPIDEMIOLOGY & DEMOGRAPHICS
INCIDENCE/PREVALENCE:
- Hyperthyroidism affects 2% of women and 0.2% of men in their lifetime.
- Toxic multinodular goiter usually occurs in women >55 yr old and is more common than Graves' disease in the elderly.

■ PHYSICAL FINDINGS & CLINICAL PRESENTATION
- Patients with hyperthyroidism generally present with the following clinical manifestations: Tachycardia, tremor, hyperreflexia, anxiety, irritability, emotional lability, panic attacks, heat intolerance, sweating, increased appetite, diarrhea, weight loss, menstrual dysfunction (oligomenorrhea, amenorrhea); the presentation may be different in elderly patients (see third bullet).
- Patients with Graves' disease may present with exophthalmos, lid retraction (Fig. 1-150, *A*), lid lag (Graves' ophthalmopathy). The following signs and symptoms of ophthalmopathy may be present: blurring of vision, photophobia, increased lacrimation, double vision, deep orbital pressure. Clubbing of fingers associated with periosteal new bone formation in other skeletal areas (Graves' acropachy) and pretibial myxedema (Fig. 1-150, *B*) may also be noted.
- In the elderly the clinical signs of hyperthyroidism may be masked by manifestations of coexisting disease (e.g., new-onset atrial fibrillation, exacerbation of CHF).

■ ETIOLOGY
- Graves' disease (diffuse toxic goiter): 80% to 90% of all cases of hyperthyroidism
- Toxic multinodular goiter (Plummer's disease)
- Toxic adenoma
- Iatrogenic and factitious
- Transient hyperthyroidism (subacute thyroiditis, Hashimoto's thyroiditis)
- Rare causes: hypersecretion of TSH (e.g., pituitary neoplasms), struma ovarii, ingestion of large amount of iodine in a patient with preexisting thyroid hyperplasia or adenoma (Jod-Basedow phenomenon), hydatidiform mole, carcinoma of thyroid, amiodarone therapy

DIAGNOSIS

■ DIFFERENTIAL DIAGNOSIS
- Anxiety disorder
- Pheochromocytoma
- Metastatic neoplasm
- Diabetes mellitus
- Premenopausal state

■ WORKUP
Suspected hyperthyroidism requires laboratory confirmation and identification of its etiology, because treatment varies with its cause. A detailed medical history will often provide clues to the diagnosis and etiology of the hyperthyroidism.

■ LABORATORY TESTS
- Elevated free thyroxine (T_4)
- Elevated free triiodothyronine (T_3): generally not necessary for diagnosis
- Low TSH (unless hyperthyroidism is a result of the rare hypersecretion of TSH from a pituitary adenoma)
- Thyroid autoantibodies useful in selected cases to differentiate Graves' disease from toxic multinodular goiter (absent thyroid antibodies)

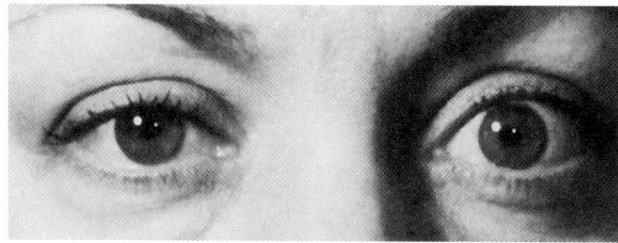
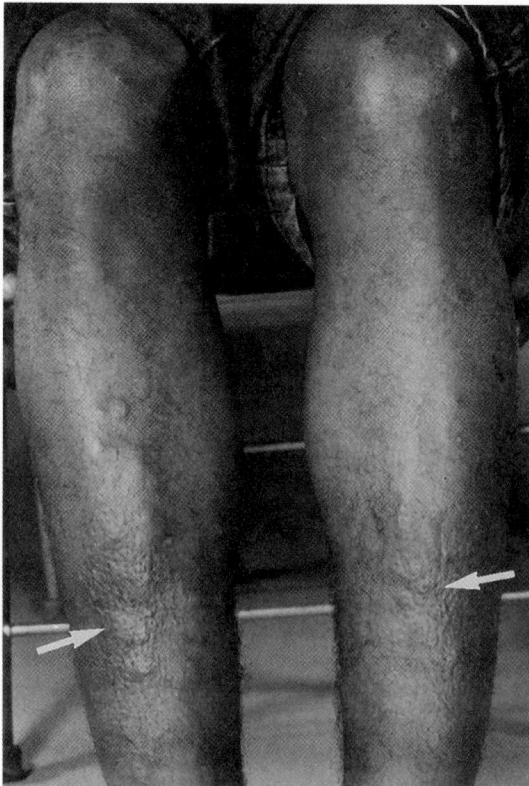

Fig. 1-150 **A,** Unilateral (*left*) lid retraction in a patient with hyperthyroidism. **B,** Pretibial myxedema (*arrows*) in a patient with Graves' disease. (From Noble J [ed]: *Textbook of primary care medicine,* ed 2, St Louis, 1996, Mosby.)

■ IMAGING STUDIES

- 24-hr radioactive iodine uptake (RAIU) is useful to distinguish hyperthyroidism from iatrogenic thyroid hormone synthesis (thyrotoxicosis factitia) and from thyroiditis.
- An overactive thyroid shows increased uptake, whereas a normal underactive thyroid (iatrogenic thyroid ingestion, painless or subacute thyroiditis) shows normal or decreased uptake.
- The RAIU results also vary with the etiology of the hyperthyroidism:
  Graves' disease: increased homogeneous uptake.
  Multinodular goiter: increased heterogeneous uptake.
  Hot nodule: single focus of increased uptake.
- RAIU is also generally performed before the therapeutic administration of radioactive iodine to determine the appropriate dose.

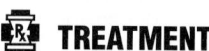

TREATMENT

■ NONPHARMACOLOGIC THERAPY

Patient education regarding thyroid disease and discussion of the therapeutic options (medications, radioactive iodine, and thyroid surgery)

■ ACUTE GENERAL Rx

ANTITHYROID DRUGS (THIONAMIDES): Propylthiouracil (PTU) and methimazole (Tapazole) inhibit thyroid hormone synthesis by blocking production of thyroid peroxidase (PTU and methimazole) or inhibit peripheral conversion of T_4 to T_3 (PTU).

1. Dosage: PTU 50 to 100 mg PO q8h; methimazole 10 to 20 mg PO q8h or 30 to 60 mg/day given as a single dose.
2. Antithyroid drugs can be used as the primary form of treatment or as adjunctive therapy before radioactive therapy or surgery or afterward if the hyperthyroidism recurs.
3. Side effects: skin rash (3% to 5% of patients), arthralgias, myalgias, granulocytopenia (0.5%). Rare side effects are aplastic anemia, hepatic necrosis from PTU, cholestatic jaundice from methimazole.
4. When antithyroid drugs are used as primary therapy, they are usually given for 6 to 24 mo; prolonged therapy may cause hypothyroidism.
5. The use of antithyroid drugs before radioactive iodine therapy is best reserved for patients in whom exacerbation of hyperthyroidism after radioactive iodine therapy is hazardous (e.g., elderly patients with coronary artery disease or significant coexisting morbidity). In these patients the antithyroid drug can be stopped 2 days before radioactive iodine therapy, resumed 2 days later, and continued for 4 to 6 wk.

RADIOACTIVE IODINE (RAI; ¹³¹I):
1. RAI is the treatment of choice for patients >21 yr of age and younger patients who have not achieved remission after 1 yr of antithyroid drug therapy. Radioiodine is also used in hyperthyroidism caused by toxic adenoma or toxic multinodular goiter.
2. Contraindicated during pregnancy (can cause fetal hypothyroidism) and lactation. Pregnancy should be excluded in women of childbearing age before radioactive iodine is administered.
3. A single dose of radioactive iodine is effective in inducing euthyroid state in nearly 80% of patients.
4. There is a high incidence of postradioactive iodine hypothyroidism (>50% within first year and 2%/yr thereafter); therefore these patients should be frequently evaluated for the onset of hypothyroidism (see Chronic Rx).

SURGICAL THERAPY (SUBTOTAL THYROIDECTOMY):
1. Indicated in obstructing goiters, in any patient who refuses radioactive iodine and cannot be adequately managed with antithyroid medications (e.g., patients with toxic adenoma or toxic multinodular goiter), and in pregnant patients who cannot be adequately managed with antithyroid medication or develop side effects to them.
2. Patients should be rendered euthyroid with antithyroid drugs before surgery.
3. Complications of surgery include hypothyroidism (28% to 43% after 10 yr), hypoparathyroidism, and vocal cord paralysis (1%).
4. Hyperthyroidism recurs after surgery in 10% to 15% of patients.

ADJUNCTIVE THERAPY: Propranolol alleviates the β-adrenergic symptoms of hyperthyroidism; initial dose is 20 to 40 mg PO q6h; dosage is gradually increased until symptoms are controlled; major contraindications to use of propranolol are CHF and bronchospasm. Diagnosis and treatment of "thyroid storm" are discussed elsewhere in Section I.

■ CHRONIC Rx

Patients undergoing treatment with antithyroid drugs should be seen every 1 to 3 mo until euthyroidism is achieved and every 3 to 4 mo while they remain on antithyroid therapy. After treatment is stopped, periodic monitoring of thyroid function tests with TSH every 3 mo for 1 yr, then every 6 mo for 1 yr, then annually is recommended.

■ DISPOSITION

Successful treatment of hyperthyroidism requires lifelong monitoring for the onset of hypothyroidism or the recurrence of thyrotoxicosis.

■ REFERRAL

- Endocrinology referral is recommended at the time of initial diagnosis and during treatment
- Surgical referral in selected patients (see Surgical Therapy)
- Hospitalization of all patients with thyroid storm

☼ PEARLS & CONSIDERATIONS

■ COMMENTS

- Elderly hyperthyroid patients may have only subtle signs (weight loss, tachycardia, fine skin, brittle nails). This form is known as **apathetic hyperthyroidism** and manifests with lethargy rather than hyperkinetic activity. An enlarged thyroid gland may be absent. Coexisting medical disorders (most commonly cardiac disease) may also mask the symptoms. These patients often have unexplained CHF, worsening of angina, or new-onset atrial fibrillation resistant to treatment. See "Graves' Disease" in Section I for additional information on the diagnosis and treatment of Graves' disease.
- **Subclinical hyperthyroidism** is defined as a normal serum free thyroxine and free triiodothyronine levels with a thyroid-stimulating hormone level suppressed below the normal range and usually undetectable. These patients usually do not present with signs or symptoms of overt hyperthyroidism. Treatment options include observation or a therapeutic trial of low-dose antithyroid agents for 6 mo to attempt to induce remission.

REFERENCES

Kearns AE, Thompson GB: Medical and surgical management of hyperthyroidism, *Mayo Clin Proc* 77:87, 2002.
Shrier DK et al: Subclinical hyperthyroidism: controversies in management, *Am Fam Physician* 65:431, 2002.
Toft AD: Subclinical hyperthyroidism, *N Engl J Med* 345:512, 2001.
Author: **Fred F. Ferri, M.D.**

BASIC INFORMATION

DEFINITION
Hypertrophic osteoarthropathy (HOA) is a syndrome of clubbing of the digits, periostitis of long bones, and arthritis. HOA may be primary or secondary to other underlying disease processes.

SYNONYMS
- Primary hypertrophic osteoarthropathy
  1. Pachydermoperiostosis
  2. Heredofamilial
  3. Idiopathic clubbing
  4. Touraine-Solente-Golé syndrome
- Secondary hypertrophic osteoarthropathy

ICD-9CM CODES
731.2 Hypertrophic osteoarthropathy

EPIDEMIOLOGY & DEMOGRAPHICS
- Primary HOA is familial autosomal dominant disease affecting young children between ages 1 and 20.
- Secondary HOA typically occurs in adults and is associated with other illnesses including:
  1. Pulmonary: Bronchogenic carcinoma, lung abscess, bronchiectasis, cystic fibrosis, pulmonary fibrosis, mesothelioma, sarcoidosis
  2. Gastrointestinal: Esophageal carcinoma, colon cancer, inflammatory bowel disease (Crohn's disease, ulcerative colitis), hepatocellular carcinoma, liver cirrhosis, amebiasis
  3. Cardiac: Infective endocarditis, right-to-left cardiac shunts, aortic aneurysm
  4. Thymoma
  5. Lymphoma
  6. Connective tissue diseases
  7. Thyroid acropachy

PHYSICAL FINDINGS & CLINICAL PRESENTATION
- Primary HOA typically presents with the insidious onset of clubbing of the hands and feet and is described as "spadelike." Other signs and symptoms include:
  1. Joint pain and swelling
  2. Decreased use of the fingers and hands
  3. Facial changes, coarse facial skin grooves
  4. Thickening of the arms and legs
  5. Oily skin, diaphoresis, gynecomastia, and acne

- Secondary HOA patients may present with clinical symptoms before the underlying disorder can be detected. Signs and symptoms are similar to the above mentioned in addition to findings related to the underlying disease (e.g., bronchogenic carcinoma, infective endocarditis).

ETIOLOGY
Unknown; immunologic, endocrine, and vascular etiologies have been suggested.

DIAGNOSIS

DIFFERENTIAL DIAGNOSIS
- Other causes of periostitis include Paget's disease, Reiter's syndrome, psoriasis, syphilis, osteoarthritis, rheumatoid arthritis, and osteomyelitis.
- Hypertrophic osteoarthropathy with the classic finding of clubbing of the digits warrants an investigation into any associated illnesses.

WORKUP
Primarily consists of blood tests, x-rays, and bone scans

LABORATORY TESTS
- CBC, electrolytes, and urine studies will typically be normal in both primary and secondary HOA.
- ESR will be elevated in secondary HOA.
- LFTs may be abnormal in patients with secondary HOA from GI pathology.
- Alkaline phosphatase may be elevated secondary to periostitis of long bones.
- Analysis of the synovial fluid from joint effusions reveals a low WBC count with normal viscosity, color, and complement levels.

IMAGING STUDIES
- X-rays of the long bones show periosteal new bone formation (Fig. 1-151).
- A chest x-ray should be obtained to rule out underlying lung cancer.
- Bone scan with technetium-99m reveals uptake along the long bones, phalanxes, and periarticular joint spaces are common findings.

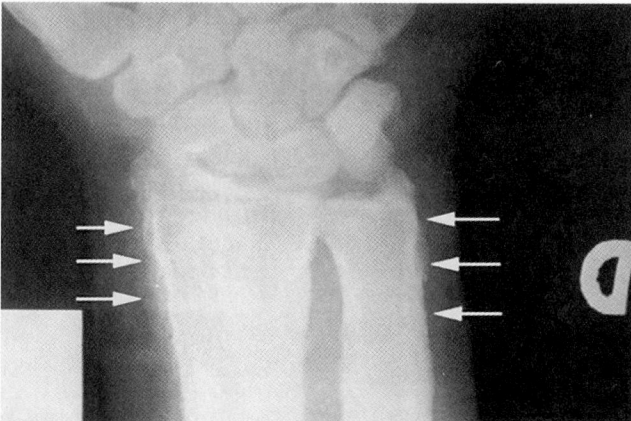

Fig. 1-151 Hypertrophic osteoarthropathy. Coarse periosteal new bone formation in the distal ulna and radius (arrows) in a patient with cyanotic congenital heart disease. (Courtesy Dr. Manuel Martinez Lavin, Mexico City. In Canoso J: *Rheumatology in primary care*, Philadelphia, 1997, WB Saunders.)

℞ TREATMENT

■ ACUTE GENERAL Rx

- Treatment of primary HOA is symptomatic. Aspirin (acetylsalicylic acid) 325 mg PO q4-6 hr prn, salicylate 750 mg bid prn, ibuprofen 400 to 800 mg tid prn, naproxen 250 to 500 mg bid prn, indomethacin 25 to 50 mg qid prn will provide bone and joint pain relief.
- For secondary HOA the treatment of choice is to eradicate the underlying disease (e.g., antibiotics for infective endocarditis, surgery for bronchogenic carcinoma).

■ CHRONIC Rx

- In patients with secondary HOA refractory to NSAIDs and aspirin, vagotomy has been tried with some success. However, the definitive treatment is to treat the underlying disease.

■ DISPOSITION

- Patients with primary HOA typically will have symptoms of joint pains and swelling for the early part of their life, but thereafter the disease becomes quiescent.
- Prognosis and disease course in patients with secondary HOA will depend on the underlying cause. The insidious development of clubbing suggests infectious process, whereas the rapid progression of clubbing may suggest underlying malignancy.

■ REFERRAL

Referral should be made to rheumatology when the diagnosis of HOA is suspected and the cause remains unclear.

☼ PEARLS & CONSIDERATIONS

■ COMMENTS

- HOA may be a marker for an underlying serious illness and a thorough investigation should be pursued. Infections and intrathoracic malignancies are the most common causes of secondary HOA.

REFERENCES

Altman RD, Tenebaum J: *Hypertrophic osteoarthropathy*. In Kelly WN et al. (eds): *Textbook of rheumatology*, ed 5, Baltimore, 1997, WB Saunders.

Martinez-Lavin M: Hypertrophic osteoarthropathy, *Curr Opin Rheumatol* 9(1):83, 1997.

Ramakrishnan S, Das SK, Mishra K: A current perspective on clubbing and hypertrophic osteoarthropathy, *J Assoc Physicians India* 49:1106, 2001.

Viola JC, Jaffe S, Brent LH: Primary hypertrophic osteoarthropathy, *J Rheumatol* 27(6):1562, 2000.

Author: **Peter Petropoulos M.D.**

BASIC INFORMATION

■ DEFINITION
Hypoaldosteronism is an aldosterone deficiency or impaired aldosterone function.

ICD-9CM CODES
255.4 Hypoadrenalism

■ EPIDEMIOLOGY AND DEMOGRAPHICS
Selective hypoaldosteronism accounts for as many as 10% of cases of unexplained hyperkalemia.

■ PHYSICAL FINDINGS & CLINICAL PRESENTATION
- Physical examination may be entirely within normal limits.
- Hypertension may be present in some patients.
- Profound muscle weakness and cardiac arrhythmias may be present.

■ ETIOLOGY
- Hyporeninemic hypoaldosteronism (renin-angiotensin dependent): decreased aldosterone production secondary to decreased renin production; the typical patient has renal disease secondary to various factors (e.g., diabetes mellitus, interstitial nephritis, multiple myeloma).
- Hyperreninemic hypoaldosteronism (renin-angiotensin independent): renin production by the kidneys is intact; the defect is in aldosterone biosynthesis or in the action of angiotensin II. Common causes of this form of hypoaldosteronism are medications (ACE inhibitors, heparin), lead poisoning, aldosterone enzyme defects, and severe illness.

DIAGNOSIS

■ DIFFERENTIAL DIAGNOSIS
Pseudohypoaldosteronism: renal unresponsiveness to aldosterone. In this condition, both renin and aldosterone levels are elevated. Pseudohypoaldosteronism can be caused by medications (spironolactone), chronic interstitial nephritis, systemic disorders (SLE, amyloidosis), or primary mineralocorticoid resistance.

■ WORKUP
Measurement of plasma renin activity following 4 hr of upright posture can differentiate hyporeninemic from hyperreninemic causes. Renin levels in the normal or low range identify cases that are renin-angiotensin dependent, whereas high renin levels identify cases that are renin-angiotensin independent. The diagnosis and etiology of hypoaldosteronism can be confirmed with the renin-aldosterone stimulation test:
- Hyporeninemic hypoaldosteronism: low stimulated renin and aldosterone levels
- End-organ refractoriness to aldosterone action: high stimulated renin and aldosterone levels
- Adrenal gland abnormality: high stimulated renin and low aldosterone levels

■ LABORATORY TESTS
- Increased potassium, normal or decreased sodium
- Hyperchloremic metabolic acidosis (caused by the absence of hydrogen-secreting action of aldosterone)
- Increased BUN and creatinine (secondary to renal disease)
- Hyperglycemia (diabetes mellitus is common in these patients)

TREATMENT

■ NONPHARMACOLOGIC THERAPY
- Low-potassium diet with liberal sodium intake (at least 4 g of sodium chloride per day)
- Avoidance of ACE inhibitors and potassium-sparing diuretics

■ ACUTE GENERAL Rx
- Judicious use of fludrocortisone (0.05 to 0.1 mg PO qam) in patients with aldosterone deficiency associated with deficiency of adrenal glucocorticoid hormones
- Furosemide 20 to 40 mg qd to correct hyperkalemia of hyporeninemic hypoaldosteronism

■ DISPOSITION
Prognosis varies with the etiology of hypoaldosteronism and presence of associated disorders.

■ REFERRAL
Endocrinology referral for renin-aldosterone stimulation test

PEARLS & CONSIDERATIONS

■ COMMENTS
Treatment of pseudohypoaldosteronism is the same as for hypoaldosteronism; however, effect is limited because of impaired renal sensitivity.
Author: **Fred F. Ferri, M.D.**

BASIC INFORMATION

■ DEFINITION
Hypopituitarism is the partial or complete loss of pituitary hormone secretion resulting from diseases of the hypothalamus or pituitary gland.

■ SYNONYMS
Panhypopituitarism
Pituitary insufficiency

ICD-9CM CODES
253.2 Panhypopituitarism

■ EPIDEMIOLOGY & DEMOGRAPHICS
- Pituitary tumors are the most common causes of hypopituitarism with an incidence of 0.2 to 2.8 cases per 100,000.
- Increased incidence of vascular or cerebrovascular disease in patients with panhypopituitarism.
- Predisposing factors for pituitary apoplexy (another cause of panhypopituitarism) include diabetes mellitus, anticoagulant therapy, head trauma, pituitary tumors, and radiation.
- Empty sella syndrome, a third cause of panhypopituitarism, can occur in both adults and children.

■ PHYSICAL FINDINGS & CLINICAL PRESENTATION
The onset of hypopituitarism is usually gradual, and symptoms are related to the lack of one or more hormones and/or mass effect if a pituitary tumor is the cause.
- Mass effect of a pituitary tumor can cause headaches and visual disturbances
- Corticotropin deficiency:
  1. Fatigue and weakness, no appetite, abdominal pain, nausea, and vomiting
  2. Hypotension, hair loss, and change in mental status
- Thyrotropin deficiency:
  1. Fatigue and weakness, weight gain, cold intolerance, and constipation
  2. Bradycardia, hung-up reflexes, pretibial edema, and hair loss
- Gonadotropin deficiency:
  1. Loss of libido, erectile dysfunction, amenorrhea, hot flashes, dyspareunia
  2. Gynecomastia with lack of hair growth and decreased muscle mass

- Growth hormone deficiency:
  1. Growth retardation in children
  2. Easy fatigue
  3. Decreased muscle mass and obesity
- Hyperprolactinemia
  1. Galactorrhea
  2. Hypogonadism
- Vasopressin deficiency:
  1. Polyuria, polydipsia and nocturia
  2. Hypotension and dehydration

■ ETIOLOGY
Hypopituitarism is the result of destruction of pituitary cells caused by:
- Pituitary tumors
  1. Macroadenomas >10 mm
  2. Microadenomas <10 mm
- Pituitary apoplexy caused by hemorrhage or infarction of the pituitary gland
- Pituitary radiation therapy
- Pituitary surgery
- Empty sella syndrome with enlargement of the sella turcica and flattening of the pituitary gland caused by extension of the subarachnoid space and filling of cerebrospinal fluid into the sella turcica
- Infiltrative disease including sarcoidosis, hemochromatosis, histiocytosis X, Wegener's granulomatosis, and lymphocytic hypophysitis
- Infection (tuberculosis, mycosis, and syphilis)
- Head trauma
- Internal carotid artery aneurysm

DIAGNOSIS

The diagnosis of hypopituitarism is suspected by clinical history and physical findings and is established by endocrine stimulation testing.

■ DIFFERENTIAL DIAGNOSIS
The differential diagnosis is as outlined under Etiology. Other rare causes include postpartum necrosis (Sheehan's syndrome), hypopituitary tumors (e.g., craniopharyngiomas and meningioma), metastatic tumors, and developmental abnormalities.

■ WORKUP
Includes basal determination of each anterior pituitary hormone followed by provocative stimulation tests and x-ray imaging

■ LABORATORY TESTS
- Corticotropin deficiency:
  1. Serum am cortisol level usually is low.
  2. Corticotropin stimulation test using 250 µg of corticotropin given IV and measuring serum cortisol before and 30 and 60 min after administration. A normal response is an increase in serum cortisol level >20 µg/dl.
- Thyrotropin deficiency:
  1. TSH and free T_4 measurements
  2. Primary hypothyroidism shows elevated TSH with low free T_4. Secondary hypothyroidism shows normal or low TSH with low free T_4
- Gonadotropin deficiency:
  1. FSH, LH, estrogen, and testosterone measurements
  2. In men, hypogonadotropic hypogonadism is seen with low testosterone levels and normal or low FSH and LH levels
  3. In premenopausal women with amenorrhea, low estrogen with normal or low FSH and LH levels is typically seen
- Growth hormone deficiency:
  1. Insulin-induced hypoglycemia stimulation test using 0.1 to 0.15 unit/kg regular insulin given IV and measuring growth hormone 30, 60, and 120 min after administration. A normal response is a growth hormone level >10 µg/dl.
  2. Serum insulin-like growth factor I can also be measured after provocative testing.
- Hyperprolactinemia:
  1. Prolactin levels may be elevated in prolactin-secreting pituitary adenomas.
- Vasopressin deficiency:
  1. Urinalysis shows low specific gravity.
  2. Urine osmolality is low.
  3. Serum osmolality is high.
  4. Fluid deprivation test over 18 hr with inability to concentrate the urine.
  5. Serum vasopressin level is low.
  6. Electrolytes may show hyponatremia and exclude hyperglycemia.

■ IMAGING STUDIES
- MRI is more sensitive than CT scan of the head in visualizing the pituitary fossa, sella turcica, optic chiasm, pituitary stalk, and cavernous sinuses. It is also more sensitive in detecting pituitary microadenomas.
- CT scan with coronal cuts through the sella turcica gives better images of bony structures.
- Skull films can be done but are not very sensitive.

℞ TREATMENT

Hormone replacement therapy and either surgery, radiation, or medications in patients with pituitary tumors.

■ NONPHARMACOLOGIC THERAPY
- IV fluid resuscitation with normal saline to maintain hemodynamic stability may be needed in some circumstances
- Correction of electrolyte and metabolic abnormalities with potassium, bicarbonate, and oxygen therapy

■ ACUTE GENERAL Rx
Acute situations like adrenal crisis or myxedema coma can occur in untreated hypopituitarism and should be treated accordingly with IV corticosteroids (e.g., hydrocortisone 100 mg IV q6h for 24 hr) and levothyroxine (e.g., 5 to 8 µg/kg IV over 15 min, then 100 µg IV q24h).

■ CHRONIC Rx
Treatment is lifelong and requires the following hormone replacement therapy:
- Hydrocortisone 20 mg PO qam and 10 mg PO qpm or prednisone 5 mg PO qam and 2.5 mg PO qpm
- Testosterone enanthate or propionate 200 to 300 mg IM q2 to 3 wk or transdermal testosterone scrotal patches can be tried
- Conjugated estrogen 0.3 to 1.25 mg/day and held the last 5 to 7 days of each month plus medroxyprogesterone 10 mg/day given during days 15 to 25
- Levothyroxine 0.05 to 0.15 mg/day
- Growth hormone is not used in adults; however, can be given at 0.04 to 0.08 mg/kg/day subcutaneously in children
- Desmopressin (DDAVP) 10 to 20 µg via intranasal spray or 0.05 to 0.1 mg PO bid is used in patients with diabetes insipidus

■ DISPOSITION
- Hormone replacement therapy is adjusted according to serum hormone blood monitoring.
- Hypopituitarism if untreated can lead to adrenal crisis, severe hyponatremia and hypothyroidism, metabolic abnormalities, and death.
- Life expectancy can be normal in patients with eradication of the pituitary disease and adequate hormone replacement therapy.

■ REFERRAL
Anyone suspected of having hypopituitarism should have an endocrine consultation. For patients with pituitary tumors, a radiation oncologist and neurosurgeon consultation should be consulted.

⚙ PEARLS & CONSIDERATIONS

■ COMMENTS
- Thyroxine supplementation increases the rate of cortisol metabolism and can lead to adrenal crisis. It is therefore recommended to supplement corticosteroids first before administering thyroid hormone replacement therapy.
- Stress doses of corticosteroids are indicated before surgery or for any medical emergency (e.g., sepsis, acute myocardial infarction, etc.).

REFERENCES

Heshmann AM et al: Hypopituitarism caused by intracellular aneurysms, *Mayo Clin Proc* 76:789, 2001.

Lamberts SWJ, de Herder WW, van der Lely AJ: Pituitary insufficiency, *Lancet* 352:127, 1998.

Vance ML: Hypopituitarism, *N Engl J Med* 330(23):1651, 1994.

Author: **Peter Petropoulos, M.D.**

BASIC INFORMATION

■ DEFINITION

Hypospadias is a developmental abnormality of the penis characterized by
- Abnormal ventral opening of the urethral meatus anywhere from the ventral aspect of the glans penis to the perineum
- Ventral curvature of the penis (chordee)
- Dorsal foreskin hood

See Fig. 1-152

ICD-9CM CODES
ICD-9-CM: 752.61
Congenital Chordee: 752.63

■ ETIOLOGY
Multifactorial
- Endocrine factors
  1. Abnormal androgen production
  2. Limited androgen sensitivity in the target tissues
  3. Premature cessation of androgenic stimulation secondary to Leydig cell dysfunction
  4. Insufficient testosterone-dihydrotestosterone synthesis as a result of deficient 5-alpha reductase enzyme activity
- Arrested development

■ EPIDEMIOLOGY & DEMOGRAPHICS
- Prevalence: 1 in 250
- Pertinent familial aspects of hypospadias include the finding of hypospadias in 6.8% of fathers of affected boys and in 14% of male siblings
- An 8.5-fold higher rate of hypospadias is reported in monozygotic twins suggesting that there is insufficient production of human chorionic gonadotropin by the single placenta

■ PHYSICAL FINDINGS & CLINICAL PRESENTATION
- Genetics: normal karyotypes are seen with glandular hypospadias; abnormal karyotypes are noted in more severe forms of hypospadias
- Cryptorchidism: 8% to 9% occurrence
- Inguinal hernia: 9% to 10% occurrence
- Hydrocele: 9% to 16% occurrence

PENILE CURVATURE (CHORDEE)
Three theories
- Abnormal development of the urethral plate
- Abnormal fibrotic mesenchymal tissue at the urethral meatus
- Corporal disproportion

DIAGNOSIS

■ WORKUP
Made by observation and examination

■ LABORATORY TESTS
Intersex evaluation should be undertaken if there is associated cryptorchidism. The evaluation should include: ultrasound, genitographic studies, chromosomal, gonadal, biochemical, and molecular studies.

TREATMENT

■ ACUTE GENERAL Rx
DESIGNATION/CLASSIFICATION
Anterior: 33%
Middle: 25%
Posterior: 41%
SPECIAL CONSIDERATION
- The only reason for operating on any hypospadias patient is to correct deformities that interfere with the function of urination and procreation
- Other reasons for interventions: Cosmetic concerns
- The American Academy of Pediatrics recommends the best time for surgical intervention is 6 to 12 mo

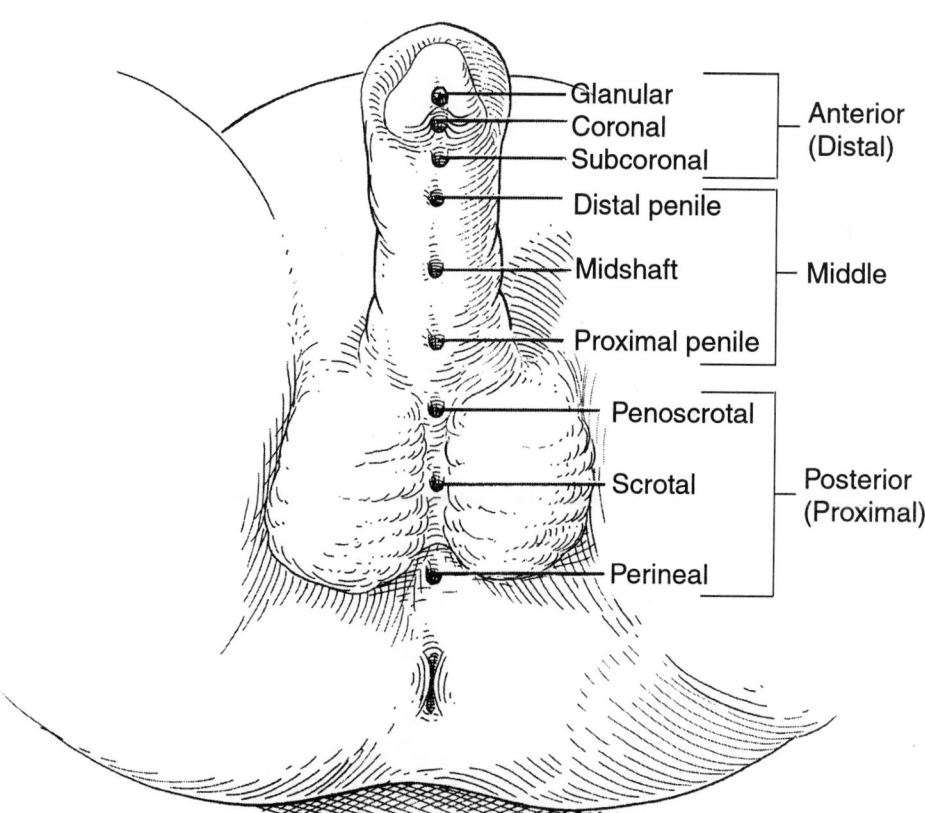

Fig. 1-152   Various locations of hypospadias. (From Walsh PC et al, eds: *Campbell's urology*, ed 8, Philadelphia, 2002, WB Saunders.)

HORMONAL MANIPULATION

- Controversial
- hCG administration is given before repair of proximal hypospadias
- The effect of the hCG administration is decreased hypospadias and chordee severity in all patients, increased vascularity and thickness of the proximal corpus spongiosum
- Application of topical testosterone increased mean penile circumference and length without any lasting side effects
- Prepubertal exogenous testosterone does not adversely effect ultimate penile growth

■ CHRONIC Rx

SURGICAL PROCEDURES

- Orthoplasty (correcting penile curvature)
- Urethroplasty
- Meatoplasty
- Glanuloplasty
- Skin coverage

There is no single universally acceptable applicable technique for hypospadias repair.

TYPES OF REPAIR

- Anterior hypospadias: MAGPI, Thiersch-Duplay urethroplasty, glans approximation procedure (GAP), tubularized incised plate (TIP) urethroplasty, Mathieu perimeatal flap, Mustarde technique, megameatus intact prepuce (MIP), pyramid procedure
- Midlevel hypospadias: TIP, Mathieu, onlay island flap (OIF), King procedure
- Posterior hypospadias:
  1. One-stage repair: OIF, double onlay preputial flap, pedicled preputial flap, transverse preputial island flap (TPIF)
  2. Two-stage repair: Orthoplasty to correct chordee followed 6 mo later or longer by Thiersch-Duplay, bladder and/or buccal mucosal hypospadias repair

COMPLICATIONS OF REPAIR

Hematoma, meatal stenosis, fistula, urethral stricture, urethral diverticulum, wound infection, impaired healing, balanitis xerotica obliterans, penile curvature

☼ PEARLS & CONSIDERATIONS

- It must be kept in mind that apparent simple isolated hypospadias may be the only visible indication of an underlying abnormality.
- The dorsal hood of redundant foreskin is used in the repair of hypospadias, and the patient with hypospadias and a dorsal hood should not be circumcised.

REFERENCES

American Academy of Pediatrics: Timing of elective surgery on the genitalia of male children with particular reference to the risks, benefits, and psychological effects of surgery and anesthesia, *Pediatrics* 97:590, 1996.

Belman AB: Hypospadias update, *Urology* 49:166, 1997.

Borer JG, Retik AB: Current trends in hypospadias repair, *Urol Clin North Am* 26:1:15, 1999.

Duckett JW, Baskin LS: Hypospadias. In Gillenwalter JY et al, eds: *Adult and pediatric urology,* ed 3, St Louis, 1996, Mosby.

Retik AB, Borer JG. In Walsh PC et al, eds: *Campbell's urology,* ed 8, Philadelphia, 2002, WB Saunders.

Zaontz MR, Packer MG: Abnormalities of the external genitalia. *Pediatr Clin North Am* 44:1267, 1997.

Author: **Philip J. Aliotta, M.D., M.S.H.A.**

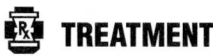
 BASIC INFORMATION

■ DEFINITION
Hypothermia is a rectal temperature <35° C (95.8° F). *Accidental hypothermia* is unintentionally induced decrease in core temperature in absence of preoptic anterior hypothalamic conditions.

■ ICD-9CM CODES
991.6 Accidental hypothermia
780.9 Hypothermia not associated with low environmental temperature

■ EPIDEMIOLOGY & DEMOGRAPHICS
Hypothermia occurs most frequently in the following groups: alcoholics, learning-impaired, patients with cardiovascular, cerebrovascular, or pituitary disorders, those using sedatives or tranquilizers, and elderly patients.

■ PHYSICAL FINDINGS & CLINICAL PRESENTATION
- The clinical presentation varies with the severity of hypothermia. Shivering may be absent if body temperature is <33.3° C (92° F) or in patients taking phenothiazines.
- Hypothermia may masquerade as CVA, ataxia, or slurred speech, or the patient may appear comatose or clinically dead.
- Physiologic stages of hypothermia:
  1. Mild hypothermia (32.2° to 35° C [90° to 95° F]): arrhythmias, ataxia
  2. Moderate hypothermia (28° to 32.2° C [82.4° to 90° F]):
     a. Progressive decrease of level of consciousness, pulse, cardiac output, and respiration
     b. Fibrillation, dysrhythmias (increased susceptibility to ventricular tachycardia)
     c. Elimination of shivering mechanism for thermogenesis

3. Severe hypothermia (≤28° C [82.4° F]):
   a. Absence of reflexes or response to pain
   b. Decreased cerebral blood flow, decreased CO₂
   c. Increased risk of ventricular fibrillation or asystole

■ ETIOLOGY
Exposure to cold temperatures for a prolonged period

🔬 DIAGNOSIS

■ DIFFERENTIAL DIAGNOSIS
- CVA
- Myxedema coma
- Drug intoxication
- Hypoglycemia

■ LABORATORY TESTS
1. Metabolic and respiratory acidosis are usually present.
   a. When blood cools, the arterial pH increases, oxygen tension (Po_2) increases, and the Pco_2 falls:
      (1) pH ↑ 0.008 U/°F (or 0.015 U/°C), ↓ in temperature.
      (2) Pao_2 ↑ 3.3%/°F, ↓ in temperature.
      (3) $Paco_2$ ↓ 2.4%/°F, ↓ in temperature.
   b. Blood gas analyzers warm the blood to 37° C, increasing the partial pressure of dissolved gases, resulting in higher oxygen and carbon dioxide levels and a lower pH than the patient's actual values. Correction of ABGs for temperature is unnecessary as a guide to therapy. The use of uncorrected values also permits reference to the standard acid-base nomograms.
2. ↓ K⁺ initially, then ↑ K⁺ with increasing hypothermia; extreme hyperkalemia indicates a poor prognosis.
3. Hematocrit (Hct) ↑ (caused by hemoconcentration), ↓ leukocytes, ↓ platelets (caused by splenic sequestration).
Blood viscosity, ↑ clotting time

■ IMAGING STUDIES
- Chest x-ray examination: generally not helpful; may reveal evidence of aspiration (e.g., intoxicated patient with aspiration pneumonia).
- ECG: prolonged PR, QT, and QRS segments, depressed ST segments, inverted T waves, AV block, hypothermic J waves (Osborne waves) may appear at 25° to 30° C; characterized by notching of the junction of the QRS complex and ST segments (Fig. 1-153).

💊 TREATMENT

■ NONPHARMACOLOGIC THERAPY
- Treatment of hypothermia varies with the following:
  1. Degree of hypothermia
  2. Existence of concomitant diseases (e.g., cardiovascular insufficiency)
  3. Patient's age and medical condition (e.g., elderly, debilitated patients vs. young, healthy patients)
- General measures:
  1. Secure an airway before warming all unconscious patients; precede endotracheal intubation with oxygenation (if possible) to minimize the risk of arrhythmias during the procedure.
  2. Peripheral vasoconstriction may impede placement of a peripheral intravenous catheter; consider femoral venous access as an alternative to the jugular or subclavian sites to avoid ventricular stimulation.

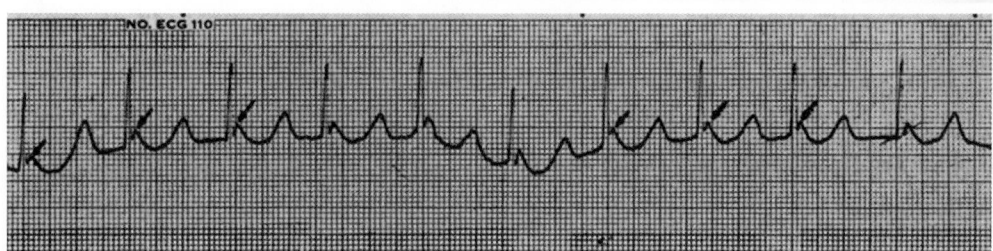

Fig. 1-153 Osborne waves (*arrows*) in an 80-year-old man with core temperature of 86° F (30° C). These waves disappeared with rewarming. (From Morse CD, Rial WY: Emergency medicine. In Rakel RE [ed]: *Textbook of family practice,* ed 4, Philadelphia, 1990, WB Saunders.)

3. A Foley catheter should be inserted, and urinary output should be monitored and maintained above 0.5 to 1 ml/kg/hr with intravascular volume replacement.

■ ACUTE GENERAL Rx
- Continuous ECG monitoring of patients is recommended; ventricular arrhythmias can be treated with bretylium; lidocaine is generally ineffective, and procainamide is associated with an increased incidence of ventricular fibrillation in hypothermic patients.
- Correct severe acidosis and electrolyte abnormalities.
- Hypothyroidism, if present, should be promptly treated (refer to "Myxedema Coma").
- If clinical evidence suggests adrenal insufficiency, administer IV methylprednisolone.

- In patients unresponsive to verbal or noxious stimuli or with altered mental status, 100 mg of thiamine, 0.4 mg of naloxone, and 1 ampule of 50% dextrose may be given.
- Warm (104° to 113° F [40° to 45° C]), humidified oxygen should also be given if it is available.
- Specific treatment:
1. Mild hypothermia (rectal temperature <32.3° C [90° F]): passive external rewarming is indicated. Place the patient in a warm room (temperature >21° C [69.8° F]), and cover with insulating material after gently removing wet clothing; recommended rewarming rates vary between 0.5° and 20° C/hr but should not exceed 0.55° C/hr in elderly persons.

2. Moderate to severe hypothermia:
   a. Active core rewarming
      (1) Delivery of heat via fluids: warm GI irrigation (with saline enemas and via NG tube); IV fluids (usually D_5NS without potassium) warmed to 104° to 107.6° F (40° to 42° C), peritoneal dialysis with dialysate heated to 40.5° to 42.5° C.
      (2) Inhalation of heated humidified oxygen
   b. Active external rewarming: immersion in a bath of warm water (40° to 41° C); active external rewarming may produce shock because of excessive peripheral vasodilation. Ideal candidates are previously healthy, young patients with acute immersion hypothermia.
   c. Extracorporeal blood warming with cardiopulmonary bypass appears to be an efficacious rewarming technique in young, otherwise healthy persons.

Author: **Fred F. Ferri, M.D.**

BASIC INFORMATION

■ DEFINITION
Hypothyroidism is a disorder caused by the inadequate secretion of thyroid hormone.

■ SYNONYMS
Myxedema

ICD-9CM CODES
244 Acquired hypothyroidism
243 Congenital hypothyroidism
244.1 Surgical hypothyroidism
244.3 Iatrogenic hypothyroidism
244.8 Pituitary hypothyroidism
246.1 Sporadic goitrous hypothyroidism

■ EPIDEMIOLOGY & DEMOGRAPHICS
INCIDENCE/PREVALENCE: 1.5% to 2% of women and 0.2% of men
PREDOMINANT AGE: Incidence of hypothyroidism increases with age; among persons older than 60 yr, 6% of women and 2.5% of men have laboratory evidence of hypothyroidism (TSH > twice normal).

■ PHYSICAL FINDINGS & CLINICAL PRESENTATION
- Hypothyroid patients generally present with the following signs and symptoms: fatigue, lethargy, weakness, constipation, weight gain, cold intolerance, muscle weakness, slow speech, slow cerebration with poor memory.
- Skin: dry, coarse, thick, cool, sallow (yellow color caused by carotenemia); nonpitting edema in skin of eyelids and hands (myxedema) secondary to infiltration of subcutaneous tissues by a hydrophilic mucopolysaccharide substance.
- Hair: brittle and coarse; loss of outer one third of eyebrows.
- Facies: dulled expression, thickened tongue, thick slow-moving lips.
- Thyroid gland: may or may not be palpable (depending on the cause of the hypothyroidism).
- Heart sounds: distant, possible pericardial effusion.
- Pulse: bradycardia.
- Neurologic: delayed relaxation phase of the DTRs, cerebellar ataxia, hearing impairment, poor memory, peripheral neuropathies with paresthesia.
- Musculoskeletal: carpal tunnel syndrome, muscular stiffness, weakness.

■ ETIOLOGY
PRIMARY HYPOTHYROIDISM (THYROID GLAND DYSFUNCTION): The cause of >90% of the cases of hypothyroidism
- Hashimoto's thyroiditis is the most common cause of hypothyroidism after 8 yr of age
- Idiopathic myxedema (nongoitrous form of Hashimoto's thyroiditis)
- Previous treatment of hyperthyroidism (radioiodine therapy, subtotal thyroidectomy)
- Subacute thyroiditis
- Radiation therapy to the neck (usually for malignant disease)
- Iodine deficiency or excess
- Drugs (lithium, PAS, sulfonamides, phenylbutazone, amiodarone, thiourea)
- Congenital (approximately 1 case per 4000 live births)
- Prolonged treatment with iodides

SECONDARY HYPOTHYROIDISM: Pituitary dysfunction, postpartum necrosis, neoplasm, infiltrative disease causing deficiency of TSH
TERTIARY HYPOTHYROIDISM: Hypothalamic disease (granuloma, neoplasm, or irradiation causing deficiency of TRH)
TISSUE RESISTANCE TO THYROID HORMONE: Rare

DIAGNOSIS

■ DIFFERENTIAL DIAGNOSIS
- Depression
- Dementia from other causes
- Systemic disorders (e.g., nephrotic syndrome, CHF, amyloidosis)

■ LABORATORY TESTS
- Increased TSH: TSH may be normal if patient has secondary or tertiary hypothyroidism, is receiving dopamine or corticosteroids, or the level is obtained following severe illness
- Decreased free T_4
- Other common laboratory abnormalities: hyperlipidemia, hyponatremia, and anemia
- Increased antimicrosomal and antithyroglobulin antibody titers: useful when autoimmune thyroiditis is suspected as the cause of the hypothyroidism

TREATMENT

■ NONPHARMACOLOGIC THERAPY
Patients should be educated regarding hypothyroidism and its possible complications. Patients should also be instructed about the need for lifelong treatment and monitoring of their thyroid abnormality.

■ ACUTE GENERAL Rx
- Start replacement therapy with levothyroxine (Synthroid, Levothroid) 25 to 100 µg/day, depending on the patient's age and the severity of the disease. The dose may be increased every 6 to 8 wk, depending on the clinical response and serum TSH level. Elderly patients and patients with coronary artery disease should be started with 12.5 to 25 µg/day (higher doses may precipitate angina). The average maintenance dose of levothyroxine is 1.7 µg/kg/day (100 to 150 µg/day in adults). The elderly may require <1 µg/kg/day, whereas children generally require higher doses (up to 3 to 4 µg/kg/day). Pregnant patients also have increased requirements. Estrogen therapy may also increase the need for thyroxine.
- After full replacement therapy with levothyroxine, the addition of triiodothyronine (0.0125 mg/day) may be beneficial in some patients with stable hypothyroidism who continue to have mood or memory problems. Recent trials have however failed to show an improvement with combination therapy.

■ CHRONIC Rx
- Periodic monitoring of TSH level is an essential part of treatment. Patients should be evaluated initially with office visit and TSH levels every 6 to 8 wk until the patient is clinically euthyroid and the TSH level is normalized. The frequency of subsequent visits and TSH measurement can then be decreased to every 6 to 12 mo. Pregnant patients should be checked every trimester.
- For monitoring therapy in patients with central hypothyroidism, measurement of serum free thyroxine (Free T_4 level) is appropriate and should be maintained in the upper half of the normal range.

■ REFERRAL
Admission to the hospital ICU is recommended in all patients with myxedema coma. Additional information on the diagnosis and treatment of this life-threatening complication of hypothyroidism is available in the topic "Myxedema Coma" in Section I.

✷ PEARLS & CONSIDERATIONS

■ COMMENTS
Subclinical hypothyroidism occurs in as many as 15% of elderly patients and is characterized by an elevated serum TSH and a normal free T_4 level. Treatment is individualized. Generally, replacement therapy is recommended for all patients with serum TSH >10 mU/L and with presence of goiter or thyroid autoantibodies.

REFERENCE
Walsh JP et al: Combined thyroxine/liothyronine treatment does not improve well being, quality of life, or cognitive function compared to thyroxine alone: a randomized controlled trial in patients with primary hypothyroidism, *J Clin Endocrinol Metab* 88:4543, 2003.
Author: **Fred F. Ferri, M.D.**

BASIC INFORMATION

DEFINITION
Specific form of fibrosing interstitial pneumonia referred to as visual interstitial pneumonia

SYNONYMS
Cryptogenetic fibrosing alveolitis
IPF

ICD-9CM CODES
516.3 Idiopathic pulmonary fibrosis

EPIDEMIOLOGY & DEMOGRAPHICS
- Presents in fifth and sixth decades and is slightly more common in men than women, mean age 66 yr
- 3% appear to cluster in families, but no clear evidence for a genetic basis
- No distinct geographic distribution, rural and urban, no prediction by race or ethnicity
- Cigarette smoking is strongly linked to idiopathic pulmonary fibrosis (IPF) and may be a cause

PHYSICAL FINDINGS & CLINICAL PRESENTATION
- Initial presentation is consistent and insidious exertional dyspnea and nonproductive cough. Over many months dyspnea is the most prominent symptom
- Associated symptoms such as fever and myalgia may be present but are not common and suggest another diagnosis
- Tachypnea to compensate for stiff noncompliant lung
- Physical examination shows fine bibasilar inspiratory crackles in more than 80% of patients, with progression upward as the disease advances
- Clubbing is seen in 25% to 50% of patients
- Cyanosis, corpulmonate, right ventricular heave, and peripheral edema may be seen
- Extrapulmonary involvement does not occur, but weight loss, malaise, and fatigue are noted

ETIOLOGY
- Unknown
- Numerous hypotheses, including contribution of environmental insults, such as metal and wood dust, infectious cause, chronic aspiration, or exposure to certain drugs

DIAGNOSIS

DIFFERENTIAL DIAGNOSIS
- Sarcoidosis and connective tissue disease with most similar clinical and pathologic presentations

- Other idiopathic interstitial pneumonias: desquamative interstitial pneumonia, respiratory bronchitis interstitial lung disease, acute interstitial pneumonia, nonspecific interstitial pneumonia, cryptogenic organizing pneumonia, bronchiolitis obliterans organizing pneumonia
It is very important to differentiate these from IPF pathologically because of an often better response to treatment
- Occupational exposures (e.g., asbestos, silica) may cause pneumoconiosis that mimics IDF

WORKUP
- Almost all patients have abnormal chest radiographs at presentation with bilateral reticular opacities most prominent in the periphery and lower lobes. Peripheral honeycombing may be seen.
- High-resolution CT scan shows patchy peripheral reticular abnormalities with intralobular linear opacities, irregular septal thickening, subplural honeycombing, and intractious bronchiectasis.
- Pulmonary function tests show restrictive impairment with reduced vital capacity and total lung capacity. An obstructive picture may also be as a result of the high prevalence of smoking.
- Laboratory abnormalities are mild and nonspecific. Mild anemia increases reactive proteins and LDH in ESR; low titers in ANA and RF are seen in up to 30% of patients.
- Limited role for bronchioalveolar lavage either in diagnosis or monitoring IPF. A lone increase in lymphocytes is uncommon, so if found, another diagnosis should be excluded.
- Gold standard for diagnosis is lung biopsy, which shows hallmark features of a heterogeneous distribution of parenchymal fibrous against a background of mild inflammation.
- Surgical lung biopsy by thoracotomy or video-assisted or thoracoscopic technique and of the options, the latter is preferred. Transbronchial lung biopsies do not provide a large enough sample to be helpful.
- Among experienced clinicians the combination of the clinical and radiographic features are often enough to establish the diagnosis.
- Lung biopsies are often not done because of other medical problems, especially severe COPD; however, they are critical to evaluate for the potential of a more treatable disease, especially in patients with any atypical features.

- The diagnosis will be missed in one third of new-onset IPF cases despite evaluations by experts with clinical diagnosis alone.

TREATMENT

- There is no proven treatment for IPF.
- Much of the focus has been on anti-inflammatory medications, especially steroids.
- Many studies that have evaluated treatment responses have grouped together several forms of idiopathic interstitial pneumonia under the IPF label.
- A trial of corticosteroids at 0.5 mg/kg × 4 wk, 0.25 mg/kg × 8 wk, then tapered down combined with azathioprine or cyclophosphamide for 3 to 6 mo is reasonable. 10% to 30% of patients may respond.
- This should only be continued if objective evidence such as improved PFT or distance able to ambulate is seen.
- Subjective improvement only may be a result of the mood-enhancing effects of the steroids.
- Complications of steroid use, especially infections, may be quite severe.
- Oral colchicine inhibits collagen formation and may be a reasonable agent to try.
  1. Much investigation into oral therapies, especially to inhibit fibrogenesis, is being done.
  2. Single lung transplantation should be considered, especially in younger, healthier patients.
- Interferon γ-1b has not been effective in IPF.

PEARLS & CONSIDERATIONS

- Spontaneous remissions do not occur
- The course is progressive with increasing fibrosis
- Mean survival after the diagnosis of biopsy-confirmed IPF is 3 yr
- 40% of patients die of respiratory failure
- The incidence of bronchiogenic carcinoma is increased

REFERENCE
Rachu G et al: A placebo-controlled trial of interferon gamma-1b in patients with idiopathic pulmonary fibrosis, *N Engl J Med* 350:12, 2004.
Author: **Lynn Bowlby, M.D.**

BASIC INFORMATION

■ DEFINITION

Immune thrombocytopenic purpura (ITP) is an autoimmune disorder characterized by a low platelet count and mucocutaneous bleeding.

■ SYNONYMS

ITP
Idiopathic thrombocytopenic purpura
Autoimmune thrombocytopenic purpura

ICD-9CM CODES

287.3 Idiopathic thrombocytopenic purpura (ITP)

■ EPIDEMIOLOGY & DEMOGRAPHICS

PREVALENCE: 5 to 10 cases/100,000 persons
INCIDENCE: 100 cases/1 million persons/yr
PREDOMINANT SEX: 72% of patients >10 yr old are female; in children, males = females
PREDOMINANT AGE: Children age 2 to 4 yr and young women (70% are <40 yr old)

■ PHYSICAL FINDINGS & CLINICAL PRESENTATION

The presentation of ITP is different in children and adults.
- Children generally present with sudden onset of bruising and petechiae from severe thrombocytopenia.
- In adults the presentation is insidious; a history of prolonged purpura may be present; many patients are diagnosed incidentally on the basis of automated laboratories that now routinely include platelet counts.
- The physical examination may be entirely normal.
- Patients with severe thrombocytopenia may have petechiae, purpura, epistaxis, or heme-positive stool from GI bleeding.
- Splenomegaly is unusual; its presence should alert to the possibility of other etiologies of thrombocytopenia.
- The presence of dysmorphic features (skeletal anomalies, auditory abnormalities) may indicate a congenital disorder as the etiology of the thrombocytopenia.

■ ETIOLOGY

Increased platelet destruction caused by autoantibodies to platelet-membrane antigens

DIAGNOSIS

■ DIFFERENTIAL DIAGNOSIS

- Falsely low platelet count (resulting from EDTA-dependent or cold-dependent agglutinins)
- Viral infections (e.g., HIV, mononucleosis, rubella)
- Drug-induced (e.g., heparin, quinidine, sulfonamides)
- Hypersplenism resulting from liver disease
- Myelodysplastic and lymphoproliferative disorders
- Pregnancy, hypothyroidism
- SLE, TTP, hemolytic-uremic syndrome
- Congenital thrombocytopenias (e.g., Fanconi's syndrome, May-Hegglin anomaly, Bernard-Soulier syndrome)

■ LABORATORY TESTS

- CBC, platelet count, and peripheral smear: platelets are decreased but are normal in size or may appear larger than normal. RBCs and WBCs have a normal morphology.
- Additional tests may be ordered to exclude other etiologies of the thrombocytopenia when clinically indicated (e.g., HIV, ANA, TSH, liver enzymes, bone marrow examination).
- The direct assay for the measurement of platelet-bound antibodies has an estimated positive predictive value of 80% to 83%. A negative test cannot be used to rule out the diagnosis.

■ IMAGING STUDIES

CT scan of abdomen in patients with splenomegaly to exclude other disorders causing thrombocytopenia

TREATMENT

■ NONPHARMACOLOGIC THERAPY

- Minimize activity to prevent injury or bruising (e.g., contact sports should be avoided).
- Avoid medications that increase the risk of bleeding (e.g., aspirin and other NSAIDs).

■ ACUTE GENERAL Rx

- Treatment varies with the platelet count, patient's age, and bleeding status.
- Observation and frequent monitoring of platelet count are needed in asymptomatic patients with platelet counts >30,000/mm³.
- Methylprednisolone 30 mg/kg/day IV infused over a period of 20 to 30 min (max dose of 1 g/day for 2 or 3 days) plus IV immunoglobulin (1 g/kg/day for 2 or 3 days) and infusion of platelets should be given to patients with neurologic symptoms, internal bleeding, or those undergoing emergency surgery.
- Prednisone 1 to 2 mg/kg qd, continued until the platelet count is normalized then slowly tapered off, is indicated in adults with platelet counts <20,000/mm³ and those who have counts <50,000/mm³ and significant mucous membrane bleeding. Response rates range from 50% to 75%, and most responses occur within the first 3 wk.
- High-dose immunoglobulins (IgG 0.4 g/kg/day IV, infused on 3 to 5 consecutive days) or high-dose parenteral glucocorticoids (methylprednisolone 30 mg/kg/day) can be used in children with platelet count <20,000/mm³ and significant bleeding or adults with severe thrombocytopenia or bleeding.
- Rituximab, a monoclonal antibody directed against the CD₂₀ antigen, has been reported useful for ITP patients resistant to conventional treatment and may help prevent serious or fatal bleeding.
- Platelet transfusion is needed only in case of life-threatening hemorrhage.
- Splenectomy should be considered in adults with platelet count <30,000/mm³ after 6 wk of medical treatment or after 6 mo if more than 10 to 20 mg of prednisone per day is required to maintain a platelet count >30,000/mm³. In children, splenectomy is generally reserved for persistent thrombocytopenia (>1 yr) and clinically significant bleeding. Appropriate immunizations (pneumococcal vaccine in adults and children, *H. influenzae* vaccine, meningococcal vaccine in children) should be administered before splenectomy.

■ CHRONIC Rx

Frequent monitoring of platelet count and symptom review in patients with chronic ITP to detect and prevent significant bleeding. A regimen of cyclophosphamide, vincristine, and prednisone (CVP) has been partially effective in chronic ITP.

■ DISPOSITION

- More than 80% of children have a complete remission within a few weeks.
- In adults, the course of the disease is chronic and only 5% of adults have spontaneous remission.
- The principal cause of death from ITP is intracranial hemorrhage (1% of children, 5% of adults).

REFERENCES

Cheng Y et al: Initial treatment of immune thrombocytopenic purpura with high dose dexamethasone, *N Engl J Med* 349:831, 2003.

Cines DB, Blanchette VS: Immune thrombocytopenic purpura, *N Engl J Med* 346:995, 2002.

Shanafelt TD et al: Rituximab for immune cytopenia in adults: idiopathic thrombocytopenic purpura, autoimmune hemolytic anemia, and Evans syndrome, *Mayo Clin Proc* 78:1340, 2003.

Zheng X et al: Remission of chronic TTP after treatment with cyclophosphamide and rituximab, *Ann Intern Med* 138:105, 2003.

Author: **Fred F. Ferri, M.D.**

BASIC INFORMATION

■ DEFINITION
Impetigo is a superficial skin infection generally secondary to *Staphylococcus aureus* and/or *Streptococcus* spp. Common presentations are bullous impetigo (generally secondary to staphylococcal disease) and nonbullous impetigo (secondary to streptococcal infection and possible staphylococcal infection); the bullous form is caused by an epidermolytic toxin produced at the site of infection.

■ SYNONYMS
Impetigo vulgaris
Pyoderma

ICD-9CM CODES
684 Impetigo

■ EPIDEMIOLOGY & DEMOGRAPHICS
- Bullous impetigo is most common in infants and children. The nonbullous form is most common in children ages 2 to 5 yr with poor hygiene in warm climates.
- The overall incidence of acute nephritis with impetigo varies between 2% and 5%.

■ PHYSICAL FINDINGS & CLINICAL PRESENTATION
- Multiple lesions with golden yellow crusts and weeping areas often found on the skin around the nose, mouth, and limbs (nonbullous impetigo) (Fig. 1-154).

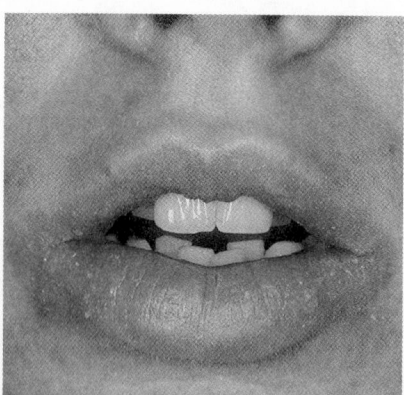

Fig. 1-154   Impetigo. Serum and crust at the angle of the mouth is a common presentation for impetigo. (From Habif TB: *Clinical dermatology: a color guide to diagnosis and therapy,* ed 3, St Louis, 1996, Mosby.)

- Presence of vesicles that enlarge rapidly to form bullae with contents that vary from clear to cloudy; there is subsequent collapse of the center of the bullae; the peripheral areas may retain fluid, and a honey-colored crust may appear in the center; as the lesions enlarge and become contiguous with the others, a scaling border replaces the fluid-filled rim (bullous impetigo); there is minimal erythema surrounding the lesions.
- Regional lymphadenopathy is most common with nonbullous impetigo.
- Constitutional symptoms are generally absent.

■ ETIOLOGY
- *S. aureus* coagulase positive is the dominant microorganism.
- *S. pyogenes* (group A β-hemolytic streptococci): M-T serotypes of this organism associated with acute nephritis are 2, 49, 55, 57, and 60.

DIAGNOSIS

■ DIFFERENTIAL DIAGNOSIS
- Acute allergic contact dermatitis
- Herpes simplex infection
- Ecthyma
- Folliculitis
- Eczema
- Insect bites
- Scabies
- Tinea corporis
- Pemphigus vulgaris and bullous pemphigoid
- Chickenpox

■ WORKUP
Diagnosis is clinical.

■ LABORATORY TESTS
- Generally not necessary
- Gram stain and C&S to confirm the diagnosis when the clinical presentation is unclear
- Sedimentation rate parallel to activity of the disease
- Increased anti-DNAse B and anti-hyaluronidase
- Urinalysis revealing hematuria with erythrocyte casts and proteinuria in patients with acute nephritis (most frequently occurring in children between 2 and 4 yr of age in the southern part of the U.S.)

TREATMENT

■ NONPHARMACOLOGIC THERAPY
Remove crusts by soaking with wet cloth compresses (crusts block the penetration of antibacterial creams).

■ GENERAL Rx
- Application of 2% mupirocin ointment (Bactroban) tid for 10 days to the affected area or until all lesions have cleared.
- Oral antibiotics are used in severe cases: commonly used agents are dicloxacillin 250 mg qid for 7 to 10 days, cephalexin 250 mg qid for 7 to 10 days, or azithromycin 500 mg on day 1, 250 mg on days 2 through 5.
- Impetigo can be prevented by prompt application of mupirocin or triple antibiotic ointment (bacitracin, Polysporin, and neomycin) to sites of skin trauma.
- Patients who are carriers of *S. aureus* in their nares should be treated with mupirocin ointment applied to their nares bid for 5 days.
- Fingernails should be kept short, and patients should be advised not to scratch any lesions to avoid spread of infection.

■ DISPOSITION
Most cases of impetigo resolve promptly with appropriate treatment. Both bullous and nonbullous forms of impetigo heal without scarring.

■ REFERRAL
Nephrology referral in patients with acute nephritis

PEARLS & CONSIDERATIONS

■ COMMENTS
- Patients should be instructed on use of antibacterial soaps and avoidance of sharing of towels and washcloths, because impetigo is extremely contagious.
- Children attending day care should be removed until 48 to 72 hr after initiation of antibiotic treatment.

Author: **Fred F. Ferri, M.D.**

BASIC INFORMATION

■ DEFINITION
Inappropriate secretion of antidiuretic hormone (SIADH) is a syndrome characterized by excessive secretion of ADH in absence of normal osmotic or physiologic stimuli (increased serum osmolarity, decreased plasma volume, hypotension).

■ SYNONYMS
SIADH

ICD-9CM CODES
276.9 Inappropriate secretion of antidiuretic hormone

■ EPIDEMIOLOGY & DEMOGRAPHICS
Nearly 50% of hyponatremia detected in the hospital setting is caused by SIADH.

■ PHYSICAL FINDINGS & CLINICAL PRESENTATION
- The patient is generally normovolemic or slightly hypervolemic; edema is absent.
- Delirium, lethargy, and seizures may be present if the hyponatremia is severe or of rapid onset.
- Manifestations of the underlying disease may be evident (e.g., fever from an infectious process or headaches and visual field defects from an intracranial mass).
- Diminished reflexes and extensor plantar responses may occur with severe hyponatremia.

■ ETIOLOGY
- Neoplasm: lung, duodenum, pancreas, brain, thymus, bladder, prostate, mesothelioma, lymphoma, Ewing's sarcoma
- Pulmonary disorders: pneumonia, TB, bronchiectasis, emphysema, status asthmaticus
- Intracranial pathology: trauma, neoplasms, infections (meningitis, encephalitis, brain abscess), hemorrhage, hydrocephalus
- Postoperative period: surgical stress, ventilators with positive pressure, anesthetic agents
- Drugs: chlorpropamide, thiazide diuretics, vasopressin, desmopressin, oxytocin, chemotherapeutic agents (vincristine, vinblastine, cyclophosphamide), carbamazepine, phenothiazines, MAO inhibitors, tricyclic antidepressants, narcotics, nicotine, clofibrate, haloperidol, SSRIs
- Other: acute intermittent porphyria, Guillain-Barré syndrome, myxedema, psychosis, delirium tremens, ACTH deficiency (hypopituitarism)

DIAGNOSIS

■ DIFFERENTIAL DIAGNOSIS
- Hyponatremia associated with hypervolemia (CHF, cirrhosis, nephrotic syndrome)
- Factitious hyponatremia (hyperglycemia, abnormal proteins, hyperlipidemia)
- Hypovolemia associated with hypovolemia (e.g., burns, GI fluid loss)

■ WORKUP
- Demonstration through laboratory evaluation (see Laboratory Tests) of excessive secretion of ADH in absence of appropriate osmotic or physiologic stimuli
- Demonstration of normal thyroid, adrenal, and cardiac function
- No recent or concurrent use of diuretics

■ LABORATORY TESTS
- Hyponatremia
- Urinary osmolarity > serum osmolarity
- Urinary sodium usually >30 mEq/L
- Normal BUN, creatinine (indicative of normal renal function and absence of dehydration)
- Decreased uric acid

■ IMAGING STUDIES
Chest x-ray examination to rule out neoplasm or infectious process

TREATMENT

■ NONPHARMACOLOGIC THERAPY
Fluid restriction to 500 to 800 ml/day

■ ACUTE GENERAL Rx
In emergency situations (seizures, coma) SIADH can be treated with combination of hypertonic saline solution (slow infusion of 250 ml of 3% NaCl) and furosemide; this increases the serum sodium by causing diuresis of urine that is more dilute than plasma; the rapidity of correction varies depending on the degree of hyponatremia and if the hyponatremia is acute or chronic; generally the serum sodium should be corrected only halfway to normal in the initial 24 hr and serum sodium should be increased by <0.5 mEq/L/hr.

■ CHRONIC Rx
- Depending on the underlying etiology, fluid restriction may be needed indefinitely. Monthly monitoring of electrolytes is recommended in patients with chronic SIADH.
- Demeclocycline (Declomycin) 300 to 600 mg PO bid may be useful in patients with chronic SIADH (e.g., secondary to neoplasm), but use with caution in patients with hepatic disease; its side effects include nephrogenic DI and photosensitivity. This medication is also very expensive.

■ DISPOSITION
- Prognosis varies depending on the cause. Generally prognosis is benign when SIADH is caused by an infectious process.
- Morbidity and mortality are high (>40%) when serum sodium concentration is <110 mEq/L.

■ REFERRAL
Hospital admission depending on severity of symptoms and degree of hyponatremia

PEARLS & CONSIDERATIONS

■ COMMENTS
- Use of hypertonic (3%) saline is contraindicated in patients with CHF, nephrotic syndrome, or cirrhosis.
- Too rapid correction of hyponatremia can cause demyelination and permanent CNS damage.

Author: **Fred F. Ferri, M.D.**

BASIC INFORMATION

■ DEFINITION
Inclusion body myositis (IBM) refers to a chronic idiopathic inflammatory myopathy with characteristics similar to polymyositis and dermatomyositis.

■ SYNONYMS
Idiopathic inflammatory myopathy

ICD-9CM CODES
729.1 Myositis

■ EPIDEMIOLOGY & DEMOGRAPHICS
- Incidence is 1/100,000 cases
- More common in men than in women (3:1)
- More common in whites than in blacks
- Usually affects persons over the age of 50 yr
- Associated with autoimmune diseases in up to 15% of the cases

■ PHYSICAL FINDINGS & CLINICAL PRESENTATION
- Most patients with IBM develop insidiously
- Usually presents with symmetric proximal muscle weakness but can be asymmetric and involve distal muscles as well (e.g., foot extensors and finger flexors)
- Patients have difficulties with buttoning a shirt, sewing, and typing
- IBM may specifically involve the quadriceps, iliopsoas, triceps, and biceps muscles
- Early loss of patellar reflex
- Like polymyositis and dermatomyositis, IBM can involve the upper esophageal muscle leading to dysphagia, aspiration, and respiratory distress

■ ETIOLOGY
The cause of IBM is not known but is believed to be a cell-mediated immune response directed against muscle fibers.

DIAGNOSIS

The diagnosis of inclusion body myositis is made by:
- History and physical findings of both proximal and distal muscle weakness
- Elevated muscle enzymes
- EMG abnormalities suggesting a myopathic process
- Muscle biopsy confirmation

■ DIFFERENTIAL DIAGNOSIS
- Polymyositis
- Muscular dystrophy
- Diabetic neuropathy
- Trichinosis
- AIDS
- Alcoholic myopathy
- Hypothyroidism
- Hypophosphatemia
- Myasthenia gravis, Eaton-Lambert syndrome
- Amyotrophic lateral sclerosis
- Guillain-Barré syndrome

■ WORKUP
Patients suspected of having IBM by clinical presentation should have an EMG, muscle biopsy, and specific blood tests to confirm the diagnosis.

■ LABORATORY TESTS
- ESR, although not specific, is elevated in the majority of cases.
- Creatine kinase is the most sensitive muscle enzyme test and can be elevated as much as 10 times above normal. In some cases of IBM, the CPK may be normal.
- Aldolase, AST, ALT, alkaline phosphatase, and LDH can be elevated.
- Anti-Jo-1 antibodies are more common in polymyositis than IBM.
- Electrolytes, TSH, Ca, and Mg should be requested to exclude other causes.
- Electromyography (EMG) is abnormal in 90% of patients and distinguishes a myopathic from neuropathic process.
- Muscle biopsy is the definitive test showing pathognomonic inclusion granules in the cytoplasm along with small "rimmed vacuoles."

■ IMAGING STUDIES
- A chest x-ray to rule out pulmonary involvement. If suspicious for pulmonary interstitial disease, a high-resolution CT scan of the chest may be helpful
- A barium swallow to look for upper esophageal dysfunction in patients with dysphagia and IBM
- MRI can help to locate sites of muscle involvement

TREATMENT

What distinguishes IBM from the other two inflammatory myopathies (polymyositis and dermatomyositis) is its lack of responsiveness to immunosuppressive treatment.

■ NONPHARMACOLOGIC THERAPY
- Physical therapy is beneficial in increasing muscle tone and strength

- Occupational therapy to assist with activities of daily living
- Speech therapy for dysphagia and swallowing problems

■ ACUTE GENERAL Rx
- Up to 90% of patients with dermatomyositis and polymyositis respond to corticosteroids. Patients with IBM generally are resistant to therapy.
- Prednisone 1 to 2 mg/kg/day for 6 mo can still be given as a therapeutic trial in patients with IBM.

■ CHRONIC Rx
- Azathioprine, methotrexate, and immunoglobulins have all been tried in patients with IBM but with little effect, if any.

■ DISPOSITION
Inclusion body myositis usually progresses slowly over years.

■ REFERRAL
Whenever the diagnosis of inflammatory myopathy is suspected and specifically inclusion body myositis, a rheumatologist and neurologist should be consulted for assistance.

PEARLS & CONSIDERATIONS

■ COMMENTS
- Inclusion body myositis is often incorrectly diagnosed as polymyositis.
- Features distinguishing IBM from polymyositis are:
  1. IBM involves distal as well as proximal muscles.
  2. IBM can be asymmetric and selectively involve quadriceps muscle.
  3. Inclusion bodies on muscle biopsy of patients with IBM.
  4. IBM is resistant to immunosuppressants.
- Unlike dermatomyositis, there is no associated increase risk of malignancy in patients with IBM.

REFERENCES
Amato AA et al: Inclusion body myositis: clinical and pathological boundaries, *Ann Neurol* 40:581, 1996.
Askansas V, Engel WK: Inclusion-body myositis and myopathies: different etiologies, possible similar pathogenic mechanisms, *Curr Opin Neurol* 15(5):525, 2002.
Hilton-Jones D: Inflammatory muscle diseases, *Curr Opin Neurol* 14(5):591, 2001.
Author: **Peter Petropoulos, M.D.**

BASIC INFORMATION

■ DEFINITION
Incontinence is the involuntary loss of urine.

ICD-9CM CODES
788.3 Incontinence
625.6 Stress incontinence
788.33 Mixed stress and urge incontinence
788.32 Male incontinence
788.39 Neurogenic incontinence
307.6 Nonorganic origin

■ EPIDEMIOLOGY & DEMOGRAPHICS
INCIDENCE AND PREVALENCE: In the general population between the ages of 15 and 64 yr, 1.5% to 5% of men and 10% to 25% of women will suffer from incontinence. In the nursing home population, 50% of the population suffers some degree of incontinence. Nearly 20% of children through the midteenage years have episodes of urinary incontinence.

■ CLINICAL, PSYCHOLOGIC, & SOCIAL IMPACT
Less than 50% of the individuals with incontinence living in the community consult health care providers, preferring to "suffer silently," turning to "home remedies," commercially available absorbent materials, and supportive aids. As their condition worsens, they become depressed, sacrifice their independence, suffer from recurrent urinary tract infection and its sequelae, limit their social interaction, refrain from sexual intimacy, and become homebound. In terms of costs, for all ages living in the community, it is estimated that $7 billion is spent for incontinence annually.

■ MAJOR TYPES OF INCONTINENCE
TRANSIENT INCONTINENCE: Incontinence occurring as a result or reaction to an acute medical problem affecting the lower urinary tract. Many of these problems can be reversed with treatment of the underlying problem.
URGE INCONTINENCE: Involuntary loss of urine associated with an abrupt and strong desire to void. It is usually associated with involuntary detrusor contractions on urodynamic investigation. In *neurologically impaired patients,* the involuntary detrusor contraction is referred to as *detrusor hyperreflexia.* In *neurologically normal patients* the involuntary contraction is called *detrusor instability.*

STRESS INCONTINENCE: The involuntary loss of urine with physical activities that increase abdominal pressure in the absence of a detrusor contraction or an overdistended bladder. Classification of stress incontinence:
Type 0: Complaint of incontinence without demonstration of leakage
Type I: Incontinence in response to stress but little descent of the bladder neck and urethra
Type II: Incontinence in response to stress with >2 cm descent of the bladder neck and urethra
Type III: Bladder neck and urethra wide open without bladder contraction; intrinsic sphincter deficiency; and denervation of the urethra. The most common causes: urethral hypermobility and displacement of the bladder neck with exertion, intrinsic sphincter deficiency from failed antiincontinence surgery, prostatectomy, radiation, cord lesions, epispadias, or myelomeningocele.
OVERFLOW INCONTINENCE: Loss of urine resulting from overdistention of the bladder with resultant "overflow" or "spilling" of the urine. Causes: hypotonic-to-atonic bladder resulting from drug effect, fecal impaction, or neurologic conditions such as diabetes, spinal cord injury, surgery, vitamin B$_{12}$ deficiency. It is also caused by obstruction at the bladder neck and urethra. In this situation, prostatism, prostatic cancer, urethral stenosis, antiincontinence surgery, pelvic prolapse, and detrusor-sphincter dyssynergia cause the incontinence.
FUNCTIONAL INCONTINENCE:
Involuntary loss of urine resulting from chronic impairments of physical and/or cognitive functioning. This is a diagnosis of exclusion. The condition can sometimes be improved or cured by improving the patient's functional status, treating comorbidities, changing medications, reducing environmental barriers, etc.
MIXED STRESS AND URGE INCONTINENCE
SENSORY URGENCY INCONTINENCE: Involuntary loss of urine as a result of decreased bladder compliance and increased intravesical pressures accompanied by severe urgency and bladder hypersensitivity without detrusor overactivity. This is seen with radiation cystitis, interstitial cystitis, eosinophilic cystitis, myelomeningocele, and radical pelvic surgery. Nephropathy can occur as a complication of this vesicoureteral reflux.

SPHINCTERIC INCONTINENCE:
Urethral Hypermobility: The basic abnormality is a weakness of pelvic floor support. Because of this weakness, during increases in abdominal pressure there is rotational descent of the vesical neck and proximal urethra. If the urethra opens concomitantly, stress urinary incontinence ensues. Urethral hypermobility is often present in women who are not incontinent. Its mere presence is not sufficient evidence to make the diagnosis of sphincteric abnormality unless incontinence is shown.
Intrinsic Sphincter Deficiency: There is an intrinsic malfunction of the sphincter itself. It is characterized by an open vesical neck at rest and a low leak point pressure (<65 cm water). Urethral hypermobility and intrinsic sphincter deficiency may coexist in the same patient. Causes of intrinsic sphincter deficiency are previous pelvic surgery, antiincontinence surgery, urethral diverticulectomy, radical hysterectomy, abdominoperineal resection of the rectum, urethrotomy, Y-V plasty of the vesical neck, myelodysplasia, anterior spinal artery syndrome, lumbo-sacral disease, aging, and hyperestrogenism.

DIAGNOSIS

■ HISTORY
- History of present illness, psychosocial factors, congenital disorders, access issues for the physically challenged, neurologic disorders, and disorders pertinent to the urologic tract
- Review of prescription and nonprescription medications
- Voiding diary to assess total voided volume, frequency of micturition, mean volume voided, largest single volume, diurnal distribution, nature and severity of incontinence

■ WORKUP
- Physical examination including general examination, gait of the patient (neuromuscular deficits), estrogen status, vaginal examination to include the periurethral region, evaluation for cystocele, rectocele, and enterocele
- Pelvic floor strength assessment
- Rectal examination to assess sphincter tone and bulbocavernosus reflex
- Neurologic examination
- Postvoid residual check using bladder scan or catheter

■ **LABORATORY TESTS**

Urinalysis, urine culture, urine cytology, BUN, and creatinine

■ **IMAGING STUDIES**

• KUB to assess bony skeleton
• IVP to rule out upper tract abnormalities, developmental anomalies, bladder configuration, and fistula
• Renal ultrasound if dye study is contraindicated

■ **SPECIALIZED STUDIES**

Simple cystometrogram, complex urodynamics including leak point pressures and uroflowmetry, endoscopic evaluation, and cystogram

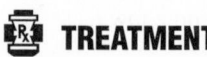 **TREATMENT**

■ **TRANSIENT INCONTINENCE**

Treatment of underlying medical conditions and behavioral therapy to include habit training and timed voiding

■ **URGE INCONTINENCE**

Bladder relaxants (i.e., tolterodine [Detrol], oxybutynin [Ditropan], imipramine), estrogen, biofeedback, Kegel exercises, and surgical removal of obstructing or other pathologic lesions

■ **STRESS INCONTINENCE**

• Pelvic floor exercises, Kegel exercises, α-adrenergic agonists (i.e., ephedrine), estrogen, biofeedback
CYSTOURETHROPEXY: Marshall-Marchetti-Krantz procedure, Burch procedure, Raz procedure, Stamey-Raz procedure, Gittes procedure, in situ

transvaginal sling, pubovaginal sling with autologous or cadaver graft, laparoscopic Burch procedure, laparoscopic sling, tension-free vaginal tape (TVT)

• For intrinsic sphincter deficiency: bulking agents (e.g., collagen), sling, and artificial sphincter

■ **OVERFLOW INCONTINENCE**

Surgical removal of any obstructing lesions, clean intermittent catheterization, and indwelling catheter

■ **FUNCTIONAL INCONTINENCE**

Behavioral training to include habit training and timed voiding, incontinence undergarments and pads, external collecting devices, and environmental manipulation

■ **MIXED URGENCY AND STRESS INCONTINENCE**

Use of measures recommended in the management of stress and urge incontinence

■ **SENSORY URGENCY**

Bladder relaxants (e.g., anticholinergics, muscle relaxants, and tricyclic antidepressants), behavior therapy to include habit training and timed voiding, cystoscopy and hydrodilation

■ **SPHINCTERIC DEFICIENCY**

Urethral bulking agents, sling procedure, artificial sphincter, mechanical clamp, and external collection devices

✿ **PEARLS & CONSIDERATIONS**

■ **COMMENTS**

Other forms of incontinence:
NOCTURNAL ENURESIS: (ICD-9CM Code: 788.3) Can be caused by sphincter abnormalities and detrusor overactivity; can occur as idiopathic, neurogenic, and with outlet obstruction
POSTVOID DRIBBLE: (ICD-9CM Code: 599.2) A postsphincteric collection of urine that is seen with urethral diverticulum and can be idiopathic
EXTRAURETHRAL INCONTINENCE: Enterovesical (ICD-9CM Codes: 596.1 and 596.2), Urethral (ICD-9CM Code: 599.1), also known as fistula
CONDITIONS THAT PREDISPOSE TO SURGICAL FAILURE: Advanced age, postmenopausal state, hysterectomy, prior failed incontinence surgery, concurrent detrusor instability, abnormal perineal electromyography, pelvic radiation

REFERENCES

Burgio UL et al: Behavioral vs. drug treatment for urge urinary incontinence in older women: a randomized controlled trial, *JAMA* 280:1995, 1998.

Holroyd-Leduc J, Straus SE: Management of urinary incontinence in women, *JAMA* 291:996, 2004.

U.S. Department of Health and Human Services, Public Health Service, Agency for Health Care Policy and Research: *Clinical practice guideline: urinary incontinence in adults,* Rockville, Md, 1996, US Department of Health and Human Services.

Author: **Philip J. Aliotta, M.D., M.S.H.A.**

BASIC INFORMATION

■ DEFINITION
Influenza is an acute febrile illness caused by infection with influenza type A or B virus.

■ SYNONYMS
Flu

ICD-9CM CODES
487.1 Influenza

■ EPIDEMIOLOGY & DEMOGRAPHICS
INCIDENCE (IN U.S.): Annual incidence of influenza-related deaths is approximately 20,000 deaths/yr
PREDOMINANT SEX: Male = female
PREDOMINANT AGE: Attack rates are higher among children than adults, although children are less prone to develop pulmonary complications
PEAK INCIDENCE: Winter outbreaks lasting 5 to 6 wk

■ PHYSICAL FINDINGS & CLINICAL PRESENTATION
- "Classic flu" is characterized by abrupt onset of fever, headache, myalgias, anorexia, and malaise after a 1- to 2-day incubation period.
- Clinical syndromes are similar to those produced by other respiratory viruses, including pharyngitis, common colds, tracheobronchitis, bronchiolitis, croup.
- Respiratory symptoms such as cough, sore throat, and nasal discharge are usually present at the onset of illness, but systemic symptoms predominate.
- Elderly patients may experience fever, weakness, and confusion without any respiratory complaints.
- Acute deterioration to status asthmaticus may occur in patients with asthma.
- Influenza pneumonia: rapidly progressive cough, dyspnea, and cyanosis may occur after typical flu onset.

■ ETIOLOGY
- Variation in the surface antigens of the influenza virus, hemagglutinin (HA) and neuraminidase (NA), leading to infection with variants to which resistance is inadequate in the population at risk

- Transmitted by small-particle aerosols and deposited on the respiratory tract epithelium

DIAGNOSIS

■ DIFFERENTIAL DIAGNOSIS
- Respiratory syncytial virus, adenovirus, parainfluenza virus infection
- Secondary bacterial pneumonia or mixed bacterial-viral pneumonia

■ WORKUP
- Virus isolation from nasal or throat swab or sputum specimens is the most rapid diagnostic method in the setting of acute illness.
- Specimens are placed into virus transport medium and processed by a reference laboratory.
- For serologic diagnosis:
  1. Paired serum specimens, acute and convalescent, the latter obtained 10 to 20 days later
  2. Fourfold rises or falls in the titer of antibodies (various techniques) considered diagnostic of recent infection

■ LABORATORY TESTS
Septic syndrome presentation: CBC, ABG analysis, blood cultures

■ IMAGING STUDIES
- Chest x-ray examination to demonstrate findings of viral pneumonia: peribronchial and patchy interstitial infiltrates in multiple lobes with atelectasis
- Possible progression to diffuse interstitial pneumonitis

TREATMENT

■ NONPHARMACOLOGIC THERAPY
- Bed rest
- Hydration

■ ACUTE GENERAL Rx
- Supportive care: antipyretics—*Avoid use of aspirin in children because of the association with Reye's syndrome*
- Antibiotics if bacterial pneumonia is proven or suspected

- Amantadine (100 mg PO bid for children >10 yr and adults <65 yr; once daily in patients >65 yr) and rimantadine (same dose schedule as amantadine)
  1. Further dose adjustments needed with renal insufficiency
  2. Fewer CNS side effects with rimantadine
- Neuraminidase inhibitors block release of virions from infected cells, resulting in shortened duration of symptoms and decrease in complications; effective against both influenza A and B
  1. Zanamivir, administered via inhaler, 10 mg bid
  2. Oseltamivir, administered orally
- Placebo-controlled studies have suggested that antiviral therapy with any of the above mentioned agents must be initiated within 1 to 2 days of the onset of symptoms and reduces the duration of illness by approximately 1 day

■ DISPOSITION
Patients are hospitalized if signs of pneumonia are present.

■ REFERRAL
Infectious disease and/or pulmonary consultation when influenza pneumonia is suspected

PEARLS & CONSIDERATIONS

■ COMMENTS
- Prevention of influenza in patients at high risk is an important goal of primary care.
- Vaccines reduce the risk of infection and the severity of illness.
  1. Antigenic composition of the vaccine is updated annually.
  2. Vaccination should be given at the start of the flu season (October) for the following groups:
     a. Adults ≥65 yr
     b. Adults and children with chronic cardiac or pulmonary disease, including asthma
     c. Adults and children with illness requiring frequent follow-up (e.g., hemoglobinopathies, diabetes mellitus)
     d. Children receiving long-term aspirin therapy

e. Immunocompromised patients
f. Household contacts of persons in the previous groups
g. Health-care workers
3. Only contraindication to vaccination is hypersensitivity to hen's eggs.
4. Special efforts should be made to vaccinate high-risk patients <65 yr, only 10% to 15% of whom are vaccinated each year.
- Chemoprophylaxis:
  1. Amantadine and rimantadine approved for prophylaxis against influenza A; they are ineffective against influenza B
  2. Consider:
     a. For high-risk patients in whom vaccination is contraindicated
     b. When the available vaccine is known not to include the circulating strain
     c. To provide added protection to immunosuppressed patients likely to have a diminished response to vaccination
     d. In the setting of an outbreak, when immediate protection of unvaccinated or recently vaccinated patients is desired
  3. Give for 2 wk in the case of late vaccination and for the duration of the flu season in all other patients

REFERENCES

Colgan R et al: Antiviral drugs in the immunocompetent host: part II. Treatment of influenza and respiratory syncytial virus infections, *Am Fam Physician* 67(4):763, 2003.

Montalto NJ: An office-based approach to influenza: clinical diagnosis and laboratory testing, *Am Fam Physician* 67(1):111, 2003.

Author: **Claudia L. Dade, M.D.**

BASIC INFORMATION

■ DEFINITION
Insemination is a therapeutic intervention designed to overcome defects preventing achieving proper concentration of functional sperm cells in the vicinity of the egg.

■ SYNONYMS
Artificial insemination

ICD-9CM CODES
606.0 Irreversible azoospermia
Husband's carrier status for genetic disease such as:
  303.1 Tay-Sachs
  286.0 Hemophilia
  333.4 Huntington's disease
  758.9 Chromosomal abnormalities
  773.0 Severe Rh disease
608.89.1 Husband's sperm frozen before orchidectomy
606.8 Husband's sperm frozen before radiation or chemotherapy

■ ETIOLOGY
See ICD-9CM Codes.

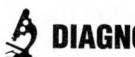

DIAGNOSIS

■ DIFFERENTIAL DIAGNOSIS
See ICD-9CM Codes.

■ WORKUP
Male: refer to urologist; ascertain that azoospermia is indeed irreversible. Individuals who were considered intractable in the recent past can now produce pregnancies with intracytoplasmic sperm injections (ICSI), even with cells obtained by testicular biopsy. Such an option should be offered to the patient before recommending a donor.

■ LABORATORY TESTS
• Testing of both partners for hepatitis, HIV, and other STDs is recommended before donor inseminations.
• Female: as described in the topic "Therapeutic Insemination (Husband/Partner)" for general infertility workup.

■ IMAGING STUDIES
As described in the topic "Therapeutic Insemination (Husband/Partner)" for general infertility workup.

TREATMENT

■ NONPHARMACOLOGIC THERAPY
SPERM SOURCE: *Use of fresh donor semen is no longer acceptable.* Semen is obtained from state-certified "sperm banks" adhering to the proper routines of donor screening for genetic and infectious diseases, and quarantining the sperm for at least 6 mo. Sperm can be shipped from the bank in containers that will maintain the sample in a frozen state for 48 hr. After this time the sample has to be transferred to another liquid nitrogen storage tank.
SPERM PREPARATION: Sperm is removed from the liquid nitrogen and allowed to thaw at room temperature, or is thawed per sperm bank instructions. Refer to "Therapeutic Insemination (Husband/Partner)" in Section I for insemination techniques. If sperm supply is not limited and the woman's age is not a factor (<35 yr), simple applications of thawed semen to the external cervical os are usually undertaken first.

■ DISPOSITION
In healthy women <34 yr of age, fecundity of approximately 10% per cycle can be expected. Fertility is age dependent. After 12 cycles, expect 75% pregnancy for women <34 yr of age.

PEARLS & CONSIDERATIONS

■ COMMENTS
• Risks: infections with STDs, including AIDS, although rare, have been reported as a result of donor semen insemination.
• Caution: observe laws applicable in the state and obtain proper consents.
• Caution: before declaring the male azoospermic, centrifuge the semen and examine sediment; several sperm cells missed on "plain" microscopic examination may suffice for ICSI.

REFERENCES

Guzick DS et al: Sperm morphology, motility, and concentration in fertile and infertile men, *N Engl J Med* 345:1388, 2001.
Hansen M et al: The risk of major birth defects after intracytoplasmic sperm injection and in vitro fertilization, *N Engl J Med* 346:725, 2002.
Schieve L et al: Low and very low birth weight in infants conceived with use of assisted reproductive technology, *N Engl J Med* 346:731, 2002.
Speroff L, Glass RH, Kase NG: *Clinical gynecologic endocrinology and infertility,* ed 6, Baltimore, 1999, Lippincott Williams & Wilkins.

Author: **John M. Wieckowski, M.D., Ph.D.**

BASIC INFORMATION

■ DEFINITION
Insemination is a therapeutic intervention designed to overcome defects preventing achieving proper concentration of functional sperm cells in the vicinity of the egg.

■ SYNONYMS
Artificial insemination

ICD-9CM CODES
628.9 Infertility (female unspecified)
606.9 Infertility (male unspecified)
302.7 Sexual/erectile dysfunction
625.1 Vaginismus
752.6 Hypospadias
792.2 Asthenospermia
606.1 Oligospermia

■ EPIDEMIOLOGY & DEMOGRAPHICS
Approximately 15% of couples experience infertility.

■ ETIOLOGY
MALE:
- Hypospadias: congenital
- Sexual/erectile dysfunction: psychogenic, vascular, neurogenic
- Asthenospermia: idiopathic, varicocele, status post vasectomy reversal, environmental (toxins, heavy metals, heat exposure, trauma to testicles)
- Antisperm antibodies, unknown, trauma to testicles, vasectomy

FEMALE:
- Cervical mucus hostility: unknown, infection
- Antisperm antibodies: unknown
- Idiopathic infertility: unknown

DIAGNOSIS

■ DIFFERENTIAL DIAGNOSIS
- Diagnosis of infertility is established by a history of 1 yr of unprotected intercourse without conception.
- Establish male vs. female infertility, or combined.
- Male: rule out congenital abnormalities, varicocele, endocrine defects.
- Female: rule out ovulatory dysfunction, tubal factors, uterine defects, endometriosis.

■ WORKUP
- Male routine: urologic examination, semen analysis
- Specialized (if indicated): sonography, vasogram, Doppler studies, testicular biopsy
- Female routine: gynecologic examination, establish ovulatory pattern by basal body temperature or endometrial biopsy
- Postcoital test
- Specialized (if indicated): diagnostic/therapeutic laparoscopy

■ LABORATORY TESTS
- Male routine: semen analysis; specialized (if indicated): antisperm antibodies, endocrine studies, testicular biopsy
- Female routine: blood type, rubella immunity, hepatitis immunity
- Selectively (>35 yr or as indicated by history): day 3 of the cycle, test FSH, LH, and estradiol to rule out occult ovarian failure, polycystic ovarian syndrome (LH/FSH inversion); androgen levels if hirsutism present; prolactin level if galactorrhea; thyroid studies if clinically indicated; anti-*Chlamydia* antibodies if tubal damage suspected or history of IUD use

■ IMAGING STUDIES
- Hysterosalpingogram: rule out hydrosalpinx, salpingitis isthmica nodosa, intramural tubal polyps, intrauterine synechiae, or polyps
- Pelvic sonography: in midcycle to rule out myomas, endometrial polyps, endometrial hypoplasia, ovarian pathology (cysts, endometriomas), or confirm dominant follicle formation
- Pituitary MRI if tumor suspected

TREATMENT

■ NONPHARMACOLOGIC THERAPY
Type of insemination depends on the nature of the fertility defect and varies in depth to which the sperm cells are delivered into the female genital tract. The following types of inseminations may be done:
- Cervical and endocervical insemination
- Intrauterine insemination
- Intratubal insemination
- Cul-de-sac insemination
- Intrafollicular insemination
- In vitro fertilization (IVF)
- IVF with intracytoplasmic sperm injection (ICSI)

Only the cervical and intrauterine inseminations can be done in a primary care setting.

CERVICAL AND INTRACERVICAL INSEMINATION: This method is indicated when normal coital sperm delivery to the cervix is prevented (e.g., coital dysfunction and hypospadias).
Semen Preparation: None; whole semen is used.
Technique: Semen is delivered to the external os or endocervical canal using a syringe with soft-tipped cannula. Cervical cap, which prolongs the contact of semen with the cervix, can be used to overcome high semen viscosity.

INTRAUTERINE INSEMINATION (IUI): This method is used for the following reasons (listed in order of decreasing effectiveness):
- Cervical mucus hostility caused by poor mucus production or quality (idiopathic or iatrogenic, such as status postcervical conization, laser treatment, etc.)
- Antisperm antibodies
- Empirical treatment for unexplained infertility
- Mild male factor defects, such as oligospermia, high semen viscosity, high or low seminal volume

Semen Preparation: Seminal fluid should not be introduced into the uterine cavity. Sperm cells have to be separated from the seminal fluid by the process of sperm "washing," and resuspended in a protein-containing medium (5% to 10% serum or synthetic serum substitute), to endow the cells with proper motility. Method that can be used without the necessity of having incubator involves centrifugation of semen through a density gradient and resuspending the pellet in the protein-containing medium. Media for the previous procedures, with or without antibiotics, are commercially available from several sources.

Technique: Internal cervical os is negotiated with one of the various commercially available "insemination catheters" and the "washed" sperm suspension is delivered to the endometrial cavity. Timing: basal body temperature graphs, cervical mucus observation, testing of urine for LH surge, or serial sonography is often used for detecting ovulation. Cervical insemination should be performed within 24 hr before anticipated ovulation. Timing of IUI should be within a few hours of ovulation, preferably before it. It is usually performed at 40 hr after the ovulation-inducing hCG injection.

■ **ACUTE GENERAL Rx:**
- Clomiphene citrate (Clomid, Serophene) is commonly used to correct ovulatory defects. It is given in doses of 50 to 200 mg qd, on days 5 through 9 after the onset of progesterone withdrawal bleeding. The higher the dose of clomiphene necessary to induce ovulation, the lower the pregnancy chance. Prolonged use of clomiphene may adversely affect the endometrium and cervical mucus.

- Tamoxifen (Nolvadex) 10 to 20 mg qd given on days 5 through 9 as described previously is also a mild ovulation-inducing agent that improves endometrial formation and cervical mucus.
- Human chorionic gonadotropin (hCG, Pregnyl, Profasi, APL) can be used to trigger ovulation when the dominant follicle size reaches 20-mm diameter.
- Use of injectable FSH (Follistim, Gonal-F, Repronex) preparations is not advisable in primary care setting.

DISPOSITION: Majority of conceptions should occur within the first 6 mo of insemination. In healthy young women a 15% to 25% pregnancy rate per cycle can be expected. The great variety of results reported in the literature indicates that the practitioner's skill in performing ovarian stimulations and sperm preparation plays a significant role in the outcome.

REFERRAL: To specialist if:
- No result after six cycles of inseminations
- Ovulatory dysfunction does not promptly respond to a low dose (50 to 100 mg) of clomiphene citrate
- Woman's age >35 yr: efficiency of treatment becomes critical
- Poor semen parameters
- Pelvic pathology needs correction

☼ PEARLS & CONSIDERATIONS

■ **COMMENTS**
- Risks of insemination: flare-up of unsuspected pelvic infection, ovarian overstimulation with gonadotropins, multifetal pregnancy.

- Caution: if sperm is in limited supply (semen frozen before orchidectomy) or woman's age is an issue, a thorough fertility evaluation is indicated to make sure that no valuable time or valuable semen is wasted. If fertility defects are found, they should be corrected, or IVF should be offered.
- IVF combined with ICSI is the ultimate insemination technique and delivers pregnancy rates of 20% to 40% per cycle.
- Results of several studies suggest that ICSI is associated with a slightly increased risk for chromosomal abnormalities.

REFERENCES

Abulghar H et al: A prospective controlled study of karyotyping for 430 consecutive babies conceived through intracytoplasmic injection, *Fertil Steril* 76:249, 2001.

Ren D et al: A sperm ion channel required for sperm motility and male fertility, *Nature* 413:603, 2001.

Speroff L, Glass RH, Kase NG: *Clinical gynecologic endocrinology and infertility,* ed 6, Baltimore, 1999, Lippincott Williams & Wilkins.

Author: **John M. Wieckowski, M.D., Ph.D.**

I

BASIC INFORMATION

■ DEFINITION
Insomnia refers to a disturbance of nocturnal sleep patterns that causes adverse daytime consequences.

■ SYNONYMS
Disorders of initiating and maintaining sleep (DIMS)

ICD-9CM CODES
780.50 Sleep disturbance, unspecified
780.51 Insomnia with sleep apnea
780.52 Other insomnia

■ EPIDEMIOLOGY & DEMOGRAPHICS
INCIDENCE (IN U.S.): 33 cases/100 persons/yr
PREVALENCE (IN U.S.): Up to 33% of the population
PREDOMINANT SEX: More common in women
PREDOMINANT AGE: >60 yr
PEAK INCIDENCE: Affects all age groups, but more common in those >60 yr old
GENETICS:
- Primary insomnia with childhood onset may be familial.
- No known genetic basis for other causes.

■ PHYSICAL FINDINGS & CLINICAL PRESENTATION
- None
- Patients usually complain of:
  1. Difficulty initiating sleep, wakefulness during sleep cycle, or early awakening
  2. Daytime fatigue, drowsiness

■ ETIOLOGY
- Psychiatric disorders (35%)
- Psychophysiologic (15%)
- Drug and alcohol abuse (12%)
- Periodic leg movements (12%)
- Sleep apnea (6%)
- Medical and toxic conditions (4%)

DIAGNOSIS

■ DIFFERENTIAL DIAGNOSIS
Insomnia is a symptom that may have numerous underlying causes (see Etiology).

■ WORKUP
- Thorough history and examination to identify possible etiology
- Sleep log

■ LABORATORY TESTS
Nighttime polysomnography in an accredited sleep laboratory may be needed to establish the etiology.

TREATMENT

■ NONPHARMACOLOGIC THERAPY
Rules of sleep hygiene may eliminate bad habits and adverse environmental factors (Box 1-18).

■ ACUTE GENERAL Rx
- Transient insomnia: benzodiazepines for no more than a week
- Acute pain: analgesics
- Zolpidem (Ambien), a nonbenzodiazepine agent, 5 to 10 mg qhs may be useful for the short-term treatment of insomnia

■ CHRONIC Rx
- Antidepressants if appropriate for underlying etiology

- Choice of a particular agent, depending on precise nature of sleep disturbance (see References for details)
- Possible tolerance and dependence with prolonged use of benzodiazepines

■ DISPOSITION
Significant improvements in sleep can be achieved in many cases.

■ REFERRAL
- If etiology uncertain
- For assessment at a sleep disorders center (recommended)

REFERENCES
Edinger ID et al: Cognitive behavior therapy for treatment of chronic primary insomnia, *JAMA* 285:1856, 2001.
Espie CA: Insomnia: conceptual issues in the development, persistence, and treatment of sleep disorder in adults, *Ann Rev Psychol* 53:215, 2002.
Lushington K, Lack L: Non-pharmacological treatments of insomnia, *J Psychiatry Relat Sci* 39(1):36, 2002.
Millman RP: Therapy of insomnia, *Med Health R I* 85(3):99, 2002.
Smith MT et al: Comparative meta-analysis of pharmacotherapy and behavior therapy for persistent insomnia, *Am J Psychiatry* 159(1):5, 2002.
Author: **Michael Gruenthal, M.D., Ph.D.**

BOX 1-18   Sleep Hygiene

- Maintain a regular sleep-wake schedule. Get out of bed early in the morning whether or not you have slept well.
- Avoid naps. Exercise during the time that you might otherwise nap.
- Preserve your bed as a haven for sleep and sex. Avoid other waking activities in bed (such as reading or watching television in the evening).
- Minimize alcohol consumption and avoid caffeine during the afternoon and evening. Don't eat heavily shortly before bed.
- Make sure your bedroom environment is conducive to sleep. It should be cool, quiet, and dark.
- If your mind is preoccupied by something such that you can't fall asleep, put the problem to rest by writing it down in a sentence or two and set it aside until morning.
- Don't try too hard to fall asleep; it will only make things worse. If you can't fall asleep after 20 to 30 minutes, get out of bed, do something relaxing, and go back to bed when you feel sleepy.

From Johnson RT, Griffin JW: *Current therapy in neurologic disease*, ed 4, St Louis, 1997, Mosby.

BASIC INFORMATION

■ DEFINITION
Insulinoma is a pancreatic insulin-secreting tumor that causes symptoms associated with hypoglycemia.

■ ICD-9CM CODES
M8151/0 Insulinoma

■ EPIDEMIOLOGY & DEMOGRAPHICS
INCIDENCE: 1 case/250,000 persons/yr
DEMOGRAPHICS: Insulinomas occur in both sexes (approximately 60% in women) and at all ages. In the Mayo Clinic series, the median age at diagnosis was 50 yr in sporadic cases but 23 yr in patients with multiple endocrine neoplasia (MEN), type 1.

■ PHYSICAL FINDINGS & CLINICAL PRESENTATION
Symptoms occur typically in the morning before breakfast (i.e., fasting hypoglycemia as opposed to reactive hypoglycemia, which is not commonly associated with insulinoma)

Neuroglycopenic symptoms	%
Various combinations of diplopia, blurred vision, sweating, palpitations, or weakness	85
Confusion or abnormal behavior	80
Unconsciousness or amnesia	53
Grand mal seizures	12
Adrenergic symptoms	**%**
Sweating	43
Tremulousness	23
Hunger, nausea	12
Palpitations	10

■ ETIOLOGY, PATHOLOGY, PATHOPHYSIOLOGY
- Insulinomas are almost always solitary. Malignant insulinomas account for 5% of the total; they tend to be larger (6 cm). Metastases are usually to the liver (47%), regional lymph nodes (30%), or both.
- Insulinomas are evenly distributed in the head, body, and tail of the pancreas; ectopic insulinomas are rare (1% to 3%). Tumor size: 5% 0.5 cm or less, 34% 0.5 to 1 cm, 53% 1 to 5 cm, 8% >5 cm.
- Histologic classification includes insulinoma in 86% of patients, adenomatosis in 5% to 15%, nesidioblastosis in 4%, and hyperplasia in 1%. Adenomatosis consists of multiple macroadenomas or microadenomas

and occurs especially in patients with MEN-1. Nesidioblastosis is also a diffuse lesion, in which islet cells form as buds on ductular structures.

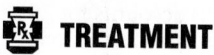

DIAGNOSIS

■ DIFFERENTIAL DIAGNOSIS (OF FASTING HYPOGLYCEMIA)
HYPERINSULINISM:
- Insulinoma
- Nonpancreatic tumors
- Severe congestive heart failure
- Severe renal insufficiency in non-insulin-dependent diabetes

HEPATIC ENZYME DEFICIENCIES OR DECREASED HEPATIC GLUCOSE OUTPUT (PRIMARILY IN INFANTS, CHILDREN):
- Glycogen storage diseases
- Endocrine hypofunction
- Hypopituitarism
- Addison's disease
- Liver failure
- Alcohol abuse
- Malnutrition

EXOGENOUS AGENTS:
- Sulfonylureas, biguanides
- Insulin
- Other drugs (aspirin, pentamidine)

FUNCTIONAL FASTING HYPOGLYCEMIA: Autoantibodies to insulin receptor or insulin

■ LABORATORY TESTS
- An overnight fasting blood sugar level combined with a simultaneous plasma insulin, proinsulin, and/or C peptide level will establish the existence of fasting organic hypoglycemia in 60% of patients.
- If single overnight fasting glucose and insulin levels are nondiagnostic, a 72-hr fast is usually done with blood glucose and insulin levels determined at 2- to 4-hr intervals: 75% of patients with insulinoma develop symptoms and a blood sugar level of less than 40 mg/dl by 24 hr, 92% to 98% develop these by 48 hr, and virtually all patients develop them by 72 hr. The test is considered positive for insulinoma if the plasma insulin/glucose ratio is more than 0.3. If, at any point, the patient becomes symptomatic, plasma insulin and glucose values should be obtained and intravenous glucose should be administered.

- Plasma proinsulin, C-peptide, antibodies to insulin, and plasma sulfonylurea levels may be used to rule out factitious use of insulin or hypoglycemic agents or autoantibodies against the insulin receptor or insulin.
- See Fig. 3-104 for a description of the diagnostic approach to patients with documented hypoglycemia and elevated insulin.

■ IMAGING STUDIES
- Abdominal CT scan or MRI detects half to two thirds of insulinomas (abdominal ultrasound is not effective). Should be done only after laboratory tests for insulinoma have confirmed the diagnosis.
- Intraoperative ultrasound
- Arteriography
- Octreotide scan

TREATMENT

■ SURGICAL TREATMENT
- Enucleation of single insulinoma
- Partial pancreatectomy for multiple adenomas

■ MEDICAL TREATMENT
- Carbohydrate administration
- Diazoxide directly inhibits insulin release and has an extrapancreatic, hyperglycemic effect that enhances glycogenolysis
- Lanreotide and octreotide (somatostatin analogs)
- Streptozotocin

■ REFERRAL
At some point in the workup the patient will probably be referred to an endocrinologist and then to a surgeon. A combination of fasting hypoglycemia and elevated insulin level is probably a good point at which to refer.

REFERENCES
Axelrod L: Insulinoma: cost-effective care in patients with rare disease, *Ann Intern Med* 123:311, 1995.

Gerich JE: Hypoglycemia. In DeGroot LS, Jameson JL, eds, *Endocrinology*, ed 4, Philadelphia, 2001, WB Saunders.

Service FJ et al: Functioning insulinoma—incidence, recurrence and long-term survival of patients, *Mayo Clin Proc* 66:711, 1991.

Author: **Tom J. Wachtel, M.D.**

BASIC INFORMATION

■ DEFINITION
Interstitial nephritis refers to a group of disorders primarily affecting the interstitium and renal tubules. Interstitial nephritis may be acute or chronic.

■ SYNONYMS
Acute interstitial nephritis (AIN)
Chronic interstitial nephritis (CIN)
Tubulointerstitial diseases

ICD-9CM CODES
583.9 Nephritis
580.89 Acute
582.89 Chronic

■ EPIDEMIOLOGY & DEMOGRAPHICS
- Approximately 1% of patients being evaluated for hematuria and proteinuria will have interstitial nephritis.
- Interstitial nephritis accounts for 25% of all cases of chronic renal failure.
- Up to 15% of all renal biopsies performed on patients with renal diseases have acute interstitial nephritis.
- Drug-induced AIN is more common in adults.
- Infection-induced AIN is more common in children.

■ PHYSICAL FINDINGS & CLINICAL PRESENTATION
Acute interstitial nephritis (AIN)
- Patients usually asymptomatic and found to have a sudden decrease in renal function
- Characteristically occurs over several days to weeks after an infection or initiation of a new medication
- Classic triad—fever, rash, and arthralgias
- Lumbar flank pain
- Gross hematuria
- Usually oliguric
Chronic interstitial nephritis (CIN)
- Usually present with symptoms related to the underlying cause (e.g., sarcoidosis, multiple myeloma, urate nephropathy)
- Symptoms of renal failure (e.g., weakness, nausea, pruritus)
- Hypertension

■ ETIOLOGY
- AIN is usually caused by drugs, infection, or is associated with immune or neoplastic disorders
- Common drugs include penicillin, methicillin, rifampin, cephalosporins, trimethoprim-sulfamethoxazole, ciprofloxacin, NSAIDs, thiazides, furosemide, triamterene, allopurinol, phenytoin, captopril, and cimetidine
- Infection (e.g., *Streptococcus, Legionella, Corynebacterium diphtheriae, Yersinia, Salmonella,* HIV, EBV, CMV, *Mycoplasma, Rickettsia,* and *Mycobacterium tuberculosis*)

- Autoimmune causes of AIN include Sjögren's syndrome, SLE, and Wegener's granulomatosis
- Common causes of CIN include polycystic kidney disease, urate nephropathy, analgesic nephropathy, sarcoidosis, multiple myeloma, lead nephropathy, hypercalcemia, and Balkan nephropathy

DIAGNOSIS

Renal biopsy is the only definitive method of establishing the diagnosis of interstitial nephritis. All other labs provide supportive evidence of interstitial nephritis.

■ DIFFERENTIAL DIAGNOSIS
The differential diagnosis includes the diseases listed under Etiology.

■ WORKUP
Any patient found to be in renal failure without evidence of prerenal or obstructive uropathy should be worked up for interstitial nephritis. Workup generally includes blood and urine studies, x-rays, and renal biopsy.

■ LABORATORY TESTS
- CBC showing anemia and eosinophilia
- BUN and creatinine are elevated and typically represent the first clue of interstitial nephritis
- Electrolytes, calcium, and phosphorus
- Uric acid
- Elevated IgE level
- Urinalysis reveals hematuria and pyuria
- Eosinophiluria by Hansen stain is suggestive of allergic interstitial nephritis
- Proteinuria <3 g/24 hr

■ IMAGING STUDIES
- Ultrasound of the kidneys shows normal size kidneys in AIN and small contracted kidneys in CIN.
- IVP findings are similar to ultrasound findings.
- Renal biopsy in AIN reveals infiltration of inflammatory cells into the interstitium with interstitial edema and sparing of the glomeruli. In CIN fibrotic scar tissue replaces the cellular infiltrate.

TREATMENT

■ NONPHARMACOLOGIC THERAPY
- Low-protein, low-potassium, low-sodium diet
- Correction of underlying electrolyte abnormalities
- IV hydration for hypercalcemia

■ ACUTE GENERAL Rx
- Corticosteroids 1 mg/kg/day are used in patients with drug-induced AIN not responding to withdrawal of the medication within 3 to 4 days. Therapy is continued for a total of 4 to 6 wk.
- Cyclophosphamide 2 mg/kg/day is added as a second agent for patients not responding to corticosteroids.
- Combined therapy is continued for 6 wk.

■ CHRONIC Rx
- Treatment of chronic interstitial nephritis is directed at the underlying cause (e.g., corticosteroids for sarcoidosis, EDTA in lead nephropathy).
- Other therapeutic measures include blood pressure control, reducing uric acid and calcium levels if indicated.

■ DISPOSITION
- Most cases of AIN resolve by withdrawing the offending drug or agent within several days.
- Dialysis is required in up to one third of patients with drug-induced AIN.
- By the time most patients with chronic interstitial nephritis present, their creatinine clearance is <50 ml/min.
- Chronic interstitial nephritis patients usually have progressive deterioration in their renal function.

■ REFERRAL
Patients with acute renal failure or chronic renal failure from interstitial nephritis should be referred to a nephrologist.

PEARLS & CONSIDERATIONS

■ COMMENTS
- There are no randomized controlled trials comparing treatment of AIN with corticosteroids versus other forms of therapy.
- If AIN has resulted from penicillin, the use of another penicillin or cephalosporins has led to recurrence.
- Patients with chronic interstitial nephritis usually have advanced renal disease with no specific therapy.

REFERENCES
Kelly CJ, Neilson EG: Tubulointerstitial diseases. In Brenner BM, Rector FC (eds): Brenner & Rector's the kidney, ed 5, Philadelphia, 1996, WB Saunders.
Kodner CM, Kudrimoti A: Diagnosis and management of acute interstitial nephritis, Amer Acad of Fam Phys 67(12):2527, 2003.
Author: **Peter Petropoulos, M.D.**

BASIC INFORMATION

DEFINITION

Irritable bowel syndrome (IBS) is a chronic functional disorder manifested by alteration in bowel habits and recurrent abdominal pain and bloating.

SYNONYMS

Irritable colon
Spastic colon
IBS

ICD-9CM CODES

564.1 Irritable bowel syndrome

EPIDEMIOLOGY & DEMOGRAPHICS

- IBS occurs in 20% of population of industrialized countries and is responsible for >50% of GI referrals. Worldwide adult prevalence is 12%. Incidence increases during adolescence and peaks in third and fourth decade of life.
- Female:male ratio is 2:1.
- Nearly 50% of patients have psychiatric abnormalities, with anxiety disorders being most common.

PHYSICAL FINDINGS & CLINICAL PRESENTATION

- The clinical presentation of IBS consists of abdominal pain and abnormalities of defecation, which may include loose stools usually after meals and in the morning, alternating with episodes of constipation.
- Physical examination is generally normal.
- Nonspecific abdominal tenderness and distention may be present.

ETIOLOGY

- Unknown
- Associated pathophysiology includes altered GI motility and increased gut sensitivity
- Risk factors: anxiety, depression, personality disorders, history of childhood sexual abuse, and domestic abuse in women

DIAGNOSIS

DIFFERENTIAL DIAGNOSIS

- IBD
- Diverticulitis
- Colon malignancy
- Endometriosis
- PUD
- Biliary liver disease
- Chronic pancreatitis

WORKUP

Diagnostic workup is aimed primarily at excluding the conditions listed in the differential diagnoses. It is important to identify "red flags" of other diseases, such as weight loss, rectal bleeding, onset in patients 50 years of age, fever, nocturnal pain, family history of malignancy.

The criteria for diagnosis of IBS are: more than 3 months of symptoms *including* abdominal pain that is relieved by a bowel movement, *or* pain accompanied by a change in bowel pattern, *and* abnormality in bowel movement 25% of the time, characterized by two of the following features:

- Abdominal distention
- Abnormal consistency
- Abnormal defecation (e.g., straining, sense of incomplete evacuation)
- Abnormal frequency
- Mucus with bowel movement

LABORATORY TESTS

- Blood work is generally normal. The presence of anemia should alert to the possibility of a colonic malignancy or IBD.
- Testing of stool for ova and parasites should be considered in patients with chronic diarrhea.

IMAGING STUDIES

- Small bowel series and barium enema are normal and not necessary for diagnosis.
- Lower endoscopy is generally normal except for the presence of some spasms.

TREATMENT

NONPHARMACOLOGIC THERAPY

- The patient should be encouraged to maintain a high-fiber diet and to eliminate foods that aggravate symptoms. Avoidance of dietary caffeine and dietary excesses is also helpful.
- Behavioral therapy is also recommended, particularly in younger patients because psychosocial stressors are important triggers of IBS.
- Importance of regular exercise and adequate fluid intake should be stressed.

GENERAL Rx

- The mainstay of treatment of IBS is high-fiber diet. Because symptoms are chronic, the use of laxatives should be avoided.
- Fiber supplementation with psyllium 1 tablespoon bid or calcium polycarbophil (FiberCon) 2 tablets one to four times daily followed by 8 oz of water may be necessary in some patients.
- Patients should be instructed that there might be some increased bloating on initiation of fiber supplementation, which should resolve within 2 to 3 wk. It is important that patients take these fiber products on a regular basis and not only prn.
- Antispasmodics-anticholinergics may be useful in refractory cases (e.g., dicyclomine [Bentyl] 10 to 20 mg up to three times daily).

- Patients who appear anxious can benefit from use of sedatives and anticholinergics such as chlordiazepoxide-clidinium (Librax) or SSRIs. Tricyclic antidepressants in low doses are also effective in some patients with IBS.
- Loperamide is effective for diarrhea. Alosetron (Lotronex), a serotonin type 3 receptor antagonist previously withdrawn because of severe constipation and ischemic colitis, has been reintroduced with limited availability. It is indicated only for women with severe chronic diarrhea-predominant IBS unresponsive to conventional therapy and not caused by anatomic or metabolic abnormality. Starting dose is 1 mg qd.
- Tegaserod (Zelnorm), a 5-HT$_4$ receptor partial agonist, increases GI motility and can be used to relieve symptoms in patients whose predominant symptom is constipation. Usual dose is 2 to 6 mg PO bid before meals. Tegaserod is contraindicated in patients with severe renal insufficiency, moderate to severe hepatic impairment, intestinal adhesions, or a history of bowel obstruction.

DISPOSITION

Greater than 60% of patients respond successfully to treatment over the initial 12 mo; however, IBS is a chronic relapsing condition and requires prolonged therapy.

REFERRAL

GI referral is recommended in patients with rectal bleeding, fever, nocturnal diarrhea, anemia, weight loss, or onset of symptoms after age 40 yr.

PEARLS & CONSIDERATIONS

COMMENTS

- Patients should be educated regarding maintenance of high-fiber diet and elimination of stressors, which can precipitate attacks of IBS. They should be reassured that their condition cannot lead to cancer.
- The modified ROME criteria define IBS as the presence of ≥12 wk of continuous or recurrent abdominal pain or discomfort that cannot be explained by structural or biochemical abnormalities and the presence of at least two of the following three features: Pain is relieved with defecation, its onset is associated with a change in the frequency of bowel movement, or its onset is associated with a change in the form of the stool.

REFERENCES

Mertz HR: Irritable bowel syndrome, *N Engl J Med* 349:22, 2003.
Viera AJ et al: Management of irritable bowel syndrome, *Am Fam Physician* 66:1867, 2002.

Author: **Fred F. Ferri, M.D.**

BASIC INFORMATION

■ DEFINITION

Kaposi's sarcoma (KS) is a vascular neoplasm most frequently occurring in AIDS patients. It can be divided into the following four subsets:
1. *Classic Kaposi's sarcoma:* most frequently found in elderly Eastern European and Mediterranean males. It consists initially of violaceous macules and papules with subsequent development of plaques and red/purple nodules. Growth is slow, and most of the patients die of unrelated causes.
2. *Epidemic or AIDS-related Kaposi's sarcoma:* most frequently occurs in homosexual men. Lesions are generally multifocal and widespread. Lymphadenopathy may be associated.
3. *Endemic Kaposi's sarcoma:* usually affects African children and adults. An aggressive lymphadenopathic form affects African children in particular.
4. *Immunosuppression-associated, or transplantation-associated, Kaposi's sarcoma:* usually associated with chemotherapy.

■ SYNONYMS

KS

ICD-9CM CODES

173.9 Malignant neoplasm of the skin

■ EPIDEMIOLOGY & DEMOGRAPHICS

• AIDS-related KS affects >35% of AIDS cases.
• Highest incidence is in homosexual men.

■ PHYSICAL FINDINGS & CLINICAL PRESENTATION

• AIDS-related KS: multifocal and widespread red-purple or dark plaques and/or nodules on cutaneous or mucosal surfaces (Fig. 1-155).
• Generalized lymphadenopathy at the time of diagnosis is present in >50% of patients with AIDS-related KS; the initial lesions have a rust-colored appearance; subsequent progression to red or purple nodules or plaques occurs.
• Most frequently affected areas are the face, trunk, oral cavity, and upper and lower extremities.

■ ETIOLOGY

A herpesvirus (HHV-8, Kaposi's sarcoma-associated herpesvirus KSHV) has been isolated from patients with most forms of KS and is believed to be the causative agent. It can be transmitted sexually (homosexual, heterosexual activities) and by other forms of nonsexual contact such as maternal-infant transmission (common in African countries).

DIAGNOSIS

■ DIFFERENTIAL DIAGNOSIS

• Stasis dermatitis
• Pyogenic granuloma
• Capillary hemangiomas
• Granulation tissue
• Postinflammatory hyperpigmentation
• Cutaneous lymphoma
• Melanoma
• Dermatofibroma
• Hematoma
• Prurigo nodularis

■ WORKUP

Diagnosis can generally be made on clinical appearance; tissue biopsy will confirm diagnosis.

■ LABORATORY TESTS

HIV in patients suspected of AIDS

TREATMENT

■ NONPHARMACOLOGIC THERAPY

Observation is a reasonable option in patients with slowly progressive disease.

■ GENERAL Rx

• Excisional biopsy often provides adequate treatment for single lesions and resected recurrences in classic Kaposi's sarcoma.
• Liquid nitrogen cryotherapy can result in complete response in 80% of lesions.
• Interlesional chemotherapy with vinblastine is useful for nodular lesions >1 cm in diameter. Intralesional injection of interferon alfa-2b has also been reported as effective and well tolerated.
• Radiation therapy is effective in non-AIDS KS and for large tumor masses that interfere with normal function.
• Systemic therapy with interferon is also effective in AIDS-related KS and is often used in combination with AZT.
• Systemic chemotherapy (vinblastine, bleomycin, doxorubicin, and dacarbazine) can be used for rapidly progressive disease and for classic and African endemic KS.
• Oral etoposide is also effective and has less myelosuppression than vinblastine.
• Paclitaxel is also effective in patients with advanced KS and represents an excellent second-line therapy.

■ DISPOSITION

• Prognosis is poor in AIDS-related KS. Death is often a result of other AIDS-defining illnesses.
• Prognosis is better in African cutaneous KS and classic sarcoma (patients usually die of unrelated causes).

PEARLS & CONSIDERATIONS

■ COMMENTS

Immunosuppression-associated Kaposi's sarcoma usually regresses with the cessation, reduction, or modification of immunosuppression therapy in most patients. Similarly in HIV patients, Kaposi's sarcoma responds concurrently with the decrease in serum HIV RNA and increase in the CD4 count.

REFERENCES

Grossma Z et al: Absence of Kaposi sarcoma among Ethiopian immigrants to Israel despite high seroprevalence of human herpesvirus 8, *Mayo Clin Proc* 77:905, 2002.

Sarid R et al: Virology, pathogenetic mechanisms, and associated diseases of Kaposi sarcoma-associated herpesvirus (human herpesvirus 8), *Mayo Clin Proc* 77:941, 2002.

Webster-Cyriaque J: Development of Kaposi's sarcoma in a surgical wound, *N Engl J Med* 346:1207, 2002.

Author: **Fred F. Ferri, M.D.**

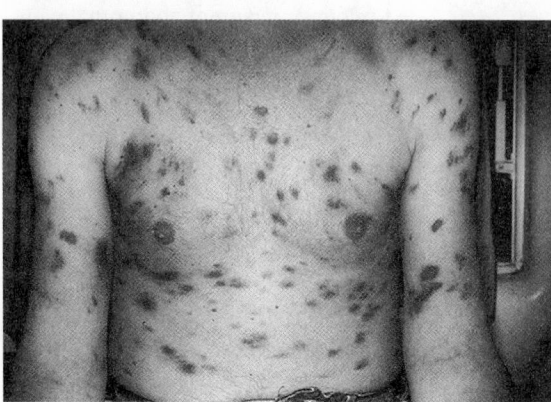

Fig. 1-155 Kaposi's sarcoma. More advanced lesions. Note widespread hemorrhagic plaques and nodules. (From Noble J [ed]: *Textbook of primary care medicine,* ed 2, St Louis, 1995, Mosby.)

BASIC INFORMATION

■ DEFINITION

Kawasaki disease (KD) refers to a generalized vasculitis of unknown etiology and characterized by cutaneous and mucous membrane edema, rash, lymphadenopathy, and involvement of multiple organs.

■ SYNONYMS

Mucocutaneous lymph node syndrome

ICD-9CM CODES

446.1 Kawasaki disease

■ EPIDEMIOLOGY & DEMOGRAPHICS

- KD is a leading cause of acquired heart disease in children.
- KD commonly occurs under the age of 5 (80%).
- KD is found more often in boys than in girls (1.5:1).
- In the United States the incidence of KD is 8.9 cases/100,000 children <5 years of age.
- Approximately 1900 new cases are diagnosed each year in the U.S.
- The incidence of KD in Japan is 80 to 90/100,000 under the age of 5.

■ PHYSICAL FINDINGS & CLINICAL PRESENTATION

A typical presentation is a young child with fever unresponsive to antibiotics for more than 5 days associated with:
- Bilateral conjunctivitis
- Erythema and edema of the hands and feet (Fig. 1-156, B)
- Periungual desquamation
- Fissuring of the lips
- Erythematous pharynx
- Strawberry tongue (Fig. 1-156, A)
- Cervical adenopathy
- Truncal scarlatiniform rash, usually nonvesicular

- Diarrhea
- Dyspnea
- Arthralgias and myalgia
- Sudden death from coronary artery involvement
- Myocardial infarction
- Congestive heart failure

■ ETIOLOGY

The cause of KD is not known although evidence substantiates an infectious etiology precipitating an immune-mediated reaction.

 DIAGNOSIS

The diagnosis of Kawasaki disease is based on a fever lasting more than 5 days along with four of the following five features:
- Bilateral conjunctival swelling
- Inflammatory changes of the lip, tongue, and pharynx
- Skin changes of the limbs
- Rash over the trunk
- Cervical lymphadenopathy

■ DIFFERENTIAL DIAGNOSIS

- Scarlet fever
- Stevens-Johnson syndrome
- Drug eruption
- Henoch-Schönlein purpura
- Toxic shock syndrome
- Measles
- Rocky Mountain spotted fever
- Infectious mononucleosis

■ WORKUP

Clinical findings in addition to lab and imaging studies are useful in searching for organ system involvement and complications (e.g., cardiac, lung, liver).

■ LABORATORY TESTS

- CBC commonly shows a normochromic normocytic anemia, a left-shift in the white blood cell count, and an elevated platelet count
- ESR is elevated
- C-reactive protein is positive
- LFTs (e.g., elevated SGOT and SGPT)
- Urinalysis may show sterile pyuria

■ IMAGING STUDIES

- Chest x-ray may reveal pulmonary infiltrates
- Echocardiogram is very helpful and may show depressed left ventricular function with regional wall motion abnormalities, pericardial effusions (30%), and abnormal coronary artery aneurysms. The echocardiogram is also useful in the long-term follow-up of patients with KD
- Intravascular ultrasound looking for coronary artery lumen irregularities
- Exercise testing with myocardial perfusion studies can be done to assess for coronary blood flow
- Cardiac catheterization with coronary angiography in the proper clinical setting is done to rule out significant obstructive coronary disease

TREATMENT

■ NONPHARMACOLOGIC THERAPY

- Oxygen in selected patients
- Salt restriction in patients with CHF

■ ACUTE GENERAL Rx

- Intravenous immunoglobulin (IVIG) 2 g/kg IV over 8 to 12 hr is the treatment of choice in children diagnosed with KD and ideally should be given within the first 10 days of the illness.

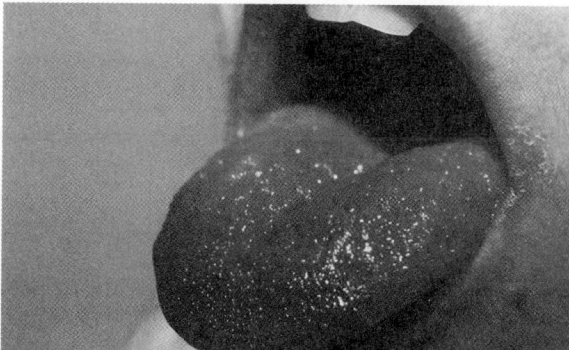
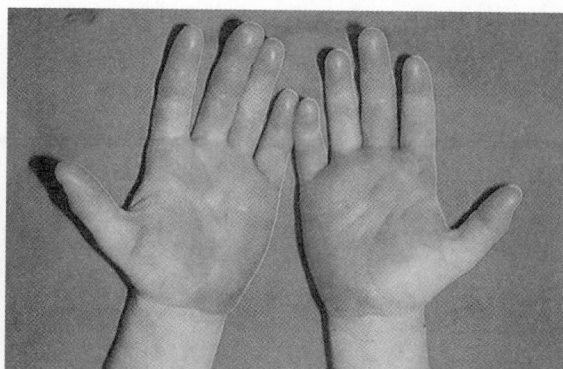

A

B

Fig. 1-156 **A,** Strawberry tongue in a patient with Kawasaki syndrome. **B,** Erythema of the hands, to be followed by desquamation. (**A** Courtesy Marshall Guill, M.D. In Goldstein B [ed]: *Practical dermatology,* ed 2, St Louis, 1997, Mosby. **B** Courtesy Department of Dermatology, University of North Carolina at Chapel Hill. In Goldstein B [ed]: *Practical dermatology,* ed 2, St Louis, 1997, Mosby.)

- Aspirin 30 to 100 mg/kg/day given in four divided doses until the patient is no longer febrile. Thereafter aspirin 3 to 5 mg/kg/day is continued until lab studies (e.g., sedimentation rate) return to normal, generally within 6 to 8 wk.
- In patients that do not defervesce within 48 hr or have recrudescent fever after initial IVIG treatment, a second dose of IVIG 2 g/kg IV over 8 to 12 hr should be considered.
- Corticosteroids and NSAIDs are not effective in the treatment of KD.

■ CHRONIC Rx
Interventional and surgical procedures can be tried in children who have developed cardiac complications of KD.
- Percutaneous transluminal coronary angioplasty
- Coronary bypass graft surgery using the internal mammary artery or the gastroepiploic artery has met with greater patency success than saphenous vein grafts
- Cardiac transplantation is an option and is indicated in patients with:
  1. Severe left ventricular failure
  2. Malignant arrhythmias
  3. Multivessel distal coronary artery disease

■ DISPOSITION
- Mortality rate of children with KD is 0.5% to 2.8%, usually from coronary artery aneurysm, coronary thrombosis, myocarditis, and pancarditis.

- Death usually occurs in the third to fourth week of the illness.
- Before the use of IVIG, approximately 20% of all patients with KD develop coronary aneurysms.
- Treatment with IVIG has reduced the incidence of coronary aneurysms by 80%.
- IVIG has also been shown to improve left ventricular function during the acute stages of the disease.
- Risk factors for the development of coronary aneurysms or giant coronary aneurysms (>8 mm) are:
  1. Fever lasting >10 days
  2. Age <1 year
  3. Male
  4. Recurrence of fever
- Between 1% to 2% of patients have recurrences of KD.

■ REFERRAL
Multiple specialists may be consulted to assist in the diagnosis of KD including dermatology, rheumatology, and infectious disease. Cardiology consultation is recommended in any patient with cardiac involvement and in the long-term follow-up of patients with KD.

☼ PEARLS & CONSIDERATIONS

■ COMMENTS
- KD was first described by Dr. Tomasaku Kawasaki in 1967 and published in the *Journal of Allergology.*

- Kawasaki disease is not transmitted from person to person.
- The mechanism of action of intravenous gamma-globulin therapy for KD remains unknown.

REFERENCES
Barron KL et al: Report of the National Institutes of Health Workshop on Kawasaki Disease, *J Rheumatol* 26(1):170, 1999.

Freeman AF, Shulran ST: Recent developments in Kawasaki disease, *Curr Opin Infect Dis* 14(3):357, 2001.

Fulton DR, Newburger JW: Long-term cardiac sequelae of Kawasaki disease, *Curr Rheumatol Rep* 2(4):324, 2000.

Gardner-Medwin JM et al: Incidence of Henoch-Schönlein purpura, Kawasaki disease, and rare vasculitides in children of different ethnic origins, *Lancet* 360:1197, 2002.

Gedalia A: Kawasaki disease: an update, *Curr Rheumatol Rep* 4(1):259, 2002.

Sundel RP: Update on the treatment of Kawasaki disease in childhood, *Curr Rheumatol Rep* 4:474, 2002.

Taubert KA, Shulman ST: Kawasaki disease, *Am Fam Physician* 59(11):3093, 1999.

Author: **Peter Petropoulos, M.D.**

BASIC INFORMATION

■ DEFINITION
Klinefelter's syndrome is a congenital disorder in which a 47,XXY chromosome complement is associated with hypogonadism and infertility.

■ SYNONYMS
47,XXY Hypogonadism

ICD-9CM CODES
758.7 Klinefelter's syndrome

■ EPIDEMIOLOGY & DEMOGRAPHICS
INCIDENCE: 1 in 500 men (most common sex chromosome disorder)
GENETICS: The most common mosaic complement is 46,XY/47,XXY. 47,XXY karyotype and occasional 48,XXYY; 48,XXXY; or 49,XXXXY have been reported. The manifestations vary in severity in patients. It is this sex chromosome mosaicism that is thought to account for the variable presentation. Fertility, although very rare, has been reported in men with Klinefelter's syndrome.

■ PHYSICAL FINDINGS
CLASSIC TRIAD: Small firm testes, azoospermia, and gynecomastia
Prepubertal: Small testes, gonadal volume <1.5 ml is a result of loss of germ cells before puberty.
Postpubertal: Gynecomastia (periductal fat growth) with small, firm, pea-sized testes. Exaggerated growth of the lower extremities results in a decreased crown-to-pubis:pubis-to-floor ratio (Fig. 1-157). There are diminished strength, diminished ability to grow a full beard or mustache, infertility; decreased intellectual development and antisocial behavior are thought to occur with high frequency.

■ ETIOLOGY
- Several postulated mechanisms: nondisjunction during meiosis and mitosis and anaphase lag during mitosis or meiosis
- Reason: maternal age
  1. The incidence of Klinefelter's rises from 0.6% when the maternal age is 35 yr or less to 5.4% when the maternal age is in excess of 45 yr.
  2. It is of interest to note that the extra X chromosome has a paternal origin as often as a maternal origin.

DIAGNOSIS

- Markedly elevated FSH levels
- Total plasma testosterone are decreased in 50% to 60% of patients

- Free testosterone levels are decreased
- Plasma estradiol is increased stimulating the increase in levels of testosterone-binding globulin with resultant decrease in the testosterone-to-estradiol ratio, which is felt to be the cause of gynecomastia

■ LABORATORY TESTS
- Normal to low serum testosterone
- Elevated sex hormone binding globulin
- Increased sex hormone binding globin (acts to further suppress any available free testosterone)
- Normal to increased estradiol (a result of augmented peripheral conversion of testosterone to estradiol)
- Testis biopsy shows azoospermia, Leydig cell hyperplasia, hyalinization, and fibrosis of the seminiferous tubules. Mosaics may have focal areas of spermatogenesis, and, on rare occasions, a sperm may appear in the ejaculate. It is the extra X chromosome that is the pivotal factor controlling spermatogenesis as well as affecting neuronal function directly leading to the behavioral abnormalities related to decreased IQ
- Buccal smear: one sex chromatin body

PREPUBERTAL MALE: Gonadotropin levels are normal.
POSTPUBERTAL MALE: Gonadotropin levels are elevated even when the testosterone level is normal.

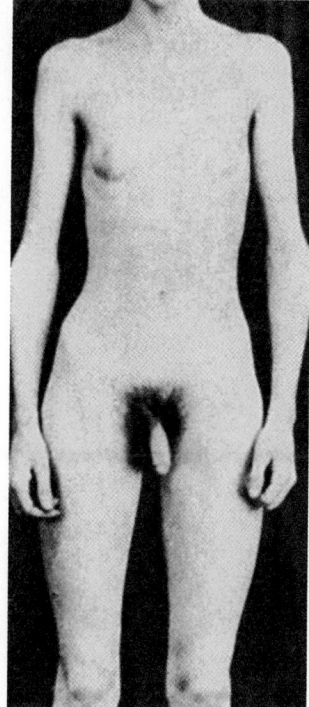

Fig. 1-157   Klinefelter's syndrome. (From Harrison JH et al: *Campbell's urology,* ed 4, Philadelphia, 1979, WB Saunders.)

DISEASE ASSOCIATIONS:
Malignancies: Breast cancer (20 times greater than XY men and 20% the rate of occurrence in women), nonlymphocytic leukemia, lymphomas, marrow dysplastic syndromes, extragonadal germ cell neoplasms
Autoimmune Disorders: Chronic lymphocytic thyroiditis, Takayasu arteritis, taurodontism (enlarged molar teeth), mitral valve prolapse, varicose veins, asthma, bronchitis, osteoporosis, and abnormal glucose tolerance testing
Others: Diabetes, varicose veins

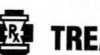

TREATMENT

Revolves around three facets of Klinefelter's syndrome:
1. Hypogonadism: androgen replacement in the form of testosterone
2. Gynecomastia: cosmetic surgery
3. Psychosocial problems: androgen therapy and educational support
4. After extensive genetic counseling intracytoplasmic sperm insertion (ICSI) has been used to treat infertility with limited success

PEARLS & CONSIDERATIONS

■ COMMENTS
- Androgen therapy should not be used in the case of severe mental retardation.
- Also, rule out breast and prostate cancer before initiating or continuing androgen therapy.
- Furthermore, androgen therapy will not improve infertility; it may suppress any spermatogenesis that is taking place within the testes.
- Other causes of primary hypogonadism:
  1. Myotonic muscular dystrophy
  2. Sertoli-cell–only syndrome
  3. Kartagener's syndrome
  4. Anorchia
  5. Acquired hypogonadism
- A 50-fold higher risk of breast cancer is reported in this population.

REFERENCES
Manning MA, Hoyme HE: Diagnosis and management of the adolescent boy with Klinefelter syndrome, *Adolescent Medicine State of the Art Reviews* 13(2):367, 2002.
Palermo GD et al: Births after intracytoplasmic sperm insertion of sperm obtained by testicular extraction from men with non-mosaic Klinefelter's syndrome, *N Engl J Med* 338:588, 1998.
Smyth CM, Bremner WJ: Klinefelter syndrome, *Arch Intern Med* 158:1309, 1998.
Author: **Philip J. Aliotta, M.D., M.S.H.A.**

BASIC INFORMATION

■ **DEFINITION**
Korsakoff's psychosis refers to a disorder of memory, out of proportion to other cognitive functions, associated with thiamine deficiency. It is classically seen in alcoholics and may follow the presentation of Wernicke's encephalopathy (see relevant entry.)

■ **SYNONYMS**
Korsakoff's syndrome
Wernicke-Korsakoff syndrome
Alcoholic polyneuritic psychosis

ICD-9CM CODES
291.1 Alcohol amnestic syndrome

■ **EPIDEMIOLOGY & DEMOGRAPHICS**
• Formerly seen most commonly in alcoholics, but declining in recent years
• Slightly more common in males
• Age of onset evenly distributed between age 30 and 70

■ **PHYSICAL FINDINGS & CLINICAL PRESENTATION**
• Impairment of ability to remember new material
• Remote memory is said to be retained but is almost universally diminished on careful testing
• Confabulation may occur

■ **ETIOLOGY**
Thiamine deficiency, commonly in alcoholics or other malnourished populations, although it may be iatrogenic from prolonged infusion of dextrose-containing fluids without thiamine repletion.

DIAGNOSIS

■ **DIFFERENTIAL DIAGNOSIS**
• Stroke, trauma, or tumor affecting the temporal lobes or hippocampus
• Cerebral anoxia
• Transient global amnesia
• Dementing illness

■ **WORKUP**
A high index of suspicion should be maintained in all alcoholics and other malnourished states.

■ **LABORATORY TESTS**
• Serum pyruvate is elevated.
• Whole-blood or erythrocyte transketolase are decreased; rapid resolution to normal in 24 hours with thiamine repletion.

■ **IMAGING STUDIES**
MRI may show diencephalic and mesencephalic lesions acutely, but there is no definitive radiologic study for diagnosis.

TREATMENT

■ **NONPHARMACOLOGIC THERAPY**
A supervised environment may be required.

■ **ACUTE GENERAL Rx**
• Thiamine 100 mg IV or IM should be given immediately.
• Thiamine given acutely during Wernicke's phase (disorders of extraocular movements, confusion, and ataxia), may prevent the development of Korsakoff's psychosis.

■ **CHRONIC Rx**
It is impossible to predict acutely the degree of recovery of an individual patient, although the vast majority will have lasting deficits. Decisions regarding long-term institutionalization should therefore be made cautiously.

■ **DISPOSITION**
Patient often must live in protected environment for rest of life.

■ **REFERRAL**
• A neurologist should assess the patient.
• Neuropsychologic testing may be helpful.

PEARLS & CONSIDERATIONS

■ **COMMENTS**
• This disease is probably underdiagnosed.
• Give thiamine if the disease is even suspected.
• A preventable cause is prolonged dextrose-containing IV fluids without supplemental thiamine.

REFERENCES
Gallucci M et al: Wernicke encephalopathy: MR findings in five patients, *Am J Roentgenol* 155(6):1309, 1990.
Zubaran C, Fernandes JG, Rodnight R: Wernicke-Korsakoff syndrome, *Postgrad Med J* 73(855):27, 1997.
Author: **Daniel Mattson, M.D., M.Sc. (Med.)**

BASIC INFORMATION

■ DEFINITION
Labyrinthitis is a peripheral vestibulopathy characterized by acute onset of vertigo usually associated with vomiting. It may or may not be associated with hearing loss.

■ SYNONYMS
Acute labyrinthitis
Acute vestibular neuronopathy
Vestibular neuronitis
Viral neurolabyrinthitis

ICD-9CM CODES
386.12 Vestibular neuronitis (active and recurrent)
386.3 Labyrinthitis

■ EPIDEMIOLOGY & DEMOGRAPHICS
INCIDENCE (IN U.S.): Most common cause of prolonged spontaneous vertigo associated with nausea at any age.
PREDOMINANT AGE: Any

■ CLINICAL PRESENTATION
- Vertigo, nausea and vomiting with onset over several hours
- Symptoms usually peak within 24 hr, then resolve gradually over several weeks
- During the first day the patient usually has difficulty focusing the eyes because of spontaneous nystagmus
- Usually has benign course, with complete recovery within 1 to 3 mo, although older patients may have intractable dizziness that persists for many months

■ PHYSICAL FINDINGS
- Nystagmus
- Nausea
- Vomiting
- Vertigo worsening with head movement
- Abnormal caloric tests
- Possible hearing loss in the affected ear
- Normal otoscopic examination typically
- Otherwise normal neurologic examination

■ ETIOLOGY
Often preceded 1-2 wk by a viral-like illness

DIAGNOSIS

■ DIFFERENTIAL DIAGNOSIS
- Acute labyrinthine ischemia (vascular insufficiency)
- Other forms of labyrinthitis (bacterial and syphilitic)
- Labyrinthine fistula
- Benign positional vertigo
- Meniere's syndrome
- Cholesteatoma
- Drug-induced
- Eighth nerve tumor
- Head trauma

■ WORKUP
- Otoscopic examination
- Neurologic examination, with close attention to cranial nerves
- Audiogram if symptoms accompanied by hearing loss
- Caloric test if presentation is atypical

■ LABORATORY TESTS
- Routine laboratory tests are generally not helpful.
- If history of significant emesis, check electrolytes, BUN, and creatinine.

■ IMAGING STUDIES
None are usually necessary, but enhancement of bony labyrinth may be seen by MRI after injection of contrast material. Head CT with fine cuts through temporal bones if history of trauma or suspect cholesteatoma. MRI of the brain with and without contrast with fine cuts through the internal auditory canal if abnormal cranial nerve examination or suspect eighth nerve tumor.

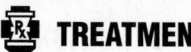 TREATMENT

■ NONPHARMACOLOGIC THERAPY
Reassurance. Initial bedrest, then encourage increase in activity as tolerated

■ ACUTE GENERAL Rx
- Phenergan or other antiemetics are effective
- Vestibular suppressant: Meclizine 12.5 to 25 mg qid often used. Scopolamine patch also effective

■ CHRONIC Rx
Important to wean off vestibular suppressant therapy as soon as possible

■ DISPOSITION
Usually does not require hospital admission unless patient is unable to tolerate oral intake of liquids

■ REFERRAL
- If symptoms persist or neurologic abnormalities are present
- Consider vestibular rehabilitation, particularly in the elderly

PEARLS & CONSIDERATIONS

■ COMMENTS
Labyrinthitis is a term that usually implies peripheral vestibulopathy associated with hearing loss. The term "vestibular neuronitis" is typically used when hearing is not affected. Despite this technical distinction, many physicians use both of these terms interchangeably.

REFERENCE
Baloh RW et al: Neurotology, *Continuum, Lifelong Learning in Neurology* 2(2):37, 1996.
Author: **Sharon S. Hartman, M.D., Ph.D.**

BASIC INFORMATION

■ DEFINITION
Lactose intolerance is the insufficient concentration of lactase enzyme, leading to fermentation of malabsorbed lactose by intestinal bacteria with subsequent production of intestinal gas and various organic acids.

■ SYNONYMS
Lactase deficiency
Milk intolerance

ICD-9CM CODES
271.3 Lactose intolerance

■ EPIDEMIOLOGY & DEMOGRAPHICS
Nearly 50 million people in the U.S. have partial or complete lactose intolerance. There are racial differences, with <25% of white adults being lactose intolerant, whereas >85% of Asian Americans and >60% of blacks have some form of lactose intolerance.

■ PHYSICAL FINDINGS & CLINICAL PRESENTATION
- Abdominal tenderness and cramping, bloating, flatulence
- Diarrhea
- Symptoms are directly related to the osmotic pressure of substrate in the colon and occur about 2 hr after ingestion of lactose
- Physical examination: may be entirely within normal limits

■ ETIOLOGY
- Congenital lactase deficiency: common in premature infants; rare in full-term infants and generally inherited as a chromosomal recessive trait
- Secondary lactose intolerance: usually a result of injury of the intestinal mucosa (Crohn's disease, viral gastroenteritis, AIDS enteropathy, cryptosporidiosis, Whipple's disease, sprue)

DIAGNOSIS

■ DIFFERENTIAL DIAGNOSIS
- IBD
- IBS
- Pancreatic insufficiency
- Nontropical and tropical sprue
- Cystic fibrosis
- Diverticular disease
- Bowel neoplasm
- Laxative abuse
- Celiac disease
- Parasitic disease (e.g., giardiasis)
- Viral or bacterial infections

■ WORKUP
- The diagnosis can usually be made on the basis of the history and improvement with dietary manipulation.
- Diagnostic workup may include confirming the diagnosis with hydrogen breath test and excluding other conditions listed in the differential diagnosis that may also coexist with lactase deficiency.

■ LABORATORY TESTS
- Lactose breath hydrogen test: A rise in breath hydrogen >20 ppm within 90 min of ingestion of 50 g of lactose is positive for lactase deficiency. This test is positive in 90% of patients with lactose malabsorption. Common causes of false-negative results are recent use of oral antibiotics or recent high colonic enema.
- The lactose tolerance test is an older and less accurate testing modality (20% rate of false positive and negative results). The patient is administered an oral dose of 1 to 1.5 gm of lactose/kg body weight. Serial measurement of blood glucose level on an hourly basis for 3 hr is then performed. The test is considered positive if the patient develops intestinal symptoms and the blood glucose level rises.

■ IMAGING STUDIES
Imaging studies are generally not indicated. A small bowel series may be useful in patients with significant malabsorption.

TREATMENT

■ NONPHARMACOLOGIC THERAPY
A lactose-free diet generally results in prompt resolution of symptoms. Lactose is primarily found in dairy products but may be present as an ingredient or component of common foods and beverages. Possible sources of lactose are breads, candies, cold cuts, dessert mixes, cream soups, bologna, commercial sauces and gravies, chocolate, drink mixes, salad dressings, and medications. Labels should be read carefully to identify sources of lactose.

■ ACUTE GENERAL Rx
- Addition of lactase enzyme supplement (Lactaid tablets, Dairy Ease) before the ingestion of milk products may prevent symptoms in some patients. However, it is not effective for all lactose-intolerant patients.
- Lactose-intolerant patients must ensure adequate calcium intake. Calcium supplementation is recommended to prevent osteoporosis.

■ CHRONIC Rx
Patient education regarding foods high in lactose, such as milk, cottage cheese, or ice cream, is recommended.

■ DISPOSITION
Clinical improvement with restriction or elimination of milk products

■ REFERRAL
GI referral for endoscopic procedures if concomant GI disorders are suspected

PEARLS & CONSIDERATIONS

■ COMMENTS
- There is great variability in signs and symptoms in patients with lactose intolerance depending on the degree of lactase deficiency.
- Most patients with lactose intolerance can ingest up to 12 oz of milk daily without symptoms.
- Nondairy synthetic drinks (e.g., Coffee-Mate) and use of rice milk are well tolerated.

REFERENCE
Swagerty DL et al: Lactose intolerance, *Am Fam Physician* 65:1845, 2002.
Author: **Fred F. Ferri, M.D.**

BASIC INFORMATION

■ DEFINITION

Lambert-Eaton myasthenic syndrome (LEMS) is a disorder of neuromuscular transmission caused by antibodies directed against presynaptic voltage-gated P/Q calcium channels on motor and autonomic nerve terminals. There are two forms: paraneoplastic (most common) and nonparaneoplastic (autoimmune).

■ SYNONYMS

Eaton-Lambert syndrome

ICD-9CM CODES

199.1 Malignant neoplasm without specification of site, other

■ EPIDEMIOLOGY & DEMOGRAPHICS

INCIDENCE (IN U.S.): Uncertain; estimated at 5 cases/1 million persons/yr
PREVALENCE (IN U.S.): Uncertain; estimated at 400 total cases
PREDOMINANT SEX: Male > female in a 2:1 ratio.
PEAK INCIDENCE: Sixth decade

■ PHYSICAL FINDINGS & CLINICAL PRESENTATION

- Weakness with diminished or absent muscle stretch reflexes
- Proximal lower extremity muscles affected most
- Ocular and bulbar muscles less commonly affected
- Transient strength improvement with brief exercise
- Autonomic dysfunction common (dry mouth in 75%, sexual dysfunction, blurred vision, constipation, orthostasis, etc.)

■ ETIOLOGY

- Antibodies directed against presynaptic voltage-gated P/Q calcium channels are present in most patients. The reduction in calcium influx causes a reduction in acetylcholine release at motor and autonomic nerve terminals.
- Paraneoplastic forms, usually small cell lung cancer, are present in 50%-70% of patients.
- Autoimmune forms, usually in patients with other autoimmune diseases, occur in 10%-30%.

DIAGNOSIS

■ DIFFERENTIAL DIAGNOSIS

Include: Myasthenia gravis, polymyositis, primary myopathies, carcinomatous myopathies, polymyalgia rheumatica, botulism, Guillain-Barré syndrome.
Section II describes the differential diagnosis of muscle weakness.

■ WORKUP

Confirm diagnosis by characteristic electrodiagnostic (EMG/NCS) findings: Reduced motor amplitudes with normal sensory studies; >10% decrement in motor amplitudes on slow repetitive nerve stimulation (RNS) at 2-3Hz, with >100% increment on fast RNS (20-30 HZ) or immediately after 10 seconds of maximum exercise (postexercise facilitation).

■ LABORATORY TESTS

Check P/Q calcium channel antibody titers (commercially available).

■ IMAGING STUDIES

Screen for an underlying malignancy. Presentation with LEMS may precede diagnosis of SCLC by up to 5 yr. Chest x-ray/CT chest may be required every 6-12 mo for small cell lung cancer.

TREATMENT

■ NONPHARMACOLOGIC THERAPY

Symptomatic treatment for autonomic dysfunction.

■ ACUTE GENERAL Rx

- Anticholinesterase agents (pyridostigmine 30-60 mg q4-6h) may yield some improvement.
- Guanidine hydrochloride: start 5-10 mg/kg/day; up to 30 mg/kg/day in 3-day intervals.
- Plasma exchange (200-250 mL/kg over 10-14 days) or IV immunoglobulins (2 g/kg over 2 to 5 days) often produce significant, temporary improvement.
- Prednisone 1.0-1.5 mg/kg/day can be gradually tapered over months to minimal effective dose.
- Azathioprine can be given alone or in combination with prednisone. Give up to 2.5 mg/kg/day. If intolerant of this, can administer cyclosporine up to 3 mg/kg/day instead.

- 3,4-diaminopyridine 10-20mg PO qid (max 100mg/day) may improve muscle strength and reduce autonomic symptoms. Available in Europe, but limited to research studies in the U.S.

■ CHRONIC Rx

Treat underlying malignancy if present.

■ DISPOSITION

- Gradually progressive weakness leading to impaired mobility if untreated
- Clinical remission may occur with chronic immunosuppressive therapy in 43% of cases
- Possible substantial improvement with successful treatment of underlying malignancy

■ REFERRAL

To a neurologist (recommended) because of infrequency of this disease and risks associated with some treatments. Referral to specialist centers for 3,4-DAP therapy may be warranted in the U.S. Surgical referral for tumor debulking in paraneoplastic forms.

PEARLS & CONSIDERATIONS

■ COMMENTS

- Prominent autonomic symptoms (dry eyes, dry mouth, impotence, orthostasis) are often the clue to the diagnosis in the appropriate clinical context.
- Many drugs may worsen weakness and should be used only if absolutely necessary. Included are succinylcholine, d-tubocurarine, quinine, quinidine, procainamide, aminoglycoside antibiotics, β-blockers, and calcium channel blockers.

REFERENCES

Dropcho EJ: Remote neurologic manifestations of cancer, *Neurol Clin* 20(1):85, 2002.

Maddison P, Newsom-Davis J: Lambert-Eaton myasthenic syndrome. In: Katirji B et al (eds): *Neuromuscular disorders in clinical practice*. Boston, 2002, Butterworth-Heinemann.

Sanders, DB: The Lambert-Eaton myasthenic syndrome, *Adv Neurol* 88:189, 2002.

Author: **Eroboghene E. Ubogu, M.D.**

BASIC INFORMATION

■ DEFINITION
Cancer of the larynx, including the vocal cords (glottis), supraglottis, and subglottis.

■ SYNONYMS
Laryngeal cancer
Head and neck cancer (subsite); other sites include oral cavity, pharynx, perinasal sinus, and salivary glands

ICD-9CM CODES
231.0 Carcinoma of larynx

■ EPIDEMIOLOGY & DEMOGRAPHICS
- 12,000 new cases per year in the U.S.
- 80% male predominance (current, with past and projected increase in female rates as a result of changing smoking habits)
- Peak incidence in sixth decade

■ PHYSICAL FINDINGS & CLINICAL PRESENTATION
Glottis
- Early diagnosis possible because of voice change (hoarseness). Any voice change of more than 2 wk duration should prompt a laryngeal examination.
- Supraglottis
  1. No early symptom
  2. Cervical lymphadenopathy
  3. Neck pain or ear pain
  4. Discomfort during swallowing
  5. Odynophagia
  6. Later: hoarseness, dysphagia, airway obstruction
- Subglottis
Even more subtle than supraglottic lesion; the same signs occur, only later in the course

■ ETIOLOGY
- Smoking (cigarette, cigar, or pipe)
- Alcohol intake/abuse
- Diet and nutritional deficiencies
- Gastroesophageal reflux
- Voice abuse
- Chronic laryngitis
- Exposure to wood dust
- Asbestosis
- Exposure to radiation
- Possible role of human papilloma virus

DIAGNOSIS

■ DIFFERENTIAL DIAGNOSIS
- Laryngitis
- Allergic and nonallergic rhinosinusitis
- Gastroesophageal reflux
- Voice abuse leading to hoarseness
- Laryngeal papilloma

- Vocal cord paralysis secondary to a neurologic condition or secondary to entrapment of the recurrent laryngeal nerve caused by mediastinal compression
- Tracheomalacia

STAGING:
Supraglottic
T1 Tumor limited to one subsite with normal cord mobility
T2 Tumor invades mucosa of more than one subsite (e.g., base of tongue, vallecula, pyriform sinus) without fixation of larynx
T3 Tumor limited to larynx with vocal cord fixation or invasion of postcricoid area or preepiglottis
T4 Tumor invades thyroid cartilage or extends into soft tissue of the neck, thyroid, or esophagus

Glottic
T1 Tumor limited to vocal cord with normal mobility
T1a Tumor limited to one vocal cord
T1b Tumor involves both vocal cords
T2 Tumor extends to supra or subglottis or impairs cord mobility
T3 Tumor limited to larynx with cord fixation
T4 Tumor invades through cartilage or other tissues beyond larynx

Stage grouping
Stage I: T1,N0,M0
Stage II: T2, N0, M0
Stage III: T3, N0, M0
T1, T2, T3, N1, M0
Stage IV: T4, N0, N1, M0
Any T, N2, N3, M0
Any T, any N or M >0

■ WORKUP
- Laboratory: none
- Endoscopic laryngeal inspection
- After (and only after) diagnosis of the malignancy, imaging with CT or MRI should be undertaken to stage the disease

HISTOLOGIC CLASSIFICATION:
Epithelial cancers
- Squamous cell carcinoma in situ
- Superficially invasive cancer
- Verrucous carcinoma
- Pseudosarcoma
- Anaplastic cancer
- Transitional cell carcinoma
- Lymphoepithelial cancer
- Adenocarcinoma
- Neuroendocrine tumors, including small cell and carcinoid
Sarcomas
Metastatic malignancies

TREATMENT

■ ACUTE GENERAL Rx
- Early Stage (T or T2): two options
  1. Conservative surgery (partial laryngectomy) with neck dissection
  2. Primary radiation

- Intermediate Stage: four options
  1. Primary radiation alone
  2. Supraglottic laryngectomy with neck dissection
  3. Supraglottic laryngectomy with postoperative radiation
  4. Chemotherapy with radiation
- Advanced Stage
Chemotherapy and radiation with total laryngectomy reserved for treatment failure
Glottis
- Carcinoma in situ
  1. Microexcision
  2. Laser vaporization
  3. Radiation
- Early Stage (T or T2): two options
  1. Voice conservation surgery
  2. Radiation
- Intermediate Stage (T3)
  1. Combined radiation and chemotherapy (cisplatin and 5FU)
  2. Total laryngectomy for treatment failure
- Advanced Stage (T4)
  1. Combined radiation and chemotherapy
  2. Total laryngectomy and neck dissection followed by postoperative radiation in unfavorable lesion or treatment failure
Subglottis
Total laryngectomy and approximate neck surgery to excise the tumor, followed by radiation
Unresected Cancers
- Induction chemotherapy and radiation followed by neck dissection in chemosensitive tumors, or by laryngectomy and neck dissection in chemoresistant tumors
- If hypopharyngeal involvement exists: laryngopharyngectomy, neck dissection, and postoperative radiation

■ DISPOSITION
Supraglottis 5-yr control
- T_1 95% to 100%
- T_2 80% to 90%
- T_3 65% to 85%
- T_4 40% to 55%
Glottis 5-yr control
- T_1 95% to 100%
- T_2 50% to 85%
- T_3 35% to 85%
- T_4 20% to 65%

REFERENCE
Sessions RB, Harrison LB, Forastiere AA: Tumors of the larynx and hypopharynx. In *Cancer: principals and practice of oncology*, ed 6, Philadelphia, 2001, Lippincott Williams & Wilkins.
Author: **Tom J. Wachtel, M.D.**

■ **BASIC INFORMATION**

■ **DEFINITION:**
Laryngitis is an acute or chronic inflammation of the laryngeal mucous membranes.

ICD-9CM CODES
464.0 Acute laryngitis
476.0 Chronic laryngitis

■ **PHYSICAL FINDINGS AND CLINICAL PRESENTATION**
ACUTE LARYNGITIS
• Clinical syndrome characterized by the onset of hoarseness, voice breaks, or episodes of aphonia. May also have accompanying sore throat, cough, nasal congestion, and rhinorrhea
• Usually associated with viral upper respiratory infection
• Larynx with diffuse erythema, edema, and vascular engorgement of the vocal folds, and occasionally mucosal ulceration
• In young children subglottis is often affected, resulting in airway narrowing with marked hoarseness, inspiratory stridor, dyspnea, and restlessness
• Respiratory compromise rare in adults

CHRONIC LARYNGITIS
Characterized by hoarseness or dysphonia persisting for longer than 2 wk

■ **ETIOLOGY**
ACUTE LARYNGITIS
• Most often associated with viral infections: influenzavirus, rhinovirus, and adenovirus are the most common, but parainfluenza virus, myxovirus, paramyxovirus, cocksackievirus, coronavirus, respiratory syncytial virus, herpesvirus, Epstein-Barr virus, varicella zoster virus, and variola virus are sometimes implicated
• Bacterial pathogens associated with acute laryngitis include group A *streptococci, Staphylococcus aureus, Streptococcus pneumoniae, Moraxella catarrhalis, Haemophilus influenzae,*
Mycoplasma pneumoniae, Chlamydia pneumoniae, and *Corynebacterium* species

CHRONIC LARYNGITIS
• Results from any of the following: tuberculosis, usually through bronchogenic spread; leprosy, from nasopharyngeal or oropharyngeal spread; syphilis, in secondary and tertiary stages; rhinoscleroma, extending from the nose and nasopharynx; actinomycosis; histoplasmosis; blastomycosis; paracoccidiomycosis; coccidiosis; candidiasis; aspergillosis; sporotrichosis; rhinosporidiosis; parasitic infections including leishmaniasis and Clinostomum infection following raw fresh-water fish ingestion
• Noninfectious causes of both acute and chronic laryngitis include malignancy, voice abuse (singers), gastroesophageal reflux disease, and chemical or environmental irritants such as cigarettes and allergens. Other causes of inflammatory or granulomatous lesions of the larynx include relapsing polychondritis, Wegener's granulomatosis, and sarcoidosis

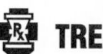 ■ **DIAGNOSIS**

■ **WORKUP**
• History and physical examination: diagnosis is usually apparent.
• Laryngoscopy for severe or persistent cases.
• Laryngeal cultures should be performed if etiology other than acute viral infection is suspected.
• Imaging not indicated unless evidence of airway compromise. Obtain plain radiographs of neck, anteroposterior and lateral views, to differentiate laryngitis from acute laryngotracheobronchitis or supraglottitis.

■ **DIFFERENTIAL DIAGNOSIS**
Young children with signs of airway obstruction:
• Supraglottitis (epiglottitis)
• Laryngotracheobronchitis
• Tracheitis
• Foreign body aspiration
Adults with persistent hoarseness consider noninfectious causes of laryngitis as listed previously

■ **TREATMENT**

■ **NONPHARMACOLOGIC THERAPY**
• Rest the voice.
• Use an air humidifier.
• Adequate hydration. Avoid alcohol and caffeine because of diuretic effect.

■ **ACUTE GENERAL Rx**
• Antibiotics and other antimicrobials: indicated only when a specific pathogen is isolated
• Avoid decongestants secondary to their drying effect
• Guaifenesin may be a useful adjunct as a mucolytic agent
• In GERD-associated laryngitis use acid-suppressive therapy (H2 blockers, proton pump inhibitors) and nocturnal antireflux precautions

■ **DISPOSITION**
Uncomplicated laryngitis is usually benign, with gradual resolution of symptoms

■ **REFERRAL**
If symptoms persist for >2 wk, refer to otolaryngologist for laryngoscopy
Consider referral to gastroenterologist if GERD is suspected

REFERENCES
Garrett CG, Osoff RH: Hoarseness, *Med Clin North Am* 83(1)115, 1999.
Nostrant TT: Gastroesophageal reflux and laryngitis: a skeptic's view, *Am J Med* 108(4A):149S, 2000.
Authors: **Jane V. Eason, M.D., and Marilyn Fabbri, M.D.**

BASIC INFORMATION

■ DEFINITION
Acute laryngotracheobronchitis is a viral infection of the upper and lower respiratory tract leading to erythema and edema of the tracheal walls and narrowing of the subglottic region.

■ SYNONYMS
Croup

ICD-9CM CODES
464.4 Croup

■ EPIDEMIOLOGY & DEMOGRAPHICS
- Croup is primarily a disease of children occurring between the ages of 1 and 6 yr.
- The peak incidence of croup is the second year of life (50 cases/1000 children).
- Most cases usually occur in the fall and represent parainfluenza type 1 viral infection.
- Winter outbreaks usually represent infection by influenza A and B viruses.
- Croup accounts for 10% to 15% of lower respiratory tract infections in young children.
- Boys are affected more often than girls.

■ PHYSICAL FINDINGS & CLINICAL PRESENTATION
- Most children with croup present with symptoms of an upper respiratory infection for several days
- Rhinorrhea
- Cough
- Low-grade fever
- Barking cough that usually occurs at night and wakes the child up
- Sore throat
- Stridor
- Apprehension
- Use of accessory muscles of respiration
- Tachypnea
- Tachycardia
- Wheezing

■ ETIOLOGY
- Parainfluenza viruses (types 1, 2, and 3) are the most common causes of croup in the U.S.
- Influenza A and B, although not a common cause of croup, does lead to more severe cases of the disease
- Adenovirus
- Respiratory syncytial virus
- *Mycoplasma pneumoniae* (rare)

DIAGNOSIS

The diagnosis of croup is usually based on the characteristic clinical presentation of a young child between the ages of 1 to 6 yr waking up with a barking cough ("seal's bark") and stridor.

■ DIFFERENTIAL DIAGNOSIS
Spasmodic croup, epiglottitis, bacterial tracheitis, angioneurotic edema, diphtheria, peritonsillar abscess, retropharyngeal abscess, smoke inhalation, foreign body

■ WORKUP
- The workup of a child with croup is to differentiate viral laryngotracheobronchitis from noninfectious causes of stridor and epiglottitis caused by *H. influenzae*.
- The clinical presentation and plain films of the soft tissues of the neck assist in differentiating viral from nonviral and noninfectious causes.

■ LABORATORY TESTS
- Laboratory tests are not often used to make the diagnosis of viral tracheobronchitis.
- CBC, viral serology, and tissue cultures can be ordered and may detect the infecting agent in up to 65% of cases.
- Pulse oximetry and arterial blood gas determination for patients with tachypnea and respiratory distress.

■ IMAGING STUDIES
- Plain (AP and lateral) films of the soft tissues of the neck may show the classic radiographic finding of subglottic stenosis or "steeple" sign.
- CT scan of the soft tissues of the neck may be performed in the cases where the differential between croup, epiglottitis, and noninfectious is more difficult.
- Direct visualization via laryngoscopy may be useful in some situations under a controlled setting.

TREATMENT

Treatment of croup focuses on airway management.

■ NONPHARMACOLOGIC THERAPY
- Oxygen
- Cool mist
- Hot steam

■ ACUTE GENERAL Rx
- Use of 0.25 to 0.75 ml of 2.25% racemic epinephrine every 20 min is used in children with severe respiratory symptoms, rest stridor, and impending intubation.
- Corticosteroids (e.g., dexamethasone 0.6 mg/kg IV or PO, prednisone 2 mg/kg/day) have been shown to be effective.
- Budesonide, a nebulized corticosteroid given at 4 mg, has been shown to improve symptoms in patients with moderate to severe croup.

■ CHRONIC Rx
Croup is an acute infectious disease with a short natural history; thus, chronic management is not usually an issue.

■ DISPOSITION
- Croup is usually benign and self-limited, resolving within 3 to 4 days.
- Complications include:
  1. Airway obstruction
  2. Otitis media
  3. Pneumonia
  4. Dehydration

■ REFERRAL
If intubation is needed (rarely), an emergency consultation with ENT and/or anesthesiology is recommended.

☼ PEARLS & CONSIDERATIONS

■ COMMENTS
- Most patients with croup can be managed at home (e.g., patients without stridor and in no respiratory distress).
- Hospitalization and observation is required for children with moderate-to-severe croup (e.g., rest stridor, respiratory distress refractory to the above mentioned acute treatments).

REFERENCES
Johnson DW, Jacobson S, Edney PC: A comparison of nebulized budesonide, intramuscular dexamethasone, and placebo for moderately severe croup, *N Engl J Med* 339(8):498, 1998.

Knutson D, Aring A: Viral croup, *Am Fam Physician* 69:535, 2004.

Rosekrans JA: Viral croup: current diagnosis and treatment, *Mayo Clin Proc* 73:1102, 1998.
Author: **Dennis Mikolich, M.D.**

BASIC INFORMATION

■ DEFINITION
Lead poisoning refers to multisystem abnormalities resulting from excessive lead exposure.

■ SYNONYMS
Plumbism

ICD-9CM CODES
984.0 Lead poisoning

■ EPIDEMIOLOGY & DEMOGRAPHICS
- Lead poisoning is most common in children ages 1 to 5 yr (17,000 cases/100,000 persons). The highest rates are among blacks, those with low income, and urban children.
- In 1991 the Centers for Disease Control and Prevention lowered the definition of a safe blood lead level to <10 μg/dl of whole blood (a blood lead level of 25 μg/dl was considered acceptable before 1991).
- It is estimated that >15% of preschoolers in the U.S. have a blood lead level >15 μg/dl.

■ PHYSICAL FINDINGS & CLINICAL PRESENTATION
- Findings vary with the degree of toxicity. Examination may be normal in patients with mild toxicity.
- Myalgias, irritability, headache, and general fatigue may be present initially.
- Abdominal cramping, constipation, weight loss, tremor, paresthesias and peripheral neuritis, seizures, and coma may occur with severe toxicity.
- Motor neuropathy is common in children with lead poisoning; learning disorders are also frequent.

■ ETIOLOGY
Chronic repeated exposure to paint containing lead, plumbing, storage of batteries, pottery, lead soldering

DIAGNOSIS

■ DIFFERENTIAL DIAGNOSIS
- Polyneuropathies from other sources
- Anxiety disorder, attention deficit disorder
- Malabsorption, acute abdomen
- Iron deficiency anemia

■ WORKUP
Laboratory screening: all U.S. children should be considered to be at risk for lead poisoning and should be screened routinely starting at 1 yr of age for low-risk children and 6 mo of age for high-risk ones.

■ LABORATORY TESTS
- Venous blood lead level: normal level: <10 μg/dl; levels of 50 to 70 μg/dl: indicative of moderate toxicity; levels >70 μg/dl: associated with severe poisoning
- Mild anemia with basophilic stippling on peripheral smear
- Elevated zinc protoporphyrin levels or free erythrocyte protoporphyrin level
- An increased body burden of lead with previous high-level exposure in patients with occupational lead poisoning can be demonstrated by measuring the excretion of lead in urine after premedication with calcium EDTA or another chelating agent

■ IMAGING STUDIES
- Imaging studies are generally not necessary.
- A plain abdominal film can visualize lead particles in the gut.
- "Lead lines" may be noted on x-ray films of long bones.

TREATMENT

■ NONPHARMACOLOGIC THERAPY
- Provide adequate amounts of calcium, iron, zinc, and protein in patient's diet
- Family education on sources of lead exposure and potential adverse health effects

■ ACUTE GENERAL Rx
- For children with blood levels of 10 to 19 μg/dl the CDC recommends nonpharmacologic interventions (see Nonpharmacologic Therapy).
- For children with blood levels between 20-44 μg/dl the CDC recommendations include case management by a qualified social worker, clinical management, environmental assessment, and lead hazard control. Chelation therapy should be considered in children with refractory blood lead levels.

Chelation therapy is indicated in children with blood lead levels 45 μg/dl:
- Succimer (DMSA) 10 mg/kg PO q8h for 5 days then q12h for 2 wk can be used in patients with levels between 45 and 70 μg/dl.
- Edetate calcium disodium (EDTA) and dimercaprol (BAL) are effective in patients with severe toxicity.
- Use of both EDTA and DMSA is indicated in children with blood levels >70 μg/dl.
- d-Penicillamine (Cuprimine) can also be used for lead poisoning, but it is not FDA approved for this condition.

■ CHRONIC Rx
- Reduce exposure, remove any potential lead sources.
- Correct iron deficiency and any other nutritional deficiencies.
- Recheck blood lead level 7 to 21 days after chelation therapy.

■ DISPOSITION
Patients with mild to moderate toxicity generally improve without any residual deficits. The presence of encephalopathy at diagnosis is a poor prognostic sign. Residual neurologic deficits may persist in these patients. Chelation therapy seems to slow the progression of renal insufficiency in patients with mildly elevated body lead burden.

■ REFERRAL
If exposure to lead is work related, it should be reported to the Office of the United States Occupational Safety and Health Administration (OSHA).

PEARLS & CONSIDERATIONS

■ COMMENTS
- Even blood lead concentrations <10 mcg/DL are inversely associated with children's IQ scores at 3 and 5 yr of age.
- Screening of household members of affected individuals is recommended.
- In children with blood lead levels ≤45 mg/dl, treatment with succimer does not improve scores on tests of cognition, behavior, or neuropsychological function.
- Lead toxicity may delay growth and pubertal development in girls.
- Low-level environmental lead exposure may accelerate progressive renal insufficiency in patients without diabetes who have chronic renal disease. Repeated chelation therapy may improve renal function and slow the progression of renal failure.

REFERENCES
Canfield RL et al: Intellectual impairment in children with blood lead concentrations below 10 mcg/deciliter, *N Engl J Med* 348:1517, 2003.

Lin JL et al: Environmental lead exposure and progression of chronic renal diseases in patients without diabetes, *N Engl J Med* 348:277, 2003.

Selevan SG et al: Blood lead concentration and delayed puberty in girls, *N Engl J Med* 348:1527, 2003.

Author: **Fred F. Ferri, M.D.**

BASIC INFORMATION

■ DEFINITION
Legg-Calvé-Perthes disease is a self-limited disorder of unknown etiology caused by ischemia of the immature femoral head that leads to bone necrosis and variable amounts of collapse during the reparative process.

■ SYNONYMS
Coxa plana
Capital femoral osteochondrosis

ICD-9CM CODES
732.1 Perthes' disease

■ EPIDEMIOLOGY & DEMOGRAPHICS
PREVALENCE: 1 case/1300 children
PREDOMINANT SEX: Male:female ratio of 4:1
PREDOMINANT AGE: 3 to 10 yr

■ PHYSICAL FINDINGS & CLINICAL PRESENTATION
- Initial complaint: usually a mildly painful limp
- Pain referred down the inner aspect of the thigh to the knee
- Moderate restriction of motion resulting from hip synovitis (abduction and internal rotation are especially limited)
- Pain at the extremes of movement and tenderness over anterior hip joint

■ ETIOLOGY
Unknown

DIAGNOSIS

■ DIFFERENTIAL DIAGNOSIS
- Toxic synovitis
- Low-grade septic arthritis
- JRA

■ WORKUP
Diagnosis is usually based on the physical findings and eventual radiographic findings.

■ IMAGING STUDIES
- Plain roentgenography to establish the diagnosis (Fig. 1-158)
- AP and frog-leg lateral radiographs
- Technetium bone scanning to assist in making the diagnosis in early cases

TREATMENT

■ ACUTE GENERAL Rx
- A brief period of bed rest followed by bracing (except in mild cases)
- Bracing possibly required for 2 to 3 yr

■ DISPOSITION
- Prognosis depends on age of patient and degree of involvement of the femoral head at onset.
- Young patients (under 6 yr) with minimal involvement do well.
- Older patients (over 8 yr) often do poorly.
- A few patients eventually develop degenerative arthritis.

■ REFERRAL
For orthopedic consultation when diagnosis is suspected

PEARLS & CONSIDERATIONS

■ COMMENTS
There is great uncertainty regarding treatment and its effect on outcome. It may be that bracing has no effect whatsoever on the end result.

REFERENCES
Adkins SB, Figler RA: Hip pain in athletes, *Am Fam Physician* 61:2109, 2000.
Gross GW, Articolo GA, Bowen JR: Legg-Calvé-Perthes disease: imaging evaluation and management, *Semin Musculoskelet Radiol* 3(4):379, 1999.
Guerado E, Garces G: Perthes disease: a study of constitutional aspects in adulthood, *J Bone Joint Surg Br* 83(4):569, 2001.
Joseph B, Mulpuri K, Varghese G: Perthes' disease in the adolescent, *J Bone Joint Surg Br* 83(5):715, 2001.
Stevens DB, Tao SS, Glueck CJ: Recurrent Legg-Calvé-Perthes disease: case report and long term follow up, *Clin Orthop* 385:124, 2001.
Thompson GH et al: Legg-Calvé-Perthes disease: current concepts, *Instr Course Lect* 51:367, 2002.
Author: **Lonnie R. Mercier, M.D.**

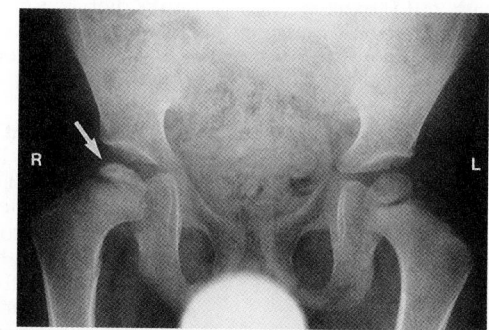
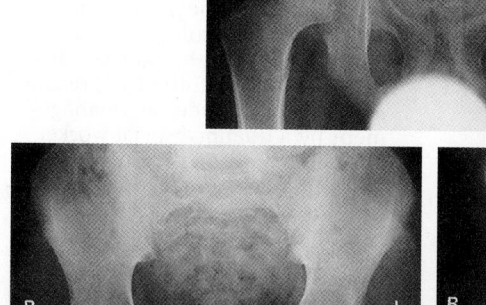
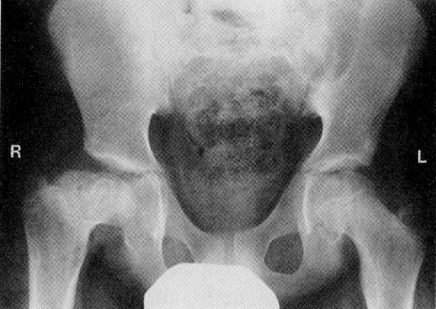

Fig. 1-158 Legg-Calvé-Perthes disease. A, An anteroposterior view of the pelvis demonstrates fragmentation and sclerosis of the right femoral epiphysis (*arrow*) in this 6-year-old male. **B,** A follow-up film obtained 8 years later shows continuing deformity resulting from the osteonecrosis. The patient developed significant degenerative arthritis (**C**) by the age of 12 years. (From Mettler FA[ed]: *Primary care radiology,* Philadelphia, 2000, WB Saunders.)

BASIC INFORMATION

■ DEFINITION
Leishmaniasis is an infectious disease caused by a heterogeneous group of protozoan parasites belonging to the genus *Leishmania* and resulting in a variety of different clinical syndromes.

ICD-9CM CODES
085.9 Leishmaniasis

■ EPIDEMIOLOGY & DEMOGRAPHICS
INCIDENCE: Approximately 400,000 new cases occur each year with almost 400 million people at risk for the disease.
- Can be classified geographically into New World versus Old World disease
- Infection can be divided into cutaneous, mucocutaneous, visceral disease
- Incubation period: from 1 wk to many months for cutaneous and mucosal leishmaniasis; 2 to 6 mo (range is 10 days to years) for visceral leishmaniasis
- Mode of transmission: by the sandfly vector; can also be spread via shared needles, blood transfusions, vertically from the mother to fetus, or sexually

■ PHYSICAL FINDINGS & CLINICAL PRESENTATION
Cutaneous Syndrome
- Localized cutaneous leishmaniasis
- Mucosal leishmaniasis
- Leishmania recidivans
- Diffuse cutaneous leishmaniasis
Visceral Syndrome
- Viscerotrophic leishmaniasis: fever, chronic fatigue, malaise, cough, intermittent diarrhea, and abdominal pain. Signs include adenopathy, hepatosplenomegaly, hyperpigmentation of skin, petechiae, jaundice, edema, and ascites
- Post–kala-azar dermal leishmaniasis: generalized cutaneous rash that is often papular or nodular; severe forms with desquamation of skin and mucosa

■ ETIOLOGY
- Old-World parasite: *Leishmania tropica, L. major, L. aethiopica, L. donovani, L. infantum*
- New-World parasite: *L. braziliensis* and *L. mexicana complex, L. chagasi, L.b. guyanensis, L.b. panamensis*

DIAGNOSIS

■ DIFFERENTIAL DIAGNOSIS
- Malaria
- African trypanosomiasis
- Brucellosis
- Enteric fever
- Bacterial endocarditis
- Generalized histoplasmosis
- Chronic myelocytic leukemia
- Hodgkin's disease and other lymphomas
- Sarcoidosis
- Hepatic cirrhosis
- Tuberculosis

■ WORKUP
- CBC
- LFTs
- Renal panel
- Serology
- Biopsy for histology and culture
- PCR

■ LABORATORY TESTS
- CBC: anemia, neutropenia, thrombocytopenia, and eosinophilia
- LFTs: hypergammaglobulinemia, hypoalbuminemia, and hyperbilirubinemia
- Elevated BUN and creatinine
- Specific diagnosis confirmed by intracellular amastigote in Giemsa-stained impression smears or sectioned tissue or culture performed in NNN (Novy, MacNeal, Nicolle) or Schneider's medium
- Serologic diagnosis: ELISA, direct agglutination tests, K39 ELISA, PCR, and monoclonal antibody staining of tissue smears
- Montenegro skin test

TREATMENT

- Nonspecific or supportive care
  1. Nutritional diet
  2. Antimicrobial agents for concurrent infections
  3. Blood transfusions
  4. Iron and vitamins
- Specific antileishmanial therapy
  1. Pentavalent antimonials: sodium stibogluconate and sodium antimonygluconate
  2. Amphotericin B
  3. Pentamidine
  4. Aminosidine
  5. Other agents: allopurinol, ketoconazole, paromomycin (combined with other regimens)

  6. Immunotherapy: IFN-γ
  7. New agent: Miltefosine
  8. Local or tropical treatments and physical therapy, including thermal treatments
  9. Plastic surgery

■ DISPOSITION
Follow-up examination is important for the early detection and treatment relapse.

■ REFERRAL
To infectious disease experts for accurate diagnosis and management

PEARLS & CONSIDERATIONS

■ COMMENTS
- Prevention by reservoir control-destruction of animal reservoir hosts, mass treatment of human in kala-azar–prevalent areas
- Prevention by vector control: insecticide spraying in domestic and peridomestic areas
- Vaccines are in various stages of development and clinical trials. None are licensed or commercially available at this time

REFERENCES
Abdeen ZA et al: Epidemiology of visceral leishmaniasis in the Jenin District, West Bank 1989-1998, *Am J Trop Med Hyg* 66(4):329, 2002.

Berman JD: Human leishmaniasis: clinical, diagnostic, and chemotherapeutic developments in the last 10 years, *Clin Infect Dis* 24:684, 1997.

Royer MA, Crowe CO: American cutaneous leishmaniasis, *Arch Pathol Lab Med* 126(4):471, 2002.

Sundar S et al: Low-dose liposomal amphotericin B in refractory Indian visceral leishmaniasis: a multicenter study, *Am J Trop Med Hyg* 66(2):143, 2002.

Sundar S et al: Oral miltefosine for Indian visceral leishmaniasis, *N Engl J Med* 347:1739, 2002.

Author: **Vasanthi Arumugam, M.D.**

■ BASIC INFORMATION

■ DEFINITION
Leprosy is a chronic granulomatous infection of humans that primarily affects the skin and peripheral nerves.

■ SYNONYMS
Hansen's disease

ICD-9CM CODES
030.9 Leprosy

■ EPIDEMIOLOGY & DEMOGRAPHICS
- The number of cases worldwide has fallen from more than 5 million cases in 1985 to less than 1 million cases in 1998.
- Nearly 75% of the cases of leprosy are found in India, Brazil, Bangladesh, Indonesia, and Myanmar.
- More than 85% of the cases diagnosed in the U.S. are found among immigrants.
- Worldwide incidence is 650,000 new cases per year.
- Annual incidence in the U.S. is 150 new cases per year.
- Leprosy is more common in men than women (2:1).
- Leprosy can occur at any age but usually is found in young children.

■ PHYSICAL FINDINGS & CLINICAL PRESENTATION
- A skin lesion: most common initial presentation
- Sensory loss
- Anhidrosis
- Neuritic pain
- Palpable peripheral nerves
- Nerve damage (most commonly affected nerves are ulnar, median, common peroneal, posterior tibial, radial cutaneous nerve of the wrist, facial, and posterior auricular)
- Muscle atrophy and weakness
- Foot drop
- Claw hand and claw toes
- Lagophthalmos, nasal septal perforation, collapse of bridge of nose (Fig. 1-159, *A*), loss of eyebrows resulting in "leonine" facies

Leprosy can present along a spectrum from simple cutaneous skin lesions with minimal sensory loss (Fig. 1-159, *B*) to severe extensive skin involvement, painful neuritis, muscle wasting and contractures, and multiple peripheral nerve damage.

■ ETIOLOGY
- Leprosy is caused by *Mycobacterium leprae,* an obligate intracellular acid-fast rod.
- The mode of transmission remains elusive. Spread in humans is thought to occur via the respiratory route or entry through broken skin.

- Zoonotic transmission from armadillos has not been proven.
- The majority of people exposed to patients with leprosy do not develop the disease because of their natural immunity.
- Incubation period is 3 to 5 yr.

■ DIAGNOSIS

- The diagnosis of leprosy relies on a detailed history and physical examination and is established by the demonstration of acid-fast bacilli in skin smears or skin biopsies of the affected sites.
- Leprosy has been classified according to the WHO system into:
  1. Paucibacillary leprosy defined as fewer than five skin lesions with no bacilli on skin smear.
  2. Multibacillary leprosy defined as six or more skin lesions and may be skin-smear positive.
- Leprosy has also been classified more specifically according to the type of skin lesions, sensory and motor deficits, and biopsy into:
  1. Indeterminate leprosy
  2. Tuberculoid leprosy

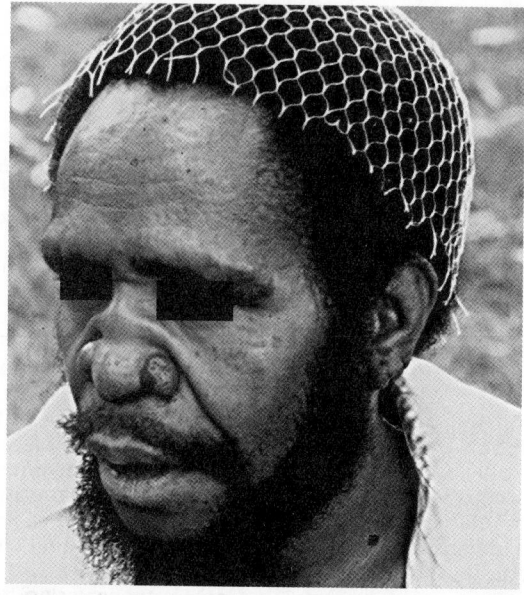

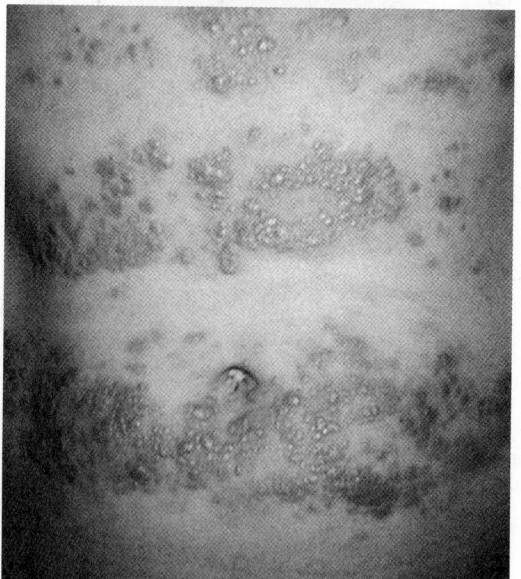

Fig. 1-159 **A,** Advanced lepromatous leprosy with collapse of the nasal septum. **B,** Lepromatous leprosy characterized by extensive papule formation over abdomen. Minimal or no sensory loss is present in the affected areas. (**A** from Gorbach SL: *Infectious diseases,* ed 2, Philadelphia, 1998, WB Saunders; **B** from Mandell GL; *Mandell, Douglas, and Bennett's principles and practice of infectious diseases,* ed 5, New York, 2000, Churchill Livingstone.)

3. Borderline tuberculoid leprosy
4. Borderline lepromatous leprosy
5. Lepromatous leprosy

■ DIFFERENTIAL DIAGNOSIS
The differential diagnosis of leprosy includes: sarcoidosis, rheumatoid arthritis, systemic lupus erythematosus, lymphomatoid granulomatosis, carpal tunnel syndrome, cutaneous leishmaniasis, fungal infections and other causes of hypopigmented, hyperpigmented, and erythematous skin lesions.

■ WORKUP
Any patient who presents with skin lesions and a sensory or muscle deficit should have a workup for leprosy.

■ LABORATORY TESTS
- *Mycobacterium leprae* cannot be cultured on artificial media. The bacteria rapidly proliferate when injected into the footpads of mice or into armadillos and sometimes is used for drug-sensitivity testing.
- Serologic tests, including the antibody to phenolic glycolipid 1 (PGL-1), are available and used for diagnostic confirmation and research epidemiologic studies.
- Lepromin intradermal skin test is not diagnostic and not for commercial use.
- Skin smears are taken from active sites or most commonly from the earlobe, elbows, or knees and are stained for acid-fast bacilli.
- Skin biopsies of active sites are stained for acid-fast bacilli.
- Peripheral nerve biopsy can be done in patients with sensory loss and no skin lesions. Common nerves biopsied are the radial cutaneous nerve of the wrist and the sural nerve of the ankle.

■ IMAGING STUDIES
X-ray studies are usually of no benefit in the diagnosis or treatment of leprosy.

TREATMENT

■ NONPHARMACOLOGIC THERAPY
- Physical therapy for patients with upper and lower extremity deformities
- Proper foot care and footwear to prevent ulcer formation

■ ACUTE GENERAL Rx
For paucibacillary leprosy:
- Dapsone 100 mg PO qd for 6 mo in an unsupervised setting is the treatment of choice.
- Rifampin 600 mg PO qd for 6 mo in a supervised setting is the recommendation by WHO.
- Ofloxacin 400 mg qd or minocycline 100 mg qd are other alternatives.

For multibacillary leprosy:
- Rifampin 600 mg PO qd and clofazimine 300 mg PO qd for 24 mo in a supervised setting.
- Rifampin 100 mg PO qd and clofazimine 50 mg PO qd for 24 mo in an unsupervised setting.
- Dapsone 100 mg PO qd is sometimes added as triple therapy in this group of patients.
- Clofazimine 50 mg daily is usually used in combination with dapsone for better bacteriocidal effect.

■ CHRONIC Rx
- If relapse occurs, the patient is treated with the same medical regimen because resistance is low.
- If relapse is from paucibacillary to multibacillary, the medical regimen for multibacillary should be used for therapy.

■ DISPOSITION
- Relapse is <1% for multibacillary and just over 1% in paucibacillary cases.
- Patients are initially followed up monthly and when treatment is completed every 3 to 6 mo for the next 5 to 10 yr.
- Some patients develop reactions known as erythema nodosum leprosum and reversal reaction, usually during treatment.
  1. Erythema nodosum leprosum results in tender nodules and is treated with either prednisolone 40 to 60 mg qd until the reaction is controlled and tapered or thalidomide 300 to 400 mg qd and tapered to 100 mg qd with monthly attempts to wean down further.

  2. Reactive reaction results in the development of new skin lesions with swelling and erythema of existing lesions. Treatment is with either NSAIDs or prednisolone.

■ REFERRAL
- National Hansen's Disease Programs (NHDP) Center in Baton Rouge, Louisiana, and 15 outpatient clinics in the U.S. offer consultations and treatment. Telephone: 1-800-642-2477.
- Any suspected case of leprosy merits an infectious disease consultation. Consultation with orthopedic, podiatry, ophthalmology, physical therapy, plastic surgery, and psychology are all in order for any of the potential sequelae of the disease.

PEARLS & CONSIDERATIONS

■ COMMENTS
- The risk of transmission is low in patients with leprosy, and therefore no infection control precautions of patients hospitalized is needed.
- Family members and close contacts need to be examined frequently for the development of lesions.
- Dapsone or rifampin prophylaxis is not recommended in the prevention of leprosy.
- BCG vaccination has a 50% protective effect in the prevention of leprosy and may be considered.

REFERENCES
Cambau E et al: Multidrug-resistance to dapsone, rifampicin, and ofloxacin in *Mycobacterium leprae, Lancet* 349:103,1997.
Jacobsen RR, Krahenbuhl JL: Leprosy, *Lancet* 353:655, 1999.
Leprosy: global target attained, *Wkly Epidemiol Rec* 20:155, 2001.
Ramos-e-Silva M, Rebello PF: Leprosy: recognition and treatment, *Am J Clin Dermatol* 2(4):203, 2001.
Authors: **Peter Petropoulos, M.D., and Dennis Mikolich, M.D.**

BASIC INFORMATION

■ DEFINITION
Leptospirosis is a zoonosis caused by the spirochete *Leptospira interrogans*.

■ SYNONYMS
Weil's disease

ICD-9CM CODES
100.9 Leptospirosis

■ EPIDEMIOLOGY & DEMOGRAPHICS
INCIDENCE (IN U.S.):
- 0.05 cases/100,000 persons
- Significant underestimation because of underreporting
- Hawaii consistently has the highest reported annual incidence rate in U.S.

PREDOMINANT SEX: Male (4:1)
PREDOMINANT AGE: Teenagers and young adults
PEAK INCIDENCE: Summer months, into the fall
GENETICS:
Neonatal Infection: Can occur

■ PHYSICAL FINDINGS & CLINICAL PRESENTATION
ANICTERIC FORM:
- Milder and more common presentation of disease
- A self-limited systemic illness with two stages:
  1. Septicemic stage: presents abruptly with fevers, headache, severe myalgias, rigors, prostration, and sometimes circulatory collapse; conjunctival suffusion is common; skin rash, pharyngitis, lymphadenopathy, hepatomegaly, splenomegaly, or muscle tenderness may occur; lasts about 1 wk with complete resolution usual.
  2. Immune stage: occurs a few days after first stage with similar symptoms; hallmark is aseptic meningitis.

ICTERIC LEPTOSPIROSIS (WEIL'S SYNDROME):
  1. Denotes severe cases, with symptoms of hepatic, renal, and vascular dysfunction
  2. Biphasic course: persistence of fever, jaundice, and azotemia
  3. Complications: oliguria or anuria, hemorrhage, hypotension, vascular collapse

■ ETIOLOGY
Caused by a spirochete, *L. interrogans*
- Infects a variety of animals, including most mammals
- Specific serotypes associated with different hosts—*pomona* in livestock, *canicola* in dogs (Fig. 1-160), and *icterohaemorrhagiae* in rodents

- Exposure to animal urine or infected water method by which organism penetrates skin or mucous membranes; most cases related to recreational swimming and canoeing; outbreak occurred in participants of triathlons in Wisconsin and Illinois; recently described cases in inner-city residents are related to exposure to rat urine

DIAGNOSIS

■ DIFFERENTIAL DIAGNOSIS
- Bacterial meningitis
- Viral hepatitis
- Influenza
- Legionnaire's disease

■ WORKUP
Culture of blood, CSF, and urine:
- Organism can be isolated from blood or CSF during first 10 days of illness.
- Urine should be cultured after first week and for up to 30 days after onset of illness.

■ LABORATORY TESTS
- Normal or elevated WBCs, at times up to 70,000/mm³
- Elevated transaminases or bilirubin
- Anemia, azotemia, hypoprothrombinemia in those with icteric illness
- Elevated CK in first phase
- Meningitis in both phases, but aseptic in second phase

■ IMAGING STUDIES
Chest radiographs to show bilateral nonlobar infiltrates

TREATMENT

■ NONPHARMACOLOGIC THERAPY
- Supportive
- Observation for dehydration, hypotension, renal failure, hemorrhage

■ ACUTE GENERAL Rx
- IV penicillin G 1 million U q4h
- Doxycycline 100 mg PO bid for 7 days
- Vitamin K administration if hypoprothrombinemia present
- Possible Jarisch-Herxheimer reaction when treated with penicillin

■ DISPOSITION
- Anicteric leptospirosis is self-limited, but administration of antibiotics can decrease severity and duration of symptoms.
- Icteric leptospirosis, even with supportive therapy, may have a mortality as high as 10%.

■ REFERRAL
- If more than mild disease
- If no response to treatment

PEARLS & CONSIDERATIONS

■ COMMENTS
Significantly underreported illness

REFERENCES
Katz AR et al: Leptospirosis in Hawaii, 1974-1998: epidemiologic analysis of 353 laboratory-confirmed cases, *Am J Trop Med Hyg* 66:61, 2002.
Tunbridge AJ et al: A breathless triathlete, *Lancet* 359:130, 2002.
Author: **Maurice Policar, M.D.**

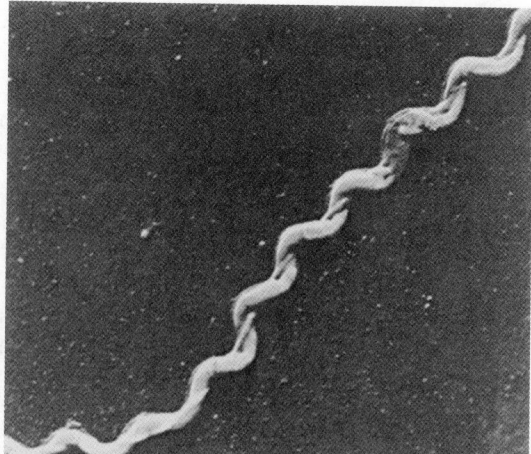

Fig. 1-160 Electron micrograph of *Leptospira interrogans* (serovar *canicola*) showing the tightly coiled helicoids rod with the periplasmic axial filament. (Courtesy Armed Forces Institute of Pathology, AFIP No. 60-10941. In Gorbach SL: *Infectious diseases,* ed 2, Philadelphia, 1998, WB Saunders.)

BASIC INFORMATION

■ DEFINITION

Acute lymphoblastic leukemia (ALL) is characterized by uncontrolled proliferation of abnormal, immature lymphocytes and their progenitors, ultimately replacing normal bone marrow elements.

■ SYNONYMS

Lymphoid leukemia
ALL

ICD-9CM CODES

204.0 Acute lymphoblastic leukemia

■ EPIDEMIOLOGY & DEMOGRAPHICS

- ALL is primarily a disease of children (peak incidence at ages 2 to 10 yr).
- It is diagnosed in 3000 to 4000 persons in the U.S. each year; two thirds are children.

■ PHYSICAL FINDINGS & CLINICAL PRESENTATION

- Skin pallor, purpura, or easy bruising
- Lymphadenopathy or hepatosplenomegaly
- Fever, bone pain, oliguria, weakness, weight loss, mental status changes

■ ETIOLOGY

- Unknown; increased risk in patients with a previous use of antineoplastic agents (e.g., chemotherapy of NHL, Hodgkin's disease, ovarian cancer, myeloma)
- Environmental factors (e.g., ionizing radiation), toxins (e.g., benzene)

DIAGNOSIS

■ DIFFERENTIAL DIAGNOSIS

Acute myeloid leukemia (AML): the distinction between ALL and AML and the classification of the various subtypes are based on the following factors:
- Cell morphology
  1. Lymphoblasts: a high nucleus/cytoplasmic ratio; usually, cytoplasmic granules are not present.
  2. Myeloblasts: abundant cytoplasm; often, cytoplasmic granules (Auer rods) are present.
- Histochemical stains
  1. Peroxidase and Sudan black stains: negative in ALL; useful to distinguish nonlymphoid from lymphoid cells
  2. Chloroacetate esterase: a pink cytoplasmic reaction identifies granulocytes; useful to distin-

guish granulocytes from monocytes in patients with AML
Lymphoblastic lymphoma
Aplastic anemia
Infectious mononucleosis
Leukemoid reaction to infection
Multiple myeloma

■ WORKUP

- Laboratory evaluation
- Bone marrow examination (with biopsy, cytochemistry, immunophenotyping, and cytogenetics)
- Lumbar puncture and imaging studies

■ LABORATORY TESTS

- CBC reveals normochromic, normocytic anemia, thrombocytopenia.
- Peripheral smear will reveal lymphoblasts.
- Initial blood work should also include BUN, creatinine, serum electrolytes, uric acid, LDH.
- Special diagnostic tests include immunophenotyping, cytogenetics, and cytochemistry.
- The French, American, British (FAB) Cooperative Study Group has classified ALL into three groups (L1-L3) based on cell size, cytoplasmic appearance, nucleus shape, and chromatin pattern; the most common form is the L2 type.
- Immunologic classification is on the basis of expression of surface antigens by blast cells: T lineage and B lineage.

■ IMAGING STUDIES

- Chest radiograph to evaluate for the presence of mediastinal mass
- CT scan or ultrasound of abdomen to assess splenomegaly or leukemic infiltration of abdominal organs

TREATMENT

■ ACUTE GENERAL Rx

- Emergency treatment is indicated in patients with intracerebral leukostasis. It consists of one or more of the following:
  1. Cranial irradiation of the whole brain in one- or two-dose fractions
  2. Leukapheresis
  3. Oral hydroxyurea (requires 48 to 72 hr to significantly lower the circulating blast count)
- Urate nephropathy can be prevented by vigorous hydration and lowering uric acid level with allopurinol and urine alkalization with acetazolamide.

- Infections must be aggressively treated with broad-spectrum antibiotics.
  1. Any febrile or neutropenic patients must have cultures taken and be properly treated with IV antibiotics.
  2. If evidence of infection persists despite adequate treatment with antibiotics, amphotericin B may be added to provide coverage against fungal infections (*Candida, Aspergillus*).
- Correct significant thrombocytopenia (platelet counts <20,000/mm³) with platelet transfusion.
- Bleeding secondary to DIC is treated with heparin and replacement of clotting factors.
- Induction therapy is intensive chemotherapy to destroy a significant number of leukemic cells and achieve remission; it usually consists of a combination of vincristine (Oncovin), prednisone, and l-asparaginase (ELSPAR) in children or an anthracene in adults.
- Consolidation therapy consists of an aggressive course of chemotherapy with or without radiotherapy shortly after complete remission has been obtained. Its purpose is to prolong the remission period or cure. Commonly used agents are VM-26, VP-16, HiDAC.
- Meningeal prophylactic therapy with intrathecal methotrexate with or without cranial irradiation is indicated to prevent meningeal sequestration of leukemic cells.
- The goal of maintenance therapy is to maintain a state of remission. In patients with ALL, intermittent therapy is continued for at least 3 yr with a combination of methotrexate and 6-mercaptopurine (Purinethol).
- Bone marrow transplantation: patients should receive allograft in the first complete remission if they are between ages 20 and 50 yr and have matched a sibling donor.

■ DISPOSITION

- Prognosis is generally poorer in adult disease compared with childhood disease (40% adult cure rate versus 80% cure rate in children).
- Five-year leukemia-free survival is <40%.
- The presence of Philadelphia chromosome (Ph⁺), monosomy 5 and 7, and abnormalities of 11q23 are bad prognostic signs.

Author: **Fred F. Ferri, M.D.**

BASIC INFORMATION

■ DEFINITION

Acute myelogenous leukemia (AML) is a disorder characterized by uncontrolled proliferation of primitive myeloid cells (blasts), ultimately replacing normal bone marrow elements frequently resulting in hematopoietic insufficiency (granulocytopenia, thrombocytopenia, or anemia) with or without leukocytosis.

■ SYNONYMS

Acute nonlymphoblastic leukemia (ANLL)
Acute nonlymphocytic leukemia
Acute myeloid leukemia (AML)

ICD-9CM CODES
205.0 Acute myelogenous leukemia

■ EPIDEMIOLOGY & DEMOGRAPHICS
- AML usually affects adults (most patients are 30 to 60 yr old; median age at presentation is 50 yr).
- Annual incidence is 2 to 4/100,000

■ PHYSICAL FINDINGS & CLINICAL PRESENTATION
Patients generally come to medical attention because of the effects of the cytopenias:
- Anemia manifests with weakness or fatigue.
- Thrombocytopenia can manifest with bleeding, petechiae, and ecchymosis.
- Neutropenia can result in infections and fever.
- Physical examination may reveal skin pallor, bruises, petechiae; abdominal examination may reveal hepatosplenomegaly; peripheral lymphadenopathy may also be present.
- Hyperleukocytosis can lead to symptoms of leukostasis, such as ocular and cerebrovascular dysfunction or bleeding.

■ ETIOLOGY
Risk factors are previous use of antineoplastic agents, chromosomal abnormalities, ionizing radiation, toxins, immunodeficiency states, and chronic myeloproliferative disorders.

DIAGNOSIS

■ DIFFERENTIAL DIAGNOSIS
- Acute lymphocytic leukemia
- Leukemoid reaction
- Myelodysplastic syndrome
- Infiltrative diseases of the bone marrow
- Epstein-Barr, other viral infection

■ LABORATORY TESTS
- CBC reveals anemia, thrombocytopenia. Peripheral WBC count varies from <5000/mm³ to >100,000/mm³.
- Additional laboratory findings may include elevated LDH and uric acid levels, decreased fibrinogen, and increased FDP secondary to DIC.
- Cytogenetic abnormalities are common (chromosome 8 is most frequently involved in AML).
- The distinction between ALL and AML and the classification of the various subtypes are based on the following factors:
  1. Cell morphology: myeloblasts reveal abundant cytoplasm; cytoplasmic granules are often present (Auer rods).
  2. Histochemical stains:
     a. Peroxidase and Sudan black stains are negative in ALL.
     b. Chloroacetate esterase: a pink cytoplasmic reaction identifies granulocytes; useful to distinguish granulocytes from monocytes in patients with AML.
- AML is diagnosed by the presence of at least 30% blast cells and positive peroxidase or Sudan black histochemical stain in the bone marrow aspirate.
- The French, American, British (FAB) Cooperative Study Group has classified AML into seven categories (M1-M7) based on the type and percentage of immature cells.

■ IMAGING STUDIES
- Chest x-ray examination is useful to evaluate for the presence of mediastinal masses.
- CT scan of the abdomen may reveal hepatosplenomegaly or leukemic involvement of other organs.

TREATMENT

■ ACUTE GENERAL Rx
- Emergency treatment consisting of one or more of the following is indicated in patients with intracerebral leukostasis:
  1. Cranial irradiation
  2. Leukapheresis
  3. Oral hydroxyurea
- Urate nephropathy can be prevented by vigorous hydration and lowering uric acid level with allopurinol and urine alkalinization with acetazolamide.
- Infections must be aggressively treated with broad-spectrum antibiotics.
- Correct significant thrombocytopenia with platelet transfusions.
- Bleeding secondary to DIC is treated with heparin and replacement of clotting factors.
- Intensive induction chemotherapy to destroy a significant number of leukemic cells and achieve remission usually consists of cytarabine (Cytosar) and daunorubicin. Alltransretinoic acid is effective for the induction of remission of AML M3 subtype (acute promyelocytic leukemia).
- High-dose cytarabine (ARA-C) (HiDAC) can be used in patients with refractory or relapsed AML. It usually takes 28 to 32 days from the start of therapy to achieve remission. The duration of remission is variable; the median duration of remission in an adult with AML is 1 yr.
- Consolidation therapy consists of an aggressive course of chemotherapy with or without radiation shortly after complete remission has been obtained; its purpose is to prolong the remission period or cure. Complications of consolidation therapy are usually secondary to severe bone marrow suppression (anemia, thrombocytopenia, granulocytopenia).
- Goal of therapy is to maintain a state of remission. A postinduction course of high-dose cytarabine can provide equivalent disease-free survival and somewhat better overall survival than autologous marrow transplantation in adults.
- Autologous bone marrow transplantation is indicated in patients <55 yr without a sibling donor. Allogeneic bone marrow transplantation is generally available to <20% of patients; usually performed only in patients <40 yr old because of higher incidence of GVHD with advancing age.

■ DISPOSITION
- Remission can be achieved in nearly 80% of patients <55 yr of age. Remission rates are highest in children.
- Cure for allogeneic bone marrow transplantation approaches 60%; cure rates with autologous transplantation are slightly lower.
- Favorable cytogenics are inv (16) (p13;q22) and t(8;21), t(15;17).

PEARLS & CONSIDERATIONS

■ COMMENTS
- The major complication of chemotherapy is profound marrow depression with pancytopenia lasting 3 to 4 wk. Treatment is aimed at RBC and platelet replacement and aggressive monitoring and treatment of suspected infections.
- Low doses of arsenic trioxide can induce complete remissions in patients with acute promyelocytic leukemia.

Author: **Fred F. Ferri, M.D.**

BASIC INFORMATION

■ DEFINITION

Chronic lymphocytic leukemia (CLL) is a lymphoproliferative disorder characterized by proliferation and accumulation of mature-appearing neoplastic lymphocytes.

■ SYNONYMS

CLL

ICD-9CM CODES

204.1 Leukemia, chronic lymphocytic

■ EPIDEMIOLOGY & DEMOGRAPHICS

- Most frequent form of leukemia in Western countries (10,000 new cases/yr in the U.S.)
- Generally occurs in middle-aged and elderly patients (median age of 65 yr)
- Male:female ratio of 2:1

■ PHYSICAL FINDINGS & CLINICAL PRESENTATION

- Lymphadenopathy, splenomegaly, and hepatomegaly in the majority of patients
- Variable clinical presentation according to stage of the disease
- Abnormal CBC: many cases are diagnosed on the basis of laboratory results obtained after routine physical examination
- Some patients come to medical attention because of weakness and fatigue (secondary to anemia) or lymphadenopathy

■ ETIOLOGY

Unknown

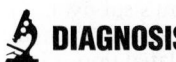

DIAGNOSIS

■ DIFFERENTIAL DIAGNOSIS

- Hairy cell leukemia
- Adult T cell lymphoma
- Prolymphocytic leukemia
- Viral infections
- Waldenström's macroglobulinemia

■ WORKUP

- Laboratory evaluation
- Bone marrow aspirate
- Chromosome analysis

■ LABORATORY TESTS

- Proliferative lymphocytosis (≥15,000/dl) of well-differentiated lymphocytes is the hallmark of CLL.
- There is monotonous replacement of the bone marrow by small lymphocytes (marrow contains ≥30% of well-differentiated lymphocytes).

- Hypogammaglobulinemia and elevated LDH may be present at the time of diagnosis.
- Anemia or thrombocytopenia, if present, indicates poor prognosis.
- Trisomy-12 is the most common chromosomal abnormality, followed by 14 q+, 13 q, and 11 q; these all indicate a poor prognosis.
- New laboratory techniques (CD 38, fluorescence in situ hybridization [FISH]) can identify patients with early-stage CLL at higher risk of rapid disease progression.

STAGING

- Rai et al divided CLL into five clinical stages:
  Stage 0—Characterized by lymphocytosis only (≥15,000/mm³ on peripheral smear, bone marrow aspirate ≥40% lymphocytes). The coexistence of lymphocytosis and other factors increases the clinical stage.
  Stage 1—Lymphadenopathy
  Stage 2—Lymphadenopathy/ hepatomegaly
  Stage 3—Anemia (Hgb <11 g/mm³)
  Stage 4—Thrombocytopenia (platelets <100,000/mm³)
- Another well-known staging system developed by Binet divides chronic lymphocytic leukemia into three stages:
  Stage A—Hgb ≥10 g/dl, platelets ≥100,000/mm³, and fewer than three areas involved (the cervical, axillary, and inguinal lymph nodes [whether unilaterally or bilaterally]; the spleen; and the liver)
  Stage B—Hgb ≥10 g/dl, platelets ≥100,000/mm³, and three or more areas involved
  Stage C—Hgb <10 g/dl, low platelets (<100,000/mm³), or both (independent of the areas involved)

■ IMAGING STUDIES

CT scan of abdomen to evaluate for hepatomegaly and splenomegaly

TREATMENT

■ NONPHARMACOLOGIC THERAPY

- Treatment goals are relief of symptoms and prolongation of life.
- Observation is appropriate for patients in Rai Stage 0 or Binet Stage A.

■ ACUTE GENERAL Rx

- Symptomatic patients in Rai Stage I and II or Binet Stage B: chlorambucil; local irradiation for isolated symptomatic lymphadenopathy and lymph nodes that interfere with vital organs

- Fludarabine is an effective treatment for CLL that does not respond to initial treatment with chlorambucil. Recent reports indicate that when used as the initial treatment for CLL, fludarabine yields higher response rates and a longer duration of remission and progression-free survival than chlorambucil; overall survival, however, is not enhanced.
- Rai Stages III and IV, Binet Stage C: chlorambucil chemotherapy with or without prednisone
  1. Fludarabine, CAP (cyclophosphamide, Adriamycin, prednisone), or cyclophosphamide, doxorubicin, vincristine, and prednisone (mini-CHOP) can be used in patients who respond poorly to chlorambucil.
  2. Splenic irradiation can be used in selected patients with advanced disease.

■ CHRONIC Rx

Treatment of systemic complications:
- Hypogammaglobulinemia is frequent in CLL and is the chief cause of infections. Immune globulin (250 mg/kg IV every 4 wk) may prevent infections but has no effect on survival. Infections should be treated with broad-spectrum antibiotics. Patients should be monitored for opportunistic infections.
- Recombinant hematopoietic cofactors (e.g., granulocyte-macrophage colony–stimulating factor and granulocyte colony–stimulating factor) may be useful to overcome neutropenia related to treatment.
- Erythropoietin may be useful to treat anemia that is unresponsive to other measures.

■ DISPOSITION

The patient's prognosis is directly related to the clinical stage (e.g., the average survival in patients in Rai Stage 0 or Binet Stage A is >120 mo, whereas for RAI Stage 4 or Binet Stage C it is approximately 30 mo). Overall 5-yr survival is 60%.

PEARLS & CONSIDERATIONS

■ COMMENTS

Long-term follow-up and frequency of follow-up are generally determined by the pace of the disease.

REFERENCE

Shanafelt TD, Call TG: Current approach to diagnosis and management of chronic lymphocytic leukemia, *Mayo Clin Proc* 79:388, 2004.
Author: **Fred F. Ferri, M.D.**

BASIC INFORMATION

■ DEFINITION

Chronic myelogenous leukemia (CML) is a malignant clonal disorder of hemopoietic stem cells characterized by abnormal proliferation and accumulation of immature granulocytes. CML is characterized by a chronic phase lasting months to years, followed by an accelerated myeloproliferative phase manifested by poor response to therapy, worsening anemia, or decreased platelet count; the second phase then evolves into a terminal phase (acute transformation), characterized by elevated number of blast cells and numerous complications (e.g., sepsis, bleeding).

■ SYNONYMS

CML
Chronic granulocytic leukemia
Chronic myeloid leukemia

ICD-9CM CODES

201.1 Chronic myelogenous leukemia

■ EPIDEMIOLOGY & DEMOGRAPHICS

- CML usually affects middle-aged patients (median age at presentation is 53 yr) and accounts for 15% of adult leukemias
- 4300 new cases/yr in the U.S.

■ PHYSICAL FINDINGS & CLINICAL PRESENTATION

- The chronic phase usually reveals splenomegaly; hepatomegaly is not infrequent, but lymphadenopathy is very unusual and generally indicates the accelerated proliferative phase of the disease.
- Common complaints at the time of diagnosis are weakness or discomfort secondary to an enlarged spleen (abdominal discomfort or pain). Splenomegaly is present in up to 40% of patients at time of diagnosis.
- 40% of patients are asymptomatic and diagnosis is based solely on an abnormal blood count.

■ ETIOLOGY

Current evidence strongly implicates the chromosome translocation t (9;22) (q34;q11.2) as the cause of chronic granulocytic leukemia. This translocation is present in >95% of patients. The remaining patients have a complex or variant translocation involving additional chromosomes that have the same end result (fusion of the BCR [break point cluster region] gene on chromosome 22 to ABL [Ableson leukemia virus] gene on chromosome 9).

DIAGNOSIS

■ DIFFERENTIAL DIAGNOSIS

- Splenic lymphoma
- CLL
- Myelodysplastic syndrome

■ LABORATORY TESTS

- Elevated WBC count (generally >100,000/mm^3) with broad spectrum of granulocytic forms.
- Bone marrow demonstrates hypercellularity with granulocytic hyperplasia, increased ratio of myeloid cells to erythroid cells, and increased number of megakaryocytes. Blasts and promyelocytes constitute <10% of all cells.
- Philadelphia chromosome (which results from the reciprocal translocation between the long arms of chromosomes 9 and 22) is present in >95% of patients with CML; its presence (Ph^1) is a major prognostic factor because survival rate of patients with Philadelphia chromosome is approximately eight times better than that of those without it. Some believe that Ph$^+$ defines CML and that those who are Ph$^-$ have another disease.
- Leukocyte alkaline phosphatase (LAP) markedly decreased (used to distinguish CML from other myeloproliferative disorders).
- Anemia and thrombocytosis are often present.
- Additional laboratory results are elevated vitamin B$_{12}$ levels (caused by increased transcobalamin 1 from granulocytes) and elevated blood histamine levels (because of increased basophils).

■ IMAGING STUDIES

Chest x-ray examination and CT scan of abdomen

TREATMENT

■ ACUTE GENERAL Rx

Imatinib mesylate (Gleevec), an oral tyrosine kinase inhibitor, is effective and indicated as first-line treatment for CML myeloid blast crisis, accelerated phase, or CML in its chronic phase. More than 60% of patients have major cytogenetic response (<35% Philadelphia chromosome-positive cells in the marrow) and more than 80% have progression-free survival after 24 mo. Complete hematologic response usually occurs in less than 1 mo.

- Symptomatic hyperleukocytosis (e.g., CNS symptoms) can be treated with leukapheresis and hydroxyurea; allopurinol should be started to prevent urate nephropathy following the rapid lysis of the leukemia cells.
- Cytotoxic chemotherapy with hydroxyurea has largely replaced busulfan as the standard cytotoxic drug.
- Allogeneic stem-cell transplantation (SCT) (following intense chemotherapy with busulfan and cyclophosphamide or combined chemotherapy with cyclophosphamide and fractionated total body irradiation to destroy residual leukemic cells) is the only curative treatment for CML in chronic phase unresponsive to imatinib. Generally only 20% of patients are candidates for SCT given the limitations of age or lack of HLA-matched related donors.
  1. It should be considered in "young" patients (increased survival in patients <55 yr) with compatible siblings.
  2. Early transplantation is also important for patient's survival.
- Transplantation of marrow from an HLA-matched, unrelated donor is also now recognized as safe and effective therapy for selected patients with chronic myelogenous leukemia.

REFERENCES

Goldman JM, Melo JV: Chronic myeloid leukemia, advances in biology and new approaches to treatment, *N Engl J Med* 349:1451, 2003.

Hughes TP et al: Frequency of major molecular responses to imatinib or interferon alfa plus cytarabine in newly diagnosed chronic myeloid leukemia, *N Engl J Med* 349:1423, 2003.

Kantarjian H et al: Hematologic and cytogenetic responses to imatinib mesylate in chronic myelogenous leukemia, *N Engl J Med* 346:645, 2002.

Author: **Fred F. Ferri, M.D.**

BASIC INFORMATION

■ DEFINITION
Hairy cell leukemia is a lymphoid neoplasm characterized by the proliferation of mature B cells with prominent cytoplasmic projections (hairs).

■ SYNONYMS
Leukemic reticuloendotheliosis

ICD-9CM CODES
202.4 Hairy cell leukemia

■ EPIDEMIOLOGY & DEMOGRAPHICS
PREVALENCE: Occurs predominantly in men between 40 and 60 yr of age. About 2% of leukemia cases are of the hairy cell type.
PREDOMINANT SEX: Male:female ratio of 4:1

■ PHYSICAL FINDINGS & CLINICAL PRESENTATION
- Usually, splenomegaly (present in >90% of cases) secondary to tumor cell infiltration
- Pallor, ecchymosis, and evidence of infection if the pancytopenia is severe
- Weakness, lethargy, and fatigue
- Infections (resulting from impaired resistance secondary to neutropenia) and easy bruising (secondary to thrombocytopenia) also common

■ ETIOLOGY
Neoplastic disease of the lymphoreticular system of unknown etiology

DIAGNOSIS

■ DIFFERENTIAL DIAGNOSIS
- Other forms of leukemia
- Lymphoma
- Viral syndrome

■ WORKUP
Comprehensive history, physical examination, and laboratory evaluation to confirm the diagnosis

■ LABORATORY TESTS
- Pancytopenia involving erythrocytes, neutrophils, and platelets is common; anemia is usually present and varies from minimal to severe.
- Hairy cells (Fig. 1-161) can account for 5% to 80% of cells in the peripheral blood. The cytoplasmic projections on the cells are redundant plasma membranes.
- Leukemic cells stain positively for tartrate-resistant acid phosphatase (TRAP) stain.
- Bone marrow may result in a "dry tap" (because of increased marrow reticulin).

TREATMENT

■ NONPHARMACOLOGIC THERAPY
Approximately 8% to 10% of patients are asymptomatic and have minimal splenomegaly and minor cytopenia. They are usually detected on routine laboratory evaluation and do not require initial therapy. They should, however, be frequently monitored for progression of their disease.

■ ACUTE GENERAL Rx
- Drugs of choice are the purine analogues 2-Chloro-2 deoxyadenosine (Cladribine) or 2-deoxycoformycin (DCF, Pentostatin). They induce complete remissions in up to 85% of patients and partial responses in 5% to 25%.
- 2-Chloro-2 deoxyadenosine (CdA) 0.14 mg/kg qd for 7 days has minimal toxicity and is able to induce complete durable responses with a single course of therapy.

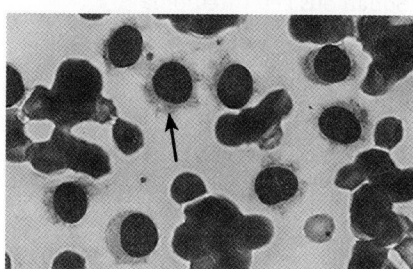

Fig. 1-161 Hairy cell leukemia. Note the lymphocytes with hairlike cytoplasmic projections surrounding the nucleus. (From Rodak BF: *Diagnostic hematology,* Philadelphia, 1995, WB Saunders.)

- Interferon-α produces a partial remission in 30% to 70% of patients and complete remission, often of short duration, in 5% to 10 % of patients.
- The anti-CD 22 recombinant immunotoxin BL 22 can induce complete remission in patients with hairy cell leukemia that is resistant to treatment with purine analogues.

■ CHRONIC Rx
Patients should be monitored with periodic examination and laboratory tests for progression of their disease.

■ DISPOSITION
Prognosis has become increasingly favorable with the newer agents. Approximately 90% of patients who are treated have a complete or partial response.

■ REFERRAL
Hematology consultation is recommended in all patients.

PEARLS & CONSIDERATIONS

■ COMMENTS
The diagnosis of hairy cell leukemia is occasionally missed and subsequently made by the histopathologist following removal of the spleen for diagnostic purposes.

REFERENCE
Kreitman RJ et al: Efficacy of the anti-CD 22 recombinant immunotoxin BL 22 in chemotherapy resistant hairy-cell leukemia, *N Engl J Med* 345:241, 2001.
Author: **Fred F. Ferri, M.D.**

BASIC INFORMATION

■ DEFINITION

Oral hairy leukoplakia (OHL) is a painless, white, plaquelike lesion typically located on the lateral aspect of the tongue.

ICD-9CM CODES

528.6 Oral hairy leukoplakia

■ ETIOLOGY

Epstein-Barr virus (EBV) is implicated in its etiology, and OHL is a result of replication EBV in the epithelium of keratinized cells.

■ EPIDEMIOLOGY & DEMOGRAPHICS

OHL is usually found in human immunodeficiency virus (HIV) seropositive individuals but may also be identified in other immunocompromised patients such as transplant recipients (particularly renal) and patients taking steroids. A diagnosis of OHL is an indication to institute a workup to evaluate and manage HIV disease. Despite a high incidence of EBV seroprevalence in HIV-seropositive individuals, OHL occurs in only 25% of these cases.

■ PHYSICAL FINDINGS & CLINICAL PRESENTATION

- Varying morphology and appearance
- May be unilateral or bilateral
- White and can be small with fine vertical corrugations on the lateral margin of the tongue (Fig. 1-162)

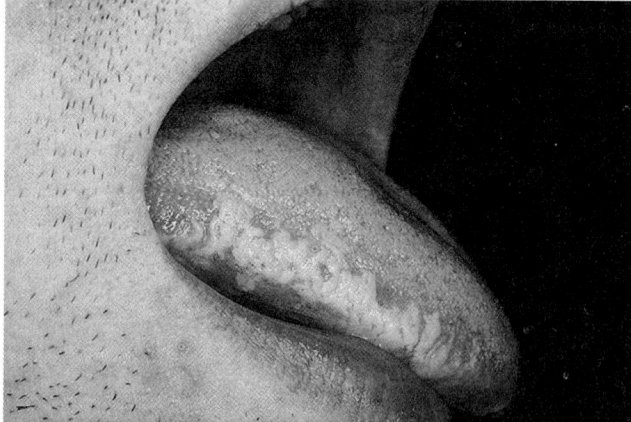

Fig. 1-162 Oral hairy leukoplakia. Note white verrucoid plaques on the lateral border of the tongue. (From Noble J: *Primary care medicine*, ed 3, St Louis, 2001, Mosby.)

- Irregular surface; may have prominent folds or projection, occasionally markedly resembling hairs
- May spread to cover the entire dorsal surface or spread onto the ventral surface of the tongue where they usually appear flat
- Rarely lesions manifest on the soft palate, buccal mucosa, and in the posterior oropharynx
- Usually asymptomatic, but some have mouth pain, soreness, or a burning sensation, impaired taste, or difficulty eating; others complain of its unsightly appearance
- OHL may progress to oral squamous cell carcinoma, which has a poor prognosis

DIAGNOSIS

■ DIFFERENTIAL DIAGNOSIS

- *Candida albicans*
- Lichen planus
- Idiopathic leukoplakia
- White sponge nevus
- Dysplasia
- Squamous cell carcinoma

■ WORKUP

Requires physical examination and evaluation of HIV disease

■ LABORATORY TESTS

The *provisional* diagnosis is clinical and based on:
- Visual inspection
- Inability to scrape the lesion off the tongue with a blade

- Failure to respond to antifungal therapy

The *presumptive* diagnosis requires biopsy and histologic demonstration of:
- Epithelial hyperplasia with hairs
- Absence of inflammatory cell infiltrate

The *definitive* diagnosis requires:
- In situ hybridization of histologic or cytologic specimens revealing EBV DNA *or*
- Electron microscopy of specimens revealing herpeslike particles
- Measurement of the DNA content in cells of oral leukoplakia may be used to predict the risk of oral carcinoma.

NOTE: Specimens obtained from lesions may demonstrate hyphae of *Candida albicans,* which may coexist and potentiate EBV-induced OHL.

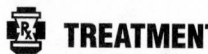 TREATMENT

■ NONPHARMACOLOGIC THERAPY

OHL is usually asymptomatic and requires no specific therapy. It may resolve spontaneously and has no known premalignant potential.

■ ACUTE GENERAL Rx

- Highly active antiretroviral (HAART) therapy has considerably changed the frequency of oral lesions caused by opportunistic infections in HIV-seropositive individuals.
- Topical retinoids (0.1% vitamin A) may improve the appearance of OHL-affected oral surfaces through their dekeratinizing and immunomodulation effects; however, they are expensive and prolonged use may result in a burning sensation over the treated area.
- Topical podophyllin resin 25% solution has been reported to induce resolution.
- Surgical excision and cryotherapy may help, but the lesions may recur.
- High-dose acyclovir or ganciclovir will cause lesions to resolve, but only temporarily.

REFERENCE

Sudbo J et al: DNA content as a prognostic marker in patients with oral leukoplakia, *N Engl J Med* 344:1270, 2001.
Author: **Sajeev Handa, M.D.**

BASIC INFORMATION

■ DEFINITION
Lichen planus refers to a papular skin eruption characteristically found over the flexor surfaces of the extremities, genitalia, and mucous membranes.

■ SYNONYMS
Lichen
Lichen planus et atrophicus

ICD-9CM CODES
697.0 Lichen planus

■ EPIDEMIOLOGY & DEMOGRAPHICS
- Incidence in the U.S.: 440/100,000
- Usually found in people between the ages of 30 to 60
- Found equally between males and females (1:1)
- Lichen planus associated with discoid lupus, SLE, pemphigus vulgaris, bullous pemphigoid, myasthenia gravis, and ulcerative colitis

■ PHYSICAL FINDINGS & CLINICAL PRESENTATION
History
- Usually starts on an extremity and may remain localized or it can spread to involve other areas over a 1- to 4-mo time period.
- Pruritic

Physical findings
- Anatomic distribution:
  1. Flexor surface of wrists, forearms, shins, and upper thighs
  2. Neck and back area
  3. Nails
  4. Scalp
  5. Oral mucosa, buccal mucosa, tongue, gingiva, and lips

Genital mucosa
- Lesion configuration:
  1. Linear
  2. Annular (more common)
  3. Reticular pattern noted on oral mucosa and genital area
- Lesion morphology:
  1. Papules (flat, smooth and shiny)—most common presentation
  2. Hypertrophic
  3. Follicular
  4. Vesicular
- Color:
  1. Dark red, bluish red, purplish-violaceous color is noted in cutaneous lichen planus
  2. Individual lesions characteristically have white lines visible (Wickham's striae)
  3. Oral and genital lichen planus have a reticular network of white lines that may be raised or annular in appearance

  4. Atrophic purplish violaceous color
- Scalp lesions may result in alopecia.

■ ETIOLOGY
- The cause of lichen planus is unknown. Leading theory is cell-mediated immune response.
- Lichenlike reactions can occur from drugs (e.g., tetracycline, quinacrine, chloroquine, penicillamine, and hydrochlorothiazide).

DIAGNOSIS

- Clinical history and physical findings usually establish the diagnosis of lichen planus.
- Skin biopsy can be done to confirm the diagnosis.

■ DIFFERENTIAL DIAGNOSIS
- Drug eruption
- Psoriasis
- Basal cell carcinoma
- Bowen's disease
- Leukoplakia
- Candidiasis
- Lupus rash
- Secondary syphilis
- Seborrheic dermatitis

■ WORKUP
No workup is necessary in patients with lichen planus. If the diagnosis is questionable, a skin biopsy is performed.

■ LABORATORY TESTS
Laboratory tests are not specific for the diagnosis of lichen planus.

■ IMAGING STUDIES
Imaging studies are not helpful in diagnosing lichen planus.

TREATMENT

There are no large, randomized trials published to date substantiating the benefit and effectiveness of treatment in lichen planus. Much of the therapeutic information is based on observational data and the personal preferences of experts.

■ NONPHARMACOLOGIC THERAPY
- Avoid scratching.
- Use mild soaps and emollients after bathing to prevent dryness.

■ ACUTE GENERAL Rx
For cutaneous lichen planus
- Topical steroids, triamcinolone acetonide 0.1% with occlusion

- Acitretin 30 mg/day PO for 8 wk can be used
- Systemic prednisone 30 to 60 mg/day as a starting dose and tapered to 15 to 20 mg/day maintenance for 6 wk has also been tried
- Intradermal steroid triamcinolone acetonide 5 mg/ml can be tried for thick hyperkeratotic lesions
- Hydroxyzine 25 mg PO q6h can be used for pruritus

For oral lichen planus
- Topical steroid fluocinonide in an adhesive base used six times/day for 9 wk
- Topical retinoids 0.1% retinoic acid in an adhesive base or gel can be used for oral or genital lesions
- Etretinate 75 mg/day for 2 mo can also be used for oral lesions

■ CHRONIC Rx
Refer to acute general treatment

■ DISPOSITION
- Spontaneous remissions of cutaneous lichen planus occur in over 65% of cases within the first year.
- Spontaneous remission of oral lichen planus usually occurs by 5 yr.
- Approximately 10% to 20% of patients will have recurrence.

■ REFERRAL
If the diagnosis of lichen planus is suspected, a dermatology consultation is recommended.

PEARLS & CONSIDERATIONS

■ COMMENTS
- Lichen planus can be remembered as purple, planar, pruritic, polygonal papules (5 Ps).
- Lesions can develop at the site of prior skin injury (Koebner's phenomenon).
- Although transformation to skin cancer has been seen in patients with lichen planus, it remains unclear if there is a true correlation.

REFERENCES
Boyd AS, Neldner KH: Lichen planus, *J Am Acad Dermatol* 25:593, 1991.
Cribier B, Rances C, Chosidow O: Treatment of lichen planus: an evidence-based medicine analysis of efficacy, *Arch Dermatol* 134(12):1521, 1998.
Katta R: Lichen planus, *Am Fam Physician* 61(11):3319, 2000.
Author: **Peter Petropoulos, M.D.**

BASIC INFORMATION

■ DEFINITION
Chronic inflammatory condition of the skin usually affecting the vulva, perianal area, and groin

ICD-9CM CODES
701.0 Lichen sclerosus

■ EPIDEMIOLOGY & DEMOGRAPHICS
- Most common in postmenopausal women and men between ages 40 and 60 yr
- More common in females
- Can occur in children (usually prepubertal girls with involvement of the vulva and perineum)

■ PHYSICAL FINDINGS & CLINICAL PRESENTATION
- Erythema may be the only initial sign. A characteristic finding is the presence of ivory-white atrophic lesions on the involved area.
- Close inspection of the affected area will reveal the presence of white-to-brown follicular plugs on the surface (dells).
- When the genitals are involved, the white parchmentlike skin assumes an hourglass configuration around the introital and perianal area ("keyhole" distribution, see Fig. 1-163). Inflammation, subepithelial hemorrhages, and chronic ulceration may develop.
- Dyspareunia, genital bleeding, and anal bleeding are common.

■ ETIOLOGY
Unknown. There may be an autoimmune association and a genetic familial component.

 DIAGNOSIS

■ DIFFERENTIAL DIAGNOSIS
- Localized scleroderma (morphea)
- Cutaneous discoid lupus erythematosus
- Atrophic lichen planus
- Psoriasis

■ WORKUP
Diagnosis is based on close examination of the lesions for the presence of ivory-white atrophic lesions and typical location.

■ LABORATORY TESTS
Punch or deep shave biopsy can be used to confirm the diagnosis when in doubt.

■ IMAGING STUDIES
Not indicated

TREATMENT

■ NONPHARMACOLOGIC THERAPY
Attention to hygiene and elimination of irritants or excessive bathing with harsh soaps

■ GENERAL Rx
- Application of clobetasol propionate 0.05% topically bid for up to 4 wk is usually effective. Repeat courses of corticosteroids may be necessary because of the chronic nature of this disorder. Continual application of topical steroids may lead to atrophy of the vulva.
- Use of topical testosterone (2%) has been found to be less effective than topical corticosteroids.
- Lubricants (e.g., Nutraplus cream) are useful to soothe dry tissues.
- Hydroxyzine 25 mg at hs is effective in decreasing nocturnal itching.
- Use of intralesional steroids, etretinate, and surgical management are usually reserved for refractory cases.

■ DISPOSITION
- The disease persists in approximately one third of patients.
- Most prepubertal girls improve spontaneously at menarche.
- Squamous cell carcinoma can develop within the lesions in 3% to 10% of older patients; therefore, periodic examination and biopsy of suspicious areas are indicated.

PEARLS & CONSIDERATIONS

■ COMMENTS
- Prepubertal lichen sclerosus may be confused with sexual abuse in prepubertal girls and may lead to false accusations and investigations.
- Lichen sclerosus of the vulva (kraurosis vulvae) usually occurs after menopause and is generally chronic. It can be painful and interfere with sexual activity.
- Lichen sclerosus of the penis (balanitis xerotica obliterans) is seen more commonly in uncircumcised males. It affects the glans and prepuce and may lead to stricture if it encroaches into the urinary meatus.

Author: **Fred F. Ferri, M.D.**

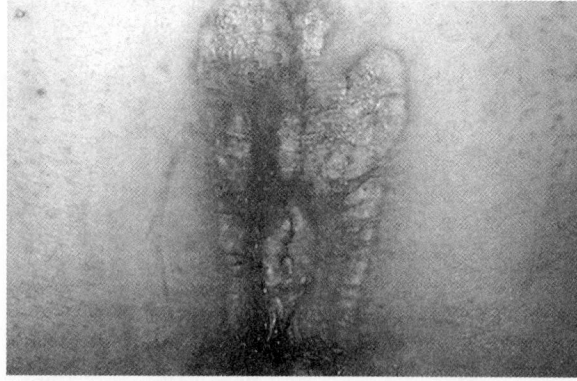

Fig. 1-163 Lichen sclerosus. Perianal area is thinned and chalk white (keyhole distribution). (Courtesy Department of Dermatology, University of North Carolina at Chapel Hill. From Goldstein BG, Goldstein AO: *Practical dermatology,* ed 2, St Louis, 1997, Mosby.)

BASIC INFORMATION

■ DEFINITION

Listeriosis is a systemic infection caused by the gram-positive aerobic bacterium *Listeria monocytogenes*.

ICD-9CM CODES

027.0 Listeriosis
771.2 Congenital listeriosis
771.2 Fetal listeriosis
665.4 Suspected fetal damage affecting management of pregnancy

■ EPIDEMIOLOGY & DEMOGRAPHICS

INCIDENCE (IN U.S.):
- Listeria meningitis: about 0.7 cases/100,000 persons (fourth most common cause of community-acquired bacterial meningitis in adults)
- Perinatal listeriosis: 8.6 cases/100,000 persons
- Nonperinatal listeriosis: 3 cases/1 million persons

PREDOMINANT SEX: Pregnant women are more susceptible to *Listeria* bacteremia, accounting for up to one third of reported cases.

PREDOMINANT AGE:
- Pregnant women
- Immunocompromised patients of any age

GENETICS
Congenital Infection:
- With transplacental transmission, syndrome termed *granulomatosis infantisepticum* in neonate
- Characterized by disseminated abscesses in multiple organs, skin lesions, conjunctivitis
- Mortality: 33% to 100%

Neonatal Infection:
- Infant becoming ill after 3 days of age; mother invariably asymptomatic
- Clinical picture of sepsis of unknown origin

■ PHYSICAL FINDINGS & CLINICAL PRESENTATION

- Infections in pregnancy
  1. More common in third trimester
  2. Usually present with fever and chills without localizing symptoms or signs of infection
- Meningoencephalitis
  1. More common in neonates and immunocompromised patients, but up to 30% of adults have no underlying condition
  2. In neonates: poor appetite with or without fever possibly the only presenting signs
  3. In adults: presentation often subacute, with low-grade fever and personality change as only signs
  4. Focal neurologic signs seen without demonstrable brain abscess on CT scan
- Cerebritis/thromboencephalitis:
  1. Headache and fever may be only presenting complaints
  2. Progressive cranial nerve palsies, hemiparesis, seizures, depressed level of consciousness, cerebellar signs, respiratory insufficiency may also be seen
- Focal infections
  1. Ocular infections (purulent conjunctivitis) and skin lesions (granulomatosis infantisepticum) as a result of inadvertent inoculation by laboratory and veterinary personnel
  2. Others: arthritis, prosthetic joint infections, peritonitis, osteomyelitis, organ abscesses, cholecystitis

■ ETIOLOGY

- Direct invasion of skin and eye has been documented, but mechanism of GI entry is unclear.
- Organism's intracellular life cycle explanatory of:
  1. Importance of cell-mediated immunity in host defense
  2. Increased incidence of infection in neonates, pregnant women, and immunocompromised hosts

DIAGNOSIS

■ DIFFERENTIAL DIAGNOSIS

- Meningitis caused by other bacteria, mycobacteria, or fungi
- CNS sarcoidosis
- Brain neoplasm or abscess
- Tuberculous and fungal (especially cryptococcal) meningitis
- Cerebral toxoplasmosis
- Lyme disease
- Sarcoidosis

■ WORKUP

Dictated by age, end-organ involvement, and immune status

■ LABORATORY TESTS

- Cultures of blood and other appropriate body fluids
- Variable CSF findings, but neutrophils usually predominate
- Organisms uncommonly seen on Gram stain and may be difficult to identify morphologically
- Monoclonal antibodies, polymerase chain reaction, and DNA probe techniques to detect *Listeria* in foods

■ IMAGING STUDIES

- If focal cerebral involvement suspected: CT scan or MRI
- MRI most sensitive for evaluation of brainstem and cerebellum

TREATMENT

Empiric therapy should be administered when diagnosis is suspected because overall mortality is 23%.

■ ACUTE GENERAL Rx

- Drugs of choice:
  1. IV ampicillin 8 to 12 g/day in divided doses
  2. IV penicillin 12 to 24 million U/day in divided doses
- Continuation of therapy for 2 wk
- Alternative: trimethoprim/sulfamethoxazole
- Gentamicin added to provide synergy

■ CHRONIC Rx

Relapses reported, especially in immunocompromised hosts, after 2 wk of therapy

■ DISPOSITION

Long-term follow-up of immunodeficiency state

■ REFERRAL

Infectious disease consultation for all patients

PEARLS & CONSIDERATIONS

■ COMMENTS

- Foodborne cases have been linked to various products: coleslaw, soft cheese, pasteurized milk, vegetables, undercooked chicken, hot dogs.
- Complete decontamination of food products is difficult because *Listeria* is resistant to pasteurization and refrigeration.

REFERENCES

De Valk H et al: Two consecutive nationwide outbreaks of listeriosis in France, October 1999-February 2000, *Am J Epidemiol* 154(10):944, 2001.

Wing EJ, Gregory SH: Listeria monocytogenes: clinical and experimental update, *J Infect Dis* 185(Suppl 1):S18, 2002.

Author: **Claudia L. Dade, M.D.**

BASIC INFORMATION

■ DEFINITION
Long QT syndrome is an electrocardiographic abnormality characterized by a corrected QT interval longer than 0.44 sec and associated with an increased risk of developing life-threatening ventricular arrhythmias.

■ SYNONYMS
Congenital forms:
- Jervell and Lange-Nielsen syndrome (associated with deafness)
- Romano-Ward syndrome (associated with normal hearing)

Sporadic forms of long QT syndrome (nonfamilial)

ICD-9CM CODES
427.9 Unspecified cardiac dysrhythmia

■ EPIDEMIOLOGY & DEMOGRAPHICS
- Familial associated with deafness: autosomal recessive
- Familial associated with normal hearing: autosomal dominant (the incidence is unknown)

■ PHYSICAL FINDINGS & CLINICAL PRESENTATION
- Syncope caused by ventricular tachycardia
- Sudden death
- Abnormal ECG (prolonged QT) in asymptomatic relatives of known case. Bazett formula; $QTc5QT/\sqrt{RR}$. Calculated QTc should be <440 ms. If patient has atrial fibrillation, take the average of the longest and shortest QTc intervals.
- Routine (baseline) ECG finding.

■ ETIOLOGY
- Cardiac repolarization abnormality
- Congenital cause (chromosome 3 or chromosome 7 abnormality)
- Acquired causes:
  Drugs (quinidine, procainamide, sotalol, amiodarone, disopyramide, phenothiazines, tricyclic antidepressants, quinolones, astemizole or cisapride given with ketoconazole or erythromycin, and antimalarials), particularly among patients with asthma or those using potassium-lowering medications

Hypokalemia, hypomagnesemia
Liquid protein diet
CNS lesions
Mitral valve prolapse

DIAGNOSIS

■ DIFFERENTIAL DIAGNOSIS
See "Syncope."
Diagnostic criteria for the congenital long QT syndrome
ECG criteria

Corrected QT >480 ms	3 points
Corrected QT 460 to 480 ms	2 points
Corrected QT 450 to 460 ms (males)	1 point
Torsades de Pointe	2 points
T-wave alternans	1 point
Notched T wave in 3 leads	1 point
Bradycardia	0.5 points
History	
Syncope with stress	2 points
Syncope without stress	1 point
Congenital deafness	0.5 points
Definite family history of long QT	1 point
Unexplained cardiac death in first-degree relative under age 30	0.5 points

Total score ≥4: definite long QT syndrome
Total score 2 to 3: intermediate probability
Total score ≤1: low probability

■ WORKUP
In relatives of known patients with long QT syndrome or in young patients with syncope:
- Stress test may prolong the QT interval or cause T-wave alternans
- Valsalva maneuver: may prolong the QT interval or cause T-wave alternans
- Prolonged ECG monitoring with various stimulations aimed at increasing catecholamines (perform in a setting that can provide resuscitation)
- Epinephrine-induced prolongation of the 2T interval (Epinephrine infusion QT stress test
- Genetic analysis
  LQT1 locus of KCNQ1 potassium channel gene
  LQT2 locus of KCNH2 potassium channel gene

LQT33 locus of SCN5A sodium channel gene

TREATMENT

- Asymptomatic sporadic forms with no complex ventricular arrhythmias: no treatment
- Risk stratification
  High risk (<50% of cardiac event): QTc >500 ms and LQT1 and LQT2 or male with LQT3
  Moderate risk (30% to 50%): QTc >500 ms in female with LQT3 or L QTc <500 ms in male with LQT3 or in female with LQT2 or 3
  Low risk (<30%): QTc <500 ms and LQT1 and or male OQT2
- General recommendations:
  Avoid competitive sports
  β-blocker at maximum tolerated dose
  Cardiology referral is recommended for all cases. Pacemaker and implantable defibrillator may be advised

REFERENCES
Ackerman MJ: The long QT syndrome: ion channel diseases of the heart, *Mayo Clin Proc* 73:250, 1998.
Ackerman MJ et al: Epinephrine-induced QT interval prolongation: a gene-specific paradoxical response in congenital long QT syndrome, *Mayo Clin Proc* 77:413, 2002.
Al-Khatib SM et al: What clinicians should know about the QT interval, *JAMA* 289:2120, 2003.
De Bruin ML, Hoes AW, Leufkens HGM: QTc-prolonging drugs and hospitalizations for cardiac arrhythmias, *Am J Cardiol* 91:59, 2003.
Priori SG et al: Risk stratification in the long-QT syndrome, *N Engl J Med* 348:1866, 2003.
Roden DM: Drug-induced prolongation of the QT interval, *N Engl J Med* 350:1013, 2004.
Wehrens HXT: Novel insights in the congenital long QT syndrome, *Ann Intern Med* 137;981, 2002.
Author: **Tom J. Wachtel, M.D.**

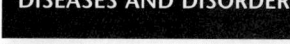
 BASIC INFORMATION

■ DEFINITION

Lumbar disk syndromes are diseases resulting from disk disorder, either herniation or degenerative change (spondylosis). Massive disk protrusion may rarely lead to paralysis in the lower extremity, a condition termed *cauda equina syndrome*. Gradual narrowing of the spinal canal (lumbar stenosis), usually from spondylosis, may also cause lower extremity symptoms.

ICD-9CM CODES
722.10 Lumbar disk displacement
724.02 Lumbar stenosis
344.60 Cauda equina syndrome
721.3 Lumbar spondylosis

■ EPIDEMIOLOGY & DEMOGRAPHICS
PREVALENCE:
- Variable
- At least one episode in 80% of adults

PREVALENT AGE:
- Herniation: 20 to 40 yr
- Stenosis: >40 to 50 yr
- Disk symptoms: rare <20 yr

PREVALENT SEX: Approximately equal

■ PHYSICAL FINDINGS & CLINICAL PRESENTATION (TABLE 1-34)
- Overlapping clinical syndromes that may result:
  1. Mild herniation without nerve root compression
  2. Herniation with nerve root compression
  3. Cauda equina syndrome
  4. Chronic degenerative disease with or without leg symptoms
  5. Spinal stenosis

- Low back pain, often worsened by activity or coughing and sneezing
- Local lumbar or lumbosacral tenderness
- Paresthesias, usually unilateral
- Restricted low back motion
- Increased pain on bending toward affected side
- Weakness and reflex changes
- Sensory examination usually not helpful
- Lumbar stenosis that possibly produces symptoms (pseudoclaudication), which are often misinterpreted as being vascular
- Positive straight leg raising test if nerve root compression is present

■ ETIOLOGY
Unknown

▲ DIAGNOSIS

■ DIFFERENTIAL DIAGNOSIS
- Soft-tissue strain/sprain
- Tumor
- Degenerative arthritis of hip
- Insufficiency fracture of hip or pelvis
Section II describes the differential diagnosis of common low back pain syndromes.

■ WORKUP
In most cases, the diagnosis can be established on a clinical basis alone.

■ IMAGING STUDIES
- Plain roentgenograms may be indicated within the first few weeks; they are usually normal in soft disk herniation, but with chronic degenerative disk disease, loss of height of the disk space and osteophyte formation can occur.

- Myelography, CT scanning, and MRI may be indicated in patients whose symptoms do not resolve or when other spinal pathology may be suspected.
- Electrodiagnostic studies may confirm the diagnosis or rule out peripheral nerve disorders.

℞ TREATMENT

■ NONPHARMACOLOGIC THERAPY
- Short course (3 to 5 days) of bed rest for severe pain; prolonged rest for acute disk herniation with leg pain
- Physical therapy for modalities plus a careful gradual exercise program
- Lumbosacral corset brace during rehabilitation process in conjunction with exercise program
- Percutaneous electrical nerve stimulation (PENS) may be beneficial in selected patients with chronic back pain

■ PHARMACOLOGIC THERAPY
- NSAIDs
- Muscle relaxants for sedative effect
- Analgesics
- Epidural steroid injection for leg symptoms in selected patients

■ DISPOSITION
- Almost all lumbar disk syndromes improve with time.
- Recurrent episodes usually respond to medical management.
- Recovery from the rare paralytic event is often incomplete.

■ REFERRAL
- For orthopedic or neurosurgical consultation for intractable pain or significant neurologic deficit
- Emergency referral for cauda equina syndrome

TABLE 1-34 Diagnosis of Lower Lumbar and Sacral Radiculopathy

	PAIN	WEAKNESS (SELECTED MUSCLES)	SENSORY LOSS	REFLEX LOSS
L4	Across thigh and medial leg to medial malleolus	Quadriceps, thigh adductors, tibialis anterior	Medial leg	Knee
L5	Posterior thigh and lateral calf, dorsum of foot	Extensor digitorum brevis and longus, peronei	Dorsum of foot	
S1	Buttock and posterior thigh, calf, and lateral foot	Extensor digitorum brevis, peronei, gastrocnemius, soleus	Sole or lateral border of foot	Ankle
S2-4	Posterior thigh, buttock, and genitalia	Gastrocnemius, soleus, abductor hallucis, abductor digiti quinti pedis, sphincter muscles	Buttocks, anal region, and genitalia	Bulbocavernosus, anal

From Goldman L, Bennett JC (eds): *Cecil textbook of medicine,* ed 21, Philadelphia, 2000, WB Saunders.

⊙ PEARLS & CONSIDERATIONS

■ COMMENTS
- Surgery is most consistently helpful when leg pain (not back pain) predominates.
- A clinical algorithm for evaluation of back pain is described in Section III, Fig. 3-26.

REFERENCES

Buchner M, Schilotenwolf M: Cauda equina syndrome caused by intervertebral lumbar disc prolapse: mid-term results of 22 patients and literature review, *Orthopedics* 25:727, 2002.

Deyo RA, Weinstein JN: Low back pain, *N Engl J Med* 344:363, 2001.

Kawaguchi Y et al: The association of lumbar disc disease with vitamin-D receptor gene polymorphism, *J Bone Joint Surg* 84(a):2022, 2002.

Linton SJ: A review of psychological risk factors in back and neck pain, *Spine* 25:1148, 2000.

Paassilta P et al: Identification of a novel common genetic risk factor for lumbar disc disease, *JAMA* 285:1843, 2001.

Papagelopoulos PJ et al: Treatment of lumbrosacral radicular pain with epidural steroid injections, *Orthopedics* 24:145, 2001.

Robinson LR: Role of neurophysiologic evaluation in diagnosis, *J Am Acad Orthop Surg* 8:190, 2000.

Silber JS et al: Advances in surgical management of lumbar degenerative disc disease, *Orthopedics* 25:767, 2002.

Simotas AC: Non-operative treatment for lumbar spinal stenosis, *Clin Orthop* 384:153, 2001.

Swenson R, Haldeman S: Spinal manipulation for low back pain, *J Am Acad Orthop Surg* 11:228, 2003.

Tribus CB: Degenerative lumbar scoliosis: evaluation and management, *J Am Acad Orthop Surg* 11:174, 2003.

Wetzel FT, McNally TA: Treatment of chronic discogenic low back pain with intradiskal electrothermal therapy, *J Am Acad Orthop Surg* 11:6, 2003.

Yoshihara K et al: Atrophy of the multifidus muscle in patients with lumbar disc herniation: histochemical and electromyographic study, *Orthopedics* 26:493, 2003.

Author: **Lonnie R. Mercier, M.D.**

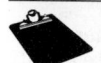

BASIC INFORMATION

■ DEFINITION

A primary lung neoplasm is a malignancy arising from lung tissue. The World Health Organization distinguishes 12 types of pulmonary neoplasms. Among them, the major types are *squamous cell carcinoma, adenocarcinoma, small cell carcinoma,* and *large cell carcinoma*. However, the crucial difference in the diagnosis of lung cancer is between small cell and non–small cell types, because the therapeutic approach is different. Selective characteristics of lung carcinomas:

ADENOCARCINOMA: Represents 35% of lung carcinomas; frequently located in mid lung and periphery; initial metastases are to lymphatics, frequently associated with peripheral scars

SQUAMOUS CELL (EPIDERMOID): 20% to 30% of lung cancers; central location; metastasis by local invasion; frequent cavitation and obstructive phenomena

SMALL CELL (OAT CELL): 20% of lung carcinomas; central location; metastasis through lymphatics; associated with lesion of the short arm of chromosome 3; high cavitation rate

LARGE CELL: 15% to 20% of lung carcinomas; frequently located in the periphery; metastasis to CNS and mediastinum; rapid growth rate with early metastasis

BRONCHOALVEOLAR: 5% of lung carcinomas; frequently located in the periphery; may be bilateral; initial metastasis through lymphatic, hematogenous, and local invasion; no correlation with cigarette smoking; cavitation rare

■ SYNONYMS

Lung cancer

ICD-9CM CODES

162.9 Malignant neoplasm of bronchus and lung, unspecified

■ EPIDEMIOLOGY & DEMOGRAPHICS

- Lung cancer is responsible for >30% of cancer deaths in males and >25% of cancer deaths in females.
- Tobacco smoking is implicated in 85% of cases; second-hand smoke is responsible for approximately 20% of cases.
- There are >180,000 new cases of lung cancer yearly in the U.S., most occurring >age 50 yr (<4% in patients <40 yr of age).

■ PHYSICAL FINDINGS & CLINICAL PRESENTATION

- Weight loss, fatigue, fever, anorexia, dysphagia

- Cough, hemoptysis, dyspnea, wheezing
- Chest, shoulder, and bone pain
- Paraneoplastic syndromes:
  1. *Eaton-Lambert syndrome:* myopathy involving proximal muscle groups
  2. Endocrine manifestations: hypercalcemia, ectopic ACTH, SIADH
  3. Neurologic: subacute cerebellar degeneration, peripheral neuropathy, cortical degeneration
  4. Musculoskeletal: polymyositis, clubbing, hypertrophic pulmonary osteoarthropathy
  5. Hematologic or vascular: migratory thrombophlebitis, marantic thrombosis, anemia, thrombocytosis, or thrombocytopenia
  6. Cutaneous: acanthosis nigricans, dermatomyositis
- Pleural effusion (10% of patients), recurrent pneumonias (secondary to obstruction), localized wheezing
- Superior vena cava syndrome:
  1. Obstruction of venous return of the superior vena cava is most commonly caused by bronchogenic carcinoma or metastasis to paratracheal nodes.
  2. The patient usually complains of headache, nausea, dizziness, visual changes, syncope, and respiratory distress.
  3. Physical examination reveals distention of thoracic and neck veins, edema of face and upper extremities, facial plethora, and cyanosis.
- *Horner's syndrome:* constricted pupil, ptosis, facial anhidrosis caused by spinal cord damage between C8 and T1 secondary to a superior sulcus tumor (bronchogenic carcinoma of the extreme lung apex); a superior sulcus tumor associated with ipsilateral Horner's syndrome and shoulder pain is known as *"Pancoast" tumor*.

■ ETIOLOGY

- Tobacco abuse
- Environmental agents (e.g., radon) and industrial agents (e.g., ionizing radiation, asbestos, nickel, uranium, vinyl chloride, chromium, arsenic, coal dust)

DIAGNOSIS

■ DIFFERENTIAL DIAGNOSIS

- Pneumonia
- TB
- Metastatic carcinoma to the lung
- Lung abscess
- Granulomatous disease
- Carcinoid tumor
- Mycobacterial and fungal diseases
- Sarcoidosis
- Viral pneumonitis

- Benign lesions that simulate thoracic malignancy:
  1. Lobar atelectasis: pneumonia, TB, chronic inflammatory disease, allergic bronchopulmonary aspergillosis
  2. Multiple pulmonary nodules: septic emboli, Wegener's granulomatosis, sarcoidosis, rheumatoid nodules, fungal disease, multiple pulmonary AV fistulas
  3. Mediastinal adenopathy: sarcoidosis, lymphoma, primary TB, fungal disease, silicosis, pneumoconiosis, drug-induced (e.g., phenytoin, trimethadione)
  4. Pleural effusion: CHF, pneumonia with parapneumonic effusion, TB, viral pneumonitis, ascites, pancreatitis, collagen-vascular disease

■ WORKUP

Workup generally includes chest x-ray examination, CT scan of chest, PET scan, and tissue biopsy.

■ LABORATORY TESTS

Obtain tissue diagnosis. Various modalities are available:

- Biopsy of any suspicious lymph nodes (e.g., supraclavicular node)
- Flexible fiberoptic bronchoscopy: brush and biopsy specimens are obtained from any visualized endobronchial lesions
- Transbronchial needle aspiration: done via a special needle passed through the bronchoscope; this technique is useful to sample mediastinal masses or paratracheal lymph nodes
- Transthoracic fine-needle aspiration biopsy with fluoroscopic or CT scan guidance to evaluate peripheral pulmonary nodules
- Mediastinoscopy and anteromedial sternotomy in suspected tumor involvement of the mediastinum
- Pleural biopsy in patients with pleural effusion
- Thoracentesis of pleural effusion and cytologic evaluation of the obtained fluid: may confirm diagnosis

■ IMAGING STUDIES

- Chest x-ray examination: The radiographic presentation often varies with the cell type. Pleural effusion, lobar atelectasis, and mediastinal adenopathy can accompany any cell types.
- CT scan of chest: to evaluate mediastinal and pleural extension of suspected lung neoplasms.
- Positron emission tomography (PET) with 18F-fluorodeoxyglucose (18 FDG-PET), a metabolic marker of malignant tissue, is superior to CT scan in detecting mediastinal and

distant metastases in non–small cell lung cancer. It is useful for preoperative staging of non–small call lung cancer.

STAGING

- Following confirmation of diagnosis, patients should undergo staging:
  1. The international staging system is the most widely accepted staging system for non–small cell lung cancer. In this system, stage 1 (N0 [no lymph node involvement], stage 2 (N1 [spread to ipsilateral bronchopulmonary or hilar lymph nodes]) include localized tumors for which surgical resection is the preferred treatment. Stage 3 is subdivided into 3A (potentially resectable) and 3B. The surgical management of stage IIIA disease (N2 [involvement of ipsilateral mediastinal nodes] is controversial). Only 20% of N2 disease is considered minimal disease (involvement of only one node) and technically resectable. Stage 4 indicates metastatic disease. The pathologic staging system uses a tumor/nodal involvement/metastasis system.
  2. In patients with small cell lung cancer, a more practical accepted staging system is the one developed by the Veterans Administration Lung Cancer Study Group (VALG). This system contains two stages:
     a. Limited stage: disease confined to the regional lymph nodes and to one hemithorax (excluding pleural surfaces)
     b. Extensive stage: disease spread beyond the confines of limited stage disease
  3. Pretreatment staging procedures for lung cancer patients, in addition to complete history and physical examination, generally include the following tests:
     a. Chest x-ray examination (PA and lateral), ECG
     b. Laboratory evaluation: CBC, electrolytes, platelets, calcium, phosphorus, glucose, renal and liver function studies, ABGs, and skin tests for TB
     c. Pulmonary function studies
     d. CT scan of chest and PET scan: A recent Dutch trial revealed a 51% relative reduction in futile thoracotomies for patients with suspected non–small cell lung cancer who underwent preoperative assessment with PET with the tracer 18FDG-PET in addition to conventional workup
     e. Mediastinoscopy or anterior mediastinotomy in patients being considered for possible curative lung resection
     f. Biopsy of any accessible suspect lesions
     g. CT scan of liver and brain; radionuclide scans of bone in all patients with small cell carcinoma of the lung and patients with non–small cell lung neoplasms suspected of involving these organs
     h. Bone marrow aspiration and biopsy only in selected patients with small cell carcinoma of the lung. In the absence of an increased LDH or cytopenia, routine bone marrow examination is not recommended

▣ TREATMENT

■ NONPHARMACOLOGIC THERAPY

- Nutritional support
- Avoidance of tobacco or other substances toxic to the lungs
- Supplemental O_2 prn

■ ACUTE GENERAL Rx
NON–SMALL CELL CARCINOMA:

- Surgery
  1. Surgical resection is indicated in patients with limited disease (not involving mediastinal nodes, ribs, pleura, or distant sites). This represents approximately 15% to 30% of diagnosed cases.
  2. Preoperative evaluation includes review of cardiac status (e.g., recent MI, major arrhythmias) and evaluation of pulmonary function (to determine if the patient can tolerate any loss of lung tissue). Pneumonectomy is possible if the patient has a preoperative $FEV_1 \geq 2$ L or if the MVV is .50% of predicted capacity.
  3. Preoperative chemotherapy should be considered in patients with more advanced disease (stage IIIA) who are being considered for surgery, because it increases the median survival time in patients with non–small cell lung cancer compared with the use of surgery alone.
- Treatment of unresectable non–small cell carcinoma of the lung:
  1. Radiotherapy can be used alone or in combination with chemotherapy; it is used primarily for treatment of CNS and skeletal metastases, superior vena cava syndrome, and obstructive atelectasis; although thoracic radiotherapy is generally considered standard therapy for stage 3 disease, it has limited effect on survival. Palliative radiotherapy should be delayed until symptoms occur since immediate therapy offers no

advantage over delayed therapy and results in more adverse events from the radiotherapy.
  2. Chemotherapy: various combination regimens are available. Current drugs of choice are paclitaxel plus either carboplatin or cisplatin; cisplatin plus vinorelbine; gemcitabine plus cisplatin; carboplatin or cisplatin plus docetaxel. The overall results are disappointing, and none of the standard regimens for non–small cell lung cancer is clearly superior to the others. Gefitinib (Iressa), an inhibitor of epidermal growth factor receptor (EGFR) tyrosine kinase, is an oral preparation currently undergoing clinical trials for advanced non–small cell lung cancer.
  3. The addition of chemotherapy to radiotherapy improves survival in patients with locally advanced, unresectable non–small cell lung cancer. The absolute benefit is relatively small, however, and should be balanced against the increased toxicity associated with the addition of chemotherapy.

TREATMENT OF SMALL CELL LUNG CANCER:

- Limited stage disease: standard treatments include thoracic radiotherapy and chemotherapy (cisplatin and etoposide)
- Extensive stage disease: standard treatments include combination chemotherapy (cisplatin or carboplatin plus etoposide or combination of irinotecan and cisplatin
- Prophylactic cranial irradiation for patients in complete remission to decrease the risk of CNS metastasis

■ DISPOSITION

- The 5-yr survival of patients with non–small cell carcinoma when the disease is resectable is approximately 30%.
- Median survival time in patients with limited stage disease and small cell lung cancer is 15 mo; in patients with extensive stage disease, it is 9 mo.

REFERENCES

Kris MG et al: Efficacy of gefitinib, an inhibitor of the epidermal growth factor receptor tyrosine kinase, in symptomatic patients with non-small cell lung cancer, *JAMA* 290:2149, 2003.

Lardinois D et al: Staging of non-small cell lung cancer with integrated positron-emission tomography and computed tomography, *N Engl J Med* 348:2500, 2003.

Spira A, Ettinger DS: Multidisciplinary management of lung cancer, *N Engl J Med* 350:379, 2004.

Author: **Fred F. Ferri, M.D.**

BASIC INFORMATION

■ DEFINITION
Lyme disease is a multisystem inflammatory disorder caused by the transmission of a spirochete, *Borrelia burgdorferi*. Lyme disease is spread by the bite of infected *Ixodes* ticks, taking 36 to 48 hr for a tick to feed and spread *B. burgdorferi*.

■ SYNONYMS
Bannworth's syndrome
Acrodermatitis chronica atrophicans

ICD-9CM CODES
088.8 Lyme disease

■ EPIDEMIOLOGY & DEMOGRAPHICS
INCIDENCE (IN U.S.): Geographic variation, 4.4 cases/100,000 persons; reported in 43 states and District of Columbia. Approximately 90% of cases in the U.S. are found in nine states: Massachusetts, Connecticut, Rhode Island, New York, New Jersey, Pennsylvania, Minnesota, Wisconsin, and California.
PREDOMINANT SEX: Male = female
PREDOMINANT AGE: Median age of 28 yr
PEAK INCIDENCE: May to November

■ PHYSICAL FINDINGS
Lyme disease may present in the following stages:
- *Early localized:* early Lyme disease, erythema chronicum migrans (ECM); skin rash, often at site of tick bite; possible fever, myalgias 3 to 32 days after tick bite
- *Early disseminated:* days to weeks later; multiorgan system involvement, including CNS, joints, cardiac; related to dissemination of spirochete

- *Late persistent:* months to years after tick exposure; affects central and peripheral nervous system, cardiac, joints

Common presenting signs and symptoms include:
- ECM (Fig. 1-164)
- Lymphadenopathy, neck pains, pharyngeal erythema, myalgias, hepatosplenomegaly often present early in the disease
- Patients will complain of malaise, fatigue, lethargy, headache, fever/chills, neck pain, myalgias, back pain

■ ETIOLOGY
B. burgdorferi transmitted from bite of an *Ixodes* tick (most commonly belonging to the species *Scapularis*)

DIAGNOSIS

Clinical presentation, exposure to ticks in endemic area, and diagnostic testing for antibody response to *B. burgdorferi*

■ DIFFERENTIAL DIAGNOSIS
- Chronic fatigue/fibromyalgia
- Acute viral illnesses
- Babesiosis
- Ehrlichiosis

■ WORKUP
- ELISA testing—Western blot
- Immunofluorescent assay
- Early disease often difficult to diagnose serologically secondary to slow immune response
- Culturing of skin lesions (ECM) and polymerase chain reaction (PCR) of skin biopsy and blood to give definitive diagnosis (available only in reference laboratories)

■ IMAGING STUDIES
- Echocardiogram if conduction abnormalities are present with cardiac involvement
- CT scan, MRI of head for CNS involvement

℞ TREATMENT

- Early Lyme disease
  Doxycycline 100 mg bid or amoxicillin 500 mg qid for 10-14 days (doxycycline should be avoided in children/pregnant females)
  Alternative treatments: cefuroxime axetil 500 mg bid for 10-14 days, azithromycin 500 mg PO qd for 1 day followed by 250 mg qd for 6 days
- Early Disseminated and late persistent infection: 30 days of treatment necessary; doxycycline and ceftriaxone appear equally effective for acute disseminated Lyme disease
- Arthritis: 30 days of doxycycline or amoxicillin plus probenecid (repeated courses of therapy are often needed)
- Neurologic involvement requires Parenteral antibiotics
  Ceftriaxone 2 g/day for 21 to 28 days
  Alternative: cefotaxime 2 g q8h
  Alternative: penicillin G 5 million U qid
- Cardiac involvement: IV ceftriaxone or penicillin plus cardiac monitoring
- Evidence from recent study suggests that prolonged treatment with IV or PO antibiotic therapy for up to 90 days did not improve symptoms more than placebo

☼ PEARLS & CONSIDERATIONS

- The U.S. Advisory Committee on immunization practices (ACIP) has recommended that "vaccination should be considered for patients 15 to 70 years of age who live, work, and recreate in high- or moderate-risk areas, and are exposed to ticks either frequently or for long periods of time."
- In some patients with Lyme disease, nonspecific complaints such as headache, fatigue, and arthralgia may persist for months after appropriate (and ultimately successful) antibiotic treatment. These patients undergo slow spontaneous resolution; further therapy for Lyme disease should not be given unless there are objective findings of active disease (including physical findings; abnormalities on cerebrospinal or synovial fluid analysis; changes on formal neuropsychologic testing).

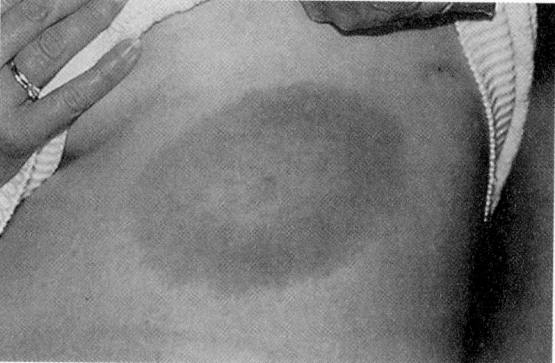

Fig. 1-164   Erythema migrans. Note expanding erythematous lesion with central clearing on trunk. (Courtesy John Cook, M.D. From Goldstein B [ed]: *Practical dermatology,* ed 2, St Louis, 1997, Mosby.)

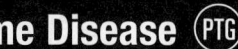
- A single dose of 200 mg doxycycline given within 72 hr of *Ixodes* tick bite can prevent development of Lyme disease.

REFERENCES

Gomes-Solecki MCJ et al: A first tier rapid assay for the serodiagnosis of *Borrelia burgdorferi* infection, *Arch Intern Med* 161:2015, 2002.

Klempner MS et al: Two controlled trials of antibiotic treatment in patients with persistent symptoms and a history of Lyme disease, *N Engl J Med* 345:85, 2001.

Nadelman RB et al: Prophylaxis with single dose doxycycline for the prevention of Lyme disease after an *Ixodes scapularis* tick bite, *N Engl J Med* 345:79, 2001.

Poland GA: Prevention of Lyme disease: a review of the evidence, *Mayo Clin Proc* 76:713, 2001.

Shadick NA et al: The cost-effectiveness of vaccination against Lyme disease, *Arch Intern Med* 161:554, 2001.

Smith RP et al: Clinical characteristics and treatment outcome of early Lyme disease in patients with microbiologically confirmed erythema migrans, *Ann Intern Med* 136:421, 2002.

Steere AC: Lyme disease, *N Engl J Med* 345:115, 2001.

Wormer GP et al: Duration of antibiotic therapy for early Lyme disease. A randomized, double-blind, placebo-controlled trial, *Ann Intern Med* 138:697, 2003.

Authors: **Joseph F. Grillo, M.D., and Dennis J. Mikolich, M.D.**

BASIC INFORMATION

■ DEFINITION

Lymphangitis refers to the inflammation of lymphatic vessels.

■ SYNONYMS

Nodular lymphangitis
Sporotrichoid lymphangitis

ICD-9CM CODES

457.2 Lymphangitis

■ EPIDEMIOLOGY & DEMOGRAPHICS

Incidence (in U.S.): Several hundred cases/yr of sporotrichoid lymphangitis

■ PHYSICAL FINDINGS & CLINICAL PRESENTATION

ACUTE LYMPHANGITIS:
- Commonly associated with a bacterial cellulitis
- May or may not recognize site of skin trauma (i.e., laceration, puncture, ulcer)
- In hours to days, distal appearance of erythema, edema, and tenderness, with linear erythematous streaks extending proximally to regional lymph nodes
- Possible lymphadenitis and fever
- Predisposition to group A streptococcal infection of the skin in those with chronic lymphedema and superficial fungal infections (e.g., tinea pedis)

"SPOROTRICHOID" OR "NODULAR" LYMPHANGITIS:
- Includes subcutaneous nodules that develop along the path of involved lymphatics
- Most commonly results from inoculation of the skin of the hand
- Usually preceded by well-defined episode of cutaneous inoculation or trauma
- Lesions apparent from one to several weeks after inoculation
- Initially, nodular or papular lesion; may ulcerate
- May have frank pus or a serosanguineous discharge
- Systemic complaints uncommon, but infection with certain microorganisms associated with fever, chills, myalgias, and headache

■ ETIOLOGY

- Acute lymphangitis: usually associated with *Streptococcus pyogenes* (group A streptococcus), but staphylococcal organisms have been implicated
- Nodular lymphangitis caused by one of several organisms
  1. *Sporothrix schenckii*
     a. Most common recognized cause in the U.S., usually in the Midwest
     b. Found in soil and plant debris
  2. *Nocardia brasiliensis:* found in soil
  3. *Mycobacterium marinum:* associated with trauma related to water (e.g., aquariums, swimming pools, fish)
  4. *Leishmania brasiliensis*
     a. Protozoal parasite transmitted to humans by sandflies, mostly to travelers in endemic areas
     b. Small endemic focus in Texas
  5. *Francisella tularensis*
     a. Most often in Midwestern states
     b. Associated with contact with infected mammals (e.g., rabbits) or tick bites

DIAGNOSIS

■ DIFFERENTIAL DIAGNOSIS

- Nodular lymphangitis
- Insect or snake bites
- Filariasis

■ WORKUP

- Acute lymphangitis: blood cultures
- Nodular lymphangitis: various stains and cultures of drainage or biopsy specimens of inoculation sites to make definitive diagnosis

■ LABORATORY TESTS

- WBCs possibly elevated with cellulitis
- Eosinophilia common with helminthic infections

TREATMENT

■ NONPHARMACOLOGIC THERAPY

Limb elevation

■ ACUTE GENERAL Rx

- Penicillin possibly sufficient, but 1 wk of dicloxacillin or cephalexin 500 mg PO qid commonly used to ensure antistaphylococcal coverage
- If allergic to penicillin:
  1. Clindamycin 300 mg PO qid for 7 days *or*
  2. Erythromycin 500 mg PO qid for 7 days
- Nodular lymphangitis: specific therapy directed at etiologic agent
- For superficial fungal infections: treatment may prevent recurrence of acute lymphangitis

■ DISPOSITION

- Acute lymphangitis: usually resolves with therapy
- Recurrent attacks: may lead to chronic lymphedema of limb, rarely resulting in elephantiasis nostras (nonfilarial elephantiasis)
- Nodular lymphangitis: usually responds to appropriate therapy

■ REFERRAL

- If acute lymphangitis is more than a mild disease or involves the face
- If nodular lymphangitis or filariasis is suspected

PEARLS & CONSIDERATIONS

■ COMMENTS

- Outside of the U.S., initial episodes of filariasis caused by *Brugia malayi* resemble acute lymphangitis.
- Chronic lymphedema or elephantiasis results from recurrent episodes.

REFERENCE

Tobin EH, Jih WW: Sporotrichoid lymphocutaneous infections: etiology, diagnosis and therapy, *Am Fam Physician* 63:326, 2001.
Author: **Maurice Policar, M.D.**

BASIC INFORMATION

■ DEFINITION
Lymphedema refers to excessive accumulation of interstitial protein rich fluid typically resulting from impaired regional lymphatic drainage.

■ SYNONYMS
Elephantiasis

ICD-9CM CODES
457.1 Lymphedema: acquired (chronic), praecox, secondary
457.1 Elephantiasis (nonfilarial)

■ EPIDEMIOLOGY & DEMOGRAPHICS
PRIMARY LYMPHEDEMA:
- Found in 1.1/100,000 people <20 yr old.
- Females outnumber males 3.5:1.
- Incidence peaks between ages 12 to 16 yr old.

SECONDARY LYMPHEDEMA: See specific etiology (e.g., filariasis, breast cancer, prostate cancer)

■ PHYSICAL FINDINGS & CLINICAL PRESENTATION
Edema:
- Painless and progressive
  1. Initially, the edema is pitting and smooth; however, with advanced cases, the edema becomes non-pitting (this depends on the extent of fibrosis that has occurred).
  2. Elevation of the leg resolves the swelling in the early stages but not in the advanced stages.
- More often unilateral but depending on the etiology can be bilateral
- Not always restricted to the lower extremities but may involve the genitals, face, or upper extremities (e.g., arm swelling after mastectomy)
- Stemmer's sign (squaring of the toes caused by edema in the digits)
- "Buffalo hump" appearance of the dorsum of the foot
- Loss of the ankle contour, giving a "tree trunk" appearance of the leg (Fig. 1-165)

Skin:
- Hard, thick, leathery skin
- Occasional drainage of lymph
- Infections (cellulitis, lymphangitis, onychomycosis)

■ ETIOLOGY
Lymphedema is caused by a reduction in lymphatic transport and is classified into primary and secondary forms. Primary idiopathic lymphedema is thought to result from developmental abnormalities including:
- Congenital lymphedema
  1. Detected at birth or recognized within first 2 yr of life; involving one or both extremities, usually the entire leg
  2. May be familial (Milroy's disease)
- Lymphedema praecox
  1. Usually unilateral; occurring in the teenage years
  2. Most common form of primary lymphedema
  3. May be familial (Meige's disease)
- Lymphedema tarda
  1. Usually occurs after the age of 30 yr
  2. Uncommon, accounting for less than 10% of cases of primary lymphedema

Secondary lymphedema develops after disruption or obstruction of the lymphatic system as a consequence of:
- Surgery for malignant tumors (e.g., breast, prostate, lymphoma)
- Edema of the arm after axillary lymph node dissection is the most common cause of lymphedema in the U.S.
- Incidence of lymphedema is ~14% in patients s/p mastectomy with adjuvant radiation treatment
- Inflammation (streptococci, filariasis)
- Filariasis is the most common cause of lymphedema in the world
- Trauma
- Radiation with lymph node removal

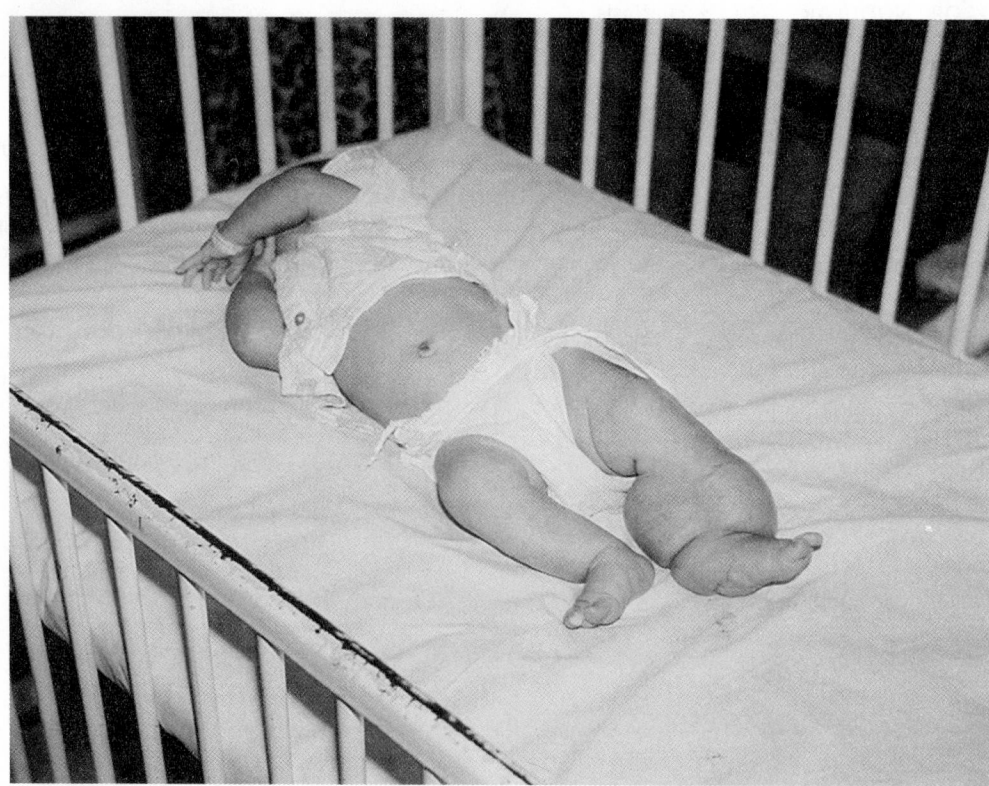

Fig. 1-165   Lymphedema. (From Seidel HM [ed]: *Mosby's guide to physical examination*, ed 4, St Louis, 1999, Mosby.)

DIAGNOSIS

DIFFERENTIAL DIAGNOSIS
Exclude other causes of edema (e.g., cirrhosis, nephrosis, CHF, myxedema, hypoalbuminemia, chronic venous stasis, reflex sympathetic dystrophy, obstruction from abdominal or pelvic malignancy).

WORKUP
A detailed history and physical examination should help exclude most of the differential diagnosis.

LABORATORY TESTS
- BUN, Cr, liver function tests, albumin, urine analysis, TFTs are obtained to exclude possible systemic causes of edema.
- Noninvasive venous studies help exclude venous insufficiency.

IMAGING STUDIES
- Lymphoscintigraphy:
  1. Diagnostic image of choice
  2. Sensitivity and specificity of 100% in diagnosing lymphedema
- CT scan: to exclude malignancy leading to obstruction
- Lymphangiography:
  1. Available but rarely used
  2. May be requested by surgeons considering repair or excision of tissue for lymphedema
  3. Difficult to perform; most information can be obtained from the nuclear lymphoscintigram

TREATMENT

NONPHARMACOLOGIC THERAPY
Reduce leg swelling and size:
- Leg elevation
- Limb massage
- Pneumatic leg compression

Maintain edema-free state:
- Elastic support stockings that are properly fitted according to compression pressure and length are essential to prevent edema from returning.

- Compression pressures are graduated; most of the pressure is distal with less and less pressure from the stockings, moving proximally.
- Compression pressures range from 20 to 30 mm Hg, 30 to 40 mm Hg, 40 to 50 mm Hg, and 50 to 60 mm Hg. Most prefer 40 to 50 mm Hg for lymphedema.
- The length should cover the edematous site. Choices include below the knee, thigh-high, and pantyhose lengths.

ACUTE GENERAL Rx
- Diuretics, including furosemide 40 to 80 mg qd, may aid in reducing leg swelling but should be used only temporarily. Hydrochlorothiazide 25 mg qd can also be used for reducing edema or preventing leg swelling.
- Treat infections, such as lymphangitis (usually caused by group A streptococcus), with penicillin VK 250 mg qid for 10 days or erythromycin 250 mg qid in penicillin-allergic patients. If recurrent episodes of infection occur, many consider prophylaxis with penicillin VK 250 mg qid for 10 days at the beginning of each month. Clotrimazole 1% cream should be applied qd to dried fissured areas in between toes to prevent fungal infections.
- In secondary lymphedema, treating the underlying cause is indicated (e.g., prostate cancer, breast cancer). If the etiology is filariasis caused by the parasites *Wuchereria bancrofti* or *Brugia malayi*, treatment is diethylcarbamazine citrate (DEC) 5 mg/kg in divided doses for 3 wk.

CHRONIC Rx
Surgery for chronic lymphedema is considered if:
- Continued increase in leg size despite medical treatment
- Impaired leg function
- Recurrent infections
- Emotional lability secondary to the cosmetic appearance

Surgical procedures are divided into two types:
- Those performed to improve lymph node drainage (e.g., anastomoses of the lymph system with the venous system)
- Those performed to excise the subcutaneous tissue (e.g., Charles' procedure, Thompson's procedure, and the modified Homans' procedure)

DISPOSITION
Lymphedema is a slowly progressive disorder that can lead to significant disfigurement of the extremities or other body parts.

REFERRAL
Consultation with vascular surgeons should be made if medical therapy for leg size reduction fails or if recurrent infections occur.

PEARLS & CONSIDERATIONS

COMMENTS
- It is important to remember that surgery is not a cure.
- Children and adolescents (along with parents and adults) should be encouraged to pursue a normal life, participating in school activities and sports (preferably noncontact, e.g., swimming).
- It should also be remembered that cases of lymphangiosarcomas have been associated, although rarely, with postmastectomy lymphedema.

REFERENCES
Caban ME: Trends in the evaluation of lymphedema, *Lymphology* 35(1):28, 2002.

Neese PY: Management of lymphedema, *Lippincotts Prim Care Pract* 4(4):390, 2000.

Rockson SG: Lymphedema, *Am J Med* 110:288, 2001.

Rockson SG et al: American Cancer Society Lymphedema Workshop. Workgroup III: diagnosis and management of lymphedema, *Cancer* 83(12 suppl):2882, 1998.

Author: **Peter Petropoulos, M.D.**

BASIC INFORMATION

■ DEFINITION

Lymphogranuloma venereum (LGV) is a sexually transmitted, systemic disease caused by *Chlamydia trachomatis*.

■ SYNONYMS

Tropical bubo
Poradenitis inguinalis
LGV

ICD-9CM CODES

099.1 Lymphogranuloma venereum

■ EPIDEMIOLOGY & DEMOGRAPHICS

- Male:female ratio is 5:1
- LGV is rare in the U.S. (285 cases reported in 1993).
- LGV is endemic in Africa, India, parts of Southeast Asia, South America, and the Caribbean.

■ PHYSICAL FINDINGS & CLINICAL PRESENTATION

Primary stage:
- Primary lesion caused by multiplication of organism at site of infection
- Papule, shallow ulcer
- Herpetiform lesion at site of inoculation (most common)
- Incubation period of 3 to 21 days
- Most common site of lesion in women: posterior wall, fourchette, or vulva
- Spontaneous healing, without scarring

Second stage:
- Inguinal syndrome: characteristic inguinal adenopathy
- Begins 1 to 4 wk after primary lesion
- Syndrome is the most frequent clinical sign of the disease
- Unilateral inguinal adenopathy in 70% of cases
- Symptoms: painful, extensive adenitis (bubo) and suppuration may occur with numerous sinus tracts
- "Groove sign" signaling femoral and inguinal node involvement (20%); most often seen in men
- Involvement of deep iliac and retroperitoneal lymph nodes in women may present as a pelvic mass

Third stage (anogenital syndrome):
- Subacute: proctocolitis
- Late: tissue destruction or scarring, sinuses, abscesses, fistulas, strictures of perineum, elephantiasis

■ ETIOLOGY

Chlamydia trachomatis is the causative agent. There are three serotypes: L1, L2, and L3.

DIAGNOSIS

■ DIFFERENTIAL DIAGNOSIS

- Inguinal adenitis, suppurative adenitis, retroperitoneal adenitis, proctitis, schistosomiasis
- Section II describes the differential diagnosis of genital sores.

■ WORKUP

- Clinical manifestation
- Screening for other STDs
- A clinical algorithm for evaluation of genital ulcer disease is described in Section III, Fig. 3-79.

■ LABORATORY TESTS

- Positive Frei test:
  1. Intradermal chlamydial antigen
  2. Nonspecific for all *Chlamydia*
  3. No longer available (historical significance only)
- Complement fixation test:
  1. Titer >1:64 in active infection
  2. Convalescent titers no difference
- Cell culture of *Chlamydia*—aspiration of fluctuant node yields highest rates of recovery
- CBC—mild leukocytosis with lymphocytosis or monocytosis
- Elevated sedimentation rate
- VDRL and HIV screening to rule out other STDs

■ IMAGING STUDIES

- Barium enema: may reveal elongated structure of LGV
- CT scan for retroperitoneal adenitis

TREATMENT

■ NONPHARMACOLOGIC THERAPY

- Avoid milk and milk products while taking medication.
- Practice sexual abstinence.
- Treat sexual partners.

■ ACUTE GENERAL Rx

- Doxycycline 100 mg PO bid × 21 days
- Erythromycin base 500 mg PO qid × 21 days
- Sulfisoxazole 500 mg PO qid × 21 days
- Surgical:
  1. Aspirate fluctuant nodes
  2. Incise and drain abscesses

■ CHRONIC Rx

- Longer course of therapy will be needed for chronic or relapsing cases, which may be caused by reinfection and/or inadequate treatment.
- A rectal stricture will require a colostomy.
- Surgery should be considered only after antibiotic treatment.

■ DISPOSITION

Good prognosis with early treatment, usually resulting in complete resolution of symptoms.

■ REFERRAL

Surgical consultation if patient develops obstruction, fistula, or rectal stricture. May need referral to plastic surgeon if patient has lymphatic obstruction.

PEARLS & CONSIDERATIONS

■ COMMENTS

- Pregnant and lactating women should be treated with erythromycin regimen.
- Congenital transmission does not occur, but infection may be acquired through an infected birth canal.
- Patient education materials may be obtained through local and state health clinics.

REFERENCE

Centers for Disease Control and Prevention: 2002 sexually transmitted diseases treatment guidelines, *MMWR Morb Mortal Wkly Rep* 51(RR-6), 2002.
Author: **George T. Danakas, M.D.**

BASIC INFORMATION

■ DEFINITION

Non-Hodgkin lymphoma is a heterogeneous group of malignancies of the lymphoreticular system.

■ SYNONYMS

NHL

ICD-9CM CODES

201.9 Lymphoma, non-Hodgkin

■ EPIDEMIOLOGY & DEMOGRAPHICS

- Median age at time of diagnosis: 50 yr
- Sixth most common neoplasm in the U.S. (56,000 new cases/yr)
- Increasing incidence with age

■ PHYSICAL FINDINGS & CLINICAL PRESENTATION

- Patients often present with asymptomatic lymphadenopathy.
- Approximately one third of NHL originates extranodally. Involvement of extranodal sites can result in unusual presentations (e.g., GI tract involvement can simulate PUD).
- NHL cases associated with HIV occur predominantly in the brain.
- Pruritus, fever, night sweats, weight loss are less common than in Hodgkin's disease.
- Hepatomegaly and splenomegaly may be present.

DIAGNOSIS

■ DIFFERENTIAL DIAGNOSIS

- Hodgkin's disease
- Viral infections
- Metastatic carcinoma
- A clinical algorithm for evaluation of lymphadenopathy is described in Section III
- The differential diagnosis of lymphadenopathy is described in Section II

■ WORKUP

Initial laboratory evaluation may reveal only mild anemia and elevated LDH and ESR. Proper staging of non-Hodgkin's lymphoma requires the following:

- A thorough history, physical examination, and adequate biopsy
- Routine laboratory evaluation (CBC, ESR, urinalysis, LDH, BUN, creatinine, serum calcium, uric acid, LFTs, serum protein electrophoresis)
- Chest x-ray examination (PA and lateral)
- Bone marrow evaluation (aspirate and full bone core biopsy)

- CT scan of abdomen and pelvis; CT scan of chest if chest x-ray films abnormal
- Bone scan (particularly in patients with histiocytic lymphoma)
- Depending on the histopathology, the results of the above studies and the planned therapy, some other tests may be performed: gallium scan (e.g., in patients with high-grade lymphomas), liver/spleen scan, PET scan, lymphangiography, lumbar puncture
- β-2 Microglobulin levels should be obtained initially (prognostic value) and serially in patients with low-grade lymphomas (useful to monitor therapeutic response of the tumor)
- Serum interleukin levels have prognostic value in diffuse large cell lymphoma

CLASSIFICATION: The Working Formulation of non-Hodgkin lymphoma for clinical usage subdivides lymphomas into low grade, intermediate grade, high grade, and miscellaneous (Table 1-35).

STAGING: The Ann Arbor classification is used to stage non-Hodgkin lymphomas (see "Hodgkin's Disease" in Section I). Histopathology has greater therapeutic implications in NHL than in Hodgkin's disease.

■ IMAGING STUDIES

See "Workup."

TREATMENT

■ ACUTE GENERAL Rx

The therapeutic regimen varies with the histologic type and pathologic stage. Following are the commonly used therapeutic modalities:

LOW-GRADE NHL (E.G., NODULAR, POORLY DIFFERENTIATED):

1. Local radiotherapy for symptomatic obstructive adenopathy
2. Deferment of therapy and careful observation in asymptomatic patients
3. Single-agent chemotherapy with cyclophosphamide or chlorambucil and glucocorticoids
4. Combination chemotherapy alone or with radiotherapy: generally indicated only when the lymphoma becomes more invasive, with poor response to less aggressive treatment; commonly used regimens: CVP, CHOP, CHOP-BLEO, COPP, BACOP; addition of recombinant alpha interferon at low doses to chemotherapy prolongs remission duration in patients with low-grade NHL

5. Monoclonal antibodies directed against B-cell surface antigens can also be used to treat follicular lymphomas that are resistant to conventional therapy. The anti-CD20 monoclonal antibody rituximab is a targeted, minimally toxic treatment effective against low-grade NHL in patients who have not received previous treatment
6. The addition of rituximab to CHOP is generally well tolerated; however, additional studies may be necessary to clarify the role of CHOP plus rituximab in patients with indolent NHL
7. Ibritumomab tiuxetan (Zevalin), an immunoconjugate that combines the linker-chelator tiuxetan with the monoclonal antibody ibritumomab, can be used as part of a two-step regimen for treatment of patients with relapsed or refractory low-grade, follicular, or transformed B-cell NHL refractory to rituximab
8. New purine analogs (FLAMP, 2CDA) can be used in salvage treatment of refractory lymphomas. They all have activity in follicular lymphomas

INTERMEDIATE- AND HIGH-GRADE LYMPHOMAS (E.G., DIFFUSE HISTIOCYTIC LYMPHOMA):

Combination chemotherapy regimens (e.g., CHOP, PRO-MACE-CYTABOM, MACOP-B, M-BACOD). An anthracycline-containing regimen (such as CHOP) given in standard doses and schedule is generally best for treatment of older patients with advanced stage, aggressive-histology lymphoma who do not have significant comorbid illness.

1. High-dose sequential therapy is superior to standard-dose MACOP-B for patients with diffuse large-cell lymphoma of the B-cell type.
2. Dose-modified chemotherapy should be considered for most HIV-infected patients with lymphoma. As compared with treatment with standard doses of cytotoxic chemotherapy (M-BACOD), reduced doses cause significantly fewer hematologic toxic effects yet have similar efficacy in patients with HIV-related lymphoma.
   - Three cycles of CHOP followed by involved-field radiotherapy may be superior to eight cycles of CHOP alone in patients with localized intermediate- and high-grade NHL.
   - The addition of rituximab against CD20 B-cell lymphoma to the CHOP regimen increases the complete response rate and prolongs event-free and overall survival in elderly patients with diffuse large B-cell lymphoma without a clinically significant increase in toxicity.

- Granulocyte-colony stimulating factor (G-CSF): may be effective in reducing the risk of infection in patients with aggressive lymphoma undergoing chemotherapy
- Radioimmunotherapy with (^{131}I) anti-B1 antibody therapy for NHL either by itself or in combination with other treatments
- Treatment with high-dose chemotherapy and autologous

bone marrow transplant: as compared with conventional chemotherapy, increases event-free and overall survival in patients with chemotherapy-sensitive non-Hodgkin lymphoma in relapse

■ DISPOSITION
- Patients with low-grade lymphoma, despite their long-term survival (6 to 10 yr average), are rarely cured, and

the great majority (if not all) eventually die of the lymphoma, whereas patients with a high-grade lymphoma may achieve a cure with aggressive chemotherapy.
- Complete remission occurs in 35% to 50% of patients with intermediate- and high-grade lymphoma. Prognostic factors include the histologic subtype, age of patient, and bulk of disease.

Author: **Fred F. Ferri, M.D.**

TABLE 1-35 Classification Systems for Grading Lymphomas

KIEL CLASSIFICATION	WORKING FORMULATION	REVISED EUROPEAN-AMERICAN CLASSIFICATION

Low-grade malignancy
  Lymphocytic, CLL
  Lymphocytic, other
  Lymphoplasmacytoid
  Centrocytic
	Low grade
	A. Malignant lymphoma, small lymphocytic
	   Consistent with chronic lymphocytic leukemia
		B-cell lymphomas
		
		B-CLL/SLL
		Lymphoplasmacytoid lymphoma

	B. Malignant lymphoma, follicular, predominantly small cleaved cell	Follicle center lymphomas

Centroblastic/Centrocytic
    Follicular without sclerosis
    Follicular with sclerosis
    Follicular and diffuse,
      without sclerosis
	Diffuse areas
	Sclerosis
	C. Malignant lymphoma, follicular mixed, small
	   cleaved and large cell
		Marginal zone lymphomas (MALT)
		Mantle cell lymphoma

Follicular and diffuse,
      with sclerosis
    Diffuse
	Diffuse areas
	
	Sclerosis
		Diffuse large B-cell lymphoma
		
		Primary mediastinal large B-cell
		  lymphoma

Low-grade malignant lymphoma, unclassified	Intermediate grade	Burkitt's lymphoma

High-grade malignancy
  Centroblastic
  Lymphoblastic, Burkitt's type
  Lymphoblastic, convoluted
    cell type
	D. Malignant lymphoma, follicular
	   Diffuse areas
	E. Malignant lymphoma, diffuse small cleaved cell
		T-cell lymphomas
		
		T-CLL

Lymphoblastic, other (unclassified) immunoblastic		Mycosis fungoides/Sézary syndrome

High-grade malignant lymphoma,
    unclassified
  Malignant lymphoma unclassified
    (unable to specify high grade
    or low grade)
	F. Malignant lymphoma, diffuse mixed, small and
	   large cell sclerosis
	G. Malignant lymphoma diffuse
		Peripheral T-cell lymphoma,
		  unspecified

Composite lymphoma	Large cell
	
	Cleaved cell
	Noncleaved cell
	Sclerosis
	High grade
	H. Malignant lymphoma large cell, immunoblastic
	   Plasmacytoid
	   Clear cell
	   Polymorphous
	   Epithelioid cell component
	I. Malignant lymphoma lymphoblastic
	   Convoluted cell
	   Nonconvoluted cell
	J. Malignant lymphoma small noncleaved cell
	   Burkitt's
	   Follicular areas
		Angioimmunoblastic T-cell
		  lymphoma
		Angiocentric lymphoma
		Intestinal T-cell lymphoma
		Adult T-cell lymphoma/leukemia
		Anaplastic large cell lymphoma
		Precursor T-lymphoid
		  lymphoma/leukemia

From Abeloff MD: *Clinical oncology,* ed 2, New York, 2000, Churchill Livingstone.
B-CLL, B-cell chronic lymphoid leukemia; *MALT,* mucosa-associated lymphoid tumor; *SLL,* lymphoid leukemia; *T-CLL,* T-cell CLL.

BASIC INFORMATION

■ DEFINITION

Macular degeneration refers to a group of diseases associated with loss of central vision and damage to the macula. Degenerative changes occur in the pigment, neural, and vascular layers of the macula. The dry macular degeneration is usually ischemic in etiology, and a wet macular degeneration is associated with leakage of fluid from blood vessels, usually referred to as age-related macular degeneration (ARMD).

ICD-9CM CODES

362.5 Degeneration of macula and posterior pole

■ EPIDEMIOLOGY & DEMOGRAPHICS

INCIDENCE (IN U.S.):
• Main cause of blindness in the U.S.
• Increases with age

PREVALENCE (IN U.S.): Varies, but approximately 5% of people <50 yr old have some signs of macular degeneration.

PREDOMINANT SEX: Male = female

PREDOMINANT AGE: >50 yr

PEAK INCIDENCE:
• 75 to 80 yr old
• Dramatic increases in incidence and prevalence with age until approximately 80% of people 75 yr or older have senile macular degeneration.

GENETICS:

• Different syndrome: senile macular degeneration is age related.
• Several rare neurologic syndromes are associated with macular degeneration.

■ PHYSICAL FINDINGS

• Decreased central vision
• The most common abnormality seen in age-related macular degeneration (AMD) is the presence of drusen, or yellowish deposits deep to the retina (Fig. 1-166)

■ ETIOLOGY

• Pigmentary and vascular changes with exudate, edema, and scar tissue development
• Early in course, possible subretinal neovascularization

DIAGNOSIS

■ DIFFERENTIAL DIAGNOSIS

• Diabetic retinopathy
• Hypertension
• Histoplasmosis
• Trauma

■ WORKUP

Complete eye examination, including visual field and fluorescein angiography

■ LABORATORY TESTS

Evaluate for diabetes and other metabolic problems, as well as vascular diseases.

■ IMAGING STUDIES

None necessary

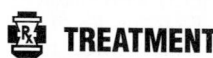

TREATMENT

■ NONPHARMACOLOGIC THERAPY

Laser treatment to stop progression of disease—photo dynamic treatment with verteporfin IV

■ ACUTE GENERAL Rx

Laser treatment

■ CHRONIC Rx

• Repeated laser treatments
• Antioxidants and zinc may slow down progression of ARMD

■ DISPOSITION

• Follow closely by ophthalmologist.
• If vision deteriorates, refer urgently to an ophthalmologist.

■ REFERRAL

To ophthalmologist early in the course of the disease if the sight is to be saved

PEARLS & CONSIDERATIONS

■ COMMENTS

The vision of only 1 out of 10 people can be saved, but the disease is so devastating that vigorous therapy should be attempted.

REFERENCES

Gottlieb JL: Age-related macular degeneration, *JAMA* 288:2233, 2002.

Jonas, JB: Verteporfin theory of subfoveal chorordial neovascularization in age-related macular degeneration, *Am J Ophthalmol* 133(6):F57, 2002.

Makenzie PJ, Chang TS: ETN assessment of vision-related emotion in patients with age related macular degeneration, *Ophthalmology* 109(4):720, 2002.

Ting TD et al: Decreased visual acuity associated with cystoid macular edema in neovascular or age-related macular degeneration, *Arch Ophthamol* 120(6):731, 2002.

Author: **Melvyn Koby, M.D.**

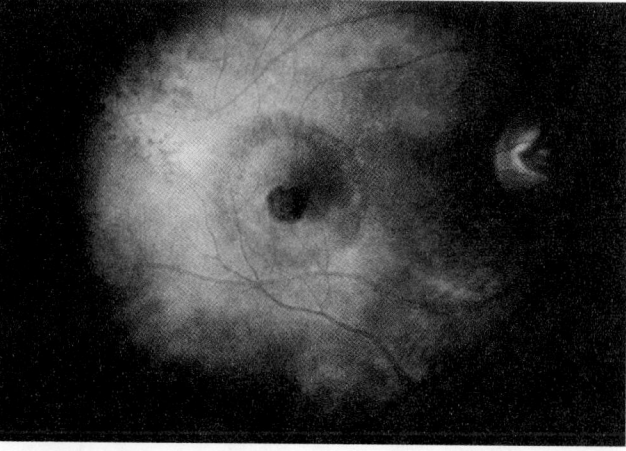

Fig. 1-166 **Wet macular degeneration.** (From Noble J: *Primary care medicine,* ed 3, St Louis, 2001, Mosby.)

BASIC INFORMATION

■ DEFINITION

Malaria is a protozoan disease caused by the genus *Plasmodium* and transmitted by female *Anopheles spp.* mosquitoes. It is characterized by hectic fever and often presents with classic malarial paroxysm. Four species of genus plasmodium usually infect humans

- *P. falciparum*
- *P. vivax*
- *P. malariae*
- *P. ovale*

ICD-9CM CODES
084.6 Malaria

■ EPIDEMIOLOGY & DEMOGRAPHICS

Global:
- 300 to 500 million cases/yr
- 1 to 3 million deaths/yr
- 41% of the world's population lives in endemic area

U.S.:
- Total 1544 cases reported by CDC in 1997
- 567 cases diagnosed as *P. falciparum*
- Most infections limited to
  1. Immigrant population
  2. Returned travelers or troops from endemic area
- Occasionally, transmission through exposure to infected blood product
- Congenital transmission is possible
- Local mosquito-borne transmission has been reported
- Competent mosquito vectors are present
  1. *A. albimanus* in eastern U.S.
  2. *A. freeborni* in western U.S.

Geographic distribution:
- *P. falciparum:* Sub-Saharan Africa, Papua New Guinea, Solomon Islands, Haiti, Indian subcontinent
- *P. vivax:* Central America, South America, North Africa, Middle East, Indian subcontinent
- *P. vivax* and *P. falciparum:* South America, Eastern Asia, Oceania
- *P. Ovale:* West Africa
- *P. malariae:* worldwide

Parasite life cycle (Fig. 1-167):
- Human infection begins when a female anopheline mosquito bites (only female anopheline mosquito takes blood meal) and inoculates plasmodial sporozoites into bloodstream
- The sporozoites then travel to liver and invade to hepatocytes
- In the hepatocytes, the sporozoites mature to tissue schizont or become dormant hypnozoites
- The tissue schizont amplify the infection by producing large number of merozoites (10,000 to 30,000)
- Each merozoite is capable of invading a RBC and can establish the asexual cycle of replication in RBC

- Asexual cycles produce and release 24 to 32 merozoites at the end of 48- or 72-hr *(P. malariae)* cycle
- The hypnozoites are only found in relapsing malaria *P. vivax* or *P. ovale* and may remain dormant up to 6 to 11 mo
- Eventually some intraerythrocytic parasites develop into gametocytes, the sexual form necessary to complete the life cycle in the anopheline mosquito vector
- The gametocytes, when taken up by a female anopheline mosquito with a blood meal, further differentiate to form male and female gametes
- They fertilize in the mosquito gut to produce a diploid zygote that matures to an ookinete
- The ookinete produce haploid sporozoites by meiotic division
- The sporozoites then migrate to the salivary gland of the mosquito, ready to infect the human

■ PHYSICAL FINDINGS & CLINICAL PRESENTATION

- Fever is the hallmark of malaria, known as malarial paroxysm, initially daily until synchronization of infection after several weeks, when fever may occur every other day (tertian) in *P. vivax, P. ovale,* or *P. falciparum* malaria or every third day (quartan) in *P. malarie* malaria.
- Classic malarial paroxysm characterized by
  1. Cold stage: abrupt onset of cold feeling associated with rigors, shakes
  2. Hot stage: high fever (~40° C) associated with restlessness
  3. Sweating stage: patient defervesces
- Nonspecific symptoms are
  1. Headache
  2. Cough
  3. Myalgia
  4. Vomiting
  5. Diarrhea
  6. Jaundice

P. Falciparum:
- Most pathogenic of the four species
- Rapidly progresses to high-level parasitemia
- Important cause of the fatal malaria
- Classic malarial paroxysm usually absent
- Incubation period after exposure is 12 days (range: 9 to 60 days)
- Cytoadherence and resetting of RBC play central role in pathogenesis
- The sequestration of RBC in vital organs leads to fatal complications
- Cerebral malaria is a feared complication

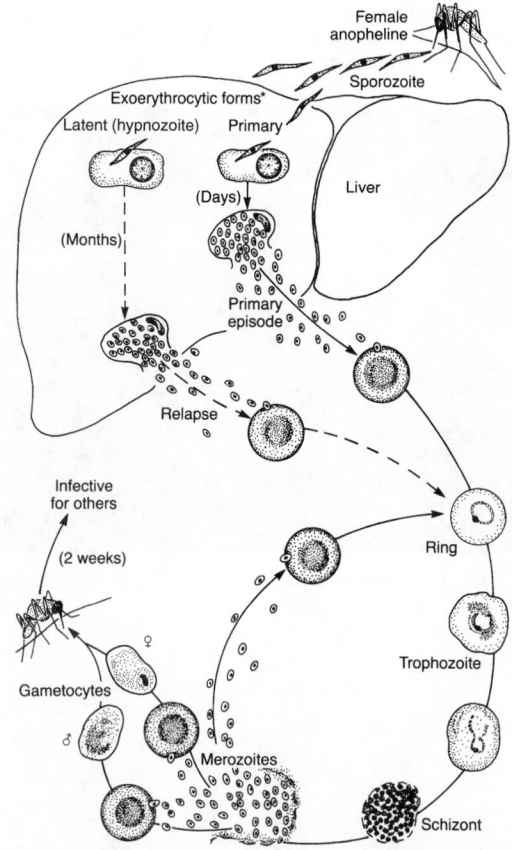

Fig. 1-167   Life cycle of plasmodia in humans. *Exoerythrocytic forms are also called tissue schizonts. (From Gorbach SL: *Infectious diseases,* ed 2, Philadelphia, 1998, WB Saunders.)

- Invades erythrocytes of all ages
- Lacks hypnozoites (intrahepatic stage), does not relapse
- Blood smear usually shows ring form only
- Pigment color is black
- Banana-shaped gametocytes; if seen in blood, smear is diagnostic
- Chloroquine resistance widely present

P. vivax:
- Known as tertian malaria: fever occurs every other day
- Duffy blood-group antigen FYA- or FYB-related receptor needed for attachment to RBC
- FyFy phenotype (most West African) individuals are resistant to *P. Vivax* malaria
- Incubation period after exposure is 14 days (range: 8 to 27 days)
- Hypnozoites may cause relapse of infection after years
- Infects mainly reticulocytes
- Irregularly shaped large rings and trophozoites, enlarged RBC, and Schüffner's dot are seen in peripheral blood smear (Fig. 1-168)
- Pigment color is yellow-brown
- *P. vivax* from Papua New Guinea have reduced sensitivity to chloroquine
- Primaquine needed to eradicate the hypnozoites

P. ovale:
- Also known as tertian malaria; fever occurs every other day
- Occurs mainly in tropical Africa
- Incubation period after exposure is 14 days (range: 8 to 27 days)
- Hypnozoits may cause relapse of infection
- Infects mainly reticulocytes
- Infected RBC seen as enlarged, oval shape containing large ring or trophozoites with Schüffner's dot
- Pigment color is dark brown
- Primaquine needed to eradicate the hypnozoites
- No chloroquine resistance encountered

P. malarie:
- Known as quartan malaria; fever occurs every third day
- Common cause of chronic malarial infection
- May persist 20 to 30 yr after leaving the endemic area
- Worldwide distribution
- Incubation period after exposure is 30 days (range: 16 to 60 days)
- Lacks hypnozoits (intrahepatic stage)
- May persist in blood for many years if treated inadequately
- Chronic infection may cause soluble immune-complex, resulting in nephritic syndrome
- Infects mainly mature RBC
- Band or rectangular forms of trophozoites are commonly seen in peripheral blood smear
- Pigment color is brown-black

cerebral malaria:
- Feared complication of *P. falciparum* infection
- Mortality ~20%
- Pathogenesis is poorly understood
- Ischemia as a result of sequestration of parasites or cytokines induced by parasite toxin(s) is the key debate
- Seizure and altered mental status leading to coma are cardinal manifestation
- Hypoglycemia, lactic acidosis, and elevated circulating TNF-α may present
- CSF studies: no increase of WBC count or protein, raised lactate concentrate, and increased opening pressure, especially in children, may present

DIAGNOSIS

■ DIFFERENTIAL DIAGNOSIS OF MALARIA
- Typhoid fever
- Dengue fever
- Yellow fever
- Viral hepatitis
- Influenza
- Brucellosis
- UTI
- Leishmaniasis
- Trypanosomiasis
- Rickettsial diseases
- Leptospirosis

■ WORKUP
- Clinical diagnosis is notoriously inaccurate
- Demonstration of malarial parasites in blood smear is essential
- Newer molecular diagnostic techniques are promising

■ LABORATORY TESTS
- The thick and thin blood film is required to identify malarial parasites
- The thick smears are more sensitive and primarily used to detect the presence of parasites
- The thin smears are used for species differentiation and parasite density estimation
- Person suspected of having malaria but no parasite seen in blood smears

should have blood smears repeated every 12 to 24 hr for 3 consecutive days

PREPARATION OF BLOOD SMEAR
- Must be prepared from fresh blood obtained by pricking the fingers
- The thin smear is fixed in methanol before staining
- The thick smear is stained unfixed
- The smear should be stained with a 3% Giemsa solution (pH of 7.2) for 30 to 45 min
- The parasite density should be estimated by counting the percentage of RBC infected, not the number of parasites, under an oil immersion lens on thin film

COMMON ERRORS IN READING MALARIAL SMEARS
- Platelets overlying an RBC
- Misreading artifacts as parasites
- Concern about missing a positive slide

MOLECULAR DIAGNOSIS OF MALARIA
- Polymerase chain reaction (PCR)
  1. It is useful in accurate species diagnosis
  2. It can detect the low-level parasitemias
  3. Is expensive and time-consuming
  4. It needs technical expertise
- Quantitative buffy cost (QBC)
  1. This test detects nuclear material of parasites using acridine orange stain
  2. It is unable to speciate the parasites accurately
  3. It cannot quantitate parasitemias
- Para Sight F and Malaria PF Test
  1. This test uses a monoclonal antibody to detect *P. falciparum*-specific, histidine-rich protein (HRP)-2
  2. It can detect *P. falciparum* only
  3. Past infection may confuse diagnosis
- OptiMal test
  1. This test detects lactage dehydrogenase (LDH) of parasites
  2. It can differentiate *falciparum* from *non-falciparum*

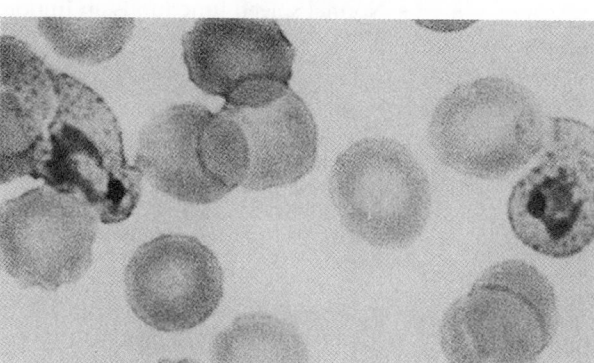

Fig. 1-168 Giemsa-stained blood smear in *Plasmodium vivax* malaria. Asexual parasites. Note that the parasites are large and ameboid, the infected erythrocytes are the largest cells in the field (because they are reticulocytes), and the erythrocytes contain numerous pink dots (Schüffner's dots) (×2000). (From Klippel JH et al [eds]: *Internal medicine*, ed 5, St Louis, 1998, Mosby.)

TREATMENT

■ NONPHARMACOLOGIC THERAPY
- ANTIMOSQUITO MEASURES
  1. Eradication of mosquito breeding places by chemical spray
  2. Use of mosquito nets properly in the endemic areas
  3. Use of protective clothing
  4. Use of insect spray (permethrin), mosquito coils, or repellents (diethyltoluamide)

■ ACUTE GENERAL THERAPY
A definitive diagnosis of malaria is essential for specific antimalarial chemotherapy

NON-*FALCIPARUM* MALARIA:
- Chloroquine 600 mg base (1000 mg chloroquine phosphate) po loading dose, 6 hr later 300 mg base (500 mg salt), then 300 mg base (500 mg salt) daily for 2 days
- In the case of *P. vivax* and *P. ovale,* treatment with primaquine 15 mg daily for 14 days is needed to eradicate the exoerythrocytic forms, especially the hypnozoites responsible for relapses
- G6PD should be measured before primaquine is given
- Chloroquine-resistant *P. vivax* has been documented; in that case, quinine is given

FALCIPARUM MALARIA:
- Chloroquine can be used cautiously for falciparum malaria acquired in chloroquine-sensitive areas (chloroquine is more rapidly effective than quinine)
- Mainstay of treatment is oral quinine sulfate 10 mg (salt)/kg (usually 650 mg) q8h for 3 to 7 days, followed by pyrimethamine with sulfadoxine (Fansider) 3 tablets (each tablets contains 500 mg sulfadoxine and 25 mg pyrimethamine) or doxycycline 200 mg loading dose, then 100 mg bid for 7 days to eradicate asexual forms of the parasite

ALTERNATIVES:
- Quinine followed by clindamycin 900 mg tid × 5 days, or
- Mefloquine 1250 mg as a single dose, or
- Halofantrine 500 mg q6 h × 3 doses, repeat a week later, or
- Atovaquone 1000 mg daily × 3 days plus proguanil 400 mg daily × 3 days, or
- Atovaquone 1000 mg daily × 3 days plus doxycycline 100 mg bid × 3 days, or
- Artesunate 4 mg/kg daily × 3 days plus mefloquine 1250 mg single dose

NOTE: Parasitemia may paradoxically rise in the first 24 to 36 hr and is not an indication of treatment failure.

SEVERE *FALCIPARUM* MALARIA:
- It is a medical emergency
- Intensive care is preferred

- Measurement of blood glucose, lactate, ABG is important
- Intravenous quinidine gluconate 10 mg salt/kg loading dose (maximum 600 mg) in NS infuse slowly over 1 to 2 hr, followed by continuous infusion of 0.02 mg/kg/min until patient can swallow
- Cardiac monitor needed for observation of QT interval
- Alternatively, artemether 3.2 mg/kg IM then 1.6 mg/kg daily × 3 days
- Plasmaparesis is an option for parasitemia >30% or in pregnant woman and in elderly with severe malaria

MULTIDRUG-RESISTANT MALARIA:
- Mefloquine 1250 mg as a single dose, or
- Halofantrine 500 mg every 6 hr for three doses, repeat same course after 1 wk
- Combination therapy usually preferred

■ DISPOSITION
RISK FACTOR FOR FATAL MALARIA:
- Failure to take chemoprophylaxis
- Delay in seeking medical care
- Misdiagnosis

COMPLICATIONS OF MALARIA:
- Anemia
- Acidosis
- Hypoglycemia
- Respiratory distress
- DIC
- Blackwater fever
- Renal failure
- Shock

☀ PEARLS & CONSIDERATIONS

HOST RESPONSE:
- The specific immune response to malaria confers protection from high-level parasitemia and disease, but not from infection
- Asymptomatic parasitemia without illness (premunition) is common among adults in endemic area
- Immunity is specific for both the species and the strain of infecting malarial parasites
- Immunity to all strains is never achieved
- Normal spleen function is an important host factor because of immunologic as well as filtering functions of the spleen
- Both humoral and cellular immunity are necessary for protection
- Polyclonal increase in serum level of IgG, IgM, and IgA occur in immune individuals
- Antibody to antigenically variant protein PfEMP1 is important for protection in case of *P. falciparum* malaria
- Passively transferred IgG from immune individual has been shown protective

- Maternal antibody confers relative protection of infants from severe disease
- Genetic disorders (sickle cell disease, thalassemia, and G6PD deficiency) confer protection from death because parasites are unable to grow efficiently in low-oxygen tensions, thus preventing high-level parasitemias
- Individuals deficient of Duffy factor in RBC are resistant to infection by P. vivax
- Nonspecific defense mechanisms, cytokines (TNF-α, IL-1, 6, 8) also play an important role in protection; it causes fever (temperatures of 40° C damage mature parasites) and other pathologic effects

PREVENTION OF MALARIA:
Prophylaxis should be taken 1 wk before travel, continue weekly for the duration of stay and for 4 wk after leaving endemic area

NON-*FALCIPARUM* MALARIA:
Chloroquine 300 mg base (500 mg chloroquine phosphate) PO/wk

FALCIPARUM MALARIA:
- Mefloquine 250 mg (228 mg base) PO/wk, or
- Doxycycline 100 mg PO/day, or
- Primaquine 0.5 mg base/kg/day, or
- Chloroquine (300 mg base) plus proguanil (200 mg) PO/day

SPECIAL CONSIDERATION:
- Long-term visitors or travelers
- Children <12 yr
- Immunocompromised host
- Pregnant women

VACCINATION:
- No effective and safe vaccine available yet
- A live, attenuated, whole sporozoite vaccine shown to work
- A synthetic peptide (SPf66) vaccine proved ineffective
- New DNA-based vaccines are in development

MALARIA INFORMATION:
- CDC Travelers' Health Hotline (877) 394-8747
- CDC Travelers' Health Fax (888) 232-3299
- CDC Malaria Epidemiology (770) 488-7788
- Internet: http://www.cdc.gov

REFERENCES
Djmide A et al: A molecular marker for chloroquine-resistant falciparum malaria, *N Engl J Med* 344(4):257, 2001.

Malaria surveillance: 1996-97, *MMWR Morb Mortal Wkly Rep* 50, 2001.

White P: The treatment of malaria, *N Engl J Med* 335:800, 1996.

Winstanley P: Modern chemotherapeutic options for malaria, *Lancet Infect Dis* 1:242, 2001.
Author: **Amar Ashraf, M.D.**

BASIC INFORMATION

■ **DEFINITION**

A Mallory-Weiss tear is a longitudinal mucosal laceration in the region of the gastroesophageal junction.

■ **SYNONYMS**

Mallory-Weiss syndrome

ICD-9CM CODES

530.7 Gastroesophageal laceration-hemorrhage syndrome
530.82 Esophageal hemorrhage

■ **EPIDEMIOLOGY & DEMOGRAPHICS**

- Accounts for 5% to 15% of cases of upper GI bleeding
- Reported from early childhood to old age; the majority of patients are in their 40s to 60s
- More common in males
- Alcohol use is present in 30% to 60% of patients

■ **PHYSICAL FINDINGS & CLINICAL PRESENTATION**

- Vomiting, retching, or vigorous coughing will often, but not always, precede hematemesis.
- Patients may be clinically stable or present with tachycardia, hypotension, melena, or hematochezia.
- Bleeding may be self-limited or severe.
- Tears may be seen in association with other upper GI tract lesions, including hiatus hernia (present in as many as 90% of patients), ulcers, and esophageal varices, particularly in alcoholics.

■ **ETIOLOGY**

- An acute increase in intraabdominal pressure is transmitted to the esophagus, resulting in mucosal laceration.
- Vomiting may be associated with alcohol use, ketoacidosis, ulcer disease, uremia, pancreatitis, cholecystitis, pregnancy, or myocardial infarction.
- Tears may be iatrogenic, related to endoscopy (especially in struggling or retching patients), esophageal dilation, lower esophageal pneumatic

disruption therapy for achalasia, transesophageal echocardiography, or in association with polyethylene glycol electrolyte colonic lavage preparation.

 DIAGNOSIS

■ **DIFFERENTIAL DIAGNOSIS**

- Esophageal or gastric varices
- Esophagitis/esophageal ulcers (peptic or pill-induced)
- Gastric erosions
- Gastric or duodenal ulcer
- Dieulafoy lesion
- Arteriovenous malformations
- Neoplasms (usually gastric)

■ **WORKUP**

Endoscopy is the diagnostic method of choice.

■ **LABORATORY TESTS**

- Complete blood count, PT, PTT
- Lytes, BUN, creatinine, LFTs, pregnancy test, or others to evaluate for predisposing conditions

■ **IMAGING STUDIES**

Upper GI series are usually insensitive for the detection of Mallory-Weiss tears.

TREATMENT

■ **NONPHARMACOLOGIC THERAPY**

- Supportive care
- Aspirin, NSAIDs, and anticoagulants should be held

■ **ACUTE GENERAL Rx**

- Patients with active bleeding or hemodynamic instability require large-bore IVs, fluid resuscitation, and transfusion of blood products (red blood cells, FFP, and platelets) as appropriate
- NG decompression and antiemetics may be considered
- Endoscopic therapy for patients with active or ongoing hemorrhage, including electrocoagulation, injection (e.g., 1:10,000 epinephrine), sclerotherapy (for bleeding associated

with esophageal varices), band ligation, or endoscopic hemoclips (therapies may be used alone or in combination)
- Arterial embolization is described in patients with active bleeding who are poor surgical candidates
- Laparotomy, with gastrotomy and oversewing of the tear, is required in a small percentage of patients with uncontrolled bleeding

■ **CHRONIC Rx**

- Healing will usually occur without specific therapy.
- H_2-blockers or proton pump inhibitors may be given to help facilitate healing, but should not be used chronically unless appropriate indications are present.
- Predisposing conditions should be identified and treated.

■ **DISPOSITION**

Prognosis is good, with spontaneous cessation of bleeding in upwards of 90% of patients. Endoscopic features can guide treatment. Delayed rebleeding is described. Death has been reported in 3% to 12% of patients, often with severe bleeding and underlying comorbid conditions, including coagulopathy, thrombocytopenia, alcohol use, and multisystem organ failure.

■ **REFERRAL**

- GI referral for endoscopy
- Surgical referral for bleeding unresponsive to endoscopic treatment, or in the setting of coexistent perforation

PEARLS & CONSIDERATIONS

■ **COMMENTS**

Detecting and treating predisposing conditions is as important as assessing and treating the bleeding itself.

REFERENCE

Kortas DY et al: Mallory-Weiss tear: predisposing factors and predictors of a complicated course. *Am J Gastro* 96:2863, 2001.

Author: **Harlan G. Rich, M.D.**

BASIC INFORMATION

■ DEFINITION

Marfan's syndrome is an inherited disorder of connective tissue involving skeleton, cardiovascular system, eyes, lungs, and central nervous system.

ICD-9CM CODES

759.82 Marfan's syndrome

■ EPIDEMIOLOGY & DEMOGRAPHICS

PREVALENCE: 1 case/10,000 persons
- Both sexes are affected equally by this autosomal dominant syndrome.
- Approximately 30% of cases are a new mutation.

■ PHYSICAL FINDINGS & CLINICAL PRESENTATION

Diagnostic criteria for Marfan's syndrome (Fig. 1-169):
- Skeleton
  Joint hypermobility, tall stature, pectus excavatum, reduced thoracic kyphosis, scoliosis, arachnodactyly, dolichostenomelia, pectus carinatum, and erosion of the lumbosacral vertebrae from dural ectasia†
- Eye
  Myopia, retinal detachment, elongated globe, ectopia lentis†

- Cardiovascular
  Mitral valve prolapse, endocarditis, arrhythmia, dilated mitral annulus, mitral regurgitation, tricuspid valve prolapse, aortic regurgitation, aortic dissection,† dilation of the aortic root†
- Pulmonary
  Apical blebs, spontaneous pneumothorax
- Skin and integument
  Inguinal hernias, incisional hernias, striae atrophicae
- Central nervous system
  Attention deficit disorder, hyperactivity, verbal-performance discrepancy, dural ectasia, anterior pelvic meningocele†
  If the family history is positive for a close relative clearly affected by Marfan's syndrome, manifestations should be present in the skeleton and one of the other organ systems, and the diagnosis confirmed by linkage analysis or mutation detection.
  If the family history is negative or unknown, the patient should have manifestations in the skeleton, the cardiovascular system, and one other system, and at least one of the manifestations indicated by †.
  Manifestations are listed within each organ system in increasing speci-

ficity for Marfan's syndrome; although none is completely specific, those indicated by † are the most specific.

■ ETIOLOGY

Mutations in the gene that encodes fibrillin-1, the major constituent of microfibrils, which form the frame for elastic fibers. All the manifestations of Marfan's syndrome can be explained by the defective microfibrils.

DIAGNOSIS

■ DIFFERENTIAL DIAGNOSIS

Each of the clinical manifestations of the syndrome may have other causes; however, if the diagnostic criteria are met, the diagnosis is made.

■ WORKUP

- Echocardiography to establish:
  Mitral valve prolapse
  Mitral regurgitation
  Tricuspid valve prolapse
  Aortic regurgitation
  Dilation of the aortic root
- Chest x-ray
- Transesophageal echocardiography, chest CT scan, chest MRI, or aortography for suspected aortic dissection
- Chest x-ray for pulmonary apical bullae
- Ophthalmologic examination by ophthalmologist

TREATMENT

- Regular cardiac and aorta monitoring by physical examination and echocardiography
- Endocarditis prophylaxis
- Restriction of contact sports, weight lifting, and overexertion
- β-Blockers
- Early use of angiotensin-converting enzyme inhibitors in young patients with Marfan syndrome and valvular regurgitation may lessen the need for mitral valve surgery
- Genetic counseling
- Monitor aorta during pregnancy (because of increased risk of dissection)

REFERENCES

Pyertiz ER: Marfan's syndrome. In Braunwald E (ed): *Heart disease: a textbook of cardiovascular medicine*, ed 6, Philadelphia, 2001, WB Saunders.

Yetman AT et al: Comparison of outcome of the Marfan syndrome in patients diagnosed at age 6 years versus those diagnosed at age >6 years of age, *Am J Cardiol* 91:102, 2003.

Author: **Tom J. Wachtel, M.D.**

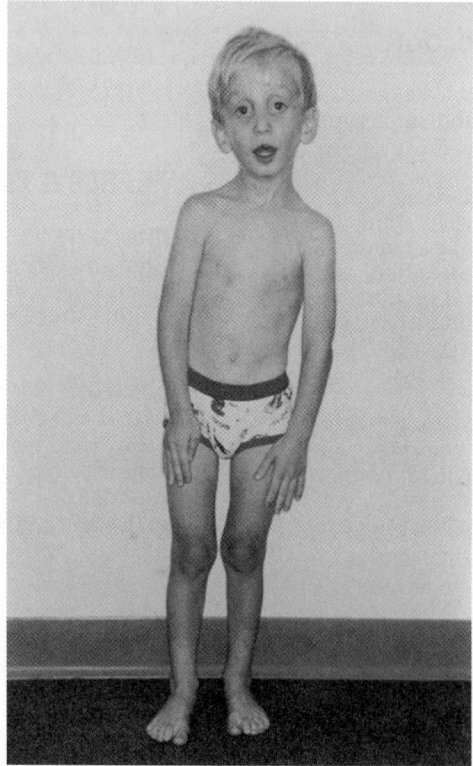

Fig. 1-169 **Marfan's syndrome.** Note the elongated facies, droopy lids, apparent dolichostenomelia, and mild scoliosis. (From Behrman RE: *Nelson's textbook of pediatrics,* Philadelphia, 1996, WB Saunders.)

BASIC INFORMATION

■ **DEFINITION**
- Pain in the breast.
- Mastodynia is synonymous with mastalgia.
- This condition is usually cyclical, but may be noncyclical or extramammary.

ICD-9CM CODES
611.71 Mastodynia

■ **EPIDEMIOLOGY & DEMOGRAPHICS**
- Mastodynia will affect up to 70% of women at some time in their reproductive lives.
- Severe cyclical mastodynia lasting more than 5 days/mo and of sufficient intensity to interfere with sexual, physical, social, and work-related activities is reported among 30% of premenopausal women.
- Underlying fear of breast cancer is the reason most of these women seek medical consultation.
- One tenth of women with mastodynia require pain-relieving therapy.

■ **PHYSICAL FINDINGS & CLINICAL PRESENTATION**
- Usually, the breasts are normal bilaterally
- Full, tender breasts
- Generalized breast nodularity without discrete lumps
- Chest wall tenderness: extramammary breast pain
- Distinguishing mammary from extramammary pain can be difficult
- With the patient lying on her side so that the breast tissue falls away from the chest wall, tenderness can then be reproduced by direct pressure over the offending site
- Cyclical mastodynia presents in the luteal phase of the menstrual cycle
- Women with cyclical mastodynia tend to have abdominal bloating, leg swelling, and other symptoms of premenstrual syndrome
- Noncyclical mastodynia, on the other hand, is unrelated to the menstrual cycle
- Extramammary breast pain simulates noncyclical mastodynia

■ **ETIOLOGY**
- Hormonal imbalance
- Abnormal lipid metabolism
- Premenstrual syndrome (20%)
- Fibrocystic breast disease
- Emotional abuse and anxiety
- Excessive caffeine intake
- Breast cancer (10%)
- Tietze syndrome (idiopathic costochondritis)

🔬 **DIAGNOSIS**

■ **DIFFERENTIAL DIAGNOSIS**
- See Etiology.
- The majority of women with mastodynia have no underlying abnormality.
- Breast fullness and tenderness associated with hormonal changes fluctuate with menstrual cycle.
- Similarly, the breast nodularity, which may or may not be the result of fibrocystic breast disease, also fluctuate with the menstrual cycle.
- Discrete breast lump needs full evaluation to rule out malignancy.
- Tietze syndrome is usually unilateral and may be associated with chest wall swelling.

■ **WORKUP**
- Complete history and thorough clinical examination.
- Pain analogue cards may be helpful in establishing the pattern of symptomatology. In patients >35 years of age, mammography should be performed as part of the baseline investigations.
- Most women presenting with severe mastodynia are <35. This group has a lower risk of subclinical breast cancer, and their breasts have increased density. In this younger group, radiologic investigations are of limited value, unless a discrete breast lump is palpated.

■ **LABORATORY TESTS**
Although hormonal imbalance and abnormal lipid metabolism have been implicated in the etiopathogenesis of mastodynia, there is no good evidence to support any consistent pattern of serum hormonal or lipid profile in women with mastodynia. These tests are therefore not recommended.

■ **IMAGING STUDIES**
- Mammography should be part of the baseline investigations if the woman is >35 yr.
- Ultrasound can be performed as needed; it is particularly helpful in the assessment of cystic breast lesions.
- In women <35 yr, imaging investigations are not helpful unless a lump has been palpated clinically.
- There are no radiologic features associated with mastodynia: rather, radiologic investigations are performed to exclude the rare presence of a subclinical carcinoma.

℞ **TREATMENT**

■ **NONPHARMACOLOGIC THERAPY**
- 85% of the women with mastodynia can be reassured after full clinical evaluation
- The remaining 15% will require some form of therapy in addition to reassurance
- Firm, supportive brassiere designed for postpartum use; this is particularly helpful if mastodynia is associated with breast swelling
- Low-fat, high-carbohydrate diet
- Reduction of caffeine intake

■ **ACUTE GENERAL Rx**
- Evening primrose oil (EPO), which contains gamma-linolenic acid, has been shown to have some effectiveness and is an acceptable treatment for mastodynia.
- Topical NSAID preparations may confer some benefit and can be prescribed for these women.
- Hormonal therapy is the mainstay of treatment.
- Danazol is the only drug approved by the FDA for the treatment of mastodynia. Danazol is an antigonadotrophin with some androgenic and peripheral antiestrogenic effects. Its efficacy is well established with significant relief of mastodynia in 70% to 93% of cases.
- Widespread use of danazol is limited because of its adverse side effects. These include menstrual irregularities, depression, acne, hirsutism, and, in severe cases, voice deepening. Women taking danazol should be advised to use effective nonhormonal contraception because of its potential adverse effects on the fetus.
- The side effects of danazol can be significantly reduced by using a low dose (100 mg daily) and confining treatment to the fortnight preceding menstruation.
- Tamoxifen, a synthetic antiestrogen, has also been shown to be effective in the treatment of mastodynia. Although effective in relieving symptoms, its use is extremely limited because of side effects. When used, it should be at a low dosage of 10 mg/day, and duration should be limited to 6 mo at a time. In the U.S., this agent has no approval for use in women with mastodynia.
- Bromocriptine is a dopamine-receptor agonist whose primary action is inhibition of prolactin release. It has been used extensively in the treatment of severe cyclical mastodynia and is effective. Again, side effects such as headache and dizziness have limited its use.

- Lisuride maleate was recently found to be effective by one study.
- Other hormonal agents that have been reported to be effective in small studies cannot be recommended. They either have unacceptable side effect profiles or their efficacy is not established. These agents include gestrinone, GnRH analogues, progesterone, and hormone replacement therapy.

■ CHRONIC Rx

- Long-standing cases of mastodynia can be managed with intermittent low-dose danazol therapy to limit side effects. In between these courses of hormone, nonpharmacologic and nonhormonal therapy can be used.
- Severe, unremitting mastodynia that fails to respond to medical treatment may require mastectomy; this is rare.

■ DISPOSITION

- Cyclical mastodynia resolves spontaneously in 20% to 30% of women.
- Up to 60% of women may develop recurrent symptoms 2 yr after treatment.
- Noncyclical mastodynia responds poorly to treatment, but may resolve spontaneously in up to 50% of women.

■ REFERRAL

- Detection of a breast lump or any other findings suggestive of neoplasm should be fully investigated. In addition, an immediate referral should be arranged.
- Women with chronic, unremitting mastodynia that fails to respond to pharmacologic therapy should be referred for possible mastectomy; this is rare.

☼ PEARLS & CONSIDERATIONS

■ COMMENTS

- There is no good evidence to support the use of vitamin B_6, diuretics, and vitamin E. Mastodynia may represent a presenting symptom of other more generalized disorder (e.g., premenstrual syndrome, psychologic disturbance).
- In these cases, treating mastodynia in isolation will not work; the underlying conditions must be appropriately addressed.

REFERENCES

Colgrave S, Holcombe C, Salmon P: Psychological characteristics of women presenting with breast pain, *J Psychosom Res* 50:303, 2001.

Fentiman IS, Hamed H: Assessment of breast problems, *Int J Clin Pract* 55:458, 2001.

Kaleli S et al: Symptomatic treatment of premenstrual mastalgia in premenopausal women with lisuride maleate: a double-blind placebo-controlled randomized study, *Fertility & Sterility* 75:718, 2001.

Marchant DJ: Benign breast disease, *Obstet Gynecol Clin North Am* 29:1-20, 2002.

Norlock FE: Benign breast pain in women: a practical approach to evaluation and treatment, *J Am Med Womens Assoc* 57:85, 2002.

Author: **Alexander Olawaiye, M.D.**

BASIC INFORMATION

■ DEFINITION
Mastoiditis is inflammation of the mastoid process and air cells, a complication of acute otitis media.

ICD-9CM CODES
383.00 Mastoiditis, acute or subacute
383.1 Mastoiditis, chronic

■ EPIDEMIOLOGY & DEMOGRAPHICS
INCIDENCE (IN U.S.): Widespread use of broad-spectrum antibiotics has led to a marked decline in the incidence of acute mastoiditis.
PREDOMINANT SEX: More common in males
PREDOMINANT AGE: 2 mo to 18 yr
PEAK INCIDENCE: Early childhood

■ PHYSICAL FINDINGS & CLINICAL PRESENTATION
- Acute mastoiditis is usually a complication of acute otitis media.
- Most common presenting symptom: pain and tenderness in the postauricular region.
- Other signs or symptoms include:
  1. Fever
  2. Postauricular erythema and edema
  3. Protrusion of the pinna inferiorly and anteriorly
  4. Tympanic membrane usually intact with signs of acute otitis media (occasionally ruptured with otorrhea)
- Complications of acute mastoiditis include:
  1. Subperiosteal abscess (most common complication)
  2. Hearing loss
  3. Facial nerve palsy
  4. Labyrinthitis
  5. Intracranial complications such as hydrocephalus, meningitis, encephalitis, intracranial abscess, and lateral sinus thrombosis
- Chronic mastoiditis (which follows a long course of recurrent otitis media, treated but never controlled completely) is characterized by chronic otorrhea and chronic tympanic membrane perforation.

■ ETIOLOGY
- All patients with otitis media exhibit some degree of mastoid inflammation because of the continuity between the middle air space and the mastoid cavity.
- Initial hyperemia and edema of the mucosal lining of the air cells results in accumulation of purulent exudate.
- Dissolution of calcium from bony septae and osteoclastic activity in the inflamed periosteum lead to bone necrosis and coalescence of air cells. This process can result in the development of a subperiosteal abscess.
- Most common bacterial isolates:
  1. *Streptococcus pneumoniae*
  2. *Streptococcus pyogenes*
  3. *Haemophilus influenzae*
  4. *Moraxella catarrhalis*
  5. *Staphylococcus aureus*
- Often, multiple organisms in chronic mastoiditis, with predominance of anaerobes and gram-negative bacteria.
- *Mycobacterium tuberculosis,* as well as nontuberculous mycobacteria, has been isolated in cases of mastoiditis.
- Unusual organisms such as *Aspergillus* and *Rhodococcus equi* have been reported in cases of mastoiditis in severely immunocompromised individuals.

DIAGNOSIS

■ DIFFERENTIAL DIAGNOSIS
- Children
  1. Rhabdomyosarcoma
  2. Histiocytosis X
  3. Leukemia
  4. Kawasaki syndrome
- Adults
  1. Fulminant otitis externa
  2. Histiocytosis X
  3. Metastatic disease

■ WORKUP
Thorough history and physical examination are important in establishing diagnosis.

■ LABORATORY TESTS
- Fluid for Gram stain and culture may be obtained by myringotomy.
- If there is a perforation in the tympanic membrane with drainage, cultures of this may be taken after carefully cleaning the external canal.

■ IMAGING STUDIES
- Plain x-rays of the mastoid region may demonstrate clouding or opacification in areas of pneumatization resulting from inflammatory swelling of the air cells.
- CT scan is the best radiologic modality for evaluating inflammation in this region.
- CT scan can demonstrate early involvement of bone (mastoiditis with bone destruction).
- MRI is more sensitive than CT scan in evaluating soft tissue involvement and is useful in conjunction with CT scan to investigate other complications of mastoiditis.

TREATMENT

■ NONPHARMACOLOGIC THERAPY
Myringotomy, if the ear is not already draining

■ ACUTE GENERAL Rx
- Initiated with IV antibiotics directed against the common organisms *S. pneumoniae* and *H. influenzae*. If the disease in the mastoid has had a prolonged course, coverage for *Staphylococcus aureus* with gram-negative enteric bacilli may be considered for initial therapy until results of cultures become available.
- Continued until all signs of mastoiditis have resolved
- Directed against enteric gram-negative organisms and anaerobes in chronic mastoiditis
- Indications for mastoidectomy:
  1. Failure to improve after 24 to 72 hr of therapy
  2. Persistent fever
  3. Imminent or overt signs of intracranial complications
  4. Evidence of a subperiosteal abscess in the mastoid bone

■ DISPOSITION
Proceed with mastoidectomy when medical therapy fails.

■ REFERRAL
- To otorhinolaryngologist:
  1. If diagnosis in doubt
  2. If aural complications present
  3. To evaluate for surgical intervention
- To neurosurgeon if intratemporal or intracranial extension of infection suspected
  1. Aural complications: bone destruction, subperiosteal abscess, petrositis, facial paralysis, labyrinthitis
  2. Intracranial complications: extradural abscess, lateral sinus thrombophlebitis or thrombosis, subdural abscess, meningitis, brain abscess, otitic hydrocephalus

REFERENCES
De S, Makura ZG, Clarke RW: Paediatric acute mastoiditis: the Alder Hey experience, *J Laryngol Otol* 116(6):440, 2002.
Vassbotn FS et al: Acute mastoiditis in a Norwegian population: a 20-year retrospective study, *Int J Pediatr Otorhinolaryngol* 62(3):237, 2002.
Authors: **Marilyn Fabbri, M.D., and Jane V. Eason, M.D.**

BASIC INFORMATION

■ DEFINITION

Measles is a childhood exanthem, caused by an RNA virus called *Morbillivirus,* belonging to the family *Paramyxoviridae.*

■ SYNONYMS

Rubeola

ICD-9CM CODES

055.9 Measles
055.0 Encephalitis
055.1 Pneumonia
V04.2 Vaccination

■ EPIDEMIOLOGY & DEMOGRAPHICS

- Before the introduction of an effective vaccine in 1963, measles was one of the most common childhood illnesses, and in developing countries, where it strikes mostly children under age 5 yr, it remains a leading cause of childhood mortality
- 30 million cases worldwide each year
- In developed countries, measles outbreaks occur occasionally in adolescents and young adults who have not been immunized (incidence 0 to 10/100,000 person-years)

■ PHYSICAL FINDINGS & CLINICAL PRESENTATION

- Incubation: 10 to 14 days (up to 3 wk in adults)
- Prodrome: 2 to 4 days; malaise, fever, rhinorrhea, conjunctivitis, cough
- Exanthem phase: 7 to 10 days
  The fever increases and peaks at 104° to 105° F together with the rash; it persists for 5 or 6 days. The patient's fever decreases over 24 hr.
  Rash: Erythematous maculopapular eruption begins behind the ears, progresses to the forehead and neck (Fig. 1-170), then spreads to face, trunk, upper extremities, buttocks, and lower extremities in that order. After 3 days the rash fades in the same sequence by becoming copper brown and then desquamates.
  Enanthem: Koplik spots are white papules of 1 to 2 mm in diameter on an erythematous base. They first appear on the buccal mucosa opposite the lower molar 2 days before the rash and spread over 24 hours to involve most of the buccal and lower labial mucosa. They fade after 3 days.
  Other symptoms and signs: malaise, anorexia, vomiting, diarrhea, abdominal pain, pharyngitis, lymphadenopathy, and occasional splenomegaly.

- Atypical measles (in vaccinated persons)
  Incubation: 10 to 14 days
  Prodrome: 1 to 3 days; high fever and headache
  Rash: maculopapular, urticarial, or petechial rash that begins peripherally and progresses centrally
- Modified measles applies to patients who have received immune serum globulin and develop a milder illness
- Complications (30% of cases):
  Otitis media
  Laryngitis, tracheitis
  Pneumonia (accounts for 90% of measles deaths)
  Encephalitis with lethargy, irritability, and seizures; 60% recover completely, 25% have neurologic sequelae (mental retardation, hemiplegia, paraplegia, epilepsy, deafness), and 15% die
  Myocarditis, pericarditis, and hepatitis
  Complications more common in immunocompromised hosts and persons with AIDS

■ ETIOLOGY & PATHOGENESIS

- The measles virus is transmitted through the respiratory tract by airborne droplets.
- It initially infects the respiratory epithelium; the patient becomes viremic during the prodromal phase and the virus is disseminated to

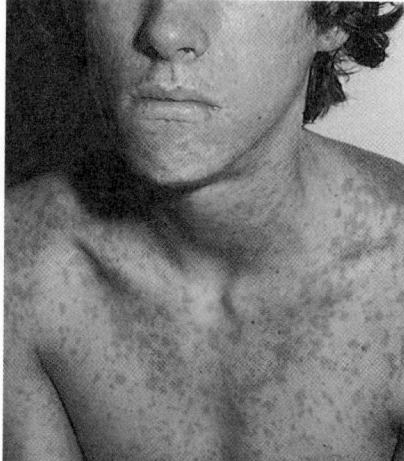

Fig. 1-170   Rubeola. (From Zitelli BJ, Davis HW: *Atlas of pediatric physical diagnosis,* ed 3, St Louis, 1997, Mosby.)

skin, respiratory tract, and other organs.
- Viral clearance is achieved via cellular immunity.

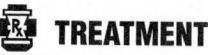

DIAGNOSIS

■ DIFFERENTIAL DIAGNOSIS

- Other viral infections by enteroviruses, adenoviruses, human parvovirus B-19, rubella
- Scarlet fever
- Allergic reaction
- Kawasaki disease

■ WORKUP

Knowledge of outbreak, history and physical findings (Koplik spots are diagnostic), laboratory tests

■ LABORATORY TESTS

- CBC: leukopenia
- ELISA for measles antibodies, which appear shortly after the onset of the rash and peak 3 to 4 wk later
- CSF analysis in encephalitis may reveal a pleocytosis (lymphocytes) and an elevated protein

■ IMAGING STUDIES

Chest x-ray if pneumonia is suspected

TREATMENT

- Supportive
- Vitamin A
- Ribavirin for severe measles pneumonitis

■ PREVENTION

- Passive immunization: Human immunoglobulin 0.25 ml/kg IM within 6 days of exposure. Double the dose for immunocompromised persons.
- Active immunization (see Section V, Table 5-6).

REFERENCES

Bernstein DI, Schiff GM: Measles. In Gorbach SL, Bartlett JG, Blacklow NR (eds): *Infectious diseases,* ed 2, Philadelphia, 1998, Saunders.
Epidemiology of measles—United States, *MMWR* 48:749, 1998.
Measles, *Clin Evid Concise* 7:55-56, 2002.
Author: **Tom J. Wachtel, M.D.**

BASIC INFORMATION

■ DEFINITION
Meckel's diverticulum is an ileal diverticulum located 100 cm proximal to the cecum. It results from failure of the omphalomesenteric duct to obliterate completely (as it should by the eighth week of gestation).

ICD-9CM CODES
751.0 Meckel's diverticulum

■ EPIDEMIOLOGY & DEMOGRAPHICS
Meckel's diverticulum, based on autopsy studies, occurs in 1% to 3% of the population. Complications occur more frequently in males.

■ PHYSICAL FINDINGS & CLINICAL PRESENTATION
- Painless lower GI bleeding (4%)
- Intestinal obstruction secondary to intussusception, volvulus, herniation, or entrapment of a loop of bowel through a defect in the diverticular mesentery (6%)
- Meckel's diverticulitis mimics acute appendicitis (5%)
- Rare primary tumor arising from diverticulum (carcinoid, sarcoma, leiomyoma, adenocarcinoma)
- Asymptomatic (80% to 95%)

■ ETIOLOGY & PATHOGENESIS
As a remnant of the omphalomesenteric duct, Meckel's diverticulum contains all layers of the intestinal wall and has its own mesentery and blood supply (branch of the superior mesenteric artery). The mucosa is usually ileal or gastric.

DIAGNOSIS

■ DIFFERENTIAL DIAGNOSIS
- Appendicitis
- Crohn's disease
- All causes of lower GI bleeding (polyp, colon cancer, AV malformation, diverticulosis, hemorrhoids)

Diagnosis is often made intraoperatively when the preoperative diagnosis is appendicitis. In the case of GI bleeding of unknown sources, a technetium scan will identify Meckel's diverticulum (sensitivity: 85% in children, 62% in adults; specificity: 95% in children, 9% in adults) (Fig. 1-171).

TREATMENT

Surgical resection

REFERENCES
Keljo DJ, Squires RH: Meckel's diverticulum. In Feldman M, Scharschmidt BF, Sleisenger MH (eds): *Gastrointestinal and liver disease*, ed 6, Philadelphia, 1998, WB Saunders.

Martin JP et al: Meckel's diverticulum, *Am Fam Physician* 61:1037, 2000.

Author: **Tom J. Wachtel, M.D.**

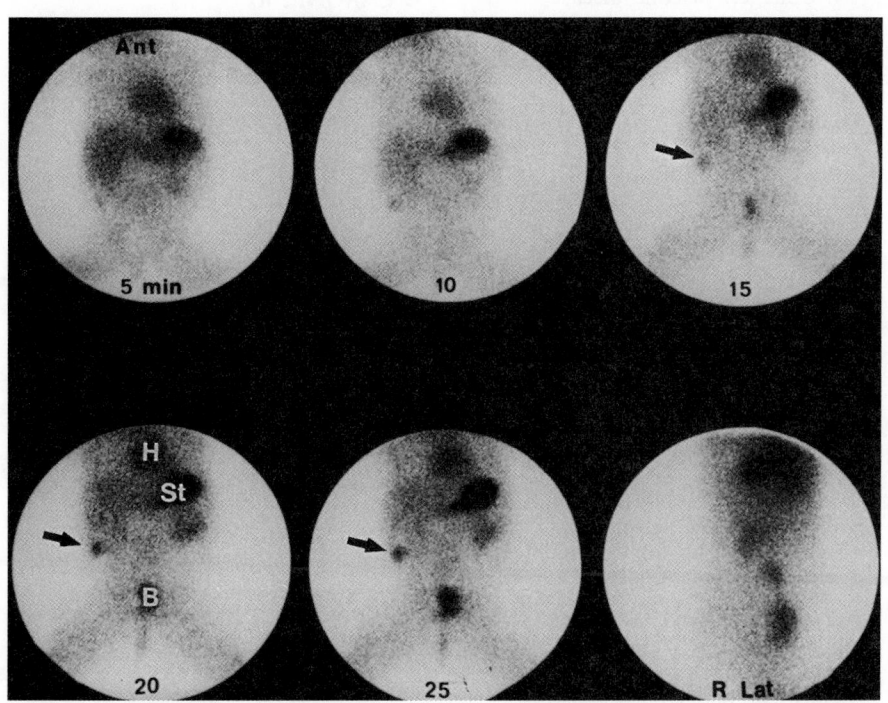

Fig. 1-171   Meckel's diverticulum. In this 2-year-old child who had unexplained rectal bleeding, a nuclear medicine study was performed using radioactive material that concentrates in gastric mucosa (technetium-99m pertechnetate). Sequential 5-minute images of the abdomen are obtained. On the 20-minute image, the heart (*H*), stomach (*St*), and bladder (*B*) are clearly seen, in addition to an ectopic focus of activity (*arrow*) representing a Meckel diverticulum. (From Mettler FA [ed]: *Primary care radiology,* Philadelphia, 2000, WB Saunders.)

BASIC INFORMATION

■ DEFINITION
Meigs' syndrome is characterized by the presence of a benign solid ovarian tumor associated with ascites and right hydrothorax that disappear after tumor removal.

■ ICD-9CM CODES
620.2 Ovarian mass (unspecified)
220.0 Benign ovarian lesion
789.5 Ascites
511.9 Pleural effusion

■ EPIDEMIOLOGY & DEMOGRAPHICS
- Occurs in <1% of ovarian fibromas (associated with approximately 0.004% of ovarian tumors)
- Most frequently encountered during middle age (average age, approximately 48 yr)

■ PHYSICAL FINDINGS & CLINICAL PRESENTATION
- Asymptomatic pelvic mass on bimanual examination
- Intermittent pelvic pain (intermittent torsion)
- Acute pelvic tenderness
- Acute abdominal tenderness
- Abdominal pelvic mass
- Abdominal bloating
- Fluid wave
- Shifting dullness
- "Puddle sign"
- Hyperresonance or flatness to chest percussion, absence of tactile and vocal fremitus
- Absent or loud bronchial breath sounds, rales, mediastinal displacement, tracheal shift
- Weight loss and emaciation

■ ETIOLOGY
- Not specifically known
- Usually associated with "edematous" fibromas (or other benign ovarian solid tumor) in excess of 10 cm
- Plausible that large fibroma with narrow stalk has inadequate lymphatic drainage; when coupled with intermittent torsion, results in back flow transudation into the peritoneal cavity; accumulated peritoneal ascites then passes to the right pleural cavity via lymphatics (overloaded thoracic duct) or via abdominal pleural commutation (i.e., foramen of Bochdalek)

DIAGNOSIS

■ DIFFERENTIAL DIAGNOSIS
- Abdominal ovarian malignancy
- Various gynecologic disorders:
  1. Uterus; endometrial tumor, sarcoma, leiomyoma ("pseudo-Meigs' syndrome")
  2. Fallopian tube: hydrosalpinx, granulomatous salpingitis, fallopian tube malignancy
  3. Ovary: benign, serous, mucinous, endometrioid, clear cell, Brenner tumor, granulosa, stromal, dysgerminoma, fibroma, metastatic tumor
- Nongynecologic (GI tract or GU tract tumor or pathology) causes of pelvic mass
  1. Ascites
  2. Portal vein obstruction
  3. IVC obstruction
  4. Hypoproteinemia
  5. Thoracic duct obstruction
  6. TB
  7. Amyloidosis
  8. Pancreatitis
  9. Neoplasm
  10. Ovarian hyperstimulation
  11. Pleural effusion
  12. CHF
  13. Malignancy
  14. Collagen-vascular disease
  15. Pancreatitis
  16. Cirrhosis

■ WORKUP
- Clinical condition characterized by ovarian mass, ascites, and right-sided pleural effusion
- Ovarian malignancy and the other causes (see "Differential Diagnosis") of pelvic mass, ascites, and pleural effusion to be considered
- History of early satiety, weight loss with increased abdominal girth, bloating, intermittent abdominal pain, dyspnea, nonproductive cough

■ LABORATORY TESTS
- CBC to rule out inflammatory process
- Tumor markers (CA-125, Hcg, AFP, CEA) to evaluate malignancy
- Chemical/LFT profile to evaluate metabolic or hepatic involvement

■ IMAGING STUDIES
- Pelvic sonography (color flow Doppler evaluation of adnexal mass) to evaluate pelvic pathology (CT scan or MRI if etiology indeterminate)
- Chest x-ray examination
- ABG if respiratory compromise

TREATMENT

■ NONPHARMACOLOGIC TREATMENT
- Informed consent and proper preparation of patient for possible staging laparotomy (TAHBSO, omentectomy, possible bowel resection, pelvic/periaortic lymphadenectomy)
- Bowel prep if considering pelvic malignancy

■ ACUTE GENERAL Rx
Depending on clinical presentation, size of pelvic mass, amount of ascites, and pleural effusion:
- If pelvic mass <10 cm, minimal ascites/pleural effusion: consider diagnostic open laparoscopy (possible exploratory laparotomy) and salpingo-oophorectomy with removal of ovarian fibroma (tumor).
- If pelvic mass >10 cm, moderate/large amount ascites/pleural effusion: consider pleurocentesis if respiratory compromise (cytology: AFB) and exploratory laparotomy with salpingo-oophorectomy and removal of ovarian fibroma (tumor).
- Treat pelvic malignancy, GI or GU tumor as indicated.

■ CHRONIC Rx
- Resolution of ascites and right-sided pleural effusion after removal of ovarian fibroma
- No long-term follow-up for benign ovarian fibroma

■ DISPOSITION
Excellent progress and complete survival are expected.

■ REFERRAL
To gynecologist or gynecologic oncologist for evaluation and treatment, especially if malignancy considered or encountered

REFERENCES
Abramov Y et al: The role of inflammatory cytokines in Meigs' syndrome, *Obstet Gynecol* 99(5 Pt 2):917, 2002.
Buttin BM et al: Meigs' syndrome with an elevated CA 125 from benign Brenner tumors, *Obstet Gynecol* 98(5 Pt 2):980, 2001.
Meigs JV, Cass JW: Fibroma of the ovary with ascites and hydrothorax: with a report of seven cases, *Am J Obstet Gynecol* 33:249, 1937.
Author: **Dennis M. Weppner, M.D.**

BASIC INFORMATION

■ DEFINITION

Melanoma is a skin neoplasm arising from the malignant degeneration of melanocytes. It is classically subdivided in four types:
- Superficial spreading melanoma (70%) (Fig. 1-172, A)
- Nodular melanoma (15% to 20%) (Fig. 1-172, B)
- Lentigo maligna melanoma (5% to 10%)
- Acral lentiginous melanoma (7% to 10%)

■ SYNONYMS

Malignant melanoma

ICD-9CM CODES

172.9 Melanoma of the skin, site unspecified

■ EPIDEMIOLOGY & DEMOGRAPHICS

- Annual incidence of melanoma is 13 cases/100,000 persons.
- Melanoma has doubled to tripled in incidence over the past 25 years.
- Lifetime risk of cutaneous melanoma for white Americans is 1/90.
- Melanoma is the leading cause of death from skin disease.
- Median age at diagnosis is 53 yr.
- Superficial spreading melanoma occurs most often in young adults on sun-exposed areas.
- Acral lentiginous melanoma is most often found in Asian Americans and African Americans and is not related to sun exposure.
- Death rate for white men with melanoma is 3/100,000.
- 8%-10% of melanomas arise in people with a family history of the disease.

■ PHYSICAL FINDINGS & CLINICAL PRESENTATION

Variable depending on the subtype of melanoma:
- *Superficial spreading melanoma* is most often found on the lower legs, arms, and upper back. It may have a combination of many colors or may be uniformly brown or black.
- *Nodular melanoma* can be found anywhere on the body, but it most frequently occurs on the trunk on sun-exposed areas. It has a dark-brown or red-brown appearance, can be dome shaped or pedunculated; they are frequently misdiagnosed because they may resemble a blood blister or hemangioma and may also be amelanotic.
- *Lentigo maligna melanoma* is generally found in older adults in areas continually exposed to the sun and frequently arising from lentigo maligna (Hutchinson's freckle) or melanoma in situ. It might have a complex pattern and variable shape; color is more uniform than in superficial spreading melanoma.
- *Acral lentiginous melanoma* frequently occurs in soles, subungual mucous membranes, and palms (sole of the foot is the most prevalent site). Unlike other types of melanoma, it has a similar incidence in all ethnic groups.
- The warning signs that the lesion may be a melanoma can be summarized with the ABCD rules:
  A: Asymmetry (e.g., lesion is bisected and halves are not identical)
  B: Border irregularity (uneven, ragged border)
  C: Color variegation (presence of various shades of pigmentation)
  D: Diameter enlargement (>6 mm)

■ ETIOLOGY

- UV light is the most important cause of malignant melanoma.
- There is a modest increase in melanoma risk in patients with small nondysplastic nevi and a much greater risk in those with dysplastic lesions.
- The CDKN2A gene, residing at the 9p21 locus, is often deleted in people with familial melanoma.

DIAGNOSIS

■ DIFFERENTIAL DIAGNOSIS

- Dysplastic nevi
- Solar lentigo
- Vascular lesions
- Blue nevus
- Basal cell carcinoma
- Seborrheic keratosis

■ WORKUP

- Perform excisional biopsy with elliptical excision that includes 1 to 2 mm of normal skin surrounding the lesion and extends to the subcutaneous tissue; incisional punch biopsy is sometimes necessary in surgically sensitive areas (e.g., digits, nose).
- The sentinel lymph node dissection (SLND) should be considered in patients with intermediate (1 to 4 mm) melanomas or high-risk skin tumors to obtain information regarding a patient's subclinical lymph node status with minimal morbidity. It involves the use of radiologic lymphoscintigraphy to map lymphatic drainage from the site of the primary melanoma to the first "sentinel" lymph node in the region. When properly performed, if the sentinel node is negative, the remaining lymph nodes in the region will not have metastases in more than 98% of cases.

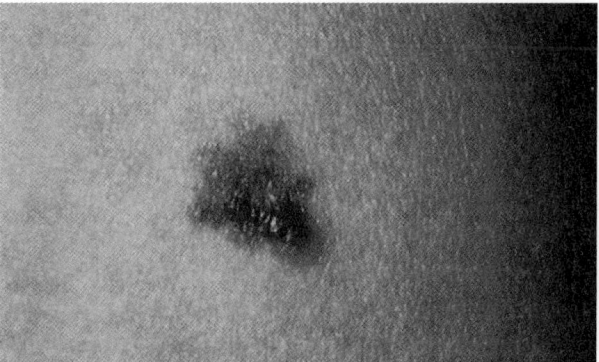
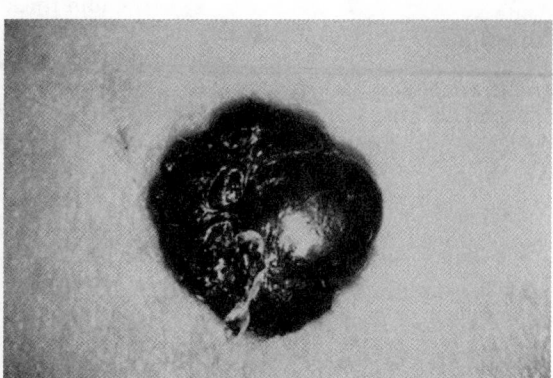

Fig. 1-172 **A,** Superficial spreading melanoma. **B,** Nodular melanoma. (From Abeloff MD [ed]: *Clinical oncology,* ed 2, New York, 2000, Churchill Livingstone.)

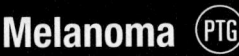
- The staging system for melanoma adapted by the American Joint Committee on Cancer (AJCC) is as follows:

T*	Thickness of primary tumor
Tis	In situ
T1	≤1.0 mm
T2	1.01-2.0 mm
T3	2.01-4.0 mm
T4	>4.0 mm
N†	Number of positive lymph nodes
N0	0
N1	1
N2	2 or 3
N3	≥4 (or combination of in-transit metastases, satellite lesions, or an ulcerated primary lesion with any number of nodes)
M	Metastases
M0	0
M1	Distant subcutaneous or lymph node metastases
M2	Lung metastases
M3	All other visceral or any distant metastases or an elevated lactate dehydrogenase level not attributable to another cause

Clinical Stage	
0	(T0N0M0)
IA	(T1aN0M0)
IB	(T1bN0M0)
	(T2aN0M0)
IIA	(T2bN0M0)
	(T3aN0M0)
IIB	(T3bN0M0)
	(T4aN0M0)
IIC	(T4bN0M0)
IIIA	(T1-T4aN1bM0)
IIIB	T1-T4aN2bM0)
IIIC	(AnyT,N2c,M0)
	(Any T, N3, M0)
IV	(Any T, Any N, >M1)

*a, without ulceration; b, with ulceration
†a, micrometastasis; b, macrometastases; c, in-transit metastases with metastatic lymph nodes

■ LABORATORY TESTS

The pathology report should indicate the following:
- Tumor thickness (Breslow microstage)
- Tumor depth (Clark level)
- Mitotic rate
- Radial growth rates vs. vertical growth rate
- Tumor infiltrating lymphocyte
- Histologic regression

- Reverse transcriptase-polymerase chain reaction (RT-PCR) assay for tyrosine messenger RNA is a useful marker for the presence of melanoma cells. It is performed on sentinel lymph node biopsy and is useful for detection of submicroscopic metastases.

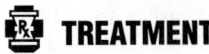

■ TREATMENT

■ NONPHARMACOLOGIC THERAPY

Avoid excessive sun exposure; liberal use of sunscreens with UBV and UVA protection (recent laboratory data suggest that melanoma is promoted by UVA; therefore UVB sunscreens may not be effective in preventing melanoma). Recent literature reports, however, reveal no association between melanoma and sunscreen use.

■ GENERAL Rx

- Initial excision of the melanoma
- Reexcision of the involved area after histologic diagnosis:
  1. The margins of reexcision depend on the thickness of the tumor.
  2. Low-risk or intermediate-risk tumors require excision of 1 to 3 cm.
  3. Melanomas of moderate thickness (0.9 to 2.0 mm) can be excised safely with 2-cm margins.
  4. A 1-cm margin of excision for melanoma with a poor prognosis (as defined by a tumor thickness of at least 2 mm) is associated with a significantly greater risk of regional recurrence than is a 3-cm margin, but with a similar overall survival rate.
- Lymph node dissection: recommended in all patients with enlarged lymph nodes.
  1. Elective lymph node dissection remains controversial.
  2. It is indicated with positive sentinel node. It may be considered in those with a primary melanoma that is between 1 and 4 mm thick (especially in patients <60 yr old).
- Adjuvant therapy with interferon alfa-2b (intron A) is considered controversial in patients with metastatic

melanoma. It is approved by the FDA for AJCC stages IIb and III melanoma; however, its statistical benefit remains unclear.
- Dacarbazine (DTIC) and interleukin 2 (IL-2) can be used in metastatic melanoma. Results are generally poor, with median survival in patients with distant metastatic melanoma approximately 6 mo.
- Patients with a history of melanoma should be followed with skin examinations every 6 mo or sooner if patient detects any new lesions; the assessments usually consist of medical history, physical examination, chest x-ray examination, and laboratory evaluation.

■ DISPOSITION

- Prognosis varies with the stage of the melanoma. The 5-yr survival related to thickness is as follows: <0.76 mm, 99% survival; 0.6 to 1.49 mm, 85%; 1.5 to 2.49 mm, 84%; 2.5 to 3.9 mm, 70%; >4 mm, 44%.
- The 5-yr survival in patients with distant metastasis is <10%.
- Treatment of advanced disease consists (in addition to surgical excision and lymph node dissection) of chemotherapy, immunotherapy, and radiation therapy.

REFERENCES

Balch CM et al: A new American Joint Committee on Cancer Staging System for cutaneous melanoma, *Cancer* 88:1484, 2000.

Dennis LK et al: Sunscreen use and the risk for melanoma: a quantitative review, *Ann Intern Med* 139:966, 2003.

Kanzler MH, Mraz-Gernhard S: Treatment of primary cutaneous melanoma, *JAMA* 285:1819, 2001.

Masci P, Borden EC: Malignant melanoma: treatment emerging, but early detection is still key, *Cleve Clin J Med* 69:529, 2002.

Thomas JM et al: Excision margins in high-risk malignant melanoma, *N Engl J Med* 350:757, 2004.

Author: **Fred F. Ferri, M.D.**

BASIC INFORMATION

■ DEFINITION

Meniere's disease is a syndrome characterized by recurrent vertigo with fluctuating hearing loss, roaring tinnitus, and fullness in the ear.

■ SYNONYMS

Endolymphatic hydrops
Lermoyez's syndrome
Meniere's syndrome

ICD-9CM CODES

386.01 Meniere's disease, cochleovestibular (active)

■ EPIDEMIOLOGY & DEMOGRAPHICS

INCIDENCE (IN U.S.): 15 cases/100,000 persons
PREVALENCE (IN U.S.): 100-200 cases/100,000 persons
PREDOMINANT SEX: Male = female
PREDOMINANT AGE: Adults
GENETICS: Not known to be genetic

■ PHYSICAL FINDINGS & CLINICAL PRESENTATION

- Hearing may be unilaterally decreased
- Pallor, sweating, and nausea may occur during a severe attack
- Usually the patient develops a sensation of fullness and pressure along with decreased hearing and tinnitus in a single ear
- Next the patient typically experiences severe vertigo, which peaks within minutes, then slowly subsides over hours
- Persistent sense of disequilibrium for days after an acute episode

■ ETIOLOGY

- Unknown; viral and autoimmune etiologies have been suggested
- Associated with endolymphatic hydrops

DIAGNOSIS

■ DIFFERENTIAL DIAGNOSIS

- Acoustic neuroma
- Migrainous vertigo
- Multiple sclerosis
- Autoimmune inner ear syndrome
- Otitis media
- Vertebrobasilar disease
- Viral labyrinthitis

■ WORKUP

- Glycerol test and electrocochleography are used by some ENT specialists.
- Electronystagmography may show peripheral vestibular deficit.

■ LABORATORY TESTS

Audiometry suggests cochlear-type hearing loss.

■ IMAGING STUDIES

MRI to rule out acoustic neuroma, especially if cerebellar or CNS dysfunction is present

TREATMENT

■ NONPHARMACOLOGIC THERAPY

Limit activity during attacks.

■ ACUTE GENERAL Rx

- Prochlorperazine 5 to 10 mg PO q6h or 25 mg PO bid
- Promethazine 12.5 to 25 mg PO q4-6h
- Diazepam 5 to 10 mg IV/PO for acute attack
- Meclizine 25 mg q6h
- Scopolamine patch

■ CHRONIC Rx

Diuretics, salt restriction, and avoidance of caffeine are traditional.

■ DISPOSITION

- Usually followed by ENT specialist
- Usual course of disease consists of alternating attacks and remissions
- Majority of patients can be managed medically; fewer than 10% of patients will undergo surgical intervention for persistent incapacitating vertigo

■ REFERRAL

If attacks persist

⚙ PEARLS & CONSIDERATIONS

■ COMMENTS

- Many variations of the classical clinical picture. Without the combination of fluctuating hearing loss and vertigo, the diagnosis remains uncertain.
- In one-third of patients both ears are eventually involved.

REFERENCES

Baloh RW, Fife TD, Furman JM, Zee DS: Recurrent spontaneous attacks of vertigo, *Continuum Lifelong Learning in Neurology* 2(2):56, 1996.

Thai-Von H, Bounaix MJ, Fraysse B: Meniere's disease: pathophysiology and treatment, *Drugs* 61(8):1089, 2001.

Weber PC, Adkins WY Jr: The differential diagnosis of Meniere's disease, *Otolaryngol Clin North Am* 30(6):977, 1997.

Author: **Sharon S. Hartman, M.D., Ph.D.**

BASIC INFORMATION

■ DEFINITION
A meningioma is an intracranial tumor arising from arachnoid cells.

ICD-9CM CODES
225.2 Cerebral meninges

■ EPIDEMIOLOGY & DEMOGRAPHICS
INCIDENCE (IN U.S.): 2.6/100,000 persons/yr. Incidence increases with increasing age.
PREVALENCE (IN U.S.): Not reported
PREDOMINANT SEX: Female:male ratio of 3:2 in adults; male > female in childhood and male = female among African Americans
PEAK INCIDENCE: Males: sixth decade, females: seventh decade; rare in childhood
GENETICS: Tumors associated with a missing sequence/loss of heterozygosity on chromosome 22.

■ PHYSICAL FINDINGS AND CLINICAL PRESENTATION
- Varies with location and size
- May be asymptomatic
- Seizures and hemiparesis common, as are headache, personality change/confusion and visual impairment
- Children are more likely to present with signs of increased intracranial pressure without further localizing features

■ TYPICAL LOCATIONS
- Parasagittal
- Convexity
- Sphenoid wing
- Spinal canal
- Others: optic nerve sheath, choroid plexus, ectopic (intraventricular)

■ ETIOLOGY
- Most are associated with an abnormality on chromosome 22, and in association with neurofibromatosis type 2 as well as in certain familial aggregates.
- Cranial radiation may be responsible for some cases where the tumor occurs in the irradiated field following an appropriate latency period from the radiation.
- The link with sex hormones is suggested by the increase in growth rate during luteal phase of the menstrual cycle and during pregnancy, as well as with breast carcinomas.

DIAGNOSIS

■ IMAGING STUDIES
- Cranial computed tomography scanning or magnetic resonance imaging can detect and determine the extent of meningiomas (Figure 1-173).
- Bone windows optimally identify bone involvement.
- On non-enhanced scans, meningiomas typically are isodense to slightly hyperdense to brain and are homogeneous in appearance. With the addition of contrast, meningiomas show homogeneous enhancement; gadolinium can facilitate imaging of smaller additional lesions that are missed on unenhanced images.

■ DIFFERENTIAL DIAGNOSIS
Other well-circumscribed intracranial tumors:
- Acoustic schwannoma (typically at the pontocerebellar junction)
- Ependymoma, lipoma, and metastases within the spinal cord

■ WORKUP
- Imaging studies followed by surgical removal with histologic confirmation if clinically indicated
- There are nine benign histologic variants and four variants associated with increased recurrence and rates of metastasis. Features suggesting increased rate of recurrence include brain invasion, high rate of mitosis, and highly anaplastic features

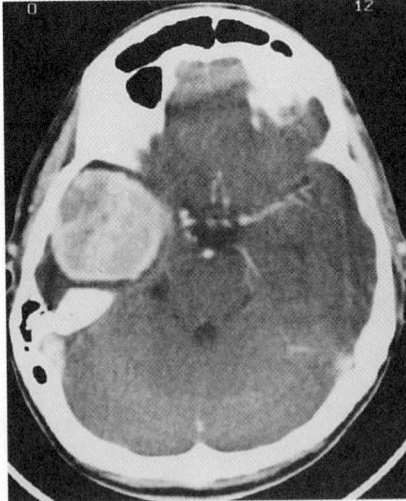

Fig. 1-173 Contrast-enhanced CT scan demonstrates a large contrast-enhancing right sphenoid wing meningioma. (From Specht N [ed]: *Practical guide to diagnostic imaging*, St Louis, 1998, Mosby.)

TREATMENT

■ NONPHARMACOLOGIC THERAPY
The mainstay of treatment for meningiomas remains surgical removal if symptomatic

■ ACUTE GENERAL Rx
- Generally none. For lesions that cause significant mass effect, steroids (Decadron) are sometimes used to decrease edema
- Anticonvulsants to control seizures

■ CHRONIC Rx
- Radiation therapy is the only validated form of adjuvant therapy and may be beneficial in patients with incomplete resections or inoperable tumors.
- Sterotactic radiosurgery has increasingly been used to treat meningiomas.
- Little information is available on the efficacy of traditional antineoplastic agents.
- Hormonal treatments are under investigation.

■ DISPOSITION
- Estimated surgical mortality is 7%.
- Long-term outcome is variable, based on location and completeness of resection.
- Most incidentally discovered meningiomas remain asymptomatic. Calcified tumors may be less likely to progress than noncalcified ones.
- Significant morbidity and mortality can be observed in meningiomas with otherwise favorable pathology secondary to unfavorable location (e.g, skull base).

■ REFERRAL
Neurosurgical consultation for all cases

REFERENCES

Gor S et al: The natural history of asymptomatic meningiomas in Olmsted County, Minnesota, *Neurology* 51:1718, 1998.
Kleihues P et al: The WHO classification of tumors of the nervous system, *J Neuropathol Exp Neurol* 61(3):215, 2002.
Sekhar LN, Levine ZT, Sarma S: Grading of meningiomas, *J Clin Neurosci* 8(suppl 1):1, 2001.
Author: **Nicole J. Ullrich, M.D., Ph.D.**

BASIC INFORMATION

■ DEFINITION
Bacterial meningitis is an inflammation of meninges with increased intracranial pressure, and pleocytosis or increased WBCs in CSF secondary to bacteria in the pia-subarachnoid space and ventricles, leading to neurologic sequelae and abnormalities.

ICD-9CM CODES
320 Bacterial meningitis

■ EPIDEMIOLOGY & DEMOGRAPHICS
INCIDENCE (IN U.S.): 3 cases/100,000 persons
PREDOMINANT SEX: Male = female
PREDOMINANT AGE: All ages, neonate to geriatric

■ PHYSICAL FINDINGS & CLINICAL PRESENTATION
- Fever
- Headache
- Neck stiffness, nuchal rigidity, meningismus
- Altered mental state, lethargy
- Vomiting, nausea
- Photophobia
- Seizures
- Coma; lethargy, stupor
- Rash: petechial associated with meningococcal infection
- Myalgia
- Cranial nerve abnormality (unilateral)
- Papilledema
- Dilated, nonreactive pupil(s)
- Posturing: decorticate/decerebrate
- Physical examination findings of Kernig's sign and Brudzinski's sign in adults with meningitis are often not helpful in determining meningeal inflammation

■ ETIOLOGY
Neisseria meningitidis is now more common than *Haemophilus influenzae* as a cause of bacterial meningitis in children as well as adults. *H. influenzae* is the cause of >30% of cases of meningitis (usually in infants and children <6 yr old). It is associated with sinusitis, otitis media.
- Neonates: group B streptococci, *Escherichia coli*, *Klebsiella* sp., *Listeria monocytogenes*
- Infants through adolescence:
  1. *N. meningitidis*
  2. *H. influenzae*
  3. *Streptococcus pneumoniae*
- Adults
  1. *N. meningitidis*
  2. *S. pneumoniae*
- Elderly
  1. *S. pneumoniae*
  2. *N. meningitidis*
  3. *L. monocytogenes*
  4. Gram-negative bacilli

DIAGNOSIS

Diagnostic approach is based on patient presentation and physical examination. Key elements to diagnosis are CSF evaluation and CT scan or MRI if the patient is in a coma or has focal neurologic deficits, pupillary abnormalities, or papilledema.

■ DIFFERENTIAL DIAGNOSIS
- Endocarditis, bacteremia
- Intracranial tumor
- Lyme disease
- Brain abscess
- Partially treated bacterial meningitis
- Medications
- SLE
- Seizures
- Acute mononucleosis
- Other infectious meningitides
- Neuroleptic malignant syndrome
- Subdural empyema
- Rocky Mountain spotted fever

■ WORKUP
CSF examination:
- Opening pressure >100 to 200 mm Hg
- WBC <5 to >100 mm³
- Neutrophilic predominance: >80%
- Gram stain of CSF: positive in 60% to 90% patients
- CSF protein: >50 mg/dl
- CSF glucose: <40 mg/dl
- Culture: positive in 65% to 90% cases
- CSF bacterial antigen: 50% to 100% sensitivity
- E-test for susceptibility of pneumococcal isolates

■ LABORATORY TESTS
Blood culturing, WBC with differential, and CSF examination (see "Workup")

■ IMAGING STUDIES
- CT scan or MRI of head: necessary with increased intracranial pressure, coma, neurologic deficits
- Sinus CT: if sinusitis suspected

TREATMENT

- Empiric therapy is necessary with IV antibiotic treatment if patient has purulent CSF fluid at time of lumbar puncture, is asplenic, or has signs of DIC/sepsis pending Gram stain and culture results. Therapy after Gram stain pending cultures is recommended for the following age and patient risk groups:
  1. Neonates: ampicillin plus cefotaxime
  2. Infants/children: ampicillin or third-generation cephalosporin (plus chloramphenicol if purulent or patient compromised)
  3. Adults (18 to 50 yr): third-generation cephalosporin
  4. Older adults (>50 yr): ampicillin plus third-generation cephalosporin

- Penicillin-resistant pneumococcus: because of an increasing incidence of this organism, empiric treatment with ceftriaxone or cefotaxime plus vancomycin (60 mg/kg/day) has been recommended.
- Table 1-36 describes common pathogens of bacterial meningitis and their empiric treatment based on age.
- Table 1-37 describes specific antibiotic treatments for known pathogens.
- Steroids: dexamethasone 0.15 mg/kg q6h for first 4 days of therapy should be used in adults with bacterial meningitis and mental status changes or acute neurologic phenomenon. Decreased mortality and neurologic sequelae are seen with adjunct therapy.
- Dexamethasone also benefits children with Hib or pneumococcal meningitis and should be given within the first 2 days of illness.

PEARLS & CONSIDERATIONS

■ COMMENTS
- Prevention of meningitis can be achieved through chemoprophylaxis of close contacts (household members and anyone exposed to oral secretions).
- Effective medications are rifampin 10 mg/kg PO bid for 2 days or ceftriaxone 250 mg IM single dose in patients over age 12; 125 mg IM if age 12 and under.
- Ciprofloxacin 500mg for prevention of Neisseria meningitis can be given to patients over the age of 18 yr who cannot tolerate rifampin to eradicate pharyngeal colonization.
- Vaccines with antibodies against serogroup A, C, Y, W-135 capsular polysaccharides are available for adults and children over the age of 2 yr.

REFERENCES
Aronin SI, Peduzzi P, Quagliarello VJ: Community-acquired bacterial meningitis: risk stratification for adverse clinical outcome an effect of antibiotic timing, *Ann Int Med* 129:862, 1998.

Choi C: Bacterial meningitis in aging adults, *Clin Infect Dis* 33:1380, 2001.

Hasbun R et al: Computed tomography of the head before lumbar puncture in adults with suspected meningitis, *N Engl J Med* 345:1727, 2001.

Rosenstein NE et al: Meningococcal disease, *N Engl J Med* 344:1378, 2001.

Thomas KE et al: The diagnostic accuracy of Kernig's sign, Brudzinski's sign, and nuchal rigidity in adults with suspected meningitis, *Clin Infect Dis* 35:46, 2002.
Authors: **Glenn G. Fort, M.D., and Dennis J. Mikolich, M.D.**

TABLE 1-36 Common Pathogens of Bacterial Meningitis and Their Empiric Treatment Based on Age

AGE	COMMON PATHOGENS	TREATMENT*	DURATION (DAYS)
0-1 mo	Group B streptococcus	Ampicillin + third-generation cephalosporin†	14-21
	Listeria monocytogenes	or ampicillin + aminoglycoside	14-21
	Escherichia coli		21
	Streptococcus pneumoniae		10-14
1-3 mo	Group B streptococcus,	Ampicillin + third-generation cephalosporin†	14-21
	E. coli, L. monocytogenes		14-21
	S. pneumoniae		10-14
	Neisseria meningitidis,		7-10
	Haemophilus influenzae		
3 mo-18 yr	H. influenzae, H. meningitidis,	Third-generation cephalosporin† or	7-10 (N. influenzae and
	S. pneumoniae	meropenem or chloramphenicol	N. meningitidis)
			10-14 (S. pneumoniae)
18-50 yr	H. influenzae, N. meningitidis,	Third-generation cephalosporin† or	Same as above
	S. pneumoniae	meropenem or ampicillin + chloramphenicol	
>50 yr	S. pneumoniae, L. monocyto-	Ampicillin + third-generation cephalosporin†	10-14 (S. pneumoniae)
	genes, gram-negative bacilli	or ampicillin + fluoroquinolone‡ or	14-21 (L. monocytogenes)
		meropenem	21 Gram-negative bacilli
			other than H. influenzae

From Rakel RE (ed): *Principles of family practice*, ed 6, Philadelphia, 2002, WB Saunders.
*Add vancomycin in areas where there is greater than 2% incidence of highly drug resistant *S. pneumoniae*.
†Ceftriaxone or cefotaxime.
‡Ciprofloxacin or levofloxacin.

TABLE 1-37 Specific Antibiotic Treatments for Known Pathogens

PATHOGEN	PRIMARY THERAPY	ALTERNATIVE*
Group B streptococcus	Penicillin G or ampicillin	Vancomycin or third-generation cephalosporin†
Streptococcus pneumoniae (MIC < 0.1)	Third-generation cephalosporin†	Meropenem, penicillin
S. pneumoniae (MIC > 0.1)	Vancomycin + third-generation cephalosporin*	Substitute rifampin for vancomycin; or meropenem; or vancomycin as monotherapy if highly allergic to other alternatives
Haemophilus influenzae (β-lactamase-negative)	Ampicillin	Third-generation cephalosporin† or chloramphenicol or aztreonam
H. influenzae (β-lactamase-positive)	Third-generation cephalosporin†	Chloramphenicol or aztreonam or fluoroquinolones‡
Listeria monocytogenes	Ampicillin + gentamicin	Trimethoprim-sulfamethoxazole
Neisseria meningitidis	Penicillin G or ampicillin	Third-generation cephalosporin†
Enterobacteriaceae	Third-generation cephalosporin† + aminoglycoside	Trimethoprim-sulfamethoxazole or aztreonam or fluoroquinolones or antipseudomonal penicillin (or ampicillin) + aminoglycoside
Pseudomonas aeruginosa	Ceftazidine + aminoglycoside	Aminoglycoside + aztreonam or aminoglycoside + antipseudomonal penicillin§
Staphylococcus aureus (methicillin-sensitive)	Antistaphylococcal penicillin¶ ± rifampin	Vancomycin + rifampin or trimethoprim-sulfamethoxazole + rifampin
S. aureus (methicillin-resistant)	Vancomycin + rifampin	
Staphylococcus epidermidis	Vancomycin + rifampin	

From Rakel RE (ed): *Principles of family practice*, ed 6, Philadelphia, 2002, WB Saunders.
MIC, Minimum inhibitory concentration.
*If patient is highly allergic or intolerant of primary therapy.
†Ceftriaxone or cefotaxime.
‡Ciprofloxacin or levofloxacin.
§Piperacillin, mezlocillin, or ticarcillin.
¶Nafcillin, oxacillin, or methicillin.

BASIC INFORMATION

■ DEFINITION
Viral meningitis is an acute aseptic meningitis usually with lymphocytic pleocytosis and negative CSF stains and cultures.

■ SYNONYMS
Aseptic meningitis

ICD-9CM CODES
047.8 Meningitis, aseptic

■ EPIDEMIOLOGY & DEMOGRAPHICS (TABLE 1-38)
INCIDENCE (IN U.S.): 11 cases/100,000 persons
PREDOMINANT SEX: Male = female
GENETICS: Those with abnormal humoral immunity and agammaglobulinemia have associated difficulty with viral clearance.

■ PHYSICAL FINDINGS & CLINICAL PRESENTATION
- Fever
- Headache
- Nuchal rigidity
- Photophobia
- Myalgias
- Vomiting
- Rash
- Diarrhea
- Pharyngitis

■ ETIOLOGY
- Enterovirus
- Mumps virus
- Measles
- Enteroviruses
- Arboviruses
- Herpes (simplex and zoster)
- HIV
- Lymphocytic choriomeningitis virus

- Adenovirus
- CMV
- Arthropod-borne viruses
- West Nile virus

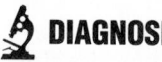

DIAGNOSIS

The diagnostic approach is similar to bacterial meningitis (see "Bacterial Meningitis"); the foremost need is to rule out bacterial meningitis with CSF evaluation. Presentation may be similar to that of meningitis with bacterial involvement.

■ DIFFERENTIAL DIAGNOSIS
- Bacterial meningitis
- Meningitis secondary to Lyme disease, TB, syphilis, amebiasis, leptospirosis
- Rickettsial illnesses: Rocky Mountain spotted fever
- Migraine headache
- Medications
- SLE
- Acute mononucleosis/Epstein-Barr virus
- Seizures
- Carcinomatous meningitis

■ WORKUP
CSF examination:
- Usually shows pleocytosis
- Lymphocytic predominance (polyps in early stages)
- Opening pressure: 200 to 250 mm Hg
- WBC: 100 to 1000 mm³
- Increased CSF protein
- Decreased or normal CSF glucose
- Negative Gram stain, cultures, CIE, latex agglutination
- No viral cultures routinely available; if patient is suspected of having mumps, serologic testing may be diagnostic; complement fixation used

- PCR for HSV, West Nile or enterovirus (which could shorten duration of antibiotic treatment and hospitalization if bacterial meningitis was suspected)

■ LABORATORY TESTS
CBC with differential, blood culturing, and CSF examination (see Workup)

■ IMAGING STUDIES
CT scan or MRI: if cerebral edema, focal neurologic findings develop

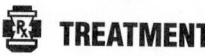

TREATMENT

No specific antiviral therapy for enterovirus, arbovirus, mumps virus; lymphocytic choriomeningitis virus is available. Treatment is supportive unless HSV is detected, which would be treated with IV acyclovir.

REFERENCES

Attia J et al: Does this adult patient have acute meningitis? *JAMA* 282:175, 1999.
Barton LL, Hyndman NJ: Lymphocyticchoriomengitis virus: reemerging central nervous system pathogen, *Pediatrics* 105:E351C, 2000.
Oostenbrink R et al: Children with meningeal signs: predicting who needs empiric antibiotic treatment, *Arch Pediatr Adolesc Med* 156(12):1189, 2002.
Ramers C et al: Impact of a diagnostic cerebrospinal fluid enterovirus polymerase chain reaction test on patient management, *JAMA* 283:2680, 2000.
Authors: **Glenn G. Fort, M.D., and Dennis J. Mikolich, M.D.**

TABLE 1-38 **Epidemiology of Acute Viral Meningitis**

	EPIDEMIOLOGIC FACTORS*				
SEASON	PATIENT'S AGE (yr)	PATIENT'S SEX	RISK FACTOR		SUGGESTED VIRAL AGENT
Summer-fall	Infant	—	Infected mother		Coxsackievirus B
	1-15	—	Swimming pools, closed communities		Enteroviruses
			Geographic area: California, southeastern United States		California serogroup virus
Winter	1-15	—	School exposure		Varicella virus, measles virus
		Male/female 3:1			Mumps virus
	16-21	—	College exposure		Measles virus
		Male/female 3:1			Mumps virus
		—			Epstein-Barr virus (mononucleosis)
	Any	—	Mice, rats, hamsters		Lymphocytic choriomeningitis virus
	Adults	—	Varicella-zoster		Varicella-zoster virus
Any	Any	—	Immunocompromise		Adenovirus
		—	Acquired immunodeficiency syndrome		Human immunodeficiency virus

From Gorbach SI: *Infectious diseases*, ed 2, Philadelphia, 1998, WB Saunders.
*Epidemiologic factors are suggestive but should not be used to exclude diagnoses in individual cases.

BASIC INFORMATION

■ DEFINITION
Meningomyelocele is the most common type of spina bifida and is characterized by herniation of the spinal cord, nerves, or both through a bony defect of the spine.

■ SYNONYMS
Myelomeningocele
Spina bifida cystica

ICD-9CM CODES
741.9 Spina bifida without mention of hydrocephalus
741.9 Meningomyelocele

■ EPIDEMIOLOGY & DEMOGRAPHICS
INCIDENCE (IN U.S.): 1 case/1000 births
PREDOMINANT SEX: Male = female
PREDOMINANT INCIDENCE: Newborn
GENETICS: Environmental and genetic factors have a joint role.

■ ETIOLOGY
- Failure of neural tube to close completely at about 4 wk gestation
- Associated with maternal valproate use

■ PHYSICAL FINDINGS & CLINICAL PRESENTATION
- Evident at birth—a sac protruding in the lumbar region (Fig. 1-174)
- Severity of neurologic deficits depends on the location of the lesion along the neuroaxis
- Motor dysfunction in the legs
- Lack of bladder or bowel control

- Often associated with Chiari II malformation and resulting obstructive hydrocephalus

DIAGNOSIS

- Physical examination provides diagnosis in most instances.
- MR imaging can provide better definition of the defect.
- Coexisting hydrocephalus is detected by measurement of head size, ultrasonography, CT, or MRI.

■ DIFFERENTIAL DIAGNOSIS
- Teratoma
- Meningocele

■ WORKUP
- Evaluate for hydrocephalus.
- Evaluate for other congenital abnormalities, such as congenital heart disease, intestinal malformation, club foot, and skeletal deformities.

■ LABORATORY TESTS
Prenatal testing often reveals elevated alpha fetoprotein in amniotic fluid or maternal serum.

■ IMAGING STUDIES
- MRI of spine
- X-ray studies of skull exhibit craniolacuna, a honeycombed pattern associated with hydrocephalus
- CT or MRI of head may reveal hydrocephalus

TREATMENT

- Surgical closure of myelomeningocele is performed soon after birth
- Control of hydrocephalus (shunt)
- Management of urinary incontinence
- Counseling of parents

■ ACUTE GENERAL Rx
- Shunt placement for obstructive hydrocephalus
- Treatment of seizures, if present

■ CHRONIC Rx
- Follow closely for development of hydrocephalus
- Bladder catheterization
- Avoid use of latex-containing products to prevent development of latex allergy

■ DISPOSITION
Followed by a team of specialists including neurosurgeons, urologists, orthopedists, and myelodysplasia nurses

PEARLS & CONSIDERATIONS

All mothers of children with neural tube defects should be instructed on nutritional supplementation with folate for future pregnancies.

■ COMMENTS
- Intrauterine repair of meningomyelocele decreases the incidence of hindbrain herniation and shunt-dependent hydrocephalus in infants, but increases the incidence of premature delivery.
- U.S. Public Health Service recommends 400 micrograms of folate intake per day for all women capable of becoming pregnant for primary prevention of neural tube defects.

REFERENCES
Botto LD et al: Neural-tube defects, *N Engl J Med* 341:1509, 2002.
Jobe AH: Fetal surgery for myelomeningocele, *N Engl J Med* 347:230, 2002.
Author: **Maitreyi Mazumdar, M.D.**

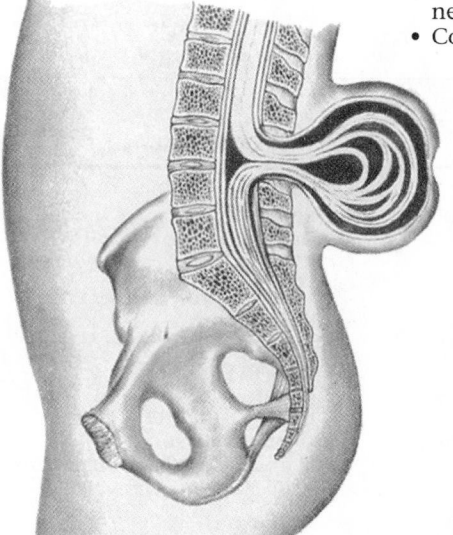

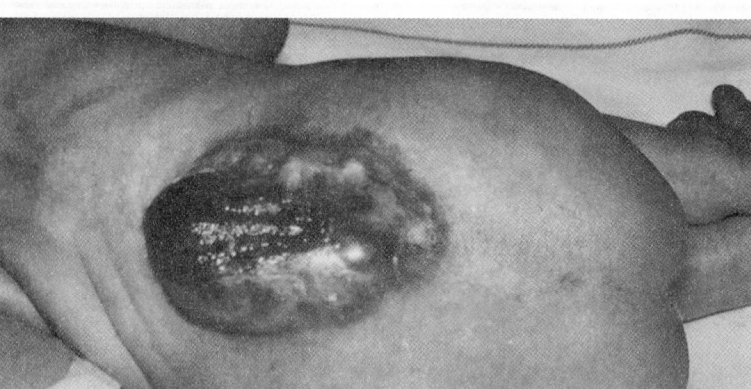

Fig. 1-174 **Meningomyelocele.** (From Wong DL: *Whaley's and Wong's nursing care of infants and children*, ed 5, St Louis, 1995, Mosby.)

BASIC INFORMATION

■ DEFINITION
Menopause is the occurrence of no menstrual periods for 1 yr after age 40 yr or permanent cessation of ovulation following lost ovarian activity. It is a climacteric reproductive stage of life marked by waxing and waning estrogen levels followed by decreasing ovarian function. Premature ovarian failure and no menstrual periods may also occur because of depletion of ovarian follicles before the age of 40 yr.

■ SYNONYMS
Change of life
Climacteric ovarian failure

ICD-9CM CODES
627 Premenopausal menorrhagia
627.2 Menopausal or female climacteric states
627.4 States associated with artificial menopause
716.3 Climacteric arthritis

■ EPIDEMIOLOGY & DEMOGRAPHICS
- Average age of menopause in the U.S. is 51 yr.
- Age at which menopause occurs is genetically determined.
- Smokers experience menopause an average of 1.5 yr earlier than non-smokers.
- More than one third of a woman's life will be spent after menopause.
- Onset of perimenopause is usually in a woman's mid- to late-40s.
- Approximately 4000 women each day begin menopause.

■ PHYSICAL FINDINGS & CLINICAL PRESENTATION
- Atrophic vaginitis, which can cause burning, itching, bleeding, dyspareunia
- Either complete cessation of menses or a period of irregular cycles and diminished or heavier bleeding
- Osteoporosis
- Psychologic dysfunction:
  1. Anxiety
  2. Depression
  3. Insomnia
  4. Nervousness
  5. Irritability
  6. Inability to concentrate
- Sexual changes, decreased libido, dyspareunia
- Urinary incontinence
- Vasomotor symptoms (hot flashes, flushes), night sweats, cardiovascular disease, coronary artery disease, atherosclerosis, headaches, tiredness, and lethargy

■ ETIOLOGY
- The most common etiology: physiologic, caused by degenerating theca cells that fail to react to endogenous gonadotropins, producing less estrogen; decreased negative feedback in the hypothalamic pituitary access, increased follicle-stimulating hormone (FSH), and increased luteinizing hormone (LH), which leads to stromal cells that continue to produce androgens as a result of the LH stimulation
- Surgical castration
- Family history of early menopause, cigarette smoking, blindness, abnormal chromosomal karyotype (Turner's syndrome, gonadal dysgenesis), precocious puberty, and left-handedness

⚗ DIAGNOSIS

■ DIFFERENTIAL DIAGNOSIS
- Asherman's syndrome
- Hypothalamic dysfunction
- Hypothyroidism
- Pituitary tumors
- Adrenal abnormalities
- Ovarian abnormalities
- Polycystic ovarian syndrome
- Pregnancy
- Ovarian neoplasm
- TB

■ WORKUP
- If the clinical picture is highly suggestive of menopause, estrogen can be prescribed. If all symptoms resolve, then diagnosis has essentially been made. Before estrogen is prescribed, a complete history and physical examination are needed. If a patient has estrogen-dependent malignancy, unexplained abnormal uterine bleeding, history of thrombophlebitis, or acute liver disease, estrogen therapy is contraindicated.
- Progesterone challenge test: progesterone 100 mg is given IM to induce withdrawal bleeding. If no withdrawal bleeding is obtained, it would be safe to assume that a hypoestrogenic state is present.
- Physical examination, height, weight, blood pressure, breast examination, and pelvic examination are needed.
- Assess risk for coronary artery disease, osteoporosis, cigarette smoking, personal history, history of breast cancer, liver disease, active coagulation disorder, or any unexplained vaginal bleeding.

■ LABORATORY TESTS
- FSH, LH, and estrogen levels: if the FSH is markedly elevated and the estrogen level is markedly depressed, constitutes laboratory diagnosis of ovarian failure; LH only if polycystic ovarian disease is to be ruled out in a younger patient
- TSH to rule out thyroid dysfunction and prolactin level if patient has symptoms of galactorrhea and if suspicion of pituitary adenoma exists
- A general chemistry profile to check for any systemic diseases
- Pap smear, endometrial biopsy, or D&C in patients who have had irregular periods or intermenstrual or postmenopausal bleeding
- Mammogram

■ IMAGING STUDIES
- CT scan or MRI of head if pituitary tumor is suspected
- Bone density studies
- Pelvic ultrasound to check endometrial stripe

℞ TREATMENT

■ NONPHARMACOLOGIC THERAPY
- A balanced diet: low in fat, with total fat intake being <30% of calories; total calories sufficient to maintain body weight or to produce weight loss if that is needed
- Avoidance of smoking, excessive alcohol or caffeine intake
- Exercise: weight-bearing exercise for osteoporosis prevention
- Kegel exercises for strengthening the pelvic floor
- Adequate calcium intake: 1500 mg qd is necessary to maintain zero calcium balance in postmenopausal women
- Change in the ambient temperature (may ameliorate hot flashes and reduce night sweats)
- Vitamin E
- Avoidance of caffeine, alcohol, and spicy foods if they trigger hot flashes
- Vaginal lubricants to help with the dyspareunia secondary to vaginal dryness (e.g., Replens, K-Y Jelly, or Gyne-Moistrin cream)

■ ACUTE GENERAL Rx
Estrogen replacement in symptomatic patients can be done in a variety of forms, including oral estrogen and transdermal estrogen patch.
- Examples of oral estrogen would include conjugated estrogens:
  1. Premarin: start with 0.625 mg qd and increase up to 1.25 mg qd, depending on symptoms. Cenestin (synthetic conjugated estrogens, A) available in 0.625-, 0.9-, and 1.25-mg doses.
  2. Estradiol (Estrace): start with 1 mg qd and increase to 2 mg qd; also available in 0.5 mg tablet for patients who experience side effects from the estrogen.
  3. Esterified estrogens (Estratab): start with 0.3 to 1.25 mg qd.
  4. Estropipate (Ogen, Ortho-Est): start with 0.625 to 1.25 mg qd.
  5. Esterified estrogen/testosterone combination: give 1.25 mg and

methyltestosterone 2.5 mg (Estratest) and esterified estrogen 0.625 mg and methyltestosterone 1.25 mg (Estratest HS). May improve sexual enjoyment and libido.

- If the patient has had a hysterectomy for benign disease, estrogen alone is sufficient. However, if she still has her uterus, progestin should be added for its protective effect against endometrial cancer. Medroxyprogesterone acetate (Provera) is the most commonly prescribed progestin. It can be prescribed in a continual daily dose of 2.5 mg or of 5 mg if continual breakthrough bleeding is encountered. This can also be prescribed in a 5-mg cyclic fashion for the first 14 days of the month or as 10-mg tablets for the first 10 days of the month. Patients need to be advised that this generally will cause withdrawal bleeding but in a fairly regular fashion. Continuous hormone replacement therapy is preferred, because after a period of time the patient should be amenorrheic. Patients should be counseled that they may experience some irregular spotting for the first 6 to 9 mo after starting the hormone replacement therapy.
- Combination oral preparations Femhrt ⅕ (1 mg norethindrone acetate/5 μg ethinyl estradiol) one pill daily. Ortho—Prefest 1 mg 17β-estradiol (white pill) alternating with 1 mg 17β-estradiol and 0.9 mg norgestimate (pink pill) q3d Prempro 0.625 mg conjugated estrogen/2.5 mg medroxyprogesterone one pill daily Prempro 0.625 mg conjugated estrogen/5.0 mg medroxyprogesterone one pill daily Activella 1 mg estradiol and 0.5 mg norethindrone acetate Premphase 0.625 mg conjugated estrogen with 5 mg medroxyprogesterone last 14 days.
- Transdermal patches can be either estradiol (Estraderm, Vivelle, Fempatch) 0.025 to 0.1 mg applied twice weekly or Climara 0.025 to 0.1 mg used once a week. With these preparations, progesterone should be used in a similar fashion. Combipatch—apply twice weekly (combination estrogen and progesterone).
- Vaginal creams can be used, and these should be reserved for local therapy of atrophic vaginitis. Systemic absorption does occur; however, blood levels are unpredictable. Start with a loading dose of 2 to 4 g of estrogen-containing cream nightly for 1 to 2 wk. When symptoms improve, once to twice weekly is adequate maintenance.
- Vagifem estradiol vaginal tablets. Initial dosage: one Vagifem tablet, inserted vaginally, once daily for 2 wk. Maintenance dose: one Vagifem tablet, inserted vaginally, twice weekly.
- Femring vaginal ring delivering the equivalent of 50 micrograms per day inserted every 3 months.
- For women in whom estrogen is contraindicated or for those who do not wish to take estrogen, the following regimens can be used:
  1. Depo-Provera 150 mg IM every month (may be helpful in alleviating hot flashes)
  2. Clonidine 0.05 to 0.15 mg qd
  3. Bellergal-S
  4. Fosamax (alendronate sodium) or Actonel (risedronate) 5 mg qd or 35 mg weekly are approved for prophylactic prevention of osteoporosis. They should be taken on an empty stomach; wait at least 30 min before ingesting any substance, including liquids, because this decreases absorption into the body. They should be swallowed on arising for the day with a full glass of water, 6 to 8 oz, and patients should not lie down for at least 30 min and until after their first food of the day.
  5. Evista (Raloxifene) 60 mg daily PO has positive bone effect, a total cholesterol–lowering effect, and LDL cholesterol–lowering effect; it is a selective estrogen receptor agonist; it does not affect estrogen receptors in the breast or uterus. It does not ameliorate vasomotor symptoms or vaginal atrophy.
- Tibolone significantly improves vasomotor symptoms, libido, and vaginal lubrication.

■ CHRONIC Rx
Hormone replacement therapy should be used only for the short term unless benefits closely outweigh the risks of long-term use.

■ DISPOSITION
If treated, the patient should have resolution of her symptoms, reduced incidence of osteoporosis and, most recently, reduction in the risk of developing Alzheimer's disease. Lifelong medical supervision is necessary to monitor adequacy of treatment and prevention of complications. This should include annual Pap smears, pelvic examinations, breast examinations, mammography, and endometrial sampling of any type of abnormal bleeding. If untreated, the vasomotor symptoms will eventually disappear; however, this takes many years, and some women who are in their 80s have experienced hot flashes. Urogenital atrophy will continue to worsen. Osteoporosis and coronary artery disease risks will increase with every passing year. Women using ERT for >10 yr may have increased risk of developing ovarian cancer.

■ REFERRAL
Most menopausal women are managed by their gynecologist. However, this condition can be managed adequately by the patient's primary care physician who has an interest in treating menopausal women.

PEARLS & CONSIDERATIONS

■ COMMENTS
- Short-term risks of HRT include an 18-fold increased rise for cholecystitis, 3.5-fold risk of a thrombocardiac event in the first year, and probably increased risk of stroke and MI.
- Results of the WHI study found that for every 10,000 women taking HRT for 1 yr (10,000 person-yr), 7 more would have coronary events, 8 more strokes, 8 more pulmonary emboli, and 8 more with early breast cancer than would 10,000 women taking placebo. Benefits of HRT were 6 fewer cases of colorectal cancer and 5 fewer hip fractures per 10,000 women.
- HRT should not be initiated or continued for the primary or secondary prevention of CHD.
- Patient education materials can be obtained through the American College of Obstetricians and Gynecologists, 409 12th Street SW, Washington, DC 20024, and *Menopause News*, 2074 Union Street, San Francisco, CA 94123; phone: 1-800-241-MENO. Multiple patient educational brochures are produced by pharmacologic companies.

REFERENCES
Han KK et al: Benefits of soy isoflavone therapeutic regimen on menopausal symptoms, *Obstet Gynecol* 99:389, 2002.

Humphrey L et al: Postmenopausal hormone replacement and the primary prevention of cardiovascular disease, *Ann Int Med* 137:273, 2002.

Lacey JV et al: Menopausal hormone replacement therapy and risk of ovarian cancer, *JAMA* 288:334, 2002.

Manson JE, Martin KA: Postmenopausal hormone-replacement therapy, *N Engl J Med* 345:34, 2001.

Nelson H et al: Postmenopausal hormone replacement therapy, *JAMA* 288:872, 2002.

Santoro N: The menopause transition: an update, *Human Reproduction Update* 8(2):155, 2002.

Speroff L: Efficacy and tolerability of a noval estradiol vaginal ring for relief of menopausal symptoms, *Obstet Gynecol* 102(4):823, 2003.

Writing Group for the Women's Health Initiative Investigators: Risks and benefits of estrogen plus progestin in healthy postmenopausal women, *JAMA* 288:321, 2002.

Author: **George T. Danakas, M.D.**

BASIC INFORMATION

■ DEFINITION
Mesenteric adenitis is a painful enlargement of mesenteric lymph nodes.

ICD-9CM CODES
289.2 Mesenteric adenitis

■ EPIDEMIOLOGY & DEMOGRAPHICS
- Incidence unknown
- Affects mostly children (under age 18 yr) with no sex preference
- When *Yersinia* enterocolitis is the cause, boys are more frequently involved

■ PHYSICAL FINDINGS & CLINICAL PRESENTATION
- Abdominal pain of variable severity (mild ache to severe colic) beginning in upper abdomen or right lower quadrant, eventually localizes in right side but not in a precise location (unlike appendicitis)
- In *Yersinia* infection outbreaks, the symptoms include abdominal pain (84%), diarrhea (78%), fever (43%), anorexia (22%), nausea (13%), and vomiting (8%)
- Physical findings:
  Other lymphadenopathy (20% of cases)
  Right lower quadrant tenderness (site of maximum tenderness may vary from one examination to the next)
  Guarding (rare)
  Mild fever

■ ETIOLOGY & PATHOGENESIS
- Reactive hyperplasia of lymph nodes that drain the ileocecal region, similar to that seen in inflammatory or allergic conditions. One study reported that approximately two thirds of cases are secondary (reactive) and one third are primary (no demonstrable associated inflammatory process).
- *Yersinia enterocolitica, Yersinia pseudotuberculosis, Salmonella* species, *E. coli,* streptococci have been implicated with mesenteric adenitis.

DIAGNOSIS

■ DIFFERENTIAL DIAGNOSIS
- Acute appendicitis (5% to 10% of patients admitted to hospitals with a diagnosis of appendicitis are discharged with a diagnosis of mesenteric adenitis)
- Crohn's disease

Section II describes the differential diagnosis of abdominal pain.

■ LABORATORY TESTS
- CBC may show leukocytosis
- Abdominal sonography and helical appendiceal CT scan may be useful
- Laparotomy if appendicitis is suspected

■ PROGNOSIS
Recurrent bouts are common; therefore if laparotomy is performed and a normal appendix is found, it should be removed.

REFERENCES
Adam JT: Nonspecific mesenteric lymphadenitis. In Schwartz SE et al (eds): *Principles of surgery,* ed 6, New York, 1994, McGraw-Hill.

Macari M et al: Mesenteric adenitis: CT diagnosis of primary versus secondary causes, incidence, and clinical significance on pediatric and adult patients, *Am J Roentgenol* 178:853, 2002.

Pearson RD, Guerrant RL: Enteric fever and other causes of abdominal symptoms with fever. In Mandell GL (ed): *Mandell, Douglas, and Bennett's principles and practice of infectious diseases,* ed 5, New York, 2000, Churchill Livingstone.

Author: **Tom J. Wachtel, M.D.**

BASIC INFORMATION

■ DEFINITION
Mesenteric venous thrombosis (MVT) is a thrombotic occlusion of the mesenteric venous system involving major trunks or smaller branches and leading to intestinal infarction in its acute form.

ICD-9CM CODES
557.0 Mesenteric venous thrombosis

■ EPIDEMIOLOGY & DEMOGRAPHICS
Between 5% and 15% of patients with acute mesenteric infarction have mesenteric venous thrombosis. MVT is slightly more common in men than women. The typical age of occurrence is 50 to 60 yr.

■ PHYSICAL FINDINGS & CLINICAL PRESENTATION
Acute MVT
- Symptoms: abdominal pain in 90% of patients, typically out of proportion to the physical findings. Nausea and vomiting occur in 50% and GI bleeding occurs in 50% (occult), 15% (gross).
- Physical findings:
  Early: abdominal tenderness, decreased bowel sounds, abdominal distention
  Later: guarding and rebound tenderness, fever, and septic shock
Subacute MVT
- Symptoms: nonspecific abdominal pain for weeks or months
- Physical findings: none
Chronic MVT
- Symptoms: upper GI hemorrhage from bleeding varices
- Physical findings: none other than signs of blood loss if significant

■ ETIOLOGY & PATHOGENESIS
Hypercoagulable states (see "Hypercoagulable States" in Section I)
- Peripheral deep venous thrombosis
- Neoplasms
- Antithrombin III, protein C, protein S deficiencies
- Lupus anticoagulant (antiphospholipid antibody)
- Oral contraceptive use, pregnancy
- Polycythemia vera
- Thrombocytosis
- Paroxysmal nocturnal hemoglobinuria
Portal hypertension
- Cirrhosis
Inflammation
- Pancreatitis
- Peritonitis (e.g., appendicitis, diverticulitis, perforated viscus)
- Inflammatory bowel disease
- Pelvic or intraabdominal abscess
- Intraabdominal cancer

Postoperative state or trauma
- Blunt abdominal trauma
- Postoperative states (abdominal surgery)
Thrombosis may begin in small mesenteric branches (e.g., in hypercoagulable states) and propagate to the major venous mesenteric trunks, or begin in large veins (e.g., in cirrhosis, intraabdominal cancer, surgery) and extend distally. If collateral drainage is inadequate, the intestine becomes congested, edematous, cyanotic, and hemorrhagic and eventually may infarct.

DIAGNOSIS

■ DIFFERENTIAL DIAGNOSIS
All other causes of abdominal pain (e.g., peritonitis, intestinal obstruction, pancreatitis, peptic ulcer disease, gastritis, inflammatory bowel disease, perforated viscus). Also to be considered in the differential diagnosis of GI hemorrhage

■ WORKUP
Laboratory tests and imaging studies

■ LABORATORY TESTS
- CBC: leukocytosis
- Electrolytes: metabolic acidosis (lactic) indicate bowel infarction
- Elevated amylase
- Tests for hypercoagulable status

■ IMAGING STUDIES
- Abdominal plain x-ray: ileus, ascites, bowel dilation, bowel wall thickening, loop separation, and thumbprinting
- Abdominal CT scan (diagnostic in 90%) (Fig. 1-175): bowel wall thickening, venous dilation, venous thrombus
- Arteriography if CT scan is not diagnostic
Occasionally the diagnosis is made by a laparotomy.

TREATMENT

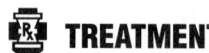

- Anticoagulation or thrombolytic therapy
- Laparotomy if intestinal infarction is suspected
Short ischemic segment: resection
Long ischemic segment:
1. Nonviable: resection or close
2. Viable: intraarterial papaverine, and/or thrombectomy followed by "second look" intervention
- The treatment of chronic MVT is the same as for portal hypertension

■ PROGNOSIS
- Mortality of acute mesenteric venous thrombosis: 20% to 50%
- Recurrence rate: 15% to 25%

REFERENCES
Brandt LJ, Smithline AE: Ischemic lesions of the bowel. In Feldman M, Scharsachmidt BF, Sleisenger MH (eds): *Gastrointestinal and liver disease,* ed 6, Philadelphia, 1998, WB Saunders.
Kumar S, Sarr MG, Kemeth PS: Mesenteric venous thrombosis, *N Engl J Med* 345:1683, 2002.
Author: **Tom J. Wachtel, M.D.**

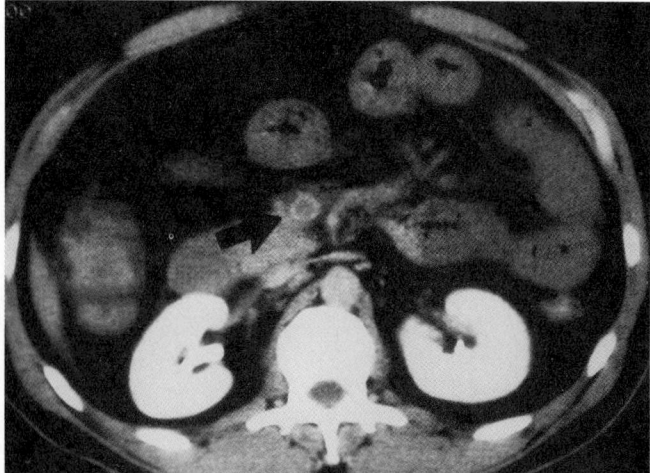

Fig. 1-175   This CT scan demonstrates thrombus within a dilated superior mesenteric vein (*arrow*). Abdominal imaging techniques such as CT scan or duplex ultrasonography provide a direct examination of the mesenteric and portal veins. (From Sabiston D: *Textbook of surgery,* ed 15, Philadelphia, 1997, WB Saunders.)

BASIC INFORMATION

■ DEFINITION
Malignant mesothelioma is a rare neoplastic lesion associated with asbestos exposure. There are three major histologic subtypes: epithelial (most common), sarcomatous, and mixed (epithelial/sarcomatous).

ICD-9CM CODES
199.1 Malignant mesothelioma, site NOS

■ EPIDEMIOLOGY & DEMOGRAPHICS
- Associated with asbestos exposure (all fiber types)
- Over 3000 new cases diagnosed in U.S. annually
- More common in men as a result of asbestos exposure in the workplace
- Right-sided involvement is more common
- Incidence of mesothelioma increases with age; median age at presentation is >60 yr
- There are currently more than 8 million persons in the U.S. who are at risk for mesothelioma because of prior asbestos exposure

■ PHYSICAL FINDINGS & CLINICAL PRESENTATION
- Dyspnea
- Nonpleuritic chest pain
- Fever, weight loss, sweats, fatigue, loss of appetite
- Dysphagia, superior vena cava syndrome, Horner's syndrome in advanced stages
- Auscultation may reveal unilateral loss of breath sounds
- Dullness on percussion may be present

■ ETIOLOGY
- Asbestos exposure
- Other reported potentially causal factors include prior radiation therapy and extravasated thorotrast, zeolite, and erionite fibers

DIAGNOSIS

■ DIFFERENTIAL DIAGNOSIS
Metastatic adenocarcinomas (from lung, breast, ovary, kidney, stomach, prostate)

■ WORKUP
- Staging evaluation includes complete history (including occupational history), physical examination, and testing to determine potential operability (CT, bone scan, PFTs)
- Thoracoscopy, pleuroscopy, and open lung biopsy are useful in obtaining adequate tissue samples for diagnosis
- Pulmonary function tests
- Staging: the UICC staging uses the TNM categories to organize mesothelioma in stages I-IV in a manner similar to that used for non–small cell lung cancer

■ LABORATORY TESTS
- Diagnostic thoracentesis is generally insufficient for diagnosis because pleural effusions may only reveal atypical mesothelial cells
- Immunohistochemistry is useful to distinguish adenocarcinoma from epithelial malignant mesothelioma (mesotheliomas are generally CEA negative and cytokeratin positive)
- Thrombocytosis and anemia may be found on initial lab evaluation

■ IMAGING STUDIES
- Chest radiographs may reveal pleural plaques or calcifications in the diaphragm
- CT scan of the chest/abdomen and bone scan are used to assess the extent of disease

TREATMENT

■ GENERAL Rx
- Operable patient (epithelial type, no positive nodes, confined to pleura, adequate PFTs): the two surgical techniques for therapeutic intervention are decortication (pleurectomy) and extrapleural pneumonectomy. Postoperative chemotherapy with cisplatin, doxorubicin, and cyclophosphamide and subsequent external beam radiation are used in some centers with limited success.

- Inoperable patient (disease too extensive, sarcomatous or mixed histology type, poor PFTs): supportive care plus/minus radiation therapy for symptoms or supportive care plus chemotherapy. Combined modality therapies (surgery, radiation therapy, chemotherapy, and biologics) have also been used to reduce both local and distant recurrences.
- Intrapleural instillation of cisplatin or biologics (e.g., interferons, interleukin-2) is generally limited to very early disease because it can only penetrate a very limited depth of the tumor and there is a propensity of the pleural space to become progressively obliterated with advancing disease.
- The role of radiation therapy in the treatment of mesotheliomas remains uncertain. It is often used for palliation of local pain despite lack of trials to prove its utility.
- Obliteration of the pleural space (pleurodesis) with instillation of tetracycline, bleomycin, or biologic substances such as C. parvum into the pleural cavity is often tried in attempting to treat recurrent symptomatic pleural effusions.

■ DISPOSITION
Median survival for patients undergoing pleurectomy ranges from 6.7 to 21 mo, for extrapleural pneumonectomy 4 to 21 mo. Survival is better for patients with epithelial form.

☼ PEARLS & CONSIDERATIONS

■ COMMENTS
- Patients with early disease should be referred to treatment centers specializing in mesothelioma treatment before attempts are made to obliterate the pleural space with pleurodesis.
- An approach to the evaluation and treatment of mesothelioma is described in Section III, Fig. 3-126.

REFERENCE
Abeloff MD: *Clinical oncology*, ed 2, New York, 2000, Churchill Livingstone.
Author: **Fred F. Ferri, M.D.**

BASIC INFORMATION

■ DEFINITION
The metabolic syndrome is the combination of four conditions: abdominal obesity, hypertension, dyslipidemia, and diabetes.
Guidelines from the National Cholesterol Education Program define the metabolic syndrome as the presence of any three of the following:
- Abdominal obesity: waist circumference >102 cm (40 inches) in men and >88 cm (35 inches) in women
- Hypertriglyceridemia: ≥150 mg/dl (1.69 mmol/L)
- Low high-density lipoprotein cholesterol:
- High blood pressure: ≥130/85 mm Hg
- High fasting glucose: ≥110 mg/dl (6.1 mmol/L)

■ SYNONYMS
Syndrome X
Insulin resistance syndrome
Obesity dyslipidemia syndrome

ICD-9CM CODES
277.7 Dysmetabolic syndrome X

■ EPIDEMIOLOGY & DEMOGRAPHICS
- 22% of U.S. adults
- Prevalence increases with age, from 6.7% for ages 20-29 yr to 42.0% for age >70 yr
- Increased prevalence in Mexican Americans (31.9%)
- Increased prevalence in Mexican-American and African American women compared with men in the respective ethnic groups
- Other risk factors include low socioeconomic status, lack of physical activity, high carbohydrate diet, no alcohol intake, smoking, postmenopausal status, and high body mass index

■ CLINICAL PRESENTATION & PHYSICAL FINDINGS
- Hypertension and obesity as defined previously
- Patients with the metabolic syndrome are at markedly increased risk for coronary artery disease and diabetes

■ ETIOLOGY
- Abdominal obesity is associated with insulin resistance and hyperinsulinemia.

- Insulin may increase blood pressure through increased activity of the sympathetic nervous system, reduction in nitric oxide production, and upregulation of angiotensin II receptors.
- Androgens may play a role in abdominal obesity and insulin resistance.
- Genetic factors may predispose patients to develop the metabolic syndrome.
- Elevations in inflammatory markers and cytokines (i.e., IL-6 and CRP) have been associated with insulin resistance and metabolic syndrome.
- Deficiency of adiponectin plays a role in the development of insulin resistance.

DIAGNOSIS

■ DIFFERENTIAL DIAGNOSIS
- Other forms of obesity (i.e., Cushing's syndrome, hypothyroidism)
- Other forms of hyperlipidemia and hypertension

■ WORKUP
- History with focus on symptoms of coronary artery disease (angina) and diabetes
- Complete physical examination, including height, weight, waist circumference, and blood pressure

■ LABORATORY TESTS
- Fasting lipid profile (total cholesterol, LDL cholesterol, HDL cholesterol, and triglyceride)
- Fasting glucose

TREATMENT

■ NONPHARMACOLOGIC THERAPY
- Dietary modifications aimed at weight loss
- Increase physical activity

■ PHARMACOLOGIC THERAPY
- Treat hypertension (see "Hypertension")
  1. Blood pressure goal: <130/80
  2. Angiotensin converting enzyme inhibitors may be preferred as initial drug

- Treat hyperlipidemia
  1. LDL goal is <130 mg/dl, or if patient has coronary heart disease (CHD) or CHD risk equivalents (peripheral arterial disease, abdominal aortic aneurysm, symptomatic carotid artery disease, diabetes, or an estimated 10-yr CHD risk >20%), LDL goal is <100 mg/dl
  2. HMG CoA reductase inhibitors (statins) commonly used as first-line agents
  3. Patients with high (200-499 mg/dl) or very high triglycerides (>500 mg/dl) may benefit from the addition of a Fibrate. Must rule out hypothyroidism
- Treat diabetes
  1. Goal fasting blood glucose <130 mg/dl
  2. Metformin and thiazolidinediones used as first line to improve insulin sensitivity
- Treat cardiovascular risk factors
  1. Aspirin therapy in patients with CAD
  2. Risk can be lowered with weight loss, exercise, blood pressure control and treatment of hyperlipidemia

■ REFERRAL
- To nutritionist for diet counseling
- To weight-loss and exercise programs

PEARLS & CONSIDERATIONS

■ COMMENTS
The metabolic syndrome is a common risk factor for cardiovascular disease. Recent findings suggest that it may also be an important factor in the cause of chronic kidney disease.

REFERENCES
Chen J et al: The metabolic syndrome and chronic kidney disease in U.S. adults, *Ann Intern Med* 140:167, 2004.
Executive summary of the third report of the national cholesterol education program (NCEP) expert panel on detection, evaluation, and treatment of high blood cholesterol in adults (adult treatment panel III), *JAMA* 287:2486, 2001.
Authors: **Mark J. Fagan, M.D., and Geeta Gopalakrishnan, M.D.**

BASIC INFORMATION

■ DEFINITION
Metatarsalgia refers to pain of the metatarsus, especially of the MTP articulation (Fig. 1-176). This is a non-specific symptom usually involving the lesser toes.

ICD-9CM CODES
726.7 Metatarsalgia

■ PHYSICAL FINDINGS & CLINICAL PRESENTATION
- Pain beneath the metatarsal heads with ambulation
- Plantar callus formation beneath the metatarsal heads, usually involving one of the middle three toes
- Local tenderness
- Deformity
- Joint stiffness

■ ETIOLOGY
- Splayfoot
- Osteoarthritis, rheumatoid arthritis
- Freiberg's disease (avascular necrosis of second metatarsal head)
- Cavus foot (high arch)
- Bunion deformity
- Hallux rigidus
- MTP synovitis
- Morton's neuroma
- Often no obvious cause

DIAGNOSIS

■ DIFFERENTIAL DIAGNOSIS
See Etiology.

■ WORKUP
Underlying cause should always be sought.

■ LABORATORY TESTS
Rheumatoid factor may be required to rule out rheumatoid synovitis.

■ IMAGING STUDIES
Plain radiography to determine presence or absence of joint disease or deformity

TREATMENT

■ NONPHARMACOLOGIC THERAPY
- Metatarsal bar or pad proximal to heads to redistribute weight
- Extra-depth shoe for contracture or deformity, if present
- Soft orthotic or well-padded liner to diffuse pressure around metatarsal heads
- Relief pads for plantar keratoses
- Soaks and pumice stone abrasion to decrease callus volume
- Rocker bottom shoe for resistant cases

■ CHRONIC Rx
- NSAIDs
- Intraarticular injection in selected cases with joint involvement

■ DISPOSITION
Prognosis is variable, depending on etiology.

■ REFERRAL
Failure to respond to medical management

REFERENCES
Chalmers AC et al: Metatarsalgia and rheumatoid arthritis—a randomized, single blind, sequential comparing 2 types of foot orthoses and supportive shoes, *J Rheumatol* 27(7):1643, 2000.

Gorter K et al: Variation in diagnosis and management of common foot problems by GPs, *Fam Pract* 18(6):569, 2001.

Morscher E, Ulrich J, Dick W: Morton's intermetatarsal neuroma: morphology and histological substrate, *Foot Ankle Int* 21(7):558, 2000.

Waldecker U: Metatarsalgia in hallux valgus deformity: a pedographic analysis, *J Foot Ankle Surg* 41(5):300, 2002.

Yu JS, Tanner JR: Considerations in metatarsalgia and midfoot pain: an MR imaging perspective, *Semin Musculoskelet Radiol* 6(2):91, 2002.

Author: **Lonnie R. Mercier, M.D.**

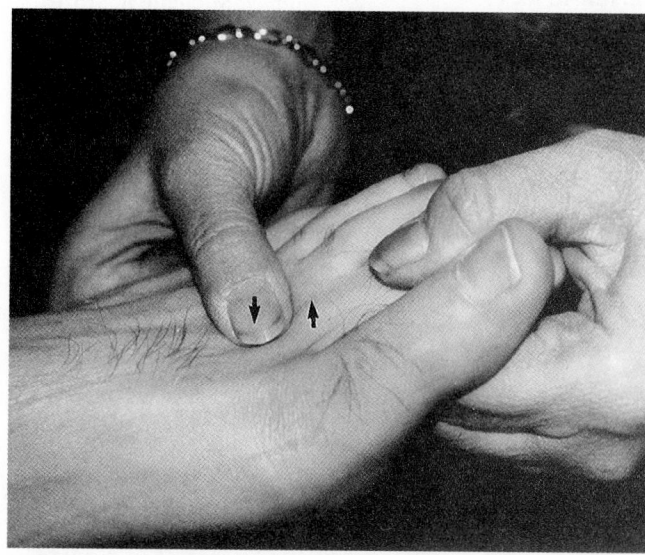

Fig. 1-176 Vertical stress test for metatarsophalangeal stability. One of the examiner's hands stabilizes the metatarsal head, whereas the other grasps the proximal phalanx. Examiner attempts to displace the proximal phalanx dorsally. A positive test result is the ability to displace dorsally while reproducing symptoms. (From Scuderi G [ed]: *Sports medicine: principles of primary care* St Louis, 1997, Mosby.)

BASIC INFORMATION

■ DEFINITION
Consumption of large amounts of calcium and alkali resulting in the triad of hypercalcemia, metabolic alkalosis, and renal insufficiency.

ICD-9CM CODES
275.42 Milk-alkali syndrome

■ EPIDEMIOLOGY & DEMOGRAPHICS
In the early 20th century the milk-alkali syndrome was associated with an antacid regimen created by F.W. Sippy that included large amounts of calcium and bicarbonate. With the development of more effective and less toxic treatments, the syndrome virtually disappeared. Since the 1980s, however, there has been a small resurgence associated with exuberant use of calcium-containing products for the prevention of osteoporosis and the use of calcium bicarbonate rather than aluminum bicarbonate in patients with chronic renal failure.

■ PHYSICAL FINDINGS & CLINICAL PRESENTATION
Symptoms range from asymptomatic (diagnosis made by the incidental finding hypercalcemia and renal failure) to symptomatic hypercalcemia.

■ ETIOLOGY
Overconsumption of calcium bicarbonate with reported ranges of 2.5 to 20 g/day

DIAGNOSIS

■ DIFFERENTIAL DIAGNOSIS
Hypercalcemia secondary to hyperparathyroidism or malignancy

■ LABORATORY TESTS
- Elevated plasma calcium (wide variation reported)
- Renal insufficiency
- Elevated plasma bicarbonate and arterial pH
- PTH, usually suppressed, may be elevated, particularly if checked after treatment has begun
- Phosphate level is variable

TREATMENT

■ NONPHARMACOLOGIC THERAPY
Hemodialysis has been indicated for some patients with significant renal failure.

■ ACUTE GENERAL Rx
- Discontinuation of calcium bicarbonate supplements
- Hydration
- Monitor for rebound hypocalcemia as a result of elevation of PTH with treatment
- Patient education

■ REFERRAL
Differentiation from hyperparathyroidism can be difficult and may require the assistance of an endocrinologist.

PEARLS & CONSIDERATIONS

■ COMMENTS
Detailed history of dietary supplements and OTC medications can provide the most important clues.

REFERENCES
Abreo K et al: The milk-alkali syndrome: a reversible form of acute renal failure, *Arch Intern Med* 153:1005, 1993.

Beall DP, Scofield RH: Milk-alkali syndrome associated with calcium carbonate consumption, *Medicine* 74:89, 1995.

Sippy BW: Gastric and duodenal ulcer: medical cure by an efficient removal of gastric juice corrosion, *JAMA* 64:1625, 1915.

Author: **Michelle A. Stozek, M.D.**

BASIC INFORMATION

■ DEFINITION
Mitral regurgitation (MR) is retrograde blood flow through the left atrium secondary to an incompetent mitral valve. Eventually there is an increase in left atrial and pulmonary pressures, which may result in right ventricular failure.

■ SYNONYMS
Mitral insufficiency
MR

ICD-9CM CODES
424.0 Mitral regurgitation

■ EPIDEMIOLOGY & DEMOGRAPHICS
The incidence of MR has increased over the past 30 yr; however, this may be because of increasing availability of echocardiography rather than any real increases in this condition.

■ PHYSICAL FINDINGS & CLINICAL PRESENTATION
- Patients with MR generally present with the following symptoms:
  1. Fatigue, dyspnea, orthopnea, frank CHF
  2. Hemoptysis (caused by pulmonary hypertension)
  3. Possible systemic emboli in patients with left atrial mural thrombi associated with atrial fibrillation
- Hyperdynamic apex, often with palpable left ventricular lift and apical thrill
- Holosystolic murmur at apex with radiation to base or to left axilla; poor correlation between the intensity of the systolic murmur and the degree of regurgitation
- Apical early- to mid-diastolic rumble (rare)

■ ETIOLOGY
- Papillary muscle dysfunction (as a result of ischemic heart disease)
- Ruptured chordae tendineae
- Infective endocarditis
- Calcified mitral valve annulus
- Left ventricular dilation
- Rheumatic valvulitis
- Primary or secondary mitral valve prolapse
- Hypertrophic cardiomyopathy
- Idiopathic myxomatous degeneration of the mitral valve
- Myxoma
- SLE
- Fenfluramine, dexfenfluramine

DIAGNOSIS

■ DIFFERENTIAL DIAGNOSIS
- Hypertrophic cardiomyopathy
- Pulmonary regurgitation
- Tricuspid regurgitation
- VSD

■ WORKUP
Diagnostic workup consists of echocardiography, ECG, and chest x-ray examination.

■ IMAGING STUDIES
- Echocardiography: enlarged left atrium, hyperdynamic left ventricle (erratic motion of the leaflet is seen in patients with ruptured chordae tendineae); Doppler electrocardiography will show evidence of MR. The most important aspect of the echocardiographic examination is the quantification of left ventricular systolic performance.
- Chest x-ray study:
  1. Left atrial enlargement (usually more pronounced in mitral stenosis)
  2. Left ventricular enlargement
  3. Possible pulmonary congestion
- ECG:
  1. Left atrial enlargement
  2. Left ventricular hypertrophy
  3. Atrial fibrillation

TREATMENT

■ NONPHARMACOLOGIC THERAPY
Salt restriction

■ ACUTE GENERAL Rx
- Medical: Medical therapy is primarily directed toward treatment of complications (e.g., atrial fibrillation) and prevention of bacterial endocarditis.
  1. Digitalis (for inotropic effect and to control ventricular response if atrial fibrillation with fast ventricular response is present)
  2. Afterload reduction (to decrease the regurgitant fraction and to increase cardiac output): may be accomplished with nifedipine, hydralazine plus nitrates or ACE inhibitors
  3. Anticoagulants if atrial fibrillation occurs

  4. Antibiotic prophylaxis before dental and surgical procedures (see Section V, Boxes 5-1 to 5-3 and Tables 5-25 and 5-26)
- Surgery: Surgery is the only definitive treatment for MR. Transesophageal echocardiography allows accurate assessment of the feasibility of valve repair and is indicated before surgical intervention. The timing of surgical repair is controversial; generally surgery should be considered early in symptomatic patients despite optimal medical therapy and in patients with moderate to severe MR and minimal symptoms if there is echocardiographic evidence of rapidly progressive increase in left ventricular end-diastolic and end-systolic dimension (echocardiographic evidence of systolic failure includes end-systolic dimension >55 mm and fractional shortening <31%). Surgery is also indicated in asymptomatic patients with preserved ventricular function if there is a high likelihood of valve repair or if there is evidence of pulmonary hypertension or recent atrial fibrillation.

■ DISPOSITION
Prognosis is generally good unless there is significant impairment of left ventricle or significantly elevated pulmonary artery pressures. Most patients remain asymptomatic for many years (average interval from diagnosis to onset of symptoms is 16 yr).

■ REFERRAL
Surgical referral in selected patients (see "Acute General Rx"); emergency surgery may be necessary in patients with MR caused by ruptured chordae tendineae following MI.

PEARLS & CONSIDERATIONS

■ COMMENTS
Patients should be counseled regarding weight reduction (if obese), avoidance of tobacco, and maintenance of normal (nonstrenuous) activities.

REFERENCE
Otto CM: Evaluation and management of chronic mitral regurgitation, *N Engl J Med* 345:740, 2001.
Author: **Fred F. Ferri, M.D.**

BASIC INFORMATION

■ DEFINITION
Mitral stenosis is a narrowing of the mitral valve orifice. The cross section of a normal orifice measures 4 to 6 cm². A murmur becomes audible when the valve orifice becomes smaller than 2 cm². When the orifice approaches 1 cm², the condition becomes critical, and symptoms become more evident.

■ SYNONYMS
MS

ICD-9CM CODES
394.0 Mitral stenosis

■ EPIDEMIOLOGY & DEMOGRAPHICS
- The occurrence of mitral valve stenosis has decreased worldwide over the past 30 yr (particularly in developed countries) as a result of declining incidence of rheumatic fever.
- The incidence of mitral stenosis is higher in women.

■ PHYSICAL FINDINGS & CLINICAL PRESENTATION
- Exertional dyspnea initially, followed by orthopnea and PND
- Acute pulmonary edema (may develop after exertion)
- Systemic emboli (caused by stagnation of blood in the left atrium; may occur in patients with associated atrial fibrillation)
- Hemoptysis (may be present as a result of persistent pulmonary hypertension)
- Prominent jugular A waves are present in patients with normal sinus rhythm.
- Opening snap occurs in early diastole; a short (<0.07-second) A_2 to opening snap interval indicates severe mitral stenosis.
- Apical middiastolic or presystolic rumble that does not radiate is present.
- Accentuated S_1 (because of delayed and forceful closure of the valve) is present.
- If pulmonary hypertension is present, there may be an accentuated P_2 and/or a soft, early diastolic decrescendo murmur (Graham Steell murmur) caused by pulmonary regurgitation (it is best heard along the left sternal border and may be confused with aortic regurgitation).
- A palpable right ventricular heave may be present at the left sternal border.
- Patients with mitral stenosis usually have symptoms of left-sided heart failure: dyspnea on exertion, PND, orthopnea.
- Right ventricular dysfunction (in late stages) may be manifested by peripheral edema, enlarged and pulsatile liver, and ascites.

■ ETIOLOGY
- Progressive fibrosis, scarring, and calcification of the valve
- Rheumatic fever (still a common cause in underdeveloped countries); heart valves most frequently affected in rheumatic heart disease (in descending order of occurrence): mitral, aortic, tricuspid, and pulmonary
- Congenital defect (parachute valve)
- Rare causes: endomyocardial fibroelastosis, malignant carcinoid syndrome, SLE

DIAGNOSIS

■ DIFFERENTIAL DIAGNOSIS
- Left atrial myxoma
- Other valvular abnormalities (e.g., tricuspid stenosis, mitral regurgitation)
- Atrial septal defect

■ WORKUP
Physical examination and echocardiography

■ IMAGING STUDIES
- Echocardiography:
  1. The characteristic finding on echocardiogram is a markedly diminished E to F slope of the anterior mitral valve leaflet during diastole; there is also fusion of the commissures, resulting in anterior movement of the posterior mitral valve leaflet during diastole (calcification in the valve may also be noted).
  Two-dimensional echocardiogram can accurately establish valve area.
- Chest x-ray study:
  1. Straightening of the left cardiac border caused by dilated left atrial appendage
  2. Left atrial enlargement on lateral chest x-ray film (appearing as double density of PA chest x-ray film)
  3. Prominence of pulmonary arteries
  4. Possible pulmonary congestion and edema (Kerley B lines)
- ECG:
  1. Right ventricular hypertrophy; right axis deviation caused by pulmonary hypertension
  2. Left atrial enlargement (broad notched P waves)
  3. Atrial fibrillation

- Cardiac catheterization to help establish the severity of mitral stenosis and diagnose associated valvular and coronary lesions. Findings on cardiac catheterization include:
  1. Normal left ventricular function
  2. Elevated left atrial and pulmonary pressures

TREATMENT

■ NONPHARMACOLOGIC THERAPY
Decrease level of activity in symptomatic patients.

■ ACUTE GENERAL Rx
- Medical:
  1. If the patient is in atrial fibrillation, control the rate response with diltiazem, digitalis, or esmolol. Although digitalis is the drug of choice for chronic heart rate control, IV diltiazem or esmolol may be acutely preferable when a rapid decrease in heart rate is required.
  2. If the patient has persistent atrial fibrillation (because of large left atrium), permanent anticoagulation is indicated to decrease the risk of serious thromboembolism.
  3. Treat CHF with diuretics and sodium restriction.
  4. Give antibiotic prophylaxis with dental and surgical procedures (see Section V, Boxes 5-1 to 5-3, and Tables 5-25 and 5-26).
- Surgical: valve replacement is indicated when the valve orifice is <0.7 to 0.8 cm² or if symptoms persist despite optimal medical therapy; commissurotomy may be possible if the mitral valve is noncalcified and if there is pure mitral stenosis without significant subvalvular disease.
- Percutaneous transvenous mitral valvotomy (PTMV) is becoming the therapy of choice for many patients with mitral stenosis responding poorly to medical therapy, particularly those who are poor surgical candidates and whose valve is not heavily calcified; balloon valvotomy gives excellent mechanical relief, usually resulting in prolonged benefit.

■ DISPOSITION
- Prognosis is generally good except in patients with chronic pulmonary hypertension.
- Operative mortality rates for mitral valve replacement are 1% to 5% in most institutions.

Author: **Fred F. Ferri, M.D.**

BASIC INFORMATION

■ DEFINITION

Mitral valve prolapse (MVP) is the posterior bulging of interior and posterior leaflets in systole. Mitral valve prolapse syndrome refers to a constellation of MVP and associated symptoms (e.g., autonomic dysfunction, palpitations) or other physical abnormalities (e.g., pectus excavatum).

■ SYNONYMS

MVP
Mitral click murmur syndrome

ICD-9CM CODES

424.0 Mitral valve disorders
394.9 Other and unspecified mitral valve diseases

■ EPIDEMIOLOGY & DEMOGRAPHICS

- MVP can be found by 2-D echocardiogram in 4% of the general population (females > males).
- Increased incidence is seen with autoimmune thyroid disorders, Ehlers-Danlos syndrome, Marfan's syndrome, pseudoxanthoma elasticum, pectus excavatum, anorexia nervosa, and bulimia.

■ PHYSICAL FINDINGS & CLINICAL PRESENTATION

- Usually, young female patient with narrow AP chest diameter, low body weight, low blood pressure
- Mid to late click, heard best at the apex
- Crescendo mid to late diastolic murmur
- Findings accentuated in the standing position
- Most patients with MVP are asymptomatic; symptoms (if present) consist primarily of chest pain and palpitations
- Neurologic abnormalities (e.g., TIA or stroke) are rare
- Patients may also complain of anxiety, fatigue, and dyspnea

■ ETIOLOGY

- Myxomatous degeneration of connective tissue of mitral valve

- Congenital deformity of mitral valve and supportive structures
- Secondary to other disorders (e.g., Ehlers-Danlos, pseudoxanthoma elasticum)

DIAGNOSIS

■ DIFFERENTIAL DIAGNOSIS

- Other valvular abnormalities
- Constrictive pericarditis
- Ventricular aneurysm

■ WORKUP

- Medical history and physical examination
- Workup consists primarily of echocardiography in patients with a systolic click or murmur on careful auscultation

■ IMAGING STUDIES

Echocardiography shows the anterior and posterior leaflets bulging posteriorly in systole.

TREATMENT

■ NONPHARMACOLOGIC THERAPY

Avoidance of stimulants (e.g., caffeine, nicotine) in patients with palpitations

■ ACUTE GENERAL Rx

- The empiric use of antiarrhythmic drugs to prevent sudden death in patients with uncomplicated MVP is not advisable; β-blockers may be tried in symptomatic patients (e.g., palpitations, chest pain); they decrease the heart rate, thus decreasing the stretch on the prolapsing valve leaflets.
- Antibiotic prophylaxis for infective endocarditis when undergoing dental, GI, or GU procedures is indicated only in patients with MVP who have a systolic murmur and echocardiographic evidence of mitral regurgitation (see Boxes 5-1 to 5-3 and Tables 5-25 and 5-26).

■ CHRONIC Rx

Monitoring for complications:
- Bacterial endocarditis (risk is three to eight times that of the general population)

- TIA or stroke secondary to embolic phenomena (from fibrin and platelet thrombi); risk in young patients: <0.05%/yr
- Cardiac arrhythmias (usually supraventricular)
- Sudden death (rare occurrence, most often caused by ventricular arrhythmias)
- Mitral regurgitation (most common complication of MVP)

■ DISPOSITION

The incidence of complications of MVP is very low (<1%/yr) and generally associated with an increase in mitral leaflet thickness to ≥5 mm; young patients (age <45) with absence of mitral systolic murmur or mitral regurgitation on Doppler echocardiography are at low risk for any complications.

■ REFERRAL

Surgical referral may be necessary in patients who develop symptomatic progressive mitral regurgitation.

PEARLS & CONSIDERATIONS

■ COMMENTS

- Recent studies suggest that the prevalence of MVP and its propensity to cause symptoms and serious complications have been overestimated in the past.
- Asymptomatic patients with MVP and mild or no mitral regurgitation can be evaluated clinically every 3 to 5 yr. High-risk patients should undergo a follow-up examination once a year.

REFERENCES

Bouknight DP, O'Rourke RA: Current management of mitral valve prolapse, Am Fam Physician 61:3343, 2000.
Freed LA: Prevalence and clinical outcome of mitral valve prolapse, N Engl J Med 341:1, 1999.
Gilon D et al: Lack of evidence of an association between MVP and stroke in young patients, N Engl J Med 341:8, 1999.
Author: Fred F. Ferri, M.D.

BASIC INFORMATION

■ DEFINITION

The term *mixed connective tissue disease* describes a set of connective tissue symptoms that sometimes overlap with other known connective tissue diseases (SLE, progressive systemic sclerosis, polymyositis) but whose exact significance remains under debate. The disorder is sometimes referred to as an "overlap syndrome," but many prefer the term *undifferentiated connective tissue disease.*

ICD-9CM CODES
710.9 Diffuse connective tissue disease

■ EPIDEMIOLOGY & DEMOGRAPHICS
PREVALENCE: Approximately 10 to 15 cases/100,000 persons
PREDOMINANT SEX: Female:male ratio of 8:1
PREDOMINANT AGE: 4 to 80 yr

■ PHYSICAL FINDINGS & CLINICAL PRESENTATION
• Polyarthritis, polyarthralgia
• Raynaud's phenomenon, hand swelling, or sclerodactyly
• Esophageal hypomotility, myalgia, and muscle weakness
• Other: pericarditis, facial erythema, psychosis

■ ETIOLOGY
Autoimmune disorder

DIAGNOSIS

■ DIFFERENTIAL DIAGNOSIS
Other connective tissue disorders (SLE, progressive systemic sclerosis, polymyositis)

■ WORKUP
• Diagnosis is not well defined.
• Commonly used diagnostic tests are described in Laboratory Tests.

■ LABORATORY TESTS (BOX 1-19)
• Rheumatoid factor is often present in low titers.
• If myositis is present, muscle enzyme (CPK) levels increase.
• Positive ANA is often present with a speckled pattern.
• ESR is elevated.
• Anti-RNP antibodies may be present.

TREATMENT

• Except for pulmonary and scleroderma-like symptoms, response to corticosteroids is excellent in most cases.
• Rheumatoid symptoms may respond to NSAIDs, but other cases may not even respond to gold or penicillamine.
• Immunosuppressive agents are used on occasion, but the best therapeutic options remain uncertain.

■ DISPOSITION
• Initially, this disorder was thought to be a mild variant of SLE, sometimes called "benign lupus," with excellent prognosis.
• Further studies suggested, however, that this was not always the case and serious renal, vascular, and neurologic complications were noted.
• Pulmonary involvement is a common clinical manifestation that may even lead to pulmonary hypertension and sometimes death.
• Whether MCTD is a separate entity continues under debate as concepts about the disorder evolve.

• Long-term outcomes remain uncertain.

PEARLS & CONSIDERATIONS

■ COMMENTS
A clinical algorithm for evaluation of a positive ANA titer is described in Section III, Fig. 3-19.

REFERENCES

Fernandes C et al: Mixed connective tissue disease presenting with pneumonitis and pneumatosis intestinalis, *Arthritis Rheum* 43:704, 2000.

Kozaka T et al: Pulmonary involvement in mixed connective tissue disease: high-resolution CT findings in 41 patients, *J Thorac Imaging* 16:94, 2001.

Ling TC, Johnson BT: Esophageal investigations in connective tissue disease: which tests are most appropriate? *J Clin Gastroenterol* 32:33, 2001.

Lopez-Longo FJ et al: Does mixed connective tissue disease have a less favorable prognosis than systemic lupus erythematosis? *Arthritis Rheum* 44(suppl):119, 2001.

Lowe D, Kredich DW, Schanberg Durham LE: Thalidomide: an effective and safe agent for the treatment of pediatric mixed connective tissue disease, *Arthritis Rheum* 43(suppl):117, 2000.
Author: **Lonnie R. Mercier, M.D.**

BOX 1-19   Guidelines for Diagnosing Mixed Connective Tissue Disease

General
Clinical features of a diffuse connective tissue disorder

Serologic
1. Positive ANA, speckled pattern, titer >1:1000
2. Antibodies to U1 RNP
3. Absence of antibodies to dsDNA, histones, Sm, Scl-70, and other specificities
4. Commonly: Hypergammaglobulinemia and positive rheumatoid factor

Clinical
1. Sequential evolution of overlap features over course of several years, including Raynaud's phenomenon, serositis, gastrointestinal dysmotility, myositis, arthritis, sclerodactyly, skin rashes, and an abnormal DL_{co} on pulmonary function tests
2. Absence of truncal scleroderma, severe renal disease, and severe central nervous system involvement
3. A nail fold capillary pattern identical to that seen in systemic sclerosis (dropout and dilated vessels)

From Bennett RM: Mixed connective tissue disease and other overlap syndromes. In Kelley WN et al (eds): *Textbook of rheumatology,* ed 3, Philadelphia, 1989, WB Saunders.
ANA, Antinuclear antibodies; *dsDNA,* double-stranded DNA; *MCTD,* mixed connective tissue disease; *RNP,* ribonucleoprotein.

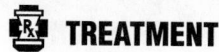
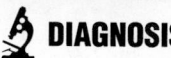 **BASIC INFORMATION**

■ DEFINITION
Viral infection characterized by discrete skin lesions with central umbilication (Fig. 1-177).

ICD-9CM CODES
078.0 Molluscum contagiosum

■ EPIDEMIOLOGY & DEMOGRAPHICS
- Molluscum contagiosum spreads by autoinoculation, scratching or touching a lesion.
- It usually occurs in young children. It is also common in sexually active adults and patients with HIV infection.
- Incubation period varies between 4 and 8 wk.
- Spontaneous resolution in immunocompetent patients can occur after several months.

■ PHYSICAL FINDINGS & CLINICAL PRESENTATION
- The individual lesion appears initially as a flesh-colored, firm, smooth-surfaced papule with subsequent central umbilication. Lesions are frequently grouped. The size of each lesion generally varies from 2 to 6 mm in diameter.
- Typical distribution in children involves the face, extremities, and trunk. Mucous membranes are spared.
- Distribution in adults generally involves pubic and genital areas.
- Erythema and scaling at the periphery of the lesions may be present as a result of scratching or hypersensitivity reaction.
- Lesions are not present on the palms and soles.

■ ETIOLOGY
Viral infection of epithelial cells caused by a pox virus

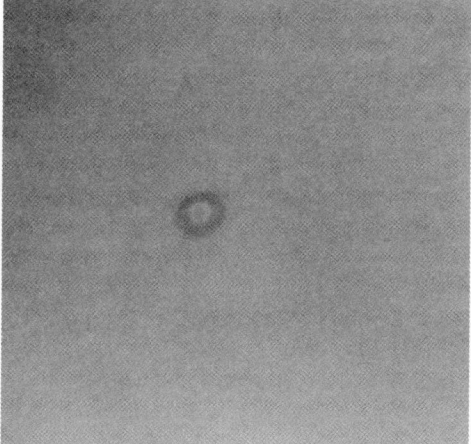

DIAGNOSIS
Diagnosis is usually established by the clinical appearance of the lesions (distribution and central umbilication). A magnifying lens can be used to observe the central umbilication. If necessary, the diagnosis can be confirmed by removing a typical lesion with a curette and examining the content on a slide after adding potassium hydroxide and gentle heating. Staining with toluidine blue will identify viral inclusions.

■ DIFFERENTIAL DIAGNOSIS
- Verruca plana (flat warts): no central umbilication, not dome shaped, irregular surface, can involve palms and soles
- Herpes simplex: lesions become rapidly umbilicated
- Varicella: blisters and vesicles are present
- Folliculitis: no central umbilication, presence of hair piercing the pustule or papule
- Cutaneous cryptococcosis in AIDS patients: budding yeasts will be present on cytologic examination of the lesions
- Basal cell carcinoma: multiple lesions are absent

■ WORKUP
Careful examination of the papules

■ LABORATORY TESTS
Generally not indicated in children. STD screening for other sexually transmitted diseases is recommended in all cases of genital molluscum contagiosum.

■ IMAGING STUDIES
Not indicated

Fig. 1-177 Molluscum contagiosum. (From Rakel RE: *Textbook of family practice,* ed 6, Philadelphia, 2002, WB Saunders.)

TREATMENT

■ NONPHARMACOLOGIC THERAPY
Prevention of autoinoculation by scratching or touching lesions

■ GENERAL THERAPY
- Therapy is individualized depending on number of lesions, immune status, and patient's age and preference.
- Observation for spontaneous resolution is reasonable in patients with few, small, not irritated, and not-spreading lesions. Genital lesions should be treated in all sexually active patients.
- Curettage following pretreatment of the area with combination prilocaine 2.5% with lidocaine 2.5% cream (EMLA) for anesthesia is useful for treatment of few lesions. Curettage should be avoided in cosmetically sensitive areas because scarring may develop.
- Treatments with liquid nitrogen therapy in combination with curettage are effective in older patients who do not object to some discomfort.
- Application of cantharidin 0.7% to individual lesions covered with clear tape will result in blistering over 24 hr and possible clearing without scarring. This medication should be avoided on facial lesions.
- Other treatment measures include use of tretinoin 0.025% gel or 0.1% cream at hs, daily use of salicylic acid (Occlusal) at hs, and use of laser therapy.
- Trichloroacetic acid peel generally repeated every 2 wk for several weeks is useful in immunocompromised patients with extensive lesions.

■ DISPOSITION
Most patients respond well to the therapeutic modalities listed previously. Spontaneous resolution can occur after 6 to 9 mo in some immunocompetent patients.

■ REFERRAL
To dermatology when diagnosis is in doubt or in patients with extensive lesions

PEARLS & CONSIDERATIONS

■ COMMENTS
Genital molluscum contagiosum in children may be indicative of sexual abuse.
Author: **Fred F. Ferri, M.D.**

BASIC INFORMATION

■ DEFINITION
Mononucleosis is a symptomatic infection caused by Epstein-Barr virus.

■ SYNONYMS
Infectious mononucleosis (IM)

ICD-9CM CODES
075 Infectious mononucleosis

■ EPIDEMIOLOGY & DEMOGRAPHICS
INCIDENCE IN U.S.: 45 cases/100,000 persons/yr
PREDOMINANT SEX: Incidence is the same, but occurs earlier in females.
PREDOMINANT AGE: Most common between the ages of 15 and 24 yr.

■ PHYSICAL FINDINGS & CLINICAL PRESENTATION
- Following an incubation period of 1 to 2 mo, a prodrome may occur, with fever, chills, malaise, and anorexia for several days. This is followed by the classic triad, which includes pharyngitis, fever, and adenopathy. Although fatigue and malaise may be prominent, pharyngitis is usually the most severe symptom. Exudates are common.
- Lymphadenopathy is most prominent in the cervical region but may be diffuse.
- Splenomegaly may occur, most commonly during the second week of illness.
- Rash is uncommon, but will occur in nearly all patients who receive ampicillin.
- At times, IM can present as fever and adenopathy without pharyngitis. Although complications may be severe, they are uncommon, and tend to resolve completely. Involvement of the hematologic, pulmonary, cardiac, or nervous system may occur; splenic rupture is rare. IM is usually a self-limited illness, but symptoms of malaise and fatigue may last months before resolving.

■ ETIOLOGY
The cause of IM is primary infection with Epstein-Barr virus (EBV). Primary infection during childhood causes little or no symptoms. Infection during childhood is more common in lower socioeconomic groups. The frequency of IM in late adolescence is attributed to the onset of social contact between the sexes. Close personal contact is usually necessary for transmission, although EBV has occasionally been transmitted by blood transfusion. Transfer via saliva while kissing may be responsible for many cases.

DIAGNOSIS

■ DIFFERENTIAL DIAGNOSIS
- Heterophile-negative infectious mononucleosis caused by cytomegalovirus (CMV); although clinical presentation may be similar, CMV more frequently follows transfusion
- Bacterial and viral causes of pharyngitis
- Toxoplasmosis
- Acute retroviral syndrome of HIV, lymphoma

■ WORKUP
Heterophile antibody (monospot) and complete blood counts should be sent.

■ LABORATORY TESTS
- Increased WBC is common, with a relative lymphocytosis and neutropenia. Atypical lymphocytes are the hallmark of IM, but are not pathognomonic. Mild thrombocytopenia is common. A falling hematocrit may signal splenic rupture. Elevated hepatocellular enzymes and cryoglobulins occur in most cases. Heterophile antibody, as measured by the Monospot test, may be positive at presentation, or may appear later in the course of illness. A negative test should be repeated if clinical suspicion is high. If this test remains negative for 8 wk, other causes of IM are likely. The monospot usually remains positive for 3 to 6 mo, but can last for 1 yr.
- A positive test has been reported with primary HIV infection.
- In addition to the heterophile antibody, virus-specific antibodies may result in response to IM. Determination of these EBV-specific antibodies is rarely necessary to diagnose IM, although early diagnosis in monospot negative cases may be made by isolating IgM to the viral capsid antigen (VCA), which is usually positive during the acute illness.

■ IMAGING STUDIES
Chest radiograph may rarely show infiltrates. An elevated left hemidiaphragm may occur in cases of splenic rupture.

TREATMENT

■ NONPHARMACOLOGIC THERAPY
- Supportive rest is advocated by some, but impact on outcome is not clear
- Splenectomy if rupture occurs. Transfusions for severe anemia or thrombocytopenia

■ ACUTE GENERAL Rx
- Pharmacologic therapy is not indicated in uncomplicated illness.
- The use of steroids is suggested in patients who have severe thrombocytopenia or hemolytic anemia, or impending airway obstruction as a result of enlarged tonsils. Prednisone, 60-80 mg PO qd for 3 days, then tapered over 1 to 2 wk. There is no role for antiviral agents such as acyclovir in the management of IM.

■ CHRONIC Rx
An extremely rare, chronic form of IM with persistent fevers and other objective findings has been described. This should be differentiated from chronic fatigue syndrome, which is not related to EBV.

■ DISPOSITION
Eventual resolution of all symptoms is the rule.

■ REFERRAL
More than mild illness

✲ PEARLS & CONSIDERATIONS

■ COMMENTS
Contact sports should be avoided during the first month of illness, because splenic rupture can occur, even in the absence of clinically detectable splenomegaly.

REFERENCES
Crawford DH et al: Sexual history and Epstein-Barr virus infection, *J Infect Dis* 186:731, 2002.

Godshall SE, Kirchner JT: Infectious mononucleosis: complexities of a common syndrome, *Postgrad Med* 107:175, 2000.

Vidrih JA et al: Positive Epstein-Barr virus heterophile antibody tests in patients with primary immunodeficiency virus infection, *Am J Med* 111:192, 2001.
Author: **Maurice Policar, M.D.**

BASIC INFORMATION

■ DEFINITION

Morton's neuroma refers to an inflammatory fibrosing process of the plantar digital nerve characterized by pain in the sole of the foot. Morton's neuroma is also described as an interdigital plantar neuropathy with or without plantar neuroma.

■ SYNONYMS

Morton's metatarsalgia
Morton's toe
Interdigital neuroma

ICD-9CM CODES

355.6 Morton's neuroma

■ EPIDEMIOLOGY & DEMOGRAPHICS

- Morton's neuroma most commonly involves the plantar digital nerve between the heads of the third and fourth metatarsals
- May also involve the second and third metatarsal and can involve both simultaneously
- Commonly occurs in people wearing tight-fitting shoes in toe region and high heels
- Morton's neuroma is usually unilateral
- Morton's neuroma is found more often in women than in men
- Can occur in both young and old

■ PHYSICAL FINDINGS & CLINICAL PRESENTATION

- Pain is usually located in a specific region, usually in the sole of the foot between the third and fourth metatarsal area and is unilateral in the majority of cases.
- Numbness may occur.
- Pain is exacerbated with exercise and relieved with rest and may radiate to the toes and to the ankle.
- Point tenderness is noted on examination, and palpation reveals fullness at the site of discomfort.
- An audible, painful click called "Murder's click" is noted in patients with Morton's neuroma after compressing and releasing the forefoot.
- Patients may have neuroma but silent lesions without symptoms.

■ ETIOLOGY

- Morton's neuroma is thought to be caused by nerve thickening from repeated injury.
- The typical finding is swelling of the plantar digital nerve that pathologically resembles other nerve entrapment syndromes (e.g., median nerve compression in carpal tunnel syndrome).

DIAGNOSIS

The diagnosis of Morton's neuroma is strictly made on clinical grounds alone as there are no laboratory tests or x-ray imaging studies that are specific for this disorder.

■ DIFFERENTIAL DIAGNOSIS

- Diabetic neuropathy
- Alcoholic neuropathy
- Nutritional neuropathy
- Toxic neuropathy
- Osteoarthritis
- Trauma (e.g., fracture)
- Gouty arthritis
- Rheumatoid arthritis

■ WORKUP

Exclude other causes as mentioned in the Differential Diagnosis.

■ LABORATORY TESTS

- Laboratory studies are not specific for the diagnosis of Morton's neuroma
- CBC and ESR are usually normal
- Blood glucose
- B_{12} and folic acid level

■ IMAGING STUDIES

- X-ray imaging is primarily done to exclude other causes of foot pain (e.g., fractures, ostearthritis, gouty arthritis).
- MRI can detect and localize a neuroma but is rarely needed to make the diagnosis. An MRI can also be performed in patients with recurrent pain after surgical excision of a Morton's neuroma.
- Ultrasound imaging is also being used to locate Morton's neuromas but is rarely needed to make the diagnosis.

TREATMENT

■ NONPHARMACOLOGIC THERAPY

- Changing the type of footwear is the first line of treatment.
- Use open footwear and custom shoe inserts and avoid weight-bearing activities.
- Metatarsal pad with arch support is helpful.
- Participate in ultrasound therapy.

■ ACUTE GENERAL Rx

- If conservative measures are unsuccessful, injection of the intermetatarsal bursa with hydrocortisone may help
- Nonsteroidal antiinflammatory agents (e.g., ibuprofen 400 to 800 mg PO tid or naproxen 250 to 500 mg bid)

■ CHRONIC Rx

- If nonpharmacologic and acute treatments do not give sufficient relief, surgical excision of the nerve has been successful in 95% of the cases.
- Surgery can be performed in the physician's office using local anesthesia.
- Numbness in the area where the nerve was excised is a common postoperative finding.

■ DISPOSITION

- Postoperative patients return to their normal activities by 3 to 6 wk.
- In cases where pain persists after surgery a "stump neuroma" may be present.
- Approximately 80% of patients who failed to have relief with the initial surgery did find relief with a second procedure.

■ REFERRAL

If surgery is being considered, a consultation with either a podiatrist or an orthopedic surgeon is indicated.

☼ PEARLS & CONSIDERATIONS

■ COMMENTS

- Dr. Thomas G. Morton is given credit for describing this disorder in 1876.
- Morton's neuroma occurs just before the nerve bifurcates at the metatarsal area to innervate sides of two adjacent toes.

REFERENCES

Bencardino J et al: Morton's neuroma: is it always symptomatic? *AJR Am J Roentgenol* 175(3):649, 2000.

Morscher E, Ulrich J, Dick W: Morton's intermetatarsal neuroma: morphology and histological substrate, *Foot Ankle Int* 21:558, 2000.

Wu J, Chin DT: Painful neuromas: a review of treatment modalities, *Ann Plast Surg* 43(6):661, 1999.

Wu KK: Morton's interdigital neuroma: a clinical review of its etiology, treatment and results, *J Foot Ankle Surg* 35(2):112, 1996.

Zanetti M et al: Morton neuroma: effect on MR imaging findings on diagnostic thinking and therapeutic decisions, *Radiology* 326:188, 1999.

Author: **Dennis J. Mikolich, M.D.**

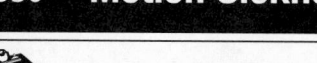
 BASIC INFORMATION

■ **DEFINITION**
Patients with motion sickness suffer perspiration, nausea, vomiting, increased salivation, and generalized malaise in response to movement.

■ **SYNONYMS**
Physiologic vertigo

ICD-9CM CODES
994.6 Motion sickness

■ **EPIDEMIOLOGY & DEMOGRAPHICS**
INCIDENCE (IN U.S.): Common
PREVALENCE (IN U.S.): Common
PREDOMINANT SEX: Male = female
PREDOMINANT AGE: Any age
PEAK INCIDENCE: Any age
GENETICS: Not known to be genetic

■ **PHYSICAL FINDINGS & CLINICAL PRESENTATION**
• Vomiting
• Sweating
• Pallor

■ **ETIOLOGY**
• Motion (e.g., amusement rides, rides in automobiles or planes)
• Exacerbated by anxiety, fumes (e.g., industrial pollutants), visual stimuli

 DIAGNOSIS

■ **DIFFERENTIAL DIAGNOSIS**
• Acute labyrinthitis
• Gastroenteritis
• Metabolic disorders
• Viral syndrome

■ **WORKUP**
None necessary in routine case

■ **LABORATORY TESTS**
None necessary

■ **IMAGING STUDIES**
None necessary

TREATMENT

■ **NONPHARMACOLOGIC THERAPY**
• Fixate on far object.
• Cease motion.
• Avoid reading.
• Avoid alcohol.

■ **ACUTE GENERAL Rx**
• Scopolamine patch (Transderm Scop) is most effective. It should be applied to hairless area behind ear every 3 days prn. It should be applied >4 hr before antiemetic effect is required.
• Over-the-counter oral preparations (e.g., Dramamine) are less effective.
• Meclizine (Antivert) 12.5 to 25 mg q6h may be effective.

■ **CHRONIC Rx**
• Rarely chronic
• Symptoms generally resolve completely with cessation of motion exposure

■ **DISPOSITION**
Follow-up is not needed.

■ **REFERRAL**
If another diagnosis is suspected (e.g., purulent ear, fever, cranial nerve abnormalities)

PEARLS & CONSIDERATIONS

■ **COMMENTS**
• Many patients with migraine report having severe motion sickness as a child.
• Improved ventilation, avoidance of large meals before travel, semirecumbent sitting, and avoidance of reading while in motion will minimize the risk of motion sickness.

REFERENCES
Koch KL: Illusory self-motion and motion sickness: a model for brain-gut interacting and nausea, *Dig Dis Sc:* 48(8 Suppl):53S, 1999.
Yates BJ, Miller AD, Lacot JB: Physiological basis and pharmacology of motion sickness: an update, *Brain Res Bull* 45(5):395, 1998.
Author: **Fred F. Ferri, M.D.**

BASIC INFORMATION

■ DEFINITION

Mucormycosis is a fungal infection by *Zygomycetes* fungi, which include *Mucorales* spp. *(Mucor, Rhizopus, Absidia, Cunninghamella, Mortierella, Saksenaea, Syncephalastrum, Apophysomyces,* and *Thamnidium)* and *Entomophthorales* spp. *(Conidiobolus* and *Basidiobolus).*

ICD-9CM CODES
117.7 Mucormycosis

■ EPIDEMIOLOGY & DEMOGRAPHICS

Infection by these ubiquitous organisms occurs in association with underlying conditions including diabetes mellitus, lymphoma, severe burns or trauma, prolonged postoperative course, multiple myeloma, hepatitis, cirrhosis, renal failure, steroid treatment, immunodeficiency states (e.g., AIDS), and use of contaminated Elastoplast bandages.
Immunocompetent hosts may become infected in tropical climates.

■ PHYSICAL FINDINGS & CLINICAL PRESENTATION

• Rhinocerebral-rhinoorbital-paranasal syndrome may present with fever, facial and orbital pain, headache, diplopia, loss of vision, facial or orbital cellulitis, facial anesthesia, cranial nerve dysfunction, black nasal discharge, epistaxis, and seizure. Physical findings in this situation include proptosis, chemosis, nasal, palatal (Fig. 1-178), or pharyngeal necrotic ulcerations, and retinal infarction. Thrombosis of the cavernous sinus or internal carotid artery may occur.
• Pulmonary mucormycosis can present with pneumonia, lung abscess,

pulmonary infarction, pleurisy, pleural effusion, hemoptysis, chills, and fever.
• Gastrointestinal zygomycosis presents with abdominal pain, diarrhea, GI hemorrhage, ulcers, peritonitis, and bowel infarction.
• Cutaneous zygomycosis presents as nodular lesions (hematogenous seeding) or a wound infection.
• Cardiac mucormycosis is a form of endocarditis.
• Septic arthritis and osteomyelitis.
• Brain abscess.
• Disseminated zygomycosis (rare but uniformly fatal).
• Physical findings depend on the location of the infection.

■ ETIOLOGY & PATHOGENESIS
The cause of mucormycosis is infection by a fungus of the *Zygomycetes* class (see Definition). Normal host defenses include leukocytes and pulmonary macrophages. Quantitative (e.g., neutropenia) or qualitative (e.g., diabetes mellitus or steroid treatment) disruption in the host defenses predisposes the patient to infection.

DIAGNOSIS

■ DIFFERENTIAL DIAGNOSIS
• Infection of the sites described previously by other organisms (bacterial [including TB and leprosy], viral, fungal, or protozoan)
• Noninfectious tissue necrosis (e.g., neoplasia, vasculitis, degenerative) of the sites described previously

■ WORKUP
• Biopsy of infected tissue with direct light microscopy examination establishes the diagnosis within minutes of the biopsy in the case of nasopharyngeal infection

• Bronchoalveolar lavage or bronchoscopy with biopsy for smear, culture, and histologic examination
• X-rays and other imaging studies of symptomatic sites may be required before infection is suspected and tissue specimens are obtained

TREATMENT

Amphotericin B given IV at a daily dose of 0.5 to 1.5 mg/kg infused over 2 to 4 hr for a total of 1 to 4 g. Adverse reactions may be managed as follows:
• Fever, chills, headache, myalgias, nausea, and vomiting: premedicate with aspirin (650 mg PO), acetaminophen (650 mg PO), diphenhydramine (25 to 50 mg IV), hydrocortisone (25 to 100 mg IV), or meperidine (25 to 50 mg IV).
• Hypokalemia and hypomagnesemia are treated with potassium and magnesium replacement.
• Nephrotoxicity and renal tubular acidosis can be mitigated to some extent with 500 ml of normal saline infusion 30 min before and after each dose of amphotericin. Amphotericin dose reduction may also be necessary.
• Renal function and electrolytes should be monitored twice a week during the entire course of amphotericin.
• Lipid preparations of amphotericin B may be less toxic (i.e., amphotericin B lipid complex, amphotericin B colloidal dispersion, and liposomal amphotericin B).
• The role of flucytosine, rifampin, and tetracycline is controversial.
• Surgical debridement or radical resection.

■ PROGNOSIS
• Sinus infection with no underlying disease: 75% survival.
• Sinus infection with diabetes: 60% survival.
• Sinus infection with renal disease: 25% survival.
• Surgery may increase survival by 5% to 20%.
• Early diagnosis improves survival as well as control of the underlying condition.

REFERENCE
Meyers BR, Gurtman AC: Phycomycetes. In Gorbach SL, Bartlett JG, Blacklow NR (eds): *Infectious diseases,* ed 2, Philadelphia, 1998, WB Saunders.
Author: **Tom J. Wachtel, M.D.**

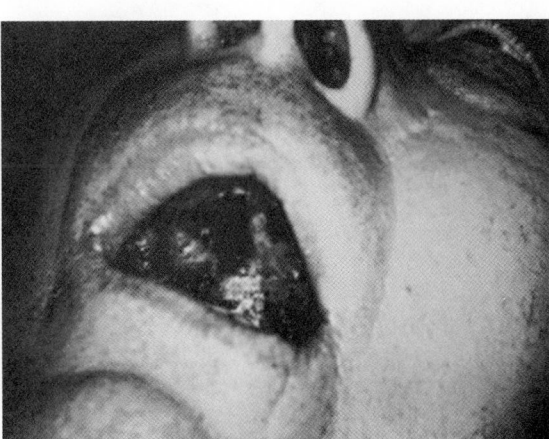

Fig. 1-178 Necrosis of the hard palate secondary to invasion by Rhizopus species in a renal transplant patient taking corticosteroids. (From Gorbach SL: *Infectious diseases,* ed 2, Philadelphia, 1998, WB Saunders.)

BASIC INFORMATION

■ **DEFINITION**
Multifocal atrial tachycardia is a supraventricular, moderately rapid arrhythmia (rate 100 to 140 bpm) with P waves having at least three or more different morphologies.

■ **SYNONYMS**
Chaotic atrial rhythm; the term "wandering pacemaker" is used for a similar arrhythmia associated with a normal or slow heart rate.

ICD-9CM CODES
427.89 Multifocal atrial tachycardia

■ **EPIDEMIOLOGY & DEMOGRAPHICS**
Same as chronic lung disease (obstructive or restrictive), which the arrhythmia may complicate

■ **PHYSICAL FINDINGS & CLINICAL PRESENTATION**
Symptoms:
• Palpitation
• Lightheadedness
• Syncope
• Symptoms of the underlying pulmonary disease
• Physical findings associated with the underlying pulmonary disease

■ **ETIOLOGY**
• Exact mechanism unknown
• Associated abnormalities include hypoxia, hypercarbia, acidosis, electrolyte disturbances, digitalis toxicity

🔬 **DIAGNOSIS**

■ **DIFFERENTIAL DIAGNOSIS**
• Atrial fibrillation
• Atrial flutter
• Sinus tachycardia
• Paroxysmal atrial tachycardia
• Extrasystoles

■ **WORKUP**
• ECG (Fig. 1-179)
• Pulmonary function tests
• Electrolytes
• Arterial blood gases
• Digoxin level (if patient on digoxin)

℞ **TREATMENT**

• Improve the pulmonary or metabolic dysfunction if possible
• Calcium blockers
• β-Blockers if not contraindicated by obstructive lung disease
• If the arrhythmia is asymptomatic, it can be left untreated

REFERENCE
Myerburg RJ, Kloosterman EM, Castellanos A: Recognition, clinical assessment, and management of arrhythmias and conduction disturbances. In Fuster V et al (eds): *Hurst's: the heart, arteries, and veins,* ed 10, New York, 2001, McGraw-Hill.
Author: **Tom J. Wachtel, M.D.**

MULTIFOCAL ATRIAL TACHYCARDIA

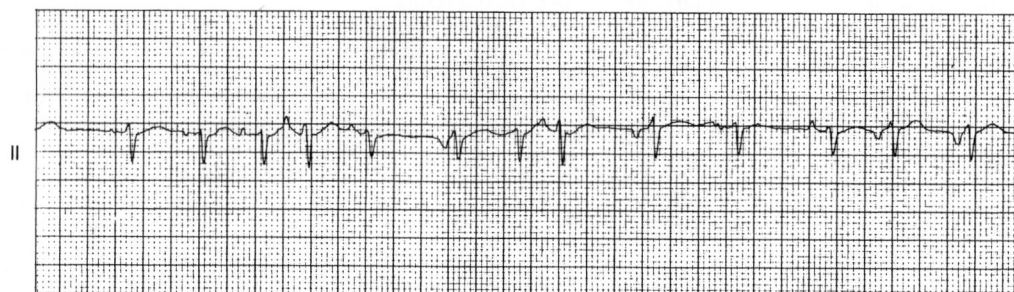

II

Fig. 1-179   The P waves show variable shapes or variable PR intervals, or both.
(From Goldberger AL: *Clinical electrocardiography,* ed 5, St Louis, 1994, Mosby.)

BASIC INFORMATION

■ DEFINITION

Multiple myeloma is a malignancy of plasma cells characterized by overproduction of intact monoclonal immunoglobulin or free monoclonal kappa or lambda chains.

ICD-9CM CODES
203.0 Multiple myeloma

■ EPIDEMIOLOGY & DEMOGRAPHICS
ANNUAL INCIDENCE: 4 cases/100,000 persons (blacks affected twice as frequently as whites); multiple myeloma accounts for 10% of all hematologic cancers
PREDOMINANT AGE: Peak incidence in the seventh decade at a median age of 69 yr

■ PHYSICAL FINDINGS & CLINICAL PRESENTATION
The patient usually comes to medical attention because of one or more of the following:
- Bone pain (back, thorax) or pathologic fractures caused by osteolytic lesions
- Fatigue or weakness because of anemia secondary to bone marrow infiltration with plasma cells
- Recurrent infections as a result of impaired neutrophil function and deficiency of normal immunoglobulins
- Nausea and vomiting caused by constipation and uremia
- Delirium secondary to hypercalcemia
- Neurologic complications, such as spinal cord or nerve root compression, blurred vision from hyperviscosity
- Pallor and generalized weakness from anemia
- Purpura, epistaxis from thrombocytopenia
- Evidence of infections from impaired immune system
- Bone pain, weight loss
- Swelling on ribs, vertebrae, and other bones

DIAGNOSIS

■ DIFFERENTIAL DIAGNOSIS
- Metastatic carcinoma
- Lymphoma
- Bone neoplasms (e.g., sarcoma)
- Monoclonal gammopathy of undetermined significance (MGUS)

■ LABORATORY TESTS
- Normochromic, normocytic anemia; rouleaux formation on peripheral smear
- Hypercalcemia is present in 15% of patients at diagnosis
- Elevated BUN, creatinine, uric acid, and total protein
- Proteinuria secondary to overproduction and secretion of free monoclonal kappa or lambda chains (Bence Jones protein)
- Tall homogeneous monoclonal spike (M spike) on protein immunoelectrophoresis (IEP) in approximately 75% of patients; decreased levels of normal immunoglobulins
  1. The increased immunoglobulins are generally IgG (75%) or IgA (15%).
  2. Approximately 17% of patients have flat level of immunoglobulins but increased light chains in the urine by electrophoresis.
  3. A very small percentage (<2%) of patients have nonsecreting myeloma (no increase in immunoglobulins and no light chains in the urine) but have other evidence of the disease (e.g., positive bone marrow examination).
- Reduced ion gap resulting from the positive charge of the M proteins and the frequent presence of hyponatremia in myeloma patients
- Hyponatremia, serum hyperviscosity (more common with production of IgA)
- Bone marrow examination: usually demonstrates nests or sheets of plasma cells, which comprise >30% of the bone marrow, and ≥10% are immature
- Serum β-2 microglobulin has little diagnostic value; it is useful for prognosis because levels >8 mg/L indicate high tumor mass and aggressive disease
- Elevated serum levels of LDH at the time of diagnosis define a subgroup of myeloma patients with very poor prognosis
- Increased interleukin-6 in serum during active stage of myeloma
- The production of DKK1, an inhibitor of osteoblast differentiation, by myeloma cells is associated with the presence of lytic bone lesions in patients with multiple myeloma.

■ IMAGING STUDIES
X-ray films of painful areas usually demonstrate punched-out lytic lesions or osteoporosis. Bone scans are not useful, because lesions are not blastic.

TREATMENT

■ NONPHARMACOLOGIC THERAPY
Prevention of renal failure with adequate hydration and avoidance of nephrotoxic agents and dye contrast studies

■ ACUTE GENERAL Rx
- Newly diagnosed patients with good performance status are best treated with autologous stem cell transplantation, resulting in improved survival. Useful guidelines (from the Hematology Disease Site Group of the Cancer Care Ontario Practice Guidelines Initiative) regarding the role of high-dose chemotherapy and stem-cell transplantation are as follows:
  1. Autologous transplantation is recommended for patients with stage II or III myeloma and good performance status.
  2. Allogenic transplantation is not recommended as routine therapy.
  3. Patients potentially eligible for transplantation should be referred for assessment early after diagnosis and should not be extensively exposed to alkylating agents before collection of stem cells.
  4. Autologous peripheral stem cells should be harvested early in the patient's treatment course (best when performed as part of initial therapy).
  5. A single transplant with high-dose melphalan, with or without total body irradiation, is suggested for patients undergoing transplantation outside a clinical trial.
  6. At this time no conclusion can be reached about the role of interferon therapy after transplantation.
- Chemotherapeutic agents effective in multiple myeloma are:
  1. Melphalan and prednisone: the rates of response to this treatment range from 40% to 60%. Adding continuous low-dose interferon to standard melphalan-prednisone therapy does not improve response rate or survival; however, response duration and plateau phase duration are prolonged by maintenance therapy with interferon.

2. Vincristine, doxorubicin (Adriamycin), and dexamethasone (VAD) can be used in patients not responding or relapsing after treatment with melphalan and prednisone; methylprednisolone is substituted for dexamethasone (VAMP) in some centers.

3. High-dose chemotherapy (HDCT) with vincristine, melphalan, cyclophosphamide, and prednisone (VMCP) alternating with vincristine, carmustine, doxorubicin, and prednisone (BVAP) combined with bone marrow transplantation improves the response rate, event-free survival, and overall survival in patients with myeloma.

4. Current HDCT regimen with autologous stem-cell support achieve complete response in approximately 20% to 30% of patients, with best results seen in good-risk patients, defined as young patients (<50 yr of age) with good performance status and a low tumor burden (β_2 microglobulin ≤2.5 mg/L).

5. Thalidomide, an agent with antiangiogenic properties, is useful to induce responses in patients with multiple myeloma refractory to chemotherapy.

6. Bortezomib (Velcade) is a newer protease inhibitor that is cytotoxic for multiple myeloma. It is indicated for treatment of refractory multiple myeloma. It is expensive, with an average course of treatment (5 cycles) costing >$20,000.

■ CHRONIC Rx

- Promptly diagnose and treat infections. Common bacterial agents are *Streptococcus pneumoniae* and *Haemophilus influenzae*. Prophylactic therapy against *Pneumocystis carinii* with trimethoprim sulfamethoxazole must be considered in patients receiving chemotherapy and high-dose corticosteroid regimens.
- Control hypercalcemia and hyperuricemia.
- Control pain with analgesics; radiation therapy and surgical stabilization may also be indicated.
- Treat anemia with epoetin alfa.
- Monthly infusions of the biphosphonate pamidronate provide significant protection against skeletal complications and improve the quality of life of patients with advanced multiple myeloma. Zoledronic acid (Zometa) can be infused over 15 min and is more effective than pamidronate for treatment of hypercalcemia of malignancy. Biphosphonates (pamidronate, zoledranate, and ibandronate) also appear to have an antitumor effect.

■ DISPOSITION

- Prognosis is better in asymptomatic patients with indolent or smoldering myeloma: median survival time is approximately 10 yr in persons with no lytic bone lesions and a serum myeloma protein concentration <3 g/dl.

- As compared with a single autologus stem-cell transplantation, double transplantation (two successive autologus stem-cell transplantations) improves survival among patients with myeloma, especially those who do not have a very good partial response after undergoing one transplantation.

REFERENCES

Attal M et al: Single versus double autologus stem-cell transplantation for multiple myeloma, *N Engl J Med* 349:2495, 2003.

Imrie K et al: The role of high dose chemotherapy and stem-cell transplantation in patients with multiple myeloma: a practice guideline of the Cancer Care Ontario Practice Guidelines Initiative, *Ann Intern Med* 136:619, 2002.

Rajkumar SV et al: Current therapy for multiple myeloma, *Mayo Clin Proc* 77:813, 2002.

Tian E et al: The role of WNT-signaling antagonist DKK1 in the development of osteolytic lesions in multiple myeloma, *N Engl J Med* 349:2483, 2003.

Author: **Fred F. Ferri, M.D.**

BASIC INFORMATION

■ DEFINITION

Multiple sclerosis (MS) is a chronic demyelinating disease of the central nervous system (CNS) characterized by demyelinating lesions in the CNS (plaques) separated in time and space.

■ SYNONYMS

Disseminated sclerosis

ICD-9CM CODES

340 Multiple sclerosis

■ EPIDEMIOLOGY & DEMOGRAPHICS

PREVALENCE: 10 to 150 cases/100,000 persons; higher in northern latitudes and with geographic clustering. It is the most common demyelinating disease in humans.
GENETICS: Increased prevalence with multiple haplotypes of the major histocompatibility complex, most commonly DR2, DR15, and DR4.
PREDOMINANT AGE: Young adults (17 to 42 yr)

■ PHYSICAL FINDINGS & CLINICAL PRESENTATION

- Common symptoms: fatigue, diplopia, visual loss, vertigo, hemiparesis, paraparesis, isolated focal weakness, numbness, paresthesias, ataxia, cognitive and urinary dysfunction.
- Visual abnormalities:
  1. Internuclear ophthalmoplegia (INO)—paresis of the adducting eye on lateral conjugate gaze with horizontal nystagmus of the abducting eye
  2. Optic neuritis (ON)—see topic "Optic neuritis"
  3. Nystagmus
- Upper motor neuron (UMN) signs—spasticity, increased deep tendon reflexes, positive Hoffmann's sign, extensor plantar responses, clonus and weakness consistent with an UMN lesion
- Sensory loss—isolated loss of pain/temp in dermatomes, dissociated loss of pain/temp from vibration/position sense, thoracic band of sensory loss (see Section II for the differential diagnosis of paresthesias)
- Ataxia—intention tremor, heel-to-shin ataxia, inability to tandem
- Bladder dysfunction—detrusor hyperreflexia, flaccidity, and dyssynergia
- Lhermitte's sign: flexion of the neck elicits an electrical sensation extending down the spine and occasionally into the extremities

■ ETIOLOGY

The exact etiology of MS is unknown. It is thought to be a combination of multiple genes and environmental factors. Evidence supporting a genetic predisposition includes concordance rates that are 25.9% in monozygotic twins, 2.3% in dizygotic twins, and 1.9% in nontwin siblings.

DIAGNOSIS

- MS is primarily a clinical diagnosis based on a consistent clinical presentation with evidence of CNS demyelinating lesions disseminated in time (separated by at least 1 mo) and space (two distinct areas of the CNS), not better explained by another disease.
- History and examination may be sufficient if both support the presence of two lesions separated in time and space. If, however, there is only evidence of one lesion on examination, MRI or paraclinical testing plus oligoclonal bands (OCBs) may be used to make the diagnosis. If there has been only one relapse, the MRI may be diagnostic if it shows dissemination in time and space (at least 6 mo for a new MS-like T2 lesion and 3 mo for a gadolinium-enhancing lesion).
- In relapsing-remitting MS (80% of patients), signs and symptoms evolve over a period of several days, stabilize, and then improve spontaneously or in response to corticosteroids. In primary progressive MS, manifestations gradually worsen from disease onset without relapses. Most patients with relapsing-remitting MS eventually transition to secondary progressive MS. In secondary progressive MS, manifestations worsen gradually with or without superimposed acute relapses.

■ DIFFERENTIAL DIAGNOSIS

- Autoimmune: acute disseminated encephalomyelitis (ADEM), postvaccination encephalomyelitis
- Degenerative: subacute combined degeneration (B_{12} deficiency), inherited spastic paraparesis
- Infections: progressive multifocal leukoencephalopathy, Lyme, syphilis, HIV, HTLV-1, Whipple's, expanded differential in immunocompromised patients
- Inflammatory: SLE, Sjögren's, Behçet's, vasculitis, sarcoidosis, celiac disease
- Inherited metabolic disorders: leukodystrophies
- Mitochondrial: Leber's hereditary optic neuropathy, mitochondrial encephalopathy lactic acidosis and strokelike episodes (MELAS)
- MS variants: recurrent optic neuropathy, neuromyelitis optica

(Devic's), acute tumor-like lesion (Marburg variant), Baló's concentric sclerosis, myelinoclastic diffuse sclerosis (Schilder's disease)
- Neoplasms: metastases, CNS lymphoma
- Vascular: subcortical infarcts, Binswanger's disease

■ WORKUP

- Lumbar puncture is indicated for all first-time relapses and recommended for all evaluations when the diagnosis of MS is not definite. Possible CSF abnormalities include a mild-moderate increase in total protein and mononuclear WBCs. Elevated CSF IgG Index and OCBs (sent with paired serum samples) are elevated in 70% and 90% respectively of patients with clinically definite MS. False positives occur with other inflammatory conditions.
- Serum: recommend CBC, ESR, CHEM 7, LFTs, ANA, B12. Consider Lyme titer, ACE, infectious and collagen-vascular serologies, very-long-chain fatty acids and arylsulfatase A.
- Consider paraclinical testing: evoked potentials (VEPs, BAERs, SSEPs) and urodynamic testing. Myelin loss will slow conduction velocities.

■ IMAGING STUDIES

MRI with gadolinium can be used to assess disease load, activity, and progression (see Fig. 1-180). A normal MRI, however, cannot be used conclusively to exclude MS.

TREATMENT

■ NONPHARMACOLOGIC THERAPY

Patient education regarding the disease, treatment options and prognosis

■ ACUTE GENERAL Rx

- Relapses: typically, high-dose IV methylprednisolone (5 days of 1000 mg/day can be used; an alternative dose is 15 mg/kg/day).
- Disease-modifying therapy: includes interferon β-1a (Avonex, Rebif), interferon β-1b (Betaseron), and glatiramer acetate (Copaxone). All four drugs have been shown to slow progression of relapsing disease and reduce the annual relapse rate by 20%-40%.
- Cytotoxic: mitoxantrone is effective in rapidly relapsing and secondary progressive MS.

■ CHRONIC Rx

- Fatigue: amantadine 100 mg bid. Modafinil (for somnolence) and fluoxetine are alternatives.

- Spasticity: may be controlled with baclofen, tizanidine, diazepam, and/or lorazepam.
- Pain: carbamazepine and gabapentin are most effective.
- Depression: frequent (20% of patients) and can be treated with antidepressants.
- Urinary urgency: oxybutynin or propantheline.
- Tremor: can generally be controlled with clonazepam 0.5 mg bid.

■ DISPOSITION
The majority of patients experience clinical improvement in weeks to months after the initial manifestations. The rate of disease progression is highly variable. The average interval from the initial clinical presentation to death is 35 yr.

■ REFERRAL
- Initial neurology referral is recommended in all patients with MS.
- Referrals to a physician specializing in rehabilitation, PT/OT, urology, and psychiatry are often needed.

REFERENCES

CHAMPS Study Group: MRI predictors of early conversion to clinically definite MS in the CHAMPS placebo group, *Neurology* 59:998, 2002.

Compston A, McAlpine D (eds): *McAlpine's multiple sclerosis.* London, Churchill Livingstone, 1998.

Ebers GC et al: A population-based study of multiple sclerosis in twins, *N Engl J Med* 315:1638, 1986. {AU: Please provide author initial.}

Galetta SL et al: Immunomodulatory agents for the treatment of relapsing multiple sclerosis, *Arch Intern Med* 162:2161, 2002.

Jacobs LD et al: Intramuscular interferon beta-1a therapy, initiated during a first demyelinating event in multiple sclerosis, *N Engl J Med* 343:898, 2000.

Author: **Alexandra Degenhardt, M.D**

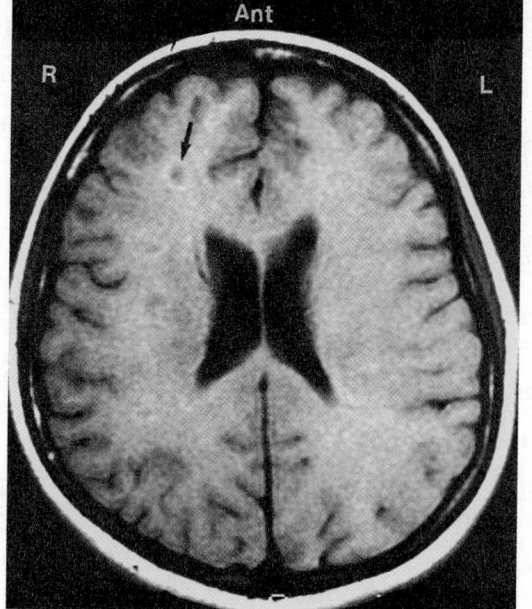

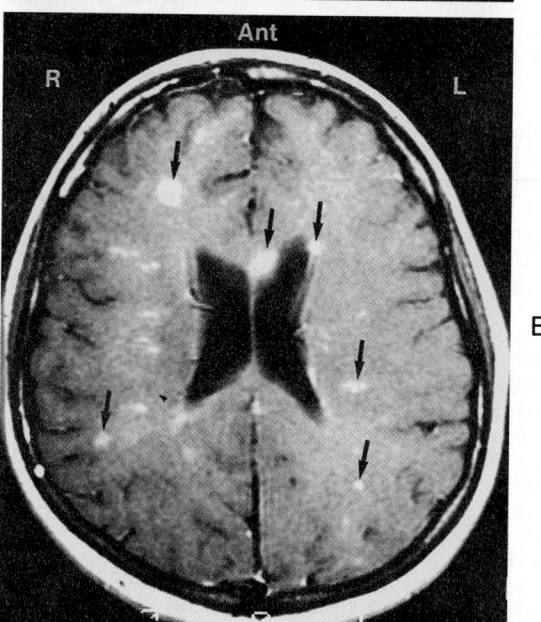

Fig. 1-180   Multiple sclerosis. The noncontrasted T1-weighted magnetic resonance scan (**A**) shows one hypodensity (black hole) in the right frontal lobe (*arrow*). A gadolinium-enhanced scan (**B**) shows many enhancing lesions, only some of which are indicated (*arrows*). (From Mettler FA [ed]: *Primary care radiology,* Philadelphia, 2000, WB Saunders.)

BASIC INFORMATION

■ DEFINITION
Mumps is an acute generalized viral infection that is usually characterized by nonsuppurative swelling and tenderness of one or both parotid glands. It is caused by mumps virus, a paramyxovirus and member of the paramyxoviridae family.

ICD-9CM CODES
072.9 Mumps

■ EPIDEMIOLOGY & DEMOGRAPHICS
INCIDENCE (IN U.S.):
- About 1600 infections/yr
- More than 150,000 cases/yr before licensure of mumps vaccine in 1967

PREDOMINANT SEX: Males = females
PREDOMINANT AGE: 75% of disease in teenage yr
PEAK INCIDENCE: Late winter and early spring months
GENITICS:
Congenital Infection:
- First-trimester infection is associated with excessive fetal deaths.
- Second- and third-trimester infection is not associated with increased fetal mortality.

Neonatal Infection:
- Uncommon
- Uncommon in infants <1 yr because of passive immunity conferred by placental transfer of maternal antibody

■ PHYSICAL FINDINGS & CLINICAL PRESENTATION
- Prodromal period:
  1. Low-grade fever
  2. Malaise
  3. Anorexia
  4. Headache
- Parotid swelling and tenderness are often first signs of infection.
  1. Progresses over 2 to 3 days, then opposite side may become involved
  2. Unilateral parotitis in 25% of cases
  3. Considerable pain with parotid swelling, causing trismus and difficulty with mastication and pronunciation
  4. Pain exacerbated by eating or drinking citrus and other acidic foods
  5. Possible fever with parotid swelling, ranging up to 40° C
  6. Parotid swelling usually resolving within 1 wk
- CNS involvement:
  1. May occur from 1 wk before to 2 wk after the onset of parotitis or even in its absence

2. Meningitis
   a. Occurs in 1% to 10% of persons with mumps parotitis
   b. Occur three times more often in males than females
   c. Symptoms: headache, fever, nuchal rigidity, and vomiting
   d. Full recovery with no sequelae
3. Encephalitis
   a. May develop early, as a result of direct viral invasion of neurons, or late, around the second week after onset of parotitis, and is a postinfectious demyelinating process
   b. Mumps accounted for only 0.5% of viral meningitis
   c. Symptoms: fever, alterations in the level of consciousness, possible seizures, paresis or paralysis, and aphasia. Fever can be quit high (40° C-41° C)
   d. Cerebellitis and hydrocephalus are serious complications of mumps encephalitis
   e. May result in permanent sequelae or death
4. Other rare neurologic complications
   a. Cerebellar ataxia
   b. Transverse myelitis
   c. Gullain-Barré syndrome
   d. Facial palsy
- Epididymoorchitis:
  1. Most common extra salivary gland complication of mumps in adult men
  2. Occurs in 38% of postpubertal males who have mumps
  3. Most often unilateral but is bilateral in 30% of males who develop this complication
  4. May precede development of parotitis
  5. May be only manifestation of mumps
  6. Two thirds of cases develop during first week of parotitis
  7. One quarter of cases develop in second week
  8. Symptoms
     a. Severe pain, swelling, and tenderness of the testes and scrotal erythema
     b. Fever and chills
  9. Some degree of testicular atrophy in 50% of cases, months to years later
  10. Sterility from bilateral orchitis is rare
- Involvement of pancreas and ovaries:
  1. Abdominal pain
  2. Fever
  3. Vomiting

4. Oophoritis
   a. Occurs in 5% of postpubertal women with mumps
   b. Symptoms include fever, nausea, vomiting, and lower abdominal pain
   c. May rarely result in decreased fertility and premature menopause
- Transient renal impairment:
  1. Common
  2. Manifest by hematuria and polyuria
- Joint involvement:
  1. Migratory polyarthritis is most frequent
  2. Infrequently affects adults with mumps
  3. Rarely in children
  4. Self-limited, with complete resolution
- Pancreatitis
  1. Uncommon as a severe illness
  2. Milder degree of upper abdominal discomfort
- Deafness:
  1. Most often unilateral, involving high frequencies; may rarely cause bilateral involvement
  2. Most patients recover
  3. Permanent unilateral deafness reported in 1 in 20,000 cases
  4. Labrynthitis and end lymphatic hydrops also reported
- Myocardial involvement:
  1. Uncommon
  2. Rarely causes progressive and culminant fatal myocarditis with dilated cardiomyopathy
  3. Refractory arrhythmia and congestive heart failure
  4. Coronary artery involvement

■ ETIOLOGY
- Virus is spread via direct contact, droplet nuclei, fomites, or secretions through the nose and mouth
- Patients are contagious from 48 hr before to 9 days after parotid swelling

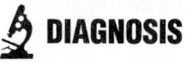

DIAGNOSIS

■ DIFFERENTIAL DIAGNOSIS
- Other viruses that may cause acute parotitis:
  1. Parainfluenza types 1 and 3
  2. Coxsackie viruses
  3. Influenza A
  4. Cytomegalovirus
- Suppurative parotitis:
  1. Most often caused by staphylococcal aureus

2. May be differentiated from mumps
   a. Extreme indurations, tenderness and erythema overlying the gland
   b. Ability to express pus from Stensen's duct or massage of parotid
- Other conditions that may occur with parotid enlargement or swelling
  1. Sjögren's syndrome
  2. Leukemia
  3. Diabetes mellitus
  4. Uremia
  5. Malnutrition
  6. Cirrhosis
- Drugs that cause parotid swelling:
  1. Phenothiazines
  2. Phenylbutazone
  3. Thiouracil
  4. Iodides
- Conditions that cause unilateral swelling:
  1. Tumors
  2. Cysts
  3. Stones causing obstruction
  4. Strictures causing obstruction

■ WORKUP
- Diagnosis based on history of exposure and physical finding of parotid tenderness with mild to moderate constitutional symptoms.
- Diagnosis is confirmed by a variety of serologic tests or isolation of the virus.

■ LABORATORY TESTS
- Diagnosis is confirmed by fourfold rise between acute and convalescent sera by CF, ELISA, or neutralization tests.
- Virus can be isolated from the saliva, usually from 2 to 3 days before to 4 to 5 days after the onset of parotitis.
- Virus can be isolated from CSF in patients with meningitis during the first 3 days of meningeal findings. More rapid confirmation of mumps in the CSF is IgM antibody capture Immunoassay and nested PCR assay.

- Virus can be detected in urine during the first 2 wk of infection.
- WBC
  1. May be normal
  2. Possible mild leucopenia with a relative lymphocytosis
  3. Leucocytosis with left shift with extra salivary gland involvement, such as meningitis, orchitis, or pancreatitis
- Serum amylase:
  1. Elevated in the presence of parititis
  2. May remain elevated for 2 to 3 wk
  3. May be differentiated from mumps and parotids by isoenzyme analysis or serum pancreatic lipase
- Mumps meningitis:
  1. CSF WBCs from 10 to 2000 WBC/mm3 with a predominance of lymphocytes
  2. In 20% to 25% of patients, predominance of polymorphonuclear cells
  3. CSF protein normal or mildly elevated
  4. CSF glucose low, >40mg/100ml, in 6% to 30% of patients

■ TREATMENT

■ NONPHARMACOLOGIC THERAPY
- Supportive treatment
- Adequate hydration and nutrition

■ ACUTE GENERAL Rx
- Analgesics and antipyretics to relieve pain and fever
- Narcotic analgesics, along with bed rest, ice packs, and a testicular bridge, to relieve pain associated with mumps orchitis
- IV fluids for patients with frequent vomiting associated with mumps pancreatitis or meningitis

■ DISPOSITION
Most patients recover without incident.

✷ PEARLS & CONSIDERATIONS

■ COMMENTS
Prevention:
- Attenuated live mumps virus vaccine has been available since 1967.
  1. Usually given in combination with measles and rubella vaccines
  2. Should be given at 15 mo of age, and again at 5 to 12 yr
  3. Seroconversion in about 100% infants given the vaccine
  4. Contraindicated in pregnant women and immunocompromised patients
  5. Patients with asymptomatic HIV infection and patients with symptomatic HIV infection, in the absence of severe immunosuppression, can safely receive MMR vaccine
  6. Adverse events of vaccination include
     a. Local pain
     b. Indurations
     c. Thrompocypenic purpura
     d. Guillain-Barré syndrome
     e. Cerebellar ataxia
- Infected patients should be isolated until parotid swelling resolves
- Because virus may be shed before the onset of parotid swelling, isolation possibly not of great value in limiting spread of infection.

REFERENCES
Centers for Disease Control and Prevention: Mumps surveillance—United States 1988-1993, *MMWR Morb Mortal Wkly Rep* 4A(No ss-3):1, 1995.

Gans H et al: Immune responses to measles and mumps vaccination of infants at 6, 9, 12 months, *J Infect Dis* 184(7):817, 2001.

Author: **Vasanthi Arumugam, M.D.**

BASIC INFORMATION

■ DEFINITION

Munchausen syndrome is marked by the willful, and often active, production of symptoms or feigning of disease, usually associated with exaggerated lying (pseudologia fantastica) and with the apparent purpose of inducing medical testing, procedures, and treatment, or assuming the patient role.

■ SYNONYMS

Factitious disorder
Munchausen by proxy
Deliberate disability
Hospital addiction syndrome
Artifactual illness
Artefaktkrankheit
Dermatitis artefacta
Surreptitious illness

ICD-9CM CODES
300.19 Factitious disorder

■ EPIDEMIOLOGY & DEMOGRAPHICS

INCIDENCE (IN U.S.): Unknown
PREVALENCE (IN U.S.): Unknown
PREDOMINANT SEX: Male:female ratio of 2:1
PREDOMINANT AGE: 30 to 40 yr
PEAK INCIDENCE: 30s
GENETICS: No genetic predisposition known

■ PHYSICAL FINDINGS & CLINICAL PRESENTATION

- False complaints or self-inflicted injury or symptoms without clear secondary gain
- Presentation often acute and dramatic
- Workup usually negative but a predisposing condition often present

■ ETIOLOGY

- Unknown
- Personality disorders and psychodynamic factors: thought to play a role

DIAGNOSIS

■ DIFFERENTIAL DIAGNOSIS

- Malingering: a clear secondary gain (e.g., financial gain or avoidance of unwanted duties) is present.
- Somatoform disorders or hypochondriasis: similar presentations, but disorder is not under the patient's control.
- Self-injurious behavior is common in many other psychiatric conditions (e.g., borderline personality disorder, psychoses, or nonfatal suicide attempt as may occur in depression); in those conditions the patients confess the intentional self-harm and describe motivating factors.
- May also present as Munchausen by proxy in which a mother (86% of time) or other caregiver induces illness in a child (52% between ages of 3 and 13 yrs) for the purpose of obtaining medical attention without other secondary gain.

■ WORKUP

- Workup is often dictated by the presenting complaints.
- No specific tests for Munchausen syndrome although Minnesota Multiphasic Personality Inventory (MMPI) may show an unreliable profile.
- Diagnosis is invariably made when the patient is caught in the act of lying or inducing an injury.

■ LABORATORY TESTS

No specific tests are required.

 TREATMENT

■ NONPHARMACOLOGIC THERAPY

- Therapy is difficult, because patients nearly always terminate the physician-patient relationship (usually in an angry manner) when discovered.
- Only one case of successful psychiatric therapy exists in the literature.

■ ACUTE GENERAL Rx

None

■ DISPOSITION

- Ultimate course is unknown.
- After confronted with their behavior, patients seek other physicians or hospitals.
- Extensive medical workups and exploratory surgery are frequent.

■ REFERRAL

Always when diagnosis is made

REFERENCES

Feldman MD, Brown RM: Munchausen by proxy in an international context, *Child Abuse Negl* 26:509, 2002.
Turner J, Reid S: Munchausen's syndrome, *Lancet* 359:346, 2002.
Author: **Rif S. El-Mallakh, M.D.**

BASIC INFORMATION

■ DEFINITION

Muscular dystrophy (MD) refers to a heterogenous group of inherited disorders resulting in characteristic patterns of muscle weakness, some with cardiac involvement even in the absence of peripheral symptoms. For the purposes of this section, only disorders with childhood or adult onset will be considered (i.e., excluding congenital myopathies).

■ ICD-9CM CODES

359 Muscular dystrophies and other myopathies
359.1 Hereditary progressive muscular dystrophy

■ EPIDEMIOLOGY & DEMOGRAPHICS

INCIDENCE:
- Most common childhood MD is Duchenne's muscular dystrophy with an incidence of 1/3500 male births
- Most common adult MD is myotonic dystrophy with an incidence as high as 1/8000

GENETICS:
- **Dystrophinopathies:** X-linked recessive defect in dystrophin gene resulting in either absence (Duchenne MD) or reduced/defective (Becker's MD) dystrophin.
- **Myotonic Dystrophy:** Autosomal dominant (AD) CTG trinucleotide repeat.
- **Limb-Girdle Muscular Dystrophy:** Autosomal recessive, also autosomal dominant forms with deficiency identified in multiple proteins (sarcoglycan, calpain, dysferlin, telethonin, lamin A/C, myotilin, and caveolin-3).
- **Emery-Dreifuss Muscular Dystrophy:** X-linked recessive defect in nuclear protein emerin or AR defect in inner nuclear lamina proteins lamin A/C.
- **Fascioscapulohumeral Muscular Dystrophy:** AD; genetic mutation causes deletion of 3.3 kb repeat.
- **Oculopharyngeal Muscular Dystrophy:** AD GCG trinucleotide repeat resulting in deficient mRNA transfer from nucleus.

■ PHYSICAL FINDINGS & CLINICAL PRESENTATION

- **Dystrophinopathies:** Proximal arm and leg weakness with hypertrophic calf muscles, delayed motor milestones, cognitive impairment, cardiac involvement, progressive course resulting in respiratory complications and respiratory failure
  Duchenne's (DMD) onset 2-3 yr old, typically wheelchair-bound by 12 yr
  Becker's (BMD) onset 5-15 yr old, ambulatory beyond age 15
- **Myotonic Dystrophy:** Variable age of onset and severity manifesting as predominately distal weakness with long face, percussion and grip myotonia, temporalis and masseter wasting, ptosis, hypersomnolence, cognitive impairment, and cardiac conduction defects. May be associated with frontal balding, cataracts, impaired glucose tolerance, male infertility.
- **Limb-Girdle Muscular Dystrophy:** Phenotypically and genetically heterogenous characterized by proximal hip and shoulder girdle weakness, some genotypes featuring cardiac involvement.
- **Emery-Dreifuss Muscular Dystrophy:** Early adulthood onset with predominately humeroperoneal weakness, early contractures, and cardiac conduction defects.
- **Fascoscapulohumeral Muscular Dystrophy:** Onset typically in late childhood or adolescence with weakness mostly in face and shoulder girdle musculature and possible later, mild involvement of lower extremities. Cardiac conduction defects and cognitive impairment may occur.
- **Oculopharyngeal Muscular Dystrophy:** Symptom onset typically in mid-adult life with ptosis, dysphagia, dysarthria, and proximal muscle weakness.

■ ETIOLOGY

Contingent upon genotype, see Genetics

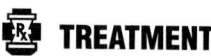

DIAGNOSIS

■ DIFFERENTIAL DIAGNOSIS

Myasthenia gravis, inflammatory myopathy, metabolic myopathy, endocrine myopathy, toxic myopathy, mitochondrial myopathy

■ WORKUP

- Creatine kinase (CK)
- ECG, Holter monitor, formal cardiac electrophysiology or echocardiography to screen for cardiac conduction defects and cardiomyopathy
- EMG
- Muscle biopsy with histochemistry useful for diagnosis of dystrophinopathies and limb-girdle muscular dystrophy (sarcoglycanopathy, dysferlinopathy)
- DNA analysis helpful is clinical suspicion is for myotonic, Emery-Drefuss, and facioscapulohumeral muscular dystrophies
- Assessment of respiratory parameters, including forced vital capacity (FVC)

TREATMENT

■ NONPHARMACOLOGIC THERAPY

- Genetic counseling
- Physical, occupational, respiratory, speech therapy as symptoms dictate
- Screening for sleep-disordered breathing with overnight polysomnogram (PSG) if daytime hypersomnolence, early morning headaches, disturbed sleep; may benefit from noninvasive positive pressure ventilation
- Pacemaker placement may be necessary if cardiac conduction defect present

■ ACUTE GENERAL Rx

Prednisone may modestly prolong ambulation in Duchenne MD and may be recommended until loss of ambulatory function.

■ CHRONIC Rx

Vigilance to avoid cardiac and respiratory complications, joint contractures

■ DISPOSITION

Variable course and severity of phenotype contingent upon diagnosis.

■ REFERRAL

- Surgical referral for correction of scoliosis or contractures may be necessary
- Assessment and follow-up in a muscular dystrophy specialty clinic

☼ PEARLS & CONSIDERATIONS

- Formal evaluation recommended by anesthetist before any operation with general anesthesia in patients with dystrophinopathy
- Gower's sign: difficulty in rising from a supine to a standing position as a result of truncal and hip-girdle weakness. Affected patients push themselves on all fours and then quickly grab their thighs and walk up the thighs to a standing position (Fig. 1-181)

■ COMMENTS

Muscular Dystrophy Association—USA National Headquarters, 3300 E. Sunrise Drive, Tucson, AZ 85718. Toll-free phone number: (800) 572-1717. Web address: www.mdausa.org/

REFERENCES

Emery AE: Muscular dystrophy into the new millennium, *Neuromuscul Disord* 12(4):843, 2002.

Emery AE: The muscular dystrophies, *Lancet* 359(9307):687, 2002.

Saperstein DS, Amato AA, Barohn RJ: Clinical and genetic aspects of distal myopathies, *Muscle Nerve* 24(11):1440, 2001.

Author: **Taylor Harrison, M.D.**

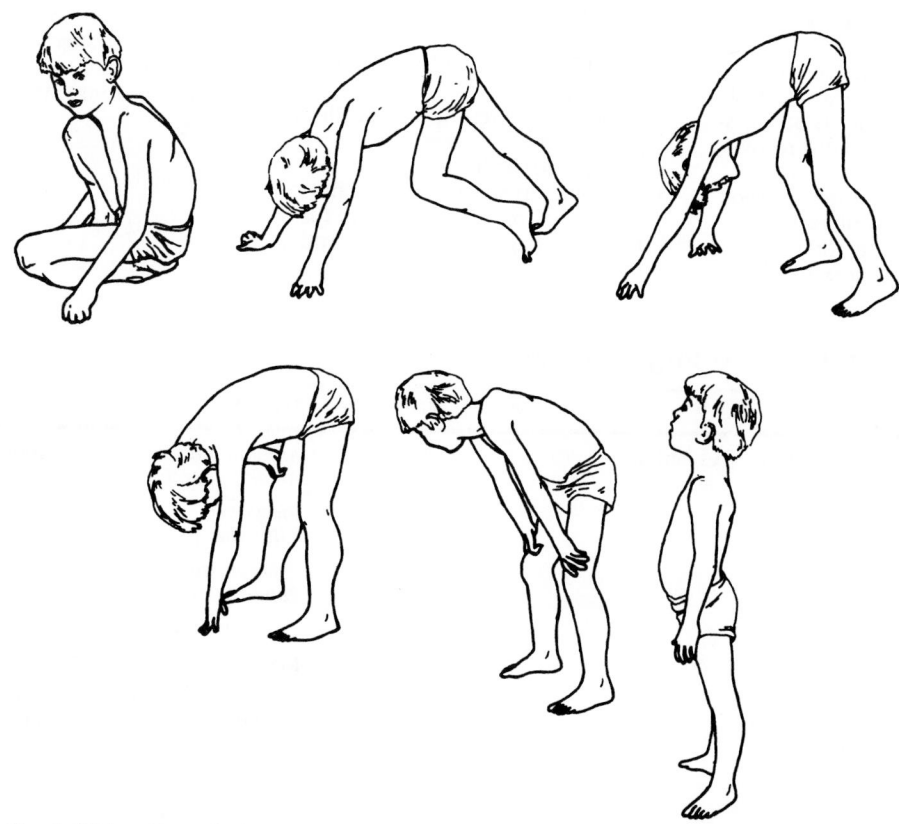

Fig. 1-181   Gower's sign in Duchenne's muscular dystrophy. (From Siegel IM: *Muscle and its diseases: an outline primer of basic science and clinical method,* Chicago, 1986, Year Book Medical.)

BASIC INFORMATION

■ DEFINITION
Mushroom poisoning is intoxication resulting from ingestion of poisonous mushrooms.

ICD-9CM CODES
988.1 Mushroom poisoning

■ EPIDEMIOLOGY & DEMOGRAPHICS
- Five percent of all mushrooms are poisonous. Distinction between poisonous and edible mushrooms may be difficult even by experienced persons.
- Common poisonous species include *Amanita, Russula, Gyromitra,* and *Omphalotus.*

■ PHYSICAL FINDINGS & CLINICAL PRESENTATION (TABLE 1-39)
- *Russula* causes confusion, delirium, visual disturbance, tachycardia, and diarrhea within a few hours of ingestion. Prognosis: spontaneous recovery (mortality <1%).
- *Amanita* and *Gyromitra* intoxication begins with symptoms of gastroenteritis (nausea, vomiting, diarrhea, abdominal cramps) approximately

10 hr following ingestion. *Amanita* then goes on to cause cardiomyopathy and hepatic and renal failure. *Gyromitra* produces jaundice and seizures. Both mushrooms are associated with a 50% mortality rate.
- *Omphalotus* causes symptoms of gastroenteritis that subside spontaneously within 24 hr.

■ PATHOPHYSIOLOGY
- *Amanita* contains cytotoxic substances and isoxazoles that are gamma-aminobutyric acid neurotransmitter analogs.
- *Gyromitra* contains a pyridoxine antagonist that disrupts the GI mucosa and causes hemolysis.
- *Russula* contains a cholinergic substance.

DIAGNOSIS

■ DIFFERENTIAL DIAGNOSIS
- Food poisoning
- Overdose of prescription or illegal drug
- Other intoxications
- See topic on specific organ failure (e.g., renal or hepatic failure) for differential diagnosis of those conditions

■ WORKUP
- History
- Inspection and identification of suspected mushrooms
- Mushroom or gastric content analysis (by thin-layer chromatography or radioimmunoassay)

TREATMENT

- Gastric lavage
- Repeated administration of activated charcoal
- Supportive care as needed (may require respiratory assistance, hemodialysis, or emergency liver transplantation)

REFERENCE
Haubrich WS: Mushroom poisoning. In Haubrich WS, Schaffner F, Berk JE (eds): *Gastroenterology,* ed 5, Philadelphia, 1995, WB Saunders.
Author: **Tom J. Wachtel, M.D.**

TABLE 1-39   Mushroom Poisoning Syndromes

SYNDROME	INCUBATION PERIOD (hr)	SPECIES	TOXIN
Confusion, restlessness, visual disturbances, lethargy	2	*Amanita muscaria* *Amanita pantherina*	Ibotenic acid, muscimol
Parasympathetic activity	2	*Inocybe* sp. *Clitocybe* sp.	Muscarine
Hallucinations	2	*Psilocybe* sp. *Panacolus* sp.	Psilocybin Psilocin
Disulfiram	2	*Coprinus atramentarius*	Disulfiram-like substances
Gastroenteritis	2	Many	Unknown
Hepatorenal failure	6-24	*Amanita phalloides* *Amanita virosa* *Amanita verna* *Galerina autumnalis* *Galerina marginata* *Galerina venenata*	Amatoxins Phallotoxins
Hepatic failure	6-24	*Gyromitra* sp.	Gyromitrin

From Gorbach SL: *Infectious diseases,* ed 2, Philadelphia, 1998, WB Saunders.

BASIC INFORMATION

DEFINITION
Myasthenia gravis (MG) is an autoimmune disorder of postsynaptic neuromuscular transmission classically directed against the nicotinic acetylcholine receptor (AChR) of the neuromuscular junction, resulting in a decrease in functional postsynaptic ACh receptors and consequent weakness.

ICD-9CM CODES
358.0 Myasthenia gravis

EPIDEMIOLOGY & DEMOGRAPHICS
INCIDENCE (IN U.S.): 2 to 5 cases/yr/1,000,000 persons
PREVALENCE (IN U.S.): 1/20,000 persons
PREDOMINANT SEX: Female > male (3:2) in adults; female = male in elderly
PEAK INCIDENCE: Female: second-third decade; male: sixth-seventh decade
GENETICS: Increased frequency of HLA-B8, DR3
Congenital MG: Related to multiple identified genetic defects of neuromuscular transmission, not an autoimmune etiology and not to be treated with immunosuppressive drugs
Neonatal MG: Occurs in 15% to 20% of infants born to mothers with MG. This condition is only temporary and is caused by transplacental passage of AChR-ab. Spontaneous recovery often occurs within 1 mo.

PHYSICAL FINDINGS & CLINICAL PRESENTATION
- The hallmark of MG is fluctuating weakness worsened with exercise and improved with rest
- Generalized weakness involving proximal muscles, diaphragm, neck extensors in 85%
- Weakness confined to eyelids and extraocular muscles in about 15% of patients
- Bulbar symptoms of ptosis, diplopia, dysarthria, dysphagia common
- Normal reflexes, sensation, and coordination

ETIOLOGY
Antibody-mediated decrease in nicotinic acetylcholine receptors in the postsynaptic neuromuscular junction resulting in defective neuromuscular transmission and subsequent muscle weakness and fatigue

DIAGNOSIS

DIFFERENTIAL DIAGNOSIS
Lambert-Eaton myasthenic syndrome, botulism, medication-induced myasthenia, chronic progressive external ophthalmoplegia, congenital myasthenic syndromes, thyroid disease, basilar meningitis, intracranial mass lesion with cranial neuropathy, Miller-Fisher variant of Guillain-Barré Syndrome

WORKUP
Tensilon test: edrophonium chloride (Tensilon), 2 mg IV; useful in MG patients with ocular symptoms; it has rapid onset (30 sec) and short duration of action (5 min). Nonspecific.
Repetitive nerve stimulation (RNS): successive stimulation shows decrement of muscle action potential in clinically weak muscle, may be negative in up to 50%.
Single-fiber electromyography (SFEMG): highly sensitive, abnormal in up to 95% of myasthenics.
Serum AChR antibodies found in up to 80% of patients.
A subset of patients with seronegative MG may have muscle-specific receptor tyrosine kinase (MuSK) antibodies.

ADDITIONAL TESTS
- Spirometry to document pulmonary function
- CT scan of anterior chest to rule out thymoma (found in 12% of patients with MG) or residual thymic tissue
- TSH, free T_4: to rule out thyroid disease (found in 5% to 15% of patients with MG) or residual thymic tissue
- PPD, chest x-ray if immunosuppressive treatment considered

TREATMENT

NONPHARMACOLOGIC THERAPY
- Patient education to facilitate recognition of worsening symptoms and impress need for medical evaluation at onset of clinical deterioration
- Avoidance of selected drugs known to provoke exacerbations of MG (β-blockers, aminoglycoside and quinolone antibiotics, class I antiarrhythmics)
- Prompt treatment of infections, diet modification, and speech evaluation with dysphagia

ACUTE GENERAL Rx
- Symptomatic treatment with acetylcholinesterase inhibitors:
  Pyridostigmine 30 to 60 mg PO q4-6h initially; onset of effects is 30 min, duration 4 hr

  Mestinon timespan, 180 mg can be given qd or bid; however, absorption may be erratic
  Major side effects are GI upset and increased salivary and bronchial secretions, which may be treated with hyoscyamine or Robinul
- Immunosuppressive treatment with corticosteroids, azathioprine, mycophenolate mofetil, cyclosporine for chronic disease-modifying therapy
  Prednisone initiated at 15-20 mg qd titrate by 5 mg increments to effect or dose of 1 mg/kg per day with improvement in 2-4 wk and maximal response by 3-6 mo
  Azathioprine initiated at 50 mg qd titrated to 2-3 mg/kg/day with clinical effect in 6-12 mo
  Mycophenolate mofetil initiated at 500 mg bid and titrated to 2-3 g per day, clinical effect in 2 wk to 2 mo
  Cyclosporine initiated at 5 mg/kg/day with clinical effect within 1-2 mo
- Plasmapheresis and intravenous immunoglobulin are effective short-term options for immunotherapy
- Mechanical ventilation is lifesaving in setting of a myasthenic crisis, defined as neuromuscular respiratory failure related to diaphragm weakness. Consider elective intubation if forced vital capacity <155 cc/kg, maximal expiratory pressure <40 cm H_2O, or negative inspiratory pressure <25 cm H_2O)

SURGICAL Rx
- In thymomatous MG, thymectomy is indicated in all patients.
- For nonthymomatous autoimmune MG: thymectomy is an option in patients less than 40 yr of age to increase probability of remission or improvement; however, benefit not conclusively established.

DISPOSITION
Course of disease is highly variable, influenced by factors such as clinical features at onset, association with thymic pathology, age, duration of symptoms at time of diagnosis.

REFERRAL
Surgical referral for thymectomy in selected cases (see Surgical Rx)

REFERENCES
Drachman DB: Medical progress: myasthenia gravis, *N Engl J Med* 330(25):1797, 1994.
Wittbrodt ET: Drugs and myasthenia gravis: an update, *Arch Int Med* 157(4):399, 1997.
Author: **Taylor Harrison, M.D.**

BASIC INFORMATION

■ DEFINITION

Mycosis fungoides refers to a T-cell lymphoproliferative disorder with characteristic cutaneous skin lesions and with the potential to disseminate into lymph nodes and viscera (Fig. 1-182).

■ SYNONYMS

Cutaneous T-cell lymphoma

ICD-9CM CODES

202.1 Mycosis fungoides

■ EPIDEMIOLOGY & DEMOGRAPHICS

- Incidence of mycosis fungoides is 4/1 million.
- Approximately 1000 new cases are diagnosed annually in the U.S.
- More commonly affects males than females (2:1).
- Blacks > whites (2:1).
- Usually found in males 40 to 60 yr of age.

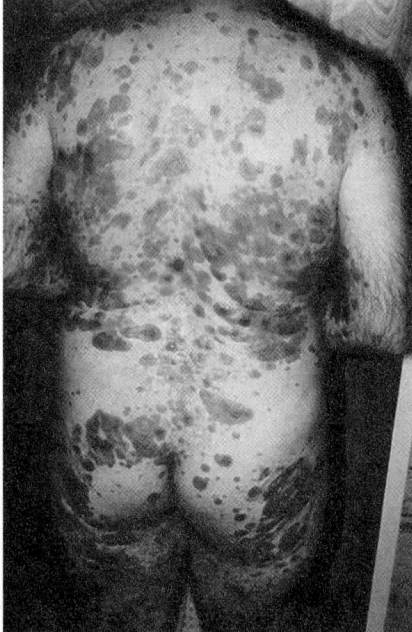

Fig. 1-182 Cutaneous T-cell lymphoma (mycosis fungoides). Note patch, plaque, and tumor stages. (From Noble J [ed]: *Textbook of primary care medicine,* ed 2, St Louis, 1996, Mosby.)

■ PHYSICAL FINDINGS & CLINICAL PRESENTATION

Mycosis fungoides characteristically progresses through three phases:
- A premycotic phase featuring scaly, erythematous patches that can last from months to years. During this stage the diagnosis can only be suspected, because the histopathologic features are not definitive for mycosis fungoides. Lesions are pruritic and can appear anywhere but are usually found in sun-shielded areas. Parapsoriasis en plaques, poikilodermatous parapsoriasis, parapsoriasis lichenoides, and variegata are skin lesions suspicious of representing premycotic cutaneous T-cell lymphoma.
- The infiltrative plaque phase features raised, indurated erythematous palpable plaques that are pruritic and may be associated with alopecia.
  1. Stage IA disease is defined as a patch or plaque skin disease involving <10% of the skin surface area.
  2. Stage IB disease is defined as a patch or plaque skin disease involving ≥10% of the skin surface area.
- The tumor phase is characterized by large, lumpy nodules arising from a premycotic patch, plaque, or unaffected skin and represents systemic infiltration and spreading. The tumors can be pruritic and large (>10 cm) and ulceration can occur.
  1. Stage II disease is defined by the presence of tumors.
- In approximately 5% of cases of mycosis fungoides, the presentation may be a diffuse, painful, pruritive erythroderma known as Sézary syndrome.
  1. Stage III disease is defined by the presence of generalized erythroderma.
- Lymphadenopathy can occur during the plaque or tumor stages and may be regional or diffuse.
  1. Stage IVA disease is defined by a lymph node biopsy showing large clusters of atypical cells, more than six cells, or showing total effacerent by atypical cells.
- Infiltration of the liver, spleen, lungs, bone marrow, kidney, stomach, and brain can occur.
  1. Stage IVB disease is defined by the presence of visceral involvement.

■ ETIOLOGY

The specific cause of mycosis fungoides is not known. Infection with the retrovirus HTLV-1 has been suspected, given the association of HTLV-1 infected individuals and T-cell leukemia. Other considerations listed but unsubstantiated include environmental toxins (e.g., tobacco, pesticides, herbicides, and solvents) and genetic predisposition.

DIAGNOSIS

The diagnosis of mycosis fungoides is established by skin biopsy. This may be difficult to differentiate from other skin lesions in the early phases of the disease (e.g., premycotic patch or early plaque lesions) and therefore the diagnosis can only be suspected.

■ DIFFERENTIAL DIAGNOSIS

- Contact dermatitis
- Atopic dermatitis
- Nummular dermatitis
- Parapsoriases
- Superficial fungal infections
- Drug eruptions
- Psoriasis
- Photodermatitis
- Alopecia mucinosa
- Lymphomatoid papulosis

■ WORKUP

- Any patient who is suspected of having mycosis fungoides should have a staging workup done. Prognosis in patients with mycosis fungoides depends on the type of skin lesions and the extent of disease.
- The workup should focus on identifying:
  1. The type of skin lesion and the extent of skin involvement of the body (e.g., skin involvement is > or <10% of the skin surface)
  2. Presence of lymphadenopathy
  3. Visceral involvement (e.g., lungs, liver)
  4. Presence of Sézary cells in the blood
- A TNM staging classification has been proposed by the Cutaneous T-Cell Lymphoma Workshop in 1979 and continues to be used today in guiding therapy.

■ LABORATORY TESTS

- CBC with differential
- Total lymphocyte count
- Measure the percentage of Sézary cells present (normal <5%)
- BUN/creatinine
- Electrolytes, calcium, and phosphorus
- LFTs
- Multiple skin biopsies over suspected areas are done to confirm the diagnosis
- If lymph nodes are present, excisional lymph node biopsy is performed

- Bone marrow and liver biopsies can be done if initial laboratory screening suggests organ involvement

■ IMAGING STUDIES
- Chest x-ray to rule out pulmonary involvement
- Chest, abdominal, and pelvic CT-scan looking for mediastinal, abdominal, and pelvic lymphadenopathy

 ## TREATMENT

Treatment is guided according to the stage of disease.

■ NONPHARMACOLOGIC THERAPY
- For dry cracking skin, emollients (e.g., lanolin and petrolatum) are applied bid.
- Moisturizing lotion (e.g., ammonium lactate) applied bid.
- Topical antibiotics (e.g., bacitracin) are used on ulcerative tumors.

■ ACUTE GENERAL Rx
- Treatment of patients with premycotic limited patch or plaque phase include:
  1. Psoralen ultraviolet light (PUVA) therapy where 0.6 mg/kg of 8-methoxypsoralen is ingested 1 to 2 hr before exposure of the skin to UV light (320 to 400 nm). This is done three times per week and tapered to two times per week until all the lesions have cleared. This is typically continued for 6 mo.
  2. Remissions can be retreated with PUVA.

- Treatment of patients with cutaneous patch and plaque lesions involving >10% of the skin surface includes:
  1. Topical chemotherapy using nitrogen mustard, carmustine, or mechlorethamine hydrochloride applied to the affected body areas.
  2. PUVA is an alternative treatment option.
- Treatment of patients with tumor phase disease includes:
  1. Total skin electron beam therapy in doses of 3000 to 3600 cGy given over 8 to 10 wk.
  2. Total skin electron beam therapy with PUVA is an alternative in recurrence tumor phase disease.

■ CHRONIC Rx
- In patients developing diffuse erythroderma (e.g., Sézary syndrome, extracorporeal photophoresis) in which 8-methoxypsoralen is ingested and peripheral blood is exposed to UVA through a membrane filter.
- Interferon and other systemic chemotherapeutic agents (e.g., methotrexate, cyclophosphamide, doxorubicin, vincristine, and prednisone) are considered in disseminated mycosis fungoides.

■ DISPOSITION
- The median survival in patients with early patch or plaque phase disease and no extradermal involvement is 12 yr.
- The median survival of patients with skin involvement, lymph node involvement, but no visceral involvement is approximately 5 yr.
- The median survival in patients with visceral involvement is 2.5 yr.

■ REFERRAL
Any patient with suspected mycosis fungoides should be referred to a dermatologist for definitive diagnosis and initial therapy. Oncology consultation is also indicated in patients with more advanced disease.

☼ PEARLS & CONSIDERATIONS

■ COMMENTS
- Mycosis fungoides is thought to represent one class of the spectrum of cutaneous T-cell lymphomas. Sézary syndrome, reticulum-cell sarcoma, and histiocytic lymphoma are also classified as T-cell neoplasias.
- Alibert was the first to describe mycosis fungoides in 1806 and named it so because of its resemblance to mushrooms.

REFERENCES
Apisarnthanarox N, Talpur R, Duvic M: Treatment of cutaneous T cell lymphoma: current status and future directions, *Am J Clin Dermatol* 3(3):195, 2002.
Kim YH, Hoppe RT: Mycosis fungoides and the Sézary syndrome, *Semin Oncol* 26(3):276, 1999.
Lorincz AL: Cutaneous T-cell lymphoma (mycosis fungoides), *Lancet* 347(9005):871, 1996.
Siegel RS, Kozel TM: Cutaneous T-cell lymphoma leukemia, *Curr Treat Options Oncol* 1(1):43, 2000.
Author: **Peter Petropoulos, M.D.**

BASIC INFORMATION

■ DEFINITION
Myelodysplastic syndromes (MDS) are a group of acquired clonal disorders affecting the hemopoietic stem cells and characterized by cytopenias with hypercellular bone marrow and various morphologic abnormalities in the hemopoietic cell lines. MDSs show abnormal (dysplastic) hemopoietic maturation. Marrow cellularity is increased, reflecting an effective hematopoiesis, but inadequate maturation results in peripheral cytopenias. Myelodysplasia encompasses several heterogenous syndromes. The French-American-British classification of myelodysplastic syndromes includes the following: refractory anemia, refractory anemia with ringed sideroblasts, refractory anemia with excess blasts, chronic myelomonocytic leukemia, and refractory anemia with excess blasts in transformation.

■ SYNONYMS
MDS
Preleukemia
Dysmyelopoietic syndrome

ICD-9CM CODES
238.7 Myelodysplastic syndrome

■ EPIDEMIOLOGY & DEMOGRAPHICS
INCIDENCE (IN U.S.): Approximately 82 cases/100,000 persons/yr
PREDOMINANT AGE: More common in elderly patients, with a median age of >65 yr

■ PHYSICAL FINDINGS & CLINICAL PRESENTATION
- Splenomegaly, skin pallor, mucosal bleeding, ecchymosis may be present.
- Patients often present with fatigue.
- Fever, infection, and dyspnea are common.

■ ETIOLOGY
Unknown. However, exposure to radiation, chemotherapeutic agents, benzene, or other organic compounds is associated with myelodysplasia.

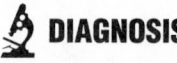 DIAGNOSIS

■ DIFFERENTIAL DIAGNOSIS
- Hereditary dysplasias (e.g., Fanconi's anemia, Diamond-Blackfan syndrome)

- Vitamin B_{12}/folate deficiency
- Exposure to toxins (drugs, alcohol, chemotherapy)
- Renal failure
- Irradiation
- Autoimmune disease
- Infections (TB, viral infections)
- Paroxysmal nocturnal hemoglobinuria

■ WORKUP
- Diagnostic workup includes laboratory evaluation and bone marrow examination.
- An algorithmic approach to patients with suspected myelodysplastic syndromes is described in Section III.

■ LABORATORY TESTS
- Anemia with variable MCV (normal or increased)
- Reduced reticulocyte count (in relation to the degree of anemia)
- Hypogranular or agranular neutrophils
- Thrombocytopenia or normal platelet count
- Hypogranular platelets may be present
- Hypercellular bone marrow, with frequent clonal chromosomal abnormalities

■ IMAGING STUDIES
Abdominal CT scan may reveal hepatosplenomegaly.

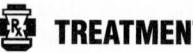 TREATMENT

■ NONPHARMACOLOGIC THERAPY
RBC transfusions in patients with severe symptomatic anemia

■ ACUTE GENERAL Rx
- Results of chemotherapy are generally disappointing.
- The role of myeloid growth factors (granulocyte colony–stimulating factor, granulocyte-macrophage colony–stimulating factor) and immunotherapy is undefined. In a recent trial, 34% of patients treated with antithymocyte globulin (40 mg/kg for 4 days) became transfusion independent. Response was also associated with a statistically significantly longer survival.
- Allogeneic stem-cell transplantation should be considered in patients <60 yr old because this is the established procedure with cure potential.

■ CHRONIC Rx
Monitor for infections, bleeding, and complications of anemia.

■ DISPOSITION
- Cure rates in young patients with allogeneic bone marrow transplantations approach 30% to 50%.
- The risk of transformation to acute myelogenous leukemia varies with the percentage of blasts in the bone marrow.
- Advanced age, male sex, and deletion of chromosomes 5 and 7 are associated with a poor prognosis.
- According to the International Myelodysplastic Syndrome Risk Analysis Workshop, the most important variables in disease outcome are the specific cytogenetic abnormalities, the percentage of blasts in the bone marrow, and the number of hematopoietic lineages involved in the cytopenias.

■ REFERRAL
Hematology referral in all patients with MDS

☼ PEARLS & CONSIDERATIONS

■ COMMENTS
- Erythropoietin (epoetin alfa) SC three times weekly may be effective in increasing the Hgb and reducing the RBC transfusion requirement in some patients.
- Patients with cytogenetic abnormalities associated with poor prognosis should be considered for aggressive treatment with high-dose chemotherapy and stem-cell transplantation.
- Nearly 50% of the deaths that result from myelodysplastic syndromes are the result of cytopenia associated with bone marrow failure.

REFERENCE
Molldrem JJ et al: Antithymocyte globulin for treatment of the bone marrow failure associated with myelodysplastic syndromes, *Ann Intern Med* 137:156, 2002.
Author: **Fred F. Ferri, M.D.**

BASIC INFORMATION

■ DEFINITION

Acute coronary syndromes are manifestations of ischemic heart disease and represent a broad clinical spectrum that includes unstable angina/non-ST elevation MI and ST-elevation MI.

1. **Myocardial infarction** is characterized by necrosis resulting from an insufficient supply of oxygenated blood to an area of the heart. According to the joint European Society of Cardiology/American College of Cardiology, either one of the following criteria for acute evolving or recent MI satisfies the diagnosis:
   a. Typical rise and gradual fall (troponin) or more rapid rise and fall (CK-MB) of biochemical markers of myocardial necrosis with at least one of the following:
      i. Ischemic symptoms
      ii. Development of pathologic Q waves on ECG
      iii. ECG changes indicative of ischemia (ST-segment elevation or depression)
      iv. Coronary artery intervention (e.g., coronary angioplasty)
   b. Pathologic findings of acute MI
2. **ST elevation MI**: area of ischemic necrosis that penetrates the entire thickness of the ventricular wall and results in ST-segment elevation.
3. **Unstable angina**: coronary arterial plaque rupture with fragmentation and distal arterial embolization resulting in myocardial necrosis. Usually occurs without ST-elevation and is thus termed **non-ST elevation MI.**

■ SYNONYMS

MI
Non-ST elevation MI
ST-elevation MI
Heart attack
Coronary thrombosis
Coronary occlusion

ICD-9CM CODES

410.9 Acute myocardial infarction, unspecified site

■ EPIDEMIOLOGY & DEMOGRAPHICS

INCIDENCE/PREVALENCE (IN U.S.):
- >500 cases/100,000 persons.
- >500,000 MIs in the U.S. yearly.
- More prominent in males between the ages of 40 and 65 yr; no predominant sex after age 65 yr.
- Women experience more lethal and severe first acute MIs than men, regardless of comorbidity, previous angina, or age.
- At least one fourth of all myocardial infections are clinically unrecognized.

■ PHYSICAL FINDINGS & CLINICAL PRESENTATION

Clinical presentation:
- Crushing substernal chest pain usually lasts longer than 30 min.
- Pain is unrelieved by rest or sublingual nitroglycerin or is rapidly recurring.
- Pain radiates to the left or right arm, neck, jaw, back, shoulders, or abdomen and is not pleuritic in character.
- Pain may be associated with dyspnea, diaphoresis, nausea, or vomiting.
- There is no pain in approximately 20% of infarctions (usually in diabetic or elderly patients).

Physical findings:
- Skin may be diaphoretic, with pallor (because of decreased oxygen).
- Rales may be present at the bases of lungs (indicative of CHF).
- Cardiac auscultation may reveal an apical systolic murmur caused by mitral regurgitation secondary to papillary muscle dysfunction; S_3 or S_4 may also be present.
- Physical examination may be completely normal.

■ ETIOLOGY

- Coronary atherosclerosis
- Coronary artery spasm
- Coronary embolism (caused by infective endocarditis, rheumatic heart disease, intracavitary thrombus)
- Periarteritis and other coronary artery inflammatory diseases
- Dissection into coronary arteries (aneurysmal or iatrogenic)
- Congenital abnormalities of coronary circulation
- MI with normal coronaries (MINC syndrome): more frequent in younger patients and cocaine addicts. The risk of acute MI is increased by a factor of 24 during the 60 min after the use of cocaine in persons who are otherwise at relatively low risk. Most patients with cocaine-related MI are young, nonwhite, male cigarette smokers without other risk factors for ASHD who have a history of repeated cocaine use. Blood and urine toxicology screen for cocaine is recommended in all young patients who present with acute MI
- Hypercoagulable states, increased blood viscosity (polycythemia vera)

DIAGNOSIS

■ DIFFERENTIAL DIAGNOSIS

The various causes of myocardial ischemia are described in Section II along with the differential diagnosis of chest pain.

■ LABORATORY TESTS

- Cardiac troponin levels: cardiac-specific troponin T (cTnT) and cardiac-specific troponin I (cTnI) are highly specific for myocardial injury. Increases in serum levels of cTnT and cTnI may occur relatively early after muscle damage (3-12 hr), peak within 24 hr, and may be present for several days after MI (up to 7 days for cTnI and up to 10-14 days for cTnT). Troponin T tests can be falsely positive in patients with renal failure. The threshold level of troponin T considered positive for MI is 0.1 ng/ml in patients with normal renal function or 0.5 ng/ml in patients with renal impairment.
- Creatine kinase MB isoenzyme is a useful marker for MI. It is released in the circulation in amounts that correlate with the size of the infarct.
- Neither CK-MB nor troponin consistently appear in the blood within 6 hr after an ischemic event; therefore serial testing (e.g., on presentation and after 8 hr) is necessary to definitely rule out MI.
- ECG
1. In ST-elevation MI, there is development of:
   a. Inverted T waves, indicating an area of ischemia
   b. Elevated ST segment, indicating an area of injury
   c. Q waves, indicating an area of infarction (usually develop over 12 to 36 hr)
2. In unstable angina/non-ST elevation MI, Q waves are absent, but the following indications are present:
   a. History and myocardial enzyme elevations are compatible with MI.
   b. ECG shows ST segment elevation, depression, or no change followed by T wave inversion.

■ IMAGING STUDIES

- Chest radiography is useful to evaluate for pulmonary congestion and exclude other causes of chest pain.
- Echocardiography can evaluate wall motion abnormalities and identify mural thrombus or mitral regurgitation, which can occur acutely after MI.

TREATMENT

■ NONPHARMACOLOGIC THERAPY

- Limit patient's activity: bed rest for the initial 24 hr; if the patient remains stable, gradually increase activity.
- Diet: NPO until stable, then no added salt and a low-cholesterol diet.
- Patient education to decrease the risk of subsequent cardiac events (proper diet, cessation of smoking, regular exercise) should be initiated when the patient is medically stable.

■ ACUTE GENERAL Rx

- Any patient with suspected acute MI should immediately receive the following:
  1. Aspirin: give 160 to 325 mg PO unless true aspirin allergy is suspected. If the first dose is chewed, a blood level is achieved more rapidly than if it is swallowed. Clopidogrel may be substituted if true allergy is present.
  2. Nitrates: they increase the supply of oxygen by reducing coronary vasospasm and decrease consumption of oxygen by reducing ventricular preload. Sublingual nitroglycerin can be administered immediately on suspicion of MI (unless systolic blood pressure is <90 mm Hg or heart rate is <50 bpm or >100 bpm); IV nitroglycerin can be subsequently used. Nitroglycerin should be used with great caution in patients with inferior wall MI; nitrate usage can result in hypotension because these patients are sensitive to change in preload. It should also be avoided in patients suspected of having right ventricular infarction (increased risk of preload reduction) and if a patient has used sildenafil (Viagra), tadalafil (Cialis), or vardenafil (Levitra) within the previous 24 hr.
  3. Adequate analgesia: morphine sulfate 2 mg IV q5min PRN can be given for severe pain unrelieved by nitroglycerin. Hypotension secondary to morphine can be treated with careful IV hydration with saline solution. If sinus bradycardia accompanies hypotension, use atropine (0.5 to 1.0 mg IV q 5 min PRN to a total dose of 2.5 mg). Respiratory depression caused by morphine can be reversed with naloxone (Narcan) 0.8 mg.
  4. Nasal oxygen: administer at 2 to 4 L/min.

- If readily available without delay, percutaneous coronary intervention (PCI) with adjunctive glycoprotein IIb/IIIa is preferred over thrombolytic therapy. It is effective and generally results in more favorable outcomes than thrombolytic therapy. When PCI is performed, use of IV heparin is recommended. Coronary stents are useful to decrease ischemia, improve long-term patency, and lower the rate of restenosis of the infarct-related artery.
- Thrombolytic therapy: if the duration of pain has been <6 hr and primary angioplasty is not readily available, recanalization of the occluded arteries should be attempted with thrombolytic agents, possibly in combination with glycoprotein IIb/IIIa inhibition. Because the effectiveness of thrombolytics is time-dependent, ideally these agents should be administered either in the field or within 30 min of the patient's arrival in the emergency department. When tPA or rPA is used, IV heparin is given to increase the likelihood of patency in the infarct-related artery. In patients receiving streptokinase or APSAC, IV heparin is not indicated, because it does not offer any additional benefit and can result in increased bleeding complications. Tenecteplase and reteplase are comparable with accelerated infusion recombinant TPA in terms of efficacy and safety, but are more convenient because they are administered by bolus injection. Lanoplase and heparin bolus plus infusion is as effective as TPA with regard to mortality, but the rate of intracranial hemorrhage is significantly higher. Absolute contraindications to thrombolytic therapy include active internal bleeding, intracranial neoplasm or arteriovenous malformation, intracranial surgery in past 6 mo, stroke in past year, head trauma with loss of consciousness in past 6 mo, surgery in noncompressible location in past 6 wk, alteration in mental status, and infectious endocarditis.
- β-adrenergic blocking agents should be given to all patients with evolving acute MI, provided that there are no contraindications (see below). β-Blockers are useful to reduce myocardial oxygen consumption and prevent tachyarrhythmias. Early IV β-blockage (in the initial 24 hr) followed by institution of an oral maintenance regimen is also effective in reducing recurrent infarction

and ischemia. Frequently used agents are:
  1. Metoprolol (Lopressor): IV 5 mg q2min × 3 doses, then PO 25 to 50 mg q6h, given 15 min after last IV dose, continued for 48 hr; maintenance dosage is 50 to 100 mg bid.
  2. Atenolol (Tenormin): IV 5 mg over 5 min, repeat in 10 min if initial dose is well tolerated, then start PO dose 10 min after the last IV dose; PO 50 mg qd, increasing to 100 mg as tolerated.
Before using β-blockers, some of the contraindications and side effects (i.e., exacerbation of asthma, CNS effects, hypertension, bradycardia) must be carefully assessed.
- ACE inhibitors reduce left ventricular dysfunction and dilation and slow the progression of CHF during and after acute MI. They should be initiated within hours of hospitalization, provided that the patient does not have hypotension or a contraindication (bilateral renal stenosis, renal failure, or history of angioedema caused by previous treatment with ACE inhibitors).
  1. Commonly used agents are captopril 12.5 mg PO bid, enalapril 2.5 mg bid, or lisinopril 2.5 to 5 mg qd initially, with subsequent titration as needed.
  2. ACE inhibitors may be stopped in patients without complications and no evidence of left ventricular dysfunction after 6 to 8 wk.
  3. ACE inhibitors should be continued indefinitely in patients with impaired left ventricular function (ejection fraction <40%) or clinical CHF.
- Glycoprotein IIb receptor inhibitors (tirofiban, eptifibatide), when administered with heparin and aspirin, further reduce the incidence of ischemic events in patients with non-Q wave MI. The use of IV glycoprotein IIb/IIIa inhibitors (e.g., abciximab) before and during PTCA also reduces the risk of closure postangioplasty.
- Initiation of statin therapy before hospital discharge.

■ CHRONIC Rx

Evaluation of post-MI patients
- Submaximal (low level) treadmill test (can be done 1 to 3 wk after MI) in stable patients without any clinical evidence of significant left ventricular dysfunction or post-MI angina
  1. Useful to assess the patient's functional capacity and formulate an at-home exercise program
  2. Helpful to determine the patient's prognosis

- Radionuclide angiography or two-dimensional echocardiography
  1. To evaluate patient's left ventricular ejection fraction
  2. To evaluate ventricular size and segmental wall motion
  3. Echocardiography to rule out presence of mural thrombi in patients with anterior wall infarction; transesophageal echo is preferred if mural thrombosis is suspected
- A 24-hr Holter monitor study to evaluate patients who have demonstrated significant arrhythmias during their hospital stay; selected patients with complex ventricular ectopy may be candidates for programmed electrical stimulation studies and antiarrhythmic therapy and/or implanted defibrillator, depending on the results of these studies

■ DISPOSITION

The prognosis after MI depends on multiple factors:

- Use of β-blockers: the mortality of patients on a regular regimen of β-blockers is significantly decreased when compared with that of control groups.
- Presence of arrhythmias, frequent ventricular ectopy (≥10/hr), or repetitive forms of ventricular ectopic beats (couplets, triplets) indicates an increased risk (two to three times greater) of sudden cardiac death. New bundle branch block, Mobitz II second-degree block, and third-degree heart block also adversely affect outcome.
- Size of infarct: the larger it is, the higher the post-MI mortality rate. Significant myocardial stunning with subsequent improvement of ventricular function occurs in most patients after anterior MI. A lower level of creatine kinase, an estimate of the extent of necrosis, is independently predictive of recovery of function.
- Site of infarct: inferior wall MI carries a better prognosis than anterior wall MI; however, patients with inferior wall MI and right ventricular involvement have a high risk for arrhythmic complications and cardiac shock.
- Type of infarct: although the in-hospital mortality rate is higher for patients with ST-elevation infarcts, the long-term prognosis for non–ST-elevation MI may be worse because some of these patients have a higher incidence of sudden cardiac death after hospital discharge.

- Ejection fraction after MI: the lower the left ventricular ejection fraction, the higher the mortality after MI.
- Presence of post-MI angina indicates a high mortality rate.
- Performance on low-level exercise test: the presence of ST segment changes during the test is a predictor of high mortality during the first year.
- Presence of pericarditis during the acute phase of MI increases mortality at 1 yr.
- Type A behavior (competitive drive, ambitiousness, hostility) is associated with a lower mortality rate after symptomatic MI.
- The Killip classification is an independent predictor of all-cause mortality in patients with non-ST elevation acute coronary syndromes.
- Self-reported moderate alcohol consumption in the year before acute MI is associated with reduced 1-yr mortality.
- Use of lipid-lowering agents in patients with hyperlipidemia unresponsive to exercise and dietary restrictions is beneficial. Statins may also lower vascular inflammation and damage by mechanisms other than reduction of LDL cholesterol. Early initiation of statin treatment in patients with acute MI is associated with reduced 1-yr mortality.
- Additional poor prognostic factors include the following: cigarette smoking, history of hypertension or prior MI, presence of ST segment depression in acute MI, increasing age, diabetes mellitus, and female sex (especially women >50 yr of age).
- Plasma myeloperoxidase measurement may be a potentially useful lab test for stratification of patients presenting with chest pain. An elevated single initial measurement of plasma myeloperoxidase in patients presenting with chest pain independently predicts the early risk of MI, and the risk of major adverse events in the following 1 mo and 6 mo periods.

REFERENCES

Andersen HR et al: A comparison of coronary angioplasty with fibrinolytic therapy in acute myocardial infarction, *N Engl J Med* 349:733, 2003.

Becker RC: Antithrombotic therapy after myocardial infarction, *N Engl J Med* 347:1019, 2002.

Birnbaum Y et al: Ventricular septal rupture after acute myocardial infarction, *N Engl J Med* 347:1426, 2002.

Brennan ML et al: Prognostic value of myeloperoxidase in patients with chest pain. N Engl J Med 349:1595, 2003

Cannon CP, Baim DS: Expanding the reach of primary percutaneous coronary intervention for the treatment of acute myocardial infarction, *J Am Coll Cardiol* 39:1720, 2002.

Dickstein K et al: Effects of losartan and captopril on mortality and morbidity in high-risk patients after acute myocardial infarction: the OPTIMAAL randomized trial, *Lancet* 360:752, 2002.

Hurlen et al: Warfarin, aspirin, or both after myocardial infarction, *N Engl J Med* 347:969, 2002.

Khot UN et al: Prognostic importance of physical examination for heart failure in Non-ST elevation acute coronary syndromes, *JAMA* 290:2174, 2003.

Meier MA et al: The new definition of myocardial infarction, *Arch Intern Med* 162:1585, 2002.

Moss AJ et al: Prophylactic implantation of a defibrillator in patients with myocardial infarction and reduced ejection fraction, *N Engl J Med* 346:877, 2002.

Newby LK et al: Early statin initiation and outcomes in patients with acute coronary syndromes, *JAMA* 287:3087, 2002.

Stenestrand U, Wallentin L: Early revascularisation and 1-year survival in 14-day survivors of acute myocardial infarction: a prospective cohort study, *Lancet* 359:1805, 2002.

Stone GW et al: Comparison of angioplasty with stenting, with or without abciximab, in acute myocardial infarction, *N Engl J Med* 346:957, 2002.

Zimetbaum PJ, Josephson ME: Use of electrocardiogram in acute myocardial infarction, *N Engl J Med* 348:933, 2003.

Author: **Fred F. Ferri, M.D.**

BASIC INFORMATION

■ DEFINITION
Myocarditis is an inflammatory condition of the myocardium.

■ ICD-9CM CODES
429.0 Myocarditis, nonspecific
391.2 Myocarditis, rheumatic
422.91 Myocarditis, viral (except coxsackie)
074.23 Myocarditis, coxsackie
422.92 Myocarditis, bacterial

■ EPIDEMIOLOGY & DEMOGRAPHICS
- The incidence of focal myocarditis reported at autopsy is 1% to 7% in asymptomatic patients.
- Myocarditis is a major cause of sudden unexpected death (15% to 20% of cases) in adults <40 years of age.

■ PHYSICAL FINDINGS & CLINICAL PRESENTATION
- Persistent tachycardia out of proportion to fever
- Faint S_1, S_4 sound on auscultation
- Murmur of mitral regurgitation
- Pericardial friction rub if associated with pericarditis
- Signs of biventricular failure (hypotension, hepatomegaly, peripheral edema, distention of neck veins, S_3)
- Patients may present with a history of recent flulike syndrome (fever, arthralgias, malaise)

■ ETIOLOGY
- Infection
  1. Viral (coxsackie B virus, CMV, echovirus, polio virus, adenovirus, mumps, HIV, EBV)
  2. Bacterial (*Staphylococcus aureus, Clostridium perfringens,* diphtheria, and any severe bacterial infection)
  3. Mycoplasma
  4. Mycotic (*Candida, Mucor, Aspergillus*)
  5. Parasitic (*Trypanosoma cruzi, Trichinella, Echinococcus,* amoeba, *Toxoplasma*)
  6. *Rickettsia rickettsii*
  7. Spirochetal (*Borrelia burgdorferi*—Lyme carditis)
- Rheumatic fever
- Secondary to drugs (e.g., cocaine, emetine, doxorubicin, sulfonamides, isoniazid, methyldopa, amphotericin B, tetracycline, phenylbutazone, lithium, 5-FU, phenothiazines, interferon alfa, tricyclic antidepressants, cyclophosphamides)
- Toxins (carbon monoxide, ethanol, diphtheria toxin, lead, arsenicals)
- Collagen-vascular disease (SLE, scleroderma, sarcoidosis, Kawasaki syndrome)
- Sarcoidosis
- Radiation
- Postpartum

DIAGNOSIS

■ DIFFERENTIAL DIAGNOSIS
- Cardiomyopathy
- Acute myocardial infarction
- Valvulopathies
The differential diagnosis of chest pain is described in Section II

■ WORKUP
- Medical history: the clinical presentation of myocarditis is nonspecific and can consist of fatigue, palpitations, dyspnea, precordial discomfort, myalgias.
- Diagnostic workup includes chest x-ray examination, ECG, laboratory evaluation, echocardiogram, cardiac catheterization, and endomyocardial biopsy (selected patients).

■ LABORATORY TESTS
- Elevated cardiac troponin T (TnT) is suggestive of myocarditis in patients with clinically suspected myocarditis. A normal level does not rule out the diagnosis
- Increased CK (with elevated MB fraction, LDH), and AST secondary to myocardial necrosis
- Increased ESR (nonspecific but may be of value in following the progress of the disease and the response to therapy)
- Increased WBC (increased eosinophils if parasitic infection)
- Viral titers (acute and convalescent)
- Cold agglutinin titer, ASLO titer, blood cultures
- Lyme disease antibody titer

■ IMAGING STUDIES
- Chest x-ray examination: enlargement of cardiac silhouette
- ECG: sinus tachycardia with nonspecific ST-T wave changes; interventricular conduction defects and bundle branch block may be present
  1. Lyme disease and diphtheria cause all degrees of heart block.
  2. Changes of acute MI can occur with focal necrosis.
- Echocardiogram:
  1. Dilated and hypokinetic chambers
  2. Segmental wall motion abnormalities
- Cardiac catheterization and angiography:
  1. To rule out coronary artery disease and valvular disease.
  2. A right ventricular endomyocardial biopsy can confirm the diagnosis, although a negative biopsy result does not exclude myocarditis. Recent studies have shown that myocardial biopsy may be unnecessary, because immunosuppression therapy based on biopsy results is generally ineffective.

TREATMENT

■ NONPHARMACOLOGIC THERAPY
- Supportive care is the first line of therapy for patients with myocarditis.
- Restrict physical activity (to decrease cardiac work). Bed rest is advisable during viremia.

■ ACUTE GENERAL Rx
- Treat underlying cause (e.g., use specific antibiotics for bacterial infection).
- Treat CHF with diuretics, ACE inhibitors, and salt restriction. A β-blocker may be added once clinical stability has been achieved. Digoxin should be used with caution and only at low doses.
- If ventricular arrhythmias are present, treat with quinidine or procainamide.
- Provide anticoagulation to prevent thromboembolism.
- Use preload and afterload reducing agents for treating cardiac decompensation.
- Corticosteroid use is contraindicated in early infectious myocarditis; it may be justified in only selected patients with intractable CHF, severe systemic toxicity, and severe life-threatening arrhythmias.
- Immunosuppressive drugs (prednisone with cyclosporine or azathioprine) do not have any significant effect on the prognosis of myocarditis and should not be used in the routine treatment of patients with myocarditis. Immunosuppression may have a role in the treatment of myocarditis from systemic autoimmune disease (e.g., SLE, scleroderma) and in patients with idiopathic giant cell myocarditis.

■ DISPOSITION
Nearly 50% of patients with myocarditis will die within 5 yr of diagnosis. Prognosis is best for patients with "fulminant" lymphocytic myocarditis (severe hemodynamic compromise, rapid onset of symptoms, or high fever). These patients tend to have complete recovery with total resolution of myocarditis on repeat biopsy

■ REFERRAL
Consider heart transplant if patient develops intractable CHF.

REFERENCE
Wu LA et al: Current role of endomyocardial biopsy in the management of dilated cardiomyopathy and myocarditis, *Mayo Clin Proc* 76:1030, 2001.
Author: **Fred F. Ferri, M.D.**

BASIC INFORMATION

■ DEFINITION

Myotonia is a type of muscular dystrophy in which relaxation of a muscle after contraction is delayed or prolonged. The most common type of muscular dystrophy with myotonia is myotonic dystrophy, which is described below.

■ SYNONYMS

Myotonic dystrophy

ICD-9CM CODES

359.2 Myotonic disorders
728.85 Muscle spasm

■ EPIDEMIOLOGY & DEMOGRAPHICS

PREVALENCE: 3 to 5 cases/100,000 persons
- Genetic disorder inherited as an autosomal dominant illness
- Symptoms usually manifest during adolescence or early adulthood. Cases of infantile myotonic dystrophy have been described.

■ PHYSICAL FINDINGS & CLINICAL PRESENTATION

- Usual first complaint is distal extremity weakness sometimes associated with muscle stiffness, cramps, or difficulty relaxing the grasp.
- Weakness spreads to eventually involve all muscle groups. Flexor neck muscle weakness and masseter and temporal wasting are often prominent features, as is dysarthria.
- Percussion of a muscle produces a slow contraction followed by prolonged relaxation. The "myotonic reflex" is best tested by percussing the thenar muscles and observing a slow flexion followed by slow relaxation of the thumb.
- As the disease progresses, generalized weakness becomes more pronounced and myotonia becomes less evident.
- Extramuscular involvement:
  Mental retardation of variable severity (may be absent)
  Frontal baldness (Fig. 1-183)
  Cataracts
  Diabetes mellitus
  Hypogonadism
  Adrenal failure
  Cardiomyopathy
- Infantile myotonic dystrophy presents as neonatal extreme hypotonia with "shark mouth" deformity (upper lip forming an inverted V).

■ ETIOLOGY & PATHOGENESIS

Genetic disorder encoded on chromosome 19 leading to sustained firing of the muscle membrane, causing prolonged muscle contraction

DIAGNOSIS

■ DIFFERENTIAL DIAGNOSIS

- Myotonia congenita (Thomsen's disease)
  May be autosomal dominant or recessive (two distinct varieties)
  The disease is limited to muscles and causes hypertrophy and stiffness after rest. Muscle function normalizes with exercise. There is no weakness. Symptoms are exacerbated by exposure to cold.
- Paramyotonia congenita
  Autosomal dominant disease
  Weakness and stiffness of facial muscles and distal upper extremities, especially or exclusively on cold exposure
- Muscular dystrophies
- Inflammatory myopathies (polymyositis)
- Metabolic muscle diseases
- Myasthenic syndromes
- Motor neuron disease

■ WORKUP

- History and physical examination usually sufficient
- Muscle enzymes usually abnormal (CPK, aldolase, AST)
- EMG: typical myotonic "dive bomber" bursts
- Muscle biopsy: type I fiber atrophy, ring fibers, and increased central nucleation

TREATMENT

- Phenytoin
- Quinine
- Quinidine
- Procainamide
- Acetazolamide
- Genetic counseling
- Assistive devices, orthotics

■ REFERRAL

To neurologist

REFERENCE

Rose M, Griggs R: Inherited muscle, neuromuscular, and neuronal disorders. In Goetz CG (ed): *Textbook of clinical neurology*, Philadelphia, 1999, WB Saunders.
Author: **Tom J. Wachtel, M.D.**

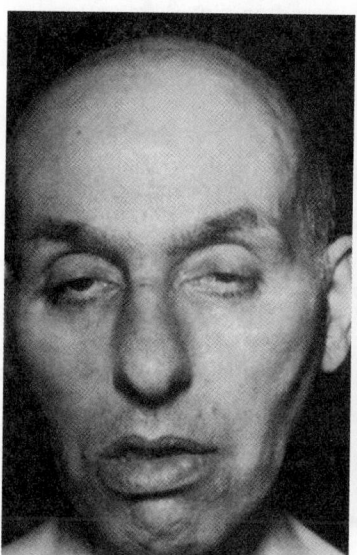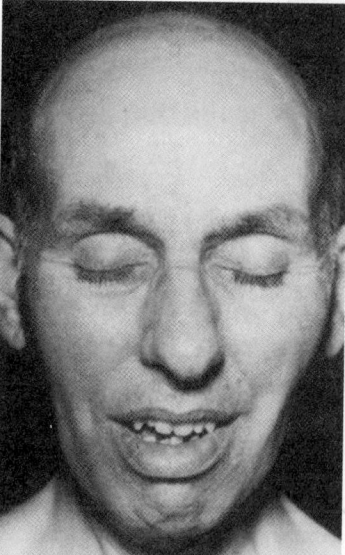

Fig. 1-183   Myotonic dystrophy with typical myopathic facies, frontal balding, and sunken cheeks. (From Dubowitz V: *Muscle disorders in childhood,* London, 1995, WB Saunders.)

BASIC INFORMATION

■ DEFINITION
Myxedema coma is a life-threatening complication of hypothyroidism characterized by profound lethargy or coma and usually accompanied by hypothermia.

ICD-9CM CODES
244.8 Myxedema, pituitary
244.1 Myxedema, primary

■ PHYSICAL FINDINGS & CLINICAL PRESENTATION
- Profound lethargy or coma
- Hypothermia (rectal temperature <35° C [95° F]); often missed by using ordinary thermometers graduated only to 34.5° C or because the mercury is not shaken below 36° C
- Bradycardia, hypotension (secondary to circulatory collapse)
- Delayed relaxation phase of DTR, areflexia
- Myxedema facies (Fig. 1-184)
- Alopecia, macroglossia, ptosis, periorbital edema, nonpitting edema, doughy skin
- Bladder dystonia and distention

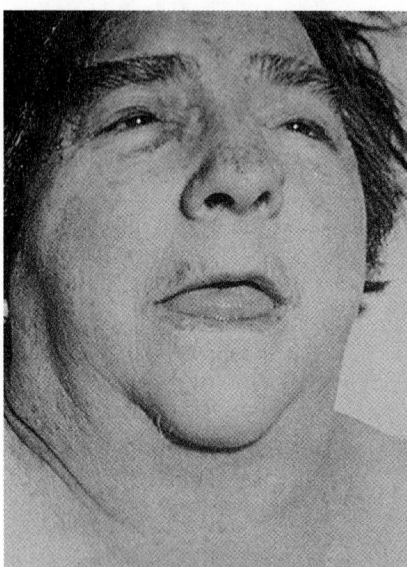

Fig. 1-184 Myxedema facies. Note dull, puffy, yellowed skin, coarse, sparse hair; temporal loss of eyebrows; periorbital edema; prominent tongue. (Courtesy Paul W. Ladenson, M.D. The Johns Hopkins University and Hospital, Baltimore: In Seidel HM [ed]: *Mosby's guide to physical examination*, ed 4, St Louis, 1999, Mosby.)

■ ETIOLOGY
Decompensation of hypothyroidism secondary to:
- Sepsis
- Exposure to cold weather
- CNS depressants (sedatives, narcotics, antidepressants)
- Trauma, surgery

DIAGNOSIS

■ DIFFERENTIAL DIAGNOSIS
- Severe depression, primary psychosis
- Drug overdose
- CVA, liver failure, renal failure
- Hypoglycemia, CO_2 narcosis, encephalitis

■ WORKUP
Diagnosis of hypothyroidism and exclusion of contributing factors (e.g., sepsis, CVA) with laboratory and radiographic studies (see Laboratory Tests)

■ LABORATORY TESTS
- Markedly increased TSH (if primary hypothyroidism), decreased serum free T_4
- CBC with differential, urine and blood cultures to rule out infectious process
- Electrolytes, BUN, creatinine, LFTs, calcium, glucose
- ABGs to rule out hypoxemia and carbon dioxide retention
- Cortisol level to rule out adrenal insufficiency
- Elevated CPK
- Hyperlipidemia

■ IMAGING STUDIES
- CT scan of head in suspected CVA
- Chest x-ray examination to rule out infectious process

TREATMENT

■ NONPHARMACOLOGIC THERAPY
- Prevent further heat loss; cover the patient but avoid external rewarming because it may produce vascular collapse.

- Support respiratory function; intubation and mechanical ventilation may be required.
- Monitor patients in the ICU.

■ ACUTE GENERAL Rx
- Give levothyroxine 5 to 8 μg/kg (300 to 500 μg) IV infused over 15 min, then 100 μg IV q24h.
- Glucocorticoids should also be administered until coexistent adrenal insufficiency can be ruled out. Hydrocortisone hemisuccinate 100 mg IV bolus is initially given, followed by 50 mg IV q12h or 25 mg IV q6h until initial plasma cortisol level is confirmed normal.
- IV hydration with D_5NS is used to correct hypotension and hypoglycemia (if present); avoid overhydration and possible water intoxication because clearance of free water is impaired in these patients.
- Rule out and treat precipitating factors (e.g., antibiotics in suspected sepsis).

■ CHRONIC Rx
Refer to "Hypothyroidism" in Section I.

■ DISPOSITION
Mortality rate in myxedema coma is 20% to 50%.

■ REFERRAL
Endocrinology consultation is appropriate in patients with myxedema coma.

PEARLS & CONSIDERATIONS

■ COMMENTS
If the diagnosis is suspected, initiate treatment immediately without waiting for confirming laboratory results.

REFERENCE
Wall CR: Myxedema coma: diagnosis and treatment, *Am Fam Physician* 62:2485, 2000.
Author: **Fred F. Ferri, M.D.**

BASIC INFORMATION

■ DEFINITION
Narcolepsy is a chronic neurologic disorder characterized by excessive daytime sleepiness and a dysregulation of rapid eye movement (REM) sleep features. Symptoms associated with the dysregulation of REM sleep include cataplexy, sleep paralysis, and hallucinations during the transition between sleep and wakefulness.

ICD-9CM CODES
347 Narcolepsy

■ EPIDEMIOLOGY & DEMOGRAPHICS
PREVALENCE: Approximately 1 in 2000 men and women in the U.S.
AGE OF ONSET: Peak 15-30 yr (range 10-55 yr)
GENETICS:
- Associated with specific human leukocyte antigen (HLA) subtypes DQB1*0602
- There is a 20-40 times higher risk of developing narcolepsy if there is an affected family member
- Monozygotic concordance rate is 17%-36%, indicating incomplete penetrance with an environmental contribution to the disease process

■ PHYSICAL FINDINGS & CLINICAL PRESENTATION
- Irresistible urges to sleep may occur during the day and lead to temporarily refreshing naps.
- Cataplexy occurs in 60%-100% of narcoleptics and is reported as a partial or total loss of voluntary muscle control with preserved consciousness that is precipitated by a strong emotion. This is the most specific symptom associated with narcolepsy.
- Sleep paralysis, which occurs in up to 80% of narcoleptics, is a loss of muscle tone during the transition between sleep and wakefulness. It may be associated with frightening or vivid hallucinations and can be interrupted by sensory stimuli.
- Hypnagogic (wake to sleep) or hypnopompic (sleep to wake) hallucinations may occur in 15%-80% of patients.
- Fragmented nighttime sleep is reported by 60%-90% of narcoleptics and may be mistaken for insomnia or other intrinsic sleep disorder.

■ ETIOLOGY
Narcolepsy is a complex disorder with no clear etiology. Research suggests that a deficient hypocretin/orexin system in the hypothalamus may be associated with the development of narcolepsy. Human cerebrospinal fluid levels of hypocretin-1 are low to undetectable in narcoleptics; however, this finding is not specific for narcolepsy.

DIAGNOSIS

■ DIFFERENTIAL DIAGNOSIS
Excessive daytime somnolence:
- Sleep apnea
- Inadequate sleep time
- Insomnia
- Hypothyroidism
- Drugs and alcohol
- Seizures
- Sleep fragmentation (multiple causes)

Cataplexy:
- Seizures
- Cardiovascular insufficiency
- Psychogenic (multiple causes)

■ WORKUP
- Medical history should include questions regarding sleep apnea, seizures, dissociated REM sleep features, and a detailed family history. Questions concerning other hypothalamic dysfunction such as unexplained weight gain, endocrinologic abnormalities, circadian dysrhythmias, and autonomic nervous system problems are also helpful.
- Overnight polysomnography followed by a multiple sleep latency test is the standard used for diagnosis. A clinical diagnosis of narcolepsy can be made with a clear history of cataplexy and excessive daytime somnolence. Without these features, the diagnosis depends upon the sleep laboratory testing.

■ LABORATORY TESTS
HLA subtyping and CSF hypocretin/orexin levels may be helpful in cases of suspected but unconfirmed narcolepsy; however, there is currently no clinical standard by which to interpret these results. Complicated cases should be referred to institutions with active narcolepsy protocols for further workup and data collection.

TREATMENT

■ NONPHARMACOLOGIC THERAPY
Scheduled daily naps can be used for symptoms of excessive daytime somnolence and to combat irresistible sleep urges.

■ CHRONIC Rx
For excessive daytime somnolence:
1. Modafinil (Provigil) 200-600 mg PO qam, or divided bid
2. Methylphenidate (Ritalin) 5-15 mg PO bid-tid
3. Dextroamphetamine (Dexedrine) 10-60 mg PO qd
4. Sodium Oxybate (Xyrem); contact the Xyrem Success Program for prescription information

For cataplexy and REM-related symptoms:
1. Fluoxetine (Prozac) 20 mg PO qd initially
2. Venlafaxine (Effexor) 25 mg PO qd initially
3. Sertraline (Zoloft) 25 mg PO qd initially
4. Clomipramine (Anafranil) 25 mg/day initially
5. Protriptyline (Vivactil) 5 mg tid initially
6. Imipramine (Tofranil) 25 to 50 mg/day initially
7. Desipramine (Norpramine) 10 mg bid initially
8. Sodium Oxybate (Xyrem); contact the Xyrem Success Program for prescription information

■ DISPOSITION
This is a chronic sleep disorder without periods of remission.

■ REFERRAL
Because this disorder is under intense investigation, patients should be referred to programs with sleep specialists who study, manage, and implement new therapies as they arise.

PEARLS & CONSIDERATIONS

Most narcoleptics report the onset of symptoms beginning in childhood to early adulthood. Often the symptoms of narcolepsy begin with excessive daytime sleepiness and progress with time to include REM-dysregulation (e.g., cataplexy, sleep paralysis, hypnagogic hallucinations).

■ COMMENTS
True narcolepsy is a relatively rare cause of excessive daytime sleepiness.

REFERENCES

Brooks SN, Guilleminault C: New insights into the pathogenesis and treatment of narcolepsy, *Curr Opin Pulm Med* 7(6):407, 2001.

Elliott AC: Primary care assessment and management of sleep disorders, *J Am Acad Nurs Pract* 13(9):409, 2001.

Greenhill LL et al: Practice parameter for the use of stimulant medications in the treatment of children, adolescents, and adults, *J Am Acad Child Adolesc Psychiatry* 41(2 suppl):26S, 2002.

Hublin C et al: Epidemiology of narcolepsy, *Sleep* 17:S7, 1994.

Krahn LE et al: Narcolepsy: new understanding of irresistible sleep, *Mayo Clin Proc* 76:185, 2001.

Mignot E: Genetic and familial aspects of narcolepsy, *Neuorology* 50:S16, 1998.

Mignot E et al: The role of cerebrospinal fluid hypocretin measurement in the diagnosis of narcolepsy and other hypersomnias, *Arch Neurol* 59:1553, 2002.

Overeem S et al: Narcolepsy: clinical features, new pathophysiologic insights, and future perspectives, *J Clin Neurophysiol* 18(2):78, 2001.

Scammell TE: The neurobiology, diagnosis, and treatment of narcolepsy, *Ann Neurol* 53:154, 2003.

Silber MH: Sleep disorders, *Neurol Clin* 19(1):173, 2001.

Thorpy M: Current concepts in the etiology, diagnosis and treatment of narcolepsy, *Sleep Med* 2:5, 2001.

Xyrem multicenter study group: A 12-month, open-label, multicenter extension trial of orally administered sodium oxybate for the treatment of narcolepsy, *Sleep* 26:31, 2003.

Author: **Jeffrey S. Durmer, M.D., Ph.D.**

BASIC INFORMATION

■ DEFINITION

Malignant renal tumor derived from primitive metanephric blastome. Most tumors are unicentric, but some are multifocal in one or both kidneys. Associated anomalies may be present.

■ SYNONYM

Wilms' Tumor

ICD-9CM CODES

189.0 Nephroblastoma

■ EPIDEMIOLOGY & DEMOGRAPHICS

- Pediatric malignancy mean presentation is at 41.5 mo in boys and 46.9 mo in girls
- Slightly more frequent in girls
- Incidence rate is 7.9 cases/yr/million white children <15 yr (a little over 500 new cases/yr in the U.S.); the incidence is double in black children
- Associated syndromes:
  1. Cryptorchidism
  2. Hypospadias
  3. Hemihypertrophy with or without the Beckwith-Wiedemann syndrome, aniridia
  4. Denys-Drash syndrome (nephroblastoma, pseudohermaphrodism, glomerulonephritis)
  5. WAGR syndrome (Wilms' tumor, aniridia, genitourinary malformations, and mental retardation)
- Familial nephroblastoma occurs in 1.5% (with younger age at diagnosis and more frequent multifocal tumors)

■ PHYSICAL FINDINGS & CLINICAL PRESENTATION

- Wilms' tumor often is discovered when a parent notices a mass while bathing or dressing a child, most commonly a child who is about 3 yr old, or during a routine physical examination. The mass is unilateral, firm, and nontender and below the costal margin
- Abdominal swelling and/or pain
- Nausea
- Vomiting
- Constipation
- Loss of appetite
- Fever of unknown origin
- Night sweats
- Hematuria (less common than in adult renal malignancies)
- Malaise
- High blood pressure that is triggered when the tumor obstructs the renal artery
- Varicocele
- Signs of associated syndromes

■ PATHOLOGY

- Three cell types: blastomal, stromal, and epithelial may be present. Structural diversity is characteristic.
- Anaplasia is evidenced by the presence of gigantic polyploid nuclei. The term *focal anaplasia* is used to describe such findings when it is confined within the primary tumor in the kidney.
- Staging

Stage I: Tumor limited to the kidney whose capsule is intact. The tumor is completely excised.

Stage II: Tumor extends beyond the kidney but is completely excised. No peritoneal involvement.

Stage III: Residual tumor confined to the abdomen following surgery. No hematogenous metastases.

Stage IV: Hematogenous metastases present.

Stage V: Bilateral renal involvement at time of initial diagnosis.

DIAGNOSIS

■ DIFFERENTIAL DIAGNOSIS

- Other renal malignancies
  1. Hypernephroma
  2. Transitional cell carcinoma
  3. Lymphoma
  4. Clear cell sarcoma
  5. Rhabdoid tumor of the kidney
- Renal cyst
- Other intraabdominal or retroperitoneal tumors.

■ LABORATORY TESTS

- CBC
- Transaminases (ALT, AST)
- Alkaline phosphatase
- BUN and creatinine
- Serum calcium
- Urinalysis

■ IMAGING STUDIES

- Renal ultrasound to confirm existence of a solid mass in a kidney
- Abdominal CT scan with contrast (Fig. 1-185)
- Chest x-ray or CT scan

TREATMENT

- Surgical resection and surgical staging
  1. Stages I and II: surgery followed by chemotherapy
  2. Stages III and IV: surgery followed by radiation and chemotherapy
- Chemotherapeutic agents used in the treatment of Wilms' tumor include vincristine, dactinomycin, and doxorubicin

■ PROGNOSIS

- Stage I: 95% survival
- Stage II: 91% survival
- Stage III: 91% survival
- Stage IV: 81% survival
- Prognosis is better for patients whose age is <2 yr

REFERENCE

Ebb DH et al: Solid tumors of childhood. In *Cancer, principles and practice of oncology*, ed 6, Philadelphia, 2001, Lippincott Williams & Wilkins.
Author: **Tom J. Wachtel, M.D.**

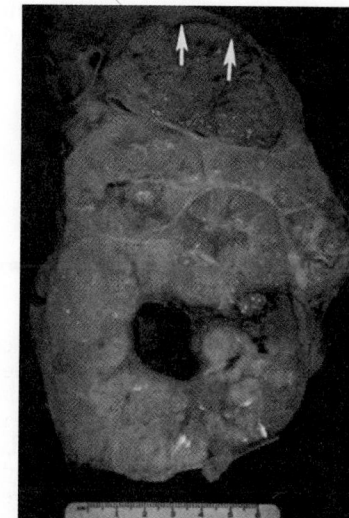
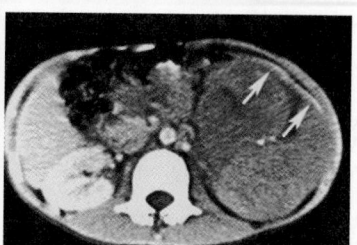

Fig. 1-185   Wilms' tumor. A, Gross specimen shows a large mass compressing a small rim of normal renal tissue (*arrows*). **B,** CT scan of kidney. A rim of compressed normal tissue represents the residual normal renal parenchyma (*arrows*). (From Behrman RE: *Nelson textbook of pediatrics,* ed 16, Philadelphia, 2000, WB Saunders.)

BASIC INFORMATION

■ DEFINITION

Nephrotic syndrome is characterized by high urine protein excretion (>3.5g/1.73 m³/24 hr), peripheral edema, and metabolic abnormalities (hypoalbuminemia, hypercholesterolemia).

ICD-9CM CODES
581.9 Nephrotic syndrome

■ EPIDEMIOLOGY & DEMOGRAPHICS

- Nephrotic syndrome occurs predominantly in children ages 2 to 6 yr (2 new cases/100,000 persons/yr) and in adults of all ages (3 to 4 new cases/100,000 persons/yr).
- Membranous glomerulonephritis is the most common cause of nephrotic syndrome.

■ PHYSICAL FINDINGS & CLINICAL PRESENTATION

- Peripheral edema
- Ascites, anasarca
- Hypertension
- Pleural effusion
- Typically patients present with severe peripheral edema, exertional dyspnea, and abdominal fullness secondary to ascites. There is a significant amount of weight gain in most patients

■ ETIOLOGY

- Idiopathic (may be secondary to the following glomerular diseases: minimal change disease [nil disease, lipoid nephrosis], focal segmental glomerular sclerosis, membranous nephropathy, membranoproliferative glomerular nephropathy)
- Associated with systemic diseases (diabetes mellitus, SLE, amyloidosis). Amyloidosis and dysproteinemias should be considered in patients older than 40 yr
- Majority of children with nephrotic syndrome have minimal change disease (this form also associated with allergy, nonsteroidals, and Hodgkin's disease)
- Focal glomerular disease: can be associated with HIV infection, heroin abuse. A more severe form of nephrotic syndrome associated with rapid progression to end-stage renal failure within months can also occur in HIV seropositive patients and is known as "collapsing glomerulopathy"
- Membranous nephropathy: can occur with Hodgkin's lymphoma, carcinomas, SLE, gold therapy
- Membranoproliferative glomerulonephropathy: often associated with upper respiratory infections

DIAGNOSIS

■ DIFFERENTIAL DIAGNOSIS

- Other edema states (CHF, cirrhosis)
- Primary renal disease (e.g., focal glomerulonephritis, membranoproliferative glomerulonephritis). Table 1-40 summarizes primary renal diseases that present as idiopathic nephrotic syndrome
- Carcinoma, infections
- Malignant hypertension
- Polyarteritis nodosa
- Serum sickness
- Toxemia of pregnancy

■ WORKUP

- Diagnostic workup consists of family history and history of drug use or toxin exposure and laboratory evaluation. Renal biopsy is generally performed in individuals with persistent proteinuria in whom the etiology of the proteinuria is unclear.

■ LABORATORY TESTS

- Urinalysis reveals proteinuria. The presence of hematuria, cellular casts, and pyuria is suggestive of nephritic syndrome. Oval fat bodies (tubular epithelial cells with cholesterol esters) are also found in the urine in patients with nephrotic syndrome.
- 24-hr urine protein excretion is >3.5 g/1.73 m³/24 hr.
- Abnormalities of blood chemistries include serum albumin <3 g/dl, decreased total protein, elevated serum cholesterol, glucose, azotemia.
- Additional tests in patients with nephrotic syndromes depending on the history and physical examination are ANA, serum and urine immunoelectrophoresis, C3, C4, CH-50, LDH, liver enzymes, alkaline phosphatase, hepatitis B and C screening, and HIV.

■ IMAGING STUDIES

- Ultrasound of kidneys
- Chest x-ray

TREATMENT

■ NONPHARMACOLOGIC THERAPY

- Bed rest as tolerated, avoidance of nephrotoxic drugs, low-fat diet, fluid restriction in hyponatremic patients; normal protein intake unless urinary protein loss exceeds 10 g/24 hr (some patients may require additional dietary protein to prevent negative nitrogen balance and significant protein malnutrition)
- Improved urinary protein excretion and serum lipid changes have been observed with a low-fat soy protein diet providing 0.7 g of protein/kg/day. However, because of increased risk of malnutrition, many nephrologists recommend normal protein intake
- Strict sodium restriction to help manage peripheral edema
- Close monitoring of patients for development of peripheral venous thrombosis and renal vein thrombosis because of hypercoagulable state secondary to loss of antithrombin III and other proteins involved in the clotting mechanism

■ ACUTE GENERAL Rx

- Furosemide is useful for severe edema.
- Use of ACE inhibitors to reduce proteinuria is generally indicated even in normotensive patients.
- Anticoagulant therapy should be administered as long as patients have nephrotic proteinuria, an albumin level <20 g/L, or both.

The mainstay of therapy is treatment of the underlying disorder:

- Minimal change disease generally responds to prednisone 1 mg/kg/day. Relapses can occur when steroids are discontinued. In these individuals, cyclophosphamide and chlorambucil may be useful.
- Focal and segmental glomerulosclerosis: steroid therapy is also recommended. However, response rate is approximately 35% to 40%, and most patients progress to end-stage renal disease within 3 yr.
- Membranous glomerulonephritis: prednisone 2 mg/kg/day may be useful in inducing remission. Cytotoxic agents can be added if there is poor response to prednisone.
- Membranoproliferative glomerulonephritis: most patients are treated with steroid therapy and antiplatelet drugs. Despite treatment, the majority of patients will progress to end-stage renal disease within 5 yr.

■ CHRONIC Rx

- Patients should be monitored for azotemia and should be aggressively treated for hypertension and hyperlipidemia. Furosemide is useful for severe edema. Anticoagulants may be necessary for thromboembolic events. Prophylactic anticoagulation should be considered in patients with membranous glomerulonephritis.
- Oral vitamin D is useful in the treatment of hypocalcemia (because of vitamin D loss).

■ REFERRAL

Nephrology consultation is recommended in all cases of nephrotic syndrome.

Author: **Fred F. Ferri, M.D.**

TABLE 1-40 Summary of Primary Renal Diseases That Present as Idiopathic Nephrotic Syndrome

	MINIMAL-CHANGE NEPHROTIC SYNDROME (MCNS)	FOCAL SEGMENTAL SCLEROSIS	MEMBRANOUS NEPHROPATHY	MEMBRANOPROLIFERATIVE GLOMERULONEPHRITIS (MPGN)	
				TYPE I	TYPE II
Frequency*					
Children	75%	10%	<5%	10%	10%
Adults	15%	15%	50%	10%	10%
Clinical Manifestations					
Age (yr)	2-6, some adults	2-10, some adults	40-50	5-15	5-15
Sex	2:1 male	1.3:1 male	2:1 male	Male-female	Male-female
Nephrotic syndrome	100%	90%	80%	60%	60%
Asymptomatic proteinuria	0	10%	20%	40%	40%
Hematuria	10%-20%	60%-80%	60%	80%	80%
Hypertension	10%	20% early	Infrequent	35%	35%
Rate of progression to renal failure	Does not progress	10 years	50% in 10-20 yr	10-20 yr	5-15 yr
Associated conditions	Allergy? Hodgkin's disease, usually none	None	Renal vein thrombosis, cancer, SLE, hepatitis B	None	Partial lipodystrophy
Laboratory Findings	Manifestations of nephrotic syndrome ↑ BUN in 15%-30%	Manifestations of nephrotic syndrome ↑ BUN in 20%-40%	Manifestations of nephrotic syndrome	Low C1, C4, C3-C9	Normal C1, C4, low C3-C9
Immunogenetics	HLA-B8, B12 (3.5)†	Not established	HLA-DRW3 (12-32)†	Not established	C3 nephritic factor Not established
Renal Pathology					
Light microscopy	Normal	Focal sclerotic lesions	Thickened GBM, spikes	Thickened GBM, proliferation	Lobulation
Immunofluorescence	Negative	IgM, C3 in lesions	Fine granular IgG, C3	Granular IgG, C3	C3 only
Electron microscopy	Foot process fusion	Foot process fusion	Subepithelial deposits	Mesangial and subendothelial deposits	Dense deposits
Response of Steroids	90%	15%-20%	May slow progression	Not established	Not established

Modified from Goldman L, Ausiello D (eds): *Cecil textbook of medicine*, ed 22, Philadelphia, 2004, WB Saunders.
*Approximate frequency as a cause of idiopathic nephrotic syndrome. About 10% of adult nephrotic syndrome is due to various diseases that usually present with acute glomerulonephritis.
†Relative risk.
↑, Elevated; *BUN*, blood urea nitrogen; *C*, complement; *GBM*, glomerular basement membrane; *hepatitis B*, hepatitis B virus; *HLA*, human leukocyte antigen; *Ig*, immunoglobulin; *SLE*, systemic lupus erythematosus.

BASIC INFORMATION

■ DEFINITION
Neuroblastomas are tumors of post-ganglionic sympathetic neurons that typically originate in the adrenal medulla or the sympathetic chain/ganglion. Often present at birth, but not diagnosed until later, when the child shows symptoms of the disease.

ICD-9CM CODES
194.0 Neuroblastoma, unspecified site

■ EPIDEMIOLOGY & DEMOGRAPHICS
INCIDENCE (IN U.S.): 8%-10% of all solid tumors of childhood; 1/10,000 children <15 yr
PREDOMINANT SEX: Male:female ratio of 1:1.3
PEAK AGE: Mean age of onset is 18 mo; 75% onset by 5 yr; 97% by 10 yr
GENETICS: N-*myc* protooncogene; loss of short arm chromosome 1 (1p36) found in some tumors. There is a small subset with an autosomal dominant pattern of inheritance.

■ PHYSICAL FINDINGS & CLINICAL PRESENTATION
- Mass in abdomen, neck, or chest (Fig. 1-186). 70%-80% of children have regional lymph node involvement or distant metastases at time of presentation
- Spinal cord/paraspinal: can present with back pain, signs of compression—paraplegia, stool/urine retention
- Thoracic: difficulty breathing, dysphagia, infections, chronic cough
- Secondary symptoms referable to metastatic disease: chronic pain, pancytopenia, periorbital ecchymosis, proptosis, weight loss, fever, multiple subcutaneous bluish nodules, irritability

■ PARANEOPLASTIC SYNDROMES
- Angiotensin → hypertension
- Catecholamines → hypertension, flushing
- Opsoclonus-Myoclonus syndrome → "dancing eyes, dancing feet," myoclonic jerks and chaotic eye movements in all directions; may be initial presentation before tumor diagnosis
- Progressive cerebellar ataxia

DIAGNOSIS

■ DIFFERENTIAL DIAGNOSIS
- Other small, round, blue-cell childhood tumors, such as lymphoma and rhabdomyosarcoma
- Wilms' tumor

■ WORKUP
- Careful general physical examination
- Biopsy and resection of tumor when possible

■ LABORATORY TESTS
- 24-hour urine for catecholamines → homovanillic acid (HVA) and vanillymandelic acid (VMA) are secreted by 90%-95% of tumors
- Bone marrow biopsy and aspirate → karyotype, DNA index, N-myc copy number

■ IMAGING STUDIES
- Chest x-ray, abdominal x-ray, skeletal survey, abdominal ultrasound
- CT scan of the chest and abdomen
- Body scan with ^{131}I-MIBG (meta-iodobenzylguanidine) → taken up by neuroblasts
- Bone scan Tc-99 MDP → visualize lytic bone lesions and metastases

■ STAGING (EVANS CLASSIFICATION)
I. Confined to single organ
II. Extension beyond organ of origin but not past midline
III. Extension across midline
IV. Distant metastases

TREATMENT

■ NONPHARMACOLOGIC THERAPY
Assure patient that there is hope for recovery with aggressive treatment.

■ ACUTE GENERAL Rx
- Overall, treatment will be determined by several factors, including age at diagnosis, stage of disease, site of primary tumor and metastases and tumor histology
- Surgery
- Radiation therapy
- Multiagent chemotherapy is mainstay (e.g., cisplatinum, etoposide, adriamycin, cyclophosphamide, carboplatin)
- Autologous bone marrow transplantation following aggressive chemotherapy for stage IV disease
- Immunotherapy using monoclonal antibodies and vaccines that attempt to initiate an immune reaction against the disease are under development

■ DISPOSITION/PROGNOSIS
- Refer immediately to a multidisciplinary oncology team
- Overall survival is >40%. Children under the age of 1 yr have a cure rate as high as 90%
- Poor prognosis associated with stage IV disease (20% survival compared with >95% in stage I), age >1 yr at diagnosis, increased number of N-myc copies, adrenal tumor, chronic 1p deletion

REFERENCES
Bown N: Neuroblastoma tumor genetics: clinical and biological aspects, *J Clin Path* 54(12):897, 2001.
Schilling FH et al: Neuroblastoma screening at one year of age, *N Engl J Med* 346:1047, 2002.
Woods WG et al: Screening of infants and mortality due to neuroblastoma, *N Engl J Med* 346:1041, 2002.
Author: **Nicole J. Ullrich, M.D., Ph.D.**

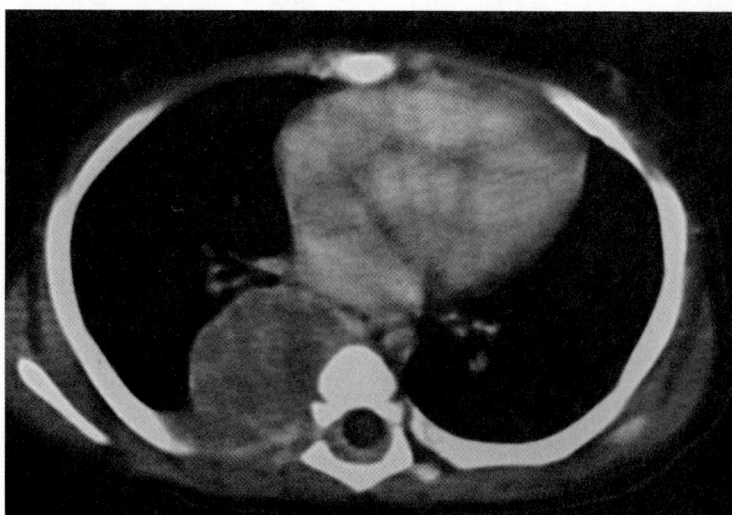

Fig. 1-186 CT scan of a thoracic neuroblastoma with intraspinal extension at diagnosis. (From Behrman RE: *Nelson textbook of pediatrics,* Philadelphia, 1996, WB Saunders.)

BASIC INFORMATION

■ DEFINITION
Neurofibromatosis (NF) is an autosomal dominant inherited neurocutaneous disorder. There are two types of neurofibromatosis disorders: NF type 1 (NF1) and NF type 2 (NF2).

■ SYNONYMS
- NF1 is also called von Recklinghausen disease
- NF2 is also called bilateral acoustic neurofibromatosis

ICD-9CM CODES
237.71 Type 1, von Recklinghausen's
237.72 Type 2, acoustic

■ EPIDEMIOLOGY & DEMOGRAPHICS
- Incidence of NF1 (1/3000), NF2 (1/33,000)
- Prevalence of NF1 (1/5000), NF2 (1/210,000)
- NF1 and NF2 are autosomal dominant, with approximately 50% of cases having no family history
- The two disorders affect approximately 100,000 people in the U.S.
- Equally affects males and females
- NF1 may be associated with optic gliomas, astrocytomas, spinal neurofibromas, pheochromocytomas, and chronic myeloid leukemia
- NF2 may be associated with meningiomas, spinal schwannomas, and cataracts

■ PHYSICAL FINDINGS & CLINICAL PRESENTATION
- Common features of NF1 include:
  1. Café-au-lait macules (100% of children by age 2)
     a. Hyperpigmented skin lesions occurring anywhere on the body except the face, palms, and soles
     b. Appear early in life and increase in size and number during puberty
     c. Focal or diffuse
  2. Axillary and inguinal freckling (70%)
  3. Multiple cutaneous and subcutaneous neurofibromas (95%) (Fig. 1-187)
     a. Firm, varying in size from mm to cm
     b. Vary in number from a few to thousands
     c. May be sessile, pedunculated, regular or irregular in shape
  4. Lisch nodule (small hamartoma of the iris) found in >90% of adult cases
  5. Visual defects possibly related to optic gliomas (2% to 5%)
  6. Neurodevelopment problems (30% to 40%)

- Common features of NF2 include:
  1. Hearing loss and tinnitus related to bilateral acoustic neuromas (>90% of adults)
  2. Cataracts (81%)
  3. Headache
  4. Unsteady gait
  5. Cutaneous neurofibromas but less than NF1
  6. Café-au-lait macules (1%)

■ ETIOLOGY
- NF1 is caused by DNA mutations located on the long arm of chromosome 17 responsible for encoding the protein neurofibromin.
- NF2 is caused by DNA mutations located in the middle of the long arm of chromosome 22 responsible for encoding the protein merlin.

DIAGNOSIS

- NF1 is diagnosed if the person has two or more of the following features:
  1. Six or more café-au-lait macules >5 mm in prepubertal patients and >15 mm in postpubertal patients
  2. Two or more neurofibromas of any type or one plexiform neurofibroma
  3. Axillary or inguinal freckling
  4. Optic glioma

  5. Two or more Lisch nodules (iris hamartomas)
  6. Sphenoid wing dysplasia or cortical thinning of long bones, with or without pseudarthrosis
  7. A first-degree relative (parent, sibling, or child) with NF1 based on the previous criteria
- NF2 is diagnosed if the person has either of the following two criteria:
  1. Bilateral eighth nerve masses seen by appropriate imaging studies
  2. A first-degree relative with NF2 and either a unilateral eighth nerve mass or two of the following: neurofibroma, meningioma, glioma, schwannoma, or juvenile posterior subcapsular lenticular opacity

■ WORKUP
The diagnosis of neurofibromatosis is usually self-evident. Workup is dictated by clinical symptoms in NF1 and usually includes MRI evaluation of the head and spine in NF2.

■ LABORATORY TESTS
- Genetic testing is possible in individuals who desire prenatal diagnosis for NF1. There is no single standard test and multiple tests are required. Results can only tell if an individual is affected but cannot predict the severity of the disease.

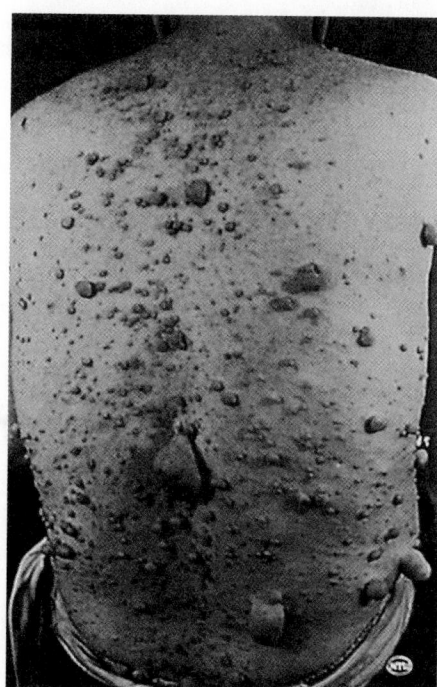

Fig. 1-187 Nodules. Solid, large (>1 cm), deep-seated mass in dermal or subcutaneous tissues. These nodules are neurofibromas in a patient with neurofibromatosis. (From Goldman L, Ausiello D [eds]: *Cecil textbook of medicine,* ed 22, Philadelphia, 2004, WB Saunders.)

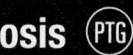
- In NF2, linkage analysis testing provides a >99% certainty the individual has NF2.

■ IMAGING STUDIES
- MRI with gadolinium is the imaging study of choice in both NF1 and NF2 patients. MRI increases detection of optic gliomas, tumors of the spine, acoustic neuromas, and "bright spots" thought to represent hamartomas.
- MRI of the spine is recommended in all patients diagnosed with NF2 to exclude intramedullary tumors.

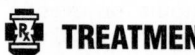

TREATMENT

Treatment is directed primarily at symptoms and complications of NF1 and NF2.

■ NONPHARMACOLOGIC THERAPY
- Counseling addressing prognosis, genetic, psychologic, and social issues
- Slit-lamp examination by an ophthalmologist searching for cataracts and hamartomas
- Hearing testing and speech pathology evaluation

■ ACUTE GENERAL Rx
- Surgery is usually not done on skin tumors unless cosmetically requested or if suspicion of malignant transformation exists.

- Surgery may be indicated for spinal or cranial neurofibromas, gliomas, or meningiomas.
- Acoustic neuromas can be treated by surgical excision.

■ CHRONIC Rx
- Radiation may be indicated in NF1 patients with optic nerve gliomas.
- Stereotactic radiosurgery using gamma knife may be an alternative approach to surgery for acoustic neuromas.

■ DISPOSITION
- Prognosis varies according to the severity of involvement.
- There is no cure for neurofibromatosis.

■ REFERRAL
A multidisciplinary team of consultants is needed in patients with neurofibromatosis including neurosurgeon, otolaryngologist, dermatologist, neurologist, audiologist, speech pathologist, and neuropsychologist.

PEARLS & CONSIDERATIONS

■ COMMENTS
- Friedrich Daniel von Recklinghausen first reported his cases in 1882, although there had been similar accounts dating back to the 1600s.
- The first report in the literature of NF2 was by Wishart in 1822.

- For additional information refer to the National Neurofibromatosis Foundation (141 Fifth Avenue, Suite 7-S, New York, NY 10010, 800-322-7838) or Neurofibromatosis Inc. (3401 Woodbridge Court, Mitchellville, MD 20716, 301-577-8984).

REFERENCES
Evans DG, Sainio M, Baser NE: Neurofibromatosis type 2, *J Med Genet* 37(12):897, 2000.

Gutmann DH et al: The diagnostic evaluation and multidisciplinary management of neurofibromatosis 1 and neurofibromatosis 2, *JAMA* 278(1):51, 1997.

Karnes PS: Neurofibromatosis: a common neurocutaneous disorder, *Mayo Clin Proc* 73(11):1071, 1998.

Korf BP: Diagnosis and management of neurofibronatosum type 1, *Curr Neurol Neurosci Rep* 1(2):162, 2001.

Lakkis MM, Tennekoon GI: Neurofibronatosin type 1: 1 general overview, *J Neurosci Res* 62(6):755, 2000.

Young H, Hyman S, North K: Neurofibromatosis 1: clinical review and exception to the rates, *J Child Neurol* 17(8):588, 2002.

Author: **Peter Petropoulos, M.D.**

BASIC INFORMATION

■ DEFINITION

Neuroleptic malignant syndrome is a disorder characterized by hyperthermia, muscular rigidity, autonomic dysfunction, and depressed/fluctuating levels of arousal that evolve over 24-72 hours. This occurs as an idiosyncratic adverse reaction most commonly to dopamine-receptor antagonists (especially D2/4 receptor) or sudden withdrawal from a dopaminergic agent or agonist, such as antiparkinsonian medications.

ICD-9CM CODES

333.92 Neuroleptic malignant syndrome

■ EPIDEMIOLOGY & DEMOGRAPHICS

INCIDENCE (IN U.S.): 0.07%-0.15% annual incidence in psychiatric population.

Incidence falling from as high as 1.4% to 12.2% in the 1980s because of better recognition of early signs, low threshold to discontinue typical neuroleptics, and more frequent use of atypical agents.

PREDOMINANT SEX: More than two thirds of patients are male.

PREDOMINANT AGE: Young and middle-aged adults

PREDISPOSING FACTORS:
- High-potency dopamine antagonists
- Long-acting depot preparations or multiple agents used
- Preexisting brain disease

■ PHYSICAL FINDINGS & CLINICAL PRESENTATION

- Muscle rigidity (hypertonia, cogwheeling, or "lead pipe" rigidity)
- Hyperthermia (38.6° to 42.3° C, usually <40° C)
- Autonomic symptoms: diaphoresis, sialorrhea, skin pallor, urinary incontinence
- Tachycardia, tachypnea
- Labile BP (Hypertension or postural hypotension)
- Mental status changes (agitation, catatonia, fluctuating consciousness, obtundation)

■ ETIOLOGY

- Unknown. Impaired thermoregulation in hypothalamus and limbic cortex may occur as a result of relative lack of dopamine activity (central dopamine-blockade hypothesis: most accepted)
- Neuroleptic drugs have different potencies for inducing NMS:
Typical neuroleptics: High potency—haloperidol; medium potency—chlorpromazine, fluphenazine; low potency—levomepromazine, loxapine

Atypical neuroleptics: Low potency—risperidone, olanzapine, clozapine, quetiapine

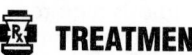

DIAGNOSIS

■ DIFFERENTIAL DIAGNOSIS

- Heatstroke, drug-induced states and overdose (ecstasy abuse, phencyclidine), thyrotoxicosis, pheochromocytoma, serotonin syndrome
- Malignant hyperthermia, catatonia, acute psychosis with agitation
- Central nervous system or systemic infections, including sepsis

■ WORKUP

Careful drug history

■ LABORATORY TESTS

- Elevated CPK (in 71% of patients, with a mean value of 3700 U/L)
- Urinary myoglobin
- Leukocytosis, usually 10,000 to 40,000/mm³
- Electrolytes and renal function
- Blood gases
- Drug levels

■ IMAGING STUDIES

None specific for this disease

TREATMENT

■ NONPHARMACOLOGIC THERAPY

- Stop all neuroleptic agents and reinstitute any recently discontinued dopaminergic agents
- Respiratory support; nutritional support in cases with dysphagia or comatose
- Careful fluid balance monitoring with adequate hydration (intravenous in severe cases)
- Active cooling (cooling blanket and antipyretics)
- Skilled nursing care to prevent decubitus ulcers in bed-confined patients

■ ACUTE GENERAL Rx

- Intravenous benzodiazepines (e.g., diazepam 2-10 mg, with total daily dose of 10-60 mg) to relax muscles and control agitation.
- Bromocriptine, a dopamine receptor agonist, is the mainstay of therapy for patients with neuroleptic malignant syndrome. Initial doses of 2.5 to 10 mg are given IV q8h and are increased by 5 mg/day until clinical improvement is seen. The drug should be continued for at least 10 days after the syndrome has been controlled and then tapered slowly.
- Amantadine, a NMDA receptor antagonist with possible dopaminergic properties, administered orally at doses of 100-200 mg PO bid, has

been shown to reduce mortality in comparison to supportive therapy alone.
- Dantrolene therapy is also effective. Initially, patients can be given 0.25 mg/kg IV q6-12h, followed by a maintenance dose up to 3 mg/kg/day. After 2 to 3 days, patients may be given the drug orally (25 to 600 mg/day in divided doses). Oral dantrolene therapy (50-600 mg/day) may be continued for several days afterwards.
- Electroconvulsive therapy with neuromuscular blockage in pharmacologically refractory cases. Succinylcholine should not be used as it may cause hyperkalemia and cardiac arrhythmias in patients with rhabdomyolysis or dysautonomia.

■ CHRONIC Rx

- Mortality rate is currently 5%-10% despite previous therapeutic measures. Serious sequelae may occur in a further 20%. Complete recovery occurs in >70% of patients. Mortality rates have declined from 15%-25% because of earlier recognition and aggressive pharmacologic and supportive care.
- Factors adversely affecting mortality are development of renal failure and core temperature >104° F (40° C).
- Respiratory care, nutritional support, and physical therapy in more severe cases.

■ DISPOSITION

Monitor closely for future complications of pharmacologic therapy.

■ REFERRAL

If patient's condition is critical, patients are preferably treated in a medical/neurologic ICU.

PEARLS & CONSIDERATIONS

■ COMMENTS

Early detection and diagnosis lead to a more favorable outcome. Treatment is a medical emergency.

REFERENCES

Buckley PF, Sajatovic M, Adityanjee. Neuroleptic malignant syndrome. In Katirji B et al: *Neuromuscular disorders in clinical practice.* Boston, 2002, Butterworth-Heinemann.

Sueman VL: Clinical management of neuroleptic malignant syndrome, *Psychiatr Q* 72(4):825, 2001.

Ty EB, Rothner AD: Neuroleptic malignant syndrome in children and adolescents, *J Child Neurol* 16(3):157, 2001.

Author: **Eroboghene E. Ubogu, M.D.**

BASIC INFORMATION

■ DEFINITION
Nocardiosis is an infection caused by aerobic actinomycetes found in soil and characterized by lung, soft tissue, or CNS involvement.

ICD-9CM CODES
039 Actinomycotic infections
039.9 Nocardiosis NOS, of unspecified site

■ EPIDEMIOLOGY & DEMOGRAPHICS
- *Nocardia* species are found worldwide in the soil.
- Nocardiosis is found most commonly in patients who are compromised (e.g., receiving steroids, immunosuppressive therapy, lymphoma, leukemia, lung cancer, and other pulmonary infections).
- Other underlying conditions associated with nocardiosis are pemphigus vulgaris, Whipple's disease, Goodpasture's syndrome, Cushing's disease, cirrhosis, ulcerative colitis, and rheumatoid arthritis.
- Use of steroids is an independent risk factor for developing Nocardiosis.
- Between 500 to 1000 new cases are diagnosed each year in the United States.
- Approximately 2% of patients with AIDS develop nocardiosis.
- Occurs more commonly in men than in women (2:1).
- Adults > children.

■ PHYSICAL FINDINGS & CLINICAL PRESENTATION
- Inhalation of *Nocardia* organisms is the most common mode of entry, and pneumonia is the most common presentation, with 75% manifesting with fever, chills, dyspnea, and a productive cough (Fig. 1-188).
  1. Presentation can be acute, subacute, or chronic.
  2. Nocardiosis should be suspected if soft tissue abscesses or CNS tumors or abscesses form in conjunction with the pulmonary infection.
  3. Pulmonary infection may spread into the pericardium, mediastinum, and superior vena cava.
- Cutaneous disease usually occurs via direct inoculation of the organism as a result of skin puncture by a thorn or splinter, surgery, IV catheter use, or animal scratches or bites manifesting in:
  1. Cellulitis
  2. Lymphocutaneous nodules appearing along lymphatic sites draining the infected puncture wound
  3. Mycetoma (Madura foot), a chronic deep nodular infection usually involving the hands or feet that can cause skin breakdown, fistula formation, and spread along the fascial planes to infect surrounding skin, subcutaneous tissue, and bone
- The CNS system is infected in approximately one third of all cases. Brain abscesses is the most common pathologic finding.
- Dissemination of nocardiosis may infect other tissues and organs including kidney, heart, skin, and bone.

■ ETIOLOGY
- The most common *Nocardia* species leading to infection in humans are:
  1. *N. asteroides* (causing more than 80% of the cases of pulmonary nocardiosis)
  2. *N. brasiliensis* (most common cause of mycetoma)
  3. *N. otitidiscaviarum*
- *N. asteroides* has two subgroups
  1. *N. farcinica*
  2. *N. nova*

DIAGNOSIS

The diagnosis of nocardiosis requires a high index of suspicion in the proper clinical setting and is confirmed by bacteriologic staining and growth of the organism in culture.

■ DIFFERENTIAL DIAGNOSIS
- There are no pathognomonic findings separating nocardiosis pneumonia from other infectious etiologies of the lung. Diagnoses presenting in a similar manner and often confused for nocardiosis are:
  1. Tuberculosis
  2. Lung abscess
  3. Lung tumor
  4. Other causes of pneumonia
  5. Actinomycosis
  6. Mycosis
  7. Cellulitis
  8. Coccidioidomycosis
  9. Histoplasmosis
  10. Aspergillosis
  11. Kaposi's sarcoma

■ WORKUP
All patients with suspected nocardiosis need laboratory identification of the microorganism by obtaining sputum in the case of pneumonia, cultures of the infected skin lesions in mycetoma or lymphocutaneous disease, or the sampling of any purulent material (e.g., brain abscess, lung abscess, and pleural effusion).

■ LABORATORY TESTS
- Blood tests are not very sensitive in the diagnosis of nocardiosis.
- Gram stain shows gram-positive beaded filaments with multiple branches.
- Gomori methenamine silver staining may detect the organism.

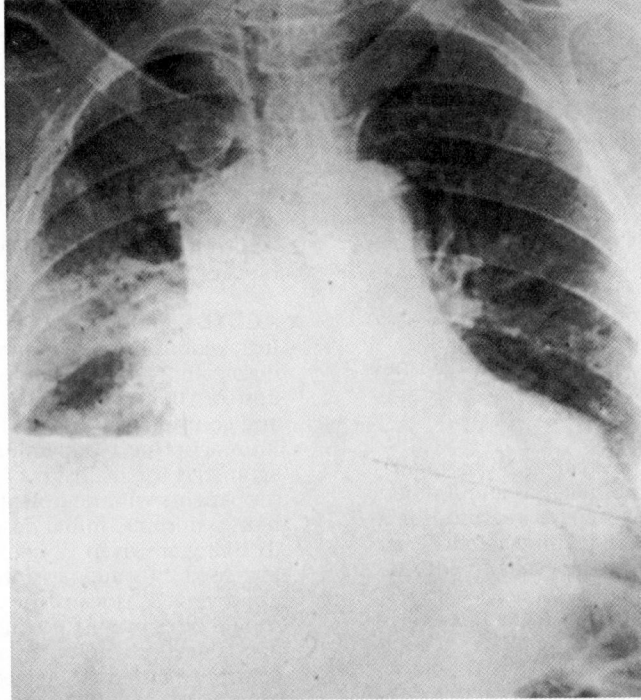

Fig. 1-188 Right lower lobe *Nocardia* pneumonia in a renal transplant recipient. (From Gorbach SL: *Infectious diseases*, ed 2, Philadelphia, 1998, WB Saunders.)

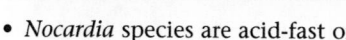
- *Nocardia* species are acid-fast on a modified Ziehl-Neelsen stain.
- *Nocardia* are slow-growing organisms and colony growth in cultures may take up to 2 to 3 wk.

■ IMAGING STUDIES
- Chest x-ray may demonstrate infiltrates, densities, nodules, cavitary masses, or multiple abscesses.
- CT scan of the brain is indicated in the appropriate clinical setting to exclude CNS brain abscesses.

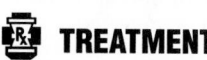 ## TREATMENT

■ NONPHARMACOLOGIC THERAPY
- Supportive therapy with oxygen in patients with pneumonia
- Chest physiotherapy
- For any abscess formation, surgical drainage indicated (e.g., skin, lung, or brain)

■ ACUTE GENERAL Rx
- There are no prospective randomized trials to date highlighting the most effective treatment of Nocardiosis. Nevertheless, sulfonamides are considered the treatment of choice. Sulfadiazine 6 to 10 g is given in 4 to 6 divided oral doses.
- Trimethoprim-sulfamethoxazole (160 mg/800 mg) given orally every 6 to 8 hr.
- Amikacin has been the IV antibiotic of choice.

- Alternative drug treatment includes:
  1. Minocycline 100 to 200 mg bid
  2. Erythromycin 500 mg qid and ampicillin 1 g qid for *N. nova* species
  3. Amoxicillin 500 mg and clavulanate 125 mg tid
  4. Ofloxacin 400 mg bid
  5. Clarithromycin 500 mg bid

■ CHRONIC Rx
- Although the optimal duration of therapy has not been determined, long-term therapy is generally recommended for all infections caused by *Nocardia*.
- Patients with cellulitis and lymphocutaneous syndrome are treated for 2 to 4 mo depending on whether there is bone involvement or not.
- Mycetomas are best treated with antibiotics for 6 to 12 mo but may require surgical drainage.
- Pulmonary and systemic nocardiosis excluding the CNS is treated for 6 to 12 mo.
- CNS involvement is treated with drainage and antibiotics for 12 mo.
- All immunosuppressed patients should receive 12 mo of antibiotic therapy.

■ DISPOSITION
- Patients with pulmonary nocardiosis have a mortality rate of 15% to 30%.
- CNS involvement carries a >40% mortality rate.
- Isolated skin lesions have a low mortality rate.

■ REFERRAL
Whenever the diagnosis of nocardiosis is suspected, consultation with infectious disease is indicated. Pulmonary evaluation and assistance may be needed in pulmonary nocardiosis. Neurosurgery consultation is indicated in patients with single or multiple brain abscesses.

⚙ PEARLS & CONSIDERATIONS

■ COMMENTS
- Tuberculosis and nocardiosis may coexist in the same patient.
- Nocardiosis does not spread from animal to animal.
- Nocardiosis is not transmitted from person to person.
- Nocardiosis is distinguished by its ability to disseminate to any organ and its tendency to relapse despite appropriate antibiotic therapy.

REFERENCES
Boiron P et al: Nocardia, nocardiosis and mycetoma, *Med Mycol* 36(Suppl 1):26, 1998.
Lerner PI: Nocardiosis, *Clin Infect Dis* 22(6):891, 1996.
Torres HA et al: Nocardiosis in cancer patients, *Medicine* 81(5):388, 2002.
Wallace RJ et al: Taxonomy of *Nocardia* species, *Clin Infect Dis* 18:476, 1994.
Author: **Peter Petropoulos, M.D.**

BASIC INFORMATION

■ DEFINITION

Liver disease occurring in patients who do not abuse alcohol and manifested histologically by mononuclear cells and/or polymorphonuclear cells, hepatocyte ballooning, and spotty necrosis.

■ SYNONYMS

- Nonalcoholic steatohepatitis (NASH)
- Fatty liver hepatitis
- Diabetes hepatitis
- Alcohol-like liver disease
- Laënnec's disease

ICD-9CM CODES

571.8 Fatty liver

■ EPIDEMIOLOGY & DEMOGRAPHICS

- Nonalcoholic fatty liver disease affects 10% to 24% of general population
- Increased prevalence in obese persons (57% to 74%), type 2 diabetes mellitus, and hyperlipidemia (primarily hypertriglyceridemia)
- Most common cause of abnormal liver test results in adults in the U.S. (accounts for up to 90% of cases of asymptomatic ALT elevations)
- 30 million obese adults have steatosis, 8.6 million may have steatohepatitis

■ PHYSICAL FINDINGS & CLINICAL PRESENTATION

- Most patients are asymptomatic
- Patients may report a sensation of fullness or discomfort on the right side of the upper abdomen
- Nonspecific complaints of fatigue or malaise may be reported
- Hepatomegaly is generally the only positive finding on physical examination
- Acanthosis nigricans may be found in children

■ ETIOLOGY

- Insulin resistance is the most reproducible factor in the development of nonalcoholic fatty liver disease
- Risk factors are obesity (especially truncal obesity), diabetes mellitus, hyperlipidemia

DIAGNOSIS

■ DIFFERENTIAL DIAGNOSIS

- Alcohol-induced liver disease (a daily alcohol intake of 20 g in females and 30 g in males [three 12-oz beers or 12 oz of wine] may be enough to cause alcohol-induced liver disease)
- Viral hepatitis
- Autoimmune hepatitis
- Toxin or drug-induced liver disease

■ WORKUP

Diagnosis is usually suspected on the basis of hepatomegaly, asymptomatic elevations of transaminases, or "fatty liver" on sonogram of abdomen in obese patients with little or no alcohol use. Liver biopsy will confirm diagnosis and provide prognostic information. It should be considered in patients with suspected advanced liver fibrosis (presence of obesity or type 2 diabetes, AST/ALT ratio 1, age 45 yr).

■ LABORATORY TESTS

- Elevated ALT, AST: AST/ALT ratio is usually <1, but can increase as fibrosis advances
- Negative serology for infectious hepatitis; generally normal GGTP, and serum alkaline phosphatase
- Hyperlipidemia (primarily hypertriglyceridemia) may be present
- Elevated glucose levels may be present
- Prolonged prothrombin time, hypoalbuminuria, and elevated bilirubin may be present in advanced stages
- Elevated serum ferritin and increased transferrin saturation may be found in up to 10% of patients; however, hepatic iron index and hepatic iron level are normal
- Liver biopsy may show a wide spectrum of liver damage, ranging from simple steatosis to advanced fibrosis and cirrhosis

■ IMAGING STUDIES

- Ultrasound generally reveals diffuse increase in echogenicity as compared with that of the kidneys; CT scan reveals diffuse low-density hepatic parenchyma.

- Occasionally patients may have focal rather than diffuse steatosis, which may be misinterpreted as a liver mass on ultrasound or CT; use of MRI in these cases will identify focal fatty infiltration.

TREATMENT

■ NONPHARMACOLOGIC THERAPY

Weight reduction in all obese patients (500 g per week in children and 1600 g per week in adults is preferred)

■ GENERAL THERAPY

- No medications have been proved to directly improve liver damage from nonalcoholic fatty liver disease.
- Medications to control hyperlipidemia (e.g., fenofibrates for elevated triglycerides) and hyperglycemia (e.g., metformin) can lead to improvement in abnormal liver test results.

■ DISPOSITION

- Patients with pure steatosis on liver biopsy generally have a relatively benign course.
- The presence of steatohepatitis or advanced fibrosis on liver biopsy is associated with a worse prognosis.

■ REFERRAL

Liver transplantation should be considered in patients with decompensated, end-stage disease; however, in these patients there may be a recurrence of nonalcoholic fatty liver disease posttransplantation.

REFERENCES

Angulo P: Nonalcoholic fatty liver disease, *N Engl J Med* 346:1221, 2002.

Clark JM: Nonalcoholic fatty liver disease, *JAMA* 289:3000, 2003.

Dixon JB et al: Nonalcoholic fatty liver disease: predictors of nonalcoholic steatohepatitis and liver fibrosis in the severely obese, *Gastroenterology* 121:91, 2001.

Author: **Fred F. Ferri, M.D.**

BASIC INFORMATION

■ DEFINITION

Nosocomial infections (NI) are infections acquired as a result of hospitalization, generally after 48 hr of admission.

■ SYNONYMS

Hospital-acquired infections

■ EPIDEMIOLOGY & DEMOGRAPHICS

INCIDENCE (IN U.S.):
- Develop in at least 5% of hospitalized patients
- Account for 88,000 deaths/yr

In 1992 these infections were estimated to add $45 billion to the annual expenditures for health care in the U.S.

PREVALENCE (IN U.S.): 2 to 4 million cases/yr

PREDOMINANT SEX:
- Overall, approximately equal
- Elderly women: predominantly nosocomial urinary tract infections

PREDOMINANT AGE:
- Elderly patients (>60 yr old) at highest risk
- High-risk patients who may develop NI at any age:
  1. ICU
  2. Intubation
  3. Chronic lung disease
  4. Renal disease
  5. Comatose
  6. Chronic urethral or vascular catheterization
  7. Malnutrition
  8. Postoperative state

PEAK INCIDENCE: Varies widely with infection site

■ PHYSICAL FINDINGS & CLINICAL PRESENTATION

Vary with specific NI

■ ETIOLOGY
- Bacteria
- Fungi
- Viruses

SOURCES AND MODES OF TRANSMISSION:
1. Patient's own flora
   a. Comprises resistant organisms acquired during hospitalization
   b. Frequently maintained thereafter by persistent GI colonization
2. Unwashed hands of staff
   a. Physicians
   b. Nurses
3. Invasion of protective defenses (intact skin, respiratory cilia, urinary sphincters, and mucosa)
   a. IV lines
   b. Catheters
   c. Respiratory equipment
   d. Surgical wounds
   e. Scopes and other imaging devices

4. Failure to provide adequate negative pressure, high-volume air flow chambers for respiratory isolation of patients with TB
5. Failure to rapidly identify and provide appropriate care (with isolation or precautions) for patients with communicable diseases
6. Inanimate environment
7. Food
8. Fomites

RISKS AMPLIFIED:
1. Use of broad-spectrum antibiotics
   a. Select highly resistant bacteria
   b. Establish highly resistant bacteria as endemic flora in microenvironments within the hospital
2. Highly vulnerable patients with specific risk factors
   a. Immunosuppression (as a result of therapy, transplantation, AIDS)
   b. Old age
   c. Postsurgery
   d. Prolonged surgery
   e. Chronic lung disease
   f. Ventilator dependence
   g. Antacid therapy
   h. Vascular lines
   i. Hyperalimentation
   j. ICU stay
   k. Recent antibiotic therapy
3. Clustering of seriously ill patients
   a. Often with wounds or drainage of contaminated materials
   b. Intensifying probability of cross-infection

HAND WASHING BETWEEN ALL PATIENT CONTACTS: Single most important method of decreasing NI
1. Regular soap
2. Chlorhexidine for methicillin-resistant *Staphylococcus aureus* (MRSA) and other resistant gram-positive organisms
3. Iodophor for resistant gram-negative organisms
4. Purpose
   a. Degrease hand surfaces
   b. Wash away oils and associated bacteria
5. Procedure
   a. Lukewarm water
   b. Must include all surfaces
   c. Special attention to areas between fingers and to the dirtier dominant hand (most people reflexively wash their cleaner, nondominant hand more vigorously)

VANCOMYCIN-RESISTANT *ENTEROCOCCUS FAECIUM* (VREF):
1. The percentage of nosocomial infections caused by VREF increased more than 20-fold between 1989 and 1993, rising from 0% to 3% to 7% to 9%.
2. A high percentage of VREF isolated, 80% are also ampicillin resistant.

3. Factors predisposing to VREF colonization or infection include percentage of hospital days receiving antimicrobial therapy, use of IV, underlying disease, immunosuppression, and abdominal surgery.
4. Evidence suggests that vehicle is the hands of medical personnel.
5. Control measures
   a. Aggressive isolation of colonized and infected patients
   b. Restraint in using broad-spectrum antibiotics

CLOSTRIDIUM DIFFICILE:
1. Causes diarrhea as a result of pseudomembranous colitis
2. May be transmitted among hospitalized patients
3. Warrants stool (contact) precautions

SURVEILLANCE:
1. Crucial for early identification of infections
   a. Enabling immediate intervention
   b. Education
2. Prospective, concurrent, total hospital surveillance
   a. Provides most complete data
   b. Feasible with sophisticated computerized data collection and analysis
3. Daily plotting of all infections on comprehensive wall maps
   a. Including all beds on all wards
   b. Enhances immediate recognition of microclusters of infections by body site and by organism
   c. Facilitates proper early control of potential outbreaks

DIAGNOSIS

■ MOST COMMON NOSOCOMIAL INFECTIONS:
- Urinary tract infections (40% to 45%)
- Surgical wound and other soft tissue infections (25% to 30%)
- Pneumonia (15% to 20%)
- Bacteremia (5% to 12%)

NOSOCOMIAL URINARY TRACT INFECTIONS:
- General associations:
  1. Foley catheters
  2. Inappropriate catheter care (including opening catheter junctions)
  3. Female sex
  4. Absence of systemic antibiotics
- Physical findings:
  1. Fever
  2. Dysuria
  3. Leukocytosis
  4. Pyuria
  5. Flank or costovertebral angle tenderness

- Usual organisms:
  1. *E. coli*
  2. *Klebsiella*
  3. *Enterobacter*
  4. *Pseudomonas*
  5. *Enterococcus*
- Sepsis in 1% to 3% of nosocomial UTIs
- Prevention:
  1. Meticulous technique during insertion and daily perineal care
  2. Never open the catheter-collection tubing junction
  3. Obtain all specimens using sterile syringe
  4. Substitute intermittent catheterization for Foley catheters

NOSOCOMIAL BACTEREMIAS:
- General associations:
  1. IV lines
  2. Arterial lines
  3. CVP lines
  4. Phlebitis
  5. Hyperalimentation
- Fever possibly only presenting sign
- Exit site of all vascular lines carefully evaluated for:
  1. Erythema
  2. Induration
  3. Tenderness
  4. Purulent drainage
- Usual organism for device-associated bacteremia
  1. *S. aureus*
  2. *Staphylococcus epidermidis* for long-term IV lines
  3. *Enterobacter*
  4. *Klebsiella*
  5. *Candida* spp.
  6. *Pseudomonas aeruginosa* may come from a water source or reflect cutaneous bacteria
- Phlebitis in 1.3 million patients yearly
- Approximately 10,000 annual deaths from IV sepsis
- Prevention:
  1. Meticulous sterile technique during IV insertion
  2. Emphasis should be placed on attention to detail, including hand washing, adherence to guidelines for catheter insertion and maintenance, appropriate use of antiseptic solutions such as chlorhexidine or iodine to prepare the skin around the catheter insertion site, and use of sterile technique for central catheter insertion
  3. Modified catheter may reduce risk for endoluminal colonization and catheter-related sepsis in subclavian lines
  4. Decrease use of routine IVs (patients would rather drink)

NOSOCOMIAL PNEUMONIAS:
- More common in ICUs
- General associations:
  1. Aspiration
  2. Intubation

  3. Altered consciousness
  4. Old age
  5. Chronic lung disease
  6. Postsurgery
  7. Antacids
- Signs of pneumonia common among patients on general wards:
  1. Cough
  2. Sputum
  3. Fever
  4. Leukocytosis
  5. New infiltrate on chest x-ray examination
- Signs more subtle in ICUs, because many patients have purulent sputum because of chronic intubation
  1. Change in sputum character or volume
  2. Small changes on chest x-ray examination
- Usual organisms:
  1. *Klebsiella*
  2. *Acinetobacter*
  3. *Enterobacter*
  4. *Pseudomonas aeruginosa*
  5. *S. aureus*
- Less common organisms:
  1. MRSA
  2. *Legionella, Flavobacterium*
  3. Respiratory syncytial virus (infants)
  4. Adenovirus
- 1% of hospitalized patients affected
- Mortality rate high (40%)
- Prevention:
  1. Meticulous sterile technique during suctioning and handling airway
  2. Do not routinely change ventilator breathing circuits and components more frequently than q48h
  3. Drain respirator tubing without allowing fluid to return to respirator
  4. Hand washing routinely to prevent colonization of patients and transfer of organisms among patients

NOSOCOMIAL SOFT TISSUE INFECTIONS:
- Associations:
  1. Decubitus ulcers
  2. Surgical wound classification (contaminated or dirty-infected)
  3. Abdominal surgery
  4. Presence of drain
  5. Preoperative length of stay
  6. Duration of surgery >2 hr
  7. Surgeon
  8. Presence of other infection
- Physical findings:
  1. Decubitus ulcer with fluctuance at margin or under firm eschar
  2. Erythema extending >2 cm beyond margin of surgical wound
  3. Tenderness
  4. Induration
  5. Erythema
  6. Fluctuance
  7. Purulent drainage

  8. Dehiscence of sutures
- Usual organisms:
  1. *S. aureus*
  2. *Enterococcus*
  3. *Enterobacter*
  4. *Acinetobacter*
  5. *E. coli*
- Prevention:
  1. Careful skin care and frequent, proper positioning of patient to prevent decubitus ulcer
  2. Meticulous sterile surgical technique
  3. Hand washing to decrease colonization when handling postoperative wound
  4. Limit prophylactic antibiotics to 24 hr perioperatively
  5. Double-wrap contaminated dressings (hold in gloved hand and evert gloves over dressings) before disposal

■ LABORATORY TESTS
- Appropriate to specific NI and specific patient's condition
- Cultures generally indicated for proper confirmation of responsible pathogens
  1. Urine
  2. Blood
  3. Sputum
  4. Soft tissue infection
- Molecular analysis of nosocomial epidemics
  1. Plasmid fingerprinting
  2. Restriction endonuclease digestion (plasmid and genomic DNA)
  3. Peptide analysis by SDS-PAGE
  4. Immunoblotting
  5. Ribosomal (rRNA) typing
  6. DNA probes
  7. Multilocus enzyme electrophoresis
  8. Restriction fragment length polymorphism (RFLP)
  9. Polymerase chain reaction (PCR)
  10. Provide confirmation of point-source or common strains
  11. Offer occasionally indispensable corroboration of hypotheses reached utilizing classic epidemiology

■ IMAGING STUDIES
Rarely needed for diagnosis of NI

℞ TREATMENT

■ ACUTE GENERAL Rx
- Appropriate to etiologic organism:
  1. Antibiotic
  2. Antifungal
  3. Antiviral
- Specific therapy determined after careful consideration of resident flora within the microenvironment in which the patient was hospitalized

1. Empiric therapy
   a. Frequently difficult to fashion accurately
   b. Often undesirable, unless the patient's clinical condition requires urgent treatment
2. Consultation for expert advice regarding antibiotic selection in view of known epidemiologic risks within the hospital
   a. Nosocomial infection control nurses
   b. Hospital epidemiologist
- Avoid unnecessary treatment for organisms that are colonizing but not infecting patients
- Prevention of spread of communicable diseases often requiring Isolation or Precautions
  1. Classic Schema (Strict, Respiratory Isolation and Contact [Skin and Wound] Precautions) being replaced by more streamlined Revised Guidelines (Airborne, Droplet, Contact Isolation Precautions)
  2. Less careful response to some diseases (e.g., hemorrhagic fevers) inadvertently induced by removal of strict isolation category
  3. Universal/Standard Precautions and Body Substance Isolation continue within a new Standard Isolation Precautions Guideline
- Universal Precautions used for all patients during all contacts with blood, body fluids, or secretions
  1. Gloves
  2. Goggles
  3. Impermeable gowns if aerosol or splash is likely
- Consider aggressive isolation to restrict spread of resistant organisms and their plasmids
  1. MRSA
  2. VREF
  3. Highly resistant gram-negative organisms

■ REFERRAL
- To nosocomial infection control nurses
- To hospital epidemiologist

⚙ PEARLS & CONSIDERATIONS

■ COMMENTS
- Sharps and splash injuries to staff relatively are rare, but nearly all are preventable.
  1. Nurses incur most injuries.
  2. Usual causes:
     a. Needle sticks
     b. Scalpel and surgical needle injuries
     c. Blood splashes
  3. Prevention:
     a. Never recap needles
     b. Needle disposal only in rigid, impermeable plastic containers
     c. Clearly announce instrument passes in operating room or during procedures and use passing trays
     d. Gloves and goggles if aerosol or splash is likely
     e. Never leave needles or other sharp items in beds
     f. Never dispose of sharp items in regular trash bags
  4. Infection control staff should be consulted immediately after exposure to determine need for prophylaxis for hepatitis B or HIV.
  5. All staff should be immune to hepatitis B (natural or vaccine).

- Fungi previously considered to be contaminants now risks for patients with cancer and organ transplantation
  1. *Candida* spp.
     a. *C. guilliermondii*
     b. *C. krusei*
     c. *C. parapsilosis*
     d. *C. tropicalis*
  2. *Aspergillus* spp.
  3. *Curvularia* spp.
  4. *Bipolaris* spp.
  5. *Exserohilum* spp.
  6. *Alternaria* spp.
  7. *Fusarium* spp.
  8. *Scopulariopsis* spp.
  9. *Pseudallescheria boydii*
  10. *Trichosporon beigelii*
  11. *Malassezia furfur*
  12. *Hansenula* spp.
  13. *Microsporum canis*
- Focused, committed efforts by the entire health care staff continuously directed toward prevention
  1. Each NI addressed as an opportunity to improve the organization and delivery of care
  2. Essential that individual staff members understand that small risks applied to large populations result in a large number of total events (i.e., NI)

REFERENCES
Goldmann DA: Blood-borne pathogens and nosocomial infections, *J Allergy Clin Immunol* S21-6, 2002.

Johanson WG, Dever LL: Nosocomial pneumonia, *Intensive Care Med* 29(1):23, 2003.

Rowin ME et al: Pediatric intensive care unit nosocomial infections: epidemiology, sources and solutions, *Crit Care Clin* 19(3):473, 2003.
Author: **Zeena Lobo, M.D.**

BASIC INFORMATION

■ DEFINITION

Obesity refers to excess body fat defined as a body mass index (BMI) ≥ 30 kg/m². Overweight is defined as BMI of 25 to 29.9 kg/m².

■ SYNONYMS

Overweight

ICD-9CM CODES

278.0 Obesity

■ EPIDEMIOLOGY & DEMOGRAPHICS

- Approximately 97 million adults in the U.S. are overweight or obese.
- From 1960 to 1999, the prevalence of excess weight (BMI ≥ 25 kg/m²) increased from 44% to 61% of the adult population, and the prevalence of obesity (BMI ≥ 30 kg/m²) doubled, from 13% to 27%.
- The Third National Health and Nutrition Examination Survey (NHANES III) estimated that 13.7% of children and 11.5% of adolescents are overweight.
- According to NHANES III data, 54.9% of U.S. adults aged 20 yr and older are either overweight or obese (32.6% are overweight with BMI 25 to 29.9; 22.3% are obese with BMI ≥ 30).
- Overweight and obesity are defined as stated previously on the basis of epidemiologic data showing increased mortality with BMIs above 25 kg/m².
- For persons with a BMI of ≥ 30 kg/m², all-cause mortality is increased by 50% to 100% above that of persons with BMIs in the range of 20 to 25 kg/m².
- Obesity is more prevalent in black and Hispanic women compared with non-Hispanic white women and men.
- Women in the U.S. with low incomes or low education are more likely to be obese than those of higher socioeconomic status.
- In 1993 the Deputy Assistant Secretary for Health (J. Michael McGinnis) and the former Director of the Centers for Disease Control and Prevention (CDC) (William Foege) coauthored a journal article, "Actual Causes of Death in the U.S." It concluded that a combination of dietary factors and sedentary activity patterns accounts for at least 300,000 deaths each year, and obesity is the second leading cause of preventable death in the United States.

■ PHYSICAL FINDINGS & CLINICAL PRESENTATION

- Obesity is self-evident on examination.
- Measuring the height in meters and weight in kilograms determines your BMI.
- Increased waist circumference (>40 inches in men and >35 inches in women) is apparent.
- Hypertension is related to obesity.
- Symptoms of diabetes (e.g., polyuria, polydipsia, retinopathy, and neuropathy) may be present.
- Joint pain and swelling are associated with osteoarthritis and obesity.
- Dyspnea may be present.

■ ETIOLOGY

- The cause of obesity is multifactorial, involving social, cultural, behavioral, physiologic, metabolic, and genetic factors.
- Supporting genetic factors come from identical twins reared apart and "obesity genes" encoding for the appetite-suppressant hormone leptin.
- Environmental factors are a major determinant of obesity with the underlying theme of excess calorie intake and lack of physical activity.

DIAGNOSIS

- Determination of the BMI establishes the diagnosis of obesity according to the previous definition and assesses the individual's risk for disease.
- BMI is defined as the weight in kilograms divided by the square of the height in meters ($W \div H^2$).

■ DIFFERENTIAL DIAGNOSIS

- Hypothalamic disorders, hypothyroidism, Cushing's syndrome, insulinoma, and chronic corticosteroid use can cause obesity.

■ WORKUP

The workup of an obese patient typically requires laboratory work to assess for risks and complications.

■ LABORATORY TESTS

- Laboratory tests are not specific in diagnosing obesity; however, they are used to identify diabetes and hyperlipidemia commonly related to excess weight.
- In the proper clinical setting, thyroid function studies (TSH, free T_4) will exclude hypothyroidism as a cause of obesity.

■ IMAGING STUDIES

- X-ray imaging studies are not specific in the diagnosis of obesity.
- Several methods are available for determining or calculating total body fat but offer no significant advantage over the BMI.
  1. Total body water
  2. Total body potassium
  3. Bioelectrical impedance
  4. Dual-energy x-ray absorptiometry

TREATMENT

- Treatment is aimed at weight reduction and risk factor modification (e.g., diabetes, lipids, hypertension).
- Once a joint decision between patient and clinician has been made to lose weight, the expert panel recommends as an initial goal the loss of 10% of baseline weight, to be lost at a rate of 1 to 2 lb/wk over a 6-mo period.

■ NONPHARMACOLOGIC THERAPY

- The three major components of weight loss therapy are:
  1. Many studies demonstrate that obese adults can lose about 0.5 kg per wk by decreasing their daily intake to 500 to 1000 kcal below the caloric intake required for the maintenance of their current weight.
  2. Increased physical activity initially by walking 30 min 3 times/wk and gradually build up to intense walking 45 min 5 days/wk. The eventual goal is at least 30 min of moderate intense walking.
  3. Behavioral therapy is also necessary.

■ ACUTE GENERAL Rx

- Medications for the treatment of obesity are currently approved as an adjunct to diet and physical activity for patients with a BMI of ≥ 30 with no concomitant obesity-related risk factors or diseases, and for patients with a BMI ≥ 27 with concomitant obesity-related risk factors or diseases.
- Medications approved for the treatment of obesity include
  - Benzphetamine 25-50 mg 1-3 times/day
  - Phendimetrazine 17.5-70 mg 2-3 times/day or 105 mg sustained-release/day
  - Phentermine 18.75-37.5 mg/day
  - Phentermine resin 15-30 mg/day
  - Diethylpropion 25 mg 3 times/day or 75 mg sustained-release/day

○ Sibutramine 5-15 mg/day
○ Orlistat 120 mg 3 times/day with or within 1 hr after fat-containing meals, plus a daily vitamin
- Benzphetamine, phendimetrazine, phentermine and diethylpropion are approved for use of a few weeks generally presumed to be 12 wk or less. Only sibutramine and orlistat are approved for long-term use. The safety and efficacy of weight loss medications beyond 2 yr of use have not been established.
- Medications are divided into appetite suppressants (e.g., sibutramine) and those that decrease nutrient absorption (e.g., orlistat).
- In 1997 both dexfenfluramine and fenfluramine were withdrawn from the market secondary to side effects of valvular heart lesions and pulmonary hypertension.
- Contraindications using benzphetamine, phendimetrazine, phentermine, and diethylpropion include hypertension, advanced cardiovascular disease, hyperthyroidism, glaucoma, and history of substance abuse.
- Side effects of sibutramine include increases in blood pressure and pulse, dry mouth, headache, insomnia, and constipation. Side effects of orlistat include oily spotting, flatus with discharge, and fecal urgency.
- Other medications in clinical trials include bupropion (Wellbutrin), topiramate (Topamax), and metformin (Glucophage).

■ **CHRONIC Rx**
- Surgery is a consideration in clinically severe obesity (e.g., BMI ≥ 40 or ≥ 35 with comorbid conditions).

- Gastroplasty, gastric banding, gastric partitioning, and gastric bypass are the surgical procedures performed.

■ **DISPOSITION**
- Obesity increases the risk of developing hypertension, hyperlipidemia, type 2 diabetes, coronary artery disease, cerebrovascular disease, osteoarthritis, sleep apnea, and endometrial, breast, prostate, and colon cancers.
- Obesity accelerates the progression of coronary atherosclerosis in young men (age range 15 to 34 yr).
- All-cause mortality is increased in obese patients.

■ **REFERRAL**
Obesity is commonly seen in the primary care setting. If pharmacologic therapy is considered, consultation with physicians specializing in obesity and experienced with the use of the drug is recommended. In addition, consultation with nutritionists and behavioral therapists is helpful. A consultation with general surgery is indicated in patients being considered for surgical intervention.

☼ PEARLS & CONSIDERATIONS

■ **COMMENTS**
- The National Heart, Lung, and Blood Institute's (NHLBI) Obesity Education Initiative in cooperation with the National Institute of Diabetes convened the Expert Panel on the Identification, Evaluation, and Treatment of Overweight and Obesity in Adults in May 1995 and have since published evidence-based clinical guidelines.

- The total cost attributable to obesity in 1995 was $99.2 billion dollars or 5.7% of the national health expenditure within the U.S.
- Despite being effective, only about 20% of adult men and women actually restrict caloric intake and increase physical activity.

REFERENCES

Blanck HM et al: Use of non-prescription weight loss products: results from a multistate survey, *JAMA* 286:930, 2001.

Clinical Guidelines on the Identification, Evaluation, and Treatment of Overweight and Obesity in Adults. The Evidence Report. National Institute of Health, National Heart, Lung, and Blood Institute. *www.nhlbi.nih.gov/guidelines/obesity/ob_gdlns.pdf*

Executive Summary of the Clinical Guidelines on the Identification, Evaluation, and Treatment of Overweight and Obesity in Adults, *Arch Intern Med* 158(17):1855, 1867, 1998.

Lyznicki JM et al: Obesity: assessment and management in primary care, *Am Fam Physician* 63:2185, 2001.

McTigue KM et al: The natural history of the development of obesity in a cohort of young US adults between 1981 and 1988, *Ann Intern Med* 136:857, 2002.

McTigue KM et al: Screening and interventions for obesity in adults: summary of the evidence for the U.S. Preventive Services Task Force, *Ann Intern Med* 139:933, 2003.

Steinbrook R: Surgery for obesity, *N Engl J Med* 350:11, 2004.

Weil E et al: Obesity among adults with disabling conditions, *JAMA* 288:1265, 2002.

Wilson PW et al: Overweight and obesity as determinants of cardiovascular risk, *Arch Intern Med* 162:1867, 2002.

Yanovski SZ, Yanovski JA: Obesity: drug therapy, *N Engl J Med* 346(8):591, 2002.

Author: **Peter Petropoulos, M.D.**

BASIC INFORMATION

■ DEFINITION

Obsessive-compulsive disorder (OCD) involves recurrent obsessions (intrusive and inappropriate thoughts, impulses, or images) or compulsions (behaviors or mental acts performed in response to obsessions or rigid application of rules) that consume >1 hr/day or cause impairment or distress.

■ SYNONYMS

Abortive insanity

ICD-9CM CODES

F42.8 Obsessive-compulsive disorder (DSM-IV 300.3)

■ EPIDEMIOLOGY & DEMOGRAPHICS

PREVALENCE (IN U.S.): 1% to 2% of adults

PREDOMINANT SEX: Approximately equal distribution between sexes.

PREDOMINANT AGE:
- Modal age of onset for females is between 20 and 29 yr.
- Modal age of onset for males is between 6 and 15 yr.
- Condition is chronic.

PEAK INCIDENCE: Mean age at onset is 19.6 yr.

GENETICS:
- There is no clear genetic pattern.
- Rate of concordance is higher in monozygotic (33%) vs. dizygotic (7%) twins.
- Rate of disorder is also higher in first-degree relatives of individuals with OCD and Tourette's disorder than the general population.

■ PHYSICAL FINDINGS & CLINICAL PRESENTATION

- Persistent and recurrent intrusive and ego-dystonic obsessive ideas, thoughts, impulses, or images that are perceived as alien and beyond one's control.
- Frequent experiencing of obsessions related to contamination (e.g., when using the telephone), excessive doubt (e.g., was the door locked?), organization (the need for a particular order), violent impulses (e.g., to yell obscenities in church), or intrusive sexual imagery.
- Obsessions possibly leading to compulsive behaviors (e.g., repeated hand washing, checking, rearrang-

ing), or mental tasks (e.g., counting, repeating phrases).
- Obsessions and compulsions almost always accompanied with high anxiety and subjective distress.

■ ETIOLOGY

- In the past, OCD was seen in context of the psychoanalytic theory in which obsessions and compulsions were viewed as arrest of psychosexual development in the anal stage, perhaps secondary to excessively restrictive or punitive parenting.
- Disorder now seen as a biologic condition closely linked with learning disabilities and Tourette's disorder.
- Serotoninergic pathways believed important in some ritualistic instinctual behaviors, with dysfunction of these pathways possibly giving rise to OCD.

DIAGNOSIS

■ DIFFERENTIAL DIAGNOSIS

- Other psychiatric disorders in which obsessive thoughts occur (e.g., body dysmorphic disorder or phobias).
- Other conditions in which compulsive behaviors are seen (e.g., trichotillomania).
- Major depression, hypochondriasis, and several anxiety disorders with predominant obsessions or compulsions; however, in these disorders the thoughts are not anxiety provoking or are extremes of normal concern.
- Delusions or psychosis, which may be mistaken for obsessive thoughts; distinguished from OCD in that the individual recognizes the ideas are not real.
- Tics and stereotypic movements that appear compulsive but are not driven by the desire to neutralize an obsession.
- Paraphilias or pathologic gambling; distinguished from compulsions in that they are usually enjoyable.

■ WORKUP

- Careful history leading to diagnosis
- Neurologic examination to rule out concomitant Tourette's or other tic disorder
- In adolescents and children: psychologic testing to reveal learning disabilities

■ LABORATORY TESTS

No specific tests are indicated.

■ IMAGING STUDIES

- No specific studies are indicated.
- There have been research reports of reversible abnormalities on PET scans.

TREATMENT

■ NONPHARMACOLOGIC THERAPY

Behavioral therapies are often quite helpful, but success is often greater for compulsions than for obsessions.

■ GENERAL Rx

- Antidepressants with serotonergic reuptake blockade, including fluoxetine, clomipramine, fluvoxamine, paroxetine, and sertraline
- No response in only 15% of patients
- Indefinite treatment

■ DISPOSITION

- OCD is a chronic condition with a waxing and waning course.
- Exacerbations are usually associated with stress.
- When untreated, 15% of patients progressively deteriorate in function.

■ REFERRAL

- If distinction from other psychiatric conditions, particularly delusional disorder, is not clear
- If patient refractory to treatment
- If treatment with antidepressants is problematic (e.g., when comorbid with bipolar illness)

REFERENCES

Abramowitz JS et al: Treatment compliance and outcome in obsessive-compulsive disorder, *Behav Mod* 26:447, 2002.

Ackerman DL, Greenland S: Multivariate meta-analysis of controlled drug studies for obsessive-compulsive disorder, *J Clin Psychopharmacol* 22:309, 2002.

Albert U et al: Management of treatment resistant obsessive-compulsive disorder: algorithms for pharmacotherapy, *Pan Minerva Medica* 44:83, 2002.

McDonough M, Kennedy N: Pharmacological management of obsessive-compulsive disorder: a review for clinicians, *Harv Rev Psychiatry* 10:127, 2002.

Author: **Rif S. El-Mallakh, M.D.**

BASIC INFORMATION

■ DEFINITION
The term *ocular foreign body* refers to a foreign body on the surface of the corneal epithelium.

■ ICD-9CM CODES
930 Foreign body in external eye

■ EPIDEMIOLOGY & DEMOGRAPHICS
INCIDENCE (IN U.S.): Universal, with a predominance in active people
PREDOMINANT SEX: Perhaps slightly more common in men
PREDOMINANT AGE: Childhood through active adult years
PEAK INCIDENCE: Childhood through active adult years

■ PHYSICAL FINDINGS & CLINICAL PRESENTATION
Most common foreign bodies:
- Grinding (Fig. 1-189)
- Drilling
- Auto mechanics
- Working beneath cars
- Airborne particles blown by fans and so forth

DIAGNOSIS

■ DIFFERENTIAL DIAGNOSIS
- Corneal abrasion
- Corneal ulceration
- Glaucoma
- Herpes ulcers
- Infection
- Other keratitis

■ WORKUP
Fluorescein stain, slit lamp examination if no foreign body is found

■ LABORATORY TESTS
Intraocular pressure to make certain that eye has not been penetrated

■ IMAGING STUDIES
Occasionally, MRI of the orbits to identify foreign bodies not found by other means

TREATMENT

■ NONPHARMACOLOGIC THERAPY
Remove foreign body.

■ ACUTE GENERAL Rx
- Saline irrigation
- Removal of foreign body with moist cotton-tipped applicator after instillation of topical anesthetic drops
- Cycloplegics, antibiotics, and pressure dressing after removal of foreign body

■ DISPOSITION
If symptoms persist 24 hr after examination, refer to an ophthalmologist.

■ REFERRAL
To ophthalmology within 24 hr if patient not completely comfortable

PEARLS & CONSIDERATIONS

■ COMMENTS
Alkaline or acidic chemical foreign bodies can be dangerous, and pH test must be performed if either of these is suspected (for all chemical foreign bodies).
Author: **Melvyn Koby, M.D.**

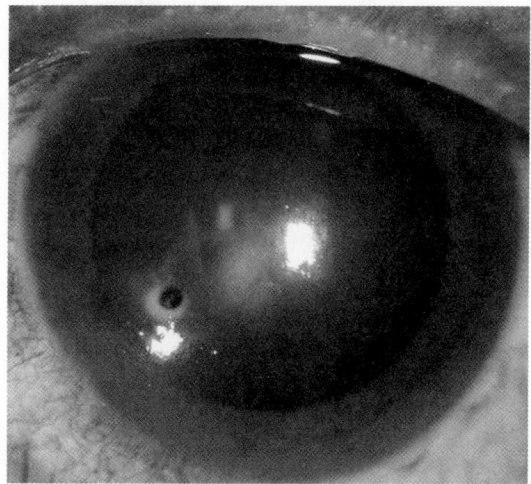

Fig. 1-189 A small, iron foreign body may be seen on external examination. (Courtesy Department of Dermatology, University of North Carolina at Chapel Hill. In Goldstein GB, Goldstein AO: *Practical dermatology,* ed 2, St Louis, 1997, Mosby.)

BASIC INFORMATION

■ DEFINITION
Onychomycosis is defined as a persistent fungal infection affecting the toenails and fingernails.

■ SYNONYMS
Tinea unguium
Ringworm of the nails

ICD-9CM CODES
110.1 Onychomycosis

■ EPIDEMIOLOGY & DEMOGRAPHICS
- Onychomycosis is most commonly found in people between the ages of 40 to 60 yr.
- Onychomycosis rarely occurs before puberty.
- Incidence: 20 to 100 cases/1000 population.
- Toenail infection is four to six times more common than fingernail infections.
- Onychomycosis affects men more often than women.
- Occurs more frequently in patients with diabetes, peripheral vascular disease, and any conditions resulting in the suppression of the immune system.
- Occlusive footwear, physical exercise followed by communal showering, and incompletely drying the feet predisposes the individual to developing onychomycosis.

■ PHYSICAL FINDINGS & CLINICAL PRESENTATION
- Onychomycosis causes nails to become thick, brittle, hard, distorted, and discolored (yellow to brown color). Eventually, the nail may loosen, separate from the nail bed, and fall off (Fig. 1-190).

- Onychomycosis is frequently associated with tinea pedis (athlete's foot).

■ ETIOLOGY
- The most common causes of onychomycosis are dermatophyte, yeast, and nondermatophyte molds.
- The dermatophyte *Trichophyton rubrum* accounts for 80% of all nail infections caused by fungus.
- *Trichophyton interdigitale* and *Trichophyton mentagrophytes* are other fungi causing onychomycosis.
- The yeast *Candida albicans* is responsible for 5% of the cases of onychomycosis.
- Nondermatophyte molds *Scopulariopsis brevicaulis* and *Aspergillus niger,* although rare, can also cause onychomycosis.
- Onychomycosis is classified according to the clinical pattern of nail bed involvement. The main types are:
  1. Distal and lateral subungual onychomycosis (DLSO)
  2. Superficial onychomycosis
  3. Proximal subungual onychomycosis
  4. Endonyx onychomycosis
  5. Total dystrophic onychomycosis

DIAGNOSIS

The diagnosis of onychomycosis is based on the clinical nail findings and confirmed by direct microscopy and culture.

■ DIFFERENTIAL DIAGNOSIS
- Psoriasis
- Contact dermatitis
- Lichen planus
- Subungual keratosis
- Paronychia
- Infection (e.g., *Pseudomonas*)

- Trauma
- Peripheral vascular disease
- Yellow nail syndrome

■ WORKUP
The workup of suspected onychomycosis is directed at confirming the diagnosis of onychomycosis by visualizing hyphae under the microscope or by growing the organism in culture.

■ LABORATORY TESTS
- Blood tests are not specific in the diagnosis of onychomycosis
- KOH prep
- Fungal cultures on Sabouraud medium

■ IMAGING STUDIES
- Imaging studies are not very specific in making the diagnosis of onychomycosis.
- If an infection is present and osteomyelitis is a consideration, an x-ray of the specific area and a bone scan may help establish the diagnosis.

TREATMENT

■ NONPHARMACOLOGIC THERAPY
- Surgical removal of the nail plate is a treatment option; however, the relapse rate is high.
- Prevention of reinfection by wearing properly fitted shoes, avoiding public showers, and keeping feet and nails clean and dry.

■ ACUTE GENERAL Rx
- Topical antifungal creams are used for early superficial nail infections.
  1. Miconazole 2% cream applied over the nail plate bid
  2. Clotrimazole 1% cream bid

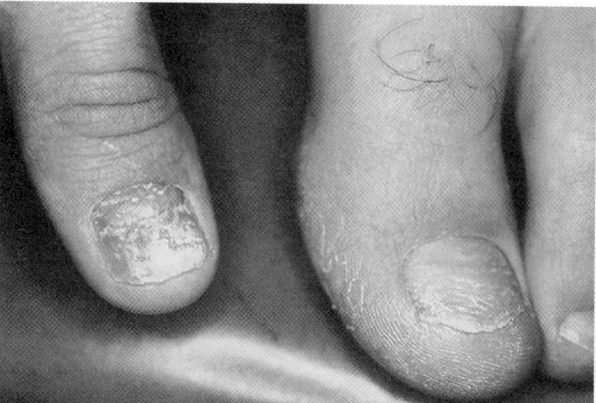

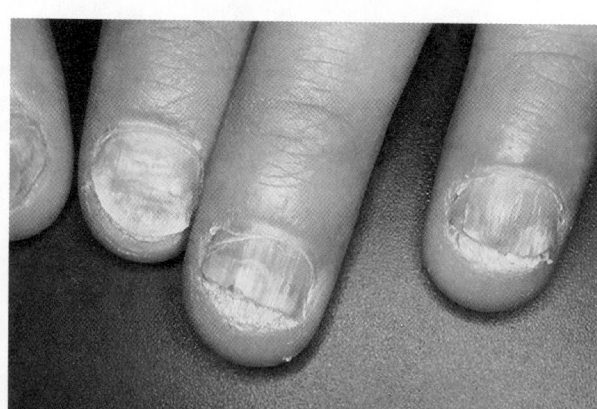

Fig. 1-190   A, Superficial white onychomycosis. **B,** Distal subungual onychomycosis.
(From Noble J [ed]: *Textbook of primary care medicine,* ed 3, St Louis, 2002, Mosby.)

- Oral agents
  1. *Itraconazole*
     a. For toenails: 200 mg qd × 3 mo
     b. For fingernails: 200 mg PO bid × 7 days, followed by 3 wk of no medicine, for two pulses
  2. *Terbinafine*
     a. For toenails: 250 mg/day for 3 mo
     b. For fingernails: 250 mg/day for 6 wk
  3. *Fluconazole*
     a. For toenails: 150 to 300 mg once weekly, until infection clears
     b. For fingernails: 150 to 300 mg once weekly until infection clears
- All oral agents used for onychomycosis require periodic monitoring of liver function blood tests.
- Itraconazole is contraindicated in patients taking cisapride, astemizole, triazolam, midazolam, and terfenadine. Statins should be discontinued during itraconazole therapy.
- Fluconazole is contraindicated in patients taking cisapride and terfenadine.
- Oral antifungal agents should not be initiated during pregnancy.
- Ciclopirox, a topical nail lacquer antifungal agent, is FDA approved for treatment of mild to moderate disease not involving the lunula.

■ CHRONIC Rx
See under "Acute General Rx."

■ DISPOSITION
- Spontaneous remission of onychomycosis is rare.
- A disease-free toenail is reported to occur in approximately 25% to 50% of patients treated with the oral antifungal agents mentioned previously.

■ REFERRAL
- Podiatry consultation is indicated in diabetic patients for proper instruction in foot care, footwear, and nail debridement or surgical removal of the toenail.
- Dermatology consultation is indicated in patients refractory to treatment or if another diagnosis is considered (e.g., psoriasis).

⚙ PEARLS & CONSIDERATIONS

■ COMMENTS
- The growth of fungus on an infected nail typically begins at the end of the nail and spreads under the nail plate to infect the nail bed as well.
- Please review informational insert regarding drug-drug interactions and contraindications before initiating oral antifungal agents.

REFERENCES

Elewski BE, Hay RJ: Update on the management of onychomycosis: highlights of the Third International Summit on Cutaneous Antifungal Therapy, *Clin Infect Dis* 23:305, 1996.

Epstein E: How often does oral treatment of toenail onychomycosis produce a disease-free nail? an analysis of published data, *Arch Dermatol* 134(12):1551, 1998.

Gupta AK: The new oral antifungal agents for onychomycosis of the toenails, *J Eur Acad Dermatol Venereol* 13(1):1, 1999.

Rodgers P, Bassler M: Treating onychomycosis, *Am Fam Physician* 63:663, 2001.

Scher RK, Coppa LM: Advances in the diagnosis and treatment of onychomycosis, *Hosp Med* 34(4):11, 1998.

Author: **Dennis Mikolich, M.D.**

BASIC INFORMATION

■ DEFINITION
Optic atrophy refers to the degeneration of the axons of the optic nerve, which can have many causes.

■ SYNONYMS
Unilateral/Bilateral optic atrophy

ICD-9CM CODES
377.10 Atrophy, optic nerve

■ EPIDEMIOLOGY & DEMOGRAPHICS
PREDOMINANT SEX: From head injury, most common in males
PREDOMINANT AGE: 21 to 40 yr
PEAK INCIDENCE: Varies depending on etiology

■ PHYSICAL FINDINGS & CLINICAL PRESENTATION
- Asymmetry of disc color is often first subtle finding
- Temporal part of optic disc is pale initially (Fig. 1-191); later the entire disc is pale/white
- Optic disc pallor occurs 4-6 wk after optic nerve injury
- Unilateral lesion produces a relative afferent pupillary defect (RAPD): swing flashlight eye to eye; abnormal pupil dilates to direct light
- Decreased visual acuity and visual field deficits (e.g., central scotoma)

■ ETIOLOGY
- Optic neuritis—multiple sclerosis, sarcoidosis, infections (syphilis, CMV, HIV)
- Vascular—ischemic optic neuropathy, central retinal artery occlusion, temporal arteritis

- Compression—glaucoma, pituitary tumor, meningioma, thyroid eye disease
- Hereditary—Leber's hereditary optic neuropathy
- Nutritional, toxic and metabolic—Amiodarone, Isoniazid, B_{12} deficiency, tobacco-alcohol
- Trauma

DIAGNOSIS

■ DIFFERENTIAL DIAGNOSIS
- Nutritional, toxic, and hereditary causes are usually bilateral.
- Unilateral optic atrophy in a young person is usually MS.
- Postviral atrophy is seen in childhood.

■ WORKUP
- Depends on suspected etiology/clinical presentation. History including age of onset, risk factors, acuity of onset of symptoms, presence of pain, family history, and other associated neurologic findings should be considered.
- Visual field testing may help identify etiology (e.g., centrocecal field defects may occur with nutritional/toxic causes), but specificity is low.
- To differentiate between optic nerve vs. macular disease an Amsler chart and/or visual evoked responses may be helpful.
- If high clinical suspicion for MS, consider MRI of brain and LP.

■ LABORATORY TESTS
- Depends on suspect etiology: none for trauma, tumor, MS

- Autoimmune diseases: ESR, ANA, and so forth

■ IMAGING STUDIES
- MRI brain with special (thin) cuts through orbits to identify compressive lesions
- MRI brain with contrast to evaluate for demyelinating plaques (MS)

TREATMENT

■ ACUTE GENERAL Rx
Treat the underlying cause—discontinue identifiable toxins, B_{12} replacement, neurosurgical intervention if tumor found; consider IV steroids if there is evidence for active demyelinating disease.

■ CHRONIC Rx
The optic nerve does not regenerate.

■ DISPOSITION
- Visual loss occurs over weeks to months
- Usually, follow-up by neurologist or ophthalmologist

■ REFERRAL
If tumor is found

PEARLS & CONSIDERATIONS

■ COMMENTS
- An experienced clinician should be able to identify pale optic discs and a relative afferent pupillar defect.
- Pupillary dilation with mydriatic agents (e.g., Pilocarpine) may be necessary for a better funduscopic examination.
- Patient education material can be obtained from the National Eye Institute, Department of Health and Human Services, 9000 Rockville Pike, Bethesda, MD 20892.

REFERENCE
Van Stavern GP, Newman NJ: Optic neuropathies. An overview, *Ophthalmol Clin North Am* 14(1):61, 2001.
Author: **Richard S. Isaacson, M.D.**

A B

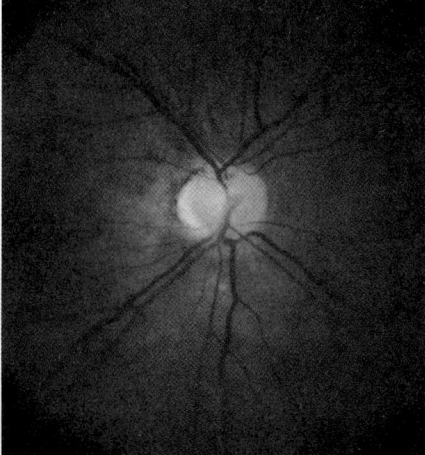 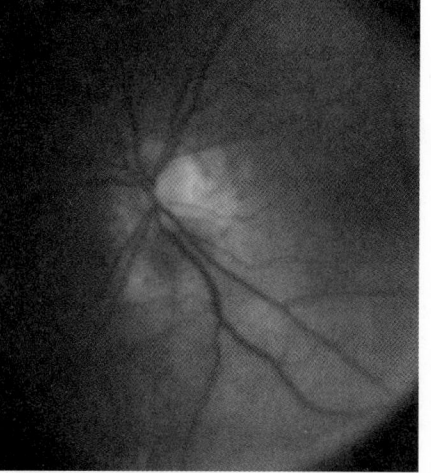

Fig. 1-191 Optic atrophy. A, Patient's right eye shows atrophy. **B,** Left eye is unaffected. (Courtesy John W. Payne, M.D., The Wilmer Ophthalmological Institute, The Johns Hopkins University and Hospital, Baltimore. From Seidel HM [ed]: *Mosby's guide to physical examination,* ed 4, St Louis, 1999, Mosby.)

BASIC INFORMATION

■ DEFINITION
Optic neuritis is an inflammation of one or both optic nerves resulting in a reduction of visual function.

■ SYNONYMS
Optic papillitis
Retrobulbar neuritis

ICD-9CM CODES
377.3 Optic neuritis

■ EPIDEMIOLOGY & DEMOGRAPHICS
INCIDENCE (IN U.S.): Relatively common, 1-5/100,000 per yr
PREVALENCE (IN U.S.): Common in patients with multiple sclerosis (MS)
PREDOMINANT SEX: Female
PEAK INCIDENCE: 20-49 yr
GENETICS: MS more common in patients with certain HLA blood types

■ PHYSICAL FINDINGS & CLINICAL PRESENTATION
- Presents with subacute (hours to days) visual loss and most often pain with movement of affected eye
- Relative afferent papillary defect (RAPD) (swing flashlight eye to eye—abnormal pupil appears to dilate to direct light)
- Decreased visual acuity
- Visual field abnormalities, most commonly central scotoma; red desaturation
- Normal orbit and fundus; occasionally there is disc edema acutely (see Fig. 1-192)

- After several months the optic disc may become pale

■ ETIOLOGY
An inflammatory response caused by a variety of diseases. MS develops in 30% of patients within 3 yr and in 52% of patients with one or more MRI brain lesions within 10 yr.

DIAGNOSIS

■ DIFFERENTIAL DIAGNOSIS
- Inflammatory: Sarcoidosis, SLE, Behçet's, postinfectious, postvaccination
- Infectious: syphilis, TB, Lyme, Bartonella, HIV
- Ischemic: giant cell arteritis, anterior and posterior ischemic optic neuropathies, diabetic papillopathy, branch or central retinal artery or vein occlusion
- Mitochondrial: Leber's hereditary optic neuropathy
- Mass lesion: aneurysm, meningioma, glioma, metastases
- Retinal migraine
- Ocular: optic drusen, retinal detachment, vitreous hemorrhage, posterior scleritis, neuroretinitis, maculopathies and retinopathies
- Acute papilledema
- Toxic/nutritional: B_{12} deficiency, tobacco-alcohol amblyopia, methanol, ethambutol

■ WORKUP
The examination, including cranial nerves and ophthalmoscopy, should otherwise be normal.

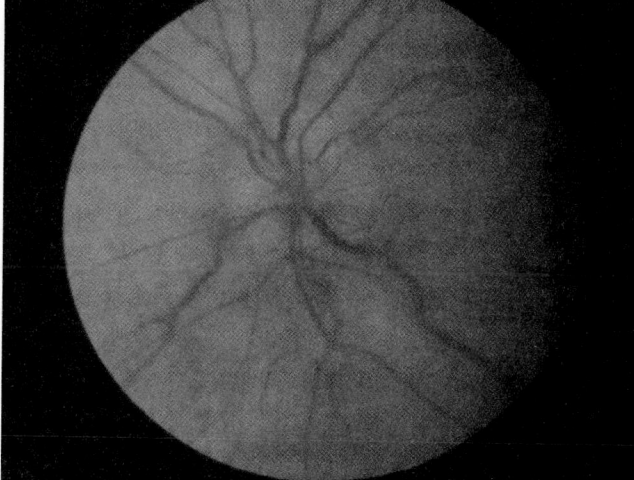

Fig. 1-192   A case of optic neuritis. The optic disc edema seen here is often not present. Note the otherwise normal fundus. (Courtesy of J. Barton, M.D., Beth Israel Deaconess Medical Center, Boston.)

■ LABORATORY TESTS
- Recommend: CBC, ANA, ESR, VDRL
- Consider HIV Ab, Lyme titer, sarcoidosis testing

■ IMAGING STUDIES
If MS is suspected, MRI of the brain may be diagnostic. Otherwise, MRI of the orbit is useful to evaluate for compressive or infiltrative etiologies.

TREATMENT

■ NONPHARMACOLOGIC THERAPY
Assure patient that most vision will return.

■ ACUTE GENERAL Rx
Not shown to improve visual outcome. Methylprednisolone 250 mg IV every 6 hr for 3 days followed by an oral prednisone taper hastens recovery and reduces the conversion rate to clinically definite MS over 2 yr.

■ CHRONIC Rx
Full visual acuity usually returns in 6 mo.

■ DISPOSITION
Follow visual acuity weekly until vision improves.

■ REFERRAL
- If patient has other neurologic signs, such as proptosis, ophthalmoplegia, or tender temporal artery
- If onset is gradual and if vision does not improve after several weeks
- If vision deteriorates as steroids are tapered

PEARLS & CONSIDERATIONS

■ COMMENTS
Bilateral ON, especially with poor recovery, suggests a diagnosis other than possible MS, such as Leber's hereditary optic neuropathy or toxic optic neuropathies. Acute bilateral loss with a severe headache or diplopia should raise concern for pituitary apoplexy.

REFERENCES
Beck R et al: The effect of corticosteroids for acute optic neuritis on the subsequent development of multiple sclerosis, *N Engl J Med* 329:1764, 1993.
Eggenber ER: Inflammatory optic neuropathies, *Ophthalmol Clin North Am* 14(1):73, 2001.
Hickman S et al: Management of acute optic neuritis, *Lancet* 360:1953, 2002.
Author: **Alexandra Degenhardt, M.D.**

BASIC INFORMATION

■ DEFINITION

Orchitis is an inflammatory process (usually infectious) involving the testicles. Infection may be viral or bacterial and can be associated with infection of other male sex organs (prostate, epididymis, bladder) or lower urogenital tract or sexually transmitted diseases often via hematogenous spread. Common causes are:
- Viral: Mumps—20% postpubertal; coxsackie B virus
- Bacterial: Pyogenic via spread from involving epididymis; bacteria include *Escherichia coli, Klebsiella pneumoniae, Staphylococcus, Streptococcus, P. aeruginosa, Rickettsia, Brucella*
- Other:
  HIV associated
  CMV
  Toxoplasmosis
  Fungi
  1. Cryptococcosis
  2. Histoplasmosis
  3. *Candida*
  4. Blastomycosis
  Mycobacteria

ICD-9CM CODES
0.72 Mumps
098.13 Acute gonococcal orchitis
095.8 Syphilitic orchitis
016.50 Tuberculous orchitis, unspecified

■ EPIDEMIOLOGY & DEMOGRAPHICS
PREDOMINANT SEX: Male
PREDOMINANT ORGANISM: The leading cause of viral orchitis is mumps. The mumps virus rarely causes orchitis in prepubertal males but involves one or both testicles in nearly 30% of postpubertal males.

■ PHYSICAL FINDINGS & CLINICAL PRESENTATION
- Testicular pain, swelling
- Unilateral or bilateral
- May have associated epididymitis, prostatitis, fever, scrotal edema, erythema cellulitis
- Inguinal lymphadenopathy
- Nausea, vomiting
- Acute hydrocele (bacterial)
- Rare development—abscess formation, pyocele of scrotum, testicular infarction
- Spermatic cord tenderness may be present

 DIAGNOSIS

Clinical presentation as described previously with possible history of acute viral illness or concomitant epididymitis.

■ DIFFERENTIAL DIAGNOSIS
- Epididymoorchitis—gonococcal
- Autoimmune disease
- Vasculitis
- Epididymyosis
- Mumps—with or without parotitis

- Neoplasm
- Hematoma
- Spermatic cord torsion

■ LABORATORY TESTS
- CBC with differential
- Urinalysis
- Viral titer—mumps
- Urine culture
- Ultrasound of testicle to rule out abscess

■ IMAGING STUDIES
Ultrasound if abscess suspected

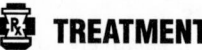 **TREATMENT**

- Dependent on etiology
- Viral (mumps)—observation
- Bacterial—empiric antibiotic treatment with parenteral antibiotic treatment for identified pathogen, including gram-negative rods, staphylococci, streptococci; treatment options are ceftriaxone (250 mg IM × 1) plus doxycycline (100 mg PO bid × 10 days), ofloxacin (300 mg PO bid × 10 days), ciprofloxacin (500 mg PO bid or 400 mg IV bid)
- Surgery for abscess, pyogenic process

REFERENCE
Cook JL, Dewbury K: The changes seen on high-resolution ultrasound in orchitis, *Clin Radiol* 55(1):13, 2000.
Author: **Dennis J. Mikolich, M.D.**

BASIC INFORMATION

■ DEFINITION

Osgood-Schlatter disease is a painful swelling of the tibial tuberosity that occurs in adolescence.

ICD-9CM CODES

732.4 Osgood-Schlatter disease

■ EPIDEMIOLOGY & DEMOGRAPHICS

PREVALENCE: 4 cases/100 adolescents
PREDOMINANT AGE: 11 to 15 yr (bilateral in 20%)
PREDOMINANT SEX: Male:female ratio of 3:1

■ PHYSICAL FINDINGS & CLINICAL PRESENTATION

- Pain at the tibial tubercle that is aggravated by activity, especially stair-walking and squatting
- Tender swelling and enlargement of the tibial tubercle
- Increased pain with knee extension against resistance

■ ETIOLOGY

- Unknown
- May be traumatically induced inflammation

🔬 DIAGNOSIS

■ DIFFERENTIAL DIAGNOSIS

- Referred hip pain (any child with hip pain should have a thorough clinical hip examination)
- Patellar tendinitis

■ WORKUP

In most cases, the diagnosis is obvious on a clinical basis.

■ IMAGING STUDIES

- Lateral roentgenogram of the upper portion of the tibia with the leg slightly internally rotated may reveal variable degrees of separation and fragmentation of the upper tibial epiphysis (Fig. 1-193).
- Occasionally, fragmented area fails to unite to the tibia and persists into adulthood.

💊 TREATMENT

■ ACUTE GENERAL Rx

- Ice, especially after exercise
- NSAIDs
- Gentle hamstring and quadriceps stretching exercises
- Abstinence from physical activity
- Temporary immobilization in a knee splint for 2 to 4 wk in resistant cases

■ DISPOSITION

- Prognosis for complete restoration of function and relief from pain is excellent.
- Condition usually heals when the epiphysis closes.
- Complications are rare.
- Symptoms in the adult:
  1. Although unusual, prominence of the tibial tubercle is usually permanent
  2. May be more susceptible to local irritation, especially when kneeling
  3. Rarely, nonunion of the epiphyseal fragment, but it is usually asymptomatic
  4. Surgery rarely required

■ REFERRAL

For orthopedic consultation when diagnosis is uncertain or when symptoms persist.

⚙ PEARLS & CONSIDERATIONS

■ COMMENTS

Larsen-Johansson disease is a similar disorder that can develop where either the quadriceps or patellar tendon inserts into the patella. Treatment and prognosis are the same as with Osgood-Schlatter disease.

REFERENCES

Blankstein A et al: Ultrasonography as a diagnostic modality in Osgood-Schlatter disease: a clinical study and review of the literature, *Arch Orthop Trauma Surg* 121(9):536, 2001.

Duri ZA, Patel DV, Aichroth PM: The immature athlete, *Clin Sports Med* 21(3):461, 2002.

Hirano A et al: Magnetic resonance imaging of Osgood-Schlatter disease: the course of the disease, *Skeletal Radiol* 31(6):334, 2002.

Tyler W, McCarthy EF: Osteochondrosis of the superior pole of the patelia: two cases with histologic correlation, *Iowa Orthop J* 22:86, 2002.

Author: **Lonnie R. Mercier, M.D.**

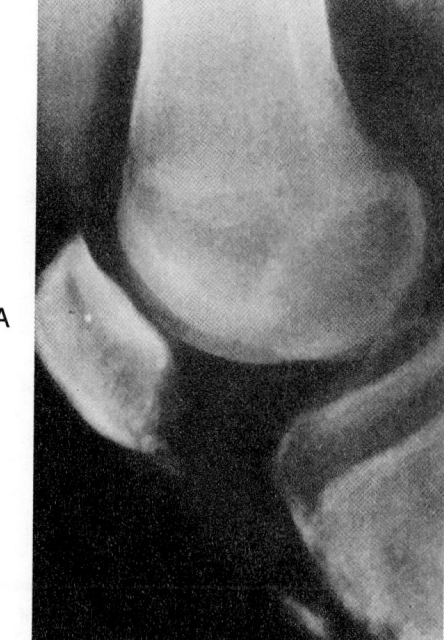
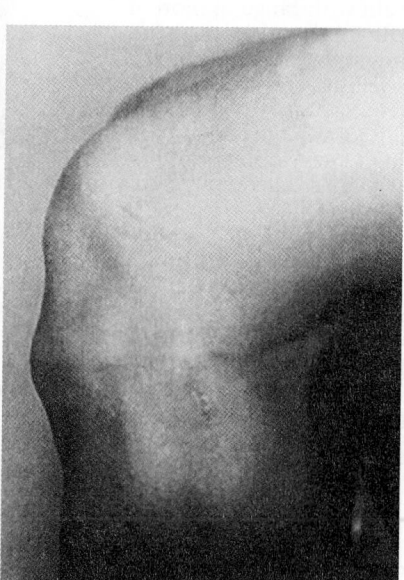

Fig. 1-193 **A,** Radiograph of Osgood-Schlatter disease demonstrating thickening of patella tendon, fragmentation of the tibial tubercle, and soft tissue swelling. **B,** Clinical picture of bony prominence anteriorly at the tibial tubercle. (From Scuderi G [ed]: *Sports medicine: principles of primary care,* St Louis, 1997, Mosby.)

BASIC INFORMATION

■ DEFINITION
Osteoarthritis is a joint condition in which degeneration and loss of articular cartilage occur, leading to pain and deformity. Two forms are usually recognized: primary (idiopathic) and secondary. The primary form may be localized or generalized.

■ SYNONYMS
Degenerative joint disease
Osteoarthrosis
Arthrosis

ICD-9CM CODES
715.0 Osteoarthrosis and allied disorders

■ EPIDEMIOLOGY & DEMOGRAPHICS
PREVALENCE: 2% to 6% of general population
PREDOMINANT SEX: Female = male
PREDOMINANT AGE: >50 yr

■ PHYSICAL FINDINGS & CLINICAL PRESENTATION
- Similar symptoms in most forms: stiffness, pain, and crepitus
- Joint tenderness, swelling
- Decreased range of motion
- Crepitus with motion
- Bony hypertrophy
- Pain with range of motion
- DIP joint involvement possibly leading to development of nodular swellings called Heberden's nodes (Fig. 1-194)
- PIP joint involvement possibly leading to development of nodular swellings called Bouchard's nodes

■ ETIOLOGY
Primary osteoarthritis is of unknown cause. Secondary osteoarthritis may result from a number of disorders including trauma, metabolic conditions, and other forms of arthritis.

DIAGNOSIS

■ DIFFERENTIAL DIAGNOSIS
- Bursitis, tendinitis
- Radicular spine pain

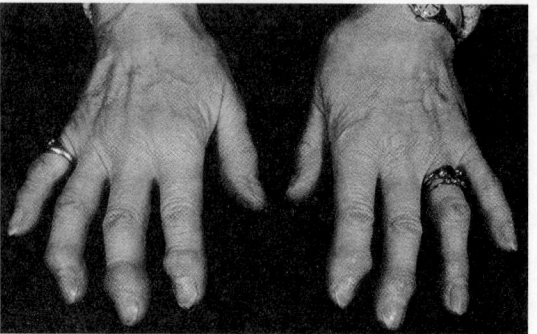

- Inflammatory arthritides
- Infectious arthritis

■ WORKUP
- No diagnostic test exists for degenerative joint disease.
- Laboratory evaluation is normal.
- Rheumatoid factor, ESR, CBC, and ANA tests may be required if inflammatory component is present.
- Synovial fluid examination is generally normal.

■ IMAGING STUDIES
- Roentgenographic evaluation reveals:
  1. Joint space narrowing
  2. Subchondral sclerosis
  3. New bone formation in the form of osteophytes
- When knee is involved, standing AP x-ray on any patient over 40.

TREATMENT

■ ACUTE GENERAL Rx
- Rest, restricted use or weight bearing, and heat
- Walking aids such as a cane (often helpful for weight-bearing joints)
- Suitable footwear
- Gentle range of motion and strengthening exercise
- Local creams and liniments to provide a counterirritant effect
- Education, reassurance

■ PHARMACOLOGIC THERAPY
- Mild analgesics for joint pain
- NSAIDs if inflammation is present
- Occasional local corticosteroid injections
- Mild antidepressants, especially at night, if depression is present
- Viscosupplementation (injection of hyaluronic acid products into the degenerative joint) is of uncertain benefit
- Nutritional supplements (glucosamine and chondroitin) are unproven

■ DISPOSITION
Progression is not always inevitable, and the prognosis is variable depending on the site and extent of the disease.

Fig. 1-194 Osteoarthritis of the distal interphalangeal (DIP) joints. This patient has the typical clinical findings of advanced osteoarthritis of the DIP joints, including large, firm swellings (Heberden's nodes), some of which are tender and red because of associated inflammation of the periarticular tissues as well as of the joint. (From Klippel J, Dieppe P, Ferri F [eds]: *Primary care rheumatology*, London, 1999, Mosby.)

■ REFERRAL
Surgical consultation for patients not responding to medical management

☼ PEARLS & CONSIDERATIONS

■ COMMENTS
Surgical intervention is generally helpful in degenerative joint disease. Arthroplasty, arthrodesis, and realignment osteotomy are the most common procedures performed. Arthroscopic debridement (of the knee) appears to be of only limited value.

REFERENCES
Brief AA, Maurer SG, Dicesare PE: Use of glucosamine and chondroitin sulfate in the management of osteoarthritis, *J Am Acad Orthop Surg* 9:71, 2001.

Buckwalter JA et al: The increasing need for nonoperative treatment of patients with osteoarthritis, *Clin Orthop* 385:36, 2001.

Felson DT: Hyaluronate sodium injections for osteoarthritis: hope, hype and hard truths, *Arch Intern Med* 162:245, 2002.

Hinton R et al: Osteoarthritis: diagnosis and therapeutic considerations, *Am Fam Physician* 65:841, 2002.

Hoaglund FT, Steinbach LS: Primary osteoarthritis of the hip: etiology and epidemiology, *J Am Acad Orthop Surg* 9:320, 2001.

Hunt SA, Jazrawi LM, Sherman OH: Arthroscopic management of osteoarthritis of the knee, *J Am Orthop Surg* 10:356, 2002.

Kelly MA et al: Osteoarthritis and beyond: a consensus on the past, present and future of hyaluronans in orthopedics, *Orthopedics* 26:1064, 2003.

Leopold S et al: Corticosteroid compared with hyaluronic acid injections for the treatment of osteoarthritis of the knee, *J Bone Joint Surg* 85:1197, 2003.

Lo HG: Intra-articular hyaluronic acid in treatment of knee osteoarthritis, *JAMA* 290:3115, 2003.

Moseley JB et al: A controlled trial of arthroscopic surgery for osteoarthritis of the knee, *N Engl J Med* 347:81, 2002.

NIH Conference, Felson DT, chair: Osteoarthritis: new insights. Parts 1-2: The disease and its risk factors and treatment approaches, *Ann Intern Med* 133:635, 2000.

Sharma L et al: The role of knee alignment in disease progression and functional decline in osteoarthritis, *JAMA* 286:188, 2001.

Wai EK, Kreder HJ, Williams JI: Arthroscopic debridement of the knee for osteoarthritis in patients fifty years of age or older, *J Bone Joint Surg* 84(A):17, 2002.

Author: **Lonnie R. Mercier, M.D.**

BASIC INFORMATION

■ DEFINITION

Osteochondritis dissecans is a disorder in which a portion of cartilage and underlying subchondral bone separates from a joint surface and may even become detached.

■ SYNONYMS

Osteochondrosis
Talar dome fracture: commonly used in describing the lesion of the talus

ICD-9CM CODES

732.7 Osteochondritis dissecans

■ EPIDEMIOLOGY & DEMOGRAPHICS

PREVALENCE: 0.3 cases/1000 persons
PREVALENT AGE: Onset at 10 to 30 yr
PREVALENT SEX: Male:female ratio of 3:1
The most common joint affected is the knee, with the lateral surface of the medial femoral condyle the most frequent area involved. The capitellum of the humerus, dome of the talus, shoulder, and hip may also be affected.

■ PHYSICAL FINDINGS & CLINICAL PRESENTATION

- Pain, stiffness, and swelling
- Intermittent locking if the fragment becomes detached
- Occasionally palpable loose body
- Tenderness at the site of the lesion
- When the knee is involved, positive Wilson's sign (pain with knee extension and internal rotation)
- Some asymptomatic cases

■ ETIOLOGY

Unknown

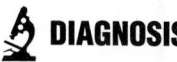 DIAGNOSIS

■ DIFFERENTIAL DIAGNOSIS

- Acute fracture
- Neoplasm

■ IMAGING STUDIES

- Plain roentgenography to confirm the diagnosis (Fig. 1-195)
- "Tunnel view" helpful in knee cases
- Typical finding: radiolucent, semilunar line outlining the oval fragment of bone (but findings variable, depending on the amount of healing and stability)
- MRI or bone scanning usually not necessary in establishing diagnosis but helpful in determining prognosis and management, especially with regards to the stability of the lesion

TREATMENT

■ ACUTE GENERAL Rx

- Observation every 4 to 6 mo for patients in whom the lesion is asymptomatic
- Symptomatic patients who are skeletally immature:
  1. Observation with an initial period of non–weight-bearing for 6 to 8 wk (in knee cases)
  2. When symptoms subside, gradual resumption of activities

■ DISPOSITION

- Juvenile cases with open epiphyses have a favorable prognosis.
- Cases developing after skeletal maturity are more likely to develop osteoarthritis.
- Large fragments, especially those in weight-bearing areas, have a more unfavorable prognosis, especially if they involve the lateral femoral condyle.
- Loose body formation and degenerative joint disease are more common when condition develops after age 20 yr.

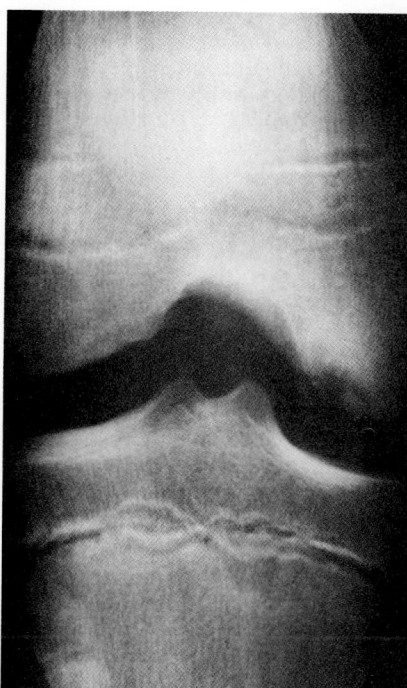

Fig. 1-195 Osteochondritis dissecans of the knee. The "tunnel" view is often helpful in visualizing the defect. This fragment may become detached and form a loose body. This area should not be confused with the normal irregularity of the distal femoral epiphysis in young children.

■ REFERRAL

For orthopedic consultation:
- For most adults with unstable lesions
- If a loose body is present
- If symptomatic care has failed

PEARLS & CONSIDERATIONS

■ COMMENTS

- Although inflammation is suggested by the name, it has not been shown to be of significance in this disorder. "Osteochondral lesion" or "osteochondrosis dissecans" may be more appropriate terms to describe these disorders.
- Repetitive trauma with ischemic necrosis is the most likely cause.
- The condition is often bilateral, especially in the knee, which could suggest the possibility of an endocrine or genetic basis.
- This condition should always be considered in the patient whose "sprained ankle" does not improve over the usual course of treatment.

REFERENCES

Cain EL, Clancy WG: Treatment algorithm for osteochondral injuries of the knee, *Clin Sports Med* 20:321, 2001.
Hixon AL, Gibbs LM: Osteochondritis dissecans: a diagnosis not to miss, *Am Fam Physician* 61:151, 2000.
Sanders RK, Crim JR: Osteochondral injuries, *Semin Ultrasound CT MRI* 22:352, 2001.
Author: **Lonnie R. Mercier, M.D.**

BASIC INFORMATION

■ DEFINITION
Osteomyelitis is an acute or chronic infection of the bone secondary to the hematogenous or contiguous source of infection or direct traumatic inoculation, which is usually bacterial.

■ SYNONYMS
Bone infection

ICD-9CM CODES
730.1 Chronic osteomyelitis
730.2 Acute or subacute osteomyelitis

■ EPIDEMIOLOGY & DEMOGRAPHICS
PREDOMINANT SEX: Male > female
PREDOMINANT AGE: All ages

■ PHYSICAL FINDINGS
HEMATOGENOUS OSTEOMYELITIS:
Usually occurs in tibia/fibula (children).
- Localized inflammation: often secondary to trauma with accompanying hematoma or cellulitis
- Abrupt fever
- Lethargy
- Irritability
- Pain in involved bone

VERTEBRAL OSTEOMYELITIS: Usually hematogenous.
- Fever: 50%
- Localized pain/tenderness
- Neurologic defects: motor/sensory

CONTIGUOUS OSTEOMYELITIS: DIRECT INOCULATION.
- Associated with trauma, fractures, surgical fixation
- Chronic infection of skin/soft tissue
- Fever, drainage from surgical site

CHRONIC OSTEOMYELITIS:
- Bone pain
- Sinus tract drainage, nonhealing ulcer
- Chronic low-grade fever
- Chronic localized pain

■ ETIOLOGY
- *Staphylococcus aureus*
- *S. aureus* (methicillin-resistant)
- *Pseudomonas aeruginosa*
- Enterobacteriaceae
- *Streptococcus pyogenes*
- *Enterococcus*
- Mycobacteria
- Fungi
- Coagulase-negative staphylococci
- *Salmonella* (in sickle cell disease)

DIAGNOSIS

■ DIFFERENTIAL DIAGNOSIS
- Brodie's abscess
- Gaucher's disease
- Bone infarction
- Charcot's joint
- Gout
- Fracture

■ WORKUP
- ESR, C-reactive protein
- Blood culturing
- Bone culture
- Pathologic evaluation of bone biopsy for acute/chronic changes consistent with necrosis or acute inflammation

■ IMAGING STUDIES
- Bone x-ray examination
- Bone scan (Fig. 1-196)
- Gallium scan
- Indium scan
- MRI (most accurate imaging study)
- Doppler studies: useful in patients with peripheral vascular disease to determine vascular adequacy

TREATMENT

Surgical debridement in biopsy-positive cases will guide direction for antibiotic therapy. This will vary with type of osteomyelitis. Duration of therapy is usually 6 wk for acute osteomyelitis; chronic osteomyelitis may need a longer course of medication.

- *S. aureus:* cefazolin IV, nafcillin IV, vancomycin IV (in patient allergic to penicillin)
- *S. aureus* (methicillin resistant): vancomycin IV
- *Streptococcus* spp.: cefazolin or ceftriaxone
- *P. aeruginosa:* piperacillin plus aminoglycoside or ceftazidime plus aminoglycoside
- Enterobacteriaceae: ceftriaxone or fluoroquinolone
- Hyperbaric oxygen therapy: may be useful in treatment of chronic osteomyelitis, especially with associated wound healing
- Surgical debridement of all devitalized bone and tissue
- Immobilization of affected bone (plaster, traction) if bone is unstable
- Bone grafts using a vascularized or open graft may be necessary if the remaining bone is inadequate

REFERENCES
Boutin RD et al: Update on imaging of orthopedic infections, *Orthop Clin North Am* 29:41, 1998.
Carek PJ et al: Diagnosis and management of osteomyelitis, *Am Fam Physician* 63:2413, 2001.
Authors: **Glenn G. Fort, M.D., and Dennis J. Mikolich, M.D.**

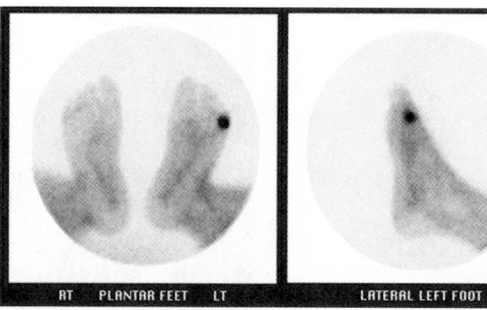

Fig. 1-196   Osteomyelitis. Intense accumulation of Tc-99m WBC in proximal phalanx of fifth digit of left foot at 4 hours after injection. (From Specht N [ed]: *Practical guide to diagnostic imaging,* St Louis, 1998, Mosby.)

BASIC INFORMATION

DEFINITION
Osteonecrosis refers to the death of bone marrow, cortex, and medullary bone caused by interruption of blood supply to the bone.

SYNONYMS
Aseptic necrosis
Avascular necrosis
Ischemic necrosis

ICD-9CM CODES
730.1 Osteonecrosis

EPIDEMIOLOGY & DEMOGRAPHICS
- Osteonecrosis accounts for 10% of all hip surgeries performed annually in the U.S.
- Osteonecrosis involves the femoral head most frequently, followed by the humeral head, femoral condyles, and distal femur.
- Between 5% to 25% of patients on chronic corticosteroid use develop osteonecrosis.
- Incidence of osteonecrosis in alcoholics is 2% to 5%.
- Osteonecrosis is found in 10% of patients with sickle cell anemia.

CLINICAL PRESENTATION & PHYSICAL FINDINGS
- May be clinically silent
- Pain in the affected bone (hip, knee or shoulder)
- Pain at rest or with use
- Decreased range of motion of the affected joint
- Joint pain with passive motion

ETIOLOGY
The etiology of osteonecrosis can be divided into:
- Atraumatic
  1. Idiopathic
  2. Alcohol
  3. Hemoglobinopathy (e.g., sickle cell disease)
  4. Connective tissue disorders (SLE, rheumatoid arthritis, vasculitis, antiphospholipid syndrome)
  5. Corticosteroid use
  6. Pregnancy
  7. Estrogen use
  8. Gaucher's disease
  9. Dysbarism
  10. Radiation therapy
- Traumatic
  1. Femoral neck fracture
  2. Septic

DIAGNOSIS

The diagnosis of avascular necrosis should be suspected in any patient with focal bone pain on corticosteroids or with any of the above mentioned comorbid conditions.

DIFFERENTIAL DIAGNOSIS
The differential diagnosis of osteonecrosis is as stated under Etiology and includes hyperlipidemias, pancreatitis, renal transplantation, chronic liver disease, obesity, and chemotherapy.

WORKUP
Radiographic imaging is the mainstay for confirming the clinical suspicion of osteonecrosis.

LABORATORY TESTS
CBC, electrolytes, BUN, creatinine, LFTs, ESR, ANA, RF, lipid profile, and other serologic tests are used as adjuncts in supporting the diagnosis of avascular necrosis.

IMAGING STUDIES
- Plain films help define and classify the disease course. Staging systems have been developed for osteonecrosis of the femoral head:
  1. Stage I: Initial x-rays are normal, but bone scan is positive.
  2. Stage II: Abnormal radiolucency is noted.
  3. Stage III: Deformity with collapse and sclerosis.
  4. Stage IV: Early osteoarthritis.
- Bone scan reveals decreased uptake at the affected site with a "doughnut sign" and can detect avascular necrosis before the plain x-rays.
- MRI scan is more sensitive and specific than bone scan, especially when looking for osteonecrosis of the femoral head.
- If a MRI is not available, CT scan of the involved bone is efficacious.

TREATMENT

Treatment of osteonecrosis of the hip can be directed at three stages:
- Before bone collapse
- After bone collapse
- After arthritic formation

NONPHARMACOLOGIC THERAPY
- Immobilization
- Non–weight-bearing with the use of crutches
- Special muscle strengthening exercise

ACUTE GENERAL Rx
- NSAIDs, ibuprofen 800 mg PO tid, naproxen 500 mg bid, or acetaminophen 500 mg (2 tabs) PO q6h can be used for symptom relief.

- For displaced hip fractures, prompt surgical reduction is indicated in attempt to reperfuse the femoral head.

CHRONIC Rx
- For patients with stage I or II osteonecrosis (before bone collapse occurs), core decompression treatment is tried to prevent bone collapse.
- In stage III osteonecrosis (after bone collapse), a hemiarthroplasty or total joint replacement is required.
- In stage IV osteonecrosis (arthritis setting in after bone collapse), a total joint replacement is usually required.

DISPOSITION
- There is no therapy to prevent avascular necrosis from occurring in patients predisposed to getting the disease.
- Patients diagnosed with avascular necrosis have a slow progressive course.
- Patients with symptoms and diagnosed by x-ray imaging to be at stage I or II (pre-bone collapse) can expect within 18 to 36 mo to develop bone collapse of the affected site.

REFERRAL
Whenever the diagnosis of avascular necrosis is suspected clinically or detected radiographically, a rheumatology and/or orthopedic consultation should be made.

PEARLS & CONSIDERATIONS

COMMENTS
- The pathogenesis of osteonecrosis is secondary to decrease perfusion of the bone elements leading to necrosis. Interruption of blood supply can occur either by arterial or venous occlusion, traumatic vascular injury, or extravascular compression.
- How each specific cause (e.g., alcohol, corticosteroids, SLE) leads to vascular interruption remains elusive.
- In approximately 70% of all patients with displaced hip fractures, there is near total loss of blood supply to the femoral head.

REFERENCES
Assouline-Dayan Y, Chang C: Pathogenesis and natural history of osteonecrosis, *Semin Arthritis Rheum* 32(2):94, 2002.
Koo K-H et al: Preventing collapse in early osteonecrosis of the femoral head, *J Bone Joint Surg* 77B:870, 1995.
Pavelka K: Osteonecrosis, *Baillieres Best Pract Res Clin Rheumatol* 14(2):399, 2000.
Author: **Peter Petropoulos, M.D.**

BASIC INFORMATION

■ DEFINITION

Osteoporosis is characterized by a progressive decrease in bone mass that results in increased bone fragility and a higher fracture risk. The various types are as follows:

PRIMARY OSTEOPOROSIS: 80% of women and 60% of men with osteoporosis
- Idiopathic osteoporosis: unknown pathogenesis; may occur in children and young adults
- Type I osteoporosis: may occur in postmenopausal women (age range: 51 to 75 yr); characterized by accelerated and disproportionate trabecular bone loss and associated with vertebral body and distal forearm fractures (estrogen withdrawal effect)
- Type II osteoporosis (involutional): occurs in both men and women >70 yr of age; characterized by both trabecular and cortical bone loss, and associated with fractures of the proximal humerus and tibia, femoral neck, and pelvis

SECONDARY OSTEOPOROSIS: 20% of women and 40% of men with osteoporosis; osteoporosis that exists as a common feature of another disease process, heritable disorder of connective tissue, or drug side effect (see "Differential Diagnosis")

ICD-9CM CODES
733.0 Osteoporosis

■ EPIDEMIOLOGY & DEMOGRAPHICS

PREVALENCE (IN U.S.):
- Approximately 25 million men and women
- Twice as common in women
- Results in 1.5 million fractures annually (70% women)
- Osteoporosis-related fractures in 50% women and 20% men >65 yr
- Results: institutionalization, mortality, and costs in excess of $10 billion annually

RISK FACTORS:
- Age: each decade after 40 yr associated with a fivefold increase risk
- Genetics:
  1. Ethnicity (white/Asian > black > Polynesian)
  2. Gender (female > male)
  3. Family history
- Environmental factors: poor nutrition, calcium deficiency, physical inactivity, medication (steroids/heparin), tobacco use, ETOH, traumatic injury
- Chronic disease states: estrogen deficiency, androgen deficiency, hyperthyroidism, hypercortisolism, cirrhosis, gastrectomy

■ PHYSICAL FINDINGS & CLINICAL PRESENTATION
- Most commonly silent with no signs and symptoms
- Insidious and progressive development of dorsal kyphosis (dowager's hump), loss of height, and skeletal pain typically associated with fracture (Fig. 1-197); other physical findings related to other conditions with associated increased risk for osteoporosis (see "Risk Factors")

■ ETIOLOGY
- Primary osteoporosis; multifactorial resulting from a combination of factors including nutrition, peak bone mass, genetics, level of physical activity, age of menopause (spontaneous vs. surgical), and estrogen status
- Secondary osteoporosis: associated decrease in bone mass resulting from an identified cause, including endocrinopathies—hypogonadism, hyperthyroidism, hyperparathyroidism, Cushing's syndrome, hyperprolactinemia, acromegaly, diabetes mellitus, gastrointestinal disease, malabsorption, primary biliary cirrhosis, gastrectomy, malnutrition (including anorexia nervosa)

DIAGNOSIS

■ DIFFERENTIAL DIAGNOSIS
- Malignancy (multiple myeloma, lymphoma, leukemia, metastatic carcinoma)
- Primary hyperparathyroidism
- Osteomalacia
- Paget's disease
- Osteogenesis imperfecta: types I, III, and IV (see also "Epidemiology and Demographics" and "Etiology")

■ WORKUP
- History and physical examination (20% of women with type I osteoporosis have associated secondary cause), with appropriate evaluation for identified risk factors and secondary causes
- Diagnosis of osteoporosis made by bone mineral density (BMD) determination (BMD should ideally evaluate the hip, spine, and wrist):
  1. Dual-energy x-ray absorptiometry (DEXA)
  2. Single-energy x-ray
  3. Peripheral dual-energy x-ray
  4. Single-photon absorptiometry
  5. Dual-photon absorptiometry
  6. Quantitative CT scan
  7. Radiographic absorptiometry

■ LABORATORY TESTS
- Biochemical profile to evaluate renal and hepatic function, primary hyperparathyroidism, and malnutrition
- CBC for nutritional status and myeloma
- TSH to rule out the presence of hyperthyroidism
- Consideration of 24-hr urine collection for calcium (excess skeletal loss, vitamin D malabsorption/deficiency), creatinine, sodium, and free cortisol (to detect occult Cushing's

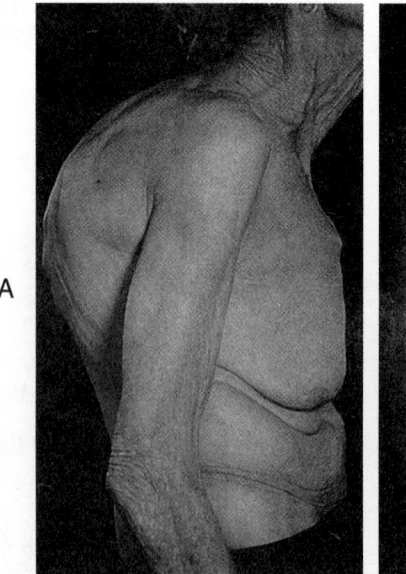
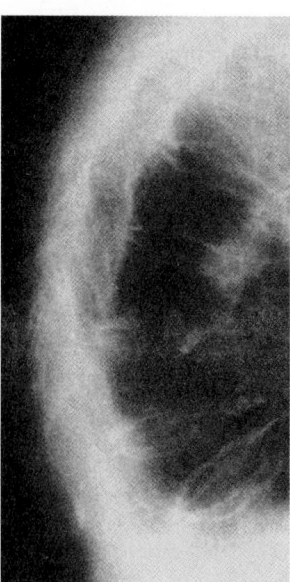

Fig. 1-197 **Dowager's hump. A,** Marked thoracic kyphosis resulting from multiple osteoporotic fractures in an elderly woman with, **B,** the corresponding radiograph. (From Klippel J, Dieppe P, Ferri F [eds]: *Primary care rheumatology,* London, 1999, Mosby.)

disease); no need to measure calcitropic hormones (PTH, calcitriol, calcitonin) unless specifically indicated

- Biochemical markers of bone remodeling; may be useful to predict rate of bone loss and/or follow therapy response; specific biochemical markers followed (e.g., 3-mo interval) to document normalization as a response to therapy
  1. High turnover osteoporosis: high levels of resorption markers (lysyl pyridinoline [LP], deoxylysyl pyridinoline [DPD], n-telopeptide of collagen cross-links [NTX], C-telopeptide of collagen cross-links [PICP]) and formation markers (osteocalcin [OCN], bone-specific alkaline phosphatase [BSAP], carboxy-terminal extension peptide of type I procollagen [PICP]); accelerated bone loss responding best to antiresorptive therapy
  2. Low-normal turnover osteoporosis: normal or low levels of the markers of resorption and formation (see "high turnover osteoporosis" above); no accelerated bone loss; responds best to drugs that enhance bone formation

■ IMAGING STUDIES

- BMD determination (see "Workup") should be performed on all women with determined risk factors and/or associated secondary causes; accepted screening criteria are currently being investigated.
  1. Normal: BMD <1 SD of the young adult reference mean
  2. Osteopenia: BMD <1 to 2.5 SD below the young adult reference mean
  3. Osteoporosis: BMD >2.5 SD below the young adult reference mean
- For patient undergoing treatment: annual BMD to follow response to therapy
- X-ray examination of appropriate part of skeleton to evaluate clinical osteoporotic fracture only

TREATMENT

■ NONPHARMACOLOGIC THERAPY

Prevention:
- Identification and minimization of risk factors
- Appropriate diagnosis and treatment of secondary causes
- Behavioral modification: proper nutrition (dietary calcium >800 mg/day, vitamin D 400 to 800 U/day), physical activity, fracture prevention strategies

■ ACUTE GENERAL Rx

- Vitamin D supplement: 400 U/day
- Calcium supplement: 1000 to 1500 mg/day
- Estrogen (conjugated equine estrogen or equivalent): 0.3 to 0.625 mg/day
- Progestin: continuous (e.g., 2.5 mg medroxyprogesterone acetate/day or equivalent) or cyclic (e.g., 10 mg medroxyprogesterone acetate days 16 to 25 each month or equivalent) coadministered in nonhysterectomized women
- Alendronate (10 mg/day) or risedronate (5 mg/day) on awakening with 8 oz water on empty stomach with no oral intake for at least 30 min
- Alendronate: 70 mg once weekly for treatment of postmenopausal osteoporosis and a 35-mg tablet for the prevention of osteogenesis in postmenopausal women
- Synthetic salmon calcitonin: 100 U/day SC or 200 U/day intranasally
- Raloxifene: 60 mg qd
- Risedronate: 35 mg once weekly on awakening with 8 oz water or empty stomach with no oral intake for at least 30 min
- Other FDA-approved drugs (without osteoporosis indication) used to treat osteoporosis:
  1. Calcitriol
  2. Etidronate
  3. Thiazide
- Combination estrogen/alendronate or estrogen-progestin/alendronate may be considered in individualized patients on HRT with identified osteoporosis
- BMD baseline obtained before onset of therapy and at 1 yr; decrease of 2% or greater results in dosage adjustment or medication change
- Baseline biochemical markers of remodeling baseline considered; identified high turnover osteoporosis patients rescreened at 3 mo to document marker return to normal

■ CHRONIC Rx

- Lifelong disorder requiring lifelong attention to behavior modification issues (nutrition, physical activity, fracture prevention strategies) and compliance with pharmacologic intervention
- Continuing need to eliminate high-risk factors where possible and to diagnose and optimally manage secondary causes of osteoporosis

■ DISPOSITION

Goal for diagnosis and treatment: identification of women at risk, initiation of preventive measures for all women lifelong, institution of treatment modalities that will result in a decrease in fracture risk, and reduction of morbidity, mortality, and unnecessary institutionalization, thereby improving quality of independent life and productivity.

■ REFERRAL

- To reproductive endocrinologist, endocrinologist, gynecologist, or rheumatologist if unfamiliar with diagnosis and management of osteoporosis
- If multidisciplinary management is required, to other specialties depending on presence of acute fracture and/or secondary associated disorders

PEARLS & CONSIDERATIONS

■ COMMENTS

Patient information is available from American College of Obstetricians and Gynecologists.

REFERENCES

Bone HG et al: Ten years' experience with alendronate for osteoporosis in postmenopausal women, *N Engl J Med* 350:12, 2004.

Fitzpatrick LA: Secondary causes of osteoporosis, *Mayo Clin Proc* 77:453, 2002.

Greenspan SL et al: Alendronate improves bone mineral density in elderly women with osteoporosis residing in long-term care facilities, *Ann Intern Med* 136:742, 2002.

Nelson H et al: Screening for postmenopausal osteoporosis: a review of the evidence for the US Preventive Task Force, *Ann Intern Med* 137:529, 2002.

NIH consensus development panel on osteoporosis prevention, diagnosis, and therapy, *JAMA* 285:785, 2001.

Peb WCG et al: Percutaneous vertebroplasty for severe osteoporotic vertebral body compression fractures, *Radiology* 223:121, 2002.

Reid IR et al: Intravenous zoledronic acid in postmenopausal women with low bone mineral density, *N Engl J Med* 346:653, 2002.

South-Paul JE: Osteoporosis: part I. Evaluation and assessment, *Am Fam Physician* 63(5):897, 2001.

South-Paul JE: Osteoporosis: part II. Nonpharmacologic and pharmacologic treatment, *Am Fam Physician* 63(6):1121, 2001.

U.S. Preventive Services Task Force: Screening for osteoporosis in postmenopausal women: recommendations and rationale, *Ann Intern Med* 137:526, 2002.

Author: **Dennis M. Weppner, M.D.**

BASIC INFORMATION

■ DEFINITION

Otitis externa is a term encompassing a variety of conditions causing inflammation and/or infection of the external auditory canal (and/or auricle and tympanic membrane). There are six subgroups of otitis externa:
- Acute localized otitis externa (furunculosis)
- Acute diffuse bacterial otitis externa (swimmer's ear)
- Chronic otitis externa
- Eczematous otitis externa
- Fungal otitis externa (otomycosis)
- Invasive or necrotizing (malignant) otitis externa (See Fig. 1-198.)

■ SYNONYMS
See "Definition."

ICD-9CM CODES
38.10 Otitis externa

■ EPIDEMIOLOGY & DEMOGRAPHICS
INCIDENCE (IN U.S.)
- Among the most common disorders
- Affects 3% to 10% of patients seeking otologic care

PREVALENCE (IN U.S.)
- Diffuse otitis externa (swimmer's ear) is most often seen in swimmers and in hot, humid climates, conditions that lead to water retention in the ear canal.
- Necrotizing otitis externa is more common in elderly, diabetics, immunocompromised patients.

PREDOMINANT SEX: None

PREDOMINANT AGE:
- Occurs at all ages
- Necrotizing otitis externa: typically occurs in elderly: mean age >65 yr

■ PHYSICAL FINDINGS & CLINICAL PRESENTATION

The two most common symptoms are otalgia, ranging from pruritus to severe pain exacerbated by motion (e.g., chewing), and otorrhea. Patients may also experience aural fullness and hearing loss secondary to swelling with occlusion of the canal. More intense symptoms may occur with bacterial otitis externa, with or without fever, and lymphadenopathy (anterior to tragus). There are also findings unique to the various forms of the infection:
- Acute localized otitis externa (furunculosis):
  1. Occurs from infected hair follicles, usually in the outer third of the ear canal, forming pustules and furuncles
  2. Furuncles are superficial and pointing or deep and diffuse
- Impetigo:
  1. In contrast to furunculosis, this is a superficial spreading infection of the ear canal that may also involve the concha and the auricle
  2. Begins as a small blister that ruptures, releasing straw-colored fluid that dries as a golden crust
- Erysipelas:
  1. Caused by group A *Streptococcus*
  2. May involve the concha and canal
  3. May involve the dermis and deeper tissues
  4. Area of cellulitis, often with severe pain
  5. Fever chills, malaise
  6. Regional adenopathy
- Eczematous otitis externa:
  1. Stems from a variety of dermatologic problems that can involve the external auditory canal

2. Severe itching, erythema, scaling, crusting, and fissuring possible
- Acute diffuse otitis externa (swimmer's ear):
  1. Begins with itching and a feeling of pressure and fullness in the ear that becomes increasingly tender and painful
  2. Mild erythema and edema of the external auditory canal, which may cause narrowing and occlusion of the canal, leading to hearing loss
  3. Minimal serous secretions, which may become profuse and purulent
  4. Tympanic membrane may appear dull and infected
  5. Usually absence of systemic symptoms such as fever, chills
- Otomycosis:
  1. Chronic superficial infection of the ear canal and tympanic membrane
  2. In primary fungal infection, major symptom is intense itching
  3. In secondary infection (fungal infection superimposed on bacterial infection), major symptom is pain
  4. Fungal growth of variety of colors
- Chronic otitis externa:
  1. Dry and atrophic canal
  2. Typically, lack of cerumen
  3. Itching, often severe, and mild discomfort rather than pain
  4. Occasionally, mucopurulent discharge
  5. With time, thickening of the walls of the canal, causing narrowing of the lumen
- Necrotizing otitis externa (also known as malignant otitis externa):
  1. Redness, swelling, and tenderness of the ear canal
  2. Classic finding of granulation tissue on the floor of the canal and the bone-cartilage junction
  3. Small ulceration of necrotic soft tissue at bone-cartilage junction
  4. Most common complaints: pain (often severe) and otorrhea
  5. Lessening of purulent drainage as infection advances
  6. Facial nerve palsy often the first and only cranial nerve defect
  7. Possible involvement of other cranial nerves

■ ETIOLOGY
- Acute localized otitis externa: *Staphylococcus aureus*
- Impetigo:
  1. *S. aureus*
  2. *Streptococcus pyogenes*
- Erysipelas: *S. pyogenes*
- Eczematous otitis externa:
  1. Seborrheic dermatitis
  2. Atopic dermatitis
  3. Psoriasis

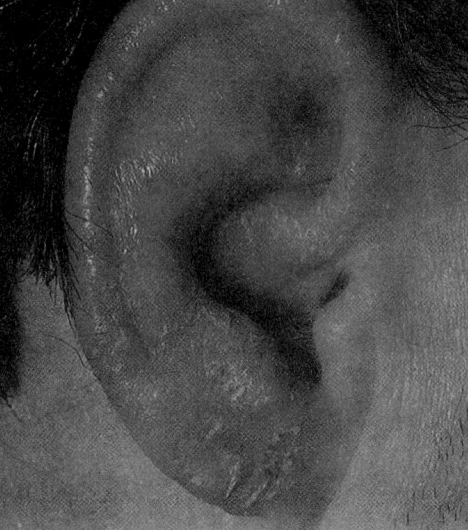

Fig. 1-198 Malignant external otitis. Severe infection of the ear has occurred after months of chronic inflammation of the pinna. (From Habif TP: *Clinical dermatology: a color guide to diagnosis and therapy*, ed 3, St Louis, 1996, Mosby.)

4. Neurodermatitis
5. Lupus erythematosus
- Acute diffuse otitis externa:
  1. Swimming
  2. Hot, humid climates
  3. Tightly fitting hearing aids
  4. Use of ear plugs
  5. *Pseudomonas aeruginosa*
  6. *S. aureus*
- Otomycosis:
  1. Prolonged use of topical antibiotics and steroid preparations
  2. *Aspergillus* (80% to 90%)
  3. *Candida*
- Chronic otitis externa: persistent low-grade infection and inflammation
- Necrotizing otitis externa (NOE):
  1. Complication of persistent otitis externa
  2. Extends through Santorini's fissures, small apertures at the bone-cartilage junction of the canal, into the mastoid and along the base of the skull
  3. *P. aeruginosa*

DIAGNOSIS

■ DIFFERENTIAL DIAGNOSIS
- Acute otitis media
- Bullous myringitis
- Mastoiditis
- Foreign bodies
- Neoplasms

■ WORKUP
Thorough history and physical examination

■ LABORATORY TESTS
- Cultures from the canal are usually not necessary unless the patient is refractory to treatment.
- Leukocyte count normal or mildly elevated.
- ESR is often quite elevated in malignant otitis externa.

■ IMAGING STUDIES
- CT scan is the best technique for defining bone involvement and extent of disease in malignant otitis externa.
- MRI is slightly more sensitive in evaluation of soft tissue changes.
- Gallium scans are more specific than bone scans in diagnosing NOE.
- Follow-up scans are helpful in determining efficacy of treatment.

NOTE: Expert opinion supports history and physical examination as the best means of diagnosis. Persistent pain that is constant and severe should raise the question of NOE (particularly in elderly, diabetics, and immunocompromised).

TREATMENT

■ NONPHARMACOLOGIC THERAPY
- Cleansing and debridement of the ear canal with cotton swabs and hydrogen peroxide or other antiseptic solution allows for a more thorough examination of the ear.
- If the canal lumen is edematous and too narrow to allow adequate cleansing, a cotton wick or gauze strip inserted into the canal serves as a conduit for topical medications to be drawn into the canal. Usually remove wick after 2 days.
- Local heat is useful in treating deep furunculosis.
- Incision and drainage is indicated in treatment of superficial pointing furunculosis.

■ ACUTE GENERAL Rx
Topical medications:
- An acidifying agent, such as 2% acetic acid, inhibits growth of bacteria and fungi
- Topical antibiotics (in the form of otic or ophthalmic solutions) or antifungals, often in combination with an acidifying agent and a steroid preparation
- The following are some of the available preparations:
  1. Neomycin otic solutions and suspensions:
     a. with polymyxin-B-hydrocortisone (Corticosporin)
     b. with hydrocortisone-thonzonium (Coly-Mycin S)
  2. Polymyxin-B-hydrocortisone (Otobiotic)
  3. Quinolone otic solutions:
     a. Ofloxacin 0.3% solution (Floxin Otic)
     b. Ciprofloxacin 0.3% with hydrocortisone (Cipro HC)
  4. Quinolone ophthalmic solutions:
     a. Ofloxacin 0.3% (Ocuflox)
     b. Ciprofloxacin 0.3% (Ciloxan)
  5. Aminoglycoside ophthalmic solutions:
     a. Gentamicin sulfate 0.3% (Garamycin)
     b. Tobramycin sulfate 0.3% (Tobrex)
     c. Tobramycin 0.3% and dexamethasone 0.1% (TobraDex)
  6. Chloramphenicol 0.5% otic solution or 0.25% ophthalmic solution (Chloromycetin)
  7. Gentian violet (methylrosaniline chloride 1%, 2%)
  8. Antifungals:
     a. Amphotericin B 3% (Fungizone lotion)
     b. Clotrimazole 1% solution (Lotrimin)
     c. Tolnaftate 1% (Tinactin)
- Topical preparations should be applied qid (bid for quinolones, antifungals), generally for 3 days after cessation of symptoms (average 10 to 14 days total).

Systemic antibiotics:
- Reserved for severe cases, most often infections with *P. aeruginosa* or *S. aureus*
- Treatment usually for 10 days with ciprofloxacin 750 mg q12h or ofloxacin 400 mg q12h, or with antistaphylococcal agent (e.g., dicloxacillin or cephalexin 500 mg q6h)

Treatment for NOE:
- Requires prolonged therapy up to 3 mo. Whether to use oral parenteral therapy is based on clinical judgment
- Oral quinolones, ciprofloxacin 750 mg q12h or ofloxacin 400 mg q12h may be appropriate initial therapy or used to shorten the course of IV therapy
- Intravenous antipseudomonals with or without aminoglycosides are also appropriate
- Local debridement

Pain control:
- May require NSAIDs or opioids
- Topical corticosteroids to reduce swelling and inflammation

■ CHRONIC Rx
- Patients prone to recurrent infections should try to identify and avoid precipitants to infection.
- Swimmers should try tight-fitting ear plugs or tight-fitting bathing caps, and remove all excess water from the ears after swimming.
- Treat underlying systemic diseases and dermatologic conditions that predispose to infection.

■ DISPOSITION
Inadequate treatment of otitis externa may lead to NOE and mastoiditis.

■ REFERRAL
To an otolaryngologist:
- NOE
- Treatment failure
- Severe pain

REFERENCES
Holten KB, Gick J: Management of the patient with otitis externa, *J Fam Practice* 50(4):353, 2001.
Sander R: Otitis externa: a practical guide to treatment and prevention, *Am Fam Physician* 63(5):927, 2001.
Author: **Jane V. Eason, M.D.**

BASIC INFORMATION

■ DEFINITION

Otitis media is the presence of fluid in the middle ear accompanied by signs and symptoms of infection.

■ SYNONYMS

Acute suppurative otitis media
Purulent otitis media

ICD-9CM CODES

382.9 Acute or chronic otitis media
382.10 381.00 Otitis media with effusion

■ EPIDEMIOLOGY & DEMOGRAPHICS

INCIDENCE (IN U.S.)
- Affects patients of all ages, but is largely a disease of infants and young children
- Occurs once in about 75% of all children
- Occurs three or more times in one third of all children by 3 yr of age
- The diagnosis of acute otitis media increased from 9.9 million in 1975 to 25.5 million in 1990
- From 1975 to 1990, office visits for acute otitis media increased three-fold for children <2 yr, doubled for children ages 2 to 5, and almost doubled for children ages 6 to 10 yr

PREDOMINANT SEX: Males
PREDOMINANT AGE:
- 47% to 60% of all children have their first episode of OM during their first year of life, 60% to 70% by their fourth birthday
- Incidence of infection declines with age; seen infrequently in adults

PEAK INCIDENCE:
- Between 6 and 36 mo
- Second peak between ages 4 and 6 yr
- Fall, winter, early spring

GENETICS:
Familial Disposition:
- Native Americans
- Eskimos
- Australian aborigines
- Those with a strong family history

Congenital Infection: High incidence in children born with cleft palates and other craniofacial abnormalities

■ PHYSICAL FINDINGS & CLINICAL PRESENTATION

- Fluid in the middle ear along with signs and symptoms of local inflammation (Figs. 1-199 and 1-200).
  1. Erythema with diminished light reflex
- Erythema of the tympanic membrane without other abnormalities is not a diagnostic criterion for acute otitis media because it may occur with any inflammation of the upper respiratory tract, crying, or nose blowing.

- As infection progresses, middle ear exudation occurs (exudative phase); the exudate rapidly changes from serous to purulent (suppurative phase).
  1. Retraction and poor motility of the tympanic membrane, which then becomes bulging and convex
- At any time during the suppurative phase the tympanic membrane may rupture, releasing the middle ear contents.
- Symptoms:
  1. Otalgia, ranging from slight discomfort to severe, spreading to the temporal region
  2. Ear stuffiness and hearing loss may precede or follow otalgia
  3. Otorrhea
  4. Vertigo
  5. Nystagmus
  6. Tinnitus
  7. Fever
  8. Lethargy
  9. Irritability
  10. Nausea, vomiting
  11. Anorexia
- After an episode of acute otitis media:
  1. Persistence of effusion for weeks or months (called secretory, serous, or nonsuppurative otitis media)
  2. Fever and otalgia usually absent
  3. Hearing loss possible (10 to 50 dB, with predominant involvement of the low frequencies)

■ ETIOLOGY

- Most common etiologic factor is an upper respiratory tract infection (often viral), which causes inflammation and obstruction of the eustachian tube. Bacterial colonization of the nasopharynx in conjunction with eustachian tube dysfunction leads to infection.
- May occasionally develop as a result of hematogenous spread or via direct invasion from the nasopharynx.
- Most common bacterial pathogens:
  1. *Streptococcus pneumoniae* causes 40% to 50% of cases and is the least likely of the major pathogens to resolve without treatment
  2. *Haemophilus influenzae* causes 20% to 30% of cases
  3. *Moraxella catarrhalis* causes 10% to 15% of cases
  4. Of increasing importance, infection caused by penicillin-

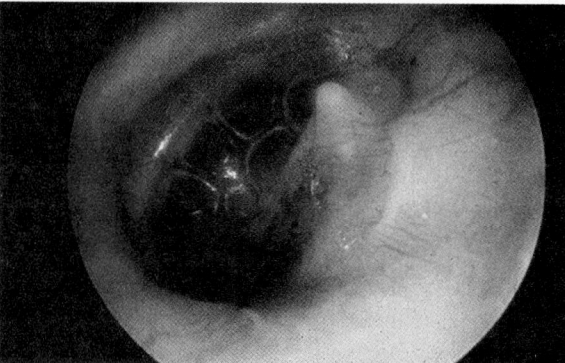

Fig. 1-199   Otitis media with effusion of left ear. Retracted eardrum, prominent short process of malleus, and air bubbles seen anteriorly through the tympanic membrane. (From Behrman RE: *Nelson textbook of pediatrics,* ed 16, Philadelphia, 1996, WB Saunders.)

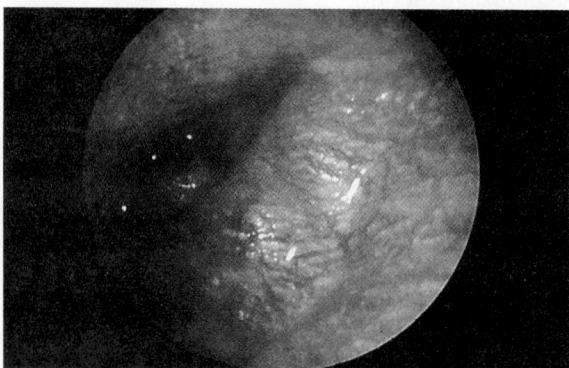

Fig. 1-200   Acute left otitis media. (From Behrman RE: *Nelson textbook of pediatrics,* ed 16, Philadelphia, 1996, WB Saunders.)

nonsusceptible *S. pneumoniae* (MIC 0.1 μg/ml), ranging from 8% to 34%. About 50% of PNSSP isolates are penicillin-intermediate (MIC 0.1 to 1.0 mg/ml)
- Viral pathogens:
  1. Respiratory syncytial virus
  2. Rhinovirus
  3. Adenovirus
  4. Influenza
- Others:
  1. *Mycoplasma pneumoniae*
  2. *Chlamydia trachomatis*

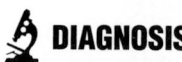 DIAGNOSIS

■ DIFFERENTIAL DIAGNOSIS
- Otitis externa
- Referred pain
  1. Mouth
  2. Nasopharynx
  3. Tonsils
  4. Other parts of the upper respiratory tract
- Section II describes the differential diagnosis of earache.

■ WORKUP
Thorough otoscopic examination; adequate visualization of the tympanic membrane requires removal of cerumen and debris.
- Tympanometry
  1. Measures compliance of the tympanic membrane and middle ear pressure
  2. Detects the presence of fluid
- Acoustic reflectometry
  1. Measures sound waves reflected from the middle ear
  2. Useful in infants >3 mo
  3. Increased reflected sound correlated with the presence of effusion

■ LABORATORY TESTS
- Tympanocentesis
  1. Not necessary in most cases as the microbiology of middle ear effusions has been shown to be quite consistent
  2. May be indicated in:
     a. Highly toxic patients
     b. Patients who fail to respond to treatment in 48 to 72 hr
     c. Immunocompromised patients
- Cultures of the nasopharynx: sensitive but not specific
- Blood counts: usually show a leukocytosis with polymorphonuclear elevation
- Plain mastoid radiographs: generally not indicated; will reveal haziness in the periantral cells that may extend to entire mastoid
- CT or MRI may be indicated if serious complications suspected (meningitis, brain abscess)

TREATMENT

■ ACUTE GENERAL Rx
Hydration, avoidance of irritants (e.g., tobacco smoke), nasal systemic decongestants, cool mist humidifier
Antimicrobials:
NOTE: Most uncomplicated cases of acute otitis media resolve spontaneously, without complications. Studies have demonstrated limited therapeutic benefit from antibiotic therapy. However, when opting to employ antibiotic therapy:
- Amoxicillin remains the drug of choice for first-line treatment of uncomplicated acute otitis media, despite increasing prevalence of drug-resistant *S. pneumoniae.*
- Treatment failure is defined by lack of clinical improvement of signs or symptoms after 3 days of therapy.
- With treatment failure, in the absence of an identified etiologic pathogen, therapy should be redirected to cover.
  1. Drug-resistant *S. pneumoniae*
  2. β-lactamase–producing strains of *H. influenzae* and *M. catarrhalis*
- Agents fulfilling these criteria include amoxicillin/clavulanate, second-generation cephalosporins (e.g., cefuroxime axetil, cefaclor); ceftriaxone (given IM). Cefaclor, cefixime, loracarbef and ceftibuten are active against *H. influenzae* and *M. catarrhalis,* but less active against *pneumococci,* especially drug resistant strains, than the agents listed previously.
- TMP/SMX and macrolides have been used as first- and second-line agents, but pneumococcal resistance to these agents is rising (up to 25% resistance to TMP/SMX, and up to 10% resistance to erythromycin).
- Cross-resistance between these drugs and the β-lactams exist; therefore patients who are treatment failures on amoxicillin are more likely to have infections resistant to TMP/SMX and macrolides.
- Newer fluoroquinolones (grepafloxacin, levofloxacin, sparfloxacin) have enhanced activity against *pneumococci* as compared with older agents (ciprofloxacin, ofloxacin).
- Treatment should be modified according to cultures and sensitivities.
- Generally treatment course is 10 to 14 days.
- Follow up approximately 4 wk after discontinuation of therapy to verify resolution of all symptoms, return to normal otoscopic findings, and restoration of normal hearing.
NOTE: Effusions may persist for 2 to 6 wk or longer in many cases of adequately treated otitis media.

■ SURGICAL Rx
- No evidence to support the routine of myringotomy, but in severe cases it provides prompt pain relief and accelerates resolution of infection.
- Purulent secretions retained in the middle ear lead to increased pressure that may lead to spread of infection to contiguous areas. Myringotomy to decompress the middle ear is necessary to avoid complications.
- Complications include mastoiditis, facial nerve paralysis, labyrinthitis, meningitis, brain abscess.
- Other procedures used for drainage of the middle ear include insertion of a ventilation tube and/or simple mastoidectomy.

■ CHRONIC Rx
- Myringotomy and tympanostomy tube placement for persistent middle ear effusion unresponsive to medical therapy for ≥3 mo if bilateral or ≥6 mo if unilateral.
- Adenoidectomy, with or without tonsillectomy, often advocated for treatment of recurrent otitis media, although indications for this procedure are controversial.
- Chronic complications include tympanic membrane perforations, cholesteatoma, tympanosclerosis, ossicular necrosis, toxic or suppurative labyrinthitis, and intracranial suppuration.

■ REFERRAL
- To otorhinolaryngologist if:
  1. Medical treatment failure
  2. Diagnosis uncertain: adults with ≥1 episode of otitis media should be referred for ENT evaluation to rule out underlying process (e.g., malignancy)
  3. Any of the above mentioned acute and chronic complications

PEARLS & CONSIDERATIONS

■ COMMENTS
Prevention:
- Multiple component conjugate vaccines hold promise for decreasing recurrent episodes of acute otitis media
- Breast-feeding, bottle-feeding infants in an upright position
- Avoidance of irritants (e.g., tobacco smoke)

REFERENCE
Zapalac JS et al: Suppurative complications of acute otitis media in the era of antibiotic resistance, *Arch Otolaryngol Head Neck Surg* 128(6):660, 2002.
Author: **Jane V. Eason, M.D.**

BASIC INFORMATION

■ DEFINITION

Otosclerosis is a conductive hearing loss secondary to fixation of the stapes resulting in gradual hearing loss. About 15% of cases affect only one ear.

ICD-9CM CODES
387.9 Otosclerosis

■ EPIDEMIOLOGY & DEMOGRAPHICS
INCIDENCE (IN U.S.): Most common cause of hearing loss in young adults
PREVALENCE (IN U.S.): 5 cases/1000 persons
PREDOMINANT SEX: Male:female ratio of 2:1
PREDOMINANT AGE: Symptoms start between 15 and 30 yr, with slowly progressive hearing loss.
PEAK INCIDENCE: Middle age
GENETICS: One half of cases are dominantly inherited.

■ PHYSICAL FINDINGS & CLINICAL PRESENTATION
- Tympanic membrane is normal in most cases (tested with tuning fork).
- Bone conduction is greater than air conduction.
- Weber localizes to affected ear.

■ ETIOLOGY
- A disease where vascular type of spongy bone is laid down
- Unknown

DIAGNOSIS

■ DIFFERENTIAL DIAGNOSIS
- Hearing loss from any cause: cochlear otosclerosis, polyps, granulomas, tumors, osteogenesis imperfecta, chronic ear infections, trauma
- A clinical algorithm for evaluation of hearing loss is described in Section III.
- Table 1-41 describes common types of conductive and sensorineural hearing loss.

■ WORKUP
Audiometry

■ LABORATORY TESTS
None, unless infection suspected

■ IMAGING STUDIES
MRI with specific cuts through inner ear

TREATMENT

■ NONPHARMACOLOGIC THERAPY
Hearing aid only of temporary use

■ CHRONIC Rx
Progresses to deafness without surgical intervention

■ DISPOSITION
Referral to ENT specialist

■ REFERRAL
To ENT specialist for surgery if moderate hearing loss suspected

PEARLS & CONSIDERATIONS

■ COMMENTS
A full ENT evaluation in a young or middle-aged person with hearing loss is mandatory unless cause is obvious (such as trauma or repeated infection).

REFERENCE
Chole RA, McKenna M: Pathophysiology of otosclerosis, *Otol Neurotol* 22(2):249, 2001.
Author: **Fred F. Ferri, M.D.**

TABLE 1-41 Common Types of Conductive and Sensorineural Hearing Loss

CONDUCTIVE HEARING LOSS	SENSORINEURAL HEARING LOSS
Otitis media with effusion	Presbycusis (hearing loss with aging)
TM perforation	Ototoxicity
Tympanosclerosis	Meniere's disease
Retracted TM (eustachian tube dysfunction)	Idiopathic loss
Ossicular problems	Noise-induced loss
Otosclerosis	Perilymphatic fistula
Foreign body in ear canal	Hereditary (congenital) loss
Cerumen impaction	Multiple sclerosis
Tumor of the ear canal or middle ear	Diabetes
Cholesteatoma	Syphilis
	Acoustic neuroma

From Rakel RE (ed): *Principles of family practice*, ed 6, Philadelphia, 2002, WB Saunders.
TM, Tympanic membrane.

BASIC INFORMATION

■ DEFINITION

Ovarian tumors can be benign, requiring operative intervention but not recurring or metastasizing; malignant, recurring, metastasizing, and having decreased survival; or borderline, having a small risk of recurrence or metastases but generally having a good prognosis.

■ SYNONYMS

Epithelial ovarian cancer
Germ cell tumor
Sex cord stromal tumor
Ovarian tumor of low malignant potential

ICD-9CM CODES

183.0 Malignant neoplasm of ovary

■ EPIDEMIOLOGY & DEMOGRAPHICS

INCIDENCE: 12.9 to 15.1 cases/100,000 persons; approximately 25,000 new cases annually
PREDOMINANCE: Median age of 61 yr, peaks at age 75 to 79 yr (54/100,000)
GENETICS: Familial susceptibility has been shown with the BRCA1 gene located on 17q12 to 21. This correlates with breast-ovarian cancer syndrome.
RISK FACTORS: Low parity, delayed childbearing, use of talc on the perineum, high-fat diet, fertility drugs (possibly), Lynch II syndrome (non-polyposis colon cancer, endometrial cancer, breast cancer, and ovarian cancer clusters in first- and second-degree relatives), breast-ovarian familial cancer syndrome, site-specific familial ovarian cancer (NOTE: Use of oral contraceptives appears to have a protective effect.)

■ PHYSICAL FINDINGS & CLINICAL PRESENTATION

- 60% present with advanced disease
- Abdominal fullness, early satiety, dyspepsia
- Pelvic pain, back pain, constipation
- Pelvic or abdominal mass
- Lymphadenopathy (inguinal)
- Sister Mary Joseph nodule (umbilical mass)

■ ETIOLOGY

- Can be inherited as site-specific familial ovarian cancer (two or more first-degree relatives have ovarian cancer)
- Breast-ovarian cancer syndrome (clusters of breast and ovarian cancer among first- and second-degree relatives)
- Lynch syndrome
- No family history and unknown etiology in the majority of ovarian cancer cases

DIAGNOSIS

■ DIFFERENTIAL DIAGNOSIS

- Primary peritoneal cancer
- Benign ovarian tumor
- Functional ovarian cyst
- Endometriosis
- Ovarian torsion
- Pelvic kidney
- Pedunculated uterine fibroid
- Primary cancer from breast, GI tract, or other pelvic organ metastasized to the ovary

■ WORKUP

- Definitive diagnosis made at laparotomy
- Careful physical and history including family history
- Exclusion of nongynecologic etiologies
- Observation of small, cystic masses in premenopausal women for regression for 2 mo

■ LABORATORY TESTS

- CBC
- Chemistry profile
- CA-125 or lysophosphatidic acid level
- Consider: hCG, Inhibin, AFP, neuron-specific enolase (NSE), and LDH in patients at risk for germ cell tumors
- Osteopontin-Potential new biomarker for ovarian cancer

■ IMAGING STUDIES

- Ultrasound (has not been shown to be effective as a screening mechanism but is useful in the evaluation of a pelvic mass)
- Chest x-ray examination
- Mammogram
- CT scan to help evaluate extent of disease
- Other studies (BE, MRI, IVP, etc.) as clinically indicated

TREATMENT

■ NONPHARMACOLOGIC THERAPY

Virtually all cases of ovarian cancer involve surgical exploration. This includes:
- Abdominal cytology
- Total abdominal hysterectomy and bilateral salpingo-oophorectomy (except in early stages where fertility is an issue)
- Omentectomy
- Diaphragm sampling
- Selective lymphadenectomy (pelvis and paraaortic)
- Primary cytoreduction with a goal of residual tumor diameter <2 cm
- Bowel surgery, splenectomy if needed to obtain optimal (<2 cm) cytoreduction

■ ACUTE GENERAL Rx

- Optimal cytoreduction is generally followed by chemotherapy (except in some early-stage disease).
- Cisplatin-based combination chemotherapy is used for stage II or greater, 6 mo treatment.
- Chemotherapy regimens continue to change as research continues.
- Consider second-look surgery when chemotherapy is complete.

■ CHRONIC Rx

- If CA-125 have recurrent disease
- Physical and pelvic examinations every 3 mo for 2 yr, every 4 mo during third year, then every 6 mo
- CA-125 every visit
- Yearly Pap smear

■ DISPOSITION

- Overall 5-yr survival rates remain low because of the preponderance of late-stage disease:
Stage I and II 80% to 100%
Stage III 15% to 20%
Stage IV 5%
- Younger patients (<50 yr) in all stages have a considerably better 5-yr survival than older patients (40% vs. 15%).

■ REFERRAL

- Studies have shown that optimal cytoreduction is most likely to occur in the hands of a gynecologic oncologist.
- Have gynecologic/oncology backup available if suspicious of malignancy.
- Always refer advanced disease.

REFERENCES

Haber D: Prophylactic oophorectomy to reduce the risk of ovarian and breast cancer in carriers of BRCA mutations, *N Engl J Med* 346:1660, 2002.
Kim JH et al: Osteopontin as a potential diagnostic biomarker for ovarian cancer, *JAMA* 287:1671, 2002.
Modan B et al: Parity, oral contraceptives and the risk of ovarian cancer among carriers and noncarriers of a brca1 or brca2 mutation, *N Engl J Med* 345:235, 2001.
Olson SH et al: Symptoms of ovarian cancer, *Obstet Gynecol* 98:212, 2001.
Author: **Gil Farkash, M.D.**

BASIC INFORMATION

DEFINITION

Benign ovarian neoplasms are clinically indistinguishable from their malignant counterparts. Therefore all persistent adnexal masses must be considered malignant until proven otherwise. Nonneoplastic tumors are as follows:

- Germinal inclusion cyst
- Follicle cyst
- Corpus luteum cyst
- Pregnancy luteoma
- Theca lutein cysts
- Sclerocystic ovaries
- Endometrioma

Neoplastic tumors that are derived from coelomic epithelium are as follows:

- Cystic tumors: serous cystoma, mucinous cystoma, mixed forms
- Tumors with stromal overgrowth: fibroma, adenofibroma, Brenner tumor

Tumors derived from germ cells are dermoids (benign cystic teratomas).

ICD-9CM CODES
220 Benign neoplasm of ovary

EPIDEMIOLOGY & DEMOGRAPHICS

- Reproductive years:
  1. Most common benign ovarian neoplasms: serous cystadenoma and benign cystic teratoma
  2. Most common adnexal mass: functional cyst
- Risk of malignancy increases after age 40 yr.
- Infants: adnexal masses are usually follicular cysts secondary to maternal hormone stimulation that regress during first few months of life.
- Childhood:
  1. Adnexal masses are rare.
  2. 8% are malignant.
  3. Almost always dysgerminomas or teratomas (germ cell origin).
  4. Frequency of malignancy is inversely correlated with age.
- Adolescence:
  1. Most common adnexal mass is a functional cyst.
  2. Most common neoplastic ovarian tumor is a benign cystic teratoma.
  3. Solid/cystic adnexal tumors are rare and almost always dysgerminomas or malignant teratomas.

PHYSICAL FINDINGS & CLINICAL PRESENTATION

- Usually asymptomatic
- Pelvic pain/pressure
- Dyspareunia
- Abdominal pain ranging from mild to severe peritoneal irritation
- Increasing abdominal girth/distention
- Adnexal mass of pelvic examination
- Children: abdominal/rectal mass

ETIOLOGY

- Physiologic
- Endometriosis
- Unknown

DIAGNOSIS

DIFFERENTIAL DIAGNOSIS

- Ovarian torsion
- Malignancy: ovary, fallopian tube, colon
- Uterine fibroid
- Diverticular abscess/diverticulitis
- Appendiceal abscess/appendicitis (especially in children)
- Tuboovarian abscess
- Paraovarian cyst
- Distended bladder
- Pelvic kidney
- Ectopic pregnancy
- Retroperitoneal cyst/neoplasm

WORKUP

- Complete history and physical examination
- Pelvic examination/rectrovaginal examination to reveal firm, irregular, mobile mass
- Laparoscopy/laparotomy to establish diagnosis

LABORATORY TESTS

- Pregnancy test
- Serum tumor markers:
  1. Cancer antigen 125 (CA 125)
  2. α-Fetoprotein (AFP) (endodermal sinus tumor, immature teratoma)
  3. β-Human chorionic gonadotropin (hCG)
  4. Lactic dehydrogenase (LDH) (dysgerminoma)

IMAGING STUDIES
Ultrasound:

- May differentiate adnexal mass from other pelvic masses
- Features that increase risk of malignancy include solid component, papillae, multiple septations/solitary thick septa, ascites, matted bowel, bilaterality, irregular borders
- CT scan with contrast or IVP
- Colonoscopy/barium enema, if symptomatic

TREATMENT

NONPHARMACOLOGIC THERAPY
Repeat pelvic examination for premenopausal women in 4 to 6 wk.

ACUTE GENERAL Rx
Indications for surgery:

- Postmenopausal or premenarcheal palpable adnexal mass
- Adnexal mass with suspicious ultrasound features
- Premenopausal woman with persistent cyst >5 cm
- Any adnexal mass >10 cm
- Suspected torsion or rupture

CHRONIC Rx

- Depends on diagnosis
- Possible suppression of formation of new cysts by oral contraceptives

DISPOSITION
Depends on diagnosis

REFERRAL

- If malignancy suspected
- If surgery required

REFERENCES

Copeland LJ, Jarrell JF: *Textbook of gynecology,* ed 2, Philadelphia, 1999, WB Saunders.

Dayal M, Barnhart KT: Noncontraceptive benefits and therapeutic uses of the oral contraceptive pill, *Semin Reprod Med* 19(4):295, 2001.

Doret M, Raudrant D: Functional ovarian cysts and the need to remove them, *Euro J Obstet Gynecol Reprod Biol* 100(1):1, 2001.

Kurjak A, Kupesic S, Simunic V: Ultrasonic assessment of the peri- and postmenopausal ovary, *Maturitas* 41(4):245, 2002.

Author: **George T. Danakas, M.D.**

BASIC INFORMATION

■ DEFINITION
Paget's disease of the bone is a non-metabolic disease of bone characterized by repeated episodes of osteolysis and excessive attempts at repair that results in a weakened bone of increased mass. Monostotic (solitary lesion) and polyostotic (numerous lesions) disease are both described.

■ SYNONYMS
Osteitis deformans

■ ICD-9CM CODES
731.0 Paget's disease (osteitis deformans)

■ EPIDEMIOLOGY & DEMOGRAPHICS
PREVALENCE: Localized lesions in 3% of patients >50 yr
PREVALENT AGE: Rare before 40 yr
PREVALENT SEX: Male:female ratio of 2:1

■ PHYSICAL FINDINGS & CLINICAL PRESENTATION
- Many lesions are asymptomatic.
- Onset is variable.
- Symptoms result mainly from the effects of complications:
  1. Skeletal pain, especially hip and pelvis
  2. Bowing of long bones, sometimes leading to pathologic fracture
  3. Increased heat of extremity (resulting from increased vascularity)
  4. Skull enlargement and spinal involvement caused by characteristic bone enlargement, which can produce neurologic complications (vision, hearing loss, radicular pain, and cord compression)
  5. Thoracic kyphoscoliosis
  6. Secondary osteoarthritis, especially of hip
  7. Heart failure as a result of chest and spine deformity and blood shunting

■ ETIOLOGY
Unknown

DIAGNOSIS

■ DIFFERENTIAL DIAGNOSIS
- Fibrous dysplasia
- Skeletal neoplasm (primary or metastatic)
- Osteomyelitis
- Hyperparathyroidism
- Vertebral hemangioma

■ LABORATORY TESTS
- Increased serum alkaline phosphatase (SAP)

- Normal serum calcium and phosphorus levels
- Increased urinary excretion of pyridinoline cross-links, although test is expensive and not usually required in routine cases
- Other: bone biopsy only in uncertain cases or if sarcomatous degeneration is suspected

■ IMAGING STUDIES
- Appropriate radiographs reflect the characteristic radiolucency and opacity (Fig. 1-201).
- Bone scanning usually reflects the activity and extent of the disease.

TREATMENT

■ ACUTE GENERAL Rx
- Counseling regarding home environment to prevent falls
- Cane for balance and weight-bearing pain

■ PHARMACOLOGIC THERAPY
- Calcitonin
- Biphosphonates
- NSAIDs for pain relief
- General indications for treatment
  1. All symptomatic patients
  2. Asymptomatic patients with high level of metabolic activity or those at risk for deformity
  3. Preoperative, if surgery involves pagetic site

■ DISPOSITION
- Many monostotic lesions probably remain asymptomatic.
- Progression of the disease is common.
- Malignant degeneration occurs in <1% of patients and should be considered when there is a sudden increase in pain.

- Sarcomatous change carries a grave prognosis.

■ REFERRAL
- For dental evaluation if there is involvement of the mandible or maxilla
- For ENT evaluation if there is hearing loss
- For ophthalmologic evaluation if there is impaired vision
- For orthopedic consultation for assessment of pain in bone or joint

PEARLS & CONSIDERATIONS

■ COMMENTS
Surgical intervention is often required for neurologic complications or joint symptoms
- Often associated with profuse blood loss
- Elective cases: benefit from preoperative treatment to suppress bone activity and vascularity

REFERENCES
Crandall C: Risedronate: a clinical review, *Arch Intern Med* 161:353, 2001.
Lin JT, Lane JM; Bisphosphonates, *J Am Acad Orthop Surg* 11:1, 2003.
Roodman GD: Studies in Paget's disease and their relevance to oncology, *Semin Oncol* 28:15, 2001.
Russell G et al: Clinical disorders of bone resorption, *Novartis Found Symp* 232:251, 2001.
Schneider D et al: Diagnosis and treatment of Paget's disease of bone, *Am Fam Physician* 65:2069, 2002.
Theriault RL, Hortobagyi GN: The evolving role of bisphosphonates, *Semin Oncol* 28:284, 2001.

Author: **Lonnie R. Mercier, M.D.**

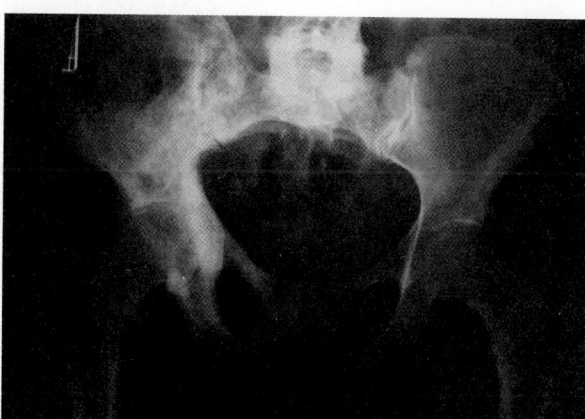

Fig. 1-201 Frontal radiograph of the pelvis shows marked prominence to the trabeculae in the right ilium, ischium, and pubic bones with small lytic areas identified compatible with the later stages of Paget's disease. (From Specht N [ed]: *Practical guide to diagnostic imaging*, St Louis, 1998, Mosby.)

BASIC INFORMATION

■ DEFINITION
Paget's disease of the breast is a malignant disease that presents itself as a scaly, sore, eroding, bleeding ulcer of the nipple. Microscopically, typical large clear cells (Paget's cells) with pale and abundant cytoplasm and hyperchromatic nuclei with prominent nucleoli are found in the epidermal layer. Paget's disease is more often associated with primary invasive or in situ carcinoma of the breast.

ICD-9CM CODES
174.0 Malignant neoplasm of female breast, nipple, and areola

■ EPIDEMIOLOGY & DEMOGRAPHICS
- Not common
- Found in 1 in 100 to 200 breast cancer patients

■ PHYSICAL FINDINGS & CLINICAL PRESENTATION
- Variable
- Itching or burning nipple and/or reported lump
- Very minimal scaly lesion that may bleed when scales are lifted
- Typical ulcer located on nipple with serous fluid weeping or small amount of bleeding coming from it (Fig. 1-202)
- Palpable carcinoma in the breast of some patients

■ ETIOLOGY
- Exact origin unknown
- Possibly migration of either in situ or invasive carcinoma cells in breast to nipple skin to produce Paget's disease

DIAGNOSIS

■ DIFFERENTIAL DIAGNOSIS
- Chronic dermatitis
- Florid papillomatosis of the nipple or nipple adenoma
- Eczema

■ WORKUP
- Clinically apparent
- Careful breast examination with diagnosis in mind
- Palpable mass or mammographic lesions in 60% to 70% of patients
- A clinical algorithm for the evaluation of nipple discharge is described in Section III, Fig. 3-36.

■ LABORATORY TESTS
Biopsy of nipple lesion

■ IMAGING STUDIES
Mammograms to search for possible primary carcinoma

TREATMENT

■ NONPHARMACOLOGIC THERAPY
- Fewer patients:
  1. Paget's disease of nipple only finding when mammographically negative breast
  2. Consideration of wide excision of nipple with or without radiation

- Other patients: additional invasive or in situ carcinoma recognized
- Either modified mastectomy or breast conservation treatment
- Presence of underlying in situ or invasive carcinoma in mastectomy specimen of majority of patients

■ ACUTE GENERAL Rx
Systemic adjuvant therapy, depending on extent of invasive carcinoma found

■ DISPOSITION
- Parallel prognosis to that of breast cancer patient without Paget's disease
- Regular follow-up as in other invasive or in situ carcinoma patients

■ REFERRAL
At outset, all suspicious nipple lesions should be referred for evaluation and treatment.

REFERENCES
Sakoratias GH et al: Paget's disease of the breast, *Canc Treat Rev* 27(1):9, 2001.
Sakoratias GH et al: Paget's disease of the breast: a clinical perspective, *Langenbecks Arch Surg* 386(6):444, 2001.
Author: **Takuma Nemoto, M.D.**

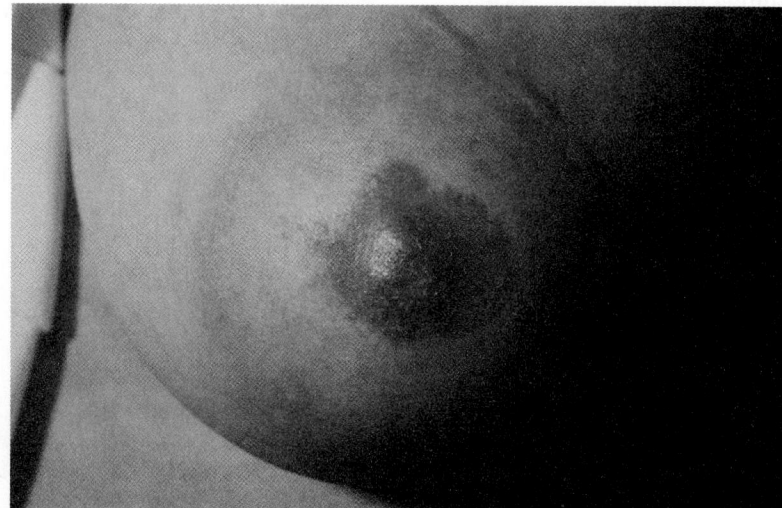

Fig. 1-202 Paget's disease of the breast. The lesion has insidiously spread for 1 year to infiltrate the areola and surrounding skin. (From Habif TP: *Clinical dermatology: a color guide to diagnosis and therapy*, ed 3, St Louis, 1996, Mosby.)

BASIC INFORMATION

■ DEFINITION
Pancreatic cancer is an adenocarcinoma derived from the epithelium of the pancreatic duct.

■ ICD-9CM CODES
157.9 Pancreatic cancer
157.0 (head)
157.1 (body)
157.2 (tail)
157.3 (duct)
230.9 (in situ)

■ EPIDEMIOLOGY & DEMOGRAPHICS
INCIDENCE: 1 case/10,000 persons/yr
PEAK AGE: Seventh and eighth decades of life
PREDOMINANT SEX: Male:female ratio of 2:1

■ PHYSICAL FINDINGS & CLINICAL PRESENTATION
Presenting symptoms:
• Jaundice
• Abdominal pain
• Weight loss
• Anorexia/change in taste
• Nausea
• Uncommonly: depression, GI bleeding, acute pancreatitis, back pain
Physical findings:
• Icterus
• Cachexia
• Excoriations from scratching pruritic skin

■ ETIOLOGY
Unknown, but several conditions have been associated with pancreatic cancer:
• Smoking
• Alcoholism
• Gallstones
• Diabetes mellitus
• Chronic pancreatitis
• Diet rich in animal fat
• Occupational exposures: oil refining, paper manufacturing, chemical industry

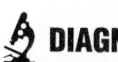

DIAGNOSIS

■ DIFFERENTIAL DIAGNOSIS
• Common duct cholelithiasis
• Cholangiocarcinoma
• Common duct stricture
• Sclerosing cholangitis
• Primary biliary cirrhosis
• Drug-induced cholestasis (e.g., phenothiazines)
• Chronic hepatitis
• Sarcoidosis
• Other pancreatic tumors (islet cell tumor, cystadenocarcinoma, epidermoid carcinoma, sarcomas, lymphomas)

■ WORKUP

Routine laboratory tests	% abnormal
Alkaline phosphatase	80
Bilirubin	55
Total protein	15
Amylase	15
Hematocrit	60

■ IMAGING STUDIES

Noninvasive imaging	% abnormal
Abdominal ultra-sonography	60
Abdominal CT scan (Fig. 1-203) (without or with contrast [IV or oral])	90
Abdominal MRI scan	90
Invasive imaging	
Endoscopic retrograde cholangiopancreatography (ERCP)	90
CT scan or ultrasonography-guided needle aspiration cytology	90-95

TREATMENT

• Surgery
Curative pancreatectomy (Whipple's procedure) appropriate for only 10% to 20% of patients whose lesion is <5 cm, solitary, and without metastases. Surgical mortality is 5%. Adjuvant chemotherapy may improve postoperative survival.
Palliative surgery (for biliary decompression/diversion)
Palliative therapeutic endoscopic retrograde cholangiopancreatography (ERCP) using stents
• Chemotherapy
The best combination chemotherapy using streptozotocin, mitomycin C, and 5-FU provides only a 19-wk median survival.
• Radiation
External beam radiation for palliation of pain.
• Combined chemotherapy and radiation provides a median survival of 11 mo.
• Celiac plexus block by an experienced anesthesiologist provides pain relief in 80% to 90% of cases.

■ DISPOSITION
Adjunct chemotherapy has a significant survival benefit in patients with resected pancreatic cancer, whereas adjuvant chemotherapy has a deleterious effect on survival.

REFERENCES

Cello JP: Pancreatic cancer. In Feldman M, Scharschmidt BF, Sleisenger MH (eds): *Gastrointestinal and liver disease,* ed 6, Philadelphia, 1998, WB Saunders.

Michaud DS et al: Physical activity, obesity, height, and the risk of pancreatic cancer, *JAMA* 286:821, 2001.

Neoptolemos JP et al: A randomized trial of chemotherapy and radiochemotherapy after resection of pancreatic cancer, *N Engl J Med* 350:1200, 2004.

Wong GY: Effect of neurolytic celiac plexus block on pain relief, quality of life, and survival in patients with unresectable pancreatic cancer, *JAMA* 291:1092, 2004.

Author: **Tom J. Wachtel, M.D.**

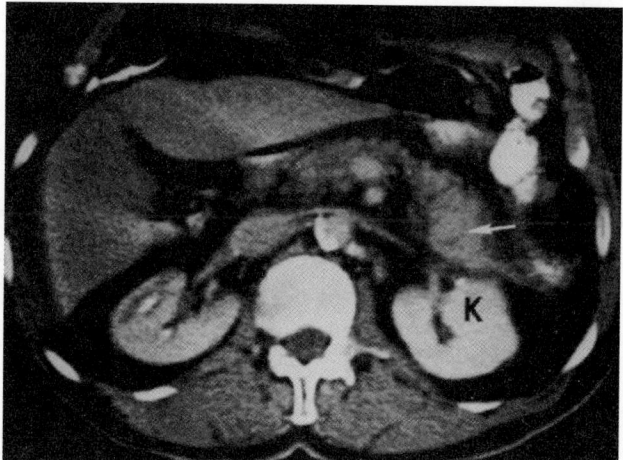

Fig. 1-203 CT scan of a patient with adenocarcinoma of the body and tail of the pancreas. The tumor *(arrow)* is seen anterior and adjacent to the left kidney *(K)*. At operation, the tumor was invading Gerota's fascia. (From Sabiston D: *Textbook of surgery,* ed 15, Philadelphia, 1997, WB Saunders.)

BASIC INFORMATION

■ DEFINITION
Acute pancreatitis is an inflammatory process of the pancreas with intrapancreatic activation of enzymes that may also involve peripancreatic tissue and/or remote organ systems.

ICD-9CM CODES
577.0 Acute pancreatitis

■ EPIDEMIOLOGY & DEMOGRAPHICS
• Acute pancreatitis is most often secondary to biliary tract disease and alcohol.
• Incidence in urban areas is twice that of rural areas (20 cases/100,000 persons in urban areas).
• 20% of patients have necrotizing pancreatitis; the remainder have interstitial pancreatitis.

■ PHYSICAL FINDINGS & CLINICAL PRESENTATION
• Epigastric tenderness and guarding; pain usually developing suddenly, reaching peak intensity within 10 to 30 min, severe and lasting several hours without relief
• Hypoactive bowel sounds (secondary to ileus)
• Tachycardia, shock (secondary to decreased intravascular volume)
• Confusion (secondary to metabolic disturbances)
• Fever
• Tachycardia, decreased breath sounds (atelectasis, pleural effusions, ARDS)
• Jaundice (secondary to obstruction or compression of biliary tract)
• Ascites (secondary to tear in pancreatic duct, leaking pseudocyst)
• Palpable abdominal mass (pseudocyst, phlegmon, abscess, carcinoma)
• Evidence of hypocalcemia (Chvostek's sign, Trousseau's sign)
• Evidence of intraabdominal bleeding (hemorrhagic pancreatitis):
  1. Gray-bluish discoloration around the umbilicus (Cullen's sign)
  2. Bluish discoloration involving the flanks (Grey Turner's sign)
• Tender subcutaneous nodules (caused by subcutaneous fat necrosis)

■ ETIOLOGY
• In >90% of cases: biliary tract disease (calculi or sludge) or alcohol
• Drugs (e.g., thiazides, furosemide, corticosteroids, tetracycline, estrogens, valproic acid, metronidazole, azathioprine, methyldopa, pentamidine, ethacrynic acid, procainamide, sulindac, nitrofurantoin, ACE inhibitors, danazol, cimetidine, piroxicam, gold, ranitidine, sulfasalazine, isoniazid, acetaminophen, cisplatin, opiates, erythromycin)
• Abdominal trauma
• Surgery
• ERCP
• Infections (predominantly viral infections)
• Peptic ulcer (penetrating duodenal ulcer)
• Pancreas divisum (congenital failure to fuse of dorsal or ventral pancreas)
• Idiopathic
• Pregnancy
• Vascular (vasculitis, ischemic)
• Hypolipoproteinemia (types I, IV, and V)
• Hypercalcemia
• Pancreatic carcinoma (primary or metastatic)
• Renal failure
• Hereditary pancreatitis
• Occupational exposure to chemicals: methanol, cobalt, zinc, mercuric chloride, creosol, lead, organophosphates, chlorinated naphthalenes
• Others: scorpion bite, obstruction at ampulla region (neoplasm, duodenal diverticula, Crohn's disease), hypotensive shock

DIAGNOSIS

■ DIFFERENTIAL DIAGNOSIS
• PUD
• Acute cholangitis, biliary colic
• High intestinal obstruction
• Early acute appendicitis
• Mesenteric vascular obstruction
• DKA
• Pneumonia (basilar)
• Myocardial infarction (inferior wall)
• Renal colic
• Ruptured or dissecting aortic aneurysm

■ LABORATORY TESTS
Pancreatic enzymes
• Amylase is increased, usually elevated in the initial 3 to 5 days of acute pancreatitis. Isoamylase determinations (separation of pancreatic cell isoenzyme components of amylase) are useful in excluding occasional cases of salivary hyperamylasemia. The use of isoamylase rather than total serum amylase reduces the risk of erroneously diagnosing pancreatitis and is preferred by some as initial biochemical test in patients suspected of having acute pancreatitis.
• Urinary amylase determinations are useful to diagnose acute pancreatitis in patients with lipemic serum, to rule out elevated serum amylase secondary to macroamylasemia, and to diagnose acute pancreatitis in patients whose serum amylase is normal.
• Serum lipase levels are elevated in acute pancreatitis; the elevation is less transient than serum amylase; concomitant evaluation of serum amylase and lipase increases diagnostic accuracy of acute pancreatitis. An elevated lipase/amylase ratio is suggestive of alcoholic pancreatitis.
• Elevated serum trypsin levels are diagnostic of pancreatitis (in absence of renal failure); measurement is made by radioimmunoassay. Although not routinely available, the serum trypsin level is the most accurate laboratory indicator for pancreatitis.
• Rapid measurement of urinary trypsinogen-2 (if available) is useful in the ER as a screening test for acute pancreatitis in patients with abdominal pain; a negative dipstick test for urinary trypsinogen-2 rules out acute pancreatitis with a high degree of probability, whereas a positive test indicates need for further evaluation.

Additional tests:
• CBC: reveals leukocytosis; Hct may be initially increased secondary to hemoconcentration; decreased Hct may indicate hemorrhage or hemolysis.
• BUN is increased secondary to dehydration.
• Elevation of serum glucose in previously normal patient correlates with the degree of pancreatic malfunction and may be related to increased release of glycogen, catecholamines, and glucocorticoid release and decreased insulin release.
• Liver profile: AST and LDH are increased secondary to tissue necrosis; bilirubin and alkaline phosphatase may be increased secondary to common bile duct obstruction. A threefold or greater rise in serum ALT concentrations is an excellent indicator (95% probability) of biliary pancreatitis.
• Serum calcium is decreased secondary to saponification, precipitation, and decreased PTH response.
• ABGs: Pao_2 may be decreased secondary to ARDS, pleural effusion(s); pH may be decreased secondary to lactic acidosis, respiratory acidosis, and renal insufficiency.
• Serum electrolytes: potassium may be increased secondary to acidosis or renal insufficiency, sodium may be increased secondary to dehydration.

■ IMAGING STUDIES
• Abdominal plain film is useful to distinguish other conditions that may mimic pancreatitis (perforated viscus); it may reveal localized ileus (sentinel loop), pancreatic calcifications (chronic pancreatitis), blurring

of left psoas shadow, dilation of transverse colon, calcified gallstones.
- Chest x-ray may reveal elevation of one or both diaphragms, pleural effusions, basilar infiltrates, platelike atelectasis.
- Abdominal ultrasonography is useful in detecting gallstones (sensitivity of 60% to 70% for detecting stones associated with pancreatitis). It is also useful for detecting pancreatic pseudocysts; its major limitation is the presence of distended bowel loops overlying the pancreas.
- CT scan is superior to ultrasonography in identifying pancreatitis and defining its extent, and it also plays a role in diagnosing pseudocysts (they appear as a well-defined area surrounded by a high-density capsule); GI fistulation or infection of a pseudocyst can also be identified by the presence of gas within the pseudocyst. Sequential contrast enhanced CT is useful for detection of pancreatic necrosis. The severity of pancreatitis can also be graded by CT scan.
- Magnetic resonance cholangiopancreatography (MRCP) is also a useful diagnostic modality if a surgical procedure is not anticipated.
- ERCP should not be performed during the acute stage of disease unless it is necessary to remove an impacted stone in the ampulla of Vater; patients with severe or worsening pancreatitis but without obstructive jaundice (biliary obstruction) do not benefit from early ERCP and papillotomy.

℞ TREATMENT

■ NONPHARMACOLOGIC THERAPY
- Bowel rest with avoidance of PO liquids or solids during the acute illness
- Avoidance of alcohol and any drugs associated with pancreatitis

■ ACUTE GENERAL Rx
General measures:
- Maintain adequate intravascular volume with vigorous IV hydration.
- Patient should remain NPO until clinically improved, stable, and hungry.
- Nasogastric suction is useful in severe pancreatitis to decompress the abdomen in patients with ileus.

- Control pain: oral analgesics may cause spasms of the sphincter of Oddi (meperidine may produce less constriction than other analgesics; however, clear evidence regarding this claim is lacking and metabolites may cause significant neurotoxic effects such as seizures, myoclonus, or tremors).
- Correct metabolic abnormalities (e.g., replace calcium and magnesium as necessary).
- TPN may be necessary in prolonged pancreatitis.

Specific measures:
- IV antibiotics should not be used prophylactically; their use is justified if the patient has evidence of septicemia, pancreatic abscess, or pancreatitis secondary to biliary calculi. Appropriate empiric antibiotic therapy should cover:
  1. *B. fragilis* and other anaerobes (cefotetan, cefoxitin, metronidazole, or clindamycin plus aminoglycoside)
  2. *Enterococcus* (ampicillin)
- Surgical therapy has a limited role in acute pancreatitis; it is indicated in the following:
  1. Gallstone-induced pancreatitis: cholecystectomy when acute pancreatitis subsides
  2. Perforated peptic ulcer
  3. Excision or drainage of necrotic or infected foci
- Identification and treatment of complications:
  1. Pseudocyst: round or spheroid collection of fluid, tissue, pancreatic enzymes, and blood.
     a. Diagnosed by CT scan or sonography
     b. Treatment: CT scan or ultrasound-guided percutaneous drainage (with a pigtail catheter left in place for continuous drainage) can be used, but the recurrence rate is high; the conservative approach is to reevaluate the pseudocyst (with CT scan or sonography) after 6 to 7 wk and surgically drain it if the pseudocyst has not decreased in size. Generally pseudocysts <5 cm in diameter are reabsorbed without intervention whereas those >5 cm require surgical intervention after the wall has matured.

  2. Phlegmon: represents pancreatic edema. It can be diagnosed by CT scan or sonography. Treatment is supportive measures, because it usually resolves spontaneously.
  3. Pancreatic abscess: diagnosed by CT scan (presence of bubbles in the retroperitoneum); Gram staining and cultures of fluid obtained from guided percutaneous aspiration (GPA) usually identify bacterial organism. Therapy is surgical (or catheter) drainage and IV antibiotics (imipenem-cilastin [Primaxin] is the drug of choice).
  4. Pancreatic ascites: usually caused by leaking of pseudocyst or tear in pancreatic duct. Paracentesis reveals very high amylase and lipase levels in the pancreatic fluid; ERCP may demonstrate the lesion. Treatment is surgical correction if exudative ascites from severe pancreatitis does not resolve spontaneously.
  5. GI bleeding: caused by alcoholic gastritis, bleeding varices, stress ulceration, or DIC.
  6. Renal failure: caused by hypovolemia resulting in oliguria or anuria, cortical or tubular necrosis (shock, DIC), or thrombosis of renal artery or vein.
  7. Hypoxia: caused by ARDS, pleural effusion, or atelectasis.

■ DISPOSITION
Prognosis varies with the severity of pancreatitis; overall mortality in acute pancreatitis is 5% to 10%; poor prognostic signs are the following:
- Age >55 yr
- Fluid sequestration >6000 ml
- Laboratory abnormalities on admission: WBC >16,000, blood glucose >200 ml/dl, serum LDH >350 IU/L, AST >250 IU/L
- Laboratory abnormalities during the initial 48 hr: decreased Hct >10% with hydration or Hct <30%, BUN rise >5 mg/dl, serum calcium <8 mg/dl, arterial Po_2 <60 mm Hg, and base deficit >4 mEq/L

■ REFERRAL
- Hospitalization is indicated in moderate/severe cases of pancreatitis.
- Surgical consultation is needed in suspected gallstone pancreatitis, perforated peptic ulcer, or presence of necrotic or infected foci.

Author: **Fred F. Ferri, M.D.**

BASIC INFORMATION

■ DEFINITION
Chronic pancreatitis is a recurrent or persistent inflammatory process of the pancreas characterized by chronic pain and by pancreatic exocrine and/or endocrine insufficiency.

ICD-9CM CODES
577.1 Chronic pancreatitis

■ EPIDEMIOLOGY & DEMOGRAPHICS
• Chronic pancreatitis occurs in approximately 5 to 10/100,000 persons in industrialized countries.
• Male:female ratio is 5:1.

■ PHYSICAL FINDINGS & CLINICAL PRESENTATION
• Persistent or recurrent epigastric and LUQ pain, may radiate to the back
• Tenderness over the pancreas, muscle guarding
• Significant weight loss
• Bulky, foul-smelling stools, greasy in appearance
• Epigastric mass (10% of patients)
• Jaundice (5% to 10% of patients)

■ ETIOLOGY
• Chronic alcoholism
• Obstruction (ampullary stenosis, tumor, trauma, pancreas divisum, annular pancreas)
• Hereditary pancreatitis
• Severe malnutrition
• Idiopathic
• Untreated hyperparathyroidism (hypercalcemia)
• Mutations of the cystic fibrosis transmembrane conductance regulator (CFTR) gene and the TF genotype
• Sclerosing pancreatitis: A form of chronic pancreatitis characterized by infrequent attacks of abdominal pain, irregular narrowing of the pancreatic duct, and swelling of the pancreatic parenchyma; these patients have high levels of serum immunoglobins (IgG4)

DIAGNOSIS

■ DIFFERENTIAL DIAGNOSIS
• Pancreatic cancer
• PUD
• Cholelithiasis with biliary obstruction
• Malabsorption from other etiologies
• Recurrent acute pancreatitis

■ WORKUP
Medical history with focus on alcohol use, laboratory tests, diagnostic imaging

■ LABORATORY TESTS
• Serum amylase and lipase may be elevated (normal amylase levels, however, do not exclude the diagnosis).
• Hyperglycemia, glycosuria, hyperbilirubinemia, and elevated serum alkaline phosphatase may also be present.
• 72-hr fecal fat determination (rarely performed) reveals excess fecal fat.
• Bentiromide test or secretin stimulation test can confirm pancreatic insufficiency.
• Elevated levels of serum IgG4 are found in sclerosing pancreatitis, but not in other disorders of the pancreas.

■ IMAGING STUDIES
• Plain abdominal radiographs may reveal pancreatic calcifications (95% specific for chronic pancreatitis).
• Ultrasound of abdomen may reveal duct dilation, pseudocyst, calcification, and presence of ascites.
• CT scan of abdomen is useful for the detection of calcifications, to evaluate for ductal dilation, and for ruling out pancreatic cancer.
• ERCP can be used to evaluate for the presence of dilated ducts, strictures, pseudocysts, and intraductal stones.
• Use of fine needle aspiration (FNA) and endoscopic ultrasound (EUS) are newer diagnostic modalities.

TREATMENT

■ NONPHARMACOLOGIC THERAPY
• Avoidance of alcohol
• Frequent, small-volume, low-fat meals

■ ACUTE GENERAL Rx
• Avoidance of narcotics if possible (simple analgesics or NSAIDs can be used)
• Treatment of steatorrhea with pancreatic supplements (e.g., Pancrease, Creon, Pancrelipase titrated prn based on the amount of steatorrhea and patient's weight loss)
• Octreotide 200 μg SC tid may be useful for pain secondary to idiopathic chronic pancreatitis
• Treatment of complications (e.g., type IDM)
• Glucocorticoid therapy in patients with sclerosing pancreatitis can induce clinical remission and significantly decrease serum concentrations of IgG4, immune complexes, and the IgG4 subclass of immune complexes

■ CHRONIC Rx
• Surgical intervention may be necessary to eliminate biliary tract disease and improve flow of bile into the duodenum by eliminating obstruction of pancreatic duct.
• ERCP with endoscopic sphincterectomy and stone extraction is useful in selected patients.
• Transduodenal sphincteroplasty or pancreaticojejunostomy in selected patients. Surgery should also be considered in patients with intractable pain.

■ DISPOSITION
• Long-term survival is poor (50% of patients die within 10 hr from chronic pancreatitis or malignancy).
• Prognosis is best in patients with recurrent acute pancreatitis resulting from cholelithiasis, hyperparathyroidism, or stenosis of the sphincter of Oddi.

■ REFERRAL
GI referral for ERCP, surgical referral in selected patients (see "Chronic Rx").

REFERENCES
Hamano H et al: High serum IgG4 concentrations in patients with sclerosing pancreatitis, *N Engl J Med* 344:732, 2001.

Hollerbach S et al: Endoscopic ultrasonography and fine needle aspiration cytology for diagnosis of chronic pancreatitis, *Endoscopy* 33:824, 2001.
Author: **Fred F. Ferri, M.D.**

BASIC INFORMATION

■ **DEFINITION**

Idiopathic Parkinson's disease is a progressive neurodegenerative disorder characterized clinically by rigidity, tremor, and bradykinesia. The major manifestations of the disease are due to loss of dopamine in the substantia nigra pars compacta. Its pathological hallmark is the Lewy body, which is a cytoplasmic eosinophilic inclusion body.

■ **SYNONYMS**

Paralysis agitans

ICD-9CM CODES

332.0 Idiopathic Parkinson's disease, primary
332.1 Parkinson's disease, secondary

■ **EPIDEMIOLOGY & DEMOGRAPHICS**

PREVALENCE:
- Affects over 1 million people in North America
- In age group, <40 yr, <5/100,000 are affected
- In those >70 yr, 700/100,000 are affected
- Highest incidence in whites, lowest incidence in Asians and black Africans

■ **PHYSICAL FINDINGS & CLINICAL PRESENTATION**
- Tremor—typically a resting tremor with a frequency of 4-6 Hz that is often first noted in the hand as a pill rolling tremor (thumb and forefinger). Can also involve the leg and lip. Tremor improves with purposeful movement. Usually starts asymmetrically but can eventually involve the other hemibody.
- Rigidity—increased muscle tone. This, too, is usually asymmetric in onset, involving the arm, leg or both. It is resistance that persists throughout the range of passive movement of a joint.
- Akinesia/Bradykinesia—slowness in initiating movement.
- Masked facies—face seems expressionless, giving the appearance of depression. Decreased blink, often there is excess drooling.
- Gait disturbance.
- Stooped posture, decreased arm swing.
- Difficulty initiating the first step; small shuffling steps that increase in speed (festinating gait) as if the patient is chasing his or her center of gravity (steps become progressively faster and shorter while the trunk inclines further forward).
- Other complaints and findings early on include micrographia—handwriting becomes smaller, and hypophonia—voice becomes softer.
- Postural instability—tested by "pull test." Ask patient to stand in place with back to examiner. Examiner pulls patient back by the shoulders, and proper response would be to take no steps back or very few steps back without falling. Retropulsion is a positive test as is falling straight back. This is not usually severe early on. If falls and postural reflexes are greatly impaired early on, then consider other disorders.

■ **ETIOLOGY**
- Unknown.
- Most cases are sporadic, with age being the most common risk factor, though there is probably a combination of both environmental and genetic factors contributing to disease expression. There are rare familial forms with at least three different genes identified. The two most well known are the parkin gene, which is a significant cause of early-onset autosomal recessive Parkinson's disease and isolated juvenile-onset Parkinson's' disease (at or before age 20), and alpha synuclein, which is responsible for autosomal dominant Parkinson's disease in isolated families.

 DIAGNOSIS

A presumptive clinical diagnosis can be made based on a comprehensive history and physical examination. The combination of asymmetric signs, resting tremor, and good response to L-dopa best differentiates idiopathic Parkinson's disease from other causes of parkinsonism (see "Differential Diagnosis").

■ **DIFFERENTIAL DIAGNOSIS**
- Multisystem atrophy—distinguishing features include autonomic dysfunction, including urinary incontinence, orthostatic hypotension, and erectile dysfunction, parkinsonism, cerebellar signs, and normal cognition.
- Diffuse Lewy Body disease—parkinsonism with concomitant dementia. Patients often have early hallucinations and fluctuations in level of alertness and mental status.
- Corticobasal degeneration—often begins asymmetrically with apraxia, cortical sensory loss in one limb, and sometimes alien limb phenomenon.
- Progressive supranuclear palsy—tends to have axial rigidity greater than appendicular (limb) rigidity. These patients have early and severe postural instability. Hallmark is supranuclear gaze palsy that usually involves vertical gaze before horizontal.
- Essential tremor
- Secondary (acquired) parkinsonism
  1. Postinfectious parkinsonism—von Economo's encephalitis
  2. Parkinson's pugilistica—after repeated head trauma
  3. Iatrogenic—any of the neuroleptics and antipsychotics. The high potency D_2-blocker neuroleptics are most likely to cause parkinsonism. Quetiapine is an atypical antipsychotic with a lower risk of causing parkinsonism. Clozaril does not cause parkinsonism. Toxins (e.g., MPTP, manganese, carbon monoxide)
- Cerebrovascular disease (basal ganglia infarcts)

■ **WORKUP**

Identification of clinical signs and symptoms associated with Parkinson's disease (see "Physical Findings") and elimination of conditions that may mimic it with a comprehensive history and physical examination

■ **IMAGING STUDIES**

CT scan has almost no role in investigations. MRI of the head may sometimes distinguish between idiopathic Parkinson's disease and other conditions that present with signs of parkinsonism (see "Differential Diagnosis").

TREATMENT

■ **NONPHARMACOLOGIC THERAPY**
- Physical therapy, patient education and reassurance, treatment of associated conditions (e.g., depression)
- Avoidance of drugs that can induce or worsen parkinsonism: neuroleptics (especially high potency), certain antiemetics (prochlorperazine, trimethobenzamide), metoclopramide, nonselective MAO inhibitors (may induce hypertensive crisis), reserpine, methyldopa

■ **ACUTE GENERAL Rx**
- There is persistent controversy whether L-dopa or dopamine agonists should be the initial treatment.
- It is appropriate to initiate pharmacotherapy when required by symptoms; prior practice of waiting for limitation of ADLs is now outdated.
- Motor complications do develop during the course of the disease and likely reflect the combination of disease progression together with the side effects of dopaminergic medications.

■ CHRONIC Rx

- Selegiline (Eldepryl), an inhibitor of MAO B, can be used early as initial therapy in those with very mild disease or as adjunctive therapy. Selegiline was once advocated as early, first-line therapy because of proposed neuroprotective effects; however, those benefits are probably less robust than once thought. Usual dose, 5 mg bid with breakfast and lunch. It can be useful in treating the fatigue that is commonly associated with PD. Concurrent use of stimulants and sympathomimetics should be avoided.
- Levodopa therapy
  1. Cornerstone of symptomatic therapy—should be used with a peripheral dopa decarboxylase inhibitor (carbidopa) to minimize side effects (nausea, mood changes, postural hypotension). The combination of the two drugs is marketed under the trade name Sinemet.
  2. Usual starting dose is 25/100 mg (carbidopa/levodopa) tid 1 hr before meals.
  3. Controlled-release preparations (Sinemet CR [200 mg levodopa/50 mg of carbidopa, or 100 mg levodopa/25 mg carbidopa]) are available, but their use should be deferred to a neurologist.
- Dopamine receptor agonists (Ropinirole, Pramipexole, Pergolide, and Bromocriptine) are not as potent as levodopa, but they are often used as initial treatment in younger patients to attempt to delay the onset of complications (dyskinesias, motor fluctuations) associated with levodopa therapy. These medications are more expensive than levodopa. In general they cause more side effects than levodopa. These include nausea, vomiting, lightheadedness, peripheral edema, confusion, and somnolence.
  1. Ropinirole (Requip): initial dose is 0.25 mg tid
  2. Pramipexole (Mirapex): initial dose of 0.125 mg tid
  3. Pergolide (Permax): initial dose, 0.05 mg for first 2 days increased by 0.1 mg every third day over

next 12 days. There have been a few cases of restrictive valvulopathy in association with Permax use. All patients on this medication need a good clinical cardiac examination, and if any concern, an echo
  4. Bromocriptine (Parlodel): initial dose, 1.25 mg qhs
- Amantadine (Symmetrel) is an antiviral agent that augments release and decreases reuptake of dopamine. It can be used alone early in the disease or in combination with levodopa; dosage is 100 mg tid (titrate q week from 100 mg qd). Must adjust for elderly and renal impairment. Most notable side effect, especially in elderly, is confusion.
- Anticholinergic agents are helpful in treating the tremor and drooling in patients with Parkinson's disease and can be used alone or in combination with levodopa; potential side effects (particularly in the elderly) include constipation, urinary retention, memory impairment, and hallucinations.
  1. Trihexyphenidyl (Artane): initial dose, 1 mg PO tid po
  2. Benztropine (Cogentin): usual dose, 0.5 to 1 mg qd or bid
- SURGICAL OPTIONS
  1. Pallidal (globus pallidus interna) and subthalamic deep brain stimulation are currently the surgical options of choice; Thalamic DBS may be useful for refractory tremor.
  2. Surgery is limited to patients with disabling, medically refractory problems, and patients must still have a good response to L-dopa to undergo surgery. DBS results in decreased dyskinesias, fluctuations, rigidity, and tremor. Bilateral DBS has better effect on midline symptoms, such as gait and balance; however, it has higher side effects, such as dysphagia and decreased cognition.

■ DISPOSITION

Parkinson's disease usually follows a slowly progressive course leading to disability over the course of several years. However, every patient will

progress individually and patients should be reassured that this diagnosis does not, by definition, result in being either wheelchair or bed bound.

■ REFERRAL

- Neurology consultation is recommended on initial diagnosis of Parkinson's disease.
- Rehabilitation medicine referral to a physiatrist or physical therapist for outpatient physical therapy is recommended for most patients with disabling symptoms. The most useful speech therapy method available is the Lee Silverman technique, which focuses on projection.

☼ PEARLS & CONSIDERATIONS

Asymmetry of symptoms at onset is very useful in distinguishing PD from other causes of parkinsonism. Though resting tremor is a common presenting symptom, up to one fourth of patients with idiopathic PD do not have classic resting tremor.

■ COMMENTS

Additional patient information on Parkinson's disease can be obtained from the Internet at www.parkinson.org and from the National Parkinson Foundation, Inc., 1501 Ninth Avenue NW, Miami, FL 33136; phone: (800) 327-4545.

REFERENCES

Ahlskog, JE: Parkinson's disease: medical and surgical treatment, in Hurtig H, Stern M (eds): *Neurologic clinics: movement disorders* 19:3, 2001.

Lang AE et al: Parkinson's disease, *N Engl J Med* 339(15):1044,

Lang AE et al: Parkinson's disease, *N Engl J Med* 339(16):1130,

Siderowf, A: Parkinson's disease: clinical features, epidemiology, and genetics, in Hurtig H, Stern M (eds): *Neurologic clinics: movement disorders* 19:3, 2001.

Author: **Cindy Zadikoff, M.D.**

BASIC INFORMATION

■ DEFINITION
Paronychia is a localized superficial infection or abscess of the lateral and proximal nail fold. Paronychia may be acute or chronic.

ICD-9CM CODES
681.9 Paronychia

■ EPIDEMIOLOGY & DEMOGRAPHICS
- Acute paronychia affects males and females equally.
- Chronic paronychia more common in females than males (9:1).
- Acute paronychia most often occurs in children.
- Chronic paronychia usually presents in the fifth or sixth decade of life.
- Paronychia is the most common infection of the hand.

■ PHYSICAL FINDINGS & CLINICAL PRESENTATION
- Acute paronychia usually presents with the sudden onset of redness, swelling, and pain with abscess or cellulitis formation in the nail fold. Fluid with purulence is often present.
- Chronic paronychia is insidious, presenting with mild swelling and erythema of the nail folds.
- Acute paronychia usually involves only one finger.
- Chronic paronychia may involve more than one finger.
- Acute paronychia usually involves the thumb.
- Chronic paronychia commonly involves the middle finger.

■ ETIOLOGY
- Any disruption of the seal between the proximal nail fold and the nail plate can cause paronychial infections.
- Acute paronychia is almost always bacterial in origin (e.g., *Staphylococcus aureus* [most common], *Streptococcus pyogenes*, *Streptococcus faecalis*, *Proteus* and *Pseudomonas* species, and anaerobes).
- Chronic paronychia is commonly caused by *Candida albicans* (70%) with bacterial organisms accounting for the remaining 30%.

- Trauma, nail biting, hangnails, diabetes, and chronic exposure to water are common predisposing features of paronychia.

DIAGNOSIS

The diagnosis of paronychia is self-evident on physical examination.

■ DIFFERENTIAL DIAGNOSIS
- Herpetic whitlow
- Pyogenic granuloma
- Viral warts
- Ganglions
- Squamous cell carcinoma

■ WORKUP
A workup is usually not pursued unless there is treatment failure.

■ LABORATORY TESTS
- Gram stain and culture any purulent drainage.
- KOH mount may show pseudohyphae.

■ IMAGING STUDIES
X-ray the digit if concerned about osteomyelitis.

TREATMENT

■ NONPHARMACOLOGIC THERAPY
- For acute paronychia without purulent drainage, warm soaks tid or qid are helpful. If pus is present, surgical drainage is required.
- For chronic paronychia, avoid chronic immersion in water or exposure to moisture.

■ ACUTE GENERAL Rx
- First-generation cephalosporin (e.g., cephalexin 250 to 500 mg qid) or penicillinase-resistant penicillin (e.g., dicloxacillin 250 to 500 mg qid) are usually the antibiotics of choice for acute paronychia.
- Alternative antibiotic choices include clindamycin and amoxicillin-clavulanate potassium
- Surgical drainage is indicated if purulent discharge is noted.
- A No. 11 blade scalpel is used to lift the lateral perionychium and proximal eponychium off the nail, facilitating drainage.

- If the pus is located beneath the nail, the lateral edge of the nail can be lifted off the nail bed and excised.

■ CHRONIC Rx
- If no fungal organism is found, tincture of iodine (2 drops bid) helps keep the nail and skin dry.
- Chronic paronychia caused by *Candida albicans* is treated with topical antifungal agents (e.g., miconazole or ketoconazole applied tid).
- Unresponsive cases may be treated with itraconazole or fluconazole but should be done in consultation with dermatology and/or infectious disease.
- Surgery may be needed in refractory cases.

■ DISPOSITION
- Most acute paronychias with appropriate treatment resolve within 7 to 10 days.
- Osteomyelitis is a potential complication of paronychia.
- Untreated chronic paronychia leads to thickening and discoloration with eventual nail loss.

■ REFERRAL
Chronic paronychia refractory to topical medical therapy is best referred to dermatology and/or infectious disease. A hand surgeon is consulted if abscess drainage is needed or if surgery is being considered.

PEARLS & CONSIDERATIONS

■ COMMENTS
- Women with chronic paronychia caused by *Candida albicans* should also be examined for candidal vaginitis.
- The GI tract, including the mouth and bowel, were the usual sources of *Candida albicans* in chronic paronychia.

REFERENCES
Rich P: Nail disorders: diagnosis and treatment of infectious, inflammatory, and neoplastic conditions, *Med Clin North Am* 82:1171, 1998.
Rockwell PG: Acute and chronic paronychia, *Am Fam Physician* 63:1113, 2001.
Authors: **Peter Petropoulos, M.D., and Dennis Mikolich, M.D.**

■ BASIC INFORMATION

■ DEFINITION
Paroxysmal atrial tachycardia (PAT) is a group of arrhythmias that generally originate as reentrant rhythm from the AV node and are characterized by sudden onset and abrupt termination.

■ SYNONYMS
PAT
SVT
Supraventricular tachycardia

ICD-9CM CODES
427.0 Paroxysmal atrial tachycardia

■ PHYSICAL FINDINGS & CLINICAL PRESENTATION
- Patient is usually asymptomatic.
- Patient may be aware of "fast" heartbeat.
- Persistent tachycardia may precipitate CHF or hypotension during acute MI.

■ ETIOLOGY
- Preexcitation syndromes (Wolff-Parkinson-White [WPW] syndrome)
- Atrial septal defect
- Acute MI

■ DIAGNOSIS

■ WORKUP
ECG:
- Absolutely regular rhythm at rate of 150 to 220 bpm is present.
- P waves may or may not be seen (the presence of P waves depends on the relationship of atrial to ventricular depolarization).
- Wide QRS complex (>0.12 sec) with initial slurring (delta wave) during sinus rhythm and short PR (≤0.12 sec) is characteristic of WPW syndrome; this syndrome is a result of an accessory AV pathway (bundle of Kent) that preexcites the ventricular muscle earlier than would be expected if the impulse reached the ventricles by way of normal conduction system; arrhythmias associated with WPW are narrow-complex SVT,

atrial fibrillation, and ventricular fibrillation; digoxin and verapamil use should be avoided because they can lead to arrhythmia acceleration through the accessory pathway. Radiofrequency catheter ablation of accessory pathways (performed in conjunction with diagnostic electrophysiology testing) is a safe and effective treatment of patients with WPW syndrome.

■ TREATMENT

■ NONPHARMACOLOGIC THERAPY
- Valsalva maneuver in the supine position is the most effective way to terminate SVT; carotid sinus massage (after excluding occlusive carotid disease) is also commonly used to elicit vagal efferent impulses.
- Synchronized DC shock is used if patient shows signs of cardiogenic shock, angina, or CHF.

■ ACUTE GENERAL Rx
- Adenosine (Adenocard), an endogenous nucleoside, is useful for treatment of paroxysmal SVT, particularly that associated with WPW; it is considered by many the first choice of therapy for treatment of almost all episodes of SVT unresponsive to vagal maneuvers; the dose is 6 mg given as a rapid IV bolus; tachycardia is usually terminated within a few seconds; if necessary, may repeat with 12 mg IV bolus. Contraindications are second- or third-degree AV block, sick sinus syndrome (SSS), atrial fibrillation, and ventricular tachycardia. Adenosine may cause bronchospasm in asthmatics. Patients receiving theophylline (a competitive antagonist of adenosine receptors) are usually refractory to treatment. Dipyridamole enhances the effect of adenosine; therefore patients receiving dipyridamole should be started at lower doses.

- Verapamil 5 to 10 mg IV is given over 5 min; if no effect, may repeat in 30 min.
  1. Verapamil should be used cautiously in patients with SVT associated with hypotension.
  2. Slow injection of calcium chloride (10 ml of a 10% solution given over 5 to 8 min before verapamil administration) decreases the hypotensive effect without compromising its antiarrhythmic effect.
- Repeat carotid massage after IV verapamil if SVT persists.
- Metoprolol (IV 5 mg/2 min up to 15 mg) or esmolol (500 μg/kg IV bolus, then 50 μg/kg/min) may be effective in the treatment of SVT.
- IV digitalization (0.75 to 1 mg slow IV loading)
  1. Repeat carotid massage 30 min later; if not successful, give additional 0.25 mg IV digoxin and repeat carotid sinus massage 1 hr later.
  2. Digoxin should be avoided in patients with WPW syndrome and narrow QRS tachycardia (increased risk of atrial fibrillation during AV reentrant tachycardia).

■ DISPOSITION
Most patients respond well with resolution of the paroxysmal atrial tachycardia with treatment (see "Acute General Rx").

■ REFERRAL
Radiofrequency ablation is the procedure of choice in patients with accessory pathways and recurrent symptomatic episodes.

☼ PEARLS & CONSIDERATIONS

■ COMMENTS
Accessory pathways occur in 0.1% to 0.3% of the general population.
Author: **Fred F. Ferri, M.D.**

BASIC INFORMATION

■ DEFINITION
Paroxysmal cold hemoglobinuria (PCH) is a type of hemolytic anemia caused by an IgG autoantibody to the erythrocyte P antigen. The PCH antibody is cold reacting and fixes complement to erythrocytes with exposure to cold in the extremities. Hemolysis occurs when these complement-fixed erythrocytes enter the warmth of the body's core.

ICD-9CM CODES
283.2 Hemoglobinuria caused by hemolysis from external causes

■ EPIDEMIOLOGY & DEMOGRAPHICS
- May occur in children following a viral infection
- In adults, may occur in setting of autoimmune disease, lymphoma, or chronic lymphocytic leukemia
- May be seen in patients with secondary or tertiary syphilis

■ PHYSICAL FINDINGS & CLINICAL PRESENTATION
- Dark-colored urine following exposure to cold
- Nonspecific symptoms include fever, chills, and pain in the back, legs, or abdomen
- Pallor or jaundice may be present
- Urine is brown or red

■ ETIOLOGY
- Caused by an IgG antibody that interacts with the erythrocyte P antigen and fixes complement to red blood cells with exposure to cold. These complement-fixed red blood cells hemolyze when they enter the body's core.
- PCH antibodies seen in association with secondary or tertiary syphilis, viral infections, autoimmune conditions, lymphoma, and chronic lymphocytic leukemia.

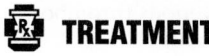

DIAGNOSIS

■ DIFFERENTIAL DIAGNOSIS
- Other causes of red or brown urine: beet ingestion, medications (phenazopyridine), myoglobinuria, hematuria
- Other causes of hemolysis: hemoglobinopathies, erythrocyte membrane defects, medications, toxins, microangiopathy, other forms of autoimmune hemolysis

■ WORKUP
Examination for signs of secondary or tertiary syphilis

■ LABORATORY TESTS
- Urinalysis to test for hemoglobinuria without red blood cells in urine sediment
- CBC and peripheral blood smear for presence of anemia, reticulocytes, and spherocytes
- Tests for hemolysis (indirect bilirubin, LDH, haptoglobin)
- Direct Coombs' test positive during hemolytic episodes

- Diagnosis established by demonstrating presence of IgG that reacts with red cells at reduced temperatures
  1. Tests using radiolabeled monoclonal anti-IgG are more sensitive than older tests

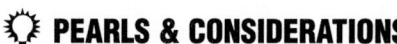

TREATMENT

■ ACUTE GENERAL THERAPY
- Avoidance of exposure to cold
- Treatment of syphilis, if present

■ CHRONIC Rx
- Prednisone 1 mg/kg/day PO to reduce antibody production
- For refractory cases, cyclophosphamide 100 mg/day for adults or azathioprine 100 mg/day for adults can be used

■ DISPOSITION
- Cases related to viral infection persist for 6 to 12 wk.
- Adult cases related to lymphomas or chronic lymphocytic leukemia may last several years.

■ REFERRAL
To hematologist for treatment and monitoring

PEARLS & CONSIDERATIONS

■ COMMENTS
Donath and Landsteiner described the syndrome of PCH in patients with syphilis in 1904.
Author: **Mark J. Fagan, M.D.**

BASIC INFORMATION

■ DEFINITION

Paroxysmal nocturnal hemoglobinuria (PNH) is a rare disease characterized by episodes of intravascular hemolysis and hemoglobinuria usually occurring at night. Thrombocytopenia, leukopenia, and recurrent venous thrombosis are also associated with PNH.

■ SYNONYMS

PNH

ICD-9CM CODES

283.2 Paroxysmal nocturnal hemoglobinuria

■ EPIDEMIOLOGY & DEMOGRAPHICS

- Affects patients of any age (reported spectrum 6 to 82 yr) but most common in patients aged 30 to 50 yr
- Affects both sexes (slight female predominance) and all races

■ PHYSICAL FINDINGS & CLINICAL PRESENTATION

Initial manifestations
- Anemia symptoms (35%)
- Hemoglobinuria (25%)
- Bleeding (20%)
- Aplastic anemia (15%)
- GI symptoms (10%)
- Hemolytic anemia (10%)
- Iron deficiency anemia (5%)
- Venous thrombosis (5%)
- Infections (5%)
- Neurologic symptoms

Hemoglobinuria
- Typically the first morning void reveals dark urine with progressive clearing during the day. The cause for the circadian rhythm is unknown.

Hemolysis
- In addition to the circadian hemolysis and resulting hemoglobinuria, episodes of hemolytic exacerbations can accompany infections, menstruation, transfusion, surgery, iron therapy, and vaccinations. Symptoms of severe hemolysis include chest, back, or abdominal pain, headache, fever, malaise, and fatigue.

Aplastic anemia
- Aplastic anemia may be the presenting manifestation of PNH (therefore PNH must be in the differential diagnosis of aplastic anemia) or may develop as a later complication of PNH.

Thrombosis
- Lower extremity DVT
- Subclavian thrombosis
- Portal or mesenteric vein thrombosis
- Hepatic vein thrombosis (Budd-Chiari syndrome)
- Cerebrovascular thromboses

Renal failure
- Acute renal failure associated with massive hemoglobinuria (acute tubular necrosis)
- Progressive renal failure associated with thrombosis within renal small veins

Dysphagia

Infections (associated with leukopenia or steroid treatment)

Physical findings include:
- Pallor (anemia)
- Jaundice (hemolysis)
- Splenomegaly
- Unilateral extremity swelling (DVT)
- Ascites (Budd-Chiari syndrome)

■ ETIOLOGY & PATHOGENESIS

- Complement-mediated hemolysis; the erythrocytes are abnormally sensitive to acidified serum.
- Patients have two populations of RBCs, some sensitive to hemolysis (PNH III cells) and others not (PNH I cells) in variable proportions (10% to 75% PNH III cells). About 20% PNH III are required for hemoglobinuria to be detectable.
- The RBC defects in PNH are in the membrane proteins as follows:
  Decay-accelerating factor deficiency
  Membrane inhibitor of reactive lysis deficiency
  C-8 binding protein deficiency
- These protein deficiencies are the result of an acquired mutation located in the X chromosome, which regulates glycosylphosphatidylinositol (GPI). GPI anchors the abovementioned proteins in the RBC membrane; GPI-deficient RBCs proliferate as an abnormal clone. Because women are affected least as frequently as men are, the mutation must be expressed as dominant gene. The mechanism whereby the mutant stem cells can dominate hematopoiesis in PNH is unknown.
- The pathophysiology of the relationship of PNH and aplastic anemia is unknown.

DIAGNOSIS

Clinical situations:
- Intravascular hemolysis
- Hemoglobinuria
- Pancytopenia associated with hemolysis
- Iron deficiency associated with hemolysis
- Recurrent venous thrombosis
- Recurrent episodes of abdominal pain, headache, or back pain associated with hemolysis

■ DIFFERENTIAL DIAGNOSIS

- See "Hemolytic Anemia" in Section I.
- See "Aplastic Anemia" in Section I.

- See "Anemia" algorithm in Section III.

■ LABORATORY TESTS

- CBC: anemia, leukopenia, thrombocytopenia
- Reticulocytosis
- RBC smear: spherocytes
- Negative Coombs' test
- Low leukocyte alkaline phosphatase
- Elevated LDH
- Low serum haptoglobin
- Low serum iron saturation, low ferritin
- Elevated urine hemoglobin
- Elevated urine urobilinogen
- Elevated urine hemosiderin
- Positive Ham test (acidified serum RBC lysis)
- Normoblastic hyperplasia on bone marrow aspirate or biopsy
- Identification of GPI-anchored protein deficiency on hematopoietic cells using monoclonal antibodies or flow cytometry
- Cytogenetic studies are not diagnostic

TREATMENT

- Androgenic steroids
- Prednisone (15 to 40 mg qod)
- Eculizumab, a humanized antibody that inhibits the activation of terminal complement components reduces intravascular hemolysis, hemoglobinuria, and need for transfusion in patients with PNH.
- Iron replacement
- Transfusions
- Treatment and prevention of thrombosis (heparin, coumarin)
- Avoidance of oral contraceptives
- Bone marrow transplantation

■ REFERRAL

To hematologist

■ PROGNOSIS

- 50% survival to 10 to 15 yr
- 25% survival to 25 yr
- If thrombosis at presentation, only 40% survival to 4 yr
- 1% incidence of leukemia
- 5% incidence of myelodysplastic syndrome

REFERENCES

Hillmen P et al: Effect of eculizumab on hemolysis and transfusion requirements in patients with paroxysmal nocturial hemoglobinuria, *N Engl J Med* 350:6, 2004.

Parker CJ, Lee GR: Paroxysmal nocturnal hemoglobinuria. In Lee GR et al (eds): *Wintrobe's clinical hematology*, ed 10, Baltimore, 1999, Williams & Wilkins.

Author: **Tom J. Wachtel, M.D.**

BASIC INFORMATION

■ DEFINITION
Pediculosis is lice infestation. Humans can be infested with three kinds of lice: *Pediculus capitis* (head louse [Fig. 1-204]), *Pediculus corporis* (body louse), and *Phthirus pubis* (pubic, or crab, louse). Lice feed on human blood and deposit their eggs (nits) on the hair shafts (head lice and pubic lice) and along the seams of clothing (body lice). Nits generally hatch within 7 to 10 days. Lice are obligate human parasites and cannot survive away from their hosts for longer than 7 to 10 days.

■ SYNONYMS
Lice

ICD-9CM CODES
132.9 Pediculosis

■ EPIDEMIOLOGY & DEMOGRAPHICS
- There are 6 million to 12 million cases of head lice in the U.S. yearly.
- Lice infestation of the scalp is most common in children (girls > boys).
- Infestation of the eyelashes is most frequently seen in children and may indicate sexual abuse.
- The chance of acquiring pubic lice from one sexual exposure with an infested partner is >90% (most contagious STD known).
- Body lice is most common in conditions of poor hygiene.

■ PHYSICAL FINDINGS & CLINICAL PRESENTATION
- Pruritus with excoriation may be caused by hypersensitivity reaction, inflammation from saliva, and fecal material from the lice.
- Nits can be identified by examining hair shafts.
- The presence of nits on clothes is indicative of body lice.
- Lymphadenopathy may be present (cervical adenopathy with head lice, inguinal lymphadenopathy with pubic lice).

- Head lice is most frequently found in the back of the head and neck, behind the ears.
- Scratching can result in pustules and crusting.
- Pubic lice may affect the hair around the anus.

■ ETIOLOGY
Lice are transmitted by close personal contact or use of contaminated objects (e.g., combs, clothing, bed linen, hats).

 ## DIAGNOSIS

■ DIFFERENTIAL DIAGNOSIS
- Seborrheic dermatitis
- Scabies
- Eczema
- Other: pilar casts, trichonodosis (knotted hair), monilethrix

■ WORKUP
Diagnosis is made by seeing the lice or their nits. Combing hair with a fine-toothed comb is recommended because visual inspection of the hair and scalp may miss more than 50% of infestations.

■ LABORATORY TESTS
Wood's light examination is useful to screen a large number of children: live nits fluoresce, empty nits have a gray fluorescence, nits with unborn louse reveal white fluorescence.

TREATMENT

■ NONPHARMACOLOGIC THERAPY
- Patients with body lice should discard infested clothes and improve their hygiene.
- Combing out nits is a widely recommended but unproven adjunctive therapy.
- Personal items such as combs and brushes should be soaked in hot water for 15 to 30 min.
- Close contacts and household members should also be examined for the presence of lice.

■ ACUTE GENERAL Rx
The following products are available for treatment of lice:
- Permethrin: available over the counter (1% permethrin [Nix]) or by prescription (5% permethrin [Elimite]); should be applied to the hair and scalp and rinsed out after 10 min. A repeat application is generally not necessary in patients with head lice.
- Lindane 1% (Kwell), pyrethrin S (Rid): available as shampoos or lotions; they are applied to the affected area and washed off in 5 min; treatment should be repeated in 7 to 10 days to destroy hatching nits.
- Malathion (Ovide) or organophosphate is effective in head lice. It is available by prescription. Use should be avoided in children ≤2 yr.
- Eyelash infestation can be treated with the application of petroleum jelly rubbed into the eyelashes three times a day for 5 to 7 days. The application of baby shampoo to the eyelashes and brows three or four times a day for 5 days is also effective. The use of fluorescein drops applied to the lids and eyelashes is also toxic to lice.
- In patients who have previously failed treatment or in whom resistance with 1% permethrin cream rinse occurs, a 10-day course of trimethoprim-sulfamethoxazole (TMP-SMX) 8 mg/kg/day of trimethoprim in divided doses is an effective treatment for head lice infestation.
- Ivermectin (Mectizan), an antiparasitic drug, given in a single oral dose of 200 µg/kg is effective for head lice resistant to other treatments (currently not FDA approved for pediculosis).

PEARLS & CONSIDERATIONS

■ COMMENTS
- Patients with pubic lice should notify their sexual contacts. Sex partners within the last month should be treated.
- Parents of patients should also be educated that head lice infestation (unlike body lice) does not indicate poor hygiene.

REFERENCES
Flinders DC, DeSchweinitz P: Pediculosis and scabies, *Am Fam Physician* 69:341, 2004.
Roberts RJ: Head lice, *N Engl J Med* 346:1645, 2002.
Author: **Fred F. Ferri, M.D.**

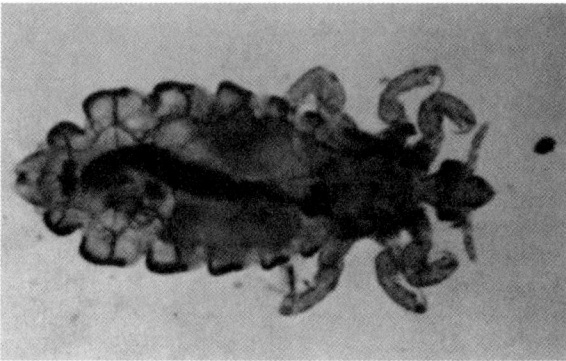

Fig. 1-204 *Pediculus humanus* var. **capitis (head louse).** (From Mandell GL [ed]: *Mandell, Douglas, and Bennett's principles and practice of infectious diseases,* ed 5, New York, 2000, Churchill Livingstone.)

BASIC INFORMATION

■ DEFINITION
Pedophilia is a sexual disorder of at least 6 mo of recurrent, intense, distressing sexual urges and/or fantasies involving prepubescent children.

■ SYNONYMS
Pedophilia erotica
Acts referred to as child sexual abuse or child molestation
One of the paraphilias

ICD-9CM CODES
302.2 Pedophilia

■ EPIDEMIOLOGY & DEMOGRAPHICS
INCIDENCE (IN U.S.): Accurate data are unavailable.
PREVALENCE (IN U.S.): Prevalence of victimization is variable, ranging from 5% to 60% of all adults reporting at least one case of sexual abuse (not necessarily penetration) before age 13 yr.
PREDOMINANT SEX:
- Majority are men: nearly 75% attracted to females exclusively; nearly 25% attracted to males exclusively; small minority attracted to both sexes
- Females: 5% to 20%

PREDOMINANT AGE: No available data
PEAK INCIDENCE:
- No available data
- Usually, onset in adolescence

GENETICS: No genetic factor has been identified.

■ PHYSICAL FINDINGS & CLINICAL PRESENTATION
- Often shy, passive, and with social and interpersonal difficulties
- Frequently, has experienced early abuse himself/herself
- Sexually excited by young children and adults with the build that resembles young children
- Do not all act on their sexual fantasies; may occasionally seek help before any sexual acts with children
- Some "belief" among those who actually molest children that their behavior is good for or welcomed by the child

■ ETIOLOGY
- Etiology is unclear.
- Personal experience with early molestation may be important, but clearly only a minority of molested children develop pedophilia.
- Influence of personality factors is possible.

DIAGNOSIS

■ DIFFERENTIAL DIAGNOSIS
- Psychosis: may present with unusual ideas or statements that may rarely be confused with pedophilia; but statements or behaviors of psychotic individuals are usually disorganized and relatively short lived.
- Incest: some is not based in pedophilia, but may instead reflect a dysfunctional family unit.
- Paraphilic sexual behavior in the setting of another condition such as mental retardation, brain injury, or drug intoxication.

■ WORKUP
- History is essential for diagnosis; however, most pedophiles are less than forthcoming even to direct questions by a physician.
- Collateral information should be obtained from family members, suspected victims, or legal and social organizations; but even experienced interviewers may be unable to diagnose pedophilia consistently.

■ LABORATORY TESTS
- Hormone profile (total testosterone, free testosterone, luteinizing hormone, follicle-stimulating hormone, prolactin, and progesterone) is sometimes recommended, but results do not guide diagnosis or treatment.
- If a medical condition with secondary CNS dysfunction is suspected, tailor laboratory investigation accordingly.

■ IMAGING STUDIES
Useful only if pedophilic behavior is believed to be a consequence of CNS damage (e.g., head trauma or mental retardation), then a head CT scan or MRI may document extent of anatomic damage.

TREATMENT

■ NONPHARMACOLOGIC THERAPY
- Usually obtain treatment under legal coercion after child molestation charge.
- Rarely, may initiate treatment request.
- Behavioral approaches are centered on aversion conditioning in which an aversive stimulus is paired with the pedophilic fantasy; when outcome is measured by repeat child molestation charges, these methods are moderately successful.
- For incestuous adult-child relationships not based in pedophilia, intensive family systems investigation and therapy are needed.

■ ACUTE GENERAL Rx & CHRONIC Rx
- Castration is an effective method of control of paraphilic behaviors, including child molestation. However, the irreversibility of the surgery and the subjective aversion to the procedure make it less than desirable.
- Chemical castration with antiandrogen compounds is more acceptable to the public; although research into the optimal dosage and the efficacy of these compounds is far from complete, they are generally believed to be safe, effective, and reversible.
- Medroxyprogesterone acetate (Provera) can be administered PO (60 mg/day) or in a depot IM form (200 to 400 mg IM once weekly).

■ DISPOSITION
- Untreated, child molesters are highly likely to be repeat offenders.
- Pedophiles who do not act on their fantasies are likely to continue these fantasies.
- NOTE: Contrary to popular belief, the majority of sexual acts are committed in the absence of alcohol.

■ REFERRAL
If pedophilia is highly suspected

REFERENCES
Murray JB: Psychological profile of pedophiles and child molesters, *J Psychol* 134:211, 2000.
Repique RJ: Assessment and treatment of persons with pedophilia, *J Psychosoc Nurs Ment Health Serv* 37:19, 1999.
Rice ME, Harris GT: Men who molest their sexually immature daughters: is a special explanation required? *J Abnorm Psychol* 111:329, 2002.
Author: Rif S. El-Mallakh, M.D.

BASIC INFORMATION

■ DEFINITION
Pelvic inflammatory disease (PID) is a spectrum of inflammatory disorders of the upper genital tract including a combination of any of the following:
- Endometritis, salpingitis, tuboovarian abscess, or pelvic peritonitis
- Resulting from an ascending lower genital tract infection
- Not related to obstetric or surgical intervention

■ SYNONYMS
Adnexitis
Pyosalpinx
Salpingitis
Tuboovarian abscess

ICD-9CM CODES
614.9 Unspecified inflammatory disease of female pelvic organs and tissue

■ EPIDEMIOLOGY & DEMOGRAPHICS
INCIDENCE/PREVALENCE:
- Estimated 600,000 to 1 million cases annually (U.S.)
- Diagnosed in 2% to 5% of women seen in STD clinics
- Most common cause of female infertility and ectopic pregnancy

RISK FACTORS:
- Adolescent sexually active in females <20 yr old (1:8)
- Previous episode of gonococcal PID
- Multiple sexual partners
- Vaginal douching
- Use of intrauterine device (threefold to fivefold increased risk of developing acute PID)

■ PHYSICAL FINDINGS & CLINICAL PRESENTATION
- Lower abdominal pain
- Abnormal vaginal discharge
- Abnormal uterine bleeding
- Dysuria
- Dyspareunia
- Nausea and vomiting (suggestive of peritonitis)
- Fever
- RUQ tenderness (perihepatitis): 5% of PID cases
- Cervical motion tenderness and adnexal tenderness
- Adnexal mass

■ ETIOLOGY
- *Chlamydia trachomatis*
- *Neisseria gonorrhoeae*
- Polymicrobial infection—*Bacteroides fragilis, Escherichia coli, Gardnerella vaginalis, Haemophilus influenzae, Mycoplasma hominis, U. urealyticum*
- *Mycobacterium tuberculosis* (an important cause in developing countries)
- Cytomegalovirus (CMV)

DIAGNOSIS

■ DIFFERENTIAL DIAGNOSIS
- Ectopic pregnancy
- Appendicitis
- Ruptured ovarian cyst
- Endometriosis
- Urinary tract infection (cystitis or pyelonephritis)
- Renal calculus
- Adnexal torsion
- Proctocolitis

■ WORKUP
DIAGNOSTIC CONSIDERATIONS:
- Clinical diagnosis is difficult and imprecise. A clinical algorithm for the evaluation of pelvic pain in the reproductive-age woman is described in Section III, Fig. 3-141; evaluation of vaginal discharge is described in Section III, Fig. 3-189.
- Clinical diagnosis of symptomatic PID has a positive predictive value of 65% to 90% when compared with laparoscopy as the standard.
- No single historical, physical, or laboratory finding is both sensitive and specific for the diagnosis of PID.

2002 CDC DIAGNOSTIC CRITERIA FOR PID:
- Empiric treatment is based on the presence of all of the following minimum criteria:
  1. Uterine tenderness
  2. Adnexal tenderness
  3. Cervical motion tenderness
- Additional criteria to increase the specificity of the diagnosis of PID in women with severe clinical signs:
  1. Oral temperature >38.3° C (101° F)
  2. Abnormal cervical or vaginal discharge
  3. Elevated ESR
  4. Elevated C-reactive protein
  5. Laboratory documentation of cervical infection with *N. gonorrhoeae* or *C. trachomatis*
- Definitive criteria for diagnosing PID, which are warranted in selected cases:
  1. Laparoscopic abnormalities consistent with PID
  2. Histopathologic evidence of endometritis on biopsy
  3. Transvaginal sonography or other imaging techniques showing thickened fluid-filled tubes with or without free pelvic fluid or tuboovarian complex

■ LABORATORY TESTS
- Leukocytosis
- Elevated acute phase reactants: ESR >15 mm/hr, C-reactive protein
- Gram stain of endocervical exudate: >30 PMNs per high-power field correlates with chlamydial or gonococcal infection
- Endocervical cultures for *N. gonorrhoeae* and *C. trachomatis*
- Fallopian tube aspirate or peritoneal exudate culture if laparoscopy performed
- hCG to rule out ectopic pregnancy

■ IMAGING STUDIES
- Transvaginal ultrasound to look for adnexal mass has sensitivity for PID of 81%, specificity 78%, accuracy 80%.
- MRI has sensitivity for PID of 95%, specificity 89%, accuracy 93%. It is useful not only for establishing the diagnosis of PID, but also for detecting other processes responsible for the symptoms. Disadvantages are its higher cost and unavailability in certain areas.

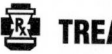 TREATMENT

■ NONPHARMACOLOGIC THERAPY
- Most patients are treated as outpatients.
- Criteria for hospitalization (2002 CDC) as follows:
  1. Surgical emergencies such as appendicitis cannot be excluded
  2. Tuboovarian abscess
  3. Pregnant patient
  4. Patient is immunodeficient
  5. Severe illness, nausea, or vomiting precluding outpatient management
  6. Patient unable to follow or tolerate outpatient regimens
  7. No clinical response to outpatient therapy

■ ACUTE GENERAL Rx
REGIMENS FOR TREATMENT OF PID RECOMMENDED BY THE CDC, 2002:
- Outpatient treatment: Regimen A:
  1. Ofloxacin 400 mg PO bid × 14 days or Levofloxacin 500 mg PO × 14 days plus metronidazole 500 mg PO bid × 14 days
- Outpatient treatment: Regimen B:
  1. Cefoxitin 2 g IM plus probenecid 1 g PO *or*
  2. Ceftriaxone 250 mg IM *or*
  3. Equivalent cephalosporin (ceftizoxime or cefotaxime) plus doxycycline 100 mg PO bid × 10 to 14 days
- Inpatient treatment: Regimen A:
  1. Cefoxitin 2 g IV q6h or cefotetan 2 g IV q12h plus doxycycline 100 mg IV or PO q12h
  2. Continuation of regimen for at least 24 hr after substantial clinical improvement, after which doxycycline 100 mg PO bid is continued for a total of 14 days

- Inpatient treatment: Regimen B:
  1. Clindamycin 900 mg IV q8h plus gentamicin loading dose IV or IM (2 mg/kg of body weight), followed by a maintenance dose (1.5 mg/kg) q8h
  2. Continuation of regimen for at least 24 hr after substantial clinical improvement, followed by doxycycline 100 mg PO bid or clindamycin 450 mg PO qid to complete a total of 14 days of therapy
- Alternative parental regimens:
  1. Ofloxacin 400 mg IV q12h or
  2. Levofloxacin 500 mg IV once daily with or without Metronidazole 500 mg IV q8h or
  3. Ampicillin/sulbactam 3 gm IV q6h plus doxycycline 100 mg PO or IV q12h

■ CHRONIC Rx

Hospitalized patients receiving IV therapy:
1. Significant clinical improvement is characterized by defervescence, decreased abdominal tenderness, and decreased uterine, adnexal, and cervical motion tenderness within 3 to 5 days.
2. If no clinical improvement occurs, further diagnostic workup is necessary, including possible surgical intervention.

■ DISPOSITION

- Long-term sequelae of PID: recurrent PID, chronic pelvic pain, ectopic pregnancy, infertility, Fitz-Hugh–Curtis syndrome (Fig. 1-205)
- Risk of tubal infertility related to episodes of PID: first episode, 8%; second episode, 20%; third episode, 40%

- Essential to evaluate and treat male sex partners

■ REFERRAL

If there is no clinical improvement with outpatient therapy observed within 72 hr, patient should be hospitalized and gynecology consult requested.

☼ PEARLS & CONSIDERATIONS

■ COMMENTS

- Maintain a low threshold for the diagnosis of PID
- Patient education material is available from local and state health departments or from the American College of Obstetricians and Gynecologists.

REFERENCES

Centers for Disease Control and Prevention: 2002 sexually transmitted diseases treatment guidelines, *MMWR Morb Mortal Wkly Rep* 51(RR-6), 2002.

Tukeva TA et al: MR imaging in pelvic inflammatory disease: comparison with laparoscopy and ultrasound, *Radiology* 210:209, 1999.

Author: **George T. Danakas, M.D.**

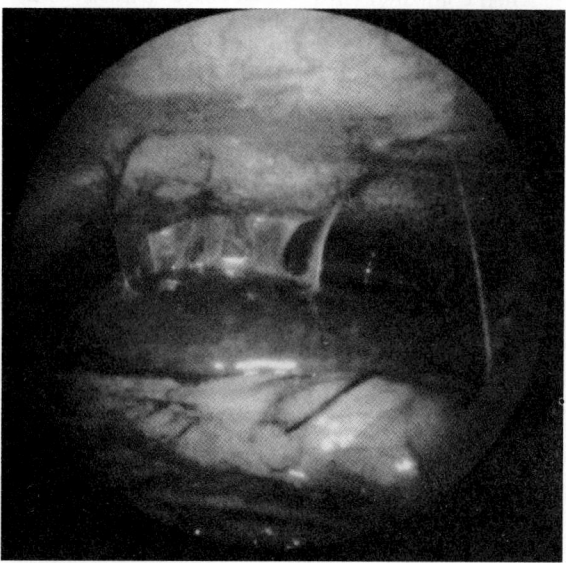

Fig. 1-205 "Violin string" adhesions are visualized in this patient with Fitz-Hugh-Curtis syndrome. (From Copeland LJ: *Textbook of gynecology,* ed 2, Philadelphia, 2000, WB Saunders.)

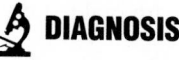

 ## BASIC INFORMATION

■ DEFINITION
- Pemphigus refers to a group of chronic, autoimmune diseases resulting in intraepidermal blister formation.
- Pemphigus has four subtypes:
  1. Pemphigus vulgaris (Fig. 1-206)
  2. Pemphigus vegetans
  3. Pemphigus foliaceus
  4. Pemphigus erythematosus
- Pemphigus vulgaris refers to an intraepidermal blistering skin disorder characterized by the formation of the flaccid blister.

■ SYNONYMS
Pemphigus

■ ICD-9CM CODES
694.4 Pemphigus

■ EPIDEMIOLOGY & DEMOGRAPHICS
- Incidence is 1/100,000
- More common in Ashkenazi Jews
- Typically occurs in the fourth and fifth decades of life
- Male = females
- Can occur in the young

■ PHYSICAL FINDINGS & CLINICAL PRESENTATION
- History
  1. Oral mucosa lesions typically occur first, followed by a generalized bullous eruption within a few months
  2. Lesions are fragile and rupture easily, leaving painful denuded lesions
  3. Usually not pruritic
- Physical findings
  1. Anatomic distribution
     a. Oral mucosa
     b. Can also involve the pharynx, larynx, vagina, penis, anus, and conjunctival mucosa
     c. Generalized cutaneous involvement
  2. Lesion configuration
     a. All stratified squamous epithelium can become involved.
  3. Lesion morphology
     a. Bullae
     b. Denuded crusting and erosion commonly occurs

■ ETIOLOGY
Pemphigus vulgaris, like all subtypes of pemphigus, is an autoimmune disease caused by autoantibodies binding to antigens within the epithelial layer of the skin.

DIAGNOSIS

The diagnosis of pemphigus vulgaris should be suspected in patients with oral lesion and flaccid bullae on the skin.

■ DIFFERENTIAL DIAGNOSIS
- Bullous pemphigoid (see Table 1-42)
- Cicatricial pemphigoid
- Behçet's disease
- Erythema multiforme
- Systemic lupus erythematosus
- Aphthous stomatitis
- Dermatitis herpetiformis
- Drug eruptions

■ WORKUP
The workup for patients with suspected pemphigus vulgaris requires specific laboratory tests and special histology and immunofluorescence testing to establish the diagnosis.

■ LABORATORY TESTS
- Autoantibodies can be detected in the serum by indirect immunofluorescence assays.
- Skin biopsy reveals intraepidermal bulla formation, also called acantholysis (loss of cell adhesion between the epidermal cells).
- Direct and indirect immunofluorescence studies of the lesion show deposits of IgG and C3 in the epidermal layers of the skin.

■ IMAGING STUDIES
X-ray imaging is not useful in the diagnosis of pemphigus vulgaris.

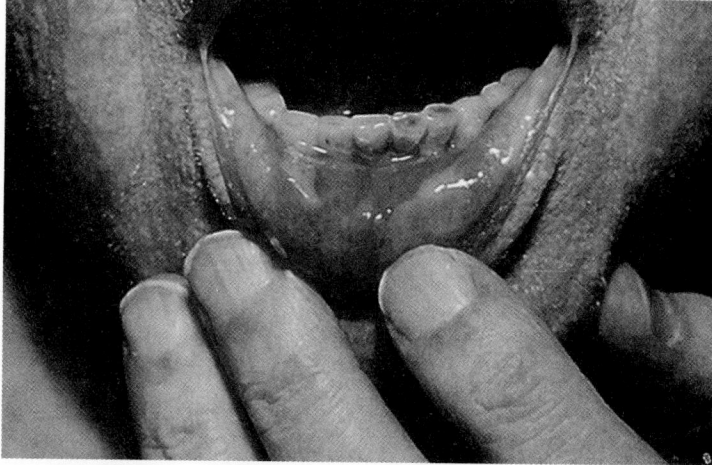

Fig. 1-206   Pemphigus vulgaris with oral lesions and no intact bullae. (Courtesy Department of Dermatology, University of North Carolina at Chapel Hill. In Goldstein BG, Goldstein AO: *Practical dermatology,* ed 2, St Louis, 1997, Mosby.)

TABLE 1-42   Differentiation of Pemphigus Vulgaris and Bullous Pemphigoid

CHARACTERISTICS	PEMPHIGUS VULGARIS	BULLOUS PEMPHIGOID
Age	≥50 years	≥60 years
Site	Oral mucosa, face, chest, groin	Flexural areas, groin, axilla, less often oral
Findings	Flaccid bullae, intraepidermal blisters, IgG autoantibodies	Intact bullae, subepidermal blisters, IgG and complement autoantibodies
Treatment	Prednisone 40-60 mg/day, immunosuppressant agents; often chronically steroid-dependent	Prednisone 1 mg/kg/day or higher initially; taper over months to years
Prognosis	>90% respond; steroid side effects significant	>90% respond; remissions and recurrences common

From Goldstein BG: *Practical dermatology,* ed 2, St Louis, 1997, Mosby.

TREATMENT

■ NONPHARMACOLOGIC THERAPY
- Use mild soaps.
- Soak lesions with Burow's solution.
- Soft diet and viscous lidocaine can be used in patients with oral lesions.

■ ACUTE GENERAL Rx
- For mild cases, topical intralesional steroids using triamcinolone acetonide 5 to 10 mg/ml can be used for individual lesions.
- For more severe cases, systemic corticosteroids are indicated at high dosages:
  1. Prednisone 200 to 400 mg/day for 6 to 8 wk, tapered to 15 mg/day
  2. Alternative approaches include prednisone 80 to 120 mg PO qd increasing the dose rapidly by 50% every 7 days until no new lesions appear; then proceed with tapering over a 6-mo period

■ CHRONIC Rx
- Adjuvant therapy is tried in patients in an attempt to decrease the amount of steroids required.
  1. Azathioprine 100 to 150 mg qd given concurrently with prednisone
  2. Cyclophosphamide 1 to 3 mg/kg/day
  3. Dapsone 25 to 100 mg/day
  4. Nicotinamide 500 mg PO qd plus tetracycline 1.5 to 3 g/day
  5. Plasmapheresis

■ DISPOSITION
- Before the use of corticosteroids, approximately 75% of patients died of pemphigus.
- Combined corticosteroids and adjuvant therapy has decreased mortality rates to <10%.
- Pemphigus vulgaris patients usually die from sepsis or complications from therapy.

■ REFERRAL
A dermatology consult is recommended for any patient with pemphigus vulgaris.

☼ PEARLS & CONSIDERATIONS

■ COMMENTS
- Pemphigus vulgaris, unlike bullous pemphigus, rarely occurs in the elderly population.
- It is important to diagnose pemphigus vulgaris early in its course.

REFERENCES

Bickle K, Roark TR, Hsu S: Autoimmune bullous dermatoses: a review, *Am Fam Physician* 65(9):1861, 2002.

Brenner S, Sasson A, Sharon O: Pemphigus and infections, *Clin Dermatol* 20(2):114, 2002.

Stanley JR: Therapy of pemphigus vulgaris, Editorial, *Arch Dermatol* 135(1):76, 1999.

Toth GG, Jonkman MF: Therapy of pemphigus, *Clin Dermatol* 19(6):761, 2001.

Author: **Peter Petropoulos, M.D.**

BASIC INFORMATION

DEFINITION
Peptic ulcer disease (PUD) is an ulceration in the stomach or duodenum resulting from an imbalance between mucosal protective factors and various mucosal damaging mechanisms (see "Etiology").

SYNONYMS
PUD
Duodenal ulcer (DU)
Gastric ulcer (GU)

ICD-9CM CODES
536.8 Peptic ulcer disease
531.3 Peptic ulcer, stomach, acute
531.7 Peptic ulcer, stomach, chronic
532.3 Peptic ulcer, duodenum, acute
532.7 Peptic ulcer, duodenum, chronic

EPIDEMIOLOGY & DEMOGRAPHICS
- Incidence: 250,000 to 500,000 (200,000 to 400,000 DU; 50,000 to 100,000 GU) annually; duodenal ulcer:gastric ulcer ratio is 4:1.
- Anatomic location: >90% of DUs occur in the first portion of the duodenum; GU occurs most frequently in the lesser curvature near the incisura angularis.

PHYSICAL FINDINGS & CLINICAL PRESENTATION
- Physical examination is often unremarkable.
- Patient may have epigastric tenderness, tachycardia, pallor, hypotension (from acute or chronic blood loss), nausea and vomiting (if pyloric channel is obstructed), board-like abdomen and rebound tenderness (if perforated), and hematemesis or melena (with a bleeding ulcer).

ETIOLOGY
Often multifactorial; the following are common mucosal damaging factors:
- *Helicobacter pylori* infection
- Medications (NSAIDs, glucocorticoids)
- Incompetent pylorus or LES
- Bile acids
- Impaired proximal duodenal bicarbonate secretion
- Decreased blood flow to gastric mucosa
- Acid secreted by parietal cells and pepsin secreted as pepsinogen by chief cells
- Cigarette smoking
- Alcohol

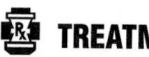 **DIAGNOSIS**

DIFFERENTIAL DIAGNOSIS
- GERD
- Cholelithiasis syndrome
- Pancreatitis
- Gastritis
- Nonulcer dyspepsia
- Neoplasm (gastric carcinoma, lymphoma, pancreatic carcinoma)
- Angina pectoris, MI, pericarditis
- Dissecting aneurysm
- Other: high small bowel obstruction, pneumonia, subphrenic abscess, early appendicitis

WORKUP
- Comprehensive history and physical examination to exclude other diagnoses. Diagnostic modalities include endoscopy or UGI series. Endoscopy is invasive and more expensive; however, it is preferred for the following reasons:
  1. Highest accuracy (approximately 90% to 95%)
  2. Useful to identify superficial or very small ulcerations
  3. Essential to diagnose gastric ulcers (1% to 4% of gastric ulcers diagnosed as benign by UGI series are eventually diagnosed as gastric carcinoma)
  4. Additional advantages over UGI series include:
     - Biopsy of suspicious looking ulcers
     - Electrocautery of bleeding ulcers
     - Measurement of gastric pH in suspected gastrinoma (e.g., patient with multiple ulcers)
     - Diagnosis of esophagitis, gastritis, duodenitis
     - Endoscopic biopsy for *H. pylori*

LABORATORY TESTS
- Routine laboratory evaluation is usually unremarkable.
- Anemia may be present in patients with significant GI bleeding.
- *H. pylori* testing via endoscopic biopsy, urea breath test, stool antigen test (*H. pylori* stool antigen), or specific antibody test is recommended:
  1. Serologic testing for antibodies to *H. pylori* is easy and inexpensive; however, the presence of antibodies demonstrates previous but not necessarily current infection. Antibodies to *H. pylori* can remain elevated for months to years after infection has cleared; therefore antibody levels must be interpreted in light of patient's symptoms and other test results (e.g., PUD seen on UGI series).

  2. The urea breath test documents active infection. The patient ingests a small amount of urea labeled with carbon 13 (^{13}C) or carbon 14. If urease is present (produced by the organism), the urea is hydrolyzed and the patient exhales labeled carbon dioxide that is then collected and measured. This test is more expensive and not as readily available. Use of proton pump inhibitors within 2 wk of the urea breath test may interfere with test results.
  3. Histologic evaluation of endoscopic biopsy samples is currently the gold standard for accurate diagnosis of *H. pylori* infection.
  4. Stool antigen test is as accurate as the urea breath test for follow-up evaluation of patients treated for *H. pylori*. This test detects the presence of infection by measuring the fecal excretion of *H. pylori* antigens. A positive result on the stool antigen test 8 wk after completion of therapy identifies patients in whom eradication of *H. pylori* was unsuccessful.
- Additional laboratory evaluation is indicated only in specific cases (e.g., amylase level in suspected pancreatitis, serum gastrin level in suspected Zollinger-Ellison [Z-E] syndrome).

IMAGING STUDIES
Conventional UGI barium studies identify approximately 70% to 80% of PUD; accuracy can be increased to approximately 90% by using double contrast.

TREATMENT

NONPHARMACOLOGIC THERAPY
- Stop cigarette smoking; cigarette smoking increases the risk of PUD, decreases the healing rate, and increases the frequency of recurrence.
- Avoid NSAIDs and alcohol.
- Special diets have been proved *unrelated* to ulcer development and healing; however, avoid foods that cause symptoms.

ACUTE GENERAL Rx
Eradication of *H. pylori,* when present, can be accomplished with various regimens:
1. Proton pump inhibitors (PPI) bid (e.g., omeprazole 20 mg bid or lansoprazole 30 mg bid) *plus* clarithromycin 500 mg bid *and* amoxicillin 1000 mg bid for 7 to 10 days

2. PPI bid *plus* amoxicillin 500 mg bid *plus* metronidazole 500 mg for 7 to 10 days
3. PPI bid *plus* clarithromycin 500 mg bid *and* metronidazole 500 mg bid for 7 days
4. Recent trials indicate that a 1-day quadruple therapy may be as effective as a 7-day triple therapy regimen. The 1-day quadruple therapy regimen consists of two tablets of 262 mg bismouth subsalicylate qid, one 500 mg metronidazole tablet qid, 2 g of amoxicillin suspension qid, and two capsules of 30 mg of lansoprazole.
5. Bismouth compound qid *plus* tetracycline 500 mg qid *and* metronidazole 500 mg qid for 14 days
6. A 5-day treatment with three antibiotics (amoxicillin 1 g bid, clarithromycin 250 mg bid, and metronidazole 400 mg bid) plus either lansoprazole 30 mg bid or ranitidine 300 mg bid is an efficacious cost-saving option for patients older than 55 yr with no history of PUD

PUD patients testing negative for *H. pylori* should be treated with antisecretory agents:

- Histamine-2 receptor antagonists (H$_2$RAs): cimetidine, ranitidine, famotidine, and nizatidine are all effective; they are usually given in split dose or at nighttime.
- Proton pump inhibitors (PPIs): can also induce rapid healing; they are usually given 30 min before meals.

Antacids and sucralfate are also effective agents for the treatment and prevention of PUD.

■ CHRONIC Rx

Maintenance therapy in duodenal ulcer patients is indicated in the following situations:

- Persistent smokers
- Recurrent ulcerations

- Chronic treatment with NSAIDs, glucocorticoids
- Elderly or debilitated patients
- Aggressive or complicated ulcer disease (e.g., perforation, hemorrhage)
- Asymptomatic bleeders

Misoprostol therapy (100 µg qid with food, increased to 200 µg qid if well tolerated) should be considered for the prevention of NSAID-induced gastric ulcers in all patients on long-term NSAID therapy; it is contraindicated in women of childbearing age because of its abortifacient properties. Proton pump inhibitors are also effective at healing ulcers and maintaining remission in patients on long-term NSAIDs.

■ DISPOSITION

- The recurrence rate for untreated PUD is approximately 60% (>70% in smokers). Treatment decreases the recurrence rate by nearly 30%.
- Patients with recurrent ulcers should be retreated for an additional 8 wk and then placed on maintenance therapy with H$_2$RAs, PPIs, sucralfate, or antacids.
- An ulcer is considered refractory to treatment if healing is not evident after 8 wk for duodenal ulcers and 12 wk for gastric ulcers. In these patients maximum acid inhibition (e.g., omeprazole 40 mg qd) is preferred over continued therapy with standard antiulcer therapy.
- Eradication of *H. pylori* (when present) is indicated in all patients. Undetectable serum antibody levels beyond the first year of therapy accurately confirm cure of *H. pylori* infection with reasonable sensitivity in initially seropositive healthy subjects.
- Screening for Zollinger-Ellison (Z-E) syndrome should also be considered in patients with multiple recurrent ulcers; in patients with Z-E, the serum gastrin level is >1000 pg/ml and the basal acid output is usually >15 mEq/hr.

- Surgery for refractory ulcers is now only rarely performed; it consists of highly selective vagotomy for duodenal ulcers or ulcer removal with antrectomy or hemigastrectomy without vagotomy for gastric ulcers.

■ REFERRAL

- GI referral for patients requiring endoscopy
- Surgical referral for patients with nonhealing ulcers despite appropriate medical therapy

✺ PEARLS & CONSIDERATIONS

■ COMMENTS

- Patients with gastric ulcers should have repeat endoscopy after 4 to 6 wk of therapy to document healing and test exfoliative cytology for gastric carcinoma.
- After endoscopic treatment of bleeding peptic ulcers, bleeding recurs in up to 20% of patients. PPI administration intravenously by continuous infusion substantially reduces the risk of recurrent bleeding.

REFERENCES

Graham DY et al: Ulcer prevention in long-term users of nonsteroidal anti-inflammatory drugs, *Arch Intern Med* 162:169, 2002.

Lai KC et al: Lansoprazole for the prevention of recurrences of ulcer complications from long-term low-dose aspirin use, *N Engl J Med* 346:2033, 2002.

Lara LF et al: One day quadruple therapy compared with 7-day triple therapy for helicobacter pylori infection, *Arch Intern Med* 163:2079, 2003.

Author: **Fred F. Ferri, M.D.**

■ BASIC INFORMATION

■ DEFINITION
Pericarditis is the inflammation (or infiltration) of the pericardium associated with a wide variety of causes (see "Etiology").

ICD-9CM CODES
420.91 Pericarditis

■ EPIDEMIOLOGY & DEMOGRAPHICS
- The incidence of acute pericarditis is 2% to 6%.
- Increased incidence in males and in adults compared with children.
- Most common cause (>40%) of constrictive pericarditis is idiopathic.
- The use of thrombolytic agents has greatly reduced the incidence of both early postinfarction pericarditis and Dressler's syndrome.

■ PHYSICAL FINDINGS & CLINICAL PRESENTATION
- Severe constant pain that localizes over the anterior chest and may radiate to arms and back; it can be differentiated from myocardial ischemia, because the pain intensifies with inspiration and is relieved by sitting up and leaning forward (the pain of myocardial ischemia is not pleuritic).
- Pericardial friction rub is best heard with patient upright and leaning forward and by pressing the stethoscope firmly against the chest; it consists of three short, scratchy sounds:
  1. Systolic component
  2. Diastolic component
  3. Late diastolic component (associated with atrial contraction)
- Cardiac tamponade may be occurring if the following are observed:
  1. Tachycardia
  2. Low blood pressure and pulse pressure
  3. Distended neck veins
  4. Paradoxical pulse

■ ETIOLOGY
- Idiopathic (possibly postviral)
- Infectious (viral, bacterial, tuberculous, fungal, amebic, toxoplasmosis)
- Collagen-vascular disease (SLE, rheumatoid arthritis, scleroderma, vasculitis, dermatomyositis)
- Drug-induced lupus syndrome (procainamide, hydralazine, phenytoin, isoniazid, rifampin, doxorubicin, mesalamine)
- Acute MI
- Trauma or posttraumatic
- After MI (Dressler's syndrome)
- After pericardiotomy
- After mediastinal radiation (e.g., patients with Hodgkin's disease)
- Uremia
- Sarcoidosis
- Neoplasm (primary or metastatic)
- Leakage of aortic aneurysm in pericardial sac
- Familial Mediterranean fever
- Rheumatic fever
- Leukemic infiltration
- Other: anticoagulants, amyloidosis, ITP

■ DIAGNOSIS

■ DIFFERENTIAL DIAGNOSIS
- Angina pectoris
- Pulmonary infarction
- Dissecting aneurysm
- GI abnormalities (e.g., hiatal hernia, esophageal rupture)
- Pneumothorax
- Hepatitis
- Cholecystitis
- Pneumonia with pleurisy

■ WORKUP
ECG, laboratory tests, and echocardiogram

■ LABORATORY TESTS
The following tests may be useful in absence of an obvious cause:
- CBC with differential
- Viral titers (acute and convalescent)
- ESR (not specific but may be of value in following the course of the disease and the response to therapy)
- ANA, rheumatoid factor
- PPD, ASLO titers
- BUN, creatinine
- Blood cultures
- Cardiac isoenzymes (usually normal, but mild elevations of CK-MB may occur because of associated epicarditis)

■ IMAGING STUDIES
- Echocardiogram to detect and determine amount of pericardial effusion; absence of effusion does not rule out the diagnosis of pericarditis. Divergence of right and left ventricular systolic pressures is present in cardiac tamponade and constrictive pericarditis.
- ECG: varies with the evolutionary stage of pericarditis
  1. Acute phase: diffuse ST-segment elevations (particularly evident in the precordial leads), which can be distinguished from acute MI by:
     a. Absence of reciprocal ST-segment depression in oppositely oriented leads (reciprocal ST-segment depression may be seen in aV_R and VI)
     b. Elevated ST segments concave upward
     c. Absence of Q waves
  2. Intermediate phase: return of ST segment to baseline, and T wave inversion in leads previously showing ST-segment elevation (Fig. 1-207)
  3. Late phase: resolution of the T wave changes
- Chest radiography
  1. Cardiac silhouette appears enlarged if more than 250 ml of fluid has accumulated
  2. Calcifications around the heart may be seen with constrictive pericarditis

■ TREATMENT

■ NONPHARMACOLOGIC THERAPY
- Limitation of activity until the pain abates
- Patient education regarding potential complications (e.g., cardiac tamponade, constrictive pericarditis)

■ ACUTE GENERAL Rx
- Antiinflammatory therapy (NSAIDs, [e.g., naproxen 500 mg bid, indomethacin 25 to 50 mg tid])
- Prednisone 30 mg bid for severe forms of acute pericarditis (before use of prednisone, tuberculous pericarditis must be excluded)
- Colchicine 0.6 mg bid may be used as an alternative in patients intolerant to NSAIDs and corticosteroids
- Consider ventricular rate control with verapamil or diltiazem because of the propensity for atrial fibrillation in these patients
- Close observation of patients for signs of cardiac tamponade
- Avoidance of anticoagulants (increased risk of hemopericardium)

TREATMENT OF UNDERLYING CAUSE:
1. Bacterial pericarditis
   a. Commonly caused by streptococci, meningococci, staphylococci, *Haemophilus*, gram-negative bacteria, anaerobic bacteria
   b. Therapy: systemic antibiotics and surgical drainage of pericardium
2. Fungal pericarditis
   a. Caused by histoplasmosis, coccidioidomycosis, candidiasis, blastomycosis, or aspergillosis
   b. Therapy: IV amphotericin B and drainage of pericardial space (if necessary)
3. Tuberculous endocarditis
   a. Therapy: antituberculous drugs for a minimum of 9 mo; concomitant corticosteroid therapy early in treatment may decrease inflammatory response and improve prognosis.
   b. Pericardiectomy may be necessary 2 to 4 wk after antituberculous drugs have been started.
4. Collagen vascular disease and idiopathic: NSAIDs, prednisone
5. Uremic: dialysis

POTENTIAL COMPLICATIONS FROM PERICARDITIS:

1. Pericardial effusion: the time required for pericardial effusion to develop is of critical importance; if the rate of accumulation is slow, the pericardium can gradually stretch and accommodate a large effusion (up to 1000 ml), whereas rapid accumulation can cause tamponade with as little as 200 ml of fluid.

2. Chronic constrictive pericarditis:
   a. Physical examination reveals jugular venous distention, Kussmaul's sign (increase in jugular venous distention during inspiration as a result of increased venous pulse), pericardial knock (early diastolic filling sound heard 0.06 to 0.1 sec after S_2), clear lungs, tender hepatomegaly, pedal edema, ascites
   b. Chest x-ray: clear lung fields, normal or slightly enlarged heart, pericardial calcification
   c. ECG: low-voltage QRS complex
   d. Echocardiography: may show pericardial thickening or may be normal
   e. Cardiac catheterization: M or W contour of the central venous pattern caused by both systolic (x) and diastolic (y) dips (this differs from cardiac tamponade, which does not display a prominent diastolic descent; in chronic constrictive pericarditis, there is also increased right ventricular and pulmonary arterial pressures)
   f. Therapy: surgical stripping or removal of both layers of the constricting pericardium

3. Cardiac tamponade:
   a. Signs and symptoms: dyspnea, orthopnea, interscapular pain.
   b. Physical examination: distended neck veins, distant heart sounds, decreased apical impulse, diaphoresis, tachypnea, tachycardia, Ewart's sign (an area of dullness at the angle of the left scapula caused by compression of the lungs by the pericardial effusion), pulsus paradoxus (decrease in systolic blood pressure >10 mm Hg during inspiration), hypotension, narrowed pulse pressure.
   c. Chest x-ray: cardiomegaly (water bottle configuration of the cardiac silhouette may be seen) with clear lungs; the chest x-ray film may be normal when acute tamponade occurs rapidly in the absence of prior pericardial effusion.
   d. ECG reveals decreased amplitude of the QRS complex, variation of the R wave amplitude from beat to beat (electrical alternans). This results from the heart's oscillating in the pericardial sac from beat to beat and frequently occurs with neoplastic effusions.
   e. Echocardiography: detects effusions as small as 30 ml; a paradoxical wall motion may also be seen.
   f. Cardiac catheterization: equalization of pressures within chambers of the heart, elevation of right atrial pressure with a prominent x but no significant y descent.
   g. MRI can also be used to diagnose pericardial effusions.
   h. Therapy for pericardial tamponade consists of immediate pericardiocentesis preferably by needle paracentesis with the use of echocardiography, fluoroscopy, or CT; in patients with recurrent effusions (e.g., neoplasms), placement of a percutaneous drainage catheter or pericardial window draining in the pleural cavity may be necessary. Aspirated fluid should be sent for analysis (protein, LDH, cytology, CBC, Gram stain, AFB stain) and cultures for AFB, fungi, and bacterial C&S.

■ DISPOSITION
- Complete resolution of pain and other signs and symptoms during the initial 3 wk of therapy
- Recurrence in 10% to 15% of patients within the initial 12 mo
- Recurrent pericarditis in 28% of patients
- Relapsing acute pericarditis and idiopathic chronic large pericardial effusion without tamponade may respond to treatment with colchicine
- Recurrence of large effusion after pericardiocentesis is common in patients with idiopathic chronic pericardial effusion. Pericardiectomy should be considered in these patients

REFERENCES

Goyle K, Walling A: Diagnosing pericarditis, *Am Fam Physician* 66:1695, 2002.
Spodick DH: Acute cardiac tamponade, *N Engl J Med* 349:7, 2003.
Author: **Fred F. Ferri, M.D.**

PERICARDITIS, EVOLVING PATTERN

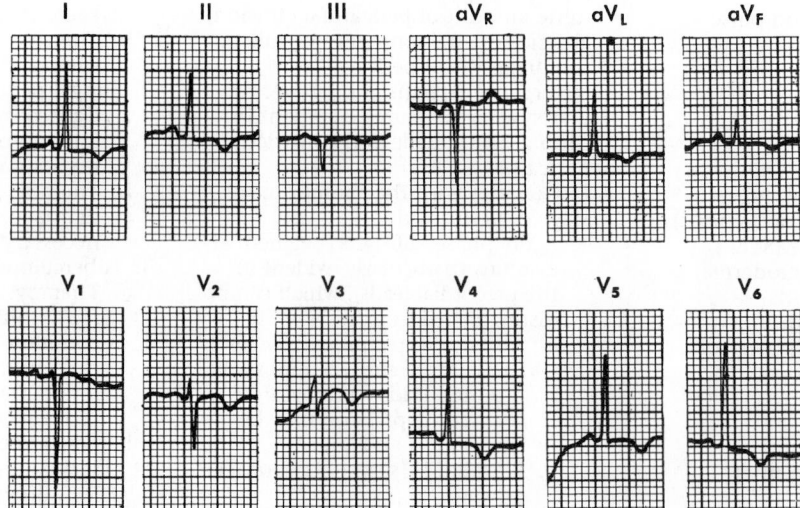

Fig. 1-207 Notice the diffuse T wave inversions in leads I, II, III, aV$_L$, aV$_F$, and V$_2$ to V$_6$. (From Goldberg AL [ed]: *Clinical electrocardiography,* ed 5, St Louis, 1994, Mosby.)

BASIC INFORMATION

■ DEFINITION

Peripheral arterial disease (PAD) usually refers to atherosclerotic obstruction of the arteries to the lower extremity.

■ ICD-9CM CODES

443.9 Peripheral vascular disease

■ EPIDEMIOLOGY & DEMOGRAPHICS

- Age-adjusted prevalence of PAD is approximately 12%.
- PAD affects men and women equally.
- Although the prevalence of PAD in Europe and North America is estimated at approximately 27 million people, PAD remains underdiagnosed and undertreated.
- An estimated 10.5 million patients are symptomatic, and the majority, 16.5 million, are asymptomatic.
- Risk factors associated with PAD are similar to coronary artery disease, including tobacco, diabetes, hyperlipidemia, and hypertension.
- Of the four risk factors, cigarette smoking is the major determinant of disease progression.
- Elevated levels of homocysteine and fibrinogen are also commonly elevated in patients with PAD and are to be considered as risk factors for PAD.

■ PHYSICAL FINDINGS & CLINICAL PRESENTATION

- Nearly 50% of the patients with PAD experience no symptoms
- Approximately one third of patients with PAD present with intermittent claudication described as an aching or cramping leg pain brought on by exertion and relieved with rest that can progress with time
- Pain at rest occurring commonly at night when the patient is supine
- Diminished pulses
- Bruits heard over the distal aorta, iliac, or femoral arteries
- Rubor with prolonged capillary refill on dependency
- Cool skin temperature
- Trophic changes of hair loss and muscle atrophy
- Nonhealing ulcers, necrotic tissue, and gangrene possible

■ ETIOLOGY

The primary cause of peripheral arterial disease is atherosclerosis: atherosclerotic lesions of the arteries to the lower extremities subsequently leading to stenosis of peripheral vessels and inability to supply oxygenated blood to working limb muscles.

DIAGNOSIS

■ DIFFERENTIAL DIAGNOSIS

- Spinal stenosis
- Degenerative joint disease of the lumbar spine and hips
- Muscle cramps
- Compartment syndrome

■ WORKUP

- The initial workup in any patient suspected of having PAD includes measuring the ankle-brachial index (ABI). The ABI is calculated by dividing the highest ankle systolic pressure using either the dorsalis pedis or posterior tibial artery by the highest systolic pressure from either arm.
- A diagnosis of PAD is based on the presence of limb symptoms or an ABI
- The severity of PAD is based on the ABI at rest and during treadmill exercise (1 to 2 mph, 5 min, or symptom-limited) and is classified as follows:
  1. Mild: ABI at rest 0.71 to 0.90 or ABI during exercise >0.50
  2. Moderate: ABI at rest 0.41 to 0.70 or ABI during exercise >0.20
  3. Severe: ABI at rest <0.40 or ABI during exercise <0.20
- As part of a noninvasive workup for patients with PAD, pulse volume recordings measuring volume of limb flow per pulse in a segment of the limb are used.
- Recording the pulse volume in different segments of the limb (e.g., thigh, calf, ankle, metatarsal, and toes), one monitors the contour of the pulse wave with significant changes occurring distal to stenotic lesions.

■ LABORATORY TESTS

- Lipid profile
- Blood glucose
- HgbA1c levels in diabetic patients
- Homocysteine
- Fibrinogen

■ IMAGING STUDIES

- Duplex ultrasound can be used to locate the occluded areas and assess the patency of the distal arterial system or prior vein grafts.
- MRA can be used as a noninvasive approach to visualize the aorta and peripheral lower extremity arteries. A major advantage of MRA is that it does not require contrast agents.
- Angiography remains the gold standard for visualizing the arterial anatomy before revascularization.

TREATMENT

■ NONPHARMACOLOGIC THERAPY

- PAD patients with no prior history of a cardiac event are to be considered as a cardiovascular "equivalent" with risks of future cardiovascular events similar to patients with prior MIs
- Tobacco counseling and smoke cessation programs are indispensable in decreasing the progression of disease as well as reducing the mortality rate from cardiovascular events in patients with PAD
- Diet counseling (e.g., salt restriction in hypertension, ADA calorie diets in diabetics)
- Exercise training walking 30 to 60 min/day at about 2 mi/hr every day improves exercise capacity, walking distance, and quality of life

■ ACUTE GENERAL THERAPY

Most patients with PAD respond to conservative management mentioned previously. If this fails, medicines can be tried (see "Chronic Rx"). Surgical reconstitution has its specific indications reserved for patient with impending limb loss (see "Chronic Rx").

■ CHRONIC Rx

- Aspirin 81 mg to 325 mg daily is recommended for secondary disease prevention in patients with cardiovascular disease.
- Clopidogrel 75 mg daily also provides protection from cardiovascular and cerebrovascular events associated with PAD.
- Pentoxyphylline (Trental, Pentoxil) 400 mg tid may provide a small benefit in walking distance when compared with placebo.
- Cilostazol (Pletal) 100 mg bid has been shown to significantly increase the distance patients with claudication can walk when compared with placebo, but should not be given to patients with congestive heart failure and an ejection fraction <40.
- Surgical reconstruction is indicated in patients with refractory rest pain, limb ischemia, nonhealing ulcers, or gangrene, and in a select group of patients with functional disability. Common surgical procedures:
  1. Aortoiliofemoral reconstruction
  2. Infrainguinal bypass (e.g., femoropopliteal, femorotibial)
  3. Extraanatomic bypass (e.g., axillofemoral or femorofemoral bypass)
- Angioplasty is used on short, discrete stenotic lesions in the iliac or femoropopliteal artery.

■ DISPOSITION

Risk factor modification with aggressive pharmacotherapy in the treatment of hyperlipidemia, diabetes, hypertension, and smoking is essential in the prevention of progression, limb ischemia, and cardiovascular events in patients with PAD.

■ REFERRAL

Consultation with a vascular surgeon is recommended in patients with PAD and rest pain, functional disability from pain, ABI less than 0.50 at rest, any signs of limb ischemia, or gangrene.

⚙ PEARLS & CONSIDERATIONS

■ COMMENTS

- PAD is a marker for generalized atherosclerosis with most patients dying from cardiovascular causes (e.g., myocardial infarction and cerebrovascular accidents).
  Asymptomatic PAD, similar to symptomatic PAD, is associated with an increased risk of atherothrombotic events (e.g., MI and CVA).
- Patients with PAD are at very high risk for an ischemic event and are six times more likely to die within 10 yr than patients without PAD.

REFERENCES

Belch JJ et al: Critical issues in peripheral arterial disease detection and management, *Arch Intern Med* 163;884, 2003.

Hiatt WR: Medical treatment of peripheral arterial disease and claudication, *N Engl J Med* 344:21, 2001.

Hirsch AT et al: Peripheral arterial disease detection, awareness, and treatment in primary care, *JAMA* 286:ll, 2001.

Lesho E et al: Management of peripheral arterial disease, *Am Fam Physician* 69:525, 2004.

Mukheijee D, Yadav JS: Update on peripheral vascular diseases: from smoking cessation to stenting, *Cleve Clinic J Med* 68:8, 2001.

Author: **Peter Petropoulos, M.D.**

■ BASIC INFORMATION

■ DEFINITION

The term *peripheral neuropathy* refers to any disorder involving the peripheral nerves. It encompasses:

- Polyneuropathy—a symmetric, usually length-dependent, disorder of peripheral nerves; a distinction is often made between predominantly small fiber (often painful) and large fiber neuropathies
- Mononeuropathy—disorder of a single peripheral nerve (e.g., median or ulnar neuropathy)
- Mononeuropathy multiplex—a multifocal disorder characterized by dysfunction of many individual peripheral nerves (when extensive, dysfunction may become confluent and resemble a generalized polyneuropathy)

ICD-9CM CODES

356.9 Unspecified idiopathic peripheral neuropathy

■ PHYSICAL FINDINGS & CLINICAL PRESENTATION

Polyneuropathy—symptoms usually begin distally in the feet and gradually spread proximally

- Sensory
  - Numbness, paresthesiae, neuropathic pain
  - Sensory ataxia (result of impairment of position sense)
  - Reduced or absent deep tendon reflexes
- Motor
  - Weakness, muscle atrophy
  - Foot deformities (high arches, hammer toes)—especially with hereditary neuropathy
- Autonomic
  - Postural hypotension

Mononeuropathy—symptoms and signs depend on the peripheral nerve affected

- Median nerve (carpal tunnel syndrome)—numbness, tingling in the thumb and adjacent two fingers; pain in the wrist and forearm; often worst at night and with activities like driving

Mononeuropathy multiplex

- Pain in the distribution of individual peripheral nerves
- Multifocal motor and sensory deficits

■ ETIOLOGY

HEREDITARY NEUROPATHIES:

- Charcot-Marie-Tooth syndrome
  1. Most common familial motor and sensory neuropathy
  2. Type I (most common) is demyelinating; Type II is axonal
  3. Foot deformities (high arches, hammer toes) are common

ACQUIRED NEUROPATHIES:

- Demyelinating
  - Guillain-Barré syndrome—acute (progression over <4 wk) ascending flaccid paralysis with areflexia; may be accompanying sensory loss, pain and autonomic dysfunction (see section entitled "Guillain-Barré Syndrome")
  - Chronic inflammatory demyelinating polyradiculoneuropathy (CIDP)—subacute to chronic (progression over >2 mo) sensorimotor polyneuropathy (may be associated with monoclonal gammopathy)
- Axonal
  1. Diabetes mellitus: frequently painful, usually affects sensory fibers more than motor
  2. Nutritional deficiency—B_{12}, folate
  3. Toxins—alcohol, drugs (e.g., isoniazid, vincristine, cisplatin, colchicines, amiodarone, phenytoin, antiretrovirals, metronidazole, dapsone, nitrofurantoin, disulfiram), chemicals (lead, arsenic, mercury)
  4. Thyroid disease (hypothyroidism)
  5. Paraproteinemia—monoclonal gammopathy of undetermined significance (MGUS), multiple myeloma, Waldenstrom's macroglobulinemia, primary systemic amyloidosis
  6. Collagen vascular disorders—SLE, rheumatoid arthritis, Sjögren's syndrome, polyarteritis nodosa (may cause polyneuropathy and mononeuropathy multiplex)
  7. Sarcoidosis: cranial nerve palsies (most common is facial nerve).
  8. Paraneoplastic
  9. Infections (leprosy, herpes zoster, TB, diphtheria, Lyme disease, HIV); may cause polyneuropathy or mononeuropathy
  10. Uremia
  11. Compression—typically causes mononeuropathy

■ DIAGNOSIS

■ WORKUP

- History should be directed toward inquiry about specific etiologies—systemic disease (e.g., diabetes mellitus, collagen disorder), alcohol intake, medication use, toxin exposure, dietary practices (e.g., veganism may cause B_{12} deficiency), risk factors for HIV infection, family history (of neuropathy or foot deformities)
- Neurophysiology (nerve conduction studies and electromyography) to determine the pattern of involvement (e.g., polyneuropathy vs. mononeuropathy multiplex) as well as the physiology (axonal vs. demyelinating)
- Lumbar puncture may be appropriate when demyelinating neuropathies suspected (e.g., GBS)
- Nerve biopsy may be indicated when vasculitis or amyloid suspected
- Section III, Fig. 3-142 describes an approach to the patient with peripheral neuropathy

■ LABORATORY TESTS

Some or all of these tests may be appropriate, depending on clinical suspicion

- Fasting blood sugar and/or 2-hr glucose tolerance test
- Serum B_{12}, homocysteine, methylmalonic acid as well as folate
- Renal function
- Thyroid function tests
- Serum protein and immunofixation electrophoresis; urine protein electrophoresis
- ANA, RF, cryoglobulins
- HIV, RPR, hepatitis serologies, Lyme titers
- Heavy metal screen; urinary porphyrins

■ IMAGING STUDIES

Usually, imaging studies are not required. Certain clinical conditions may require the following:

- Chest x-ray—when sarcoid or underlying lung cancer suspected
- Skeletal survey (long bone x-rays) to identify plasmacytoma
- MRI of lumbosacral (and/or cervical spine) if spinal cord pathology or polyradiculopathy suspected

TREATMENT

■ NONPHARMACOLOGIC THERAPY
- Stop offending agent (drugs or toxins) if any identified
- Surgical referral for entrapment neuropathy
- Physical and/or occupational therapy as well as splinting (e.g., ankle-foot orthosis) as appropriate

■ ACUTE GENERAL Rx
1. Treatment of underlying systemic disease (e.g., diabetes, uremia, multiple myeloma, etc.)
2. Nutritional replacement when appropriate (e.g., B_{12} injections)
3. Symptomatic treatment of neuropathic pain—many options available
   a. Nortriptyline—start 10 mg qhs, increase to 25 mg, 50 mg or 75 mg qhs as tolerated
   b. Amitriptyline—start 10 mg qhs, increase to 25 mg, 50 mg or 75 mg qhs as tolerated
   c. Neurontin—start 300 mg tid (more slowly in the elderly); gradually increase as needed and as tolerated, aiming initially for 900 mg tid
   d. Topamax—start 25 mg qd, then 25 mg bid, then 50 mg bid, increasing as tolerated and needed
   e. Lamictal—start 50 mg qd for 2 wk, then 50 mg bid for 2 wk; then increase by 50 mg per week as tolerated and needed (Stevens Johnson rash may occur if dose escalated too quickly)
   f. Narcotic analgesics—may be used, but the aforementioned agents should be tried first

REFERENCES

Hughes RAC: Peripheral neuropathy, *BMJ* 324:466, 2002.

Mendell JR, Sahenk Z: Clinical practice—painful sensory neuropathy, *N Engl J Med* 348:1243, 2003.

Stevens JC et al: Symptoms of 100 patients with electromyographically verified carpal tunnel syndrome, *Muscle Nerve* 22:1448, 1999.

Author: **Michael Benatar, M.B.Ch.B., D.Phil.**

BASIC INFORMATION

■ **DEFINITION**

Peritonitis refers to the acute onset of severe abdominal pain secondary to peritoneal inflammation.

■ **SYNONYMS**

Acute abdomen
Surgical abdomen

■ **ICD-9CM CODES**

567.2 Peritonitis

■ **EPIDEMIOLOGY & DEMOGRAPHICS**

Common presentation as a result of diverse etiologies; for example, 5% to 10% of the population have acute appendicitis at some point in their life.

■ **PHYSICAL FINDINGS**

• Acute abdominal pain
• Abdominal distention and ascites
• Abdominal rigidity, rebound, and guarding
• Fever, chills
• Exacerbation with movement
• Anorexia, nausea, and vomiting
• Constipation
• Decreased bowel sounds
• Hypotension and tachycardia
• Tachypnea, dyspnea

■ **ETIOLOGY**

Although acute peritonitis can be caused by a wide variety of problems, similar clinical presentation is a result of stimulation of pain receptors within the peritoneum by purulent exudates, bleeding, inflammation, or the release of caustic materials such as pancreatic juice, bile, and gastric secretions.

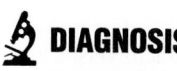 **DIAGNOSIS**

■ **DIFFERENTIAL DIAGNOSIS**

• Postoperative: abscess, sepsis, bowel obstruction, injury to internal organs
• Gastrointestinal: perforated viscus, appendicitis, IBD, infectious colitis, diverticulitis, acute cholecystitis, peptic ulcer perforation, pancreatitis, bowel obstruction
• Gynecologic: ruptured ectopic pregnancy, PID, ruptured hemorrhagic ovarian cyst, ovarian torsion, degenerating leiomyoma
• Urologic: nephrolithiasis, interstitial cystitis
• Miscellaneous: abdominal trauma, penetrating wounds, infections secondary to intraperitoneal dialysis

■ **WORKUP**

• Acute peritonitis is mainly a clinical diagnosis based on patient history and physical examination.
• Laboratory and imaging studies (see "Laboratory Tests") assist in determining the need for and type of intervention.
• If patient is hemodynamically unstable, immediate diagnostic laparotomy should be performed in lieu of adjuvant diagnostic studies.

■ **LABORATORY TESTS**

• CBC: leukocytosis, left shift, anemia
• SMA7: electrolyte imbalances, kidney dysfunction
• LFT: ascites secondary to liver disease, cholelithiasis
• Amylase: pancreatitis
• Blood cultures: bacteremia, sepsis
• Peritoneal cultures: infectious etiology
• Blood gas: respiratory vs. metabolic acidosis
• Ascitic fluid analysis: exudate vs. transudate
• Urinalysis and culture: urinary tract infection
• Cervical cultures for gonorrhea and *Chlamydia*
• Urine/serum hCG

■ **IMAGING STUDIES**

• Abdominal series: free air secondary to perforation, small or large bowel dilation secondary to obstruction, identification of fecalith
• Chest x-ray examination: elevated diaphragm, pneumonia
• Pelvic/abdominal ultrasound: abscess formation, abdominal mass, intrauterine vs. ectopic pregnancy, identify free fluid suggestive of hemorrhage or ascites
• CT: mass, ascites

TREATMENT

■ **NONPHARMACOLOGIC THERAPY**

• IV hydration to correct dehydration, hypovolemia
• Blood transfusion to correct anemia secondary to hemorrhage
• Nasogastric decompression, especially if obstruction is present
• Oxygen: intubation if necessary
• Bed rest

■ **ACUTE GENERAL Rx**

• Surgery to correct underlying pathology, such as controlling hemorrhage, correct perforation, drain abscess, and so forth.
• Broad-spectrum antibiotics:
  1. Single agent: ceftriaxone 1 to 2 g IV q24h, cefotaxime 1 to 2 g IV q4-6h
  2. Multiple agents:
     a. Ampicillin 2 g IV q4-6h; gentamicin 1.5 mg/kg/day; clindamycin 600 to 900 mg IV q8h
     b. Ampicillin 2 g IV q4-6h; gentamicin 1.5 mg/kg/day; metronidazole 500 mg IV q6-8h
• Pain control: morphine or meperidine as needed (hold until diagnosis confirmed)

■ **DISPOSITION**

Dependent on etiology of peritonitis, age of patient, coexisting medical disease, and duration of process before presentation

■ **REFERRAL**

Surgical consultation is required in all cases of acute peritonitis.

Author: **Matthew L. Withiam-Leitch, M.D., Ph.D.**

BASIC INFORMATION

■ DEFINITION
Spontaneous bacterial peritonitis (SBP) is an inflammatory reaction of the peritoneum secondary to the presence of bacteria or other microorganisms. More specifically, SBP is defined as an ascitic fluid infection without an evident intraabdominal surgically treatable source occurring primarily in patients with advanced cirrhosis of the liver.

■ SYNONYMS
Primary peritonitis
SBP

ICD-9CM CODES
567.2 Peritonitis

■ EPIDEMIOLOGY & DEMOGRAPHICS
PREDOMINANT SEX: Male > female

■ PHYSICAL FINDINGS & CLINICAL PRESENTATION
- Acute fever with accompanying abdominal pain/ascites, nausea, vomiting, diarrhea
- In cirrhotic patients, presentation may be subtle when low-grade temperature (100° F) with or without abdominal abnormalities
- In patients with ascites, a heightened degree of awareness is necessary for detection
- Jaundice and encephalopathy
- Deterioration of mental status and/or renal function

■ ETIOLOGY
- *Escherichia coli*
- *Klebsiella pneumoniae*
- *Streptococcus pneumoniae*
- *Streptococcus* spp., including *Enterococcus*
- *Staphylococcus aureus*
- Anaerobic pathogens: *Bacteroides, Clostridium* organisms
- Other: fungal, mycobacterial, viral

DIAGNOSIS

The diagnosis of SBP is established by a positive ascitic fluid bacterial culture and an elevated ascitic fluid absolute polymorphonuclear leukocyte (PMN) count (> or = 250 cells/mm³).

■ DIFFERENTIAL DIAGNOSIS
- Appendicitis (in children)
- Perforated peptic ulcer
- Secondary peritonitis
- Peritoneal abscess
- Splenic, hepatic, or pancreatic abscess
- Cholecystitis
- Cholangitis

■ WORKUP
Paracentesis and ascitic fluid analysis (see "Laboratory Tests") will confirm diagnosis.

■ LABORATORY TESTS
Ascitic fluid analysis reveals the following:
- Polymorphonuclear (PMN) cell count: >250/mm³
- Presence of bacteria on Gram stain
- pH: <7.31
- Lactic acid: >32/dl
- Protein: <1 g/dl
- Glucose: >50 mg/dl
- LDH: <225 mU/ml
- Positive culture of peritoneal fluid
- Measurement of the serum-ascites albumin gradient: The serum-ascites albumin gradient indirectly measures portal pressure. The albumin concentration of ascitic fluid and serum must be obtained on the same day. The ascitic fluid value is subtracted from the serum value to obtain the gradient. If the difference (not a ratio) is >1.1 g/dL, the patient has portal hypertension, with 97% accuracy. If the difference is <1.1 g/dL, portal hypertension is not present. The vast majority of patients with SBP have portal hypertension secondary to cirrhosis.

■ IMAGING STUDIES
- Abdominal ultrasound: if there is clinical difficulty in performing paracentesis
- CT scan: to rule out secondary peritonitis (if indicated) and to exclude abscess, mass

TREATMENT

■ ACUTE GENERAL Rx
Cefotaxime 1 to 2 g IV q8h or ceftriaxone 2 g IV q24h in patients with normal renal function; duration of treatment is generally 7 to 10 days. Oral quinolone therapy (ofloxacin 400 to 800 mg/day) or ciprofloxacin may be an acceptable alternative in selected patients.

■ PROPHYLAXIS
Give double-strength trimethoprim/sulfamethoxazole qd 5 days/wk or ciprofloxacin 750 mg/wk PO. Both have been shown to decrease occurrence of SBP in patients with cirrhosis.

✪ PEARLS & CONSIDERATIONS

■ COMMENTS
- Renal failure is a major cause of morbidity in cirrhotic patients with SBP. The use of IV albumin (1.5 g/kg at the time of diagnosis and 1 g/kg on day 3) may lower the rate of renal failure and mortality in patients with SBP.
- The criteria for the diagnosis of SBP require that abdominal paracentesis be performed and ascitic fluid be analyzed before a diagnosis of SBP can be made.
- Culturing ascitic fluid as if it were blood (with bedside inoculation of ascitic fluid into blood culture bottles) has been shown to significantly increase the culture-positivity of the ascitic fluid.
- Laparotomy may be life threatening in end-stage cirrhosis.
- Positive blood cultures in an individual with ascites require exclusion of a peritoneal source by paracentesis.

REFERENCES
Garcia-Tsao G: Current management of the complications of cirrhosis and portal hypertension: variceal hemorrhage, ascites, and spontaneous bacterial peritonitis, *Gastroenterology* 120(3):726, 2001.

Navassa M et al: Randomized, comparative study of oral ofloxacin versus intravenous cefotoxin in spontaneous bacterial peritonitis, *Gastroenterology* 111:1011, 1996.

Runyon BA et al: The serum-ascites albumin gradient is superior to the exudates-transudate concept in the differential diagnosis of ascites, *Ann Intern Med* 117:215, 1992.

Sort P et al: Effects of intravenous albumin on renal impairment and mortality in patients with cirrhosis and SBP, *N Engl J Med* 341:403, 1999.

Such J, Runyon BA: Spontaneous bacterial peritonitis, *Clin Infect Disease* 27:669, 1998.
Authors: **Joseph F. Grillo, M.D., and Dennis J. Mikolich, M.D.**

BASIC INFORMATION

■ DEFINITION

Pertussis is a prolonged bacterial infection of the upper respiratory tract characterized by paroxysms of an intense cough.

■ SYNONYMS

Whooping cough

ICD-9CM CODES

033.9 Pertussis

■ EPIDEMIOLOGY

INCIDENCE (IN U.S.): Approximately 5000 new cases/yr (Fig. 1-208)
PREDOMINANT AGE:
- 50% in children <1 yr of age
- 20% in children >15 yr of age
PEAK INCIDENCE:
- Childhood
- Usually affects children <1 yr of age

■ PHYSICAL FINDINGS & CLINICAL PRESENTATION

- Usually begins with a 1- to 2-wk prodrome that resembles a common cold
- Following this initial phase, increased production of mucus is noted
- Increased mucus production is followed by an intense, paroxysmal cough, ending with gasps and an inspiratory whoop
- In some children, cyanosis and anoxia are noted
- When prolonged, frank exhaustion and even apnea occur
- Pertussis is characterized by the finding of intense cough with a marked lymphocytosis
- Improvement during the later stage is possible
- High fever may be an indication of secondary bacterial pneumonia, which may be a later complication of pertussis

■ ETIOLOGY

Gram-negative rod, *Bordetella pertussis*, which adheres to human cilia

DIAGNOSIS

■ DIFFERENTIAL DIAGNOSIS

- Croup
- Epiglottitis
- Foreign body aspiration
- Bacterial pneumonia

■ WORKUP

- Blood cultures
- Chest x-ray examination
- Culture of bacteria, usually from nasopharynx
- Immunofluorescent staining of nasopharyngeal secretions
- ELISA for detection of antibody to pertussis

■ LABORATORY TESTS

CBC, which usually demonstrates marked lymphocytosis:
1. Up to 18,000 WBCs
2. 70% to 80% lymphocytes

■ IMAGING STUDIES

Chest x-ray examination is of value if secondary bacterial pneumonia is suspected.

TREATMENT

■ ACUTE GENERAL Rx

- Intensive supportive care:
  1. Adequate hydration
  2. Control of secretions
  3. Maintenance of airway
- Antibiotics are indicated even though their ability to alter the course of the disease is controversial.
  1. Erythromycin 50 mg/kg/day for 14 days. Recent literature reports indicate that a 7-day treatment regimen may be as effective as a 14-day course of erythromycin
  2. Although unproved, dexamethasone 1 mg/kg/day in 4 doses for severe, life-threatening paroxysms
  3. Ceftriaxone 75 mg/kg/day in 2 doses for broad coverage of secondary bacterial pneumonias
  4. Nafcillin or vancomycin when staphylococcal pneumonia is suspected
- Vaccination is successful in preventing the disease: universal vaccination is advised for all children <7 yr of age.
- Erythromycin is recommended for all close contacts in the household: TMP/SMX in two oral doses per day for those intolerant to erythromycin.
- Systemic steroids and nebulized steroids reduce length of hospital stay and improve symptoms.
- One small study showed nebulized epinephrine improves symptoms within 30 min, but found no difference after 2 hr.

■ DISPOSITION

Close attention to accepted vaccination schedules is the best prevention.

■ REFERRAL

To intensive care setting for life-threatening infections:
1. Pulmonologist
2. Infectious disease specialist

REFERENCES

He Q et al: Whooping cough caused by *Bordetella pertussis* and *Bordetella parapertussis* in an immunized population, *JAMA* 280:635, 1998.
MMWR: Pertussis—United States 1997-2000, *MMWR* 51-4, 73-75, 2002.
Tanaka M et al: Trends in pertussis among infants in the United States, 1980–1999, *JAMA* 290:2968, 2003.
Yaari E et al: Clinical manifestations of *Bordetella pertussis* infection in immunized children and young adults, *Chest* 115:1254, 1999.
Author: Joseph J. Lieber, M.D.

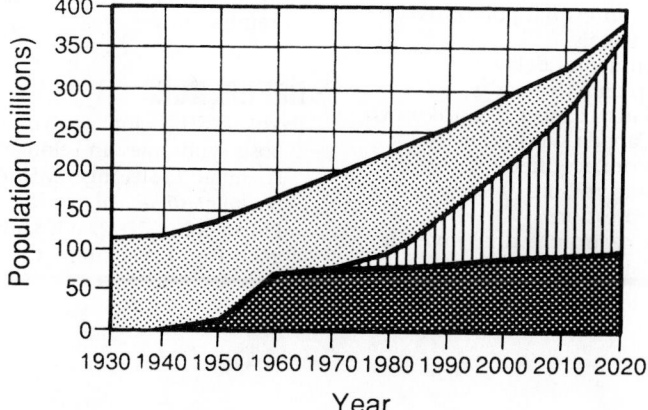

Pertussis post disease immune

Adult pertussis susceptibles

Pertussis vaccine immune (1 to 20 years old)

Fig. 1-208 Projected pertussis epidemiology in the United States through the year 2020 with continued use of present-day whole-cell pertussis vaccines. (Modified from Bass JW, Stephenson SR: *Pediatr Infect Dis J* 6:141, 1987.)

BASIC INFORMATION

■ DEFINITION
A hamartomatous polyp is a benign intestinal growth that may contain all components of the intestinal mucosa. In gastrointestinal polyposis, multiple such polyps coexist within the intestinal tract, and associated manifestations are usually also present. Commonly recognized syndromes are Peutz-Jeghers syndrome, juvenile polyposis syndrome, Cowden's disease, Bannagan-Ruvalcaba-Riley syndrome, and Cronkhite-Canada syndrome. Other lesser known inherited hamartomatous polyposis syndromes are hereditary mixed polyposis syndrome, intestinal ganglioneuromatosis and neurofibromatosis (variant of Von Recklinghausen's syndrome), Devon family syndrome, basal cell nevus syndrome, and tuberous sclerosis (may involve GI tract).

ICD-9CM CODES
ICD 9 CM Code: 759.6 (Peutz-Jeghers syndrome)
ICD 9 CM Code: 211.3 (Cronkhite-Canada syndrome)

■ PHYSICAL FINDINGS & CLINICAL PRESENTATION
Peutz-Jeghers Syndrome:
- Transmission: autosomal dominant with incomplete penetrance
- Disease expression
  1. Stomach, small and large intestinal hamartomas with bands of smooth muscle in the lamina propria
  2. Pigmented lesions around mouth (lips and buccal mucosa), nose, hands, feet, genital, and perineal areas
  3. Ovarian tumors
  4. Sertoli cell testicular tumors
  5. Airway polyps
  6. Pancreatic cancer
  7. Breast cancer
  8. Urinary tract polyps
- Cumulative lifetime cancer risk
  1. Colon cancer: 39%
  2. Stomach cancer: 29%
  3. Small intestine cancer: 13%
  4. Pancreatic cancer: 36%
  5. Breast cancer: 54%
  6. Ovarian cancer: 10%
  7. Sertoli cell tumor: 9%
  8. Overall cancer risk: 93%
- Clinical manifestation
  1. Gastrointestinal, small bowel obstruction, intussusception, GI bleeding
  2. See chapters on relevant malignancies for their signs and symptoms.

Juvenile Polyposis Syndrome:
- Transmission: autosomal dominant
- Disease expression
  1. Solitary juvenile polyps numbering 10 or more in the rectum or throughout the gastrointestinal tract; the polyps are smooth and covered with normal epithelium
  2. Various congenital abnormalities coexist in 20%
- Cumulative cancer risk is increased (may be as high as 50%)
- Clinical manifestation
  1. Intestinal obstruction
  2. Intussusception
  3. GI bleeding

Cowden's Disease:
- Transmission: autosomal dominant, rare
- Disease expression
  1. Juvenile intestinal polyposis
  2. Orocutaneous hamartomas
  3. Fibrocystic breast disease and breast cancer
  4. Goiter and thyroid cancer
  5. Facial tricholemmomas (papules) in 83%
- Cumulative cancer risk
  1. GI: same as general population
  2. Thyroid: 3% to 10%
  3. Breast: 25% to 50%

Bannagan-Ruvalcaba-Riley Syndrome:
- Transmission: autosomal dominant, rare
- Disease expression
  1. Juvenile intestinal polyposis
  2. Macrocephaly
  3. Developmental delay
  4. Penile pigmented spots
  5. Cumulative cancer risk unknown

Cronkhite-Canada syndrome:
- Transmission: acquired
- Age of onset: midlife
- Disease expression
  1. Diffuse gastrointestinal juvenile polyposis (50% to 95% of cases)
  2. Chronic diarrhea and protein-losing enteropathy (the entire intestinal mucosa may be inflamed), which leads to abdominal pain, weight loss, and various complications of malnutrition
  3. Dystrophic nails
  4. Alopecia
  5. Hyperpigmentation
- Cumulative cancer risk: same as the average population

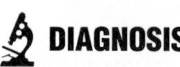

DIAGNOSIS

Diagnosis is suggested in many cases by family history and confirmed by colonoscopy and physical findings described previously.

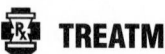

TREATMENT

■ GENERAL Rx
Peutz-Jeghers Syndrome:
- Colonoscopies with polypectomies
- Screening for breast cancer, testicular cancer, possibly ovarian cancer

Juvenile Polyposis Syndrome:
- Colonoscopies with polypectomies if few colon polyps
- Total colectomy if numerous polyps
- Esophagogastroscopies and polypectomies

Cowden's Disease: Rigorous breast cancer screening or prophylactic simple bilateral mastectomy with reconstruction

Cronkhite-Canada syndrome: Progressive malabsorption syndrome is the hallmark of this syndrome, and no specific treatment exists for it. Enteral or parenteral feeding is the cornerstone of management and can result in remission.

REFERENCE
Itzkowitz SH: Colonic polyps and polyposis syndromes. In Feldman M, Friedman L, Sleisinger MH (eds): *Gastrointestinal and liver disease*, ed 7, Philadelphia, 2002, WB Saunders.
Author: **Tom J. Wachtel, M.D.**

BASIC INFORMATION

■ DEFINITION

Peyronie's disease is an abnormal curvature and shortening of the penis during an erection (Fig. 1-209). This is caused by scarring of the tunica albuginea of the corpora cavernosa.

■ SYNONYMS

Plastic induration of the penis
Penile fibromatosis

ICD-9CM CODES

607.89 Peyronie's disease

■ EPIDEMIOLOGY & DEMOGRAPHICS

- Peyronie's disease occurs in approximately 1% of men (7:700).
- It is commonly seen between the ages of 45 to 60.
- A genetic predisposition has been suggested.
- There are no incidence and prevalence data available in the literature.

■ PHYSICAL FINDINGS & CLINICAL PRESENTATION

- Painful erections
- Tenderness over the scar tissue area
- Erectile dysfunction
- Curvature of the erected penis interfering with penetration
- Dupuytren's contracture is a commonly associated finding in patients with Peyronie's disease

■ ETIOLOGY

- The specific cause of the disease is not known. It is thought that scar tissue forms on either the dorsal or ventral midline surface of the penile shaft. The scar restricts expansion at the involved site, causing the penis to bend or curve in one direction.

- The precipitating factor appears to be trauma either from repetitive microvascular injury caused by vigorous sexual intercourse, accidents, or from prior surgeries (e.g., transurethral prostatectomy or radical prostatectomy, cystoscopy).

DIAGNOSIS

■ DIFFERENTIAL DIAGNOSIS

- The history differentiates congenital from acquired curvature of the penis.
- Other causes of erectile dysfunction must be excluded including metabolic, diabetes, thyroid, renal, hypogonadism, and hyperprolactinemia.

■ WORKUP

History and physical examination alone usually will establish the diagnosis of Peyronie's disease.

■ LABORATORY TESTS

There are no specific blood tests to diagnose Peyronie's disease. Electrolytes, BUN, creatinine, glucose, thyroid function tests (TSH, T_3U, T_4), testosterone, and prolactin level are blood tests to obtain to exclude other medical causes of erectile dysfunction.

■ IMAGING STUDIES

Imaging studies are not specific.

TREATMENT

■ NONPHARMACOLOGIC THERAPY

A conservative approach of reassurance and observation is taken at first because the disease process may be self-limiting.

■ ACUTE GENERAL Rx

Although not substantiated by direct randomized, controlled clinical trials, the following treatment modalities have been tried:
- Vitamin E 400 mg bid
- Paraaminobenzoic acid 12 g/day
- Colchicine 0.6 mg bid for 2 to 3 wk
- Fexofenadine 60 mg bid for 3 mo
- Steroid injection into the scar tissue
- Collagenase injection into the scar tissue
- Radiation to the scar tissue area

■ CHRONIC Rx

In patients who have progressed to intractable pain with erection or erectile dysfunction, surgical treatment with excision of the plaque and skin grafting may be indicated.

■ DISPOSITION

Peyronie's disease evolves slowly and in some cases can resolve on its own. Waiting for 1 yr before proceeding with surgical attempts is recommended.

■ REFERRAL

A urologic consultation is recommended in patients with progressive symptoms and erectile dysfunction.

PEARLS & CONSIDERATIONS

■ COMMENTS

- Peyronie's disease is not commonly seen in younger patients because they are able to sustain intracorporeal pressures high enough to stretch the scar tissue, preventing it from deforming the penis during erection.
- Trauma from buckling of the erected penis is thought to be the precipitant cause of scar formation and Peyronie's disease. It is found more often in men who are sexually very active and vigorous, having sexual intercourse daily or almost daily.
- Sexual positions with the women being on top or thrusting the penis into the anterior vaginal wall is thought to increase the chances of developing Peyronie's disease.

REFERENCES

Gholami SS, Lue TF: Peyronie's disease, *Urol Clin North Am* 28(2):377, 2001.
Kadloglu A et al: A retrospective review of 307 men with Peyronie's disease, *J Urol* 168(3):1075, 2002.
Tunugunthla HS: Management of Peyronie's disease—a review, *World J Urol* 19(4):244, 2001.
Author: **Peter Petropoulos, M.D.**

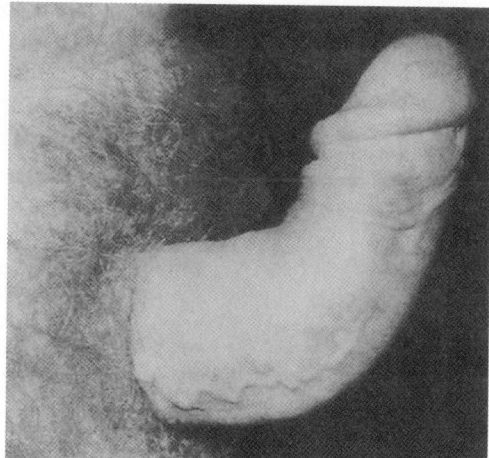

Fig. 1-209   Peyronie's disease. (Courtesy Patrick C. Walsh, M.D., The Johns Hopkins University School of Medicine, Baltimore. In Seidel HM [ed]: *Mosby's guide to physical examination,* ed 4, St Louis, 1999, Mosby.)

BASIC INFORMATION

■ DEFINITION
Pharyngitis/tonsillitis is inflammation of the pharynx or tonsils.

■ SYNONYMS
Sore throat

ICD-9CM CODES
462 Pharyngitis

■ EPIDEMIOLOGY & DEMOGRAPHICS
PREDOMINANT SEX: Female = male
PREDOMINANT AGE:
- All ages affected
- Streptococcal pharyngitis most common among school-age children
PEAK INCIDENCE: Late winter/early spring (group A streptococcal infections)
GENETICS:
Neonatal Infection: Pharyngitis below the age of 3 yr is almost always of viral etiology.

■ PHYSICAL FINDINGS & CLINICAL PRESENTATION
- Pharynx (Fig. 1-210):
  1. May appear normal to severely erythematous
  2. Tonsillar hypertrophy and exudates commonly seen but do not indicate etiology
- Viral infection:
  1. Rhinorrhea
  2. Conjunctivitis
  3. Cough
- Bacterial infection, especially group A *Streptococcus:*
  1. High fever
  2. Systemic signs of infection
- Herpes simplex or enterovirus infection: vesicles
- Streptococcal infection:
  1. Rare complications:
     a. Scarlet fever
     b. Rheumatic fever
     c. Acute glomerulonephritis

2. Extension of infection: tonsillar, parapharyngeal, or retropharyngeal abscess presenting with severe pain, high fever, trismus

■ ETIOLOGY
- Viruses:
  1. Respiratory syncytial virus
  2. Influenza A and B
  3. Epstein-Barr virus
  4. Adenovirus
  5. Herpes simplex
- Bacteria:
  1. *Streptococcus pyogenes*
  2. *Neisseria gonorrhoeae*
  3. *Arcanobacterium haemolyticum*
- Other organisms:
  1. *Mycoplasma pneumoniae*
  2. *Chlamydia pneumoniae*

DIAGNOSIS

■ DIFFERENTIAL DIAGNOSIS
- Sore throat associated with granulocytopenia, thyroiditis
- Tonsillar hypertrophy associated with lymphoma
- Section II describes the differential diagnosis of sore throat.

■ WORKUP
- Throat swab for culture to exclude *S. pyogenes, N. gonorrhoeae* (requires specific transport medium)
- Rapid streptococcal antigen test (culture should be performed if rapid test negative)
- Monospot

■ LABORATORY TESTS
- CBC with differential
  1. May help support diagnosis of bacterial infection
  2. Streptococcal infection suggested by leukocytosis >15,000/mm³
- Viral cultures, serologic studies rarely needed

■ IMAGING STUDIES
Seldom indicated

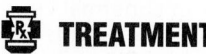

TREATMENT

■ NONPHARMACOLOGIC THERAPY
- Fluids
- Salt water gargles

■ ACUTE GENERAL Rx
- Aspirin (acetaminophen culture)
- If streptococcal infection proven or suspected:
  1. Penicillin V 500 mg PO bid for 10 days or benzathine penicillin 1.2 million U IM once (adults)
  2. Erythromycin 500 mg PO bid or 250 mg qid for 10 days if penicillin allergic
- If gonococcal infection proven or suspected: ceftriaxone 125 mg IM once

■ CHRONIC Rx
- Recurrent streptococcal infections are common and may represent reinfection from other household.
- There is no conclusive evidence from randomized clinical trials that tonsillectomy is superior to antibiotic therapy for recurrent tonsillitis in adults.

■ REFERRAL
- To otolaryngologist:
  1. If peritonsillar or other abscess is suspected
  2. If tonsillar hypertrophy persists
- To infectious diseases expert if unusual pathogen is suspected

PEARLS & CONSIDERATIONS

■ COMMENTS
Antibiotic therapy should be avoided unless bacterial etiology is suspected or proven, especially in adults.

REFERENCES
Bisno AL: Acute pharyngitis, *N Engl J Med* 344:205, 2001.
McKerrow W: Tonsillectomy versus antibiotics, *Clin Evid Concise* 7:88, 2002.
Snow V et al: Principles of appropriate antibiotic use for acute pharyngitis in adults, *Ann Intern Med* 134:506, 2001.
Vincent M et al: Pharyngitis, *Am Fam Physician* 69:1465, 2004.
Author: **Joseph R. Masci, M.D.**

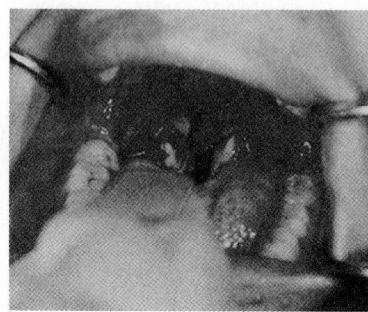
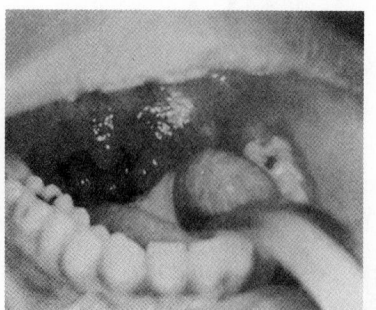

Fig. 1-210   Findings of the oropharynx. **A,** Tonsillitis and pharyngitis. **B,** Acute viral pharyngitis. (Courtesy Edward L. Applebaum, M.D., Head, Department of Otolaryngology, University of Illinois Medical Center, Chicago. In Barkauskas VH et al: *Health and physical assessment,* ed 2, St Louis, 1998, Mosby.)

BASIC INFORMATION

■ DEFINITION
Pheochromocytomas are catecholamine-producing tumors that originate from chromaffin cells of the adrenergic system. They generally secrete both norepinephrine and epinephrine, but norepinephrine is usually the predominant amine.

■ SYNONYMS
Paraganglioma

ICD-9CM CODES
194.0 Pheochromocytoma

■ EPIDEMIOLOGY & DEMOGRAPHICS
• Incidence: 0.05% of population; peak incidence in 30s and 40s.
• "Rough" rule of 10: 10% are extraadrenal, 10% are malignant, 10% are familial, 10% occur in children, 10% involve both adrenals, 10% are multiple (other than bilateral adrenal).
• Approximately 25% of patients with apparently sporadic pheochromocytoma may be carriers of mutations.
• Pheochromocytoma is a feature of two disorders with autosomal dominant pattern of inheritance:
  1. Multiple endocrine neoplasia II
  2. Von Hippel-Lindau disease: angioma of the retina, hemangioblastoma of the CNS, renal cell carcinoma, pancreatic cysts, and epididymal cystoadenoma
• Pheochromocytomas occur in 5% of patients with neurofibromatosis type 1.

■ PHYSICAL FINDINGS & CLINICAL PRESENTATION
• Hypertension: can be sustained (55%) or paroxysmal (45%).
• Headache (80%): usually paroxysmal in nature and described as "pounding" and severe.
• Palpitations (70%): can be present with or without tachycardia.
• Hyperhidrosis (60%): most evident during paroxysmal attacks of hypertension.
• Physical examination may be entirely normal if done in a symptom-free interval; during a paroxysm the patient may demonstrate marked increase in both systolic and diastolic pressure, profuse sweating, visual disturbances (caused by hypertensive retinopathy), dilated pupils (secondary to catecholamine excess), paresthesias in the lower extremities (caused by severe vasoconstriction), tremor, tachycardia.

■ ETIOLOGY
• Catecholamine-producing tumors that are usually located in the adrenal medulla.
• Specific mutations of the RET protooncogene cause familial predisposition to pheochromocytoma in Men II.
• Mutations in the von Hippel-Lindau tumor suppressor gene (VHL gene) cause familial disposition to pheochromocytoma in von Hippel-Lindau disease.
• Recently identified genes for succinate dehydrogenase subunit D (SDHD) and succinate dehydrogenase subunit B (SDHB) predispose carriers to pheochromocytoma and globus tumors.

DIAGNOSIS

■ DIFFERENTIAL DIAGNOSIS
• Anxiety disorder
• Thyrotoxicosis
• Amphetamine or cocaine abuse
• Carcinoid
• Essential hypertension

■ WORKUP
Laboratory evaluation and imaging studies to locate the neoplasm.

■ LABORATORY TESTS
• Plasma-free metanephrines are the best test for excluding or confirming pheochromocytoma and should be the test of first choice for diagnosis of the tumor. Plasma concentrations of normetanephrines >2.5 pmol/ml or metanephrine levels >1.4 pmol/ml indicate a pheochromocytoma with 100% specificity.
• 24-hr urine collection for metanephrines (100% sensitive) will also show increased metanephrines; the accuracy of the 24-hr urinary levels for metanephrines can be improved by indexing urinary metanephrine levels by urine creatinine levels.
• The clonidine suppression test is useful for distinguishing between high levels of plasma norepinephrine caused by release from sympathetic nerves and those caused by release from a pheochromocytoma. A decrease <50% in plasma norepinephrine levels after clonidine administration is normal, whereas persistent elevations are indicative of pheochromocytoma.

■ IMAGING STUDIES
• Abdominal CT scan (88% sensitivity) is useful in locating pheochromocytomas >0.5 inch in diameter (90% to 95% accurate).
• MRI: pheochromocytomas demonstrate a distinctive MRI appearance (100% sensitivity); MRI may become the diagnostic imaging modality of choice.
• Scintigraphy with ^{131}I-MIBG (100% sensitivity): this norepinephrine analog localizes in adrenergic tissue; it is particularly useful in locating extraadrenal pheochromocytomas.
• 6 [^{18}F] Fluorodopamine positron emission tomography is reserved for cases in which clinical symptoms and signs suggest pheochromocytoma and results of biochemical tests are positive but conventional imaging studies cannot locate the tumor. An alternative approach is to use vena caval sampling for plasma catecholamines and metanephrines.

TREATMENT

■ ACUTE GENERAL Rx
Laparoscopic removal of the tumor (surgical resection for both benign and malignant disease):
1. Preoperative stabilization with combination of phenoxybenzamine, β blocker, metyrosine, and liberal fluid and salt intake starting 10 to 14 days before surgery.
   a. Volume expansion is done to prevent postoperative hypotension.
   b. α-Blockade to control hypertension: phenoxybenzamine (Dibenzyline) 5 mg PO bid initially, gradually increased to 10 mg q3d up to 50-100 mg bid; prazosin may be used when phenoxybenzamine therapy alone is not effective or not well tolerated.
   c. β-Blockade with propranolol 20 to 40 mg PO q6h (to be used only after α-blockade) is useful to prevent catecholamine-induced arrhythmias and tachycardia.
   d. Metyrosine reduces tumor stores of catecholamines, decreases need for intraoperative medication to control blood pressure, and lowers intraoperative fluid requirements.
2. Hypertensive crisis preoperatively and intraoperatively should be controlled with phentolamine (Regitine) 2 to 5 mg IV q1-2h prn or nitroprusside used in combination with β-adrenergic blockers.

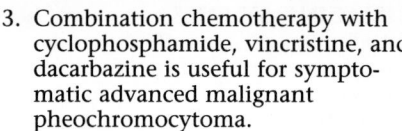
3. Combination chemotherapy with cyclophosphamide, vincristine, and dacarbazine is useful for symptomatic advanced malignant pheochromocytoma.

■ **DISPOSITION**
- The 5-yr survival rate is approximately 95% with benign disease, 40% for malignant pheochromocytoma (malignancy is determined by metastasis).
- Pheochromocytomas are three times more likely to be malignant in women.
- Postoperative follow-up of patients with sporadic and familial forms should include plasma metanephrine levels after 6 wk, 6 mo, and then annually.

☼ **PEARLS & CONSIDERATIONS**

■ **COMMENTS**
- Obtaining a detailed family history is important because 10% of pheochromocytomas are familial.
- Screening for pheochromocytoma should be considered in patients with any of the following:
  1. Malignant hypertension
  2. Poor response to antihypertensive therapy
  3. Paradoxical hypertensive response
  4. Hypertension during induction of anesthesia, parturition, surgery, or thyrotropin-releasing hormone testing
  5. Hypertension associated with imipramine or desipramine
  6. Neurofibromatosis (increased incidence of pheochromocytoma)

- All patients with pheochromocytoma should be screened for MEN-II and von Hippel-Lindau disease with pentagastrin test, serum PTH, ophthalmoscopy, MRI of the brain, CT scan of the kidneys and pancreas, and ultrasonography of the testes.
- In patients with pheochromocytoma, routine analysis for mutations of RET, VHL, SDHD, and SDHB is indicated to identify pheochromocytoma-associated syndromes.

REFERENCES

Lenders JW et al: Biochemical diagnosis of pheochromocytoma, which test is best? *JAMA* 287:1427, 2002.

Neumann HP et al: Germ-line mutations in nonsyndromic pheochromocytoma, *N Engl J Med* 346:1459, 2002.

Pacak R: Recent advances in genetics, diagnosis, localization, and treatment of pheochromocytoma, *Ann Intern Med* 134:315, 2001.

Author: **Fred F. Ferri, M.D.**

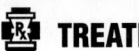
BASIC INFORMATION

■ DEFINITION

A phobia is severe anxiety that is elicited by a specific object or situation and that often leads to avoidance behavior. The provoking stimuli may be social or performance situations (social phobia) or any other stimulus (specific phobia of animals, natural environments, blood, or situational).

■ SYNONYMS

Simple phobia (obsolete name for specific phobia)

Phobias named according to the inducing stimulus, for example, arachnophobia (fear of spiders), claustrophobia (fear of tight spaces)

Social anxiety disorder (obsolete name for social phobias)

ICD-9CM CODES

F40.2 Specific phobia (DSM-IV: 300.29)
F40.1 Social phobia (DMS-IV: 300.23)

■ EPIDEMIOLOGY & DEMOGRAPHICS

PREVALENCE (IN U.S.):
- For specific phobias, the 1-yr prevalence rate is 9% and the lifetime rates range from 10% to 11.3%.
- For social phobias, prevalence rates of 3% to 13% have been reported, but only about 2% experience a significant degree of impairment to warrant clinical concern or intervention.

PREDOMINANT SEX:
- Females with specific phobias outnumber males.
- Rates vary according to the phobia (e.g., of individuals with animal or nature phobias, 75% to 90% are female; of individuals who fear blood, 55% to 70% are female; of people with situational fears, 75% to 70% are female). Similarly, more women are affected with social phobia; however, men are more likely to seek treatment.

PREDOMINANT AGE:
- Onset of most specific phobias is in childhood.
- Major exceptions: situational phobias, which have two peaks—the first in childhood and the second in the mid-20s.
- Once developed, fears are stable.
- Roots of social phobia may be in childhood, with described shyness or social inhibition, but onset usually in the midteens or into late adulthood; disorder is generally lifelong.

PEAK INCIDENCE:
- Specific phobias: lifelong condition
- Social phobia: may alternate in mid-to-late adulthood

GENETICS: Both specific phobias and social phobias are more common in first-degree relatives than the general population; however, this does not necessarily mean a genetic etiology.

■ PHYSICAL FINDINGS & CLINICAL PRESENTATION
- Specific phobias: frequently have other anxiety disorders, particularly panic and agoraphobias; most phobias are associated with sinus tachycardia on exposure to the stimulus, although blood phobias frequently (in 75% of those afflicted) are associated with sinus bradycardia, hypotension, and fainting.
- Social phobias: usually have low self-esteem and fear of evaluation from others; avoid or are fearful of any situation in which others may assess or evaluate them directly or indirectly; concurrent anxiety disorders are common, but these persons are less likely to develop panic than panic disorder patients when challenged with panicogenic lactate infusion or CO_2 inhalation.

■ ETIOLOGY
- Unknown
- Biologic features probably a relatively small component

DIAGNOSIS

■ DIFFERENTIAL DIAGNOSIS
- Panic attacks: anxiety symptoms seen in specific phobia may resemble panic attacks, but the stimulus in specific phobias or social phobias is clear, whereas panic attacks seem more random.
- Generalized anxiety disorder: difficult to distinguish from social phobia, but in social phobia the cognitive focus is fear of embarrassment or humiliation, whereas in generalized anxiety disorder the focus is more internal on the subjective sensations of discomfort.

■ WORKUP
- History: usually diagnostic
- Physical examination: to confirm absence of cardiovascular abnormalities (e.g., a chronic sinus arrhythmia)

■ LABORATORY TESTS
No specific laboratory tests are indicated.

■ IMAGING STUDIES
If phobias are associated with fainting, a cardiac workup (EEG, Holter) may be indicated.

TREATMENT

■ NONPHARMACOLOGIC THERAPY
- Treatment of choice for specific phobias is desensitization.
- Cognitive-behavioral therapy and other psychotherapeutic approaches are effective.
- Success rates are higher when the phobia is not complicated by other anxiety disorders.
- Social phobia is more problematic to treat because the psychologic difficulties are more pervasive, but cognitive-behavioral therapy and other psychotherapies are quite effective.
- For social phobia, psychotherapy is almost always required, at least as adjunct.

■ ACUTE GENERAL Rx
- Benzodiazepines: provide rapid, effective relief of anxiety associated with exposure to fearful stimuli
- Alprazolam or lorazepam: both administered sublingually to increase rate of absorption
- β-Blockers: given before exposure to the fearful stimulus (e.g., before a public speech); the lipophilic β-blockers are preferred
- Acute management of anxiety symptoms: not advisable in view of chronicity of the symptoms of social phobia

■ CHRONIC Rx
- If the phobic stimulus is encountered rarely and unexpectedly, benzodiazepines may be appropriate long-term treatment.
- If the phobic stimulus can be anticipated, β-blockers may be appropriate long-term treatment.
- Social phobia is a chronic condition. Individuals with social phobia often underachieve, drop out of school, avoid seeking work as a result of anxiety about interviews, refrain from dating and remain with family of origin, and are less likely to marry. In addition to this social and occupational dysfunction, these individuals lead very unfulfilled lives.
- Paroxetine is effective in social anxiety disorder.

■ REFERRAL
If psychotherapy advised

REFERENCES

Blanco C et al: Pharmacotherapy of social anxiety disorder, *Bio C Psychiatry* 51:109, 2002.

Kendler KS et al: The etiology of phobias: an evaluation of the stress-diathesis model, *Arch Gen Psychiatry* 59:242, 2002.

Authors: **Rif S. El-Mallakh, M.D., and Peggy L. El-Mallakh, B.S.N.**

BASIC INFORMATION

■ DEFINITION

A *pilonidal sinus* is a short tract that extends from the skin surface, is most commonly found in the intergluteal fold, and most likely represents a distended hair follicle. An *acute pilonidal abscess*, which consists of pus and a wall of edematous fat, results from rupture of an infected follicle into fat. A *chronic pilonidal abscess* results when an infected follicle ruptures directly into surrounding tissues; the wall of a chronic pilonidal abscess consists of fibrous tissue. A *pilonidal cyst* develops from a chronic abscess of long duration as a thin and flat lining of epithelium grows into the cavity from the skin surface.

■ SYNONYMS

Jeep disease

ICD-9CM CODES

685.1 Pilonidal cyst

■ EPIDEMIOLOGY & DEMOGRAPHICS

INCIDENCE: 26 cases/100,000 persons
PREDOMINANT SEX: Male > female (2.2:1)
AVERAGE AGE OF PRESENTATION: 21 yr
GENETICS: Theory of congenital origin is now disfavored.
RISK FACTORS:
- Male sex
- Caucasian race
- Family predisposition
- Obesity
- Sedentary lifestyle
- Occupation requiring prolonged sitting
- Local hirsutism
- Poor hygiene
- Increased sweat activity

■ PHYSICAL FINDINGS & CLINICAL PRESENTATION

- May manifest as asymptomatic pits or pores in the natal cleft
- Tenderness after physical activity or prolonged sitting
- Acute pilonidal abscess in 20% of patients with pilonidal disease
- Presents as a hot, tender, fluctuant swelling just lateral to the midline over the sacrum that may exude pus through the midline pit
- Chronic pilonidal abscess in 80% of patients with pilonidal disease
- Acute suppuration, tenderness, swelling, and heat
- Infrequently, systemic reaction: occasionally fever, leukocytosis, and malaise

■ ETIOLOGY

- Currently, thought to be acquired rather than congenital.
- Drilling of hair shed from the perineum or the head into sebaceous or hair follicles in the natal cleft.
- Drilling is facilitated by the friction of the natal cleft.
- Subsequent infection by skin organisms leads to pilonidal abscess.

DIAGNOSIS

■ DIFFERENTIAL DIAGNOSIS

- Perianal abscess arising from the posterior midline crypt
- Hidradenitis suppurativa
- Carbuncle
- Furuncle
- Osteomyelitis
- Anal fistula
- Coccygeal sinus

■ WORKUP

- Diagnosis is based on history and physical examination.
- Midline pits present behind the anus overlying the sacrum and coccyx.
- Broken hairs are often seen extruding from the midline pits.
- Insert probe in pilonidal sinus in path away from the anus.
- Complicated anal fistula may be angulating posteriorly before passing into a retrorectal abscess, but thorough examination of the anal cavity usually discloses point of origin.

■ LABORATORY TESTS

CBC

■ IMAGING STUDIES

CT scan in advanced recurrent cases

TREATMENT

■ NONPHARMACOLOGIC THERAPY

Prevention of exacerbations:
1. Local hygiene
2. Avoidance of prolonged sitting position
3. Weight reduction

■ ACUTE GENERAL Rx

- Procedure of choice for first-episode acute abscess: simple incision and drainage in an outpatient setting
- Cure rate of 76% after 18 mo
- Antibiotics: generally not indicated unless the patient has a medical condition such as rheumatic heart disease or is immunosuppressed

■ CHRONIC Rx

Elective treatment of pilonidal disease:
1. Minimal surgery

   a. Remove hair from midline pits and shave buttocks.
   b. May use a fine wire brush with local anesthesia to clear the pits and any lateral openings of granulation tissue and hair.
   c. Keep area clean.
2. Opening of sinus tracts
   a. Used when minimal surgery does not control episodes of suppuration
   b. Pass probe to outline the pilonidal sinus and open tract surgically
   c. Curette granulation tissue at the base of the sinus and excise edges of the skin
   d. Keep open granulating wound meticulously clean and allow to heal
   e. If complete healing does not take place, use a skin graft or advancement flap to close the defect
3. Excision
   a. This is the treatment of choice for chronic pilonidal disease.
   b. Wide excision of the pilonidal area is performed, including all affected skin and subcutaneous tissues down to the presacral fascia.
   c. Wound is left open, allowed to marsupialize, or closed as a primary procedure.
   d. Give antibiotics for 24 hr (particularly those directed against *Staphylococcus* and *Bacteroides* spp).

■ DISPOSITION

Recurrence rate for excision (most definitive procedure): 1% to 6%

■ REFERRAL

- Emergency room for incision and drainage for an acute abscess
- To a surgeon for elective treatment or management of chronic or recurrent disease

PEARLS & CONSIDERATIONS

■ COMMENTS

Because of significant associated morbidity, the elective surgical procedures outlined are performed only after the potential risks vs. benefits are carefully weighed.

REFERENCE

Church JM: Pilonidal cyst: cause and treatment, *Dis Colon Rectum* 43(8):1146, 2000.
Author: **Wan J. Kim, M.D.**

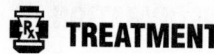

 BASIC INFORMATION

■ **DEFINITION**
Pinworms are a noninvasive infestation of the intestinal tract by *Enterobius vermicularis,* a helminth of the nematode family.

■ **SYNONYMS**
Enterobiasis

ICD-9CM CODES
127.4 Enterobiasis

■ **EPIDEMIOLOGY & DEMOGRAPHICS**
• Most common intestinal nematode with approximately 30,000 cases/yr in the U.S.
• Worldwide distribution, but most common in temperate climates.
• Highest infection rate in school-age children.
• Clusters are found in families, institutionalized persons, and homosexual men.

■ **PHYSICAL FINDINGS & CLINICAL PRESENTATION**
• Most infested persons are asymptomatic.
• Perianal itching is the most common reported symptom, with scratching leading to excoriation and sometimes secondary infection.
• Rarely insomnia, irritability, anorexia, and weight loss are described.
• Granulomas have been described in various organs resulting from worms wandering outside the intestines and dying there.

■ **ETIOLOGY & PATHOGENESIS**
Humans are the only host for this worm. Infestation is by fecal-oral route; ingested eggs hatch in the stomach and the larvae migrate to the colon where they mature. Gravid female worms migrate to the perianal skin at night, lay their eggs there, and die. The eggs cause itching; scratching causes egg deposition under fingernails, from which they can contaminate food or lead to autoreinfection.

■ **DIAGNOSIS**

■ **DIFFERENTIAL DIAGNOSIS**
• Perianal itching related to poor hygiene
• Hemorrhoidal disease and anal fissures
• Perineal yeast/fungal infections
• Section II describes the causes of pruritus ani

■ **WORKUP**
Identification of adult worms or eggs (Fig. 1-211) on transparent tape placed on the perianal skin upon awakening (NOTE: Five consecutive negative tests rule out the diagnosis.)

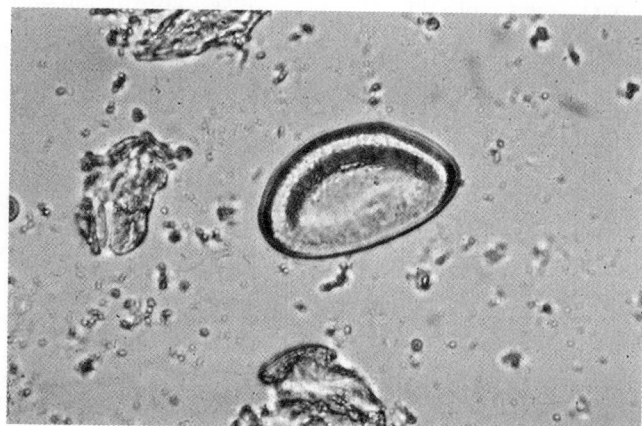
Fig. 1-211 *Enterobius vermicularis* embryonated egg. Note larva inside (40 × 10 μm). (From Gorbach SL, Bartlett JG, Blacklow NR (eds): *Infectious diseases,* ed 2, Philadelphia, 1998, WB Saunders.)

■ **TREATMENT**
Single dose of mebendazole or pyrantel pamoate repeated after 2 to 3 wk

REFERENCE
Hamer DH, Despommier DD: Intestinal nematodes. In Gorbach SL, Bartlett JG, Blacklow NR (eds): *Infectious diseases,* ed 2, Philadelphia, 1998, WB Saunders.
Author: **Tom J. Wachtel, M.D.**

BASIC INFORMATION

■ DEFINITION

Pituitary adenoma is a benign neoplasm of the anterior lobe of the pituitary that causes symptoms, either by excess secretion of hormones or by a local mass effect as the tumor impinges on other, nearby structures (e.g., optic chiasm, hypothalamus, pituitary stalk). Pituitary adenomas are classified by their size, function, and features that characterize their appearance. Microadenomas are <10 mm in size, and macroadenomas are >10 mm in size.

- *Acromegaly* is the disease state characterized by a pituitary adenoma that secretes growth hormone (GH).
- A *prolactinoma* secretes prolactin (PRL).
- *Cushing's disease* is a disease state in which there is hypersecretion of adrenocorticotropic hormone (ACTH).
- *Thyrotropin-secreting pituitary adenomas* secrete primarily thyroid-stimulating hormone (TSH).
- *Nonsecretory pituitary adenomas* are those in which the neoplasm is a space-occupying lesion whose secretory products do not cause a specific disease state.

ICD-9CM CODES
253 Pituitary adenoma
253.0 Acromegaly
253.1 Prolactinoma

■ EPIDEMIOLOGY & DEMOGRAPHICS
CLASSIFICATION (BY HORMONE SECRETED):
- PRL only ~35%
- No hormone ~30%
- GH only ~20%
- PRL and GH ~7%
- ACTH ~7%
- LF/FSH/TSH ~1%

PREVALENCE/INCIDENCE:
Pituitary Adenomas: Up to 10% to 15% of all intracranial neoplasms; 3% to 27% autopsy series
Prolactinomas: Up to 20% in women with unexplained primary or secondary amenorrhea
Growth Hormone–Secreting Pituitary Adenoma: 50 to 60 cases/1,000,000 persons
Thyrotropin-Secreting Pituitary Adenoma: 2.8% of pituitary adenomas with a slight female:male predominance of 1.7:1
Corticotropin-Secreting Pituitary Adenomas: Female:male predominance of 8:1

■ PHYSICAL FINDINGS
PROLACTINOMAS:
- Females:
  1. Galactorrhea
  2. Amenorrhea
  3. Oligomenorrhea with anovulation
  4. Infertility
  5. Estrogen deficiency leading to hirsutism
  6. Decreased vaginal lubrication
  7. Osteopenia
- Males:
  1. Large tumors more common secondary to delayed diagnosis
  2. Possible impotence or decreased libido or hypogonadism
  3. Galactorrhea rare because males lack the estrogen-dependent breast growth and differentiation

GROWTH HORMONE–SECRETING PITUITARY ADENOMA: Acromegaly
- Coarse facial features
- Oily skin
- Prognathism
- Carpal tunnel syndrome
- Osteoarthritis
- History of increased hat, glove, or shoe size
- Decreased exercise capacity
- Visual field deficits
- Diabetes mellitus

CORTICOTROPIN-SECRETING PITUITARY ADENOMA: Cushing's disease
- Usually present when the tumor is small (1 to 2 mm)
- 50% of the tumors <5 mm
- Other symptoms:
  1. Truncal obesity
  2. Round facies (moon face)
  3. Dorsocervical fat accumulation (buffalo hump)
  4. Hirsutism
  5. Acne
  6. Menstrual disorders
  7. Hypertension
  8. Striae
  9. Bruising
  10. Thin skin
  11. Hyperglycemia

THYROTROPIN-SECRETING PITUITARY ADENOMA:
- In males, larger, more invasive, and more rapidly growing tumors that present later in life
- Other symptoms: thyrotoxicosis, goiter, visual impairment

NONSECRETORY PITUITARY ADENOMAS (ENDOCRINE INACTIVE PITUITARY ADENOMA):
- Usually large at the time of diagnosis
- Symptoms:
  1. Bitemporal hemianopia secondary to compression of the optic chiasm
  2. Hypopituitarism secondary to compression of the pituitary gland
  3. Hypogonadism in men and in premenopausal women
  4. Cranial nerve deficits, secondary to extension into the cavernous sinus
  5. Hydrocephalus, secondary to extension into the third ventricle, compressing the foramen of Monro
  6. Diabetes insipidus, secondary to compression of the hypothalamus or pituitary stalk (a rare complication)

■ ETIOLOGY
Benign neoplasms of epithelial origin

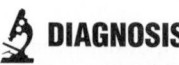

DIAGNOSIS

■ DIFFERENTIAL DIAGNOSIS
PROLACTINOMA:
- Pregnancy
- Postpartum puerperium
- Primary hypothyroidism
- Breast disease
- Breast stimulation
- Drug ingestion (especially phenothiazines, antidepressants, haloperidol, methyldopa, reserpine, opiates, amphetamines, and cimetidine)
- Chronic renal failure
- Liver disease
- Polycystic ovarian disease
- Chest wall disorders
- Spinal cord lesions
- Previous cranial irradiation

ACROMEGALY: Ectopic production of growth hormone–releasing hormone from a carcinoid or other neuroendocrine tumor

CUSHING'S DISEASE:
- Diseases that cause ectopic sources of ACTH overproduction (including small cell carcinoma of the lung, bronchial carcinoid, intestinal carcinoid, pancreatic islet cell tumor, medullary thyroid carcinoma, or pheochromocytoma)
- Adrenal adenomas, adrenal carcinoma
- Nelson's syndrome

THYROTROPIN-SECRETNG PITUITARY ADENOMAS: Primary hypothyroidism
NONSECRETORY PITUITARY ADENOMA: Nonneoplastic mass lesions of various etiologies (e.g., infectious, granulomatous)

■ WORKUP (Section III, Fig. 3-144)
PROLACTINOMA: First step: Measurement of basal PRL levels
- Elevated PRL levels are correlated with tumor size.
- Levels >200 ng/ml are diagnostic, with levels of 100 to 200 ng/ml being equivocal.
- Basal PRL levels between 20 and 100 suggest a microprolactinoma, as well as other conditions such as drug ingestion

- Basal level <20 is normal.

ACROMEGALY:
- First screening test is the measurement of the serum IGF-I level, post serum GH, TRH stimulation test.
- Follow with an oral glucose tolerance test.
- Failure to suppress serum GH to <2 ng/ml with an oral load of 100 g glucose is considered conclusive.
- A GHRH level >300 ng/ml is indicative of an ectopic source of GH.

CUSHING'S DISEASE:
- Normal or slightly elevated corticotropin levels ranging from 20 to 200 pg/ml; normal is 10 to 50 pg/ml.
- Levels <10 pg/ml usually indicate an autonomously secreting adrenal tumor.
- Levels >200 pg/ml suggest an ectopic corticotropin-secreting neoplasm.
- Cushing's disease is confirmed by demonstration of low-dose dexamethasone, which shows presence of abnormal cortisol suppressibility.
- 24-hr urine collection should demonstrate an increased level of cortisol excretion.

THYROTROPIN-SECRETING PITUITARY ADENOMA:
- Highly sensitive thyrotropin assays, which evaluate the presence of thyrotoxicosis, are one way to detect a thyrotropin-secreting tumor.
- Free alpha subunit is secreted by >80% of tumors with the ratio of the alpha subunit to thyrotropin >1.
- With central resistance to thyroid hormone, ratio is <1 and the sella is normal.
- Laboratory tests show elevated serum levels of both T_3 and T_4.

NONSECRETORY PITUITARY ADENOMA:
- Visual field testing
- Assessment of the pituitary and organ function to determine if there is hypopituitarism or hypersecretion of hormones (even if the effects of hypersecretion are subclinical)
- TRH to provoke secretion of FSH, LH, and LH-beta-subunit; will not elicit response in normal persons
- Exclusion of Klinefelter's syndrome in patient with long-standing primary hypogonadism, elevated gonadotropin levels, and enlargement of the sella

■ IMAGING STUDIES
- Study of choice: MRI of the pituitary and hypothalamus
  1. When evaluating Cushing's disease, small size at the onset of symptoms noted

- MRI, in this case, only 60% sensitive at best and may yield false positive results
- CT scan only when MRI is unavailable or is otherwise contraindicated

℞ TREATMENT

■ NONPHARMACOLOGIC THERAPY
SURGERY:
- Selective transsphenoidal resection of the adenoma is the treatment of choice for prolactinoma, acromegaly, Cushing's disease, and thyrotropin-secreting pituitary adenomas, which all tend to be microadenomas at the time of onset of symptoms.
- Macroadenomas, such as the nonsecretory pituitary adenoma, may also be surgically removed, but risk of recurrence is greater with these tumors, and adjunctive therapy such as irradiation may also be necessary.
- Radiotherapy is reserved for patients who have failed surgical treatment and who still experience the symptoms of their adenoma.
- Bilateral adrenalectomy has been done in patients with Cushing's disease on failure of other therapies; complications requiring lifelong hormone replacement or Nelson's syndrome may occur.

RADIOTHERAPY:
- Generally reserved for patients who have failed surgical treatment
- Used with varying degrees of success in all of the different pituitary adenomas

■ PHARMACOLOGIC THERAPY
PROLACTINOMA:
- Bromocriptine, a dopamine analog, is generally given orally in divided doses of 1.5 to 10 mg.
- Side effects include orthostatic hypotension, nausea, and dizziness; avoided by beginning with low-dose therapy.
- Other compounds under investigation include pergolide mesylate, a long-acting ergot derivative with dopaminergic properties, as well as other nonergot derivatives.

ACROMEGALY:
- Octreotide, a somatostatin analog, 100 μg SC, is the medical therapy of choice but is limited by side effects such as biliary sludge and gallstones, nausea, cramps, steatorrhea, and its parenteral administration.
- Bromocriptine 10 to 20 mg PO tid-qid is less effective than octreotide, but has the advantage of oral administration.

CUSHING'S DISEASE:
- Ketoconazole, which inhibits the cytochrome P-450 enzymes involved in steroid biosynthesis, is effective in managing mild to moderate disease in daily oral dosages of 600 to 1200 mg.
- Metyrapone and aminoglutethimide can be used to control hypersecretion of cortisol but are generally used when preparing a patient for surgery or while waiting for a response to radiotherapy.

THYROTROPIN-SECRETING PITUITARY ADENOMA:
- Ablative therapy with either radioactive iodide or surgery is indicated.
- Treatment directed to the thyroid alone may accelerate growth of the pituitary adenoma.
- Octreotide has been shown to be effective in doses similar to those used for acromegaly.

NONSECRETORY PITUITARY ADENOMA:
- There is no role for medical therapy at this time
- Surgery and radiotherapy are indicated.

■ CHRONIC Rx
For all pituitary adenomas:
- Careful follow-up is important. Patients undergoing transsphenoidal microsurgical resection should be seen in 4 to 6 wk to ensure that the adenoma has been completely removed and that the endocrine hypersecretion is resolved.
- If there is good clinical response, patient should be monitored yearly for recurrence and to follow the level of the hypersecreted hormone.
- Patients who have undergone irradiation should have close follow-up with backup medical therapy because response to radiotherapy may be delayed; incidence of hypopituitarism also increases with time.

REFERENCES
Davis AK, Farrell WE, Clayton RN: Pituitary tumors, *Reproduction* 121(3):363, 2001.

Kovacs K, Horvath E, Vidal S: Classification of pituitary adenomas, *J Neurooncol* 54(2):121, 2001.

Shimon I, Melmed S: Management of pituitary tumors, *Ann Intern Med* 129:472, 1998.

Author: **Beth J. Wutz, M.D.**

BASIC INFORMATION

■ DEFINITION
Pityriasis is a common self-limiting skin eruption of unknown etiology.

ICD-9CM CODES
696.3 Pityriasis rosea

■ EPIDEMIOLOGY & DEMOGRAPHICS
- Most cases of pityriasis rosea occur between ages 10 and 35 yr; mean age is 23 yr.
- The incidence of disease is highest in the fall and spring.
- Female:male ratio is 1.5:1.

■ PHYSICAL FINDINGS & CLINICAL PRESENTATION
- Initial lesion (herald patch) precedes the eruption by approximately 1 to 2 wk; typically measures 3 to 6 cm; it is round to oval in appearance and most frequently located on the trunk.
- Eruptive phase follows within 2 wk and peaks after 7 to 14 days.
- Lesions are most frequently located in the lower abdominal area. They have a salmon-pink appearance in whites and a hyperpigmented appearance in blacks.

- Most lesions are 4 to 5 mm in diameter; center has a "cigarette paper" appearance; border has a characteristic ring of scale (collarette).
- Lesions occur in a symmetric distribution and follow the cleavage lines of the trunk (Christmas tree pattern [Fig. 1-212]).
- The number of lesions varies from a few to hundreds.
- Most patients are asymptomatic; pruritus is the most common symptom.
- History of recent fatigue, headache, sore throat, and low-grade fever is present in approximately 25% of cases.

■ ETIOLOGY
Unknown, possibly viral (picornavirus)

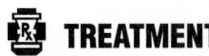 **DIAGNOSIS**

■ DIFFERENTIAL DIAGNOSIS
- Tinea corporis (can be ruled out by potassium hydroxide examination)
- Secondary syphilis (absence of herald patch, positive serologic test for syphilis)
- Psoriasis
- Nummular eczema
- Drug eruption

- Viral exanthem
- Eczema
- Lichen planus
- Tinea versicolor (the lesions are more brown and the borders are not as ovoid)

■ WORKUP
Presence of herald lesion and characteristic rash are diagnostic. Skin biopsy is generally reserved for atypical cases.

■ LABORATORY TESTS
Generally not necessary; serologic test for syphilis if clinically indicated

TREATMENT

■ NONPHARMACOLOGIC THERAPY
The disease is self-limited and generally does not require any therapeutic intervention.

■ ACUTE GENERAL Rx
- Use calamine lotion or oral antihistamines in patients with significant pruritus.
- Use prednisone tapered over 2 wk in patients with severe pruritus.
- Direct sun exposure or use of ultraviolet light within the first week of eruption is beneficial in decreasing the severity of disease.

■ DISPOSITION
- Spontaneous complete resolution of the rash within 4 to 8 wk
- Recurrence rare (<2% of cases)

☼ PEARLS & CONSIDERATIONS

■ COMMENTS
Reassure patient that the disease is not contagious and its course is benign.
Author: Fred F. Ferri, M.D.

REFERENCE
Stulberg D, Wolfrey J: Pityaris rosea, *Am Fam Physician*, 69:87, 2004.

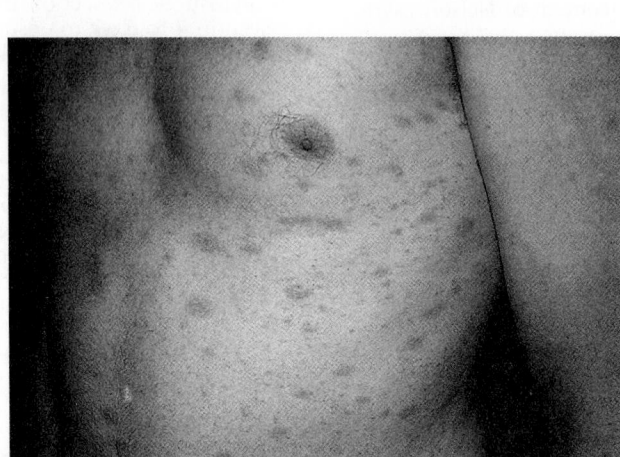

Fig. 1-212 Scale (pityriasis rosea). Shows example of how unique scaling (collarette of fine scale within several lesions), distribution and shape of lesions (oval lesions with long axis paralleling natural skin cleavage lines), and color (salmon-pink) help in diagnosing skin disease. (From Noble J [ed]: *Textbook of primary care medicine*, ed 3, St Louis, 2001, Mosby.)

BASIC INFORMATION

■ DEFINITION
Placenta previa is the implantation of the placenta over the internal os. Four degrees of this abnormality have been defined:
- Total placenta previa: the internal os is covered completely.
- Partial placenta previa: the internal os is partially covered.
- Marginal placenta previa: the edge of the placenta is at the margin of the internal os.
- Low-lying placenta: the placenta is implanted in the lower uterine segment, and although its edge does not reach the internal os, it is in close proximity to it.

See Fig. 1-213.

ICD-9CM CODES
641.1 Placenta previa

■ EPIDEMIOLOGY & DEMOGRAPHICS INCIDENCE
0.26% to 0.7% of pregnancies

■ RISK FACTORS
Previous cesarean delivery (after one such delivery, the risk is 1% to 4%; after four or more cesarean deliveries, the risk approaches 10%). Multiparity has also been associated with placenta previa.

■ PHYSICAL FINDINGS & CLINICAL PRESENTATION
The classic presentation of placenta previa is painless vaginal bleeding, usually in the second or third trimester. Uterine contractions may or may not be present. On physical examination, the uterus is soft and pain-free. The fetus is often in breech, transverse lie, or high. Fetal distress is usually not present.

■ ETIOLOGY
Uncertain

DIAGNOSIS

■ DIFFERENTIAL DIAGNOSIS
- Placenta accreta
- Placenta percreta
- Placenta increta
- Vasa previa
- Abruptio placentae
- Vaginal or cervical trauma
- Labor
- Local malignancy

■ WORKUP
- Do NOT perform a digital vaginal examination.
- The diagnosis of placenta previa can seldom be firmly established by physical examination alone. A speculum examination in a hospital setting to exclude any local bleeding may be performed.

- This diagnosis should not be dismissed until thorough evaluation, including sonography, has completely excluded its presence.

■ LABORATORY TESTS
- A complete blood count (CBC) can be used to monitor hemoglobin and hematocrit
- A Kleihauer-Betke preparation of maternal blood in all Rh-negative women and Rh-immune globulin when indicated

■ IMAGING STUDIES
- The simplest, most precise, and safest method of placental localization is transabdominal sonography with confirmatory imaging by transvaginal ultrasonography. Transperineal sonography has also proven effective in detection.
- Magnetic resonance imaging has also been effective in detecting placenta previa, although sonography remains the preferred method of diagnosis.

TREATMENT

■ NONPHARMACOLOGIC THERAPY
- In preterm pregnancies with no active bleeding, close observation and expectant management are indicated. In those with active bleeding, conservative management, including blood transfusions for severe bleeds, is appropriate. The woman should stay in the hospital for at least 48 hr after the bleeding has stopped.
- Bedrest, preferably in a hospital setting, should be prescribed.

■ ACUTE GENERAL Rx
- Initial assessment for signs of maternal hemodynamic compromise or hemorrhagic shock; large-bore intravenous access with crystalloid fluid resuscitation
- Assess fetal status and gestational age using sonogram and continuous fetal heart rate monitoring
- Cross-matched blood should be made available during bleeding episodes; if the hemorrhage is severe, cesarean delivery is indicated despite fetal immaturity
- Tocolytic therapy may be considered in those women in preterm labor, as well as the administration of corticosteroids to enhanced fetal lung maturity

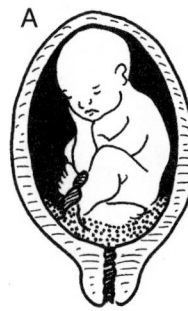
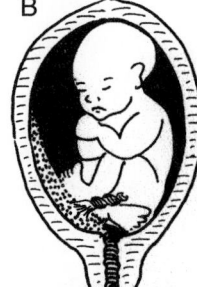
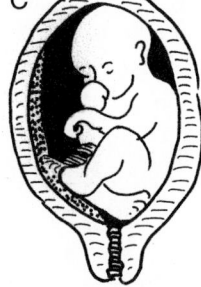

TOTAL **PARTIAL** **MARGINAL**

Fig. 1-213 Various types of placenta previa. **A,** The cervical os is completely covered by placenta. **B,** The cervical os is partially covered by placenta. **C,** The placenta extends to the edge of the cervical os. (From Rakel RE: *Textbook of family practice,* ed 6, Philadelphia, 2002, WB Saunders.)

■ **CHRONIC Rx**

- Cesarean delivery is necessary in nearly all cases of placenta previa.
- Uncontrollable hemorrhage after placental removal should be anticipated secondary to the poorly contractile nature of the lower uterine segment. The need for hysterectomy to control bleeding should be discussed with the patient before delivery, if possible.

■ **DISPOSITION**

Because of the unpredictable nature of placenta previa, not all women with placenta previa can be treated expectantly.

■ **REFERRAL**

Affected women and their families should be aware of all signs and symptoms that would necessitate immediate transport to the hospital. The possibility of hysterectomy should also be discussed early during pregnancy.

REFERENCES

Baron F, Hill WC: Placenta previa, placenta abruptio, *Clin Obstet Gynecol* 41(3):527, 1998.

Chamberlain G, Steer P: ABC of labour care: obstetric emergencies, *BMJ* 318(7194):1342, 1999.

Cunningham FG et al: *Williams obstetrics,* ed 21, New York, 2001, McGraw-Hill.

Faiz AS, Ananth CV: Etiology and risk factors for placenta previa: an overview and meta-analysis of observational studies, *J Matern Fetal Neonatal Med* 13(3):175, 2003.

Gabbe SG et al: *Obstetrics: normal and problem pregnancies,* ed 3, Philadelphia, 1996, Churchill Livingstone.

Author: **Sonya S. Abdel-Razeq, M.D**

BASIC INFORMATION

■ **DEFINITION**
Plantar fasciitis is a common, painful inflammation or degeneration of the plantar fascia, a tissue that extends from the calcaneus to the proximal phalanges of each toe.

■ **SYNONYMS**
Painful heel syndrome
Painful heel spur

ICD-9CM CODES
728.71 Plantar fasciitis
726.73 Calcaneal spur

■ **EPIDEMIOLOGY & DEMOGRAPHICS**
PREVALENT AGE: Middle age
PREVALENT SEX: Males = females
Bilateral in 10% to 20% of cases

■ **PHYSICAL FINDINGS & CLINICAL PRESENTATION**
- Pain is characteristically worse on arising and after periods of rest; "warming up" often lessens the pain
- Local tenderness at site involvement, usually the medial tubercle of the calcaneus, sometimes in the midfascia
- Pain sometimes elicited by passive dorsiflexion of toes and ankle, which stretches the plantar fascia
- A tight heel cord may be present

■ **ETIOLOGY**
- Uncertain
- Inflammation, microscopic tears, and/or degeneration
- The role of the calcaneal traction osteophyte (spur) is unclear
- May be associated with tight heel cord

 DIAGNOSIS

■ **DIFFERENTIAL DIAGNOSIS**
- Other regional tendonitis
- Stress fracture
- Tarsal tunnel syndrome
- Tumor, infection

■ **IMAGING STUDIES**
Traction osteophyte or minor soft tissue calcification may be present on plain radiography. Other studies are usually not required.

TREATMENT

- Sensible activity restriction
- Gentle stretching exercises
- NSAIDS
- Local steroid/lidocaine injections (Fig. 1-214)
- Heel lift
- Night brace, daytime cast brace

■ **DISPOSITION**
Disorder is usually self-limited, although full recovery may take 1 to 2 yr.

■ **REFERRAL**
- If symptoms fail to respond to medical management
- For surgical consideration (plantar fascia release, excision of osteophyte)

PEARLS & CONSIDERATIONS

■ **COMMENTS**
- Various cushions and heel cups are generally ineffective because stretching, not heel strikes, is probably cause of disorder.
- Surgical intervention is rarely necessary.
- Shock wave therapy is of unproven benefit.

REFERENCES

Bachbinder R et al: Ultrasound-guided extracorporeal shockwave therapy for plantar fasciitis, *JAMA* 288:1364, 2002.
DiGiovanni BF et al: Tissue specific plantar fascia stretching exercises enhances outcomes in patients with chronic heel pain, *J Bone Joint Surg* 85:1270, 2003.
Riddle DL et al: Risk factors for plantar fasciitis: a matched case-control study, *J Bone Joint Surg* 85:872, 2003.
Rompe JD et al: Evaluation of low-energy extracorporeal shockwave application for chronic plantar fasciitis, *J Bone Joint Surg* 84(A):335, 2002.
Young CC et al: Treatment of plantar fasciitis, *Am Fam Physician* 63:467, 2001.
Author: **Lonnie R. Mercier, M.D.**

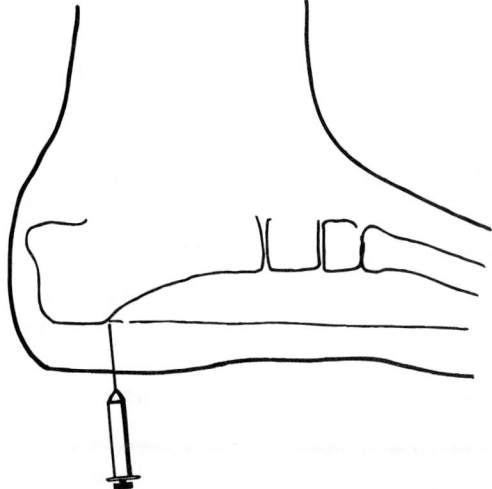

Fig. 1-214 Injection site for plantar fasciitis. Injection should be through the sole into the area of maximum tenderness. A 25- or 27-gauge needle should be used and the medication injected slowly as some pain may occur. The total volume should be no greater than 1.5 ml. (From Mercier L: *Practical orthopedics,* ed 5, St Louis, 2002, Mosby.)

BASIC INFORMATION

■ DEFINITION

Aspiration pneumonia is a lung infection caused by bacterial organisms aspirated from nasopharyngeal space.

ICD-9CM CODES

507.0 Aspiration pneumonia

■ EPIDEMIOLOGY & DEMOGRAPHICS

INCIDENCE (IN U.S.):
- Few reliable data
- 20% to 35% of all pneumonias
- 5% to 15% of all community acquired pneumonias

PREVALENCE (IN U.S.): Unreliable data
PREDOMINANT SEX: Equal
PREDOMINANT AGE: Elderly
PEAK INCIDENCE: Elderly patients in hospitals or nursing homes

■ PHYSICAL FINDINGS & CLINICAL PRESENTATION

- Shortness of breath, tachypnea, cough, sputum, fever after vomiting, or difficulty swallowing
- Rales, rhonchi, often diffusely throughout lung

■ ETIOLOGY

Complex interaction of etiologies, ranging from chemical (often acid) pneumonitis following aspiration of sterile gastric contents (generally not requiring antibiotic treatment) to bacterial aspiration

COMMUNITY-ACQUIRED ASPIRATION PNEUMONIA:
- Generally results from predominantly anaerobic mouth bacteria (anaerobic and microaerophilic streptococci, fusobacteria, gram-positive anaerobic non–spore-forming rods), *Bacteroides* species *(melaninogenicus, intermedius, oralis, ureolyticus)*, *Haemophilus influenzae,* and *Streptococcus pneumoniae*
- Rarely caused by *Bacteroides fragilis* (of uncertain validity in published studies) or *Eikenella corrodens*
- High-risk groups: elderly, alcoholics, IV drug users, patients who are obtunded, those with esophageal disorders, seizures, poor dentition, stroke victims, or recent dental manipulations

HOSPITAL-ACQUIRED ASPIRATION PNEUMONIA:
- Often occurs among elderly patients and others with diminished gag reflex; those with nasogastric tubes, intestinal obstruction, or ventilator support; and especially those exposed to contaminated nebulizers or unsterile suctioning
- High-risk groups: seriously ill hospitalized patients (especially patients with coma, acidosis, alcoholism, uremia, diabetes mellitus, nasogastric intubation, or recent antimicrobial therapy, who are frequently colonized with aerobic gram-negative rods); patients undergoing anesthesia; those with strokes, dementia, swallowing disorders; the elderly; and those receiving antacids or H_2 blockers (but not sucralfate)
- Hypoxic patients receiving concentrated O_2 have diminished ciliary activity, encouraging aspiration
- Causative organisms:
  1. Anaerobes listed previously, although in many studies gram-negative aerobes (60%) and gram-positive aerobes (20%) predominate
  2. *E. coli, P. aeruginosa, S. aureus, Klebsiella, Enterobacter, Serratia,* and *Proteus* spp. *H. influenzae, S. pneumoniae, Legionella,* and *Acinetobacter* spp. (sporadic pneumonias) in two thirds of cases
  3. Fungi, including *Candida albicans,* in fewer than 1%

DIAGNOSIS

■ DIFFERENTIAL DIAGNOSIS

- Other necrotizing or cavitary pneumonias (especially tuberculosis, gram-negative pneumonias)
- See "Pulmonary Tuberculosis"

■ WORKUP

- Chest x-ray examination
- CBC, blood cultures
- Sputum Gram stain and culture
- Consideration of tracheal aspirate

■ LABORATORY TESTS

- CBC: leukocytosis often present
- Sputum Gram stain
  1. Often useful when carefully prepared immediately after obtaining suctioned or expectorated specimen, examined by experienced observer.
  2. Only specimens with multiple WBCs and rare or absent epithelial cells should be examined.
  3. Unlike nonaspiration pneumonias (e.g., pneumococcal), multiple organisms may be present.
  4. Long, slender rods suggest anaerobes.
  5. Sputum from pneumonia caused by acid aspiration may be devoid of organisms.
  6. Cultures should be interpreted in light of morphology of visualized organisms.

■ IMAGING STUDIES

- Chest x-ray examination often reveals bilateral, diffuse, patchy infiltrates, and posterior segment upper lobes.

- Aspiration pneumonias of several days' or longer duration may reveal necrosis (especially community-acquired anaerobic pneumonias) and even cavitation with air-fluid levels, indicating lung abscess.

TREATMENT

■ NONPHARMACOLOGIC THERAPY

- Airway management to prevent repeated aspiration
- Ventilatory support if necessary

■ ACUTE GENERAL Rx

Acute aspiration of acidic gastric contents without bacteria may not require antibiotic therapy; consult infectious diseases or pulmonary expert.
FOR COMMUNITY-ACQUIRED ANAEROBIC ASPIRATION PNEUMONIA:
- Levofloxacin 500 mg qd or ceftriaxone 1 to 2 g/day
NURSING HOME ASPIRATIONS:
- Levofloxacin 500 mg qd or piperacillin-tazobactam 3.375 g q6h or ceftazidime 2 g q8h
HOSPITAL-ACQUIRED ASPIRATION PNEUMONIA:
- Piperacillin-tazobactam 3.375 g IV q6h, or clindamycin 450-900 mg IV q8h, or cefoxitin 2 g IV q8h
- Knowledge of resident flora in the microenvironment of the aspiration within the hospital is crucial to intelligent antibiotic selection; consult infection control nurses or hospital epidemiologist.
- Confirmed *Pseudomonas* pneumonia should be treated with antipseudomonal β-lactam agent plus an aminoglycoside until antimicrobial sensitivities confirm that less toxic agents may replace aminoglycoside.
- Do not use metronidazole alone for anaerobes.

■ DISPOSITION

Repeat chest x-ray examination in 6 to 8 wk.

■ REFERRAL

For consultation with infectious disease and/or pulmonary experts for patients with respiratory distress, hypoxia, ventilatory support, pneumonia in more than one lobe, necrosis or cavitation on x-ray examination, or not responding to antibiotic therapy within 2 to 3 days

REFERENCE

Marik PE: Aspiration pneumonitis and aspiration pneumonia, *N Engl J Med* 344:665, 2001.
Author: **Beth J. Wutz, M.D.**

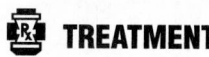
 BASIC INFORMATION

■ **DEFINITION**

Bacterial pneumonia is an infection involving the lung parenchyma

ICD-9CM CODES

486.0 Pneumonia, acute
507.0 Pneumonia, aspiration
482.9 Pneumonia, bacterial
481 Pneumonia, pneumococcal
482.1 Pneumonia, *Pseudomonas*
482.4 Pneumonia, staphylococcal
428.0 Pneumonia, *Klebsiella*
482.2 Pneumonia, *Haemophilus* influenzae

■ **EPIDEMIOLOGY & DEMOGRAPHICS**

- Incidence of community-acquired pneumonia is 1/100 persons.
- Incidence of nosocomial pneumonia is 8 cases/1000 persons/yr.
- Primary care physicians see an average of 10 cases of pneumonia annually.
- Hospitalization rate for pneumonia is 15% to 20%.
- Most cases of pneumonia occur in the winter and in elderly patients.

■ **PHYSICAL FINDINGS & CLINICAL PRESENTATION**

- Fever, tachypnea, chills, tachycardia, cough
- Presentation varies with the cause of pneumonia, the patient's age, and the clinical situation:
  1. Patients with streptococcal pneumonia usually present with high fever, shaking chills, pleuritic chest pain, cough, and copious production of purulent sputum.
  2. Elderly or immunocompromised hosts may initially present with only minimal symptoms (e.g., low-grade fever, confusion); respiratory and nonrespiratory symptoms are less commonly reported by older patients with pneumonia.
  3. Generally, auscultation reveals crackles and diminished breath sounds.
  4. Percussion dullness is present if the patient has pleural effusion.

■ **ETIOLOGY**

- *Streptococcus pneumoniae*
- *Haemophilus influenzae*
- *Legionella pneumophila* (1% to 5% of adult pneumonias)
- *Klebsiella, Pseudomonas, E. coli*
- *Staphylococcus aureus*

- Pneumococcal infection is responsible for 50% to 75% of community-acquired pneumonias, whereas gram-negative organisms cause >80% of nosocomial pneumonias
- Predisposing factors are:
  1. COPD: *H. influenzae, S. pneumoniae, Legionella*
  2. Seizures: aspiration pneumonia
  3. Compromised hosts: *Legionella,* gram-negative organisms
  4. Alcoholism: *Klebsiella, S. pneumoniae, H. influenzae*
  5. HIV: *S. pneumoniae*
  6. IV drug addicts with right-sided bacterial endocarditis: *S. aureus*

■ **DIAGNOSIS**

■ **DIFFERENTIAL DIAGNOSIS**

- Exacerbation of chronic bronchitis
- Pulmonary embolism or infarction
- Lung neoplasm
- Bronchiolitis
- Sarcoidosis
- Hypersensitivity pneumonitis
- Pulmonary edema
- Drug-induced lung injury
- Viral pneumonias
- Fungal pneumonias
- Parasitic pneumonias
- Atypical pneumonia
- Tuberculosis

■ **WORKUP**

Laboratory evaluation and chest x-ray examination

■ **LABORATORY TESTS**

- In hospitalized patients, attempt to obtain an adequate sputum specimen for Gram stain and cultures.
  1. An expectorated sputum sample is often inadequate because of many false positive results (secondary to contamination from oral flora) and many false negative results; a specimen may be considered adequate if the Gram stain shows >25 PMNs and <10 epithelial cells per low-power field.
  2. Aerosol induction with hypertonic saline solution (3% to 10%) may increase the diagnostic yield of sputum.
  3. The use of fiberoptic bronchoscopy to obtain a sputum sample is generally reserved for critically ill patients responding poorly to initial antimicrobial therapy.

  4. Gram stain of sputum may reveal the following:
     Lancet-shaped, gram-positive cocci indicate streptococcal pneumonia. Pleomorphic, small coccobacillary, gram-negative organisms indicate *H. influenzae.*
     Encapsulated gram-negative bacilli: *K. pneumoniae*
- WBC count is elevated, usually with left shift
- Blood cultures: positive in approximately 20% of cases of pneumococcal pneumonia
- Pulse oximetry or ABGs: hypoxemia with partial pressure of oxygen <60 mm Hg while the patient is breathing room air is a standard criterion for hospital admission
- Direct immunofluorescent examination of sputum when suspecting Legionella (e.g., direct fluorescent antibody [DFA] stain is a highly specific and rapid test for detecting legionellae in clinical specimen)
- Serologic testing for HIV in selected patients

■ **IMAGING STUDIES**

Chest x-ray study: findings vary with the stage and type of pneumonia and the hydration of the patient (Fig. 1-215).

- Classically, pneumococcal pneumonia presents with a segmental lobe infiltrate.
- Diffuse infiltrates on chest x-ray can be seen with *L. pneumophila, M. pneumoniae,* viral pneumonias, *P. carinii,* miliary TB, aspiration, aspergillosis.
- An initial chest x-ray film is also useful to rule out the presence of any complications (pneumothorax, empyema, abscesses).

■ **TREATMENT**

■ **NONPHARMACOLOGIC THERAPY**

- Avoidance of tobacco use
- Oxygen to maintain partial oxygen pressure in arterial blood >60 mm Hg
- IV hydration, correction of dehydration
- Assisted ventilation in patients with significant respiratory failure

■ ACUTE GENERAL Rx

- Initial antibiotic therapy should be based on clinical, radiographic, and laboratory evaluation.
- Macrolides (azithromycin or clarithromycin) or levofloxacin is recommended for empirical out-patient treatment of community-acquired pneumonia; cefotaxime or a beta-lactam/beta-lactamase inhibitor can be added in patients with more severe presentation who insist on out-patient therapy. Duration of treatment ranges from 7 to 14 days.
- In the hospital setting, patients admitted to the general ward can be treated empirically with a second- or third-generation cephalosporin (ceftriaxone, ceftizoxime, cefotaxime, or cefuroxime) plus a macrolide (azithromycin or clarithromycin) or doxycycline. An antipseudomonal quinolone (levofloxacin, moxifloxacin, or gatifloxacin) may be substituted in place of the macrolide or doxycycline.
- In hospitalized patients at risk for *P. aeruginosa* infection, empirical treatment should consist of an antipseudomonal beta-lactam (cefepime or piperacillin-tazobactam) *plus* an aminoglycoside *plus* an antipseudomonal quinolone or macrolide.

■ CHRONIC Rx

Parapneumonic effusion-empyema can be managed with chest tube placement for drainage. Instillation of fibrinolytic agents (streptokinase, urokinase) via the chest tube may be necessary in resistant cases.

■ DISPOSITION

- Most patients respond well to antibiotic therapy.
- Indications for hospital admission are:
  1. Hypoxemia (oxygen saturation <90% while patient is breathing room air)
  2. Hemodynamic instability
  3. Inability to tolerate medications
  4. Active co-existing condition requiring hospitalization

☼ PEARLS & CONSIDERATIONS

■ COMMENTS

Causes of slowly resolving or nonresolving pneumonia:
- Difficult to treat infections: viral pneumonia, *Legionella*, pneumococci, or staphylococci with impaired host response, TB, fungi
- Neoplasm: lung, lymphoma, metastasis
- CHF
- Pulmonary embolism
- Immunologic or idiopathic: Wegener's granulomatosis, pulmonary eosinophilic syndromes, SLE
- Drug toxicity (e.g., amiodarone)

REFERENCES

Davidson R et al: Resistance to levofloxacin and failure of treatment of pneumococcal pneumonia, *N Engl J Med* 346:747, 2002.

Halm EA, Teirstein AS: Management of community-acquired pneumonia, *N Engl J Med* 347:2039, 2002.

Author: **Fred F. Ferri, M.D.**

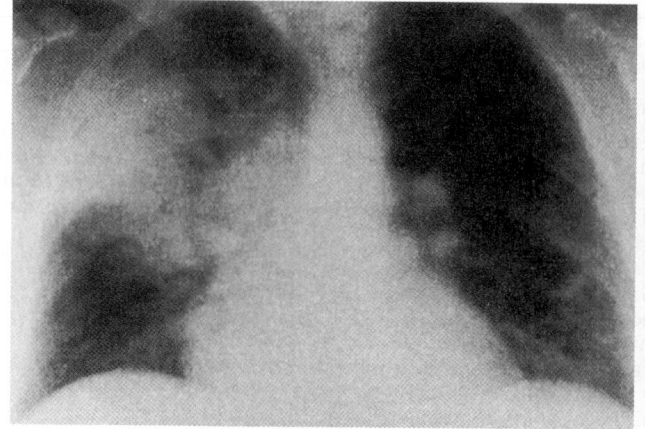
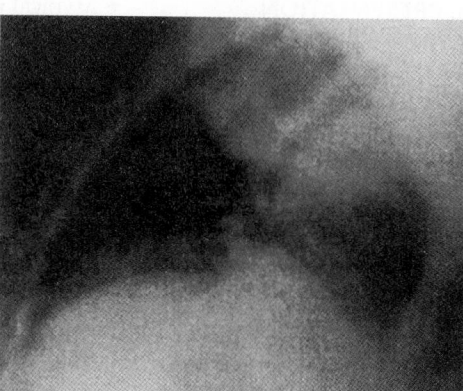

Fig. 1-215   A, PA and, **B,** lateral chest radiographs reveal right upper lobe pneumonia and patchy left lower lobe infiltrate. A variety of organisms can produce this pattern, including *S. pneumoniae* and *H. influenzae*. (From Marx J [ed]: Rosen's *Emergency medicine*, ed 5, St Louis, 2003, Mosby.)

BASIC INFORMATION

■ DEFINITION
Mycoplasma pneumonia is an infection of the lung parenchyma caused by *Mycoplasma pneumoniae*.

■ SYNONYMS
Primary atypical pneumonia
Eaton's pneumonia
Walking pneumonia

■ ICD-9CM CODES
483 *Mycoplasma* pneumonia

■ EPIDEMIOLOGY & DEMOGRAPHICS
INCIDENCE (IN U.S.):
- Hard to determine incidence precisely because of difficulty in making the diagnosis, but it is a frequent cause of community-acquired pneumonia.
- Probably many cases resolve without coming to medical attention.
- Incidence is estimated at 1 case/1000 persons/yr.
- Incidence is estimated to at least triple every (approximately) 5 yr during epidemics.

PREVALENCE (IN U.S.):
- Estimated to be present in 1 of 5 patients hospitalized for pneumonia (generally a self-limited disease, so its true prevalence is unknown)
- Estimated to cause 7% of all pneumonias and about half in those age 5 to 20 yr

PREDOMINANT SEX: Equal distribution

PREDOMINANT AGE:
- Most commonly affected: school-age children and young adults (ages 5 to 20 yr)
- Occurs in older adults as well, especially with household exposure to a young child
- More severe infections in affected elderly patients

PEAK INCIDENCE:
- Some increased incidence in fall to early winter
- Seems more prevalent in temperate climates

GENETICS:
Familial Disposition:
- None known
- May be more severe in patients with sickle cell anemia

Neonatal Infection: Severe respiratory distress, sometimes requiring intubation, attributed to this disease in infants.

■ PHYSICAL FINDINGS & CLINICAL PRESENTATION
- Nonexudative pharyngitis (common)

- Rhonchi or rales, without evidence of consolidation (common) in lower lung zones
- Associated with bullous myringitis (perhaps no more frequently than in other pneumonias)
- Skin rashes in up to one fourth of patients
  1. Morbilliform
  2. Urticaria
  3. Erythema nodosum (unusual)
  4. Erythema multiforme (unusual)
  5. Stevens-Johnson syndrome (rare)
- Muscle tenderness (<50% of the patients)
- On examination (and confirmed with testing):
  1. Mononeuritis or polyneuritis
  2. Transverse myelitis
  3. Cranial nerve palsies
  4. Meningoencephalitis
- Lymphadenopathy and splenomegaly
- Conjunctivitis

■ ETIOLOGY
Infection is spread by droplet infection from respiratory tract secretions.

DIAGNOSIS

■ DIFFERENTIAL DIAGNOSIS
- *Chlamydia pneumoniae*
- *C. psittaci*
- *Legionella* spp.
- *Coxiella burnetii*
- Several viral agents
- Q fever
- *Pneumococcus pneumoniae*
- Pleuritic pain
- Pulmonary embolism/infarction

■ WORKUP
- Chest x-ray examination
- Thorough history and physical examination
- Laboratory tests
- Evaluation guided by symptoms and findings

■ LABORATORY TESTS
- WBC:
  1. WBC count >10,000/mm³ in about a quarter of patients
  2. Differential count nonspecific
  3. Leukopenia rare
- Cold agglutinins:
  1. Detected in about half of the patients
  2. Also may be found in:
     a. Lymphoproliferative diseases
     b. Influenza
     c. Mononucleosis
     d. Adenovirus infections
     e. Occasionally, Legionnaires' disease

  3. Titers typically >1:64
     a. May be detectable with bedside testing
     b. Appear between days 5 and 10 of the illness (so may be demonstrable when patient is first examined) and disappear within about 1 mo
- Uncommonly, hemolysis
- Complement fixation testing of paired sera (fourfold rise) in patients with pneumonia and a compatible history:
  1. Considered diagnostic
  2. Not specific for the disease
- Culture of the organism from specimens
  1. Only truly specific test for infection
  2. Technically difficult and done reliably by few laboratories
  3. May require weeks to get results
- Sputum
  1. Often no sputum produced for laboratory testing
  2. When present, gram-stained specimens show polyps without organisms
- Infection occasionally complicated by pancreatitis or glomerulitis
- Disseminated intravascular coagulation is a rare complication.
- Electrocardiographic evidence of pericarditis or myocarditis may be present.

■ IMAGING STUDIES
- Predilection for lower lobe involvement (upper lobes involved in less than a fourth), with radiographic abnormalities frequently out of proportion to those on physical examination (Fig. 1-216)
- Small pleural effusions in about 30% of patients
- Large effusions: rare
- Infiltrates: patchy, unilateral, and with a segmental distribution, although multilobe involvement may be seen
- Evidence of hilar adenopathy on chest films in 20% to 25%
- Rare cases reported:
  1. Associated lung abscess
  2. Residual pneumatoceles
  3. Lobar collapse
  4. Hyperlucent lung syndrome

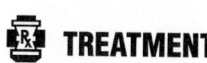 ## TREATMENT

■ ACUTE GENERAL Rx
- Therapy (10 to 14 days) with erythromycin (500 mg qid), azithromycin (500 mg daily), or clarithromycin (500 mg bid) is preferred to tetracycline, especially in young children or women of childbearing age.

- Therapy shortens the duration and severity of symptoms and may hasten radiographic clearing, but the disease is self-limiting.

■ CHRONIC Rx

- Effective antimicrobial therapy does not eliminate the organism from the respiratory secretions, which may be positive for weeks.
- Serum antibody response does not necessarily provide lifelong immunity.
- Chronic symptoms do not occur, although clinical relapses may occur 7 to 10 days following the initial response and may be associated with new areas of infiltration.

■ DISPOSITION

- Clinical improvement is almost universal within 10 days.
- Infiltrates generally clear within 5 to 8 wk.
- Rare deaths are likely attributable to underlying medical diseases.
- Person-to-person spread can be minimized by avoiding open coughing, especially in enclosed areas.

■ REFERRAL

- Not responding to treatment
- Severe infection
- Severe extrapulmonary manifestations
- Multilobe involvement accompanied by respiratory embarrassment (very rare)

🔆 PEARLS & CONSIDERATIONS

■ COMMENTS

X-ray resolution complete by 8 wk in about 90% of patients.

REFERENCES

Falguera M et al: Nonsevere community-acquired pneumonia: correlation between cause and severity or comorbidity, *Arch Intern Med* 161(15):1866, 2001.

Hyde TB et al: Azithromycin prophylaxis during a hospital outbreak of *Mycoplasma pneumoniae* pneumonia, *J Infect Dis* 183(6):907, 2001.

Author: **Harvey M. Shanies, M.D., Ph.D.**

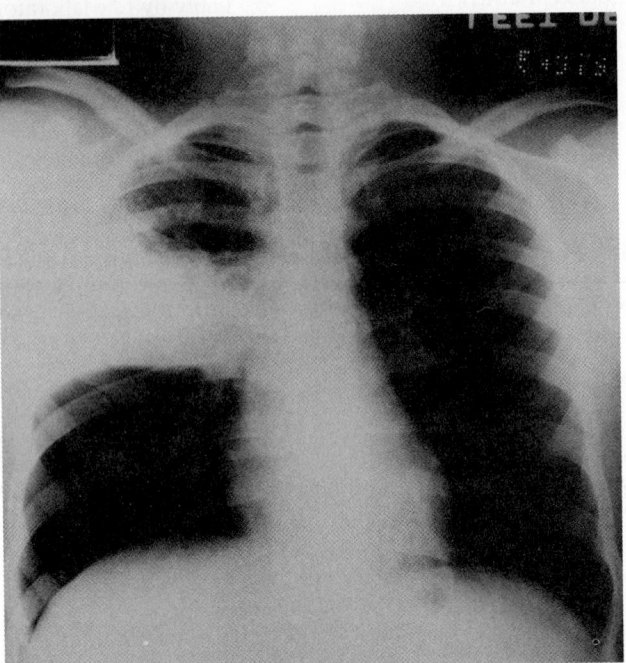

Fig. 1-216   Localized airspace opacification secondary to *Mycoplasma pneumoniae.* (From Specht N [ed]: *Practical guide to diagnostic imaging,* St Louis, 1998, Mosby.)

BASIC INFORMATION

■ DEFINITION
Pneumocystis carinii pneumonia is a serious respiratory infection caused by the fungal or protozoal organism *Pneumocystis carinii*.

■ SYNONYMS
PCP

■ ICD-9CM CODES
136.3 *Pneumocystis carinii* pneumonia

■ EPIDEMIOLOGY & DEMOGRAPHICS
INCIDENCE (IN U.S.):
- Seen primarily in the setting of acquired immunodeficiency syndrome (AIDS)
- Approximately 11 cases/100 patient-years among HIV-infected patients with CD4 lymphocyte counts <100/mm³

PREDOMINANT SEX: Equal incidence when corrected for HIV status
PREDOMINANT AGE:
- <2 yr
- 20 to 40 yr

PEAK INCIDENCE: 20 to 40 yr (parallel to AIDS epidemic)
GENETICS:
Neonatal Infection:
- Most frequent opportunistic infection among HIV-infected children, occurring in approximately 30%
- Neonatal occurrence unusual

■ PHYSICAL FINDINGS & CLINICAL PRESENTATION
- Fever, cough, shortness of breath present in almost all cases
- Lungs frequently clear to auscultation, although rales occasionally present
- Cyanosis and pronounced tachypnea in severe cases
- Hemoptysis unusual
- Spontaneous pneumothorax

■ ETIOLOGY
- *Pneumocystis carinii*, recently reclassified as a fungal organism
- Reactivation of dormant infection
- Extrapulmonary involvement rare

DIAGNOSIS

■ DIFFERENTIAL DIAGNOSIS
- Other opportunistic respiratory infections:
  1. Tuberculosis
  2. Histoplasmosis
  3. Cryptococcosis

- Nonopportunistic infections:
  1. Bacterial pneumonia
  2. Viral pneumonia
  3. Mycoplasmal pneumonia
  4. Legionellosis
- Occurs virtually exclusively in the setting of profound depression of cellular immunity

■ WORKUP
- Chest x-ray examination
- ABG
- Sputum examination for cysts of PCP and to exclude other pathogens
- Bronchoscopy with bronchoalveolar lavage or lung biopsy for diagnosis if sputum examination is negative or equivocal

■ LABORATORY TESTS
- ABG monitoring
- Elevated lactate dehydrogenase (LDH) in majority of cases
- HIV antibody test if cause of underlying immune deficiency state is unclear

■ IMAGING STUDIES
Diffuse uptake on gallium scanning of the lungs is suggestive but not diagnostic.

TREATMENT

■ NONPHARMACOLOGIC THERAPY
- Supplemental oxygen
- Ventilatory support if needed
- Prompt thoracotomy if pneumothorax develops

■ ACUTE GENERAL Rx
For confirmed or suspected PCP:
- Trimethoprim-sulfamethoxazole (20 mg/kg trimethoprim and 100 mg/kg sulfamethoxazole qd) PO or IV
- Pentamidine (4 mg/kg IV qd)
- Either regimen with prednisone (40 mg PO bid):
  1. If arterial oxygen pressure <70 mm Hg
  2. If arterial-alveolar oxygen pressure difference >35 mm Hg
  3. Dose tapered to 20 mg bid after 5 days and 20 mg qd after 10 days
- Therapy continued for 3 wk
- Alternative therapies available for patients unable to tolerate conventional therapy:
  1. Dapsone/trimethoprim
  2. Clindamycin/primaquine
  3. Atovaquone
- Alternative therapies should be given in consultation with a physician experienced in the management of PCP

■ CHRONIC Rx
- After completion of therapy, lifelong prophylaxis should be maintained with trimethoprim-sulfamethoxazole (one single-strength tablet PO qd or double-strength three times weekly).
- Patients intolerant of this therapy should be treated with dapsone (50 mg PO qd) plus pyrimethamine (50 mg PO weekly) plus leucovorin (25 mg PO weekly).
- Inhaled pentamidine (300 mg monthly by standardized nebulizer) is less effective and is reserved for patients intolerant to other forms of prophylaxis.
- Same approach taken to all HIV-infected patients with CD4 lymphocyte counts <200 to 250/mm³ or <20% of the total lymphocyte count because of their high risk of PCP.

■ DISPOSITION
- Patients should be hospitalized unless infection mild.
- After completion of therapy, long-term ambulatory follow-up is mandatory to provide secondary prevention of PCP (see "Chronic Rx") and management of the underlying immunodeficiency syndrome.

■ REFERRAL
To pulmonologist for bronchoscopy if diagnosis cannot be confirmed by sputum examination

PEARLS & CONSIDERATIONS

■ COMMENTS
All patients, especially those with severe infection or intolerant of conventional therapy, should be followed by a physician experienced in the management of PCP and, if appropriate, in the long-term management of HIV infection or other underlying disease.

REFERENCES
Kaplan JE et al: Epidemiology of human immunodeficiency virus: associated opportunistic infections in the United States in the era of highly active antiretroviral therapy, *Clin Infect Dis* 30(suppl 1):S5, 2000.

Russian DA, Levine SJ: *Pneumocystis carinii* pneumonia in patients without HIV infection, *Am J Med Sci* 321(1):56, 2001.

Author: **Joseph R. Masci, M.D.**

BASIC INFORMATION

■ DEFINITION
Viral pneumonia is infection of the pulmonary parenchyma caused by any of a large number of viral agents. The most important viruses are discussed in the following sections.

■ SYNONYMS
Nonbacterial pneumonia
Atypical pneumonia

ICD-9CM CODES
480.9 Viral pneumonia

■ EPIDEMIOLOGY & DEMOGRAPHICS
INCIDENCE (IN U.S.):
- Influenza virus:
  1. 10% to 20% of population in temperate zones infected during 1- to 2-mo epidemics occurring yearly during winter months.
  2. Up to 50% infected during pandemics.
  3. Pneumonia develops in small percentage of infected persons.
- Incidence of other important viral pneumonias is not known precisely.

PREVALENCE (IN U.S.):
- Often related to immune status of the population or presence of an epidemic
- Normal hosts (estimates):
  1. 86% of cases of pneumonia resulting in hospitalization in American adults
  2. 16% of pediatric pneumonias managed as outpatients
  3. 49% of hospitalized infants with pneumonia
- Important problem in hosts with impaired immunity

PREDOMINANT SEX:
- None generally
- Male sex may predispose to more severe respiratory disease in respiratory syncytial virus (RSV) infection

PREDOMINANT AGE:
Influenza:
- Overall incidence greatest at age 5 yr
- Falls with increasing age
- The most serious sequelae in those with chronic medical illnesses, especially cardiopulmonary disease
- Hospitalizations greatest in infants and adults >64 yr of age
RSV:
- Young children (as the major cause of pneumonia)
- Occurs throughout life
Adenoviruses:
- Young children
- Adults, primarily military recruits
Varicella:
- About 16% of adults (not infected in childhood) who contract chickenpox

- Acute varicella during pregnancy more likely to be complicated by severe pneumonia
- 90% of reported varicella pneumonia cases are in adults (highest incidence 20 to 60 yr old)
Measles:
- Young adults and older children who received a single vaccination (5% failure rate)
- Measles during pregnancy more likely to be complicated by pneumonia
- Underlying cardiopulmonary diseases and immunosuppression predispose to serious pneumonia complicating measles
- Before availability of measles vaccine, 90% of pneumonias in those <10 yr
- Currently more than a third of U.S. patients >14 yr old
- 3% to 50% of measles cases are complicated by pneumonia
CMV:
- Neonatal through adult
- Immunosuppression is key predisposing factor

PEAK INCIDENCE:
Influenza:
- Winter months for influenza A
- Year round for influenza B
- Peak of pneumonia seen weeks into the outbreak of infection
RSV: Winter and spring
Adenovirus: Endemic (military)
Varicella: Spring in temperate zones
Measles: Year round
CMV: Year round

GENETICS:
Familial Disposition:
- Close contact, not genetics, is important in acquisition
- Congenital anomalies and immunosuppression worsen course of RSV pneumonia
Congenital Infection:
- CMV is the most common intrauterine infection in the U.S.
- Pneumonia occurs occasionally in infants with symptomatic congenital infection.
Neonatal Infection:
- Severe RSV pneumonia
- Adenovirus pneumonia
  1. 5% to 20% fatality rate
  2. Can lead to residual restrictive or obstructive functional abnormalities
- "Varicella neonatorum"
  1. Disseminated visceral disease including pneumonia
  2. May develop in neonates whose mothers develop peripartum chickenpox
- CMV pneumonia
  1. Generally fatal
  2. Associated with severe cerebral damage in this population

■ PHYSICAL FINDINGS & CLINICAL PRESENTATION
INFLUENZA:
- Fever
- Uncomfortable or lethargic appearance
- Prominent dry cough (rarely hemoptysis)
- Flushed integument and erythematous mucous membranes
- Rales or rhonchi
RSV:
- Fever
- Tachypnea
- Prolonged expiration
- Wheezes and rales
ADENOVIRUSES:
- Hoarseness
- Pharyngitis
- Tachypnea
- Cervical adenitis
MEASLES:
- Conjunctivitis
- Rhinorrhea
- Koplik's spots
- Exanthem
- Pneumonitis
  1. May occur as a complication in 3% to 4% of adolescents and young adults
  2. Coincident with rash
  3. May also develop following apparent recovery from measles
- Fever
- Dry cough
VARICELLA:
- Fever
- Maculopapular or vesicular rash
  1. Becomes encrusted
  2. Pneumonia typical 1 to 6 days after rash appears
  3. Pneumonia accompanied by cough, and occasionally hemoptysis
- Few auscultatory abnormalities noted on examination of the lungs
CMV:
- Fever
- Paroxysmal cough
- Occasional hemoptysis
- Diffuse adenopathy when pneumonia occurs after transfusion

■ ETIOLOGY
Viral infection can lead to pneumonia in both immunocompetent and immunocompromised hosts.

DIAGNOSIS

■ DIFFERENTIAL DIAGNOSIS
- Bacterial pneumonia, which frequently complicates (i.e., can follow or be simultaneous with) viral (especially influenza) pneumonia
- Other causes of atypical pneumonia:
  1. *Mycoplasma*
  2. *Chlamydia*
  3. *Coxiella*

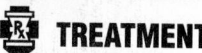

4. Legionnaires' disease
- ARDS
- Physical findings and associated hypoxemia confused with pulmonary emboli

■ WORKUP
- Information about the prevalent strain of influenza virus can be obtained from local health departments or from the Centers for Disease Control and Prevention.
- Viral diagnostic tests are usually not necessary once an outbreak has been defined.
- Influenza and other viruses can be cultured from respiratory secretions during the initial few days of the illness (special media and techniques necessary).
- Paired sera antibody titers are also useful.
- Monoclonal antibody tests are available for influenza and other respiratory viruses.
- Measles and adenovirus pneumonia are usually diagnosed clinically.
- Polymerase chain reaction may be able to rapidly detect and identify viral nucleic acid.
- Open lung biopsy is required for definite diagnosis of CMV pneumonia.

■ LABORATORY TESTS
- Sputum Gram stain (usually produced in scanty amounts) typically shows few polymorphonuclear leukocytes and few bacteria.

- WBC count may vary from leukopenic to modest elevation, usually without a leftward shift.
- Disseminated intravascular coagulation has occasionally complicated adenovirus type 7 pneumonia.
- Multinucleated giant cells on Tzanck preparation of an unroofed vesicular lesion are useful in diagnosing varicella in a patient with an infiltrate (also found in herpes simplex).
- Severe immunosuppression is associated with symptomatic CMV pneumonia (usually reactivation of latent infection, or in previously seronegative recipients from the donor).
- Hypoxemia may be profound.
- Cultures may be helpful in identifying superinfecting bacterial pathogens.
- When they occur, parapneumonic pleural effusions are exudative.

■ IMAGING STUDIES
- Chest x-ray examination may demonstrate a spectrum of findings from ill-defined, patchy, or generalized interstitial infiltrates, which can be associated with ARDS.
- A localized dense alveolar infiltrate suggests a superimposed bacterial pneumonia.
- Small calcified nodules may develop as a radiographic residual of varicella pneumonia (Fig. 1-217).

℞ TREATMENT

■ NONPHARMACOLOGIC THERAPY
GENERAL:
- Measures to diminish person-to-person transmission
- Modified bed rest
- Maintenance of adequate hydration
- Possible ventilatory support for severe pneumonia or ARDS
INFLUENZA:
- Yearly prophylactic strain-specific influenza vaccination (only subvirion vaccine should be used in children <13 yr) can be given to prevent infection.
- Live, attenuated influenza vaccines administered by nose drops may be more effective than the injected inactivated viral vaccines now available (under investigation).
RSV:
- Isolation techniques are important in limiting spread of RSV infections.
- Immunoglobulins with a high RSV-neutralizing antibody titer are beneficial in treatment.
ADENOVIRUSES:
- Intestinal inoculation of respiratory adenoviruses has been used to successfully immunize military recruits.
- Although they produce no disease in recipients, the viruses may be shed chronically and may infect others at a later date.
- These vaccines are not available for civilian populations.

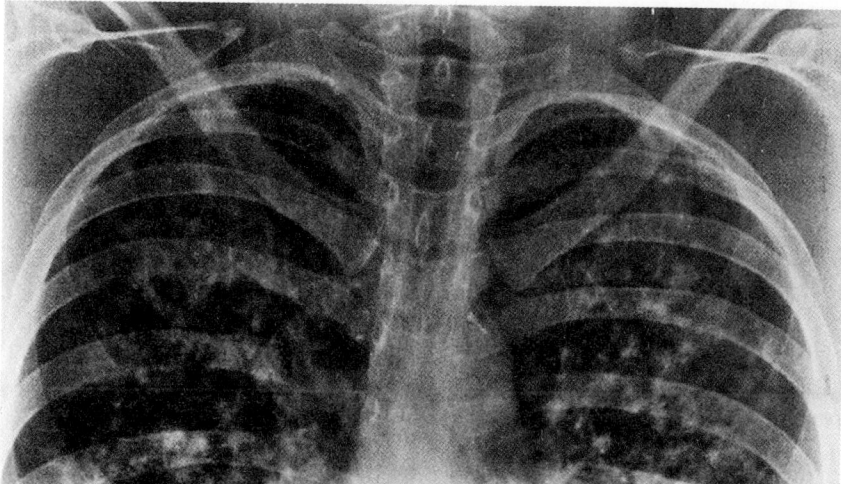

Fig. 1-217 Chickenpox—varicella pneumonia. Coned-down view of the upper lobes shows multiple ill-defined nodules in both upper lobes. (From McLoud TC: *Thoracic radiology: the requisites,* St Louis, 1998, Mosby.)

VARICELLA:
- Live, attenuated varicella vaccine has been successfully used in clinical trials.
- Varicella-zoster immune globulin should be administered within 4 days of exposure to prevent or modify the disease in susceptible persons.
- Nonimmunized persons exposed to varicella are potentially infectious between 10 and 21 days after exposure.

MEASLES:
- Effective measles vaccine is available:
  1. The vaccine should be administered at 15 mo.
  2. A second dose should be administered at the time of school entry.
- Live, attenuated vaccine or γ-globulin can prevent measles in unvaccinated persons if administered early following exposure.
- Vitamin A given PO for 2 days reduces morbidity and mortality from measles in exposed children.

■ ACUTE GENERAL Rx

GENERAL: Administer appropriate antibiotics for bacterial superinfections.
INFLUENZA:
- Amantadine and rimantadine (not commercially available) for influenza A. Early use can speed recovery from small airways dysfunction, but whether it influences the development or course of pneumonia is uncertain.
- Amantadine is also effective prophylactically during the time it is administered.

- Aerosolized ribavirin or amantadine may have a role in severe influenza pneumonia but have not been approved for this indication.
RSV: Ribavirin aerosol is effective for severe RSV pneumonia.
ADENOVIRUSES: No effective antiadenovirus agent.
VARICELLA:
- Varicella pneumonia can be treated with IV acyclovir.
- Adults who develop chickenpox should be considered for acyclovir treatment, which may prevent the development of pneumonia.
MEASLES: No effective antimeasles agent.
CMV:
- Acyclovir can prevent CMV infection in renal transplant recipients.
- Ganciclovir and foscarnet, with or without CMV hyperimmune globulin, show promise in the treatment of serious CMV infection, including pneumonia, in compromised hosts.

■ DISPOSITION
- Supportive therapy is useful.
- Deaths are possible during acute illness.
- Residual functional abnormalities may be persistent, develop into, or predispose to chronic respiratory diseases in later life.
- Morbidity and mortality following most viral pneumonias are increased by bacterial superinfection.

■ REFERRAL
- Uncertainty about the diagnosis in a compromised host
- Symptoms or findings progressive
- Severe respiratory compromise, diffuse infiltrates, or the development of ARDS

☼ PEARLS & CONSIDERATIONS

■ COMMENTS
- Influenza spreads by close contact and by small droplets transmitted by cough, which typifies the illness.
- RSV is effectively transmitted by fomites and by direct contact (little by aerosol).
- Varicella is transmitted by direct contact or by aerosol.
- Measles is transmitted by aerosol and possibly by fomites.

REFERENCES

Chien JW, Johnson JL: Viral pneumonias: multifaceted approach to an elusive diagnosis, *Postgrad Med* 107:67, 2000.

Colacino JM, Staschke KA, Laver WG: Approaches and strategies for the treatment of influenza virus infections, *Antivir Chem Chemother* 10:155, 1999.

Glezen WP et al: Impact of respiratory virus infections on persons with chronic underlying conditions, *JAMA* 283:499, 2000.

Author: **Harvey M. Shanies, M.D., Ph.D.**

BASIC INFORMATION

■ DEFINITION

A spontaneous pneumothorax (SP) is defined as the accumulation of air into the pleural space, collapsing the lung (Fig. 1-218). This can be primary SP (i.e., without any obvious underlying lung disease) or secondary SP (i.e., with underlying lung disease).

■ SYNONYMS

Primary spontaneous pneumothorax
Secondary spontaneous pneumothorax

ICD-9CM CODES

512.0 Spontaneous tension pneumothorax
512.8 Other spontaneous pneumothorax

■ EPIDEMIOLOGY & DEMOGRAPHICS

- Primary SP occurs in healthy individuals whereas secondary SP occurs in patients who have underlying lung disease.
- Approximately 20,000 new cases of spontaneous pneumothoraces occur each year in the U.S.
- SP is more common in men than women (6:1).
- Incidence of primary SP is 7.4/100,000 in men and 1.2/100,000 in women.
- Incidence of secondary SP is 6.3/100,000 in men and 2.0/100,000 in women.
- SP is commonly seen in tall, thin young men 20 to 40 yr of age.
- Tobacco increases the risk of SP.

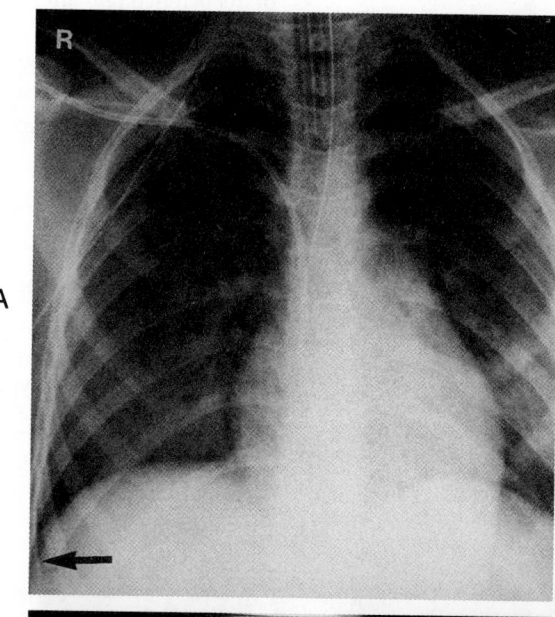

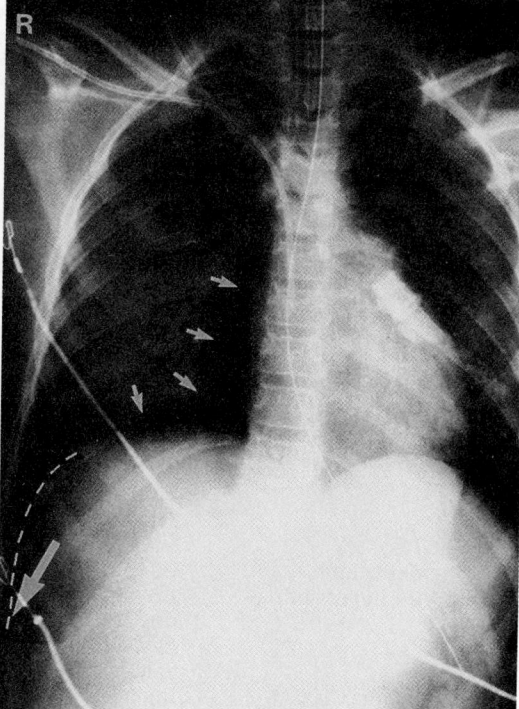

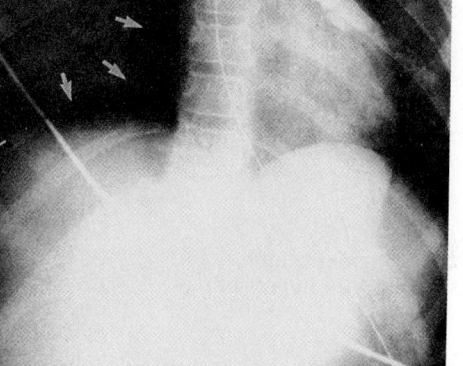

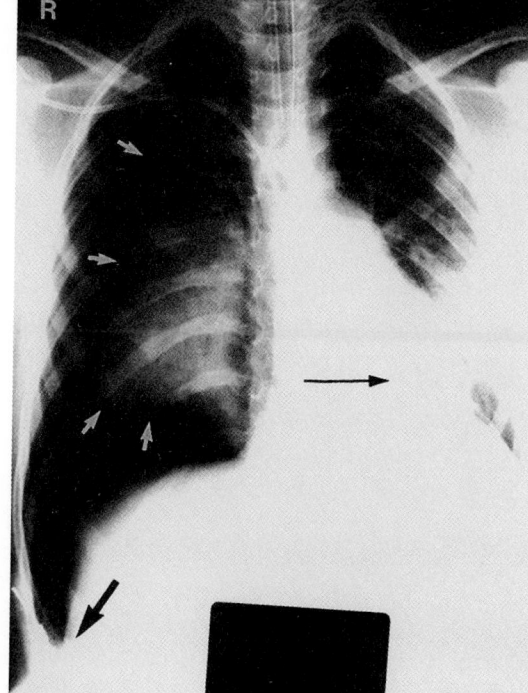

Fig. 1-218   Deep sulcus sign of pneumothorax. On a PA chest radiograph **(A)** the costophrenic angle is normally acute (*arrow*). In a supine patient, a pneumothorax will often be anterior, medical, and basilar. On a subsequent supine film **(B)** the dark area along the right cardiac border and lung base angle became much deeper and more acute than normal (*large arrow*). These findings were not recognized, and as a result, the same patient developed a tension pneumothorax **(C)** with an extremely deep costophrenic angle (*large black arrow*) and almost completely collapsed right lung (*small white arrows*) and shift of the mediastinum to the left. (From Mettler FA [ed]: *Primary care radiology*, Philadelphia, 2000, WB Saunders.)

■ **PHYSICAL FINDINGS & CLINICAL PRESENTATION**
- Sudden onset of pleuritic chest pain (90%)
- Dyspnea (80%)
- Tachycardia
- Diminished breath sounds
- Decreased tactile fremitus
- Hyperresonance

■ **ETIOLOGY**
- In primary SP, rupture of small blebs usually located near the apex of the upper lobes is a common cause.
- In secondary SP, COPD is the most common cause but can also be associated with pneumonia, bronchogenic carcinoma, mesothelioma, sarcoidosis, tuberculosis, cystic fibrosis, and many other lung diseases.

 DIAGNOSIS

Established by the chest x-ray

■ **DIFFERENTIAL DIAGNOSIS**
- Pleurisy
- Pulmonary embolism
- Myocardial infarction
- Pericarditis
- Asthma
- Pneumonia

■ **WORKUP**
Includes arterial blood gases, chest x-ray, and in some cases, CT scan of the chest

■ **LABORATORY TESTS**
ABGs may show hypoxemia and hypocapnia secondary to hyperventilation.

■ **IMAGING STUDIES**
- Spontaneous pneumothorax is usually confirmed by chest x-ray. X-ray findings include:
  1. Pleural line with absence of vessel markings peripheral to this line
  2. Expiratory films are better at demarcating the pneumothorax pleural line

3. Films should be done with patient standing and not supine
- CT scan can be done in suspected but difficult-to-visualize pneumothoraces.

 TREATMENT

■ **NONPHARMACOLOGIC THERAPY**
- Supplemental oxygen increases the rate of pneumothorax absorption.
- Cautious observation in the asymptomatic patient with <15% pneumothorax can be done but requires close daily outpatient monitoring.

■ **ACUTE GENERAL Rx**
- Aspiration using a small IV catheter in the second intercostal space midclavicular line attached to a three-way stopcock and a large syringe. Air is aspirated until resistance, excess cough by the patient, or >2.5 L is taken out. Repeat films are done immediately after aspiration and again in 24 hr.
- Chest tube insertion has been recommended for patients with primary SP who failed observation and simple aspiration and for all patients with secondary SP.

■ **CHRONIC Rx**
- Chest tube with pleurodesis has been used to prevent recurrence of both primary and secondary SP. Sclerosing agents commonly instilled through the chest tube into the pleural cavity are minocycline 5 mg/kg in 50 ml of normal saline or doxycycline 500 mg in 50 ml of normal saline.
- Talc has also been used as a sclerosing agent.
- Thoracoscopy or video-assisted thoracoscopy (VAT) is indicated in patients who have not responded to chest tube suctioning in 7 days, patients who have persistent bronchopleural fistula, and patients who have recurrent pneumothorax after chemical pleurodesis.

- Open thoracotomy is done in patients who fail VAT.

■ **DISPOSITION**
- Approximately 25% of patients with primary SP will have recurrence within 2 yr.
- The rates of recurrence after the second and third episode of spontaneous pneumothorax are 60% and 80%, respectively, with the majority of recurrences occurring on the same side as the first pneumothorax.
- Death from primary SP is uncommon. In patients with secondary SP and COPD, mortality ranges from 1% to 16%.
- The recurrence rate after open thoracotomy is <2%.

■ **REFERRAL**
A pulmonary specialist and general surgeon consultation is recommended.

✿ **PEARLS & CONSIDERATIONS**

■ **COMMENTS**
- The rate of pleural air absorption is about 1.25%/day.
- Patients with AIDS and *Pneumocystis carinii* infection have a high incidence of SP. Treatment typically requires chest tube placement and either thoracoscopy or open thoracotomy.

REFERENCES
Baumann NH et al: Management of spontaneous pneumothorax: an American College of Chest Physicians Delphi consensus statement, *Chest* 119(2):590, 2001.

Sahn SA, Heffner JE: Spontaneous pneumothorax, *N Engl J Med* 342(12)868, 2000.

Authors: **Hemchand Ramberan, M.D., and Peter Petropoulos, M.D.**

BASIC INFORMATION

■ DEFINITION
Poliomyelitis is a symptomatic infection caused by poliovirus, which (on rare occasions) may result in paralysis.

■ SYNONYMS
Polio
Infantile paralysis

ICD-9CM CODES
045.9 Poliomyelitis

■ EPIDEMIOLOGY & DEMOGRAPHICS
INCIDENCE (IN U.S.):
- Approximately 8 cases/yr.
- All cases in the U.S. and Western Hemisphere are now vaccine associated (because of oral polio vaccine [OPV]).
PREDOMINANT AGE: Almost always infants or young children
GENETICS:
Neonatal Infection: Most cases occur in otherwise healthy infants who receive OPV, or their contacts.

■ PHYSICAL FINDINGS & CLINICAL PRESENTATION
- Exposure of a nonimmune host to poliovirus usually results in asymptomatic infection.
- A small percentage of individuals may have one of three presentations:
  1. Abortive poliomyelitis: a flulike illness
     a. Fever
     b. Malaise
     c. Headache
     d. Sore throat
  2. Nonparalytic poliomyelitis: an aseptic meningitis that correlates with invasion of the CNS
     a. Headache
     b. Neck stiffness
     c. Change in mental status
  3. Paralytic poliomyelitis
     a. Most commonly affects the lumbar or bulbar regions
     b. Following paralysis, a period of variable degrees of recovery, the majority of which occurs in 2 to 6 mo
     c. Paralysis from involvement of motor neurons in the spinal cord
     d. Flaccid paralysis without sensory defects
     e. Postpolio syndrome late sequela, which may occur many years after the acute illness
     f. Functional deterioration of muscle groups that had recovered from initial paralysis thought to result from failure of reinnervation, which initially was able to restore function to weakened or paralyzed areas

■ ETIOLOGY
- Virus of genus *Enterovirus*
- Classic endemic and epidemic disease caused by wild-type poliovirus
- All cases in the U.S. currently caused by a live, attenuated virus in the OPV
  1. Extremely rare complication that occurs in vaccine recipients or their contacts
  2. Paralysis from lower motor neuron damage caused by viral infection

DIAGNOSIS

■ DIFFERENTIAL DIAGNOSIS
- Guillain-Barré syndrome
- CVA
- Spinal cord compression
- Other enteroviruses:
  1. Aseptic meningitis
  2. Paralysis (rare)

■ WORKUP
- Isolation of virus:
  1. Stool or a rectal swab
  2. Throat swabs
  3. Rarely CSF
- Paired sera for antibody titer determinations

■ LABORATORY TESTS
CSF:
- Aseptic meningitis
- Elevated WBCs
- Elevated protein
- Normal glucose

■ IMAGING STUDIES
MRI may show involvement of anterior horn of the spinal cord.

TREATMENT

■ NONPHARMACOLOGIC THERAPY
- Maintenance of respiration and hydration
- Early mobilization and exercise once fever subsides

■ ACUTE GENERAL Rx
- Aimed at reduction of pain and muscle spasm
- No agent to alter the course of disease

■ CHRONIC Rx
Physical therapy

■ DISPOSITION
- In the abortive and nonparalytic forms, complete recovery
- Paralytic disease:
  1. Variable degrees of recovery
  2. 80% usually in the first 6 mo following illness

■ REFERRAL
Always refer to an infectious disease consultant. Cases should be reported to public health agencies.

PEARLS & CONSIDERATIONS

■ COMMENTS
- Risk of disease in recipients of OPV is approximately 1 in 2.5 million.
- Use of inactivated polio vaccine (IPV) is not associated with disease:
  1. Does not confer local (mucosal) immunity
  2. Will not immunize nonvaccinated contacts
  3. Requires boosters
  4. Is given by injection
- To decrease the incidence of vaccine-associated polio, the routine childhood vaccination schedule has been changed. A recent recommendation for use of a sequential IPV-OPV schedule has again been modified. Exclusive use of IPV is now recommended. OPV use is limited to unvaccinated persons with plans for imminent (<4 wk) travel to polio-endemic areas.

REFERENCE
Centers for Disease Control and Prevention: Poliomyelitis prevention in the United States: updated recommendations of the Advisory Committee on Immunization Practices (ACIP), *MMWR Morb Mortal Wkly Rep* 49(RR-05):1, 2000.
Author: **Maurice Policar, M.D.**

BASIC INFORMATION

■ DEFINITION

Polyarteritis nodosa is a vasculitic syndrome involving medium-size to small arteries, characterized histologically by necrotizing inflammation of the arterial media and inflammatory cell infiltration.

■ SYNONYMS

Periarteritis nodosa
PAN
Necrotizing arteritis

ICD-9CM CODES

446.0 Polyarteritis nodosa

■ EPIDEMIOLOGY & DEMOGRAPHICS

- Incidence is 1:100,000 annually.
- Male:female ratio is 2:1.
- Increased incidence in patients with hepatitis B surface antigen, hepatitis C virus.

■ PHYSICAL FINDINGS & CLINICAL PRESENTATION

- Typical presentation is subacute, with the onset of constitutional symptoms over weeks to months
- Weight loss, nausea, vomiting
- Testicular pain or tenderness
- Myalgias, weakness, or leg tenderness
- Neuropathy (mononeuritis multiplex), foot drop
- Livedo reticularis, ulceration of digits, abdominal pain after meals, hematemesis, hematochezia, hypertension, asymmetric polyarthritis (tending to involve large joints of lower extremities); true synovitis occurs only in a minority of patients
- Fever may be present (polyarteritis nodosa is often a cause of fever of unknown origin) and can range from intermittent, low-grade fevers to high fevers with chills
- Tachycardia is common and often striking

■ ETIOLOGY

- Unknown
- Hepatitis B virus-associated PAN appears to be an immune complex-mediated disease

DIAGNOSIS

■ DIFFERENTIAL DIAGNOSIS

Cryoglobulinemia, SLE, infections (e.g., SBE, trichinosis, *Rickettsia*), lymphoma

■ WORKUP

- Laboratory evaluation, arteriography, and biopsy of small or medium-size arteries can confirm diagnosis. Clinical manifestations are variable and depend on the arteries involved and the organs affected (e.g., kidney involvement occurs in >80% of cases).
- The presence of any three of the following ten items allows the diagnosis of polyarteritis nodosa with a sensitivity of 82% and a specificity of 86%:
    1. Weight loss >4 kg
    2. Livedo reticularis
    3. Testicular pain or tenderness
    4. Myalgias, weakness, or leg tenderness
    5. Neuropathy
    6. Diastolic blood pressure >90 mm Hg
    7. Elevated BUN or creatinine
    8. Positive test for hepatitis B virus
    9. Arteriography revealing small or large aneurysms and focal constrictions between dilated segments
    10. Biopsy of small or medium-size artery containing WBC

■ LABORATORY TESTS

- Elevated BUN or creatinine, positive test for hepatitis B virus or hepatitis C
- Elevated ESR and C-reactive protein, anemia, elevated platelets, eosinophilia, proteinuria, hematuria

- Biopsy of small or medium-size artery of symptomatic sites (muscle, nerve) is >90% specific. Biopsy of the gastrocnemius muscle and sural nerve are commonly performed
- Assays for ANA and RF are negative; however, low, nonspecific titers may be detected

■ IMAGING STUDIES

Arteriography can be done in patients with negative biopsies or if there are no symptomatic sites. Visceral angiography will reveal aneurysmal dilation of the renal, mesenteric, or hepatic arteries.

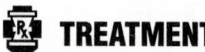 **TREATMENT**

■ NONPHARMACOLOGIC THERAPY

Low-sodium diet in hypertensive patients

■ ACUTE GENERAL Rx

Prednisone 1 to 2 mg/kg/day; cyclophosphamide in refractory cases

■ CHRONIC Rx

Monitoring for infections and potential complications such as thrombosis, infarction, or organ necrosis

■ DISPOSITION

The 5-yr survival is <20% in untreated patients. Treatment with corticosteroids increases survival to approximately 50%. Usage of both corticosteroids and immunosuppressive drugs may increase 5-yr survival >80%. Poor prognostic signs are severe renal or GI involvement.

■ REFERRAL

Surgical referral for biopsy

REFERENCE

Stone JH: Polyarteritis nodosa, *JAMA* 288:1632, 2002.
Author: **Fred F. Ferri, M.D.**

BASIC INFORMATION

■ DEFINITION
Polycystic kidney disease refers to a systemic hereditary disorder characterized by the formation of cysts in the cortex and medulla of both kidneys (Fig. 1-219).

■ SYNONYMS
Autosomal dominant polycystic kidney disease (ADPKD)

ICD-9CM CODES
753.1 Polycystic kidney, unspecified type
753.13 Polycystic kidney, autosomal dominant

■ EPIDEMIOLOGY & DEMOGRAPHICS
- Occurs in 1:400 to 1:1000 people
- Incidence: 6000 new cases per year
- Approximately 500,000 people with ADPKD in the U.S.
- Found in all ages
- Accounts for 10% of end-stage renal disease
- Associated with liver cysts (50% to 70%), pancreatic cysts (10%), splenic cysts (5%), and CNS arachnoid cysts (5%)
- Also associated with cerebral aneurysms (20%); 6% of patients with berry aneurysms have polycystic kidney disease
- Increased incidence of diverticular disease and mitral valve prolapse

■ PHYSICAL FINDINGS & CLINICAL PRESENTATION
- Usually presents in the third to fourth decade of life
- Pain (abdominal, flank, or back)
- Palpable flank mass
- Hypertension
- Headache
- Nocturia
- Hematuria
- Nephrolithiasis (20%)
- Urinary tract infection

■ ETIOLOGY
- Approximately 90% of cases are inherited as an autosomal dominant trait.
- Spontaneous mutations occur in 10% of cases.
- The abnormal gene in the majority of cases has been located to the short arm of chromosome 16. In the minority of cases the defect is located on chromosome 4.
- All cysts develop from preexisting renal tubules segments and only a small portion of the nephrons (1%) undergoes cystic formation.

DIAGNOSIS

A person is considered to have polycystic kidney disease if three or more cysts are noted in both kidneys and there is a positive family member with ADPKD.

■ DIFFERENTIAL DIAGNOSIS
- Simple cysts
- Autosomal recessive polycystic kidney disease in children
- Tuberous sclerosis
- Von Hippel-Lindau syndrome
- Acquired cystic kidney disease

■ WORKUP
The workup to establish the diagnosis of ADPKD includes a detailed family history and either an ultrasound or a CT scan of the abdomen to visualize bilateral renal cysts.

■ LABORATORY TESTS
- Hemoglobin and hematocrit is elevated because of increased secretion of erythropoietin from functioning renal cysts. This also explains the relatively mild anemia found in patients with ADPKD and renal insufficiency.
- Electrolyte abnormalities commonly seen in any patients with renal insufficiency may be present.
- BUN and creatinine can be elevated.
- Urinalysis can show microscopic hematuria, WBC casts in pyelonephritis, or proteinuria (seldom >1 g/24 hr).
- Increased erythropoietin level.
- Patients with a strong positive family history of ADPKD and no cysts detected by imaging studies can undergo genetic linkage analysis.

■ IMAGING STUDIES
- Abdominal renal ultrasound is the easiest and more cost-efficient test for renal cysts. Renal ultrasound can detect cysts from 1 to 1.5 cm.
- Abdominal CT scan is more sensitive than ultrasound and can detect cysts as small as 0.5 cm.
- Both studies can detect associated hepatic, splenic, and pancreatic cysts.
- MRI is more sensitive than ultrasound and may help in distinguishing renal cell carcinomas from simple cysts.

TREATMENT

■ NONPHARMACOLOGIC THERAPY
- Nephrolithiasis is treated in a similar manner with either IV or PO hydration. If stones remain lodged, lithotripsy or percutaneous nephrostolithotomy can be done.
- Hypertension treatment is initiated with salt restriction, weight loss, and daily walking exercise.
- Avoidance of physical contact sports is advised.

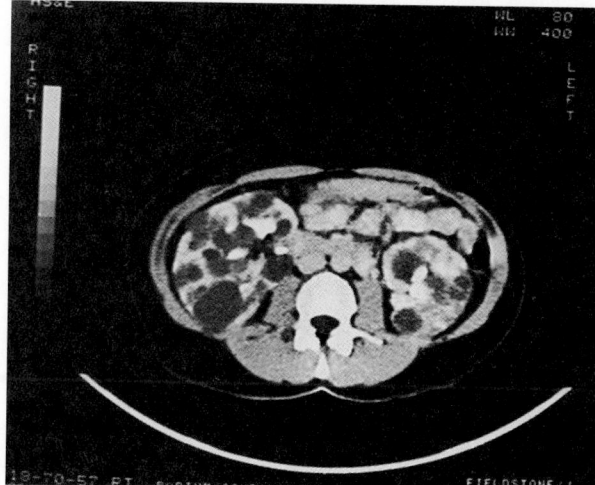

Fig. 1-219   Tomogram of autosomal dominant polycystic kidney disease. Kidney cysts. (From Stein JH [ed]: *Internal medicine,* ed 5, St Louis, 1998, Mosby.)

■ ACUTE GENERAL Rx

- Kidney infections should be treated with antibiotics known to penetrate the cyst (e.g., trimethoprim-sulfamethoxazole 1 tablet PO bid or ciprofloxacin 250 mg PO bid).
- Angiotensin-converting enzyme inhibitors (e.g., captopril 25 mg bid or tid, lisinopril 10 mg PO qd, fosinopril 10 mg PO qd, or enalapril 10 mg qd) are effective in the treatment of hypertension associated with ADPKD.
- Calcium channel blockers (e.g., nifedipine 30 to 90 mg PO qd, amlodipine 5 to 10 mg PO qd, or felodipine 5 to 10 mg PO qd) can be used with or without ACE inhibitors in the treatment of hypertension.
- α-Blockers and diuretics can be added as adjunctive therapy for hypertension.
- Blood pressure <130/85 is the goal for patients with renal disease. If there is >1 g of urinary protein per 24 hr, the target blood pressure is <125/75 mm Hg.

■ CHRONIC Rx

- Dialysis for end-stage renal failure
- Renal transplantation
- Cystic decompression in patients with intractable pain caused by enlarging cysts

■ DISPOSITION

- Approximately half the patients with ADPKD will progress to renal failure.
- Gross hematuria is usually self-limited.
- Complications of ADPKD include:
  1. End-stage renal failure
  2. Infected cysts and urinary tract infections
  3. Pyelonephritis
  4. Nephrolithiasis
  5. Electrolyte abnormalities
  6. Cerebral aneurysm rupture
  7. Intractable pain from enlarging cysts

■ REFERRAL

Nephrology consultation should be made in patients with renal insufficiency, difficult-to-control hypertension, recurrent infections, or renal stones. Urology can also be consulted in patients with nephrolithiasis, recurrent episodes of gross hematuria, or consideration for nephrectomy before transplantation.

☼ PEARLS & CONSIDERATIONS

■ COMMENTS

- A cyst is considered to be present if it measures >2 mm in diameter.
- A positive family history of ADPKD is found in approximately 60% of the cases. Renal ultrasound performed on patient's parents reveals ADPKD in about 30% of the cases.
- Up to 25% of patients may not have cysts present before the age of 30.
- Screening patients with ADPKD for cerebral aneurysms is not recommended unless there is a positive family history of cerebral aneurysms or family member with ruptured cerebral aneurysm.

REFERENCES

Beebe DK: Autosomal dominant polycystic kidney disease, *Am Fam Physician* 53(3):925, 1996.

Chapman AB, Johnson AM, Gabow PA: Intracranial aneurysms in patients with autosomal dominant polycystic kidney disease: how to diagnose and who to screen, *Am J Kidney Dis* 22:526, 1993.

Gabow PA: Autosomal dominant polycystic kidney disease, *N Engl J Med* 329(5):332, 1993.

Gibson P, Watson ML: Managing the patient with polycystic kidney disease, *Practitioner* 246(1638):450, 2002.

Welling LW, Grantham JJ: Cystic and developmental diseases of the kidney. In Brenner BM, Rector FC: *Brenner & Rector's the kidney,* ed 5, Philadelphia, 1996, WB Saunders.

Wilson PD: Polycystic kidney disease, *N Engl J Med* 350:2, 2004.

Author: **Peter Petropoulos, M.D.**

BASIC INFORMATION

■ DEFINITION

Polycystic ovary syndrome (PCOS) in its complete form associates polycystic ovaries, amenorrhea, hirsutism, and obesity.

■ SYNONYMS

Stein-Leventhal syndrome
PCOS

ICD-9CM CODES

256.4 Polycystic ovary syndrome

■ EPIDEMIOLOGY & DEMOGRAPHICS

PREVALENCE: 3% of adolescent and adult women.
- Symptoms usually begin around the time of menarche, and the diagnosis is often made during adolescence or young adulthood.
- Increased risk of endometrial and ovarian cancers.

■ PHYSICAL FINDINGS & CLINICAL PRESENTATION

- Oligomenorrhea or amenorrhea
- Dysfunctional uterine bleeding
- Infertility
- Hirsutism
- Acne
- Obesity (40% only)
- Insulin resistance (type 2 diabetes mellitus)

■ ETIOLOGY & PATHOGENESIS

- PCOS is probably a genetic disorder, but in most cases no family history is evident. Whether transmission is autosomal or X-linked is still unclear.
- Elevated serum LH concentrations and an increased serum LH:FSH ratio result either from an increased GnRH hypothalamic secretion or less likely from a primary pituitary abnormality. This results in dysregulation of androgen secretion and increased intraovarian androgen, the effect of which in the ovary is follicular atresia, maturation arrest, polycystic ovaries, and anovulation. Hyperinsulinemia is a contributing factor to ovarian hyperandrogenism, independent of LH excess. A role for insulin growth factor (IGF) receptors has been postulated for the association of PCOS and diabetes.

DIAGNOSIS

Clinical:
- PCOS is the most common cause of chronic anovulation with estrogen present. A positive progesterone withdrawal test establishes the presence of estrogen. Medroxyprogesterone (Provera) 10 mg qd is administered for 5 days and bleeding occurs if estrogen is present.

- The presence of oligomenorrhea, hirsutism, obesity, and documentation of polycystic ovaries establishes the diagnosis.

■ DIFFERENTIAL DIAGNOSIS

Causes of amenorrhea:
- Primary (unusual in PCOS)
Genetic disorder (Turner's syndrome)
Anatomic abnormality (e.g., imperforate hymen)
- Secondary
Pregnancy
Functional (cause unknown, anorexia nervosa, stress, excessive exercise, hyperthyroidism, less commonly hypothyroidism, adrenal dysfunction, pituitary dysfunction, severe systemic illness, drugs such as oral contraceptives, estrogens, or dopamine agonists)
Abnormalities of the genital tract (uterine tumor, endometrial scarring, ovarian tumor)

■ LABORATORY TESTS

Fasting blood glucose to rule out diabetes
Elevated LH/FSH ratio >2.5
Prolactin level elevation in 25%
Elevated androgens (testosterone, DHEA-S)

■ IMAGING STUDIES

Pelvic ultrasound (or CT scan) reveals the presence of twofold to fivefold ovarian enlargement with a thickened tunica albuginea, thecal hyperplasia, and 20 or more subcapsular follicles from 1 to 15 mm in diameter (Fig. 1-220).

TREATMENT

The goal is to interrupt the self-perpetuating abnormal hormone cycle:

- Reduction of ovarian androgen secretion by laparoscopic ovarian wedge resection
- Reduction of ovarian androgen secretion by using oral contraceptives or LHRH analogs
- Weight reduction for all obese women with PCOS
- FSH stimulation with clomiphene HMG, or pulsatile LHRH
- Urofollitropin (pure FSH) administration
- Glitazones may improve ovulation and hirsutism in the polycystic ovary syndrome
Choice of treatment:
- The management of hirsutism without risking pregnancy includes oral contraceptives, glucocorticoids, LHRH analogs, or spironolactone (an antiandrogen)
- Pregnancy can be achieved with clomiphene (alone or with glucocorticoids, hCG, or bromocriptine), HMG, urofollitropin, pulsatile LHRH, or ovarian wedge resection

■ REFERRAL

Gynecologist or endocrinologist

REFERENCES

Azziz R et al: Troglitazone improves ovulation and hirsutism in the polycystic ovary syndrome: a multicenter, double blind, placebo-controlled trial, *J Clin Endocrinol Metab* 86:1626, 2001.
Marx TL, Mehta AE: Polycystic ovary syndrome: pathogenesis and treatment over the short and long term, *Cleve Clin J Med* 70:31, 2003.
Richardson MR: Current perspectives in polycystic ovary syndrome, *Am Fam Physician* 68:697, 2003.
Author: **Tom J. Wachtel, M.D.**

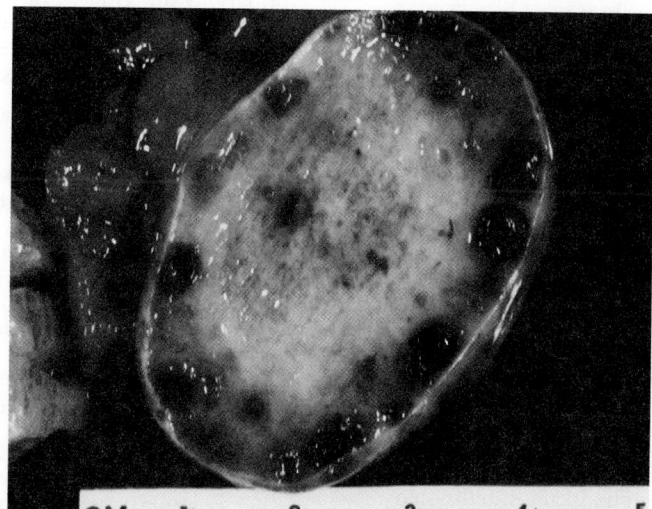

Fig. 1-220 Sagittal section of a polycystic ovary illustrating large number of follicular cysts and thickened stroma. (From Mishell DR: *Comprehensive gynecology*, ed 3, St Louis, 1997, Mosby.)

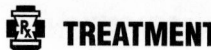
▪ BASIC INFORMATION

▪ DEFINITION
Polycythemia vera is a chronic myelo-proliferative disorder characterized mainly by erythrocytosis (increase in RBC mass).

▪ SYNONYMS
Primary polycythemia
Vaquez disease

▪ ICD-9CM CODES
238.4 Polycythemia vera

▪ EPIDEMIOLOGY & DEMOGRAPHICS
INCIDENCE/PREVALENCE: 0.5 cases/100,000 persons; mean age at onset is 60 yr; men are more affected than women.

▪ PHYSICAL FINDINGS & CLINICAL PRESENTATION
The patient generally comes to medical attention because of symptoms associated with increased blood volume and viscosity or impaired platelet function:
- Impaired cerebral circulation resulting in headache, vertigo, blurred vision, dizziness, TIA, CVA
- Fatigue, poor exercise tolerance
- Pruritus, particularly following bathing (caused by overproduction of histamine)
- Bleeding: epistaxis, UGI bleeding (increased incidence of PUD)
- Abdominal discomfort secondary to splenomegaly; hepatomegaly may be present
- Hyperuricemia may result in nephrolithiasis and gouty arthritis
The physical examination may reveal:
Facial plethora, congestion of oral mucosa, ruddy complexion
Enlargement and tortuosity of retinal veins
Splenomegaly (found in >75% of patients)

▪ DIAGNOSIS

▪ DIFFERENTIAL DIAGNOSIS
SMOKING:
- Polycythemia is secondary to increased carboxyhemoglobin, resulting in left shift in the Hgb dissociation curve.
- Laboratory evaluation shows increased Hct, RBC mass, erythropoietin level, and carboxyhemoglobin.
- Splenomegaly is not present on physical examination.
HYPOXEMIA (SECONDARY POLYCYTHEMIA): Living for prolonged periods at high altitudes, pulmonary fibrosis, congenital cardiac lesions with right-to-left shunts

- Laboratory evaluation shows decreased arterial oxygen saturation and elevated erythropoietin level.
- Splenomegaly is not present on physical examination.
ERYTHROPOIETIN-PRODUCING STATES: Renal cell carcinoma, hepatoma, cerebral hemangioma, uterine fibroids, polycystic kidneys
- The erythropoietin level is elevated in these patients; the arterial oxygen saturation is normal.
- Splenomegaly may be present with metastatic neoplasms.
STRESS POLYCYTHEMIA (GAISBÖCK'S SYNDROME, RELATIVE POLYCYTHEMIA):
- Laboratory evaluation demonstrates normal RBC mass, arterial oxygen saturation, and erythropoietin level; plasma volume is decreased.
- Splenomegaly is not present on physical examination.
HEMOGLOBINOPATHIES ASSOCIATED WITH HIGH OXYGEN AFFINITY: An abnormal oxyhemoglobin-dissociation curve (P50) is present.

▪ WORKUP
Serum erythropoietin level is the best initial test for the diagnosis of polycythemia vera. A low serum erythropoietin level is highly suggestive of polycythemia vera. A normal level does not exclude the diagnosis. If the erythropoietin level is elevated, obtain abdominal and pelvic CT to rule out renal cercal carcinoma and other causes of polycythemia.
In patients with elevated erythropoietin level, evaluate for secondary erythrocytosis:
- Measure RBC mass by isotope dilution using ^{51}Cr-labeled autologous RBCs (expensive test); a high value eliminates stress polycythemia.
- Measure arterial saturation; a normal value eliminates polycythemia secondary to smoking.
- The diagnosis of hemoglobinopathy with high affinity is ruled out by a normal oxyhemoglobin dissociation curve.

▪ LABORATORY TESTS
- Elevated RBC count (>6 million/mm³), elevated Hgb (>18 g/dl in men, >16 g/dl in women), elevated Hct (>54% in men, >49% in women)
- Increased WBC (often with basophilia); thrombocytosis in the majority of patients
- Elevated leukocyte alkaline phosphatase, serum vitamin B$_{12}$, and uric acid levels
- Low serum erythropoietin level
- Bone marrow aspiration revealing RBC hyperplasia and absent iron stores

▪ TREATMENT

▪ NONPHARMACOLOGIC THERAPY
Phlebotomy to keep Hct <45% in men and <42% in women is the mainstay of therapy.

▪ ACUTE GENERAL RX
- Hydroxyurea can be used in conjunction with phlebotomy to decrease the incidence of thrombotic events.
- Interferon α-2b is also effective in controlling RBC values without significant side effects.
- Myelosuppressive therapy with chlorambucil is effective but not routinely used because of its leukemogenic potential.

▪ CHRONIC RX
- Patient education regarding need for lifelong monitoring and treatment
- Adjunctive therapy: treatment of pruritus with antihistamines, control of significant hyperuricemia with allopurinol, reduction of gastric hyperacidity with antacids of H$_2$ blockers, low-dose aspirin to treat vasomotor symptoms in patients without bleeding diathesis

▪ DISPOSITION
- The median survival time without treatment is 6 to 18 mo following diagnosis; phlebotomy extends the average survival time to 12 yr.
- Prognosis is worse in patients >60 yr of age and those who have a history of thrombosis.

⚙ PEARLS & CONSIDERATIONS

▪ COMMENTS
The diagnosis of polycythemia vera generally requires the following three major criteria or the first two major criteria plus two minor criteria:
- Major criteria
  1. Increased RBC mass (>36 ml/kg in men, >32 ml/kg in women)
  2. Normal arterial oxygen saturation (>92%)
  3. Splenomegaly
- Minor criteria
  1. Thrombocytosis (>400,000/mm³)
  2. Leukocytosis (>12,000/mm³)
  3. Elevated leukocyte alkaline phosphatase (>100)
  4. Elevated serum vitamin B$_{12}$ (>900 pg/ml) or vitamin B$_{12}$ binding protein (>2200 pg/ml)

REFERENCE
Tefferi A: Polycythemia vera: a comprehensive review and clinical recommendations, *Mayo Clin Proc* 78:174, 2003.
Author: **Fred F. Ferri, M.D.**

BASIC INFORMATION

■ DEFINITION

Polymyalgia rheumatica is a disorder of unknown cause affecting older patients. It is characterized by shoulder and hip stiffness and an elevated erythrocyte sedimentation rate (ESR).

■ SYNONYMS

Anarthritic rheumatoid syndrome

ICD-9CM CODES

725.0 Polymyalgia rheumatica

■ EPIDEMIOLOGY & DEMOGRAPHICS

PREVALENCE: 1 case/135 persons >50 yr old
PREDOMINANT SEX: Female:male ratio of 2:1
PREDOMINANT AGE: Rare under age 50 yr; average age at onset: 70 yr

■ PHYSICAL FINDINGS & CLINICAL PRESENTATION

- Symptoms are frequently of sudden onset but are often present for months before the diagnosis is made.
- Neck, shoulder, low back, and thigh pain are common complaints.
- Morning stiffness lasting 2 to 3 hr is typical, and patients often have difficulty getting out of bed.
- Malaise, weight loss, depression, and a low-grade fever are common constitutional symptoms and may suggest systemic inflammation.

- Physical findings are usually limited. Synovitis may be present in peripheral joints and may also be responsible for the proximal girdle symptoms in spite of the fact that they appear to be "muscular" in nature.
- Mild soft tissue tenderness may be present.
- Distal extremity manifestations (knee, wrist, metacarpophalangeal joints) may occur in 25% to 45% of patients.
- The temporal arteries should be carefully examined because of the strong relation of polymyalgia rheumatica with temporal or giant cell arteritis.

■ ETIOLOGY

Unknown

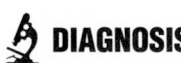

DIAGNOSIS

■ DIFFERENTIAL DIAGNOSIS

(Table 1-43)
- Rheumatoid arthritis: rheumatoid factor is negative in polymyalgia.
- Polymyositis: enzyme studies are negative in polymyalgia.
- Fibromyalgia

■ WORKUP

The diagnosis of polymyalgia rheumatica is suggested by the following findings:
- Pain and stiffness of pectoral and pelvic musculature
- Patient >50 yr old
- Morning stiffness >1 hr
- Normal motor strength
- Symptoms for at least 4 to 6 wk
- Elevated ESR (>45)
- Rapid clinical response to low-dose corticosteroid therapy

■ LABORATORY TESTS

- CBC, ESR, and rheumatoid factor should be performed.
- Mild anemia may be present.

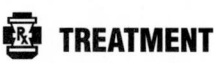

TREATMENT

■ ACUTE GENERAL RX

- Prednisone 10 to 20 mg/day is given. The response is often so dramatic that it can be used to confirm the diagnosis. Improvement is usually noted within 24 to 48 hr. Generally, if the initial prednisone dose is 20 mg/day, reduce by 2.5 mg every wk to 10 mg/day, then by 1 mg/day every month if tolerated.
- Steroids are gradually tapered over the next few weeks as soon as symptoms permit, but small doses (5 mg/day) may be needed for 2 yr.
- NSAIDs may be tried in mild cases.
- Physical therapy is usually unnecessary.

TABLE 1-43 Differential Features in Polymyalgia Rheumatica and Similar Disorders

SIGNS/SYMPTOMS	POLYMYALGIA RHEUMATICA	GIANT CELL ARTERITIS	RHEUMATOID ARTHRITIS	DERMATOMYOSITIS	FIBROMYALGIA
Morning stiffness >30 min	+	±	+*	±	Variable
Headache and/or scalp tenderness	0	+	0	0	Variable
Pain with active joint movement	+	0	+*	0	Inconstant
Tender joints	±	0	+*	0	Tender spots
Swollen joints	±	±	+	0	0
Muscle weakness	±†	0	+*	+	0
Normochromic anemia	+	+	+	0	0
Elevated erythrocyte sedimentation rate	+	+	+	±	0
Elevated serum creatine kinase	0	0	0	+	0
Serum rheumatoid factor	0	0	70%	0	0
Distinct electromyographic abnormality	0	0	0	+	0
Response to nonsteroidal antiinflammatory drug	±	0	+	0	0

From Goldman L, Ausiello D, (eds): *Cecil textbook of medicine*, ed 22, Philadelphia, 2004, WB Saunders.
0, Absent; +, present; ±, present in minority of cases.
*Associated with affected joints
†Pain inhibits movement. Disuse atrophy may occur.

PEARLS & CONSIDERATIONS

■ **COMMENTS**

The prognosis is generally favorable. Relapse occasionally occurs in several years, but again responds well to prednisone.

REFERENCES

Cohen MD, Abril A: Polymyalgia rheumatica revisited, *Bull Rheum Dis* 50:1, 2001.

De Jager JP: Polymyalgia rheumatica and giant cell arteritis: avoiding management traps, *Aust Fam Physician* 30:643, 2001.

Meskimen S, Cook TD, Blake RL: Management of giant cell arteritis and polymyalgia rheumatica, *Am Fam Physician* 61:2061, 2000.

Salvarani C et al: Distal musculoskeletal manifestations in PMR, *Arthritis Rheum* 41:1221, 1998.

Salvarani C et al: Polymyalgia rheumatica and giant-cell arteritis, *N Engl J Med* 347:261, 2002.

Weyland CM et al: Corticosteroid requirements in polymyalgia rheumatica, *Arch Intern Med* 159:577, 1999.

Author: **Lonnie R. Mercier, M.D.**

BASIC INFORMATION

■ DEFINITION

Polymyositis is a chronic idiopathic inflammatory myopathy.

■ SYNONYMS

Primary idiopathic polymyositis

ICD-9CM CODES

710.4 Polymyositis

■ EPIDEMIOLOGY & DEMOGRAPHICS

- Incidence: 5 cases/1 million/yr
- More common in females than males (2:1)

■ PHYSICAL FINDINGS & CLINICAL PRESENTATION

- Most patients with polymyositis have a subacute onset, over weeks to months
- Symmetric proximal muscle weakness involving initially the shoulders and pelvic girdle resulting in difficulty rising from a chair, walking up stairs, or combing one's hair
- Dysphagia and dysphonia result from pharyngeal muscle involvement
- Dyspnea
- Nonproductive cough
- Rales
- Aspiration pneumonia
- Respiratory failure
- Fever
- "Mechanic's hand" (fissured and coarse skin over the area between the thumb and the index finger)
- Raynaud's phenomenon

■ ETIOLOGY

- The exact cause of polymyositis is not known.
- An immunologic cause is suggested with increased frequency of HLA-DR3 and DRw52 antigens in patients with polymyositis.
- A viral etiology has been proposed secondary to the presence of autoantibodies to histidyl transferase antibody, anti-Jo-1 antibody, and signal recognition particle.

DIAGNOSIS

The diagnosis of polymyositis is made by:
- History and physical findings of proximal muscle weakness
- Elevated muscle enzyme tests
- EMG
- Muscle biopsy

■ DIFFERENTIAL DIAGNOSIS

- Dermatomyositis
- Muscular dystrophies
- Amyotrophic lateral sclerosis
- Myasthenia gravis or Eaton-Lambert syndrome
- Guillain-Barré syndrome
- Alcoholic myopathy
- Fibromyalgia
- Drug-induced myopathies (e.g., HMG- reductase inhibitors, gemfibrozil)
- Diseases associated with polymyositis (e.g., sarcoidosis, HIV)
- Inclusion body myositis

■ WORKUP

Patients suspected of having polymyositis by clinical presentation should have an EMG, muscle biopsy, and specific blood tests to confirm the diagnosis.

■ LABORATORY TESTS

- ESR although not specific is elevated in the majority of cases.
- Creatine kinase is the most sensitive muscle enzyme test and can be elevated as much as 50 times above normal.
- Aldolase, AST, ALT, alkaline phosphatase, and LDH can be elevated.
- Anti-Jo-1 antibodies are more common in polymyositis.
- Electrolytes, TSH, Ca, and Mg should be requested to exclude other causes.
- Electromyography (EMG) is abnormal in 90% of patients and distinguishes a myopathic from a neuropathic process.
- Muscle biopsy is the definitive test. Characteristic findings separate polymyositis from dermatomyositis, inclusion body myositis, and neuromuscular disorders mimicking polymyositis.

■ IMAGING STUDIES

- A chest x-ray to rule out pulmonary involvement. If suspicious for pulmonary interstitial disease, a high-resolution CT scan of the chest may be helpful
- A barium swallow to look for upper esophageal dysfunction in patients with dysphagia and polymyositis
- MRI can help to locate sites of muscle involvement

TREATMENT

■ NONPHARMACOLOGIC THERAPY

- Physical therapy is beneficial in increasing muscle tone and strength
- Occupational therapy to assist with activities of daily living
- Speech therapy for dysphagia and swallowing problems

■ ACUTE GENERAL RX

- Prednisone 1 to 2 mg/kg/day is the treatment of choice in patients with polymyositis. The dose is continued until muscle enzymes have returned to normal for 4 wk. Thereafter taper by 10 mg/mo until off of prednisone.
- Immunosuppressive agents (azathioprine, cyclophosphamide, or methotrexate) should be used if the patient fails to improve on prednisone or muscle enzymes begin rising when tapering off prednisone. See "Chronic Rx" for specific dosage.

■ CHRONIC RX

- Chronic prednisone therapy may be needed for years.
- Azathioprine (2.5 to 3.5 mg/kg/day) or methotrexate (0.5 mg/kg/wk) can be added as stated previously.

■ DISPOSITION

- As treatment is initiated, one should see the muscle enzymes return to normal before symptoms improve.
- During exacerbations, enzymes will rise first before symptoms appear.
- Approximately 50% of patients will go into remission and stop therapy within 5 yr. The remaining will either have active disease requiring ongoing treatment or inactive disease with permanent muscle atrophy and contractures.
- The 5-year mortality rate is 20%.

■ REFERRAL

For any suspected cases of polymyositis, a rheumatology referral should be made to help establish the diagnosis and implement treatment.

☼ PEARLS & CONSIDERATIONS

■ COMMENTS

- When assessing response to treatment, it is best to follow clinical muscle strength over muscle enzyme tests.
- Concern of malignancies (ovary, lung, breast, GI) associated with myositis is legitimate and merits screening patients over the age of 40, particularly patients with dermatomyositis.

REFERENCES

Hilton-Jones D: Inflammatory muscle diseases, *Curr Opin Neurol* 14(5):591, 2001.

Medsger TA et al: Classification and diagnostic criteria for polymyositis and dermatomyositis. *J Rheumatol* 22:581, 1995.

Oddis CV: Current approach to the treatment of polymyositis and dermatomyositis, *Curr Opin Rheumatol* 12(6):492, 2000.

Author: **Peter Petropoulos, M.D.**

DEFINITION

Clinically significant portal hypertension is defined as a portal vein pressure >10 mm Hg.

ICD-9CM CODES
572.3 Portal hypertension

■ EPIDEMIOLOGY & DEMOGRAPHICS
- Incidence of portal hypertension is not known.
- Cirrhosis is the most common cause of portal hypertension in the U.S.
- More than 90% of patients with cirrhosis develop portal hypertension.
- Alcoholic and viral liver diseases are the most common causes of cirrhosis and portal hypertension in the U.S.
- Schistosomiasis is the main cause of portal hypertension outside of the U.S.
- Esophageal varices may appear when portal vein pressures rise above 10 mm Hg.
- Variceal hemorrhage is the most serious complication of portal hypertension and may occur when portal pressures rise above 12 mm Hg.

■ PHYSICAL FINDINGS & CLINICAL PRESENTATION
- Jaundice
- Ascites
- Spider angiomata
- Testicular atrophy
- Gynecomastia
- Palmar erythema
- Dupuytren's contracture
- Asterixis (with advanced liver failure)
- Irritability
- Splenomegaly
- Dilated veins in the anterior abdominal wall
- Venous pattern on the flanks
- Caput medusae (tortuous collateral veins around the umbilicus)
- Hemorrhoids
- Hematemesis
- Melena
- Pruritus

■ ETIOLOGY
- Pathophysiologically caused by:
  1. Conditions resulting in an increased resistance to flow *or*
  2. Conditions leading to increase portal blood flow
- Conditions causing increased resistance to flow:
  1. Prehepatic (e.g., portal vein thrombosis, splenic vein thrombosis, congenital stenosis)
  2. Hepatic (e.g., cirrhosis, alcoholic liver disease, primary biliary cirrhosis, schistosomiasis)

  3. Posthepatic (e.g., Budd-Chiari syndrome, constrictive pericarditis, inferior vena cava obstruction)
- Conditions causing increased portal blood flow include arterial-portal venous fistula

DIAGNOSIS

- The diagnosis of portal hypertension is made on clinical grounds after a comprehensive history and physical examination.
- Noninvasive and invasive procedures serve to confirm diagnosis and determine the severity of portal hypertension.

■ DIFFERENTIAL DIAGNOSIS
- Cirrhosis
- Portal vein obstruction
- Portal vein thrombosis
- Hepatic vein thrombosis (Budd-Chiari syndrome)
- Schistosomiasis
- Right-sided heart failure
- Tricuspid regurgitation
- Constrictive pericarditis

■ WORKUP
The workup of portal hypertension includes blood tests and noninvasive imaging studies to determine if the cause of portal hypertension is prehepatic, hepatic, or posthepatic in origin.

■ LABORATORY TESTS
- CBC
- Platelet count
- LFTs
- PT/PIT
- Albumin
- Hepatitis B surface antigen and antibody
- Hepatitis C antibody
- Iron, TIBC, and ferritin
- ANA
- Anti-smooth muscle antibodies (ASMA)
- Antimitochondrial antibody (AMA)
- Ceruloplasmin
- α-1 antitrypsin
- Ascitic fluid analysis: a serum-ascites albumin gradient (SAAG) > 1.1 mg/dL suggests portal hypertension

■ IMAGING STUDIES
- Duplex-Doppler ultrasound is effective in screening for portal hypertension.
- Liver spleen scan looking for a colloidal shift from liver to spleen or bone marrow is suggestive of portal hypertension.
- CT scan can be used in the diagnosis of portal hypertension when results from Duplex-Doppler are equivocal.

- MRI provides information when Duplex-Doppler is inconclusive.
- MRA aids in the detection of portal vein obstruction.
- Measuring hepatic venous pressure gradient, although invasive and not commonly done, can be performed to estimate portal venous pressures.
- Upper endoscopy is the most reliable test documenting the presence of esophageal varices.

TREATMENT

- The treatment of portal hypertension primarily focuses on three strategies in the treatment of its major complication, variceal bleeding:
  1. Prevention of first-time variceal bleeding
  2. Treating the acute variceal bleed
  3. Prevention of rebleeding from esophageal varices

■ NONPHARMACOLOGIC THERAPY
Treatment of acute variceal bleeding requires immediate volume resuscitation with fluids and blood products.

■ ACUTE GENERAL THERAPY
- For acute variceal bleeds:
  1. Octreotide acetate 50 to 100 μg IV bolus followed by an infusion at 25 to 50 μg/hr
  2. Terlipressin 2 mg IV q4h is used until bleeding stops for 24 hr and then continued at 1 mg IV q4h for 5 days
- Endoscopic sclerotherapy and elastic band ligation can be used if the aforementioned acute pharmacotherapy fails or in combination with pharmacotherapy.
- Transjugular intrahepatic portosystemic shunt (TIPS) or surgery is used in patients failing medical and endoscopic therapy. Can be complicated by hepatic encephalopathy, as the shunt bypasses the liver and hepatic metabolism of portal blood.

■ CHRONIC RX
- Propranolol in dosages sufficient to reduce the resting heart rate by 25% has been shown to be effective in primary prophylaxis for first-time variceal bleeding and for preventing recurrent variceal bleeding.
  1. Dosages are usually given bid and decreased if heart rate falls <55 beats/min or systolic BP <90 mm Hg.
  2. Nadolol usually given on a once-daily dosing schedule can be used in place of propranolol and adjusted according to heart rate and blood pressure.

- Combination therapy with-long acting nitroglycerine, isosorbide-5-mononitrate (ISMN) 20 mg q HS added to β-blockers has been shown to improve the therapeutic benefit in preventing recurrent variceal bleeding.
- Sclerotherapy using sclerosing agents, 5% ethanolamine, 1% to 2% polidocanol, or ethanol stimulates an inflammatory fibrous reaction and variceal thrombosis and eradicates esophageal varices in 70% of patients.
- Endoscopic banding ligation of varices can be used in preventing recurrent variceal bleeding.
- TIPS is an endoscopic procedure that decompresses the portal vein and is used as a "rescue" therapy in patients who have failed medical management.

■ DISPOSITION
- The most common complication associated with portal hypertension is variceal bleeding.
- The risk of bleeding from varices is approximately 15% at 1 yr.

- Of those who have bled from esophageal varices, approximately 30% will die; among the survivors, the risk of rebleeding is 70%, with a similar third of these patients dying from this complication.

■ REFERRAL
Consultation with a gastroenterologist is recommended in patients with portal hypertension and variceal bleeding.

☼ PEARLS & CONSIDERATIONS

■ COMMENTS
- The portal vein is formed from the convergence of the superior mesenteric vein and the splenic vein and serves as a gate into which the splanchnic circulatory system connects with the liver.
- The normal portal vein carries 1500 ml/min of blood from the stomach, spleen, and small and large intestine to the liver at a pressure of 5 to 10 mm Hg.

- Clinical complications of portal hypertension (e.g., bleeding from esophageal varices, ascites, and hepatic encephalopathy) can occur when portal vein pressures rise above 12 mm Hg.

REFERENCES
De Franchis R: Updating consensus in portal hypertension: report of the Baveno III Consensus Workshop on definitions, methodology and therapeutic strategies in portal hypertension, *J Hepatol* 33:846, 2000.

Garcia-Pagan JC, Bosch J: Medical treatment of portal hypertension, *Bailliere's Clin Gastroenterol* 14(6):895, 2000.

Krige JEJ, Beckingham IJ: ABC of diseases of liver, pancreas, and biliary system: portal hypertension—1: varices, *BMJ* 322:348, 2001.

Wongcharatrawee S, Groszmann RJ: Diagnosing portal hypertension, *Bailliere's Clin Gastroenterol* 14(6):881, 2000.

Authors: **Peter Petropoulos, M.D., and Mel Anderson, M.D.**

BASIC INFORMATION

■ DEFINITION
Portal vein thrombosis is thrombotic occlusion of the portal vein.

■ SYNONYMS
Pylethrombosis

ICD-9CM CODES
452 Portal vein thrombosis
572.1 Septic portal vein thrombosis

■ EPIDEMIOLOGY & DEMOGRAPHICS
Occurs with equal frequency in children (peak age: 6 yr) and adults (peak age: 40 yr)

■ PHYSICAL FINDINGS & CLINICAL PRESENTATION
Upper GI hemorrhage (hematemesis and/or melena) caused by esophageal varices. If abdominal pain is present, mesenteric venous thrombosis should be suspected (see "Mesenteric Venous Thrombosis" in Section I).

■ ETIOLOGY AND PATHOPHYSIOLOGY
In children: umbilical sepsis (pathophysiology unknown)
In adults:
1. Hypercoagulable states
- Antiphospholipid syndrome
- Neoplasm (common cause)
- Paroxysmal nocturnal hemoglobinuria
- Myeloproliferative diseases
- Oral contraceptives
- Polycythemia vera
- Pregnancy
- Protein S or C deficiency
- Sickle cell disease
- Thrombocytosis
2. Inflammatory diseases
- Crohn's disease
- Pancreatitis
- Ulcerative colitis
3. Complications of medical intervention
- Ambulatory dialysis
- Chemoembolization
- Liver transplantation
- Partial hepatectomy
- Sclerotherapy
- Splenectomy
- Transjugular intrahepatic portosystemic shunt

4. Infections
- Appendicitis
- Diverticulitis
- Cholecystitis
5. Miscellaneous
- Cirrhosis (common cause)
- Bladder cancer

Pathophysiology: portal vein thrombosis results in portal hypertension leading to esophageal and gastrointestinal varices. The liver sustained by the hepatic artery maintains normal function.

DIAGNOSIS

■ DIFFERENTIAL DIAGNOSIS
Causes of upper GI hemorrhage are covered in Section II.

■ WORKUP
- Esophagogastroscopy shows esophageal varices.

- Abdominal ultrasound (Fig. 1-221) or MRI may show the portal vein thrombosis.

TREATMENT

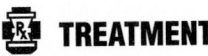

- Variceal sclerotherapy or banding
- Surgical mesocaval or splenorenal shunt

■ REFERRAL
To gastroenterologist, surgeon, or both

REFERENCE
Schafter DF, Sorrell MF: Vascular diseases of the liver. In Feldman M et al (eds): *Gastrointestinal and liver disease*, ed 6, Philadelphia, 1998, WB Saunders.
Author: **Tom J. Wachtel, M.D.**

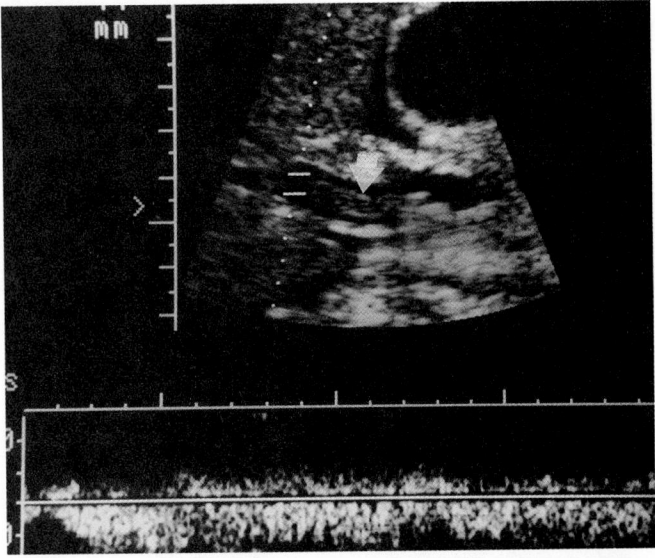

Fig. 1-221 Thrombus in portal vein evident on pulsed Doppler ultrasonography. An echogenic thrombus (*arrow*) is within the lumen of the portal vein. Doppler tracing indicates flow within portal vein. (From Sabiston D: *Textbook of surgery*, ed 15, Philadelphia, 1997, WB Saunders.)

BASIC INFORMATION

■ DEFINITION

- Postconcussive syndrome (PCS) refers to persistent neurologic symptoms that result from mild traumatic brain injury or concussion.
- Concussion may be defined as an acute trauma-induced alteration of mental function lasting fewer than 24 hr, with or without preceding loss of consciousness.
- Concussion is graded by the Colorado Medicine Society (Table 1-44) as:
  1. Grade 1 concussion (mild): No loss of consciousness (LOC), no posttraumatic amnesia but with confusion.
  2. Grade 2 concussion (moderate): No LOC, but posttraumatic amnesia and confusion.
  3. Grade 3 concussion (severe): LOC of any duration along with posttraumatic amnesia and confusion.

ICD-9CM CODES
310.2 Postconcussive syndrome

■ EPIDEMIOLOGY & DEMOGRAPHICS
- PCS incidence is 27/100,000.
- Approximately 15% of patients with mild traumatic brain injury will have persistent neurologic symptoms 1 yr after the injury.
- More often seen in men than in women.
- Usually seen in the young 20 to 30 yr of age.

■ PHYSICAL FINDINGS & CLINICAL PRESENTATION
- PCS patients usually present with neurologic symptoms and no focal neurologic deficits on examination. Symptoms start within a few days after the head injury with 15% of patients having persistent symptoms 1 yr later.
- Symptoms include:
  1. Headache (migraine type)
  2. Neck pain
  3. Dizziness and vertigo
  4. Paresthesias
  5. Difficulty in concentrating and with memory
  6. Insomnia
  7. Irritability

■ ETIOLOGY
- PCS by definition is caused by traumatic brain injury from falls, motor vehicle accidents, contact sports, and so forth.
- Postmortem findings reveal diffuse axonal injury as the primary pathologic finding along with small petechial hemorrhages and local edema.

- Diffuse axon injury is thought to lead to altered neurotransmitters and possibly to clinical manifestations.

DIAGNOSIS

A careful history, a nonfocal neurologic examination, and normal neurologic testing usually will establish the diagnosis of postconcussive syndrome.

■ DIFFERENTIAL DIAGNOSIS
- Headache (vascular or tension)
- Epidural hematoma
- Subdural hematoma
- Skull fracture
- Cervical spine disk disease
- Whiplash
- Seizure
- Cerebrovascular accident
- Depression
- Anxiety

TABLE 1-44   Concussion Guidelines and Recommendations

Acute head injuries are usually divided into two categories:
1. Diffuse brain injuries—concussion and diffuse axonal injuries.
2. Focal brain injuries—all fractures and intracranial injuries.

It is not necessary to have loss of consciousness to have a concussion.* Several severity grading scales for concussion exist; one that is commonly used is the following:

COLORADO MEDICAL SOCIETY GUIDELINES

GRADE	CONFUSION	AMNESIA	LOSS OF CONSCIOUSNESS
I	+	–	–
II	+	+	–
III	+	+	+

Return-to-Play Criteria

Return-to-play criteria are based on prevention of the *second impact syndrome*. This syndrome is characterized by a loss of autoregulation of cerebral blood flow, manifest as a rapid increased intracranial pressure following a second head injury before full recovery from the initial head injury has occurred. Return to contact sports is based on the grade of the injury.

RECOMMENDATIONS FOR RETURN TO CONTACT SPORTS FOLLOWING A CONCUSSION†

GRADE	MINIMUM TIME TO RETURN	TIME ASYMPTOMATIC‡
I	20 min	When examined
II	1 wk	1 wk
III	1 mo	1 wk

RECOMMENDATIONS FOR RETURN TO CONTACT SPORTS FOLLOWING REPEATED CONCUSSIONS

GRADE	MINIMUM TIME TO RETURN	TIME ASYMPTOMATIC‡
I (second time)	2 wk	1 wk
II (second time)	1 mo	1 wk
I (× 3), II (× 2), III (× 2)	Season over	1 wk

From Behrman RE: *Nelson textbook of pediatrics*, ed 16, Philadelphia, 2000, WB Saunders.
*In animal studies, there is evidence that there are microscopic changes in the brain after a concussion. These may not be evident in imaging studies, so the clinician must rely on history and neuropsychologic examination to follow a patient's progress. In college football players who experienced their first concussion, the neuropsychologic testing normalized in 5 days and symptoms of headache and memory resolved in 10 days.
The chronic effects of repetitive boxing injuries include cortical atrophy and a cavum septum pellucidum (identified radiographically). Whether this occurs in other sports in which head injuries are common (football, ice hockey, wrestling) or in which the head is used as part of the game (soccer) is debatable. However, there appears to be no danger in the young soccer player occasionally heading the ball.
†Contact sports means any situation in which contact is possible, including practice.
‡A symptomatic athlete should not return to contact sports regardless of the initial diagnosis. Athletes with focal brain injuries are excluded from contact sports indefinitely. Patients with a neck injury can return to contact sports when they have full, pain-free range of motion, strength and sensation, and normal lordosis of the cervical spine.

■ **WORKUP**

A patient presenting with PCS merits a workup to exclude other causes of neurologic symptoms following traumatic brain injury.

■ **LABORATORY TESTS**

Blood tests are not very specific in diagnosing PCS.

■ **IMAGING STUDIES**

- CT scan of the head is normal.
- MRI of the head is often normal but may show petechial hemorrhages or cerebral contusions.
- EEG is normal.
- Evoked potentials are normal.
- Neuropsychologic testing may reveal difficulties in concentration, memory, and executive function but is not very specific for PCS.

 TREATMENT

Postconcussive syndrome must be recognized as a physiologic and psychologic problem and treated accordingly.

■ **NONPHARMACOLOGIC THERAPY**

- Heat
- Physical therapy
- Avoidance of alcohol, narcotics, and sleep deprivation

■ **ACUTE GENERAL RX**

- Headaches can be treated with NSAIDs, ibuprofen 800 mg tid or naproxen 500 mg bid.
- Neck pain can be treated in a similar fashion.

■ **CHRONIC RX**

- Psychotherapy
- Behavioral therapy
- Vocational rehabilitation
- Depression can be treated with SSRIs but may not respond as well when compared with non-PCS patients with depression

■ **DISPOSITION**

- Most patients after mild traumatic brain injury improve without any residual deficits.
- Neuropsychologic testing may be abnormal but usually improves during the first 6 mo after injury.
- If related to contact sports, see Table 1-44.
- Predictors for the development of persistent postconcussive syndrome (>1 yr) include:
  1. Female
  2. Ongoing litigation
  3. Low socioeconomic status
  4. Prior headaches
  5. Prior mild traumatic brain injury
  6. Prior psychiatry illnesses

■ **REFERRAL**

Postconcussive syndrome patients may benefit from consultations with psychologists, psychiatrists, and neurologists.

⚙ **PEARLS & CONSIDERATIONS**

■ **COMMENTS**

- PCS syndrome starts within a few days after the injury. Recognizing depression and treating pain symptoms early in the course may help prevent the development of persistent postconcussive syndrome (>1 yr).
- The severity of the fall, duration of unconsciousness, and amnesia helps assess the severity of axonal injury.
- Attempts to determine how much of a role psychologic and neurologic factors play in the PCS are important but very difficult.

REFERENCES

Alexander MP: Mild traumatic brain injury: pathophysiology, natural history, and clinical management, *Neurology* 45:1253, 1995.

Evans RW: The postconcussive syndrome: 130 years of controversy, *Semin Neurol* 14:32, 1994.

Koshner DS: Concussion in sports: minimizing the risk for complications, *Am Fam Physician* 64:1007, 2001.

Marguiles S: The postconcussion syndrome after mild head trauma: Is brain damage overdiagnosed? Part 1, *J Clin Neuroses* 7(5):400, 2000.

Mittenberg S, Strauman S: Diagnosis of mild head injury and the postconcussion syndrome, *J Head Trauma Rehabil* 15(2):783, 2000.

Author: **Peter Petropoulos, M.D.**

BASIC INFORMATION

■ DEFINITION

Posttraumatic stress disorder (PTSD) is an anxiety disorder that arises when an individual has witnessed or experienced a potentially fatal or serious injurious condition during which he or she felt helpless or horrified. After resolution of the event the individual continues to experience the event in the form of flashbacks (reliving the trauma), intrusive recollections, dreams, or physiologic reactivity or psychologic distress in response to cues symbolizing the event. These responses are associated with persistent hyperarousal (e.g., hypervigilance, exaggerated startle, sleep disturbance, irritability, and difficulty concentrating) and avoidance (both physically and cognitively) of stimuli associated with the traumatic event.

■ SYNONYMS

Soldier's heart
Effort syndrome
Shell shock
Irritable heart
Traumatic necrosis
Survivor syndrome
Concentration camp syndrome
Gross stress reaction (DSM-I, published in 1952)

ICD-9CM CODES

308.3 Posttraumatic stress syndrome, acute
309.81 Posttraumatic stress syndrome, chronic

■ EPIDEMIOLOGY & DEMOGRAPHICS

INCIDENCE (IN U.S.): Occurs in some 50% of people experiencing a severe life-threatening event (e.g., PTSD was diagnosed in 85% of Nazi concentration camp survivors, 57% of Coconut Grove fire survivors, 67% of WWII prisoners of war, and 50% of Cambodian children subjected to various atrocities). Motor vehicle accidents are associated with PTSD 7.5% of the time.
PREVALENCE (IN U.S.):
- Lifetime prevalence estimates range from 1% to 15% of the American population.
- Prevalence estimates among high-risk populations (e.g., combat veterans or victims of violent crimes) range from 3% to 58%.

PREDOMINANT SEX: 5% to 6% of men and 10% to 14% of women; more than 50% of women's cases are related to sexual assault.
PREDOMINANT AGE:
- Development in children is possible, but presentation may be slightly different.
- No predisposing age factors have been identified.

PEAK INCIDENCE: Symptoms may begin immediately after the trauma and peak within 4 to 5 mo of the event.
GENETICS: No specific factors have been identified.

■ PHYSICAL FINDINGS & CLINICAL PRESENTATION

- After severe life-threatening event, complaints of derealization, depersonalization, detachment, dissociation, or being dazed, in association with a marked increase in anxiety and arousal
- Within 3 mo, signs of persistent hyperarousal, anxiety, and distressing memories or reexperiences of the traumatic event in most patients; symptoms may be disabling

■ ETIOLOGY

- There is a "dose-response" relationship between intensity and duration of the stress and severity of PTSD, with duration of the stress the most important factor.
- Human-made disasters cause more intense reactions than natural disasters.
- Premorbid factors (dysthymia, introversion, personality types, alcohol abuse, and family psychiatric history) may predispose to PTSD.
- Symptoms are mediated, in part, by the autonomic nervous system and the hypothalamic-pituitary-adrenal system.

⚗ DIAGNOSIS

■ DIFFERENTIAL DIAGNOSIS

- Diagnosis is made when a dysfunctional response occurs to any stress, so although most people with PTSD technically suffer from an adjustment disorder, the stress to which they are responding is usually extreme.
- Acute stress disorder is similar to PTSD but occurs within the first 4 wk of the stress.
- If symptoms of acute stress disorder persist longer than 4 wk, PTSD is possible.
- Malingering is sometimes difficult to rule out when there is secondary gain.

■ WORKUP

- History to determine symptoms
- Physical examination to look for signs of autonomic hyperactivity
- NOTE: Only the history is required for diagnosis

℞ TREATMENT

■ NONPHARMACOLOGIC THERAPY

- Various forms of individual psychotherapy are effective in reducing severity of symptoms.

- Group therapy is the mainstay treatment for many PTSD victims, particularly among combat veterans.
- Psychotherapy in the acute setting may reduce development of PTSD.

■ ACUTE GENERAL Rx

- Purely symptomatic and generally aimed at alleviating distress
- Benzodiazepines for reducing the symptoms of anxiety
- β-Blockers to alleviate some of the autonomic symptoms
- Sedating antidepressants (e.g., amitriptyline) to treat initial insomnia and suppress nightmares; in low doses may also alleviate daytime anxiety

■ CHRONIC Rx

- Antidepressants (both tricyclics and serotonin reuptake inhibitors) and nonbenzodiazepine anxiolytic buspirone are mainstay of chronic pharmacologic management.
- Although these agents provide relief, patients frequently have persisting residual and often troubling symptoms.
- Alternative approaches:
  1. Monoamine oxidase inhibiting antidepressants
  2. Chronic use of β-blockers or α_2-agonists (e.g., clonidine)
  3. Anticonvulsants such as carbamazepine

■ DISPOSITION

- Spontaneous remission in 6 mo for nearly half of patients
- Possible chronic symptoms for years
- Predictors of chronic course:
  1. Premorbid psychiatric function
  2. Acute response to stress (e.g., individuals who experience an acute stress disorder immediately after the trauma do better in the long term)

■ REFERRAL

Because early intervention improves outcome, referral to psychotherapy as soon as diagnosis made

REFERENCES

Davidson J: Recognition and treatment of posttraumatic stress disorder, *JAMA* 286:584, 2001.
Davidson J et al: Efficacy of sertraline in preventing relapse of posttraumatic stress disorder, *Am J Psych* 158:1974, 2001.
Grinage BD: Diagnosis and management of post-traumatic stress disorder, *Am Fam Physician* 68:2401, 2003.
Yehuda R: Post-traumatic stress disorder, *N Engl J Med* 346:108, 2002.
Author: **Rif S. El-Mallakh, M.D.**

BASIC INFORMATION

■ DEFINITION
Precocious puberty is defined as sexual development occurring before 8 yr of age in males and 9 yr of age in females.

■ SYNONYMS
Pubertas praecox

ICD-9CM CODES
259.1 Precocious puberty

■ EPIDEMIOLOGY & DEMOGRAPHICS
INCIDENCE: Estimated to be between 1:5000 and 1:10,000
PREDOMINANT SEX: Females > males for the idiopathic variant; for other causes, dependent on the underlying etiology.
GENETICS: The genetics for some of the etiologies of precocious puberty are known.

■ PHYSICAL FINDINGS & CLINICAL PRESENTATION
- In females: breast development, pubic hair development, accelerated growth, and menarche
- In males: increase in testicular volume and penile length, pubic hair development, accelerated growth, muscular development, acne, change in voice, and penile erections

■ ETIOLOGY
- Idiopathic or true: diagnosis of exclusion
- CNS pathology: tumors, hydrocephalus, ventricular cysts, benign lesions
- Severe hypothyroidism
- Posttraumatic head injury
- Genetic disorders: neurofibromatosis, tuberous sclerosis, McCune-Albright syndrome, congenital adrenal hyperplasia
- Gonadal tumors
- Nongonadal tumors: hepatoblastoma
- Exposure to exogenous sex steroids

DIAGNOSIS

■ DIFFERENTIAL DIAGNOSIS
- Most common diagnoses to consider: premature thelarche and premature adrenarche

- Gonadotropin hormone–releasing hormone (GnRH)–dependent precocious puberty: idiopathic, CNS tumors, hypothalamic hamartomas, neurofibromatosis, tuberous sclerosis, hydrocephalus, post acute head injury, ventricular cysts, post CNS infection
- GnRH-independent precocious puberty: congenital adrenal hyperplasia, adrenocortical tumors (males), McCune-Albright syndrome (females), gonadal tumors, ectopic hCG-secreting tumors (chorioblastoma, hepatoblastoma), exposure to exogenous sex steroids, severe hypothyroidism

■ WORKUP
Thorough history and physical examination are essential to determine if the patient has true precocious puberty. Particular attention should be paid to growth, development, order of appearance of the secondary sexual characteristics, pubertal development in family members, medications, neurologic symptoms, Tanner staging, abdominal and neurologic examination. Section III, Fig. 3-152 describes a clinical approach to precocious puberty.

■ LABORATORY TESTS
- GnRH testing will help determine if dependent or independent cause
- Sex hormone studies: LH, FSH, hCG, testosterone (males), estrogen (females)
- T_4, TSH

■ IMAGING STUDIES
- CT scan or MRI of the brain to evaluate for CNS pathology
- Consideration of pelvic ultrasound in female patients to evaluate for cysts/tumors
- Abdominal imaging with CT scan if intraabdominal pathology suspected

TREATMENT

■ NONPHARMACOLOGIC THERAPY
- Good communication with the parents is essential to care.
- Psychologic support for the child may be needed with regard to self-image and problems with peer acceptance.

■ ACUTE GENERAL Rx
There is no acute therapy for precocious puberty.

■ CHRONIC Rx
Therapy depends on the etiology of precocious puberty:
- For true precocious puberty and some CNS lesions, the treatment of choice is leuprolide 0.25 to 0.3 mg/kg with a 7.5 mg minimum IM every 4 wk.
- For other CNS lesions and extragonadal tumors, therapy is dependent on the type of lesion, location of the lesion, and the overall prognosis of the underlying problem.
- For severe hypothyroidism, treatment with thyroid hormone will result in regression of the sexual development. The child will subsequently undergo appropriate pubertal development later in life.
- For familial male gonadotropin-independent precocious puberty, ketoconazole can be used at doses of 600 mg/day divided tid, or a combination of testolactone and spironolactone can be used.

■ DISPOSITION
- For true precocious puberty and some CNS lesions, long-term outcome is usually very good. When drug therapy is instituted, it is continued until a time when further pubertal development is appropriate. It is then discontinued, allowing the child to progress through puberty.
- For other cases, long-term outcomes are dependent on the prognosis of the underlying cause.

■ REFERRAL
- Initial workup can be instituted by the primary care provider.
- Referral to an endocrinologist is indicated for most children because they will need long-term management, monitoring, and treatment.

REFERENCE
Root AW: Precocious puberty, *Pediatr Rev* 21(1):10, 2000.
Author: **Beth J. Wutz, M.D.**

BASIC INFORMATION

DEFINITION

Preeclampsia involves a triad of hypertension, proteinuria, and edema that develops after the twentieth week of gestation. Mild preeclampsia is defined as a blood pressure of <140/90 mm Hg. Severe preeclampsia is associated with a blood pressure >160/110 mm Hg, proteinuria >5 g in a 24-hr urine collection, oliguria (<400 ml/24 hr), cerebral or visual disturbances, epigastric pain, pulmonary edema, thrombocytopenia, hepatic dysfunction, or severe intrauterine growth retardation.

SYNONYMS

Pregnancy-induced hypertension
Toxemia of pregnancy

ICD-9CM CODES
642.6 Preeclampsia

EPIDEMIOLOGY & DEMOGRAPHICS
INCIDENCE: 10% to 14% in primigravidas, 5.7% to 7.3% in multigravidas
RISK FACTORS: Increased incidence and severity with multiple gestations, renal or collagen-vascular diseases. Extremes of reproductive age, <20 or >35 yr of age, obesity, African Americans, thrombophilia, previous preeclampsia.
GENETICS: Positive correlation with maternal and paternal family history.

PHYSICAL FINDINGS & CLINICAL PRESENTATION
- Generalized swelling or nondependent edema, possibly manifested by rapid weight gain (>4 lb/wk) even in the absence of edema
- Auscultation of pulmonary rales
- RUQ pain (HELLP syndrome or subcapsular liver hematoma)
- Hyperreflexia or clonus
- Vaginal bleeding (placental abruption)
- Acute or chronic fetal compromise manifested by intrauterine growth restriction or fetal tachycardia with late decelerations, respectively
- Wide range of symptoms attributable to multiorgan system dysfunction, involving hepatic, hematologic, renal, pulmonary, and CNS
- Possibility of severe disease despite "normal" blood pressure readings, so a high index of suspicion must be maintained in high-risk situations

ETIOLOGY
- Exact etiology or toxic substance is unknown

- Theories
  1. Imbalance between thromboxane A_2 (vasoconstrictor and platelet aggregator) and prostacyclin (vasodilator)
  2. Abnormal trophoblastic invasion of spiral arteries
  3. Increased sensitivity to angiotensin II by the muscular walls of the arteries
  4. Excess circulating soluble fms-like tyrosine kinase 1 (SFlT-1), which binds placental growth factor (PlGF) and vascular endothelial growth factor (VEGF), may have a pathogenic role

DIAGNOSIS

DIFFERENTIAL DIAGNOSIS
- Acute fatty liver of pregnancy
- Appendicitis
- Diabetic ketoacidosis
- Gallbladder disease
- Gastroenteritis
- Glomerulonephritis
- Hemolytic-uremic syndrome
- Hepatic encephalopathy
- Hyperemesis gravidarum
- Idiopathic thrombocytopenia
- Thrombotic thrombocytopenic purpura
- Nephrolithiasis
- Pyelonephritis
- PUD
- SLE
- Viral hepatitis

WORKUP
- Two blood pressure measurements in lateral recumbent position 6 hr apart, with an absolute pressure >140/90 mm Hg or an increase of 30 mm Hg systolic or 15 mm Hg diastolic from baseline, an increase in the mean arterial pressure (MAP) of 20 mm Hg, or an absolute MAP >105 mm Hg
- Evaluation for proteinuria as defined by >0.1 g/L on urine dipstick or >300 mg protein on a 24-hr urine collection
- Evaluation of fetal status for evidence of intrauterine growth restriction, oligohydramnios, alteration in umbilical or uterine artery Doppler flow, or acute compromise, such as abruption
- Because of the insidious nature of the disease with potential for multiple organ involvement, complete evaluation for preeclampsia in any pregnant patient presenting with CNS derangement or GI complaints after 20 wk of gestation

- Evaluation for associated conditions such as disseminated intravascular coagulation, hepatic dysfunction, or subcapsular hematoma

LABORATORY TESTS
- High-risk patients: baseline assessment of renal function (24-hr urine collection for protein and creatinine clearance), platelets, BUN, creatinine, LFTs, and uric acid should be obtained at the first prenatal visit.
- CBC (Hgb, Hct, platelets) may show signs of volume contraction or HELLP syndrome.
- LFTs (AST, ALT, LDH) are useful in evaluation for HELLP syndrome or to exclude important differentials.
- Hyperuricemia or increased creatinine may indicate decreasing renal function.
- PT, PTT, and fibrinogen should be checked to rule out disseminated intravascular coagulation.
- Peripheral smear may demonstrate microangiopathic hemolytic anemia.
- Complement levels can be used to differentiate from an acute exacerbation of a collagen-vascular disease.
- Increased levels of SFlT-1 and reduced levels of PlGF predict subsequent development of preeclampsia.

IMAGING STUDIES
- CT scan of head if atypical presentation of eclampsia, possibility of intracerebral bleed, or prolonged post-ictal state
- Sonogram of fetus to evaluate for IUGR, amniotic fluid, placenta
- Sonogram of maternal liver if suspect subcapsular hematoma

TREATMENT

NONPHARMACOLOGIC THERAPY
Bed rest in left lateral decubitus position

ACUTE GENERAL RX
Delivery is the treatment of choice and the only cure for the disease. This must be taken in the context of the gestational age of the fetus, severity of the preeclampsia, and the likelihood of a successful induction and reliability of patient.
- Administer magnesium sulfate 6 g IV loading dose, with 2 to 3 g maintenance or phenytoin at 10 to 15 mg/kg loading dose, then 200 mg IV q8h starting 12 hr after loading dose.

- Hydralazine 10 mg IV, labetalol hydrochloride 20 to 40 mg IV, nifedipine 20 mg SL can be used for acute blood pressure control.
- Continuous fetal monitoring is needed.
- Epidural is anesthesia of choice for pain management in labor or C-section.
- All patients undergoing induction of labor should receive antiseizure medications regardless of severity of disease.

■ CHRONIC RX

- Mild preeclampsia <37 wk: close observation for worsening maternal or fetal condition, with delivery at ≥37 wk with favorable cervix or at 40 wk regardless of cervical status.
- Severe preeclampsia: delivery in the presence of maternal or fetal compromise, labor, or >34 wk; at 28 to 34 wk consider steroids with close monitoring, and at <24 wk consider termination of pregnancy.
- Methyldopa is drug of choice for chronic blood pressure control during pregnancy.

■ DISPOSITION

Preeclampsia is a progressive and unpredictable disease process; a course of expectancy should be managed with caution. Up to 20% of patients who have seizures are normotensive.

■ REFERRAL

Obstetric management is indicated because of the insidious nature of the disease, with transfer of all cases <34 wk to a facility with a level three nursery.

✺ PEARLS & CONSIDERATIONS

■ COMMENTS

- Low-dose aspirin 81 mg qd and calcium supplementation 1500 mg qd can be considered in high-risk patients to decrease the risk of recurrence.
- Begin after first trimester.

REFERENCES

Creasy RT, Resnik R: *Maternal-fetal medicine,* ed 4, Philadelphia, 1999, WB Saunders.

Duley L et al: Antiplatelet drugs for prevention of pre-eclampsia and its consequences: systematic review, *BMJ* 322:329, 2001.

Esplin MS et al: Paternal and maternal components of the predisposition to preeclampsia, *N Engl J Med* 344:867, 2001.

Lain KY, Roberts JM: Contemporary concepts of the pathogenesis and management of preeclampsia, *JAMA* 287:3183, 2002.

Levine RJ et al: Circulating angiogonic factors and risk of preeclampsia, *N Enl J Med* 350:672, 2004.

Skjaerven R et al: The interval between pregnancies and the risk of preeclampsia, *N Engl J Med* 346:33, 2002.

Author: **Scott J. Zuccala, D.O.**

BASIC INFORMATION

■ DEFINITION

The *Diagnostic and Statistical Manual of Mental Disorders,* 4th ed classifies the premenstrual dysphoric disorder (PMDD) as a "depressive disorder not otherwise specified" and requires as criteria for definition the presence of ≥5 of the following symptoms in most menstrual cycles for the past year.

A. The symptoms should be present most of the time during the last week of the luteal phase, with remission beginning within a few days after the onset of the follicular phase, and absent during the week after menses, with at least one of the symptoms being either (1), (2), (3), or (4):

1. Marked depressed mood, feeling of hopelessness, or self-deprecating thoughts
2. Marked anxiety, tension, feeling of being "keyed up" or "on edge"
3. Marked affective lability (e.g., feeling suddenly sad or tearful or increased sensitivity to rejection)
4. Persistent and marked anger or irritability or increased interpersonal conflicts
5. Decreased interest in usual activities (e.g., work, school, friends, hobbies)
6. Subjective sense of difficulty in concentrating
7. Lethargy, easy fatigability, or marked lack of energy
8. Marked change in appetite, overeating, or specific food cravings
9. Hypersomnia or insomnia
10. A subjective sense of being overwhelmed or out of control
11. Other physical symptoms, such as breast tenderness or swelling, headaches, joint or muscle pain, a sensation of "bloating," or weight gain

B. The disturbance markedly interferes with work or school or with usual social activities and relationships with others (e.g., avoidance of social activities, decreased production and efficiency at work or school).

C. The disturbance is not merely an exacerbation of the symptoms of another disorder, such as major depressive disorder, panic disorder, dysthymic disorder, or a personality disorder (although it may be superimposed on any of these disorders).

D. Criteria A, B, and C must be confirmed by prospective daily ratings during at least two consecutive symptomatic cycles (diagnosis may be made provisionally before such confirmation).

NOTE: In menstruating women the luteal phase corresponds to the period between ovulation and the onset of menses, and the follicular phase begins with menses. In non-menstruating women (e.g., women who have had a hysterectomy), determination of the timing of the luteal and follicular phases may require measurement of circulating reproductive hormones.

ICD-CM CODES

625.4 Premenstrual dysphoric syndrome

■ EPIDEMIOLOGY & DEMOGRAPHICS

- PMDD affects 3% to 10% of women of reproductive age.
- Genetic factors play a significant role (increased incidence in monozygotic twins and in women whose mothers had PMDD).
- 30%-76% of women with PMDD have a lifetime history of depression.

■ PHYSICAL FINDINGS AND CLINICAL PRESENTATION

- Physical examination may be completely normal
- Depressed mood, tachycardia, sweating from comorbid disorders (e.g., panic disorder, major depression) may be present

■ ETIOLOGY

Unknown. Serotonin deficiency and altered sensitivity in serotoninergic system in response to phasic hormone fluctuations in the menstrual cycle are believed to play a role.

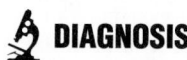 DIAGNOSIS

■ DIFFERENTIAL DIAGNOSIS

- Premenstrual syndrome
- Dysthymic syndrome
- Personality disorder
- Panic disorder
- Major depressive disorder
- Hyperthyroidism
- Polycystic ovarian syndrome

■ WORKUP

- Diagnosis is based on obtaining a detailed history and ruling out the presence of physical or psychiatric disorders.
- The diagnosis should be confirmed using a symptom checklist prospectively for two consecutive menstrual cycles. Commonly used diagnostic instruments include the Calendar of Premenstrual experiences (see reference Mortola et al.) and the Premenstrual Syndrome Diary (see reference Endicott).

TREATMENT

■ NONPHARMACOLOGIC THERAPY

- Reduction in intake of caffeine, refined sugars, or sodium may be helpful in some patients.
- Increased aerobic exercise, smoking cessation, alcohol restriction, and regular sleep are often beneficial.
- Stress reduction and management will decrease severity of symptoms.

■ GENERAL THERAPY

- Selective serotonin reuptake inhibitors (SSRIs) are first-line agents for the treatment of PMDD. Commonly used agents and initial doses are fluoxetine 10 mg qd, sertraline 50 mg qd, paroxetine 10 mg qd, and citalopram 20 mg qd. Many patients will require titration to significantly higher doses to achieve therapeutic benefit. These medications can be administered continuously during the menstrual cycle or only when the patients experience symptoms. Luteal-phase or intermittent administration involves initiating medication at the time of ovulation and stopping it at the beginning of menses.
- Second-line agents are benzodiazepines (alprazolam 0.25 mg tid prn) and the tricyclic antidepressant (clomipramine 25 mg qd as starting dose).
- Hormonal intervention with monthly IM injections of leuprolide have been reported effective in some patients; however, it should be reserved only for patients unresponsive to first- and second-line agents.
- Nutritional supplementation (Vitamin B_6 up to 100 mg/day, Vitamin E, up to 600 IU/day, calcium carbonate 1200 mg/day, and magnesium up to 500 mg/day) is also commonly used and effective in symptom reduction in some patients.

PEARLS & CONSIDERATIONS

■ COMMENTS

- Patients should complete a course of medication for at least a couple of menstrual cycles before switching to other therapeutic options.

REFERENCES

American Psychiatric Association: *Diagnostic and statistical manual of mental disorders,* ed 4, Washington, DC, American Psychiatric Association, 1994.

Bhatia SC, Bhatia SK: Diagnosis and treatment of premenstrual dysphoric disorder, *Am Fam Physician* 66:1239, 2002.

Endicott J: Severe premenstrual dysphoria: differential diagnosis and treatment, *J Am Med Women's Assoc* 53(4):170, 1998.

Grady-Weliky TA: Premenstrual dysphoric disorder, *N Engl J Med* 348:433, 2003.

Mortola JF et al: Diagnosis of premenstrual syndrome by a simple, prospective, and reliable instrument: the Calendar of Premenstrual Experiences, *Obstet Gynecol* 76:302, 1990.

Author: **Fred F. Ferri, M.D.**

BASIC INFORMATION

■ DEFINITION
Premenstrual syndrome (PMS) is a cyclic recurrence during the luteal phase of the menstrual cycle of somatic, affective, and behavioral disturbances that are of sufficient severity to affect interpersonal relationships adversely or interfere with normal activities (Fig. 1-222).

■ SYNONYMS
PMS
PMDD

ICD-9CM CODES
625.4 Premenstrual tension syndromes

■ EPIDEMIOLOGY & DEMOGRAPHICS
- PMS is thought to be extremely prevalent, intermittently affecting approximately one third of all premenopausal women.
- Severe cases occur in approximately 2% to 10% of women with PMS.
- Those seeking treatment for PMS are usually in their 30s or 40s.
- The natural history of PMS has not been clearly elucidated.

■ PHYSICAL FINDINGS & CLINICAL PRESENTATION
- Diverse and potentially disabling symptoms
- Associated with >150 psychologic, physical, and behavioral symptoms
- Most frequent reason for seeking treatment: emotional symptoms

- Most common emotional symptoms: depression, irritability, anxiety, labile moods, anger, crying easily, sadness, overly sensitive, nervous tension
- Most common physical complaints: headache, bloating, cramps, breast tenderness, migraines, fatigue, weight gain, aches and pains, palpitations
- Most common behavior symptom: food cravings
- Other behavioral symptoms: increased appetite, increased alcohol intake, decreased motivation, decreased efficiency, avoidance of activities, staying home, sleep changes, libido changes, forgetfulness, decreased concentration

■ ETIOLOGY
- Etiology remains obscure.
- Because of multifactorial-multiorgan nature of PMS, a single etiologic cause is unlikely.

DIAGNOSIS

■ DIFFERENTIAL DIAGNOSIS
- A diagnosis of exclusion, so other medical or psychologic disorders should be ruled out
- Most common disorders: depression or anxiety, thyroid disease
- Section II describes the differential diagnosis of menstrual pain

■ WORKUP
- History
- Physical examination
- Laboratory studies to rule out alternative diagnosis
- If no alternative diagnosis confirms diagnosis of PMS, basal body temperature charting is used to determine if the patient is ovulating:
  1. If she is not ovulating, it is not PMS.
  2. If she is ovulating, symptoms should be charted for at least two cycles to determine if the symptoms occur in the luteal phase.
  3. If symptoms are not occurring in the luteal phase, it is not PMS, and further investigation is needed.
     a. If symptoms occur in the follicular phase, patient has premenstrual exacerbation of another condition.
     b. If symptoms do not occur in the follicular phase, diagnosis of PMS is confirmed.

■ LABORATORY TESTS
- None available to specifically confirm the diagnosis of PMS
- Thyroid function tests to rule out thyroid disease

TREATMENT

■ NONPHARMACOLOGIC THERAPY
- Individualization of the treatment plan to maximize therapeutic response
- Psychosocial intervention:
  1. Education
  2. Stress management
  3. Environmental changes
  4. Adequate rest and sleep
  5. Regular exercise
- Nutritional recommendations:
  1. Regularly eaten, well-balanced meals
  2. Adequate amounts of protein, fiber, and complex carbohydrates; low fat
  3. Avoidance of foods that are high in salt and simple sugars; may promote water retention, weight gain, and physical discomfort
  4. Avoidance of caffeine-containing beverages; stimulant effects of caffeine may worsen tension, irritability, and insomnia
  5. Avoidance of alcohol and illicit drugs; may worsen emotional lability
  6. Calcium supplementation (1000 mg/day for women 19 to 50 yr, 1300 mg/day for girls 14 to 18 yr) to reduce the physical and emotional symptoms

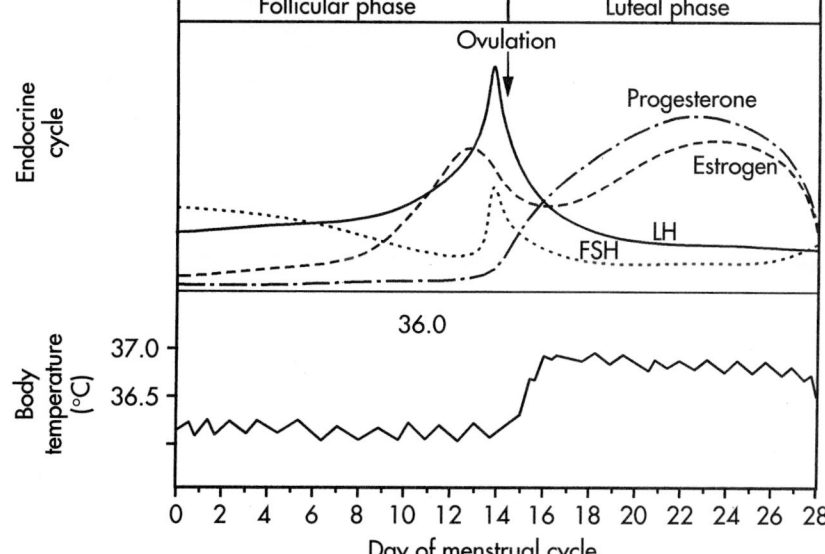
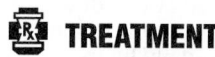

Fig. 1-222   The female hormonal cycle. (From Noble J [ed]: *Textbook of primary care medicine,* ed 2, St Louis, 1996, Mosby.)

7. Magnesium (360 mg/day) to reduce water retention and the negative effect associated with PMS.
8. Pyridoxine (vitamin B₆) 50 mg bid to improve depression, fatigue, irritability and natural diuretic ability; neurotoxicity observed at higher dosages

■ ACUTE GENERAL Rx
SUPPRESSION OF OVULATION:
- Oral contraceptives—one pill per day
- Progestin-only oral contraceptive—one pill per day
- Oral micronized progesterone—100 mg qam and 200 mg qpm on days 17 through 28 of menstrual cycle
- Progestin suppository—200 to 400 mg bid on days 17 through 28 of menstrual cycle
- Oral contraceptive containing arosperenone/ethinyl estradiol—very effective in decreasing physical symptoms
- Medroxyprogesterone (depot)—150 mg IM every 3 mo
- Levonorgestrel implants—surgical insertion every 5 yr
- Transdermal estradiol—one or two 100-μg patches every 3 days
- Danazol—100 to 200 mg/day (ovulation not suppressed at this dose)
- Gonadotropin-releasing hormone (GnRH) agonists—daily by intranasal spray or monthly by depot injection

SUPPRESSION OF PHYSICAL SYMPTOMS:
- Spironolactone—25 to 50 mg bid on days 14 through 28 of menstrual cycle
- Mefenamic acid
  1. For fluid retention: 250 mg tid on days 24 through 28 of cycle
  2. For pain: 500 mg tid on days 19 through 28 of cycle
- Bromocriptine—5 mg/day on days 10 through 26 of cycle
- Danazol—200 mg/day on days 19 through 28 of cycle

- Naproxen (Anaprox)—550 mg bid on days 17 through 28 of cycle; Naprosyn—500 mg bid on days 17 through 28 of cycle.

SUPPRESSION OF PSYCHOLOGIC SYMPTOMS:
- Nortriptyline—50 to 125 mg/day
- Fluoxetine (Prozac)—20 mg/day or 90 mg weekly (this medication has indications for premenstrual dysphoric disorder)
- Buspirone—10 mg bid or tid on days 16 through 28 of cycle, then taper drug
- Alprazolam—25 mg tid on days 16 through 28 of cycle, then taper drug
- Clonidine—0.1 mg bid
- Naltrexone—0.25 mg/day on days 9 through 18 of cycle
- Atenolol—50 mg/day
- Paroxetine (Paxil)—20 mg/day
- Sertraline (Zoloft)—50 to 100 mg/day
- Nefazodone (Serzone)—Initial dosage 100 mg bid; after 1 wk increase to 150 mg bid
- Propranolol—20 to 40 mg bid
- Verapamil—100 to 320 mg qd

■ CHRONIC Rx
- Therapy is largely trial and error, with the goal of providing effective treatment with the safest and most simple therapy.
- For severe intractable PMS: hysterectomy with bilateral oophorectomy; give trial of GnRH therapy or danazol before surgery.
- Estrogen replacement therapy recommended postoperatively to reduce the risk of osteoporosis, heart disease, and genitourinary atrophy.

■ DISPOSITION
Improved symptoms in 90% of women over time.

■ REFERRAL
- For counseling with a psychologist or psychiatrist if underlying psychiatric disorder is discovered (cognitive behavioral therapy)
- To a gynecologist if surgical therapy is contemplated

☼ PEARLS & CONSIDERATIONS

■ COMMENTS
Patient educational material is available through bookstores and pharmaceutical companies.

REFERENCES
Brown C: A new monophasic oral contraceptive containing drospirenone: effect on premenstrual symptoms, *J Reprod Med* 47(1):14, 2002.

Dimmock PW et al: Efficacy of selective serotonin-reuptake inhibitors in premenstrual syndrome: a systematic review, *Lancet* 356:1131, 2000.

Miner C, Brown E: Weekly luteal-phase dosing with enteric-coated fluoxetine 90 mg in premenstrual dysphoric disorder: a randomized, double blind, placebo-controlled clinical trial, *Clin Therapeut* 24(3):417, 2002.

Pearlstein T: Selective serotonin reuptake inhibitors for premenstrual dysphoric disorder: the emerging gold standard? *Drugs* 62(13):1869, 2002.

Thys-Jacobs S et al: Calcium carbonate and the premenstrual syndrome: effects on premenstrual and menstrual symptoms, *Am J Obstet Gynecol* 179:444, 1998.

Wyatt K: Premenstrual syndrome, *Clin Evid* 7:338, 2002.

Wyatt KM et al: Efficacy of vitamin B-6 in the treatment of premenstrual syndrome: systematic review, *BMJ* 318:1375, 1999.

Author: **George T. Danakas, M.D.**

BASIC INFORMATION

■ DEFINITION
Priapism is the persistent, usually painful, erection associated or unassociated with sexual stimulation.

ICD-9CM CODES
607.3 Priapism

■ EPIDEMIOLOGY & DEMOGRAPHICS
- Incidence and prevalence unavailable because of relative rarity
- Can affect male of any age, including children

■ PHYSICAL FINDINGS & CLINICAL PRESENTATION
- In idiopathic priapism the initial erection is associated with prolonged sexual excitement. Previous transient episodes are frequently reported. The erection involves the corpora cavernosa alone. Detumescence does not occur spontaneously.
- In secondary priapism, sexual excitement need not be involved. Otherwise the clinical picture is the same as in idiopathic priapism.
- Table 1-45 compares normal erection and priapism.

■ ETIOLOGY
Idiopathic: prolonged sexual arousal
Secondary or associated causes:
- Sickle cell disease
- Diabetes
- Leukemia
- Solid tumor penile infiltration

Iatrogenic
- TPN, which includes a fat emulsion
- Anticoagulant therapy
- Phenothiazines
- Trazodone
- Intracorporeal injection therapy for impotence
- Sildenafil (Viagra)

■ PATHOPHYSIOLOGY
- Low-flow priapism: prolonged erection leads to edema of the cavernosal trabeculae, resulting in a sequence of statis, thrombosis, venous occlusion, fibrosis, scarring, and possibly impotence
- High-flow priapism: cavernosal artery rupture leading to an arterio-cavernous fistula

DIAGNOSIS

■ WORKUP
None if the associated underlying causes are known to be present. Otherwise they should be ruled out.

TREATMENT

Goal: achieve detumescence with preservation of potency
1. Medical therapies:
- Ice packs
- Ice water enemas
- Hot water enemas
- Pressure dressing
- Sedatives
- Analgesics
- Antispasmodic/anticholinergic drugs

- Estrogens
- Anticoagulants
- Procaine
- Amyl nitrite
- Local or general anesthesia
- Ketamine (1 mg/lb)
2. In the patient with sickle cell disease: intravenous hydration, alkalinization, transfusion or exchange-transfusion, oxygen
3. Corpora cavernosa aspiration followed by injection of an α-adrenergic agonist (e.g., phenylephrine 50 μg)
4. Surgery
- Cavernospongiosum shunt
- Glans-cavernosum shunt
- Cavernosaphenous shunt
- In the less common situation of high-flow priapism (diagnosed by the finding of bright red arterial blood on aspiration), arterial embolization or surgical ligation is recommended

■ PROGNOSIS
Impotence is associated with the duration of priapism, with 36 hr being an important threshold.

■ REFERRAL
To urologist

REFERENCE
Benson GS, Boileau MA: Priapism. In Gillenwater JY et al (eds): *Adult and pediatric urology*, St Louis, 1996, Mosby.
Author: **Tom J. Wachtel, M.D.**

TABLE 1-45 **Comparison of Normal Erection and Priapism**

FACTOR	NORMAL ERECTION	PRIAPISM
Portion of penis involved	Corpora cavernosa and corpus spongiosum and glans	Corpora cavernosa
Cause	Vasodilatation of penile arteries	Obstruction of venous outflow
		Disturbance of neuroarterial mechanism (imbalance between it and adrenergic activity)
		Increased viscosity
Sexual desire	Present	Absent
Pain	Absent	Present
Duration	Minutes to hours	Hours to days

From Nseyo UO (ed): *Urology for primary care physicians*, Philadelphia, 1999, WB Saunders.

BASIC INFORMATION

■ DEFINITION
Prolactinomas are monoclonal tumors that secrete prolactin.

■ ICD-9CM CODES
253.1 Forbes-Albright syndrome

■ EPIDEMIOLOGY & DEMOGRAPHICS
INCIDENCE: Most common pituitary tumor; nearly 30% of all pituitary adenomas secrete enough prolactin to cause hyperprolactinemia.
PREDOMINANT SEX: Microadenomas are more common in women; macroadenomas are more frequent in men.

■ PHYSICAL FINDINGS & CLINICAL PRESENTATION
MEN: Decreased facial and body hair, small testicles; may also have decreased libido, impotence, and delayed puberty (caused by decreased testosterone secondary to inhibition of gonadotropin secretion).
WOMEN: Physical examination may be normal; history may reveal amenorrhea, galactorrhea, oligomenorrhea, and anovulation.
BOTH SEXES: Visual field defects and headache may occur depending on size of tumor and its expansion.

■ ETIOLOGY
Prolactin-secreting pituitary adenomas: microadenomas (<10 mm diameter) or macroadenomas (>10 mm diameter)

DIAGNOSIS

■ DIFFERENTIAL DIAGNOSIS
Hyperprolactinemia may be caused by the following:
- Drugs: phenothiazines, methyldopa, reserpine, MAO inhibitors, androgens, progesterone, cimetidine, tricyclic antidepressants, haloperidol, meprobamate, chlordiazepoxide, estrogens, narcotics, metoclopramide, verapamil, amoxapine, cocaine, oral contraceptives
- Hepatic cirrhosis, renal failure, primary hypothyroidism
- Ectopic prolactin-secreting tumors (hypernephroma, bronchogenic carcinoma)
- Infiltrating diseases of the pituitary (sarcoidosis, histiocytosis)
- Head trauma, chest wall injury, spinal cord injury
- Polycystic ovary disease, pregnancy, nipple stimulation
- Idiopathic hyperprolactinemia, stress, exercise

■ WORKUP
- The diagnosis of prolactinoma is established by demonstration of an elevated serum prolactin level (after exclusion of other causes of hyperprolactinemia) and radiographic evidence of a pituitary adenoma.
  1. Normal mean prolactin levels are 8 ng/ml in women and 5 ng/ml in men.
  2. Levels >300 ng/ml are virtually diagnostic of prolactinomas.
  3. Prolactin levels can vary with time of day, stress, sleep cycle, and meals. More accurate measurements can be obtained 2 to 3 hr after awakening, preprandially, and when patient is not distressed.
  4. Serial measurements are recommended in patients with mild prolactin elevations.
- TRH stimulation test may be useful in equivocal cases. The normal response is an increase in serum prolactin levels by 100% within 1 hr of TRH infusion; failure to demonstrate an increase in prolactin level is suggestive of pituitary lesion.
- All patients with prolactinomas should undergo visual field testing. Serial evaluation is recommended, particularly during pregnancy in patients with macroadenomas.

■ IMAGING STUDIES
- MRI with gadolinium enhancement is the procedure of choice in the radiographic evaluation of pituitary disease.
- In absence of MRI, a radiographic diagnosis is best accomplished with a high-resolution CT scanner and special coronal cuts through the pituitary region.

TREATMENT

■ NONPHARMACOLOGIC THERAPY
Pregnancy and breast-feeding should be avoided, because they can encourage tumor growth.

■ ACUTE GENERAL RX
- Management of prolactinomas depends on their size and encroachment on the optic chiasm and other vital structures, the presence or absence of gonadal dysfunction, and the patient's desires with respect to fertility.

- Medical therapy is preferred when fertility is an important consideration.
  1. Bromocriptine (Parlodel): Initial dose is 0.625 at hs for the first week. After 1 wk, add AM dose of 1.25 mg. Gradually increase dose by 1.25 mg/wk until dose of 5 to 10 mg/day is achieved; Bromocriptine decreases size of the tumor and generally lowers the prolactin level into the normal range when the initial serum prolactin is <500 ng/ml. Side effects of bromocriptine are nausea, constipation, dizziness, and nasal stuffiness. Bromocriptine appears to be safe during pregnancy.
  2. Cabergoline (Dostinex) is a longer-acting dopamine agonist that is more expensive but may be more effective and better tolerated than bromocriptine; initial dose is 0.25 mg twice weekly.
- Transsphenoidal resection: option in an infertile patient who cannot tolerate bromocriptine or cabergoline or when medical therapy is ineffective. The success rate depends on the location of the tumor (entirely intrasellar), experience of the neurosurgeon, and size of the tumor (<10 mm in diameter); the recurrence rate may reach 80% within 5 yr. Possible complications of transsphenoidal surgery include transient diabetes insipidus, hypopituitarism, CSF rhinorrhea, and infections (meningitis, wound infection).
- Pituitary irradiation is useful as adjunctive therapy of macroadenomas (>10 mm in diameter) and in patients with persistent hypersecretion following surgery. Potential complications include cranial nerve damage, radionecrosis, and cognitive abnormalities.
- Stereotactic radiosurgery (gamma knife) is a newer modality in the treatment of prolactinomas. A high dose of ionizing radiation is delivered to the tumor through multiple ports. Its advantage is minimal irradiation to surrounding tissues. Proximity of the tumor to the optic chiasm limits this therapeutic modality.

■ CHRONIC RX
- Patients on medical therapy require periodic measurement of prolactin levels. An attempt to reduce the dose of bromocriptine or cabergoline can be made after the prolactin level has been normal for 2 yr. An MRI scan of the pituitary should be obtained to rule out tumor enlargement within 6 mo of initiation of tapering regimen.
- Evaluation and monitoring of pituitary function are recommended following transsphenoidal surgery.

■ DISPOSITION
- Transsphenoidal surgery will result in a cure in nearly 50% to 75% of patients with microadenomas and 10% to 20% of patients with macroadenomas.
- Nearly 20% of microprolactinomas resolve during long-term dopamine agonist treatment.

☼ PEARLS & CONSIDERATIONS

■ COMMENTS
Patients must be monitored for several years after surgery, because up to 50% of microadenomas and nearly 90% of macroadenomas can recur.

REFERENCE
Schlechte JA: Prolactinoma, *N Engl J Med* 349:2035, 2003.
Author: **Fred F. Ferri, M.D.**

BASIC INFORMATION

■ DEFINITION

A form of compression neuropathy of the median nerve in the proximal forearm caused primarily by the pronator teres muscle. Occasionally, only the anterior interosseus motor branch is affected, sometimes causing a very specific separate clinical presentation.

■ SYNONYMS

Kiloh-Nevin syndrome (anterior interosseus syndrome)

ICD-9CM CODES

354.1 Median nerve entrapment
354.9 Mononeuritis of upper limb

■ EPIDEMIOLOGY & DEMOGRAPHICS

- Males = females
- Most common in dominant arm
- Rare (<1% median nerve entrapment disorders)

■ PHYSICAL FINDINGS & CLINICAL PRESENTATION

- Forearm discomfort and fatigue, often resulting from repetitive pronation
- Insidious onset
- Nocturnal paresthesias are not typical
- Vague numbness in hand, primarily in thumb and index finger, may be present
- Tenderness and enlargement of the pronator teres may be present
- Tinel's sign may be positive at the site of compression
- Although there are no reliable provocative tests, painful paresthesias may occasionally be elicited with forced pronation of the forearm against resistance
- Motor impairment is rare

Anterior interosseus nerve syndrome:
- Forearm pain and weakness
- Patient may be unable to form a circle when trying to pinch the index finger and thumb because of inability to flex distal phalanges of thumb and index finger
- Sensation to the hand is not affected

■ ETIOLOGY

- Localized anatomic compression
- Trauma
- Traumatic cut down or phlebotomy

DIAGNOSIS

■ DIFFERENTIAL DIAGNOSIS

- Carpal tunnel syndrome
- Cervical disc syndrome with radiculopathy
- Tendon rupture
- Tendinitis

■ WORKUP

- Electrodiagnostic studies may be helpful
- Plain radiography to rule out bony abnormalities causing compression

TREATMENT

- Rest, bracing of forearm, sling
- Stretching exercises, physical therapy
- NSAIDs

■ REFERRAL

Surgical referral in cases of failed medical management or when motor weakness is present

REFERENCES

Asami A, Takayama G, Hotokebuchi T: Pronator teres syndrome associated with mononeuritis multiplex in polyarteritis nodosa, *Hand Surg* 4(2):189, 1999.

Joist A et al: Anterior interosseous nerve compression after supracondylar fracture of the humerus: a metaanalysis, *J Neurosurg* 90(6):1053, 1999.

Rehak DC: Pronator syndrome, *Clin Sports Med* 20(3):531, 2001.

Author: **Lonnie R. Mercier, M.D.**

BASIC INFORMATION

■ DEFINITION AND CLASSIFICATION

Prostate cancer is a neoplasm involving the prostate; various classifications have been developed to evaluate malignancy potential and prognosis:

- The degree of malignancy varies with the stage

  Stage A: Confined to the prostate, no nodule palpable

  Stage B: Palpable nodule confined to the gland

  Stage C: Local extension

  Stage D: Regional lymph nodes or distant metastases

- In the Gleason classification, two histologic patterns are independently assigned numbers 1 to 5 (best to least differentiated). These numbers are added to give a total tumor score:

  1. Prognosis is generally good if score is <5.
  2. Score 6 to 10 carries an intermediate prognosis.
  3. Score >10 correlates with anaplastic lesions with poor prognosis.

- Another commonly used classification is the Tumor-Node-Metastasis (TNM) classification of prostate cancer.

ICD-9CM CODES

185 Malignant neoplasm of prostate

■ EPIDEMIOLOGY & DEMOGRAPHICS

- Prostate cancer has surpassed lung cancer as the most common non-skin cancer in men.
- More than 100,000 cases are diagnosed yearly, and nearly 30,000 males die from prostate cancer each year (second leading cause of death from cancer in U.S. men).
- Incidence of prostate cancer increases with age: uncommon <50 yr; 80% of new cases are diagnosed in patients ≥65 yr.
- Average age at time of diagnosis is 72 yr.
- Blacks in the U.S. have the highest incidence of prostate cancer in the world (1 in every 9 males).
- Incidence is low in Asians.
- Approximately 9% of all prostate cancers may be familial.

■ PHYSICAL FINDINGS & CLINICAL PRESENTATION

- Generally silent disease until it reaches advanced stages.
- Bone pain and pathologic fractures may be initial symptoms of prostate cancer.
- Local growth can cause symptoms of outflow obstruction.
- Digital rectal examination (DRE) may reveal an area of increased firmness; 10% of patients will have a negative DRE.
- Prostate may be hard, fixed, with extension of tumor to the seminal vesicles in advanced stages.

 DIAGNOSIS

■ DIFFERENTIAL DIAGNOSIS

- Benign prostatic hypertrophy
- Prostatitis
- Prostate stones

■ LABORATORY TESTS

- Measurement of PSA is useful in early diagnosis of prostate cancer and in monitoring efficacy of therapy. Normal PSA is found in >20% of patients with prostate cancer, whereas only 20% of men with PSA levels between 4 ng/ml and 10 ng/ml have prostate cancer. The American Cancer Society recommends offering the PSA test and digital rectal examination yearly to men 50 years or older who have a life expectancy of at least 10 years. Earlier testing, starting at age 45, is recommended for men at high risk (e.g., blacks, men with family history of prostate cancer).
- The use of serum-free PSA for prostate screening has been proposed by some urologists as a means to decrease unwarranted biopsies without missing a significant number of prostate cancers. This approach is based on the higher free PSA in men with benign prostatic hyperplasia and the higher protein-bound PSA levels in men with prostate cancer. For example, in men with total PSA levels of 4 to 10 ng/ml, the cancer probability is 0.25, but if the percent free PSA is ≤17%, the probability of cancer increases to 0.45.

- Prostatic acid phosphatase (PAP) can be used for evaluation of nonlocalized disease.
- Transrectal biopsy and fine-needle aspiration of prostate can confirm the diagnosis.

■ IMAGING STUDIES

- Bone scan is useful to evaluate bone metastasis (present or eventually develops in almost 80% of patients). However, according to the American Urological Association (AUA), the routine use of bone scanning is not required for staging of prostate cancer in asymptomatic men with clinically localized cancer if the PSA level is ≤20 ng/ml.
- CT scan, MRI, and transrectal ultrasonography may be useful in selected patients to assess extent of prostate cancer. High-resolution MRI with magnetic nanoparticles has been used for the detection of small and otherwise undetectable lymph-node metastases in patients with prostate cancer. However, according to the AUA, transrectal ultrasonography adds little to the combination of PSA and digital rectal examination. Similarly, CT and MRI imaging are generally not indicated for cancer staging in men with clinically localized cancer and PSA <25 ng/ml. With regard to pelvic lymph node dissection in staging, the AUA states that it may not be required in patients with PSA levels <10 ng/ml and when PSA level is <20 ng/ml and the Gleason score is <6.

TREATMENT

■ NONPHARMACOLOGIC THERAPY

Watchful waiting is reasonable in patients with early stage (T-IA) and projected life expectancy <10 yr or in patients with focal and moderately differentiated carcinoma.

■ ACUTE GENERAL RX

- Therapeutic approach varies with the following:
  1. Stage of the tumor
  2. Patient's life expectancy
  3. General medical condition
  4. Patient's treatment preference (e.g., patient may be opposed to orchiectomy)

- The optimal treatment of clinically localized prostate cancer is unclear.
  1. Radical prostatectomy is generally performed in patients with localized prostate cancer and life expectancy >10 yr.
  2. Radiation therapy (external beam irradiation or implantation of radioactive pellets [seeds]) represents an alternative in patients with localized prostate cancer, especially poor surgical candidates or patients with a high-grade malignancy.
  3. Watchful waiting is reasonable in patients who are too old or too ill to survive longer than 10 yr. If the cancer progresses to the point where it becomes symptomatic, palliation can be attempted with several methods.
- Patients with advanced disease and projected life expectancy <10 yr are candidates for radiation therapy and hormonal therapy (DES, LHRH analogs, antiandrogens, bilateral orchiectomy).
- Recommended treatment of patients with regional metastatic prostate cancer with projected life expectancy ≥10 yr includes radical prostatectomy, radiation therapy, hormonal therapy.
- Androgen-deprivation therapy with a gonadotropin-releasing hormone agonist is the mainstay of treatment for metastatic prostate cancer. Adjuvant treatment with GnRH agonists (goserelin leuprolide, or triptorelin) plus antiandrogens (flutamide, bicalutamide, or nilutamide), when started simultaneously with external irradiation, improves local control and survival in patients with locally advanced prostate cancer. Pamidronate inhibits osteoclast-mediated bone resorption and prevents bone loss in the hip and lumbar spine in men receiving treatment for prostate cancer with a GnRH.

■ CHRONIC RX
- Patients should be monitored at 3- to 6-mo intervals with clinical examination, and PSA for the first year, then every 6 mo for the second year, then yearly if stable. For patients who have undergone radical prostatectomy, a rising PSA level suggests evidence of residual or recurrent prostate cancer. Salvage radiotherapy may potentially cure patients with disease recurrence after radical prostatectomy.
- Chest x-ray examination, bone scan should be performed yearly or sooner if patient develops symptoms.

■ DISPOSITION
- Prognosis varies with the stage of the disease (see "Definition") and the Gleason classification (see "Definition").
- The ploidy of the tumor also has prognostic value: prognosis is better with diploid tumor cells, worse with aneuploid tumor cells.
- For grade 1 tumors, the extended 10-yr, disease-specific survival is similar for patients with prostatectomy (94%), radiotherapy (90%), and conservative management (93%); survival rate is better with surgery than with radiotherapy or conservative management in patients with grade 2 or 3 localized prostate cancer.
- Expression of the gene EZH2 has been identified as an important factor in the determination of the aggressiveness of prostate cancer. A recent study revealed that expression of the EZH2 gene may be a better predictor of clinical failure than Gleason score, tumor stage, or surgical margin status. Testing for EZH2 protein in prostate cancer tissue may be useful to determine prognosis and direct treatment.

REFERENCES

Gann PH et al: Strategies combining total and percent free prostate specific antigen for detecting prostate cancer: a perspective evaluation, *J Urol* 167:2427, 2002.

Harisinghani MG et al: Noninvasive detection of clinically occult lymph-node metastases in prostate cancer, *N Engl J Med* 348:2491, 2003.

Homberg L et al: A randomized trial comparing radical prostatectomy with watchful waiting in early prostate cancer, *N Engl J Med* 347:781, 2002.

Makinen T et al: Family history and prostate cancer screening with prostate specific antigen, *J Clin Oncol* 20:2658, 2002.

Nelson WG: Prostate cancer, *N Engl J Med* 349:366, 2003.

Rubin MA et al: α-Methylacyl coenzyme a racemase as a tissue biomarker for prostate cancer, *JAMA* 287:1662, 2002.

Steineck G et al: Quality of life after radical prostatectomy or watchful waiting, *N Engl J Med* 347:790, 2002.

Stephenson AJ et al: Salvage radiotherapy for recurrent prostate cancer after radical prostatectomy, *JAMA* 291:1325, 2004.

Varambally S et al: The polycarb group protein EZH2 is involved in progression of prostate cancer, *Nature* 419:624, 2002.

Author: **Fred F. Ferri, M.D.**

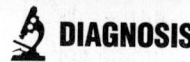
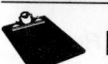 **BASIC INFORMATION**

■ DEFINITION
Benign prostatic hyperplasia is the benign growth of the prostate, generally originating in the periureteral and transition zones, with subsequent obstructive and irritative voiding symptoms.

■ SYNONYMS
BPH
Prostatic hypertrophy

ICD-9CM CODES
600 Benign prostatic hyperplasia

■ EPIDEMIOLOGY & DEMOGRAPHICS
- 80% of men have evidence of benign prostatic hypertrophy by age 80 yr.
- Medical and surgical intervention for problems caused by BPH is required in >20% of males by age 75 yr.
- Transurethral resection of the prostate (TURP) is the tenth most common operative procedure (>400,000/yr in U.S.).
- 10% to 30% of men with BPH have occult prostate cancer.

■ PHYSICAL FINDINGS & CLINICAL PRESENTATION
- Digital rectal examination (DRE) reveals enlargement of the prostate.
- Focal enlargement may be indicative of malignancy.
- There is poor correlation between size of prostate and symptoms (BPH may be asymptomatic if it does not encroach on the urethral lumen).
- Most patients with BPH complain of difficulty in initiating urination (hesitancy), decrease in caliber and force of stream, incomplete emptying of bladder often resulting in double voiding (need to urinate again a few minutes after voiding), postvoid "dribbling," and nocturia.

■ ETIOLOGY
Multifactorial; a functioning testicle is necessary for development of BPH (as evidenced by the absence in males who were castrated before puberty).

🔬 DIAGNOSIS

■ DIFFERENTIAL DIAGNOSIS
- Prostatitis
- Prostate cancer
- Strictures (urethral)
- Medication interfering with the muscle fibers in the prostate and also with bladder function

■ WORKUP
Symptom assessment (use of American Urological Association [AUA] Symptom Index for BPH [Table 1-46]), laboratory tests, and imaging studies

■ LABORATORY TESTS
- Prostate specific antigen (PSA): protease secreted by epithelial cells of the prostate; elevated in 30% to 50% of patients with BPH. Testing for PSA increases detection rate for prostate cancer and tends to detect cancer at an earlier stage. However, the PSA test does not discriminate well between patients with symptomatic BPH and those with prostate cancer, particularly if the cancers are pathologically localized and curable. The test may also trigger additional evaluation, including ultrasound biopsy of the prostate. Recent data

TABLE 1-46   International Prostate Symptom Score (I-PSS)

SYMPTOM	NOT AT ALL	LESS THAN 1 TIME IN 5	LESS THAN HALF THE TIME	ABOUT HALF THE TIME	MORE THAN HALF THE TIME	ALMOST ALWAYS	TOTAL SCORE
Incomplete emptying: Over the past month, how often have you had a sensation of not emptying your bladder completely after you finished urinating?	0	1	2	3	4	5	
Frequency: Over the past month, how often have you had to urinate again <2 hr after you finished urinating?	0	1	2	3	4	5	
Intermittency: Over the past month, how often have you found you stopped and started again several times when you urinated?	0	1	2	3	4	5	
Urgency: Over the past month, how often have you found it difficult to postpone urination?	0	1	2	3	4	5	
Weak stream: Over the past month, how often have you had a weak urinary stream?	0	1	2	3	4	5	
Straining: Over the past month, how often have you had to push or strain to begin urination?	0	1	2	3	4	5	
	NONE	1 TIME	2 TIMES	3 TIMES	4 TIMES	5 OR MORE TIMES	
Nocturia: Over the past month, how many times did you most typically get up to urinate from the time you went to bed at night until the time you got up in the morning?	0	1	2	3	4	5	

Total I-PSS score =

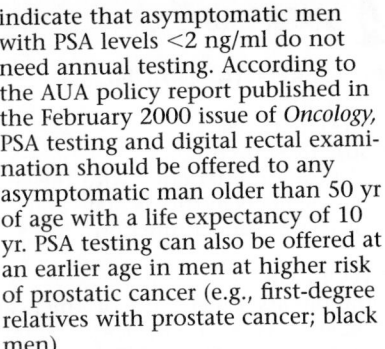

indicate that asymptomatic men with PSA levels <2 ng/ml do not need annual testing. According to the AUA policy report published in the February 2000 issue of *Oncology*, PSA testing and digital rectal examination should be offered to any asymptomatic man older than 50 yr of age with a life expectancy of 10 yr. PSA testing can also be offered at an earlier age in men at higher risk of prostatic cancer (e.g., first-degree relatives with prostate cancer; black men)

- Measurement of "free" PSA is useful to assess the probability of prostate cancer in patients with normal digital rectal examination and total PSA between 4 and 10 ng/ml. In these patients the global risk of prostate cancer is 25%; however, if the free PSA is >25%, the risk of prostate cancer decreases to 8%, whereas if the free PSA is <10%, the risk of cancer increases to 56%. Free PSA is also useful to evaluate the aggressiveness of prostate cancer. A low free PSA percentage generally indicates a high-grade cancer, whereas a high free PSA percentage is generally associated with a slower growing tumor

- Urinalysis, urine C&S to rule out infection (if suspected)
- BUN and creatinine to rule out postrenal insufficiency

■ IMAGING STUDIES
- Transrectal ultrasound may be indicated in patients with palpable nodules or significant elevation of PSA. It is also useful to estimate prostate size.
- Uroflowmetry may be used to determine relative impact of obstruction on urine flow. Urethral pressure profile is useful to predict prostatic hypertrophy within the urethral lumen.
- Pressure flow studies, although invasive, are particularly helpful in patients whose history and/or examination suggest primary bladder dysfunction as a cause of symptoms of prostatism. They are also useful in patients for whom a distinction between prostatic obstruction and impaired detrusor contractility may affect the choice of therapy. However, pressure flow studies may not be useful in the workup of the usual patient with symptoms of prostatism.
- Postvoid residual urine measurement has not been proved useful in predicting the need for or response to treatment; may be useful in monitoring the course of the disease in patients who elect nonsurgical treatment.

- Urethral cystoscopy is an option during later evaluation if invasive treatment is being planned.

TREATMENT

■ NONPHARMACOLOGIC THERAPY
- Avoidance of caffeine or any other foods that may exacerbate symptoms
- Avoidance of medications that may exacerbate symptoms (e.g., most cold and allergy remedies)

■ GENERAL RX
- Asymptomatic patients with prostate enlargement caused by BPH generally do not require treatment. Patients with mild to moderate symptoms are candidates for pharmacologic treatment (see below). For those patients who have specific complications from BPH, prostate surgery is usually the most appropriate form of treatment. However, surgery may result in significant complications (e.g., incontinence, infection).
- TURP is the most commonly used surgical procedure for BPH. Transurethral incision of the prostate (TUIP), a procedure almost equivalent in efficacy, is limited to patients whose estimated resection tissue weight would be 30 g or less. TUIP can be performed in an ambulatory setting or during a 1-day hospitalization. Open prostatectomy is typically performed on patients with very large prostates.
- Laser therapy for BPH is a less invasive alternative to TURP; however, recent studies indicate that at least in the initial 7 mo after surgery, TURP is moderately more effective than laser therapy in relieving symptoms of BPH.
- Surgery need not be treatment of last resort for most patients; that is, patients need not undergo other treatments for BPH before they can have surgery. However, recommending surgery on the grounds that a patient's surgical risk will "only increase with age" is generally inappropriate.
- Balloon dilation of the prostatic urethra is less effective than surgery for relieving symptoms but is associated with fewer complications. It is a reasonable treatment option for patients with smaller prostates and no middle lobe enlargement.
- The dietary supplement saw palmetto is effective in relieving BPH symptoms in patients with mild obstruction.

- α-Blockers (e.g., tamsulosin [Flomax], alfuzosin [Uroxatral], doxazosin, prazosin, and terazosin) relax smooth muscle of the bladder neck and prostate and can increase peak urinary flow rate. They have no effect on the size of the prostate. α-1 blockers are useful in symptomatic patients to relieve symptoms of obstruction by causing relaxation of smooth muscle tone in the prostatic capsule and urethra and bladder neck.
- Hormonal manipulation with finasteride (Proscar), a 5α-reductase inhibitor that blocks conversion of testosterone to dihydrotestosterone, can reduce the size of the prostate. Usual dose is 5 mg qd. Treatment requires 6 mo or more for maximal effect.
- Dutasteride (Avodart) is also a 5 α-reductase inhibitor useful to decrease prostate size and improve urinary flow. In addition to inhibiting the isoform of 5-α reductase located in the prostate, the medication also inhibits a second isoform and reduces DHT formation in the skin and liver. Usual dose is 0.5 mg qd.

■ CHRONIC RX
- Avoid medications and foods that exacerbate symptoms.
- Symptomatic improvement occurs in >70% of patients with proper treatment.

■ DISPOSITION
With appropriate therapy, symptoms improve or stabilize in >70% of patients with BPH.

■ REFERRAL
Urology referral for patients with severe or intolerable symptoms and for any patient suspected of having prostate cancer (10% to 30% of men with BPH).

☼ PEARLS & CONSIDERATIONS

■ COMMENTS
- Emerging technologies for treating BPH include lasers, coils, stents, thermal therapy, and hyperthermia. Laser prostatectomy appears promising; however, long-term effectiveness has not yet been demonstrated.
- The increase in the use of pharmacologic management has resulted in more than 30% reduction in the total number of transurethral resections of the prostate.

REFERENCE
Dull P et al: Managing benign prostatic hyperplasia, *Am Fam Physician* 66:77, 2002.
Author: **Fred F. Ferri, M.D.**

BASIC INFORMATION

■ DEFINITION

Prostatitis refers to inflammation of the prostate gland. There are four major categories:
- Acute bacterial prostatitis
- Chronic bacterial prostatitis
- Nonbacterial prostatitis
- Prostatodynia

ICD-9CM CODES
601.0 Prostatitis (acute)
601.1 Prostatitis (chronic)
099.54 Prostatitis (chlamydial)

■ EPIDEMIOLOGY & DEMOGRAPHICS
- 50% of men experience symptoms of prostatitis in their lifetime
- Acute bacterial prostatitis is uncommon
- The relative prevalence of the other three entities among men with inflammatory prostatic symptoms is:
  1. 5% to 10% chronic bacterial prostatitis
  2. 10% to 65% nonbacterial prostatitis
  3. 30% to 80% prostatodynia

The figures are imprecise because nonbacterial prostatitis and prostatodynia are very difficult to differentiate.

■ PHYSICAL FINDINGS & CLINICAL PRESENTATION
ACUTE BACTERIAL PROSTATITIS:
- Sudden or rapidly progressive onset of:
  1. Dysuria
  2. Frequency
  3. Urgency
  4. Nocturia
  5. Perineal pain that may radiate to the back, the rectum, or the penis
- Hematuria or a purulent urethral discharge may occur.
- Occasionally urinary retention complicates the course.
- Fever, chills, and signs of sepsis can also be part of the clinical picture.
- On rectal examination the prostate is typically tender.

CHRONIC BACTERIAL PROSTATITIS:
- May be asymptomatic when the infection is confined to the prostate
- May present as an increase in severity of baseline symptoms of benign prostatic hypertrophy
- When cystitis is also present, urinary frequency, urgency, and burning may be reported
- Hematuria may be a presenting complaint
- In elderly men, new onset of urinary incontinence may be noted

NONBACTERIAL PROSTATITIS AND PROSTATODYNIA:
- Present similarly with symptoms of bladder irritation (urinary frequency, urgency, dysuria, increase in nocturia episodes) and perineal discomfort
- The symptoms can be of variable severity, but tend to be more bothersome in prostatodynia

■ ETIOLOGY
ACUTE BACTERIAL PROSTATITIS:
- Acute usually gram-negative infection of the prostate gland
  1. Generally associated with cystitis
  2. Resulting from the ascent of bacteria in the urethra
- Occasionally the route of infection is hematogenous or a lymphatogenous spread of rectal bacteria
- The condition is seen in young or middle-aged men

CHRONIC BACTERIAL PROSTATITIS:
- Often asymptomatic
- Exacerbation of symptoms of benign prostatic hypertrophy caused by the same mechanism as in acute bacterial prostatitis

NONBACTERIAL PROSTATITIS:
- Refers to symptoms of prostatic inflammation associated with the presence of WBCs in prostatic secretions with no identifiable bacterial organism
- Chlamydia infection may be etiologically implicated in some cases

PROSTATODYNIA:
- Refers to symptoms of prostatic inflammation with no or few WBCs in the prostatic secretion
- Spasm in the bladder neck or urethra is felt to be the cause of symptoms

 DIAGNOSIS

■ DIFFERENTIAL DIAGNOSIS
- Benign prostatic hypertrophy with lower urinary tract symptoms
- Prostate cancer
- Also see differential diagnosis of hematuria

■ WORKUP
- Rectal examination
  1. Tender prostate most suggestive of acute bacterial prostatitis
  2. Enlarged prostate common in chronic bacterial prostatitis
  3. Normal prostate is consistent with chronic bacterial and nonbacterial prostatitis and is typical in prostatodynia
- Expression of prostatic secretions (EPS) by prostate massage is contraindicated in acute bacterial prostatitis but is appropriate in the other three situations

■ LABORATORY TESTS
- Urinalysis
- Urine culture and sensitivity
- Bacterial localization studies can be performed but are cumbersome and impractical in most clinical settings
- Cell count and culture of expressed prostatic secretions
- The yield of a urine culture may be increased if the specimen is obtained after a prostatic massage
- PSA is not used to diagnose prostatitis; however, a rapid rise over baseline should raise the possibility of prostatitis even in the absence of symptoms. In such cases, a follow-up PSA after treatment of prostatitis is appropriate
- CBC and blood cultures if fever, chills, or signs of sepsis exist
- If hematuria is present, a workup to rule out a urologic malignancy should be considered if the hematuria does not clear after treatment of prostatitis

TREATMENT

ACUTE BACTERIAL PROSTATITIS:
Culture guided antibiotic therapy for 4 wk (beginning with a few days of intravenous antibiotics if the infection is serious or if the patient is bacteremic).

CHRONIC BACTERIAL PROSTATITIS:
- Trimethoprim-sulfamethoxazole is first-line choice for 4 wk if the organism is sensitive.
- Second-line choice for treatment failure or organisms resistant to TMP-SMX is with a fluoroquinolone
- Patient with refractory infection or with multiple relapses may be offered long-term suppressive therapy.

NONBACTERIAL PROSTATITIS AND PROSTATODYNIA:
- No specific treatment
- Antibiotics are not effective
- A trial of treatment with an α-adrenergic blocker (terazosin, doxazosin, or tamsulosin) may be considered
- Any underlying bladder pathology should be ruled out by cystoscopy and treated if identified

REFERENCES

Fowler JE: Prostatitis. In Gillenwater JY et al (eds): *Adult and pediatric urology,* St Louis, 1996, Mosby.

McNaughton Collins M, MacDonald R, Wilt TJ: Diagnosis and treatment of chronic abacterial prostatitis: a systemic review, *Ann Intern Med* 133:367, 2000.

Author: **Tom J. Wachtel**

BASIC INFORMATION

■ DEFINITION
Pruritus ani refers to an intense chronic itching of the anus and perianal skin.

■ ICD-9CM CODES
698.0 Pruritus ani

■ EPIDEMIOLOGY & DEMOGRAPHICS
- Any age can be affected.
- Occurs in 1% to 5% of the population.
- Male to female predominance of 4:1.

■ PHYSICAL FINDINGS & CLINICAL PRESENTATION
- Anal itching
- Anal fissures
- Hemorrhoids
- Excoriations
- Pinworms
- Fecal incontinence

■ ETIOLOGY
ANORECTAL DISEASES AND FECAL CONTAMINATION:
- Diarrhea
- Anal incontinence
- Hemorrhoids
- Fissures
- Fistulae
- Rectal prolapse
- Malignancy: Bowen's disease, epidermoid cancer, perianal Paget's disease

INFECTIONS:
- Fungal: candidiasis, dermatophytes
- Parasitic: pinworms, scabies
- Bacterial: *Staphylococcus aureus,* erythrasma
- Lymphogranuloma venereal
- Granuloma
- Inguinale
- Chancroid
- Molluscum contagiosa
- Trichomoniasis
- Venereal: herpes, gonococcal syphilis, human papillomavirus

LOCAL IRRITANTS:
- Moisture, obesity, excessive perspiration
- Soaps, hygiene products
- Toilet paper: perfumed, dyed
- Underwear: irritating fabrics, detergents
- Anal creams, suppositories
- Dietary: coffee, beer, acidic foods
- Drugs: mineral oil, ascorbic acid, hydrocortisone sodium succinate, quinine, colchicine

DERMATOLOGIC DISEASES:
- Psoriasis
- Atopic dermatitis
- Seborrheic dermatitis

Section II also describes the various causes of pruritus ani.

DIAGNOSIS

■ DIFFERENTIAL DIAGNOSIS
- Allergies
- Anxiety
- Dermatologic conditions
- Infections
- Parasites
- Diabetes mellitus
- Chronic liver disease
- Neoplasia
- Proctalgia fugax

■ WORKUP
- Detailed history regarding bowel habits, hygiene, use of perfumed products, and medical history
- Inspection of perianal area
- Possible biopsy to exclude neoplasia
- Microscopic inspection of scrapings
- Colposcopy of perineum

■ LABORATORY TESTS
- Chemistry profile
- Urinalysis
- Cultures
- Stool for ova and parasites
- Tape test
- Glucose tolerance test, if necessary

TREATMENT

■ NONPHARMACOLOGIC THERAPY
- Avoidance of tight, nonporous clothing and underclothing
- Discontinuation or curtailment of coffee, beer, citrus fruits, tomatoes, chocolate, and tea
- Cleansing of anal area after bowel movements with a premoistened pad or tissue and avoidance of perfumes and dyes present in toilet paper and soaps
- Avoidance of excessive perspiration
- Aggressive management of fecal leakage or incontinence to avoid soiling of perianal skin

■ ACUTE GENERAL RX
- Minimization of frequent loose stools with antidiarrheals and fiber agents if appropriate
- Use of a 1% hydrocortisone cream sparingly bid during the acute phase of pruritus ani but not for >2 wk to avoid atrophy
- Treatment of predisposing factors, such as parasites, diabetes, liver disease, hemorrhoids, and other infections

■ CHRONIC RX
- Possible complications: excoriation and secondary bacterial infection; must be treated aggressively
- Long-standing, intractable pruritus ani: good response to intracutaneous injections of methylene blue and other agents, steroid injection

■ DISPOSITION
- Usually good results with total resolution of symptoms
- In some, persistent and recurrent symptoms

■ REFERRAL
To colorectal specialist if conservative measures fail

REFERENCES
Fardi A, Rath W: Infections of the perianal region, *Gynakoloe* 34(10):907, 2001.

Gerdom LE, Dixon D, DiPalma JA: Hemorrhoids, genital warts and other perianal complaints, *JAAPA* 14(9):37, 2001.

Pfenninger JL, Zainea GG: Common anorectal conditions: part I: symptoms and complaints, *Am Fam Physician* 63(12):2391, 2001.

Watson AJ, Loudon M: Diagnosing minor anorectal conditions, *Practitioner* 245(1627):790, 2001.

Yamada T, Alpers DH, Laine L: *Textbook of gastroenterology,* ed 3, Baltimore, 1999, Lippincott Williams & Wilkins.

Author: **Maria A. Corigliano, M.D.**

BASIC INFORMATION

■ DEFINITION
Pruritus vulvae refers to intense itching of the female external genitalia.

■ SYNONYMS
Vulvodynia

ICD-9CM CODES
698.1 Pruritus of genital organs

■ EPIDEMIOLOGY & DEMOGRAPHICS
- A female disorder that can affect women at any age
- Young girls: infection is usually causative
- Postmenopausal women: frequently affected because of hypoestrogenic state

■ PHYSICAL FINDINGS & CLINICAL PRESENTATION
Constant intense itching or burning of the vulva

■ ETIOLOGY
- About 50% are caused by monilial infection or trichomoniasis.
- Other infectious causes are herpes simplex, condylomata acuminata, and molluscum contagiosum.
- Other causes:
  1. Infestations with scabies, pediculosis pubis, and pinworms
  2. Dermatoses such as hypertrophic dystrophy, lichen sclerosus, lichen planus, and psoriasis
  3. Neoplasms such as Bowen's disease, Paget's disease, and squamous cell carcinoma
  4. Allergic or chemical dermatitis caused by dyes in clothing or toilet paper, detergents, contraceptive gels, vaginal medications, douches, or soaps
  5. Vulva or vaginal atrophy
- Severe pruritus is probably caused by degeneration and inflammation of terminal nerve fibers.
- Most intense itching occurs with hyperplastic lesions.
- Children (75%) nonspecific pruritus, lichen sclerosus, bacterial infections, yeast infection, and pinworm infestation.

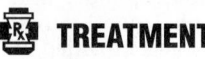 **DIAGNOSIS**

■ DIFFERENTIAL DIAGNOSIS
- Vulvitis
- Vaginitis
- Lichen sclerosus
- Squamous cell hyperplasia
- Pinworms
- Vulvar cancer
- Syringoma of the vulva

■ WORKUP
- Inspection of vulva, vagina, and perianal area looking for infection, fissures, ulcerations, induration, or thick plaques
- Must rule out trichomoniasis, candidiasis, allergy, vitamin deficiencies, diabetes

■ LABORATORY TESTS
- Wet prep of saline and KOH of vaginal discharge
- Tape test to look for pinworms
- Vaginal cultures
- Biopsy when needed

■ TREATMENT

■ NONPHARMACOLOGIC THERAPY
- Keep vulva clean and dry.
- Wear white cotton panties.
- Avoid perfumes and body creams over vulvar area because they can cause irritation.
- Reduce stress.
- Apply wet dressings with aluminum acetate (Burow's) solution frequently.
- Avoid coffee and caffeine-containing beverages, chocolate, tomatoes.
- Sitz baths may be helpful.

■ ACUTE GENERAL Rx
Need to treat underlying problem:
- Yeast infection: any of the vaginal creams or Diflucan 150-mg one-time dose
- Trichomoniasis or *Gardnerella vaginalis:* Flagyl 500 mg or 375 mg PO bid for 7 days
- Urinary tract infection: treatment of specific organism
- Estrogen replacement therapy if atrophy is the cause of pruritus
- Pinworms: mebendazole (Vermox) 100 mg one tablet at diagnosis and repeated in 1 to 2 wk; also treat other members in family >2 yr of age

- Squamous cell hyperplasia: local application of corticosteroids
  1. One of the high- or medium-potency corticosteroids (0.025% or 0.01% fluocinolone acetonide or 0.01% triamcinolone acetonide) can be used to relieve itching.
  2. Rub into vulva bid or tid for 4 to 6 wk.
  3. Once itching is controlled, fluorinated steroid can be discontinued and patient can be switched to hydrocortisone preparation.
- Lichen sclerosus: topical 2% testosterone in petrolatum massaged into the vulvar tissue bid or tid; Temovate (clobetasol propionate gel 0.05%) cream tid × 5 days is very effective
- Treatment with immune response modifiers

■ CHRONIC Rx
- If not relieved by topical measures: intradermal injection of triamcinolone (10 mg/ml diluted 2:1 saline) 0.1 ml of the suspension injected at 1-cm intervals and tissue gently massaged
- If symptoms still uncontrollable: SC injection of absolute alcohol 0.1 ml at 1-cm intervals

■ DISPOSITION
Usually controlled with conservative measures and topical steroids

■ REFERRAL
To a gynecologist for further workup if conservative measures do not give relief

REFERENCES
Copeland L: *Textbook of gynecology,* ed 2, Philadelphia, 1999, WB Saunders.

Foster DC: Vulvar disease, *Obstet Gynecol* 100(1):145, 2002.

Gerdsen R et al: Periodic genital pruritus caused by syringoma of the vulva, *Acta Obstet Gynecol Scand Suppl* 81(4):369, 2002.

Mead P: *Protocols for infectious diseases in obstetrics and gynecology,* ed 2, Cambridge, Mass, 2000, Blackwell Science.

Palk SC, Merritt DF, Mallory SB: Pruritus vulvae in prepubertal children, *J Am Acad Dermatol* 44(5):795, 2001.

Author: **Maria A. Corigliano, M.D.**

BASIC INFORMATION

DEFINITION
Pseudogout is one of the clinical patterns associated with a crystal-induced synovitis resulting from the deposition of calcium pyrophosphate dehydrate (CPPD) crystals in joint hyaline and fibrocartilage. The cartilage deposition is termed *chondrocalcinosis*.

SYNONYMS
Calcium pyrophosphate dehydrate crystal deposition disease (CPDD)
Chondrocalcinosis
Pyrophosphate arthropathy

ICD-9CM CODES
275.4 Chondrocalcinosis

EPIDEMIOLOGY & DEMOGRAPHICS
PREVALENCE:
• Uncertain
• Probably similar to gout (3/1000 persons)
• Chondrocalcinosis is present in >20% of all people at age 80 yr, but most are asymptomatic
PREDOMINANT SEX: Female:male ratio of approximately 1.5:1
PREVALENT AGE: 60 to 70 yr at onset

PHYSICAL FINDINGS & CLINICAL PRESENTATION
• Symptoms are similar to those of gouty arthritis with acute attacks and chronic arthritis
• Knee joint is most commonly affected
• Swelling, stiffness, and increased heat in affected joint

ETIOLOGY
• Unknown
• Often associated with various medical conditions, including hyperparathyroidism and amyloidosis

DIAGNOSIS

DIFFERENTIAL DIAGNOSIS
• Gouty arthritis
• Rheumatoid arthritis
• Osteoarthritis
• Neuropathic joint
Section II describes the differential diagnosis of acute monoarticular and oligoarticular arthritis and crystal-induced arthritides. An algorithm for evaluation of arthralgia limited to one or few joints is described in Section III, Fig. 3-20.

WORKUP
• Variable clinical presentation
• Diagnosis dependent on the identification of CPPD crystals

• The American Rheumatism Association revised diagnostic criteria for CPPD crystal deposition disease (pseudogout) are often used:
1. Criteria
   I. Demonstration of CPPD crystals (obtained by biopsy, necroscopy, or aspirated synovial fluid) by definitive means (e.g., characteristic "fingerprint" by x-ray diffraction powder pattern or by chemical analysis)
   II. (a) Identification of monoclinic and/or triclinic crystals showing either no or only a weakly positive birefringence by compensated polarized light microscopy
   (b) Presence of typical calcifications in roentgenograms
   III. (a) Acute arthritis, especially of knees or other large joints, with or without concomitant hyperuricemia
   (b) Chronic arthritis, especially of knees, hips, wrists, carpus, elbow, shoulder, and metacarpophalangeal joints, especially if accompanied by acute exacerbations; the following features are helpful in differentiating chronic arthritis from osteoarthritis:
      1. Uncommon site—for example, wrist, MCP, elbow, shoulder
      2. Appearance of lesion radiologically—for example, radiocarpal or patellofemoral joint space narrowing, especially if isolated (patella "wrapped around" the femur)
      3. Subchondral cyst formation
      4. Severity of degeneration—progressive, with subchondral bony collapse (microfractures), and fragmentation, with formation of intraarticular radiodense bodies
      5. Osteophyte formation—variable and inconstant
      6. Tendon calcifications, especially Achilles, triceps, obturators
2. Categories
   Definite—Criteria I or II (a) plus (b) must be fulfilled.
   Probable—Criteria II(a) or II(b) must be fulfilled.
   Possible—Criteria III(a) or (b) should alert the clinician to the possibility of underlying CPPD deposition.

LABORATORY TESTS
Crystal analysis of the synovial fluid aspirate to reveal rhomboid calcium pyrophosphate crystals

IMAGING STUDIES
Plain radiographs to reveal the following:
• Stippled calcification in bands running parallel to the subchondral bone margins
• Crystal deposition in menisci, synovium, and ligament tissue; triangular wrist cartilage and symphysis pubis are often affected

TREATMENT

NONPHARMACOLOGIC THERAPY
General measures such as heat, rest, and elevation as needed

ACUTE GENERAL Rx
• NSAIDs (as for gout)
• Colchicine
• Aspiration/steroid injection

DISPOSITION
Structural joint damage may occasionally occur, requiring arthroplasty in rare cases.

REFERRAL
For orthopedic consultation for destructive joint changes

PEARLS & CONSIDERATIONS

COMMENTS
As with gout, acute attacks may be triggered by various surgical or medical events.

REFERENCES
Agudelo CA, Wise CM: Crystal-associated arthritis in the elderly, *Rheum Dis Clin North Am* 26:527, 2000.
Canhao H et al: Cross-sectional study of 50 patients with calcium pyrophosphate dihydrate crystal arthropathy, *Clin Rheumatol* 20:119, 2001.
Halverson PB, Derfus BA: Calcium crystal-induced inflammation, *Curr Opin Rheumatol* 13:221, 2001.
Sagarin MJ: Pseudogout, *Emerg Med* 18:373, 2000.
Author: **Lonnie R. Mercier, M.D.**

BASIC INFORMATION

■ DEFINITION
Pseudomembranous colitis is the occurrence of diarrhea and bowel inflammation associated with antibiotic use.

■ SYNONYMS
Antibiotic-induced colitis

ICD-9CM CODES
008.45 *Clostridium difficile*, pseudomembranous colitis

■ EPIDEMIOLOGY & DEMOGRAPHICS
- Cephalosporins are the most frequent offending agent in pseudomembranous colitis because of their high rates of use.
- The antibiotic with the highest incidence is clindamycin (10% incidence of pseudomembranous colitis with its use).
- *Clostridium difficile* causes more than 250,000 cases of diarrhea and colitis in the U.S. every year.

■ PHYSICAL FINDINGS & CLINICAL PRESENTATION
- Abdominal tenderness (generalized or lower abdominal)
- Fever
- In patients with prolonged diarrhea, poor skin turgor, dry mucous membranes, and other signs of dehydration may be present

■ ETIOLOGY
Risk factors for *C. difficile* (the major identifiable agent of antibiotic-induced diarrhea and colitis):
- Administration of antibiotics: can occur with any antibiotic, but occurs most frequently with clindamycin, ampicillin, and cephalosporins
- Prolonged hospitalization
- Advanced age
- Abdominal surgery
- Hospitalized, tube-fed patients are at risk for *C. difficile*–associated diarrhea. Clinicians should consider testing for *C. difficile* in tube-fed patients with diarrhea unrelated to the feeding solution

DIAGNOSIS

The clinical signs of pseudomembranous colitis generally include diarrhea, fever, and abdominal cramps following use of antibiotics.

■ DIFFERENTIAL DIAGNOSIS
- GI bacterial infections (e.g., *Salmonella, Shigella, Campylobacter, Yersinia*)
- Enteric parasites (e.g., *Cryptosporidium, Entamoeba histolytica*)
- IBD
- Celiac sprue
- Irritable bowel syndrome

■ WORKUP
- All patients with diarrhea accompanied by current or recent antibiotic use should be tested for *C. difficile* (see "Laboratory Tests").
- Sigmoidoscopy (without cleansing enema) may be necessary when the clinical and laboratory diagnosis is inconclusive and the diarrhea persists.
- In antibiotic-induced pseudomembranous colitis, the sigmoidoscopy often reveals raised white-yellow exudative plaques adherent to the colonic mucosa (Fig. 1-223).

■ LABORATORY TESTS
- *C. difficile* toxin can be detected by cytotoxin tissue-culture assay (gold standard for identifying *C. difficile* toxin in stool specimen) and by enzyme-linked immunoabsorbent assay (ELISA) for *C. difficile* toxins A and B. The latter is used most widely in the clinical setting. It has a sensitivity of 85% and a specificity of 100%.
- Fecal leukocytes (assessed by microscopy or lactoferrin assay) are generally present in stool samples.
- CBC usually reveals leukocytosis.

■ IMAGING STUDIES
Abdominal film (flat plate and upright) is useful in patients with abdominal pain or evidence of obstruction on physical examination.

TREATMENT

■ NONPHARMACOLOGIC THERAPY
- Discontinue offending antibiotic
- Fluid hydration and correct electrolyte abnormalities

■ ACUTE GENERAL Rx
- Metronidazole 250 mg PO qid for 10 to 14 days
- Vancomycin 125 mg PO qid for 10 to 14 days in cases resistant to metronidazole
- Cholestyramine 4 g PO qid for 10 days in addition to metronidazole to control severe diarrhea (avoid use with vancomycin)
- When parenteral therapy is necessary (e.g., patient with paralytic ileus), IV metronidazole 500 mg qid can be used. It can also be supplemented with vancomycin 500 mg via NG tube or enema

■ CHRONIC Rx
Judicious future use of antibiotics to prevent recurrences (e.g., avoid prolonged antibiotic therapy)

■ DISPOSITION
Most patients recover completely with appropriate therapy. Fever resolves within 48 hr and diarrhea within 4 to 5 days. Mortality exceeds 10% in untreated patients.

■ REFERRAL
Hospital admission and IV hydration in severe cases

☼ PEARLS & CONSIDERATIONS

■ COMMENTS
Possible complications of pseudomembranous colitis include dehydration, bowel perforation, toxic megacolon, electrolyte imbalance, and reactive arthritis.

REFERENCES
Bartlett JG: Antibiotic-associated diarrhea, *N Engl J Med* 346:334, 2002.
Hurley BW, Nguyen CC: The spectrum of pseudomembranous enterocolitis and antibiotic-associated diarrhea, *Arch Intern Med* 162:2177, 2002.
Author: **Fred F. Ferri, M.D.**

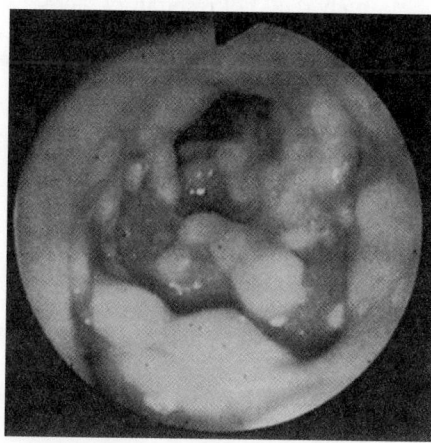

Fig. 1-223 Pseudomembranous plaques seen with colonoscopy in a patient with *C. difficile*-associated PMC. (From Gorbach SL: *Infectious diseases,* ed 2, Philadelphia, 1998, WB Saunders.)

BASIC INFORMATION

■ DEFINITION

Psittacosis is a systemic infection caused by *Chlamydia psittaci*.

■ SYNONYMS

Ornithosis

ICD-9CM CODES

073.9 Psittacosis

■ EPIDEMIOLOGY & DEMOGRAPHICS

INCIDENCE (IN U.S.):
- 45 cases reported in 1996
- True incidence possibly higher because infections may be subclinical
- Highest incidence among pet owners and people working in contact with birds

PREVALENCE (IN U.S.):
- Low among humans
- Organism carried in 5% to 8% of birds

PREDOMINANT SEX: Equal sex distribution

PREDOMINANT AGE: More common in adults

PEAK INCIDENCE: 30 to 60 yr of age

■ PHYSICAL FINDINGS & CLINICAL PRESENTATION

- Incubation period of 5 to 15 days
- Subclinical infection
- Onset abrupt or insidious
- Most common symptoms:
  1. Fever
  2. Myalgias
  3. Chills
  4. Cough
- Most common clinical syndrome: atypical pneumonia with fever, headache, dry cough, and a chest x-ray more dramatically abnormal than the physical examination
- Ranges from mild disease to respiratory failure and death, although this is extremely unusual
- Other clinical presentations:
  1. Mononucleosis-like syndrome
  2. Typhoidal form
- Most frequent physical findings:
  1. Fever
  2. Pharyngeal erythema
  3. Rales
  4. Hepatomegaly
- Less common findings:
  1. Somnolence
  2. Confusion
  3. Relative bradycardia
  4. Pleural rub
  5. Adenopathy
  6. Splenomegaly
  7. Horder's spots (pink blanching maculopapular rash)

- Besides the lungs, other specific end-organ involvement:
  1. Pericarditis
  2. Myocarditis
  3. Endocarditis
  4. Hepatitis
  5. Joints
  6. Kidneys (glomerulonephritis)
  7. CNS

■ ETIOLOGY

- *Chlamydia psittaci* is an obligate intracellular bacterium.
- Infection is usually spread by the respiratory route from infected birds.
- There is a history of exposure to birds in 85% of patients.
- Strains from turkeys and psittacine birds are most virulent for humans.
- Cows, goats, and sheep are occasionally implicated.

DIAGNOSIS

■ DIFFERENTIAL DIAGNOSIS

- *Legionella*
- *Mycoplasma*
- *Chlamydia pneumoniae* (TWAR)
- Viral respiratory infections
- Bacterial pneumonia
- Typhoid fever
- Viral hepatitis
- Aseptic meningitis
- Fever of unknown origin
- Mononucleosis

■ WORKUP

- CBC, renal and liver function tests
- *Chlamydia* serology
- Chest x-ray examination
- Special immunostaining of respiratory secretions

■ LABORATORY TESTS

- WBC count is normal or slightly elevated.
- Mild liver function abnormalities are common (50%).
- Blood cultures are almost always negative.
- Studies on respiratory secretions:
  1. Direct immunofluorescent antibody (DFA) of respiratory secretions with monoclonal antibodies to chlamydial antigens
  2. Chlamydial LPS (lipopolysaccharide) antigen by enzyme immunoassay (EIA)
  3. Polymerase chain reaction (PCR)
- Serologic studies:
  1. Complement-fixing antibodies
  2. Microimmunofluorescence
  3. Possible false-negative results and cross-reaction with other chlamydial species with both techniques

■ IMAGING STUDIES

- Chest x-ray examination is abnormal in 50% to 90% with a variety of patterns.
- Pleural effusions are common.

TREATMENT

■ NONPHARMACOLOGIC THERAPY

Oxygen supplementation as needed

■ ACUTE GENERAL Rx

- Tetracycline (500 mg PO qid) *or*
- Doxycycline (100 mg PO bid) *or*
- Erythromycin (500 mg PO qid): less effective

■ CHRONIC Rx

In the rare cases of endocarditis, combination of heart valve replacement and prolonged antibiotic course may be the treatment of choice.

■ DISPOSITION

- Mortality low (0.7%)
- Poor prognostic factors:
  1. Advanced age
  2. Leukopenia
  3. Severe hypoxemia
  4. Renal failure
  5. Confusion
  6. Multilobe pulmonary involvement
- Possible reinfection

■ REFERRAL

- To infectious disease expert:
  1. Complicated atypical pneumonia or other end-organ involvement
  2. Suspicion of an outbreak
- To pulmonologist for diagnostic bronchoscopy

PEARLS & CONSIDERATIONS

■ COMMENTS

- Hospitalized patients do not require specific isolation precautions.
- Any confirmed or suspected case of psittacosis should be reported to public health authorities.

REFERENCES

Centers for Disease Control and Prevention: Compendium of measures to control *Chlamydia psittaci* and pet birds (avian chlamydiosis), 1998, *MMWR* 47(RR-10):1, 1998.

Elliott JH: Psittacosis: a flu-like syndrome, *Aust Fam Physician* 30(8):739, 2001.

Author: **Michele Halpern, M.D.**

BASIC INFORMATION

■ DEFINITION

Psoriasis is a chronic skin disorder characterized by excessive proliferation of keratinocytes, resulting in the formation of thickened scaly plaques, itching, and inflammatory changes of the epidermis and dermis. The various forms of psoriasis include guttate, pustular, and arthritis variants.

ICD-9CM CODES

696.0 Psoriasis, arthritis, arthropathic
696.1 Psoriasis, any type except arthropathic

■ EPIDEMIOLOGY & DEMOGRAPHICS

- Psoriasis affects 1% to 3% of the world's population. Most patients have limited psoriasis involving <5% of their body surface.
- There is a strong association between psoriasis and HLA B13, B17, and B27 (pustular psoriasis).
- Peak age of onset is bimodal (adolescents and at 60 yr of age).
- Men and women are equally affected.

■ PHYSICAL FINDINGS & CLINICAL PRESENTATION

- The primary psoriatic lesion is an erythematous papule topped by a loosely adherent scale. Scraping the scale results in several bleeding points (Auspitz sign).
- Chronic plaque psoriasis generally manifests with symmetric, sharply demarcated, erythromatous, silver-scaled patches affecting primarily the intergluteal folds, elbows, scalp, fingernails, toenails, and knees (Fig. 1-224, *A*). This form accounts for 80% of psoriasis cases.
- Psoriasis can also develop at the site of any physical trauma (sunburn, scratching). This is known as Koebner's phenomenon.
- Nail involvement is common (pitting of the nail plate), resulting in hyperkeratosis, onychodystrophy with onycholysis (Fig. 1-224, *B*).

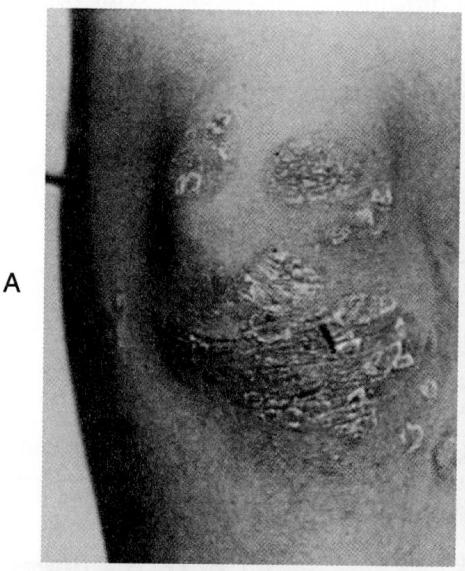

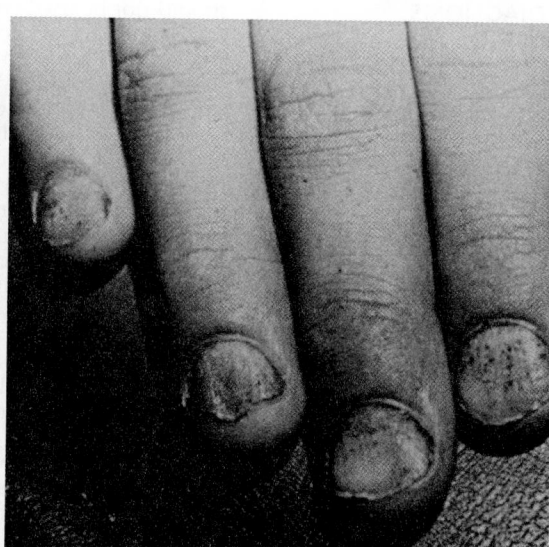

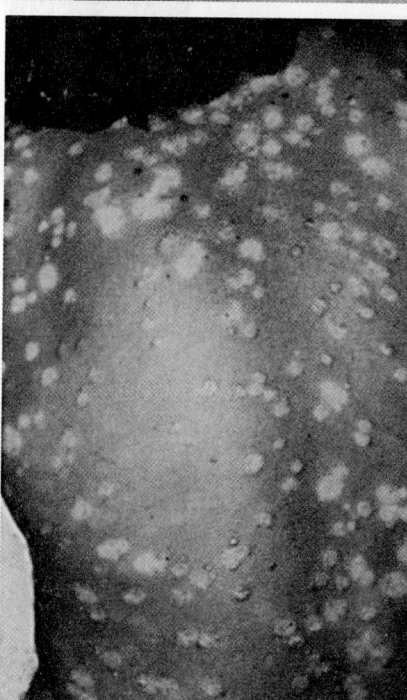

Fig. 1-224 **A,** Chronic psoriatic plaques on the knee. **B,** Psoriatic nail changes of pitting and dystrophy. **C,** Guttate psoriasis in widespread distribution over the trunk. (From Behrman RE: *Nelson textbook of pediatrics,* ed 16, Philadelphia, 2000, WB Saunders.)

- Pruritus is variable.
- Joint involvement can result in sacroiliitis and spondylitis.
- Guttate psoriasis is generally preceded by streptococcal pharyngitis and manifests with multiple drop-like lesions on the extremities and the trunk (Fig. 1-224, C).

■ ETIOLOGY
- Unknown
- Familial clustering (genetic transmission with a dominant mode with variable penetrants)
- One third of persons affected have a positive family history

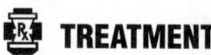 DIAGNOSIS

■ DIFFERENTIAL DIAGNOSIS
- Contact dermatitis
- Atopic dermatitis
- Stasis dermatitis
- Tinea
- Nummular dermatitis
- Candidiasis
- Mycosis fungoides
- Cutaneous SLE
- Secondary and tertiary syphilis
- Drug eruption

■ WORKUP
- Diagnosis is clinical.
- Skin biopsy is rarely necessary.

■ LABORATORY TESTS
Generally not necessary for diagnosis

℞ TREATMENT

■ NONPHARMACOLOGIC THERAPY
- Sunbathing generally leads to improvement.
- Eliminate triggering factors (e.g., stress, certain medications [e.g., lithium, β-blockers, antimalarials]).
- Patients with psoriasis benefit from a daily bath in warm water followed by application of a cream or ointment moisturizer. Regular use of an emollient moisturizer limits evaporation of water from the skin and allows the stratum corneum to rehydrate itself.

■ GENERAL Rx
Therapeutic options vary according to the extent of disease.

- Patients with limited disease (<20% of the body) can be treated with the following:
  1. Topical steroids: disadvantages are brief remissions, expense, and decreased effect with continued use. Salicylic acid can be compounded by pharmacist in concentrations of 2% to 10% and used in combination with a corticosteroid to decrease amount of scale.
  2. Calcipotriene (Dovonex): a vitamin D analogue, is effective for moderate plaque psoriasis; adults should comb the hair, apply solution to the lesions, and rub it in, avoiding uninvolved skin; disadvantages are its cost and potential burning and skin irritation. It should not be used concurrently with salicylic acid because calcipotriene is inactivated by the acidic nature of salicylic acid.
  3. Tar products (Estar, LCD, psoriGel) can be used overnight and are most effective when combined with UVB light (Goeckerman regimen).
  4. Anthralin (Drithocreme): useful for chronic plaques, can result in purple/brown staining; best used with UVB light.
  5. Retinoids such as tazarotene 0.05%, 0.1% cream or gel, are effective in thinning plaques but are expensive and can produce irritation.
  6. Other useful measures include tape or occlusive dressing, UVB and lubricating agents, interlesional steroids.
- Therapeutic options for persons with generalized disease (affecting >20% of the body):
  1. UVB light exposure three times a week
  2. Oral PUVA (psoralen plus ultraviolet A) administered two to three times weekly is effective for generalized disease. However, many treatments are required, necessitating frequent office visits, and it may be associated with phototoxicity, such as erythema and blistering, and increased risk of skin cancer
- Systemic treatments include methotrexate 25 mg every week for severe psoriasis. Etretinate (Tegison) (a synthetic retinoid) is most effective for palmar-plantar pustular psoriasis. Dose is 0.5 to 1 mg/kg/day. It can cause liver enzyme and lipid abnormalities and is teratogenic.

- Cyclosporine is also effective in severe psoriasis; however, relapses are common.
- Chronic plaque psoriasis may be treated with alefacept, a recombinant protein that selectively targets T lymphocytes. Treatment with alefacept for 12 wk (0.025, 0.075, or 0.150 mg/kg of body weight IV weekly) may result in significant improvement. Some patients also experience a sustained clinical response after the cessation of treatment. This medication is very expensive (a 12-wk course costs >$8,000). Treatment with etanercept, a tumor necrosis factor (TNF) antagonist, for 24 wk can also lead to a reduction in severity of plaque psoriasis. Efalizumab, a humanized monoclonal antibody that inhibits the activation of T cells, has also been reported to produce significant improvement in plaque psoriasis over a 24-wk treatment period.

■ DISPOSITION
The course of psoriasis is chronic, and the disease may be refractory to treatment.

■ REFERRAL
- Dermatology referral is recommended in all patients with generalized disease.
- Hospital admission may be necessary for severe diffuse or poorly responsive psoriasis. The Goeckerman regimen combines daily application of tar with UVB exposure and can result in prolonged remissions.

✷ PEARLS & CONSIDERATIONS

■ COMMENTS
Psoriasis is more emotionally than physically disabling for most patients. Counseling may be indicated, particularly when it affects younger patients.

REFERENCES
Gordon KB et al: Efalizumab for patients with moderate to severe plaque psoriasis, *JAMA* 290:3073, 2003.
Leonardi CL et al: Etanercept as monotherapy in patients with psoriasis, *N Engl J Med* 349: 2014, 2003.
Author: **Fred F. Ferri, M.D.**

BASIC INFORMATION

■ DEFINITION
Cardiogenic pulmonary edema is a life-threatening condition caused by severe left ventricular decompensation.

■ SYNONYMS
Cardiogenic pulmonary edema

ICD-9CM CODES
428.1 Acute pulmonary edema with heart disease

■ PHYSICAL FINDINGS & CLINICAL PRESENTATION
- Dyspnea with rapid, shallow breathing
- Diaphoresis, perioral and peripheral cyanosis
- Pink, frothy sputum
- Moist, bilateral pulmonary rales
- Increased pulmonary second sound, S_3 gallop (in association with tachycardia)
- Bulging neck veins

■ ETIOLOGY
Increased pulmonary capillary pressure secondary to:
- Acute myocardial infarction
- Exacerbation of CHF
- Valvular regurgitation
- Ventricular septal defect
- Severe myocardial ischemia
- Mitral stenosis
- Other: cardiac tamponade, endocarditis, myocarditis, arrhythmias, cardiomyopathy, hypertensive crisis

DIAGNOSIS

■ DIFFERENTIAL DIAGNOSIS
- Noncardiogenic pulmonary edema
- Pulmonary embolism
- Exacerbation of asthma
- Exacerbation of COPD
- Sarcoidosis
- Pulmonary fibrosis
- Viral pneumonitis and other pulmonary infections

■ LABORATORY TESTS
ABGs: respiratory and metabolic acidosis, decreased Pao_2, increased Pco_2, low pH.
NOTE: The patient may initially show respiratory alkalosis secondary to hyperventilation in attempts to maintain Pao_2.

■ IMAGING STUDIES
- Chest x-ray examination:
  1. Pulmonary congestion with Kerley B lines; fluffy perihilar infiltrates in the early stages; bilateral interstitial alveolar infiltrates
  2. Pleural effusions
- Echocardiogram:
  1. Useful to evaluate valvular abnormalities, diastolic vs. systolic dysfunction

2. Can aid in differentiation of cardiogenic vs. noncardiogenic pulmonary edema
  3. Can also estimate pulmonary capillary wedge pressure and rule out presence of myxoma or atrial thrombus
- Right heart catheterization (selected patients): cardiac pressures and cardiogenic pulmonary edema reveal increased PADP and PCWP ≥25 mm Hg

TREATMENT

■ NONPHARMACOLOGIC THERAPY
Patients should be placed in a sitting position with legs off the side of the bed to improve breathing and decrease venous return.

■ ACUTE GENERAL Rx
All the following steps can be performed concomitantly:
- 100% oxygen by face mask. Both CPAP and BiPAP systems can improve oxygenation and lower carbon dioxide tensions. Check ABGs; if marked hypoxemia or severe respiratory acidosis, intubate the patient and place on a ventilator. Positive end-expiratory pressure (PEEP) increases functional capacity and improves oxygenation.
- Furosemide: 1 mg/kg IV bolus (typically 40 to 100 mg) to rapidly establish diuresis and decrease venous return through its venodilator action; may double the dose in 30 min if no effect.
- Vasodilator therapy:
  1. Nitrates: particularly useful if the patient has concomitant chest pain.
     a. Nitroglycerin: 150 to 600 μg SL or nitroglycerin spray (Nitrolingual) may be given immediately on arrival and repeated multiple times if the patient remains symptomatic and blood pressure remains stable.
     b. 2% nitroglycerin ointment: 1 to 3 inches out of the tube applied continuously; absorption may be erratic.
     c. IV nitroglycerin: 100 mg in 500 ml of D_5W solution; start at 6 μg/min (2 ml/hr).
  2. Nitroprusside: useful for afterload reduction in hypertensive patients with decreased cardiac index (CI).
     a. Increases the CI and decreases left ventricular filling pressure.
     b. Vasodilator and diuretic therapy should be tailored to achieve PCWP ≤18 mm Hg, RAP ≤8 mm Hg, systolic blood pressure >90 mm Hg, SVR >1200 dynes/sec/cm⁻5. The

use of nitroprusside in patients with acute MI is controversial because it may intensify ischemia by decreasing the blood flow to the ischemic left ventricular myocardium.
  3. Nesiritide (Natrecor) is a B-type natriuretic peptide has venous, arterial, and coronary vasodilatory properties that decrease preload and afterload and increase cardiac output without direct inotropic effects. It is effective in cardiogenic pulmonary edema.
  4. Morphine: 2 to 4 mg IV/SC/IM, may repeat q15min prn. It decreases venous return, anxiety, and systemic vascular resistance (naloxone should be available at bedside to reverse the effects of morphine if respiratory depression occurs). Morphine may induce hypotension in volume-depleted patients.
  5. Afterload reduction with ACE inhibitors. Captopril 25 mg PO tablet can be used for SL administration (placing a drop or two of water on the tablet and placing it under the tongue helps dissolve it), onset of action is <10 min, peak effect can be reached in 30 min. ACE inhibitors can also be given IV (e.g., enalaprilat 1 mg IV given q2h prn).
  6. Dobutamine: parenteral inotropic agent of choice in severe cases of cardiogenic pulmonary edema. It can be administered at a dosage of 2.5 to 10 μg/kg/min IV. IV phosphodiesterase inhibitors (amrinone, milrinone) may be useful in refractory cases.
  7. Aminophylline: useful *only* if patient has concomitant severe bronchospasm.
  8. Digitalis: limited use in acute pulmonary edema caused by MI, may be useful in pulmonary edema resulting from atrial fibrillation or flutter with a fast ventricular response.
  9. Acute cardiogenic pulmonary edema caused by IHSS must be treated with IV normal saline solution and negative inotropic agents such as verapamil and β-blockers.

■ DISPOSITION
- Mortality for cardiogenic pulmonary edema is approximately 60% to 80%.

REFERENCE
Gandhi SU et al: The pathogenesis of acute pulmonary edema associated with hypertension, *N Engl J Med* 344:17, 2001.
Author: **Fred F. Ferri, M.D.**

BASIC INFORMATION

■ **DEFINITION**

Pulmonary embolism (PE) refers to the lodging of a thrombus or other embolic material from a distant site in the pulmonary circulation.

■ **SYNONYMS**

Pulmonary thromboembolism
PE

ICD-9CM CODES

415.1 Pulmonary embolism and infarction

■ **EPIDEMIOLOGY & DEMOGRAPHICS**

• 650,000 cases of PE occur in the U.S. each year; 50,000 result in death (increased incidence in women and with advanced age).
• More than 90% of pulmonary emboli originate in the deep venous system of the lower extremities.
• Pulmonary thromboembolism is associated with >200,000 hospitalizations each year in the U.S.
• 8% to 10% of victims of PE die within the first hour.

■ **PHYSICAL FINDINGS & CLINICAL PRESENTATION**

• Most common symptom: dyspnea
• Chest pain: may be nonpleuritic or pleuritic (infarction)
• Syncope (massive PE)
• Fever, diaphoresis, apprehension
• Hemoptysis, cough
• Evidence of DVT may be present (e.g., swelling and tenderness of extremities)
• Cardiac examination: may reveal tachycardia, increased pulmonic component of S_2, murmur of tricuspid insufficiency, right ventricular heave, right-sided S_3
• Pulmonary examination: may demonstrate rales, localized wheezing, friction rub
• Most common physical finding: tachypnea

■ **ETIOLOGY**

• Thrombus, fat, or other foreign material
• Risk factors for PE:
  1. Prolonged immobilization
  2. Postoperative state
  3. Trauma to lower extremities
  4. Estrogen-containing birth control pills
  5. Prior history of DVT or PE
  6. CHF
  7. Pregnancy and early puerperium
  8. Visceral cancer (lung, pancreas, alimentary and genitourinary tracts)
  9. Trauma, burns
  10. Advanced age
  11. Obesity
  12. Hematologic disease (e.g., antithrombin III deficiency, protein C deficiency, protein S deficiency, lupus anticoagulant, polycythemia vera, dysfibrinogenemia, paroxysmal nocturnal hemoglobinuria, factor V Leiden mutation, G20210A prothrombin mutation)
  13. COPD, diabetes mellitus
  14. Prolonged air travel

🔬 **DIAGNOSIS**

■ **DIFFERENTIAL DIAGNOSIS**

• Myocardial infarction
• Pericarditis
• Pneumonia
• Pneumothorax
• Chest wall pain
• GI abnormalities (e.g., peptic ulcer, esophageal rupture, gastritis)
• CHF
• Pleuritis
• Anxiety disorder with hyperventilation
• Pericardial tamponade
• Dissection of aorta
• Asthma

■ **WORKUP**

• It is important to remember that no single noninvasive test has both high sensitivity and high specificity for PE. Consequently, in addition to clinical assessment, most patients will require several noninvasive tests or pulmonary angiography to diagnose PE.
• Spiral CT of chest or lung scan may be diagnostic. Pulmonary angiogram (when indicated) will confirm the diagnosis.
• Serial compressive duplex ultrasonography of lower extremities can be used in patients with "low-probability" lung scan and high clinical suspicion (see "Imaging Studies"). It is useful if positive, negative results do not exclude pulmonary embolism.

■ **LABORATORY TESTS**

• ABGs generally reveal decreased Pao_2 and $Paco_2$ and increased pH; normal results do not rule out PE.
• Alveolar-arteriolar (A-a) oxygen gradient, a measure of the difference in oxygen concentration between alveoli and arterial blood, is a more sensitive indicator of the alteration in oxygenation than Pao_2; it can easily be calculated using the information from ABGs; a normal A-a gradient among patients without history of PE or DVT makes the diagnosis of PE unlikely.
• Plasma D-dimer measurement: D-dimer assays by ELISA detect the presence of plasmin-mediated degradation products of fibrin that contain cross-linked D fragments in the whole blood or plasma. A normal plasma D-dimer level is useful to exclude pulmonary embolism in patients with a nondiagnostic lung scan and a low pretest probability of PE. However, it cannot be used to "rule in" the diagnosis because it increases with many other disorders (e.g., metastatic cancer, trauma, sepsis, postoperative state). Plasma D-dimer can also be used in conjunction with lower-extremity compression ultrasonography in patients with indeterminate V/Q and spiral CT scans. Absence of DVT and presence of a normal D-dimer level in these settings generally rules out clinically significant pulmonary embolism.
• Elevated cardiac troponin levels also occur in patients with pulmonary embolism because of right ventricular dilation and myocardial injury; therefore, PE should be considered in the differential diagnosis of all patients presenting with chest pain or dyspnea and elevated cardiac troponin levels.
• ECG is abnormal in 85% of patients with acute PE. Frequent abnormalities are sinus tachycardia; nonspecific ST-segment or T wave changes; S-I, Q-III, T-III pattern (10% of patients); S-I, S-II, S-III pattern; T wave inversion in V_1 to V_6; acute RBBB; new-onset atrial fibrillation; ST segment depression in lead II; right ventricular strain.

■ **IMAGING STUDIES**

• Chest x-ray film may be normal; suggestive findings include elevated diaphragm, pleural effusion, dilation of pulmonary artery, infiltrate or consolidation, abrupt vessel cut-off, or atelectasis. A wedge-shaped consolidation in the middle and lower lobes is suggestive of a pulmonary infarction and is known as "Hampton's hump."
• Lung scan (in patient with normal chest x-ray examination):
  1. A normal lung scan rules out PE.
  2. A ventilation-perfusion mismatch is suggestive of PE, and a lung scan interpretation of high probability is confirmatory.
  3. If the clinical suspicion of PE is high and the lung scan is interpreted as low probability, moderate probability, or indeterminate, a pulmonary arteriogram is diagnostic; a positive arteriogram confirms diagnosis; a positive compressive duplex ultrasonogra-

phy for DVT obviates the need for an arteriogram, because treatment with IV anticoagulants is indicated in these patients; the overall sensitivity of compressive ultrasonography for DVT in patients with PE is 29%, specificity 97%; adding ultrasonography in patients with a nondiagnostic lung scan prevents 9% of angiographies; however, this improvement in efficacy is achieved at the cost of unnecessary anticoagulant therapy in 26% of patients who have false-positive ultrasonography results.

- Spiral CT is an excellent modality for diagnosing PE. It may be used in place of the lung scan and is favored in patients with baseline lung abnormalities on initial chest x-ray. It has the added advantage of detecting other pulmonary pathology that can mimic pulmonary embolism.

- Angiography: pulmonary angiography is the gold standard; however, it is invasive, expensive, and not readily available in some clinical settings. False-positive pulmonary angiograms may result from mediastinal disorders such as radiation fibrosis and tumors. CT angiography is an accurate, noninvasive tool in the diagnosis of PE at the main, lobar, and segmental pulmonary artery levels. A major advantage of CT angiography over standard pulmonary angiography is its ability to diagnose intrathoracic disease other than PE that may account for the patient's clinical picture. It is also less invasive, less costly, and more widely available. Its major shortcoming is its poor sensitivity for subsegmental emboli. Gadolinium-enhanced magnetic resonance angiography of the pulmonary arteries has a moderate sensitivity and high specificity for the diagnosis of PE; MRA is best reserved for selected patients when CT scan and/or lung scan are inconclusive and the risk of pulmonary angiography is high.

℞ TREATMENT

■ NONPHARMACOLOGIC THERAPY
Correction of risk factors (see "Etiology") to prevent future PE

■ ACUTE GENERAL Rx
- Heparin by continuous infusion for at least 5 days; many experts recommend a larger initial IV heparin bolus (15,000 to 20,000 U) to block platelet aggregation and thrombi and subsequent release of vasoconstrictive substances.
- Thrombolytic agents (urokinase, tPA, streptokinase): provide rapid resolution of clots; thrombolytic agents are the treatment of choice in patients with massive PE who are hemodynamically unstable and with no contraindication to their use. The use of thrombolytic agents in the treatment of hemodynamically stable patients with acute submassive pulmonary embolism remains controversial. Use of the thrombolytic agents alteplase (100 mg IV over a 2-hr period) in normotensive patients with moderate or severe right ventricular dysfunction identified by echocardiography has been advocated by some physicians. Use of alteplase in conjunction with heparin has been shown to improve the clinical course of stable patients who have acute submassive PE without internal bleeding. Additional studies are needed to confirm these findings before recommending routine use of this therapeutic approach.
- Long-term treatment is generally carried out with warfarin therapy started on day 1 or 2 and given in a dose to maintain the INR at 2 to 3.
- If thrombolytics and anticoagulants are contraindicated (e.g., GI bleeding, recent CNS surgery, recent trauma) or if the patient continues to have recurrent PE despite anticoagulation therapy, vena caval interruption is indicated by transvenous placement of a Greenfield vena caval filter.
- Acute pulmonary artery embolectomy may be indicated in a patient with massive pulmonary emboli and refractory hypotension.

■ CHRONIC Rx
Elimination of risk factors (see "Etiology") and monitoring of warfarin dose with INR on a routine basis

■ DISPOSITION
- Mortality can be reduced to <10% by rapid and effective treatment.
- Mortality from recurrent pulmonary emboli is 8% with effective treatment and >30% in patients with untreated pulmonary emboli.

☼ PEARLS & CONSIDERATIONS

■ COMMENTS
- The duration of oral anticoagulant treatment is 6 mo in patients with reversible risk factors and indefinitely in patients with persistence of risk factors that caused the initial PE.
- Patients should be educated about the need for compliance with long-term anticoagulation therapy.

REFERENCES

Agnelli G et al: Extended oral anticoagulant therapy after a first episode of pulmonary embolism, *Ann Intern Med* 139:19, 2003.

Almoosa K: Is thrombolytic therapy effective for pulmonary embolism? *Am Fam Physician* 65:1097, 2002.

Douketis JD et al: Elevated cardiac troponin levels in patients with submassive pulmonary embolism, *Arch Intern Med* 162:79, 2002.

Fedullo PF, Tapson VF: The evaluation of suspected pulmonary embolism, *N Engl J Med* 349:1247, 2003.

Goldhaber SZ: Echocardiography in the management of pulmonary embolism, *Ann Intern Med* 136:691, 2002.

Konstantinides S et al: Heparin plus alteplase compared with heparin alone in patients with submassive pulmonary embolism, *N Engl J Med* 347:1143, 2002.

Konstantinides S et al: Importance of cardiac troponins I and T in risk stratification of patients with acute pulmonary embolism, *Circulation* 106:1263, 2002.

Kruip MJ et al: Use of a clinical decision rule in combination with d-dimer concentration in diagnostic workup of patients with suspected pulmonary embolism, *Arch Intern Med* 162:1631, 2002.

Oudkerk M et al: Comparison of contrast-enhanced magnetic resonance angiography and conventional pulmonary angiography for the diagnosis of pulmonary embolism: a prospective study, *Lancet* 359:1643, 2002.

Author: **Fred F. Ferri, M.D.**

BASIC INFORMATION

■ DEFINITION
The normal pulmonary arterial systolic pressure ranges from 18 to 30 mm Hg and the diastolic pressure ranges from 4 to 12 mm Hg. Pulmonary hypertension is a hemodynamic diagnosis. Pulmonary hypertension is diagnosed when pulmonary arterial systolic and mean pressures exceed 30 and 20 mm Hg, respectively. Pulmonary hypertension is classified as primary or secondary.

■ SYNONYMS
Primary pulmonary hypertension (PPH)
Secondary pulmonary hypertension

ICD-9CM CODES
416.0 Primary pulmonary hypertension
416.8 Secondary pulmonary hypertension

■ EPIDEMIOLOGY & DEMOGRAPHICS
• Primary pulmonary hypertension (PPH) is rare, occurring in 2 cases per 1 million people.
• PPH is more common in women than men (1.7:1), usually presenting in the third to fourth decade of life.
• PPH can be associated with portal hypertension and liver cirrhosis, appetite-suppressant drugs, and HIV disease.
• PPH may be familial.
• Secondary pulmonary hypertension is more common than PPH.
• Secondary pulmonary hypertension is the common pathophysiologic mechanism leading to cor pulmonale in patients with underlying pulmonary disease (e.g., COPD, pulmonary embolism).

■ PHYSICAL FINDINGS & CLINICAL PRESENTATION
Primary pulmonary hypertension:
• PPH is insidious and may go undetected for years
• Dyspnea is the most common presenting symptom (60%)
• Syncope
• Chest pain
• Loud P_2 component of the second heart sound
• Right-sided S_4
• Jugular venous distention
• Prominent parasternal (RV) impulse
• Holosystolic tricuspid regurgitation murmur heard best along the left fourth parasternal line that increases in intensity with inspiration
• Peripheral edema
Secondary pulmonary hypertension:
• Similar to PPH but depends on the underlying cause (e.g., left-sided CHF, mitral stenosis, COPD)

■ ETIOLOGY
• The etiology of PPH is unknown. Most cases are sporadic, but there is a 6% to 12% familial incidence.
• The pathogenesis of PPH is not known; however, an emerging theory involves abnormal membrane potassium channels modulating calcium kinetics.
• Secondary pulmonary hypertension is primarily caused by underlying pulmonary and cardiac conditions including:
  1. Pulmonary thromboembolic disease
  2. Chronic obstructive pulmonary disease (COPD)
  3. Interstitial lung disease
  4. Obstructive sleep disorder
  5. Neuromuscular diseases causing hypoventilation (e.g., ALS)
  6. Collagen-vascular disease (e.g., SLE, CREST, systemic sclerosis)
  7. Pulmonary venous disease
  8. Left ventricular failure resulting from hypertension, cad, aortic stenosis, and cardiomyopathy
  9. Valvular heart disease (e.g., mitral stenosis, mitral regurgitation)
  10. Congenital heart disease with left to right shunting (e.g., ASD)

DIAGNOSIS

Primary pulmonary hypertension is a diagnosis of exclusion; all secondary causes as mentioned under "Etiology" must be excluded.

■ DIFFERENTIAL DIAGNOSIS
The differential diagnosis is as listed under "Etiology."

■ WORKUP
The workup of a patient suspected of having PPH includes a detailed evaluation of the heart and lungs. Blood tests, chest x-ray, pulmonary function tests, CT scan of the chest, radionuclide studies of the heart and lungs, echocardiogram, electrocardiograms, pulmonary angiogram, and right and left heart catheterization are all required to exclude secondary causes of pulmonary hypertension.

■ LABORATORY TESTS
• CBC is usually normal in PPH but may show secondary polycythemia.
• ABGs show low PO_2 and oxygen saturation.
• PFT is done to exclude obstructive or restrictive lung disease.
• ECG may show evidence of both right atrial enlargement (tall P wave >2.5 mV in leads II, III, aVF) and right ventricular enlargement (right axis deviation >100 and R wave > S wave in lead V1).

■ IMAGING STUDIES
• Chest x-ray shows increase in central arteries with rapid tapering of the distal vessels (Fig. 1-225).
• Lung perfusion scan (V/Q scan) aids in excluding chronic pulmonary embolism.
• Echocardiogram including M-mode, 2 D, pulse, continuous and color Doppler assesses ventricular function, excludes significant valvular pathology, and visualizes abnormal shunting of blood between heart chambers if present.
• Pulmonary angiogram is done in patients with suspicious V/Q scans.
• Cardiac catheterization is performed to directly measure pulmonary artery pressures and to detect any shunting of blood.

TREATMENT

■ NONPHARMACOLOGIC THERAPY
• Oxygen therapy to improve alveolar oxygen flow in both primary and secondary pulmonary hypertension
• Avoidance of vigorous exercise
• Chest physiotherapy

■ ACUTE GENERAL Rx
• PPH
  1. Diuretics (e.g., furosemide 40 mg to 80 mg qd) improve dyspnea and peripheral edema.
  2. Digoxin 0.25 mg qd has been used in patients with PPH.
  3. Vasodilator treatment is usually done with hemodynamic monitoring and includes IV adenosine, prostacyclin, or nitric oxide.
• Secondary pulmonary hypertension treatment is aimed at the underlying cause (see specific disease in text for treatment).

■ CHRONIC Rx
• Chronic anticoagulation with warfarin is recommended to prevent thromboses and has been shown to prolong life in patients with PPH.
• Calcium channel blockers may alleviate pulmonary vasoconstriction and prolong life in about 20% of patients with PPH.
• Continuous infusion of epoprostenol, or prostacyclin, a short-acting vasodilator and inhibitor of platelet aggregation, improves exercise capacity, quality of life, hemodynamics, and long-term survival in patients with class III or IV function.
• Inhaled aerosolized prostacyclin, iloprost, 2.5 or 5.0 μg taken 6 to 9 × day improves exercise capacity, NYHA class, and clinical deterioration in patients with primary pulmonary hypertension and selected

forms of nonprimary pulmonary hypertension.

- The endothelin-receptor antagonist bosentan taken orally at a dose of 80-160 mg bid has been approved for the treatment of PPH and scleroderma pulmonary hypertension showing improvement in clinical class and exercise capacity. Newer selective and nonselective endothelin receptor antagonists are undergoing clinical trials.
- Combination therapy using inhaled iloprost taken 1 hr before oral sildenafil 12.5 or 50 mg causes pulmonary vasodilations and, pending future trials, may be considered treatment for pulmonary hypertension.
- Lung transplantation and heart-lung transplantation are other options in end-stage class IV patients.
- Lung transplant recipients with PPH had survival rates of 73% at 1 yr, 55% at 3 yr, and 45% at 5 yr.

■ DISPOSITION
- Class II and III patients with PPH have a mean survival of 3.5 yr.
- Class IV patients have a mean survival of 6 mo.

■ REFERRAL
If the diagnosis of PPH is suspected, a consultation with a pulmonary specialist is recommended. Secondary causes of pulmonary hypertension may require consultations with rheumatology, neurology, and cardiology.

☼ PEARLS & CONSIDERATIONS

■ COMMENTS
Factors contributing to pulmonary arterial hypertension are:
- Alveolar hypoxia
- Acidosis
- Thromboemboli occluding arterial blood vessels (e.g., pulmonary embolism)
- Scarring or destruction of alveolar walls (e.g., COPD, infiltrative disease)
- Primary thickening of arterial walls as occurs in PPH

REFERENCES
Chatterjee K, De Marco T, Alpert JS: Pulmonary hypertension: hemodynamic diagnosis and management, *Arch Intern Med* 162:1925, 2002.

Ghofrani HA et al: Combination therapy with oral sildenafil and inhaled iloprost for severe pulmonary hypertension, *Ann Intern Med* 136:515, 2002.

Krowka MJ: Pulmonary hypertension: diagnosis and therapeutics, *Mayo Clin Proc* 75:625, 2000.

Nauser T, Stites S: Diagnosis and treatment of pulmonary hypertension, *Am Fam Physician* 63:1789, 2001.

Olschewski H et al: Inhaled iloprost for severe pulmonary hypertension, *N Engl J Med* 347:322, 2002.

Rubin LJ et al: Bosentan therapy for pulmonary arterial hypertension, *N Engl J Med* 346:896, 2002.

Author: **Peter Petropoulos, M.D.**

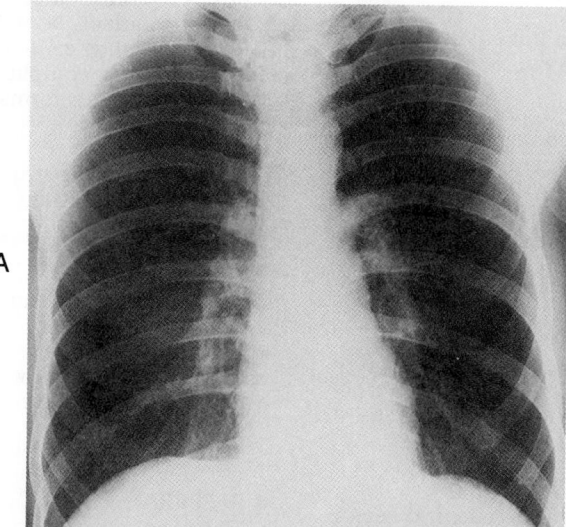

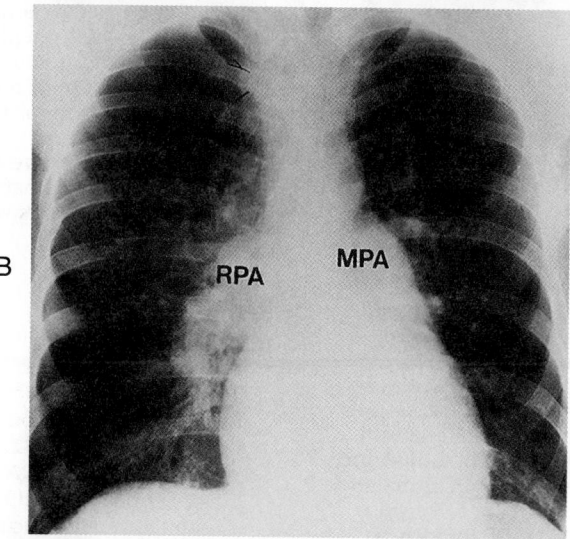

Fig. 1-225 Progressive pulmonary arterial hypertension. This patient initially presented with a relatively normal chest radiograph (**A**). However, several years later (**B**), there is increasing heart size as well as marked dilation of the main pulmonary artery *(MPA)* and right pulmonary artery *(RPA)*. Rapid tapering of the arteries as they proceed peripherally is suggestive of pulmonary hypertension and is sometimes referred to as pruning. (From Mettler FA [ed]: *Primary care radiology*, Philadelphia, 2000, WB Saunders.)

BASIC INFORMATION

■ DEFINITION
Pyelonephritis is an infection, usually bacterial in origin, of the upper urinary tract.

■ SYNONYMS
Acute pyelonephritis
Pyonephrosis
Renal carbuncle
Lobar nephronia
Acute bacterial nephritis

ICD-9CM CODES
590.81 Pyelonephritis
599.0 Urinary tract infection
595.9 Cystitis

■ EPIDEMIOLOGY & DEMOGRAPHICS
INCIDENCE (IN U.S.): Extremely common
PREDOMINANT SEX: Female
PREDOMINANT AGE:
- Sexually active years in women
- Usually >50 yr of age in men
PEAK INCIDENCE: See "Incidence."
GENETICS:
Congenital Infection: Congenital urologic structural disorders may predispose to infections at an early age.

■ PHYSICAL FINDINGS & CLINICAL PRESENTATION
- Fever
- Rigors
- Chills
- Flank pain
- Dysuria
- Polyuria
- Hematuria
- Toxic feeling and appearance
- Nausea and vomiting
- Headache
- Diarrhea
- Physical examination notable
  1. Costovertebral angle tenderness
  2. Exquisite flank pain

■ ETIOLOGY
- Gram-negative bacilli such as *E. coli* and *Klebsiella* spp. in more than 95% of cases
- Other, more unusual gram-negative organisms, especially if instrumentation of the urinary system has occurred
- Resistant gram-negative organisms or even fungi in hospitalized patients with indwelling catheters
- Gram-positive organisms such as enterococci
- *Staphylococcus aureus:* presence in urine indicates hematogenous origin
- Viruses: rarely, but these are usually limited to the lower tract

DIAGNOSIS

■ DIFFERENTIAL DIAGNOSIS
- Nephrolithiasis
- Appendicitis
- Ovarian cyst torsion or rupture
- Acute glomerulonephritis
- PID
- Endometritis
- Other causes of acute abdomen
- Perinephric abscess
- Hydronephrosis

■ WORKUP
- No workup in sexually active women
- Poorly responding infections, especially with azotemia and frank bacteremia
  1. Renal sonogram
  2. IVP
  3. To assess for underlying urologic pathology such as hydronephrosis
- Urologic imaging studies in all young men and boys
- Prostate assessment in older men

■ LABORATORY TESTS
- CBC with differential
- Renal panel
- Blood cultures
- Urine cultures
- Urinalysis
- Gram stain of urine
- Urgent renal sonography if obstruction or closed space infection suspected
- CT scans may better define the extent of collections of pus
- Helical CT scans excellent to detect calculi

TREATMENT

■ ACUTE GENERAL Rx
- Hospitalization for:
  1. Toxic patients
  2. Complicated infections
  3. Diabetes
  4. Suspected bacteremia
- Keep patients well hydrated.
- IV fluids are indicated for those unable to take adequate amounts of liquids.
- Give antipyretics such as acetaminophen when necessary.
- Antibiotic therapy should be initiated after cultures are obtained and guided by the results of culture and sensitivity testing.
  1. Oral TMP-SMX DS (bid for 10 days) or ciprofloxacin (500 mg orally bid for 10 days): adequate for stable patients who can tolerate oral medications with sensitive pathogens
  2. TMP-SMX or ciprofloxacin IV for more toxic patients

3. Ceftazidime 1 g IV q6-8h
4. Aminoglycosides such as gentamicin (2 mg/kg IV load followed by 1 mg/kg IV q8h adjusted for renal function) added but nephrotoxic especially in diabetics with azotemia
5. Vancomycin 1 g IV q12h to cover gram-positive cocci such as enterococci or staphylococci
6. Ampicillin 1 to 2 g IV q4-6h to cover enterococci, but an aminoglycoside is needed for synergy
7. Oral ampicillin or amoxicillin: no longer adequate for therapy of gram-negative infections because of resistance
- Prompt drainage with nephrostomy tube placement for obstruction
- Surgical drainage of large collections of pus to control infection
- Diabetic patients, as well as those with indwelling catheters, are especially prone to complicated infections and abscess formation

■ CHRONIC Rx
- Repair underlying structural problems, especially when renal function is compromised.
  1. Reflux
  2. Obstruction
  3. Nephrolithiasis should be considered
- Patients with diabetes mellitus and indwelling urinary catheters are at particular risk of severe and complicated infections.
- When possible, remove catheters.

■ REFERRAL
- To surgeon: surgical correction of underlying urologic problems, such as reflux and hydronephrosis
- To pediatrician: in young children, prompt correction of reflux to avoid recurrent infections as well as loss of renal function
- To internist: aggressive metabolic as well as urologic evaluation and treatment for patients with nephrolithiasis

REFERENCES
Benador D et al: Randomised controlled trial of three day versus 10 day intravenous antibiotics in acute pyelonephritis: effect on renal scarring, *Arch Dis Child* 84(3):241, 2001.
Foresman WH, Hulbert WC, Rabinowitz R: Does urinary tract ultrasonography at hospitalization for acute pyelonephritis predict vesicoureteral reflux? *J Urol* 165(6 pt 2):2232, 2001.
Vosti KL: Infections of the urinary tract in women: a prospective, longitudinal study of 235 women observed for 1-19 years, *Medicine* 81(5):369, 2002.

Author: **Joseph J. Lieber, M.D.**

BASIC INFORMATION

■ DEFINITION

Pyogenic granuloma is a benign vascular lesion of the skin and mucus membranes. They are a result of capillary proliferation generally secondary to trauma.

ICD-9CM CODES

686.1 Pyogenic granuloma

■ EPIDEMIOLOGY & DEMOGRAPHICS

• Common in children and young adults
• Caused by trauma or surgery
• Occur more frequently during pregnancy

■ PHYSICAL FINDINGS & CLINICAL PRESENTATION

• Small (<1 cm), yellow-to-red, dome-shaped lesions (Fig 1-226)
• May have surrounding scale at base
• Most commonly found on the head, neck, and extremities
• Often found on the gingiva during pregnancy (called *epulis*)

■ ETIOLOGY

Trauma causing focal capillary growth

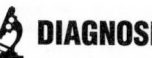 **DIAGNOSIS**

■ DIFFERENTIAL DIAGNOSIS

Amelanotic melanoma

■ WORKUP

Diagnosis is based on clinical history and appearance. Generally begins with trauma followed by the development of an erythematous papule. The lesion tends to bleed easily and develops over several days to weeks.

■ LABORATORY TESTS

Pathologic examination should be performed after excision to rule out melanoma

 TREATMENT

■ ACUTE GENERAL Rx

• Excision: using 1% lidocaine for anesthesia, shave or curette at base and border. Follow with electrocauterization or cryotherapy.

• Pregnancy epulis generally resolve spontaneously following childbirth.

■ REFERRAL

Dermatology referral recommended if lesion recurs or multiple satellite lesions occur after excision.

✸ PEARLS & CONSIDERATIONS

■ ACUTE GENERAL Rx

• Removal of entire lesion is essential because lesions may recur at the site of residual tissue.

Author: **Jennifer R. Souther, M.D.**

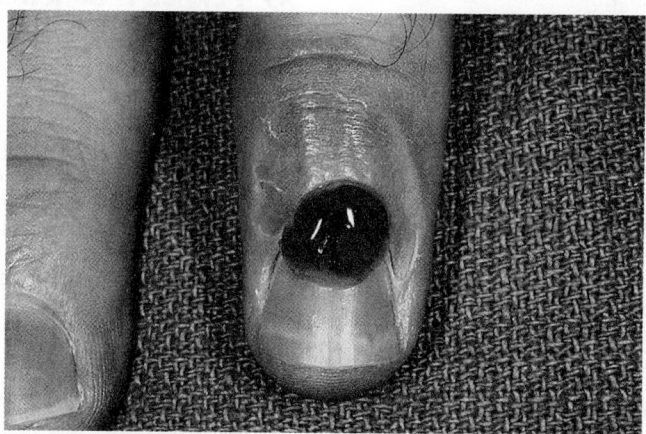

Fig. 1-226   Pyogenic granuloma. Often the lesions have a collar or moat. (From Callen JP [ed]: *Color atlas of dermatology,* ed 2, Philadelphia, 2000, WB Saunders.)

BASIC INFORMATION

■ DEFINITION
Q fever is a systemic febrile illness caused by *Coxiella burnetii* that may be acute or chronic.

■ SYNONYMS
C. burnetii infection

■ ICD-9CM CODES
083.0 Q fever

■ EPIDEMIOLOGY & DEMOGRAPHICS
- *C. burnetii* is found worldwide.
- Common animal reservoirs are cattle, sheep, and goats.
- Most cases are found in individuals who have direct contact with infected animals (e.g., farmers, veterinarians) or who are exposed to contaminated animal urine, feces, milk, or placental tissues.
- Q fever is seen more in men than in women (3:1).

■ PHYSICAL FINDINGS & CLINICAL PRESENTATION
Acute Q fever presentation:
- Fever
- Pneumonia
- Hepatitis
- Meningoencephalitis

Chronic Q fever presentation:
- Endocarditis

Most common clinical symptoms:
- Chills
- Sweats
- Nausea
- Vomiting
- Cough, nonproductive
- Headache
- Fatigue

Most frequent physical findings:
- Fever
- Inspiratory rales
- Purpuric rash
- Hepatomegaly
- Splenomegaly

■ ETIOLOGY
- Q fever is caused by the rickettsial organism *C. burnetii*.
- *C. burnetii* is a gram-negative coccobacillus that is transmitted from arthropods to animals to humans.
- The disease is acquired most often via inhalation of aerosols. In the lungs, it proliferates in macrophases and then gains access to the blood, producing a transient bacteria. Thereafter it can invade many organs, but most commonly invades the lungs and liver.

- There is an incubation period between 3 to 30 days before systemic symptoms manifest.

DIAGNOSIS

■ DIFFERENTIAL DIAGNOSIS
Q fever can have various presentations and must be in the differential diagnosis of fever, hepatitis, pneumonia, endocarditis, and meningitis.

■ WORKUP
- CBC, ESR, and LFTs
- Urinalysis
- Serology
- Chest x-ray

■ LABORATORY TESTS
In acute Q fever:
- CBC and white blood cell count is usually normal.
- Thrombocytopenia can occur (25%).
- Elevation of hepatic transaminases (two to three times the abnormal range) may be seen.
- Complement fixation (CF) shows a fourfold rise in titer between acute and convalescent samples.

In chronic Q fever (almost always endocarditis):
- ESR is elevated
- Anemia is present
- Microscopic hematuria
- Blood cultures are almost always negative
- Complement fixation (CF) titer of >1:200 to phase I antigen is diagnostic

■ IMAGING STUDIES
- Chest x-ray examination is abnormal, showing segmental lobe consolidation
- Pleural effusions (35%)

TREATMENT

■ NONPHARMACOLOGIC THERAPY
Oxygen as needed in patients with pneumonia

■ ACUTE GENERAL Rx
- Acute Q fever can be treated with doxycycline (100 mg bid) for 14 to 21 days *or*
- Erythromycin (500 mg qid) for 14 days *or*
- Ofloxacin 200 mg PO q8h for 14 to 21 days

- Hydroxychloroquine plus doxycycline for endocarditis associated with Q fever
- Fluoroquinolones are recommended for suspected meningoencephalitis

■ CHRONIC Rx
- Chronic Q fever is treated with a combination of two antibiotics, doxycycline 100 mg bid and rifampin 300 mg qd *or*
- Doxycycline 100 mg bid and Ofloxacin 200 mg po q8h *or*
- Doxycycline 100 mg bid and hydroxychloroquine 200 mg PO tid
- Duration of treatment: 2 to 3 yr

■ DISPOSITION
- Patients with acute Q fever respond well with antibiotics, with rare deaths reported.
- Mortality rate in chronic Q fever endocarditis is high (24%). Most patients will come to valve replacement surgery.

■ REFERRAL
Referral to an infectious disease expert is recommended in any cases of suspected acute or chronic Q fever.

PEARLS & CONSIDERATIONS

■ COMMENTS
- No vaccines are available.
- Infected patients do not require specific isolation precautions.
- Q fever derived its name in 1935 from Derrick, who was suspicious of a new disease during a series of acute febrile illness in abattoir workers of Queensland, Australia, justifying the name of Q fever (for query).

REFERENCES
Caron F et al: Acute Q fever pneumonia: a review of 80 hospitalized patients, *Chest* 114(3):808, 1998.

Choi E: Tularemia and Q fever, *Med Clin North Am* 86(2):393, 2002.

Gami AS et al: Q fever ondocarditis in the United States, *Mayo Clin Proc* 79:253, 2004.

Raoult, D et al: Q fever 1985-1998. Clinical and epidemiologic features of 1,383 infections, *Medicine* 79:109, 2000.

Authors: **Peter Petropoulos, M.D., and Dennis J. Mikolich, M.D.**

BASIC INFORMATION

■ DEFINITION
Rabies is a fatal illness caused by the rabies virus and transmitted to humans by the bite of an infected animal.

■ SYNONYMS
Hydrophobia

ICD-9CM CODES
071 Rabies

■ EPIDEMIOLOGY & DEMOGRAPHICS
INCIDENCE (IN U.S.): Approximately 2 cases/yr
PREDOMINANT SEX: Men (70% of cases)
PREDOMINANT AGE: <16 yr and >55 yr

■ PHYSICAL FINDINGS & CLINICAL PRESENTATION
- Incubation period of 10 to 90 days
  1. Shorter with bites of the face
  2. Longer if extremities involved
- Prodrome
  1. Fever
  2. Headache
  3. Malaise
  4. Pain or anesthesia at exposure site
  5. Sore throat
  6. GI symptoms
  7. Psychiatric symptoms
- Acute neurologic period, with objective evidence of CNS involvement
  1. Extreme hyperactivity and bizarre behavior alternating with periods of relative calm
  2. Hallucinations
  3. Disorientation
  4. Seizures
  5. Paralysis may occur
  6. Spasm of the pharynx and larynx, accompanied by severe pain, caused by drinking
  7. Fear elicited by seeing water
  8. Paralysis
  9. Coma
- Possible death from respiratory arrest

■ ETIOLOGY
- Rabies virus
- Cases in U.S. are associated with:
  1. Bats
  2. Raccoons
  3. Foxes
  4. Skunks

- In 8 of the 32 cases occurring in the U.S. since 1980, there was a history of exposure to bats without an actual bite or scratch.
- Imported cases are usually associated with dogs.
- Unusual acquisition:
  1. Via corneal transplantation
  2. Via aerosol transmission in laboratory workers and spelunkers

DIAGNOSIS

■ DIFFERENTIAL DIAGNOSIS
- Delirium tremens
- Tetanus
- Hysteria
- Psychiatric disorders
- Other viral encephalitides
- Guillain-Barré syndrome
- Poliomyelitis

■ WORKUP
- Rabies antibody
  1. Serum
  2. CSF
- Viral isolation
  1. Saliva
  2. CSF
  3. Serum
- Rabies fluorescent antibody: skin biopsy from the hair-covered area of the neck
- Characteristic eosinophilic inclusions (Negri bodies) in infected neurons

■ LABORATORY TESTS
See "Workup."

TREATMENT

■ NONPHARMACOLOGIC THERAPY
- Isolation of the patient to prevent transmission to others
- Supportive therapy (although this has not been shown to change outcome except in three cases in which the patients had received prophylaxis before onset of symptoms)

■ ACUTE GENERAL Rx
- No beneficial therapy
- Emphasis placed on prophylaxis of potentially exposed individuals as soon as possible following an exposure:
  1. Thorough wound cleansing
  2. Both active and passive immunization is most effective when used within 72 hr of exposure

- Vaccinations:
  1. Human diploid cell vaccine (HDCV) or rhesus monkey diploid cell vaccine (RVA), 1 ml IM (deltoid) on days 0, 3, 7, 14, and 28
  2. Human rabies hyperimmune globulin (RIG) 20 IU/kg, administered to persons not previously vaccinated. If anatomically feasible, the full dose should be infiltrated around the wounds and any remaining volume should be administered IM at an anatomically distant site from vaccine administration
- Preexposure prophylaxis using HDCV or RVA (1 ml IM days 0, 7, and 21 or 28) in individuals at high risk for acquisition:
  1. Veterinarians
  2. Laboratory workers working with rabies virus
  3. Spelunkers
  4. Visitors to endemic areas

■ DISPOSITION
Virtually always fatal

■ REFERRAL
- To infectious disease consultant
- To local health authorities

PEARLS & CONSIDERATIONS

■ COMMENTS
- Most cases in the U.S. are caused by:
  1. Wild animal bites (bats)
  2. Dog bites occurring outside the U.S.
  3. Some unknown exposure
- Rare cases can be transmitted by mucous membrane contact of aerosolized virus.

REFERENCES
National Association of State Public Health Veterinarians, Inc.: Compendium of animal rabies prevention and control, 2001, *MMWR* 50(RR-8):1, 2001.
Noah DL et al: Epidemiology of human rabies in the United States, 1980 to 1996, *Ann Intern Med* 128:922, 1998.
Plotkin SA: Rabies, *Clin Infect Dis* 30:4, 2000.
U.S. Department of Health: Human rabies prevention, *MMWR* 48:RR-1, 1999.
Author: **Maurice Policar, M.D.**

BASIC INFORMATION

■ DEFINITION

Exposure to ionizing radiation has the potential for radiation injury. Radionuclides present a danger to humans through the particles emitted during radioactive decay. These particles can damage cellular structures and may result in mutation, cancer, or cell death.

PRINCIPLES OF RADIOACTIVITY, ADDITIONAL DEFINITIONS:
Particles of radiation

- Photons: massless particles that travel at the speed of light and produce electromagnetic radiation. Their wavelength determine their energy; the longer the wavelength the lower the energy. In order of increasing energy, they are called ultraviolet, visible light, infrared, microwave, gamma, and x-rays. X-rays consist of a spectrum of wavelengths while gamma rays have a fixed wavelength specific to the radioactive material that produces them. X-rays and gamma rays are highly penetrating.
- β particles are electrons. They may be emitted during decay of a radionuclide (atom) that disintegrates. Positrons (positively charged electrons) may also be produced during radioactive decay. β particles are less penetrating than x-rays and gamma rays, but can still pass through several centimeters of human tissue. Nonetheless, their main toxic effect is through inhalation.
- α particles are helium nuclei (2 protons and 2 neutrons) stripped of their electrons. They are stopped by clothing; therefore, they need to be "incorporated" to cause health problems.
- Neutrons are released during nuclear fission, not during natural radionuclide decay. They can cause a stable atom to become radioactive by collision (e.g., during nuclear fallout).
- Cosmic rays are streams of electrons, protons, and α particles that come from outer space. Most of their energy is dissipated by the earth's atmosphere.
- Ionizing radiation describes any radiation with sufficient energy to break up an atom or molecule with which it collides. This is the mechanism of radiation toxicity.
- Nonionizing radiation has insufficient energy to break up atoms; nonetheless sufficient energy in the form of heat may be produced to cause localized tissue damage.

- Radioactive decay: process of transformation of unstable nuclei into more stable ones via the emissions of various particles. Decay is described by half-life, which is a characteristic of every radioisotope.
- Radiation units of measure:
  1. Roentgen: amount of radiation to which an object is exposed.
  2. Rad (radiation absorbed dose): amount of radiation absorbed by tissue.
  3. Rem (roentgen equivalent man) and Sievert (SV, the same concept in the International System): a measure that standardizes the amount of cellular damage produced by different types of radiation. One Rem (or 0.01 SV) is the dose of radiation that produces damage equivalent to one Rad of X-ray.

IRRADIATION, CONTAMINATION, AND INCORPORATION:
- Irradiation: exposure to ionizing radiation
- Contamination: an object or person covered with a radioactive substance
- Incorporation: exposure to a radionuclide by inhalation, ingestion, intravenous infusion, or percutaneously

STOCHASTIC EFFECTS OF IONIZING RADIATION:
Any dose of ionizing radiation can alter DNA, causing mutations or carcinogenic changes that may take years to be expressed. There is no dose threshold, and the effect is cumulative. The stochastic effects of radiation are mostly a concern with small but prolonged exposure to radiation.

DETERMINISTIC EFFECTS OF IONIZING RADIATION:
The dose of radiation is sufficient to kill cells; the higher the dose, the greater the number of killed cells and the greater the impact on an organ system. The deterministic effects of radiation are the consequence of a large whole-body exposure.

ICD-9CM CODE
990 Radiation exposure

■ PHYSICAL FINDINGS & ACUTE PRESENTATION
ACUTE RADIATION SYNDROME:
Follows a large, whole-body exposure of 2Sv or more (500 times the average annual exposure)
Sequence of events: four stages:
- Stage 1: nausea and vomiting begins within a few minutes to hours and lasts several hours to a few days depending on the dose.

- Stage 2: latent (asymptomatic), lasting several days to weeks, again depending on the dose.
- Stage 3: third to fifth week following exposure: abdominal pain, diarrhea, hair loss, bleeding, infection. During this stage, several subsyndromes may coexist, overlap, or occur in sequence.
  1. CNS syndrome: fever, ataxia, apathy, lethargy, and seizures
  2. Cardiovascular (CV) syndrome: arrhythmias, hypotension, myocardial injury
  3. GI syndrome: anorexia, nausea, vomiting, diarrhea, dehydration, superinfection, and sepsis
  4. Hematopoietic syndrome: pancytopenia with bleeding diathesis and sepsis
  5. Pneumonitis leading to pulmonary fibrosis
  6. Any of the syndromes has the potential to be lethal
- Stage 4: recovery, lasting weeks to months.

DOSE ESTIMATION AND PROGNOSIS:
Because radiation is often mixed and because body parts may be exposed to different amounts of radiation, the dose received is difficult to estimate in the field. Therefore, it is usually the acute radiation syndrome itself that allows prognosis. At a dose received under 3 Sv a lymphocyte count >1200/mm³ at 48 hr confers a favorable prognosis; if the count is <1200/mm³, a fatal dose is possible and more aggressive medical management is warranted. A drop in the number of granulocytes or platelets also portends a severe exposure. Patients exposed to less than 2 Sv will survive with no or minimal care. Patients exposed to 2 to 5 Sv are likely to survive with medical care. A dose of 5 to 20 Sv is survivable. A dose above 20 Sv is supralethal, and the patient will die within 24 to 48 hr from CNS or CV syndrome. At the Chernobyl nuclear reactor accident, mortality was 33% among those receiving 4 to 6 Sv and 95% among those receiving 6 to 16 Sv.

CARCINOGENESIS:
Leukemia, breast cancer, lung cancer, and thyroid cancer incidence increase following exposure to ionizing exposure. This is a stochastic effect that can occur with or without a history of acute radiation syndrome.

■ ETIOLOGY
SOURCE OF RADIATION:
- Natural
  1. Radon (domestic and mining industry)
  2. Cosmic
  3. Terrestrial
  4. Ingested (from food)
- Industrial
  1. X-ray diagnosis
  2. Nuclear medicine
  3. Consumer products
  4. Occupational (e.g., nuclear energy)
  5. Weapons

TREATMENT

- Decontamination
  1. Perform at site of exposure unless there is ongoing radiation
  2. Remove all clothing (and treat those as radioactive waste)
  3. Wash patient with soap and water. Dispose of the used water as radioactive waste
  4. Scrub any open wound
  5. Depending on the situation, the regional emergency response system should be called for additional measures such as evacuation
- Management of the acute radiation syndrome
  1. Establish IV access
  2. Manage the airway if needed
  3. Manage burns
  4. Identify and treat other injuries
  5. Provide analgesia
  6. Give antiemetics (e.g., ondansetron)
  7. Manage bleeding and transfuse if necessary
  8. Diagnose and treat sepsis
  9. Consider colony-stimulating factors
  10. Consider bone marrow transplantation

REFERENCE
Rella J: Radiation. In Goldfrank LR et al (eds): *Toxicologic emergencies,* ed. 7, New York, 2002, McGraw-Hill.
Author: **Tom J. Wachtel, M.D.**

BASIC INFORMATION

■ DEFINITION
Ramsay Hunt syndrome is a localized herpes zoster infection involving the seventh nerve and geniculate ganglia, resulting in hearing loss, vertigo, and facial nerve palsy.

■ SYNONYMS
Herpes zoster oticus
Geniculate herpes
Herpetic geniculate ganglionitis

ICD-9CM CODES
053.11 Ramsay Hunt syndrome

■ EPIDEMIOLOGY & DEMOGRAPHICS
PREDOMINANT SEX: Equal sex distribution
PREDOMINANT AGE:
- Increasingly common with advancing age
- Rare in childhood

■ PHYSICAL FINDINGS & CLINICAL PRESENTATION
- Characteristic vesicles:
  1. On pinna
  2. In external auditory canal
  3. In distribution of the facial nerve and, occasionally, adjacent cranial nerves
- Facial paralysis on the involved side

■ ETIOLOGY
Reactivation of dormant infection with varicella-zoster virus following primary varicella (usually in childhood)

DIAGNOSIS

- Usually made by recognition of the clinical features detailed previously

- Viral culture and/or microscopic examination of specimens taken from active vesicles

■ DIFFERENTIAL DIAGNOSIS
- Herpes simplex
- External otitis
- Impetigo
- Enteroviral infection
- Bell's palsy of other etiologies
- Acoustic neuroma (before appearance of skin lesions)
- The differential diagnosis of headache and facial pain is described in Section II.

■ WORKUP
If the diagnosis is in doubt, confirmation of varicella-zoster virus infection should be sought.

■ LABORATORY TESTS
- Viral culture of specimens of vesicular fluid and scrapings of the vesicle base
- Tzanck preparation, which may reveal multinucleated giant cells
- Direct immunofluorescent staining of scrapings

■ IMAGING STUDIES
MRI may demonstrate enhancement of the facial and vestibulocochlear nerves before appearance of vesicles.

TREATMENT

■ ACUTE GENERAL Rx
- Prednisone (40 mg PO for 2 days; 30 mg for 7 days; followed by tapering course) is recommended by some authors.

- Acyclovir (800 mg PO five times qd for 10 days), famciclovir (500 mg tid for 7 days), or valacyclovir (1 g every 8 hr for 7 days) may hasten healing.
- Analgesics should be used as indicated.

■ CHRONIC Rx
- Amitriptyline is effective in some cases of postherpetic pain.
- Narcotic analgesics may occasionally be necessary.

■ DISPOSITION
Recurrences are unusual.

■ REFERRAL
To otolaryngologist: patients with persistent facial paralysis for potential surgical decompression of the facial nerve

PEARLS & CONSIDERATIONS

■ COMMENTS
Immunodeficiency states, particularly infection with the human immunodeficiency virus (HIV), should be considered in:
- Younger patients
- Severe cases
- Patients with a history of specific risk behavior

REFERENCES
Hato N et al: Ramsay Hunt syndrome in children, *Ann Neurol* 48(2):254, 2000.
Ko JY, Sheen TS, Hsu MM: Herpes zoster oticus treated with acyclovir and prednisolone: clinical manifestations and analysis of prognostic factors, *Clin Otolaryngol* 25(2):139, 2000.
Author: **Joseph R. Masci, M.D.**

BASIC INFORMATION

■ DEFINITION
Raynaud's phenomenon is a vasospastic disorder usually affecting the digital arteries precipitated by exposure to cold temperatures or emotional distress and manifesting in a triphasic discoloration of the fingers or toes.

■ SYNONYMS
Primary Raynaud's phenomenon or Raynaud's disease
Secondary Raynaud's phenomenon

ICD-9CM CODES
443.0 Raynaud's syndrome, Raynaud's disease, Raynaud's phenomenon (secondary)
785.4 If gangrene present

■ EPIDEMIOLOGY & DEMOGRAPHICS
- Raynaud's phenomenon (either primary [idiopathic] or secondary [see "Etiology"]) is found in 5% to 20% of the population.
- Primary Raynaud's phenomenon is more common than secondary Raynaud's and occurs in women more often than men (4:1) and in the young (<40 yr of age) more than the old.
- Between 5% and 15% of patients thought to have primary Raynaud's will develop a secondary cause (commonly scleroderma or CREST syndrome).

■ PHYSICAL FINDINGS & CLINICAL PRESENTATION
- The classic manifestation is the triphasic color response to cold exposure (Fig. 1-227):
  1. Pallor of the digit resulting from vasospasm.
  2. Blue discoloration (cyanosis) secondary to desaturated venous blood.
  3. Red (rubor) along with pain and paresthesia when vasospasm resolves and blood returns to the digit.
- Color changes are well delineated, symmetric, and usually bilateral.
- Fingertips are most often involved, but feet, ears, and nose can be affected.
- Ulcerations and rarely gangrene may occur.
- Secondary Raynaud's phenomenon may be associated with typical findings of the underlying disease (e.g., sclerodactyly and telangiectasia in CREST syndrome).

■ ETIOLOGY
- Primary Raynaud's phenomenon is generally referred to as Raynaud's disease when no cause can be found.
- Secondary Raynaud's phenomenon has many causes:
  1. CREST syndrome (calcinosis, Raynaud's phenomenon, esophageal dysmotility, sclerodactyly, and telangiectasia)
  2. Scleroderma
  3. Mixed connective tissue disease, polymyositis, and dermatomyositis
  4. SLE
  5. Rheumatoid arthritis
  6. Thromboangiitis obliterans (Buerger's disease)
  7. Drug induced (β-blockers, ergotamine, methysergide, vinblastine, bleomycin, oral contraceptives)
  8. Polycythemia, cryoglobulinemia, and certain vasculitides
  9. Carpal tunnel syndrome
  10. Tools causing vibration
  11. Estrogen replacement therapy without progesterone

DIAGNOSIS

- The diagnosis of Raynaud's phenomenon can be made by a history of well-demarcated digit discoloration induced by cold exposure and a physical examination looking for possible secondary causes.
- The digit triphasic color changes can sometimes be induced in the office by placing the hand in an ice bath.
- Color photos and questionnaires may be useful in assisting in the diagnosis.

■ DIFFERENTIAL DIAGNOSIS
See "Etiology."

■ WORKUP
- Once the diagnosis of Raynaud's phenomenon is established, differentiating primary from secondary is helpful in treatment and prognosis. History and physical examination usually make this distinction, whereas certain laboratory studies may predict secondary causes (see "Laboratory Tests").
- A test available but not commonly used is the nailfold microscopy; if positive, it may be associated with certain collagen-vascular diseases.

■ LABORATORY TESTS
- CBC, electrolytes, BUN, Cr, ESR, ANA, urinalysis should be included in the initial evaluation.
- If the history, physical examination, and initial laboratory tests suggest a possible secondary cause, specific serologic testing (e.g., anticentromere antibodies, anti-Scl 70, cryoglobulins, complement testing, and protein electrophoresis) may be indicated.

■ IMAGING STUDIES
- Chest x-ray examination may be helpful if a secondary cause, such as scleroderma, is suggested.

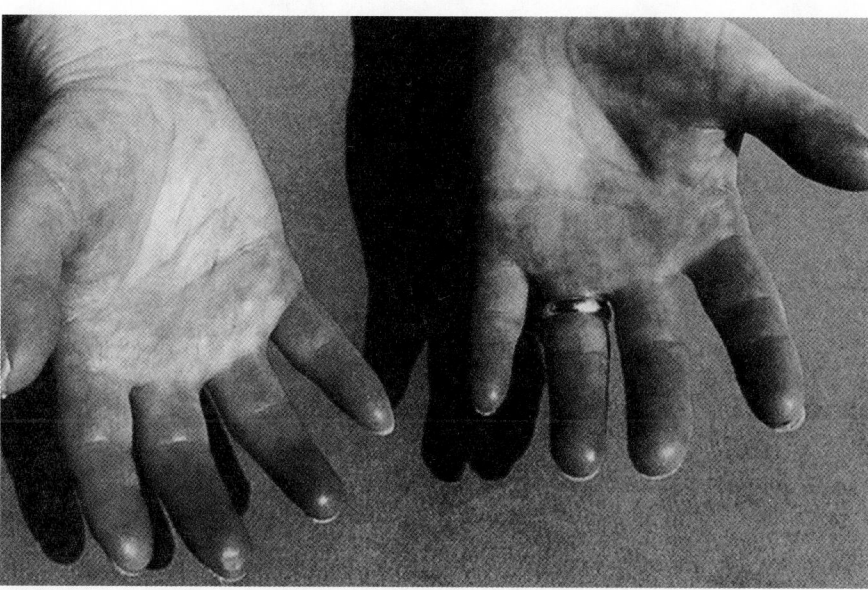

Fig. 1-227   Raynaud's phenomenon. Sharply demarcated cyanosis of the fingers with proximal venular congestion (livedo reticularis) is seen. (From Klippel J, Dieppe P, Ferri F [eds]: *Primary care rheumatology*, London, 1999, Mosby.)

- Barium swallow may be helpful if CREST syndrome is suspected.
- Angiography is rarely needed for Raynaud's phenomenon but may be helpful in diagnosing Buerger's disease as a possible etiology.

TREATMENT

■ NONPHARMACOLOGIC THERAPY

- Avoid medications that may precipitate Raynaud's phenomenon (see "Etiology").
- Avoid cold exposure. Use warm gloves, hats, and garments during the winter months or before going into cold environments (e.g., air-conditioned rooms).
- Avoid stressful situations.
- Avoid nicotine, caffeine, and over-the-counter decongestants.

■ ACUTE GENERAL Rx

- Typically, patients with Raynaud's phenomenon respond well to nonpharmacologic measures.
- Medications should be used if the above mentioned treatment does not work.
- Goal is to prevent digital ulcers and gangrene.
- Medications commonly used are described in "Chronic Rx."

■ CHRONIC Rx

- Calcium channel blockers are the most effective treatment for Raynaud's phenomenon.
  1. Nifedipine is most often prescribed at a dose of 10 to 20 mg 30 min before going outside. If symptoms occur with long duration, nifedipine XL 30 to 90 mg PO qd is effective.

  2. If side effects occur with nifedipine, other calcium blockers can be used (e.g., diltiazem 30 mg qid and gradually increased to a maximum dose of 120 mg qid). Felodipine 2.5 mg qd up to 10 mg qd can also be used.
  3. Verapamil has not been shown to be effective with Raynaud's phenomenon.
- Prazosin 1 mg bid up to 4 mg bid has been effective with Raynaud's phenomenon.
- Reserpine and guanethidine, although effective, have a high side effect profile.
- Other agents that have been tried with limited results include aspirin, pentoxifylline, captopril, and topical nitrates.
- The prostaglandins, including inhaled iloprost, IV epoprostenol, and alprostadil, may be promising in severe Raynaud's phenomenon.

■ DISPOSITION

The prognosis of patients with Raynaud's phenomenon depends on the etiology.
- Primary Raynaud's phenomenon is fairly benign, usually remaining stable and controlled with nonpharmacologic medical treatment.
- Patients with secondary Raynaud's phenomenon, specifically those with scleroderma, CREST syndrome, and thromboangiitis obliterans, may develop severe ischemic digits with ulceration, gangrene, and autoamputation.

■ REFERRAL

- Rheumatology consult is indicated if secondary collagen-vascular disease is diagnosed.
- Vascular surgery consult is indicated if ulcers, gangrene, or threatened digit loss is noted.

☼ PEARLS & CONSIDERATIONS

■ COMMENTS

Most patients with Raynaud's phenomenon can be managed by the primary care provider; however, it is important to differentiate primary from secondary forms. Secondary forms may become manifest as far out as 10 yr from the diagnosis of Raynaud's phenomenon. Periodic follow-up visits and reassessment to exclude secondary forms are important toward future treatment options and outcome.

REFERENCES

Spencer-Green G: Outcomes in primary Raynaud's phenomenon, *Arch Intern Med* 158:595, 1998.

Sturgill MG, Seibold JR: Rational use of calcium-channel antagonists in Raynaud's phenomenon, *Curr Opin Rheumatol* 10:584, 1998.

Wigley FM: Raynaud's phenomenon, *N Engl J Med* 347:1001, 2002.

Wigley FM, Flavahan NA: Raynaud's phenomenon, *Rheum Dis Clin North Am* 22(4):765, 1996.

Author: **Peter Petropoulos, M.D.**

BASIC INFORMATION

■ DEFINITION

Reflex sympathetic dystrophy (RSD) refers to a painful neuropathic symptom complex affecting an extremity following trauma, surgery, or nerve injury to that limb.

■ SYNONYMS

Causalgia
Shoulder-hand syndrome
Sudeck's atrophy
Posttraumatic pain syndrome

ICD-9CM CODES

337.20 Dystrophy sympathetic (post-traumatic) (reflex)

■ EPIDEMIOLOGY & DEMOGRAPHICS

- The incidence and prevalence of RSD is not known.
- RSD is usually initiated by trauma.
- RSD can occur in adults and children.
- RSD is often associated with psychiatric emotional lability, anxiety, and depression.

■ PHYSICAL FINDINGS & CLINICAL PRESENTATION

RSD is divided into three stages:
- Acute stage (occurring within hours to days after the injury)
  1. Burning or aching pain occurring over the injured extremity
  2. Hyperalgesia (exquisitely sensitive to touch)
  3. Edema
  4. Dysthermia
  5. Increased hair and nail growth
- Dystrophic stage (3 to 6 mo after the injury)
  1. Burning pain radiating both distal and proximally from the site of injury
  2. Brawny edema
  3. Hyperhidrosis
  4. Hypothermia and cyanosis
  5. Muscle tremors and spasms
  6. Increase muscle tone and reflexes
- Atrophic stage (6 mo after injury)
  1. Spread of pain proximally
  2. Cold, pale cyanotic skin
  3. Trophic skin changes with subcutaneous atrophy
  4. Fixed joints
  5. Contractures

■ ETIOLOGY

- The cause of RSD is unknown. It is thought to represent dysfunction of the sympathetic nervous system.
- Any injury can precipitate RSD including:
  1. Crush blunt trauma, burns, frostbite
  2. Surgery (Fig. 1-228)
  3. Parkinson's disease

4. Cerebrovascular accident
5. Myocardial infarction
6. Osteoarthritis, cervical and lumbar disk disease
7. Carpal tunnel and tarsal tunnel syndrome
8. Diabetes
9. Hyperthyroidism
10. Isoniazid therapy

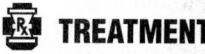 **DIAGNOSIS**

The diagnosis of RSD is primarily clinical, based on the patient's history and physical presentation.

■ DIFFERENTIAL DIAGNOSIS

The differential diagnosis includes all the causes mentioned under "Etiology."

■ WORKUP

In patients with RSD, no workup is needed because there are no specific diagnostic tests establishing the diagnosis.

■ LABORATORY TESTS

Blood tests are not specific in the diagnosis of RSD.

■ IMAGING STUDIES

- No imaging studies are diagnostic of RSD. Three-phase bone imaging may be helpful.

- Autonomic testing, although not commonly done, has been proposed.
  1. Measuring resting sweat output
  2. Measuring resting skin temperature
  3. Quantitative sudomotor axon reflex test
- X-ray studies of the affected limb may show osteoporosis from disuse.

TREATMENT

Treatment is aimed at relieving the pain and improving disuse atrophy with physical therapy.

■ NONPHARMACOLOGIC THERAPY

- Physical therapy
- Transcutaneous nerve stimulation

■ ACUTE GENERAL Rx

- The following has been tried for neuropathic pain relief:
- Amitriptyline 10 mg to 150 mg qd
- Phenytoin 300 mg qd
- Carbamazepine 100 mg bid
- Calcium channel blockers, nifedipine extended release 30 to 60 mg qd
- Prednisone 60 to 80 mg qd × 2 wk and then tapered over 1 to 2 wk to a maintenance dose of 5 mg qd for 2 to 3 mo.

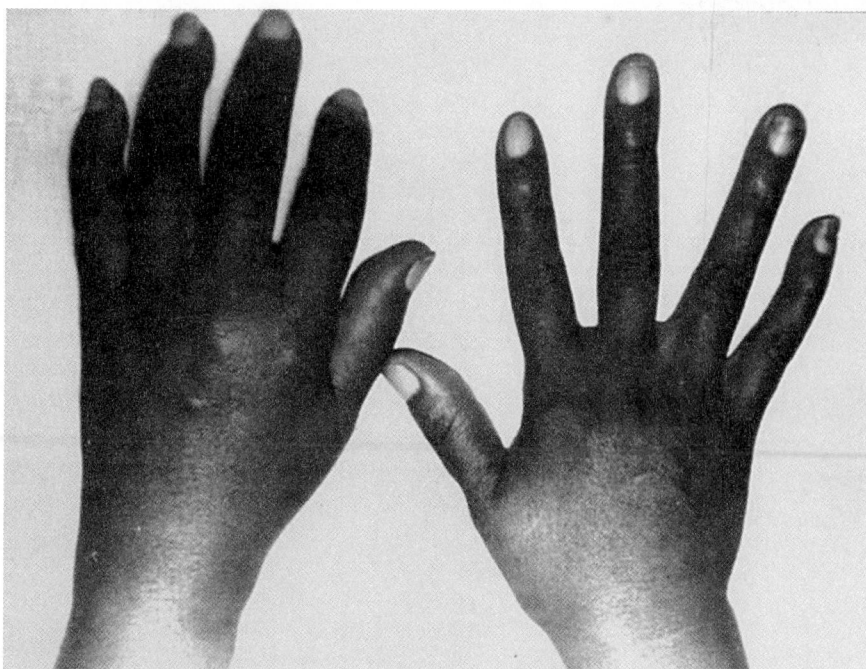

Fig. 1-228 **Sympathetic dystrophy.** Swollen, painful left hand after carpal tunnel release. This patient, a 40-year-old woman, had open release of the left carpal tunnel for idiopathic carpal tunnel syndrome 1 month prior. She was treated with several stellate ganglion blocks and intensive physiotherapy. She was well 3 months later. (From Canoso J: *Rheumatology in primary care,* Philadelphia, 1997, WB Saunders.)

■ **CHRONIC Rx**
- Stellate ganglion and lumbar sympathetic blocks can be tried
- IV qd α-adrenergic blockade with phentolamine is thought to be a good predictor of response to subsequent sympatholytic treatment
- Surgical sympathectomy

■ **DISPOSITION**
- Spontaneous remission can occur after several weeks to months.
- Patients with RSD variably will progress through all stages leading to atrophy and contractures.

■ **REFERRAL**
RSD is a very difficult diagnosis to make and referral to either rheumatology, neurology, orthopedic, or physiatry is recommended.

☼ PEARLS & CONSIDERATIONS

■ **COMMENTS**
- RSD is a common clinical entity without clear definition, pathophysiologic features, or treatment.
- Pain is the most disabling symptom for most patients with RSD and is usually out of proportion to the extent of the injury.

REFERENCES

Ochoa JL: Reflex sympathetic dystrophy: a disease of medical understanding, *Clin J Pain* 8:363, 1992.

Raja SN, Grabow TS: Complex regional pain syndrome 1 (reflex sympathetic dystrophy), *Anesthesiology* 96(5):1254, 2002.

Schwartzman RJ: New treatments for reflex sympathetic dystrophy, *N Engl J Med* 343:654, 2000.

Schwartzman RJ, Maleki J: Postinjury neuropathic pain syndromes, *Med Clin North Am* 83(3):597, 1999.

Author: **Peter Petropoulos, M.D.**

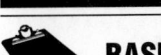

BASIC INFORMATION

■ DEFINITION
Reiter's syndrome is one of the seronegative spondyloarthropathies, so called because serum rheumatoid factor is not present in these forms of inflammatory arthritis. Reiter's syndrome is an asymmetric polyarthritis that affects mainly the lower extremities and is associated with one or more of the following:
- Urethritis
- Cervicitis
- Dysentery
- Inflammatory eye disease
- Mucocutaneous lesions

■ SYNONYMS
Reiter's disease
Reactive arthritis
Seronegative spondyloarthropathy

ICD-9CM CODES
099.3 Reiter's syndrome

■ EPIDEMIOLOGY & DEMOGRAPHICS
INCIDENCE (IN U.S.): 0.0035% annually of men <50 yr
PREDOMINANT SEX: Male
PREDOMINANT AGE: 20 to 40 yr
PEAK INCIDENCE: Most common in the third decade
GENETICS:
Familial Disposition: Strongly associated with HLA-B27 (63% to 96%)

■ PHYSICAL FINDINGS & CLINICAL PRESENTATION
- Polyarthritis
  1. Affecting the knee and ankle
  2. Commonly asymmetric
- Heel pain and Achilles tendinitis, especially at the insertion of the Achilles tendon
- Plantar fasciitis
- Large effusions
- Dactylitis or "sausage toe"
- Urethritis
- Uveitis or conjunctivitis; uveitis can progress to blindness without treatment
- Keratoderma blennorrhagicum
  1. Hyperkeratotic lesions on soles of the feet, toes, penis, hands
  2. Closely resembles psoriasis
- Aortic regurgitation similar to that seen in ankylosing spondylitis

■ ETIOLOGY
- Epidemic Reiter's syndrome following outbreaks of dysentery has been well described.
- Genetically susceptible HLA-B27–positive individuals are at risk for developing Reiter's syndrome following infection with certain pathogens:
  1. *Salmonella*
  2. *Shigella*
  3. *Yersinia enterocolitica*
  4. *Chlamydia trachomatis*
  5. Molecular mimicry mechanism suspected
- Symptom complex indistinguishable from Reiter's syndrome has been described in association with HIV infection.

DIAGNOSIS

■ DIFFERENTIAL DIAGNOSIS
- Ankylosing spondylitis
- Psoriatic arthritis
- Rheumatoid arthritis
- Gonococcal arthritis-tenosynovitis
- Rheumatic fever

■ WORKUP
- X-ray examination of affected joints
- Synovial fluid examination and culture
- Careful examination of eyes and skin
- Cultures for gonococcus (urethral, cervical, stool)

■ LABORATORY TESTS
- Elevated but nonspecific ESR
- No specific laboratory tests to diagnose Reiter's syndrome

■ IMAGING STUDIES
Plain radiographs:
- Juxtaarticular osteopenia of affected joints
- Erosions and joint space narrowing in more advanced disease
- Periostitis and reactive new bone formation at the insertions of the Achilles tendon and the plantar fascia
- Sacroiliitis:
  1. Unilateral or bilateral
  2. Indistinguishable from ankylosing spondylitis
- Vertebral bridging osteophytes

TREATMENT

■ NONPHARMACOLOGIC THERAPY
Physical therapy to maintain range of motion of the back and other joints

■ ACUTE GENERAL Rx
Flares treated with NSAIDs such as indomethacin (25 to 50 mg PO tid)
- Enteric or urethral infection should be treated with appropriate antibiotic coverage.
- Uveitis should be treated with steroid eye drops in consultation with an ophthalmologist.
- Achilles tendinitis and plantar fasciitis should be treated with injections of methylprednisolone (40 to 80 mg).
- Sulfasalazine (2 to 3 g PO tid) may be effective.
- Careful monitoring for the following is essential:
  1. GI toxicity
  2. Hypersensitivity
  3. Bone marrow suppression
- Persistent and uncontrolled disease should be managed with cytotoxic drugs (methotrexate, azathioprine) in consultation with a rheumatologist.

■ CHRONIC Rx
Chronic disease is best managed by a team approach with the collaboration of a rheumatologist or other experienced physician and physical therapist.

■ DISPOSITION
- Recurrences are frequent, even with treatment.
- Long-term sequelae:
  1. Persistent polyarthritis
  2. Chronic back pain
  3. Heel pain
  4. Progressive iridocyclitis
  5. Aortic regurgitation

■ REFERRAL
- To ophthalmologist if uveitis is suspected
- To rheumatologist if arthritis and tendinitis fail to improve rapidly after a course of NSAIDs

PEARLS & CONSIDERATIONS

■ COMMENTS
- Infection with HIV is associated with particularly severe cases of Reiter's syndrome.
- HIV testing is recommended, especially if risk factors such as unprotected sexual activity or IV drug use are identified.

REFERENCE
Al-Arfaj A: Profile of Reiter's disease in Saudi Arabia, *Clin Exp Rheumatol* 19(2):184, 2001.
Author: **Deborah L. Shapiro, M.D.**

BASIC INFORMATION

■ DEFINITION
Renal artery stenosis is the narrowing or occlusion of a renal artery, which can occur acutely (thrombosis or embolism) and cause renal infarction or progressively (e.g., atheroma or fibromuscular dysphasia) and cause renovascular hypertension and/or lead to ischemic nephropathy. In addition, renal atheroembolism caused by showers of cholesterol microemboli can lead to progressive renal failure if sustained or recurrent.

■ SYNONYMS
Acute:
Renal artery thrombosis
Renal artery embolism
Chronic:
Renovascular hypertension

ICD-9CM CODES
593.81 Renal artery occlusion
440.1 Renal artery stenosis
405.01 Renovascular hypertension, secondary
447.9 Renal artery hyperplasia

■ EPIDEMIOLOGY & DEMOGRAPHICS
- In acute renal artery occlusion, the epidemiology depends on the underlying cause (see below).
- Renovascular hypertension:
Prevalence of 0.2% to 5% of all hypertensive patients.
The prevalence is higher in patients with severe hypertension, reaching 43% of white patients and 7% of black patients with malignant hypertension.
- Approximately 1 in 6 patients with end-stage renal disease has ischemic nephropathy, and survival of patients with end-stage renal disease associated with ischemic nephropathy is half that of patients with end-stage renal disease from other causes.
- The demographics of atheromatous renal artery stenosis mirrors the pattern seen in other arteriosclerotic conditions (coronary artery disease, cerebrovascular disease, peripheral vascular disease) and is influenced by the usual risk factors (smoking, family history, diabetes, hyperlipidemia). For example, the prevalence of renal artery stenosis among hypertensive patients undergoing coronary catheterization is high (47%), with 19% having a stenosis of 50% or more. Fibromuscular dysplasia is most likely to be seen in young adult women. Takayasu's arteritis can involve the renal arteries and is also seen in young to middle-aged women.

■ PHYSICAL FINDINGS & CLINICAL PRESENTATION
Acute renal artery occlusion
- Flank or abdominal pain
- Fever

- Nausea or vomiting
- Leukocytosis
- Hematuria (microscopic or gross)
- Elevated AST, LDH, and alkaline phosphatase
- Oliguric renal failure if occlusion is bilateral; normal or near normal renal function in unilateral occlusion
Cholesterol emboli
- Multisystem manifestations resembling vasculitis (visual disturbance, painful distal extremities, abdominal pain, signs of organ or limb ischemia). Laboratory findings include eosinophiluria, proteinuria, renal failure, elevated ESR.
Progressive renal artery stenosis
- Hypertension in a young, white woman without a family history of such (fibromuscular dysplasia)
- Hypertension in a middle-aged man with other evidence of atheromatous disease
- Abdominal bruit (40% of cases)
- Renal failure
- Hypertensive retinopathy
- Pulmonary edema in a hypertensive patient
- Hypokalemia
- Renal failure following the administration of an angiotensin-converting enzyme inhibitor (if bilateral renal artery stenosis)

■ ETIOLOGY & PATHOGENESIS
Etiology of renal artery thrombosis
- Atherosclerosis
- Fibromuscular dysphasia
- Arteritis
- Aneurysm
- Arteriography
- Syphilis
- Hypercoagulable state
- Complication of renal transplantation (role of cyclosporine)
Etiology of renal artery embolism (cardiac conditions [90%])
- Myocardial infarction
- Atrial fibrillation
- Cardiomyopathy
- Endocarditis
- Paradoxical emboli from DVT in patient with cardiac septal defect
- Atheromatous plaques (cholesterol emboli)
PATHOGENESIS: Renal hypoperfusion or ischemia produces an increase in plasma renin that stimulates the conversion of angiotensin I to angiotensin II, causing vasoconstriction and aldosterone secretion, sodium retention, and potassium wasting. Hypertension results and can be self-sustaining after some time, even in the case of unilateral renal artery stenosis because of hypertensive damage to the other kidney.

DIAGNOSIS

■ WORKUP
- Documentation of hypertension
- Hypertensive workup (see "Hypertension" in Section I)

■ LABORATORY TESTS
- Creatinine
- Potassium level
- Urinalysis
- Peripheral plasma renin activity
- Captopril test (stimulation of excessive renin secretion)

■ IMAGING STUDIES
- Renal scan (70% sensitivity and 79% specificity)
- Captopril renal scan (92% sensitivity and 93% specificity)
- Hypertensive IVP (75% sensitivity and 85% specificity)
- Intravenous digital substraction angiography (88% sensitivity and 90% specificity)
- Magnetic resonance angiography
- Exercise renal scan (still being evaluated)
- Renal artery ultrasound (still being evaluated)

■ INVASIVE STUDIES
- Renal arteriography
- Selective renal vein renin measurements
- Renal biopsy for cholesterol emboli

TREATMENT

Acute renal artery thrombosis or embolism
- Thrombolytic therapy
- Anticoagulation
- Revascularization (surgery)
- Blood pressure control
Cholesterol emboli
- No treatment
Renal artery stenosis
- Blood pressure control (role of ACE inhibitors and angiotensin receptor blockers is controversial, but neither should be continued if renal function worsens)
- Angioplasty or revascularization should be reserved for patients whose blood pressure control with medication is difficult and for patients with progressive renal failure

■ NATURAL HISTORY
- Renal artery stenosis caused by fibromuscular dysplasia does not progress.
- Renal artery stenosis associated with atherosclerosis is progressive. Of patients with >60% stenosis, 5% progress to total occlusion in 1 yr and 11% progress in 2 yr.

REFERENCES
Higashi Y et al: Endothelial function and oxidative stress in renovascular hypertension, *N Engl J Med* 346:1954, 2002.
Rihal CS et al: Incidental renal artery stenosis among a prospective cohort of hypertensive patients undergoing coronary angiography, *Mayo Clin Proc* 77:309, 2002.
Author: **Tom J. Wachtel, M.D.**

BASIC INFORMATION

■ DEFINITION
Renal cell adenocarcinoma (RCA) is a primary adenocarcinoma originating in the renal parenchyma from the malignant transformation of proximal renal tubular epithelial cells.

■ SYNONYMS
Hypernephroma
Clear cell carcinoma of the kidney
Grawitz tumor

■ ICD-9CM CODES
189.0 adenocarcinoma of kidney
189.1 (renal pelvis)

■ EPIDEMIOLOGY & DEMOGRAPHICS
INCIDENCE: Approximately 1:10,000 persons/yr (3% of all adult malignancies)
AGE: Peak in age 50 to 70 yr
SEX: Male:female ratio of 2:1

■ PHYSICAL FINDINGS & CLINICAL PRESENTATION
Presenting findings in RCA patients:

Hematuria	50% to 60%
Elevated erythrocyte sedimentation rate	50% to 60%
Abdominal mass	25% to 45%
Anemia	20% to 40%
Flank pain	35% to 40%
Hypertension	20% to 40%
Weight loss	30% to 35%
Fever	5% to 15%
Hepatic dysfunction	10% to 15%
Classic triad (hematuria, abdominal mass, flank pain)	5% to 10%
Hypercalcemia	3% to 6%
Erythrocytosis	3% to 4%
Varicocele	2% to 3%

■ ETIOLOGY
Hereditary forms
• Familial renal carcinoma
• Renal carcinoma associated with von Hippel-Lindau disease
• Hereditary papillary renal cell carcinoma
Risk factors
• Cigarette smoking
• Obesity
• Use of diuretics
• Phenacetin-containing analgesics
• Asbestos exposure
• Gasoline and other petroleum products
• Lead
• Cadmium
• Thorotrast
• Role of the VHL gene located on chromosome 3

DIAGNOSIS

■ DIFFERENTIAL DIAGNOSIS
• Transitional cell carcinomas of the renal pelvis (8% of all renal cancers)
• Wilms' tumor
• Other rare primary renal carcinomas and sarcomas
• Renal cysts
• All causes of hematuria (see Section II)
• Retroperitoneal tumors

■ WORKUP
• Laboratory tests and imaging studies
• Section III, Fig. 3-158 describes the evaluation of patients with a renal mass

■ LABORATORY TESTS
• CBC: anemia or erythrocytosis
• Elevated sedimentation rate
• Nonmetastatic hepatic dysfunction with elevated alkaline phosphatase, prolonged prothrombin time, and hypoalbuminemia
• Hypercalcemia (secondary to parathyroid related protein)
• Other: elevated ferritin, elevated insulin and glucagon levels, elevated alpha-fetoprotein, and elevated beta-human chorionic gonadotropin

■ IMAGING STUDIES
• Intravenous pyelography (IVP)
• Renal ultrasound
• Abdominal CT scan with contrast (Fig. 1-229)
• MRI
• Renal arteriogram

■ STAGING
See Table 1-47.

■ COMMON SITES OF METASTASES

Lung	50% to 60%
Bone	30% to 40%
Regional nodes	15% to 30%
Main renal vein	15% to 20%
Perirenal fat	10% to 20%
Adrenal (ipsilateral)	10% to 15%
Vena cava	10% to 15%
Brain	10% to 15%
Adjacent organs (colon, pancreas)	10%
Kidney (contralateral)	2%

TREATMENT

• Surgery
  Surgical nephrectomy is the only effective management for stages I, II, and some stage III tumors.
  Various forms of partial nephrectomy may be available for patients with bilateral cancers or with a solitary kidney.
  The role of nephrectomy in patients with metastatic renal cell carcinoma is controversial and should probably be reserved for patients who have a solitary metastasis amenable to surgical resection.
• Angioinfarction (for palliation)
• Radiotherapy (for palliation)
• Chemotherapy (only 5% response rate)
• Hormonal therapy (high-dose progesterone may achieve a 15% to 20% response rate)

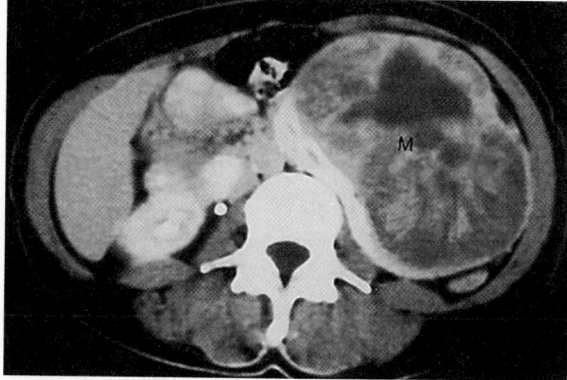

Fig. 1-229 Large renal cell carcinoma. Large mass *(M)* containing areas of high enhancement, low enhancement, and necrosis. (From Stein JH [ed]: *Internal medicine,* ed 5, St Louis, 1998, Mosby.)

- Immunotherapy (interleukin-2 may achieve a 15% to 30% response rate; alpha, beta, and gamma interferons are somewhat less effective; for example, interferon alfa-2b increased postnephrectomy median survival by 30% in one recent trial)
- Antivascular endothelial growth factor antibody Bevacizumab slows disease progression in metastatic renal cancer.

■ **PROGNOSIS**

Prognosis of surgically treated patients

TNM stage	5-year survival (%)
I	80 to 100
II	70 to 80
III (renal vein or vena cava)	50 to 60
III (nodal involvement)	15 to 25
IV	5 to 10

■ **REFERRAL**

To urologist

REFERENCES

Flanigan RC et al: Nephrectomy followed by interferon alfa-2b compared with interferon alfa-2b alone for metastatic renal-cell cancer, *N Engl J Med* 345:1655, 2002.

Jennings SB, Linehan WM: Renal, perirenal, and ureteral neoplasms. In Gillenwater JY et al: *Adult and pediatric urology*, ed 3, St Louis, 1996, Mosby.

Yang CJ: A randomized trial of Bevacizumab, an anti-vascular endothelial growth factor antibody, for metastatic renal cancer, *N Engl J Med* 349:427, 2003.

Author: **Tom J. Wachtel, M.D.**

TABLE 1-47 **Comparison of Conventional and TNM Staging Classification of RCC**

ROBSON STAGE	T	N	M
I: Tumor confined by capsule	T_1 (tumor 2.5 cm or less) T_2 (tumor >2.5 cm, limited to kidney)		
II: Tumor extension to perirenal fat or ipsilateral adrenal but confined by Gerota's fascia	T_3a (tumor invades adrenal gland or perinephric fat but not beyond Gerota's fascia)		
IIIa: Renal vein or inferior vena caval involvement	T_3b (renal vein or caval involvement below diaphragm) T_3c (caval involvement above diaphragm)	N_0 (nodes negative)	M_0 (no distant metastases)
IIIb: Lymphatic involvement	T_{1-4}	N_1 (single lymph node 2 cm or less) N_2 (single node between 2 and 5 cm, or multiple nodes <5 cm) N_3 (single or multiple nodes >5 cm)	
IIIc: Combination of IIIa and IIIb	$T_{3, 4}$		
IVa: Spread to contiguous organs except ipsilateral adrenal	T_4 (tumor extends beyond Gerota's fascia)		
IVb: Distant metastases	T_{1-4}		M_1 (distant metastases)

BASIC INFORMATION

■ DEFINITION

Acute renal failure (ARF) is the rapid impairment in renal function resulting in retention of products in the blood that are normally excreted by the kidneys.

■ SYNONYMS

ARF

ICD-9CM CODES

584.9 Acute renal failure, unspecified

■ EPIDEMIOLOGY & DEMOGRAPHICS

- ARF requiring dialysis develops in 5/100,000 persons annually.
- >10% of ICU patients develop ARF.
- >40% of hospital ARF is iatrogenic.
- The most common cause of ARF in hospitalized patients is intrinsic renal failure caused by acute tubular necrosis (ATN).

■ PHYSICAL FINDINGS & CLINICAL PRESENTATION

- The physical examination should focus on volume status. The physical findings noted below vary with the duration and rapidity of onset of renal failure
- Peripheral edema
- Skin pallor, ecchymoses
- Oliguria (however, patients can have nonoliguric renal failure), anuria
- Delirium, lethargy, myoclonus, seizures
- Back pain, fasciculations, muscle cramps
- Tachypnea, tachycardia
- Weakness, anorexia, generalized malaise, nausea

■ ETIOLOGY

- Prerenal: inadequate perfusion caused by hypovolemia, CHF, cirrhosis, sepsis. Sixty percent of community-acquired cases of ARF are due to prerenal conditions.
- Postrenal: outlet obstruction from prostatic enlargement, ureteral obstruction (stones), bilateral renal vein occlusion. Postrenal causes account for 5% to 15% of community-acquired ARF.
- Intrinsic renal: glomerulonephritis, acute tubular necrosis, drug toxicity, contrast nephropathy.
- Causes of acute renal failure are described in Section II.

DIAGNOSIS

■ DIFFERENTIAL DIAGNOSIS

Refer to "Etiology."

■ WORKUP

A thorough review of the patient's history is necessary to identify contributing factors (e.g., nephrotoxin exposure, hypertension, diabetes mellitus). Laboratory evaluation to quantify degree of abnormality; radiographic studies to exclude prerenal and postrenal factors. Categorization of renal failure into oliguric (urinary output <400 ml/day) or nonoliguric is important. Anuria is common in obstructive uropathy and acute cortical necrosis.

■ LABORATORY TESTS

- Elevated serum creatinine: the rate of rise of creatinine is approximately 1 mg/dl/day in complete renal failure.
- Elevated BUN: BUN/creatinine ratio is >20:1 in prerenal azotemia, postrenal azotemia, and acute glomerulonephritis; it is <20:1 in acute interstitial nephritis and acute tubular necrosis (Table 1-48).
- Electrolytes (potassium, phosphate) are elevated; bicarbonate level and calcium are decreased.
- CBC may reveal anemia because of decreased erythropoietin production, hemoconcentration, or hemolysis.
- Urinalysis may reveal the presence of hematuria (GN), proteinuria (nephrotic syndrome), casts (e.g., granular casts in ATN, RBC casts in acute GN, WBC casts in acute interstitial nephritis), eosinophiluria (acute interstitial nephritis).
- Urinary sodium and urinary creatinine should also be obtained to calculate the fractional excretion of sodium (FE_{Na}) (FE_{Na} = Urine sodium/plasma sodium × Plasma creatinine/urine creatinine × 100). The fractional excretion of sodium is <1 in prerenal failure, >1 in intrinsic renal failure in patients with urine output <400 ml/day.
- Urinary osmolarity is 250 to 300 mOsm/kg in ATN, <400 mOsm/kg in postrenal azotemia, and >500 mOsm/kg in prerenal azotemia and acute glomerulonephritis (Table 1-49).
- Additional useful studies are blood cultures for patients suspected of sepsis, LFTs, immunoglobulins, and protein electrophoresis in patients suspected of myeloma, creatinine kinase in patients with suspected rhabdomyolysis.

TABLE 1-48 Serum and Radiographic Abnormalities in Renal Failure

	PRERENAL	POSTRENAL (ACUTE)	INTRINSIC RENAL (ACUTE)	INTRINSIC RENAL (CHRONIC)
BUN	↑10:1 > Cr	↑ 20-40/d	↑ 20-40/d	Stable, ↑ varies with protein intake
Serum creatinine	N/moderate ↑	↑ 2-4/d	↑ 2-4/d	Stable ↑ (production equals excretion)
Serum potassium	N/moderate ↑	↑ varies with urinary volume	↑↑ (particularly when patient is oliguric) ↑↑↑ with rhabdomyolysis	Normal until end stage, unless tubular dysfunction (type 4 RTA)
Serum phosphorus	N/moderate ↑	Moderate ↑ ↑↑ with rhabdomyolysis	↑ Poor correlation with duration of renal disease	Becomes significantly elevated when serum creatinine level surpasses 3 mg/dl
Serum calcium	N	N/↓ with PO_4^{-3} retention	↓ (poor correlation with duration of renal failure)	Usually ↓
Renal size				
By ultrasound	N/↑	↑ and dilated calyces	N/↑	↓ and with ↑ echogenicity
FE_{Na}*	<1	<1 → >1	>1	>1

From Kiss B: Renal failure. In Ferri FF (ed): *Practical guide to the care of the medical patient,* ed 6, St Louis, 2004, Mosby.
↑, Increase; ↓, decrease; ↑↑, large increase, *Cr,* creatinine; *N,* normal; *Na,* sodium; *P,* plasma; *RTA,* renal tubular acidosis; *U,* urine.
*$FE_{Na} = U_{Na}/P_{Na}U_{Cr}/P_{cr} \times 100$.

- Renal biopsy may be indicated in patients with intrinsic renal failure when considering specific therapy; major uses of renal biopsy are differential diagnosis of nephrotic syndrome, separation of lupus vasculitis from other vasculitis and lupus membranous from idiopathic membranous, confirmation of hereditary nephropathies on the basis of the ultrastructure, diagnosis of rapidly progressing glomerulonephritis, separation of allergic interstitial nephritis from ATN, separation of primary glomerulonephritis syndromes. The biopsy may be performed percutaneously or by open method. The percutaneous approach is favored and generally yields adequate tissue in >90% of cases. Open biopsy is generally reserved for uncooperative patients, those with solitary kidney, and patients at risk for uncontrolled bleeding.

■ IMAGING STUDIES
- Chest x-ray examination is useful to evaluate for CHF and for pulmonary renal syndromes (Goodpasture's syndrome, Wegener's granulomatosis).
- Ultrasound of kidneys is used to evaluate for kidney size (useful to distinguish ARF from CRF), to evaluate for the presence of obstruction, and to evaluate renal vascular status (with Doppler evaluation).

- Anterograde and/or retrograde pyelogram can be used for ruling out obstruction; useful in patients at high risk of obstruction.

TREATMENT

■ NONPHARMACOLOGIC THERAPY
- Stop all nephrotoxic medications
- Dietary modification to supply adequate calories while minimizing accumulation of toxins; appropriate control of fluid balance. Physicians should recommend a nutrition program with an energy prescription of 120 to 150 KJ/kg per day and restriction of potassium (60 mEq/day), sodium (90 mEq/day), and phosphorus (800 mg/day). Ideal protein supplementation ranges from 0.6 to 1.4 g/kg depending on whether dialysis is required
- Daily weight
- Modifications of dosage of renally excreted drugs

■ ACUTE GENERAL Rx
Treatment is variable with etiology of ARF:
- Prerenal: IV volume expansion in hypovolemic patients
- Intrinsic renal: discontinuation of any potential toxins and treatment of condition causing the renal failure
- Postrenal: removal of obstruction

■ CHRONIC Rx
- Monitoring of renal function and electrolytes
- Prevention of further insults to the kidneys with proper hydration, especially before contrast studies, and avoidance of nephrotoxic agents
- Refer to topic on chronic renal failure for indications for initiation of dialysis. Daily hemodialysis is superior to every-other-day hemodialysis in patients with acute tubular necrosis and ARF.

■ DISPOSITION
- Prognosis is variable depending on the etiology of the renal failure, degree of renal failure, multiorgan involvement, and patient's age.
- Renal function recovery (ability to discontinue dialysis) varies from 50% to 75% in survivors of ARF.
- Overall mortality rate in ARF is nearly 50%, varying from 60% in patients with ATN to 35% in patients with prerenal or postrenal ARF.

■ REFERRAL
- Nephrology consultation is recommended in renal failure.
- General indications for initiation of dialysis are:
  1. Florid symptoms of uremia (encephalopathy, pericarditis)
  2. Severe volume overload
  3. Severe acid-base imbalance

TABLE 1-49   Urinary Abnormalities in Renal Failure

	PRERENAL	POSTRENAL (ACUTE)	INTRINSIC RENAL (ACUTE)	INTRINSIC RENAL (CHRONIC)
Urinary volume	↓	Absent-to-wide fluctuation	Oliguric or nonoliguric	1000 ml + until end stage
Urinary creatinine	↑ (U/P Cr ±40)	↓ (U/P Cr ±20)	↓ (U/P Cr <20)	↓ (U/P Cr <20)
Osmolarity	↑ (±400 mOsm/kg)	(<350 mOsm/kg)	(<350 mOsm/kg)	(<350 mOsm/kg)
Degree of proteinuria	Minimum	Absent	Varies with cause of renal failure: Modest with ATN Nephrotic range common with acute glomerulopathies, usually <2 g/24 hr with interstitial disease*	Varies with cause of renal disease (from 1-2 g/d to nephrotic range)
Urinary sediment	Negative, or occasional hyaline cast	Negative or hematuria with stones or papillary necrosis Pyuria with infectious prostatic disease	ATN: muddy brown Interstitial nephritis: lymphocytes, eosinophils (in stained preparations), and WBC casts RPGN: RBC casts Nephrosis: oval fat bodies	Broad casts with variable renal "residual" acute findings

From Kiss B: Renal failure. In Ferri FF (ed): *Practical guide to the care of the medical patient*, ed 6, St Louis, 2004, Mosby.
*Except NSAID-induced allergic interstitial nephritis with concomitant "nil disease."

↑, Increased; ↓, decreased; *ATN*, acute tubular necrosis; $clearance = \dfrac{\text{Urinary concentration} \times \text{Urinary volume}}{\text{Plasma concentration}}$; *Cr*, creatinine; *RBC*, red blood cell;

RPGN, rapidly progressive glomerulonephritis; *U/P*, urine/plasma; *WBC*, white blood cell.

4. Significant derangement in electrolyte concentrations (e.g., hyperkalemia, hyponatremia)
- Surgical consult may be necessary in patients with obstruction.

PEARLS & CONSIDERATIONS

COMMENTS
- It is important for physicians to recognize the growing list of medications that can result in ARF.

REFERENCES
Albright RC: Acute renal failure: a practical update, *Mayo Clin Proc* 76:67, 2001.
Kellum JA, Decker JM: Use of dopamine in acute renal failure: a meta analysis, *Crit Care Med* 29:1526, 2001.
Klassen PS et al: Association between pulse pressure and mortality in patients undergoing maintenance hemodialysis, *JAMA* 287:1548, 2002.
Nally JV: Acute renal failure in hospitalized patients, *Cleve Clin J Med* 69:569, 2002.
Schiffel H et al: Daily hemodialysis and the outcome of acute renal failure, *N Engl J Med* 346:305, 2002.
Teng M et al: Survival of patients undergoing hemodialysis with paricalcitol or calcitriol therapy, *N Engl J Med* 349:446, 2003.

Author: **Fred F. Ferri, M.D.**

BASIC INFORMATION

■ DEFINITION
Chronic renal failure (CRF) is a progressive decrease in renal function (CFR <60 ml/min for ≥3 mo) with subsequent accumulation of waste products in the blood, electrolyte abnormalities, and anemia.

■ SYNONYMS
CRF
End-stage renal disease

ICD-9CM CODES
585 Chronic renal failure

■ EPIDEMIOLOGY & DEMOGRAPHICS
- The number of patients with ESRD is increasing at the rate of 7% to 9%/yr in the U.S. Each year 2/10,000 persons develop end-stage CRF.
- In the U.S., >250,000/yr receive dialysis treatment for ESRD.

■ PHYSICAL FINDINGS & CLINICAL PRESENTATION
- Skin pallor, ecchymoses
- Edema
- Hypertension
- Emotional lability and depression
- The clinical presentation varies with the degree of renal failure and its underlying etiology. Common symptoms are generalized fatigue, nausea, anorexia, pruritus, insomnia, taste disturbances

■ ETIOLOGY
- Diabetes (37%), hypertension (30%), chronic glomerulonephritis (12%)
- Polycystic kidney disease
- Tubular interstitial nephritis (e.g., drug hypersensitivity, analgesic nephropathy), obstructive nephropathies (e.g., nephrolithiasis, prostatic disease)
- Vascular diseases (renal artery stenosis, hypertensive nephrosclerosis)

DIAGNOSIS

- CRF is primarily distinguished from ARF by the duration (progression over several months).
- Sonographic evaluation of the kidneys reveals smaller kidneys with increased echogenicity in CRF.

■ WORKUP
- Laboratory evaluation and imaging studies should be aimed at identifying reversible causes of acute decrements in GFR (e.g., volume depletion, urinary tract obstruction, CHF) superimposed on chronic renal disease

- Kidney biopsy: generally not performed in patients with small kidneys or with advanced disease

■ LABORATORY TESTS
- Elevated BUN, creatinine, creatinine clearance
- Urinalysis: may reveal proteinuria, RBC casts
- Serum chemistry: elevated BUN and creatinine, hyperkalemia, hyperuricemia, hypocalcemia, hyperphosphatemia, hyperglycemia, decreased bicarbonate
- Measure urinary protein excretion. The finding of a ratio of protein to creatinine of >1000 mg/g suggests the presence of glomerular disease
- Special studies: serum and urine immunoelectrophoresis (in suspected multiple myeloma), ANA (in suspected SLE)

■ IMAGING STUDIES
Ultrasound of kidneys to measure kidney size and to rule out obstruction

TREATMENT

■ NONPHARMACOLOGIC THERAPY
- Provide adequate nutrition and calories (147 to 168 kJ/kg/day in energy intake, chiefly from carbohydrate and polyunsaturated fats). Referral to a dietician for nutritional therapy for patients with GFR <50 ml/1.73 m² is recommended and is now a covered service by Medicare.
- Restrict sodium (approximately 100 mmol/day), potassium (≤60 mmol/day), and phosphate (<800 mg/day).
- Adjust drug doses to correct for prolonged half-lives.
- Restrict fluid if significant edema is present.
- Protein restriction (≤0.8 g/kg/day) may slow deterioration of renal function; however, recent studies have not confirmed this benefit. There is insufficient evidence to recommend or advise against routine restriction of protein intake
- Resistance exercise training can preserve lean body mass, nutritional status, and muscle function in patients with moderate chronic kidney disease.
- Avoid radiocontrast agents.
- Smoking cessation.
- Initiate hemodialysis or peritoneal dialysis (see "Acute General Rx").
- Prompt to nephrologist is essential. Late evaluation of patients with chronic renal disease is associated with greater burden and severity of comorbid disease and shorter survival.

- Kidney transplantation in selected patients.

■ GENERAL Rx
- ACE inhibitors, ARBs, and nondihydropyridine calcium channel blockers (diltiazem or verapamil) are useful in reducing proteinuria and slowing the progression of chronic renal disease, especially in hypertensive diabetic patients. A systolic blood pressure between 110 and 129 mm Hg may be beneficial in patients with urine protein excretion >1.0 g/day. Systolic BP <110 mm Hg may be associated with a higher risk for kidney disease progression.
- Initiation of dialysis
  1. Urgent indications: uremic pericarditis, neuropathy, neuromuscular abnormalities, CHF, hyperkalemia, seizures.
  2. Judgmental indications: creatinine clearance 10 to 15 ml/min; progressive anorexia, weight loss, reversal of sleep pattern, pruritus, uncontrolled fluid gain with hypertension and signs of CHF.
- Erythropoietin for anemia: 2000 to 3000 U three times a week IV/SC to maintain Hct 30% to 33%.
- Diuretics for significant fluid overload (loop diuretics are preferred).
- Correction of hypertension to at least 130/85 mm Hg with ACE inhibitors (avoid in patients with significant hyperkalemia), ARBs, and/or nondihydropyridene calcium channel blockers (verapamil, diltiazem) can be used in patients intolerant to ACE inhibitors or when other agents are needed to control blood pressure.
- Correction of electrolyte abnormalities (e.g., calcium chloride, glucose, sodium polystyrene sulfonate for hyperkalemia), sodium bicarbonate in patients with severe metabolic acidosis.
- Lipid-lowering agents in patients with dyslipidemia, target LDL cholesterol is <100 mg/dl.
- Control of renal osteodystrophy with calcium supplementation and vitamin D. Starting dose of calcium carbonate is 0.5 g with each meal, increased until the serum phosphorus concentration is normalized (most patients require 5 to 10 g/day). Calcitriol 0.125 to 0.25 μg/day PO is effective in increasing serum calcium concentration. Paricalcitol, a new vitamin-D analogue, appears to lessen the elevations in serum calcium and phosphorus levels as compared with calcitriol and may offer a significant survival advantage.
- Sevelamer (Renagel) is a useful phosphate binder to reduce serum phosphate levels.

■ DISPOSITION

- Prognosis is influenced by comorbidity of multisystem diseases.
- Kidney transplantation in selected patients improves survival. The 2-yr kidney graft survival rate for living related donor transplantations is >80%, whereas the 2-yr graft survival rate for cadaveric donor transplantation is approximately 70%.

REFERENCES

Jafar TH et al: Progression of chronic kidney disease: the role of blood pressure control, proteinuria, and angiotensin-converting enzyme inhibition, *Ann Intern Med* 139:244, 2003.

Kinchen KS et al: The timing of specialist evaluation in chronic kidney disease and mortality, *Ann Intern Med* 137:479, 2003.

Levey AS: Nondiabetic kidney disease, *N Engl J Med* 347:1505, 2002.

Lewey AS et al: National Kidney Foundation practice guidelines for chronic kidney disease: evaluation, classification, and stratification, *Ann Intern Med* 139:137, 2003.

Lewinsky NG: Specialist evaluation in chronic kidney disease: too little too late, *Ann Intern Med* 137:542, 2002.

Remuzzi G et al: Chronic renal diseases: renoprotective benefits of renin-angiotensin system inhibition, *Ann Intern Med* 136:604, 2002.

Teng M et al: Survival of patients undergoing hemodialysis with paracalcitol or calcitriol therapy, *N Engl J Med* 349:446, 2003.

Yu HT: Progression of chronic renal failure, *Arch Intern Med* 163:1417, 2003.

Author: **Fred F. Ferri, M.D.**

BASIC INFORMATION

■ DEFINITION

Renal tubular acidosis (RTA) is a disorder characterized by inability to excrete H^+ or inadequate generation of new HCO_3^-. There are four types of renal tubular acidosis:

- Type I (classic, distal RTA): abnormality in distal hydrogen secretion resulting in hypokalemic hyperchloremic metabolic acidosis.
- Type II (proximal RTA): decreased proximal bicarbonate reabsorption resulting in hypokalemic hyperchloremic metabolic acidosis.
- Type III (RTA of glomerular insufficiency): normokalemic hyperchloremic metabolic acidosis as a result of impaired ability to generate sufficient NH_3 in the setting of decreased glomerular filtration rate (<30 ml/min). This type of RTA is described in older textbooks and is considered by many not to be a distinct entity.
- Type IV (hyporeninemic hypoaldosteronemic RTA): aldosterone deficiency or antagonism resulting in decreased distal acidification and decreased distal sodium reabsorption with subsequent hyperkalemic hyperchloremic acidosis.

■ SYNONYMS

RTA

ICD-9CM CODES

588.8 Renal tubular acidosis

■ EPIDEMIOLOGY & DEMOGRAPHICS

RTA type IV affects mostly adults, whereas RTA type I and II are more frequent in children.

■ PHYSICAL FINDINGS & CLINICAL PRESENTATION

- Examination may be normal.
- Poor skin turgor may be present from dehydration.
- Muscle weakness and muscle aches from hypokalemia may occur.
- Low back pain and bone pain may be present in patients with abnormalities of calcium metabolism (RTA II).
- There is failure to thrive in children (RTA II).

■ ETIOLOGY

- Type I RTA: primary biliary cirrhosis and other liver diseases, medications (amphotericin, nonsteroidals), SLE, Sjögren's syndrome
- Type II RTA: Fanconi's syndrome, primary hyperparathyroidism, multiple myeloma, medications (acetazolamide)
- Type IV RTA: diabetes mellitus, sickle cell disease, Addison's disease, urinary obstruction

DIAGNOSIS

■ DIFFERENTIAL DIAGNOSIS

- Diarrhea with significant bicarbonate loss
- Other causes of metabolic acidosis
- Respiratory acidosis

■ WORKUP

Detection of hyperchloremic metabolic acidosis with ABGs and serum electrolytes and evaluation of potential causes (see "Etiology")

■ LABORATORY TESTS

- ABGs reveal metabolic acidosis; serum potassium is low in RTA types I and II, normal in type III, and high in type IV.
- Minimal urine pH is >5.5 in RTA type I, <5.5 in types II, III, and IV.
- Urinary anion gap is 0 or positive in all types of RTA.
- Additional useful studies include serum calcium level and urine calcium.
- Anion gap is normal.
- PTH measurement is useful in patients suspected of primary hyperparathyroidism (may be associated with type II RTA).

■ IMAGING STUDIES

- Plain abdominal radiography is useful to evaluate for nephrocalcinosis
- Renal sonogram can be used to evaluate renal size or presence of stones
- IVP in patients with nephrocalcinosis or nephrolithiasis

TREATMENT

■ ACUTE GENERAL Rx

- Type I and type II are treated with oral sodium bicarbonate (1 to 2 mEq/kg/day in RTA 1, 2 to 4 mEq/kg/day in RTA type II) titrated to correct acidosis.
- Potassium supplementation is needed in hypokalemic patients.
- Type IV RTA can be treated with furosemide to lower elevated potassium levels and sodium bicarbonate to correct significant acidosis. Fludrocortisone 100 to 300 µg/day can be used to correct mineralocorticoid deficiency.

■ CHRONIC Rx

- Frequent monitoring of potassium levels in type IV RTA
- Monitoring for bone disease in RTA type II
- Monitoring for nephrocalcinosis and nephrolithiasis in RTA type I

■ DISPOSITION

- Prognosis varies with the presence of associated conditions (see "Etiology").
- Untreated distal RTA may result in hypercalcemia, hyperphosphaturia, nephrolithiasis, and nephrocalcinosis.

PEARLS & CONSIDERATIONS

■ COMMENTS

Patient education material can be obtained from the National Kidney and Urologic Diseases Information Clearinghouse, Box NKUDIC, Bethesda, MD 20893.

Author: **Fred F. Ferri, M.D.**

BASIC INFORMATION

■ DEFINITION
Renal vein thrombosis is the thrombotic occlusion of one or both renal veins.

ICD-9CM CODES
453.3 Renal vein thrombosis

■ EPIDEMIOLOGY & DEMOGRAPHICS
- Incidence unknown, probably an underdiagnosed condition
- May occur at any age with no gender preference
- Epidemiology tied to the underlying cause

■ PHYSICAL FINDINGS & CLINICAL PRESENTATION
Acute bilateral renal vein thrombosis
- Back and bilateral flank pain
- Acute renal failure

Acute unilateral renal vein thrombosis
- Flank pain
- Decline in renal function
- Hematuria
- Increase in the amount of proteinuria if associated with nephrotic syndrome

Chronic unilateral renal vein thrombosis
- May be silent
- Pulmonary emboli and hemolysis
- Back pain
- DVT in lower extremities
- Edema
- Glycosuria
- Hyperchloremic acidosis
- Left varicocele (if the left renal vein is thrombosed)
- Dilated abdominal veins

■ ETIOLOGY & PATHOGENESIS
- Extrinsic compression by a tumor or retroperitoneal mass
- Invasion of the renal vein or inferior vena cava by tumor (almost always renal cell cancer)
- Trauma
- Hypercoagulable states
- Dehydration
- Glomerulopathies (membranous glomerulonephritis, crescenting glomerulonephritis, SLE, amyloidosis) especially in the presence of nephrotic syndrome when the serum albumin is lower than 2 g/dl
- NOTE: For unknown reasons, diabetic nephropathy is not commonly associated with renal vein thrombosis even if the nephrotic syndrome is present

A controversy has existed as to whether the renal vein thrombosis association with nephrotic syndrome is a complication of nephrotic syndrome or whether renal vein thrombosis occurring in the setting of increased renal vein pressure (e.g., with congestive heart failure, constrictive pericarditis, or extrinsic compression) can independently cause proteinuria. Current evidence is that renal vein thrombosis does not cause nephrotic syndrome.

DIAGNOSIS

■ DIFFERENTIAL DIAGNOSIS
The diagnosis of renal vein thrombosis does not include any differential consideration. The differential diagnosis is that of proteinuria. Renal vein thrombosis should be considered if proteinuria worsens or if renal function worsens in a patient with glomerulonephritis. Renal vein thrombosis should also be considered in patients with pulmonary emboli and no lower-extremity DVT.

■ WORKUP
Clinical suspicion (see "Differential Diagnosis") and imaging studies

■ IMAGING STUDIES
- Abdominal ultrasound
- Abdominal MRI
- Renal arteriography (delayed films during venous phase)
- Selective renal vein venography (inferior venacavogram images should be obtained before advancing the catheter in the vena cava because clots, if present, could be dislodged)
- Renal biopsy may be indicated if evidence of nephritis is present (e.g., active urinary sediment)

TREATMENT

- Anticoagulation in acute renal vein thrombosis to prevent pulmonary emboli and in attempt to improve renal function and decrease proteinuria
- Thrombolytic therapy or surgical thrombectomy has also been reported to be effective
- The value of anticoagulation in chronic renal vein thrombosis is dubious except in nephrotic patients with membranous glomerulonephritis with profound hypoalbuminemia where prolonged prophylactic anticoagulation may be of benefit even if renal vein thrombosis has not been documented

■ PROGNOSIS
Probable worsening of the underlying glomerulonephritis by acute renal vein thrombosis; the effect of chronic renal vein thrombosis is unclear.

REFERENCE
Yudd M, Llach F: Renal vein thrombosis. In Brenner BM (ed): *The kidney*, ed 5, Philadelphia, 2000, WB Saunders.
Author: **Tom J. Wachtel, M.D.**

BASIC INFORMATION

■ DEFINITION
Restless legs syndrome is a primary neurologic disorder of unknown cause that manifests with both sensory and motor symptoms usually involving the lower extremities and disrupting sleep.

■ SYNONYMS
"Crazy legs" (lay term)
Nocturnal myoclonus

ICD-9CM CODES
333.99 Nocturnal myoclonus

■ EPIDEMIOLOGY & DEMOGRAPHICS
PREVALENCE: 5% to 15%
DEMOGRAPHICS: Age 2 yr to no upper limit
- Age 18 to 29: 3%
- Age 30 to 79: 10%
- Age 80 and above: 19%
- Prevalence increases with age (may explain a slight female overrepresentation)
- Symptoms worsen with age

■ PHYSICAL FINDINGS & CLINICAL PRESENTATION
- Sensory nocturnal complaints usually affecting both lower extremities:
Crawly feeling or fizzle under the skin
Itching under the skin
Pain or ache
Electric shocks
Irresistible urge to move the symptomatic leg
- Other words used by patients to describe the leg symptoms: creeping, burning, searing, tugging, pulling, drawing, like water flowing, worms or bugs under the skin, restless, indescribable
- Consistent symptom relief or improvement with leg movement or walking

- Sleep disruption
- Leg movements during sleep may occur but are not the prevailing complaint (unlike the urge to move). These movements are short bursts lasting <5 sec
- Physical examination is normal

■ ETIOLOGY
- Unknown/idiopathic
- Hereditary (30% to 60%)
- Associated with iron deficiency
- Associated with renal failure (end-stage)
- Associated with pregnancy
- Associated with peripheral neuropathy or radiculopathy
- Associated with rheumatologic conditions (rheumatoid arthritis, fibromyalgia)
- Medication induced (selective serotonin reuptake inhibitors)

DIAGNOSIS

■ DIFFERENTIAL DIAGNOSIS
- Periodic limb movement disorder (PLMD) (repetitive limb movements [lower extremities > upper extremities] occurring during sleep; associated with arousals from sleep and daytime sleeping; patient is typically unaware, but bed partner reports restlessness or kicking during sleep)
- Peripheral neuropathy and radiculopathy
- Anxiety and mood disorders
- Chronic fatigue
- Other sleep disorders
- Neuroleptic-induced akathisia
- Dyskinesias while awake
- Nocturnal leg cramps with or without peripheral artery disease

■ WORKUP
- History is typically diagnostic with sensitivity and specificity both >90%
- Sleep logs
- Polysomnography
- Ambulatory recording of leg activity

TREATMENT

- Dopaminergic drugs are first line: Levodopa/carbidopa (Sinemet) Pergolide or pramipexole
- Benzodiazepines
- Trazodone
- Opioids
- Gabapentin (Neurontin)

■ PROGNOSIS
Tendency to worsen with age

REFERENCES
Allen RP: Restless legs syndrome: epidemiology and diagnosis, *Med Behav* 1:36, 1998.

Earley CJ: Restless legs syndrome, *N Engl J Med* 348:2103, 2003.

Lin SC et al: Effect of pramipexole in treatment of resistant restless legs syndrome, *Mayo Clin Proc* 73:497, 1998.

National Heart, Lung, and Blood Institute Working Group on Restless Legs Syndrome: Restless legs syndrome: detection and management in primary care, *Am Fam Physician* 62:108, 2000.

Phillips B, Young T, Finn L, et al: Epidemiology of restless legs symptoms in adults, *Arch Intern Med* 160:2137, 2000.

Author: **Tom J. Wachtel, M.D.**

BASIC INFORMATION

■ DEFINITION
Retinal detachment is a retinal separation where the inner or neural layer of the retina separates from the pigment epithelial layer and results from numerous causes.

■ SYNONYMS
Inflammatory lesions of choroid
Uveitis
Tumor
Vascular lesions
Congenital disorders

ICD-9CM CODES
361 Retinal detachment and defects

■ EPIDEMIOLOGY & DEMOGRAPHICS
INCIDENCE (IN U.S.):
- 0.02% of the population
- Particularly common in patients with high myopia of 5 diopters or more

PREVALENCE (IN U.S.): Busy ophthalmologist may see one or two acute retinal detachments per month
PREDOMINANT SEX: None
PREDOMINANT AGE:
- Congenital in younger patients
- Usually trauma in patients 30 to 40 yr and older
- High myopia a predisposition

PEAK INCIDENCE: Incidence increases with increasing age or increasing myopia.

■ PHYSICAL FINDINGS & CLINICAL PRESENTATION
Elevation of retina and vessels associated with tears in the retina, with fluid, and/or with hemorrhage beneath the retina and changes in the vitreous (Fig. 1-230).
Complaints of flashing lights and floaters

■ ETIOLOGY
- Trauma
- Tears in the retina
- Uveitis
- Fluid accumulation beneath the retina
- Tumors
- Scleritis
- Inflammatory disease
- Diabetes
- Collagen-vascular disease
- Vascular abnormalities

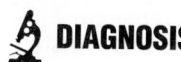

DIAGNOSIS

■ DIFFERENTIAL DIAGNOSIS
- Detachment
- Hemorrhage
- Tumors

■ WORKUP
- Full eye examination
- Fluorescein angiography
- Visual fields
- Ultrasonography to show the retinal detachment or tumors beneath it

- Medical workup only when inflammation or systemic disease considered

■ LABORATORY TESTS
Usually not necessary

■ IMAGING STUDIES
B scan of the eye

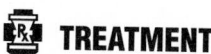

TREATMENT

■ NONPHARMACOLOGIC THERAPY
Immediate surgery

■ ACUTE GENERAL Rx
- Early surgery to repair the detachment
- Treatment of the underlying disorder

■ CHRONIC Rx
Occasionally, steroids or other treatment of underlying disease is indicated.

■ DISPOSITION
- Make an immediate referral to an ophthalmologist.
- Early intervention improves outcomes.

■ REFERRAL
Immediately

☼ PEARLS & CONSIDERATIONS

■ COMMENTS
If treated early, most patients will recover a substantial portion of their vision.

REFERENCES
Carpineto P et al: Retinal detachment prophylaxis, *Ophthalmology* 109(2):217, 2002.
Yazici B et al: Prediction of visual outcome after retinal detachment surgery using the Lotmar visometer, *Br J Ophthalmol* 86(3):278, 2002.
Author: **Melvyn Koby, M.D.**

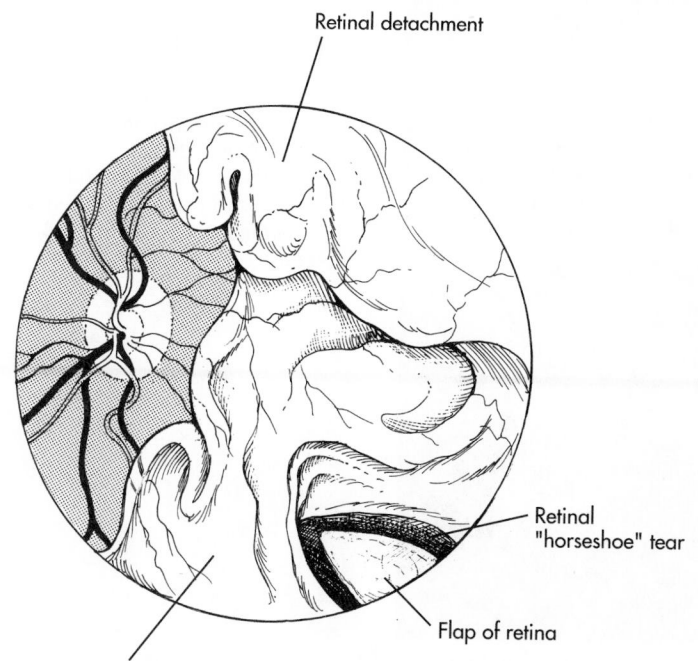

Fig. 1-230   Retinal detachment. (From Scuderi G [ed]: *Sports medicine: principles of primary care,* St Louis, 1997, Mosby.)

BASIC INFORMATION

■ **DEFINITION**

In a retinal hemorrhage, blood accumulates in the retinal and subretinal areas.

■ **SYNONYMS**

Pseudoxanthoma elasticum
Coats' disease
Retinal trauma
High-altitude retinopathy

■ **ICD-9CM CODES**

362.81 Retinal hemorrhage

■ **EPIDEMIOLOGY & DEMOGRAPHICS**

INCIDENCE (IN U.S.): Busy ophthalmologist sees one or two cases a month.
PREDOMINANT AGE: Degenerative disease in older patients
PEAK INCIDENCE:
• Children—associated primarily with trauma and hematologic disorders
• Increases with age

■ **PHYSICAL FINDINGS & CLINICAL PRESENTATION**

• Hemorrhage within the retina or subretinal area (Fig. 1-231)
• Evidence of retinal tears, tumors, and inflammation

■ **ETIOLOGY**

• Diabetes
• Hypertension
• Trauma
• Inflammation
• Tumors
• Subretinal neovascularization
• Associated with diabetes and aging

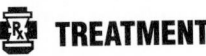 **DIAGNOSIS**

■ **DIFFERENTIAL DIAGNOSIS**

• Evaluate patients for local and systemic diseases.
• Either venous or arterial occlusion may cause retinal hemorrhage, and such occlusion is associated with atherosclerotic or heart disease, so look for these.
• Rule out malignant melanoma, trauma, hypertensive cardiovascular disease.
Section II describes the differential diagnosis of acute painless loss of vision.

■ **WORKUP**

Complete general physical examination

■ **LABORATORY TESTS**

• Minimum: CBC, sedimentation rate, and complete blood chemistries
• Fluorescein

• Angiography
• Visual field testing

■ **IMAGING STUDIES**

Usually not necessary

TREATMENT

■ **NONPHARMACOLOGIC THERAPY**

Laser or treatment of underlying disorder

■ **ACUTE GENERAL Rx**

• Laser is often indicated.
• Steroids may be indicated, depending on etiology.
• Treat underlying disease.
• Repair damage if from trauma.

■ **CHRONIC Rx**

Laser if hemorrhage is recurrent

■ **DISPOSITION**

Consider this an emergency.

■ **REFERRAL**

• Immediate referral to an ophthalmologist
• An emergency, with early treatment significantly affecting outcome

PEARLS & CONSIDERATIONS

■ **COMMENTS**

• Vision may return substantially.
• Complete recovery dependent on amount of scar tissue formed.

REFERENCES

Duncan BB et al: Hypertensive retinopathy and incident coronary heart disease in high risk men, *Br J Ophth* 86(9):1002, 2002.
Schloff S et al: Retinal findings in children with intracranial hemorrhage, *Ophthalmology* 109(8):1472, 2002.
Author: **Melvyn Koby, M.D.**

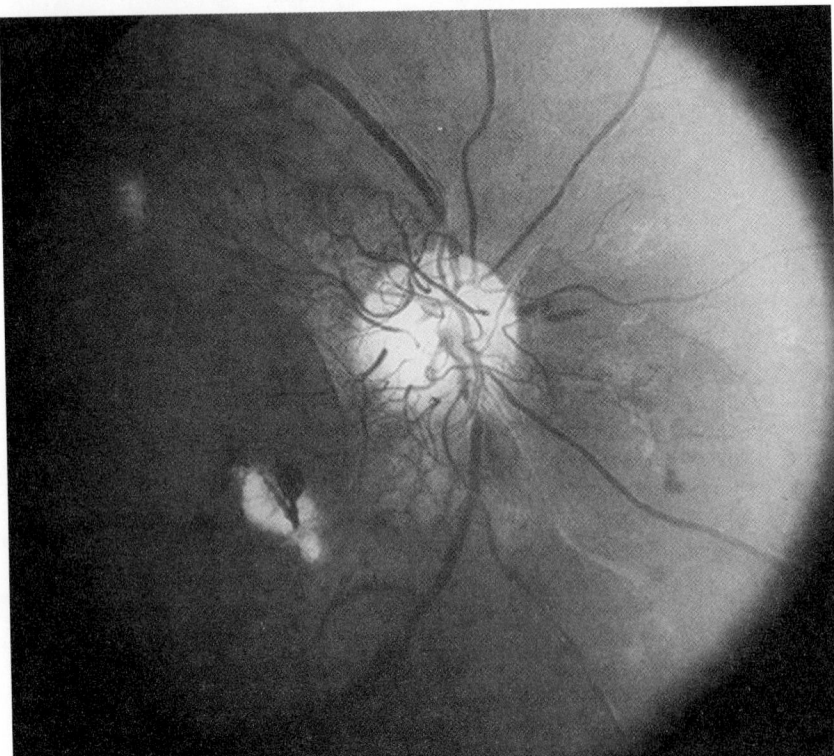

Fig. 1-231 Fronds of neovascularization on the disc are present in this right eye. Temporally, two cotton-wool spots have adjacent intraretinal hemorrhage and preretinal hemorrhage. Native retinal arteries are narrowed and show evidence of sclerosis. (From Palay D [ed]: *Ophthalmology for the primary care physician*, St Louis, 1997, Mosby.)

BASIC INFORMATION

■ DEFINITION
Retinitis pigmentosa is a generalized retinal pigment degeneration associated with a variety of inheritance patterns resulting in decreased vision. A simple recessive pattern is most severe. It may be associated with some rare neurologic syndromes.

ICD-9CM CODES
362.74 Retinitis pigmentosa, pigmentary retinal dystrophy

■ EPIDEMIOLOGY & DEMOGRAPHICS
PREVALENCE (IN U.S.): 1 in 4000 people
PREDOMINANT SEX: Depends on inheritance
PREDOMINANT AGE: 60 yr
PEAK INCIDENCE:
- Recessive incidence: in the 20s
- Dominant form: in the 40s
GENETICS:
- 19% dominant
- 19% recessive
- 8% X-linked
- 46% not known to be genetically related (mutations)
- 8% undetermined cause

■ PHYSICAL FINDINGS & CLINICAL PRESENTATION
- Deposition of retinal pigment in midperiphery and centrally in the retina with a pale optic nerve and narrowing of blood vessels (Fig. 1-232)
- Possible cataracts and macular edema
- Decrease in night vision and peripheral vision

■ ETIOLOGY
Usually hereditary

DIAGNOSIS

■ DIFFERENTIAL DIAGNOSIS
- Syphilis
- Old inflammatory scars
- Old hemorrhage
- Diabetes
- Toxic retinopathies (phenothiazines, chloroquine)

■ WORKUP
- Electrophysiologic studies
- Dark adaptation studies
- Visual fields

■ LABORATORY TESTS
- Usually not necessary
- VDRL, glucose (selected patients)

■ IMAGING STUDIES
Usually not necessary

TREATMENT

■ CHRONIC Rx
- No proven effective therapy
- Sometimes vitamin E or vitamin A may be helpful

■ DISPOSITION
Disease may be either mild or severe, but if the patient is expected to progress to total blindness, counseling and early education are important.

■ REFERRAL
To ophthalmologist to confirm diagnosis

PEARLS & CONSIDERATIONS

■ COMMENTS
- The spiderweb-like appearance of macular degeneration should not be confused with the extra pigments sometimes seen in dark-skinned individuals.
- Patient education material can be obtained from the Retinitis Pigmentosa Foundation Fighting Blindness, 1401 Mt. Royal Avenue, 4th Floor, Baltimore, MD 21217.

REFERENCES
Berson E et al: Disease progression in patients with dominant retinitis pigmentosa and rhodopsin mutations, *Invest Ophthalmol Vis Sci* (43)9:3027, 2002.
Holopigiam K et al: Local cone and rod system function in patients with retinitis pigmentosa, *Invest Ophthal Vis Sci* 43(3):779, 2001.
Author: **Melvyn Koby, M.D.**

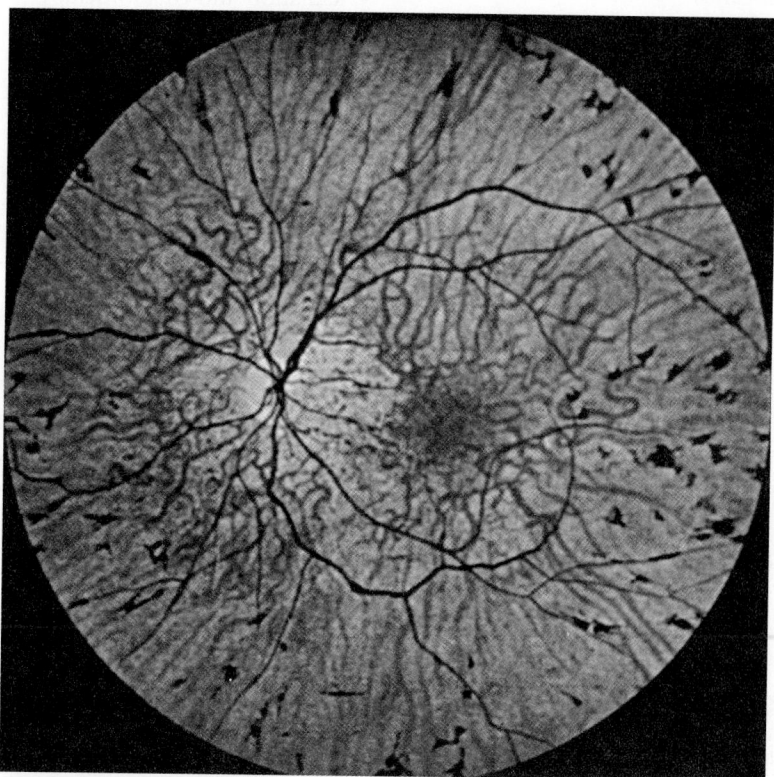

Fig. 1-232 Retinitis pigmentosa. (From Behrman RE [ed]: *Nelson textbook of pediatrics*, Philadelphia, 1996, WB Saunders.)

BASIC INFORMATION

■ DEFINITION

Retinoblastoma is an inherited, highly malignant congenital neoplasm arising from the neural layers of the retina.

ICD-9CM CODES

190.5 Retinoblastoma, malignant neoplasm of eyes, retina

■ EPIDEMIOLOGY & DEMOGRAPHICS

INCIDENCE (IN U.S.): 1 in every 23,000 to 34,000 births
PREDOMINANT AGE: 8 mo
PEAK INCIDENCE:
- 6 to 13 mo
- 72% diagnosed by 3 yr of age
- 90% diagnosed by 4 yr of age

GENETICS:
- Gene mutation or an autosomal dominant gene with 80% to 95% penetration
- 5% mutations

■ PHYSICAL FINDINGS & CLINICAL PRESENTATION
- White pupils (Fig. 1-233)
- White elevated retinal masses
- Strabismus
- Glaucoma
- Uveitis

■ ETIOLOGY
Genetic

DIAGNOSIS

■ DIFFERENTIAL DIAGNOSIS
- Strabismus
- Retinal detachment
- Uveitis
- Other tumors
- Glaucoma
- Endophthalmitis
- Cataract

■ WORKUP
Ophthalmologic examination

■ IMAGING STUDIES
- MRI: may show calcifications in retina
- Ultrasonography: good delineation of mass

TREATMENT

■ NONPHARMACOLOGIC THERAPY
- Surgical enucleation of the eye
- Radiation and chemotherapy

■ DISPOSITION
Usually treated by an ophthalmologist/oncologist

■ REFERRAL
To ophthalmologist/oncologist

PEARLS & CONSIDERATIONS

■ COMMENT
With early aggressive treatment, some patients may survive.

REFERENCES

Brichand B et al: Combined chemotherapy and local treatment in the management of intra ocular retinoblastoma, *Med Pediatr Oncol* 38(6):411, 2002.

Butros LJ et al: Delayed diagnosis of retinoblastoma analysis of degree, cause, and potential consequences, *Pediatric* 109(3):E45, 2002.

Schouten-Van Meeteren AY et al: Overview: chemotherapy for retinoblastoma: an expanding area of clinical research, *Med Pediatr Oncol* 38(6):428, 2002.

Author: **Melvyn Koby, M.D.**

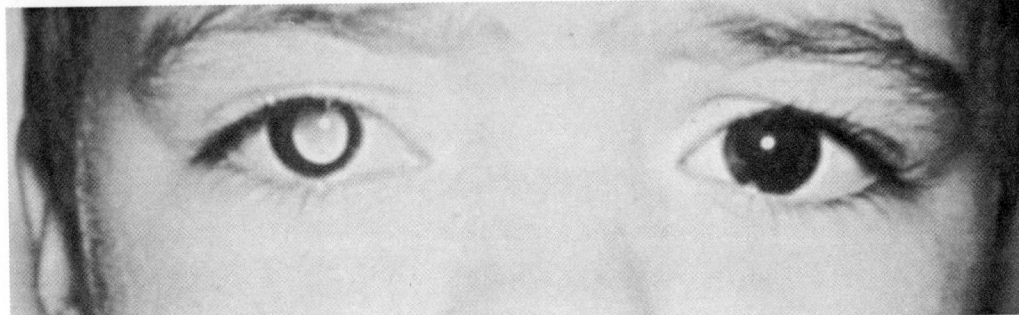

Fig. 1-233 Leukocoria. White papillary reflex in a child with retinoblastoma. (From Behrman RE [ed]: *Nelson textbook of pediatrics,* Philadelphia, 1996, WB Saunders.)

BASIC INFORMATION

■ DEFINITION

Diabetic retinopathy is an eye abnormality associated with diabetes and consisting of microaneurysms, punctate hemorrhages, white and yellow exudates, flame hemorrhages, and neovascular vessel growth (Fig. 1-234).

■ SYNONYMS

NPDR—nonproliferative diabetic retinopathy
PDR—proliferative (advanced) diabetic retinopathy

ICD-9CM CODES

250.5 Diabetes with ophthalmic manifestations
362.1 Retinopathy, diabetic, background
362.02 Retinopathy, diabetic, proliferative

■ EPIDEMIOLOGY & DEMOGRAPHICS

INCIDENCE (IN U.S.):
• Affects 11 million persons
• A leading cause of blindness in people 20 to 70 yr old
• 5000 new cases annually
PREVALENCE (IN U.S.): Prevalence of retinopathy increases with duration of diabetes. Found in 18% of people diagnosed with diabetes for 3- to 4-yr duration and in up to 80% of diabetics with a diagnosis of 15 yr or more.
PREDOMINANT SEX: Male:female
PREDOMINANT AGE: 30 yr or older
PEAK INCIDENCE: Begins 10 yr after onset of diabetes
GENETICS: Diabetes is usually hereditary.

■ PHYSICAL FINDINGS & CLINICAL PRESENTATION
• See "Definition"
• Microaneurysms
• Hemorrhages
• Exudates
• Macular edema
• Neovascularization
• Retinal detachment
• Hemorrhages in the vitreous
• In early cases, patient may not complain of a visual disturbance

■ ETIOLOGY
Associated with diabetes mellitus

DIAGNOSIS

■ DIFFERENTIAL DIAGNOSIS
• Retinal inflammatory diseases
• Tumor
• Trauma
• Arteriosclerotic vascular disease

■ WORKUP
Fluorescein angiogram

■ LABORATORY TESTS
Those appropriate for diabetes mellitus

TREATMENT

■ NONPHARMACOLOGIC THERAPY
Laser treatment with proliferative disease or macular edema
Photo coagulation of neovascular areas

■ ACUTE GENERAL Rx
• Laser therapy
• Vitrectomy
• Repair of retinal detachment
• Medical control of disease and complications and associated diseases (hypertension, etc.)

■ CHRONIC Rx
Repeated laser treatments may be necessary.

■ DISPOSITION
• Retinal examination should be performed on all routine medical visits.
• Prognosis is improved with early diagnosis and treatment.

■ REFERRAL
If diabetic retinopathy is severe enough to interfere with vision, follow-up is best done by an ophthalmologist.

PEARLS & CONSIDERATIONS

■ COMMENTS
• Early laser treatment of severe, non-proliferative, and proliferative retinopathy may minimize complications and visual loss.
• Patient education information can be obtained from the American Academy of Ophthalmology (655 Beach Street, San Francisco, CA 94109-1336) and from the American Diabetes Association (1-800-232-3472).

REFERENCES
Aiello LP et al: Systemic considerations in the management of diabetic retinopathy, *Am J Ophthal* 131(5):760, 2001.
Klein R et al: The association of atherosclerosis, vascular risk factors, and retinopathy in adults with diabetes, *Ophthalmology* 109(7):1225, 2002.
Raman V et al: Retinopathy screening in children and adolescents with diabetes, *Am NY Acad Sci* 958:387, 2002.
Author: **Melvyn Koby, M.D.**

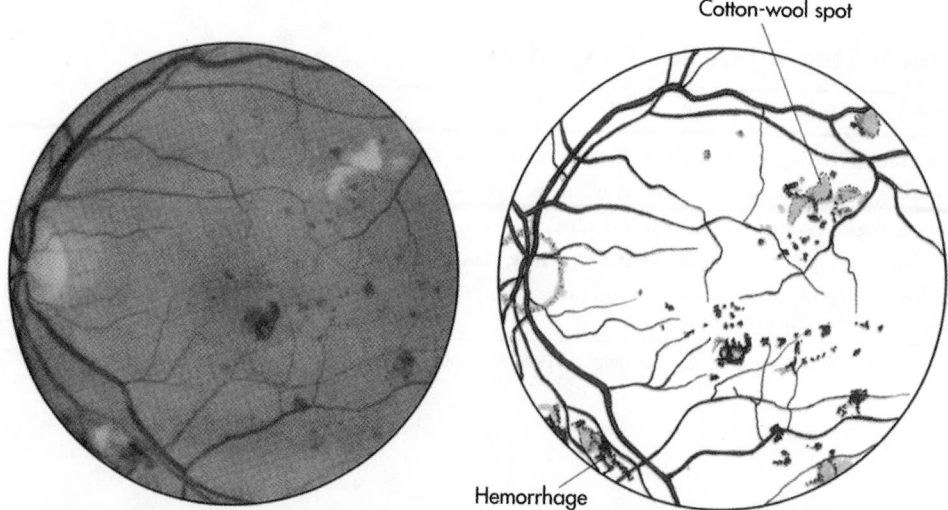

Fig. 1-234 Background diabetic retinopathy. Note flame-shaped and dot-blot hemorrhages, cotton-wool spots, and microaneurysms. (From Barkaukas VH et al: *Health and physical assessment*, ed 2, St Louis, 1998, Mosby.)

BASIC INFORMATION

■ **DEFINITION**

Reye's syndrome is a postinfectious triad consisting of encephalopathy, fatty liver degeneration, and transaminase elevation.

ICD-9CM CODES
331.81 Reye's syndrome

■ **EPIDEMIOLOGY & DEMOGRAPHICS**
• During the 1970s, 300 to 600 cases were being reported yearly in the U.S
• Since the mid-1980s, following the understanding that aspirin is associated with Reye's syndrome, the yearly count has fallen to <20 cases
• Seasonal relation with influenza and varicella outbreaks
• Age: rare in persons over age 18 yr; peak age (in the U.S.) is 6 to 8 yr
• Case fatality rate: 25% to 50%

■ **PHYSICAL FINDINGS & CLINICAL PRESENTATION**

Shortly following recovery from a viral infection (flu or chicken pox) an afebrile child begins to vomit intractably. Hepatomegaly is often present. The vomiting can lead to dehydration. Occasionally, symptoms of hypoglycemia are present. After 2 days, symptoms of encephalopathy dominate the clinical picture (lethargy, confusion, stupor, coma, seizures, decorticate or decerebrate posture) (Table 1-50).

■ **ETIOLOGY**
• Temporal association with influenza and varicella infection
• Epidemiologic association with aspirin or other salicylate use to treat the viral infection

• Possible association with aflatoxin and pesticides
• Pathology
Liver: no inflammation; the striking finding is panlobular microvesicular hepatocyte infiltration on light microscopy and mitochondrial injury on electron microscopy.
Brain: no inflammation; there are cerebral edema and anoxic degeneration.
• Pathogenesis: not fully understood but mitochondrial dysfunction is clearly at the center stage

■ **DIAGNOSIS**

■ **DIFFERENTIAL DIAGNOSIS**
• Inborn errors of metabolism
Carnitine deficiency
Ornithine transcarbamylase deficiency
Others
• Salicylate or amiodarone intoxication
• Jamaican vomiting sickness
• Hepatic encephalopathy of any cause

■ **WORKUP**

According to the CDC's case definition, the following conditions must be met for consideration as a Reye's syndrome case:
• Acute noninflammatory encephalopathy documented by:
Alteration in the level of consciousness and, if available, a record of cerebrospinal fluid containing ≤8 leukocytes per mm³ *or*
Histologic specimen demonstrating cerebral edema without perivascular or meningeal inflammation
• Hepatopathy documented either by a liver biopsy or autopsy considered to be diagnostic of Reye's syndrome

or by a threefold or greater rise in the levels of serum aspartate aminotransferase, serum alanine aminotransferase, or serum ammonia *and*
• No more reasonable explanation for the cerebral and hepatic abnormalities

■ **LABORATORY TESTS**
• Elevated transaminase (ALT and AST)
• Elevated ammonia level
• Occasional elevation of CPK, LDH, and bilirubin and prolongation of prothrombin time
• Occasional hypoglycemia (in patients under the age of 4 yr)
• Cerebrospinal fluid is normal or contains <8 WBCs/ml
• Rarely a liver biopsy is indicated (in infants or in recurrent cases)

■ **TREATMENT**

• Supportive
• Mannitol, glycerol, or hyperventilation for cerebral edema if present
• Interferon alfa (experimental)
• Prevention
Influenza vaccine
Varicella vaccine
Avoidance of aspirin in children, especially during influenza and varicella outbreaks

REFERENCES
Gellin BG, LaMontagne JR: Reye's syndrome. In Gorbach SL, Bartlett JG, Blacklow NR (eds): *Infectious diseases,* ed 2, Philadelphia, 1998, WB Saunders.
Reye syndrome—United States, 1985, *MMWR* 35:66, 1986.
Author: **Tom J. Wachtel, M.D.**

TABLE 1-50   Clinical Staging of Reye's Syndrome

GRADE	SYMPTOMS AT TIME OF ADMISSION
I	Usually quiet, **lethargic** and sleepy, vomiting, laboratory evidence of liver dysfunction
II	Deep lethargy, **confusion,** delirium, combative, hyperventilation, hyperreflexic
III	Obtunded, **light coma,** seizures, decorticate rigidity, intact pupillary light reaction
IV	Seizures, deepening coma, **decerebrate rigidity,** loss of oculocephalic reflexes, fixed pupils
V	Coma, loss of deep tendon reflexes, respiratory arrest, fixed dilated pupils, **flaccidity/decerebrate** intermittent isoelectric electroencephalogram

From Behrman RE: *Nelson textbook of pediatrics,* ed 15, Philadelphia, 1996, WB Saunders.

BASIC INFORMATION

■ DEFINITION
Rh incompatibility occurs when an absence of the D antigen on maternal RBCs and its presence on fetal RBCs causes risk of Rh isoimmunization.

ICD-9CM CODES
656.1 Rh incompatibility

■ EPIDEMIOLOGY & DEMOGRAPHICS
INCIDENCE:
- The absence of the D antigen (Rh⁻ blood type) occurs in 15% of whites, 8% of blacks, and virtually no Asians or Native Americans. If the father's blood type is not known, the chance that an Rh⁻ pregnant woman is bearing an Rh⁺ fetus is about 60%.
- Of those pregnancies complicated by Rh incompatibility, the risk of maternal isoimmunization to the D antigen is about 8% for each ABO compatible pregnancy *if no prophylaxis is given.*
- Maternal-fetal ABO incompatibility is somewhat protective against Rh isoimmunization.

GENETICS: Five major loci determine Rh status: C, D, E, c, e. The presence of the D antigen results in an Rh⁺ individual. Its absence results in an Rh⁻ individual. Of Rh⁺ fathers, 45% are homozygotes, 55% are heterozygotes. For homozygous Rh⁺ fathers, the probability of an Rh⁺ offspring is 100%. The probability for heterozygotes is about 50%.

RISK FACTORS FOR ISOIMMUNIZATION:
- Antepartum: fetal-to-maternal transfusion
- Intrapartum: fetal-to-maternal transfusion, spontaneous abortion, ectopic pregnancy, abruptio placentae, abdominal trauma, chorionic villus sampling, amniocentesis, percutaneous umbilical blood sampling (PUBS), external cephalic version, manual removal of the placenta, therapeutic abortion, autologous blood product administration

■ ETIOLOGY
The initial response to D antigen exposure is production of IgM (MW 900,000) that does not cross the placenta. With a repeated exposure, IgG (MW 160,000) is produced. IgG can cross the placenta and enter the fetal circulation, producing hemolysis in the fetus. This may produce erythroblastosis fetalis or hemolytic disease in the newborn, resulting in antepartum or neonatal death or neurologic damage to the fetus because of hyperbilirubinemia and kernicterus.

DIAGNOSIS

■ LABORATORY TESTS
ABO and Rh blood type and an antibody screen as part of the initial prenatal profile
- If antibody screen negative:
  1. Repeat antibody screen at 28 wk gestation.
  2. Obtain neonatal blood type after delivery.
  3. If Rh incompatibility is confirmed by the neonatal blood type, a Kleihauer-Betke or rosette test should be performed to determine the amount of fetomaternal transfusion in the following high-risk circumstances: abruptio placentae, placenta previa, cesarean delivery, intrauterine manipulation, manual removal of the placenta.
- If anti-D antibody screen is positive:
  1. Maternal indirect Coombs' test is needed to determine antibody titer.
  2. Determine paternal Rh status and zygosity.
  3. If father is heterozygous, PUBS or amniotic fluid is needed to determine fetal Rh status.

■ IMAGING STUDIES
Ultrasound evaluation can diagnose hydrops fetalis, but it cannot predict it.

TREATMENT

■ PREVENTION OF D ISOIMMUNIZATION
- Give 50 µg of D immunoglobulin: after spontaneous or induced abortion or ectopic pregnancy <13 wk gestation.

- Give 300 µg of D immunoglobulin (protects against 30 ml of fetal blood):
  1. After spontaneous or induced abortion >13 wk gestation, amniocentesis, CVS, PUBS, external cephalic version or other intrauterine manipulation.
  2. As antepartum prophylaxis at 28 wk gestation. Maternal anti-D prophylaxis does not cause hemolysis in the fetus or newborn.
  3. At delivery if the neonate is D- or Du-positive.
  4. If Kleihauer-Betke or rosette test confirms >30 ml of fetal red blood in maternal circulation, additional D immunoglobulin is indicated. Confirm adequacy of therapy by a maternal indirect Coombs' test 48 to 72 hr after Rh immune globulin is given.

■ MANAGEMENT OF D ISOIMMUNIZED PREGNANCIES
- Serial amniocentesis for assessment of OD_{450} after 25 wk gestation with interpretation of the Delta OD_{450} according to criteria established by Liley
- PUBS if ultrasonographic evidence of hydrops, rising zone II Delta OD_{450} values on amniocentesis, maternal history of a severely affected child
- Intrauterine exchange transfusion if severe anemia is documented remote from term
- Initiation of steroids for lung maturation at 28 wk in severely affected pregnancies with delivery at lung maturity
- Delivery as soon as lung maturation is achieved in mild to moderately affected pregnancies

■ DISPOSITION
Survival of nonhydropic infants is 90%. Of infants with hydrops, 82% survive.

■ REFERRAL
Refer all Rh isoimmunized pregnancies to a tertiary care center before 18 to 20 wk gestation.

REFERENCE
Maayan-Metzger A et al: Maternal anti-D prophylaxis during pregnancy does not cause neonatal haemolysis, *Arch Dis Child* 84:60, 2001.
Author: **Laurel M. White, M.D.**

BASIC INFORMATION

■ DEFINITION

Rhabdomyolysis is the dissolution or disintegration of muscle, which causes membrane lysis and leakage of muscle constituents, resulting in the excretion of myoglobin in the urine. Renal damage can occur as a result of tubular obstruction by myoglobin as well as hypovolemia.

■ ICD-9CM CODES
728.89 Rhabdomyolysis

■ EPIDEMIOLOGY & DEMOGRAPHICS
PREDOMINANT AGE: Rare in children

■ PHYSICAL FINDINGS & CLINICAL PRESENTATION
- Variable muscle tenderness
- Weakness
- Muscular rigidity
- Fever
- Altered consciousness
- Muscle swelling
- Malaise
- Dark urine

■ ETIOLOGY
- Exertion (exercise-induced)
- Electrical injury
- Drug-induced (statins, combination of statins with fibrates, amphetamines, haloperidol)
- Compartment syndrome
- Multiple trauma
- Malignant hyperthermia
- Limb ischemia
- Reperfusion after revascularization procedures for ischemia
- Extensive surgical (spinal) dissection
- Tourniquet ischemia
- Prolonged static positioning during surgery
- Infectious and inflammatory myositis
- Metabolic myopathies
- Hypovolemia and urinary acidification are important precipitating causes in the development of acute renal failure.

DIAGNOSIS

■ DIFFERENTIAL DIAGNOSIS
Section III, Fig. 3-51 describes a clinical algorithm for the evaluation of CPK elevation.

■ LABORATORY TESTS
- Screening for myoglobinuria with a simple urine dipstick test using orthotoluidine or benzidine
- BUN, creatinine
- Increased CPK (Fig. 1-235)
- Hyperkalemia
- Hypocalcemia
- Hyperphosphatemia
- Increased urinary myoglobin
- Pigmented granular casts
- Hyperuricemia

TREATMENT

■ ACUTE GENERAL Rx
- Early, aggressive high-volume IV fluid replacement with mannitol, to induce diuresis to prevent acute renal failure
- Treatment of electrolyte imbalances
- Alkalinization of urine is controversial but appears helpful in research models

■ DISPOSITION
The condition is easily treatable, but early diagnosis and management are necessary to avoid renal failure, which occurs in 30% of cases.

☼ PEARLS & CONSIDERATIONS

■ COMMENTS
A clinical algorithm for the evaluation of muscle cramps and aches is described in Fig. 3-130.

REFERENCES
Garcia-Valdecasas-Campelo E et al: Acute rhabdomyolysis associated with cerivastatin therapy, *Arch Intern Med* 161:893, 2001.
Halachanova V, Sansone RA, McDonald S: Delayed rhabdomyolysis after ecstasy use, *Mayo Clin Proc* 76:112, 2001.
Sauret JM et al: Rhabdomyolysis, *Am Fam Physician* 65:907, 2002.
Schenk MR et al: Continuous venovenous hemofiltration for the immediate management of massive rhabdomyolysis after fulminant malignant hyperthermia in a bodybuilder, *Anesthesiology* 94:1139, 2001.
Wappler F et al: Evidence for susceptibility to malignant hyperthermia in patients with exercise-induced rhabdomyolysis, *Anesthesiology* 94:95, 2001.
Author: **Lonnie R. Mercier, M.D.**

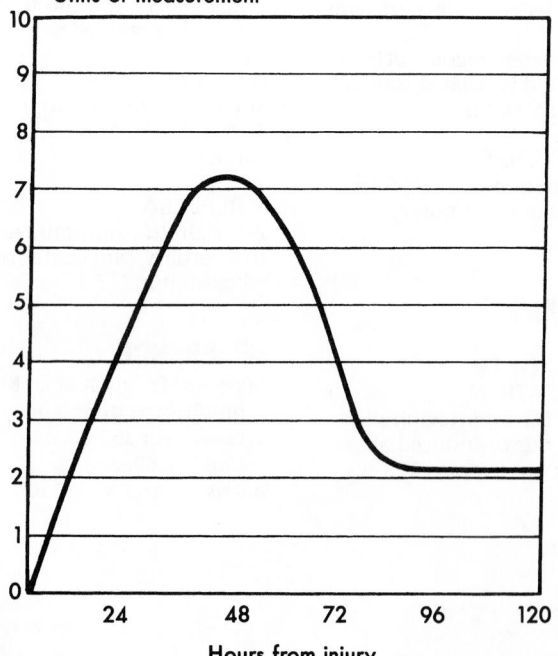

Fig. 1-235 Typical CK elimination curve. (From Rosen P [ed]: *Emergency medicine,* ed 4, St Louis, 1998, Mosby.)

BASIC INFORMATION

■ DEFINITION

Rheumatic fever is a multisystem inflammatory disease that occurs in the genetically susceptible host after a pharyngeal infection with group A streptococci.

■ SYNONYMS

Acute rheumatic fever
Rheumatic carditis

ICD-9CM CODES

390; 716.9 Rheumatic fever

■ EPIDEMIOLOGY & DEMOGRAPHICS

INCIDENCE (IN U.S.):
- 0.1% to 3% in patients with untreated streptococcal pharyngitis
- Higher incidence of streptococcal pharyngitis with:
  1. Crowding
  2. Poverty
  3. Young age

PREDOMINANT AGE:
- Age 5 to 15 yr for first attack
- Possible relapses later

PEAK INCIDENCE: School-age children
GENETICS:
Familial Disposition: Predisposition to the disease is likely to be genetically determined.

■ PHYSICAL FINDINGS & CLINICAL PRESENTATION

- Acute streptococcal pharyngitis, which may be subclinical and not reported by the patient
- After latent period of 1 to 5 wk (average, 19 days), acute rheumatic attack
- Patient is febrile, with a migratory polyarthritis of knees, ankles, wrists, elbows; typically severe for 1 wk, remits by 3 to 4 wk
- Carditis
  1. New heart murmur
     a. Mitral regurgitation
     b. Aortic insufficiency
     c. Diastolic mitral murmur
  2. Cardiomegaly
  3. CHF
  4. Pericardial friction rub or effusion
- Rarely, pancarditis is severe and fatal.
- Subcutaneous nodules can be palpated over extensor tendon surfaces or bony prominences, such as the skull.
- Chorea (Sydenham's chorea) is characterized by rapid involuntary movements affecting all muscles.
  1. Muscular weakness
  2. Emotional lability
  3. Rarely seen after adolescence and almost never in adult males
- Erythema marginatum
  1. Evanescent, pink, well-demarcated spreading to trunk and proximal extremities
  2. Not specific
- Arthralgias (joint pain without swelling)
- Abdominal pain

■ ETIOLOGY

- Group A streptococci not recovered from tissue lesions.
- It does not occur in the absence of a streptococcal antibody response.
- Immunologic cross-reactivity between certain streptococcal antigens and human tissue antigens suggests an autoimmune etiology.
- Both initial attacks and recurrences can be completely prevented by prompt treatment of streptococcal pharyngitis with penicillin.

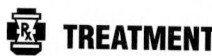

DIAGNOSIS

■ DIFFERENTIAL DIAGNOSIS

- Rheumatoid arthritis
- Juvenile rheumatoid arthritis (Still's disease)
- Bacterial endocarditis
- Systemic lupus
- Viral infections
- Serum sickness

■ WORKUP

- "Jones Criteria (revised) for Guidance in the Diagnosis of Rheumatic Fever" published by the American Heart Association

One major and two minor criteria if supported by evidence of an antecedent group A streptococcal infection
- Major criteria
  1. Increased titer of antistreptococcal antibodies such as ASO
  2. Positive throat culture
  3. Recent scarlet fever
- Minor criteria
  1. Previous rheumatic fever or rheumatic heart disease
  2. Fever
  3. Arthralgia
  4. Increased acute-phase reactants
     a. ESR
     b. C-reactive protein
     c. Leukocytosis
  5. Prolonged P-R interval

■ LABORATORY TESTS

- Throat cultures are usually negative.
- Streptococcal antibody tests are more useful in establishing the diagnosis.
  1. Peak at the beginning of the attack
  2. Can document a recent streptococcal infection
- ASO (antistreptolysin O) titers peak:
  1. 4 to 5 wk after a streptococcal throat infection
  2. During the second or third week of illness
- Anti-DNase B (Streptozyme) is also commonly used but is less reliable.
- High-titer streptococcal antibodies:
  1. Are supportive of diagnosis, but not proof
  2. Should be interpreted in the context of clinical criteria

■ IMAGING STUDIES

- Chest x-ray to assess heart size
- Echocardiogram:
  1. To evaluate murmurs
  2. To rule out pericardial effusion

TREATMENT

■ ACUTE GENERAL Rx

- Course of penicillin to eradicate throat carriage of group A streptococci
- Arthralgia or arthritis without carditis: aspirin 40 mg/lb/day for 2 wk, followed by 20 mg/lb/day for 4 to 6 wk
- Carditis and heart failure:
  1. Prednisone 40 to 60 mg/day
  2. IV corticosteroids, such as methylprednisolone, 10 to 40 mg/day for severe carditis

■ CHRONIC Rx

Secondary prevention (prevention of recurrences):
- Monthly treatment with benzathine penicillin 1.2 million U IM
- Erythromycin in patients with penicillin allergy

■ DISPOSITION

- Damage of heart valves because of fibrosis
  1. Late sequela of recurrent attacks
  2. Frequent cause of valvular heart disease in developing countries
- May progress to heart failure

■ REFERRAL

To cardiologist for management of severe carditis

REFERENCES

Carapetis JR, Currie BJ: Rheumatic fever in a high incidence population: the importance of monoarthritis and low grade fever, *Arch Dis Child* 85(30):223, 2001.

Figueroa FE et al: Prospective comparison of clinical and echocardiographic diagnosis of rheumatic carditis: long term follow up of patients with subclinical disease, *Heart* 85(40):407, 2001.

Thatai D, Turi ZG: Current guidelines for the treatment of rheumatic fever, *Drugs* 57(4):545, 1999.

Author: **Deborah L. Shapiro, M.D.**

BASIC INFORMATION

■ DEFINITION

Allergic rhinitis is an IgE-mediated hypersensitivity response to nasally inhaled allergens that causes sneezing, rhinorrhea, nasal pruritus, and congestion.

■ SYNONYMS

Hay fever
IgE-mediated rhinitis

ICD-9CM CODES

477.9 Allergic rhinitis

■ EPIDEMIOLOGY & DEMOGRAPHICS

- Allergic rhinitis affects approximately 10% to 20% of the U.S. population.
- Mean age of onset is 8 to 12 yr.

■ PHYSICAL FINDINGS & CLINICAL FINDINGS

- Pale or violaceous mucosa of the turbinates caused by venous engorgement (this can distinguish it from erythema present in viral rhinitis)
- Nasal polyps
- Lymphoid hyperplasia in the posterior oropharynx with cobblestone appearance
- Erythema of the throat, conjunctival and scleral injection
- Clear nasal discharge
- Clinical presentation: usually consists of sneezing, nasal congestion, cough, postnasal drip, loss of or alteration of smell, and sensation of plugged ears

■ ETIOLOGY

- Pollens in the springtime, ragweed in fall, grasses in the summer
- Dust, mites, animal allergens
- Smoke or any irritants
- Perfumes, detergents, soaps
- Emotion, changes in atmospheric pressure or temperature

DIAGNOSIS

■ DIFFERENTIAL DIAGNOSIS

- Infections (sinusitis; viral, bacterial, or fungal rhinitis)
- Rhinitis medicamentosa (cocaine, sympathomimetic nasal drops)
- Vasomotor rhinitis (e.g., secondary to air pollutants)
- Septal obstruction (e.g., deviated septum), nasal polyps, nasal neoplasms

- Systemic diseases (e.g., Wegener's granulomatosis, hypothyroidism [rare])

■ WORKUP

- Workup is often unnecessary if the diagnosis is apparent. A detailed medical history is useful in identifying the culprit allergen.
- Selected patients with allergic rhinitis that is not controlled with standard therapy may benefit from allergy testing to target allergen avoidance measures or guide immunotherapy. Allergy testing can be performed using skin testing or radioallergosorbent (RAST) testing. In vitro tests also can assess serum levels of specific IgE antibodies. Overall, skin tests show greater sensitivity than serum assays. In vitro tests should be considered in rare patients who fear skin tests, must take medication that interferes with skin testing, or have generalized dermatographism.
- Examination of nasal smears for the presence of neutrophils to rule out infectious causes and the presence of eosinophils (suggestive of allergy) may be useful in selected patients.
- Peripheral blood eosinophil counts are not useful in allergy diagnosis.

TREATMENT

■ NONPHARMACOLOGIC THERAPY

- Maintain allergen-free environment by covering mattresses and pillows with allergen-proof casings, eliminating carpeting, eliminating animal products, and removing dust-collecting fixtures.
- Use of air purifiers and dust filters is helpful.
- Maintain humidity in the environment below 50% to prevent dust mites and mold.
- Use air conditioners, especially in the bedroom.
- Remove pets from homes of patients with suspected sensitivity to animal allergens.

■ ACUTE GENERAL Rx

- Determine if the patient is troubled by swollen turbinates (best treated with decongestants) or blockages secondary to mucus (effectively treated by antihistamines).

- Most first-generation antihistamines can cause considerable sedation and anticholinergic symptoms. The second-generation antihistamines (loratadine, fexofenadine, cetirizine, desloratadine) are preferred because they do not have any significant anticholinergic or sedative effects; however, they are more expensive.
- Montelukast (Singulair), a leukotriene receptor antagonist commonly used for asthma, is also effective for allergic rhinitis. Usual adult dose is 10 mg qd.
- Azelastine (Astelin) is an antihistamine nasal spray effective for seasonal allergic rhinitis.
- Topical nasal steroids are very effective and are preferred by many as first-line treatment for allergic rhinitis in adults. Patients should be instructed on proper use and informed that improvement might not occur for at least 1 wk after initiation of therapy. Commonly available inhalers are:
  1. Beclomethasone dipropionate (Beconase AQ): one to two sprays in each nostril bid
  2. Fluticasone (Flonase): initially two sprays in each nostril qd or one spray in each nostril bid, decreasing to one spray in each nostril qd based on response
  3. Flunisolide (Nasalide): initially two sprays in each nostril bid
  4. Budesonide (Rhinocort): two sprays in each nostril bid or four sprays in each nostril qam

■ CHRONIC Rx

- Cromolyn sodium (Nasalcrom): one spray to each nostril three to four times daily can be used for prophylaxis (mast cell stabilizer).
- Immunotherapy is generally reserved for patients responding poorly to the above treatments.

■ DISPOSITION

Most patients experience significant relief with avoidance of allergens and proper use of medications.

■ REFERRAL

Allergy testing in patients with severe symptoms that are unresponsive to therapy or when the diagnosis is uncertain

REFERENCE

Rinne J et al: Early treatment of perennial rhinitis with budesonide or cetirizine and its effect on long-term outcome, *J Allergy Clin Immunol* 109:426, 2002.
Author: **Fred F. Ferri, M.D.**

BASIC INFORMATION

■ DEFINITION

Rickets is a systemic disease of infancy and childhood in which mineralization of growing bone is deficient as a result of abnormal calcium, phosphorus, or vitamin D metabolism. *Osteomalacia* is the same condition in the adult. *Renal osteodystrophy* is a term used to describe a similar condition in patients with chronic kidney disease. Certain forms of the disorder may respond only to high doses of vitamin D and are referred to as vitamin D–resistant rickets (VDRR).

ICD-9CM CODES
268.0 Active rickets
275.3 Vitamin D–resistant rickets
588.0 Renal rickets (renal osteodystrophy)
268.2 Osteomalacia

■ PHYSICAL FINDINGS & CLINICAL PRESENTATION

The child with classic rickets usually develops a number of specific abnormalities:
* Softening of the skull bones (craniotabes) early in the disorder
* Enlargement of the ribs at the costochondral junctions, producing the "rachitic rosary"
* Limb deformities and epiphyseal swelling (Fig. 1-236)
* Height below normal range
* Irritability and easy fatigability
* Pigeon breast deformity and an indentation of the lower ribcage at the insertion of the diaphragm, sometimes referred to as Harrison's groove; possible decrease in thoracic volume, resulting in diminished pulmonary ventilation

Physical findings in the adult with osteomalacia are more subtle:
* Possible malaise and bone pain
* Many patients presumed to have osteoporosis but may also have osteomalacia

■ ETIOLOGY
* Deficiency states
  1. True classic VDDR is rare in Western society.
  2. Absorption of vitamin D, however, may be blocked in several GI disorders.
  3. Similar disorders may also prevent absorption of calcium and phosphorus, but in the absence of these other diseases, deficiencies of calcium and phosphorus are also rare.
* Acquired or inherited renal tubular abnormalities that cause resorptive defects and result in rickets and osteomalacia; syndromes include classical VDRR (probably the most common form of rickets seen in general practice)
* Chronic renal failure:
  1. Can produce renal rickets or renal osteodystrophy
  2. Results in the retention of phosphate

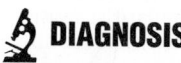

DIAGNOSIS

■ DIFFERENTIAL DIAGNOSIS
* Osteoporosis
* Hyperparathyroidism
* Hyperthyroidism

■ LABORATORY TESTS
* Requires a high degree of interest because many of the conditions are so similar that only a complicated laboratory evaluation may establish the diagnosis
* BUN, creatinine, alkaline phosphatase, calcium, and phosphorus levels in any patient suspected of having metabolic bone disease

■ IMAGING STUDIES
* In rickets:
  1. Characteristic radiographic changes in the ends of growing long bones caused by the lack of calcification of the cartilage matrix
  2. Typically widening and irregularity of the epiphyseal plate
* Radiographs in the adult with osteomalacia:
  1. More subtle and often confused with osteoporosis
  2. Possible pseudofractures (Looser's zones) where major arteries cross bone
  3. Insufficiency compression deformities in the vertebral bodies

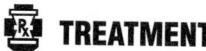

TREATMENT

* Because of the complex nature of many of these disorders, a qualified endocrinologist and nephrologist should be consulted for treatment.
* The need for orthopedic intervention is rare.
* Surgical care is indicated for slipped capital femoral epiphysis, which is fairly common in renal rickets.
* Deformity may require bracing.

REFERENCES

Abrams SA: Nutritional rickets: an old disease returns, *Nutr Rev* 60(4):111, 2002.
Ashraf S, Mughal MZ: The prevalence of rickets among non-Caucasian children, *Arch Dis Child* 87(3):263, 2002.
Caksen HN et al: Reports of osteopenia/rickets of prematurity are on the increase because of improved survival rates of low birthweight infants, *J Emerg Med* 23(3):305, 2002.
Hochberg Z: Vitamin-D-dependent rickets type 2, *Horm Res* 58(6):297, 2002.
Joiner TA et al: Primary care pediatrician knowledge of nutritional rickets, *J Natl Med Assoc* 94(11):971, 2002.
Tortolani PJ, McCarthy EF, Sponseller PD: Bone mineral density deficiency in children, *J Am Acad Orthop Surg* 10(1):57, 2002.
Author: **Lonnie R. Mercier, M.D.**

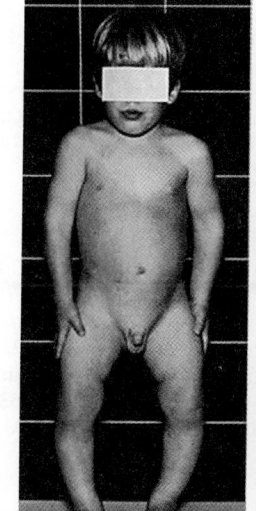
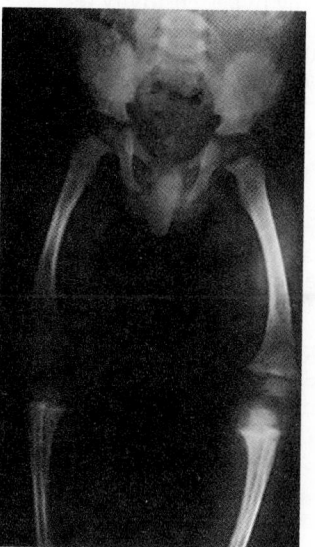

Fig. 1-236 **A,** Clinical and, **B,** radiographic appearance of a young boy with X-linked hypophosphatemic rickets. Note the striking bowing of the legs, apparent in both femora and tibiae, with flaring of the ends of the bones at the knee. (Courtesy Dr. Sara B. Arnaud. From Bikle DB: Osteomalacia and rickets. In Wyngaarden JB, Smith LH Jr, Bennett JB [eds]: *Cecil textbook of medicine,* ed 19, Philadelphia, 1992, WB Saunders.)

BASIC INFORMATION

■ DEFINITION

Rocky Mountain spotted fever (RMSF) is a febrile illness caused by infection with *Rickettsia rickettsii*.

ICD-9CM CODES

082.0 Rocky Mountain spotted fever

■ EPIDEMIOLOGY & DEMOGRAPHICS

INCIDENCE: 0.18 to 0.32 cases/100,000 person-years
DEMOGRAPHICS: Affects both genders equally and occurs at any age, but more likely in children aged 5 to 14 yr
GEOGRAPHY: Most prevalent in the Southeast, followed by the South Central states, but seen anywhere

■ PHYSICAL FINDINGS & CLINICAL PRESENTATION

- Incubation: 3 to 12 days
- First symptoms: fever, headache, malaise, and myalgias

Common history, signs, or symptoms	%
Tick bite	65
Fever	100
Rash	90
Rash on palms and soles	80
Headache	90
Myalgia	75
Nausea or vomiting	60
Abdominal pain	40
Conjunctivitis	30
Edema	20
Pneumonitis	15
Any severe neurologic complication (including stupor, delirium, seizures, ataxia, papilledema, focal neurologic deficits, and coma)	30

Rash:

- Appears during first 3 days in 50%; by day 5, 80% have it. No rash in 10%.
- Initial appearance: blanching erythematous macules on wrists and ankles that then spread to trunk, palms, and soles.
- Lesions may evolve into papules and eventually become nonblanching (petechiae or palpable purpura).

Gastrointestinal symptoms:

- Nausea, vomiting, and abdominal pain are common
- Occasionally may mimic an "acute abdomen" (e.g., appendicitis, cholecystitis)
- Mild hepatitis

Cardiopulmonary involvement:

- Interstitial pneumonitis
- Myocarditis

Renal problems:

- Prerenal azotemia
- Interstitial nephritis
- Glomerulonephritis

Neurologic involvement:

- Encephalitis (confusion, lethargy, delirium)
- Ataxia
- Convulsion
- Cranial nerve palsy
- Speech impediment
- Hemiparesis or paraparesis
- Spasticity

Fulminant Rocky Mountain spotted fever

- Early, widespread vascular necrosis leading to multisystem illness and death

■ ETIOLOGY & PATHOGENESIS

- Infectious agent: *Rickettsia rickettsii* (an intracellular bacterium).
- Vector: dog tick and wood tick (vertical transmission exists in ticks, but horizontal transmission involving rodents represents an important reservoir for the agent).
- Pathogenesis: the spread of *R. rickettsii* is hematogenous with attachment to the vascular endothelium, causing a vasculitis. The manifestations of this illness are caused by increased vascular permeability.

DIAGNOSIS

■ DIFFERENTIAL DIAGNOSIS

Influenza A, enteroviral infection, typhoid fever, leptospirosis, infectious mononucleosis, viral hepatitis, sepsis, ehrlichiosis, gastroenteritis, acute abdomen, bronchitis, pneumonia, meningococcemia, disseminated gonococcal infection, secondary syphilis, bacterial endocarditis, toxic shock syndrome, scarlet fever, rheumatic fever, measles, rubella, typhus, rickettsialpox, Lyme disease, drug hypersensitivity reactions, idiopathic thrombocytopenic purpura, thrombotic thrombocytopenic purpura, Kawasaki disease, immune complex vasculitis, connective tissue disorders

■ WORKUP

Consider RMSF in any patient with an acute febrile illness with headache and myalgia, especially with an associated history of tick exposure. Absence of rash does not rule the diagnosis.

■ LABORATORY TESTS

Routine tests	%
White cell count	
<10,000/mm³	72
>10% bands	69
Platelet count	
<150,000/mm³	52
<99,000/mm³	32
Serum sodium value <132 mEq/L	56
Aspartate aminotransferase ≥2× normal	62
Alanine aminotransferase ≥2× normal	39
Bilirubin value >1.4 mg/dl	30
Cerebrospinal fluid	
Opening pressure ≥250 mm H₂O	14
Glucose value ≤50 mg/dl	8
Protein value ≥50 mg/dl	35
White cell count ≥5/mm³	38
Mononuclear cell predominance	46
Polymorphonuclear cell predominance	50

Etiologic tests

- Antibody titers to *R. rickettsii* (by indirect fluorescent antibody test). The diagnosis of RMSF requires a fourfold increase 2 wk apart and thus is not helpful in the care of the patients despite a sensitivity and specificity of near 100%.
- The only test that can provide a timely diagnosis is the immunohistologic demonstration of *R. rickettsii* in skin biopsy specimens.

TREATMENT

- Oral or intravenous doxycycline, 200 mg/day in two divided doses
- Oral tetracycline, 25 to 50 mg/kg/day in four divided doses
- Chloramphenicol, 50 to 75 mg/kg/day in four divided doses; therapy continued for at least 2 days after defervescence

■ PROGNOSIS

Fatality rate: 1% to 4% (five times greater if treatment is initiated after day 5 of illness, which is more likely in absence of rash and during seasonal nonpeak tick activity). Long-term sequelae seen in patients who recover from severe RMSF: paraparesis, hearing loss; peripheral neuropathy; bladder and bowel incontinence; cerebellar, vestibular, and motor dysfunction; language disorders; limb amputation; and scrotal pain after cutaneous necrosis.

REFERENCES

Dumler JS: Rocky Mountain spotted fever. In Gorbach SL, Bartlett JG, Blacklow NR (eds): *Infectious diseases*, ed 2, Philadelphia, 1998, WB Saunders.

Masters EJ: Rocky Mountain spotted fever, *Arch Intern Med* 163:769, 2003.

Author: **Tom J. Wachtel, M.D.**

BASIC INFORMATION

■ DEFINITION

Rosacea is a chronic skin disorder characterized by papules and pustules affecting the face and often associated with flushing and erythema.

■ SYNONYMS

Acne rosacea

ICD-9CM CODES

695.3 Rosacea

■ EPIDEMIOLOGY & DEMOGRAPHICS

- Rosacea occurs in 1 in 20 Americans
- Onset often between age 30 and 50 yr
- More common in people of Celtic origin; however, this disease may be overlooked in nonwhites because skin pigmentation results in atypical presentation
- Female:male ratio of 3:1

■ PHYSICAL FINDINGS & CLINICAL PRESENTATION

- Facial erythema, presence of papules, pustules, and telangiectasia.
- Excessive facial warmth and redness is the predominant presenting complaint.
- Itching is generally absent.
- Comedones are absent (unlike acne).
- Women are more likely to show symptoms on the chin and cheeks, whereas in men the nose is commonly involved.
- Ocular findings (conjunctival injection, burning, stinging, tearing, eyelid inflammation, swelling, and redness) are present in >20% of patients.

■ ETIOLOGY

- Unknown.
- Hot drinks, alcohol, and sun exposure may accentuate the erythema by causing vasodilation of the skin.
- Flare-ups may also result from reactions to medications (e.g., simvastatin, ACE inhibitors, vasodilators, fluorinated corticosteroids), stress, extreme heat or cold, spicy drinks.

DIAGNOSIS

■ DIFFERENTIAL DIAGNOSIS

- Drug eruption
- Acne vulgaris
- Contact dermatitis
- SLE
- Carcinoid flush
- Idiopathic facial flushing
- Seborrheic dermatitis
- Facial sarcoidosis
- Photodermatitis
- Mastocytosis

■ WORKUP

Diagnosis is based on clinical findings.

■ LABORATORY TESTS

Not indicated

TREATMENT

■ NONPHARMACOLOGIC THERAPY

- Avoid alcohol, excessive sun exposure, and hot drinks of any type.
- Use of mild, nondrying soap is recommended; local skin irritants should be avoided.
- Reassure patient that rosacea is completely unrelated to poor hygiene.

■ GENERAL Rx

- Topical therapy with metronidazole aqueous gel (MetroGel) applied bid is effective as initial therapy for mild cases or following the use of oral antibiotics. A new 1% formulation of metronidazole (Noritate) applied qd may improve patient compliance. Clindamycin lotion (Cleocin) and sulfacetamide may also be effective.
- Systemic antibiotics: tetracycline 250 mg qid until symptoms diminish, then taper off; doxycycline 100 mg bid is also effective.
- Minocycline 50 to 100 mg qd should be used only in resistant cases, because this medication is expensive.
- Isotretinoin (Accutane) 0.5 to 1 mg/kg/day in two divided doses for 15 to 20 wk can be used for refractory papular and pustular rosacea; use of retinoids may however worsen erythema and telangiectasis.

- Laser treatment is an option for progressive telangiectasias or rhinophyma.
- Erythema and flushing may respond to low dose clonidine (0.05 mg bid).
- Another topical treatment modality for pustular and papular forms of rosacea is the use of azelaic acid (Finacea, Azelex). Azelex is available in a 20% cream base, Finacea as a 15% gel. Azelaic acid is as least as effective as topical metronidazole but may be more irritating.

■ DISPOSITION

- Rosacea is often resistant to initial treatment and recurrent. Periods of remission and relapse are common.
- The progression of rosacea is variable. Typical stages include:
  1. Facial flushing
  2. Erythema and/or edema and ocular symptoms
  3. Papules and pustules
  4. Rhinophyma

PEARLS & CONSIDERATIONS

■ COMMENTS

- Patients with resistant cases may have *Demodex folliculorum* mite infestation or tinea infection (diagnosis can be confirmed with potassium hydroxide examination); the role of *D. folliculorum* in rosacea is unclear. These mites can sometimes be found in large numbers in the lesions; however, their numbers do not generally decline with treatment.
- Rosacea can result in emotional and social stigmas, especially because many people associate rosacea and rhinophyma with alcohol abuse.
- Early consultation with an ophthalmologist is recommended in patients with suspected ocular involvement.

REFERENCE

Rosacea: a common, yet commonly overlooked condition, *Am Fam Physician* 66:435, 2002.

Author: **Fred F. Ferri, M.D.**

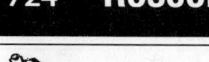

BASIC INFORMATION

■ DEFINITION
Roseola is a benign viral illness found in infants and is characterized by high fevers, followed by a rash.

■ SYNONYMS
Exanthem subitum
Sixth disease
Roseola infantum

ICD-9CM CODES
057.8 Roseola

■ EPIDEMIOLOGY & DEMOGRAPHICS
• Nearly one third of all infants develop roseola before the age of 2 yr.
• More than 90% of children older than 2 yr of age are seropositive for the virus causing roseola.
• Roseola is spread from person to person, but it is not known how.
• It is not known how contagious roseola is.
• There is no predilection for gender or time of year.

■ PHYSICAL FINDINGS & CLINICAL PRESENTATION
• Typically the child develops a high fever, usually up to 104° F (40° C) that lasts for 3 to 5 days
• Fever may be associated with a runny nose, irritability, and fatigue
• A rash appears within 48 hr of defervescence, mainly on the face, neck, trunk, arms, and legs
• The rash is a faint pink maculopapular rash that blanches when palpated
• The rash usually fades away within 48 hr
• Anorexia
• Seizures
• Cervical adenopathy

■ ETIOLOGY
• Roseola is caused by human herpesvirus-6 (HHV-6).
• The incubation period is between 5 to 15 days.

DIAGNOSIS

The diagnosis of roseola is usually made by the clinical presentation as stated previously.

■ DIFFERENTIAL DIAGNOSIS
• Measles
• Rubella
• Fifth disease
• Drug eruption
• Mononucleosis
• All causes of fever (e.g., otitis media, pneumonia, and urinary tract infection)
• Meningitis
• Other causes of seizures

■ WORKUP
• If unsure of the diagnosis of roseola in a febrile infant, a fever workup is done to rule out other infectious causes.
• The decision to proceed with a fever workup is a clinical judgment call.

■ LABORATORY TESTS
• CBC with differential
• Erythrocyte sedimentation rate (ESR)
• Blood cultures
• Urinalysis and urine cultures
• Stool cultures if diarrhea is present
• Lumbar puncture

■ IMAGING STUDIES
• Chest x-ray to rule out pneumonia

TREATMENT

■ NONPHARMACOLOGIC
• Supportive care
• Maintain hydration by drinking clear fluids: water, fruit juice, lemonade, and so forth
• Sponge bathe with lukewarm water if febrile

■ ACUTE GENERAL Rx
• Acetaminophen 10 to 15 mg/kg per dose at 4-hr intervals for fever
• Ibuprofen 5 to 10 mg/kg per dose at 6-hr intervals (maximal dose 600 mg)

■ CHRONIC Rx
Roseola is a viral disease that is short lasting; chronic treatment is usually not an issue.

■ DISPOSITION
• Roseola is generally a benign, self-limited disease that usually lasts approximately 1 wk.
• Complications, although rare, can occur and include:
  1. Febrile seizures
  2. Meningitis
  3. Encephalitis
  4. Pneumonitis
  5. Hepatitis

■ REFERRAL
Subspecialty consultation is made with the appropriate discipline if any of the above mentioned complications occur (e.g., neurology for seizures).

PEARLS & CONSIDERATIONS

■ COMMENTS
• A child with fever and rash should be excluded from daycare.
• Human herpesvirus 6 is named accordingly because it is the sixth herpesvirus discovered after herpes simplex 1 (HSV-1), HSV-2, cytomegalovirus (CMV), Epstein-Barr virus (EBV), and varicella-zoster virus (VZV).
• Roseola is called sixth disease because it represents one of six "exanthems" that occurs during childhood. The other five exanthems included in this old classification are measles, scarlet fever, rubella, Dukes disease, and erythema infectiosum (fifth disease).

REFERENCES
Asano Y et al: Clinical features of infants with primary human herpesvirus 6 infection (exanthem subitum, roseola infantum), *Pediatrics* 93:104, 1994.
Dockrell DH, Smith TF, Paya C: Human herpesvirus 6, *Mayo Clin Proc* 74:163, 1999.
Stoeckle MY: The spectrum of human herpesvirus 6 infection: from roseola infantum to adult disease, *Annu Rev Med* 51:423, 2000.
Author: **Dennis Mikolich, M.D.**

BASIC INFORMATION

■ DEFINITION
Rotator cuff syndrome refers to a spectrum of afflictions involving the tendons of the rotator cuff (primarily the supraspinatus), ranging from simple strains and tendinitis to complete rupture with cuff-tear arthropathy.

■ SYNONYMS
Impingement syndrome
Painful arc syndrome
Internal derangement of the subacromial joint
Supraspinatus syndrome

ICD-9CM CODES
726.10 Rotator cuff syndrome
727.61 Rotator cuff rupture

■ EPIDEMIOLOGY & DEMOGRAPHICS
PREVALENCE: 5% to 10% of the general population
PREDOMINANT AGE: Uncommon under 20 yr of age
PREDOMINANT SEX: More common in males than females

■ PHYSICAL FINDINGS & CLINICAL PRESENTATION
- Pain, often at night
- Rotator cuff tenderness
- Referred pain down deltoid, especially with abduction between 70 and 120 degrees ("the painful arc") (Fig. 1-237)
- Weakness in abduction or forward flexion
- Increased pain with overhead activities
- Atrophy in long-standing cases of complete tear
- Positive "drop-arm" test

■ ETIOLOGY
- Microtrauma from repetitive use
- Abnormally shaped acromion
- Shoulder instability
- Worsening of process by the overhead throwing motion

DIAGNOSIS

■ DIFFERENTIAL DIAGNOSIS
- Shoulder instability
- Degenerative arthritis
- Cervical radiculopathy
- Avascular necrosis
- Suprascapular nerve entrapment

■ WORKUP
- In chronic tendinitis, clinical findings similar to those seen in partial rupture
- Even with complete rupture, may have full, active range of motion in shoulder

■ IMAGING STUDIES
- Plain radiography to rule out other causes of shoulder pain; special views (if needed) to detect abnormally shaped acromion
- Shoulder arthrogram to diagnose full-thickness rotator cuff tear
- Ultrasonography to diagnose full-thickness rotator cuff tears
- MRI to evaluate full- or partial-thickness tears, chronic tendinitis, and other causes of shoulder pain

TREATMENT

■ ACUTE GENERAL Rx
- Rest to avoid overhead activity
- Ice or heat for comfort
- Carefully supervised program of stretching and strengthening
- Medication: NSAIDs, subacromial corticosteroid injection

■ DISPOSITION
- All forms are likely to respond to nonsurgical management.
- Even many complete rotator cuff tears have minimal pain and little loss of function.

■ REFERRAL
For orthopedic consultation in cases that fail to respond to medical management or in which rotator cuff tear is suspected

PEARLS & CONSIDERATIONS

■ COMMENTS
- There is considerable disagreement regarding the likelihood of recovery once a significant rotator cuff rupture has developed.
- Indications for surgery vary among surgeons.

REFERENCES
Goldberg BA, Nolvinski RJ, Matsen FA: Outcome of nonoperative management of full-thickness rotator cuff tears, *Clin Orthop* 382:99, 2001.
Gorski JM, Schwartz LH: Shoulder impingement presenting as neck pain, *J Bone Joint Surg* 85:635, 2003.
Granger AJ et al: MR anatomy of the subcoracoid bursa and the association of subcoracoid effusion with tears of the anterior rotator cuff and the rotator interval, *Am J Roentgenol* 174:1377, 2000.
Green A: Chronic massive rotator cuff tears: evaluation and management, *J Am Acad Orthop Surg* 11:321, 2003.
Murrell GA, Walton JR: Diagnosis of rotator cuff tears, *Lancet* 357:769, 2001.
Pradhan RL, Itoi E: Rotator interval lesions of the shoulder joint, *Orthopedics* 24:798, 2001.
Author: **Lonnie R. Mercier, M.D.**

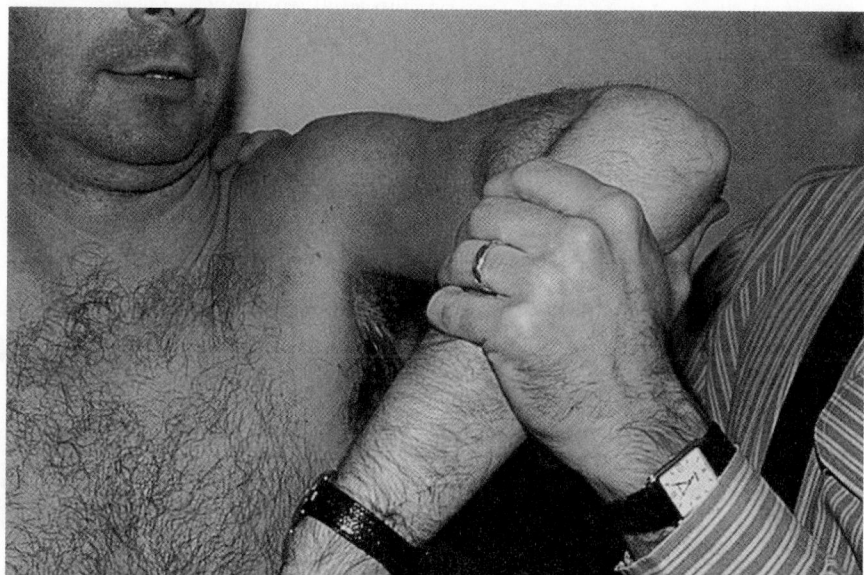

Fig. 1-237 Rotator cuff lesions are often accompanied by painful impingement of the upwardly subluxating humerus onto the acromion. Evidence for this as a cause of pain is elicited by impingement tests, for example, by forced, passive, internal rotation and abduction of the shoulder, as shown here. (From Klippel J, Dieppe P, Ferri F [eds]: *Primary care rheumatology,* London, 1999, Mosby.)

BASIC INFORMATION

■ DEFINITION

Rubella is a mild illness caused by the rubella virus that can cause severe congenital problems via in vitro transmission to the fetus when a pregnant woman becomes infected.

■ SYNONYMS

German measles

ICD-9CM CODES
056.9 Rubella
771.0 (congenital)
V04.3 (vaccination)

■ EPIDEMIOLOGY & DEMOGRAPHICS

- Before vaccination (i.e., before 1969):
  28 reported cases per 100,000 person-years, 8 of which were in persons over age 15 yr
  Four cases of congenital rubella syndrome per 100,000 live births
- After mass vaccination (i.e., after 1980) most cases have occurred in unimmunized people, with fewer than 1 case/100,000 person-years (acquired and congenital).
- Currently, 10% to 20% of childbearing-age women are susceptible.
- The highest risk of developing long-term complications of congenital infection exists during the first trimester of gestation; both risk of congenital infection and long-term complications drop during the second trimester, and although the risk of congenital infection increases during the third trimester, there is no risk of long-term complication at that point.

■ PHYSICAL FINDINGS & CLINICAL PRESENTATION

Acquired infection
- Incubation: 14 to 21 days
- Prodrome: 1 to 5 days; low-grade fever, headache, malaise, anorexia, mild conjunctivitis, coryza, pharyngitis, cough, and cervical, suboccipital, and postauricular lymphadenopathy
- Rash: 1 to 5 days
Enanthema: palatal macules
Exanthema (rash): blotchy eruption beginning on face and neck and then spreading to trunk and limbs
- Occasional splenomegaly and hepatitis (during rash)
- Complications: arthritis (15%, mostly in adult women), thrombocytopenia, myocarditis, optic neuritis, encephalitis (all less than 0.1%)

Congenital infection
- Deafness: 85%
- Intrauterine growth retardation: 70%
- Cataracts: 35%
- Retinopathy: 35%
- Patent ductus arteriosus: 30%
- Pulmonary artery hypoplasia: 25%
- In utero death: 20%
- Mental retardation: 10% to 20%
- Meningoencephalitis: 10% to 20%
- Behavior disorder: 10% to 20%
- Hepatosplenomegaly: 10% to 20%
- Bone radiolucencies: 10% to 20%
- Diabetes mellitus (type 1): 10% to 20% by age 35 yr
- Other congenital heart defects: 2% to 5%

■ ETIOLOGY & PATHOGENESIS

Acquired infection
- Viral portal of entry is upper respiratory tract.
- Viral replication occurs in lymph nodes, then hematogenous dissemination occurs to many organs, including placenta if present.
- Immune complexes may be cause of rash and arthritis.
Congenital infection
- Fetus is infected via placenta during maternal acquired infection.
- Cellular damage in the fetus results from cytolysis of fetal cells, mostly via a fetal vasculitis or from an immune-mediated inflammation and damage.

DIAGNOSIS

■ DIFFERENTIAL DIAGNOSIS

Acquired rubella syndrome
- Other viral infections by enteroviruses, adenoviruses, human parvovirus B-19, measles
- Scarlet fever
- Allergic reaction
- Kawasaki disease
Congenital rubella syndrome
- Congenital syphilis, toxoplasmosis, herpes simplex, cytomegalovirus, and enterovirus can cause a similar set of problems.

■ WORKUP

Acquired infection
- Serologic test (hemagglutination inhibition, neutralization tests, complement fixation tests, passive agglutination, enzyme immunoassay [EIA], enzyme-linked immunosorbent assay [ELISA])
- IgM antibodies (by EIA) are detected early: second to fourth week

- IgG antibodies (by ELISA) can be measured as acute phase (7 days after rash onset) and convalescent phase (14 days later)
Congenital infection
- Viral culture (from nasopharynx)
- Serologic studies: IgM antirubella virus detection by EIA is the method of choice (after the newborn is 5 mo old)

■ IMMUNIZATION

Four existing vaccines provide persisting immunity in 92% of vaccinees.
Indications:
- All children 12 mo or older (as part of the measles-mumps-rubella vaccine)
- Postpubertal women
Vaccinate if not known to be immunized (advise not to become pregnant within 3 mo of vaccination)
Premarital serologic screening for rubella immunity
Prenatal or antepartum serologic screening for rubella
Vaccinate susceptible women postpartum
Serologic screening for female workers likely to be exposed to rubella (e.g., teachers, child care employees, health care workers)
Contraindications
- Pregnancy
- Recent receipt of immune globulin or blood transfusion (2 wk before to 3 mo after)
- Immunodeficiency (except AIDS)
Adverse reaction
- Fever, rash, or lymphadenopathy: 5% to 15%
- Arthralgias: 0.5% in children; 25% in adult women
- Transient peripheral neuropathy (rare)

TREATMENT

- No known effective antiviral therapy
- Management of specific congenital problems as appropriate

REFERENCES

Rakowsky A, Sever JL: Rubella. In Gorbach SL, Bartlett JG, Blacklow NR (eds): *Infectious diseases,* ed 2, Philadelphia, 1998, WB Saunders.
U.S. Department of Health: Control and prevention of rubella: evaluation and management of suspected outbreaks, rubella in pregnant women, and surveillance for congenital rubella syndrome, *MMWR* 50(RR-12):1, 2001.
Author: **Tom J. Wachtel, M.D.**

BASIC INFORMATION

■ DEFINITION

Salivary gland neoplasms are benign or malignant tumors of a salivary gland (parotid, submandibular, or sublingual).

■ SYNONYMS

These tumors are often named according to their histologic type (see below).
ICD-9CM CODES
142.9 Salivary gland neoplasm
142.0 (Parotid)
142.1 (Submandibular)
142.2 (Sublingual)

■ EPIDEMIOLOGY & DEMOGRAPHICS

INCIDENCE: 1 to 2 cases/100,000 person-years (1% of all head and neck tumors)
DISTRIBUTION:
- Parotid gland 85% (80% are benign)
- Submandibular gland 10% (55% are benign)
- Sublingual and minor glands 5% (35% are benign)

■ PHYSICAL FINDINGS & CLINICAL PRESENTATION

- Parotid gland (Fig. 1-238):
  1. Painless swelling overlying the masseter muscle (under the temporomandibular joint)
  2. Pain
  3. Facial nerve palsy
  4. Cervical lymph nodes
  5. Mass in oral cavity
- Submandibular gland: swelling under anterior portion of the mandible
- Sublingual gland: intraoral swelling under the tongue, medial to the mandible

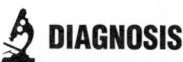 **DIAGNOSIS**

■ PATHOLOGY

History
BENIGN TUMORS:
- Mixed tumor (usually parotid)
- Adenolymphoma (Warthin's tumor)
- Adenoma
- Hemangioma, lymphangioma (in children)
- Other
MALIGNANT TUMORS:
- Mucoepidermoid carcinoma
- Adenoid cystic carcinoma
- Adenocarcinoma
- Malignant mixed tumor
- Squamous cell carcinoma
- Other

Stage (TNM)
T_0 No evidence of primary tumor
T_1 Tumor <2 cm
T_2 Tumor 2 to 4 cm
T_3 Tumor 4 to 6 cm
T_4 Tumor >6 cm
All subdivided into
- Without local extension
- With local extension
N_0 No lymph node metastasis
N_1 Single ipsilateral node <3 cm
N_2 Ipsilateral, contralateral, or bilateral node <6 cm
N_3 Any node >6 cm
M_0 No distant metastasis
M_1 Distant metastasis
Stage I T_{1a} or $_{2a}N_0M_0$
Stage II $T_{1b,2b,3a}$ N_0M_0
Stage III $T_{3b,4a}$ N_0M_0 or any T except $_{4b}N_1M_0$
Stage IV T_{4b} any N any M or any T $N_{2,3}M_0$ or any T, any N_1M_1

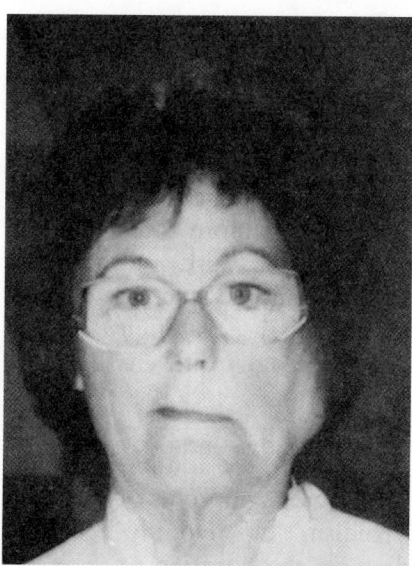

Fig. 1-238   Parotid gland tumor. This woman has a tumor in the left parotid gland, characterized by enlargement of the gland and asymmetry of the left jaw. There appear to be additional lesions present in the left mandible and below the left zygomatic arch. The patient also has paresis of the left facial nerve with drooping of the mouth. That finding raises the concern that the tumor has invaded facial nerve as it passes through the parotid gland. (Courtesy John P. Saunders, Jr., M.D. Department of Surgery, Johns Hopkins University and Hospital, Baltimore. In Seidel HM [ed]: *Mosby's guide to physical examination,* ed 4, St Louis, 1999, Mosby.)

■ WORKUP

- Fine-needle aspiration
- Imaging by CT scan or MRI
- Open biopsy (rarely indicated)

 TREATMENT

Malignant tumors:
- Surgery is the mainstay of treatment; gland resection and neck dissection if lymph nodes are involved
- Postoperative radiation
- Chemotherapy
Benign tumors: surgery for tumor resection

■ PROGNOSIS OF MALIGNANT TUMORS

Five-year survival rates:
- Mucoepidermoid carcinoma: 75% to 95%
- Adenoid cystic carcinoma: 40% to 80%
- Adenocarcinoma: 20% to 75%
- Malignant mixed tumor: 35% to 75%
- Squamous cell carcinoma: 25% to 60%

REFERENCE

Kaplan MJ, Johns ME: Malignant salivary neoplasms. In Cummings CW (ed): *Otolaryngology: head and neck surgery,* St Louis, 1992, Mosby.
Author: **Tom J. Wachtel, M.D.**

BASIC INFORMATION

■ DEFINITION
Salmonellosis is an infection caused by one of several serotypes of *Salmonella*.

■ SYNONYMS
Typhoid
Typhoid fever
Enteric fever

ICD-9CM CODES
003.0 Salmonellosis

■ EPIDEMIOLOGY & DEMOGRAPHICS
INCIDENCE (IN U.S.):
- Estimated 1 million cases/yr of non-typhoidal salmonellosis
- Approximately 500 cases of *Salmonella typhi* infection reported each year
- Largest outbreak: 200,000 persons who ingested contaminated milk

PREDOMINANT AGE:
- <20 yr old
- >70 yr old
- Highest rates of infection in infants, especially neonates

PEAK INCIDENCE: Summer and fall
GENETICS:
Neonatal Infection: Highly susceptible to infection with nontyphoidal Salmonella

■ PHYSICAL FINDINGS & CLINICAL PRESENTATION
- Infections
  1. Localized to GI tract (gastroenteritis)
  2. Systemic (typhoid fever)
  3. Localized outside of GI tract
- Gastroenteritis
  1. Accounts for majority of disease in humans
  2. Incubation period: generally 12 to 48 hr
  3. Nausea
  4. Vomiting
  5. Diarrhea
  6. Abdominal cramps
  7. Fever
  8. Bacteremia
     a. Uncommon
     b. Occurs mostly in the immunocompromised host or those with underlying conditions
  9. Self-limited illness lasting 3 or 4 days
  10. Colonization of GI tract persistent for months, especially in those treated with antibiotics
- Typhoid fever
  1. Incubation period of few days to several months, usually several weeks
  2. Prolonged fever
  3. Myalgias
  4. Headache
  5. Cough

6. Sore throat
7. Malaise
8. Anorexia
9. Abdominal pain
10. Hepatosplenomegaly
11. Diarrhea or constipation early in the course of illness
12. Rose spots (faint, maculopapular, blanching lesions) sometimes seen on chest or abdomen
- Untreated disease
  1. Fever lasting 1 to 2 mo
  2. Main complication of untreated disease: GI bleeding caused by perforation from ulceration of Peyer's patches in the ileum (Fig. 1-239)
  3. Rare complications:
     a. Mental status changes
     b. Shock
  4. Relapse rate of approximately 10%
- Infections outside GI tract
  1. Can occur in virtually any location
  2. Rare
  3. Usually occur in patients with underlying diseases
  4. Endovascular infections are caused by seeding of atherosclerotic plaques or aneurysms

5. Endocarditis is a rare complication
6. Hepatic or splenic abscesses in patients with underlying disease in these organs
7. Urinary tract infections in patients with renal TB or schistosomiasis
8. Salmonellae are a frequent cause of gram-negative meningitis in neonates
9. Osteomyelitis in children with hemoglobinopathies may be caused by these organisms

■ ETIOLOGY
- More than 2000 serotypes of *Salmonella* exist, but only a few cause disease in humans.
- Some found only in humans are the cause of enteric fever.
  1. *S. typhi*
  2. *S. paratyphi*
- Some responsible for gastroenteritis and frequently isolated from raw meat and poultry and uncooked or undercooked eggs.
  1. *S. typhimurium*
  2. *S. enteritidis*

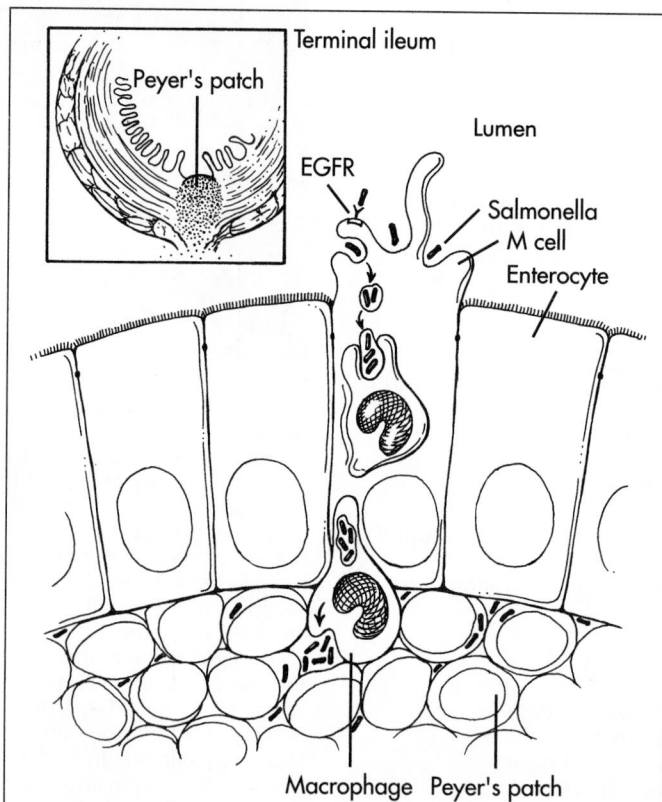

Fig. 1-239 *Salmonella typhi* invade M cells through membrane ruffling and EGF receptor-dependent pathways. Macrophages originating from Peyer's patch take up *S. typhi* in close association with M cells. *S. typhi* replicate in Peyer's patches and then enter the lymphatic system, leading to bacteremia. Replication in Peyer's patches causes hypertrophy followed by necrosis, which can cause intestinal perforation. (From Stein JH [ed]: *Internal medicine*, ed 5, St Louis, 1998, Mosby.)

- *S. cholerae-suis* is a prototype organism that causes extraintestinal nontyphoidal disease.
- Transmission generally via ingestion of contaminated food or drink.
- Outbreaks of gastroenteritis related to contaminated poultry, meat, and dairy products.
- Typhoid fever is a systemic illness caused by serotypes exclusive to humans.
  1. Acquisition by ingestion of food or water contaminated by other humans
  2. Most cases in the U.S. are:
     a. Acquired during foreign travel
     b. Acquired by ingestion of food prepared by chronic carriers, many of whom have acquired the organism outside of the U.S.

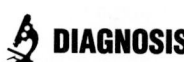 **DIAGNOSIS**

■ DIFFERENTIAL DIAGNOSIS
- Other causes of prolonged fever:
  1. Malaria
  2. TB
  3. Brucellosis
  4. Amebic liver abscess
- Other causes of gastroenteritis:
  1. Bacterial: *Shigella, Yersinia, Campylobacter*
  2. Viral: Norwalk virus, rotavirus
  3. Parasitic: *Amoeba histolytica, Giardia lamblia*
  4. Toxic: enterotoxigenic *E. coli, Clostridium difficile*

■ WORKUP
- Typhoid fever
  1. Cultures of blood, stool, urine; repeat if initially negative.
  2. Blood cultures are more likely to be positive early in the course of illness.
  3. Stool and urine cultures are more commonly positive in the second and third week of illness.
  4. Highest yield with bone marrow biopsy cultures:
     a. 90% positive
     b. Usually not necessary
  5. Serology using Widal's test is helpful in retrospect, showing a fourfold increase in convalescent titers.
- Gastroenteritis: stool cultures
- Extraintestinal localized infection:
  1. Blood cultures
  2. Cultures from the site of infection

■ LABORATORY TESTS
- Neutropenia is common
- Transaminitis is possible
- Culture to grow organism: blood, body fluids, biopsy specimens

■ IMAGING STUDIES
- Radiographs of bone may be suggestive of osteomyelitis.
- CT scan or sonogram of abdomen:
  1. May reveal hepatic or splenic abscesses
  2. May reveal aortic aneurysm

■ TREATMENT

■ NONPHARMACOLOGIC THERAPY
Adequate hydration and electrolyte replacement in persons with diarrhea

■ ACUTE GENERAL Rx
- Typhoid fever:
  1. Ciprofloxacin 500 mg PO bid or 400 mg IV bid for 14 days
  2. Ceftriaxone 2 g IV qd for 14 days
  3. If sensitive, may switch therapy to TMP/SMX 1 to 2 DS tabs PO bid or amoxicillin 2 g PO q8h to complete 14 days
  4. Dexamethasone 3 mg IV initially, followed by 1 mg IV q6h for eight doses for patients with shock or mental status changes
- Gastroenteritis:
  1. Usually not indicated for gastroenteritis alone because this illness usually self-limited
  2. May prolong the carrier state
  3. Prophylactic treatment for patients who are at high risk of developing complications from bacteremia
     a. Neonates
     b. Patients with hemoglobinopathies
     c. Patients with atherosclerosis
     d. Patients with aneurysms
     e. Patients with prosthetic devices
     f. Immunocompromised patients
  4. Treatment can be oral or parenteral, with the same regimens used for typhoid, but only for 48 to 72 hr
- Intravascular infections require 6 wk of parenteral therapy.

■ CHRONIC Rx
- Carrier states are possible in those with typhoid fever.
- More common in persons >60 yr of age and in persons with gallstones.
- Usual site of colonization is the gallbladder.

- Treatment should be considered for those with persistently positive stool cultures and for food handlers.
- Suggested regimens for eradication of carrier state:
  1. Ciprofloxacin 500 mg PO bid for 4 wk
  2. SMX/TMP one to two DS tabs PO bid for 6 wk (if susceptible)
  3. Amoxicillin 2 g PO q8h for 6 wk (if susceptible)
- Cholecystectomy may be required in carriers with gallstones who fail medical therapy.
- Prolonged course of oral therapy or lifetime suppression for:
  1. Patients with AIDS who have chronic infection
  2. Patients with AIDS who relapse after therapy

■ DISPOSITION
- Typhoid fever
  1. Treated patients usually respond to therapy; small percentage of chronic carriers.
  2. Untreated patients may have serious complications.
- Gastroenteritis
  1. Usually self-limited
  2. May be recurrent or persistent in AIDS patients

■ REFERRAL
- If gastroenteritis is persistent or recurrent
- If there is evidence of extraintestinal infection
- For typhoid fever
- For chronic carriers

☿ PEARLS & CONSIDERATIONS

■ COMMENTS
- Quinolones should not be used in children or pregnant women.
- Infections should be reported to local health departments.

REFERENCES

Benenson S et al: The risk of vascular infections in adult patients with nontyphi *Salmonella bacteremia, Am J Med* 110(1):60, 2001.

Outbreaks of multi-drug resistant *Salmonella typhimurium* associated with veterinary facilities. *MMWR* 50(33):701, 2001.

Soravia-Dunand VA et al: Aortitis due to Salmonella: report of 10 cases and comprehensive review of the literature, *Clin Infect Dis* 29:862, 1999.

Author: **Maurice Policar, M.D.**

BASIC INFORMATION

■ DEFINITION

Sarcoidosis is a chronic systemic granulomatous disease of unknown cause, characterized histologically by the presence of nonspecific, noncaseating granulomas.

■ SYNONYMS

Boeck's sarcoid

ICD-9CM CODES

135.0 Sarcoidosis

■ EPIDEMIOLOGY & DEMOGRAPHICS

• Incidence in U.S.: 10.9/100,000 whites, 35.5/100,000 blacks
• Increased incidence in females and patients 20 to 40 yr old
• Presents most commonly in the winter and early spring

■ PHYSICAL FINDINGS & CLINICAL PRESENTATION

• Clinical manifestations often vary with the stage of the disease and degree of organ involvement; patients may be asymptomatic, but a chest x-ray film may demonstrate findings consistent with sarcoidosis (see "Imaging Studies").
• Frequent manifestations:
  1. Pulmonary manifestations: dry, nonproductive cough, dyspnea, chest discomfort
  2. Constitutional symptoms: fatigue, weight loss, anorexia, malaise
  3. Visual disturbances: blurred vision, ocular discomfort, conjunctivitis, iritis, uveitis
  4. Dermatologic manifestations: erythema nodosum, macules, papules, subcutaneous nodules, hyperpigmentation, lupus pernio
  5. Myocardial disturbances: arrhythmias, cardiomyopathy
  6. Splenomegaly, hepatomegaly
  7. Rheumatologic manifestations: arthralgias have been reported in up to 40% of patients
  8. Neurologic and other manifestations: cranial nerve palsies, diabetes insipidus, meningeal involvement, parotid enlargement, hypothalamic and pituitary lesions, peripheral adenopathy

DIAGNOSIS

■ DIFFERENTIAL DIAGNOSIS

• TB
• Lymphoma
• Hodgkin's disease
• Metastases

• Pneumoconioses
• Enlarged pulmonary arteries
• Infectious mononucleosis
• Lymphangitic carcinomatosis
• Idiopathic hemosiderosis
• Alveolar cell carcinoma
• Pulmonary eosinophilia
• Hypersensitivity pneumonitis
• Fibrosing alveolitis
• Collagen disorders
• Parasitic infection

Section II describes the differential diagnosis of granulomatous lung disease and a classification of granulomatous disorders.

■ WORKUP

• Chest x-ray examination and biopsy
• Biopsy should be done on accessible tissues suspected of sarcoid involvement (conjunctiva, skin, lymph nodes); bronchoscopy with transbronchial biopsy is the procedure of choice in patients without any readily accessible site

■ LABORATORY TESTS

Laboratory abnormalities:
• Hypergammaglobulinemia, anemia, leukopenia
• LFT abnormalities
• Hypercalcemia, hypercalciuria (secondary to increased GI absorption, abnormal vitamin D metabolism, and increased calcitriol production by sarcoid granuloma)
• Cutaneous anergy to *Trichophyton, Candida,* mumps, and tuberculin
• Angiotensin-converting enzyme (ACE): elevated in approximately 60% of patients with sarcoidosis; nonspecific and generally not useful in following the course of the disease

■ IMAGING STUDIES

• Chest x-ray film (Fig. 1-240): adenopathy of the hilar and paratracheal nodes is a frequent finding; parenchymal changes may also be present, depending on the stage of the disease (stage 0, normal x-ray; stage I, bilateral hilar adenopathy; stage II, stage I plus pulmonary infiltrate; stage III, pulmonary infiltrate without adenopathy); stage IV, advanced fibrosis with evidence of honey-combing, hilar retraction, bullae, cysts, and emphysema.
• PFTs: may be normal or may reveal a restrictive pattern and/or obstructive pattern.
• Gallium-67 scan: will localize in areas of granulomatous infiltrates; however, it is not specific. The "panda" sign (localization in the lacrimal and salivary glands, giving a "panda" appearance to the face) is suggestive of sarcoidosis.

TREATMENT

■ GENERAL Rx

• Corticosteroids (Table 1-51) remain the mainstay of therapy when treatment is required (e.g., prednisone 40 mg qd for 8 to 12 wk with gradual tapering of the dose to 10 mg qod over 8 to 12 mo); corticosteroids should be considered in patients with severe symptoms (e.g., dyspnea, chest pain), hypercalcemia, ocular, CNS, or cardiac involvement, and progressive pulmonary disease.
• Patients with progressive disease refractory to corticosteroids may be treated with methotrexate 7.5 to 15 mg once/week or azathioprine.
• Hydroxychloroquine is effective for chronic disfiguring skin lesions.
• NSAIDs are useful for musculoskeletal symptoms and erythema nodosum.
• Pulmonary rehabilitation in patients with significant respiratory insufficiency.

■ DISPOSITION

The majority of patients with sarcoidosis have spontaneous remission within 2 yr and do not require treatment. Their course can be followed by periodic clinical evaluation, chest x-ray studies, and PFTs.

■ REFERRAL

Ophthalmologic examination is indicated in all patients with suspected sarcoidosis, because ocular findings (iridocyclitis, uveitis, conjunctivitis, and keratopathy) are found in >25% of documented cases.

PEARLS & CONSIDERATIONS

■ COMMENTS

Approximately 15% to 20% of patients with lung involvement advance to irreversible lung impairment (bronchiectasis, cavitation, progressive fibrosis, pneumothorax, and respiratory failure). Death from pulmonary failure occurs in 5% to 7% of patients with sarcoidosis.

REFERENCES

Paramothayan S, Jones PW: Corticosteroid therapy in pulmonary sarcoidosis, *JAMA* 287:1301, 2002.
Thomas KW, Hunninghake GW: Sarcoidosis, *JAMA* 289:3300, 2003.
Author: **Fred F. Ferri, M.D.**

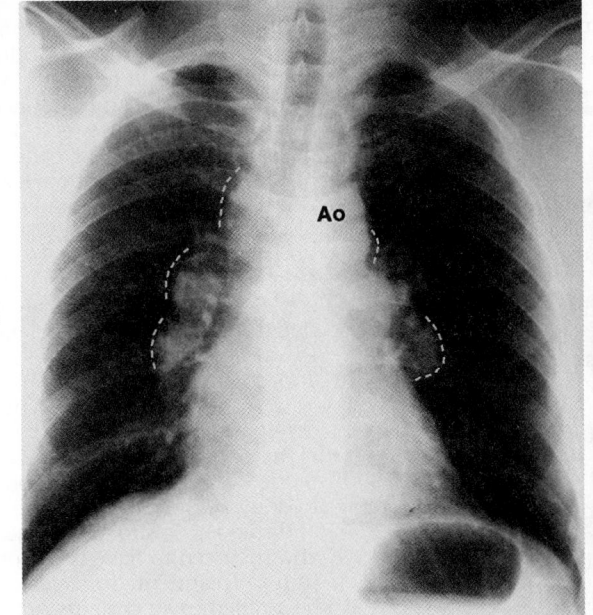

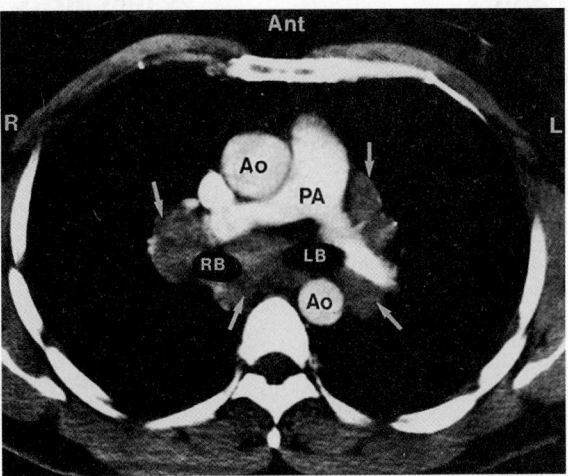

Fig. 1-240 Sarcoid. Marked lymphadenopathy (*dotted lines*) is seen in the region of both hila in the right paratracheal region **(A)**. The transverse contrast-enhanced CT scan of the upper chest **(B)** clearly shows the ascending and descending aorta (*Ao*) as well as the pulmonary artery (*PA*) and superior vena cava. The right and left mainstem bronchus area is also seen. The arrows indicate the extensive lymphadenopathy. *LB,* Left bronchus; *RB,* right bronchus. (From Mettler FA [ed]: *Primary care radiology,* Philadelphia, 2000, WB Saunders.)

TABLE 1-51   Indications for Use of Corticosteroids in Sarcoidosis

DISORDER	TREATMENT
Iridocyclitis	Corticosteroid eyedrops Local subjunctival deposit of cortisone
Posterior uveitis	Oral prednisone
Pulmonary involvement	Steroids rarely recommended for stage I; usually employed if infiltrate remains static or worsens over 3-mo period or the patient is symptomatic
Upper airway obstruction	Rare indication for intravenous steroids
Lupus pernio	Oral prednisone shrinks the disfiguring lesions
Hypercalcemia	Responds well to corticosteroids
Cardiac involvement	Corticosteroids usually recommended if patient has arrhythmias or conduction disturbances
CNS involvement	Response is best in patients with acute symptoms
Lacrimal/salivary gland involvement	Corticosteroids recommended for disordered function, *not* gland swelling
Bone cysts	Corticosteroids recommended if symptomatic

From Andreoli TE (ed): *Cecil essentials of medicine,* ed 5, Philadelphia, 2001, WB Saunders.
CNS, Central nervous system.

BASIC INFORMATION

■ DEFINITION
Scabies is a contagious disease caused by the mite *Sarcoptes scabiei*.

ICD-9CM CODES
133.0 Scabies

■ EPIDEMIOLOGY & DEMOGRAPHICS
- Scabies is generally acquired by sleeping with or in the bedding of infested individuals.
- It is generally associated with poor living conditions and is also common in hospitals and nursing homes.

■ PHYSICAL FINDINGS & CLINICAL PRESENTATION
- Primary lesions are caused when the female mite burrows within the stratum corneum, laying eggs within the tract she leaves behind; burrows (linear or serpiginous tracts) end with a minute papule or vesicle.
- Primary lesions are most commonly found in the web spaces of the hands, wrists, buttocks, scrotum, penis, breasts, axillae, and knees.
- Secondary lesions result from scratching or infection.
- Intense pruritus, especially nocturnal, is common; it is caused by an acquired sensitivity to the mite or fecal pellets and is usually noted 1 to 4 wk after the primary infestation.
- Examination of the skin may reveal burrows, tiny vesicles, excoriations, inflammatory papules.
- Widespread and crusted lesions (Norwegian or crusted scabies) may be seen in elderly and immunocompromised patients.

■ ETIOLOGY
Human scabies is caused by the mite *Sarcoptes scabiei,* var. *hominis* (Fig. 1-241).

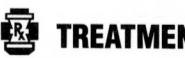 DIAGNOSIS

■ DIFFERENTIAL DIAGNOSIS
- Pediculosis
- Atopic dermatitis
- Flea bites
- Seborrheic dermatitis
- Dermatitis herpetiformis
- Contact dermatitis
- Nummular eczema
- Syphilis
- Other insect infestation

■ WORKUP
Diagnosis is made on the clinical presentation and on the demonstration of mites, eggs, or mite feces.

■ LABORATORY TESTS
- Microscopic demonstration of the organism, feces, or eggs: a drop of mineral oil may be placed over the suspected lesion before removal; the scrapings are transferred directly to a glass slide; a drop of potassium hydroxide is added and a cover slip is applied.
- Skin biopsy is rarely necessary to make the diagnosis.

TREATMENT

■ NONPHARMACOLOGIC THERAPY
Clothing, underwear, and towels used in the 48 hr before treatment must be laundered.

■ ACUTE GENERAL Rx
- Following a warm bath or shower, Lindane (Kwell, Scabene) lotion should be applied to all skin surfaces below the neck (can be applied to the face if area is infested); it should be washed off 8 to 12 hr after application. Repeat application 1 wk later is usually sufficient to eradicate infestation.
- Pruritus generally abates 24 to 48 hr after treatment, but it can last up to 2 wk; oral antihistamines are effective in decreasing postscabietic pruritus.
- Topical corticosteroid creams may hasten the resolution of secondary eczematous dermatitis.
- If the patient is a resident of an extended care facility, it is important to educate the patients, staff, family, and frequent visitors about scabies and the need to have full cooperation in treatment. Scabicide should be applied to all patients, staff, and frequent visitors, whether symptomatic or not; symptomatic family members of staff and visitors should also receive treatment.
- Permethrin 5% cream (Elimite) is also effective with usually one treatment; it should be massaged into the skin from head to soles of feet; remove 8 to 14 hr later by washing. If living mites are present after 14 days, treat again.
- A single dose (150-200 mg/kg in 6-mg tablets) of ivermectin, an antihelminthic agent, is as effective as topical lindane for the treatment of scabies. It is the best treatment for generalized crusted scabies.

■ DISPOSITION
Refractory cases usually are seen with immunocompromised hosts or patients with underlying skin diseases.

PEARLS & CONSIDERATIONS

■ COMMENTS
- Lindane is potentially neurotoxic and should not be used for infants and pregnant women (permethrin is safe and effective in these situations).
- Sexual partners should be notified and treated.

REFERENCE
Flinders DC, DeSchweinitz P: Pediculosis and scabies, *Am Fam Physician* 341:8, 2004.
Author: **Fred F. Ferri, M.D.**

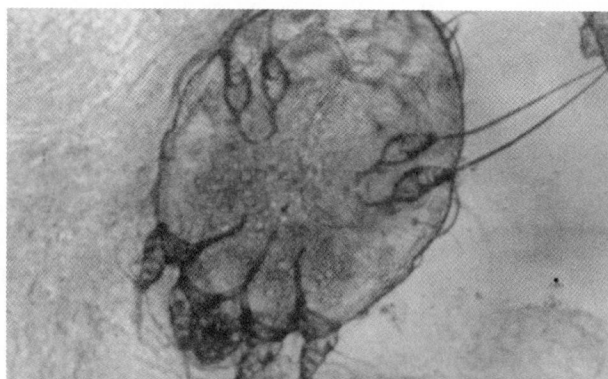

Fig. 1-241   Scabies organism in a wet mount preparation. (From Mandell GL: *Mandell, Douglas, and Bennett's principles and practice of infectious diseases,* ed 5, New York, 2000, Churchill Livingstone.)

BASIC INFORMATION

■ DEFINITION
Scarlet fever is a rash involving skin and tongue and complicating a streptococcal group A pharyngitis.

ICD-9CM CODES
034.1 Scarlet fever

■ EPIDEMIOLOGY & DEMOGRAPHICS
Same as streptococcal pharyngitis; namely, children aged 5 to 15 yr. May also complicate impetigo.

■ PHYSICAL FINDINGS & CLINICAL PRESENTATION
CLINICAL PRESENTATION:
- Febrile illness with headache, malaise, anorexia, and pharyngitis begins after a 2- to 4-day incubation period.
- Scarlatinal rash begins 1 or 2 days after the onset of pharyngitis (Fig. 1-242).

PHYSICAL FINDINGS:
- Diffuse erythema, beginning on face and spreading to neck, back, chest, rest of trunk, and extremities. Most intense on inner aspects of arms and thighs
- Erythema blanches, but nonblanching petechiae may be present or produced by a tourniquet
- Strawberry or raspberry tongue
- Rash lasts about 1 wk and then desquamates

■ ETIOLOGY
Caused by group A β-hemolytic *Streptococcus* infection, which produces one of three erythrogenic toxins (NOTE: Some streptococcal species have the ability to cause both scarlet fever and rheumatic fever)

⚗ DIAGNOSIS

■ DIFFERENTIAL DIAGNOSIS
- Viral exanthems (covered in Section II)
- Kawasaki disease
- Toxic shock syndrome
- Drug rashes
See differential diagnosis of Pharyngitis in Section I.

■ WORKUP
- Identification of group A *Streptococcus* by throat culture
- SLO antibody titers

℞ TREATMENT

- Penicillin 250 mg PO qid for 10 days or erythromycin 250 mg PO qid for 10 days in penicillin-allergic patients
- Benzathine penicillin 1 to 2 million U IM once; may be used for a patient who cannot swallow

■ COMPLICATIONS (RARE)
- Peritonsillar abscess
- Mastoiditis
- Otitis media
- Pneumonia
- Sepsis and distant foci of infection
- Acute rheumatic fever
- Inability to swallow liquids or upper airway obstruction require hospitalization

NOTE: Failure to respond to penicillin should raise doubt about the diagnosis because *Streptococcus* may be carried in the pharynx without causing infection.

REFERENCE
Stollerman GH: *Streptococcus pyogenes* (group A streptococci). In Gorbach SL, Bartlett JG, Blacklow NR (eds): *Infectious diseases,* ed 2, Philadelphia, 1998, WB Saunders.
Author: **Tom J. Wachtel, M.D.**

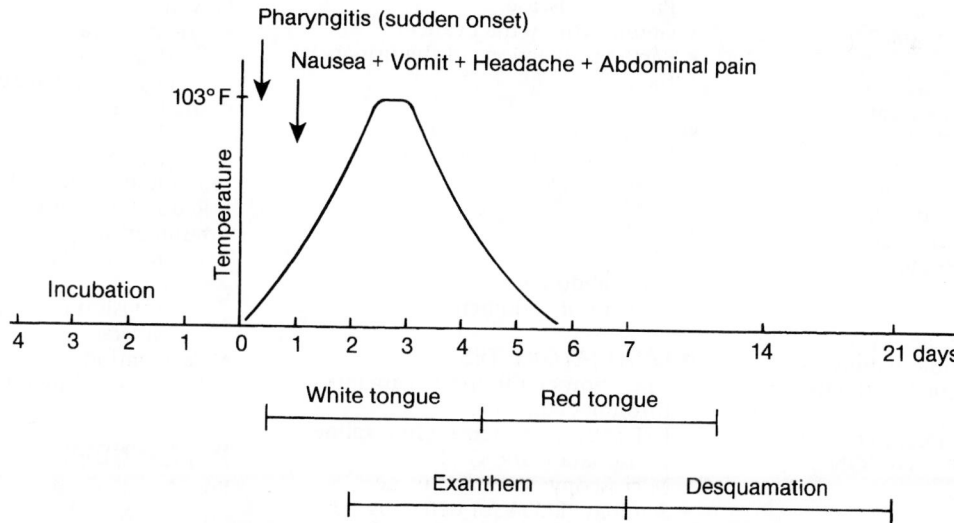

Fig. 1-242 Scarlet fever. Evolution of signs and symptoms. (From Habif TP: *Clinical dermatology: a color guide to diagnosis and therapy,* ed 3, St Louis, 1996, Mosby.)

BASIC INFORMATION

■ DEFINITION
Schistosomiasis is caused by infection with parasite blood flukes known as schistosomes.

ICD-9CM CODES
120.9 Schistosomiasis

■ EPIDEMIOLOGY & DEMOGRAPHICS
INCIDENCE
- More than 200 million people worldwide and more than 200,000 deaths annually. In U.S., estimated to exceed 400,000 persons.
- Geographic distribution of schistosomiasis is confined to an area between 36° north and 34° south latitude, where fresh water temperatures averages 25° C to 30° C.

PREVALENCE
The greatest cercarial exposure usually occurs in boys aged 5 to 10 yr

DISTRIBUTION
- *S. mansoni* in tropical and subtropical areas of sub-Saharan Africa, the Middle East, South America, and the Caribbean
- *S. haematobium* in North Africa, sub-Saharan Africa, the Middle East, and India
- *S. japonicum* in Asia, particularly in China, the Philippines, Thailand, and Indonesia
- *S. intercalatum* in central and west Africa
- *S. mekonki* in Cambodia

■ ETIOLOGY
- Human infections are caused by *S. mansoni, S. haematobium, S. japonicum, S. mekonki,* and *S. intercalatum.*
- Acquisition of disease via contact with fresh water containing infectious free-living cercarial larvae.
- In U.S., most cases are acquired during foreign travel.

PATHOGENESIS
Human disease is primarily associated with the host's granulomatous response to eggs retained in the tissue.

■ PHYSICAL FINDINGS & CLINICAL PRESENTATION
ACUTE SYMPTOMS:
- Swimmers itch
- Katayama fever

CHRONIC SYMPTOMS:
- Intestinal schistosomiasis
  1. Abdominal pain
  2. Bloody diarrhea
  3. Iron deficiency anemia
  4. Intestinal polyp
  5. Bowel ulcer and strictures

- Hepatic schistosomiasis
  1. Hepatomegaly
  2. Splenomegaly
  3. Portal hypertension
  4. Esophageal varices
- Urinary schistosomiasis
  1. Hematuria
  2. Dysuria
  3. Urinary frequency
  4. Fibrosis of bladder and ureters
  5. Squamous cell ca of bladder
  6. Proteinuria
  7. Nephrotic syndrome

COMPLICATION:
- Neurologic complication
  1. Granuloma of spinal cord or brain
  2. Transverse myelitis
  3. Epilepsy or focal neurologic deficit
- Pulmonary complication
  1. Granulomatous pulmonary endarteritis
  2. Pulmonary hypertension
  3. Cor pulmonale
- Other complications include tubal obstruction and infertility
- Recurrent bacteremia and recurrent UTI

DIAGNOSIS

■ DIFFERENTIAL DIAGNOSIS
- Amebiasis
- Bacillary dysentery
- Bowel polyp
- Prostatic disease
- Genitourinary tract cancer
- Bacterial infections of the urinary tract

■ WORKUP
- Microscopy in urine or stool
- Tissue biopsy
- Serology
- CBC
- LFT
- US of abdomen
- CT scan of abdomen

■ LABORATORY TESTS
- CBC shows eosinophilia, anemia, thrombocytopenia
- LFT with mild increase in alkaline phosphatase and GGT
- Microscopy: stool and urine
- Serology: ELISA for detecting both schistosomal antibodies and antigen
- Rectal biopsy or bladder mucosal biopsy

■ IMAGING STUDIES
- X-ray of abdomen shows "fetal head" calcification.
- Sonography also documents a thickened bladder wall, hydronephrosis and hydroureter, and bladder polyps or calcification. It also demonstrates the thickened fibrosed portal tracts.
- Esophagoscopy documents esophageal varices.
- Liver biopsy may also demonstrate granuloma and clay pipestem fibrosis.

TREATMENT

- Praziquantel 40 mg/kg of body weight in one or two doses
- Oxamniquine 15 mg/kg
- Metrifonate 7.5 to 10 mg/kg of body weight given in three doses at 2-wk intervals
- Amoscanate
- Oltipraz

■ DISPOSITION
Treated patients usually respond to therapy. Definitive cure has occurred only when there is total disappearance of viable eggs from the excreta for a total of 6 mo after treatment.

PEARLS & CONSIDERATIONS

■ COMMENTS
Prevention:
- Chemotherapy
  1. Mass
  2. Targeted population
- Snail control
  1. Mollusciciding
  2. Environmental modification
  3. Biologic control
- Reduction of water contact and contamination
  1. Provision of domestic water supplies
  2. Provision for sanitary disposal of excreta
- Vaccination
  - Improved living standards

REFERENCES
Ross A et al: Current concepts: schistosomiasis, *N Engl J Med* 346:1212, 2002.
Schwartz E et al: Schistosomiasis, *N Engl J Med* 347:766, 2002.
Author: **Vasanthi Arumugam, M.D.**

BASIC INFORMATION

■ DEFINITION

Schizophrenia is diagnosed when an individual has experienced at least 1 mo of hallucinations, delusions, thought disorder, or catatonia and at least 6 mo of decreased function and negative symptoms (avolition, anhedonia, social isolation, affective flattening).

■ SYNONYMS

Dementia praecox

ICD-9CM CODES

295.9 Schizophrenia

■ EPIDEMIOLOGY & DEMOGRAPHICS

PREVALENCE: World: 0.2% to 2%, U.S.: 1%

PREDOMINANT SEX: Males have a more severe illness and therefore skew the gender distribution toward higher in males; however, distribution is probably equal.

PREDOMINANT AGE:
• Age at onset of psychotic symptoms is in the early 20s for males and late 20s for females.
• Age of onset of the negative symptoms is usually earlier (midteenage years).

PEAK INCIDENCE: 20 to 40 yr

GENETICS:
• First-degree relatives of schizophrenics have 10 times greater chance of becoming schizophrenic than the general population.
• Discordant rates among identical twins are higher than expected with simple inheritance pattern.
• Associations with several chromosomes have been described, but none have been replicated.
• Evidence exists that triplet nucleotide repeat expansion (such as seen with Huntington's disease) may play a role in inheritance of the disease.

■ PHYSICAL FINDINGS & CLINICAL PRESENTATION

• Best defined as a dementing illness beginning in early life and progressing slowly throughout the lifetime.
• Initial "negative" symptoms of adolescence—cognitive decline, social withdrawal and awkwardness, loss of motivation and pleasure, and loss of emotional expressiveness—begin after a period of normal development.
• In early adulthood, positive symptoms of psychosis and thought disturbance occur; psychotic symptoms then wax and wane throughout life; treatment ameliorates positive symptoms but generally does little for negative ones.

• Greatest chunk of occupational and social desirability is secondary to negative symptoms.

■ ETIOLOGY

• Unknown
• Basic distinction of whether this is a degenerative or a developmental condition is not settled
• Loss of cortical tissue has been established in a series of landmark studies of discordant identical twins
• Major hypothesis: generation of the mesocortical pathways produce the hypofrontality and negative symptoms, along with a compensatory hyperactivation of the mesolimbic pathways, which produce the positive symptoms of psychosis

DIAGNOSIS

■ DIFFERENTIAL DIAGNOSIS

• Any medical condition, medicine, or substance of abuse that can affect brain homeostasis and cause psychosis: distinguished from schizophrenia by their relatively brief course and the alteration in mental status that could suggest an underlying delirium
• Other neurologic conditions (e.g., Huntington's) that have psychosis as the initial presentation
• Other psychiatric disorders: source of greatest confusion
• Mood disorders with psychosis: indistinguishable from schizophrenia cross-sectionally, but have a longitudinal course that includes full recovery
• Delusional disorder: has non-bizarre delusions and lacks the thought disturbance, hallucinations, and negative symptoms of schizophrenia
• Autism in the adult: has an early age at onset and lacks significant hallucinations or delusions

■ WORKUP

• History and physical examination to aid in determining if psychosis is secondary or primary
• Neurologic examination to uncover soft neurologic signs (clumsy, cortical thumb, loss of fine motor movements) common in schizophrenia

■ LABORATORY TESTS

• No laboratory tests are specific for schizophrenia.
• Laboratory examinations (chemistry profile, blood count, sedimentation rate, toxicology screen, and urinalysis) are geared toward excluding a primary medical condition.

■ IMAGING STUDIES

• CT scan or MRI of brain during initial workup; repeated if the course of the illness varies from expected
• Sometimes EEG to reveal slowing when psychosis is secondary to an encephalopathy
• Chest x-ray examination during initial workup to rule out a primary medical condition

TREATMENT

■ NONPHARMACOLOGIC THERAPY

• Significant social support is required by most schizophrenic patients; available support services are grossly inadequate, and schizophrenia patients constitute nearly one third of all homeless individuals. They usually require help with basic social, occupational, and interactive skills.
• For schizophrenic patients who continue to live with their families, relapse rates are related to the degree of emotionality in the family (i.e., schizophrenics living in families with high expressed emotion levels relapse with greater rates), so family interventions can sometimes reduce morbidity.
• Traditional psychotherapy is usually not useful in schizophrenia, but supportive psychotherapy may reduce suicide rate.

■ ACUTE GENERAL Rx

• Acute psychosis is usually adequately controlled by antipsychotic agents.
• Mainstay of therapy is the newer, atypical antipsychotics (risperidone, olanzapine, quetiapine, ziprasidone, aripiprazole, and clozapine). Traditional neuroleptic (e.g., haloperidol, perphenazine, fluphenazine, chlorpromazine) use is decreasing in part as a result of their propensity to cause a parkinsonian state and eventual tardive dyskinesia (rate of tardive dyskinesia 15% to 30%). Antiparkinsonian drugs (benztropine, amantidine) are used to ameliorate the parkinsonism. Risperidone has been shown to be superior to haloperidol in preventing acute psychotic relapse.
• Sedatives (benzodiazepines, and to a lesser degree, barbiturates) can be used transiently if there is an agitated state.

■ CHRONIC Rx

• Compliance is long-term focus of treatment; relapse rates are quite high in noncompliant patients. Antipsychotic agents usually must be continued at the same doses that controlled psychosis. For noncompliant patients, depot preparations that are given biweekly or monthly can be used.

- Antiparkinsonian agents may also need to be continued chronically.
- Tardive dyskinesia (choreoathetoid movements of the muscles of tongue, face, and occasionally other muscle groups) can occur in as many as 30% of patients with long-term use of the neuroleptics.
- The negative symptoms of schizophrenia can resemble depression. Additionally, depressive disorders may occur in schizophrenic patients. Antidepressant treatment of the negative symptoms is usually without effect. However, antidepressants can improve the symptoms of a discrete comorbid depressive episode.
- Mood stabilizers, such as lithium, valproate, or carbamazepine, are of little use unless there is a comorbid impulse control disorder.

- Substance abuse is a major problem in more than one third of schizophrenics. Unfortunately, these patients do poorly in traditional substance abuse treatment programs. Specialized "dual diagnosis" programs with highly structured aftercare are required.

■ DISPOSITION

- The positive symptoms of as many as 20% to 30% of schizophrenic patients do not respond to available treatments. A much higher fraction relapse as a result of poor compliance.
- The negative symptoms are responsible for the 50% to 70% of cases in which deterioration in occupational and social function continues.
- More than 10% of patients will complete suicide.

■ REFERRAL

- If hospitalization is required
- If patient is noncompliant
- If patient is resistant to treatment

REFERENCES

Csernansky JG et al: A comparison of risperidone and haloperidol for the prevention of relapse in patients with schizophrenia, *N Engl J Med* 346:16, 2002.

Freedman R: Schizophrenia, *N Engl J Med* 349:1738, 2003.

Mortensen PB et al: Effects of family history and place and season of birth on the rise of schizophrenia, *N Engl J Med* 340:603, 1999.

Authors: **Rif S. El-Mallakh, M.D., and Peggy L. El-Mallakh, B.S.N.**

BASIC INFORMATION

■ DEFINITION

Scleritis is inflammation of the sclera.

■ SYNONYMS

Anterior scleritis
Diffuse nodular, necrotizing scleritis
Scleromalacia perforans

ICD-9CM CODES

379.0 Scleritis and episcleritis

■ EPIDEMIOLOGY & DEMOGRAPHICS

INCIDENCE (IN U.S.): Busy ophthalmologist may see one or two cases a year
PREVALENCE (IN U.S.): Relatively rare
PREDOMINANT SEX: 61% women
PREDOMINANT AGE: 52 yr
PEAK INCIDENCE: Increases with increasing age

■ PHYSICAL FINDINGS & CLINICAL PRESENTATION

- Deep, boring eye pain
- Photophobia
- Tearing
- Conjunctival injection (Fig. 1-243)
- Thinning of the sclera

■ ETIOLOGY

- Inflammatory
- Allergic
- Toxic

DIAGNOSIS

■ DIFFERENTIAL DIAGNOSIS

- Most common causes are rheumatoid arthritis and collagen-vascular disease.
- Occasionally, there are allergic, infectious, or traumatic causes.
- Conjunctivitis, iritis, and episcleritis should be considered in the differential diagnosis.

■ WORKUP

- Fluorescein angiography
- Eye examination
- Visual field examination
- Workup for autoimmune disease

■ LABORATORY TESTS

- Usually not necessary
- RF, ANA, ESR may be useful

■ IMAGING STUDIES

Usually not necessary; CT scan of orbit may be useful in selected patients

TREATMENT

■ NONPHARMACOLOGIC THERAPY

- Patching
- Bandage lenses
- Surgery if thinning of the sclera is severe

■ ACUTE GENERAL Rx

- Steroids (topical, periocular, and systemic)
- Cycloplegic drops
- NSAIDs (topical and systemic)
- Other immunosuppressive drugs

■ CHRONIC Rx

- Systemic steroids can be given for the underlying disease.
- Local steroids may be helpful.

■ DISPOSITION

Urgent referral to ophthalmologist

■ REFERRAL

If not referred to an ophthalmologist early, patients may develop uveitis and other complications.

PEARLS & CONSIDERATIONS

■ COMMENTS

An ominous diagnosis because these patients often have other severe underlying debilitating disease processes.

REFERENCES

Paresio CG et al: Systemic disorders associated with episcleritis and scleritis, *Curr Opin Ophthalmal* 12(6):471, 2001.
Sainz de la Maza M et al: Ocular characteristics and disease associations in scleritis: associated peripheral keatopathy, *Arch Ophth* 120(1):15, 2002.
Author: Melvyn Koby, M.D.

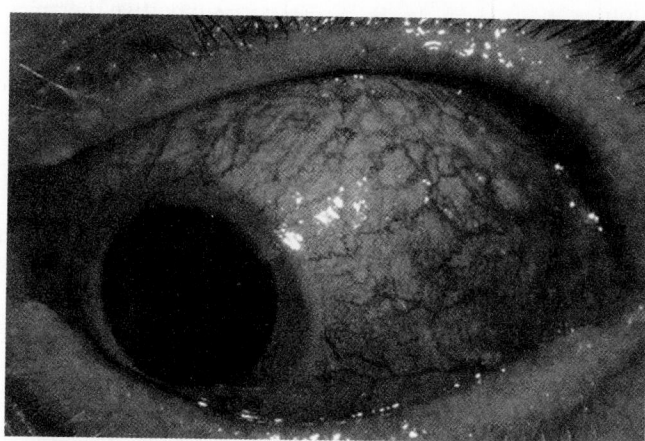

Fig. 1-243 In diffuse anterior scleritis, widespread injection of the conjunctival and deep episcleral vessels occurs. (From Palay D [ed]: *Ophthalmology for the primary care physician,* St Louis, 1997, Mosby.)

BASIC INFORMATION

■ DEFINITION
Scleroderma is a connective tissue disorder characterized by thickening and fibrosis of the skin and variably severe involvement of diverse internal organs.

■ SYNONYMS
Systemic sclerosis; morphea applies to localized scleroderma affecting only the skin. Scleredema is a disease of the skin distinct from scleroderma.

ICD-9CM CODES
710.1 (morphea: 701.0)

■ EPIDEMIOLOGY & DEMOGRAPHICS
INCIDENCE: 4 to 12 cases/million persons per year, but many mild cases go unrecognized
DEMOGRAPHICS: Female:male ratio of 4:1
PEAK AGE: 30 to 50 yr
DISTRIBUTION: Worldwide

■ PHYSICAL FINDINGS & CLINICAL PRESENTATION
CLINICAL PRESENTATION:
- Raynaud's phenomenon: initial complaint in 70% (NOTE: The prevalence of Raynaud's is 5% to 10% of the general population; most do not progress to scleroderma)
- Finger or hand swelling, sometimes associated with carpal tunnel syndrome
- Arthralgias/arthritis
- Internal organ involvement

PHYSICAL FINDINGS:
Skin
- Begins on hands, then face; skin is shiny, taut, sometimes red with loss of creases and hair
- Later skin tightening may limit movement
- Pigmentary changes occur
- Skin atrophy occurs in late stages
Musculoskeletal
- Symmetric inflammatory arthritis
- Myopathy
GI involvement
- Esophageal dysmotility with heartburn, dysphagia, odynophagia
- Delayed gastric emptying
- Small bowel dysmotility with abdominal cramps and diarrhea
- Colon dysmotility with constipation
- Primary biliary cirrhosis (see "Primary Biliary Cirrhosis" in Section I)

Pulmonary manifestations
- Pulmonary fibrosis with symptoms of dyspnea and nonproductive cough and fine inspiratory crackles on examination
- Pulmonary hypertension
Cardiac involvement
- Myocardial fibrosis leading to congestive heart failure
Renal involvement
- Malignant hypertension
- Rapidly progressive renal failure
Other organ involvement
- Hypothyroidism
- Erectile dysfunction
- Sjögren's syndrome
- Entrapment neuropathies
CREST syndrome
- Calcinosis, Raynaud's syndrome, esophageal dysmotility, sclerodactyly, telangiectasias (in CREST scleroderma is limited to distal extremities)

■ ETIOLOGY
Etiology is unknown. Unifying features exist in spite of heterogenous patterns of organ involvement and disease progression:
- Extracellular connective tissue activation
- Frequent immunologic abnormalities
- Inflammation
- Vasoconstriction

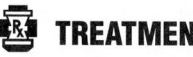
DIAGNOSIS

■ DIFFERENTIAL DIAGNOSIS
Dermatologic
- Mycosis fungoides
- Amyloidosis
- Porphyria cutanea tarda
- Eosinophilic fasciitis
- Reflex sympathetic dystrophy
Systemic
- Idiopathic pulmonary fibrosis
- Primary pulmonary hypertension
- Primary biliary cirrhosis
- Cardiomyopathies
- GI dysmotility problems
- SLE and overlap syndromes

■ WORKUP
Laboratory tests and imaging studies

■ LABORATORY TESTS
- Antinuclear antibodies (homogeneous, speckled, or nucleolar patterns)
- Negative antibody to native DNA
- Negative anti-Sm antibody
- Anti-nRNP positive in 20%
- Rheumatoid factor positive in 30%
- Anticentromere antibodies in fewer than 10% with systemic illness and in 50% to 95% with limited scleroderma (i.e., good prognosis if positive)

- Positive extractable nuclear antibody to SCL 70 in 30%
- Routine biochemistry tests may indicate specific organ involvement (e.g., liver, kidney, muscle)

■ IMAGING AND OTHER STUDIES
Arthritis: joint x-rays
GI
- Barium swallow
- Cine esophagography
- Endoscopy
- Esophageal manometry
Pulmonary
- Chest x-ray
- PFTs
- Chest CT scan
- Bronchoscopy with biopsy
- Gallium lung scan
- Bronchoalveolar lavage
Heart
- ECG
- Ambulatory (Holter) ECG monitoring
- Echocardiography
- Cardiac catheterization
Kidney: renal biopsy
Skin: skin biopsy

TREATMENT

D-penicillamine; recombinant human relaxin; supportive therapies used.
Raynaud's syndrome:
- Calcium channel blockers
- Peripheral α_1-adrenergic blockers
Arthralgias: NSAIDs
Skin: moisturizing agents
Esophageal reflux
- H_2-receptor blockers
- Proton pump inhibitors
Pulmonary hypertension and fibrosis
- Oxygen
- Lung transplant
Renal involvement
- Angiotensin-converting enzyme inhibitors
- Dialysis
- Renal transplantation

■ REFERRAL
To rheumatologist

REFERENCES
Seibold JR: Scleroderma. In Kelley WN et al (eds): *Textbook of rheumatology,* ed 5, Philadelphia, 1997, WB Saunders.
Seibold JR, Koan JH, Simms R, et al: Recombinant human relaxin in the treatment of scleroderma, *Ann Intern Med* 132:871, 2000.
Author: **Tom J. Wachtel, M.D.**

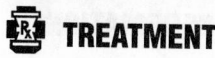
 BASIC INFORMATION

DEFINITION

Scoliosis is a lateral curvature of the spine in the upright position, usually 10 degrees or greater. Scoliosis may be classified as either structural (fixed, nonflexible) or nonstructural (flexible, correctable).

ICD-9CM CODES

737.30 Idiopathic scoliosis
737.39 Paralytic scoliosis
754.2 Congenital scoliosis
724.3 Sciatic scoliosis
737.43 Associated with neurofibromatosis

EPIDEMIOLOGY & DEMOGRAPHICS (IDIOPATHIC FORM)

PREVALENCE: 4 cases/1000 persons
PREVALENT AGE:
- Onset is variable.
- Most curves are found in adolescents (age 11 yr and over).

PREDOMINANT SEX: Females > male (7:1)

PHYSICAL FINDINGS & CLINICAL PRESENTATION

- Record patient age (in years plus months) and height.
- Perform neurologic examination to rule out neuromuscular disease.
- Inspect the shoulders and iliac crests to determine if they are level.
- Palpate the spinous processes to determine their alignment.
- Have the patient bend forward symmetrically at the waist with the arms hanging free (Adams' position); observe from the back or front to detect abnormal spine rotation (Fig. 1-244).

ETIOLOGY

- 90% unknown, usually referred to as idiopathic (genetic)
- Congenital spine deformity
- Neuromuscular disease
- Leg length inequality
- Local inflammation or infection
- Acute pain (disk disease)
- Chronic degenerative disc disease with a symmetric disc narrowing

Curves of an idiopathic nature or those accompanying congenital deformity or neuromuscular disease are those associated with structural changes. The nonstructural types (leg length discrepancy, inflammation, or acute pain) disappear when the offending disorder is corrected.

DIAGNOSIS

WORKUP

- Curvatures associated with congenital spine abnormalities, neuromuscular disease, and the other less common forms of scoliosis can usually be identified by history or associated radiographic or physical findings.
- Section III, Fig. 3-163 describes an approach to scoliosis screening.

IMAGING STUDIES

- Diagnosis of idiopathic scoliosis is confirmed by a standing roentgenogram of the spine.
- Severity of the curve is measured in degrees, usually by the Cobb method.
- MRI is usually not indicated unless there is: (1) pain, (2) a neurologic deficit, or (3) a left thoracic curve (which is often associated with an underlying spinal disorder).

TREATMENT

ACUTE GENERAL Rx

- Treatment or correction of cause if curve is nonstructural
- Early detection is key in treating genetic curve
- Regular observation for curves <20 degrees
- Bracing for idiopathic curves of 20 to 40 degrees to prevent progression
- Surgery for idiopathic curves >40 to 50 degrees in immature patient

DISPOSITION

- The larger the curve at detection, the greater the chance of progression.
- Progression is more common in young children who are beginning their growth spurt.
- Curves in females are more likely to progress.
- Curves <20 degrees will improve spontaneously more than 50% of the time.
- Failure to diagnose and treat these curves may allow progressive deformity, pain, and cardiopulmonary compromise to develop.
- Spinal deformities >50 degrees in adults may progress and eventually become painful.
- There is no difference in the rate of back pain in the general population and patients with adolescent idiopathic scoliosis.

REFERRAL

For orthopedic consultation if structural curve is present

PEARLS & CONSIDERATIONS

COMMENTS

Congenital scoliosis has a high incidence of cardiac and urinary tract abnormalities.

REFERENCES

Greiner KA: Adolescent idiopathic scoliosis: radiologic decision-making, *Am Fam Physician* 65:1817, 2002.
Lenke LG et al: Adolescent idiopathic scoliosis, *J Bone Joint Surg* 83(A):1169, 2001.
Mooney V, Brigham A: The role of measured resistance exercises in adolescent scoliosis, *Orthopedics* 26:167, 2003.
Reamy BV, Slakey JB: Adolescent idiopathic scoliosis: review and current concepts, *Am Fam Physician* 64:111, 2001.
Yawn BP: Population-based study of school scoliosis screening; *JAMA* 282:1427, 1999.

Author: **Lonnie R. Mercier, M.D.**

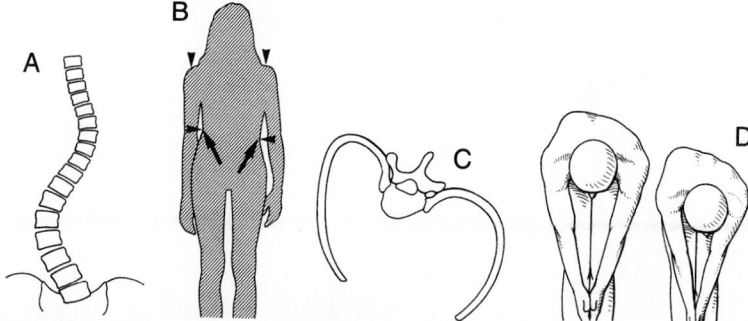

Fig. 1-244   Structural changes in idiopathic scoliosis. A, As curvature increases, alterations in body configuration develop in both the primary and compensatory curve regions. **B,** Asymmetry of shoulder height, waistline, and the elbow-to-flank distance are common findings. **C,** Vertebral rotation and associated posterior displacement of the ribs on the convex side of the curve are responsible for the characteristic deformity of the chest wall in scoliosis patients. **D,** In the school screening examination for scoliosis, the patient bends forward at the waist. Rib asymmetry of even a small degree is obvious. (From Scoles PV: Spinal deformity in childhood and adolescence. In Behrman RE, Vaughn VC III [eds]: *Nelson textbook of pediatrics*, ed 5, Philadelphia, 1989, WB Saunders.)

BASIC INFORMATION

■ DEFINITION
Recurrent depressive episodes during autumn and winter alternating with nondepressive episodes during spring and summer.

ICD-9CM CODES
296.30 Seasonal affective disorder

■ EPIDEMIOLOGY & DEMOGRAPHICS
Climate, genetic vulnerability, and social-cultural factors all play a role. Prevalence is higher in North America than in Europe.

■ PHYSICAL FINDINGS & CLINICAL PRESENTATION
Presentation typical for depression, including sleep disturbance, loss of interest in day-to-day activities, decreased libido.

■ ETIOLOGY
Probable serotonergic and catecholaminergic deficit in the CNS.

DIAGNOSIS

An interview with the patient will elicit signs of depression, and similar symptoms will occur during fall and winter.

■ DIFFERENTIAL DIAGNOSIS
Other causes of depression, such as excessive alcohol intake, drugs (e.g., propranolol), manic-depressive disorder, depressive disorder, should be considered.

■ WORKUP
Endocrine evaluation, especially thyroid, sleep studies, toxicology screen, might be considered.

■ LABORATORY TESTS
See workup. None necessary in the typical case

■ IMAGING STUDIES
None necessary

TREATMENT

■ NONPHARMACOLOGIC THERAPY
Light therapy has been shown to be effective.

■ ACUTE GENERAL Rx
None necessary unless patient is suicidal; immediate hospitalization necessary if suicide potential is present.

■ CHRONIC Rx
Serotonergic and noradrenergic antidepressants are effective.

■ DISPOSITION
Psychiatric referral if patient does not respond relatively quickly

☼ PEARLS & CONSIDERATIONS

Light therapy is often a novel approach that avoids pharmacologic intervention.

REFERENCES
Magnussen A: An overview of epidemiological studies on seasonal affective disorder, *Acta Psychiatr Scand* 101(3):176, 2000.

Neumeister A et al: Monoaminergic function in the pathogenesis of seasonal affective disorder, *Int J Neuropharm* 4(4):409, 2001.

Shaw L: Genetic studies of seasonal affective disorder and seasonality, *Compr Psychiatry* 42(2):105, 2001.
Author: **Rif S. El-Mallakh, M.D.**

BASIC INFORMATION

■ DEFINITION

Absence seizures are a type of generalized nonconvulsive seizure characterized by episodes of loss of awareness (typically ≤10 sec) associated with a 3 Hz generalized spike and slow wave EEG pattern, followed by abrupt return to full consciousness.

■ SYNONYMS

Petit mal seizures (obsolete)

ICD-9CM CODES

345.0 Generalized nonconvulsive epilepsy

■ EPIDEMIOLOGY & DEMOGRAPHICS

INCIDENCE (IN U.S.): 11 cases/100,000 persons from ages 1 through 10 yr, rare after age 14 yr
PREVALENCE (IN U.S.): Accounts for 2%-15% of the cases of childhood epilepsy
PREDOMINANT AGE: 4 to 8 yr
PEAK INCIDENCE: 6 to 7 yr
GENETICS: Clear genetic predisposition; undetermined mode of inheritance

■ PHYSICAL FINDINGS & CLINICAL PRESENTATION

- Findings are normal between seizures in children with typical absence epilepsy.
- During seizure, patient typically appears awake but abruptly ceases ongoing activity and does not respond to or recall stimuli.
- More prolonged episodes may be associated with automatisms and therefore mistaken for complex partial seizures.

■ ETIOLOGY

- Idiopathic with a presumed genetic cause
- Absence seizures can also be seen with some types of generalized epilepsy syndromes such as juvenile absence epilepsy or juvenile myoclonic epilepsy
- Experimental data: seizures arise from impaired regulation of rhythmic thalamic discharges

 DIAGNOSIS

■ DIFFERENTIAL DIAGNOSIS

- Complex partial seizures
- Daydreaming
- Psychogenic unresponsiveness

■ WORKUP

- EEG is the most powerful tool for identification of this seizure type.
- In the vast majority of untreated individuals, vigorous hyperventilation for 3 to 5 min provokes characteristic EEG finding.

■ IMAGING STUDIES

None needed for typical presentation

TREATMENT

■ NONPHARMACOLOGIC THERAPY

Avoid sleep deprivation and hyperventilation.

■ ACUTE GENERAL Rx

Not indicated for individual typical seizures

■ CHRONIC Rx

- Drug of choice is ethosuximide or sodium valproate.
- Lamotrigine is also effective.

■ DISPOSITION

- Favorable prognosis in typical childhood absence epilepsy without other seizure types
- Excellent response to medication
- Subsidence of seizures with advancing age in 70% to 90% of patients

■ REFERRAL

If uncertain about diagnosis

⚙ PEARLS & CONSIDERATIONS

■ COMMENTS

- Absence seizures may be mistakenly diagnosed as complex partial seizures based on clinical descriptions. The EEG is essential for making this distinction.
- Administering other anticonvulsants (particularly carbamazepine or phenytoin) to patients with typical absence epilepsy may exacerbate seizures.
- Patient education information can be obtained from the Epilepsy Foundation of America, 4351 Garden City Drive, Landover, MD 20785; phone: (800) EFA-1000.

REFERENCES

Mattson RH: Overview: idiopathic generalized epilepsies, *Epilepsia* 44(2):2, 2003.

Panayiotopoulos CP: Treatment of typical absence seizures and related epileptic syndromes, *Paediatr Drugs* 3(5):379, 2001.

Author: **John E. Croom, M.D., Ph.D.**

BASIC INFORMATION

■ DEFINITION

Generalized tonic-clonic seizures are marked by paroxysmal hypersynchronous neuronal activity involving both cerebral hemispheres resulting in loss of consciousness with tonic muscle contraction followed by rhythmic clonic contractions. The seizure may start focally in one region or hemisphere of the brain with subsequent or secondary generalization.

■ SYNONYMS

All obsolete:
Grand mal seizure
Major motor seizure

ICD-9CM CODES

345.1 Generalized convulsive epilepsy

■ EPIDEMIOLOGY & DEMOGRAPHICS

INCIDENCE (IN U.S.): 50-70 cases/100,000 persons/yr with highest rates during early childhood and those over 65 years of age
PREVALENCE (IN U.S.): Approximately 6.5 cases/1000 persons for all types of epilepsy
PREDOMINANT SEX: Males slightly higher than females
GENETICS: Genetic predisposition exists for the idiopathic generalized epilepsies; mode of transmission varies with the particular epilepsy syndrome.

■ PHYSICAL FINDINGS & CLINICAL PRESENTATION

- Generally normal neurologic examination. Focal deficits may be found in patients with an underlying lesion causing the seizures
- Sequence of motor events during the seizure typically includes widespread tonic muscle contraction evolving to clonic jerking
- Typically associated with postictal confusion lasting up to several hours
- May be associated with tongue, cheek, or lip biting and/or urinary incontinence

■ ETIOLOGY

- Seizures are a symptom of an underlying abnormality affecting the CNS, not a disease.
- Etiology of generalized tonic-clonic seizures can be divided into idiopathic, symptomatic, or cryptogenic causes.
- With idiopathic generalized tonic-clonic seizures, there is a postulated inherited basis for the disorder. This includes some epilepsy syndromes such as juvenile myoclonic epilepsy and Lennox-Gastaut syndrome.
- Symptomatic generalized tonic-clonic seizures result from an underlying cause such as inborn errors of metabolism, acquired metabolic or

toxic abnormalities, CNS infection or tumor, and trauma.
- Cryptogenic seizures are those without a presumed genetic etiology or clear underlying cause.

DIAGNOSIS

■ DIFFERENTIAL DIAGNOSIS

- Syncope
- Psychogenic events
- Section II describes the differential diagnosis of epilepsy.

■ WORKUP

New-onset seizures: a detailed history and physical examination with the goal of determining the underlying etiology

■ LABORATORY TESTS

- Serum glucose and electrolytes
- Additional blood studies and lumbar puncture as indicated by history and physical examination
- EEG: most valuable diagnostic tool for identifying seizure type and predicting the likelihood of recurrence

■ IMAGING STUDIES

- Generally not necessary in well-documented cases of idiopathic generalized tonic-clonic seizures
- MRI: modality of choice if history, examination, or EEG suggest partial (focal) onset

TREATMENT

■ NONPHARMACOLOGIC THERAPY

Avoid sleep deprivation or environmental precipitants (e.g., photosensitive epilepsy).

■ ACUTE GENERAL Rx

- Individual seizures lasting <5 min generally require no acute pharmacologic intervention.
- See "Status Epilepticus" in Section I for management of recurrent or prolonged seizures.

■ CHRONIC Rx

- A single seizure with an identifiable and easily correctable provoking factor (e.g., hyponatremia) does not warrant long-term use of anticonvulsants.
- If there is significant risk of recurrence (Table 1-52) or more than one unprovoked seizure, treatment is indicated.
- Sodium valproate and phenytoin are common first-line therapeutic agents (see Table 1-53).
- Newer agents such as lamotrigine and topiramate may be better tolerated.
- For each patient, anticonvulsant choice is influenced by factors such as effectiveness, cost, adverse effects, ease of administration, and type of epilepsy syndrome if present.

■ DISPOSITION

- Varies with underlying etiology
- Excellent outcome for most patients with idiopathic generalized tonic-clonic seizures

■ REFERRAL

If uncertain about diagnosis or seizure type or if the seizures fail to respond to anticonvulsant treatment. Also, refer if the patient is considering becoming pregnant.

PEARLS & CONSIDERATIONS

■ CAUTION

EEG is normal in as many as 50% of patients; thus diagnosis is primarily by history. Usually, a single seizure is not treated with chronic anticonvulsants.

REFERENCES

Browne TR, Holmes GL: Epilepsy, *N Engl J Med* 344:1145, 2001.
Chang BS, Lowenstein DH: Mechanisms of Disease: Epilepsy, *N Engl J Med* 349:1257, 2003.
Author: **John E. Croom, M.D., Ph.D.**

TABLE 1-52   Risk of Recurrence After a First Tonic-Clonic Seizure

HIGH	LOW
Abnormal neurologic findings	Febrile seizure in a child
Mental retardation	Febrile status epilepticus (child)
Abnormal EEG findings	Transient metabolic and toxic states
Myoclonic jerks, absences, or atonic seizures	Benign rolandic seizures
Structural brain lesions	Impact seizures in early nonsevere head trauma
Family history of epilepsy	
Elderly individuals	

From Johnson RT, Griffin JW: *Current therapy in neurologic disease,* ed 5, St Louis, 1997, Mosby.
EEG, Electroencephalogram.

BASIC INFORMATION

■ DEFINITION

In partial seizures, the onset of abnormal electrical activity originates in a focal region or lobe of the brain. Clinical manifestations may involve sensory, motor, autonomic, or psychic symptoms. Consciousness may be preserved (simple partial seizures) or impaired (complex partial seizures).

■ SYNONYMS

Localization-related seizures
Focal epilepsy
Obsolete terms include:
Minor motor seizures
Jacksonian seizures
Psychomotor seizures

ICD-9CM CODES

345.4 Partial epilepsy, with impairment of consciousness
345.5 Partial epilepsy, without impairment of consciousness

■ EPIDEMIOLOGY & DEMOGRAPHICS

INCIDENCE (IN U.S.): 20 cases/100,000 persons through age 65 yr, then rises sharply
PREVALENCE (IN U.S.): 6.5 cases/1000 persons for all types of epilepsy
PREDOMINANT SEX: Males slightly higher than females
GENETICS: Most acquired, but several distinct inherited syndromes have been identified.

■ PHYSICAL FINDINGS & CLINICAL PRESENTATION

- Range from normal to focal neurologic deficits, depending on underlying cause.
- Clinical presentation is varied and depends on the site of origin of the abnormal electrical discharges.
- Symptoms of simple partial seizures can include focal motor or sensory symptoms; language disturbance; olfactory, visual or auditory hallucinations; visceral sensations, or fear or panic.
- With complex partial seizures, there is a loss or reduction of awareness. This may be preceded by an aura (simple partial seizure). There may be associated automatisms or alterations in behavior.
- There may be a relatively quick "march" or progression of symptoms over seconds to minutes as the ictal focus spreads along the cortex.

■ ETIOLOGY

- Seizures are a symptom of an underlying abnormality affecting the CNS, not a disease.
- Partial-onset seizures may be caused by underlying disorders including stroke, tumor, infection, trauma, vascular malformations, or genetic factors.

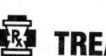 **DIAGNOSIS**

■ DIFFERENTIAL DIAGNOSIS

- Migraine
- TIA
- Presyncope
- Psychogenic phenomena
- Section II describes the differential diagnosis of epilepsy

■ WORKUP

Because partial seizures are manifestations of an underlying focal CNS disturbance that must be identified if possible, imaging studies, preferably MRI, are essential.

■ LABORATORY TESTS

EEG is the most powerful tool for localization of the seizure focus.

■ IMAGING STUDIES

- MRI with contrast: modality of choice because of its high sensitivity for stroke, tumor, abscess, atrophy, and vascular malformations
- CT scan without contrast if hemorrhage is suspected

TREATMENT

■ NONPHARMACOLOGIC THERAPY

Avoid sleep deprivation.

■ ACUTE GENERAL Rx

- Individual seizures lasting <5 min generally require no acute pharmacologic intervention.
- For management of recurrent or prolonged seizures, see "Status Epilepticus" in Section I.

■ CHRONIC Rx

- Carbamazepine or phenytoin are common first-line therapeutic agents (Table 1-53).

- Sodium valproate may also be effective.
- Newer agents such as lamotrigine or oxcarbazepine may be better tolerated.
- For each patient, anticonvulsant choice is influenced by factors such as effectiveness, cost, adverse effects, and ease of administration.

■ DISPOSITION

- Determined by underlying cause
- Approximately 70% of patients are controlled with medication

■ REFERRAL

If uncertain about diagnosis or patient fails to respond to appropriate medication, refer to a neurologist or epilepsy specialist for further evaluation. In addition, some types of partial seizures, particularly temporal lobe epilepsy, are amenable to surgical resection.

PEARLS & CONSIDERATIONS

■ COMMENTS

- Patient education information can be obtained from the Epilepsy Foundation of America, 4351 Garden City Drive, Landover, MD 20785; phone: (800) EFA-1000.
- This is the most underdiagnosed, yet the most common, type of seizure in adults.

REFERENCES

Chabolla DR: Characteristics of the epilepsies, *Mayo Clin Proc* 77:981, 2002.
Wiebe S et al: A randomized controlled trial of surgery for temporal-lobe epilepsy, *N Engl J Med* 345:311, 2001.
Author: **John E. Croom, M.D., Ph.D.**

TABLE 1-53 Drugs of Choice in Treatment of Epilepsy

SEIZURE TYPE	DRUGS OF CHOICE
Generalized tonic clonic, simple, and complex partial	Phenytoin, valproic acid Carbamazepine Levetiracetam, zonisamide
Absence	Ethosuximide Valproic acid
Benign centrotemporal epilepsy	Phenytoin, gabapentin
Neonatal seizures	Phenobarbital
Febrile seizures	Treatment generally not indicated
Infantile spasms	ACTH, vigabatrin
Lennox-Gastaut syndrome	Clonazepam, lamotrigine, topiramate
Newer drugs	
Generalized tonic clonic, simple, partial, and complex partial	Lamotrigine Tigabine Topiramate Zonisamide Oxcarbazepine Levetiracetam Gabapentin

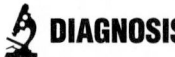

 BASIC INFORMATION

■ **DEFINITION**
A febrile seizure is a seizure in infancy or childhood, usually occurring between 3 mo and 5 yr of age, associated with fever but without evidence of intracranial infection or defined cause.

■ **SYNONYMS**
Benign febrile seizure

ICD-9CM CODES
780.3 Convulsions

■ **EPIDEMIOLOGY & DEMOGRAPHICS**
INCIDENCE (IN U.S.): Not reported
PREVALENCE (IN U.S.): 2% to 4% in children <5 yr of age
PREDOMINANT SEX: Male = female
PREDOMINANT AGE: 18 to 24 mo of age
GENETICS:
• Family history increases risk two- to threefold.
• Mode of inheritance is unknown.

■ **PHYSICAL FINDINGS & CLINICAL PRESENTATION**
• Typically occurs early in the course of an illness when temperature is rising.
• Most commonly associated with a viral upper respiratory or gastrointestinal infection.
• Simple febrile seizures are single events lacking focality and lasting less than 15 min.
• Features of complex febrile seizures include: duration longer than 15 min, focal seizures, seizure recurrence within 24 hr, or abnormal neurologic examination.
• Physical and neurologic examination and developmental history may be normal especially with simple febrile seizures.

■ **ETIOLOGY**
Unknown

DIAGNOSIS

■ **DIFFERENTIAL DIAGNOSIS**
• Epilepsy
• Meningitis
• Encephalitis

■ **WORKUP**
• In children with simple febrile seizures, no further evaluation is usually required.
• In children with complex febrile seizures, more aggressive investigation is required.

■ **LABORATORY TESTS**
• Lumbar puncture is indicated in children under 6 mo of age, in children with complex febrile seizures, or if signs or symptoms of meningitis are present.
• Complex febrile seizures may warrant EEG, toxicology screening, assessment of electrolytes, and so forth, depending on history and examination findings.

■ **IMAGING STUDIES**
• Not needed in simple febrile seizures
• Complex febrile seizures warrant head imaging studies

TREATMENT

■ **NONPHARMACOLOGIC THERAPY**
• Avoid excessive clothing.
• Encourage fluids.
• Apply tepid sponge bath to control fever.

■ **ACUTE GENERAL Rx**
• Antipyretics
• Possibly rectal diazepam in some instances of recurrent febrile seizures
• For prolonged seizures, can use parenteral diazepam or lorazepam.

■ **CHRONIC Rx**
• Prophylactic treatment with anticonvulsants is not indicated in children with typical simple febrile seizures.
• May consider anticonvulsant use in children with complex febrile seizures, but risks and benefits must be considered.

■ **DISPOSITION**
• Risk of recurrent benign febrile seizures is 30% up to the age of 5 yr.
• Risk of subsequent epilepsy is estimated at 1% to 2.5%. Risk of developing subsequent epilepsy is highest in children with complex febrile seizures and can be up to 13%-50%.
• Available data: there is no risk reduction with prophylactic anticonvulsants.

■ **REFERRAL**
If uncertain about diagnosis or with atypical presentation

REFERENCES
Baumann RJ: Prevention and management of febrile seizures, *Paediatr Drugs* 3(8):585, 2001.
Knudsen FU: Febrile Seizures: Treatment and prognosis, *Epilepsia* 41(1):2, 2000.
Shinnar S, Glauser TA: Febrile seizures, *J Child Neurol* 17(Suppl 1):S44, 2002.
Author: **John E. Croom, M.D., Ph.D.**

BASIC INFORMATION

■ DEFINITION

Septicemia is a systemic illness caused by generalized bacterial infection and characterized by evidence of infection, fever or hypothermia, hypotension, and evidence of end-organ compromise.

■ SYNONYMS

Sepsis
Sepsis syndrome
Systemic inflammatory response syndrome
Septic shock

ICD-9CM CODES
038.9 Sepsis
038.40 Sepsis, gram-negative bacteremia
038.1 Sepsis, *Staphylococcus*

■ EPIDEMIOLOGY & DEMOGRAPHICS
INCIDENCE (IN U.S.):
- Exact incidence is unknown
- Approximately 300,000 cases of gram-negative bacteremia among hospitalized patients each year
- Complicates a minority of bacteremia cases and may occur in the absence of documented bacteremia
PREDOMINANT SEX: Male = female
PREDOMINANT AGE:
- Neonatal period
- Patients >70 yr of age
GENETICS:
Familial Disposition: A great variety of congenital immunodeficiency states and other inherited disorders may predispose to septicemia.
Neonatal Infection: Incidence is high in neonatal period.

■ PHYSICAL FINDINGS & CLINICAL PRESENTATION
- Fever or hypothermia
- Hypotension
- Tachycardia
- Tachypnea
- Altered mental status
- Bleeding diathesis
- Skin rashes
- Symptoms that reflect primary site of infection: urinary tract, GI tract, CNS, respiratory tract

■ ETIOLOGY
- Disseminated infection with a great variety of bacteria:
  1. Gram-negative bacteria
  2. *E. coli*
  3. *Klebsiella* spp.
  4. *Pseudomonas aeruginosa*
  5. *Proteus* spp.
  6. *Staphylococcus aureus*
  7. *Streptococcus* spp.
  8. *Neisseria meningitidis*
- Less common infections:
  1. Fungal
  2. Viral
  3. Rickettsial
  4. Parasitic
- Activation of coagulation, complement, and kinin cascades with release of a variety of vasoactive endogenous mediators
- Predisposing host factors:
  1. General medical condition
  2. Age
  3. Immunosuppressive therapy
  4. Recent surgery
  5. Granulocytopenia
  6. Hyposplenism
  7. Diabetes
  8. Instrumentation

DIAGNOSIS

■ DIFFERENTIAL DIAGNOSIS
- Cardiogenic shock
- Acute pancreatitis
- Pulmonary embolism
- Systemic vasculitis
- Toxic ingestion
- Exposure-induced hypothermia
- Fulminant hepatic failure
- Collagen-vascular diseases

■ WORKUP
- Evaluation should focus on identifying a specific pathogen and localizing the site of primary infection.
- Hemodynamic, metabolic, coagulation disorders should be carefully characterized.
- Intensive monitoring, including the use of central venous or Swan-Ganz catheters, may be necessary.

■ LABORATORY TESTS
- Cultures of blood and examination and culture of sputum, urine, wound drainage, stool, CSF
- CBC with differential, coagulation profile
- Routine chemistries, LFTs
- ABGs
- Urinalysis

■ IMAGING STUDIES
- Chest x-ray examination
- Other radiographic and radioisotope procedures according to suspected site of primary infection

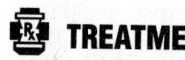 TREATMENT

■ NONPHARMACOLOGIC THERAPY
- Tissue oxygenation: oxygen saturation maintained as high as possible; early mechanical ventilation
- Focal infection drained, if possible

■ ACUTE GENERAL Rx
- Blood pressure support
  1. IV hydration
  2. Therapy with pressors (e.g., dopamine) if mean blood pressure of 70 to 75 mm Hg cannot be maintained by hydration alone
- Correction of acidosis
  1. IV bicarbonate
  2. Mechanical ventilation
- Antibiotics
  1. Directed at the most likely sources of infection
  2. Should generally provide broad coverage of gram-positive and gram-negative bacteria
  3. Typical regimens:
     a. For hospital-acquired septicemia (pending culture results): vancomycin plus ceftazidime, imipenem, aztreonam, quinolones, or an aminoglycoside
     b. For community-acquired infection in the absence of granulocytopenia: above or single-drug therapy with third-generation cephalosporin
     c. For infection in the granulocytopenic host: above or dual gram-negative coverage (e.g., cephalosporin and aminoglycoside)

4. Biological treatment Drotrecogin alfa (Xigris), a genetically engineered form of activated protein C, has recently been approved for use in patients with severe sepsis; when combined with conventional therapy, there may be a reduction in mortality
5. The role of corticosteroids in the acute management of septicemia has long been debated. Although most well-constructed clinical trials have demonstrated no benefit, recent data suggest that patients with relative adrenal insufficiency may benefit from low-dose therapy with hydrocortisone (50 mg IV q6h) and fludrocortisone (50 mg daily PO) given together for 7 days

■ CHRONIC Rx
• Adjust antibiotic therapy on the basis of culture results.
• In general, continue therapy for a minimum of 2 wk.

■ DISPOSITION
All patients with suspected septicemia should be hospitalized and given access to intensive monitoring and nursing care.

■ REFERRAL
• To infectious diseases expert
• To physician experienced in critical care

⚙ PEARLS & CONSIDERATIONS

■ COMMENTS
Mortality rises quickly if antibiotic therapy is not instituted promptly and metabolic derangements are not treated aggressively.

REFERENCES
Angus DC and Wax RS: Epidemiology of sepsis: an update, *Crit Care Med* 29(7 Suppl):S109, 2001.
Annane D et al: Effect of treatment with low doses of hydrocortisone and fludrocortisone on mortality in patients with septic shock, *JAMA* 288:862, 2002.
Balk RA: Severe sepsis and septic shock: definitions, epidemiology, and clinical manifestations, *Crit Care Clin* 16(2):179, 2000.
Author: **Joseph R. Masci, M.D.**

BASIC INFORMATION

■ DEFINITION
Serotonin syndrome (SS) refers to a group of symptoms resulting from increased activity of serotonin (5-hydroxytryptamine) in the central nervous system. Serotonin syndrome is a drug-induced disorder that is characterized by a change in mental status and alteration in neuromuscular activity and autonomic function.

■ SYNONYMS
SS

ICD-9CM CODES
333.99 Syndrome serotonin

■ EPIDEMIOLOGY & DEMOGRAPHICS
- The incidence of serotonin syndrome is not known.
- Serotonin syndrome affects males and females from ages 20 to 70 yr.
- Serotonin syndrome commonly occurs in patients receiving two or more serotonergic drugs.
- Concomitant use of a selective serotonin reuptake inhibitor (SSRI) with a monoamine oxidase inhibitor (MAOI) poses the greatest risk of developing SS.
- Combination of SSRIs with other serotonergic drugs (e.g., tryptophan) or drugs with serotonin properties (e.g., lithium, meperidine) can also lead to SS.

■ PHYSICAL FINDINGS & CLINICAL PRESENTATION
- Symptoms usually start within minutes to hours after starting a new psychopharmacologic treatment or after administering a second serotonergic drug.
- Confusion, agitation, hypomania
- Fever, tachycardia, and tachypnea
- Nausea, vomiting, abdominal pain, and diaphoresis
- Diarrhea, tremors, shivering, and seizures
- Ataxia, myoclonus, and hyperreflexia

■ ETIOLOGY
- Hyperstimulation of the brainstem and spinal cord serotonin receptors because of blocking reuptake of serotonin and catecholamines is believed to be the underlying mechanism leading to the neuromuscular and autonomic symptoms seen in SS.
- Psychopharmacologic drugs, in particular, fluoxetine and sertraline coadministered with MAOI (e.g., tranylcypromine and phenelzine), have been cited in the literature as a common cause of SS.

 DIAGNOSIS

The diagnosis of SS is made on clinical grounds. There are no specific laboratory tests for SS. A high index of suspicion along with a detailed medication history is the mainstay of diagnosis.

■ DIFFERENTIAL DIAGNOSIS
Neuroleptic malignant syndrome, substance abuse (e.g., cocaine, amphetamines), thyroid storm, infection, alcohol and opioid withdrawal

■ WORKUP
- Other causes described in the differential diagnosis must be excluded to make the diagnosis of SS. Thus all patients should have blood tests and diagnostic imaging studies to rule out infectious, toxic, and metabolic etiologies.
- Additional laboratory tests are performed to exclude complicating features of SS (e.g., renal failure secondary to rhabdomyolysis).

■ LABORATORY TESTS
- CBC with differential to rule out sepsis
- Electrolytes, BUN, and creatinine to rule out acidosis and renal failure
- Blood and urine toxicology screen
- Thyroid function tests
- CPK with isoenzymes
- Urine and blood cultures
- ECG, because ventricular rhythm disturbance is a potentially fatal complication

■ IMAGING STUDIES
Imaging studies are not very specific in the diagnosis of SS and are only ordered to exclude other causes with similar clinical presentations as SS.

TREATMENT

There is no specific antidote for excess serotonin.

■ NONPHARMACOLOGIC THERAPY
- Discontinuation of the drug is the mainstay of therapy
- Treatment is supportive: maintaining oxygenation and blood pressure and monitoring respiratory status
- Cooling blankets for patients with hyperthermia
- Mechanical intubation for patients unable to protect their airways as a result of mental status changes or seizures

■ ACUTE GENERAL Rx
- Cyproheptadine 4 mg tablet is given in 4- to 8-mg doses q1-4h (up to 32 mg for adults, 12 mg in children) until a therapeutic response is achieved.
- Benzodiazepines—lorazepam 1 to 2 mg IV q30min—has been used effectively in treating muscle rigidity, myoclonus, and seizure complications. Diazepam is an alternative choice.
- Methysergide has also been reported to be effective.
- Propranolol has serotonin-blocking properties and is given 1 to 3 mg q5min up to 0.1 mg/kg.

■ CHRONIC Rx
For patients not requiring hospital admission, cyproheptadine, lorazepam, or propranolol can be given in an oral dose on a prn basis with close follow-up.

■ DISPOSITION
- Serotonin syndrome is a potentially life-threatening condition if not recognized early.
- Prompt diagnosis and withdrawal of the medication results in improvement of symptoms within 24 hr.
- Seizures, rhabdomyolysis, hyperthermia, ventricular arrhythmia, respiratory arrest, and coma are all complicating features of SS.

■ REFERRAL
All cases of SS secondary to psychotropic medications should be referred to a psychiatrist.

PEARLS & CONSIDERATIONS

■ COMMENTS
- The use of SSRIs and MAOIs is contraindicated.
- The use of SSRIs and other serotonergic agents is not an absolute contraindication; however, prompt withdrawal of the medication is recommended if any symptoms suggesting SS occur.
- Serotonin syndrome is usually found in patients being treated for depression, bipolar disorders, obsessive-compulsive disorder, attention-deficit disorder, and Parkinson's disease.

REFERENCES
Carbone JR: The neuroleptic malignant and serotonin syndromes, *Emerg Med Clin North Am* 18(2):317, 2000.
Gillman PK: The serotonin syndrome and its treatment, *J Psychopharmacol* 13(1):100, 1999.
Mason PJ, Morris VA, Balcezak TJ: Serotonin syndrome presentation of 2 cases and review of the literature, *Medicine* 79(4):201, 2000.
Author: **Peter Petropoulos, M.D.**

BASIC INFORMATION

■ DEFINITION
Severe acute respiratory syndrome (SARS) is a respiratory illness caused by a novel coronavirus, called SARS-associated coronavirus (SARS-CoV).

CLINICAL CRITERIA
- Asymptomatic or mild respiratory illness
- Moderate respiratory illness
  - Temperature of >100.4°F (>38°C)*, and
  - One or more clinical findings of respiratory illness (e.g., cough, shortness of breath, difficulty breathing, or hypoxia)
- Severe respiratory illness
  - Temperature of >100.4°F (>38°C)*, and
  - One or more clinical findings of respiratory illness (e.g., cough, shortness of breath, difficulty breathing, or hypoxia), and
  - Radiographic evidence of pneumonia, or
  - Respiratory distress syndrome, or
  - Autopsy findings consistent with pneumonia or respiratory distress syndrome without an identifiable cause

EPIDEMIOLOGIC CRITERIA
- Travel (including transit in an airport) within 10 days of onset of symptoms to an area with current or previously documented or suspected community transmission of SARS or
- Close contact† within 10 days of onset of symptoms with a person known or suspected to have SARS

---

* A measured documented temperature of >100.4°F (>38°C) is preferred. However, clinical judgment should be used when evaluating patients for whom a measured temperature of >100.4°F (>38°C) has not been documented. Factors that might be considered include patient self-report of fever, use of antipyretics, presence of immunocompromising conditions or therapies, lack of access to health care, or inability to obtain a measured temperature. Reporting authorities should consider these factors when classifying patients who do not strictly meet the clinical criteria for this case definition.
† Close contact is defined as having cared for or lived with a person known to have SARS or having a high likelihood of direct contact with respiratory secretions and/or body fluids of a patient known to have SARS. Examples of close contact include kissing or embracing, sharing eating or drinking utensils, close conversation (<3 feet), physical examination, and any other direct physical contact between persons. Close contact does not include activities such as walking by a person or sitting across a waiting room or office for a brief period of time.

LABORATORY CRITERIA
- Confirmed
  - Detection of antibody to SARS-associated coronavirus (SARS-CoV) in a serum sample, or
  - Detection of SARS-CoV RNA by RT-PCR confirmed by a second PCR assay, by using a second aliquot of the specimen and a different set of PCR primers, or
  - Isolation of SARS-CoV
- Negative
  - Absence of antibody to SARS-CoV in a convalescent–phase serum sample obtained >28 days after symptom onset‡
- Undetermined
  - Laboratory testing either not performed or incomplete.

CASE CLASSIFICATION
- Probable case: meets the clinical criteria for severe respiratory illness of unknown etiology and epidemiologic criteria for exposure; laboratory criteria confirmed or undetermined.
- Suspect case: meets the clinical criteria for moderate respiratory illness of unknown etiology, and epidemiologic criteria for exposure; laboratory criteria confirmed or undetermined.

EXCLUSION CRITERIA
A case may be excluded as a suspect or probable SARS case if:
- An alternative diagnosis can fully explain the illness.§
- The case has a convalescent-phase serum sample (i.e., obtained >28 days after symptom onset), which is negative for antibody to SARS-CoV.‡
- The case was reported based on contact with an index case that was subsequently excluded as a case of SARS, provided other possible epidemiologic exposure criteria are not present.

■ SYNONYMS
SARS

ICD-CM CODES
Not available

■ EPIDEMIOLOGY & DEMOGRAPHICS
- The disease was first recognized in Asia in February 2003, and over the next several months spread to more

---

‡ The WHO has specified that the surveillance period for China should begin on November 1; the first recognized cases in Hong Kong, Singapore and Hanoi (Vietnam) had onset in February 2003. The date for Toronto is linked to the occurrence of a laboratory confirmed case of SARS in a U.S. resident who had traveled to Toronto; the date for Taiwan is linked to CDC's issuance of travel recommendations.

than two dozen countries in North and South America, Europe, and Asia, affecting more than 8000 patients and resulting in more than 750 deaths. In July 2003, cases were no longer being reported, and SARS outbreaks worldwide were considered contained.
- Most reported cases of SARS in the United States were exposed through foreign travel to countries with community transmission of SARS with only limited secondary spread to close contacts such as family members and health care workers.
- Incubation period is 2 to 10 days.

■ PHYSICAL FINDINGS & CLINICAL PRESENTATION
- Early manifestations: fever, myalgias, and headache. Fever is often high and associated with chills or rigors. Fever may be absent in elderly patients.
- Dry nonproductive cough occurs within 2 to 4 days of onset of fever.
- Diarrhea may occur in up to 25% of cases.
- Dyspnea and hypoxemia follow the cough and may require intubation in nearly 20% of patients.
- A biphasic course of illness may occur with initial improvement followed by subsequent deterioration in some patients.

■ ETIOLOGY
SARS-associated coronavirus

DIAGNOSIS

■ DIFFERENTIAL DIAGNOSIS
- Legionella pneumonia
- Influenza A and B
- Respiratory syncytial virus
- Acute Respiratory Distress Syndrome (ARDS)

■ WORKUP
- Initial diagnostic testing for suspected SARS patients should include chest radiograph, pulse oximetry, blood cultures, sputum Gram stain and culture, and testing for viral respiratory pathogens, notably influenza A and B and respiratory syncytial virus. A specimen for Legionella and pneumococcal urinary antigen testing should also be considered.

---

§ Factors that may be considered in assigning alternate diagnoses include the strength of the epidemiologic exposure criteria for SARS, the specificity of the diagnostic test, and the compatibility of the clinical presentation and course of illness for the alternative diagnosis.

■ LABORATORY TESTS
WHEN TO TEST FOR SARS
In the absence of documented SARS transmission, diagnostic testing for SARS-associated coronavirus (SARS-CoV) should NOT be considered unless the clinician and health department have a high index of suspicion for SARS (e.g., a hospitalized pneumonia patient has a possible SARS exposure during travel and no other explanation for his or her pneumonia).

- Respiratory specimens should be collected as soon as possible in the course of the illness. The likelihood of recovering most viruses diminishes markedly >72 hr after symptom onset.
- Three types of specimens may be collected for viral or bacterial isolation and PCR. These include (1) nasopharyngeal wash/aspirates, (2) nasopharyngeal swabs, or (3) oropharyngeal swabs. Nasopharyngeal aspirates are the specimen of choice for detection of respiratory viruses and are the preferred collection method among children aged <2 yr.
- Collection of bronchioalveolar lavage, tracheal aspirate, pleural tap: If these specimens have been obtained, half should be centrifuged and the cell-pellet fixed in formalin. Remaining unspun fluid should be placed in sterile vials with external caps and internal O-ring seals. If there are no internal O-ring seals, then cap securely and seal with parafilm.
- Acute serum specimens should be collected and submitted as soon as possible. If the patient meets the case definition, convalescent specimens should be collected and submitted no sooner than 29 days after the onset of fever.
- Laboratory assays for SARS-CoV are based on either the detection of the virus or virus products, or detection of an antibody response to viral infection.
- Isolation in Vero E6 cells and electron microscopy plays a critical role in the early identification of SARS-CoV; however, these methods are not suitable for routine diagnoses because they lack sensitivity, and viral culture requires biosafety level III containment.
- Current detection methods for SARS-CoV include real-time reverse transcription polymerase chain reaction (RT-PCR) assay for detection of viral RNA and enzyme immunoassay (EIA) for detection of antibodies to SARS-CoV. The real-time RT-PCR assay is highly sensitive, detecting between 1 and 10 RNA transcript copies per reaction, and utilizes primer and probe sets to three independent sites along the SARS-CoV genome to assure specific detection of SARS CoV.
- Serology is the gold standard for diagnosis of SARS-CoV infection. The SARS EIA uses a lysate of SARS-CoV infected Vero E6 cells as antigen. Serosurveys with the SARS EIA have demonstrated low or undetectable levels of antibody to the SARS-CoV in the general population. No cross-reactivity has been observed in validation studies with serum specimens containing antibodies to other human coronaviruses.
- The CDC real-time RT-PCR assay has proven both sensitive and specific for detection of SARS-CoV. However, as with all PCR assays, there is potential for both false-positive and false-negative results. False-positive results can occur from contamination with previously amplified DNA during specimen processing or preparation of the amplification reaction. Cross-contamination between patient specimens can also occur during the course of collection, transport, storage, and processing.
- Detecting SARS-CoV antibodies by EIA is a less ambiguous approach to diagnosing SARS-CoV infection than is RT-PCR, but antibodies are often not detectable early in the course of illness or the patient may be immune suppressed and unable to mount a good antibody response. Seroconversion from negative to positive or a fourfold rise in antibody titer from acute to convalescent serum specimens confirms recent infection.
- When prior infection is exceedingly rare, a positive serology result is also considered indicative of acute infection with SARS-CoV in a patient with a SARS-like illness. Although many SARS patients develop antibodies to SARS-CoV within as few as 8 to 10 days, some patients do not test positive until more than 28 days after the onset of illness.
- For patients with a negative antibody test result with specimens collected <28 days after illness onset, an additional serum specimen collected >28 days after onset should be tested. A negative antibody test after 28 days from onset of illness can be used to rule out SARS-CoV infection.
- Lab testing on initial evaluation should also include CBC with differential, platelet count, liver enzymes, LDH, and CPK. Common lab abnormalities in SARS include thrombocytopenia, lymphopenia, elevated LDH, and elevated CPK, ALT, AST.

■ IMAGING STUDIES
- Chest x-ray: patchy focal infiltrates or consolidation with peripheral distribution
- Chest x-ray may be normal in up to 25% of patients
- Pleural effusions are generally not present

℞ TREATMENT

■ NONPHARMACOLOGIC THERAPY
- Supportive care
- Nearly 25% of cases will require ventilator assistance
- Nutritional support

■ ACUTE GENERAL THERAPY
- There is no specific treatment currently available for SARS.
- Broad-spectrum antibiotics (quinolone or macrolide) are generally started pending laboratory testing.
- Use of corticosteroids (methylprednisolone 40 mg bid or doses up to 2 mg/kg/day) is controversial but may be beneficial in patients with significant hypoxemia and progressive pulmonary infiltrates.

■ DISPOSITION
- Case fatality rate is 3% to 12%.
- Mortality rate is higher in elderly and immunocompromised patients and lower in pediatric age group.

■ REFERRAL
- Infectious disease consultation and pulmonary consultation is recommended in all cases.
- Notification of state Department of Health is mandatory.

☼ PEARLS & CONSIDERATIONS

- Available information related to the spread of SARS suggests that only symptomatic patients transmit the virus to others. The following infection control measures are recommended for patients with suspected SARS in households or residential settings.
  1. SARS patients should limit interactions outside the home and should not go to work, school, out-of-home child care, or other public areas until 10 days after the resolution of fever, provided respiratory symptoms are absent or improving. During this time, infection control precautions should be used, as described following, to minimize the potential for transmission.

2. All members of a household with a SARS patient should carefully follow recommendations for hand hygiene (e.g., frequent hand washing or use of alcohol-based hand rubs), particularly after contact with body fluids (e.g., respiratory secretions, urine, or feces).
3. Use of disposable gloves should be considered for any direct contact with body fluids of a SARS patient. However, gloves are not intended to replace proper hand hygiene. Immediately after activities involving contact with body fluids, gloves should be removed and discarded and hands should be cleaned. Gloves must never be washed or reused.
4. Each patient with SARS should be advised to cover his or her mouth and nose with a facial tissue when coughing or sneezing. If possible, a SARS patient should wear a surgical mask during close contact with uninfected persons to prevent spread of infectious droplets. When a SARS patient is unable to wear a surgical mask, household members should wear surgical masks when in close contact with the patient.
5. Sharing of eating utensils, towels, and bedding between SARS patients and others should be avoided, although such items can be used by others after routine cleaning (e.g., washing with soap and hot water). Environmental surfaces soiled by body fluids should be cleaned with a household disinfectant according to manufacturer's instructions; gloves should be worn during this activity.
6. Household waste soiled with body fluids of SARS patients, including facial tissues and surgical masks, may be discarded as normal waste.
7. Household members and other close contacts of SARS patients should be actively monitored by the local health department for illness.
8. Household members or other close contacts of SARS patients should be vigilant for fever (i.e., measure temperature bid) or respiratory symptoms and, if these develop, should immediately seek health care evaluation. In advance of evaluation, health care providers should be informed that the individual is a close contact of a SARS patient so arrangements can be made, as necessary, to prevent transmission to others in the health care setting. Household members or other close contacts with symptoms of SARS should follow the same precautions recommended for SARS patients.
9. In the absence of fever or respiratory symptoms, household members or other close contacts of SARS patients need not limit their activities outside the home.

■ COMMENTS

- Persons who may have been exposed to SARS should be vigilant for fever (i.e., measure temperature bid) and respiratory symptoms over the 10 days following exposure. During this time, in the absence of both fever and respiratory symptoms, persons who may have been exposed to SARS patients need not limit their activities outside the home and should not be excluded from work, school, out-of-home child care, church or other public areas.
- Exposed persons should notify their health care provider immediately if fever or respiratory symptoms develop.
- Symptomatic persons exposed to SARS should follow the following infection control precautions:
  1. If fever or respiratory symptoms develop, the person should limit interactions outside the home and not go to work, school, out-of-home child care, church, or other public areas. In addition, the person should use infection control precautions in the home to minimize the risk for transmission, and continue to measure temperature bid.
  2. If symptoms improve or resolve within 72 hr after first symptom onset, the person may be allowed, after consultation with local public health authorities, to return to work, school, out-of-home child care, church or other public areas, and infection control precautions can be discontinued.
  3. For persons who meet or progress to meet the case definition for suspected SARS (e.g., develop fever and respiratory symptoms), infection control precautions should be continued until 10 days after the resolution of fever, provided respiratory symptoms are absent or improving.
  4. If the illness does not progress to meet the case definition, but the individual has persistent fever or unresolving respiratory symptoms, infection control precautions should be continued for an additional 72 hr, at the end of which time a clinical evaluation should be performed. If the illness progresses to meet the case definition, infection control precautions should be continued as described previously. If case definition criteria are not met, infection control precautions can be discontinued after consultation with local public health authorities and the evaluating clinician.
- Persons who meet or progress to meet the case definition for suspected SARS (e.g., develop fever and respiratory symptoms) or whose illness does not meet the case definition, but who have persistent fever or unresolving respiratory symptoms over the 72 hr following onset of symptoms should be tested for SARS coronavirus infection.

REFERENCES

Ksiazek TG et al: A novel coronavirus associated with severe acute respiratory syndrome, *N Engl J Med* 348:1953, 2003.

MMRW: Severe acute respiratory syndrome—Taiwan, 2003, *MMWR* 52:20, May 23, 2003.

Poutanen SM et al: Identification of severe acute respiratory syndrome in Canada, *N Engl J Med* 348:1995-2005.

Sampathkumar P et al: SARS: epidemiology, clinical presentation, management, and infection control measures, *Mayo Clin Proc* 78:882, 2003.

Author: **Fred F. Ferri, M.D.**

BASIC INFORMATION

■ DEFINITION

Sheehan's syndrome is a state of hypopituitarism resulting from an infarct of the pituitary secondary to postpartum hemorrhage or shock, causing partial or complete loss of the anterior pituitary hormones (i.e., ACTH, FSH, LH, GH, PRL, TSH) and their target organ functions.

■ ICD-9CM CODES

253.2 Sheehan's syndrome

■ EPIDEMIOLOGY & DEMOGRAPHICS

INCIDENCE: 1 case/10,000 deliveries (perhaps more rare in the U.S.)
PREDOMINANT SEX: Affects only females
RISK FACTORS:
- Hypovolemic shock
- Type I (insulin-dependent) diabetes mellitus (secondary to microvascular disease)
- Sickle cell anemia (secondary to occlusion of the small vessels in the pituitary)

ONSET OF SYMPTOMS: Average delay of 5 to 7 yr between onset of symptoms and diagnosis of disease.

■ PHYSICAL FINDINGS & CLINICAL PRESENTATION

- Failure of lactation
- Infertility
- Failure to resume menses after delivery
- Failure to regrow shaved pubic or axillary hair
- Skin depigmentation (including areola)
- Rapid breast involution
- Superinvolution of the uterus
- Hypothyroidism
- Adrenal cortical insufficiency
- Diabetes insipidus (rare)

■ ETIOLOGY

- Compromise of the blood supply to the low-pressure pituitary sinusoidal system may occur with postpartum hemorrhage or shock, resulting in pituitary infarct and/or necrosis.
- It is hypothesized that locally released factors may mediate vascular spasm of the pituitary blood supply.
- Severity of postpartum hemorrhage does not always correlate with the presence of Sheehan's syndrome.

■ DIAGNOSIS

■ DIFFERENTIAL DIAGNOSIS

- Chronic infections
- HIV
- Sarcoidosis
- Amyloidosis
- Rheumatoid disease
- Hemachromatosis
- Metastatic carcinoma
- Lymphocytic hypophysitis

■ WORKUP

- Target gland deficiency should be investigated by measuring levels of ACTH, FSH, LH, TSH (which may be normal or low), and T_4. Cortisol and estradiol (which may be low) should also be measured.
- Provocative testing of pituitary hormone reserves (e.g., metyrapone test, insulin tolerance test, and cosyntropin test): normal, subnormal, or delayed responses may suggest the presence of islands of pituitary cells that no longer have the support of the hypothalamic-portal circulation.
- Measurement of IGF-I to screen for GH deficiency: subnormal levels suggest decreased GH.
- Impaired prolactin response to TRH or dopamine antagonist stimulation is frequently found.
- During pregnancy, adjustments must be made in interpreting both hormone levels and responses to various stimuli because of normal physiologic changes.

■ IMAGING STUDIES

- Study of choice: MRI of the pituitary
  1. Sella turcica partially or totally empty
  2. Rules out mass lesion
- CT scan of the pituitary when MRI is unavailable or contraindicated

■ TREATMENT

■ ACUTE GENERAL Rx

- Acute form can be lethal, presenting with hypotension, tachycardia, failure to lactate, and hypoglycemia.
- A high degree of suspicion is required with any woman who has undergone postpartum hemorrhage and shock.
- Intravenous corticosteroids and fluid replacement should be given initially.
- Diagnosis is confirmed with a full endocrinologic workup as noted previously.
- Thyroid hormone is replaced as l-thyroxin in doses of 0.1 to 0.2 mg qd.

■ CHRONIC Rx

- With late-onset disease (symptoms of general hypopituitarism, such as oligomenorrhea or amenorrhea, vaginal atrophic changes, and loss of libido): a full endocrinologic workup and replacement of the appropriate hormones are needed.
- With symptoms of adrenal insufficiency: corticosteroids should be given.
  1. A maintenance dose of cortisone acetate or prednisone may be given.
  2. Because adrenal production of cortisol is not entirely dependent on ACTH, replacement of mineralocorticoids is rarely necessary.
  3. Stress doses of glucocorticoids should be administered during surgery or during labor and delivery.

■ DISPOSITION

Patients who receive early diagnosis and adequate hormonal replacement may expect favorable outcomes, including subsequent pregnancy.

■ REFERRAL

Patients should have yearly examinations by endocrinologist.

REFERENCES

Dejagter S et al: Sheehan's syndrome: differential diagnosis in the acute phase, *J Intern Med* 244(3):261, 1998.
Kovacs K: Sheehan's syndrome, *Lancet* 361(9356):520, 2003.
Author: **Beth J. Wutz, M.D.**

BASIC INFORMATION

■ DEFINITION

Shigellosis is an inflammatory disease of the bowel caused by one of several species of *Shigella*. It is the most common cause of bacillary dysentery in the U.S.

■ SYNONYMS

Bacillary dysentery

ICD-9CM CODES

004.9 Shigellosis

■ EPIDEMIOLOGY & DEMOGRAPHICS

INCIDENCE (IN U.S.): Approximately 15,000 cases/yr
PREDOMINANT SEX: Male homosexuals at increased risk
PREDOMINANT AGE: Young children
PEAK INCIDENCE: Summer
GENETICS:
Neonatal Infection: Rare but severe

■ PHYSICAL FINDINGS & CLINICAL PRESENTATION

- Possibly asymptomatic
- Mild illness that is usually self-limited, resolving in a few days
- Fever
- Watery diarrhea
- Bloody diarrhea
- Dysentery (abdominal cramps, tenesmus, and numerous, small-volume stools with blood, mucus, and pus)
- Descending intestinal tract illness, reflecting infection of small bowel first and then the colon
- Severe disease is more common in children and elderly and outside of U.S.
- Complications of severe illness:
  1. Seizures
  2. Megacolon
  3. Intestinal perforation
  4. Death
- Extraintestinal manifestations are rare
- Bacteremia described in patients with AIDS
- Hemolytic-uremic syndrome: usually occurs as the initial illness seems to be resolving
- Reactive arthritis, sometimes as part of Reiter's syndrome

■ ETIOLOGY

- *Shigella*
  1. *S. flexneri*
  2. *S. dysenteriae*
  3. *S. sonnei*
  4. *S. boydii*
- *S. sonnei* is the most commonly isolated species in the U.S., and it usually causes a mild watery diarrhea.
- Direct person-to-person transmission is thought to be the most common route. Outbreaks among men who have sex with men have occurred because of direct or indirect oral-anal contact.
- Contaminated food or water may transmit disease.
- A recent outbreak occurred at a community wading pool frequented by toddlers.

DIAGNOSIS

■ DIFFERENTIAL DIAGNOSIS

- May mimic any bacterial or viral gastroenteritis
- Dysentery also caused by *Entamoeba histolytica*
- Bloody diarrhea may resemble disease caused by enterotoxigenic *E. coli*

■ LABORATORY TESTS

- Total WBCs may be low, normal, or high.
- Stool should be cultured from fresh samples, because the yield is increased by processing the specimen soon after passage.
- Serology is available but rarely useful.
- Polymerase chain reaction may be diagnostic.
- Fecal leukocyte preparation may show WBCs.

■ IMAGING STUDIES

Abdominal radiographs may suggest megacolon or perforation in rare, severe cases.

TREATMENT

■ NONPHARMACOLOGIC THERAPY

- Adequate hydration
- Electrolyte replacement

■ ACUTE GENERAL Rx

Antibiotics:
- To shorten course of illness
- To limit transmission of illness
- SMX/TMP, one DS tablet PO bid for 5 days
- Ciprofloxacin 500 mg PO bid for 5 days

■ DISPOSITION

- Most disease is self-limited.
- Severe illness may be fatal.

■ REFERRAL

For severe illness or complications

☼ PEARLS & CONSIDERATIONS

■ COMMENTS

- *Shigella* is one cause of "gay bowel syndrome."
- Illness is worsened by agents that decrease intestinal motility.
- Food handlers, child-care providers, and health-care workers should have a negative stool culture documented following treatment.

REFERENCES

Centers for Disease Control and Prevention: *Shigelia sonnei* outbreak among men who have sex with men, San Francisco, California, 200-2001, *MMWR*, 50:922, 2001.

Centers for Disease Control and Prevention, Shigellosis outbreak associated with an unchlorinated fill-and-drain wading pool, Iowa, 2001, *MMWR*, 50:797, 2001.

Author: **Maurice Policar, M.D.**

BASIC INFORMATION

■ DEFINITION
Short bowel syndrome is a malabsorption syndrome that results from extensive small intestinal resection.

■ SYNONYMS
Short bowel

ICD-9CM CODES
579.3 (postsurgical malabsorption)

■ EPIDEMIOLOGY & DEMOGRAPHICS
- Parallels Crohn's disease (see "Crohn's Disease" in Section I), which is the most common cause of the syndrome in adults
- In children, two thirds of short bowels are related to congenital abnormalities (intestinal atresia, gastroschisis, volvulus, aganglionosis) and one third are related to necrotizing enterocolitis
- Prevalence: 10,000 to 20,000 cases are estimated to exist in the U.S.

■ PHYSICAL FINDINGS & CLINICAL PRESENTATION
- Diarrhea and steatorrhea
- Weight loss
- Anemia related to iron or vitamin B_{12} absorption
- Bleeding diathesis related to vitamin K malabsorption
- Osteoporosis/osteomalacia related to vitamin D and calcium malabsorption
- Hyponatremia, hypokalemia
- Hypovolemia
- Other macronutrient or micronutrient deficiency states

■ ETIOLOGY
- Extensive bowel resection for treatment of the conditions mentioned previously (see "Epidemiology").
- Pathogenesis (Fig. 1-245).

The human intestine is 3 to 8 m in length. Removal of up to one half of the small intestine produces no disruption in nutrient absorption, and most patients can maintain nutritional balance on oral feeding if they have more than 100 cm (3 ft) of jejunum. Similarly, 100 cm of intact jejunum can maintain a normal water, sodium, and potassium balance under normal circumstances. The presence of an intact colon can compensate for some small intestine loss.

Site-specific functions:
- Calcium, magnesium, phosphorus, iron, and vitamins are absorbed in the duodenum and proximal jejunum.

- Vitamin B_{12} and bile acids are absorbed in the ileum. The resection of more than 60 cm of ileum results in vitamin B_{12} malabsorption. The loss of more than 100 cm results in fat malabsorption (from the loss of bile acids).
- The loss of gastrointestinal endocrine hormones can affect intestinal motility.
- Intestinal bacterial overgrowth may also occur, especially if the ileocecal valve is lost.

 DIAGNOSIS

Presence of macronutrient and/or micronutrient loss in a patient with a known history of bowel resection

■ DIFFERENTIAL DIAGNOSIS
Because the history of significant bowel resection is typically known, there is no differential diagnosis. If that history is not known, all causes of weight loss, malabsorption, and diarrhea must be considered (see respective chapters).

 TREATMENT

Extensive small bowel resection with colectomy (<100 cm of jejunum)
- Rx: long-term parenteral nutrition (TPN). Some patients can switch to oral intake after 1 to 2 yr of TPN. In jejunostomy patients, excessive fluid loss can be reduced with H_2 blockers, proton pump inhibitors, or octreotide. Micronutrients are supplemented.

Extensive small bowel resection with partial colectomy (usually patients with Crohn's disease)
- Rx: oral intake alone is possible in all patients with >100 cm of jejunum. In addition to vitamin B_{12} deficiency, these patients often have diarrhea. Consider lactose malabsorption and bacterial overgrowth treated, respectively, with lactose restriction and antibiotics (tetracycline 250 mg tid or metronidazole 500 mg tid for 2 wk). Nonspecific antidiarrheal agents may also be indicated (e.g., Imodium or codeine). The patient must be monitored for micronutrient losses.

■ COMPLICATIONS
- Oxalate kidney stones
- Cholesterol gallstones
- D-Lactic acidosis

■ PROGNOSIS
Directly dependent on the extent of the bowel resection and in the case of Crohn's disease by the underlying illness

REFERENCE
Westergaard H: Short bowel syndrome. In Feldman M, Scharschmidt BF, Sleisenger MH (eds): *Gastrointestinal and liver disease,* ed 6, Philadelphia, 1998, WB Saunders.
Author: Tom J. Wachtel, M.D.

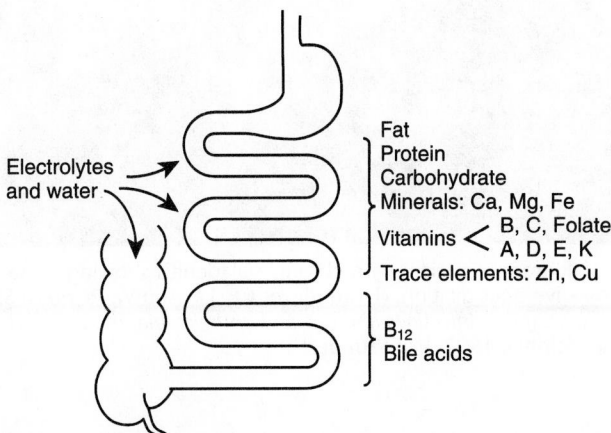

Fig. 1-245 Specific areas of absorption of constituents of diet and secretions in the gastrointestinal tract. Macronutrients and micronutrients are predominantly absorbed in the proximal jejunum. Bile acids and vitamin B_{12} are only absorbed in the ileum. Electrolytes and water are absorbed in both the small and the large intestine. (From Feldman M, Scharschmidt BF, Sleisenger MH [eds]: *Sleisenger and Fordtran's gastrointestinal and liver disease: pathophysiology, diagnosis, and management,* ed 6, Philadelphia, 1998, WB Saunders.)

BASIC INFORMATION

■ DEFINITION
Sialadenitis is an inflammation of the salivary glands.

ICD-9CM CODES
527.2 Sialadenitis

■ EPIDEMIOLOGY & DEMOGRAPHICS
Parotid or submandibular glands are most frequently affected (Fig. 1-246).

■ PHYSICAL FINDINGS & CLINICAL PRESENTATION
- Pain and swelling of the affected salivary gland
- Increased pain with meals
- Erythema, tenderness at the duct opening
- Purulent discharge from duct orifice
- Induration and pitting of the skin with involvement of the masseteric and submandibular spatial planes in severe cases

■ ETIOLOGY
- Ductal obstruction is generally secondary to a mucus plug caused by stasis of saliva with increased viscosity with subsequent stasis and infection.
- Most frequent infecting organisms are *Staphylococcus aureus*, *Pseudomonas*, *Enterobacter*, *Klebsiella*, *Enterococcus*, *Proteus*, and *Candida* spp.
- Sjögren's syndrome, trauma, radiation therapy, chemotherapy, dehydration, and chronic illness are predisposing factors.

DIAGNOSIS

■ DIFFERENTIAL DIAGNOSIS
- Salivary gland neoplasm
- Ductal stricture
- Sialolithiasis
- Decreased salivary secretion secondary to medications (e.g., amitriptyline, diphenhydramine, anticholinergics)

■ WORKUP
- Generally not necessary
- Ultrasound or CT scan in patients not responding to medical treatment (see "Imaging Studies")

■ LABORATORY TESTS
- Generally not indicated
- CBC with differential to possibly reveal leukocytosis with left shift

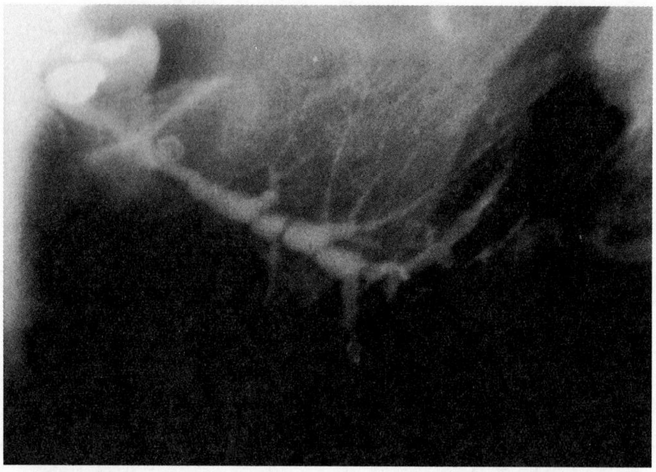

■ IMAGING STUDIES
- Ultrasound or CT scan may be needed in patients not responding to medical therapy.
- Sialography should not be performed during the acute phase.

TREATMENT

■ NONPHARMACOLOGIC THERAPY
- Massage of the gland: may express pus and relieve some of the pressure
- Rehydration
- Warm compresses
- Oral cavity irrigations

■ ACUTE GENERAL Rx
- Amoxicillin-clavulanate 500 to 875 mg or cefuroxime 250-500 mg bid should be given for 10 days. Clindamycin is an alternative choice in patients allergic to penicillin.
- IV antibiotics (e.g., cefoxitin, nafcillin) can be given in severe cases.

■ DISPOSITION
Complete recovery unless the patient has underlying obstruction (e.g., ductal stricture, tumor, or stone)

■ REFERRAL
- To ENT for nonresolving cases despite appropriate antibiotic therapy
- For salivary gland incision and drainage, which may be necessary in resistant cases

PEARLS & CONSIDERATIONS

■ COMMENTS
Prevention of dehydration will decrease the risk of sialadenitis.
Author: **Fred F. Ferri, M.D.**

Fig. 1-246 Sialogram of patient with chronic sialadenitis showing sausage link-like patterns and massive duct dilation. (From Blitzer CE, Lawson W, Reino A: Sialadenitis. In Johnson JT, Yu VL [eds]: *Infectious diseases and antimicrobial therapy of the ears, nose, and throat*, Philadelphia, 1997, WB Saunders.)

BASIC INFORMATION

■ **DEFINITION**

Sialolithiasis is the existence of hardened intraluminal deposits in the ductal system of a salivary gland.

■ **SYNONYMS**

Salivary gland stone
Salivary calculus

ICD-9CM CODES

527.5 Sialolithiasis

■ **EPIDEMIOLOGY & DEMOGRAPHICS**

Affects patients mostly in their fifth to eighth decade and occurs most commonly in the submandibular gland (80%); only 14% are located in a parotid gland.

■ **PHYSICAL FINDINGS & CLINICAL PRESENTATION**

• Symptoms: colicky postprandial pain and swelling of a salivary gland. Tends to have a remitting/relapsing course.
• Signs: swelling and tenderness of a salivary gland. The stone may be felt by palpation of the floor of the mouth (Fig. 1-247).

■ **ETIOLOGY**

• The cause is unknown. Contributing factors include saliva stagnation, sialadenitis (inflammation of a salivary gland), ductal inflammation or injury.
• Salivary calculus composition is mainly calcium phosphate and carbonate, often combined with small proportions of magnesium, zinc, ammonium salts, and organic materials/debris.

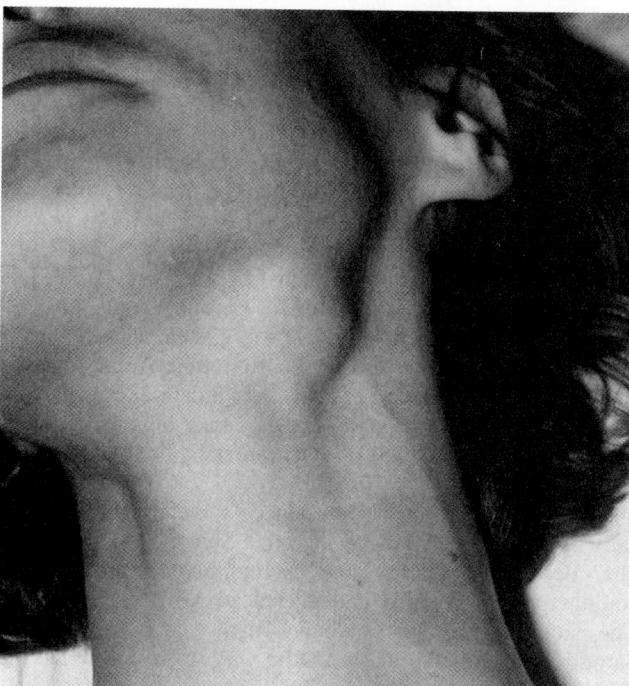

Fig. 1-247 Patient with large calculus and obstruction of the left submandibular gland. (From Blitzer CE, Lawson W, Reino A: Sialadenitis. In Johnson JT, Yu VL [eds]: *Infectious diseases and antimicrobial therapy of the ears, nose, and throat,* Philadelphia, 1997, WB Saunders.)

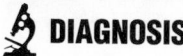 **DIAGNOSIS**

■ **DIFFERENTIAL DIAGNOSIS**

• Lymphadenitis
• Salivary gland tumor
• Salivary gland bacterial (Staphylococcus or *Streptococcus*), viral (mumps), or fungal infection (sialadenitis)
• Noninfectious salivary gland inflammation (e.g., Sjögren's syndrome, sarcoidosis, lymphoma)
• Salivary duct stricture
• Dental abscess

■ **IMAGING**

• Plain x-ray
• Sialography

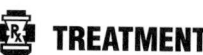 **TREATMENT**

• Warm soaks to area
• Antibiotics if associated bacterial sialadenitis is present
• Bland diet—avoid citrus fruit and spices
• Manual stone extraction sometimes associated with incisional enlargement of the ductal orifice
• Surgical salivary gland removal for retained hilar calculi

■ **REFERRAL**

To otorhinolaryngologist

REFERENCE

Kane WJ, McCaffrey TV: Sialolithiasis. In Cummings CW (ed): *Otolaryngology: head and neck surgery,* ed 2, St Louis, 1992, Mosby.

Author: **Tom J. Wachtel, M.D.**

BASIC INFORMATION

■ DEFINITION
Sick sinus syndrome is a group of cardiac rhythm disturbances characterized by abnormalities of the sinus node including (1) sinus bradycardia, (2) sinus arrest or exit block, (3) combinations of sinoatrial or atrioventricular conduction defects, and (4) supraventricular tachyarrhythmias. These abnormalities may coexist in a single patient so that a patient may have episodes of bradycardia and episodes of tachycardia.

■ SYNONYMS
Bradycardia-tachycardia syndrome

ICD-9CM CODES
427.81 Sick sinus syndrome

■ EPIDEMIOLOGY & DEMOGRAPHICS
- In children: associated with congenital heart disease
- In adults: typically associated with ischemic heart disease but may occur in the presence of a normal heart

■ PHYSICAL FINDINGS & CLINICAL PRESENTATION
- Lightheadedness, dizziness, syncope, palpitation
- Arterial embolization (e.g., stroke) associated with atrial fibrillation

- Physical examination may be normal or reveal abnormalities (e.g., heart murmurs or gallop sounds) associated with the underlying heart disease

■ ETIOLOGY
- Fibrosis or fatty infiltration involving the sinus node, atrioventricular node, the His bundle, or its branches
- In addition, inflammatory or degenerative changes of the nerves and ganglia surrounding the sinus nodes and other sclerodegenerative changes may be found

DIAGNOSIS

■ DIFFERENTIAL DIAGNOSIS
- Bradycardia: atrioventricular block
- Tachycardia: atrial fibrillation
- Atrial flutter
- Paroxysmal atrial tachycardia
- Sinus tachycardia
- Syncope (see "Syncope" in Section I)

■ WORKUP
- ECG
- Ambulatory cardiac rhythm monitoring
- 24-hour ambulatory ECG (Holter) (Fig. 1-248)
- Event recorder

- Electrophysiologic testing including sinus nodal recovery time and sinoatrial conduction time

TREATMENT

- Permanent pacemaker placement if symptoms are present
- The drug treatment of the tachycardia (e.g., with digitalis or calcium channel blockers) may worsen or bring out the bradycardia and become the reason for pacemaker requirement

■ REFERRAL
To cardiologist

REFERENCE
Zipes DP, Olgin JE: Sick sinus syndrome. In Braunwald E (ed): *Heart disease: a textbook of cardiovascular medicine*, ed 6, Philadelphia, 2001, WB Saunders.
Author: **Tom J. Wachtel, M.D.**

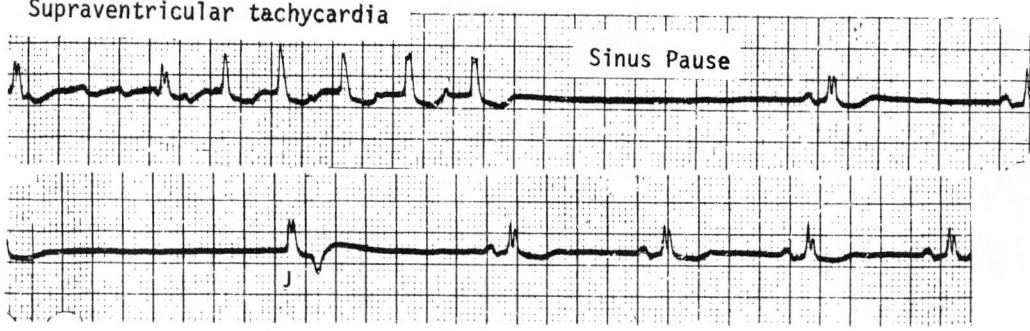

Fig. 1-248 Brady-tachy (sick sinus) syndrome. This rhythm strip shows a narrow-complex tachycardia (probably atrial flutter) followed by a sinus pause, an AV junctional escape beat *(J)*, and then sinus rhythm. (From Goldberger AL: *Clinical electrocardiography*, ed 5, St Louis, 1994, Mosby.)

BASIC INFORMATION

■ DEFINITION

Sickle cell disease is a hemoglobinopathy characterized by the production of hemoglobin S caused by substitution of the amino acid valine for glutamic acid in the sixth position of the γ-globin chain. When exposed to lower oxygen tension, RBCs assume a sickle shape resulting in stasis of RBCs in capillaries. Painful crises are caused by ischemic tissue injury resulting from obstruction of blood flow produced by sickled erythrocytes.

■ SYNONYMS

Sickle cell anemia
Hemoglobin S disease

ICD-9CM CODES

286.60 Sickle cell anemia

■ EPIDEMIOLOGY & DEMOGRAPHICS

- Sickle cell hemoglobin S is transmitted by an autosomal recessive gene. It is found mostly in blacks (1 in 400 black Americans).
- Sickle cell trait occurs in nearly 10% of black Americans.
- There is no predominant sex.

■ PHYSICAL FINDINGS & CLINICAL PRESENTATION

- Physical examination is variable depending on the degree of anemia and presence of acute vasoocclusive syndromes or neurologic, cardiovascular, GU, and musculoskeletal complications.
- There is no clinical laboratory finding that is pathognomonic of painful crisis of sickle cell disease. The diagnosis of a painful episode is made solely on the basis of the medical therapy and physical examination.
- Bones are the most common site of pain. Dactylitis, or hand-foot syndrome (acute, painful swelling of the hands and feet), is the first manifestation of sickle cell disease in many infants. Irritability and refusal to walk are other common symptoms. After infancy, musculoskeletal pain can be symmetric, asymmetric, or migratory, and it may or may not be associated with swelling, low-grade fever, redness, or warmth.
- In both children and adults, sickle vasoocclusive episodes are difficult to distinguish from osteomyelitis, septic arthritis, synovitis, rheumatic fever, or gout.
- When abdominal or visceral pain is present, care should be taken to exclude sequestration syndromes (spleen, liver) or the possibility of an acute condition such as appendicitis, pancreatitis, cholecystitis, urinary tract infection, PID, or malignancy.
- Pneumonia develops during the course of 20% of painful events and can present as chest and abdominal pain. In adults chest pain may be a result of vasoocclusion in the ribs and often precedes a pulmonary event. The lower back is also a frequent site of painful crisis in adults.
- The "acute chest syndrome" manifests with chest pain, fever, wheezing, tachypnea, and cough. Chest x-ray reveals pulmonary infiltrates. Common causes include infection (mycoplasma, chlamydia, viruses), infarction, and fat embolism.
- Musculoskeletal and skin abnormalities seen in sickle cell anemia include leg ulcers (particularly on the malleoli) and limb-girdle deformities caused by avascular necrosis of the femoral and humeral heads.
- Endocrine abnormalities include delayed sexual maturation and late physical maturation, especially evident in boys.
- Neurologic abnormalities on examination may include seizures and altered mental status.
- Infections, particularly involving *Salmonella, Mycoplasma,* and *Streptococcus,* are relatively common.
- Severe splenomegaly secondary to sequestration often occurs in children before splenic atrophy.

DIAGNOSIS

■ DIFFERENTIAL DIAGNOSIS

- Thalassemia
- Iron deficiency anemia, leukemia
- The differential diagnosis of patients presenting with a painful crisis is discussed in "Physical Findings."

■ WORKUP

- Screening of all newborns regardless of racial background is recommended. Screening can be performed with sodium metabisulfite reduction test (Sickledex test).
- Hemoglobin electrophoresis will also confirm the diagnosis and is useful to identify hemoglobin variants such as fetal hemoglobin and hemoglobin A2.

■ LABORATORY TESTS

- Anemia (resulting from chronic hemolysis), reticulocytosis, leukocytosis, and thrombocytosis are common.
- Elevations of bilirubin and LDH are also common.
- Peripheral blood smear may reveal sickle cells, target cells, poikilocytosis, and hypochromia (Fig. 1-249).
- Elevated BUN and creatinine may be present in patients with progressive renal insufficiency.
- Urinalysis may reveal hematuria and proteinuria.

■ IMAGING STUDIES

- Chest x-ray examination is useful in patients presenting with "chest syndrome." Cardiomegaly may be present on chest x-ray examination.
- Bone scan is useful to rule out osteomyelitis (usually secondary to salmonella). MRI scan is also effective in diagnosing osteomyelitis.
- CT scan or MRI of brain is often needed in patients presenting with neurologic complications such as TIA, CVA, seizures, or altered mental status.
- Transcranial Doppler is a useful commodity to identify children with sickle cell anemia who are at risk for stroke.

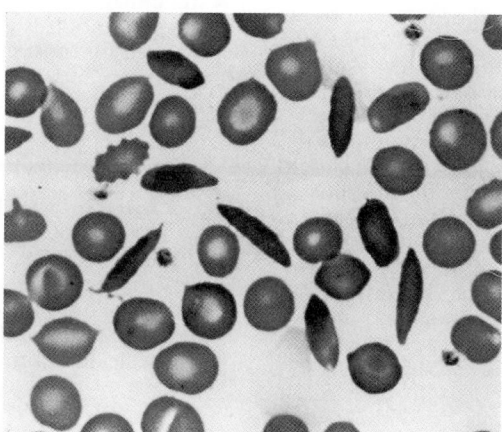

Fig. 1-249 Photomicrograph of peripheral blood smear, sickle cells, typical of sickle cell anemia. (From Andreoli TE [ed]: *Cecil essential of medicine,* ed 4, Philadelphia, 1997, WB Saunders.)

℞ TREATMENT

■ NONPHARMACOLOGIC THERAPY
- Patients should be instructed to avoid conditions that may precipitate sickling crisis, such as hypoxia, infections, acidosis, and dehydration.
- Maintain adequate hydration (PO or IV).
- Correct hypoxia.

■ ACUTE GENERAL ℞
- Aggressively diagnose and treat suspected infections (*Salmonella* osteomyelitis and pneumococcal infections occur more often in patients with sickle cell anemia because of splenic infarcts and atrophy). Combination therapy with a cephalosporin and erythromycin plus incentive spirometry and bronchodilators are useful in patients with acute chest syndrome.
- Provide pain relief during the vasoocclusive crisis. Medications should be administered on a fixed time schedule with a dosing interval that does not extend beyond the duration of the desired pharmacologic effect.
  1. Meperidine is contraindicated in patients with renal dysfunction or CNS disease because its metabolite, normeperidine (which is excreted by the kidneys) can cause seizures.
  2. Narcotics (e.g., morphine 0.1 mg/kg IV q 3-4 h or 0.3 mg/kg PO q 4 h) should be given on a fixed schedule (not prn for pain), with rescue dosing for breakthrough pain as needed.
  3. Except when contraindications exist, concomitant use of NSAIDs should be standard treatment.
  4. Nurses should be instructed not to give narcotics if the patient is heavily sedated or respirations are depressed.
  5. When the patient shows signs of improvement, narcotic drugs should be tapered gradually to prevent withdrawal syndrome. It is advisable to observe the patient on oral pain relief medications for 12 to 24 hr before discharge from the hospital.
  6. Analgesic medications should be used in combination with psychologic, behavioral, and physical modalities in the management of sickle cell disease.
- Aggressively diagnose and treat any potential complications (e.g., septic necrosis of the femoral head, priapism, bony infarcts, and acute "chest syndrome").
- Avoid "routine" transfusions but consider early transfusions for patients at high risk for complications. Indications for transfusion: aplastic crises, severe hemolytic crises (particularly during third trimester of pregnancy), acute chest syndrome, and high risk of stroke.
- Hydroxyurea (500 to 750 mg/day) increases hemoglobin F levels and reduces the incidence of vasoocclusive complications. It is generally well tolerated. Side effects consist primarily of mild reversible neutropenia.
- Replace folic acid (1 mg PO qd).

■ CHRONIC ℞
- Guidelines for prompt management of fever, infections, pain, and specific complications should be reviewed.
- Genetic counseling is recommended in all cases.
- Avoid unnecessary transfusions. Exchange transfusions may be necessary for patients with acute neurologic signs, in aplastic crisis, or undergoing surgery.
- Allogeneic stem cell transplantation can be curative in young patients with symptomatic sickle cell disease; however, the death rate from the procedure is nearly 10%, the marrow recipients are likely to be infertile, and there is an undefined risk of chemotherapy-induced malignancy.
- Penicillin V 125 mg PO bid should be administered by age 2 mo and increased to 250 mg bid by age 3. Penicillin prophylaxis can be discontinued after age 5 except in children who have had splenectomy.

■ REFERRAL
- Hospitalization is generally recommended for most crises and complications.
- Psychosocial counseling and support structures should be developed.

☼ PEARLS & CONSIDERATIONS

■ COMMENTS
- Patients and their families should receive genetic counseling and should be made aware of the difference between sickle cell trait and sickle cell disease.
- Regular immunizations and pneumococcal vaccination are recommended. The prophylactic administration of penicillin soon after birth and the timely administration of pneumococcal and *H. influenzae* type b vaccines have resulted in a significant decline in the incidence of these infections. The heptavalent conjugated pneumococcal vaccine (Prevan) should be administered from 2 mo of age. The 23-valent unconjugated pneumococcal vaccine is given from age 2 and can be boosted once 3 yr later. Influenza vaccination can be given after 6 mo of age.
- Patients should be instructed on a well-balanced diet and appropriate folic acid supplementation.
- The presence of dactylitis, Hb 7, or leukocytosis in the absence of infection during the first 2 yr of life, indicates a higher risk of severe sickle cell disease later in life.
- Among patients with sickle cell disease, the acute chest syndrome is commonly precipitated by fat embolism and infection, especially community-acquired pneumonia. Among older patients and those with neurologic symptoms, the syndrome often progresses to respiratory failure.
- Poloxamer 188, a nonionic surfactant with hemorrheologic and antithrombotic properties, has been reported to produce a significant but relatively small decrease in the duration of painful episodes and an increase in the proportion of patients who achieved resolution of the symptoms. A more significant effect was observed in patients who received concomitant hydroxyurea.

REFERENCES

Orringer E et al: Purified poloxamer 188 for treatment of acute vaso-occlusive crisis of sickle cell disease, *JAMA* 286:2099, 2001.

Vichinski EP et al: Causes and outcomes of the acute chest syndrome in sickle cell disease, *N Engl J Med* 342:1855, 2000.

Wethers DL: Sickle cell disease in childhood, *Am Fam Physician* 62:1013, 2000.

Author: Fred F. Ferri, M.D.

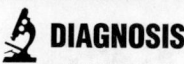

BASIC INFORMATION

■ DEFINITION

Silicosis is a lung disease attributable to the inhalation of silica (silicon dioxide) in crystalline form (quartz) or in cristobalite or tridymite forms.

■ SYNONYMS

Pneumoconiosis caused by silica

ICD-9CM CODES

502 Silicosis, occupational
503 Pneumoconiosis caused by other inorganic dust

■ EPIDEMIOLOGY & DEMOGRAPHICS

- Occupational disease affecting men and women involved in gathering, milling, processing, or using silica-containing rock or sand
- An estimated 1 million Americans are exposed (Table 1-54)

■ PHYSICAL FINDINGS & CLINICAL PRESENTATION

- Dyspnea
- Cough
- Wheezing
- Abnormal chest x-ray in an asymptomatic person
- See Table 1-55 for clinicopathologic types of silicoses

■ PATHOGENESIS

- Silica particles are ingested by alveolar macrophages, which in turn release oxidants causing cell injury and cell death, attract fibroblasts, and activate lymphocytes, increasing immunoglobulins in the alveolar space.
- Hyperplasia of alveolar epithelial cells occurs.
- Collagen accumulates in the interstitium.
- Neutrophils also accumulate and secrete proteolytic enzymes, which leads to tissue destruction and emphysema.
- Silica dust may be carcinogenic (not proven).
- Exposure to silicosis predisposes to tuberculosis.
- Some patients develop rheumatoid silicotic pulmonary nodules and may have arthritic symptoms of rheumatoid arthritis (Caplan's syndrome). Scleroderma has also been associated with silicosis.

DIAGNOSIS

■ DIFFERENTIAL DIAGNOSIS

- Other pneumoconiosis, berylliosis, hard metal disease, asbestosis
- Sarcoidosis
- Tuberculosis
- Interstitial lung disease
- Hypersensitivity pneumonitis
- Lung cancer
- Langerhans' cell granulomatosis (histiocytosis X)
- Granulomatous pulmonary vasculitis

■ WORKUP

- History of occupational exposure
- Chest x-ray (Fig. 1-250)
Chronic silicosis
- Characteristic finding: small, rounded lung parenchymal opacities
- Hilar lymphadenopathy with "eggshell" calcifications
- Pleural plaques (uncommon)
Accelerated silicosis (progressive massive fibrosis)
- Large parenchymal lesions resulting from coalesced small nodules
Acute silicosis
- Ground-glass appearance of the lung fields
- Chest CT scan
- Pulmonary function tests
Combination of obstructive and restrictive changes with or without reduction in diffusing capacity
- Bronchoscopy with lung biopsy in uncertain cases

TABLE 1-54 Industries and Occupations

INDUSTRIES	OCCUPATIONS
Mining, tunneling, and excavating	
Underground: gold, copper, iron, tin, uranium, civil engineering projects	Miner, driller, tunneler, developer, stoper
Surface: coal, iron, excavation of foundations	Mobile rig drill operator
Quarrying	
Granite, sandstone, slate, sand, china, stone/clay	Driller, hammer, digger
Stonework	
Granite sheds, monumental masonry	Cutter, dresser, driller, polisher, grinder, mason
Foundries	
Ferrous and nonferrous metals	Molder, knockout man, fettler, coremaker, caster
Abrasives	
Production: silica flour, metal polish, sandpapers, fillers in paint, rubber, and plastics	Crusher, pulverizer, and mixer; workers in the manufacture of abrasives
Sandblasting: oil rigs, tombstones	Operators of high-speed jets
Ceramics	
Manufacture of pottery, stoneware, refractory bricks for ovens and kilns	Workers at any stage of process if products are dry
Others	
Glass making, boiler scaling, traditional crafts, stone grinders, gemstone workers, dental technicians	

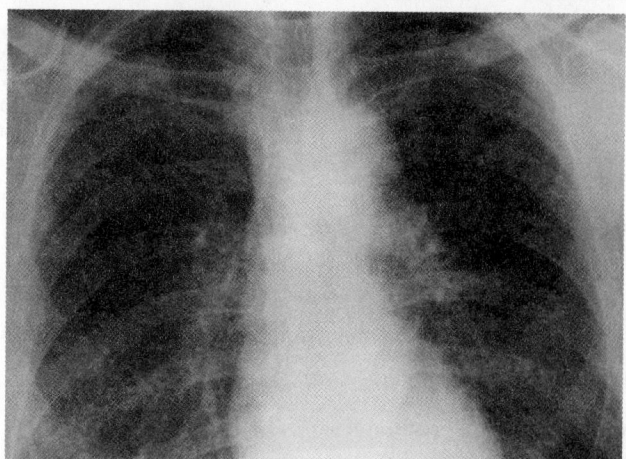

Fig. 1-250 **Simple silicosis.** There are multiple small (2- to 4-mm) nodules distributed throughout the lungs, with an upper lobe predominance. (From McLoud TC: *Thoracic radiology: the requisites,* St Louis, 1998, Mosby.)

■ COURSE
CHRONIC SILICOSIS:
- May not progress with absence of further exposure
- Accelerated silicosis: progressive respiratory failure and cor pulmonale

ACUTE SILICOSIS: Fatal course from respiratory failure over several months to a few years

TREATMENT

- Prevention (industrial hygiene)
- Treatment of associated tuberculosis if present
- Supportive measures (oxygen, bronchodilators)
- Lung transplant

REFERENCE
Becklake MR: Silicosis. In Murray JF, Nadel JA (eds): *Textbook of respiratory medicine,* ed 2, Philadelphia, 1994, WB Saunders.
Author: **Tom J. Wachtel, M.D.**

TABLE 1-55 Clinicopathologic Types of Silicosis

TYPE	EXPOSURE	PATHOLOGIC FEATURES	CLINICAL FEATURES
Chronic	Usually over 20 yr, often to dust containing <30% quartz	Mainly the classic silicotic islet or nodule; usually involving hilar nodes first, then upper lobes to which it may be limited	Small, rounded opacities on roentgenogram not necessarily associated with increased morbidity or mortality; impairment of pulmonary function may occur
Accelerated	5-15 yr, usually to fiber dusts of higher quartz content	Numerous nodules at various stages of development, sometimes with irregular interstitial fibrosis	Irregular upper zone fibrosis with a nodular component; symptomatic with impairment and often progression to respiratory failure and death; cavitation with infection by atypical mycobacteria not unusual
Acute	Several months, usually to very fine dusts of high quartz content	Alveoloproteinosis (airspaces filled with neutrophils, epithelial cells, and proteinaceous materials) with interstitial reactions and early, loosely organized nodules	Resembles acute airspace disease on chest roentgenogram, rapid progression to acute respiratory failure; fulminating tuberculosis is a possible terminal complication

BASIC INFORMATION

■ **DEFINITION**

Sinusitis is inflammation of the mucous membranes lining one or more of the paranasal sinuses. The various presentations are:
- Acute sinusitis: infection lasting <30 days, with complete resolution of symptoms.
- Subacute infection: lasts from 30 to 90 days, with complete resolution of symptoms.
- Recurrent acute infection: episodes of acute infection lasting <30 days, with resolution of symptoms, which recur at intervals at least 10 days apart.
- Chronic sinusitis: inflammation lasting >90 days, with persistent upper respiratory symptoms.
- Acute bacterial sinusitis superimposed on chronic sinusitis: new symptoms that occur in patients with residual symptoms from prior infection(s). With treatment, the new symptoms resolve but the residual ones do not.

ICD-9CM CODES

473.9 Sinusitis (accessory) (nasal) (hyperplastic) (nonpurulent) (purulent) (chronic)
461.9 Acute sinusitis

■ **SYNONYMS**

Rhinosinusitis: Sinusitis is almost always accompanied by inflammation of the nasal mucosa; thus it is now the preferred term.

■ **EPIDEMIOLOGY & DEMOGRAPHICS**

INCIDENCE (IN U.S.): Seems to correlate with the incidence of upper respiratory tract infections
PEAK INCIDENCE: Fall, winter, spring: September through March

■ **PHYSICAL FINDINGS & CLINICAL PRESENTATION**
- Patients often give a history of a recent upper respiratory illness with some improvement, then a relapse
- Mucopurulent secretions in the nasal passage
  1. Purulent nasal and postnasal discharge lasting >7 to 10 days
  2. Facial tightness, pressure, or pain
  3. Nasal obstruction
  4. Headache
  5. Decreased sense of smell
  6. Purulent pharyngeal secretions, brought up with cough, often worse at night
- Erythema, swelling, and tenderness over the infected sinus in a small proportion of patients
  1. Diagnosis cannot be excluded by the absence of such findings.
  2. These findings are not common, and do not correlate with number of positive sinus aspirates.

- Intermittent low-grade fever in about half of adults with acute bacterial sinusitis
- Toothache is a common complaint when the maxillary sinus is involved
- Periorbital cellulitis and excessive tearing with ethmoid sinusitis
  1. Orbital extension of infection: chemosis, proptosis, impaired extraocular movements
- Characteristics of acute sinusitis in children with upper respiratory tract infections:
  1. Persistence of symptoms
  2. Cough
  3. Bad breath
- Symptoms of chronic sinusitis (may or may not be present)
  1. Nasal or postnasal discharge
  2. Fever
  3. Facial pain or pressure
  4. Headache
- Nosocomial sinusitis is typically seen in patients with nasogastric tubes or nasotracheal intubation.

■ **ETIOLOGY**
- Each of the four paranasal sinuses is connected to the nasal cavity by narrow tubes (ostia), 1 to 3 mm diameter; these drain directly into the nose through the turbinates. The sinuses are lined with a ciliated mucous membrane (mucoperiosteum).
- Acute viral infection
  1. Infection with the common cold or influenza
  2. Mucosal edema and sinus inflammation
  3. Decreased drainage of thick secretions/obstruction of the sinus ostia
  4. Subsequent entrapment of bacteria
     a. Multiplication of bacteria
     b. Secondary bacterial infection
- Other predisposing factors
  1. Tumors
  2. Polyps
  3. Foreign bodies
  4. Congenital choanal atresia
  5. Other entities that cause obstruction of sinus drainage
  6. Allergies
  7. Asthma
- Dental infections lead to maxillary sinusitis
- Viruses recovered alone or in combination with bacteria (in 16% of cases):
  1. Rhinovirus
  2. Coronavirus
  3. Adenovirus
  4. Parainfluenza virus
  5. Respiratory syncytial virus
- The principal bacterial pathogens in sinusitis are *Streptococcus pneumoniae*, nontypeable *Haemophilus influenzae*, and *Moraxella catarrhalis*.
- In the remainder of cases find *Streptococcus pyogenes, Staphylococcus aureus*, α-hemolytic streptococci, and mixed anaerobic infections (*Peptostreptococcus, Fusobacterium, Bacteroides, Prevotella*).

- Infection is polymicrobial in about one third of cases.
- Anaerobic infections seen more often in cases of chronic sinusitis and in cases associated with dental infection; anaerobes are unlikely pathogens in sinusitis in children.
- Fungal pathogens are isolated with increasing frequency in immunocompromised patients:
  1. *Aspergillus*
  2. *Pseudallescheria*
  3. *Sporothrix*
  4. Phaeohyphomycoses
  5. Hyalohyphomycoses
  6. Zygomycetes
- Nosocomial infections: occur in patients with nasogastric tubes, nasotracheal intubation, cystic fibrosis, immunocompromised
  1. *S. aureus*
  2. *Pseudomonas aeruginosa*
  3. *Klebsiella pneumoniae*
  4. *Enterobacter spp.*
  5. *Proteus mirabilis*
- Organisms typically isolated in chronic sinusitis:
  1. *S. aureus*
  2. *S. pneumoniae*
  3. *H. influenzae*
  4. *P. aeruginosa*
  5. Anaerobes

🔬 **DIAGNOSIS**

■ **DIFFERENTIAL DIAGNOSIS**
- Temporomandibular joint disease
- Migraine headache
- Cluster headache
- Dental infection
- Trigeminal neuralgia

■ **WORKUP**
- In the normal healthy host the paranasal sinuses should be sterile. Although the contiguous structures are colonized with bacteria and likely contaminate the sinuses, the mucociliary lining functions to remove these bacteria.
- Gold standard for diagnosis: recovery of bacteria in high density ($\geq 10^4$ colony-forming units/ml) from a paranasal sinus, in the setting of a patient with history of upper respiratory infection and symptoms persisting 7 to 10 days. Sinus aspiration is the best method for obtaining cultures; however, it must be performed by an otorhinolaryngologist and is not practical for the primary care practitioner. Therefore most diagnoses are based on the clinical history and presentation, possibly supported by radiologic evaluations.
  1. Standard four-view sinus radiographs (Fig. 1-251)
     a. Complete opacification and air-fluid levels are most specific findings (average 85% and 80%, respectively)

b. Mucosal thickening has low specificity (40% to 50%)

c. Absence of all three of the previous findings has estimated sensitivity of 90%

d. Overall, standard radiographs are of limited use in diagnosis, although negative films are strong evidence against the diagnosis

2. CT scans:
   a. Much more sensitive than plain radiographs in detecting acute changes and disease in the sinuses
   b. Recommended for patients requiring surgical intervention, including sinus aspiration; it is a useful adjunct to guide therapy

3. Transillumination:
   a. Used for diagnosis of frontal and maxillary sinusitis
   b. Place transilluminator in the mouth or against cheek to assess maxillary sinuses, under medial aspect of the supraorbital ridge to assess frontal sinuses
   c. Absence of light transmission indicates that sinus is filled with fluid
   d. Dullness (decreased light transmission) is less helpful in diagnosing infection

4. Endoscopy:
   a. Used to visualize secretions coming from the ostia of infected sinuses
   b. Culture collection via endoscopy often contaminated by nasal flora; not nearly as good as sinus puncture

5. Sinus puncture:
   a. Gold standard for collecting sinus cultures
   b. Generally reserved for treatment failures, suspected intracranial extension, and nosocomial sinusitis

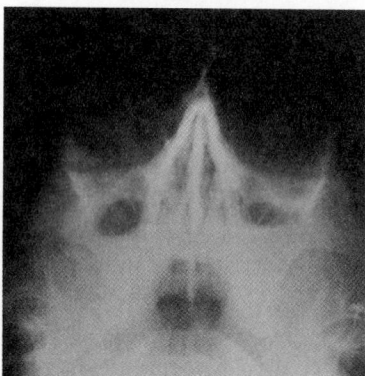

Fig. 1-251   Waters' view of maxillary sinus with air-fluid level. (From Noble J [ed]: *Primary care medicine*, ed 3, St Louis, 2001, Mosby.)

℞ TREATMENT

■ NONPHARMACOLOGIC THERAPY

To help promote sinus drainage:
- Air humidification with vaporizers (for steam) or humidifiers (for a cool mist)
- Application of hot, wet towel over the face
- Sipping hot beverages
- Hydration

■ ACUTE GENERAL Rx
- Sinus drainage:
  1. Nasal vasoconstrictors, such as phenylephrine nose drops, 0.25% or 0.5%
  2. Topical decongestants should not be used for more than a few days because of the risk of rebound congestion
  3. Systemic decongestants
  4. Nasal or systemic corticosteroids, such as nasal beclomethasone, short course oral prednisone
  5. Nasal irrigation, with hypertonic or normal saline (saline may act as a mild vasoconstrictor of nasal blood flow)
  6. Use of antihistamines has no proven benefit, and the drying effect on the mucous membranes may cause crusting, which blocks the ostia, thus interfering with sinus drainage
- Analgesics, antipyretics
Antimicrobial therapy:
- Most cases of acute sinusitis have a viral etiology and will resolve within 2 wk without antibiotics.
- Current treatment recommendations favor symptomatic treatment for those with mild symptoms.
- Antibiotics should be reserved for those with moderate to severe symptoms who meet the criteria for diagnosis of sinusitis.
- Antibiotic therapy is usually empiric, targeting the common pathogens:
  1. First-line antibiotics include amoxicillin, erythromycin, TMP/SMX.
  2. Second-line antibiotics include the newer macrolides: clarithromycin, azithromycin, amoxicillin/clavulanate, cefuroxime axetil, cefprozil, cefaclor, loracarbef, ciprofloxacin, levofloxacin, clindamycin, metronidazole, others.
  3. For patients with uncomplicated acute sinusitis, the less expensive first-line agents appear to be as effective as the costlier second-line agents.
- Hospitalization and IV antibiotics may be required for more severe infection and those with suspected in-

tracranial complications. Broader-spectrum antibiotic coverage may be indicated in severe cases, to cover for MRSA, *Pseudomonas,* and fungal pathogens.
Duration of therapy generally 10 to 14 days, although some have success with much shorter regimens
Surgery:
- Surgical drainage indicated
  1. If intracranial or orbital complications suspected
  2. Many cases of frontal and sphenoid sinusitis
  3. Chronic sinusitis recalcitrant to medical therapy
- Surgical debridement imperative in the treatment of fungal sinusitis
Complications:
- Untreated, sinusitis may lead to a number of serious, life-threatening complications.
- Intracranial complications include meningitis, brain abscess, epidural and subdural empyema.
- Intracranial sequelae are more common with frontal and ethmoid infections.
- Extracranial complications include orbital cellulitis, blindness, orbital abscess, osteomyelitis.
- Extracranial sequelae are more commonly seen with ethmoid sinusitis.

■ CHRONIC Rx
- Broad-spectrum antibiotics that cover both aerobes and anaerobes
- Duration of therapy not clearly established: range 3 to 6 wk
- Adjunctive therapy: one or more of the various options listed previously
- Surgical intervention may be necessary in nonresponders

■ DISPOSITION
Appropriate diagnosis and treatment necessary to avoid the various sequelae that can occur without proper therapy

■ REFERRAL
- To infectious disease specialist if failure to respond to initial therapy
- To otorhinolaryngologist for:
  1. Failure to respond to therapy
  2. Fungal infection suspected
  3. Intracranial or orbital complications suspected

REFERENCES
Brook I: Bacteriology of acute and chronic frontal sinusitis, *Arch Otolaryngol Head Neck Surg* 128(5):583, 2002.

Jiang RS, Lin JF, Hsu CY: Correlation between bacteriology of the middle meatus and ethmoid sinus in chronic sinusitis, *J Laryngol Otgol* 116(6):443, 2002.
Author: **Jane V. Eason, M.D.**

BASIC INFORMATION

■ DEFINITION

Sjögren's syndrome (SS) is an autoimmune disorder characterized by lymphocytic and plasma cell infiltration and destruction of salivary and lacrimal glands with subsequent diminished lacrimal and salivary gland secretions.

- *Primary:* dry mouth (xerostomia) and dry eyes (xerophthalmia) develop as isolated entities.
- *Secondary:* associated with other disorders.

■ SYNONYMS

SS
Sicca syndrome

ICD-9CM CODES

710.2 Sjögren's syndrome

■ EPIDEMIOLOGY & DEMOGRAPHICS

INCIDENCE/PREVALENCE: 1 case/2500 persons; secondary SS is just as common and can affect up to one third of SLE patients and nearly 20% of RA patients.

PREDOMINANT AGE: Peak incidence is in the sixth decade.

PREDOMINANT SEX: Female > male

■ PHYSICAL FINDINGS & CLINICAL PRESENTATION

- Dry mouth with dry lips (cheilosis), erythema of tongue (Fig. 1-252), and other mucosal surfaces, carious teeth
- Dry eyes (conjunctival injection, decreased luster, and irregularity of the corneal light reflex)
- Possible salivary gland enlargement and dysfunction with subsequent difficulty in chewing and swallowing food and in speaking without frequent water intake

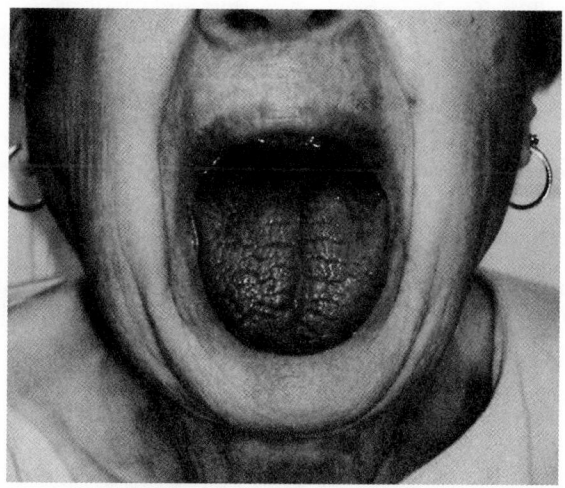

Fig. 1-252 "Crocodile tongue" in SS patient. (From Noble J: *Primary care medicine,* ed 3, St Louis, 2001, Mosby.)

- Purpura (nonthrombocytopenic, hyperglobulinemic, vasculitic) may be present
- Evidence of associated conditions (e.g., RA or other connective disease, lymphoma, hypothyroidism, COPD, trigeminal neuropathy, chronic liver disease, polymyopathy)

■ ETIOLOGY

Autoimmune disorder

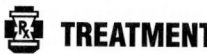

DIAGNOSIS

■ DIFFERENTIAL DIAGNOSIS

- Medication-related dryness (e.g., anticholinergics)
- Age-related exocrine gland dysfunction
- Mouth breathing
- Anxiety
- Other: sarcoidosis, primary salivary hypofunction, radiation injury, amyloidosis

■ WORKUP

Workup involves the demonstration of the following criteria for diagnosis of primary and secondary Sjögren's syndrome:

PRIMARY:
- Symptoms and objective signs of ocular dryness:
  1. Schirmer's test: <8 mm wetting per 5 min
  2. Positive rose bengal or fluorescein staining of cornea and conjunctiva to demonstrate keratoconjunctivitis sicca
- Symptoms and objective signs of dry mouth:
  1. Decreased parotid flow using Lashley cups or other methods
  2. Abnormal biopsy result of minor salivary gland (focus score >2 based on average of four assessable lobules)

- Evidence of systemic autoimmune disorder:
  1. Elevated titer of rheumatoid factor >1:320
  2. Elevated titer of ANA >1:320
  3. Presence of anti-SS A (Ro) or anti-SS B (La) antibodies

SECONDARY:
- Characteristic signs and symptoms of SS (described in "Physical Findings")
- Clinical features sufficient to allow a diagnosis of RA, SLE, polymyositis, or scleroderma

■ LABORATORY TESTS

- Positive ANA (>60% of patients) with autoantibodies anti-SS A and anti-SS B may be present.
- Additional laboratory abnormalities may include elevated ESR, anemia (normochromic, normocytic), abnormal liver function studies, elevated serum β_2 microglobulin levels, rheumatoid factor.
- A definite diagnosis SS can be made with a salivary gland biopsy.

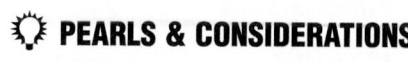

TREATMENT

■ NONPHARMACOLOGIC THERAPY

- Adequate fluid replacement
- Proper oral hygiene to reduce the incidence of caries

■ ACUTE GENERAL Rx

- Use artificial tears frequently.
- Pilocarpine 5 mg PO qid is useful to improve dryness. A cyclosporine 0.05% ophthalmic emulsion (Restasis) may also be useful for dry eyes. Recommended dose is one drop bid in both eyes.
- Cevimeline (Evoxac), a cholinergic agent with muscarinic agonist activity, 30 mg PO tid is effective for the treatment of dry mouth in patients with Sjögren's syndrome.

■ CHRONIC Rx

Periodic dental and ophthalmology evaluations to screen for complications

☼ PEARLS & CONSIDERATIONS

■ COMMENTS

Unusual presentations of SS may occur in association with polymyalgia rheumatica, chronic fatigue syndrome, FUO, and inflammatory myositis.

REFERENCE

Fife RS et al: Cevimeline for the treatment of xerostomia in patients with Sjögren syndrome, *Arch Intern Med* 162:1293, 2002.

Author: **Fred F. Ferri, M.D.**

BASIC INFORMATION

■ DEFINITION

The American Academy of Sleep Disorders defines obstructive sleep apnea as "characterized by repetitive episodes of upper airway obstruction that occur during sleep, usually associated with a reduction in blood oxygen saturation."

■ SYNONYMS

Sleep apnea syndrome
Obstructive sleep apnea-hypopnea syndrome

ICD-9CM CODE

780.53-0 Obstructive sleep apnea syndrome

■ EPIDEMIOLOGY & DEMOGRAPHICS

Obstructive sleep apnea (OSA) occurs most frequently in 40- to 65-year-old men (4%) and women (2%). The prevalence is higher in obese and hypertensive individuals. Pediatric OSA most frequently occurs in preschool-aged children (2%) and is associated with hypertrophy of the tonsils and adenoids.

■ PHYSICAL FINDINGS & CLINICAL PRESENTATION

- Systemic hypertension
- History of snoring, witnessed apneas and excessive daytime somnolence
- Obesity with body mass index >27 kg/m², neck circumference >43 cm (17") in men
- Working memory impairment, inability to concentrate, short tempered
- Examination of oropharynx may reveal erythema caused by snoring and narrowing secondary to large tonsils, pendulous uvula, excessive soft tissue, prominent tongue and retrognathia
- Patient's bed partner may report loud, snoring, episodic choking sounds, disrupted sleep with repetitive arousals, thrashing movements of extremities during sleep
- Decreased libido, mood swings, and depression

■ ETIOLOGY

Narrowing of upper airway secondary to:
- Obesity
- Macroglossia
- Tonsillar and adenoid hypertrophy
- Micrognathia
- Muscular weakness
- Use of alcohol or sedatives at bedtime

DIAGNOSIS

■ DIFFERENTIAL DIAGNOSIS

- Excessive Daytime Somnolence
  Inadequate sleep time
  Pulmonary disease
  Parkinsonism
  Sleep-related epilepsy
  Narcolepsy
  Hypothyroidism
- Sleep Fragmentation
  Sleep-related asthma
  Sleep-related GERD
  Periodic limb movement disorder
  Parasomnias
  Psychophysiologic insomnia
  Panic disorder
  Narcolepsy

■ WORKUP

- Medical history should include questions about snoring, witnessed apneas, and excessive daytime sleepiness. Additional history concerning morning headaches, alcohol intake, weight gain, and mood/personality changes also may help to implicate apnea.
- Sleep apnea can be confirmed by overnight polysomnography (gold standard). Testing is performed during the patient's habitual sleep hours and ideally includes all stages of sleep and body positions. Patients with sleep apnea have >5 apneic/hypopneic episodes per hour (termed respiratory disturbance index, or RDI) with desaturations of at least 4% by oximetry or coincidental arousals. Overnight oximetry tests can suggest the presence of sleep apnea but are not sufficient to rule out sleep apnea.
- Portable monitors that measure RDI are available but they lack the EEG, EMG, and technical observations necessary to diagnose sleep apnea with reliable accuracy. The use of such devices is usually related to limited availability of polysomnography.

■ LABORATORY TESTS

- TSH level is indicated in suspected hypothyroidism.
- CBC (with iron studies) is indicated for detecting anemia.
- Pulmonary function tests are indicated for detecting related pulmonary disorders.
- ECG is indicated for detecting related heart disease.

■ IMAGING STUDIES

Radiography of soft tissues in the neck in patients with suspected anatomic abnormalities

TREATMENT

■ NONPHARMACOLOGIC THERAPY

- Weight loss in overweight patients
- Avoidance of sedating medications and alcohol
- Sleep hygiene training
- Elimination of the supine sleeping position
- For mild obstructive sleep apnea in select patient populations (e.g., retrognathia) an oral appliance (constructed by a qualified dentist) may be useful to push the mandible forward
- Uvulopalatopharyngoplasty (UPPP, both standard and laser-assisted [LAUP]) in patients with significant obstruction of retropalatal airway
- Nasal septoplasty in patients with nasoseptal deformity

■ ACUTE GENERAL Rx

- Nighttime treatment with continuous positive airway pressure (CPAP) provides immediate resolution of sleep apnea. Symptoms of excessive daytime somnolence may linger and necessitate further investigation or medical therapy
- Tracheostomy: reserved for life-threatening cases that are unresponsive to other treatments
- Nasal steroids in allergy or sinusitis patients

■ CHRONIC Rx

- CPAP therapy
- Weight loss

■ DISPOSITION

- Most patients improve with weight loss and CPAP.
- Overall success rate for UPPP is about 40%.
- Weight loss over time may reduce the need for CPAP pressure or obviate its use entirely.

■ REFERRAL

- Sleep physician for proper study type(s) and/or complex symptoms
- Surgical referral for patients unresponsive to weight loss and CPAP
- Dental referral for oral devices

PEARLS & CONSIDERATIONS

- In a primary care setting, patients with high risk of sleep apnea are those who meet two of the following three criteria: (1) snoring, (2) persistent daytime sleepiness or drowsiness while driving, (3) obesity or hypertension.
- Children with OSA may have symptoms of excessive daytime somnolence, hyperactivity, insomnia, declining academic performance, and a history of recurrent ear or throat infections.
- Some patients with sleep apnea experience nocturnal dysrhythmias (bradycardia, paroxysmal tachyarrhythmias). In cardiac patients, trials using atrial overdrive pacing have demonstrated a significant reduction in the number of episodes of sleep apnea without reduction in the total sleep time.

- The use of vagal nerve stimulators (VNS) in epilepsy patients has been associated with an increase in apneas and hypopneas. VNS-related respiratory events may be reduced by altering VNS stimulation parameters or by initiating CPAP.

REFERENCES

American Academy of Pediatrics: Clinical practice guideline: diagnosis and management of childhood obstructive sleep apnea syndrome, *Pediatrics* 109:704, 2002.

Arens, R: Obstructive sleep apnea in childhood, clinical features. In Loughlin G, Carroll J, Marcus C (eds): *Sleep and breathing in children,* New York, 2000, Marcel Dekker.

Flemons WW: Obstructive sleep apnea, *N Engl J Med* 347:498, 2002.

Garrigue A et al: Benefit of atrial pacing in sleep apnea syndrome, *N Engl J Med* 346:404, 2002.

Marzec M et al: Effects of vagal nerve stimulation on sleep-related breathing in epilepsy patients, *Epilepsia* 44:930, 2003.

Partinen M, Hublin C: Epidemiology of sleep disorders. In Kryger M, Roth T, Dement W (eds): *Principles and practice of sleep medicine,* ed 3, Philadelphia, 2000, WB Saunders.

Schroeder BM: Obstructive sleep apnea syndrome in children, *Am Fam Physician* 66:1338, 2002.

The International Classification of Sleep Disorders Revised, Diagnostic and Coding Manual. American Academy of Sleep Medicine, 2000.

Author: **J.S. Durmer, M.D., Ph.D.**

BASIC INFORMATION

■ DEFINITION
Smallpox infection is due to the variola virus, a DNA virus member of the genus *Orthopoxvirus*. It is a human virus with no known nonhuman reservoir of disease. Natural infection occurs following implantation of the virus on the oropharyngeal or respiratory mucosa.

ICD-9CM CODES
050.9 Smallpox NOS
V01.3 Smallpox exposure
050.0 Smallpox, hemorrhagic (pustular)
050.1 Variola minor (alastrim)
050.0 Variola major

■ EPIDEMIOLOGY & DEMOGRAPHICS
- Smallpox infection was eliminated from the world in 1977. The last cases of smallpox, from laboratory exposure, occurred in 1978. The threat of bioterrorism has brought on renewed interest in smallpox virus.
- Routine vaccination against smallpox ended in 1972.
- Smallpox is spread from one person to another by infected saliva droplets that expose a susceptible person who has face-to-face contact with the ill person.
- Persons with smallpox are most infectious during the first wk of illness, when the largest amount of virus is present in saliva; however, some risk of transmission lasts until all scabs have fallen off.
- The incubation period is about 12 days (range: 7 to 17 days) following exposure.
- Contaminated clothing or bed linen could also spread the virus. Special precautions need to be taken to ensure that all bedding and clothing of patients are cleaned appropriately with bleach and hot water. Disinfectants such as bleach and quaternary ammonia can be used for cleaning contaminated surfaces.

■ PHYSICAL FINDINGS & CLINICAL PRESENTATION
- Initial symptoms include high fever, fatigue, and headaches and back aches. A characteristic rash, most prominent on the face, arms, and legs, follows in 2 to 3 days (Fig. 1-253).
- The rash starts with flat red lesions that evolve at the same rate. The rash follows a centrifugal pattern.
- Lesions are firm to the touch, domed, or umbilicated. They become pus-filled and begin to crust early in the second wk.

- Scabs develop and then separate and fall off after about 3 to 4 wk. Depigmentation persists at the base of the skin lesions for 3 to 6 mo after illness. Scarring is usually most extensive on the face.
- Associated with the rash may be fever, headache, generalized malaise, vomiting, and colicky abdominal pain.
- Variola major may produce a rapidly fatal toxemia in some patients.
- Complications of smallpox include dehydration, pneumonia, blepharitis, conjunctivitis, and corneal ulcerations.

■ ETIOLOGY
Smallpox is caused by the variola virus. There are at least two strains of the virus, the most virulent known as *variola major* and a less virulent strain known as *variola minor* (elastrim).

DIAGNOSIS

■ DIFFERENTIAL DIAGNOSIS
- Rash from other viral illnesses (e.g., hemorrhagic chicken pox, measles, coxsackievirus)
- Abdominal pain may mimic appendicitis
- Meningococcemia
- Insect bites
- Impetigo
- Dermatitis herpetiformis
- Pemphigus
- Papular urticaria

■ WORKUP & LABORATORY TESTS
- Laboratory examination requires high-containment (BL-4) facilities.
- Electron microscopy of vesicular scrapings can be used to distinguish poxvirus particles from varicella-zoster virus or herpes simplex. To obtain vesicular or pustular fluid it may be necessary to open lesions with the blunt edge of a scalpel. A cotton swab may be used to harvest the fluid.
- In absence of electron microscopy, light microscopy can be used to visualize variola viral particles (Guarnieri bodies) following Giemsa staining.
- Polymerase chain reaction (PCR) techniques and restriction fragment-length polymorphisms can rapidly identify variola.

■ IMAGING STUDIES
Chest x-ray in patients with suspected pneumonia

TREATMENT

■ NONPHARMACOLOGIC THERAPY
- Supportive therapy
- IV hydration in severe cases
- A suspect case of smallpox should be placed in strict respiratory and contact isolation

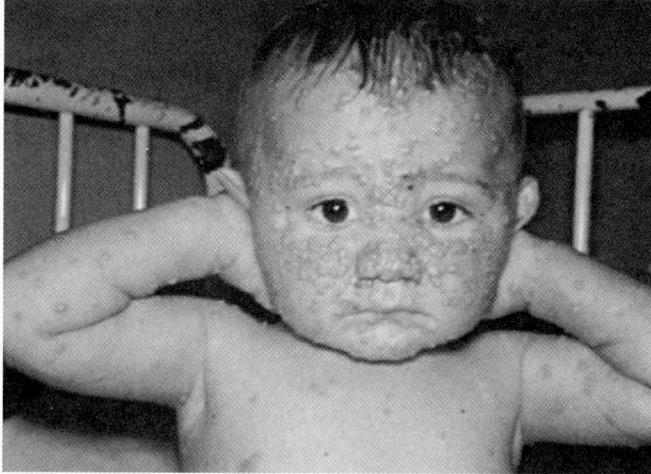

Fig. 1-253 Appearance of the rash of smallpox on day 6 to 7. All of the lesions are in the same stage of development. (From Gorbach SL: *Infectious diseases*, ed 2, Philadelphia, 1998, WB Saunders.)

■ ACUTE GENERAL Rx

- There is no proven treatment for smallpox. Vaccination administered within 3 to 4 days may prevent or significantly ameliorate subsequent illness. Vaccinia immune globulin can be used for treatment of vaccine complications and for administration with vaccine to those for whom vaccine is otherwise contraindicated.
- Patients can benefit from supportive therapy (e.g., IV fluids, acetaminophen for pain or fever).
- Antibiotics are indicated only if secondary bacterial infections occur. Penicillase-resistant antimicrobial agents should be used if smallpox lesions are secondarily infected.
- Topical idoxuridine should be considered for corneal lesions.

■ DISPOSITION

- Mortality for variola major is 20% to 50%. Variola minor has a mortality rate of 1%.
- After severe smallpox, pitted lesions (most commonly on the face) are seen in up to 80% of survivors.
- Panophthalmitis and blindness from viral keratitis or secondary eye infection occur in 1% of patients.
- Arthritis caused by viral infection of the metaphysis of growing bones occurs in 2% of children.

■ REFERRAL

- ID consultation and notification of local health authorities is mandatory in all cases of smallpox.

☼ PEARLS & CONSIDERATIONS

- The smallpox virus is fragile and in the event of an aerosol release of smallpox, all viruses will be inactivated or dissipated within 1 to 2 days. Buildings exposed to the initial aerosol release of the virus do not need to be decontaminated. By the time the first cases are identified, typically 2 wk after release, the virus in the building will be gone. Infected patients, however, will be capable of spreading the virus and possibly contaminating surfaces while they are sick. Standard hospital-grade disinfectants such as quaternary ammonias are effective in killing the virus on surfaces and should be used for disinfecting hospitalized patients' rooms or other contaminated surfaces. In the hospital setting, patients' linens should be autoclaved or washed in hot water with bleach added. Infectious waste should be placed in biohazard bags and autoclaved before incineration.

- Symptomatic patients with suspected or confirmed smallpox are capable of spreading the virus. Patients should be placed in medical isolation to avoid spread of the virus. In addition, people who have come into close contact with smallpox patients should be vaccinated immediately and closely watched for symptoms of smallpox.

■ COMMENTS

- In people exposed to smallpox, the vaccine can lessen the severity of or even prevent illness if given within 4 days of exposure.
- Vaccine against smallpox contains another live virus called vaccinia. The vaccine does not contain smallpox virus.
- Primary vaccination confers full immunity to smallpox in more than 95% of persons for up to 10 yr.

REFERENCES

Breman JG, Henderson DA: Diagnosis and management of smallpox, *N Engl J Med* 346:1300, 2002.

Frey SE et al: Clinical responses to undiluted and diluted smallpox vaccine, *N Engl J Med* 346:1265, 2002.

Henderson DA et al: Smallpox as a biological weapon, *JAMA* 281:2127, 1999. www.bt.cdc.gov/Agent/Smallpox/SmallpoxGen.asp

Author: **Fred F. Ferri, M.D.**

BASIC INFORMATION

■ DEFINITION
Somatization disorder refers to a pattern of recurring multiple somatic complaints that begin before the age of 30 yr and persist over several years. Patients complain of multiple sites of pain (a minimum of four), GI symptoms (a minimum of two), a sexual or reproductive symptom, and a pseudoneurologic symptom. These cannot be explained by a medical condition or are in excess to expected disability from a coexisting medical condition.

■ SYNONYMS
Briquet's syndrome
Nonorganic physical symptoms
Medically unexplained symptoms
Functional somatic symptoms
AICD-9CM CODES
300.81 Somatization disorder

■ EPIDEMIOLOGY & DEMOGRAPHICS
PREVALENCE (IN U.S.): Lifetime rates of 0.25% to 2% in women, <0.2% in men
PREDOMINANT SEX:
- Women are more commonly affected in the U.S.
- Males of other cultures (e.g., Greece and Puerto Rico) are more commonly affected.

PREDOMINANT AGE: By definition, onset occurs before age 30 yr.
PEAK INCIDENCE: Typically before age 25 yr
GENETICS:
- Genetic and environmental factors may be involved.
- There is a high risk of associated substance abuse or antisocial personality disorder.

■ PHYSICAL FINDINGS & CLINICAL PRESENTATION
- Typical patient is unmarried, non-white, poorly educated, and from rural setting.
- Onset is frequently in the teens; course is marked by frequent, unexplained, and frequently disabling pain and physical complaints.
- Patient frequently undergoes multiple procedures and seeks treatment from multiple physicians.

- Patient meets criteria for at least one other psychiatric condition, most commonly substance abuse disorders and personality disorders (antisocial disorder is the most common); anxiety and depressive disorders are also common.

■ ETIOLOGY
- Believed to be the physical expression of psychologic distress
- May be more common in individuals without sufficient verbal or intellectual capacity to communicate psychologic distress, individuals with alexithymia (inability to describe emotional states), or individuals from cultural backgrounds that consider emotional distress as an undesirable weakness
- Some aspects of somatization behavior possibly learned from somatizing patients

🔬 DIAGNOSIS

■ DIFFERENTIAL DIAGNOSIS
- Undifferentiated somatoform disorder (ICD-10 F45.1, DMS-IV 300.81): one or more physical complaints that cannot be explained by a medical condition are present for at least 6 mo (NOTE: Somatization is more severe and less common).
- Conversion disorder: there is an alteration or loss of voluntary motor or sensory function with demonstrable physical cause and related to a psychologic stress or a conflict (NOTE: With multiple complaints, the diagnosis of conversion is not made).
- Pain disorder: distinguished from somatization disorder by the presence of other somatic complaints.
- Munchausen's (factitious disorder) and malingering: the psychologic basis of the complaints in somatization disorder is not conscious as in factitious disorder (Munchausen's) and malingering, in which symptoms are produced intentionally.

■ WORKUP
- Rule out a general medical condition.
- If somatization is suspected on the basis of a history of repeated, multiple, unexplained complaints, restraint in ordering tests is recommended.

■ LABORATORY TESTS
No specific laboratory tests are required.

■ IMAGING STUDIES
No specific imaging studies are required.

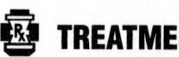 **TREATMENT**

■ NONPHARMACOLOGIC THERAPY
- Legitimize patient's complaints; when this is not done, there is frequently an increase in complaints and associated disability.
- Minimize diagnostic investigation and symptomatic treatment.
- Set attainable treatment goals.
- Treat coexisting psychiatric conditions.

■ ACUTE GENERAL Rx
- No specific pharmacologic therapy is available.
- Antidepressants may be useful for coexisting anxiety and depression.

■ CHRONIC Rx
- A trusting relationship based on mutual respect between the patient and the physician is the best long-term treatment.
- If there is coexisting anxiety or depression, chronic use of antidepressants may be warranted.

■ DISPOSITION
A chronic condition with frequent exacerbations

■ REFERRAL
If therapy is required and the patient has the psychologic mindedness to participate

REFERENCES
De Gucht V, Fischler B: Somatization: A critical review of conceptual and methodological issues, *Psychosomatics* 43:1, 2002.
Epstein RC et al: Somatization reconsidered, *Arch Intern Med* 159:215, 1999.
Author: **Rif S. El-Mallakh, M.D.**

BASIC INFORMATION

■ DEFINITION

Spinal cord compression is the neurologic loss of spine function. Lesions may be complete or incomplete and develop gradually or acutely. Incomplete lesions often present as distinct syndromes, as follows:
- Central cord syndrome
- Anterior cord syndrome
- Brown-Séquard syndrome
- Conus medullaris syndrome
- Cauda equina syndrome

ICD-9CM CODES
344.89 Brown-Séquard syndrome
344.60 Cauda equina syndrome
336.8 Conus medullaris syndrome
Other lesions listed by site

■ PHYSICAL FINDINGS & CLINICAL PRESENTATION

Clinical features reflect the amount of spinal cord involvement (Fig. 1-254):
- Motor loss and sensory abnormalities
- Babinski testing usually positive
- Clonus
- Gradual compression, often manifested by progressive difficulty walking, clonus with weight bearing, and involuntary spasm; development of sensory symptoms; bladder dysfunction (late)
- Central cord syndrome: results in a variable quadriparesis with the upper extremities more severely involved than the lower extremities; some sensory sparing
- Anterior cord syndrome: results in motor, pain, and temperature loss below the lesion

- Brown-Séquard syndrome:
  1. Spinal cord syndrome caused by injury to either half of the spinal cord and resulting in the loss of motor function, position, vibration, and light touch on the affected side
  2. Pain and temperature sense lost on the opposite side
- Conus medullaris syndrome: results in variable motor loss in the lower extremities with loss of bowel and bladder function
- Cauda equina syndrome: typical low back pain, weakness in both lower extremities, saddle anesthesia, and loss of voluntary bladder and bowel control

■ ETIOLOGY
- Trauma
- Tumor
- Infection
- Inflammatory processes
- Degenerative disk conditions with spinal stenosis
- Acute disk herniation
- Cystic abnormalities

DIAGNOSIS

■ DIFFERENTIAL DIAGNOSIS
- See "Etiology."
- Section II describes the differential diagnosis of paraplegia.

■ WORKUP
- Spinal cord compression: requires an immediate referral for radiographic and neurologic assessment
- Laboratory results usually unremarkable unless infectious or inflammatory causes suspected

■ IMAGING STUDIES
- Depend on the suspected etiology
- MRI usually required

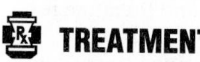

TREATMENT

Urgent surgical decompression is usually indicated as soon as the etiology is established.

■ DISPOSITION
Important indicators regarding prognosis (Leventhal):
- The greater the distal motor and sensory sparing, the greater the expected recovery.
- When a plateau of recovery is reached, no further improvement is expected.
- The quicker the recovery, the greater the recovery

■ REFERRAL
Immediate referral for radiographic and neurologic evaluation and treatment in all suspected cases of spinal cord compression

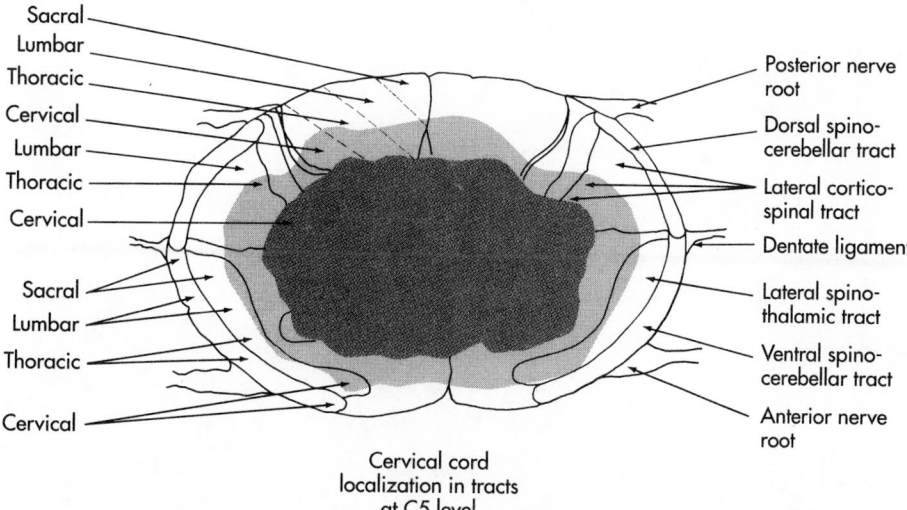

Fig. 1-254 Diagrammatic description of the spinal pathways at the lower cervical level showing the usual distribution of the contusion hemorrhage that causes a central cord syndrome. (From Goldman L, Ausiello D [eds]: *Cecil textbook of medicine*, ed 22, Philadelphia, 2004, WB Saunders.)

REFERENCES

Baines MJ: Spinal cord compression—a personal and palliative care perspective, *Clin Oncol (R Coll Radiol)* 14(2):135, 2002.

Benjamin R: Neurologic complications of prostate cancer, *Am Fam Physician* 65(9):1834, 2002.

Buchner M, Schiltenwolf M: Cauda equina syndrome caused by intervertebral lumbar disc prolapse: mid-term results of 22 patients and literature review, *Orthopedics* 25:727, 2002.

Carlson GD et al: Sustained spinal cord compression. Part I: time-dependent effect on long-term pathophysiology, *J Bone Joint Surg* 85:86, 2003.

Carlson GD et al: Sustained spinal cord compression. Part II: effect of methylprednisolone on regional blood flow and recovery of somatosensory evoked potentials, *J Bone Joint Surg* 85:95, 2003.

Casey AT et al: Rheumatoid arthritis of the cervical spine: current techniques for management, *Orthop Clin North Am* 33(2):291, 2002.

Kadanka Z et al: Approaches to spondylotic cervical myelopathy: conservative versus surgical in a 3-year follow-up study, *Spine* 27(20):2205, 2002.

Malcolm GP: Surgical disorders of the cervical spine: presentation and management of common disorders, *J Neurosurg Psychiatry* 73(Suppl 1):134, 2002.

Matsunaga S et al: Trauma-induced myelopathy in patients with ossification of the posterior longitudinal ligament, *J Neurosurg* 97(2 Suppl):172, 2002.

Mohanty SP, Venkatram N: Does neurological recovery in thoracolumbar and lumbar burst fractures depend on the extent of canal compromise? *Spinal Cord* 40(6):295, 2002.

Tang HJ et al: Spinal epidural abscess—experience with 46 patients and evaluation of prognostic factors, *J Infect* 45(2):76, 2002.

Author: **Lonnie R. Mercier, M.D.**

BASIC INFORMATION

■ DEFINITION
A spinal epidural abscess (SEA) is a focal suppurative infection occurring in the spinal epidural space.

ICD-9CM CODES
324.1 Spinal epidural abscess

■ EPIDEMIOLOGY & DEMOGRAPHICS
INCIDENCE IN U.S.:
- 2 to 25 cases/100,000 hospitalized patients/yr
- May be increasing over the past three decades

PREDOMINANT AGE:
- Median age of onset approximately 50 yr (35 yr in intravenous drug users)
- Peak incidence in seventh and eighth decades of life

■ PHYSICAL FINDINGS
The presentation of SEA can be nonspecific. Fever, malaise, and back pain are the most consistent early symptoms. Pain is often focal. It may initially be mild but can progress to become severe. As the disease progresses, root pain can occur, followed by motor weakness, sensory changes, bladder and bowel dysfunction, and paralysis. Physical findings may be limited to fever or spinal tenderness. The evolution to neurologic deficits can occur as quickly as a few hours, or over weeks to months. Once paralysis occurs, it may quickly become irreversible without the appropriate intervention.

■ ETIOLOGY
- Bacteria account for the majority of cases in the U.S. Immigrants from tuberculosis-endemic areas may present with tuberculous SEAs. Fungi and parasites can also cause this condition. The most common causative organism is *Staphylococcus aureus*. Most posterior EAs thought to originate from distant focus (e.g., skin and soft tissue infections), while anterior EAs commonly associated with diskitis or vertebral osteomyelitis. No source found in approximately one third of cases.
- Associated predisposing conditions include a compromised immune system such as occurs in patients with diabetes mellitus, alcoholism, cancer, AIDS, and chronic renal failure, or following epidural anesthesia, spinal surgery or trauma, or intravenous drug use. No predisposing condition can be found in approximately 20% of patients.
- Damage to the spinal cord can be caused by direct compression of the spinal cord, vascular compromise, bacterial toxins, and inflammation.

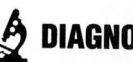 **DIAGNOSIS**

■ DIFFERENTIAL DIAGNOSIS
- Herniated disc
- Vertebral osteomyelitis and diskitis
- Metastic tumors
- Meningitis

■ LABORATORY TESTS
- WBC may be normal or elevated.
- ESR usually elevated over 30 mm/hr.
- Blood cultures are positive in approximately 60% of patients with SEA.
- CSF cultures positive in 19%, but lumbar puncture unnecessary, and may be contraindicated.
- Once imaging is done, CT-guided aspiration or open biopsy should be done to determine causative organism. Abscess content culture positive in 90%.

■ IMAGING STUDIES
- MRI with gadolinium is the imaging modality of choice; CT scan with contrast may show the abscess.
- CT with myelography is more sensitive for cord compression.

 TREATMENT

■ NONPHARMACOLOGIC THERAPY
- Surgical decompression is the mainstay of treatment. Decompression within the first 24 hr has been related to an improved prognosis.
- Nonsurgical treatment is effective in some patients, but failure rate may be excessive. This approach should not be considered in most patients.

■ ACUTE GENERAL Rx
- In addition to surgery, antibiotics directed at the most likely organism should be initiated.
- If the organism is unknown, broad coverage against staphylococci, streptococci and gram-negative bacilli should be initiated. The regimen can be adjusted according to culture results. Therapy should continue for at least 4 to 6 wk.

■ CHRONIC Rx
Neurologic deficits may remain despite aggressive treatment.

■ DISPOSITION
Irreversible paralysis and death can occur in up to 25% of patients.

■ REFERRAL
All cases should be referred to a neurosurgeon and an infectious diseases specialist.

REFERENCE
Chao D, Nanda A: Spinal epidural abscess: a diagnostic challenge, *Am Fam Physician* 65:1341, 2002.
Author: **Maurice Policar, M.D.**

BASIC INFORMATION

■ DEFINITION
Spinal stenosis is the pathologic condition compressing or narrowing the spinal canal, nerve root canal, or intervertebral foramina.

■ SYNONYMS
Central spinal stenosis
Lateral spinal stenosis
Spondylosis

ICD-9CM CODES
724.02 Spinal stenosis lumbar, lumbosacral

■ EPIDEMIOLOGY & DEMOGRAPHICS
- More common in the elderly >65 yr
- More than 30,000 patients underwent surgery for spinal stenosis in 1994

■ CLINICAL PRESENTATION & PHYSICAL FINDINGS
- Neurogenic claudication: leg, buttock, or back pain precipitated by walking and relieved by sitting
- Radicular leg pain
- Paresthesias
- Difficulty standing or lying in an erect position
- Decreased lumbar extension
- Normal peripheral pulses
- Positive Romberg
- Wide-based gait
- Reduced knee and ankle reflex
- Urine incontinence

■ ETIOLOGY
Spinal stenosis may be primary or secondary
- Primary stenosis (congenital or developmental narrowing) (Fig. 1-255)
  1. Idiopathic
  2. Achondroplasia
  3. Morquio-Ullrich syndrome
- Secondary stenosis (acquired)
  1. Degenerative (hypertrophy of the articular processes, disk degeneration, ligamentum flavum hypertrophy, spondylolisthesis)
  2. Fracture/trauma
  3. Postoperative (postlaminectomy)
  4. Paget's disease
  5. Ankylosing spondylitis
  6. Tumors
  7. Acromegaly

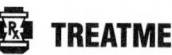

DIAGNOSIS

■ DIFFERENTIAL DIAGNOSIS
Spinal stenosis must be differentiated from other common causes of back and leg pain; osteoarthritis of the knee or hip, osteomyelitis, epidural abscess, metastatic tumors, multiple myeloma, intermittent claudication secondary to peripheral vascular disease, neuropathy, scoliosis, herniated nucleus pulposus, spondylolisthesis, acute cauda equina syndrome, ankylosing spondylitis, Reiter's syndrome, fibromyalgia.

■ WORKUP
The workup of spinal stenosis consists of a detailed history, physical examination, and specific imaging studies.

■ IMAGING STUDIES
- Lumbar spine film
- CT scan of the lumbosacral spine: sensitivity (75% to 85%), specificity (80%)
- MRI of the lumbosacral spine: sensitivity (80% to 90%), specificity (95%)
- Myelogram: sensitivity (77%), specificity (72%). Absolute stenosis is defined as the anterior-posterior (AP) diameter of the spinal canal <10 mm. Relative stenosis: 10 to 12 mm AP diameter
- CT and MRI can visualize both the central and lateral canals

Electromyography (EMG) and nerve conduction velocity (NCV) are additional studies particularly useful in differentiating peripheral neuropathy from lumbar spinal stenosis.

TREATMENT

■ NONPHARMACOLOGIC THERAPY
- Physiotherapy
- Lumbar corsets
- Back exercises
- Abdominal muscle strengthening
- Aquatic exercises

■ ACUTE GENERAL Rx
- Surgery is indicated in patients with significant compression of nerve roots as determined by MRI or CT and incapacitating symptoms limiting activities of daily living or bladder and bowel incontinence.
- Surgical procedures include decompressive laminectomy, arthrodesis, hemilaminectomy, and medial facetectomy.

■ CHRONIC Rx
- Conservative therapy with NSAIDs, (ibuprofen 800 mg PO tid, naproxen 500 mg PO bid) may be tried for symptomatic relief in addition to acetaminophen 1 g PO qid.
- Epidural steroid injections may provide temporary relief.

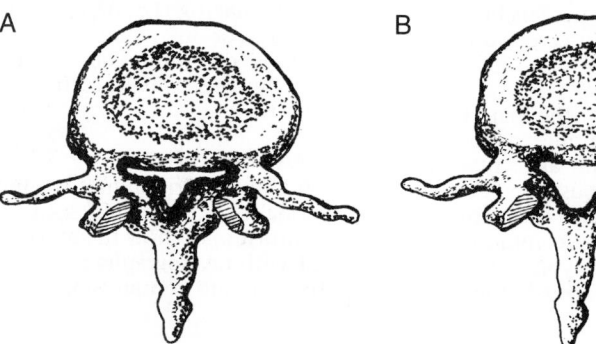

Fig. 1-255 Spinal stenosis. A, A trefoil spinal canal, with reduced diameters, is a frequent predisposing factor of spinal stenosis. Trefoil changes are present through development and become magnified from facet joint hypertrophy, ligamentum flavum hypertrophy, or other impingement mechanisms(s). **B,** A normal spinal canal. (From Canoso J: *Rheumatology in primary care,* Philadelphia, 1997, WB Saunders.)

■ DISPOSITION
- Approximately 20% of patients having surgery require repeat surgery within 10 yr. Nearly a third of the patients continue to experience pain.
- The natural history of spinal stenosis is one of slow progression. In some cases symptoms improve. Although not very common, cord compression with resultant bowel and bladder incontinence and paresis can occur.

■ REFERRAL
- Patients who have spinal stenosis should be referred to an orthopedic surgeon specializing in back surgery or to a neurosurgeon.
- Pain clinic referrals should be made if surgery is contraindicated or if the patient does not want surgery.

☼ PEARLS & CONSIDERATIONS

■ COMMENTS
Approximately a third of the patients with neurogenic claudication have co-existing peripheral vascular disease. Spinal stenosis not only is found in the elderly but also can be a common cause of chronic low back pain in the young and merits an evaluation.

REFERENCES

Fritz JM et al: Lumbar spinal stenosis: a review of current concepts in evaluation, management, and outcome measurements, *Arch Phys Med Rehabil* 79:700, 1998.

Katz JN et al: Degenerative spinal stenosis, diagnostic value of the history and physical examination, *Arthritis Rheum* 38:1236, 1995.

Katz JN et al: Seven to ten years outcome of decompressive surgery for degenerative lumbar spinal stenosis, *Spine* 21:92, 1996.

Postacchini F: Management of lumbar spinal stenosis, *J Bone Joint Surg* 78-B(1):154, 1996.

Schonstrom N, Willen J: Imaging lumbar spinal stenosis, *Radiol Clin North Am* 39(1):31, 2001.

Sheehan JM, Shaffrey CI, Jane JA: Degenerative lumbar stenosis: the neurosurgical perspective, *Clin Orthop* 384:61, 2001.

Author: **Peter Petropoulos, M.D.**

BASIC INFORMATION

DEFINITION

Spontaneous miscarriage is fetal loss before wk 20 of pregnancy, calculated from the patient's last menstrual period or the delivery of a fetus weighing <500 g. *Early loss* is before menstrual wk 12, while *late loss* refers to losses from 12 to 20 wk.

Miscarriage can also be classified as *incomplete* (partial passage of fetal tissue through partially dilated cervix), *complete* (spontaneous passage of all fetal tissue), *threatened* (uterine bleeding without cervical dilation or passage of tissue), *inevitable* (bleeding with cervical dilation without passage of fetal tissue), or *missed abortion* (intrauterine fetal demise without passage of tissue). *Recurrent miscarriage* involves three or more spontaneous pregnancy losses before wk 20.

ICD-9CM CODES
634.0 Spontaneous abortion

SYNONYMS
Abortion

EPIDEMIOLOGY & DEMOGRAPHICS
INCIDENCE: 15% to 20% of clinically recognized pregnancies, with 80% of miscarriages occurring in the first trimester

RISK FACTORS: Prior pregnancy history (risk after live birth = 5%, prior pregnancy aborted = 20% subsequent risk) is the most significant risk factor. Vaginal bleeding, especially >3 days, carries with it a 15% to 20% chance of miscarriage.

GENETICS:
- Distribution of abnormal karyotypes: autosomal trisomy (50%), monosomy 45,X (20%), triploidy (15%), tetraploidy (10%), structural chromosomal abnormalities (5%).
- With two or more spontaneous miscarriages, a karyotype should be performed to evaluate for balanced translocation, which has 80% risk for abortion, and, if the pregnancy is carried to term, has 3% to 5% risk for unbalanced karyotype.
- After 9 wk, the later in gestation, the greater the chance of a normal karyotype.

PHYSICAL FINDINGS & CLINICAL PRESENTATION
- Profuse bleeding and cramping has a higher association with miscarriage than bleeding without cramping, which is more consistent with a threatened miscarriage.
- Cervical dilation with history or finding of fetal tissue at cervical os may be present.
- In cases of missed abortion, uterine size may be smaller than menstrual dating, in contrast to molar gestation, where size may be greater than dates.

ETIOLOGY
- In a general overview the etiology can be classified in terms of maternal (environmental) and fetal (genetic) factors, with the majority of miscarriages being related to genetic or chromosomal causes
- Causes: uterine anomalies (unicornuate uterus risk = 50%, bicornuate or septate uterus risk = 25% to 30%), incompetent cervix (iatrogenic or congenital, associated with 20% of midtrimester losses), diethylstilbestrol exposure in utero (T-shaped uterus), submucous leiomyomas, intrauterine adhesions or synechiae, luteal phase or progesterone deficiency, autoimmune disease such as anticardiolipin antibodies, uncontrolled diabetes mellitus, HLA associations between mother and father, infections such as TB, *Chlamydia, Ureaplasma,* smoking and alcohol use, irradiation, and environmental toxins

DIAGNOSIS

DIFFERENTIAL DIAGNOSIS
- Normal pregnancy
- Hydatidiform molar gestation
- Ectopic pregnancy
- Dysfunctional uterine bleeding
- Pathologic endometrial or cervical lesions

WORKUP
- Because of the potential for morbid maternal sequelae, all patients with bleeding in the first trimester should have an evaluation for possible ectopic pregnancy.
- Prior pregnancy history guides the workup, such that if there are three early, prior pregnancy losses a workup and treatment for recurrent miscarriage should begin before next conception, or if there is a strong history for second-trimester loss, consideration for cerclage should be given.
- Many of the treatments require preconceptual therapy, including control of disease processes, such as diabetes, and thus a careful workup can begin after the prior pregnancy loss but before conception.

LABORATORY TESTS
- Type and antibody screen is used to evaluate for the need for Rh immune globulin.
- In circumstances in which an ectopic gestation is considered, quantitative serum hCG can be used with transvaginal sonogram to assign a level of risk; 2000 mIU/ml (third reference standard) is the discriminatory zone above which an intrauterine gestational sac should be demonstrated.
- During the preconception period, Hgb A1C, anticardiolipin antibody, lupus anticoagulant, karyotyping, endometrial biopsy with progesterone level, and cervical cultures or serum antibodies can be checked for suspected disease processes.
- Progesterone level <5 mg/dl indicates nonviable gestation vs. >25 mg/dl, which confers a good prognosis.

IMAGING STUDIES
Transabdominal or transvaginal sonogram can be used in combination with menstrual dating and serum quantitative hCG to document pregnancy location, fetal heart presence, gestational sac size, and adnexal pathology and, if used serially, can help confirm a missed abortion.

TREATMENT

■ NONPHARMACOLOGIC THERAPY

Depending on the patient's clinical status, desire to continue the pregnancy, and certainty of the diagnosis, expectancy can be considered. In pregnancies <6 wk or >14 wk, complete expulsion of fetal tissue occurs and surgical intervention such as dilation and curettage (D&C) can be avoided.

■ ACUTE GENERAL Rx

- *Incomplete miscarriage* between 6 and 14 wk can be associated with large amounts of blood loss, and thus these patients should undergo D&C.
- In cases of *missed abortion,* if fetal demise has occurred >6 wk before or gestational age is >14 wk, there is an increased risk of hypofibrinogenemia with disseminated intravascular coagulation, and thus D&C should be performed early in the disease course. Can consider use of misoprostol (Cytotec) 200 mg po q6h × 4 doses
- *Threatened abortions* may be managed expectantly, watching for signs of cervical dilation or sonographic evidence of missed abortion. Hormonal therapy, such as progesterone, is contraindicated during this time because it may increase the chance of missed abortion.
- If surgical intervention is required, preoperative use of 40 U of oxytocin (Pitocin) in 1000 ml lactated Ringer's solution may be used to decrease the amount of bleeding and shorten the operative time.
- Postoperatively all patients undergoing a D&C should receive antibiotics (doxycycline 100 mg bid for 7 days), methylergonovine (Methergine) 0.2 mg q6h for four doses, and Motrin or NSAIDs prn for pain.
- Preoperative laminaria is useful in cases of nondilated or primigravida cervices.
- In all cases of first- or second-trimester bleeding in Rh-negative patients, Rh immune globulin 300 μg should be given to prevent Rh sensitization.

■ CHRONIC Rx

Expectancy may be considered for those pregnancies <6 menstrual weeks depending on the clinical situation and the patient's desire.

■ DISPOSITION

In most cases it is important to document the resolution of the pregnancy, in terms of either a pathology specimen from a D&C or documentation of decreasing quantitative hCGs. If the pathology report does not confirm a miscarriage or the quantitative hCG value plateaus or rises after evacuation, the diagnosis of ectopic or molar gestation must be examined.

■ REFERRAL

In cases of ectopic gestation, incomplete or missed abortion, surgical evacuation of the uterus and possible laparoscopic evaluation of the adnexa should be undertaken by qualified personnel.

REFERENCES

Luise C et al: Outcome of expectant management of spontaneous first trimester miscarriage, *BMJ* 324:873, 2002.

Ness RB et al: Cocaine and tobacco use and the risks of spontaneous abortion, *N Engl J Med* 340:333, 1999.

Author: **Scott J. Zuccala, D.O.**

BASIC INFORMATION

■ DEFINITION
Sporotrichosis is a granulomatous disease caused by *Sporothrix schenckii*.

ICD-9CM CODES
117.1 Sporotrichosis

■ EPIDEMIOLOGY & DEMOGRAPHICS
PREDOMINANT SEX: The most common form, lymphocutaneous sporotrichosis, occurs equally in both sexes. Males predominate in both pulmonary and osteoarticular sporotrichosis.
PREDOMINANT AGE: Generally, lymphocutaneous sporotrichosis occurs in persons 35 yr of age or younger, and pulmonary sporotrichosis occurs in persons between the ages of 30 to 60 yr.
GENETICS:
Neonatal Infection: At least one case of transmission from the cheek lesion of the mother to the skin of the infant has been reported.

■ PHYSICAL FINDINGS & CLINICAL PRESENTATION
• Cutaneous disease
1. Arises at the site of inoculation
2. Initial lesion usually located on the distal part of an extremity, although any area may be affected, including the face
3. Variable incubation period of approximately 3 wk once introduced into the skin
4. Granulomatous reaction provoked
5. Lesion becomes papulonodular, erythematous, elastic, variable in size
6. Subsequently, nodule becomes fluctuant, undergoes central necrosis, breaks down, discharges mucoid pus from which fungus may be isolated
7. Indolent ulcer with raised erythematous or violaceous borders
8. Secondary lesions:
   a. Develop along superficial lymphatic channels
   b. Evolve in the same manner as the primary lesion, with subsequent inflammation, induration, and suppuration
• Fixed, or plaque form
1. Erythematous verrucous, ulcerated, or crusted lesions
2. Does not spread locally
3. Does not involve lymphatic vessels
4. Rarely undergoes spontaneous resolution
5. More often persists for years without systemic symptoms and within a setting of normal laboratory examinations

• Osteoarticular involvement
1. Most common extracutaneous form
2. Usually presents as monoarticular arthritis
3. Left untreated, may progress to:
   a. Synovitis
   b. Osteitis
   c. Periostitis
   d. All involving elbows, knees, wrists, and ankles
4. Joint inflamed
   a. Associated with an effusion
   b. Painful on motion
• Early pulmonary disease
1. Usually associated with a paucity of clinical findings
   a. Low-grade fever
   b. Cough
   c. Fatigue
   d. Malaise
   e. Weight loss
2. Untreated
   a. Cavitary pulmonary disease
   b. Frank pulmonary dysfunction
3. Meningitis uncommon
   a. Except perhaps in the immunocompromised patient
   b. Presents with few signs or symptoms of neurologic involvement
4. Few reported cases
   a. Infection of the ocular adnexa
   b. Endophthalmitis without antecedent trauma
   c. Infection of the testes and epididymis

■ ETIOLOGY
• *Sporothrix schenckii*
1. Global in distribution
2. Often isolated from soil, plants, and plant products
3. Majority of case reports from tropical and subtropical regions of the Americas
• Occupational or recreational exposure
1. Hay
2. Straw
3. Sphagnum moss
4. Timber
5. Thorny plants (e.g., roses and barberry bushes)
• Animal contact
1. Armadillos
2. Cats
3. Squirrels
• Human-to-human transmission
• Tattooing

DIAGNOSIS

■ DIFFERENTIAL DIAGNOSIS
• Fixed, or plaque, sporotrichosis
1. Bacterial pyoderma
2. Foreign body granuloma
3. Tularemia
4. Anthrax

5. Other mycoses: blastomycosis, chromoblastomycosis
• Lymphocutaneous sporotrichosis
1. *Nocardia brasiliensis*
2. *Leishmania braziliensis*
3. Atypical mycobacterial disease: *M. marinum, M. kansasii*
• Pulmonary sporotrichosis
1. Pulmonary TB
2. Histoplasmosis
3. Coccidioidomycoses
• Osteoarticular sporotrichosis
1. Pigmented villonodular synovitis
2. Gout
3. Rheumatoid arthritis
4. Infection with *M. tuberculosis*
5. Atypical mycobacteria: *M. marinum, M. kansasii, M. avium-intra-cellulare*
• Meningitis
1. Histoplasmosis
2. Cryptococcosis
3. TB

■ WORKUP
• The diagnosis should be considered in individuals who are occupationally exposed to soil, decaying plant matter, and thorny plants (gardeners, horticulturists, farmers) who present with chronic nonhealing ulcers or lesions with or without associated arthritis or pulmonary symptoms.
• Diagnosis is made by culture:
1. Pus
2. Joint fluid
3. Sputum
4. Blood
5. Skin biopsy
• Isolation of the fungus from any site is considered diagnostic of infection.
• Saprophytic colonization of the respiratory tract has been described.
• A positive blood culture may indicate infection in an immunocompromised host.
• Increasingly sensitive laboratory culturing systems may detect the fungus in the normal host.
• Biopsy specimens are diagnostic if characteristic cigar-shaped, round, oval, or budding yeast forms are seen.
• Despite special staining, the yeast may remain difficult to detect unless multiple sections are examined.
• No standard method of serologic testing is available.
• Previously described techniques have been hampered by the presence of antibody in the absence of infection.

■ LABORATORY TESTS
• CBCs and serum chemistries are generally normal.
• Elevated ESR is seen with extracutaneous disease.

- CSF analysis in meningeal disease reveals:
  1. Lymphocytic pleocytosis
  2. Elevated protein
  3. Hypoglycorrhachia
- Nested PCR assays represent future clinical modality to rapidly detect *Sporothrix schenckii.*

IMAGING STUDIES
- Chest x-ray examination: unilateral or bilateral upper lobe cavitary or noncavitary lesions
- Radiographic findings of affected joints:
  1. Loss of articular cartilage
  2. Periosteal reaction
  3. Periarticular osteopenia
  4. Cystic changes

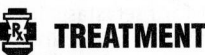 TREATMENT

NONPHARMACOLOGIC THERAPY
Local heat and prevention of bacterial superinfection in cutaneous or plaque form

ACUTE GENERAL Rx
CUTANEOUS AND LYMPHOCUTANEOUS SPOROTRICHOSIS:
- Itraconazole at doses of 100 to 200 mg/day is the drug of choice and should be given for 3 to 6 mo.
- Use saturated solution of potassium iodide (SSKI) 5 to 10 drops PO tid or 1.5 ml PO tid, gradually increasing to 40 to 50 drops PO tid or 3 ml PO tid after meals.
- Maximum tolerated dose should be continued until cutaneous lesions have resolved, approximately 6 to 12 wk.
- Adjunctive therapy with heat is useful and occasionally curative.
- Side effects:
  1. Nausea
  2. Anorexia
  3. Diarrhea
  4. Parotid or lacrimal gland hypertrophy
  5. Acneiform rash

DEEP-SEATED MYCOSES (E.G., OSTEOARTICULAR, NONCAVITARY PULMONARY DISEASE)
- Itraconazole
  1. Appropriate initial chemotherapy
  2. Probably as effective as amphotericin B
  3. Less toxic than amphotericin B
  4. Better tolerated than ketoconazole

5. 100 to 200 mg bid for 1 to 2 yr with continued lifelong suppressive therapy in selected patients
6. Absence of relapses from 40 to 68 mo has been documented when at least 200 mg/day administered for 24 mo
7. Insufficient data for use in disseminated disease (e.g., fungemia and meningitis)
- Parenteral amphotericin B, total course of 2 to 2.5 g or more, results in cure in approximately two thirds of cases
  1. Relapses are common.
  2. Amphotericin B–resistant isolates of *Sporothrix schenckii* have been reported.
  3. Remains the drug of choice for severely ill patients with disseminated disease.
  4. In cavitary pulmonary disease, given perioperatively as an adjunct to surgical resection.
  5. In meningitis, amphotericin B may be used alone or in combination with 5-fluorocytosine.
- Fluconazole
  1. Less effective than itraconazole
  2. Requires daily doses of 400 mg/day for lymphocutaneous disease and 800 mg/day for visceral or osteoarticular disease

CHRONIC Rx
For lymphocutaneous and visceral disease, therapy with itraconazole 200 mg/day for periods of 24 mo or greater

DISPOSITION
- Prognosis for cutaneous disease is good.
- Prognosis is less satisfactory for extracutaneous disease, especially if associated with abnormal immunologic states or other underlying systemic diseases.

REFERRAL
To surgeon; with an established diagnosis of pulmonary sporotrichosis, cavitary lesions require resection of involved tissue

PEARLS & CONSIDERATIONS

COMMENTS
- In patients with underlying immunosuppression (e.g., hematologic malignancy or infection with HIV), progression of the initial infection may develop into multifocal extracutaneous sporotrichosis.

- In this subset of patients, dissemination of cutaneous lesions is accompanied by hematogenous spread to lungs, bone, mucous membranes, CNS.
- Osteoarticular and pulmonary manifestations predominate with the development of polyarticular arthritis and osteolytic bone lesions.
- In the absence of therapy, the infection is ultimately fatal.
- Patients with underlying immunosuppressive states should be carefully evaluated even when presenting with single cutaneous lesions.
- Diagnostic modalities should include:
  1. Radiographic examination of chest
  2. Technetium pyrophosphate bone scan
  3. Culture of synovial fluid, blood, skin lesion(s)
- In patients with AIDS, itraconazole appears to be the drug of choice, although meningitis and pulmonary disease may warrant the use of amphotericin B.
- In patients with AIDS, lifetime suppressive therapy with itraconazole should follow initial therapy given the potential for relapse and dissemination.

REFERENCES
Curi AL et al: Retinal granuloma caused by *Sporothrix schenckii, Am J Ophthalmol* 136(1):205, 2003.
de Lima Barros MB et al: Sporotrichosis with widespread cutaneous lesions: report of 24 cases related to transmission by domestic cats in Rio de Janeiro, Brazil, *Int J Dermatol* 42(9):677, 2003.
Gottlieb GS et al: Disseminated sporotrichosis associated with treatment with immunosuppressants and tumor necrosis factor-alpha antagonists, *Clin Infect Dis* 37(6):838, 2003.
Hu S et al: Detection of *Sporothrix schenckii* in clinical samples by a nested PCR assay, *J Clin Microbiol* 41(4):1414, 2003.
Queiroz-Telles F et al: Subcutaneous mycoses, *Infect Dis Clin North Am* 17(1):59, 2003.
Zhou CH et al: Laryngeal and respiratory tract sporotrichosis and steroid inhaler use, *Arch Pathol Lab Med* 127(7):893, 2003.

Author: **George O. Alonso, M.D.**

BASIC INFORMATION

■ DEFINITION
Squamous cell carcinoma (SCC) is a malignant tumor of the skin arising in the epithelium.

■ SYNONYMS
SCC
Skin cancer

ICD-9CM CODES
173.9 Skin neoplasm, site unspecified

■ EPIDEMIOLOGY & DEMOGRAPHICS
- SCC is the second most common cutaneous malignancy, comprising 20% of all cases of nonmelanoma skin cancer.
- Incidence is highest in lower latitudes (e.g., southern U.S., Australia).
- Male:female ratio of 2:1.
- Incidence increases with age and sun exposure.
- Average age at diagnosis is 66 yr.

■ PHYSICAL FINDINGS & CLINICAL PRESENTATION
- SCC commonly affects scalp, neck region, back of hands, superior surface of the pinna, and the lip.
- The lesion may have a scaly, erythematous macule or plaque.
- Telangiectasia, central ulceration may also be present (Fig. 1-256).

- Most SCC present as exophytic lesions that grow over a period of months.

■ ETIOLOGY
Risk factors include UVB radiation and immunosuppression (renal transplant recipients have a threefold increased risk).

DIAGNOSIS

■ DIFFERENTIAL DIAGNOSIS
- Keratoacanthomas
- Actinic keratosis
- Amelanotic melanoma
- Basal cell carcinoma
- Benign tumors
- Healing traumatic wounds
- Spindle cell tumors
- Warts

■ WORKUP
Diagnosis is made with full-thickness skin biopsy (incisional or excisional).

TREATMENT

■ ACUTE GENERAL Rx
- Electrodesiccation and curettage for small SCCs (<2 cm in diameter), superficial tumors and lesions located in extremity and trunk.

- Tumors thinner than 4 mm can be managed by simple local removal.
- Lesions between 4 and 8 mm thick or those with deep dermal invasion should be excised.
- Tumors penetrating the dermis can be treated with several modalities, including excision and Mohs' surgery, radiation therapy, and chemotherapy.
- Metastatic SCC can be treated with cryotherapy and combination of chemotherapy using 13-*cis*-retinoic acid and interferon α-2A.

■ DISPOSITION
- Survival is related to size, location, degree of differentiation, immunologic status of the patient, depth of invasion, and presence of metastases. Risk factors for metastasis include lesions on the lip or ear, increasing lesion depth, and poor cell differentiation.
- Patients whose tumors penetrate through the dermis or exceed 8 mm in thickness are at risk of tumor recurrence.
- The most common metastatic locations are regional lymph nodes, liver, and lung.
- Tumors on the scalp, forehead, ears, nose, and lips also carry a higher risk.
- SCCs originating in the lip and pinna metastasize in 10% to 20% of cases.
- Five-year survival for metastatic squamous cell carcinoma is 34%.

■ REFERRAL
Oncology referral for metastatic SCC

PEARLS & CONSIDERATIONS

■ COMMENTS
SCC arising in areas of prior radiation, thermal injury, and areas of chronic ulcers or chronic draining sinuses are more aggressive and have a higher frequency of metastases than those originating in actinic damaged skin.
Author: **Fred F. Ferri, M.D.**

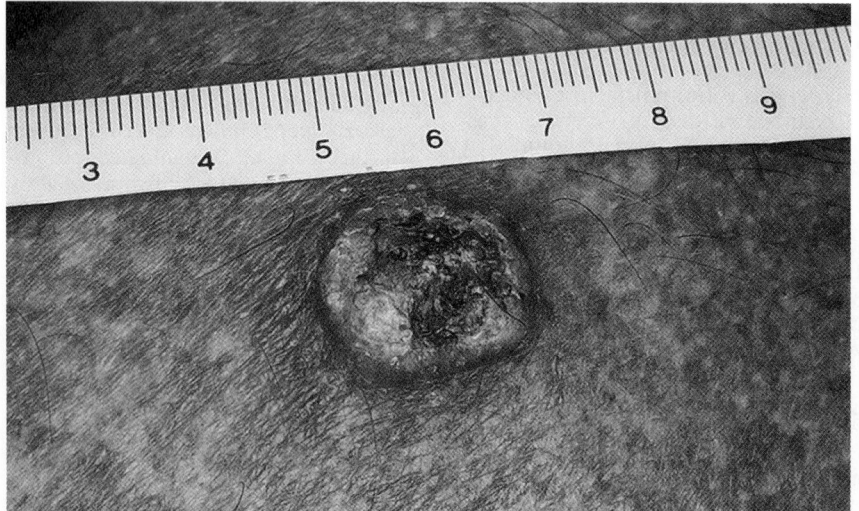

Fig. 1-256 Squamous cell carcinoma. Nodular hyperkeratotic lesion with central erosion. (From Noble J et al: *Textbook of primary care medicine,* ed 3, St Louis, 2001, Mosby.)

BASIC INFORMATION

■ DEFINITION

Stasis dermatitis refers to an inflammatory skin disease of the lower extremities, commonly seen in patients with chronic venous insufficiency. (Fig. 1-257)

ICD-9CM CODES
459.81 Stasis dermatitis

■ EPIDEMIOLOGY & DEMOGRAPHICS
- Stasis dermatitis occurs more frequently in the elderly
- Rarely seen before the age of 50 yr
- Estimated to occur in up to 6% to 7% of the patients >50 yr
- Occurs in woman more often than men, perhaps related to lower extremity venous impairment aggravated through pregnancy

■ PHYSICAL FINDINGS & CLINICAL PRESENTATION
- Insidious onset
- Pruritus
- Chronic edema usually described as "brawny" edema as stasis dermatitis pathologically is associated with dermal fibrosis
- Erythema
- Scaly
- Eczematous patches
- Commonly located over the medial malleolus
- Progressive pigment changes can occur as a result of extravasation of red blood cells and hemosiderin deposition within the cutaneous tissue.
- Secondary infections can occur

■ ETIOLOGY
- Stasis dermatitis is thought to occur as a direct result from any insult or injury of the lower extremity venous system leading to venous insufficiency including:
  1. Deep vein thrombosis
  2. Trauma
  3. Pregnancy
  4. Vein stripping
  5. Vein harvesting in patients requiring coronary artery bypass grafting (CABG)

- Venous insufficiency subsequently results in venous hypertension, causing skin inflammation and the aforementioned physical findings and clinical presentation.

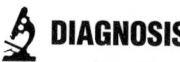 **DIAGNOSIS**

The diagnosis of stasis dermatitis is primarily made by a detailed history and physical examination.

■ DIFFERENTIAL DIAGNOSIS
- Contact dermatitis
- Atopic dermatitis
- Cellulitis
- Tinea dermatophyte infection
- Pretibial myxedema
- Nummular eczema
- Lichen simplex chronicus
- Xerosis
- Asteatotic eczema
- Deep vein thrombosis

■ WORKUP
The workup of a patient with stasis dermatitis is directed at excluding potential life-threatening causes (e.g., deep vein thrombosis) and complications (e.g., cellulites and sepsis).

■ LABORATORY TESTS
Blood tests are generally not very helpful unless a secondary infection is present.

■ IMAGING STUDIES
- X-rays, CT scans, and MRIs are generally not very helpful.
- Doppler studies are indicated in any patient suspected of having a deep vein thrombosis.

RX **TREATMENT**

■ NONPHARMACOLOGIC THERAPY
- Leg elevation
- Compression stocking with a gradient of at least 30 to 40 mm Hg
- For weeping skin lesions, wet to dry dressing changes are helpful

■ ACUTE GENERAL Rx
- In patients with acute stasis dermatitis, a compression (Unna) boot can be applied. An Unna boot consists of a roll of gauze that is saturated with zinc oxide ointment supported with an elastic wrap.
- Topical corticosteroid creams or ointments (e.g., triamcinolone 0.1% bid) are used frequently to help reduce inflammation and itching.
- Secondary infections should be treated with appropriate antibiotics. Most secondary infections are the result of *Staphylococcus* or *Streptococcus* organisms, thus dicloxacillin 250 mg qid, cephalexin 250 mg qid or levofloxacin 250 mg qd are appropriate antibiotics of choice.

■ CHRONIC Rx
- Patients with chronic stasis dermatitis can be treated with topical emollients (e.g., white petrolatum, lanolin, Eucerin).
- Topical dressings (e.g., DuoDerm) are effective in the treatment of chronic venous stasis ulcers.

■ DISPOSITION
- The mainstay of treatment of stasis dermatitis is to control leg edema and prevent venous stasis ulcers from developing.
- Chronic venous stasis ulcers may take months to heal and may require skin grafting.

■ REFERRAL
- Dermatology referral is made if the diagnosis is unclear.
- Vascular surgery referral is made for assistance in the management of chronic venous insufficiency and chronic venous stasis ulcers.

☼ PEARLS & CONSIDERATIONS

■ COMMENTS
Inflammatory skin changes from stasis dermatitis are thought to result from poor oxygen perfusion to the lower-extremity skin tissue. Various theories, including venous pooling, arteriovenous shunting, increased venous hydrostatic pressure affecting microcirculation, fibrin barriers preventing oxygen diffusion, and leukocyte trapping with resultant microvascular damage, have all been hypothesized as causes of stasis dermatitis.

REFERENCES
Flugman SL et al: Stasis dermatitis, www.emedicine.com.
Yuwono HS: Diagnosis and treatment in the management of chronic venous insufficiency, *Clin Hemorheol Microcirc* 23(2-4):233, 2000.
Author: **Peter Petropoulos, M.D.**

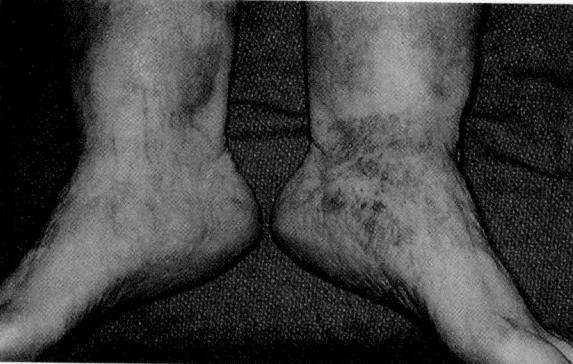

Fig. 1-257 Moderate stasis dermatitis with hyperpigmentation and bilateral venous insufficiency. (Courtesy Department of Dermatology, University of North Carolina at Chapel Hill. From Goldstein BG, Goldstein AO: *Practical dermatology,* ed 2, St Louis, 1997, Mosby.)

BASIC INFORMATION

■ DEFINITION

The term *status epilepticus* refers to continuous seizure activity lasting at least 5 min, or two or more discrete seizures between which there is incomplete recovery of consciousness.

ICD-9CM CODES
345.3 Grand mal status

■ EPIDEMIOLOGY & DEMOGRAPHICS
INCIDENCE (IN U.S.): 100,000 to 152,000 cases per year
PREDOMINANT SEX: Male = female
GENETICS: Familial predisposition is rare.

■ PHYSICAL FINDINGS & CLINICAL PRESENTATION
• Patients are typically unresponsive and usually have obvious tonic, clonic, or tonic-clonic movements of the extremities (convulsive status epilepticus).
• Some patients are unresponsive or have an altered level of consciousness with no clear observable repetitive motor activity (nonconvulsive status epilepticus).
• Clinical manifestations can evolve and can become subtle with only small amplitude twitching movements of the face, limbs, or eyes.

■ ETIOLOGY
• Preexisting epilepsy with breakthrough seizures or low anticonvulsant drug levels
• CNS infection or tumor
• Drug toxicity or metabolic disturbance
• Hypoxia
• Head trauma
• Stroke

DIAGNOSIS

■ DIFFERENTIAL DIAGNOSIS
• Coma
• Encephalopathic states
• Psychogenic unresponsiveness

■ WORKUP
Because convulsive status epilepticus is an emergency with substantial morbidity and mortality, treatment must be early and aggressive, not postponed until an etiology is determined.

■ LABORATORY TESTS
• While treatment is being initiated: glucose, electrolytes, BUN, ABG, drug levels, CBC, UA, toxicology screen
• Lumbar puncture in children with fever and adults suspected to have meningitis

■ IMAGING STUDIES
Unless the etiology is known, CT or MRI of the brain is recommended as soon as possible after seizures have been controlled.

TREATMENT

■ NONPHARMACOLOGIC THERAPY
• Give oxygen by nasal cannula or nonrebreathing mask.
• Maintain blood pressure.
• Maintain body temperature.
• Monitor ECG.
• Obtain IV access.

■ ACUTE GENERAL Rx
• Thiamine 100 mg IV and glucose 50 mg D_{50} by IV push (2 ml/kg D_{25} in children) unless hyperglycemic
• Lorazepam 0.1 mg/kg IV at 2 mg/min
• If seizures persist, phosphenytoin 20 mg/kg IV at 150 mg/min (if not available, use phenytoin 20 mg/kg IV at up to 50 mg/min as tolerated)
• If seizures persist, phenobarbital 20 mg/kg IV at 50-75 mg/min; will likely require intubation
• If seizures persist, emergency neurologic consultation for management of additional doses of phenobarbital and/or general anesthesia with midazolam, propofol, or pentobarbital

■ CHRONIC Rx
Chronic treatment with anticonvulsants is indicated if there is significant risk of recurrence (i.e., known epilepsy, brain lesion, epileptiform EEG abnormalities).

■ DISPOSITION
• Favorable if status is treated promptly and there is no underlying acute symptomatic cause such as an underlying CNS lesion or systemic metabolic insult.
• Overall mortality is 22%; higher in the elderly (38%) and substantially lower in children (2.5%). Difference in mortality is mainly because status epilepticus in the elderly is more often the result of an acute symptomatic cause.

■ REFERRAL
If seizures do not respond to initial management as outlined, or if the patient is in nonconvulsive status epilepticus, because there is debate regarding the need for aggressive management

PEARLS & CONSIDERATIONS

■ COMMENTS
• Because of varied clinical presentations of status epilepticus, there is no clinical basis for being certain that seizures have stopped unless the patient regains full consciousness.
• EEG provides definitive information about seizure cessation. If available, use of EEG in the management of status epilepticus is recommended highly.

REFERENCES
Logroscino G et al: Long-term mortality after a first episode of status epilepticus, *Neurology* 58:537, 2002.
Lowenstein DH, Alldredge B: Status epilepticus, *N Engl J Med* 338:970, 1998.
Treiman DM et al: A comparison of four treatments for generalized convulsive status epilepticus, *N Engl J Med* 339:792, 1998.
Author: **John E. Croom, M.D., Ph.D.**

BASIC INFORMATION

DEFINITION
Stevens-Johnson syndrome (SJS) is a severe vesiculobullous form of erythema multiforme affecting skin, mouth, eyes, and genitalia.

SYNONYMS
SJS
Herpes iris
Febrile mucocutaneous syndrome

ICD-9CM CODES
695.1 Stevens-Johnson syndrome

EPIDEMIOLOGY & DEMOGRAPHICS
- SJS affects predominantly children and young adults.
- Male:female ratio of 2:1.

PHYSICAL FINDINGS & CLINICAL PRESENTATION
- The cutaneous eruption is generally preceded by vague, nonspecific symptoms of low-grade fever and fatigue occurring 1 to 14 days before the skin lesions. Cough is often present. Fever may be high during the active stages.
- Bullae generally occur on the conjunctiva, mucous membranes of the mouth, nares, and genital regions.
- Corneal ulcerations may result in blindness.
- Ulcerative stomatitis results in hemorrhagic crusting.
- Flat, atypical target lesions or purpuric maculae may be distributed on the trunk or be widespread (Fig. 1-258).

- The pain from oral lesions may compromise fluid intake and result in dehydration.
- Thick, mucopurulent sputum and oral lesions may interfere with breathing.

ETIOLOGY
- Drugs (e.g., phenytoin, penicillins, phenobarbital, sulfonamides) are the most common cause.
- Upper respiratory tract infections (e.g., *Mycoplasma pneumoniae*) and herpes simplex viral infections have also been implicated in SJS.

DIAGNOSIS

DIFFERENTIAL DIAGNOSIS
- Toxic erythema (drugs or infection)
- Pemphigus
- Pemphigoid
- Urticaria
- Hemorrhagic fevers
- Serum sickness
- *Staphylococcus* scalded-skin syndrome
- Behçet's syndrome

WORKUP
- Diagnosis is generally based on clinical presentation and characteristic appearance of the lesions.
- Skin biopsy is generally reserved for when classic lesions are absent and diagnosis is uncertain.

LABORATORY TESTS
CBC with differential, cultures in cases of suspected infection

IMAGING STUDIES
Chest x-ray examination may show patchy changes in patients with pulmonary involvement.

TREATMENT

NONPHARMACOLOGIC THERAPY
- Withdrawal of any potential drug precipitants
- Careful skin nursing to prevent secondary infection

ACUTE GENERAL Rx
- Treatment of associated conditions, (e.g., acyclovir for herpes simplex virus infection, erythromycin for mycoplasma infection)
- Antihistamines for pruritus
- Treatment of the cutaneous blisters with cool, wet Burow's compresses
- Relief of oral symptoms by frequent rinsing with lidocaine (Xylocaine Viscous)
- Liquid or soft diet with plenty of fluids to ensure proper hydration
- Treatment of secondary infections with antibiotics
- Corticosteroids: use remains controversial; when used, prednisone 20 to 30 mg bid until new lesions no longer appear, then rapidly tapered
- Topical steroids: may use to treat papules and plaques; however, should not be applied to eroded areas
- Vitamin A: may be used for lacrimal hyposecretion

DISPOSITION
- Prognosis varies with severity of disease. It is generally good in patients with limited disease; however, mortality may approach 10% in patients with extensive involvement.
- Oral lesions may continue for several months.
- Scarring and corneal abnormalities may occur in 20% of patients.

REFERRAL
- Hospital admission in a unit used for burn care is recommended in severe cases.
- Urethral involvement may necessitate catheterization.
- Ocular involvement should be monitored by an ophthalmologist.

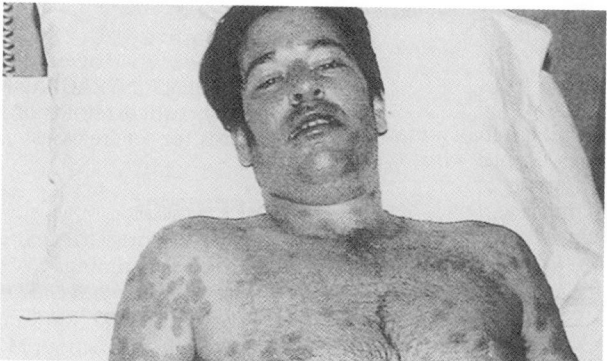

Fig. 1-258   Stevens-Johnson syndrome. (From Stein JH: *Internal medicine*, ed 5, St Louis, 1998, Mosby.)

PEARLS & CONSIDERATIONS

COMMENTS
Risk of recurrence of SJS is 30% to 40%.
Author: **Fred F. Ferri, M.D.**

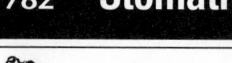 **BASIC INFORMATION**

■ **DEFINITION**

Stomatitis is inflammation involving the oral mucous membranes.

■ **SYNONYMS**

Heterogeneous grouping of unrelated illnesses, each with their own designation(s)

ICD-9CM CODES
528.0 Stomatitis
054.2 (herpetic)
528.2 (aphthous)
112.0 (monilial)

■ **CLASSIFICATION**

WHITE LESIONS: Candidiasis (thrush)
Caused by yeast infection (Candida albicans)
Examination: white, curdlike material that when wiped off leaves a raw bleeding surface
Epidemiology: seen in the very young and the very old, those with immunodeficiency (AIDS, cancer), persons with diabetes, and patients treated with antibacterial agents
Other
- Leukoedema: filmy opalescent-appearing mucosa, which can be reverted to normal appearance by stretching. This condition is benign.
- White sponge nevus: thick, white corrugated folds involving the buccal mucosa. Appears in childhood as an autosomal dominant trait. Benign condition.
- Darier's disease (keratosis follicularis): white papules on the gingivae, alveolar mucosa, and dorsal tongue. Skin lesions also present (erythematous papules). Inherited as an autosomal dominant trait.
- Chemical injury: white sloughing mucosa.
- Nicotine stomatitis: whitened palate with red papules.
- Lichen planus: linear, reticular, slightly raised striae on buccal mucosa. Skin is involved by pruritic violaceous papules on forearms and inner thighs.
- Discoid lupus erythematosus: lesion resembles lichen planus.
- Leukoplakia: white lesions that cannot be scraped off; 20% are premalignant epithelial dysplasia or squamous cell carcinoma.
- Hairy leukoplakia: shaggy white surface that cannot be wiped off; seen in HIV infection, caused by EBV.

RED LESIONS:
- Candidiasis may present with red instead of the more frequent white lesion (see "White Lesions"). Median rhomboid glossitis is a chronic variant.
- Benign migratory glossitis (geographic tongue): area of atrophic depapillated mucosa surrounded by a keratotic border. Benign lesion, no treatment required.
- Hemangiomas.
- Histoplasmosis: ill-defined irregular patch with a granulomatous surface, sometimes ulcerated.
- Allergy.
- Anemia: atrophic reddened glossal mucosa seen with pernicious anemia.
- Erythroplakia: red patch usually caused by epithelial dysplasia or squamous cell carcinoma.
- Burning tongue (glossopyrosis): normal examination; sometimes associated with denture trauma, anemia, diabetes, vitamin B_{12} deficiency, psychogenic problems.

DARK LESIONS (BROWN, BLUE, BLACK):
- Coated tongue: accumulation of keratin; harmless condition that can be treated by scraping
- Melanotic lesions: freckles, lentigines, lentigo, melanoma, Peutz-Jeghers syndrome, Addison's disease
- Varices
- Kaposi's sarcoma: red or purple macules that enlarge to form tumors; seen in patients with AIDS

RAISED LESIONS:
- Papilloma
- Verruca vulgaris
- Condyloma acuminatum
- Fibroma
- Epulis
- Pyogenic granuloma
- Mucocele
- Retention cyst

BLISTERS:
- Primary herpetic gingivostomatitis
Caused by herpes simplex virus type 1 or less frequently type 2
Course: day 1—malaise, fever, headache, sore throat, cervical lymphadenopathy; days 2 and 3—appearance of vesicles that develop into painful ulcers of 2 to 4 mm in diameter; duration of up to 2 wk
Recurrent intraoral herpes: rare, recurrences typically involve only the keratinized epithelium (lips)

- Pemphigus and pemphigoid
- Hand-foot-mouth disease: caused by coxsackievirus group A
- Erythema multiforme
- Herpangina: caused by echovirus
- Traumatic ulcer
- Primary syphilis
- Perlèche (or angular cheilitis)
- Recurrent aphthous stomatitis (canker sores)
- Behçet's syndrome (aphthous ulcers, uveitis, genital ulcerations, arthritis, and aseptic meningitis)
- Reiter's syndrome (conjunctivitis, urethritis, and arthritis with occasional oral ulcerations)
- Unknown cause
Course: solitary or multiple painful ulcers may develop simultaneously and heal over 10 to 14 days. The size of the lesions and the frequency of recurrences are variable.

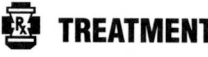 **DIAGNOSIS**

WHITE LESIONS: Candidiasis (thrush) diagnosis: ovoid yeast and hyphae seen in scrapings treated with KOH culture
BLISTERS:
- Exfoliative cytology
- Viral culture
- Immunofluorescence for herpes antigen

TREATMENT

WHITE LESIONS: Candidiasis (thrush) treatment:
- Topical with nystatin or clotrimazole
- Systemic with ketoconazole or fluconazole
BLISTERS:
- Supportive
- Consider acyclovir
RECURRENT INTRAORAL HERPES:
Topical corticosteroids or systemic steroids for severe cases

REFERENCE

Allen CM, Blozis GG: Oral mucosal lesions. In Cummings CW (ed): Otolaryngology: head and neck surgery, ed 2, St Louis, 1992, Mosby.
Author: **Tom J. Wachtel, M.D.**

BASIC INFORMATION

■ **DEFINITION**

Strabismus is a condition of the eyes in which the visual axes of the eyes are not straight in the primary position or in which the eyes do not follow each other in the different positions of gaze.

■ **SYNONYMS**

Esotropia
Exotropia
Restrictive eye movement

ICD-9CM CODES

378.9 Strabismus

■ **EPIDEMIOLOGY & DEMOGRAPHICS**

INCIDENCE (IN U.S.): 2% of all children
PREDOMINANT SEX: None
PREDOMINANT AGE: Birth to 5 yr of age
PEAK INCIDENCE: Childhood
GENETICS: None known

■ **PHYSICAL FINDINGS & CLINICAL PRESENTATION**

Conjugate gaze loss in both eyes with the eyes focusing independently (Fig. 1-259)

■ **ETIOLOGY**

• Most cases are congenital.
• Rarely, there is neurologic disease or severe refractive errors.

 DIAGNOSIS

■ **DIFFERENTIAL DIAGNOSIS**

• Refractive errors
• CNS tumors
• Orbital tumors
• Brain and CNS dysfunction

■ **WORKUP**

• Eye examination
• Visual field

■ **LABORATORY TESTS**

Generally not needed

■ **IMAGING STUDIES**

Necessary only if other neurologic findings are found

R **TREATMENT**

■ **NONPHARMACOLOGIC THERAPY**

• Glasses
• Patching
• Prisms

■ **CHRONIC Rx**

• Glasses
• Alternate eye patching
• Surgery

■ **DISPOSITION**

• The earlier the condition is treated, the more likely it is that the child will have normal vision in both eyes.
• After age 5 yr, visual loss is usually permanent.

■ **REFERRAL**

• If surgery is contemplated
• To an ophthalmologist for management (usually)

☼ **PEARLS & CONSIDERATIONS**

■ **COMMENTS**

• If properly treated, this easily recognizable and treatable condition results in normal vision.
• If not treated, this condition can result in decrease in vision in one eye (amblyopia).

REFERENCES

Kushmer BJ: Recently acquired diploxin in adults with long-standing strabismus, *Arch Ophth* 119(12):1795, 2001.
Rubin SE: Management of strabismus in the first year of life, *Pediatr Ann* 30(8):474, 2001.
Ziakas NG: A study of heredity as a risk factor in strabismus eye, 16(5):519, 2002.

Author: **Melvyn Koby, M.D.**

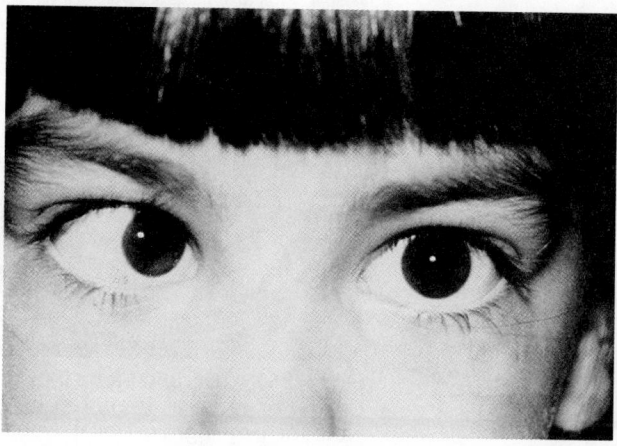
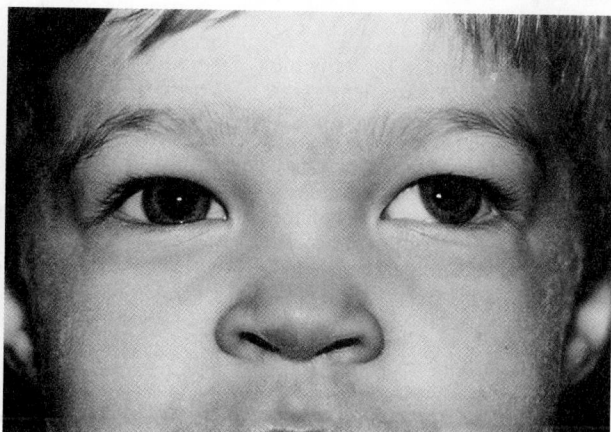

Fig. 1-259   **A,** Note the nasal deviation of the right eye with the corneal light reflection temporally displaced on the right eye and centered in the left pupil, indicating an esotropia. **B,** Divergent strabismus of the left eye, defining an exotropia. (From Hodkelman [ed]: *Primary pediatric care,* ed 3, St Louis, 1997, Mosby.)

BASIC INFORMATION

■ DEFINITION
Stroke describes acute brain injury caused by decreased blood supply or hemorrhage.

■ SYNONYMS
Cerebrovascular accident (CVA)

ICD-9CM CODES
436 Acute stroke

■ EPIDEMIOLOGY & DEMOGRAPHICS
INCIDENCE (IN U.S.):
- Occurs in 5 to 10/100,000 persons <40 yr of age
- Occurs in 10 to 20/100,000 persons >65 yr of age

PREVALENCE (IN U.S.): Estimated at 2 million persons
PREDOMINANT SEX: Incidence is 30% higher in males
PREDOMINANT AGE: 60+ yr
PEAK INCIDENCE: 80 to 84 yr

■ PHYSICAL FINDINGS & CLINICAL PRESENTATION
Motor and/or sensory and/or cognitive deficits, depending on distribution and extent of involved vascular territory. More common manifestations include contralateral motor weakness or sensory loss, as well as language difficulties (aphasia; predominantly left-sided lesions) and visuospatial/neglect phenomena (predominantly right-sided lesions). Onset is usually sudden; however, this depends on specific etiology.

■ ETIOLOGY
- 70% to 80% are caused by ischemic infarcts; 20% to 30% are hemorrhagic.
- 80% of ischemic infarcts are from occlusion of large or small vessels caused by atherosclerotic vascular disease, 15% are caused by cardiac embolism, 5% are from other causes, including hypercoagulable states and vasculitis.

- Small vessel occlusion is most often caused by lipohyalinosis precipitated by chronic hypertension.
- Risk factors for ischemic stroke are described in Box 1-20.

DIAGNOSIS

■ DIFFERENTIAL DIAGNOSIS
- TIA (Transient ischemic attack, traditionally defined as focal neurologic deficits lasting <24 hr [usually lasting <60 min])
- Migraine
- Seizure
- Mass lesion

■ WORKUP
- Thorough history and physical examination, including detailed neurologic and cardiovascular evaluation to identify vascular territory and likely etiology (Table 1-56). Infectious, toxic, and metabolic causes should be excluded because each may cause clinical deterioration of old stroke symptoms.
- Cardiac: mandatory ECG, telemetry, consider serial enzymes; transthoracic and/or transesophageal echocardiography, Holter monitor, or carotid Doppler should be seriously considered especially in setting of suspected embolic etiology.

■ LABORATORY TESTS
- CBC
- Platelet count
- PT (INR)
- PTT
- BUN, creatinine
- Lipid panel
- Glucose
- Electrolytes
- Urinalysis
- Additional tests, depending on suspected etiology (in younger patients; e.g., coagulopathies)

■ IMAGING STUDIES
- CT scan without contrast to distinguish hemorrhage from infarct (Figs. 1-260 and 1-261)

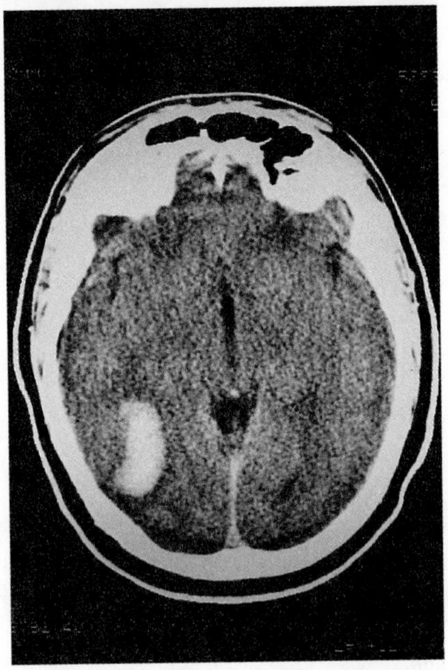

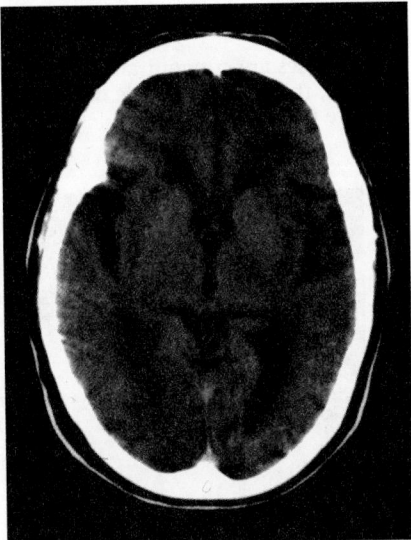

Fig. 1-260   Intracerebral hemorrhage. Noncontrast CT scan demonstrates an intracerebral hemorrhage in the right occipital lobe. (From Specht N [ed]: *Practical guide to diagnostic imaging*, St Louis, 1998, Mosby.)

Fig. 1-261   Occipital lobe infarct (posterior cerebral artery territory). Note the large right occipital hypodensity with mass effect caused by infarction and subsequent edema. (From Cwinn AA, Grahovac SZ [eds]: *Emergency CT scans of the head: a practical atlas*, St Louis, 1998, Mosby.)

BOX 1-20   Risk Factors for Ischemic Stroke

Diabetes
Hypertension
Smoking
Family history of premature vascular disease
Hyperlipidemia
Atrial fibrillation
History of transient ischemic attack (TIA)
History of recent myocardial infarction
History of congestive heart failure (left ventricular [LV] ejection fraction <25%)
Drugs (sympathomimetics, oral contraceptive pill, cocaine)

From Andreoli TE (ed): *Cecil essentials of medicine*, ed 5, Philadelphia, 2001, WB Saunders.

TABLE 1-56   Neurologic Signs Associated with Cerebrovascular Accident by Location

ARTERY AFFECTED	NEUROLOGIC SIGNS
Internal Carotid Artery	
(Supplies the cerebral hemispheres and diencephalon by the ophthalmic and ipsilateral hemisphere arteries)	Occasional unilateral blindness Severe contralateral hemiplegia, hemianesthesia, and hemianopia Profound aphasia if left hemisphere involved
Middle Cerebral Artery	
(Supplies structures of higher cerebral processes of communication; language interpretation; perception and interpretation of space, sensation, form, and voluntary movement)	Alterations in communication, cognition, mobility, and sensation Homonymous hemianopia Contralateral hemiplegia or hemiparesis
Anterior Cerebral Artery	
(Supplies medial surfaces and upper convexities of frontal and parietal lobes and medial surface of hemisphere, which includes motor and somesthetic cortex serving the legs)	Emotional lability Confusion, amnesia, personality changes Urinary incontinence Impaired mobility, with weakness greater in lower extremities than in upper
Posterior Cerebral Artery	
(Supplies medial and inferior temporal lobes, medial occipital lobe, thalamus, posterior hypothalamus, and visual receptive area)	Homonymous hemianopia Hemianesthesia Cortical blindness Memory deficits
Vertebral or Basilar Arteries	
(Supply the brainstem and cerebellum) Incomplete occlusion	Drop attacks Unilateral and bilateral weakness of extremities Diplopia, homonymous hemianopia Nausea, vertigo, tinnitus, and syncope Dysphagia Dysarthria Sometimes confusion and drowsiness
Anterior portion of pons	"Locked-in" syndrome—no movement except eyelids; sensation and consciousness preserved
Complete occlusion or hemorrhage	Coma Miotic pupils Decerebrate rigidity Respiratory and circulatory abnormalities Death
Posterior Inferior Cerebellar Artery	
(Supplies the lateral and posterior portion of the medulla)	Wallenberg syndrome Dysphagia, dysphonia Ipsilateral anesthesia of face and cornea for pain and temperature (touch preserved) Ipsilateral Horner syndrome Contralateral loss of pain and temperature sensation in trunk and extremities Ipsilateral decompensation of movement (cerebellar signs)
Anterior Inferior and Superior Cerebellar Arteries	
(Supply the cerebellum)	Difficulty in articulation, swallowing, gross movements of limbs; nystagmus (cerebellar signs)
Anterior Spinal Artery	
(Supplies the anterior spinal cord)	Flaccid paralysis, below level of lesion Loss of pain, touch, temperature sensation (proprioception preserved, sensory level)
Posterior Spinal Artery	
(Supplies the posterior spinal cord)	Sensory loss, particularly proprioception, vibration, touch, and pressure (movement preserved)

Adapted from Seidel HM (ed): *Mosby's guide to physical examination,* ed 4, St Louis, 1999, Mosby.

- An MRI is superior to CT in identifying abnormalities in the posterior fossa and, in particular, lacunar (small vessel) infarcts. Diffusion weighted imaging (DWI) is best to determine hyperacute ischemia (positive within 15-30 min of symptom onset). MRA is recommended to help identify vascular pathology (e.g., extent of intracranial atherosclerosis or vascular distribution of ischemia)
- In select cases (e.g., hemorrhagic stroke), conventional angiography may identify aneurysms or other vascular malformations

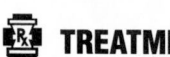 **TREATMENT**

■ **NONPHARMACOLOGIC THERAPY**
- To prevent pulmonary emboli, above-the-knee elastic stockings, pneumatic boots, or SQ Heparin if nonhemorrhagic etiology and patient is immobile in bed
- Carotid endarterectomy (CEA) is recommended in patients with carotid territory stroke associated with 70% to 99% ipsilateral carotid stenosis, performed by an experienced surgeon who has demonstrated low morbidity and mortality

- Modification of risk factors (e.g., smoking cessation, exercise, diet)

■ **ACUTE GENERAL Rx**
- Box 1-21 describes initial considerations for patients with stroke.
- Judicious control of blood pressure; patients with chronic hypertension may extend the area of infarction if the blood pressure is lowered into the "normal" range. It is best not to lower blood pressure too aggressively in the acute setting unless it is very markedly elevated. Adequate hydration and bed rest (e.g., head of bed down in pressure dependent ischemia vs. head of bed up if patient is aspiration risk). Tight glycemic control is also recommended (e.g., sliding scale insulin).
- Patients presenting <3 hr after onset of a nonhemorrhagic stroke, thrombolytic therapy in a specialized stroke center is beneficial in selected populations.

■ **ACUTE SPECIFIC Rx**
- Depends on several factors, including etiology, vascular territory involved, risk factors, and elapsed time from symptom onset to arrival at hospital.

- Box 1-22 describes criteria for thrombolytic therapy in patients with thromboembolic stroke (IV tPA inclusion criteria includes clearly defined symptom onset within 3 hr of onset of treatment, measurable deficit with NIH Stroke Scale >4, and no evidence for bleed on neuroimaging).
- If atrial fibrillation and/or a cardiac mural thrombus is found on echocardiography, heparin may be considered.
- If a subarachnoid or intracerebral hemorrhage is found on CT, MR angiography and/or cerebral angiography may be indicated to identify aneurysm. If no aneurysm is found and clot is expanding, neurosurgical evacuation of clot may be attempted, but outcomes are generally poor.
- In select cases of patients presenting >3 hr but <6 hr, an *interventional* neuroradiologist or neurosurgeon may be able to offer either direct injection of a clot-busting agent (such as intraarterial tPA) or direct extraction of the clot. However, this remains investigational and yet has to be studied in the setting of a controlled trial. Intracranial angioplasty/stenting may also be a consideration.

BOX 1-21   Initial Considerations for Patients with Strokes

Initial care
    Stabilize the patient, secure the airway, and provide adequate oxygenation
    Assess level of consciousness, language, visual fields, eye movements, and pupillary movements
    Obtain history and perform physical examination
    Perform CT of head without contrast
    Obtain CBC with platelets and differential, electrolytes, creatinine, BUN, glucose, PT/PTT, arterial blood gas, or oxygen saturation
    Consider a toxicology screen
    Consider special coagulation studies such as antiphospholipid antibodies, factor V Leiden assay, protein C and protein S, antithrombin III, ANA, fibrinogen, RPR, homocysteine, serum protein electrophoresis
Consider acute intervention with t-PA if symptoms for less than 3 hr
Consider the following with admission orders
    Transthoracic echocardiogram (consider transesophageal echocardiogram if transthoracic echocardiogram is equivocal or there is a high suspicion of cardiogenic thromboembolism)
    Carotid duplex ultrasonography
    Telemetry
    Supplemental oxygen and appropriate oxygen saturation monitoring
    Antiplatelet therapy
    Fluid restriction if infarct is large, to reduce cerebral edema
    Close monitoring of intake and output
    Regular determinations of blood glucose levels to avoid hyperglycemia
    NPO if there are concerns about the pharyngeal reflex pending swallowing evaluation
    Elevate the head of the bed 20-30 degrees to reduce cerebral edema
    Bed rest for the first 24 hr with fall precautions, then advance as appropriate
    Vital signs and neurologic checks every 2 hr times four until stable
    Prophylaxis for DVT if immobile (elastic stockings at a minimum)
    Speech therapy consultation to evaluate swallowing
    Neurology, physical therapy, occupational therapy, nutrition, and social services consultations

From Rakel RE (ed): *Principles of family practice*, ed 6, Philadelphia, 2002, WB Saunders.
ANA, Antinuclear antibodies; *BUN,* blood urea nitrogen; *CBC,* complete blood count; *CT,* computed tomography; *DVT,* deep vein thrombosis; *NPO,* nothing by mouth; *PT/PTT,* cerothrombin time/partial thromboplastin time; *RPR,* rapid plasma reagin; *t-PA,* tissue plasminogen activator.

■ CHRONIC Rx

- Antiplatelet therapy (aspirin, dipyridamole/aspirin [Aggrenox], clopidogrel [Plavix], or ticlopidine) reduces the risk of subsequent stroke.
- If patient presents with first TIA/stroke and was on no prior antiplatelet agent, aspirin (325 mg vs. 81 mg each day) is usually chosen initially. Another agent may be added later if another event occurs. Coumadin is usually reserved for patients with cardioembolic stroke.
- Warfarin for patients with atrial fibrillation or cardiogenic embolism.

■ DISPOSITION

Prognosis depends on severity of deficits, etiology, and other concurrent medical/surgical illness. A polymodality physical medicine and rehabilitative approach is an integral part of poststroke recovery. This includes physical, occupational, and speech therapy individualized depending on deficits.

■ REFERRAL

- Neurology/neurosurgical referral depending on etiology and resources available; depending on time of symptom onset, transfer of patient to institution able to provide more specific acute treatment is recommended
- Vascular surgery if patient is candidate for CEA

REFERENCES

American Heart Association Scientific Statement: Primary prevention of ischemic stroke: a statement for health care professionals from the stroke council of the American Heart Association, *Circulation* 103:167, 2001.

Barnett HJM: A modern approach to posterior circulation ischemic stroke, *Arch Neurol* 59:359, 2002.

Benevante D, Hart RG: Stroke: management of acute ischemic stroke, *Am Fam Physician* 59:2828, 1999.

Caplan LR: Stroke treatment: promising but still struggling, *JAMA* 279:1304, 1998.

Green DM et al: Serum potassium level and dietary potassium intake as risk factors for stroke, *Neurology* 59:314, 2002.

Halperin JL, Fuster V: Patent foramen ovale and recurrent stroke: another paradoxical twist, *Circulation* 105:2580, 2002.

Meschia JF et al: Thrombolytic treatment of acute ischemic stroke, *Mayo Clin Proc* 77:542, 2002.

Qureshi A et al: Spontaneous intracranial hemorrhage, *N Engl J Med* 344:1450, 2001.

Sacco RL et al: High-density lipoprotein cholesterol and ischemic stroke in the elderly, *JAMA* 285:2729, 2001.

Strauss SE et al: New evidence for stroke prevention, clinical applications and scientific review, *JAMA* 288:1388, 2002.

Author: **Richard S. Isaacson, M.D.**

BOX 1-22 **Criteria for Tissue Plasminogen Activator (alteplase [Activase]) Use in Patients with Thromboembolic Stroke**

Criteria for considering t-PA as a treatment option

Age ≥18 yr

Noncontrast CT without evidence of hemorrhage

Time since onset of symptoms clearly <3 hr before t-PA administration would begin

Criteria for excluding t-PA as a treatment option

Historical and clinical findings

  Clinical presentation suggests subarachnoid hemorrhage, even if CT is normal

    Sudden, severe headache, often with loss of consciousness at onset

    Vomiting common

  Active internal bleeding, increased risk of bleeding, or known bleeding diathesis, including:

    Recent use of warfarin with a prolonged international normalized ratio (INR)—some would add current use of warfarin regardless of INR

    Use of heparin within 48 hr with a prolonged aPTT

    Platelet count <100,000/mm³

    History of intracranial hemorrhage

    Known arteriovenous malformation or aneurysm

    GI or GU bleeding within the past 21 days

    Arterial puncture within the past 7 days

  Recent lumbar puncture

  Stroke, intracranial surgery, or head trauma within the previous 3 mo

  Major surgery or serious trauma within the preceding 14 days

  Persistent systolic blood pressure >185 mm Hg or diastolic blood pressure >110 mm Hg

  Seizure at stroke onset

  Rapidly improving neurologic signs

  Isolated, mild neurologic deficits

  Acute myocardial infarction

  Post–myocardial infarction pericarditis

  Blood glucose <50 mg/dl or >400 mg/dl

  Patient pregnant or lactating

CT findings

  Evidence of intracranial hemorrhage

  Hypodensity or effacement of the sulci in ⅓ of the territory of the middle cerebral artery

From Rakel RE (ed): *Principles of family practice*, ed 6, Philadelphia, 2002, WB Saunders.

aPTT, Activated partial thromboplastin time; *CT,* computed tomography; *GI,* gastrointestinal; *GU,* genitourinary; *t-PA,* tissue plasminogen activator.

BASIC INFORMATION

■ DEFINITION
Subarachnoid hemorrhage is the presence of active bleeding into the subarachnoid space usually secondary to a spontaneous ruptured aneurysm or after head trauma.

ICD-9CM CODES
430 Subarachnoid hemorrhage

■ EPIDEMIOLOGY & DEMOGRAPHICS
INCIDENCE (IN U.S.): 6 to 28 cases/100,000 persons/yr
PREDOMINANT SEX: Males > females in persons <40 yr of age; then female:male ratio of 3:2 in persons >40 yr old
PREDOMINANT AGE: >50 yr
PEAK INCIDENCE: 50 to 60 yr
GENETICS:
- First-degree relatives have a 4%-9% risk of intracranial aneurysms (as compared with about 2% in the general population) and these may tend to rupture at a younger age and at a smaller size than sporadic ones. Recommendations on screening unaffected family members depend on the number of relatives with aneurysms. There may also be a familial predisposition to multiple aneurysms.
- Increased incidence in some inherited systemic diseases (e.g., autosomal dominant polycystic kidney disease and connective tissue diseases such as Ehlers-Danlos syndrome).

■ PHYSICAL FINDINGS & CLINICAL PRESENTATION
- Patients typically present with sudden onset of a severe headache with maximal intensity at onset. Classically described by the patient as "the worst headache of my life," however, this is not always the case. Additional findings may include nuchal rigidity, nausea, and vomiting.
- Transient loss of consciousness occurs in 45% of patients.
- Focal neurologic deficits may be present.
- Funduscopic examination may reveal subhyaloid hemorrhage.

■ ETIOLOGY
- Key distinction is aneurysmal (nontraumatic etiology in >60% of cases, most commonly after rupture of saccular "berry" aneurysms) vs. nonaneurysmal (traumatic) SAH
- Others: Arteriovenous malformation (AVM), angioma, fusiform or mycotic aneurysm, dissecting and tumor-related aneurysms

DIAGNOSIS

■ DIFFERENTIAL DIAGNOSIS
- Intraparenchymal hemorrhage
- Subarachnoid extension of an extracranial arterial dissection or intracerebral hemorrhage
- Meningoencephalitis (e.g., hemorrhagic meningoencephalitis caused by HSV)
- Headache associated with sexual activity (e.g., coital/postcoital headache; usually acute onset of severe headache around time of orgasm)

■ WORKUP
- CT scan without contrast is initial test of choice, with a sensitivity of about 90% in the first 24 hr. If CT is negative and there is a high clinical suspicion for SAH, lumbar puncture must be considered as there is an approximately 7% (or 1 in 14) chance of having a SAH. Spinal fluid is considered positive if there is xanthochromia and if there is a constant amount of red cells in each LP tube. LP performed <2 hr after onset of headache may be falsely negative for xanthochromia.
- If CT scan is unavailable, transfer patient immediately to a facility that has one.
- ECG (nonspecific ST-and T-wave changes, "cerebral T-waves").

■ LABORATORY TESTS
PT, PTT, platelet count at a minimum for clotting abnormality

■ IMAGING STUDIES
CT scan (Fig. 1-262) followed by cerebral angiography if hemorrhage is confirmed. May also use Transcranial Doppler (TCD) as a baseline to later more adequately assess for vasospasm

TREATMENT

■ NONPHARMACOLOGIC THERAPY
- Intubation as necessary
- Bed rest, isotonic fluids

■ ACUTE GENERAL Rx
- Short-acting analgesics (e.g., morphine 1 to 4 mg IV) and sedation (e.g., midazolam 1 to 5 mg IV); avoid oversedation and watch neurologic examination closely
- Seizure prophylaxis controversial (consider phenytoin 15 to 20 mg/kg IV load, 100 mg TID maintenance)
- Vasospasm prophylaxis (nimodipine 60 mg PO q4h); see "Chronic Rx"
- BP control (e.g., labetalol 10 to 40 mg IV q30min); lower BP for unprotected aneurysms vs. higher BP if protected (post coiling/clipping)
- Stool softeners
- Neurosurgical or interventional neuroradiologic referral mandatory if aneurysm or arteriovenous malformation demonstrated by angiogra-

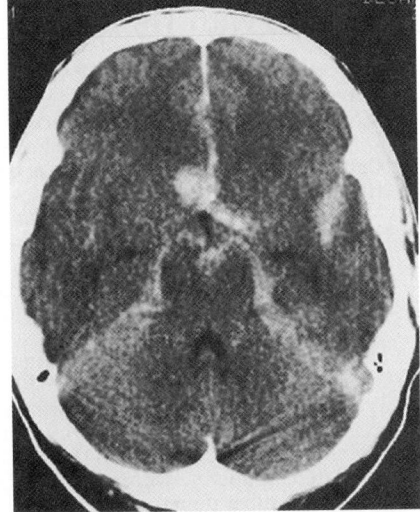

Fig. 1-262 Noncontrast CT demonstrates diffuse subarachnoid hemorrhage. The rounded area of hyperdensity anterior to the suprasellar cistern represents an aneurysm of the anterior communicating artery. (From Specht N [ed]: *Practical guide to diagnostic imaging,* St Louis, 1998, Mosby.)

phy; also, invasive ICP monitoring and/or ventriculostomy may be required on an emergent basis (e.g., deteriorating level of consciousness and/or development of hydrocephalus)

■ CHRONIC Rx

Vasospasm occurs in 20%-30% of patients and peaks at about 1 wk; monitor closely for this. Consider TCD monitoring in high-risk patients. "Triple H" therapy for prevention of vasospasm includes hemodilution, hypertension (consider pressors), and hypervolemia. Intraarterial papaverine and/or balloon angioplasty may be necessary in some cases.

■ DISPOSITION

Approximately 35% early mortality, 45% at 1 mo

■ REFERRAL

Transfer as soon as possible to a facility with neurosurgical care.

☼ PEARLS & CONSIDERATIONS

■ COMMENTS

About 20% of patients experience warning signs within 3 mo before aneurysm rupture, including moderate or severe headache ("sentinel headache"), dizziness, nausea and vomiting, transient motor or sensory deficits, loss of consciousness, or visual disturbances.

REFERENCES

Bederson JB et al: Recommendations for the management of patients with unruptured intracranial aneurysms: a statement for healthcare professionals from the Stroke Council of the American Heart Association, *Circulation* 102(18):2300, 2000.

Edlow JA, Caplan LR: Avoiding pitfalls in the diagnosis of subarachnoid hemorrhage, *N Engl J Med* 342:29, 2000.

Edlow JA, Wyer PC: How good is a negative cranial computed tomographic scan result in excluding subarachnoid hemorrhage? *Ann Emerg Med* 36:507, 2000.

Morgenstern LB et al: Worst headache and subarachnoid hemorrhage: prospective modern computed tomography and spinal fluid analysis, *Ann Emerg Med* 32:297, 1998.

Raaymakers TW, and the MARS Study Group: Aneurysms in relatives of patients with subarachnoid hemorrhage. Frequency and risk factors, *Neurology* 53:982, 1999.

Treggiari, MM et al: Systematic review of the prevention of delayed ischemic neurological deficits with hypertension, hypervolemia, and hemodilution therapy following subarachnoid hemorrhage, *J Neurosurg* 98:978, 2003.

Author: **Richard S. Isaacson, M.D.**

BASIC INFORMATION

■ DEFINITION

Subclavian steal syndrome is an occlusion or severe stenosis of the proximal subclavian artery leading to decreased antegrade flow or retrograde flow in the ipsilateral vertebral artery and neurologic symptoms referable to the posterior circulation.

■ SYNONYMS

Proximal subclavian (or innominate) artery stenosis or occlusion

ICD-9CM CODES

435.2 Subclavian steal syndrome

■ EPIDEMIOLOGY & DEMOGRAPHICS

• Similar to that of other manifestations of atherosclerosis (coronary artery disease, cerebrovascular disease, or peripheral vascular disease)
• Affects middle-aged persons (men somewhat younger than women on average) with arteriosclerotic risk factors including family history, smoking, diabetes mellitus, hyperlipidemia, hypertension, sedentary lifestyle

■ PHYSICAL FINDINGS & CLINICAL PRESENTATION

Symptoms:
• Many patients are asymptomatic.
• Upper extremity ischemic symptoms: fatigue, exercise-related aching, coolness, numbness of the involved upper extremity.
• Neurologic symptoms are reported by 25% of patients with known unilateral subclavian steal. These include brief spells of:
  1. Vertigo
  2. Diplopia
  3. Decreased vision
  4. Oscillopsia
  5. Gait unsteadiness

These spells are only occasionally provoked by exercising the ischemic upper extremity (classic subclavian steal). Left subclavian steal is more common than right, but the latter is more serious.
• Posterior circulation stroke related to subclavian steal is rare.
• Innominate artery stenosis can cause decreased right carotid artery flow and cerebrovascular symptoms of the anterior cerebral circulation, but this is uncommon.
Physical findings:
• Delayed and smaller volume pulse (wrist or antecubital) in the affected upper extremity
• Lower blood pressure in the affected upper extremity
• Supraclavicular bruit
NOTE: Inflating a blood pressure cuff will increase the bruit if it originates from a vertebral artery stenosis and decrease the bruit if it originates from a subclavian artery stenosis.

■ ETIOLOGY & PATHOGENESIS

Etiology:
• Atherosclerosis
• Arteritis (Takayasu's disease and temporal arteritis)
• Embolism to the subclavian or innominate artery
• Cervical rib
• Chronic use of a crutch
• Occupational (baseball pitchers and cricket bowlers)
Pathogenesis: The vertebral artery originates from the subclavian artery. For subclavian steal to occur, the occlusion must be proximal to the takeoff of the vertebral artery. On the right side, only a small distance separates the bifurcation of the innominate artery and the takeoff of the vertebral artery, explaining why the condition occurs less commonly on the right side. Occlusion of the innominate artery must affect right carotid artery flow.

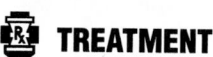

DIAGNOSIS

• See "History," "Physical Findings," and "Imaging Studies."
• The carotid arteries should be evaluated at least noninvasively in all cases.

■ DIFFERENTIAL DIAGNOSIS

• Posterior circulation TIA (and stroke)
• Upper extremity ischemia
  1. Distal subclavian artery stenosis/occlusion
  2. Raynaud's syndrome
  3. Thoracic outlet syndrome

■ IMAGING STUDIES

• Noninvasive upper extremity arterial flow studies
• Doppler sonography of the vertebral, subclavian, and innominate arteries
• Arteriography

TREATMENT

• In most patients the disease is benign and requires no treatment other than atherosclerosis risk factor modification and aspirin. Symptoms tend to improve over time as collateral circulation develops.
• Vascular surgical reconstruction requires a thoracotomy; it may be indicated in innominate artery stenosis or when upper extremity ischemia is incapacitating.

REFERENCE

Caplan LR: Large-vessel occlusive disease of the posterior circulation. In Caplan LR (ed): *Stroke: a clinical approach,* ed 2, New York, 1993, Butterworth-Heinemann.
Author: **Tom J. Wachtel, M.D.**

BASIC INFORMATION

■ DEFINITION

A subdural hematoma is bleeding into the subdural space, caused by rupture of bridging veins between the brain and venous sinuses.

ICD-9CM CODES

432.1 Subdural hematoma

■ EPIDEMIOLOGY & DEMOGRAPHICS

Nearly all cases are caused by trauma, although the trauma may be quite trivial and easily overlooked. Victims are commonly at the extremes of age. Coagulation abnormalities, especially the increasing use of anticoagulation in the elderly, is a significant risk factor.

■ PHYSICAL FINDINGS & CLINICAL PRESENTATION

- Vague headache, is often worse in morning than evening.
- Some apathy, confusion, and clouding of consciousness is common, although frank coma may complicate late cases. Chronic subdural hematomas may cause a dementia picture.
- Neurologic symptoms may be transient, simulating TIA.
- Almost any sign of cortical dysfunction may occur, including hemiparesis, sensory deficits, or language abnormalities, depending on which part of the cortex the hematoma presses on.
- New-onset seizures should raise the index of suspicion.

■ ETIOLOGY

Traumatic rupture of cortical bridging veins, especially where stretched by underlying cerebral atrophy.

DIAGNOSIS

■ DIFFERENTIAL DIAGNOSIS

- Epidural hematoma
- Subarachnoid hemorrhage
- Mass lesion
- Ischemic stroke
- Intraparenchymal hemorrhage

■ WORKUP

- CT scan has revolutionized the diagnosis of subdural hematoma (see Fig. 1-263)
- Hematocrit, platelet count, PTT, and PT/INR should be routinely checked.

TREATMENT

■ NONPHARMACOLOGIC THERAPY

Small subdural hematomas may be observed, but if there is an underlying cause, such as anticoagulation, this should be rapidly corrected to prevent further accumulation of blood.

■ ACUTE THERAPY

- Neurosurgical drainage of blood from subdural space via burr hole is the definitive procedure, although it is common for the hematoma to reaccumulate.
- If seizures occur, they should be treated appropriately.

■ DISPOSITION

Referral to neurosurgery for possible evacuation

PEARLS & CONSIDERATIONS

- The very young and very old are particularly susceptible to subdural hematomas.
- Relatively minor trauma may cause a subdural hematoma.
- Caution should be taken in interpreting CT findings in the subacute stage, where blood appears as isodense to brain, and therefore the distance from the cortical sulci to the skull needs to be evaluated.

REFERENCES

Chen JC, Levy ML: Causes, epidemiology, and risk factors of chronic subdural hematoma, *Neurosurg Clin N Am* 11(3):399, 2000.
Voelker JL: Nonoperative treatment of chronic subdural hematoma, *Neurosurg Clin N Am* 11(3):507, 2000.
Author: **Daniel Mattson, M.D., M.Sc.(Med.)**

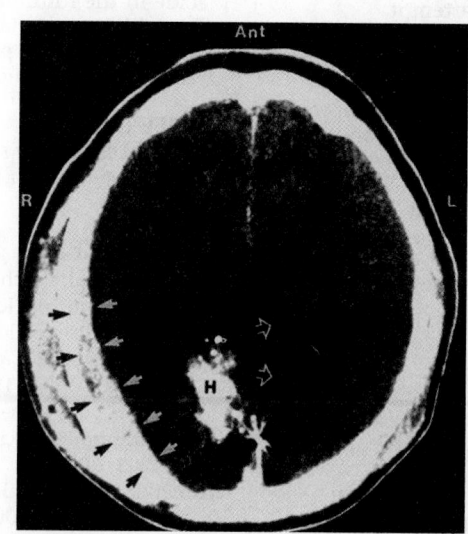 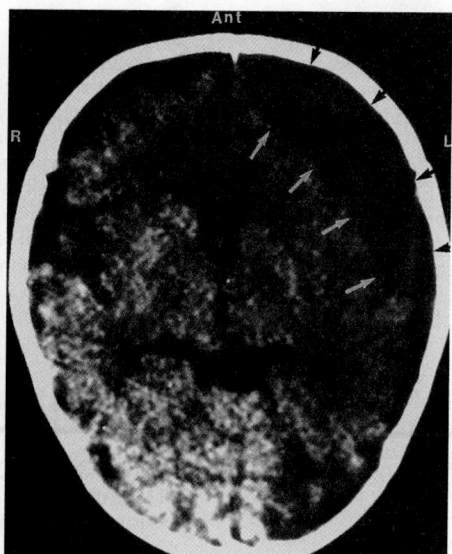

Fig. 1-263   Subdural hematomas. A noncontrasted computed tomography scan of an acute subdural hematoma **(A)** shows a crescentic area of increased density in the right posterior parietal region between the brain and the skull (*black and white arrows*). An area of intraparenchymal hemorrhage *(H)* is also seen; a chronic subdural hematoma for a different patient is shown in **(B).** There is an area of decreased density in the left frontoparietal region *(arrows)* effacing the sulci, compressing the anterior horn of the left lateral ventricle, and shifting the midline somewhat to the right. (From Mettler FA [ed]: *Primary care radiology,* Philadelphia, 2000, WB Saunders.)

BASIC INFORMATION

■ DEFINITION
Suicide refers to successful and unsuccessful attempts to kill oneself.

■ SYNONYMS
Self-murder

ICD-9CM CODES
Categorized by method (e.g., poisoning)

■ EPIDEMIOLOGY & DEMOGRAPHICS
INCIDENCE (IN U.S.):
- 10.42 cases/100,000 persons; 1.4% of total deaths
- 18.7/100,000 men
- 4.4/100,000 women

PREDOMINANT AGE: Increases with age (e.g., 13.1 cases/100,000 persons aged 15 to 24 yr, 16.9 cases/100,000 persons aged 65 to 74 yr, and 23.5 cases/100,000 persons aged 75 to 84 yr); 41 suicides/100,000 men >75 yr)

PEAK INCIDENCE: >65 yr of age

GENETICS:
- Biologic factors may increase the risk of suicide directly (e.g., by increasing impulsivity) or indirectly (e.g., by predisposing to a mental illness).
- Family history of suicide is associated with suicidal behavior.
- Risk in whites is double the risk of nonwhites.

■ PHYSICAL FINDINGS & CLINICAL PRESENTATION
Methods used in attempted (unsuccessful) suicides differ from those used in completed suicides.
- Overdose used in >70% of attempted suicides. Cutting of wrists or other parts of the body is the second most common form.
- About 60% of completed suicides are accomplished with firearms. Hanging is the second most common method for completed suicides. Suffocation (e.g., carbon monoxide) and overdose are also relatively common forms of completing suicide.
- Several risk factors are usually present concurrently, including a psychiatric illness such as depression or anxiety, middle age or advanced age, white race, male gender, a recent divorce or separation, comorbid substance abuse (particularly when intoxicated), previous history of suicide attempts, fatal plan (e.g., firearms or hanging), history of violence, and family history of suicide. Concurrent chronic physical illness

increases the risk for suicide greatly (e.g., the risk for suicide among AIDS or renal dialysis patients is nearly 30 times that of the general population).

■ ETIOLOGY
- Individuals with a mental or a substance abuse disorder are responsible for >90% of all suicides.
- The concurrence of more than one condition (e.g., depression and alcohol abuse) greatly increases the risk of suicide.
- Hopelessness is a strong predictor of suicide potential.

DIAGNOSIS

■ DIFFERENTIAL DIAGNOSIS
- Some disorders are associated with self-injurious behavior that is not suicidal. Borderline personality disorder, for example, manifests with self-mutilation without active suicidal intent. Eating disorders are harmful and may be fatal, but death is never the goal.
- Some suicidal behavior is intended as a "call for help." In these situations individuals usually design the suicide so that they will be discovered before significant damage has been done.

■ WORKUP
- Suicidal patients present in one of four ways:
  1. Covert suicidal ideation
  2. Overt suicidal ideation
  3. After a suicide attempt
  4. Dead from a suicide attempt
- Covert suicidal ideation occurs in patients primarily with multiple vague physical complaints, depression, anxiety, or substance abuse.
- As part of the history, the physician must directly inquire into the presence of suicidal ideation.
- The concurrence of multiple psychiatric problems, substance abuse, and multiple physical problems increases the risk.

TREATMENT

■ NONPHARMACOLOGIC THERAPY
- Major immediate intervention: placement of the patient in a safe environment (usually hospitalization in a psychiatric unit or a medical unit with continuous observation)

- Long-term: psychotherapy aimed at factors that underlie the decision to pursue suicide or at the risk factors contributing to suicidal behavior
- Substance abuse treatment (e.g., AA, NA) when substance abuse is present

■ ACUTE GENERAL Rx
- Benzodiazepines are useful in reducing the extreme anxiety and dysphoria in a suicidal patient; however, these agents are depressive and should be used only when patient is in safe environment.
- Antipsychotics can be used if psychosis is present (e.g., voices telling patient to hurt self).
- Mood stabilizers and antidepressants should be started in the acute setting but may have up to a 2-wk latency period.

■ CHRONIC Rx
- Therapy should be aimed at the underlying condition (e.g., antidepressants for depression, anxiolytics or antidepressants for anxiety, ongoing substance abuse treatment for substance abuse history, or psychotherapy for chronic low self-esteem, hopelessness).
- In elderly, loneliness and medical disability are major reasons for suicide and therefore major targets for intervention.

■ DISPOSITION
- Prior suicide attempt is the best predictor for completed suicides (i.e., patients who attempt suicide once are at high risk for completing suicide in the future).
- Conditions associated with suicide (e.g., depression, physical ailments) are usually chronic and recurring.

■ REFERRAL
If patient is acutely suicidal and requires protection in hospital

REFERENCES
Gould MS et al: Psychopathology associated with suicidal ideation and attempts among children and adolescents, *J Am Acad Child Adolesc Psychiatry* 37:915, 1998.

Mann JJ: A current perspective of suicide and attempted suicide, *Ann Intern Med* 136:302, 2002.

Zametkin AJ et al: Suicide in teenagers, *JAMA* 286:3120, 2001.

Author: **Rif S. El-Mallakh, M.D.**

BASIC INFORMATION

■ DEFINITION
Superior vena cava syndrome is a set of symptoms that results when a mediastinal mass compresses the superior vena cava (SVC) or the veins that drain into it.

ICD-9CM CODES
453.2 (vena cava thrombosis)

■ EPIDEMIOLOGY & DEMOGRAPHICS
Mirrors lung cancer (especially small cell carcinoma) and lymphoma: see "Lung Neoplasm" and "Lymphoma" in Section I

■ PHYSICAL FINDINGS & CLINICAL PRESENTATION
Symptoms:
- Shortness of breath
- Chest pain
- Cough
- Dysphagia
- Headache
- Syncope
- Visual trouble

Signs:
- Chest wall vein distention
- Neck vein distention
- Facial edema
- Upper extremity swelling
- Cyanosis

■ ETIOLOGY
- Lung cancer (80% of all cases, of which half are small cell lung cancer)
- Lymphoma (15%)
- Tuberculosis
- Goiter
- Aortic aneurysm (arteriosclerotic or syphilitic)
- SVC thrombosis
    1. Primary: associated with a central venous catheter
    2. Secondary: as a complication of SVC syndrome associated with one of the above mentioned causes

DIAGNOSIS

■ DIFFERENTIAL DIAGNOSIS
The syndrome is characteristic enough to exclude other diagnoses. The differential diagnosis concerns the underlying etiologies listed previously.

■ WORKUP
- Chest x-ray
- Venography
- Chest CT scan or MRI
- Ultrasonography
- Sputum cytology
- Bronchoscopy
- Mediastinoscopy
- Thoracotomy

TREATMENT

Although invasive procedures such as mediastinoscopy or thoracotomy are associated with higher than usual risk of bleeding, a tissue diagnosis is usually needed before commencing therapy.

Emergency empiric radiation is indicated in critical situations such as respiratory failure or central nervous system signs associated with increased intracranial pressure.
- Treatment of the underlying malignancy
    1. Radiation
    2. Chemotherapy
- Anticoagulant or fibrinolytic therapy in patients who do not respond to cancer treatment within a week or if an obstructing thrombus has been documented
- Diuretics
- Steroids

■ REFERRAL
To a thoracic surgeon, pulmonary specialist, and/or oncologist

REFERENCE
Markman M: Diagnosis and management of superior vena cava syndrome, *Cleveland Clin J Med* 66:59, 1999.
Author: **Tom J. Wachtel, M.D.**

BASIC INFORMATION

■ DEFINITION

Syncope is the temporary loss of consciousness resulting from an acute global reduction in cerebral blood flow.

ICD-9CM CODES
720.2 Syncope

■ EPIDEMIOLOGY & DEMOGRAPHICS

- Syncope accounts for 3% to 5% of emergency room visits.
- 30% of the adult population will experience at least one syncopal episode during their lifetime.
- Incidence of syncope is highest in elderly men and young women.

■ PHYSICAL FINDINGS & CLINICAL PRESENTATION

- Blood pressure: if low, consider orthostatic hypotension; if unequal in both arms (difference >20 mm Hg), consider subclavian steal or dissecting aneurysm. (NOTE: Blood pressure and heart rate should be recorded in the supine and standing positions.) If there is drop in BP but no change in HR, the patient may be on a beta blocker or may have an autonomic neuropathy.
- Pulse: if patient has tachycardia, bradycardia, or irregular rhythm, consider arrhythmia.
- Heart: if there are murmurs present suggestive of AS or IHSS, consider syncope secondary to left ventricular outflow obstruction; if there are JVD and distal heart sounds, consider cardiac tamponade.
- Carotid sinus pressure: can be diagnostic if it reproduces symptoms and other causes are excluded; a pause >3 sec or a systolic BP drop >50 mm Hg without symptoms or <30 mm Hg with symptoms when sinus pressure is applied separately on each side for <5 sec is considered abnormal. This test should be avoided in patients with carotid bruits or cerebrovascular disease; ECG monitoring, IV access, and bedside atropine should be available when carotid sinus pressure is applied.

■ ETIOLOGY

- Neurally mediated syncope
  1. Psychophysiologic (emotional upset, panic disorders, hysteria)
  2. Visceral reflex (micturition, defecation, food ingestion, coughing, ventricular contraction; glossopharyngeal neuralgia)
  3. Carotid sinus pressure
  4. Reduction of venous return caused by Valsalva maneuver
- Orthostatic hypotension
  1. Hypovolemia
  2. Vasodilator medications

  3. Autonomic neuropathy (diabetes, amyloid, Parkinson's disease, multisystem atrophy)
  4. Pheochromocytoma
  5. Carcinoid syndrome
- Cardiac
  1. Reduced cardiac output
     a. Left ventricular outflow obstruction (aortic stenosis, hypertrophic cardiomyopathy)
     b. Obstruction to pulmonary flow (pulmonary embolism, pulmonic stenosis, primary pulmonary hypertension)
     c. MI with pump failure
     d. Cardiac tamponade
     e. Mitral stenosis
     f. Reduction of venous return (atrial myxoma, valve thrombus)
     g. β-blockers
  2. Arrhythmias or asystole
     a. Extreme tachycardia (>160 to 180 bpm)
     b. Severe bradycardia (<30 to 40 bpm)
     c. Sick sinus syndrome
     d. AV block (second- or third-degree)
     e. Ventricular tachycardia or fibrillation
     f. Long QT syndrome
     g. Pacemaker malfunction
     h. Psychotropic medications and beta blockers
  3. Other causes
     a. Hypoxia
     b. Hypoglycemia
     c. Anemia
     d. Hyperventilation

DIAGNOSIS

■ DIFFERENTIAL DIAGNOSIS

1. Seizure (see "Workup")
2. Vertebrobasilar TIA usually manifests as diplopia, vertigo, ataxia but not loss of consciousness. Isolated syncopal episodes without accompanying neurologic symptoms are unlikely to be a TIA
3. Recreational drugs/alcohol
4. Psychologic stress

■ WORKUP

The history is crucial to diagnosing the cause of syncope and may suggest a diagnosis that can be evaluated with directed testing:
- Sudden loss of consciousness: consider cardiac arrhythmias.
- Gradual loss of consciousness: consider orthostatic hypotension, vasodepressor syncope, hypoglycemia.
- History of aura before loss of consciousness (LOC) or prolonged confusion (>1min), amnesia or lethargy after LOC suggests seizure rather than syncope.

- Patient's activity at the time of syncope:
  1. Micturition, coughing, defecation: consider syncope secondary to decreased venous return.
  2. Turning head or while shaving: consider carotid sinus syndrome.
  3. Physical exertion in a patient with murmur: consider aortic stenosis.
  4. Arm exercise: consider subclavian steal syndrome.
  5. Assuming an upright position: consider orthostatic hypotension.
- Associated events:
  1. Chest pain: consider MI, pulmonary embolism.
  2. Palpitations: consider arrhythmias.
  3. Incontinence (urine or fecal) and tongue biting are associated with seizure or syncope.
  4. Brief, transient shaking after LOC may represent myoclonus from global cerebral hypoperfusion and not seizures. However, sustained tonic/clonic muscle action is more suggestive of seizure.
  5. Focal neurologic symptoms or signs point to a neurologic event such as a seizure with residual deficits (e.g. Todd's paralysis) or cerebral ischemic injury.
  6. Psychologic stress: syncope may be vasovagal.
- Review current medications, particularly antihypertensive and psychotropic drugs.

■ LABORATORY TESTS

Routine blood tests rarely yield diagnostically useful information and should be done only if they are specifically suggested by the results of the history and physical examination. The following are commonly ordered tests.
- Pregnancy test should be considered in women of childbearing age
- CBC to rule out anemia, infection
- Electrolytes, BUN, creatinine, magnesium, calcium to rule out electrolyte abnormalities and evaluate fluid status
- Serum glucose level
- Cardiac isoenzymes should be obtained if the patient gives a history of chest pain before the syncopal episode
- ABGs to rule out pulmonary embolus, hyperventilation (when suspected)
- Evaluate drug and alcohol levels when suspecting toxicity

■ IMAGING STUDIES

- Echocardiogram is useful in patients with a heart murmur to rule out AS, IHSS, or atrial myxoma.
- If seizure is suspected, CT scan and/or MRI of the head and EEG may be useful.
- If head trauma or neurologic signs on examination, CT or MRI may be helpful.

- If pulmonary embolism is suspected, ventilation-perfusion scan should be done.
- If arrhythmias are suspected, a 24-hr Holter monitor and admission to a telemetry unit is appropriate. Generally, Holter monitoring is rarely useful, revealing a cause for syncope in <3% of cases. Loop recorders that can be activated after syncopal episode to retrieve information about the cardiac rhythm during the preceding 4 min add considerable diagnostic yield in patients with unexplained syncope.
- Implantable cardiac monitors that function as permanent loop recorders or implantable cardioverter-defibrillators, which are placed subcutaneously in the pectoral region with the patient under local anesthesia, are useful in patients with cardiac syncope.
- Electrophysiologic studies may be indicated in patients with structural heart disease and/or recurrent syncope.
- ECG to rule out arrhythmias; may be diagnostic in 5% to 10% of patients.

■ TILT-TABLE TESTING
- Useful to support a diagnosis of neurally mediated syncope. Patients older than age 50 should have stress testing before tilt-table testing. Positive results would preclude tilt-table testing.
- Indicated in patients with recurrent episodes of unexplained syncope as well as for patients in high-risk occupations (e.g., pilots, bus drivers) (Fig. 1-264). The test is also useful for identifying patients with prominent bradycardic response who may benefit from implantation of a permanent pacemaker.
- It is performed by keeping the patient in an upright posture on a tilt table with footboard support. The angle of the tilt table varies from 60 to 80 degrees. The duration of upright posture during tilt-table testing varies from 25 to 45 min.
- The hallmark of neurally mediated syncope is severe hypotension associated with a paradoxical bradycardia triggered by a specific stimulus. The diagnosis of neurally mediated syncope is likely if upright tilt testing reproduces these hemodynamic changes in <15 min and causes presyncope or syncope.

■ PSYCHIATRIC EVALUATION
- May be indicated in young patients without heart disease who have frequently recurring syncope and other somatic symptoms.
- Generalized anxiety disorder, pain disorder, and major depression predispose patients to neurally mediated reactions and may result in syncope.

- Alcohol and drug dependence can also lead to syncope.

℞ TREATMENT

■ NONPHARMACOLOGIC THERAPY
- Ensure proper hydration; consider TED stockings and salt tablets.
- Eliminate medications that may induce hypotension.

■ ACUTE GENERAL Rx
- Varies with the underlying etiology of syncope (e.g., pacemaker in patients with syncope secondary to complete heart block)
- Syncope caused by orthostatic hypotension is treated with volume replacement in patients with intravascular volume depletion. Also consider midodrine to promote venous return via adrenergic-mediated vasoconstriction and Florinef for its mineralocorticoid effects to increase intravascular volume

■ DISPOSITION
Prognosis varies with the age of the patient and the etiology of the syncope. Generally:
- Benign prognosis (very low 1-yr morbidity) in patients:
  1. Age <30 yr and having noncardiac syncope
  2. Age <70 yr and having vasovagal/psychogenic syncope or syncope of unknown cause
- Poor prognosis (high mortality and morbidity) in patients with cardiac syncope

- Patients with the following risk factors have a higher 1-yr mortality: abnormal ECG, history of ventricular arrhythmia, history of CHF

■ REFERRAL
Hospital admission in elderly patients without prior history of syncope or unknown etiology of their syncope and in any patients suspected of having cardiac syncope.

☼ PEARLS & CONSIDERATIONS

■ COMMENTS
- Section III, Fig. 3-173 describes an algorithmic approach to the patient with syncope.
- The etiology of syncope is identified in <50% of cases during the initial evaluation.
- A thorough history and physical examination are the most productive means of establishing a diagnosis in patients with syncope.

REFERENCES
Fenton AM et al: Vasovagal syncope, *Ann Intern Med* 133:722, 2000.
Kapoor WN: Syncope, *N Engl J Med* 343:1856, 2000.
Menozzi C et al: Mechanism of syncope in patients with heart disease and negative electrophysiologic test, *Circulation* 105:2741, 2002.
Soteriades ES et al: Incidence and prognosis of syncope, *N Engl J Med* 347:878, 2002.
Author: **Sean I. Savitz, M.D.**

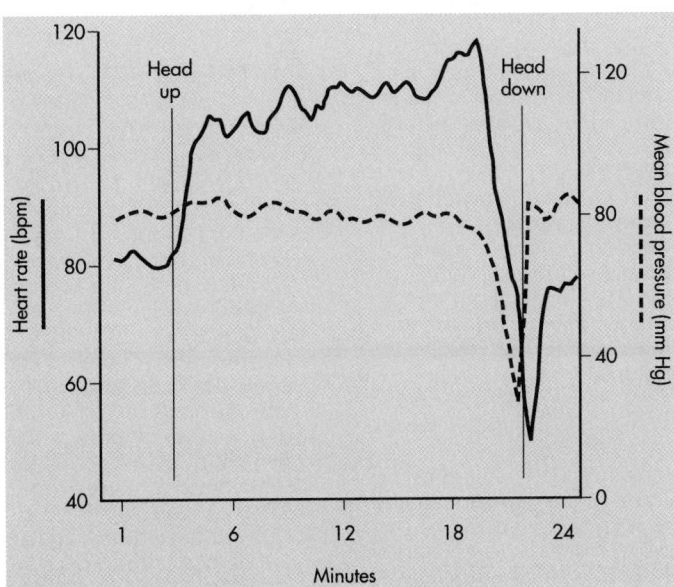

Fig. 1-264 Head-up tilt test performed on an 18-year-old woman with a history of syncope associated with pain, preceded by a prodrome of dizziness, graying vision, and diaphoresis. A similar prodrome preceded syncope during the test. Note the precipitous, nearly simultaneous, decline of heart rate and blood pressure after an initial rise in heart rate. Vital signs returned to normal rapidly after the head was lowered. (Courtesy Robert F. Sprung, University of Utah. In Goldman L, Ausiello D [eds]: *Cecil textbook of medicine*, ed 22, Philadelphia, 2004, WB Saunders.)

BASIC INFORMATION

■ DEFINITION

Syphilis is a sexually transmitted treponemal disease, acute and chronic, characterized by primary skin lesion, secondary eruption involving skin and mucous membranes, long periods of latency, and late lesions of skin, bone, viscera, CNS, and cardiovascular system.

■ SYNONYMS

Lues

ICD-9CM CODES

097.9 Syphilis, acquired unspecified

■ EPIDEMIOLOGY & DEMOGRAPHICS

- Widespread, primarily involving ages 20 to 35 yr. Racial differences in incidence are related to social factors. Usually more prevalent in urban areas. Estimated annual incidence of 90,000 cases in the U.S. Increase in incidence in the late 1980s to 1990s, likely related to illicit drug use and prostitution. Increase occurred primarily in lower socioeconomic groups.
- Communicability is indefinite and variable. Communicable during primary, secondary, and latent mucocutaneous lesions in up to first 4 yr of latency. Most probable congenital transmission occurs in early maternal syphilis. Adequate penicillin treatment ends infectivity within 24 to 48 hr.

■ PHYSICAL FINDINGS & CLINICAL PRESENTATION

PRIMARY SYPHILIS: Characteristic lesion is a painless chancre on genitalia, mouth, or anus; atypical primary lesions may occur. Usually appears 3 wk after exposure and may spontaneously involute.

SECONDARY SYPHILIS:

- Localized or diffuse mucocutaneous lesions and generalized lymphadenopathy. Common to have constitutional symptoms, flulike symptoms. May begin about 4 to 6 wk after appearance of primary lesion. Manifestations may resolve in 1 wk to 12 mo.
- 60% to 80% of patients have maculopapular lesions on their palms and soles.
- Condylomata lata intertriginous papules form at areas of friction and moisture, such as the vulva.
- 21% to 58% have mucocutaneous or mucosal lesions (pharyngitis, tonsillitis, "mucous patch" lesion on oral and genital mucosa).

EARLY LATENT (<1 YR): Generally asymptomatic

LATE LATENT (>1 YR):

- Characterized by gummas (nodular, ulcerative lesions) that can involve the skin, mucous membranes, skeletal system, and viscera.
- Manifestations of cardiovascular syphilis include aortitis, aneurysm, or aortic regurgitation.
- Neurosyphilis may be asymptomatic or symptomatic. Tabes dorsalis, meningovascular syphilis, general paralysis, or insanity may occur. Iritis, choroidoretinitis, and leukoplakia may also occur.

■ ETIOLOGY

- *Treponema pallidum,* a spirochete
- Spread by sexual intercourse or by intrauterine transfer

DIAGNOSIS

■ DIFFERENTIAL DIAGNOSIS

- Other genitoulcerative diseases such as herpes, chancroid (see Section II)
- See Section III for a clinical algorithm for the evaluation of genital ulcer disease

■ WORKUP

Confirmation is primarily through laboratory diagnosis.

■ LABORATORY TESTS

- Dark-field microscopy of fluid from lesion to look for treponeme
- Serologic testing, both nontreponemal (VDRL, RPR) and treponemal (FTA, MHA)
- Lumbar puncture for CSF VDRL in patients with evidence of latent syphilis

TREATMENT

■ ACUTE GENERAL Rx

- Early (primary, secondary, early latent): penicillin G benzathine 2.4 million U IM × 1 or doxycycline 100 mg PO bid × 14 days
- Late (late latent, cardiovascular, gumma): penicillin G benzathine 2.4 million U IM qwk × 3 wk or doxycycline 100 mg PO bid × 4 wk
- Neurosyphilis: aqueous crystalline penicillin G 18 to 24 million U/day, administered as 3 to 4 million U IV q4h × 10 to 14 days or procaine penicillin 2.4 million U IM/day plus probenecid 500 mg PO qid, both for 10 to 14 days
- Congenital syphilis: aqueous crystalline penicillin G 50,000 U/kg/dose IV q12h × first 7 days of life and q8h after that for total of 10 days or procaine penicillin G 50,000 U/kg/dose IM/day × 10 days

- Penicillin-allergic patients with primary or secondary syphilis: doxycycline 100 mg PO bid × 14 days, or tetracycline 500 mg PO qid × 14 days, or ceftriaxone 1 g IM or IV × 8 to 10 days, or azithromycin 2 g PO stat (preliminary data only)
- Latent syphilis in penicillin-allergic patient: doxycycline 100 mg PO bid or tetracycline 500 mg qid for 28 days
- Tetracyclines are contraindicated in pregnancy. If pregnant and penicillin allergic, must be desensitized

■ DISPOSITION

- Repeat quantitative nontreponemal tests at 3, 6, and 12 mo. Pregnancy requires monthly tests until delivery.
- If a fourfold increase in titer occurs, if initial high titer fails to drop by fourfold within a year, or persistent signs, retreatment may be indicated. Use treatment regimen for late syphilis.
- Pregnant women without a fourfold drop in titer in a 3-mo period need to be retreated.
- Cases should be reported to local or state health department for referral, follow-up, and partner notification.

■ REFERRAL

- Pregnant and possible congenital syphilis
- Pregnant and allergic to penicillin, with need to be desensitized
- Late latent syphilis with serious CNS, cardiovascular, or other organ system compromise

PEARLS & CONSIDERATIONS

■ COMMENTS

- Jarisch-Herxheimer reaction (fever, myalgia, tachycardia, hypotension) may occur within 24 hr of treatment.
- One third of untreated patients develop CNS and/or cardiovascular sequelae.
- Up to 80% of those treated during late stages remain seropositive indefinitely.
- Treponemal tests remain positive even after adequate therapy.

REFERENCES

Centers for Disease Control and Prevention: Primary and secondary syphilis—United States, 1999, *MMWR Morb Mortal Wkly Rep* 50(7):113, 2001.

Centers for Disease Control and Prevention: 2002 sexually transmitted diseases treatment guidelines, *MMWR Morb Mortal Wkly Rep* 51(RR-6), 2002.

Golden MR, Marra CM, Holmes KK: Update on syphilis: resurgence of an old problem, *JAMA* 290(11):1510, 2003.

Author: **Maria A. Corigliano, M.D.**

BASIC INFORMATION

■ DEFINITION

Syringomyelia is a disease of the spine characterized by the formation of fluid-filled cavities within the spinal cord, sometimes extending into the brainstem.

ICD-9CM CODES

336.0 Syringomyelia

■ EPIDEMIOLOGY & CLINICAL PRESENTATION

- Often a history of birth injury exists.
- Onset is usually insidious, with symptoms often not beginning until the third or fourth decade.
- Cervical spine is the most commonly affected area.
  1. Intrinsic hand atrophy, weakness, and anesthetic sensory loss may develop.
  2. The latter may lead to unnoticed burns or other injuries in the hand.
  3. Loss of pain and temperature sensation may occur, but tactile sense in the upper extremity is preserved.
  4. Sharp testing elicits no pain, but patient often perceives the sharpness of the object.
  5. A Charcot joint in the shoulder or elbow may develop.
- Reflexes are absent in the upper extremity.
- Spasticity and hyperreflexia are present in the lower extremity.
- Scoliosis is common.
- Nystagmus and Horner's syndrome may also occur.
- Trophic skin changes eventually develop in many cases.

■ ETIOLOGY

- Cause is unknown, but condition is thought to result from obstruction of the outlet of the fourth ventricle, often associated with a Chiari I malformation, which causes fluid to be diverted down the central cord.
- Syringes later in life may be the result of trauma or an intramedullary tumor.

DIAGNOSIS

■ DIFFERENTIAL DIAGNOSIS

- ALS
- MS
- Spinal cord tumor
- Tabes dorsalis
- Progressive spinal muscular atrophy

■ IMAGING STUDIES

- Plain radiographs usually reveal widening of the bony canal in the region of involvement.
- Bony anomalies are often present at the base of the skull and at the C1-C2 spinal segments.
- Myelography, MRI (Fig. 1-265), and other imaging studies are recommended.

TREATMENT

Drainage and operative repair of any bony anomalies are undertaken, often with decompression laminectomy of C1 and C2.

■ DISPOSITION

- Condition is slowly progressive in most cases, but course may be quite variable, ranging from death in a few months to slow incapacitation over several years: progression may halt at any time.
- Surgical intervention often stops progression but frequently does not lead to improvement in neurologic findings.

■ REFERRAL

For neurosurgical consultation when diagnosis is suspected

REFERENCES

Klekamp J: The pathophysiology of syringomyelia: historical overview and current concepts, *Acta Neurochir* 144(7):649, 2002.

Riente L, Frigelli S, Delle SA: Neuropathic shoulder arthropathy associated with syringomyelia and Arnold-Chiari malformation (type I), *J Rheumatol* 29(3):638, 2002.

Silber JS, Vaccaro AR, Green B: Summary statement: chronic long-term sequelae after spinal cord injury: post-traumatic spinal deformity and post-traumatic myelopathy associated with syringomyelia, *Spine* 26(24 Suppl):S128, 2001.

Vannemreddy SS, Rowed DW, Bharatwal N: Posttraumatic syringomyelia: predisposing factors, *Br J Neurosurg* 16(3):276, 2002.

Author: **Lonnie R. Mercier, M.D.**

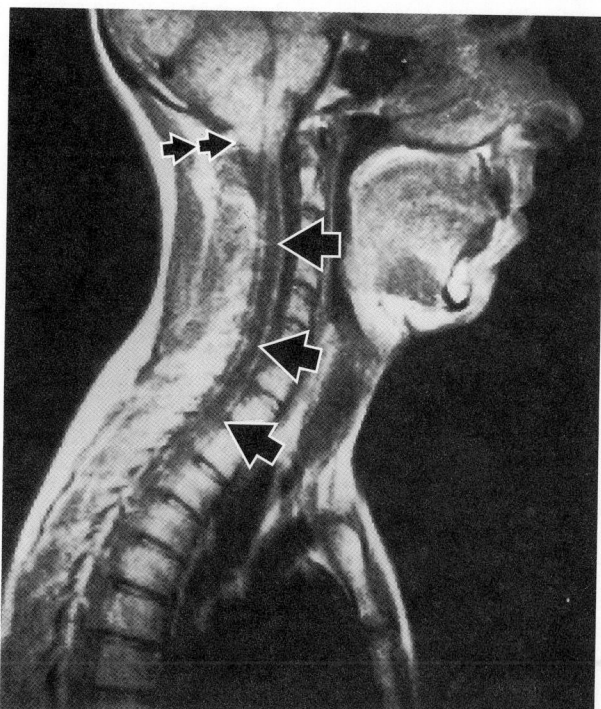

Fig. 1-265 Midsagittal magnetic resonance image of Arnold-Chiari malformation *(small black arrows)* and syringomyelia *(three large black arrows)* in a 31-year-old man. Note the cerebellar tonsils extending below the posterior rim of the foramen magnum *(dark structure immediately above the black arrow).* The syrinx extends from the medulla well into the thoracic cord. (From Andreoli TE [ed]: *Cecil essentials of medicine,* ed 4, Philadelphia, 1997, WB Saunders.)

BASIC INFORMATION

■ DEFINITION
Systemic lupus erythematosus (SLE) is a chronic multisystemic disease characterized by production of autoantibodies and protean clinical manifestations.

■ SYNONYMS
SLE

ICD-9CM CODES
710.0 Systemic lupus erythematosus

■ EPIDEMIOLOGY & DEMOGRAPHICS
PREVALENCE: 20 cases/100,000 persons
PREDOMINANT SEX: Female:male ratio of 7:1
PREDOMINANT AGE: 20 to 45 yr (childbearing years)

■ PHYSICAL FINDINGS & CLINICAL PRESENTATION
- Skin: erythematous rash over the malar eminences (Fig. 1-266), generally with sparing of the nasolabial folds (butterfly rash); alopecia; raised erythematous patches with subsequent edematous plaques and adherent scales (discoid lupus); leg, nasal, or oropharyngeal ulcerations; livedo reticularis; pallor (from anemia); petechiae (from thrombocytopenia)

- Joints: tenderness, swelling, or effusion, generally involving peripheral joints
- Cardiac: pericardial rub (in patients with pericarditis), heart murmurs (if endocarditis or valvular thickening or dysfunction)
- Other: fever, conjunctivitis, dry eyes, dry mouth (sicca syndrome), oral ulcers, abdominal tenderness, decreased breath sounds (pleural effusions)

■ ETIOLOGY
Unknown. Autoantibodies are typically present many years before the diagnosis of SLE.

DIAGNOSIS

■ DIFFERENTIAL DIAGNOSIS
- Other connective tissue disorders (e.g., RA, MCTD, progressive systemic sclerosis)
- Metastatic neoplasm
- Infection

■ WORKUP
The diagnosis of SLE can be made by demonstrating the presence of any four or more of the following criteria of the American Rheumatism Association:
1. Butterfly rash
2. Discoid rash

3. Photosensitivity (particularly leg ulcerations)
4. Oral ulcers
5. Arthritis
6. Serositis (pleuritis, pericarditis)
7. Renal disorder (persistent proteinuria >0.5 g/day or 3+ if quantitation not performed, cellular casts)
8. Neurologic disorder (seizures, psychosis [in absence of offending drugs or metabolic derangement])
9. Hematologic disorder:
   a. Hemolytic anemia with reticulocytosis
   b. Leukopenia ($<4000/mm^3$ total on two or more occasions)
   c. Lymphopenia ($<1500/mm^3$ on two or more occasions)
   d. Thrombocytopenia ($<100,000/mm^3$ in the absence of offending drugs)
10. Immunologic disorder:
   a. Positive SLE cell preparation
   b. Anti-DNA (presence of antibody to native DNA in abnormal titer)
   c. Anti-Sm (presence of antibody to Smith nuclear antigen)
   d. False-positive STS known to be positive for at least 6 mo and confirmed by negative TPI or FTA tests
11. ANA: an abnormal titer of ANA by immunofluorescence or equivalent assay at any time in the absence of drugs known to be associated with "drug-induced lupus" syndrome

■ LABORATORY TESTS
Suggested initial laboratory evaluation of suspected SLE:
- Immunologic evaluation: ANA, anti-DNA antibody, anti-Sm antibody
- Other laboratory tests: CBC with differential, platelet count (Coombs' test if anemia detected), urinalysis (24-hr urine collection for protein if proteinuria is detected), PTT and anticardiolipin antibodies in patients with thrombotic events, BUN, creatinine to evaluate renal function

■ IMAGING STUDIES
- Chest x-ray for evaluation of pulmonary involvement (e.g., pleural effusions, pulmonary infiltrates)
- Echocardiogram to screen for significant valvular heart disease (present in 18% of patients with SLE); echocardiography can identify a subset of lesions (valvular thickening and dysfunction) other than verrucous (Libman-Sacks) endocarditis that are prone to hemodynamic deterioration

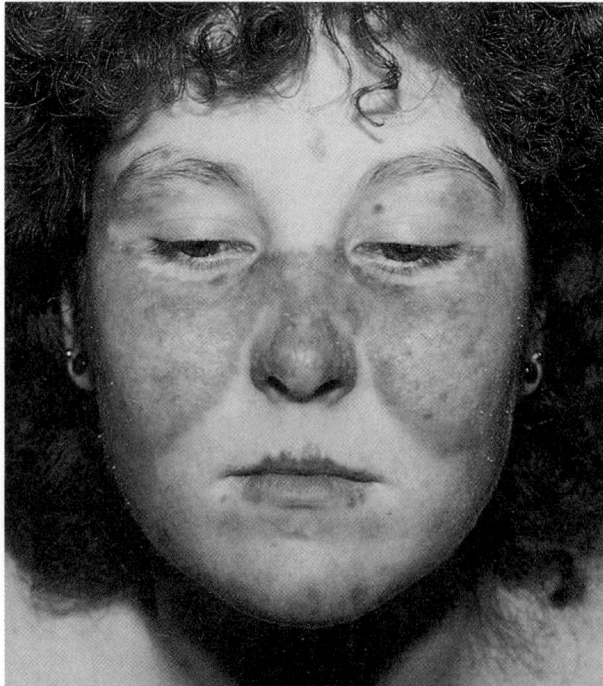

Fig. 1-266 Acute cutaneous LE (systemic LE). The classic butterfly rash occurs in 10% to 50% of patients with acute LE. (From Habif TP: *Clinical dermatology: a color guide to diagnosis and therapy,* ed 3, St Louis, 1996, Mosby.)

℞ TREATMENT

■ NONPHARMACOLOGIC THERAPY

Patients with photosensitivity should avoid sunlight and use high-factor sunscreen.

■ GENERAL Rx

- Joint pain and mild serositis are generally well controlled with NSAIDs; antimalarials are also effective (e.g., hydroxychloroquine [Plaquenil]).
- Cutaneous manifestations are treated with the following:
  1. Topical corticosteroids; intradermal corticosteroids are helpful for individual discoid lesions, especially in the scalp
  2. Antimalarials (e.g., hydroxychloroquine [Plaquenil] and quinacrine)
  3. Sunscreens that block ultraviolet (UV) A and UVB radiation
  4. Immunosuppressive drugs (methotrexate or azathioprine) are used as steroid-sparing drugs
- Renal disease
  1. The use of high-pulsed doses of cyclophosphamide given at monthly intervals is more effective in preserving renal function than is treatment with glucocorticoids alone. The combination of methylprednisolone and cyclophosphamide is superior to bolus therapy with methylprednisolone or cyclophosphamide alone in patients with lupus nephritis.
  2. The use of plasmapheresis in combination with immunosuppressive agents (to prevent the rebound phenomenon of antibody levels after plasmapheresis) is generally reserved for rapidly progressive renal failure or life-threatening systemic vasculitis.
- CNS involvement: treatment generally consists of corticosteroid therapy; however, its efficacy is uncertain, and it is generally reserved for organic brain syndrome. Anticonvulsants and antipsychotics are also indicated in selected cases; headaches are treated symptomatically.

- Hemolytic anemia: treatment of Coombs'-positive hemolytic anemia consists of high doses of corticosteroids; nonhemolytic anemia (secondary to chronic disease) does not require specific therapy.
- Thrombocytopenia
  1. Initial treatment consists of corticosteroids.
  2. In patients with poor response to steroids, encouraging results have been reported with the use of danazol, vincristine, and immunoglobulins. Combination chemotherapy with cyclophosphamide and prednisone combined with vincristine, vincristine and procarbazine, or etoposide may be useful in patients with severe refractory idiopathic thrombocytopenic purpura.
  3. Splenectomy generally does not cure the thrombocytopenia of SLE, but it may be necessary as an adjunct in managing selected cases.
- Infections are common because of compromised immune function secondary to SLE and the use of corticosteroid, cytotoxic, and antimetabolite drugs; pneumococcal bacteremia is associated with high mortality rate.
- Close monitoring for exacerbation of the disease and for potential side effects from medications (corticosteroids, cytotoxic agents) with frequent laboratory evaluation and office visits is necessary in all patients with SLE.
- Valvular heart disease is present in 18% of patients with SLE. The prevalence of infective endocarditis is approximately 1% (similar to the prevalence after prosthetic valve surgery, but greater than that following rheumatic valvulitis). Valvular heart disease in patients with SLE frequently changes over time (e.g., vegetations can appear unexpectedly for the first time, resolve, or change in size or appearance). These frequent changes are temporarily unrelated to other clinical features of SLE and can be associated with substantial morbidity and mortality.

■ DISPOSITION

- Most patients with lupus experience remissions and exacerbations.
- The leading cause of death in SLE is infection (one third of all deaths); active nephritis causes approximately 18% of deaths, and CNS disease causes 7% of deaths; the survival rate is 75% over the first 10 yr. Blacks and Hispanics generally have a worse prognosis.
- Symptomatic pericarditis occurs in one fourth of patients with SLE at some point during the course of the disease. Asymptomatic involvement is estimated to be more than 60% based on autopsy reports.
- Renal histologic studies and evaluation of renal function are useful in determining disease activity and predicting disease outcome (e.g., serum creatinine levels >3 mg/dl or evidence of diffuse proliferative involvement on renal biopsy are poor prognostic factors).

■ REFERRAL

- Rheumatology consultation in all patients with SLE
- Hematology consultation in patients with significant hematologic abnormalities (e.g., severe hemolytic anemia or thrombocytopenia)
- Nephrology consultation in patients with significant renal involvement

REFERENCES

Arbuckle MR et al: Development of autoantibodies before the clinical onset of systemic lupus erythematosus, *N Engl J Med* 349:1526, 2003.

Illei GG et al: Combination therapy with pulse cyclophosphamide plus methylprednisolone improves long-term renal outcome without adding toxicity in patients with lupus nephritis, *Ann Intern Med* 135:248, 2001.

Author: **Fred F. Ferri, M.D.**

BASIC INFORMATION

■ DEFINITION

Tabes dorsalis is a form of tertiary neurosyphilis affecting the dorsal columns of the spinal cord and peripheral nerves, characterized by paroxysmal pain, particularly in the abdomen and legs; sensory ataxia; normal strength; autonomic dysfunction, and Argyll-Robertson pupils.

■ SYNONYMS

Posterior spinal sclerosis
Tabetic neurosyphilis
Syphilitic myeloneuropathy

ICD-9CM CODES

094.0 Tabes dorsalis, ataxia, locomotor

■ EPIDEMIOLOGY & DEMOGRAPHICS

INCIDENCE (IN U.S.): Rare, but increasing with HIV/AIDS
PREVALENCE (IN U.S.): Rare; more common with HIV/AIDS epidemic
PREDOMINANT SEX: Male
PEAK INCIDENCE: 15-20 yr after initial infection

■ PHYSICAL FINDINGS & CLINICAL PRESENTATION

- Argyll-Robertson pupil in 50% (pupil reacts poorly to light but well to accommodation)
- Loss of position and vibration at ankles (wide-based gait; inability to walk in the dark: sensory ataxia)
- Loss of deep pain sensation, resulting in deep foot ulcers
- Degenerative joint disease, especially in knees caused by severe neuropathy (Charcot joints)
- Normal strength with areflexia in the legs
- Lightning pains in the legs
- Severe intermittent visceral pains, such as gastrointestinal, laryngeal (visceral crises)
- Autonomic dysfunction (urinary and fecal incontinence)

■ ETIOLOGY

Infectious *(Treponema pallidum)*

DIAGNOSIS

■ DIFFERENTIAL DIAGNOSIS

- Vitamin B_{12} deficiency (subacute combined degeneration of the spinal cord)
- Vitamin E deficiency
- Chronic nitrous oxide abuse
- Spinal cord neoplasm (involving conus medullaris)
- Lyme disease

■ WORKUP

Thorough neurologic history and examination

■ LABORATORY TESTS

- Lumbar puncture for elevated VDRL and FTA-ABS titers. False-positive CSF VDRL titers may occur with traumatic tap. CSF mononuclear pleocytosis (>5 white cells/microL) with increased protein support the diagnosis.
- Serum venereal disease research laboratory test (VDRL). This may be normal in 25%-30% of patients. Serum microhemagglutination-Treponema Pallidum (MHA-TP) or Fluorescent Treponemal Antigen-Antibody test (FTA-ABS) is necessary if clinical suspicion high.
- False-positive serum VDRL may occur in Lyme disease, nonvenereal treponematoses, genital herpes simplex, pregnancy, SLE, alcoholic cirrhosis, scleroderma, and mixed connective tissue disease.

■ IMAGING STUDIES

Not necessary if diagnosis confirmed

TREATMENT

■ ACUTE GENERAL Rx

Procaine penicillin 2 to 4 million U IM qd, along with probenecid 500 mg PO qid, for 14 days, or Aqueous penicillin G 3 to 4 million U IV q4h for 10-14 days.
If penicillin allergic, doxycycline 200 mg PO bid for 4 wk.

Many of the symptoms—degenerative neuropathic joint disease, lightning pains—persist after treatment.

■ CHRONIC Rx

- Physical therapy
- Analgesics, carbamazepine, gabapentin, or steroids may help "lightning" pain
- Supportive care (wheelchair, toileting issues, etc.)

■ DISPOSITION

Close follow-up required. Repeat lumbar puncture every 6 mo until CSF pleocytosis normalizes. If pleocytosis does not normalize in 6 mo or CSF is still abnormal in 2 yr, repeat treatment.
Further indication for retreatment: if there is a fourfold increase in titers or a failure of titers >1:32 to decrease at least fourfold by 12-24 mo.

■ REFERRAL

Joint replacement in moderate cases

REFERENCES

Centers for Disease Control and Prevention: 2002 sexually transmitted diseases treatment guidelines, *MMWR Morb Mortal Wkly Rep* 51(RR-6), 2002.
Solbrig MV, Healy JF, Jay CA: Infections of the nervous system. In Bradley WG, Daroff RB, Fenichel GM, Marsden CD: *Neurology in clinical practice. The neurological disorders. Vol II,* Boston, 2000, Butterwoth-Heinemann.
Author: **Eroboghene E. Ubogu, M.D.**

BASIC INFORMATION

■ DEFINITION
Takayasu's arteritis refers to a chronic systemic granulomatous vasculitis primarily affecting large arteries (aorta and its branches).

■ SYNONYMS
Pulseless disease
Aortitis syndrome
Aortic arch arteritis

■ ICD-9CM CODES
446.7 Takayasu disease or syndrome

■ EPIDEMIOLOGY & DEMOGRAPHICS
- Most cases have been reported from Japan, China, India, and Mexico
- Exact incidence and prevalence is not known
- Incidence in the U.S. 2.6/1 million
- Females > males 9:1
- Seen predominantly in patients <30 yr old

■ PHYSICAL FINDINGS & CLINICAL PRESENTATION
Takayasu's arteritis most frequently involves the aortic arch and its branches and can manifest as:
- Arm claudication, weakness, and numbness
- Amaurosis fugax, diplopia, headache, and dizziness
- Systemic symptoms
  1. Low-grade fever
  2. Malaise
  3. Weight loss
  4. Fatigue
- Vascular bruits of the carotid artery, subclavian artery, and aorta
- Discrepancy of blood pressures between the upper extremities
- Absence pulses
- Hypertension
- Retinopathy
- Aortic insufficiency murmur

■ ETIOLOGY
- The cause of Takayasu's arteritis is unknown. A delayed hypersensitivity to mycobacteria and spirochetes is a theory but remains to be substantiated.
- Infiltration of inflammatory cells into the vasa vasorum and media of large elastic arteries leads to thickening and narrowing or obliteration.

DIAGNOSIS

Criteria have been established for the diagnosis of Takayasu's arteritis by the American College of Rheumatology in 1990 and include:
- Age of disease <40 yr
- Claudication of extremities

- Decreased brachial artery pulse
- BP difference >10 mm Hg
- Bruit over subclavian arteries or aorta
- Abnormal arteriogram
- Takayasu's arteritis is diagnosed if at least three of the six criteria are present, giving a sensitivity of 90% and a specificity of 98%

■ DIFFERENTIAL DIAGNOSIS
Other causes of inflammatory aortitis must be excluded: giant cell arteritis, syphilis, tuberculosis, SLE, rheumatoid arthritis, Buerger's disease, Behçet's disease, Cogan's syndrome, Kawasaki disease, and spondyloarthropathies.

■ WORKUP
Any young patient with findings of absence pulses and loud bruits merits a workup for Takayasu's arteritis. The workup generally includes blood testing to look for signs of inflammation and imaging studies with the angiogram being the diagnostic gold standard.

■ LABORATORY TESTS
- CBC may reveal an elevated WBC count
- ESR is elevated in active disease

■ IMAGING STUDIES
- Ultrasound: Carotid, thoracic, and abdominal ultrasound are useful adjunctive imaging studies in diagnosing occlusive disease resulting from Takayasu's arteritis (Fig. 1-267).
- Doppler and noninvasive upper and lower extremity studies are helpful in assessing blood flow and absent pulses.
- CT scan is used to assess the thickness of the aorta.
- Angiogram can show narrowing of the aorta and/or branches of the aorta, aneurysm formation, and poststenotic dilation. Angiographic findings are classified as four types:
  1. Type I: Lesions involve only the aortic arch and its branches.
  2. Type II: Lesions only involving the abdominal aorta and its branches.
  3. Type III: Lesions involving the aorta above and below the diaphragm.
  4. Type IV: Lesions involving the pulmonary artery.

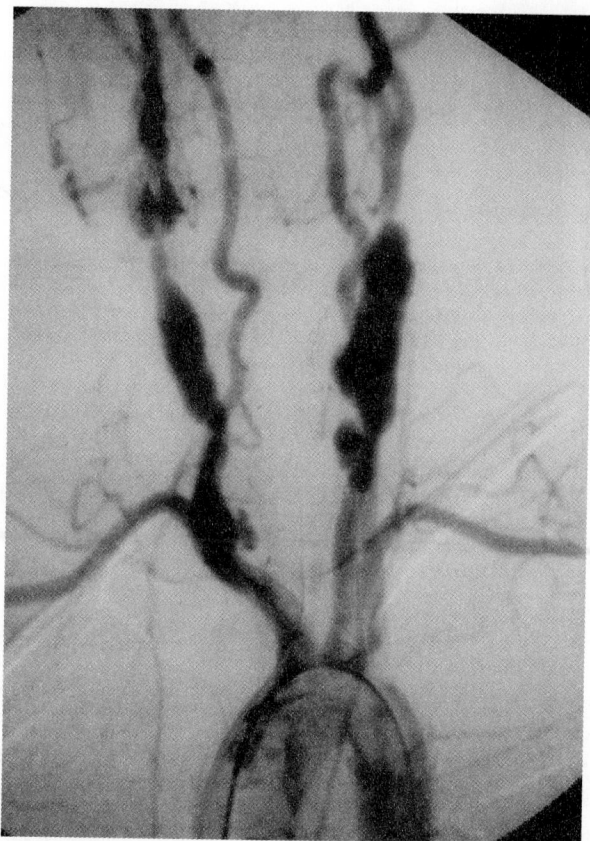

Fig. 1-267 Angiogram of a child with Takayasu's arteritis showing massive bilateral carotid dilation, stenosis, and poststenotic dilation. (From Behrman RE: *Nelson textbook of pediatrics*, ed 16, Philadelphia, 2000, WB Saunders.)

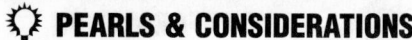

℞ TREATMENT

■ ACUTE GENERAL Rx
- Corticosteroids are the treatment of choice. Prednisone 40 to 60 mg PO qd or 1 mg/kg/day is used for 3 mo.
- Patients are monitored for symptoms and by following the ESR. If symptoms have resolved and the ESR is normal, attempts to taper prednisone are made.

■ CHRONIC RX
- Patients who cannot be tapered off the corticosteroids or who have relapse of the disease are given methotrexate 0.15 to 0.35 mg/kg or approximately 15 mg/wk.
- Cyclophosphamide 1 to 2 mg/kg/day can be given with glucocorticoids as adjunctive therapy in relapse or treatment-resistant patients.

■ DISPOSITION
- Treatment improves symptoms within days with relief of ischemic claudication, return of pulses on examination, and reversal of lumen narrowing on angiograms. However, some patients may continue to have progression of arterial lesions despite therapy.

- With the addition of a second agent in patients with treatment resistance or relapse, 50% remission has been seen.
- Mortality results are mixed, showing high rates in reports from Asia and lower rates in studies done in the U.S. (2%).
- Death can occur suddenly from ruptured aneurysm, myocardial infarction, and stroke.

■ REFERRAL
Whenever the diagnosis of vasculitis is suspected, a rheumatology consult is appropriate. Vascular surgery and cardiology consultations are recommended for any evidence of carotid, peripheral, and coronary artery disease or if a large abdominal aneurysm is found.

☼ PEARLS & CONSIDERATIONS

■ COMMENTS
The long-term prognosis of treated patients with Takayasu's disease is good, with >90% of patients surviving more than 15 yr.

REFERENCES

Arend WP et al: American College of Rheumatology 1990 criteria for the classification of Takayasu's arteritis, *Arthr Rheum* 33:1129, 1990.

Fraga A, Medina F: Takayasu's arteritis, *Curr Rheumatol Rep* 4(1):30, 2002.

Giordano JM: Surgical treatment of Takayasu's disease, *Clev Clin J Med* 69(Suppl 2):S11, 2002.

Kerr GS et al: Takayasu arteritis, *Ann Intern Med* 120:919, 1994.

Weyend CM, Goronzy JJ: Mechanisms of disease: medium and large vessel vasculitis, *N Engl J Med* 349:160, 2003.

Authors: **Peter Petropoulos, M.D., and Mel Anderson, M.D.**

BASIC INFORMATION

■ DEFINITION
Four species of adult tapeworm may infect humans as the definitive host: *Taenia saginata* (beef tapeworm), *Taenia solium* (pork tapeworm), *Diphyllobothrium latum* (fish tapeworm), and *Hymenolepis nana*. In addition, *T. solium* may infect humans in its larval form (cysticercosis), and several animal tapeworms (see "Echinococcosis" in Section I) may cause infection in an analogous manner.

■ SYNONYMS
Cysticercosis (larval infection by *T. solium*)

ICD-9CM CODES
123.9 Tapeworm infestation

■ EPIDEMIOLOGY & DEMOGRAPHICS
INCIDENCE (IN U.S.):
- Diagnosed primarily in immigrants
- Varies widely by country of origin and dietary practices

PREVALENCE (IN U.S.):
- *T. saginata:* <0.1%
- *D. latum:* <0.05%
- *T. solium:* <0.1%
- *H. nana:* sporadic, often in setting of outbreak

PREDOMINANT SEX: Equal sex distribution

PREDOMINANT AGE:
- *T. saginata, T. solium, D. latum:* 20 to 39 yr of age
- *H. nana* in setting of institution outbreaks: children

■ PHYSICAL FINDINGS & CLINICAL PRESENTATION
- Adult worms
  1. Attach to bowel mucosa
  2. Feed and grow
  3. Cause minimal or no symptoms or sequelae
- Cysticercosis
  1. Mass lesions of brain (neurocysticercosis), soft tissue, viscera
  2. Neurocysticercosis may cause seizures, hydrocephalus
- Prolonged infection with *D. latum*
  1. Vitamin B_{12} deficiency
  2. Megaloblastic anemia

■ ETIOLOGY
TAPEWORM
- Adult worm resides in small or large bowel; proglottids and eggs passed in stool.
- Eggs are ingested by the animal intermediate host.
- Eggs hatch into larvae.
- Larvae disseminate largely in skeletal muscle, brain, viscera.
- Humans eat infected beef *(T. saginata)*, infected pork *(T. solium)*, or infected fish *(D. latum)*.
- Larvae mature into adults within the GI lumen.
- *H. nana* infection is acquired by ingesting eggs in human or rodent feces.

CYSTICERCOSIS
- Humans ingest eggs of *T. solium* in food contaminated with human feces that contain the eggs.
- Eggs hatch into larvae in gut.
- Larvae disseminate widely through tissues (particularly soft tissue and CNS) forming cystic lesions containing either viable or nonviable larvae.

⚗ DIAGNOSIS

■ DIFFERENTIAL DIAGNOSIS
Section II describes the differential diagnosis of intestinal helminths.

■ WORKUP
- Stool examination for eggs or proglottids (tapeworm)
- Cerebral CT scan (neurocysticercosis)
- Serum antibody (neurocysticercosis)

■ IMAGING STUDIES
- Tapeworm: incidental finding on upper GI series
- Neurocysticercosis:
  1. Cerebral cysts are readily demonstrated by CT scan or MRI.
  2. Calcified lesions are an incidental finding.

℞ TREATMENT

■ ACUTE GENERAL Rx
- All patients with intestinal tapeworm infections should be treated with a single oral dose of praziquantel.
  1. *T. solium:* 5 mg/kg
  2. *T. saginata:* 20 mg/kg
  3. *D. latum:* 10 mg/kg
  4. *H. nana:* 25 mg/kg
- Therapy that may be considered for symptomatic cysticercosis:
  1. May regress spontaneously
  2. Surgery
  3. Albendazole 15 mg/kg PO qd in three doses for 28 days
  4. Praziquantel 50 mg/kg PO qd in three doses for 15 days
- Therapy contraindicated with:
  1. Ocular infections
  2. Cerebral infections in which local inflammation caused by destruction of the parasite may cause significant damage

■ CHRONIC Rx
- Retreatment if required
- Avoidance of undercooked pork, meat, or fish
- Cysticercosis: proper hand washing, proper disposal of human waste

■ DISPOSITION
- Neurologic follow-up for patients with neurocysticercosis
- Ophthalmologic follow-up for patients with ocular involvement

■ REFERRAL
Patients treated for neurocysticercosis should be evaluated by a physician experienced in managing this infection, if possible.

☼ PEARLS & CONSIDERATIONS

■ COMMENTS
T. solium is the most dangerous of the tapeworms because of the potential for cysticercosis by means of autoinfection.

REFERENCE
Garcia HH, Del Brutto OH: *Taenia solium* cysticercosis, *Infect Dis Clin North Am* 14(1):97, 2000.
Author: **Joseph R. Masci, M.D.**

BASIC INFORMATION

■ DEFINITION
Tardive dyskinesia is a movement disorder associated with the long-term use of antipsychotics, particularly dopamine-blocking neuroleptics.

ICD-9CM CODES
333.82 Tardive dyskinesia

■ EPIDEMIOLOGY & DEMOGRAPHICS
The disorder is caused by dopamine-blocking neuroleptics (e.g., Haldol). The incidence is declining with the use of newer generation antipsychotics.

■ PHYSICAL FINDINGS & CLINICAL PRESENTATION
- Typically appears with the reduction or withdrawal of the antipsychotics
- Characterized by:
  1. Slow, writhing movements of the arms and legs
  2. Grimacing at the face
  3. Symptoms subside when the antipsychotic is reintroduced

■ ETIOLOGY
Prolonged use of dopamine-blocking neuroleptics

DIAGNOSIS

■ DIFFERENTIAL DIAGNOSIS
- Huntington's chorea
- Excessive treatment with L-dopa

■ WORKUP
Careful documentation of drug history

■ IMAGING STUDIES
CT, MRI are normal

TREATMENT

■ NONPHARMACOLOGIC THERAPY
None

■ CHRONIC Rx
Olanzapine and amisulpride may be of symptomatic help, but long-term efficacy is unproven.

■ REFERRAL
Movement disorder specialist if symptoms are severe

PEARLS & CONSIDERATIONS

- Tardive dyskinesia in the elderly and mentally deficient seem to be especially difficult to manage.

REFERENCES
Caroff SN et al: Movement disorders associated with atypical antipsychotic drugs, *J Clin Psychiatry* 63(Suppl 4):12, 2002.
Casey DE: Tardive dyskinesia: Pathophysiology and animal models, *J Clin Psychiatry* 61 (Suppl 4):5, 2000.
Author: **Fred F. Ferri, M.D.**

BASIC INFORMATION

■ DEFINITION

Tarsal tunnel syndrome is a rare entrapment neuropathy that develops as a result of compression of the posterior tibial nerve in the tunnel formed by the flexor retinaculum behind the medial malleolus of the ankle (Fig. 1-268).

ICD-9CM CODES

355.5 Tarsal tunnel syndrome

■ EPIDEMIOLOGY & DEMOGRAPHICS

PREVALENCE: Unknown
PREDOMINANT SEX: Female = male

■ PHYSICAL FINDINGS & CLINICAL PRESENTATION

- Neuritic symptoms along the course of the posterior tibial nerve in the sole and heel
- Swelling over tarsal tunnel
- Possible positive Tinel's sign
- Possible reproduction of symptoms with sustained eversion of hindfoot or digital compression of tunnel
- Sensory and motor changes unusual

■ ETIOLOGY

Space-occupying lesions (ganglia, varicosities, lipomas, synovial hypertrophy)

DIAGNOSIS

■ DIFFERENTIAL DIAGNOSIS

- Plantar fasciitis
- Peripheral neuropathy
- Proximal radiculopathy
- Local tendinitis
- Peripheral vascular disease
- Morton's neuroma

■ ELECTRICAL STUDIES

Electrodiagnostic testing is often inconclusive. Delayed sensory conduction or increased motor latency may be seen.

TREATMENT

- NSAIDs
- Immobilization
- Medial heel wedge or orthotic to minimize heel eversion
- Local steroid injection into tunnel

■ REFERRAL

For surgical decompression if needed

REFERENCES

Burks JB, DeHeer PA: Tarsal tunnel syndrome secondary to an accessory muscle: a case report, *J Foot Ankle Surg* 40(6):401, 2001.

Garchar DJ, Lewis JE, DiDomenico LA: Hypertrophic sustentaculum tali causing a tarsal tunnel syndrome: a case report, *J Foot Ankle Surg* 40(2):110, 2001.

Gorter K et al: Variation in diagnosis and management of common foot problems by GPs, *Fam Pract* 18(6):569, 2001.

Labib SA et al: Heel pain triad (HPT): the combination of plantar fasciitis, posterior tibial tendon dysfunction and tarsal tunnel syndrome, *Foot Ankle Int* 23(3):212, 2002.

Pecina M: Diagnostic tests for tarsal tunnel syndrome, *J Bone Joint Surg Am* 84-A(9):1714, 2002.

Author: **Lonnie R. Mercier, M.D.**

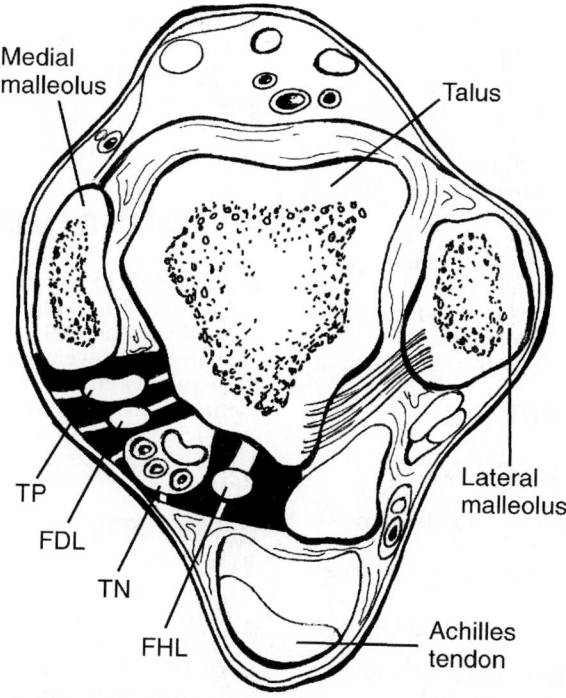

Fig. 1-268   Anatomy of tarsal tunnel syndrome. Transverse view of ankle. *FDL,* Flexor digitorum longus; *FHL,* flexor hallucis longus tendon; *TN,* tibial nerve (single contour), posterior tibial artery, veins; *TP,* tibialis posterior tendon. Tendons and neurovascular elements are included into individual fibrous septa that connect periosteum with the deep fascia. (From Canoso J: *Rheumatology in primary care,* Philadelphia, 1997, WB Saunders.)

BASIC INFORMATION

■ **DEFINITION**

Temporomandibular joint (TMJ) syndrome refers to a group of disorders leading to symptoms of the temporomandibular joint.

■ **SYNONYMS**

Temporomandibular dysfunction
Painful temporomandibular joint

ICD-9CM CODES

524.60 Temporomandibular joint pain-dysfunction syndrome

■ **EPIDEMIOLOGY & DEMOGRAPHICS**

• 15% of the population have TMJ disorders
• Females > males 4:1
• Occurs between the second and fourth decades of life
• Usually unilateral, affecting either side with equal frequency

■ **PHYSICAL FINDINGS & CLINICAL PRESENTATION**

• Otalgia
• Odontalgia
• Headaches (frontal, temporal, retroorbital)
• Tinnitus
• Dizziness
• Clicking or popping sounds with movement of the TMJ
• Joint locking
• Tender to palpation
• Limited range of motion of the TMJ

■ **ETIOLOGY**

Causes of TMJ syndrome are multifactorial, encompassing local anatomic anomalies to familiar disease processes that can involve the TMJ.

• Myofascial pain-dysfunction syndrome (MPD): the most common cause of TMJ syndrome and results from teeth grinding and clenching the jaw (bruxism)
• Internal TMJ derangement: abnormal connection of the articular disk to the mandibular condyle
• Degenerative joint disease
• Rheumatoid arthritis
• Gouty arthritis
• Pseudogout
• Ankylosing spondylitis
• Trauma
• Prior surgery (orthodontic, intraarticular steroid injection)
• Tumors

■ **DIAGNOSIS**

■ **DIFFERENTIAL DIAGNOSIS**

The differential diagnosis of TMJ syndrome is thought of in terms of etiology and includes the list as mentioned previously under Etiology. Myofascial pain-dysfunction syndrome, internal TMJ derangement, and degenerative joint disease represent >90% of all causes of TMJ syndrome.

■ **WORKUP**

Includes a detailed history and physical examination, followed by radiographic imaging evaluation.

■ **LABORATORY TESTS**

Laboratory examination is not very helpful in the diagnosis of TMJ syndrome.

■ **IMAGING STUDIES**

• Plain x-rays: The most common x-rays are the panoramic, transorbital, and transpharyngeal views in both opened and closed positions.
• Arthrography is helpful in looking for meniscus involvement.
• CT scan is very accurate in diagnosing meniscal and osseous derangements of the TMJ.
• MRI can better visualize soft tissue inflammation, if present.

■ **TREATMENT**

■ **NONPHARMACOLOGIC THERAPY**

• Soft diet to rest the muscles of mastication
• Heat 15 to 20 min four to six times per day
• Massage of the masseter and temporalis muscles
• Formed splints or bite appliances
• Range-of-motion exercises

■ **ACUTE GENERAL Rx**

• Nonsteroidal antiinflammatory drugs (NSAIDs): ibuprofen 800 PO mg tid prn, naproxen 500 PO mg bid prn, titrated to relieve symptoms
• Muscle relaxants: diazepam 2.5 to 5 mg PO tid prn
• In degenerative joint disease of the TMJ, intraarticular steroid injection can be tried

■ **CHRONIC Rx**

• Most of the above mentioned treatment is used for myofascial pain-dysfunction syndrome; however, it can be applied to other causes of TMJ syndrome. Surgery is usually a measure of last resort in patients who are refractory to nonpharmacologic and acute general treatment.
• Surgical procedures include:
  1. Meniscoplasty
  2. Meniscectomy
  3. Subcondylar osteotomy
  4. TMJ reconstruction

■ **DISPOSITION**

The course depends on the underlying etiology; however, a lengthy course with exacerbations of symptoms can be expected.

■ **REFERRAL**

All patients with TMJ syndrome refractory to conservative nonpharmacologic and acute therapy should be referred to a periodontist, oral maxillofacial surgeon, or ENT surgeon.

✿ PEARLS & CONSIDERATIONS

■ **COMMENTS**

• Patients with rheumatoid arthritis involving the TMJ usually will have bilateral involvement.
• Frequently emotional stress initiates the myofascial pain-dysfunction, which accounts for 85% of all cases of TMJ syndrome.

REFERENCES

Baba K, Tsukiyama Y et al: A review of temporomandibular disorder diagnostic techniques, *J Prosthet Dent* 86(2):184, 2001.
Blank LW: Clinical guidelines for managing mandibular dysfunction, *Gen Dentist* 46(6):592, 1998.
Dierks EJ: Temporomandibular disorders and facial pain syndromes. In Kelly WN et al: *Textbook of rheumatology,* ed 5, Philadelphia, 1997, WB Saunders.
Pankhurst CL: Controversies in the aetiology of temporomandibular disorders. Part I. Temporomandibular disorders: all in the mind? *Prim Dent Care* 4(1):25, 1997.

Author: **Peter Petropoulos, M.D.**

BASIC INFORMATION

■ DEFINITION
Testicular neoplasms are primary cancers originating in a testis (Fig. 1-269).

■ SYNONYMS
Testis tumor
Testicular cancer

ICD-9CM CODES
186.9 Testicular neoplasm
M906/3 (seminoma)
M9101/3 (embryonal carcinoma or teratoma)
M9100/3 (choriocarcinoma)

■ EPIDEMIOLOGY & DEMOGRAPHICS
- Incidence: 2 to 3 cases/100,000 men/yr
- 1% to 2% of all cancers in males
- Age: can occur in any age but most common in young adults; average age for embryonal cell carcinoma: 30 yr; average age for seminoma: 36 yr

■ PHYSICAL FINDINGS & CLINICAL PRESENTATION
- Any mass within the testicle should be considered cancer until proven otherwise. It may be found by the patient who brings it to the attention of a physician or it may be found by a physician on a routine examination.
- Symptoms other than scrotal or testicular swelling are typically absent unless the cancer has metastasized. Occasionally a patient may complain of scrotal fullness or heaviness.
- Testicular palpation should be performed with two hands. Transillumination may distinguish a solid mass (e.g., cancer) and a fluid-filled lesion (e.g., hydrocele or spermatocele). The mass is nontender, indeed less sensitive than a normal testicle.

■ ETIOLOGY & PATHOLOGY
- Cryptorchidism (undescended testes) even if corrected by orchiopexy
- Pathology

Cell type	Frequency %
Seminoma	42
Embryonal cell carcinoma	26
Teratocarcinoma	26
Teratoma	5
Choriocarcinoma	1
Other rare types:	
Yolk sac carcinoma	
Mixed germ cell tumors	
Carcinoid tumor	
Sertoli cell tumors	
Leydig cell tumors	
Lymphoma	
Metastatic cancer to the testes	

- TNM staging system for testicular cancer

T_0 No apparent primary
T_1 Testis only (excludes rete testis)
T_2 Beyond the tunica albuginea
T_3 Rete testis or epididymal involvement
T_4 Spermatic cord
    1. Spermatic cord
    2. Scrotum
N_0 No nodal involvement
N_1 Ipsilateral regional nodal involvement
N_2 Contralateral or bilateral abdominal or groin nodes
N_3 Palpable abdominal nodes or fixed groin nodes
N_4 Juxtaregional nodes
M_0 No distant metastases
M_1 Distant metastases present

The clinical stages consist of stage A, with tumor confined to the testis and cord structures; stage B, with tumor confined to the retroperitoneal lymph nodes; and stage C, with tumor involving the abdominal viscera or disease above the diaphragm.

DIAGNOSIS

■ DIFFERENTIAL DIAGNOSIS
- Spermatocele
- Varicocele
- Hydrocele
- Epididymitis
- Epidermoid cyst of the testicle
- Epididymis tumors

■ WORKUP
Physical examination, laboratory tests, and imaging studies (Section III, Fig. 3-176)

■ LABORATORY TESTS
- Serum human chorionic gonadotropin (hCG)
- Serum alpha-fetoprotein (AFP)
One or both of these tumor markers will be elevated in 70% of cases of testicular cancer.
- Testicular biopsy is contraindicated.

■ IMAGING STUDIES
- Ultrasound (Fig. 1-270)
- CT scan or MRI of pelvis and abdomen
- Chest x-ray

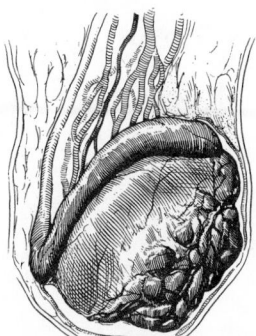

Fig. 1-269   Testicular tumor causing an irregular mass intrinsic to the testis. (From Sabiston D: *Textbook of surgery,* ed 15, Philadelphia, 1997, WB Saunders.)

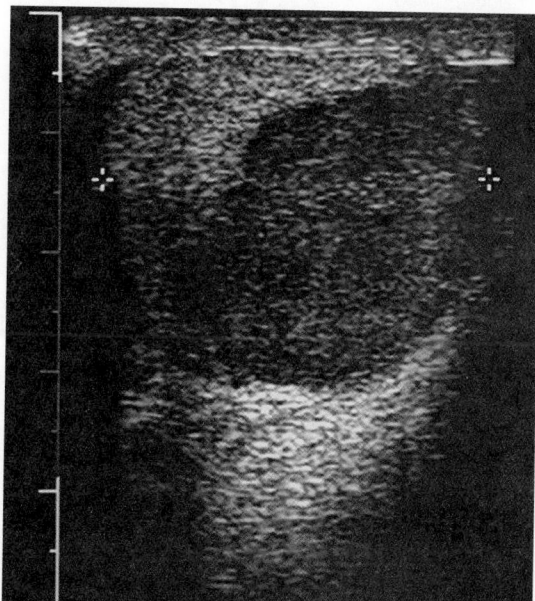

Fig. 1-270   Testicular ultrasound showing an intratesticular solid neoplasm. (From Nseyo UO [ed]: *Urology for primary care physicians,* Philadelphia, 1999, WB Saunders.)

TREATMENT

- Surgical exploration of the testicle through an inguinal incision with a noncrushing clamp placed on the cord before direct testicular examination. If a mass is confined within the body of the testicle, an orchiectomy is performed
- Retroperitoneal lymph node dissection for clinical stage A and low stage B (lymph nodes under 6 cm in greatest diameter) provides cure in 70%
- Chemotherapy: cisplatin, vinblastine, and bleomycin
  1. Not indicated in clinical stage A
  2. Controversial in low stage B
  3. Cornerstone of treatment in high stage B or stage C
- Radiation therapy for stage A and low stage B seminoma provides cure in 85%
- Posttreatment surveillance for testicular cancer survivors (annually)
  1. General maintenance
  2. Fertility assessment
  3. Sexuality status
  4. Skin examination (increased risk of dysplastic nivi)
  5. Testicular examination (3% to 4% risk of second testicular cancer)
  6. Serum tumor markers (hCG, AFP)
  7. Chest x-ray (for late relapse)
  8. Complications of cisplatin: hypertension, hyperlipidemia, renal failure, hypomagnesemia, hearing loss, tinnitus, peripheral neuropathy, and infertility

■ **REFERRAL**
To urologist

REFERENCES

Rowland RG, Foster RS, Donohue JP: Testis tumors. In Gillenwater JY et al (eds): *Adult and pediatric urology,* vol 2, ed 3, St Louis, 1998, Mosby.

Vaughn D et al: Long-term medical care of testicular cancer survivors, *Ann Intern Med* 136:463, 2002.

Author: **Tom J. Wachtel, M.D.**

BASIC INFORMATION

■ DEFINITION

Testicular torsion is a twisting of the spermatic cord leading to cessation of testicular blood flow, ischemia, and infarction if left untreated (Fig. 1-271).

■ SYNONYMS

Spermatic cord torsion

ICD-9CM CODES

608.2 Testicular torsion

■ EPIDEMIOLOGY & DEMOGRAPHICS

- Affects 1:4000 males
- Two thirds of all cases occur between the ages of 12 and 18 yr, but may occur at any age, including antenatally

■ PHYSICAL FINDINGS & CLINICAL PRESENTATION

- Typical sequence is sudden onset of hemiscrotal pain, then swelling, nausea, and vomiting without fever or urinary symptoms.
- Painless testicular swelling occurs in 10%.
- One out of three patients reports previous episodes of spontaneously remitting scrotal pain.
- In the neonate, testicular torsion should be presumed in patients with a painless, discolored hemiscrotal swelling.
- In rare cases, torsion may involve an undescended testicle. In such situations an empty hemiscrotum is palpated together with a tender lump in the inguinal area.

■ ETIOLOGY

Testicular torsion may occur without any underlying abnormality but is more likely when the tunica vaginalis extends high on the spermatic cord (bell-clapper deformity).

DIAGNOSIS

■ DIFFERENTIAL DIAGNOSIS (SEE ALSO SECTION II)

- Torsion of the testicular appendages
- Testicular tumor
- Epididymitis
- Incarcerated inguinoscrotal hernia
- Orchitis
- Spermatocele
- Hydrocele

■ WORKUP

The diagnosis is usually based on history and physical examination.

■ IMAGING STUDIES

- Radionuclide scrotal scanning (technetium-99m): cold testicle
- Doppler ultrasonic stethoscope (Doppler flowmetry)

TREATMENT

Surgical derotation of the spermatic cord followed by bilateral testicular fixation with nonabsorbable sutures

■ PROGNOSIS

- There is an 80% testicular salvage rate if detorsion occurs within 12 hr of onset.
- After 24 hr, irreversible testicular infarction is expected.
- Because the contralateral testes can be affected (immunologic process), when treatment is delayed and return of blood flow does not occur after detorsion, some recommend orchiectomy of the infarcted testicle.

■ REFERRAL

To urologist

REFERENCE

Kogan S et al: Spermatic cord torsion. In Gillenwater JY et al (eds): *Adult and pediatric urology*, ed 3, St Louis, 1996, Mosby.
Author: **Tom J. Wachtel, M.D.**

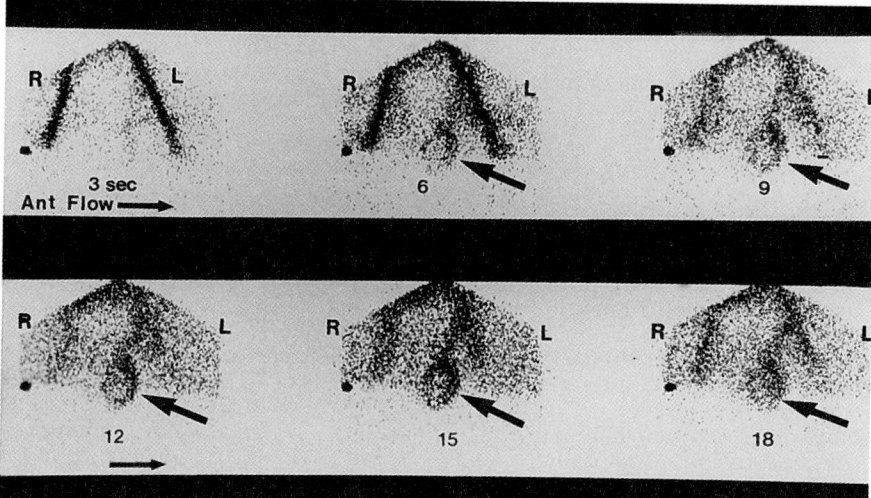

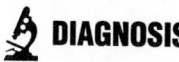

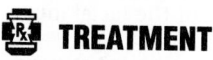

Fig. 1-271   Testicular torsion. Evaluation of blood flow to the testicle has been done by giving an intravenous bolus of radioactive material. The right and left iliac vessels are clearly identified, and sequential images are obtained every 3 sec. Here, increased flow is seen to the rim of the left testicle *(arrows)*, and there is no blood flow centrally. This is the appearance of a testicular torsion in which the torsion has been present for more than approximately 24 hr. (From Mettler FA [ed]: *Primary care radiology,* Philadelphia, 2000, WB Saunders.)

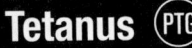
 BASIC INFORMATION

■ DEFINITION
Tetanus is a life-threatening illness manifested by muscle rigidity and spasms; it is caused by a neurotoxin (tetanospasmin) produced by *Clostridium tetani*.

ICD-9CM CODES
037 Tetanus

■ EPIDEMIOLOGY & DEMOGRAPHICS
INCIDENCE (IN U.S.): 48 to 64 cases reported annually since 1986
PREDOMINANT AGE: >60 yr of age
GENETICS:
Neonatal Infection:
- Rare in U.S.
- Among the leading causes of neonatal mortality in many parts of the world (caused by infection of the umbilical cord stump)

■ PHYSICAL FINDINGS & CLINICAL PRESENTATION
- Trismus ("lockjaw")
- Risus sardonicus (peculiar grin), characteristic grimace that results from contraction of the facial muscles
- Generalized muscle spasms causing severe pain and, at times, respiratory compromise and death
- Rigid abdominal muscles, flexed arms, and extended legs
- Autonomic dysfunction several days after onset of illness
- Leading cause of death: fluctuations in heart rate and blood pressure
- Usually, absence of fever
- Localized tetanus
  1. Rigidity of muscles near the injury
  2. Weakness as a result of lower motor neuron injury
  3. May be self-limited and resolve spontaneously
  4. More often progresses to generalized tetanus
  5. Cephalic tetanus:
     a. May occur with head injuries
     b. Can manifest as cranial nerve dysfunction

■ ETIOLOGY
- *C. tetani* is a gram-positive, spore-forming bacillus that resides primarily in the soil.
- Majority of cases are caused by punctures and lacerations.
- Toxin is elaborated from organisms in a contaminated wound.
- Local symptoms are caused by inhibition of neurotransmitter at presynaptic sites.
  1. Over the next 2 to 14 days, the toxin travels up the neurons to the CNS, where it acts on inhibitory neurons to prevent neurotransmitter release.
  2. Unopposed motor activity results in tonic contractions of muscles.

 DIAGNOSIS

■ DIFFERENTIAL DIAGNOSIS
- Strychnine poisoning
- Dystonic reaction caused by neuroleptic agents
- Local infection (dental or masseter muscle) causing trismus
- Severe hypocalcemia
- Hysteria

■ WORKUP
- Positive wound culture is not helpful in diagnosis.
- Isolation of organism is possible in patients without the illness.

■ LABORATORY TESTS
- Usually, normal blood counts and chemistries
- Toxicology of serum and urine to rule out strychnine poisoning

TREATMENT

■ NONPHARMACOLOGIC THERAPY
- Monitoring in a hospital ICU: keep surroundings dark and quiet
- Intubation or tracheostomy for severe laryngospasm
- Debridement of wound

■ ACUTE GENERAL Rx
- Human tetanus immunoglobulin (HTIg) 500 U via IM injection
- Tetanus toxoid (Td) 0.5 ml by IM injection at a different site
- Metronidazole 500 mg IV q6h, or penicillin G 1 million U IV q4h for 10 days
- IV diazepam to control muscle spasms
- Neuromuscular blockade if necessary

■ CHRONIC Rx
- Supportive care
- Possible mechanical ventilation
- Minimal external stimuli
- Control of heart rate and blood pressure:
  1. Labetalol for sympathetic hyperactivity
  2. Pacemaker for sustained bradycardia
- Physical therapy once spasms subside

■ DISPOSITION
Full recovery over weeks to months if complications can be avoided

■ REFERRAL
- To emergency department
- To infectious disease specialist

PEARLS & CONSIDERATIONS

■ COMMENTS
- Illness is preventable.
- Boosters of Td should be given every 10 yr to maintain immune status.
- Passive as well as active immunization (HTIg + Td) should be given for patients with tetanus-prone wounds who have not been adequately immunized in the previous 5 yr.
- A recent U.S. study showed that only 72% of people >6 yr had protective levels of antibody.

REFERENCES
Hsu SS et al: Tetanus in the emergency department: a current review, *J Emerg Med* 20(4):357, 2001.
McQuillam GM et al: Serologic immunity to diphtheria and tetanus in the United States, *Ann Intern Med* 136:660, 2002.
Author: **Maurice Policar, M.D.**

BASIC INFORMATION

■ DEFINITION

Tetralogy of Fallot (TOF) is a congenital heart deformity consisting of the following four features:
- Ventricular septal defect (VSD)
- Infundibular stenosis leading to obstruction to the right ventricular (RV) outflow tract
- Overriding aorta
- Right ventricular hypertrophy (RVH)

See Fig. 1-272.

ICD-9CM CODES
745.2 Tetralogy of Fallot

■ EPIDEMIOLOGY & DEMOGRAPHICS
- TOF is the most common cyanotic congenital heart malformation after age 1 yr.
- TOF accounts for nearly 10% of all congenital heart disease.
- TOF occurs in approximately 3000 newborns/yr.

■ PHYSICAL FINDINGS & CLINICAL PRESENTATION
- Of the four major features of TOF, infundibular stenosis leading to right ventricular outflow tract obstruction and VSD are the primary defects leading to:
  1. Right-to-left shunting and hypoxemia
  2. Altered RV hemodynamics
  3. Decreased pulmonary blood flow
- The aforementioned pathophysiologic concepts subsequently result in common manifestations of TOF, including:
  1. Cyanosis secondary to increased RV pressures from infundibular stenosis resulting in the shunting of deoxygenated blood from the RV through the VSD into the left ventricle, thus bypassing the lungs
  2. Dyspnea on exertion
  3. Clubbing
  4. Child assuming a squatting position after exercise increasing systemic vascular resistance, thereby decreasing right-to-left shunting
  5. Low birth weight and growth rate
  6. Palpable RV impulse
  7. Systolic thrill along the left sternal border
  8. Single second heart sound, inaudible P2 component
  9. Systolic ejection murmur resulting from RV outflow tract obstruction

■ ETIOLOGY
Unknown

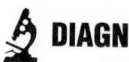

DIAGNOSIS

The diagnosis of TOF is suspected in any neonate, infant, or child presenting with cyanosis and a heart murmur.

■ DIFFERENTIAL DIAGNOSIS
- Asthma
- Isolated VSD
- Pulmonary atresia
- Patent ductus arteriosus
- Aortic stenosis
- Pneumothorax

■ WORKUP
The initial workup of TOF like any cardiac disease requires a detailed history and physical examination along with an echocardiography, chest x-ray, ECG, and simple laboratory tests.

■ LABORATORY TESTS
- CBC with polycythemia resulting from longstanding cyanosis
- ABGs with hypoxemia, normal pH, and pCO_2
- Pulse oximetry
- ECG commonly demonstrating RVH defined as right axis deviation >90 degrees with an R wave greater than S wave in lead V1. Right atrial enlargement with peaked p wave amplitude >2.5 mm in the inferior leads or initial portion of the p wave >1.5 mm in lead V1

■ IMAGING STUDIES
- CXR revealing boot-shaped heart commonly described as "coeur en sabot"; prominent RV with decreased pulmonary vascularity
- Echocardiography demonstrating VSD with a stenotic RV outflow tract and an overriding aorta
- Cardiac catheterization and angiography aid in the determination of the severity of right-to-left shunting, localization of the VSD, and anatomic assessment of the RV outflow tract, pulmonary artery, and coronary artery anatomy

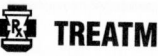

TREATMENT

■ NONPHARMACOLOGIC THERAPY
- Oxygen
- Knee-chest position in hypoxemic spells helps reduce venous return and increase systemic vascular resistance, thus decreasing right-to-left shunting

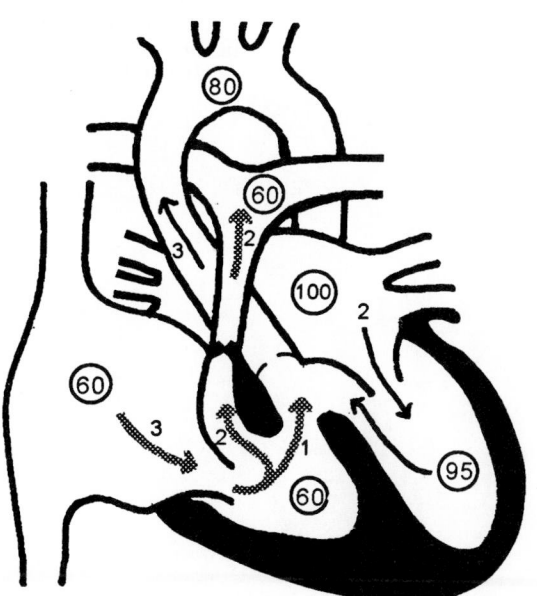

Fig. 1-272 Physiology of tetralogy of Fallot (TOF). The circled numbers represent oxygen saturations. The numbers next to the arrows represent volumes of blood flow (in L/min/m²). The atrial (mixed venous) oxygen saturation is decreased secondary to the systemic hypoxemia. Three L/min/m² of desaturated blood enter the right atrium and traverse the tricuspid valve. Two liters flow through the right ventricular outflow tract into the lungs, whereas 1 L shunts right to left through the VSD into the ascending aorta. Thus the pulmonary blood flow is two-thirds normal (Qp:Qs of 0.7:1). Blood returning to the left atrium is fully saturated. Only 2 L of blood flow across the mitral valve. The oxygen saturation in the left ventricle may be slightly decreased owing to right-to-left shunting across the VSD. Two liters of saturated left ventricular blood, mixing with 1 L of desaturated right ventricular blood, are ejected into the ascending aorta. The aortic saturation is decreased, and the cardiac output is normal. (From Behrman RE: *Nelson textbook of pediatrics,* ed 16, Philadelphia, 2000, WB Saunders.)

■ ACUTE GENERAL THERAPY

Acute treatment of any infant or child with TOF who is cyanotic with respiratory distress is aimed at increasing systemic vascular resistance and decreasing right-to-left shunting (e.g., phenylephrine 0.1 to 0.5 µg/kg/min IV).

■ CHRONIC Rx

- Palliative repair includes procedures increasing pulmonary blood flow, thus reducing right-to-left shunting. Examples of palliative procedures include the Blalock-Taussig shunt whereby a shunt is made between the subclavian artery and the pulmonary artery, the Waterston shunt attaching the ascending aorta to right pulmonary artery, and the Potts shunt attaching the descending aorta to left pulmonary artery.
- Complete surgical repair has good success and involves closing the VSD with a Dacron patch and relieving the RV outflow tract obstruction. It is recommended for nearly every patient with TOF.

■ DISPOSITION

- Almost all TOF patients will have had either palliative or complete surgical repair before reaching adulthood.
- Less than 3% of patients with TOF reach 40 yr of age without having surgery.
- Survival after complete operative repair for TOF is excellent provided the RV outflow tract obstruction has been relieved and the VSD has been closed. Most adults lead unrestricted lives and are asymptomatic.

- 85% of patients who have operative repair of TOF survive ≥36 yr.
- Early and late postoperative complications can occur and generally manifest in arrhythmias from atrial and ventricular tachycardias and diminished exercise tolerance from RV failure. The latter is usually secondary to chronic pulmonary regurgitation and/or residual RV outflow tract obstruction.

■ REFERRAL

- Infants and children with cyanotic heart disease should be referred to a pediatric cardiologist for further diagnostic evaluation. On diagnosing TOF, patients should be referred to centers experienced in palliative and complete surgical repair.
- Adult patients with repaired TOF should be comanaged with cardiology.

☼ PEARLS & CONSIDERATIONS

- Tetralogy of Fallot was first described and published by the French physician Etienne Fallot in 1888.
- The first surgical treatment for TOF was performed by Dr. Alfred Blalock at Johns Hopkins University in 1945.

■ COMMENTS

- The severity of right ventricular outflow tract obstruction is the primary determinant of clinical symptoms and outcome.
- Coexisting cardiac abnormalities occur in nearly 40% of patients with TOF, including patent ductus arteriosus, atrial septal defect (ASD), multiple VSDs, absence of a pulmonary artery, and complete AV septal defects.
- Children with TOF require SBE prophylaxis before any dental work or surgery on the bowel or bladder.

REFERENCES

Braunwald *Heart disease: a textbook of cardiovascular medicine,* ed 6, Philadelphia, 2001, WB Saunders.

Hirsch JC, Mosca RS, Bove EL: Complete repair of tetralogy of Fallot in the neonate: results in the modern era, *Ann Surg* 232(4), 2000.

Nollert G et al: Long-term survival in patients with repair of tetralogy of Fallot: 36-year follow-up of 490 survivors of the first year after surgical repair, *J Am Coll Cardiol* 30:1374, 1997.

Therrien J, Marx GR, Gatzoulis MA: Late-problems in tetralogy of Fallot—recognition, management and prevention, *Cardiol Clin* 20(3), 2002.

Authors: **Wen-Chih Wu, M.D., and Peter Petropoulos, M.D.**

■ **BASIC INFORMATION**

■ **DEFINITION**

Thalassemias are a heterogeneous group of disorders of hemoglobin synthesis that have in common a deficient synthesis of one or more of the polypeptide chains of the normal human hemoglobin, resulting in a quantitative abnormality of the hemoglobin thus produced. There are no qualitative changes such as those encountered in the hemoglobinopathies (e.g., sickle cell disease).

■ **SYNONYMS**

Mediterranean anemia
Cooley's anemia

ICD-9CM CODES
282.4 Thalassemia

■ **EPIDEMIOLOGY & DEMOGRAPHICS**

- Thalassemia is the most common genetic disorder worldwide.
- The highest concentration of alpha-thalassemia is found in Southeast Asia and the African west coast. For example, in Thailand the prevalence is 5% to 10%. It is also common among blacks, with a prevalence of approximately 5%.
- The worldwide prevalence of beta-thalassemia is approximately 3%; in certain regions of Italy and Greece the prevalence reaches 15% to 30%. This high prevalence can be found in Americans of Italian or Greek descent.
- The distribution of thalassemia in Europe and Africa parallels that of malaria, suggesting that thalassemic persons are thus more resistant to the parasite, thus permitting evolutionary survival advantage.

■ **CLASSIFICATION**
BETA THALASSEMIA:

- Beta (+) thalassemia (suboptimal beta-globin synthesis)
- Beta (o) thalassemia (total absence of beta-globin synthesis)
- Delta-beta thalassemia (total absence of both delta-globin and beta-globin synthesis)
- Lepore hemoglobin (synthesis of small amounts of fused delta-beta-globin and total absence of delta- and beta-globin)
- Hereditary persistence of fetal hemoglobin (HPHF) (increased hemoglobin F synthesis and reduced or absence of delta- and beta-globin)

ALPHA THALASSEMIA:

- Silent carrier (three alpha-globin genes present)
- Alpha thalassemia trait (two alpha-globin genes present)

- Hemoglobin H disease (one alpha-globin gene present)
- Hydrops fetalis (no alpha-globin gene)
- Hemoglobin Constant Sprint (elongated alpha-globin chain)

THALASSEMIC HEMOGLOBINOPATHIES: Hb Terre Haute, Hb Quong Sze, HbE, Hb Knossos

■ **PHYSICAL FINDINGS & CLINICAL PRESENTATION**
BETA THALASSEMIA:

- Heterozygous beta thalassemia (thalassemia minor): no or mild anemia, microcytosis and hypochromia, mild hemolysis manifested by slight reticulocytosis and splenomegaly
- Homozygous beta thalassemia (thalassemia major): intense hemolytic anemia; transfusion dependency; bone deformities (skull and long bones); hepatomegaly; splenomegaly; iron overload leading to cardiomyopathy, diabetes mellitus, and hypogonadism; growth retardation; pigment gallstones; susceptibility to infection
- Thalassemia intermedia caused by combination of beta and alpha thalassemia or beta thalassemia and Hb Lepore: resembles thalassemia major but is milder

ALPHA THALASSEMIA:

- Silent carrier: no symptoms.
- Alpha thalassemia trait: microcytosis only.
- Hemoglobin H disease: moderately severe hemolysis with microcytosis and splenomegaly.
- The loss of all four alpha-globin genes is incompatible with life (stillbirth of hydropic fetus). NOTE: Pregnancies with hydrops fetalis are associated with a high incidence of toxemia.

■ **PATHOGENESIS**

- Beta thalassemia: The reduction of beta-globin synthesis results in redundant alpha-globin chains (Heinz bodies), which are cytotoxic and cause intramedullary hemolysis and ineffective erythropoiesis. More than 100 mutations have been identified. Fetal hemoglobin may be increased.
- Alpha thalassemia: Several mutations can result in insufficient amounts of alpha globin available for combination with non–alpha globins.

■ **DIAGNOSIS**

■ **DIFFERENTIAL DIAGNOSIS**

Usually the diagnosis is straightforward; iron deficiency must be ruled out in the presence of microcytosis; if iron deficiency is not present, the cause of microcytosis is probably thalassemia.

■ **LABORATORY TESTS**
BETA THALASSEMIA:

- Microcytosis (MCV: 55 to 80 FL)
- Normal RDW (RBC distribution width)
- Smear: nucleated RBCs, anisocytosis, poikilocytosis, polychromatophilia, Pappenheimer and Howell-Jolly bodies
- Hemoglobin electrophoresis: absent or reduced hemoglobin A, increased fetal hemoglobin, variable increase in the amount of hemoglobin A_2
- Markers of hemolysis: elevated indirect bilirubin and LDH, decreased haptoglobin

ALPHA THALASSEMIA:

- Microcytosis in the absence of iron deficiency
- Hemoglobin electrophoresis is normal, except for the presence of hemoglobin H in hemoglobin H disease

■ **TREATMENT**

- Thalassemia minor: no treatment but avoid iron administration for incorrect diagnosis of iron deficiency
- Beta thalassemia major (and hemoglobin H disease)
  1. Transfusion as required together with chelation of iron with desferrioxamine (by intravenous or subcutaneous administration, 8 to 12 hr nightly, 5 to 6 days a week at a dose of 2 to 6 g/day using a portable infusion pump)
  2. Splenectomy for hypersplenism if present
  3. Bone marrow transplantation
  4. Hydroxyurea may increase the level of hemoglobin F

■ **REFERRAL**
To hematologist

REFERENCE

Olivieri NF: The beta-thalassemias, *N Engl J Med* 341:99, 1999.
Author: **Tom J. Wachtel, M.D.**

BASIC INFORMATION

■ DEFINITION
Thoracic outlet syndrome is the term used to describe a condition producing upper extremity symptoms thought to result from neurovascular compression at the thoracic outlet. Three types are described based on the point of compression: (1) cervical rib and scalenus syndrome, in which abnormal scalene muscles or the presence of a cervical rib may cause compression; (2) costoclavicular syndrome, in which compression may occur under the clavicle; and (3) hyperabduction syndrome, in which compression may occur in the subcoracoid area.

ICD-9CM CODES
353.0 Thoracic outlet syndrome

■ EPIDEMIOLOGY & DEMOGRAPHICS
PREVALENCE: Varies from source to source; presence of cervical ribs in 0.5% to 1% of population (50% bilateral), but most are asymptomatic
PREDOMINANT AGE: Rare under 20 yr of age
PREDOMINANT SEX: Female > male (3.5:1)

■ PHYSICAL FINDINGS & CLINICAL PRESENTATION
- Symptoms and signs are related to the degree of involvement of each of the various structures at the level of the first rib.
- True venous or arterial involvement is rare.
- Diagnosis is most often used in the consideration of neural pain affecting the arm, which would suggest involvement of the brachial plexus.
  1. *Arterial compression:* pallor, paresthesias, diminished pulses, coolness, digital gangrene, and a supraclavicular bruit or mass
  2. *Venous compression:* edema and pain; thrombosis causing superficial venous dilation about the shoulder
  3. *"True" neural compression:* lower trunk (C8, T1) findings with intrinsic weakness and diminished sensation to the finger and small fingers and ulnar aspect of the forearm
  4. Possible supraclavicular tenderness
  5. Provocative tests (Adson's, Wright's): may reproduce pain but are of disputed usefulness

■ ETIOLOGY
- Congenital cervical rib or fibrous extension of cervical rib (Fig. 1-273)
- Abnormal scalene muscle insertion

- Drooping of shoulder girdle resulting from generalized hypotonia or trauma
- Narrowed costoclavicular interval as a result of downward and backward pressure on shoulder (sometimes seen in individuals who carry heavy backpacks)
- Acute venous thrombosis with exercise (effort thrombosis)
- Bony abnormalities of first rib
- Abnormal fibromuscular bands
- Malunion of clavicle fracture

DIAGNOSIS

■ DIFFERENTIAL DIAGNOSIS
- Carpal tunnel syndrome
- Cervical radiculopathy
- Brachial neuritis
- Ulnar nerve compression
- Reflex sympathetic dystrophy
- Superior sulcus tumor

■ WORKUP
Except for venous or arterial pathology, no ancillary diagnostic tests are reliable for diagnostic confirmation.

■ IMAGING STUDIES
- Arteriography or venography when vascular pathology is strongly suspected clinically
- Cervical spine radiographs to rule out cervical disk disease
- Chest film to rule out lung tumor
- EMG, NCV studies to rule out carpal tunnel syndrome, cervical radiculopathy

TREATMENT

■ ACUTE GENERAL Rx
- Sling for pain relief
- Physical therapy modalities plus shoulder girdle–strengthening exercises

- Postural reeducation
- NSAIDs

■ DISPOSITION
- Surgery: generally successful for vascular disorders
- Nonsurgical treatment: often successful for patients with pain as the primary symptom

■ REFERRAL
For vascular surgery consultation when venous or arterial impairment is present

PEARLS & CONSIDERATIONS

■ COMMENTS
- True thoracic outlet syndrome is probably an uncommon condition.
- Diagnosis is often used to describe a wide variety of clinical symptoms.
- Considerable disagreement exists regarding the frequency of this disorder.

REFERENCES
Gillard J et al: Diagnosing thoracic outlet syndrome: contribution of provocative tests, ultrasonography, electrophysiology and helical computed tomography in 48 patients, *J Bone Joint Surg* 68:416, 2001.

Pascarelli EF, Hsu YP: Understanding work-related upper extremity disorders: clinical findings in 485 computer users, musicians and others, *J Occup Rehab* 11:1, 2001.

Sheth RN, Belzberg AJ: Diagnosis and treatment of thoracic outlet syndrome, *Neurosurg Clin North Am* 12:295, 2001.
Author: **Lonnie R. Mercier, M.D.**

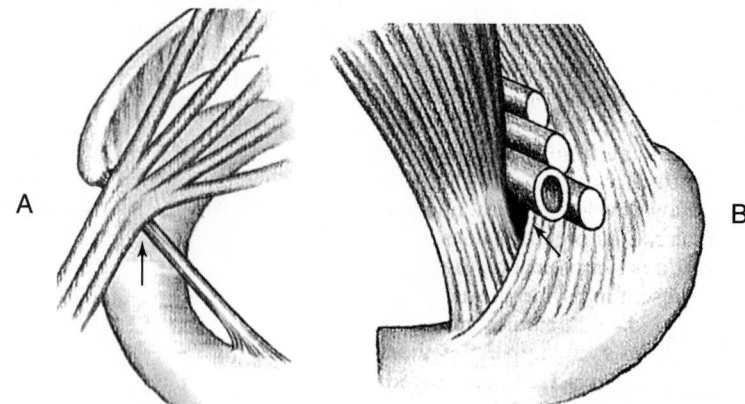

Fig. 1-273 **A,** Compression caused by a cervical rib *(arrow).* **B,** Abnormal scalene muscle insertions that may cause compression at the cervicobrachial region *(arrow).* (From Mercier LR: *Practical orthopedics,* ed 5, St Louis, 2000, Mosby.)

BASIC INFORMATION

■ DEFINITION
Thromboangiitis obliterans (Buerger's disease) is an occlusive inflammatory disease of the small- to medium-size arteries of the upper and lower extremities.

■ SYNONYMS
Buerger's disease
Presenile gangrene

■ ICD-9CM CODES
443.1 Thromboangiitis obliterans (Buerger's disease)

■ EPIDEMIOLOGY & DEMOGRAPHICS
- Since 1950, the incidence of thromboangiitis obliterans has fallen significantly.
- The prevalence of thromboangiitis obliterans is higher in Japan, India, and Southeast Asia when compared with the U.S.
- Thromboangiitis obliterans is rare in women.
- The disease typically occurs before the age of 50 yr and is found predominantly in men who smoke.

■ PHYSICAL FINDINGS & CLINICAL PRESENTATION
- Paresthesias, coldness, skin ulcers, gangrene, along with pain at rest or with walking (claudication)
- Prolonged capillary refill with dependent rubor
- Necrotic skin ulcers at the tips of the digits
- Pathognomonic migratory thrombophlebitis

■ ETIOLOGY
- Unknown.
- The remarkable feature is the close association between tobacco smoking and disease exacerbation. If abstinence from tobacco is adhered to, thromboangiitis obliterans takes a favorable course. If smoking is continued, the disease progresses, leading to gangrene and small-digit amputations.
- There is some thought of a genetic predisposition because the prevalence is higher in the Far East.

DIAGNOSIS

■ DIFFERENTIAL DIAGNOSIS
Thromboangiitis obliterans must be distinguished from arteriosclerotic peripheral vascular disease by the criteria mentioned in "Workup."

■ WORKUP
The diagnosis of thromboangiitis obliterans is made on:
- Clinical criteria
  1. Peripheral vascular disease occurring predominantly in men before the age of 50 yr
  2. Typically, affects the arms and the legs and not just the lower extremities as arteriosclerosis does
  3. Found solely in tobacco smokers, with improvement in those who abstain
  4. Associated with migratory thrombophlebitis
  5. No other atherosclerotic risk factors (e.g., diabetes, cholesterol, or hypertension)
- Angiographic criteria (see "Imaging Studies")
- Pathologic criteria: fresh inflammatory thrombus within both small- and medium-size arteries and veins, along with giant cells around the thrombus

■ IMAGING STUDIES
- Noninvasive vascular studies help differentiate proximal occlusive disease characteristic of arteriosclerosis from distal disease typical of thromboangiitis obliterans.
- Angiography findings in thromboangiitis obliterans include:
  1. Involvement of distal small- and medium-size vessels
  2. Occlusions are segmental, multiple, smooth, and tapered
  3. Collateral circulation gives a "tree root" or "spider leg" appearance
  4. Both upper and lower extremities are involved

TREATMENT

■ NONPHARMACOLOGIC THERAPY
Abstaining from smoking is the only way to stop the progression of the disease. Medical and surgical treatments will prove to be futile if the patient continues to smoke. Exacerbation of ischemic ulcers is directly related to tobacco use.

■ ACUTE GENERAL Rx
- The goal of medical treatment is to provide relief of ischemic pain and healing of ischemic ulcers. If the patient does not completely abstain from tobacco, medical measures will not be helpful.
- Prostaglandin vasodilator therapy given IV or intraarterially provides some relief of pain but does not change the course of the disease.

- Epidural anesthesia and hyperbaric oxygen have a vasodilator effect and have been shown to aid in pain relief from ischemic ulcers.

■ CHRONIC Rx
- Surgical bypass procedures and sympathectomy, as with medical treatment, will not be efficacious unless the patient stops smoking.
- Surgical bypass may be difficult because the occlusions of thromboangiitis obliterans are distal. Nevertheless, if successfully done, this can lead to rapid healing of ischemic ulcers.
- Sympathectomy leads to increased flow by decreasing the vasoconstriction of distal vessels and also has been shown to aid in the healing and relief of pain from ischemic ulcers.
- Debridement must be done on necrotic ulcers if needed.
- Amputation is frequently required for gangrenous digits; however, below-knee or above-knee amputations are rarely necessary.

■ DISPOSITION
The course of thromboangiitis obliterans can be dramatically changed by the cessation of tobacco smoking. If the patient continues to smoke, recurrent exacerbation of ischemic ulcers, necrosis, and gangrene leading to small digit amputations will be inevitable.

■ REFERRAL
Vascular surgical consultation is recommended in any young smoker with claudication and ischemic ulcers, especially if both the upper and lower extremities are involved.

PEARLS & CONSIDERATIONS

■ COMMENTS
Smoking cessation is mandatory. In individuals who quit smoking, prognosis is markedly improved.

REFERENCE
Olin JW: Thromboangiitis obliterans (Buerger's disease), *N Engl J Med* 343(12):864, 2000.
Author: **Peter Petropoulos, M.D.**

BASIC INFORMATION

■ DEFINITION
Superficial thrombophlebitis is inflammatory thrombosis in subcutaneous veins.

■ SYNONYMS
Phlebitis

ICD-9CM CODES
451.0 Thrombophlebitis, superficial

■ EPIDEMIOLOGY & DEMOGRAPHICS
• 20% of superficial thrombophlebitis cases are associated with occult DVT.
• Catheter-related thrombophlebitis incidence is 100:100,000.

■ PHYSICAL FINDINGS & CLINICAL PRESENTATION
• Subcutaneous vein is palpable, tender; tender cord is present with erythema and edema of the overlying skin and subcutaneous tissue.
• Induration, redness, and tenderness are localized along the course of the vein. This linear appearance rather than circular appearance is useful to distinguish thrombophlebitis from other conditions (cellulitis, erythema nodosum).
• There is no significant swelling of the limb (superficial thrombophlebitis generally does not produce swelling of the limb).
• Low-grade fever may be present. High fever and chills are suggestive of septic phlebitis.

■ ETIOLOGY
• Trauma to preexisting varices
• Intravenous cannulation of veins (most common cause)
• Abdominal cancer (e.g., carcinoma of pancreas)
• Infection (*Staphylococcus* is the most common pathogen)
• Hypercoagulable state
• DVT

DIAGNOSIS

■ DIFFERENTIAL DIAGNOSIS
• Lymphangitis
• Cellulitis
• Erythema nodosum
• Panniculitis
• Kaposi's sarcoma

■ WORKUP
Laboratory evaluation to exclude infectious etiology and imaging studies to rule out DVT in suspected cases

■ LABORATORY TESTS
CBC with differential, blood cultures, culture of IV catheter tip (when secondary to intravenous cannulation)

■ IMAGING STUDIES
• Serial ultrasound or venography in patients with suspected DVT
• CT scan of abdomen in patients with suspected malignancy (Trousseau's syndrome: recurrent migratory thrombophlebitis)

TREATMENT

■ NONPHARMACOLOGIC THERAPY
• Warm, moist compresses
• It is not necessary to restrict activity; however, if there is extensive thrombophlebitis, bed rest with the leg elevated will limit the thrombosis and improve symptoms.

■ ACUTE GENERAL Rx
• NSAIDs to relieve symptoms
• Treatment of septic thrombophlebitis with antibiotics with adequate coverage of *Staphylococcus*
• Ligation and division of the superficial vein at the junction to avoid propagation of the clot in the deep venous system when the thrombophlebitis progresses toward the junction of the involved superficial vein with deep veins

■ DISPOSITION
Clinical improvement within 7 to 10 days

■ REFERRAL
Surgical referral in selected cases (see "Acute General Rx")

PEARLS & CONSIDERATIONS

■ COMMENTS
• Patients with positive cultures should be evaluated and treated for endocarditis.
• Septic thrombophlebitis is more common in IV drug addicts.

Author: **Fred F. Ferri, M.D.**

BASIC INFORMATION

■ DEFINITION
Deep vein thrombosis (DVT) is the development of thrombi in the deep veins of the extremities or pelvis.

■ SYNONYMS
DVT
Deep venous thrombophlebitis

ICD-9CM CODES
451.1 Thrombosis of deep vessels of lower extremities
451.83 Thrombosis of deep veins of upper extremities
541.9 Deep vein thrombosis of unspecified site

■ EPIDEMIOLOGY & DEMOGRAPHICS
Annual incidence in urban population is 1.6 cases/1000 persons.

■ PHYSICAL FINDINGS & CLINICAL PRESENTATION
- Pain and swelling of the affected extremity
- In lower extremity DVT, leg pain on dorsiflexion of the foot (Homans' sign)
- Physical examination may be unremarkable

■ ETIOLOGY
The etiology is often multifactorial (prolonged stasis, coagulation abnormalities, vessel wall trauma). The following are risk factors for DVT:
- Prolonged immobilization (≥3 days)
- Postoperative state
- Trauma to pelvis and lower extremities
- Birth control pills, high-dose estrogen therapy
- Visceral cancer (lung, pancreas, alimentary tract, GU tract)
- Age >60 yr
- History of thromboembolic disease
- Hematologic disorders (e.g., antithrombin III deficiency, protein C deficiency, protein S deficiency, heparin cofactor II deficiency, sticky platelet syndrome, G20210A prothrombin mutation, lupus anticoagulant, dysfibrinogenemias, anticardiolipin antibody, hyperhomocystinemia, concurrent homocystinuria, high levels of factors VIII, XI, and factor V Leiden mutation)
- Pregnancy and early puerperium
- Obesity, CHF
- Surgery, fracture, or injury involving lower leg or pelvis
- Surgery requiring >30 min of anesthesia
- Gynecologic surgery (particularly gynecologic cancer surgery)
- Recent travel (within 2 wk, lasting >4 hr)
- Smoking and abdominal obesity
- Central venous catheter or pacemaker insertion
- Superficial vein thrombosis, varicose veins

DIAGNOSIS

■ DIFFERENTIAL DIAGNOSIS
- Postphlebitic syndrome
- Superficial thrombophlebitis
- Ruptured Baker's cyst
- Cellulitis, lymphangitis, Achilles tendinitis
- Hematoma
- Muscle or soft tissue injury, stress fracture
- Varicose veins, lymphedema
- Arterial insufficiency
- Abscess
- Claudication
- Venous stasis

■ WORKUP
The clinical diagnosis of DVT is inaccurate. Pain, tenderness, swelling, or color changes are not specific for DVT. Compression ultrasonography is preferred as the initial study to diagnose DVT. An initial negative test should be repeated after 5 days (if the clinical suspicion of DVT persists) to detect propagation of any thrombosis to the proximal veins.

■ LABORATORY TESTS
- Laboratory tests are not specific for DVT. Baseline PT (INR), PTT, and platelet count should be obtained on all patients before starting anticoagulation.
- Use of d-dimer assay by ELISA may be useful in the management of suspected DVT. The combination of a normal d-dimer study on presentation together with a normal compression venous ultrasound is useful to exclude DVT and generally eliminate the need to do repeat ultrasound at 5 to 7 days. Recent trials indicate that DVT can be ruled out in patients who are clinically unlikely to have DVT and who have a negative d-dimer test. Compressive ultrasonography can be safely omitted in such patients.
- Laboratory evaluation of young patients with DVT, patients with recurrent thrombosis without obvious causes, and those with a family history of thrombosis should include protein S, protein C, fibrinogen, antithrombin III level, lupus anticoagulant, anticardiolipin antibodies, factor V Leiden, factor VIII, factor IX, and plasma homocysteine levels.

■ IMAGING STUDIES
- Compression ultrasonography is generally preferred as the initial study because it is noninvasive and can be repeated serially (useful to monitor suspected acute DVT); it offers good sensitivity for detecting proximal vein thrombosis (in the popliteal or femoral vein). Its disadvantages are poor visualization of deep iliac and pelvic veins and poor sensitivity in isolated or nonocclusive calf vein thrombi.
- Contrast venography is the gold standard for evaluation of DVT of the lower extremity. It is, however, invasive and painful. Additional disadvantages are the increased risk of phlebitis, new thrombosis, renal failure, and hypersensitivity reaction to contrast media; it also gives poor visualization of deep femoral vein in the thigh and internal iliac vein and its tributaries.
- Magnetic resonance direct thrombus imaging (MRDTI) is an accurate noninvasive test for diagnosis of DVT. Current limitations are its cost and lack of widespread availability.

TREATMENT

■ NONPHARMACOLOGIC THERAPY
- Initial bed rest for 1 to 4 days followed by gradual resumption of normal activity
- Patient education on anticoagulant therapy and associated risks

■ ACUTE GENERAL Rx
- Traditional treatment consists of IV unfractionated heparin for 4 to 7 days followed by warfarin therapy. Low–molecular-weight heparin enoxaparin (Lovenox) is also effective for initial management of DVT and allows outpatient treatment. Recommended dose is 1 mg/kg q12h SC and continued for a minimum of 5 days and until a therapeutic INR (2 to 3) has been achieved with warfarin. Warfarin therapy should be initiated when appropriate (usually within 72 hr of initiation of heparin). A 5 mg loading dose of warfarin is recommended in inpatients because it produces less excess anticoagulation than does a 10 mg dose; the smaller dose also avoids the development of a potential hypercoagulable state caused by precipitous decreases in levels of protein C during the first 36 hr of warfarin therapy. In the outpatient setting, a warfarin nomogram using 10 mg loading doses may be more effective in reaching a therapeutic INR.

- Low–molecular-weight heparin, when used, should be overlapped with warfarin for at least 5 days and until the INR has exceeded 2 for 2 consecutive days.
- Exclusions from outpatient treatment of DVT include patients with potential high complication risk (e.g., HB <7, platelet count <75,000, guaiac-positive stool, recent CVA or noncutaneous surgery, noncompliance).
- Insertion of an inferior vena cava filter to prevent pulmonary embolism is recommended in patients with contraindications to anticoagulation.
- Thrombolytic therapy (streptokinase) can be used in rare cases (unless contraindicated) in patients with extensive iliofemoral venous thrombosis and a low risk of bleeding.

■ CHRONIC Rx

The optimal duration of anticoagulant therapy varies with the cause of DVT and the patient's risk factors:

1. Therapy for 3 to 6 mo is generally satisfactory in patients with reversible risk factors (low-risk group).
2. Anticoagulation for at least 6 mo is recommended for patients with idiopathic venous thrombosis or medical risk factors for DVT (intermediate-risk group)
3. Indefinite anticoagulation is necessary in patients with DVT associated with active cancer; long-term anticoagulation is also indicated in patients with inherited thrombophilia (e.g., deficiency of protein C or S antibody), antiphospholipid, and those with recurrent episodes of idiopathic DVT (high-risk group).

☼ PEARLS & CONSIDERATIONS

■ COMMENTS

- When using heparin, there is a risk of heparin-induced thrombocytopenia (with unfractionated more so than with LMWH). Platelet count should be obtained initially and repeated every 3 days while on heparin.

- Prophylaxis of DVT is recommended in all patients at risk (e.g., low––molecular-weight heparin [enoxaparin 30 mg SC bid] after major trauma, post surgery of hip and knee; enoxaparin 40 mg SC qd post–abdominal surgery in patients with moderate to high DVT risk; gradient elastic stockings alone or in combination with intermittent pneumatic compression [IPC] boots following neurosurgery).
- Ximelagatran is an oral direct thrombin inhibitor. For prophylaxis of venous thromboembolism, ximelagatran 24 mg PO bid started the morning after total knee arthroplasty is well tolerated and at least as effective as warfarin, but it does not require coagulation monitoring or dose adjustment.
- Fondaparinux (Arixtra), a synthetic analog of heparin, can also be used for prevention of DVT after hip fracture surgery, hip replacement, or knee replacement. Initial dose is 2.5 mg SC given 6 to 8 hr postoperatively and continued daily. Its bleeding risk is similar to enoxaparin; however, it is more effective in preventing DVT.
- The risk of recurrent venous thromboembolism in heterozygous carriers of factor V Leiden and a first spontaneous venous thromboembolism is similar to that of noncarriers of factor V Leiden; therefore heterozygous patients should receive secondary thromboprophylaxis for a similar length of time as patients without factor V Leiden.

REFERENCES

Baarslag et al: Prospective study of color duplex ultrasonography compared with contrast venography in patients suspected of having deep venous thrombosis of the upper extremities, *Ann Intern Med* 136:865, 2002.

Berquist D et al: Duration of prophylaxis against venous thromboembolism with enoxaparin after surgery for cancer, *N Engl J Med* 346:975, 2002.

Chunilal SD et al: The sensitivity and specificity of a red blood cell agglutination D-dimer assay for venous thromboembolism when performed on venous blood, *Arch Interen Med* 162:217, 2002.

Francis CW et al: Ximelagatran versus warfarin for the prevention of venous thromboembolism after total knee arthroplasty, *Ann Intern Med* 137:648, 2002.

Fraser DG et al: Diagnosis of lower-limb deep venous thrombosis: a prospective blinded study of magnetic resonance direct thrombus imaging, *Ann Intern Med* 136:89, 2002.

Kelly et al: Plasma D-Dimers in the diagnosis of venous thromboembolism, *Arch Intern Med* 162:747, 2002.

Kovacs MJ et al: Comparison of 10-mg and 5mg warfarin initiation nomograms together with low-molecular-weight heparin for outpatient treatment of acute venous thromboembolism. A randomized, double-blind, controlled trial, *Ann Intern Med* 138:714, 2003.

Kraaijenhagen RA et al: Simplification of the diagnostic management of suspected deep vein thrombosis, *Arch Intern Med* 162:907, 2002.

Meyer G et al: Comparison of low-molecular-weight heparin and warfarin for the secondary prevention of venous thromboembolism in patients with cancer, *Arch Intern Med* 162:1729, 2002.

Schulman S et al: Secondary prevention of venous thromboembolism with the oral direct thrombin inhibitor ximelagran, *N Engl J Med* 349:1713, 2003.

Wells PS et al: Evaluation of d-dimer in the diagnosis of suspected deep vein thrombosis, *N Engl J Med* 349:1227, 2003.

Author: **Fred F. Ferri, M.D.**

🗒 BASIC INFORMATION

■ DEFINITION
Thrombotic thrombocytopenic purpura (TTP) is a rare disorder characterized by thrombocytopenia (often accompanied by purpura) and microangiopathic hemolytic anemia; neurologic impairment, renal dysfunction, and fever may also be present.

■ SYNONYMS
TTP

ICD-9CM CODES
446.6 Thrombotic thrombocytopenic purpura

■ EPIDEMIOLOGY & DEMOGRAPHICS
- TTP primarily affects females between 10 and 50 yr of age.
- Frequency is 3.7 cases/yr/1 million persons.

■ PHYSICAL FINDINGS & CLINICAL PRESENTATION
- Purpura (secondary to thrombocytopenia)
- Jaundice, pallor (secondary to hemolysis)
- Mucosal bleeding
- Fever
- Fluctuating levels of consciousness (secondary to thrombotic occlusion of the cerebral vessels)

■ ETIOLOGY
- The exact cause of TTP remains unknown. Recent studies reveal that there is platelet aggregation as a result of abnormalities in circulating von Willebrand factor caused by endothelial injury.
- Many drugs, including clopidogrel, penicillin, antineoplastic agents, oral contraceptives, quinine, and ticlopidine, have been associated with TTP. Other precipitating causes include infectious agents, pregnancy, malignancies, allogenic bone marrow transplantation, and neurologic disorders.

🔬 DIAGNOSIS

■ DIFFERENTIAL DIAGNOSIS
- DIC
- Malignant hypertension
- Vasculitis
- Eclampsia or preeclampsia
- Hemolytic-uremic syndrome (typically encountered in children, often following a viral infection)
- Gastroenteritis as a result of a serotoxin-producing serotype of *Escherichia coli*
- Medications: clopidogrel, ticlopidine, penicillin, antineoplastic chemotherapeutic agents, oral contraceptives

■ WORKUP
- A comprehensive history, physical examination, and laboratory evaluation usually confirms the diagnosis.
- The disease often begins as a flulike illness ultimately followed by clinical and laboratory abnormalities.

■ LABORATORY TESTS
- Severe anemia and thrombocytopenia
- Elevated BUN and creatinine
- Evidence of hemolysis: elevated reticulocyte count, indirect bilirubin, LDH, decreased haptoglobin
- Urinalysis: hematuria (red cells and red cell casts in urine sediment) and proteinuria
- Peripheral smear: severely fragmented RBCs (schistocytes)
- No laboratory evidence of DIC (normal FDP, fibrinogen)

🧪 TREATMENT

■ ACUTE GENERAL Rx
- Discontinue potential offending agents.
- Plasmapheresis with fresh frozen plasma (FFP) replacement; cryosupernatant may be substituted for FFP in patients who fail to respond to this treatment. Daily plasma exchange is generally performed until hemolysis has ceased and the platelet count has normalized.
- Corticosteroids (prednisone 1 to 2 mg/kg/day) may be effective alone in patients with mild disease or may be administered concomitantly with plasmapheresis plus plasma exchange with FFP.
- Vincristine has been used in patients refractory to plasmapheresis.

- Use of antiplatelet agents (ASA, dipyridamole) is controversial.
- Platelet transfusions are contraindicated except in severely thrombocytopenic patients with documented bleeding.
- Splenectomy is performed in refractory cases.

■ CHRONIC Rx
- Relapsing TTP may be treated with plasma exchange.
- Remission of chronic TTP that is unresponsive to conventional therapy has been reported after treatment with cyclophosphamide and the monoclonal antibody rituximab.
- Splenectomy done while the patients are in remission has been used in some centers to decrease the frequency of relapse in TTP.

■ DISPOSITION
- Survival of patients with TTP currently exceeds 80% with plasma exchange therapy.
- Relapse occurs in 20% to 40% of patients who have TTP in remission.

■ REFERRAL
Surgical referral for splenectomy in selected patients (see "Acute General Rx" and "Chronic Rx")

💡 PEARLS & CONSIDERATIONS

■ COMMENTS
Thrombotic microangiopathy can also be associated with administration of cyclosporine and mitomycin C, and with HIV infection.

REFERENCES
Bennett CL et al: Thrombotic thrombocytopenic purpura associated with clopidogrel, *N Engl J Med* 342:1773, 2000.

Elliot MA, Nichols WL: Thrombotic thrombocytopenic purpura and hemolytic uremic syndrome, *Mayo Clin Proc* 76:1154, 2001.

Kojouri K et al: Quinine-associated thrombotic thrombocytopenic purpura-hemolytic uremic syndrome: frequency, clinical features, and long-term outcomes, *Ann Intern Med* 135:1047, 2001.
Author: **Fred F. Ferri, M.D.**

BASIC INFORMATION

■ DEFINITION
Thyroid carcinoma is a primary neoplasm of the thyroid. There are four major types of thyroid carcinoma: papillary, follicular, anaplastic, and medullary.

■ SYNONYMS
Papillary carcinoma of thyroid
Follicular carcinoma of thyroid
Anaplastic carcinoma of thyroid
Medullary carcinoma of thyroid

ICD-9CM CODES
193 Malignant neoplasm of thyroid

■ EPIDEMIOLOGY & DEMOGRAPHICS
• Thyroid cancer is the most common endocrine cancer, with an annual incidence of 14,000 new cases in the U.S. and about 1100 deaths.
• Female:male ratio of 3:1.
• Most common type (50% to 60%) is papillary carcinoma.
• Median age at diagnosis: 45 to 50 yr.

■ PHYSICAL FINDINGS & CLINICAL PRESENTATION
• Presence of thyroid nodule
• Hoarseness and cervical lymphadenopathy
• Painless swelling in the region of the thyroid

■ ETIOLOGY
• Risk factors: prior neck irradiation
• Multiple endocrine neoplasia II (medullary carcinoma)

DIAGNOSIS

■ DIFFERENTIAL DIAGNOSIS
• Multinodular goiter
• Lymphocytic thyroiditis
• Ectopic thyroid

■ WORKUP
The workup of thyroid carcinoma includes laboratory evaluation and diagnostic imaging. However, diagnosis is confirmed with fine-needle aspiration (FNA) or surgical biopsy. The characteristics of thyroid carcinoma vary with the type:
• Papillary carcinoma
  1. Most frequently occurs in women during second or third decades
  2. Histologically, psammoma bodies (calcific bodies present in papillary projections) are pathognomonic; they are found in 35% to 45% of papillary thyroid carcinomas

  3. Majority are not papillary lesions but mixed papillary follicular carcinomas
  4. Spread is via lymphatics and by local invasion
• Follicular carcinoma
  1. More aggressive than papillary carcinoma
  2. Incidence increases with age
  3. Tends to metastasize hematogenously to bone, producing pathologic fractures
  4. Tends to concentrate iodine (useful for radiation therapy)
• Anaplastic carcinoma
  1. Very aggressive neoplasm
  2. Two major histologic types: small cell (less aggressive, 5-yr survival approximately 20%) and giant cell (death usually within 6 mo of diagnosis)
• Medullary carcinoma
  1. Unifocal lesion: found sporadically in elderly patients
  2. Bilateral lesions: associated with pheochromocytoma and hyperparathyroidism; this combination is known as MEN-II and is inherited as an autosomal dominant disorder

■ LABORATORY TESTS
• Thyroid function studies are generally normal. TSH, T_4, and serum thyroglobulin levels should be obtained before thyroidectomy in patients with confirmed thyroid carcinoma
• Increased plasma calcitonin assay in patients with medullary carcinoma (tumors produce thyrocalcitonin)

■ IMAGING STUDIES
• Thyroid scanning with iodine-123 or technetium-99m can identify hypofunctioning (cold) nodules, which are more likely to be malignant. However, warm nodules can also be malignant.
• Thyroid ultrasound can detect solitary solid nodules that have a high risk of malignancy. However, a negative ultrasound does not exclude diagnosis of thyroid carcinoma.
• FNA biopsy is the best method to assess a thyroid nodule (refer to "Thyroid Nodule" in Section I).

TREATMENT

■ ACUTE GENERAL Rx
• Papillary carcinoma
  1. Total thyroidectomy is indicated if the patient has:
     a. Extrapyramidal extension of carcinoma
     b. Papillary carcinoma limited to thyroid but a positive history of irradiation to the neck
     c. Lesion >2 cm

  2. Lobectomy with isthmectomy may be considered in patients with intrathyroid papillary carcinoma <2 cm and no history of neck or head irradiation; most follow surgery with suppressive therapy with thyroid hormone because these tumors are TSH responsive. The accepted practice is to suppress serum TSH concentrations to <0.1 μU/ml.
  3. Radiotherapy with iodine-131 (after total thyroidectomy), followed by thyroid suppression therapy with triiodothyronine, can be used in metastatic papillary carcinoma.
• Follicular carcinoma
  1. Total thyroidectomy followed by TSH suppression as noted previously
  2. Radiotherapy with iodine-131 followed by thyroid suppression therapy with triiodothyronine is useful in patients with metastasis
• Anaplastic carcinoma
  1. At diagnosis, this neoplasm is rarely operable; palliative surgery is indicated for extremely large tumor compressing the trachea.
  2. Management is usually restricted to radiation therapy or chemotherapy (combination of doxorubicin, cisplatin, and other antineoplastic agents); these measures rarely provide significant palliation.
• Medullary carcinoma
  1. Thyroidectomy should be performed.
  2. Patients and their families should be screened for pheochromocytoma and hyperparathyroidism.

■ DISPOSITION
Prognosis varies with the type of thyroid carcinoma: 5-yr survival approaches 80% for follicular carcinoma and is approximately 5% with anaplastic carcinoma.

PEARLS & CONSIDERATIONS

■ COMMENTS
Family members of patients with medullary carcinoma should be screened; DNA analysis for the detection of mutations in the RET gene structure permits the identification of MEN IIA gene carriers.
Author: **Fred F. Ferri, M.D.**

BASIC INFORMATION

■ DEFINITION

A thyroid nodule is an abnormality found on physical examination of the thyroid gland; nodules can be benign (70%) or malignant.

■ ICD-9CM CODES

241.0 Nodule, thyroid

■ EPIDEMIOLOGY & DEMOGRAPHICS

- Palpable thyroid nodules occur in 4% to 7% of the population.
- Thyroid nodules can be found in 50% of autopsies; however, only 1 in 10 is palpable.
- Malignancy is present in 5% to 30% of palpable nodules.
- Incidence of thyroid nodules increases after 45 yr of age. They are found more frequently in women.
- History of prior head and neck irradiation increases the risk of thyroid cancer.
- Increased likelihood that nodule is malignant: nodule increasing in size or >2 cm, regional lymphadenopathy, fixation to adjacent tissues, age <40 yr, symptoms of local invasion (dysphagia, hoarseness, neck pain, male sex, family history of thyroid cancer or polyposis [Gardner syndrome]).

■ PHYSICAL FINDINGS & CLINICAL PRESENTATION

- Palpable, firm, and nontender nodule in the thyroid area should prompt suspicion of carcinoma. Signs of metastasis are regional lymphadenopathy, inspiratory stridor.
- Signs and symptoms of thyrotoxicosis can be found in functioning nodules.

■ ETIOLOGY

- History of prior head and neck irradiation
- Family history of pheochromocytoma, carcinoma of the thyroid, and hyperparathyroidism (medullary carcinoma of the thyroid is a component of MEN-II)

DIAGNOSIS

■ DIFFERENTIAL DIAGNOSIS

- Thyroid carcinoma
- Multinodular goiter
- Thyroglossal duct cyst
- Epidermoid cyst
- Laryngocele
- Nonthyroid neck neoplasm
- Branchial cleft cyst

■ WORKUP

- Fine-needle aspiration (FNA) biopsy is the best diagnostic study; the accuracy can be >90%, but it is directly related to the level of experience of the physician and the cytopathologist interpreting the aspirate.
- FNA biopsy is less reliable with thyroid cystic lesions; surgical excision should be considered for most thyroid cysts not abolished by aspiration.
- A diagnostic approach to thyroid nodule is described in Section III.

■ LABORATORY TESTS

- TSH, T_4, and serum thyroglobulin levels should be obtained before thyroidectomy in patients with confirmed thyroid carcinoma on FNA biopsy.
- Serum calcitonin at random or after pentagastrin stimulation is useful when suspecting medullary carcinoma of the thyroid and in anyone with a family history of medullary thyroid carcinoma.
- Serum thyroid autoantibodies (see "Thyroiditis" in Section I) are useful when suspecting thyroiditis.

■ IMAGING STUDIES

- Thyroid ultrasound is done in some patients to evaluate the size of the thyroid and the number, composition (solid vs. cystic), and dimensions of the thyroid nodule; solid thyroid nodules have a higher incidence of malignancy, but cystic nodules can also be malignant.
- The introduction of high-resolution ultrasonography has made it possible to detect many nonpalpable nodules (incidentalomas) in the thyroid (found at autopsy in 30% to 60% of cadavers). Most of these lesions are benign. For most patients with nonpalpable nodules that are incidentally detected by thyroid imaging, simple follow-up neck palpation is sufficient.
- Thyroid scan with technetium-99m pertechnetate:
  1. Classifies nodules as hyperfunctioning (hot), normally functioning (warm), or nonfunctioning (cold); cold nodules have a higher incidence of malignancy.
  2. Scan has difficulty evaluating nodules near the thyroid isthmus or at the periphery of the gland.
  3. Normal tissue over a nonfunctioning nodule might mask the nodule as "warm" or normally functioning.
- Both thyroid scan and ultrasound provide information about the risk of malignant neoplasia based on the characteristics of the thyroid nodule, but their value in the initial evaluation of a thyroid nodule is limited because neither provides a definite tissue diagnosis.

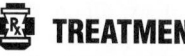 TREATMENT

■ GENERAL Rx

- Evaluation of results of FNA
  1. Normal cells: may repeat biopsy during present evaluation or reevaluate patient after 3 to 6 mo of suppressive therapy (l-thyroxine, prescribed in doses to suppress the TSH level to 0.1 to 0.5)
     a. Failure to regress indicates increased likelihood of malignancy.
     b. Reliance on repeat needle biopsy is preferable to routine surgery for nodules not responding to thyroxine.
  2. Malignant cells: surgery
  3. Hypercellularity: thyroid scan
     a. Hot nodule: ^{131}I therapy if the patient is hyperthyroid
     b. Warm or cold nodule: surgery (rule out follicular adenoma vs. carcinoma)

■ DISPOSITION

Variable with results of FNA biopsy. Refer to "Thyroid Carcinoma" in Section I for prognosis in patients with malignant nodules diagnosed with biopsy.

■ REFERRAL

Surgical referral for FNA biopsy

PEARLS & CONSIDERATIONS

■ COMMENTS

- Most solid, benign nodules grow, therefore an increase in nodule volume alone is not a reliable predictor of malignancy.
- Surgery is indicated in hard or fixed nodule, presence of dysphagia or hoarseness, and rapidly growing solid masses regardless of "benign" results on FNA.
- Suppressive therapy of malignant thyroid nodules postoperatively with thyroxine is indicated. The use of suppressive therapy for benign solitary nodules is controversial.

REFERENCES

Alexander EK et al: Natural history of benign solid and cystic thyroid nodules, *Ann Intern Med* 138:315, 2003.
Welker MJ, Orlov D: Thyroid nodules, *Am Fam Physician* 67:559, 2003.
Author: **Fred F. Ferri, M.D.**

BASIC INFORMATION

■ DEFINITION
Thyroiditis is an inflammatory disease of the thyroid. It is a multifaceted disease with varying etiology, different clinical characteristics (depending on the stage), and distinct histopathology. Thyroiditis can be subdivided into three common types (Hashimoto's, painful, painless) and two rare forms (suppurative, Riedel's). To add to the confusion, there are various synonyms for each form, and there is no internationally accepted classification of autoimmune thyroid disease.

■ SYNONYMS
Hashimoto's thyroiditis: *chronic lymphocytic thyroiditis, chronic autoimmune thyroiditis, lymphadenoid goiter*
Painful subacute thyroiditis: subacute thyroiditis, *giant cell thyroiditis, de Quervain's thyroiditis, subacute granulomatous thyroiditis, pseudogranulomatous thyroiditis*
Painless postpartum thyroiditis: *subacute lymphocytic thyroiditis, postpartum thyroiditis*
Painless sporadic thyroiditis: *silent sporadic thyroiditis, subacute lymphocytic thyroiditis*
Suppurative thyroiditis: *acute suppurative thyroiditis, bacterial thyroiditis microbial inflammatory thyroiditis, pyogenic thyroiditis*
Riedel's thyroiditis: *fibrous thyroiditis*

ICD-9CM CODES
245.2 Hashimoto's thyroiditis
245.1 Subacute thyroiditis
245.9 Silent thyroiditis
245.0 Suppurative thyroiditis
245.3 Riedel's thyroiditis

■ PHYSICAL FINDINGS & CLINICAL PRESENTATION
- Hashimoto's: patients may have signs of hyperthyroidism (tachycardia, diaphoresis, palpitations, weight loss) or hypothyroidism (fatigue, weight gain, delayed reflexes) depending on the stage of the disease. Usually there is diffuse, firm enlargement of the thyroid gland; thyroid gland may also be of normal size (atrophic form with clinically manifested hypothyroidism).
- Painful subacute: exquisitely tender, enlarged thyroid, fever; signs of hyperthyroidism are initially present; signs of hypothyroidism can subsequently develop.
- Painless thyroiditis: clinical features are similar to subacute thyroiditis except for the absence of tenderness of the thyroid gland.
- Suppurative: patient is febrile with severe neck pain, focal tenderness of the involved portion of the thyroid, erythema of the overlying skin.

- Riedel's: slowly enlarging hard mass in the anterior neck; often mistaken for thyroid cancer; signs of hypothyroidism occur in advanced stages.

■ ETIOLOGY
- Hashimoto's: autoimmune disorder that begins with the activation of CD4 (helper) T-lymphocytes specific for thyroid antigens. The etiologic factor for the activation of these cells is unknown.
- Painful subacute: possibly postviral; usually follows a respiratory illness; it is not considered to be a form of autoimmune thyroiditis.
- Painless thyroiditis: it frequently occurs postpartum.
- Suppurative: infectious etiology, generally bacterial, although fungi and parasites have also been implicated; it often occurs in immunocompromised hosts or following a penetrating neck injury.
- Riedel's: fibrous infiltration of the thyroid; etiology is unknown.
- Drug induced: lithium, interferon alfa, amiodarone, interleukin-2.

DIAGNOSIS

■ DIFFERENTIAL DIAGNOSIS
- The hyperthyroid phase of Hashimoto's, subacute, or silent thyroiditis can be mistaken for Graves' disease.
- Riedel's thyroiditis can be mistaken for carcinoma of the thyroid.
- Painful subacute thyroiditis can be mistaken for infections of the oropharynx and trachea or for suppurative thyroiditis.
- Factitious hyperthyroidism can mimic silent thyroiditis.

■ WORKUP
- The diagnostic workup includes laboratory and radiologic evaluation to rule out other conditions that may mimic thyroiditis (see "Differential Diagnosis") and to differentiate the various forms of thyroiditis.
- The patient's medical history may be helpful in differentiating the various types of thyroiditis (e.g., presentation following childbirth is suggestive of silent [postpartum, painless] thyroiditis; occurrence following a viral respiratory infection suggests subacute thyroiditis; history of penetrating injury to the neck indicates suppurative thyroiditis).

■ LABORATORY TESTS
- TSH, free T_4: may be normal, or indicative of hypo- or hyperthyroidism depending on the stage of the thyroiditis.
- WBC with differential: increased WBC with "shift to the left" occurs

with subacute and suppurative thyroiditis.
- Antimicrosomal antibodies: detected in >90% of patients with Hashimoto's thyroiditis and 50% to 80% of patients with silent thyroiditis.
- Serum thyroglobulin levels are elevated in patients with subacute and silent thyroiditis; this test is nonspecific but may be useful in monitoring the course of subacute thyroiditis and distinguishing silent thyroiditis from factitious hyperthyroidism (low or absent serum thyroglobulin level).

■ IMAGING STUDIES
24-hr radioactive iodine uptake (RAIU) is useful to distinguish Graves' disease (increased RAIU) from thyroiditis (normal or low RAIU).

TREATMENT

■ ACUTE GENERAL Rx
- Treat hypothyroid phase with levothyroxine 25 to 50 μg/day initially and monitor serum TSH initially every 6 to 8 wk.
- Control symptoms of hyperthyroidism with β-blockers (e.g., propranolol 20 to 40 mg PO q6h).
- Control pain in patients with subacute thyroiditis with NSAIDs. Prednisone 20 to 40 mg qd may be used if NSAIDs are insufficient, but it should be gradually tapered off over several weeks.
- Use IV antibiotics and drain abscess (if present) in patients with suppurative thyroiditis.

■ DISPOSITION
- Hashimoto's thyroiditis: long-term prognosis is favorable; most patients recover their thyroid function.
- Painful subacute thyroiditis: permanent hypothyroidism occurs in 10% of patients.
- Painless thyroiditis: 6% of patients have permanent hypothyroidism.
- Suppurative thyroiditis: there is usually full recovery following treatment.
- Riedel's thyroiditis: hypothyroidism occurs when fibrous infiltration involves the entire thyroid.

■ REFERRAL
Surgical referral in patients with compression of adjacent neck structures and in some patients with suppurative thyroiditis

REFERENCE
Pearce EN et al: Thyroiditis, *N Engl J Med* 348:2646, 2003.
Author: **Fred F. Ferri, M.D.**

BASIC INFORMATION

■ DEFINITION
Thyrotoxic storm is the abrupt and severe exacerbation of thyrotoxicosis.

ICD-9CM CODES
242.9 Thyrotoxic storm
242.0 With goiter
242.2 Multinodular
242.3 Adenomatous
242.8 Thyrotoxicosis factitia

■ PHYSICAL FINDINGS & CLINICAL PRESENTATION
- Goiter
- Tremor, tachycardia, fever
- Warm, moist skin
- Lid lag, lid retraction, proptosis
- Altered mental status (psychosis, coma, seizures)
- Other: evidence of precipitating factors (infection, trauma)

■ ETIOLOGY
- Major stress (e.g., infection, MI, DKA) in an undiagnosed hyperthyroid patient
- Inadequate therapy in a hyperthyroid patient

 DIAGNOSIS

The clinical presentation is variable. The patient may present with the following signs and symptoms:
- Fever
- Marked anxiety and agitation, psychosis
- Hyperhidrosis, heat intolerance
- Marked weakness and muscle wasting
- Tachyarrhythmias, palpitations
- Diarrhea, nausea, vomiting
- Elderly patients may have a combination of tachycardia, CHF, and mental status changes

■ DIFFERENTIAL DIAGNOSIS
- Psychiatric disorders
- Alcohol or other drug withdrawal
- Pheochromocytoma
- Metastatic neoplasm

■ WORKUP
- Laboratory evaluation to confirm hyperthyroidism (elevated free T_4, decreased TSH)
- Evaluation for precipitating factors (e.g., ECG and cardiac enzymes in suspected MI, blood and urine cultures to rule out sepsis)

- Elimination of disorders noted in the differential diagnosis (e.g., psychiatric history, evidence of drug and alcohol abuse)

■ LABORATORY TESTS
- Free T_4, TSH
- CBC with differential
- Blood and urine cultures
- Glucose
- Liver enzymes
- BUN, creatinine
- Serum calcium
- CPK

■ IMAGING STUDIES
Chest x-ray examination to exclude infectious process, neoplasm, CHF in suspected cases

TREATMENT

■ NONPHARMACOLOGIC THERAPY
- Nutritional care: replace fluid deficit aggressively (daily fluid requirement may reach 6 L); use solutions containing glucose and add multivitamins to the hydrating solution.
- Monitor for fluid overload and CHF in the elderly and in those with underlying cardiovascular or renal disease.
- Treat significant hyperthermia with cooling blankets.

■ ACUTE GENERAL Rx
- Inhibition of thyroid hormone synthesis
  1. Administer propylthiouracil (PTU) 300 to 600 mg initially (PO or via NG tube), then 150 to 300 mg q6h.
  2. If the patient is allergic to PTU, use methimazole (Tapazole) 80 to 100 mg PO or PR followed by 30 mg PR q8h.
- Inhibition of stored thyroid hormone
  1. Iodide can be administered as sodium iodine 250 mg IV q6h, potassium iodide (SSKI) 5 gtt PO q8h, or Lugol's solution, 10 gtt q8h. It is important to administer PTU or methimazole 1 hr *before* the iodide to prevent the oxidation of iodide to iodine and its incorporation in the synthesis of additional thyroid hormone.

2. Corticosteroids: dexamethasone 2 mg IV q6h or hydrocortisone 100 mg IV q6h for approximately 48 hr is useful to inhibit thyroid hormone release, impair peripheral conversion of T_3 from T_4, and provide additional adrenocortical hormone to correct deficiency (if present).
- Suppression of peripheral effects of thyroid hormone
  1. β-Adrenergic blockers: Administer propranolol 80 to 120 mg PO q4-6h. Propranolol may also be given IV 1 mg/min for 2 to 10 min under continuous ECG and blood pressure monitoring. β-Adrenergic blockers must be used with caution in patients with CHF or bronchospasm. Cardioselective β-blockers (e.g., esmolol or metoprolol) may be more appropriate for patients with bronchospasm, but these patients must be closely monitored for exacerbation of bronchospasm because these agents lose their cardioselectivity at high doses.
- Control of fever with acetaminophen 325 to 650 mg q4h; avoidance of aspirin because it displaces thyroid hormone from its binding protein
- Digitalization of patients with CHF and atrial fibrillation (these patients may require higher than usual digoxin doses)
- Treatment of any precipitating factors (e.g., antibiotics if infection is strongly suspected)

■ DISPOSITION
Patients with thyrotoxic crisis should be treated and appropriately monitored in the ICU.

■ REFERRAL
Endocrinology referral is appropriate in patients with thyrotoxic crisis.

✵ PEARLS & CONSIDERATIONS

■ COMMENTS
If the diagnosis is strongly suspected, therapy should be started immediately without waiting for laboratory confirmation.
Author: **Fred F. Ferri, M.D.**

BASIC INFORMATION

■ DEFINITION
Tinea corporis is a dermatophyte fungal infection caused by the genera *Trichophyton* or *Microsporum*.

■ SYNONYMS
Ringworm
Body ringworm
Tinea circinata

ICD-9CM CODES
110.5 Tinea corporis

■ EPIDEMIOLOGY & DEMOGRAPHICS
- The disease is more common in warm climates.
- There is no predominant age or sex.

■ PHYSICAL FINDINGS & CLINICAL PRESENTATION
- Typically appears as single or multiple annular lesions with an advancing scaly border; the margin is slightly raised, reddened, and may be pustular.
- The central area becomes hypopigmented and less scaly as the active border progresses outward (Fig. 1-274).
- The trunk and legs are primarily involved.
- Pruritus is variable.

- It is important to remember that recent topical corticosteroid use can significantly alter the appearance of the lesions.

■ ETIOLOGY
Trichophyton rubrum is the most common pathogen.

DIAGNOSIS

■ DIFFERENTIAL DIAGNOSIS
- Pityriasis rosea
- Erythema multiforme
- Psoriasis
- SLE
- Syphilis
- Nummular eczema
- Eczema
- Granuloma annulare
- Lyme disease
- Tinea versicolor
- Contact dermatitis

■ WORKUP
Diagnosis is usually made on clinical grounds. It can be confirmed by direct visualization under the microscope of a small fragment of the scale using wet mount preparation and potassium hydroxide solution; dermatophytes appear as translucent branching filaments (hyphae) with lines of separation appearing at irregular intervals.

■ LABORATORY TESTS
- Microscopic examination of hyphae
- Mycotic culture is usually not necessary
- Biopsy is indicated only when the diagnosis is uncertain and the patient has failed to respond to treatment

TREATMENT

■ NONPHARMACOLOGIC THERAPY
Affected areas should be kept clean and dry.

■ ACUTE GENERAL Rx
- Various creams are effective; the application area should include normal skin about 2 cm beyond the affected area:
  1. Miconazole 2% cream (Monistat-Derm) applied bid for 2 wk
  2. Clotrimazole 1% cream (Mycelex) applied and gently massaged into the affected areas and surrounding areas bid for up to 4 wk
  3. Naftifine 1% cream (Naftin) applied qd
  4. Econazole 1% (Spectazole) applied qd
- Systemic therapy is reserved for severe cases and is usually given up to 4 wk; commonly used agents:
  1. Ketoconazole (Nizoral), 200 mg qd
  2. Fluconazole (Diflucan), 200 mg qd
  3. Terbinafine (Lamisil), 250 mg qd

■ DISPOSITION
Majority of cases resolve without sequelae within 3 to 4 wk of therapy.

■ REFERRAL
Dermatology referral in patients with persistent or recurrent infections

REFERENCES
Friedlander SF et al: Terbinafine in the treatment of trichophytin tinea capitis, *Pediatrics* 109:602, 2002.
Hainer BL: Dermatophyte infections, *Am Fam Physician* 67:101, 2003.
Weinstein A, Berman B: Topical treatment of common superficial tinea infections, *Am Fam Physician* 65:2095, 2002.
Author: **Fred F. Ferri, M.D.**

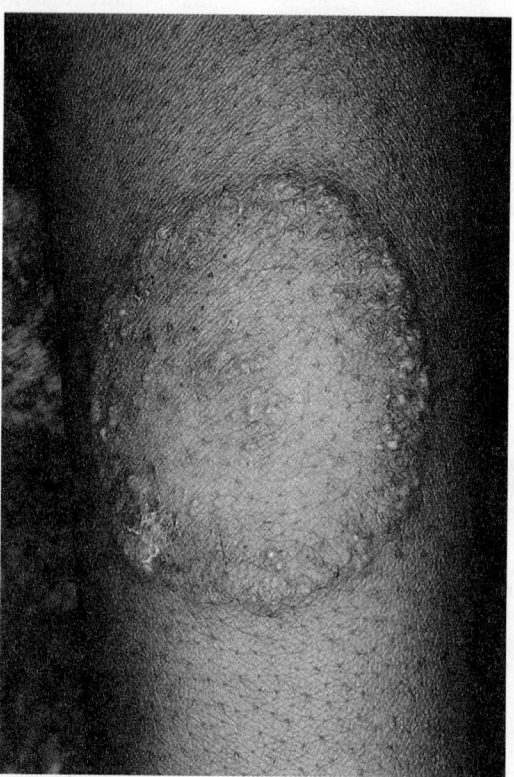

Fig. 1-274 Annular lesion (tinea corporis). Note raised erythematous scaling border and central clearing. (From Noble J et al: *Textbook of primary care medicine,* ed 3, St Louis, 2001, Mosby.)

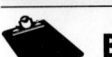

BASIC INFORMATION

■ DEFINITION
Tinea cruris is a dermatophyte infection of the groin.

■ SYNONYMS
Jock itch
Ringworm

ICD-9CM CODES
110.3 Tinea cruris

■ EPIDEMIOLOGY & DEMOGRAPHICS
- Most common during the summer
- Men are affected more frequently than women

■ PHYSICAL FINDINGS & CLINICAL PRESENTATION
- Erythematous plaques have a half-moon shape and a scaling border.
- The acute inflammation tends to move down the inner thigh and usually spares the scrotum; in severe cases the fungus may spread onto the buttocks.
- Itching may be severe.
- Red papules and pustules may be present.
- An important diagnostic sign is the advancing well-defined border with a tendency toward central clearing (Fig. 1-275).

■ ETIOLOGY
- Dermatophytes of the genera *Trichophyton, Epidermophyton,* and *Microsporum. T. rubrum* and *E. floccosum* are the most common causes.
- Transmission from direct contact (e.g., infected persons, animals). The patient's feet should be evaluated as a source of infection because tinea cruris is often associated with tinea pedis.

DIAGNOSIS

■ DIFFERENTIAL DIAGNOSIS
- Intertrigo
- Psoriasis
- Seborrheic dermatitis
- Erythrasma
- Candidiasis
- Tinea versicolor

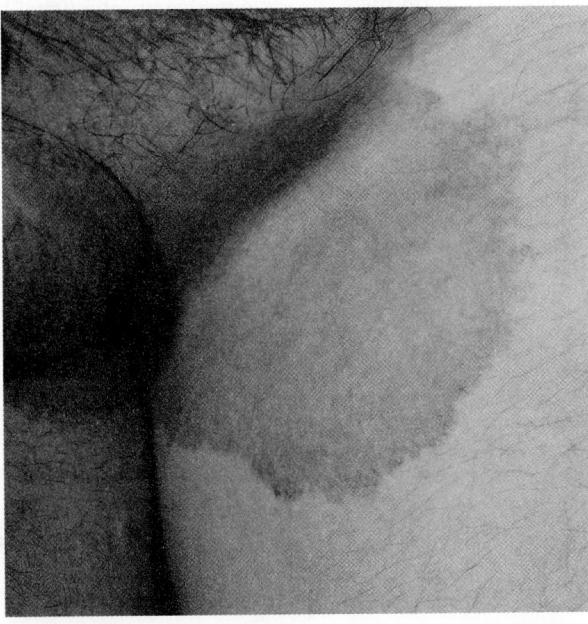

Fig. 1-275   Tinea cruris. A halfmoon-shaped plaque has a well-defined, scaling border. (From Habif TB: *Clinical dermatology: a color guide to diagnosis and therapy,* ed 3, St Louis, 1996, Mosby.)

■ WORKUP
Diagnosis is based on clinical presentation and demonstration of hyphae microscopically using potassium hydroxide.

■ LABORATORY TESTS
- Microscopic examination
- Cultures are generally not necessary

TREATMENT

■ NONPHARMACOLOGIC THERAPY
- Keep infected area clean and dry.
- Use of boxer shorts is preferred to regular underwear.

■ ACUTE GENERAL Rx
- Drying powders (e.g., Miconazole nitrate [Zeasorb AF]) may be useful in patients with excessive perspiration.
- Various topical antifungal agents are available: miconazole (Lotrimin), terbinafine (Lamisil), sulconazole nitrate (Exelderm), betamethasone dipropionate/clotrimazole (Lotrisone).
- Oral antifungal therapy is generally reserved for cases unresponsive to topical agents. Effective medications are itraconazole (Sporonax) 100 mg/day for 2 to 4 wk, ketoconazole (Nizoral) 200 mg qd, fluconazole (Diflucan) 200 mg qd, and terbinafine (Lamisil) 250 mg qd.

■ DISPOSITION
Most cases respond promptly to therapy with complete resolution within 2 to 3 wk.

REFERENCE
Hainer BL: Dermatophyte infections, *Am Fam Physician* 67:101, 2003.
Author: **Fred F. Ferri, M.D.**

I

BASIC INFORMATION

■ DEFINITION
Tinea pedis is a dermatophyte infection of the feet.

■ SYNONYMS
Athlete's foot

ICD-CM CODES
110.4 Tinea pedis

■ EPIDEMIOLOGY & DEMOGRAPHICS
- Most common dermatophyte infection
- Increased incidence in hot humid weather. Occlusive footwear is a contributing factor
- Occurrence is rare before adolescence
- More common in adult males

■ PHYSICAL FINDINGS & CLINICAL PRESENTATION
- Typical presentation is variable and ranges from erythematous scaling plaques (see Fig. 1-276) and isolated blisters to interdigital maceration.
- The infection usually starts in the interdigital spaces of the foot. Most infections are found in the toe webs or in the soles.
- Fourth or fifth toes are most commonly involved.

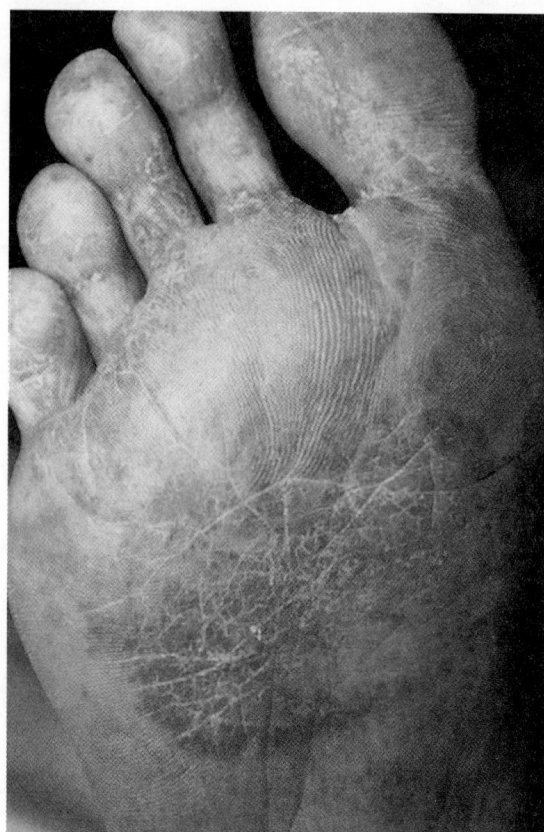

- Pruritus is common and is most intense following removal of shoes and socks.
- Infection with *tinea rubrum* often manifests with a moccasin distribution affecting the soles and lateral feet.

■ ETIOLOGY
Dermatophyte infection caused by *T. rubrum*, *T. mentagrophytes*, or less commonly *E. floccosum*

DIAGNOSIS

■ DIFFERENTIAL DIAGNOSIS
- Contact dermatitis
- Toe web infection
- Eczema
- Psoriasis
- Keratolysis exfoliativa
- Juvenile plantar dermatosis

■ WORKUP
- Diagnosis is usually made by clinical observation.
- Laboratory testing, when performed, generally consists of a simple potassium hydroxide (KOH) preparation with mycologic examination under a light microscope to confirm the presence of dermatophytes.

■ LABORATORY TESTS
- Microscopic examination of a scale or the roof of a blister with 10% KOH under low or medium power will reveal hyphae.
- Mycologic culture is rarely indicated in the diagnosis of tinea pedis.
- Biopsy is reserved for when the diagnosis remains in question after testing or failure to respond to treatment.

■ IMAGING STUDIES
- None

TREATMENT

■ NONPHARMACOLOGIC THERAPY
- Keep infected area clean and dry. Aerate feet by using sandals when possible.
- Use 100% cotton socks rather than nylon socks to reduce moisture.
- Areas likely to become infected should be dried completely before being covered with clothes.

■ ACUTE GENERAL THERAPY
- Butenafine Hcl 1% (Mentax) cream applied bid for 1 wk or qd for 4 wk is effective in interdigital tinea pedis.
- Ciclopirox 0.77 % (Loprox) cream applied bid for 4 wk is also effective.
- Clotrimazole 1% (Lotrimin AF) cream is an OTC treatment. It should be applied to affected and surrounding area bid for up to 4 wk.
- Naftifine (Naftin) 1 % cream applied qd or gel applied bid for 4 wk also produces a significantly high cure rate.
- When using topical preparations, the application area should include normal skin about 2 cm beyond the affected area.
- Areas of maceration can be treated with Burow's solution soaks for 10-20 min bid followed by foot elevation.
- Oral agents (fluconazole 150 mg once/week for 4 wk) can be used in combination with topical agents in resistant cases.

☼ PEARLS & CONSIDERATIONS

Combination therapy of antifungal and corticosteroid (clotrimazole/betamethasone [Lotrisone]) should only be used when the diagnosis of fungal infection is confirmed and inflammation is a significant issue.

REFERENCE
Weinstein A, Berman B: Topical treatment of common superficial tinea infections, *Am Fam Physician* 65:2095, 2002.
Author: **Fred F. Ferri, M.D.**

Fig. 1-276 Tinea pedis. (From Goldstein BG, Goldstein AO: *Practical dermatology*, ed 2, St Louis, 1997, Mosby.)

BASIC INFORMATION

■ **DEFINITION**
Tinea versicolor is a fungal infection of the skin caused by the yeast *Pityrosporum orbiculare (Malassezia furfur)*.

■ **SYNONYMS**
Pityriasis versicolor

ICD-9CM CODES
111.0 Tinea versicolor

■ **EPIDEMIOLOGY & DEMOGRAPHICS**
• Increased incidence in adolescence and young adulthood
• More common during the summer (hypopigmented lesions are more evident when the skin is tanned)

■ **PHYSICAL FINDINGS & CLINICAL PRESENTATION**
• Most lesions begin as multiple small, circular macules of various colors.
• The macules may be darker or lighter than the surrounding normal skin and will scale with scraping.
• Most frequent site of distribution is trunk.
• Facial lesions are more common in children (forehead is most common facial site).

• Eruption is generally of insidious onset and asymptomatic.
• Lesions may be hyperpigmented in blacks.
• Lesions may be inconspicuous in fair-complexioned individuals, especially during the winter.
• Most patients become aware of the eruption when the involved areas do not tan (Fig. 1-277).

■ **ETIOLOGY**
The infection is caused by the lipophilic yeast *P. orbiculare* (round form) and *P. ovale* (oval form); these organisms are normal inhabitants of the skin flora; factors that favor their proliferation are pregnancy, malnutrition, immunosuppression, oral contraceptives, and excess heat and humidity.

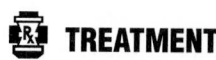 **DIAGNOSIS**

■ **DIFFERENTIAL DIAGNOSIS**
• Vitiligo
• Pityriasis alba
• Secondary syphilis
• Pityriasis rosea
• Seborrheic dermatitis

■ **WORKUP**
Diagnosis is based on clinical appearance; identification of hyphae and budding spores (spaghetti and meatballs appearance) with microscopy confirms diagnosis.

■ **LABORATORY TESTS**
Microscopic examination using potassium hydroxide confirms diagnosis when in doubt.

TREATMENT

■ **NONPHARMACOLOGIC THERAPY**
Sunlight accelerates repigmentation of hypopigmented areas.

■ **ACUTE GENERAL Rx**
• Topical treatment: selenium sulfide 2.5% suspension (Selsun or Exsel) applied daily for 10 min for 7 consecutive days results in a cure rate of 80% to 90%.
• Antifungal topical agents (e.g., miconazole, ciclopirox, clotrimazole) are also effective but generally expensive.
• Oral treatment is generally reserved for resistant cases. Effective agents are ketoconazole (Nizoral) 200 mg qd for 5 days, or single 400-mg dose (cure rate >80%), fluconazole (Diflucan) 400 mg given as a single dose (cure rate >70% at 3 wk after treatment), or itraconazole 200 mg/day for 5 days.

■ **DISPOSITION**
The prognosis is good, with death of the fungus usually occurring within 3 to 4 wk of treatment; however, recurrence is common.

PEARLS & CONSIDERATIONS

■ **COMMENTS**
Patients should be informed that the hypopigmented areas will not disappear immediately after treatment and that several months may be necessary for the hypopigmented areas to regain their pigmentation.
Author: **Fred F. Ferri, M.D.**

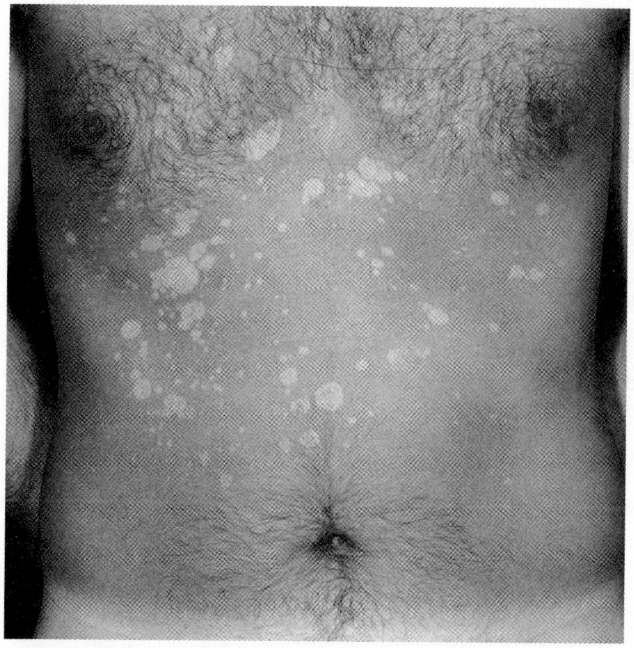

Fig. 1-277 The classic presentation of tinea versicolor with white, oval, or circular patches on tan skin. (From Habif TB: *Clinical dermatology: a color guide to diagnosis and therapy,* ed 3, St Louis, 1996, Mosby.)

BASIC INFORMATION

■ DEFINITION

Tinnitus is the false perception of sound in the absence of an acoustic stimulus.

■ SYNONYM

Ringing in the ear(s)

ICD-9CM CODES

388.30 Tinnitus

■ EPIDEMIOLOGY & DEMOGRAPHICS

- Prevalence: <45 yr: <1% in men and women; 45 to 65 yr old: 7% in men, 4% in women; above age 65: 10% in men, 5% in women
- More common in whites than in blacks
- More common in the southern U.S.
- Frequent association with hearing loss

SYMPTOMS (ALWAYS SUBJECTIVE)

- Ringing (35.5%)
- Buzzing (11.2%)
- Cricket-like (8.5%)
- Hissing (7.8%)
- Whistling (6.6%)
- Humming (5.3%)
- The pitch is high in most cases
- Tinnitus is reported to be unilateral (34%), bilateral with lateral dominance (44%), or equal in both ears (22%)
- Patients typically wait for several years before seeking medical attention
- Most patients report that the tinnitus is much louder subjectively than it is when matched with audible sounds

■ ETIOLOGY

OTOLOGIC:

- Noise-induced hearing loss
- Presbycusis
- Otosclerosis
- Otitis
- Ceruminosis
- Meniere's disease

NEUROLOGIC:

- Head and neck injury
- Multiple sclerosis
- Acoustic neuroma
- Other brain tumors

INFECTIONS:

- Otitis media
- Meningitis
- Lyme disease
- Syphilis

TOXIC (DRUGS):

- Aspirin
- NSAIDs
- Aminoglycosides
- Loop diuretics
- Vincristine

OTHER:

- Facial and dental disorders

DIAGNOSIS

■ DIFFERENTIAL DIAGNOSIS

- Objective tinnitus: hearing real sounds
  1. Pulsatile sounds: carotid stenosis, aortic valve disease, high cardiac output, arteriovenous malformations
  2. Muscular sounds: palatal myoclonus, spasm of stapedius or tensor tympani muscle
  3. Spontaneous autoacoustic emissions auditory hallucinations

■ WORKUP

- Description of the sound
  1. Constant or episodic
  2. Unilateral or bilateral
  3. Gradual or sudden onset
  4. Duration
  5. Hearing loss present or not
  6. Vertigo present or not
  7. Precipitating factors (e.g., background noise, alcohol, stress, sleep)
  8. Impact in daily life

PHYSICAL EXAMINATION

- Focus on head and neck
- Vital signs
- Signs of associated illnesses

LABORATORY

- CBC, FBS, creatinine, ALT, Alk Phos, TSH, lipids, ESR, Lyme titer
- Comprehensive audiologic evaluation
- In selected cases: brain magnetic resonance imaging with contrast

TREATMENT

- Prevent (further) hearing loss with appropriate ear protection and avoidance of noise exposure.
- Treat any identified etiologic factor and avoid ototoxic drugs
- Medications:
  1. Antiarrhythmic drugs (lidocaine, tocainide, flecainide) probably ineffective
  2. Benzodiazepines may help, but tinnitus recurs upon cessation of therapy
  3. Carbamazepine and other anticonvulsants are ineffective
  4. Antidepressants may be helpful and are worth a trial (most studies involve tricyclics)
  5. Gingko biloba may be helpful
- Acupuncture is ineffective
- Tinnitus retraining (habituation) may lead to improvement in as many of 75% of patients. Programs include counseling combined with low-level broadband noise exposure and usually take 1.5 years to complete
- Masking devices that cover up the unwanted sounds may be helpful in selected patients
- Surgical treatment is controversial
- Self-help groups (e.g., the American Tinnitus Association) provide useful information and support
- Patient education and reassurance

■ REFERRAL

ENT

REFERENCES

Lockwood AH, Salvi RJ, Burkard RF: Tinnitus, *N Engl J Med* 347:904, 2002.

Noell CA, Meyeroff WL: Tinnitus: diagnosis and treatment of this elusive symptom, *Geriatrics* 58:28, 2003.

Author: **Tom J. Wachtel, M.D.**

BASIC INFORMATION

■ DEFINITION
Torticollis is a contraction or contracture of the muscles of the neck that causes the head to be tilted to one side. It is usually accompanied by rotation of the chin to the opposite side with flexion. Usually it is a symptom of some underlying disorder. This term is often used incorrectly in cases when the torticollis may simply be positional.

■ SYNONYMS
Twisted neck
"Wry neck"

ICD-9CM CODES
723.5 Spastic (intermittent) torticollis
754.1 Congenital muscular (sternocleidomastoid)
300.11 Hysterical
714.0 Rheumatoid
333.83 Spasmodic

■ PHYSICAL FINDINGS & CLINICAL PRESENTATION
- Congenital muscular torticollis:
  1. Palpable soft tissue "mass" in the sternocleidomastoid shortly after birth
  2. Mass gradually subsides, leaving a shortened, contracted sternocleidomastoid muscle
  3. Head characteristically tilted toward the side of the mass and rotated in the opposite direction
  4. Facial asymmetry and other secondary changes persisting into adulthood
- Spasmodic torticollis:
  1. "Spasms" in the cervical musculature; may be bilateral and uncontrollable
  2. Head often tilted toward the affected side
- Findings in other cases depend on etiology.

■ ETIOLOGY
Torticollis has been attributed to more than 50 different causes:
- Localized fibrous shortening of unknown cause involving the sternocleidomastoid, leading to the condition termed *congenital muscular torticollis*
- Spasmodic torticollis: of uncertain etiology, possibly a variant of dystonia musculorum deformans
- Infection, specifically pharyngitis, tonsillitis, retropharyngeal abscess
- Miscellaneous rare causes: congenital musculoskeletal deformities, trauma, inflammation from rheumatoid arthritis, vestibular disturbances, posterior fossa tumor, syringomyelia, neuritis of spinal accessory nerve, and drug reactions

DIAGNOSIS

■ DIFFERENTIAL DIAGNOSIS
- Usually involves separating each disorder from the others
- Acquired positional disorders (e.g., ocular disturbances, acute disk herniation)

■ WORKUP
- Workup is dependent on the clinical situation.
- Laboratory studies are usually not helpful unless infection or rheumatoid disease is suspected.
- Section II describes a differential diagnosis for the evaluation and therapy of neck pain.
- Any child with a gradually increasing torticollis should have a complete eye examination.

■ IMAGING STUDIES
- Plain radiographs in cases of trauma or to rule out congenital abnormalities
- MRI in appropriate cases
- Electrodiagnostic studies: only rarely indicated to rule out neurologic causes

TREATMENT

- Congenital muscular torticollis: gentle stretching exercises carried out by the parent
- Spasmodic torticollis: physical therapy, psychotherapy, cervical braces, biofeedback, and pain control

- Other forms: treated according to etiology

■ DISPOSITION
- Most patients with congenital muscular torticollis respond well to conservative treatment.
- Spasmodic torticollis is often resistant to normal conservative treatment.
- Prognosis of other forms of torticollis is dependent on etiology.

■ REFERRAL
- Torticollis often requires a multidisciplinary approach unless the etiology is obvious.
- Children usually do not require any specific studies; however, an orthopedic consultation is recommended.

REFERENCES
Braun V, Richter HP: Selective peripheral denervation for spasmodic torticollis: 13 year experience with 155 patients, *J Neurosurg* 97:207, 2002.
Cheng JC et al: Clinical determinants of the outcome of manual stretching in the treatment of congenital muscular torticollis infants, *J Bone Joint Surg* 83(A):679, 2001.
McGuire KJ et al: Torticollis in children: can dynamic computed tomography determine severity and treatment, *J Pediatr Orthop* 22:766, 2002.
Tang SF et al: Longitudinal followup study of ultrasonography in congenital muscular torticollis, *Clin Orthop* 403:179, 2002.
Author: **Lonnie R. Mercier, M.D.**

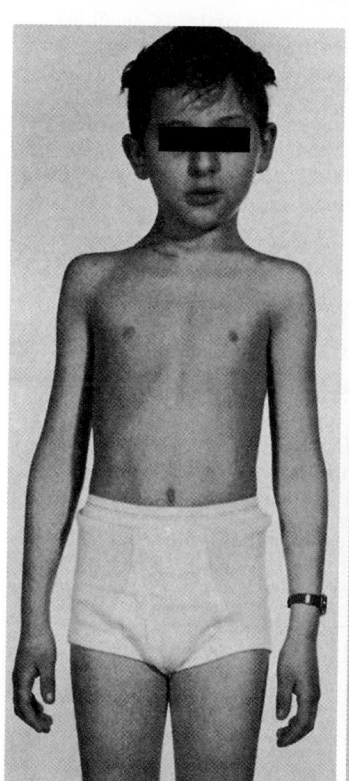 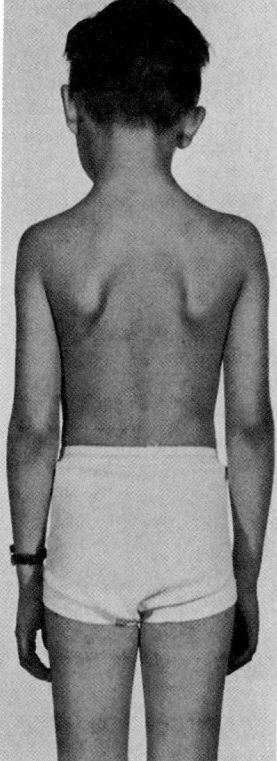

Fig. 1-278 Torticollis. In this child, the right sternocleidomastoid muscle is contracted. (From Brinker MR, Miller MD: *Fundamentals of orthopaedics,* Philadelphia, 1999, WB Saunders.)

BASIC INFORMATION

■ DEFINITION

Tics are sudden, brief, intermittent involuntary or semivoluntary movements (motor tics) or sounds (phonic or vocal tics) that mimic fragments of normal behavior.
Tourette's syndrome is an inherited neuropsychiatric disorder characterized by multiple motor and vocal tics that change during the course of the illness. Onset is before age 18.

■ SYNONYMS

Gilles de la Tourette syndrome
Motor-verbal tic disorder

ICD-9CM CODES

307.23 Gilles de la Tourette disorder

■ EPIDEMIOLOGY & DEMOGRAPHICS

PREVALENCE (IN U.S.): True prevalence is difficult to determine because of different ascertainment methods. Estimates range from 0.7% to 5%.
SEX: Male:female ratio is 3:1
AGE: Typical age of onset is between 2-15 yr. Mean is 5-7 yr.
INCIDENCE: Childhood/adolescence

■ PHYSICAL FINDINGS & CLINICAL PRESENTATION

Neurologic examination is normal.
- Vocal tics (clearing of throat, repetitive short phrases, e.g., "You bet," swearing [coprolalia]).
- Motor tics can be simple (e.g., blinking, grimacing, head jerking) or complex (e.g., gesturing). Tics wax, wane, and change over time. Often they can be suppressed for short periods. Commonly they are preceded by an urge to perform the tic.
- Often TS is associated with a variety of behavioral symptoms, most commonly ADHD and OCD. Incidence of OCD in TS patients is >30% and reaches its peak as tics are beginning to recede. 50%-75% of TS patients meet the criteria for ADHD and often this is what brings the patient to a doctor's attention (See Box 1-23).

■ ETIOLOGY

TS is at least in part genetic. There is a strong family history of OCD and/or TS in patients with tics, and twin studies provide evidence for importance of genetic factors. However, no candidate genes have been identified thus far. Underlying "tic generator" is not known. Based on beneficial effects of dopamine antagonists, dopamine is thought to be one of the major neurotransmitters involved.

DIAGNOSIS

■ DIFFERENTIAL DIAGNOSIS

- Sydenham's chorea—occurs after infection with Group A Streptococcus
- PANDAS—pediatric autoimmune neurolopsychiatric disorder associated with streptococcal infection
- Sporadic tic disorders—these tend to be motor or vocal but not both
- Head trauma
- Drug intoxication—there are many drugs that are known to induce or exacerbate tic disorder, including methylphenidate, amphetamines, pemoline, anticholinergics, and antihistamines
- Postinfectious encephalitis
- Inherited disorders—these include Huntington's disease, Hallervorden Spatz, and neuroacanthocytosis. All of these should have other abnormalities on neurologic examination

■ WORKUP

Clinical observation and history to confirm diagnosis

■ LABORATORY TESTS

No definitive laboratory tests

■ IMAGING STUDIES

CT scan and MRI of brain are normal and unnecessary in the absence of abnormal neurologic examination.

TREATMENT

■ NONPHARMACOLOGIC THERAPY

Multidisciplinary: parents, teachers, psychologists, school nurses

■ ACUTE GENERAL Rx

Dopamine-blocking agents may be used to reduce severity of tics acutely (e.g., haloperidol 0.25 mg PO qhs initially).

■ CHRONIC Rx

Tics only require treatment when they interfere with psychosocial, educational, and occupational functioning of a person. Often it is the behavioral problems that are associated with more significant disability and thus may need to be addressed first.
TREATMENT OF TICS:
- Clonidine—many choose to use this as first-line agent because of fewer long-term side effects. Start at 0.05 mg and slowly titrate to about 0.45 mg daily (needs tid/qid dosing). May also help with symptoms of ADHD.
- Guanfacine (Tenex), another alpha agonist similar to clonidine but can be administered once daily. Typical starting dose is 0.5 mg titrating to 1-3 mg qd.
- Tetrabenazine—dopamine-depleting agent that is not currently available in the U.S. Avoids many of the typical side effects of the neuroleptics.
- Atypical antipsychotics such as Ziprasidone (Geodon) and Olanzapine (Zyprexa). These have fewer side effects than typical neuroleptics.
- Dopamine-blocking agents—neuroleptics. Many physicians use Pimozide before Haldol because it is thought to have fewer side effects. It can prolong the QT interval and so the patient must have an ECG before starting therapy, 3 mo after starting, and at least yearly after that. Usual starting dose 0.5 to 1 mg qhs titrating to 2-4 mg/daily. Other agents include Fluphenazine (Prolixin).
TREATMENT OF ADHD:
Often treatment of this is needed before treatment of tics. Some of these stimulants can increase the frequency and intensity of tics and they may need to be combined with dopamine-depleting agents.
- Dextroamphetamine
- Methylphenidate

BOX 1-23 Evaluation of Tourette's Syndrome

Core clinical manifestations
    Axial motor and vocal tics
    Obsessions and compulsions
Common clinical manifestations
    Distractibility, hyperactivity, and impulsivity
    Learning difficulties or disorders
Psychiatric manifestations
    Mood disorders, especially depression
    Anxiety disorders, especially separation and/or phobias

From Johnson RT, Griffin JW: *Current therapy in neurologic disease,* ed 5, St Louis, 1997, Mosby.

TREATMENT OF OCD:
SSRIs, such as fluoxetine, are the most effective.

■ DISPOSITION

- In the later teen years, intensity and frequency of tics diminish.
- One third of patients will achieve significant remission. Though complete, lifelong remission is rare.
- One third will have mild, persistent, but "unimpairing" tics.

■ REFERRAL

To neurologist to confirm initial diagnosis

☼ PEARLS & CONSIDERATIONS

- Must emphasize that tics do not need treatment unless they interfere with an individual's ability to function.
- Coprolalia, one of the most recognizable and distressing symptoms, is present in less than half of patients with Tourette's and typically appears a few years after disease onset.

■ COMMENTS

- Patient education may be obtained from the Tourette's Syndrome Association (TSA), 4240 Bell Blvd., Bayside, NY, 11361-2864; phone: (800) 237-0717, (718) 224-2999. www.tsa-usa.org.

REFERENCES

Jankovic J: Tourette's syndrome, *N Engl J Med* 345:1184, 2001.

Jankovic J: Tics and Tourette's syndrome. In Jankovic J, Tolosa E (eds): *Parkinson's disease and movement disorders*, Philadelphia, 2002, Lippincott Williams & Wilkins.

Jimenez-Jimenez FJ, Garcia-Ruiz DJ: Pharmacological options for the treatment of Tourette's disorder, *Drugs* 61(15):2007, 2001.

Marcus D, Kurlan R: Tics and its disorders. In Hurtig H, Stern M (eds): *Neurologic clinics: movement disorders*, 19:3, 2001.

Author: **Cindy Zadikoff, M.D.**

BASIC INFORMATION

■ DEFINITION

Toxic shock syndrome is an acute febrile illness resulting in multiple organ system dysfunction caused most commonly by a bacterial exotoxin. Disease characteristics also include hypotension, vomiting, myalgia, watery diarrhea, vascular collapse, and an erythematous sunburnlike cutaneous rash that desquamates during recovery.

ICD-9CM CODES
040.89 Toxic shock syndrome

■ EPIDEMIOLOGY & DEMOGRAPHICS
- Case reported incidence peak: 14 cases/100,000 menstruating women/yr in 1980; has since fallen to 1 case/100,000 persons
- Occurs most commonly between ages 10 and 30 yr in healthy, young menstruating white females
- Case fatality ratio of 3%

■ ETIOLOGY (FIG. 1-279)
- Menstrually associated TSS: 45% of cases associated with tampons, diaphragm, or vaginal sponge use

- Nonmenstruating associated TSS: 55% of cases associated with puerperal sepsis, post–cesarean section endometritis, mastitis, wound or skin infection, insect bite, pelvic inflammatory disease, and postoperative fever
- Causative agent: *S. aureus* infection of a susceptible individual (10% of population lacking sufficient levels of antitoxin antibodies), which liberates the disease mediator TSST-1 (exotoxin)
- Other causative agents: coagulase-negative streptococci producing enterotoxins B or C, and exotoxin A producing group A β-hemolytic streptococci

■ PHYSICAL FINDINGS & CLINICAL PRESENTATION
- Fever (≥38.9° C)
- Diffuse macular erythrodermatous rash that desquamates 1 to 2 wk after disease onset in survivors
- Orthostatic hypotension
- GI symptoms: vomiting, diarrhea, abdominal tenderness
- Constitutional symptoms: myalgia, headache, photophobia, rigors, altered sensorium, conjunctivitis, arthralgia

- Respiratory symptoms: dysphagia, pharyngeal hyperemia, strawberry tongue
- Genitourinary symptoms: vaginal discharge, vaginal hyperemia, adnexal tenderness
- End-organ failure
- Severe hypotension and acute renal failure
- Hepatic failure
- Cardiovascular symptoms: DIC, pulmonary edema, ARDS, endomyocarditis, heart block

DIAGNOSIS

■ DIFFERENTIAL DIAGNOSIS
- Staphylococcal food poisoning
- Septic shock
- Mucocutaneous lymph node syndrome
- Scarlet fever
- Rocky Mountain spotted fever
- Meningococcemia
- Toxic epidermal necrolysis
- Kawasaki's syndrome
- Leptospirosis
- Legionnaires' disease
- Hemolytic-uremic syndrome
- Stevens-Johnson syndrome
- Scalded skin syndrome

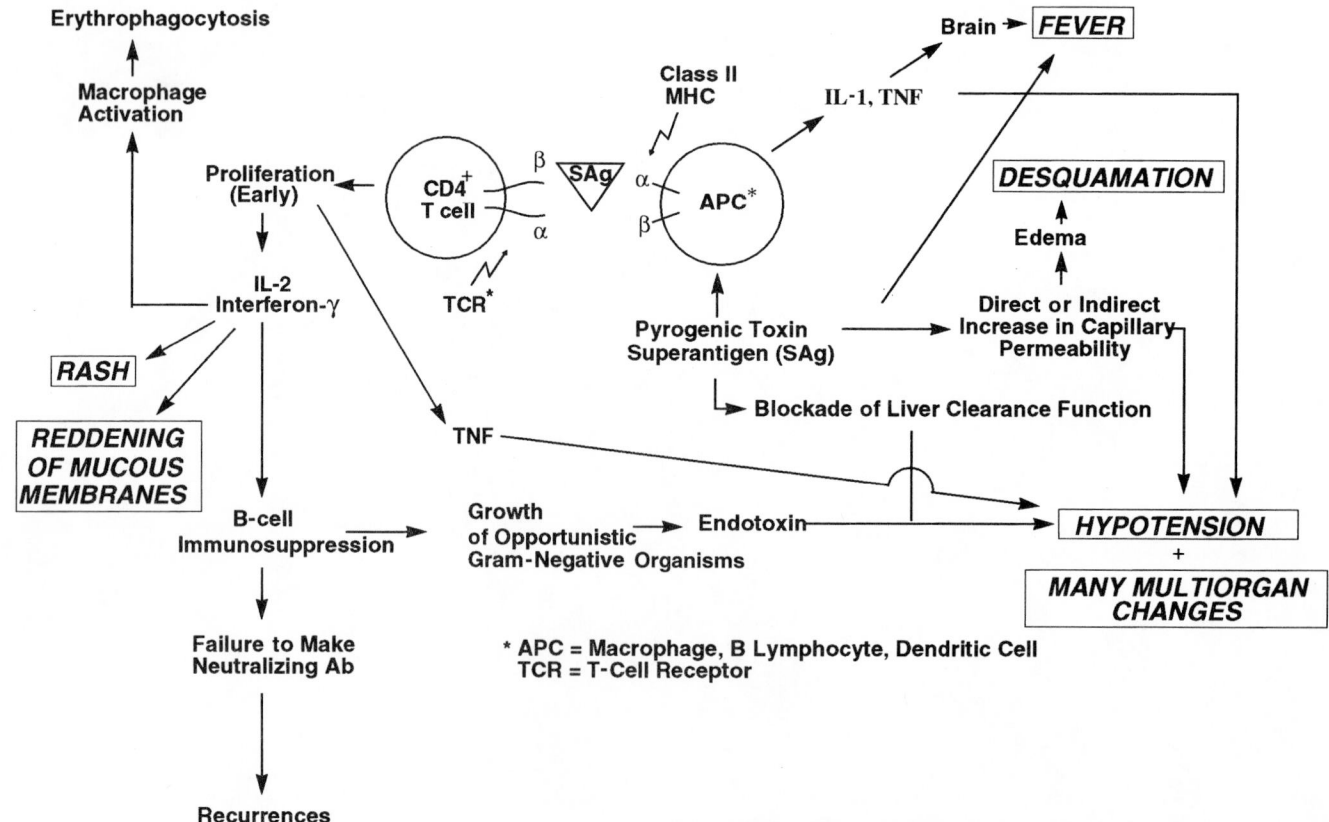

Fig. 1-279 Model for the development of toxic shock syndrome and related illnesses. *Ab,* Antibody; *IL1,* interleukin-1; *IL2,* interleukin-2; *MHC,* major histocompatibility complex; *Sag,* superantigen; *TNF,* tumor necrosis factor. (From Gorbach SL, Bartlett JG, Blacklow NR [eds]: *Infectious diseases,* ed 2, Philadelphia, 1998, WB Saunders.)

- Erythema multiforme
- Acute rheumatic fever

■ WORKUP

Broad-spectrum syndrome with multi-organ system involvement and variable but acute clinical presentation, including the following:

1. Fever ≥38.1° C
2. Classic desquamating (1 to 2 wk) rash
3. Hypotension/orthostatic SBP 90 or less
4. Syncope
5. Negative throat/CSF cultures
6. Negative serologic test for Rocky Mountain spotted fever, rubeola, and leptospirosis
7. Clinical involvement of three or more of the following:
   a. Cardiopulmonary: ARDS, pulmonary edema, endomyocarditis, second- or third-degree AV block
   b. CNS: altered sensorium without focal neurologic findings
   c. Hematologic: thrombocytopenia (PLT <100 k)
   d. Liver: elevated LFT results
   e. Renal: >5/HPF, negative urine cultures, azotemia, and increased creatinine double normal
   f. Mucous membrane involvement: vagina, oropharynx, conjunctiva
   g. Musculoskeletal: myalgia, CPK twice normal
   h. GI: vomiting, diarrhea

■ LABORATORY TESTS

- Pan culture (cervix/vagina, throat, nasal passages, urine, blood, CSF, wound) for *Staphylococcus, Streptococcus,* or other pathogenic organisms
- Electrolytes to detect hypokalemia, hyponatremia
- CBC with differential and clotting profile for anemia (normocytic/normochromic), thrombocytopenia, leukocytosis, coagulopathy, and bacteremia
- Chemistry profile to detect decreased protein, increased AST, increased ALT, hypocalcemia, elevated BUN/creatinine, hypophosphatemia, increased LDH, increased CPK
- Urinalysis to detect WBC (>5/HPF), proteinemia, microhematuria
- ABGs to assess respiratory function and acid-base status
- Serologic tests considered for Rocky Mountain spotted fever, rubeola, and leptospirosis

■ IMAGING STUDIES

- Chest x-ray examination to evaluate pulmonary edema
- ECG to evaluate arrhythmia
- Sonography/CT scan/MRI considered if pelvic abscess or TOA suspected

■ TREATMENT

■ NONPHARMACOLOGIC THERAPY

- For optimal outcome: high index of suspicion and early and aggressive supportive management in an ICU setting
- Aggressive fluid resuscitation (maintenance of circulating volume, CO, SBP)
- Thorough search for a localized infection or nidus: incision and drainage, debridement, removal of tampon or vaginal sponge
- Central hemodynamic monitoring, Swan-Ganz catheter and arterial line for surveillance of hemodynamic status and response to therapy
- Foley catheter to monitor hourly urine output
- Possible MAST trousers as temporary measure
- Acute ventilator management if severe respiratory compromise
- Renal dialysis for severe renal impairment
- Surgical intervention for indicated conditions (i.e., ruptured TOA, wound abscess, mastitis)

■ ACUTE GENERAL Rx

- Isotonic crystalloid (normal saline solution) for volume replacement following "7-3" rule
- Electrolyte replacement (K+, Ca+)
- PRBC/coagulation factor replacement/FFP to treat anemia or D&C
- Vasopressor therapy for hypotension refractory to fluid volume replacement (i.e., dopamine beginning at 2 to 5 µg/kg/min)
- Naloxone infusion (i.e., 0.5 mg/kg/hr) to improve SBP by blocking endogenous endorphin effects
- Parenteral antibiotic therapy; β-lactamase resistant antibiotic (methicillin, nafcillin, or oxacillin) initiated early
- Broad-spectrum antibiotic added if concurrent sepsis suspected
- Tetracycline added if considering Rocky Mountain spotted fever

■ CHRONIC Rx

- Severely ill patient: may require prolonged hospitalization and supportive management with gradual recovery and/or sequelae from severe end-organ involvement (ARDS or renal failure requiring dialysis)
- Majority of patients: complete recovery
- Early late-onset complications (within 2 wk):
  1. Skin desquamation
  2. Impaired digit sensation
  3. Denuded tongue
  4. Vocal cord paralysis

5. ATN
6. ARDS

- Late-onset complications (after 8 wk):
  1. Nail splitting/loss
  2. Alopecia
  3. CNS sequelae
  4. Renal impairment
  5. Cardiac dysfunction
- Recurrent TSS:
  1. More common in menstrually related cases
  2. Less common in patient treated with β-lactamase–resistant antistaphylococcal antibiotics
  3. Patients with history of TSS: if suspect signs and symptoms occur, should have high index of suspicion and low threshold for evaluation and treatment

■ PREVENTION

- Avoidance of tampons or use of low-absorbency tampons only (<4 hr in situ) and alternate with napkins
- Education for patients concerning signs and symptoms of TSS
- Avoidance of tampons for patients with history of TSS

■ DISPOSITION

- Complete recovery for most patients
- Long-term management of early- and late-onset complications for minority of patients

■ REFERRAL

- For multidisciplinary management, involving primary physician, gynecologist, internist, infectious disease specialist, and other supportive care specialists
- To tertiary level hospital

☼ PEARLS & CONSIDERATIONS

■ COMMENTS

Patient information available from American College of Gynecologists and Obstetricians.

REFERENCES

Davis D et al: Toxic shock syndrome: case report of a postpartum female and a literature review, *J Emerg Med* 16(4):607, 1998.

Hajjeh RA et al: Toxic shock syndrome in the United States: surveillance update, 1979-1996, *Emerg Infect Dis J* 5(6), 1999.

Issa NC et al: Staphylococcal toxic shock syndrome: suspicion and prevention are keys to control, *Postgrad Med* 110(4):55, 2001.

Miche CA, Shah V: Managing toxic shock syndrome. *Nursing Times* 99(5):26, 2003.

Author: **Dennis M. Weppner, M.D.**

BASIC INFORMATION

■ DEFINITION
Toxoplasmosis is an infection caused by the protozoal parasite *Toxoplasma gondii.*

ICD-9CM CODES
130.9 Toxoplasmosis

■ EPIDEMIOLOGY & DEMOGRAPHICS
INCIDENCE (IN U.S.):
- Increases with age
- Increases with certain activities
  1. Slaughterhouse workers
  2. Cat owners
- Increases with certain geographic locations: high prevalence of cats

INCIDENCE (IN U.S.): 3% to 70% of healthy adults

PREDOMINANT SEX: Equal gender distribution

PREDOMINANT AGE:
- Infancy (congenital infection)
- Prevalence increases with age

PEAK INCIDENCE: Temperate climates

GENETICS:
Congenital Infection:
- Incidence and severity vary with the trimester of gestation during which the mother acquired infection.
  1. 10% to 25% (first trimester)
  2. 30% to 54% (second trimester)
  3. 60% to 65% (third trimester)
- Congenital infection occurring in the first trimester is the most severe.
- 89% to 100% of infections in the third trimester are asymptomatic.
- Risk to the fetus is not correlated with symptoms in the mother.

■ PHYSICAL FINDINGS & CLINICAL PRESENTATION
- Acquired (immunocompetent host)
  1. 80% to 90% asymptomatic
  2. Adenopathy (usually cervical)
  3. Fever
  4. Myalgias
  5. Malaise
  6. Sore throat
  7. Maculopapular rash
  8. Hepatosplenomegaly
  9. Chorioretinitis rare
- Acquired (in patients with AIDS)
  1. 89% of symptomatic cases
     a. Encephalitis
     b. Intracerebral mass lesions
  2. Pneumonitis
  3. Chorioretinitis
  4. Other end organ
- Acquired (immunocompromised patients)
  1. Encephalitis
  2. Myocarditis (especially in heart transplant patients)
  3. Pneumonitis

- Ocular infection in the immunocompetent host
  1. Congenital infection
  2. Blurred vision
  3. Photophobia
  4. Pain
  5. Loss of central vision if macula involved
  6. Focal necrotizing retinitis
  7. Typically presents in second or third decade
- Congenital
  1. Results from acute infection acquired by the mother within 6 to 8 wk before conception or during gestation
  2. Usually, asymptomatic mother
  3. No sign of disease
  4. Chorioretinitis
  5. Blindness
  6. Epilepsy
  7. Psychomotor or mental retardation
  8. Intracranial calcifications
  9. Hydrocephalus
  10. Microcephaly
  11. Encephalitis
  12. Anemia
  13. Thrombocytopenia
  14. Hepatosplenomegaly
  15. Lymphadenopathy
  16. Jaundice
  17. Rash
  18. Pneumonitis
  19. Most infected infants are asymptomatic at birth

■ ETIOLOGY
- *Toxoplasma gondii*
  1. Ubiquitous intracellular protozoan
  2. Present worldwide
  3. Cat is definitive host
- Human infection
  1. Ingestion of oocysts shed by cats
  2. Ingestion of meat containing tissue cysts
  3. Vertical transmission

DIAGNOSIS

■ DIFFERENTIAL DIAGNOSIS
- Lymphadenopathy
  1. Infectious mononucleosis
  2. CMV mononucleosis
  3. Cat-scratch disease
  4. Sarcoidosis
  5. Tuberculosis
  6. Lymphoma
  7. Metastatic cancer
- Cerebral mass lesions in immunocompromised host
  1. Lymphoma
  2. Tuberculosis
  3. Bacterial abscess
- Pneumonitis in immunocompromised host
  1. *Pneumocystis carinii* pneumonia
  2. Tuberculosis
  3. Fungal infection

- Chorioretinitis
  1. Syphilis
  2. Tuberculosis
  3. Histoplasmosis (competent host)
  4. CMV
  5. Syphilis
  6. Herpes simplex
  7. Fungal infection
  8. Tuberculosis (AIDS patient)
- Myocarditis
  1. Organ rejection in heart transplant recipients
- Congenital infection
  1. Rubella
  2. CMV
  3. Herpes simplex
  4. Syphilis
  5. Listeriosis
  6. Erythroblastosis fetalis
  7. Sepsis

■ WORKUP
- Acute infection, immunocompetent host
  1. CBC
  2. *Toxoplasma* serology (IgG, Ig) in serial blood specimens 3 wk apart
  3. Lymph node biopsy if diagnosis uncertain
- Immunocompromised host
  1. CNS symptoms
     a. Cerebral CT scan or MRI if CNS symptoms present
     b. Spinal tap, if safe
     c. Brain biopsy if no response to empiric therapy
  2. Ocular symptoms
     a. Funduscopic examination
     b. Serologic studies
     c. Rarely, vitreous tap
  3. Pulmonary symptoms
     a. Chest x-ray examination
     b. Bronchoalveolar lavage
     c. Transbronchial or open lung biopsy
  4. Myocarditis
     a. Cardiac enzymes
     b. Electrocardiogram
     c. Endomyocardial biopsy for definitive diagnosis
- Toxoplasmosis in pregnancy
  1. Initial maternal screening with IgM and IgG
     a. If negative, mother at risk of acute infection and should be retested monthly
     b. If both IgG and IgM positive, obtain IgA and IgE ELISA, AC/HS test
     c. IgA and IgE ELISA, AC/HS test elevated in acute infection
     d. Ig high for 1 yr or more
     e. IgG repeated 3 to 4 wk later to determine if titer is stable
  2. Acute maternal infection not excluded or documented
     a. Fetal blood sampling (for culture, Ig, IgA, IgE)
     b. Amniotic fluid PCR
  3. Fetal ultrasound every other week if maternal infection documented

- Congenital toxoplasmosis
  1. Placental histology
  2. Specific IgM or IgA in infant's blood

■ LABORATORY TESTS
- Antibody studies
  1. More than one test necessary to establish diagnosis of acute toxoplasmosis
  2. IgM antibody
     a. Appears 5 days into infection
     b. Peaks at 2 wk
     c. Falls to low level or disappears within 2 mo
     d. May persist at low levels for 1 yr or more
  3. Antibody not measurable
     a. Ocular toxoplasmosis
     b. Reactivation
     c. Immunocompromised hosts
  4. IgA ELISA, IgE ELISA, and IgE ASAGA
     a. More sensitive tests
     b. Disappear more rapidly than Ig, establishing diagnosis of acute infection
  5. IgG antibody
     a. Appears 1 to 2 wk after infection
     b. Peaks at 6 to 8 wk
     c. Gradually declines over months to years

■ IMAGING STUDIES
- Chest x-ray examination if pulmonary involvement suspected
- Cerebral CT scan or MRI if encephalitis suspected

TREATMENT

■ NONPHARMACOLOGIC THERAPY
- Selected cases of ocular infection
  1. Photocoagulation
  2. Vitrectomy
  3. Lentectomy
- Selected cases of congenital cerebral infection
  1. Ventricular shunting

■ ACUTE GENERAL Rx
- Acute infection, immunocompetent host
  1. No treatment, unless severe and persistent symptoms or vital organ damage
- Acute infection, immunocompromised host, non-AIDS
  1. Treat even if asymptomatic
  2. Duration
     a. Until 4 to 6 wk after resolution of all signs and symptoms
     b. Usually 6 mo or longer
- Reactivated infection, immunocompromised host, non-AIDS
  1. Treat if symptomatic

- Acute or reactivated infection, AIDS
  1. Treat in all cases
  2. Induction course
     a. 3 to 6 wk
     b. Maintenance therapy continued for life
  3. Empiric therapy
     a. AIDS with positive IgG
     b. Multiple ring-enhancing lesions on cerebral CT scan or MRI
     c. Response seen by day 7 in 71% and day 14 in 91%
- Ocular infection
  1. Treat in all cases
  2. Therapy continued for 1 mo or longer if needed
  3. Response seen in 70% within 10 days
  4. Retreat as needed
  5. Steroids may be indicated
  6. Surgical treatment in selected cases
- Treatment regimens
  1. Pyrimethamine 100 to 200 mg loading dose once PO, then 25 mg PO qd (50 to 75 mg in AIDS) *plus*
  2. Leucovorin 10 to 20 mg PO qd *plus*
  3. Sulfadiazine 1 to 1.5 g PO q6h
- Acute infection in pregnancy
  1. Treat immediately
  2. Risk of fetal infection reduced by 60% with treatment
     a. First trimester
        i. Spiramycin 3 g PO qd in two to four divided doses
        ii. Sulfadiazine 4 g PO qd in four divided doses
     b. Second and third trimester
        i. Sulfadiazine as above *plus*
        ii. Pyrimethamine 25 mg PO qd *plus*
        iii. Leucovorin 5 to 15 mg PO qd
        iv. Spiramycin as above
- Congenital infection
  1. Sulfadiazine 50 mg/kg PO bid *plus*
  2. Pyrimethamine 2 mg/kg PO for 2 days, then 1 mg/kg PO, three times weekly *plus*
  3. Leucovorin 5 to 20 mg PO three times weekly
  4. Minimum duration of treatment: 12 mo

■ CHRONIC Rx
- Maintenance therapy in AIDS patients because of the high risk (80%) of relapse
  1. Pyrimethamine 25 mg PO qd
  2. Sulfadiazine 500 mg PO qid
  3. Leucovorin 10 to 20 mg PO qd

■ DISPOSITION
- Prognosis
  1. Excellent in the immunocompetent host
  2. Good in ocular infection (although relapses are common)
- Treatment of acute infection in pregnancy
  1. Reduces incidence and severity of congenital toxoplasmosis
- Treatment of congenital infection
  1. Improvement in intellectual function
  2. Regression of retinal lesions
- AIDS
  1. 70% to 95% response to therapy

■ REFERRAL
- To infectious disease expert:
  1. Immunocompromised hosts
  2. Pregnant women
  3. Difficulty in making a diagnosis or deciding on treatment
- To pediatric infectious disease expert:
  1. Congenital infection
- To obstetrician:
  1. Pregnant seronegative mother
  2. Acute seroconversion
- To ophthalmologist:
  1. Congenital infection
  2. Any case of ocular infection

☼ PEARLS & CONSIDERATIONS

■ COMMENTS
- Prevention of toxoplasmosis is most important in seronegative pregnant women and immunocompromised hosts.
- Patient instructions:
  1. Cook meat to 66° C.
  2. Cook eggs.
  3. Do not drink unpasteurized milk.
  4. Wash hands thoroughly after handling raw meat.
  5. Wash kitchen surfaces that come in contact with raw meat.
  6. Wash fruits and vegetables.
  7. Avoid contact with materials potentially contaminated with cat feces.

REFERENCES
Beazley DM, Egerman RS: Toxoplasmosis, *Semin Perinatol* 22(4):332, 1998.
Boyer KM: Diagnostic testing for congenital toxoplasmosis, *Pediatr Infect Dis J* 20(1):59, 2001.
Jones JL et al: Congenital toxoplasmosis: a review, *Obstet Gynecol Surv* 56(50):296, 2001.
Author: **Michele Halpern, M.D.**

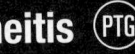
 BASIC INFORMATION

■ DEFINITION
Bacterial tracheitis is an acute infectious disease affecting the trachea and large conducting airways. Tracheal inflammation may be caused by a large number of inhaled stimuli, but bacterial infection is a life-threatening illness associated with viscous purulent secretions and subglottic edema.

■ SYNONYMS
Bacterial tracheobronchitis
Pseudomembranous croup
Membranous laryngotracheobronchitis

ICD-9CM CODES
464.10 Tracheitis

■ EPIDEMIOLOGY & DEMOGRAPHICS
INCIDENCE (IN U.S.):
- Uncommon
- May be the most common cause of acute upper airway obstruction requiring admission to pediatric ICUs

PREDOMINANT SEX: Boys > girls in one series

PREDOMINANT AGE:
- 1 mo to 8 yr
- Almost all <13 yr (most <3 yr)

PEAK INCIDENCE: Three fourths of cases reported in winter

GENETICS: Down syndrome is a possible predisposing factor.

Congenital Infection: Some cases found in those with anatomic abnormalities of the upper airways.

■ PHYSICAL FINDINGS & CLINICAL PRESENTATION
- Croupy or "brassy" cough
- Inspiratory stridor (frequent)
- Wheezing (unusual)
- Fever (often >102° F)
- Thick, purulent secretions expectorated
  1. Minority of patients expectorate "rice-like" pellets.
  2. Most patients are unable to mobilize secretions.
     a. Become inspissated
     b. Form pseudomembranes

■ ETIOLOGY
- *Staphylococcus aureus*
- *Haemophilus influenzae*
- β-Hemolytic streptococcal infection
- Secondary to viral infections of the respiratory tract
  1. Primary influenza
  2. RSV
  3. Parainfluenza
- Many cases follow measles
  1. Especially when accompanied by chest radiographic infiltrates
  2. Sometimes fatal outcome

⚕ DIAGNOSIS

■ DIFFERENTIAL DIAGNOSIS
- Viral croup
- Epiglottitis
- Diphtheria
- Necrotizing herpes simplex infection in the elderly
- CMV in immunocompromised patients
- Invasive *Aspergillosis* in immunocompromised patients

■ WORKUP
- Direct laryngoscopy
  1. Typical secretions
     a. May form pseudomembranes
     b. Airway obstruction
  2. Normal epiglottis rules out epiglottitis
  3. Possible subglottic edema

■ LABORATORY TESTS
- WBC is sometimes elevated.
- On differential, left shift is almost universal.
- Gram stain and culture of tracheal secretions confirm diagnosis.
- Blood cultures are positive in a minority.

■ IMAGING STUDIES
- Lateral x-ray examination of neck
  1. Normal epiglottis
  2. Vague density or a "dripping candle" appearance of tracheal mucosa
     a. Secretions
     b. Pseudomembranes
- Films
  1. Not diagnostic
  2. Should not be performed on patients in acute respiratory distress, because severe or fatal upper airway obstruction can develop suddenly
- Pneumonic infiltrates frequent
- Atelectasis
  1. Unusual
  2. May involve an entire lung

℞ TREATMENT

■ NONPHARMACOLOGIC THERAPY
- Aggressive maintenance of a patent airway
  1. Laryngoscopy or bronchoscopy used diagnostically and therapeutically to strip away pseudomembranes
  2. Voluminous and tenacious secretions suctioned from the underlying friable mucosa
     a. May extend from between the vocal cords to the main carina
     b. Larger channels of rigid instruments for more effective suctioning

- Prevention of complete large airway obstruction
  1. Nasotracheal intubation
  2. Humidification of inspired gas
  3. Frequent saline instillation and suctioning
  4. Intubation with general anesthesia, performed in the operating room, is preferred by some
- Ventilatory support necessary
- Initial management in ICU

■ ACUTE GENERAL Rx
- Antibiotic therapy
  1. Start immediately
  2. Continue for 2 wk
- Initial therapy
  1. β-Lactamase–producing *H. influenzae*
  2. β-Lactamase–producing staphylococci
- Oral therapy is usually sufficient after 5 or 6 days of IV administration

■ DISPOSITION
- Most patients are extubated in 5 to 6 days after initiating antibiotic therapy.
- Anoxic encephalopathy is reported in 7% of survivors.

■ REFERRAL
Suspected diagnosis

☼ PEARLS & CONSIDERATIONS

■ COMMENTS
- Infants are at increased risk of airway obstruction because of the small transverse area of the upper airway.
- Presence of pneumonia and a staphylococcal etiology are thought to worsen prognosis.
- Reported complications:
  1. Toxic shock syndrome
  2. Persistent postextubation stridor
  3. Pneumothorax
  4. Volutrauma

REFERENCES
Ahmed QA, Niederman MS: Respiratory infection in the chronically critically ill patient, *Clin Chest Med* 22(10):71, 2001.

Bernstein T, Brilli R, Jacobs B: Is bacterial tracheitis changing? A 14-month experience in a pediatric intensive care unit, *Clin Infect Dis* 27:458, 1998.

Brook I: Aerobic and anaerobic microbiology of bacterial tracheitis in children, *Pediatr Emerg Care* 13:16, 1997.

Stroud RH, Friedman NR: An update on inflammatory disorders of the pediatric airway: epiglottitis, croup and tracheitis, *Am J Otolaryngol* 22(40):268, 2001.

Author: **Harvey M. Shanies, M.D., Ph.D.**

BASIC INFORMATION

■ DEFINITION

Hemolytic transfusion reaction is an acute intravascular hemolysis caused by mismatches in the ABO system. It is caused by complement-fixing Ig and IgG antibodies to group A and B RBCs. Hemolytic transfusion reactions can also be caused by minor antigen systems; however, they are usually less severe. In delayed serologic transfusion reactions, hemolysis with hemoglobinemia is unusual; in these delayed reactions the only manifestations may be the development of a newly positive Coombs' test and fever.

■ ICD-9CM CODES

999.8 Other transfusion reaction

■ EPIDEMIOLOGY & DEMOGRAPHICS

Acute intravascular hemolysis occurs in <1 in 50,000 transfusions.

■ PHYSICAL FINDINGS & CLINICAL PRESENTATION (TABLE 1-57)

• Hypotension
• Pain at the infusion site
• Fever, tachycardia, chest or back pain, dyspnea
• Often, severe reactions occur in surgical patients under anesthesia who are unable to give any warning signs

■ ETIOLOGY

Most fatal hemolytic reactions are caused by clerical errors and mislabeled specimens.

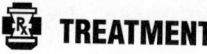 **DIAGNOSIS**

■ DIFFERENTIAL DIAGNOSIS

• Bacterial contamination of blood
• Hemoglobinopathies

■ WORKUP

The transfusion must be stopped immediately. The blood bank must be notified, and the donor transfusion bag must be returned to the blood bank along with a freshly drawn post-transfusion specimen.

■ LABORATORY TESTS

• Positive Coombs' test, elevated BUN, creatinine, and bilirubin
• Hemoglobinuria (wine-colored urine), hemoglobinemia (pink plasma)
• Decreased Hct, decreased serum haptoglobin

TREATMENT

■ NONPHARMACOLOGIC THERAPY

• Stop transfusion immediately. Test anticoagulated blood from the recipient for the presence of free Hgb in the plasma.
• Monitor vital signs.

■ ACUTE GENERAL Rx

• Vigorous IV hydration to maintain urine flow at >100 ml/hr until hypotension is corrected and hemoglobinuria clears. IV furosemide may be necessary to maintain adequate renal flow.
• The addition of mannitol may prevent renal damage (controversial).
• Monitor for the presence of DIC.
• Use of IV steroids is controversial.

■ DISPOSITION

Mortality exceeds 50% in severe transfusion reactions.

PEARLS & CONSIDERATIONS

■ COMMENTS

Hemolysis caused by minor antigen systems is generally less severe and may be delayed 5 to 10 days after transfusion.
Author: **Fred F. Ferri, M.D.**

TABLE 1-57 Signs and Symptoms of Acute Adverse Reactions to Blood Transfusion

REACTION	FEVER	CHILLS/ RIGORS	NAUSEA/ VOMITING	CHEST DISCOMFORT/ PAIN	FACIAL FLUSHING	WHEEZING/ DYSPNEA	BACK/ LUMBAR PAIN	DISCOMFORT AT INFUSION SITE	HYPOTENSION
Acute hemolytic	X	X	X	X	X	X	X	X	X
Febrile nonhemolytic	X	X		X	X				
Nonimmune hemolysis									
Acute lung injury	X			X		X			X
Allergic									
Massive transfusion complications									
Anaphylaxis	X	X	X	X	X	X	X	X	X
Passive cytokine infusion	X	X	X						
Hypervolemia						X			
Bacterial sepsis	X	X	X				X	X	X
Air embolus				X		X			

From Goldman L, Bennett JC (eds): *Cecil textbook of medicine,* ed 21, Philadelphia, 2000, WB Saunders.

BASIC INFORMATION

■ DEFINITION

The term *transient ischemic attack* (TIA) refers to a transient neurologic dysfunction caused by focal brain or retinal ischemia with symptoms typically lasting less than 60 min but always less than 24 hr and is followed by a full recovery of function. Acute brain ischemia is a medical emergency requiring prompt neurologic evaluation and potential intervention.

■ SYNONYMS

TIA

ICD-9CM CODES

435.9 Unspecified transient cerebral ischemia

■ EPIDEMIOLOGY & DEMOGRAPHICS

INCIDENCE (IN U.S.): 49 cases/100,000 persons/yr
PREDOMINANT SEX: Males > females
PEAK INCIDENCE: >60 yr

■ PHYSICAL FINDINGS & CLINICAL PRESENTATION

- During an episode, neurologic abnormalities are confined to discrete vascular territory.
- Typical carotid territory symptoms are ipsilateral monocular visual disturbance, contralateral homonymous hemianopsia, contralateral hemimotor or sensory dysfunction, and language dysfunction (dominant hemisphere) alone or in combination.
- Typical vertebrobasilar territory symptoms are binocular visual disturbance, vertigo, diplopia, dysphagia, dysarthria, and motor or sensory dysfunction involving the ipsilateral face and contralateral body.

■ ETIOLOGY

- Cardioembolic
- Large vessel atherothrombotic disease
- Lacunar disease
- Hypoperfusion with fixed distal small vessel disease
- Hypercoagulable states

DIAGNOSIS

■ DIFFERENTIAL DIAGNOSIS

- Hypoglycemia
- Seizures
- Migraine
- Subdural hemorrhage
- Mass lesions
- Vestibular disease
- Section II describes the differential diagnosis of neurologic deficits, focal and multifocal.

■ WORKUP

- Thorough history and physical examination
- Ancillary investigations including neuroimaging aimed at identifying the etiology quickly

■ LABORATORY TESTS

- CBC with platelets
- PT (INR) and PTT
- Glucose
- Lipid profile
- ESR (if clinical suspicion for infectious or inflammatory process)
- Urinalysis
- Chest x-ray
- ECG and consider cycling cardiac enzymes
- Other tests as dictated by suspected etiology

■ IMAGING STUDIES

- Head CT scan to exclude hemorrhage including a chronic subdural hemorrhage
- MRI and MRA. (In several studies, MRI with diffusion-weighted imaging has identified early ischemic brain injury in up to 50% of patients with TIA). MRA of the brain and neck can identify large vessel intracranial and extracranial stenoses, arteriovenous malformations, and aneurysms
- Carotid Doppler studies identify carotid stenosis
- Echocardiography if cardiac source is suspected
- Telemetry for hospitalized patients for at least 24 hr. May consider 24-hr Holter if patient is being discharged
- Four-vessel cerebral angiogram if considering carotid endarterectomy or carotid stent

TREATMENT

■ NONPHARMACOLOGIC THERAPY

- Carotid endarterectomy for carotid territory TIA associated with an ipsilateral stenosis of 70% to 99%: should be done by a surgeon who is experienced with and performs this procedure frequently
- Modification of risk factors

■ ACUTE GENERAL Rx

- Depends on etiology
- If the time of the onset of symptoms is clear, and there are significant deficits on neurologic examination, and brain hemorrhage has been ruled out, then the patient may be a candidate for thrombolytic therapy, but this should be discussed with a neurologist or a specialist in cerebrovascular disease.
- Acute anticoagulation: no data supporting benefits in the acute setting. Heparin is considered for new-onset atrial fibrillation and atherothrombotic carotid disease causing recurrent transient neurologic symptoms especially in the setting before carotid endarterectomy or carotid stenting.
- Section III, Fig. 3-183 describes an algorithm for the treatment of transient ischemic attacks.

■ CHRONIC Rx

- No data supporting the use of long-term anticoagulation in the management of TIA, although stroke patients with atrial fibrillation or demonstrated cardiac thrombi have been shown to benefit from long-term warfarin therapy.
- First line of treatment has traditionally been aspirin. No significant benefit of high-dose aspirin (up to 1500 mg/day) has been conclusively found over lower doses (75 mg to 325 mg/day).
- Also consider aspirin/dipyridamole extended-release capsules (Aggrenox, 1 capsule po bid) as a first-line therapy. In a study of patients with TIA or stroke, Aggrenox reduced subsequent cerebrovascular events to a greater extent than either drug alone. Recommend Aggrenox or oral anticoagulation for patients who continue to have TIAs while on aspirin (aspirin failures), but there are no data to support this recommendation.

■ DISPOSITION

- According to one study, 10% to 20% of patients have a stroke in the next 90 days, and in 50% of these patients, stroke occurs in the first day or two after the TIA.
- Another study showed a stroke risk of 4.4% in the first month and 11.6% in the first year.
- The annual risk of myocardial infarction is 2.4%.
- One-year and 3-yr survival rates are 98% and 94%, respectively.

■ REFERRAL

Recommend referring all patients with TIA for an urgent neurologic evaluation and management.

☼ PEARLS & CONSIDERATIONS

■ CAVEAT

Urgently evaluate all patients who present with symptoms suggestive of acute brain ischemia. Do not wait for symptoms to resolve to distinguish TIA versus stroke.

Many TIAs are simply lacunar infarcts secondary to hypertension. Control the hypertension.

REFERENCES

Alamowitch S et al: Risk, causes, and prevention of ischaemic stroke in elderly patients with symptomatic internal-carotid-artery stenosis, *Lancet* 357:1154, 2001.

Albers GW et al: Transient ischemic attack—proposal for a new definition, *N Engl J Med* 347:1713, 2002.

Algra A et al: Oral anticoagulants versus antiplatelet therapy for preventing further vascular events after transient ischaemic attack or minor stroke of presumed arterial origin, *Cochrane Database Syst Rev* (4):CD001342, 2001.

Gorelick PB et al: Prevention of a first stroke, *JAMA* 281:1112, 1999.

Johnston SC: Clinical practice. Transient ischemic attack, *N Engl J Med* 347:1687, 2002.

Sacco RL, Elkind MS: Update on antiplatelet therapy for stroke prevention, *Arch Intern Med* 160(11):1579, 2000.

Sarasin FP, Gaspoz JM, Bounameaux H: Cost-effectiveness of new antiplatelet regimens used as secondary prevention of stroke or transient ischemic attack, *Arch Intern Med* 160(18):2773, 2000.

Author: **Sean I. Savitz, M.D.**

BASIC INFORMATION

■ DEFINITION
Trichinosis is an infection by one of various species of *Trichinella*.

ICD-9CM CODES
124 Trichinosis

■ EPIDEMIOLOGY & DEMOGRAPHICS
INCIDENCE (IN U.S.): <100 cases/yr
GENETICS:
Congenital Infection:
- Abrupt delivery of stillbirths in infected pregnant women
- Vertical infection of the fetus

■ PHYSICAL FINDINGS
- Symptoms
  1. May vary widely depending on the time from ingestion of contaminated meat and on worm burden
  2. Most persons asymptomatic
- Enteral phase
  1. Correlates with penetration of ingested larvae into the intestinal mucosa
  2. May last from 2 to 6 wk
  3. Mild, transient diarrhea and nausea
  4. Abdominal pain
  5. Diarrhea or constipation
  6. Vomiting
  7. Malaise
  8. Low-grade fevers
- Migratory or parenteral phase
  1. In the intestine, maturation and mating
  2. Newborn larvae
     a. Penetrate into lymphatic and blood vessels
     b. Migrate to muscles where they penetrate into muscle cells, enlarge, coil, and develop a cyst wall
  3. Patients may present with
     a. Fever
     b. Myalgias
     c. Periorbital or facial edema
     d. Headache
     e. Skin rash
     f. Other symptoms caused by the penetration of tissues by the newborn migrating larvae
  4. Peak in symptoms 2 to 3 wk after infection, then slowly subside

- Severe complications
  1. Brain damage by granulomatous inflammation or occlusion of arteries
  2. Cardiac involvement
  3. Can lead to death

■ ETIOLOGY
- The nematode responsible for this illness is an obligate intracellular parasite belonging to the genus *Trichinella*.
- It is one of the most ubiquitous parasites in the world and may be found in virtually all warm-blooded animals.
- Infection in humans occurs by the ingestion of contaminated animal meat that is raw or partially cooked and contains viable cysts.
- Most cases are now related to the consumption of poorly processed pork or wild game (bear, wild boar, cougar, and walrus).

DIAGNOSIS

■ DIFFERENTIAL DIAGNOSIS
- Different presentations have different differential diagnoses.
- Early illness may resemble gastroenteritis.
- Later symptoms may be confused with:
  1. Measles
  2. Dermatomyositis
  3. Glomerulonephritis
- The differential diagnosis of nematode tissue infections is described in Section II.

■ WORKUP
- Antibody assay of serum is usually positive by approximately 2 wk after infection.
- Muscle biopsy is used to detect the larva in muscle tissue if diagnosis unclear; best done by placing the tissue between two slides.

■ LABORATORY TESTS
- CBC: leukocytosis with prominent eosinophilia
- ESR: usually normal
- Elevation of muscle enzymes common (i.e., CPK, aldolase)

■ IMAGING STUDIES
Soft-tissue radiographs may show calcified cyst walls.

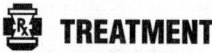 TREATMENT

■ NONPHARMACOLOGIC THERAPY
Bed rest for myalgias

■ ACUTE GENERAL Rx
- Thiabendazole to treat persons within 24 hr of ingesting contaminated meat, at the dose of 25 mg/kg/day for 1 wk
- Salicylates to decrease muscle discomfort
- Steroids in critically ill patients
- A recent study showed clinical improvement of myositis significantly more often in patients treated with thiabendazole or mebendazole versus those treated with fluconazole or placebo

■ DISPOSITION
- Most symptoms subside over time.
- Reports of long-term sequelae:
  1. Myalgias
  2. Headaches
- Occasionally, death occurs.

■ REFERRAL
Diagnosis uncertain

PEARLS & CONSIDERATIONS

■ COMMENTS
- Prevention by thorough cooking of meats
- Inadequate to smoke, cure, or dry meats

REFERENCES
Moorhead A et al: Trichinellosis in the United States, 1991-1996: declining but not gone, *Am J Trop Med Hyg* 60:66, 1999.
Watt G et al: Blinded, placebo-controlled trial of antiparasitic drugs for trichinosis myositis, *J Infect Dis* 182:371, 2000.
Author: **Maurice Policar, M.D.**

■ BASIC INFORMATION

■ DEFINITION
Tricuspid regurgitation (TR) refers to abnormal flow of blood from the right ventricle to the right atrium during systole (Fig. 1-280).

■ SYNONYMS
Tricuspid insufficiency

ICD-9CM CODES
397.0 Disease of the tricuspid valve
424.2 Tricuspid valve insufficiency (nonrheumatic)

■ EPIDEMIOLOGY & DEMOGRAPHICS
- Isolated TR is more common than tricuspid stenosis (TS).
- In patients with rheumatic heart disease, TR rarely occurs alone and is usually associated with mitral and/or aortic valve disease.
- Trivial TR is frequently detected by echocardiogram and is considered a normal variant.

■ PHYSICAL FINDINGS & CLINICAL PRESENTATION
- Symptoms of TR are determined by the underlying cause (e.g., pulmonary hypertension, left ventricular failure, and mitral stenosis)
- Dyspnea
- Orthopnea
- Paroxysmal nocturnal dyspnea
- Signs of right-sided heart failure:
  1. Elevated jugular venous distention with large V waves
  2. Right ventricular lift
  3. Right-sided S_3

  4. Holosystolic murmur heard best along the left parasternal line and fourth intercostal space and is louder during inspiration
  5. Pulsatile liver
  6. Hepatomegaly
  7. Ascites
  8. Edema

■ ETIOLOGY
- TR is usually functional rather than structural.
- Functional TR refers to conditions leading to dilation of the tricuspid annulus and/or right ventricle and includes:
  1. Any cause of pulmonary hypertension (e.g., COPD, pulmonary embolism, restrictive lung disease, collagen vascular disease, and primary pulmonary hypertension)
  2. Coronary artery disease with right ventricular infarction
  3. Left-sided congestive heart failure leading to right-sided heart failure
  4. Dilated cardiomyopathy (e.g., alcohol, idiopathic)
- Structural TR refers to conditions directly affecting the tricuspid valve and includes:
  1. Rheumatic fever
  2. Infective endocarditis
  3. Congenital (e.g., Ebstein's anomaly)
  4. Carcinoid
  5. Marfan's syndrome
  6. Tricuspid valve prolapse
  7. Traumatic (e.g., pacemaker insertion)
  8. Right atrial myxoma

  9. Collagen-vascular disease (e.g., SLE)
  10. Radiation

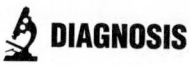 DIAGNOSIS

The diagnosis of TR is made by clinical history, physical examination, and adjunctive studies including ECG, chest x-ray, echocardiography, and rarely, right-sided heart catheterization.

■ DIFFERENTIAL DIAGNOSIS
The differential diagnosis of TR is as stated under "Etiology."

■ WORKUP
- Any patient suspected of having significant TR should undergo the following:
  1. Chest x-ray
  2. Electrocardiogram
  3. Echocardiogram (confirmatory)
  4. Right-sided cardiac catheterization

■ LABORATORY TESTS
- Blood tests are not very specific in diagnosing TR.
- ECG may show evidence of:
  1. Right atrial enlargement (e.g., P-wave height in leads II, III, aVF >2.5 mV)
  2. Right ventricular enlargement/hypertrophy (e.g., R wave > S wave in lead V_1)
  3. Right axis deviation >100 degrees
  4. Atrial fibrillation

■ IMAGING STUDIES
- Chest x-ray can show:
  1. Evidence of COPD with flattened diaphragms, barrel chest, dilated pulmonary arteries, and increased retrosternal air space
  2. Enlarged right atrium
  3. Enlarged right ventricle
- Echocardiogram, M-mode, 2-D with continuous wave, pulse wave, and color Doppler will:
  1. Detect TR
  2. Estimate the severity of TR
  3. Estimate the pulmonary artery pressure
  4. Exclude vegetation, mass, or prolapse
  5. Assess overall ventricular function
- Right-sided catheterization shows:
  1. Elevated right atrial and right ventricular end-diastolic pressures
  2. Large V waves

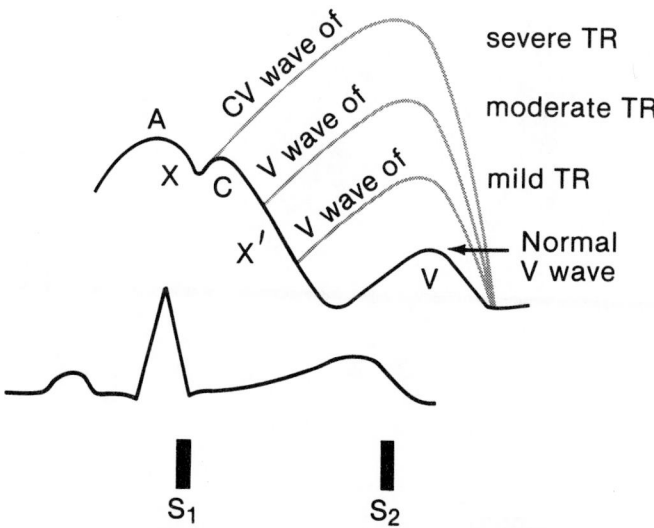

Fig. 1-280   The jugular venous pulse in tricuspid regurgitation. The jugular venous pulse wave normally drops during ventricular systole. As TR becomes more severe, the CV wave becomes more obvious during ventricular systole. (From Conn R: *Current diagnosis,* ed 9, Philadelphia, 1997, WB Saunders.)

TREATMENT

Treatment of TR is directed at the underlying cause.

NONPHARMACOLOGIC THERAPY

Oxygen therapy is beneficial in patients with functional TR secondary to underlying pulmonary hypertension provoked by alveolar hypoxia.

ACUTE GENERAL Rx

- Functional TR caused by left-sided heart failure is treated in similar fashion with preload and afterload reduction with or without inotrope therapy:
  1. Digoxin 0.25 mg PO qd
  2. Furosemide 40 to 80 mg PO qd for edema
  3. Angiotensin-converting enzyme inhibitors (e.g., lisinopril 10 to 40 mg PO qd, fosinopril 10 to 40 mg PO qd, enalapril 10 mg PO bid, and captopril 50 mg PO tid).
- Structural TR treatment depends on the underlying cause (e.g., antibiotics for infective endocarditis).

CHRONIC Rx

- Tricuspid valve surgery is considered in patients with severe TR from rheumatic mitral stenosis and pulmonary hypertension, structural valve damage from carcinoid, congenital anomalies, or infective endocarditis.
- Surgical procedures may include:
  1. Total valve replacement
  2. Annuloplasty
  3. Converting the tricuspid valve from three leaflets to two leaflets

DISPOSITION

- The natural history of TR will depend on the underlying etiology.
- Patients with rheumatic valve disease requiring replacement of both the mitral and tricuspid valve have a high 30-day morbidity/mortality rate of 15% to 20%.

REFERRAL

For patients with significant symptomatic TR, a cardiology consultation is recommended.

PEARLS & CONSIDERATIONS

COMMENTS

- Antibiotic prophylaxis for dental, GI, or GU procedures is recommended in patients with structural tricuspid valve abnormalities.
- TR secondary to tricuspid valve prolapse may also be associated with mitral valve prolapse.

REFERENCES

Frater R: Tricuspid insufficiency, *J Thorac Cardiovasc Surg* 122(3):427, 2001.

Raman SV et al: Tricuspid valve disease: tricuspid valve complex perspective, *Curr Prob Cardiol* 27(3):103, 2002.

Trichon BH, O'Connor CM: Secondary mitral and tricuspid regurgitation accompanying left ventricular systolic function: is it important, and how is it treated? *Am Heart J* 144(3):373, 2002.

Waller BF et al: Pathology of tricuspid valve stenosis and pure tricuspid regurgitation—Part I, *Clin Cardiol* 18(2):97, 1995.

Waller BF et al: Pathology of tricuspid valve stenosis and pure tricuspid regurgitation—Part II, *Clin Cardiol* 18(3):167, 1995.

Authors: **Wen-Chih Wu, M.D., and Peter Petropoulos, M.D.**

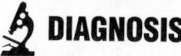

 BASIC INFORMATION

■ **DEFINITION**

Tricuspid stenosis (TS) is narrowing of the orifice of the tricuspid valve, resulting in a diastolic pressure gradient between the right atrium and right ventricle restricting right atrial emptying (Fig. 1-281).

■ **SYNONYMS**

Tricuspid valve stenosis
TS

■ **ICD-9CM CODES**

397.0 Disease of the tricuspid valve

■ **EPIDEMIOLOGY & DEMOGRAPHICS**

• TS is more common in women than in men and is seen in patients between the ages of 20 to 60.
• TS is more common in India than in the U.S.
• In patients who have rheumatic heart disease, TS is present at autopsy in 15%, but was clinically significant in only 5%.
• Rheumatic TS very seldom occurs alone; it is usually associated with mitral and/or aortic valve disease.

■ **PHYSICAL FINDINGS & CLINICAL PRESENTATION**

• Patients with severe symptomatic TS usually present with symptoms of fatigue, abdominal swelling, and anasarca. They may complain of right upper quadrant abdominal pain secondary to passive congestive hepatomegaly from elevated systemic venous pressures.
• Jugular venous distention with a prominent a wave is noted along with a palpable hepatic pulsation.
• Right atrial pulsation may be palpated to the right of the sternum and a diastolic thrill may be felt over the left sternal edge that is increased with inspiration.
• An opening snap and diastolic murmur is best heard along the left sternal border of the fourth intercostal space and is augmented by inspiration.

■ **ETIOLOGY**

Rheumatic heart disease is the primary cause of TS, resulting in scarring of the valve leaflets and fusion of the commissures. This, along with shortening of the chordae tendineae and immobility of the valve leaflets, results in narrowing of the tricuspid valve orifice. Other causes of TS are congenital TS, right atrial myxoma, metastatic tumor (e.g., lymphoma), carcinoid syndrome, systemic lupus endocarditis, and tricuspid valve bacterial endocarditis.

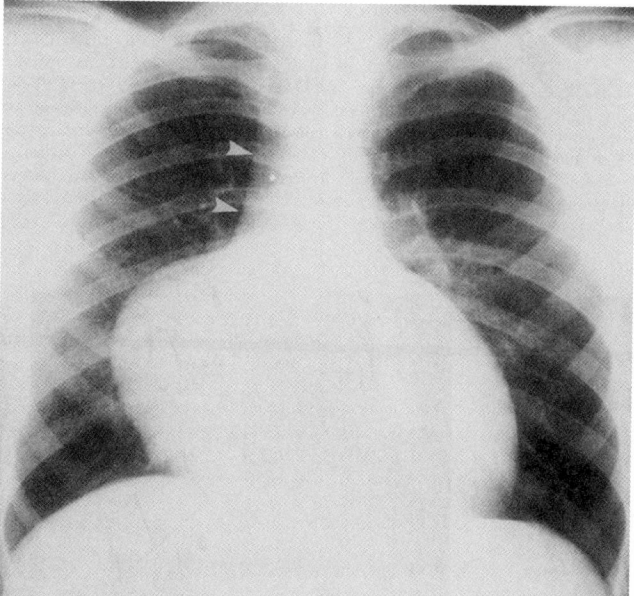

Fig. 1-281 Right atrial enlargement in congenital tricuspid stenosis. The right heart border is prominent; the superior vena cava is dilated (arrowheads). (From Rubens MB: Chest x-ray in adult heart disease. In Julian DG et al [eds]: *Diseases of the heart,* ed 2, London, 1996, WB Saunders.)

■ **DIAGNOSIS**

■ **DIFFERENTIAL DIAGNOSIS**

• Congenital tricuspid atresia
• Endomyocardial fibrosis
• Right atrial thrombi
• Constrictive pericarditis

■ **WORKUP**

• Echocardiography (first choice)
• Chest x-ray examination
• ECG
• Cardiac angiography in selected patients

■ **IMAGING STUDIES**

• Echocardiography reveals doming of the anterior tricuspid leaflet with restriction of movement of the leaflet tip along with reduced excursion of the posterior and septal leaflets. Doppler is used to calculate the diastolic gradient across the tricuspid.
• Chest x-ray reveals an enlarged right atrium and pulmonary oligemia.
• ECG in many cases will show atrial fibrillation secondary to an enlarged right atrium. However, in patients who are in normal sinus rhythm, the ECG will show criteria for right atrial enlargement (tall peaked P waves >2.5 mm in height in leads II, III, or aVF).
• Cardiac catheterization will measure simultaneous pressures in the right atrium and right ventricle giving the gradient across the valve (normal gradient <1 mm Hg). Tricuspid valve area can also be determined (severe: <1 cm²).

■ **TREATMENT**

■ **NONPHARMACOLOGIC THERAPY**

Most patients with severe TS will have peripheral edema and therefore salt restriction is essential.

■ **ACUTE GENERAL Rx**

• Furosemide 40 mg qd; gradually increased according to symptoms and edema.
• Digoxin 0.25 mg qd and warfarin (maintaining the INR between 2 to 3) is used in patients who develop atrial fibrillation.

■ **CHRONIC Rx**

• Balloon dilation of the stenosed tricuspid valve has been described in both rheumatic and congenital TS with some success, but experience is limited and complications may occur (e.g., advanced heart block, significant tricuspid regurgitation).

- It must be remembered that rheumatic TS is usually associated with mitral disease. The decision to proceed with surgery for TS typically occurs in the setting of significant symptomatic mitral valve disease requiring surgery and there is a mean diastolic gradient across the tricuspid valve of >5 mm Hg with a tricuspid valve area of <2 cm^2.
- Surgical procedures for significant tricuspid stenosis include closed commissurotomy, open commissurotomy, and tricuspid valve replacement. This is usually determined during surgery.
- Tricuspid valve replacement carries a high 30-day operative morbidity/mortality of 15% to 20% in addition to the high risk of thrombus formation.

■ DISPOSITION

The natural course of severe TS is not very well known.

■ REFERRAL

TS is difficult to diagnose and therefore consultation with a cardiology specialist is recommended.

☼ PEARLS & CONSIDERATIONS

■ COMMENTS

- Rheumatic TS almost always occurs in association with either mitral valve disease and/or aortic valve disease.
- Unlike mitral stenosis patients, TS patients typically do not complain of dyspnea, orthopnea, or paroxysmal nocturnal dyspnea.

REFERENCES

Chrissos D et al: One-year follow-up of a patient with reversible tricuspid valve stenosis due to lymphomatic mass into the right atrioventriuclar wall, *Echocardiography*19(7 pt 1):565, 2002.

Krishnamoorthy KM: Balloon dilatation of isolated congenital tricuspid stenosis, *Int J Cardiol* 89(1):119, 2003.

Mehra MR et al: Difficult cases in heart failure: isolated tricuspid stenosis and heart failure: a focus on carcinoid heart disease, *Congest Heart Fail* 9(5):294, 2003.

Raman SV et al: Tricuspid valve disease: tricuspid valve complex perspective, *Curr Prob Cardiol* 27(3):103, 2002.

Roguin A et al: Long-term follow-up of patients with severe rheumatic tricuspid stenosis, *Am Heart J* 136(1):103, 1998.

Waller BF et al: Pathology of tricuspid valve stenosis and pure tricuspid regurgitation—Part I, *Clin Cardiol* 18(2):97, 1995.

Waller BF et al: Pathology of tricuspid valve stenosis and pure tricuspid regurgitation—Part II, *Clin Cardiol* 18(3):167, 1995.

Authors: **Wen-Chih Wu, M.D., and Peter Petropoulos, M.D.**

■ BASIC INFORMATION

■ DEFINITION
Tricyclic antidepressants (TCAs) are secondary or tertiary amines that have variable abilities to inhibit reuptake of neurotransmitters (norepinephrine, dopamine, and serotonin) and to be anticholinergic, antihistaminic, and sedating. These properties are important to consider when prescribing these agents and when managing an intentional or accidental overdose.

■ SYNONYMS
Tricyclic antidepressant intoxication or poisoning
TCA OD

ICD-9CM CODES
969.0

■ EPIDEMIOLOGY & DEMOGRAPHICS
- TCAs are the most common cause of death resulting from prescription drug overdose in the U.S.
- Available TCAs: amitriptyline, imipramine, desipramine, nortriptyline, doxepin, amoxapine, clomipramine, protriptyline, and others

■ PHYSICAL FINDINGS & CLINICAL PRESENTATION
Cardiovascular
- Intraventricular conduction delay (QRS prolongation)
- Sinus tachycardia
- Atrioventricular block
- Prolongation of the QT interval (Fig. 1-282)
- Ventricular tachycardia
- Wide complex tachycardia without P waves
- Refractory hypotension (the most common cause of death from TCA OD)
- Late arrhythmias or sudden death (in addition to the previous, which occur during the first 24 to 48 hr: late problems can occur up to 5 days after the OD)

Central nervous system
- Coma
- Delirium
- Myoclonus
- Seizures

Other
- Hyperthermia
- Ileus
- Urinary retention
- Pulmonary complications (e.g., aspiration pneumonitis)
- Life-threatening overdose exists with the ingestion of more than 1 g of TCA. Among patients who reach a hospital, most deaths occur within the first 24 hr; lack of initial symptoms can be deceptive

■ PATHOGENESIS
Mechanisms of tricyclic antidepressant cardiovascular toxicity (Table 1-58)
CNS toxicity
- Cholinergic blockade is believed to cause hyperthermia, ileus, urinary retention, pupillary dilation, delirium, and coma.
- The mechanism of myoclonus and seizures is not fully understood.

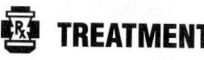

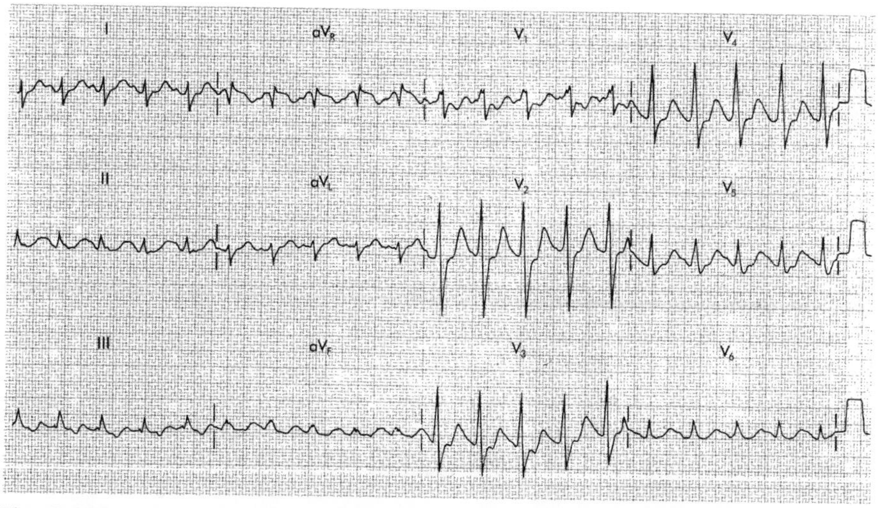

■ DIAGNOSIS

■ DIFFERENTIAL DIAGNOSIS
Cardiotoxicity from TCA can be confused with intoxication by drugs that cause QRS prolongation. These include class Ia antiarrhythmic agents (disopyramide, procainamide, quinidine), class Ic antiarrhythmic agents (encainide, flecainide, propafenone), cocaine, propranolol, quinine, chloroquine, neuroleptics, propoxyphene, and digoxin. Other causes of QRS prolongation include hyperkalemia, ischemic heart disease, cardiomyopathy, and cardiac conduction system dysfunction.

■ WORKUP
- Clinical presentation
- Knowledge of the overdose
- Serum drug levels (TCA concentration >1 μg/ml is life threatening and TCA concentration >3 μg/ml is often fatal)
- Baseline CBC, prothrombin time, BUN, creatinine, and electrolytes

■ TREATMENT

■ MANAGEMENT
Initial measures
- Hospitalization with cardiac monitoring as well as monitoring of vital signs and temperature
- Initiate intravenous access
- Administer activated charcoal with sorbitol
- Large-bore tube gastric lavage is of unproven benefit
- Ipecac is contraindicated
- 12-Lead ECG
- If no evidence of cardiotoxicity has been noted during the first 6 hr of observation, further monitoring is not necessary; if there is evidence of cardiotoxicity, monitoring should continue for 24 hr after all signs of toxicity have resolved

Treatment of specific complications of TCA toxicity: See Table 1-59
When the patient is medically stable, psychiatric evaluation should be obtained.

REFERENCES
Glauser J: Tricyclic antidepressant poisoning, *Cleve Clin J Med* 67:704, 2000.
Pentel PR, Keyler DE, Haddad LM: Tricyclic antidepressants. In Haddad LM, Shannon MW, Winchester JF (eds): *Clinical management of poisoning and drug overdose*, ed 3, Philadelphia, 1998, WB Saunders.
Author: **Tom J. Wachtel, M.D.**

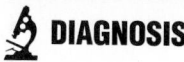

Fig. 1-282 The ECG from a patient with tricyclic antidepressant overdose shows three major findings: sinus tachycardia (from anticholinergic and adrenergic effects), prolongation of the QRS (from slowed ventricular conduction), and prolongation of the QT (from delayed repolarization). (From Goldberger AL: *Clinical electrocardiography*, ed 5, St Louis, 1994, Mosby.)

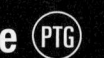

TABLE 1-58 Mechanism of Tricyclic Antidepressant Cardiovascular Toxicity

TOXIC EFFECT	MECHANISM
Conduction Delays, Arrhythmias	
QRS prolongation atrioventricular block	Cardiac sodium channel → slowed depolarization in atrioventricular node, His-Purkinje fibers, and ventricular myocardium
Sinus tachycardia	Cholinergic blockade, inhibition of norepinephrine reuptake
Ventricular tachycardia Monomorphic	Cardiac sodium channel inhibition → reentry
Torsades de pointes	Cardiac potassium channel inhibition → prolonged repolarization
Ventricular bradycardia	Impaired cardiac automaticity
Hypotension	
Vasodilation	Vascular α-adrenergic receptor blockade
Decreased cardiac contractility	Cardiac sodium channel inhibition → impaired excitation-contraction coupling

TABLE 1-59 Treatment of Complications of Tricyclic Antidepressant Toxicity

TOXIC EFFECT	TREATMENT
Cardiovascular	
QRS prolongation	Hypertonic $NaHCO_3$ if QRS prolongation is marked or progressing; not clear if treatment is needed in the absence of hypotension or arrhythmias
Hypotension	Intravascular volume expansion, $NaHCO_3$ Vasopressors (norepinephrine) or inotropic agents (dopamine) Correct hyperthermia, acidosis, seizures Consider mechanical support
Ventricular tachycardia	$NaHCO_3$, lidocaine, overdrive, pacing Correct hypotension, hypothermia, acidosis, seizures
Torsades de pointes	Overdrive pacing
Ventricular bradycardia	Chronotropic agent (epinephrine), pacemaker
Sinus tachycardia	Treatment rarely needed
Atrioventricular block type II second or third degree	Pacemaker
Hypertension	Rapidly titratable antihypertensive agent (nitroprusside)
Central Nervous System	
Delirium	Restraints, benzodiazepine Neuromuscular blockade for hyperthermia, acidosis
Seizures	Benzodiazepine Neuromuscular blockade for hyperthermia, acidosis
Coma	Intubation, ventilation if needed
Other	
Hyperthermia	Control seizures, agitation Cooling measures
Acidosis	$NaHCO_3$ Correct hypotension, hypoventilation

 BASIC INFORMATION

■ **DEFINITION**
Trigeminal neuralgia is a syndrome characterized by recurrent excruciating paroxysms of lancinating pain in the distribution of one or more divisions of the trigeminal (fifth) nerve.

■ **SYNONYMS**
Tic douloureux

ICD-9CM CODES
350.1 Trigeminal neuralgia

■ **EPIDEMIOLOGY & DEMOGRAPHICS**
INCIDENCE (IN U.S.): 3-5/100 000
PREVALENCE (IN U.S.): 155/1 million persons
PREDOMINANT SEX: Slight predominance of females to males
PEAK INCIDENCE: Median age 67 years
GENETICS: Uncommonly familial and possibly caused by underlying genetic etiology (see below in "Etiology" under "Rare causes")

■ **PHYSICAL FINDINGS & CLINICAL PRESENTATION**
• Each attack lasts only seconds but may cluster.
• Often, attacks are brought on by mild stimulation of trigger zones, located in the affected division of the fifth nerve. These triggers include light touching, eating, drinking, shaving and draught of air.

■ **ETIOLOGY**
• It is thought that 80%-90% of cases are due to compression of the trigeminal nerve root at the cerebellopontine angle by an aberrant loop of artery or vein, and rarely a saccular aneurysm or arteriovenous malformation
• Compressive lesions such as schwannomas, epidermoid cysts and meningiomas, also typically at the cerebellopontine angle
• Bony compression of the fifth nerve (e.g., from an osteoma or deformity resulting from osteogenesis imperfecta)

• Primary demyelinating disorders: multiple sclerosis (2%-4% of patients) and rarely Charcot-Marie-Tooth disease. In multiple sclerosis, usually there is a plaque of demyelination at the root entry zone of the fifth nerve in the pons
• Rare causes: (a) infiltrative disorders such as carcinomatous or amyloid deposits in the fifth nerve root, nerve proper, or ganglion; (b) familial occurrence has been reported in Charcot-Marie-Tooth disease

🔬 **DIAGNOSIS**

■ **DIFFERENTIAL DIAGNOSIS**
• Dental pathology
• The differential diagnosis of headache and facial pain is described in Section II.

■ **WORKUP**
MRI scans (CT scan with thin posterior fossa cuts if MRI not available) for all patients to exclude mass lesions or evidence of central demyelination as in multiple sclerosis

■ **IMAGING STUDIES**
See "Workup."

℞ **TREATMENT**

■ **NONPHARMACOLOGIC THERAPY**
• In refractory cases, surgical options, including percutaneous radiofrequency gangliolysis and microvascular decompression
• Gamma-knife radiosurgery is an increasingly popular alternative to conventional surgery for trigeminal neuralgia

■ **ACUTE GENERAL Rx**
None, episodes are too brief

■ **CHRONIC Rx**
• Carbamazepine is the treatment of choice, providing relief to at least 75% of patients. Begin with 100 mg

bid and increase gradually as tolerated using a tid regimen.
• If carbamazepine is not tolerated or effective, use gabapentin, 400 mg PO tid. Doses as high as 3600 mg/day are easily tolerated. Topiramate (Topamax) 25 mg qhs gradually titrated up to 100 mg bid is also effective.

■ **DISPOSITION**
Spontaneous remissions occur after months to years.

■ **REFERRAL**
If uncertain about diagnosis or if surgical treatment is necessary

☼ **PEARLS & CONSIDERATIONS**

Even in patients with multiple sclerosis, a vascular compression may be the source of symptoms and thus may benefit from intervention such as surgery.

■ **COMMENTS**
Because prolonged remission may occur, drug tapering at yearly intervals is recommended.

REFERENCES
Elias WJ and Burchiel KJ: Trigeminal neuralgia and other neuropathic pain syndromes of the head and face, *Curr Pain Headache Rep* 6(2):115, 2002.
Kitt CA et al. Trigeminal neuralgia: opportunities for research and treatment, *Pain* 85: 3, 2000.
Loeser JD: Tic douloureux, *Pain Res Manag* 6(3):156, 2001.
Love S, Coakham HB: Trigeminal neuralgia: pathology and pathogenesis, *Brain* 124(Pt 12):2347, 2001.
Maesawa S et al: Clinical outcomes after stereotactic radiosurgery for idiopathic trigeminal neuralgia, *J Neurosurg* 94:16, 2001.
Author: U. Shivraj Sohur, M.D., Ph.D.

BASIC INFORMATION

■ DEFINITION
Digital stenosing tenosynovitis refers to an inflammatory process of the digital flexor tendon sheath.

■ SYNONYMS
Trigger finger

ICD-9CM CODES
727.03 Trigger finger (acquired)

■ EPIDEMIOLOGY & DEMOGRAPHICS
- Trigger finger can be found in all age groups but is commonly found in patients older than 45 yr
- More frequently affects females (4:1)
- Occupational risk groups: meat cutters, seamstress, tailors, and dentists
- In adults the middle finger is most often affected (Fig. 1-283)
- In children the thumb is most often affected

■ PHYSICAL FINDINGS & CLINICAL PRESENTATION
- Hand pain
- Painful triggering or snapping with flexion and extension of the affected digit
- Locking or loss of active digital extension is the most common symptom
- The digit possibly fixed in flexion (trapped or incarcerated)
- Usually affects one digit
- If more digits are involved, a systemic cause most likely present (e.g., diabetes, rheumatoid arthritis)
- A palpable tender nodule noted at the MCP joint of the affected digit
- Pain over the flexor tendon with resisted flexion

- Pain with passive stretching

■ ETIOLOGY
Trigger finger is described as being primary or secondary:
- Primary (idiopathic)
- Secondary
  1. Diabetes
  2. Rheumatoid arthritis
  3. Hypothyroidism
  4. Histiocytosis
  5. Amyloidosis
  6. Gout

DIAGNOSIS

The diagnosis of trigger finger is usually made by the clinical historical presentation and by physical examination.

■ DIFFERENTIAL DIAGNOSIS
- Dupuytren's contracture
- De Quervain's tenosynovitis
- Acute digital tenosynovitis
- Proliferative tenosynovitis
- Carpal tunnel syndrome
- Flexion tendon rupture
- Trauma

■ WORKUP
If a secondary cause of trigger finger is suspected, a workup should be pursued.

■ LABORATORY TESTS
- CBC with differential
- Electrolytes, BUN, and creatinine
- Blood glucose
- Thyroid function tests
- Uric acid
- Rheumatoid factor

■ IMAGING STUDIES
X-ray studies are not very helpful unless a secondary cause has affected other organs (e.g., rheumatoid lung).

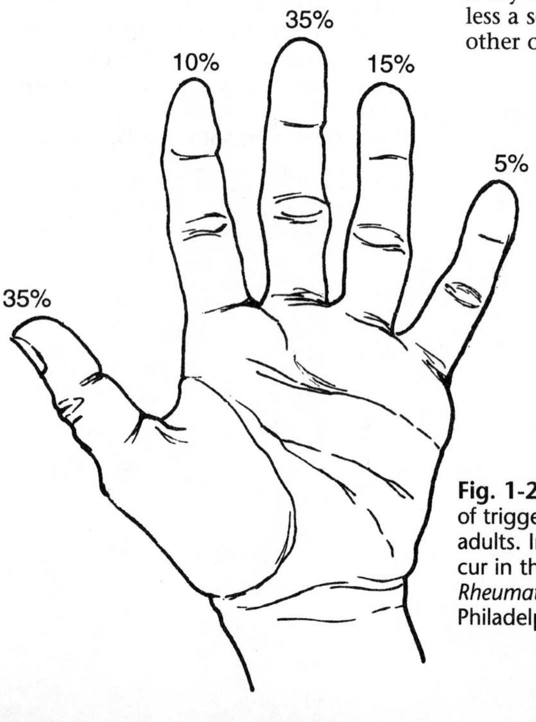

35%
10%   15%
5%
35%

Fig. 1-283   Trigger finger. Frequency of trigger finger according to digit in adults. In children, virtually all cases occur in the thumb. (From Canoso J: *Rheumatology in primary care*, Philadelphia, 1997, WB Saunders.)

TREATMENT

■ NONPHARMACOLOGIC THERAPY
Splinting can be tried early in the course but has been very successful.

■ ACUTE GENERAL Rx
- In primary idiopathic trigger finger steroid injection, 15 to 20 mg depomethylprenisolone acetate in 1 ml 1% Xylocaine has been used with success.
- Triamcinolone 10 mg with 1 ml of 1% Xylocaine is an alternative steroid choice to be used in patients who do not respond to the first injection.
- If symptoms do not resolve in 3 wk, a repeat injection can be tried.

■ CHRONIC Rx
- Surgical release is indicated in patients with refractory symptoms (e.g., locked digits) despite nonpharmacologic and acute treatment.
- Surgery is also indicated in patients with recurrent symptoms despite steroid injection therapy.

■ DISPOSITION
- Following steroid injection, symptoms usually resolve in 3 to 5 days, and locking resolves in 60% of the cases in 2 to 3 wk.
- If symptoms recur, a repeat steroid injection improves the symptoms in >80% of patients.
- Diabetic patients do not have the same success rate with steroid injections as the primary idiopathic group.

■ REFERRAL
If steroid injection therapy is considered, a rheumatology consult is requested.

PEARLS & CONSIDERATIONS

■ COMMENTS
If more than one digit is involved, a workup for a secondary systemic cause is in order.

REFERENCES
Canoso JJ: Trigger finger. In *Rheumatology in primary care,* Philadelphia, 1997, Saunders.

Chin DH, Jones NF: Repetitive motion hand disorder, *J Calif Dent Assoc* 30(2):49, 2002.

Moore JS: Flexor tendon entrapment of the digits (trigger finger and trigger thumb), *J Occup Environ Med* 42(5):526, 2000.

Saldana MJ: Trigger digits: diagnosis and treatment, *J Am Acad Orthop Surg* 9(4):246, 2001.
Author: **Peter Petropoulos, M.D.**

BASIC INFORMATION

■ DEFINITION
Trochanteric bursitis is a presumed inflammation or irritation of the gluteus maximus bursa or the bursa separating the greater trochanter from the gluteus medius and gluteus minimus (Fig. 1-284).

■ SYNONYMS
Greater trochanteric pain syndrome

■ ICD-9CM CODES
726.5 Bursitis trochanteric area

■ EPIDEMIOLOGY & DEMOGRAPHICS
• Trochanteric bursitis is commonly associated with other conditions:
  1. Osteoarthritis of the hip
  2. Lumbar spinal degenerative joint disease
  3. Rheumatoid arthritis
• Incidence peaks between the fourth and sixth decades of life but can occur at any age group
• Occurs in females > males (4:1)

■ PHYSICAL FINDINGS & CLINICAL PRESENTATION
• Hip pain is the most common complaint. The pain is chronic, intermittent, and located over the lateral thigh.
• Numbness is present.
• Pain is precipitated with prolonged lying or standing on the affected side.
• Walking, climbing, and running exacerbate the pain.
• Point tenderness over the greater trochanter is noted.
• Pain is reproduced with resisted hip abduction.

■ ETIOLOGY
• The specific cause of trochanteric bursitis is not known although repetitive high-intensity use of the hip joint, trauma, infection (tuberculosis and bacterial), and crystal deposition can precipitate the disease.
• Trochanteric bursitis can occur when other conditions such as osteoarthritis of the knee and hip and bunions of the feet cause changes in the patient's gait, placing excess stress on the hip joint.

DIAGNOSIS

A detailed physical examination and clinical presentation usually make the diagnosis of trochanteric bursitis. Laboratory tests and x-ray images are helpful adjunctive studies used to exclude other conditions either associated with or mimicking trochanteric bursitis.

■ DIFFERENTIAL DIAGNOSIS
• Osteoarthritis of the hip
• Osteonecrosis of the hip
• Stress fracture of the hip
• Osteoarthritis of the lumbar spine
• Fibromyalgia
• Iliopsoas bursitis
• Trochanteric tendonitis
• Gout
• Pseudogout
• Trauma
• Neuropathy

■ WORKUP
A workup is indicated if suspected associated conditions exist; otherwise treatment can be started on clinical grounds alone.

■ LABORATORY TESTS
CBC with differential may show elevated white count if infection is present.
ESR is elevated in an infectious process.
Uric acid may be elevated in patients with gout.

■ IMAGING STUDIES
• Plain x-rays of the hip are not very helpful in diagnosing trochanteric bursitis. Sometimes calcifications may be seen around the greater trochanter.
• Bone scan can be done but is usually not necessary.
• CT and MRI may show bursitis but are usually not warranted because it will not alter treatment.

TREATMENT

■ NONPHARMACOLOGIC THERAPY
• Heat 15 to 20 min four to six times per day
• Ultrasound therapy
• Rest
• Partial weight bearing
• Physical therapy to strengthen back, hip, and knee muscles

■ ACUTE GENERAL Rx
• NSAIDs, ibuprofen 800 mg PO tid, or naproxen 500 mg PO bid is used for pain relief.
• Acetaminophen 500-mg tablet, 1 to 2 tablets PO q6h prn can be used with NSAIDs or alternating with NSAIDs.
• Corticosteroid injection (30 to 40 mg depomethylprednisolone acetate mixed with 3 ml 1% Xylocaine)

■ CHRONIC Rx
Although rarely done, surgical removal of the bursa is possible for patients with refractory symptoms or infection.

■ DISPOSITION
• Most patients respond to NSAIDs and/or nonpharmacologic therapy.
• If steroid injection is used, approximately 70% of patients respond after the first injection and more than 90% respond to two injections.
• 25% of patients receiving steroid injection may develop a relapse.

■ REFERRAL
A rheumatology or orthopedics referral is made if steroid injection therapy is needed or if the etiology is thought to be infectious.

PEARLS & CONSIDERATIONS

■ COMMENTS
• The absence of pain with flexion and extension differentiates trochanteric bursitis from degenerative joint disease of the hip.
• Localization of pain over the lateral thigh differentiates trochanteric bursitis from pain caused by meralgia paresthetica located over the anterolateral thigh and pain from osteoarthritis located over the inner thigh groin area.

REFERENCES
Adkins SB, Figler RA: Hip pain in athletes, *Am Fam Physician* 61(7):2109, 2000.
Canoso JJ: Hip pain. In Canoso JJ, Kersey R (eds): *Rheumatology in primary care.* Philadelphia, 1997, WB Saunders.
Authors: **Peter Petropoulos, M.D., and Mel Anderson, M.D.**

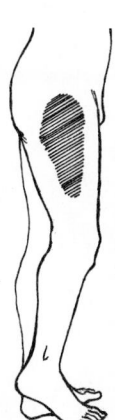

Fig. 1-284 Typical location of pain in trochanteric bursitis syndrome. This is also a frequent pain radiation site for lumbar spine lesion, various nerve compression syndromes, and hip disease, particularly in osteonecrosis of the femoral head. (From Canoso J: *Rhematology in primary care,* Philadelphia, 1997, WB Saunders.)

BASIC INFORMATION

■ DEFINITION
Tropical sprue is a malabsorption syndrome occurring primarily in tropical regions, including Puerto Rico, India, and Southeast Asia.

■ SYNONYMS
"Tropical enteropathy" refers to a subclinical form of tropical sprue.

ICD-9CM CODES
579.1 Tropical sprue

■ EPIDEMIOLOGY & DEMOGRAPHICS
Tropical sprue is endemic in tropical regions, the Middle East, the Far East, the Caribbean, and India.

■ PHYSICAL FINDINGS & CLINICAL PRESENTATION
• Diffuse, nonspecific abdominal tenderness and distention
• Low-grade fever
• Glossitis, cheilosis, hyperkeratosis, hyperpigmentation
• Diarrhea

■ ETIOLOGY
• Unknown
• Associated with overgrowth of predominantly coliform bacteria in the small intestine

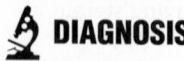

DIAGNOSIS

The clinical features of tropical sprue include anorexia, diarrhea, weight loss, abdominal pain, and steatorrhea; these symptoms can develop in expatriates even several months after immigrating to temperate regions.

■ DIFFERENTIAL DIAGNOSIS
• Celiac disease
• Parasitic infestation
• Inflammatory bowel disease
• Other causes of malabsorption (e.g., Whipple's disease)

■ WORKUP
Diagnostic workup includes a comprehensive history (especially travel history), physical examination, laboratory evidence of malabsorption (see "Laboratory Tests"), and jejunal biopsy; the biopsy results are nonspecific, with blunting, atrophy, and even disappearance of the villi and subepithelial lymphocytic infiltration.

■ LABORATORY TESTS
• Megaloblastic anemia (>50% of cases)
• Vitamin B_{12} deficiency, folate deficiency
• Steatorrhea, abnormal D-xylose absorption

■ IMAGING STUDIES
GI series with small bowel follow-through may reveal coarsening of the jejunal folds.

TREATMENT

■ NONPHARMACOLOGIC THERAPY
Monitoring of weight and calorie intake

■ ACUTE GENERAL Rx
• Folic acid therapy (5 mg bid for 2 wk followed by a maintenance dose of 1 mg tid) will improve anemia and malabsorption in more than two thirds of patients
• Tetracycline 250 mg qid for 4 to 6 wk in individuals who have returned to temperate zones, up to 6 mo in patients in endemic areas; ampicillin 500 mg bid for at least 4 wk in patients intolerant to tetracycline
• Correction of vitamin B_{12} deficiency: vitamin B_{12} 1000 µg IM weekly for 4 wk, then monthly for 3 to 6 mo
• Correction of other nutritional deficiencies (e.g., calcium, iron)

■ DISPOSITION
Complete recovery with appropriate therapy

■ REFERRAL
GI referral for jejunal biopsy

PEARLS & CONSIDERATIONS

■ COMMENTS
Additional patient education information can be obtained from National Digestive Diseases Information Clearinghouse, Box NDDIC, Bethesda, MD 20892; phone: (301) 654-3810.
Author: **Fred F. Ferri, M.D.**

■ BASIC INFORMATION

■ DEFINITION
Miliary tuberculosis (TB) is an infection of disseminated hematogenous disease, caused by the bacterium *Mycobacterium tuberculosis,* and is often characterized as resembling millet seeds on examination.
Extrapulmonary disease may occur in virtually every organ site.

■ SYNONYMS
Disseminated TB

ICD-9CM CODES
018.94 Miliary tuberculosis

■ EPIDEMIOLOGY & DEMOGRAPHICS
INCIDENCE (IN U.S.): >38% of AIDS patients with TB have disseminated disease, often with concurrent pulmonary and extrapulmonary active sites. (See "Pulmonary Tuberculosis" in Section I.)
PREVALENCE (IN U.S.):
- Undetermined
- Highest prevalence
  1. AIDS patients
  2. Minorities
  3. Children
  4. Foreign-born persons
  5. Elderly
PREDOMINANT SEX:
- No specific predilection
- Male predominance in AIDS, shelters, and prisons reflected in disproportionate male TB incidence
PREDOMINANT AGE: Predominantly among 24- to 45-yr-olds
PEAK INCIDENCE: HIV-positive patients, regardless of age

■ PHYSICAL FINDINGS & CLINICAL PRESENTATION
- See also "Etiology"
- Common symptoms
  1. High intermittent fever
  2. Night sweats
  3. Weight loss
- Symptoms referable to individual organ systems may predominate
  1. Meninges
  2. Pericardium
  3. Liver
  4. Kidney
  5. Bone
  6. GI tract
  7. Lymph nodes
  8. Serous spaces
     a. Pleural
     b. Pericardial
     c. Peritoneal
     d. Joint
  9. Skin
  10. Lung: cough, shortness of breath

- Adrenal insufficiency possible caused by infection of adrenal gland
- Pancytopenia
  1. With fever and weight loss *or*
  2. Without other localizing symptoms or signs *or*
  3. With only splenomegaly
- TB hepatitis
  1. Tender liver
  2. Obstructive enzymes (alkaline phosphatase) elevated out of proportion to minimal hepatocellular enzymes (SGOT, SGPT) and bilirubin
- TB meningitis
  1. Gradual-onset headache
  2. Minimal meningeal signs
  3. Malaise
  4. Low-grade fever (may be absent)
  5. Sudden stupor or coma
  6. Cranial nerve VI palsy
- TB pericarditis
  1. Effusions resembling TB pleurisy
  2. Cardiac tamponade
- Skeletal TB
  1. Large joint arthritis (with effusions resembling TB pericarditis)
  2. Bone lesions (especially ribs)
  3. Pott's disease
     a. TB spondylitis, especially of lower thoracic spine
     b. Paraspinous TB abscess
     c. Possible psoas abscess
     d. Frequent cord compression (often relieved by steroids)
- Genitourinary TB
  1. Renal TB
     a. Papillary necrosis
     b. Destruction of renal pelvis
     c. Strictures of upper third of ureters
     d. Hematuria
     e. Pyuria with misleading bacterial cultures
     f. Preserved renal function
  2. TB orchitis or epididymitis
     a. Scrotal mass
     b. Draining abscess
  3. Chronic prostatic TB
- Gastrointestinal TB
  1. Diarrhea
  2. Pain
  3. Obstruction
  4. Bleeding
  5. Especially common with AIDS
  6. Bowel lesions
     a. Circumferential ulcers
     b. Short strictures
     c. Calcified granulomas
     d. TB mesenteric caseous adenitis
     e. Abscess, but rare fistula formation
     f. Often difficult to distinguish from granulomatous bowel disease (Crohn's disease)

- TB peritonitis
  1. Fluid resembles TB pleurisy
  2. PPD often negative
  3. Tender abdomen
  4. Doughy peritoneal consistency, often with ascites
  5. Peritoneal biopsy indicated for diagnosis
- TB lymphadenitis (scrofula)
  1. May involve all node groups
  2. Common adenopathies
     a. Cervical
     b. Supraclavicular
     c. Axillary
     d. Retroperitoneal
  3. Biopsy generally needed for diagnosis
  4. Surgical resection of nodes may be necessary
  5. Especially common with AIDS
- Cutaneous TB
  1. Skin infection from autoinoculation or dissemination
  2. Nodules or abscesses
  3. Tuberculids (possibly allergic reactions)
  4. Erythema nodosum
- Miscellaneous presentations
  1. TB laryngitis
  2. TB otitis
  3. Ocular TB
     a. Choroidal tubercles
     b. Iritis
     c. Uveitis
     d. Episcleritis
  4. Adrenal TB
  5. Breast TB

■ ETIOLOGY
- See also "Pulmonary Tuberculosis" in Section I
- *Mycobacterium tuberculosis* (Mtb), a slow growing, aerobic, non–spore-forming, nonmotile bacillus
- Humans are the only reservoir for Mtb
- Pathogenesis:
  1. AFB (Mtb) are ingested by macrophages in alveoli, then transported to regional lymph nodes where spread is contained.
  2. Some AFB reach the bloodstream and disseminate widely.
  3. Immediate active disseminated disease may ensue or a latent period may develop.
  4. During latent period, T-cell immune mechanisms contain infection in granulomas until later reactivation occurs as a result of immunosuppression or other undefined factors in conjunction with reactivated pulmonary TB or alone.

- Miliary TB may occur as a consequence of the following:
  1. Primary infection: inability to contain primary infection leads to a hematogenous spread and progressive disseminated disease.
  2. In late chronic TB and in those with advanced age or poor immunity, a continuous seeding of the blood may develop and lead to disseminated disease.

DIAGNOSIS

DIFFERENTIAL DIAGNOSIS
- Widespread sites of possible dissemination associated with myriad differential diagnostic possibilities
- Lymphoma
- Typhoid fever
- Brucellosis
- Other tumors
- Collagen-vascular disease

WORKUP
- Prompt evaluation is essential
- Sputum for AFB stain and culture
- Chest x-ray examination
- PPD
- Fluid analysis and culture wherever available
  1. Sputum
  2. Blood: particularly helpful in patients with AIDS
  3. Urine
  4. CSF
  5. Pleural
  6. Pericardial
  7. Peritoneal
  8. Gastric aspirates
- Biopsy of any involved tissue is advisable to make immediate diagnosis
  1. Transbronchial biopsy preferred and easily accessible
  2. Bone marrow
  3. Lymph node
  4. Scrotal mass if present
  5. Any other involved site
  6. Positive granuloma or AFB on biopsy specimen is diagnostic
- Imaging studies as needed

LABORATORY TESTS
- Culture and fluid analysis as described previously
- Smear-negative sputum often is positive weeks later on culture
- CBC is usually normal
- ESR is usually elevated

IMAGING STUDIES
- Chest x-ray examination (may or may not be positive) (See "Pulmonary Tuberculosis" in Section I)
- CT scan or MRI of brain
  1. Tuberculoma
  2. Basilar arachnoiditis
- Barium studies of bowel

TREATMENT

NONPHARMACOLOGIC THERAPY
- Bed rest during acute phase of treatment
- High-calorie, high-protein diet to reverse malnutrition and enhance immune response to TB
- Isolation in negative-pressure rooms with high-volume air replacement and circulation (with health care provider wearing proper protective 0.5- to 1-micron filter respirators)
  1. Until three consecutive sputum AFB smears are negative, if pulmonary disease coexists
  2. Isolation not required for closed-space TB infections

ACUTE GENERAL Rx
- See "Pulmonary Tuberculosis" in Section I.
- Therapy should be initiated immediately. Do not wait for definitive diagnosis.
- More rapid response to chemotherapy by disseminated TB foci than cavitary pulmonary TB.
- Treatment for 6 mo with INH plus rifampin plus PZA.
  1. Treatment for 12 mo often required for bone and renal TB.
  2. Prolonged treatment often required for CNS and pericardial.
  3. Prolonged treatment often required for all disseminated TB in infants.
- Compliance (rigid adherence to treatment regimen) is the chief determinant of success.
  1. Supervised DOT is recommended for all patients.
  2. Supervised DOT is mandatory for unreliable patients.
- Steroids are often helpful additions in fulminant miliary disease with the hypoxemia and DIC.

CHRONIC Rx
- Generally not indicated beyond treatment described previously
- Prolonged treatment supervised by ID expert required in a few complicated infections caused by resistant organisms

DISPOSITION
- Monthly follow-up by physician experienced in TB treatment
- Confirm sensitivity testing, and alter treatment appropriately (see "Pulmonary Tuberculosis" in Section I)

REFERRAL
- To infectious disease expert for:
  1. HIV-positive patient
  2. Patient with suspected drug-resistant TB
  3. Patients previously treated for TB
  4. Patients whose fever has not decreased and sputum (if positive) has not converted to negative in 2 to 4 wk
  5. Patients with overwhelming pulmonary or extrapulmonary tuberculosis
- To pulmonary, orthopedic, or GI physicians for examinations or biopsy

PEARLS & CONSIDERATIONS

COMMENTS
- All contacts (especially close household contacts and infants) should be properly tested for PPD conversions >3 mo following exposure
- Those with positive PPD should be evaluated for active TB and properly treated or given prophylaxis.

REFERENCES

American Thoracic Society: Diagnostic standards and classification of tuberculosis in adults and children, *Am J Respir Crit Care Med* 161:1376, 2000.

Del-Giudice P et al: Unusual cutaneous manifestations of miliary tuberculosis, *Clin Infect Dis* 30(1):201, 2000.

Goto S et al: A successfully treated case of disseminated tuberculosis-associated hemophagocytic syndrome and multiple organ dysfunction syndrome, *Am J Kidney Dis* 38(4):E19, 2001.

Kuo PH et al: Severe immune hemolytic anemia in disseminated tuberculosis with response to antituberculosis therapy, *Chest* 119(6):1961, 2001.

Mert A et al: Spontaneous pneumothorax: a rare complication of miliary tuberculosis, *Ann Thorac Cardiovasc Surg* 7(1):45, 2001.

Small P, Fujiwara P: Management of tuberculosis in the United States, *N Engl J Med* 345:189, 2001.

Author: **George O. Alonso, M.D.**

BASIC INFORMATION

■ DEFINITION
Pulmonary tuberculosis (TB) is an infection of the lung and, occasionally, surrounding structures, caused by the bacterium *Mycobacterium tuberculosis*.

■ SYNONYMS
TB

ICD-9CM CODES
011.9 Pulmonary tuberculosis

■ EPIDEMIOLOGY & DEMOGRAPHICS
INCIDENCE (IN U.S.):
- Approximately 7 cases/100,000 persons—lowest in reported history
- >90% of new cases each year from reactivated prior infections
- 9% newly infected
- Only 10% of patients with PPD conversions (higher [8%/yr] in HIV-positive patients) will develop TB, most within 1 to 2 yr
- Two thirds of all new cases in racial and ethnic minorities
- 80% of new cases in children in racial and ethnic minorities
- Occurs most frequently in geographic areas and among populations with highest AIDS prevalence
  1. Urban blacks and Hispanics between 25 and 45 yr old
  2. Poor, crowded urban communities
- Nearly 36% of new cases from new immigrants

PREVALENCE (IN U.S.):
- Estimated 10 million people infected
- Varies widely among population groups

PREDOMINANT SEX:
- No specific predilection
- Male predominance in AIDS, shelters, and prisons reflected in disproportionate male incidence

PREDOMINANT AGE:
- 24 to 45 yr old
- Childhood cases common among minorities
- Nursing home outbreaks among elderly

PEAK INCIDENCE:
- Infancy
- Teenage years
- Pregnancy
- Elderly
- HIV-positive patients, regardless of age, at highest risk

GENETICS:
- Populations with widespread low native resistance have been intensely infected when initially exposed to TB.
- Following elimination of those with least native resistance, incidence and prevalence of TB tend to decline.

■ PHYSICAL FINDINGS & CLINICAL PRESENTATION
- See "Etiology"
- Primary pulmonary TB infection generally asymptomatic
- Reactivation pulmonary TB
  1. Fever
  2. Night sweats
  3. Cough
  4. Hemoptysis
  5. Scanty nonpurulent sputum
  6. Weight loss
- Progressive primary pulmonary TB disease: same as reactivation pulmonary TB
- TB pleurisy
  1. Pleuritic chest pain
  2. Fever
  3. Shortness of breath
- Rare massive, suffocating, fatal hemoptysis secondary to erosion of pulmonary artery within a cavity (Rasmussen's aneurysm)
- Chest examination
  1. Not specific
  2. Usually underestimates extent of disease
  3. Rales accentuated following a cough (posttussive rales)

■ ETIOLOGY
- *Mycobacterium tuberculosis* (Mtb), a slow-growing, aerobic, non–spore-forming, nonmotile bacillus, with a lipid-rich cell wall
  1. Lacks pigment
  2. Produces niacin
  3. Reduces nitrate
  4. Produces heat-labile catalase
  5. Mtb staining, acid-fast and acid-alcohol fast by Ziehl-Neelsen method, appearing as red, slightly bent, beaded rods 2 to 4 microns long (acid-fast bacilli [AFB]), against a blue background
  6. Polymerase chain reaction (PCR) to detect <10 organisms/ml in sputum (compared with the requisite 10,000 organisms/ml for AFB smear detection)
  7. Culture
     a. Growth on solid media (Löwenstein-Jensen; Middlebrook 7H11) in 2 to 6 wk
     b. Growth in liquid media (BACTEC, using a radioactive carbon source for early growth detection) often in 9 to 16 days
     c. Enhanced in a 5% to 10% carbon dioxide atmosphere
  8. DNA fingerprinting (based on restriction fragment length polymorphism [RFLP])
     a. Facilitates immediate identification of Mtb strains in early growing cultures

     b. False-negatives possible if growth suboptimal
  9. Humans are the only reservoir for Mtb
  10. Transmission
     a. Facilitated by close exposure to high-velocity cough (unprotected by proper mask or respirators) from patient with AFB-positive sputum and cavitary lesions, producing aerosolized droplets containing AFB, which are inhaled directly into alveoli
     b. Occurs within prisons, nursing homes, and hospitals
- Pathogenesis
  1. AFB (Mtb) ingested by macrophages in alveoli, then transported to regional lymph nodes where spread is contained
  2. Some AFB may reach bloodstream and disseminate widely
  3. Primary TB (asymptomatic, minimal pneumonitis in lower or midlung fields, with hilar lymphadenopathy) essentially an intracellular infection, with multiplication of organisms continuing for 2 to 12 wk after primary exposure, until cell-mediated hypersensitivity (detected by positive skin test reaction to tuberculin purified protein derivative [PPD]) matures, with subsequent containment of infection
  4. Local and disseminated AFB thus contained by T-cell–mediated immune responses
     a. Recruitment of monocytes
     b. Transformation of lymphocytes with secretion of lymphokines
     c. Activation of macrophages and histiocytes
     d. Organization into granulomas, where organisms may survive within macrophages (Langhans' giant cells), but within which multiplication essentially ceases (95%) and from which spread is prohibited
  5. Progressive primary pulmonary disease
     a. May immediately follow the asymptomatic phase
     b. Necrotizing pulmonary infiltrates
     c. Tuberculous bronchopneumonia
     d. Endobronchial TB
     e. Interstitial TB
     f. Widespread miliary lung lesions
  6. Postprimary TB pleurisy with pleural effusion
     a. Develops after early primary infection, although often before conversion to positive PPD

b. Results from pleural seeding from a peripheral lung lesion or rupture of lymph node into pleural space

c. May produce a large (sometimes hemorrhagic) exudative effusion (with polymorphonuclear cells early, rapidly replaced by lymphocytes), frequently without pulmonary infiltrates

d. Generally resolves without treatment

e. Portends a high risk of subsequent clinical disease, and therefore must be diagnosed and treated early (pleural biopsy and culture) to prevent future catastrophic TB illness

f. May result in disseminated extrapulmonary infection

7. Reactivation pulmonary TB
a. Occurs months to years following primary TB
b. Preferentially involves the apical posterior segments of the upper lobes and superior segments of the lower lobes
c. Associated with necrosis and cavitation of involved lung, hemoptysis, chronic fever, night sweats, weight loss
d. Spread within lung occurs via cough and inhalation

8. Reinfection TB
a. May mimic reactivation TB
b. Ruptured caseous foci and cavities, which may produce endobronchial spread

9. Mtb in both progressive primary and reactivation pulmonary TB
a. Intracellular (macrophage) lesions (undergoing slow multiplication)
b. Closed caseous lesions (undergoing slow multiplication)
c. Extracellular, open cavities (undergoing rapid multiplication)
d. INH and rifampin are cidal in all three sites
e. PZA especially active within acidic macrophage environment
f. Extrapulmonary reactivation disease also possible

10. Rapid local progression and dissemination in infants with devastating illness before PPD conversion occurs

11. Most symptoms (fever, weight loss, anorexia) and tissue destruction (caseous necrosis) from cytokines and cell-mediated immune responses

12. Mtb has no important endotoxins or exotoxins

13. Granuloma formation related to tumor necrosis factor (TNF) secreted by activated macrophages

🔬 DIAGNOSIS

■ DIFFERENTIAL DIAGNOSIS
- Necrotizing pneumonia (anaerobic, gram-negative)
- Histoplasmosis
- Coccidioidomycosis
- Melioidosis
- Interstitial lung diseases (rarely)
- Cancer
- Sarcoidosis
- Silicosis
- Paragonimiasis
- Rare pneumonias
  1. *Rhodococcus equi* (cavitation)
  2. *Bacillus cereus* (50% hemoptysis)
  3. *Eikenella corrodens* (cavitation)

■ WORKUP
- Sputum for AFB stains
- Chest x-ray examination
- PPD
  1. Recent conversion from negative to positive within 3 mo of exposure is highly suggestive of recent infection.
  2. Single positive PPD is not helpful diagnostically.
  3. Negative PPD never rules out acute TB.
  4. Be certain that positive PPD does not reflect "booster phenomenon" (prior positive PPD may become negative after several years and return to positive only after second repeated PPD; repeat second PPD within 1 wk), which thus may mimic skin test conversion.
  5. Positive PPD reaction is determined as follows:
     a. Induration after 72 hr of intradermal injection of 0.1 ml of 5 TU-PPD
     b. 5-mm induration if HIV-positive, close contact of active TB, fibrotic chest lesions
     c. 10-mm induration if in high–medical risk groups (immunosuppressive disease or therapy, renal failure, gastrectomy, silicosis, diabetes), foreign-born high-risk group (Southeast Asia, Latin America, Africa, India), low socioeconomic groups, IV drug addict, prisoner, health care worker
     d. 15-mm induration if low risk
  6. Anergy antigen testing (using mumps, *Candida*, tetanus toxoid) may identify patients who are truly anergic to PPD and these antigens, but results are often confusing. Not recommended.
  7. Patients with TB may be selectively anergic only to PPD.
  8. Positive PPD indicates prior infection but does not itself confirm active disease.

■ LABORATORY TESTS
- Sputum for AFB stains and culture
  1. Induced sputum if patient not coughing productively
- Sputum from bronchoscopy if high suspicion of TB with negative expectorated induced sputum for AFB
  1. Positive AFB smear is essential before or shortly after treatment to ensure subsequent growth for definitive diagnosis and sensitivity testing
  2. Consider lung biopsy if sputum negative, especially if infiltrates are predominantly interstitial
- AFB stain-negative sputum may grow Mtb subsequently
- Gastric aspirates reliable, especially in HIV-negative patients
- CBC
  1. Variable values
     a. WBCs: low, normal, or elevated (including leukemoid reaction: >50,000)
     b. Normocytic, normochromic anemia often
  2. Rarely helpful diagnostically
- ESR usually elevated
- Thoracentesis
  1. Exudative effusion
     a. Elevated protein
     b. Decreased glucose
     c. Elevated WBCs (polymorphonuclear leukocytes early, replaced later by lymphocytes)
     d. May be hemorrhagic
  2. Pleural fluid usually AFB-negative
  3. Pleural biopsy often diagnostic—may need to be repeated for diagnosis
  4. Culture pleural biopsy tissue for AFB
- Bone marrow biopsy is often diagnostic in difficult-to-diagnose cases, especially miliary tuberculosis

■ IMAGING STUDIES
- Chest x-ray examination
  1. Primary infection reflected by calcified peripheral lung nodule with calcified hilar lymph node
  2. Reactivation pulmonary TB
     a. Necrosis
     b. Cavitation (especially on apical lordotic views)
     c. Fibrosis and hilar retraction
     d. Bronchopneumonia
     e. Interstitial infiltrates
     f. Miliary pattern
     g. Many of previous may also accompany progressive primary TB
  3. TB pleurisy
     a. Pleural effusion, often rapidly accumulating and massive
  4. TB activity not established by single chest x-ray examination
  5. Serial chest x-ray examinations are excellent indicators of progression or regression

℞ TREATMENT

■ NONPHARMACOLOGIC THERAPY
- Bed rest during acute phase of treatment
- High-calorie, high-protein diet to reverse malnutrition and enhance immune response to TB
- Isolation in negative-pressure rooms with high-volume air replacement and circulation, with health care provider wearing proper protective 0.5- to 1-micron filter respirators, until three consecutive sputum AFB smears are negative

■ ACUTE GENERAL Rx
- Compliance (rigid adherence to treatment regimen) chief determinant of success
  1. Supervised directly observed therapy (DOT) recommended for all patients and mandatory for unreliable patients
- Preferred adult regimen: DOT
  1. Isoniazid (INH) 15 mg/kg (max 900 mg) + rifampin 600 mg + ethambutol (EMB) 30 mg/kg (max 2500 mg) + pyrazinamide (PZA) (2 g [<50 kg]; 2.5 g [51 to 74 kg]; 3 g [>75 kg]) thrice weekly for 6 mo
  2. Alternative, more complicated DOT regimens
- Rifapentine, a rifampin derivative with a much longer serum half-life, was shown to be as effective when administered weekly (with weekly isoniazid) as conventional regimens for drug-sensitive pulmonary tuberculosis in non-HIV-infected patients.
- Short-course daily therapy: adult
  1. HIV-negative patient: 6 mo total therapy (2 mo INH 300 mg + rifampin 600 mg + EMB 15 mg/kg [max 2500 mg]) + PZA (1.5 g [<50 kg]; 2 g [51 to 74 kg]; 2.5 g [>75 kg]) daily and until smear negative and sensitivity confirmed; then INH + rifampin daily × 4 mo)
  2. HIV-positive patient: 9 mo total therapy (2 mo INH + rifampin + EMB + PZA daily until smear negative and sensitivity confirmed; then INH + rifampin qd × 7 mo)
  3. Continue treatment at least 3 mo following conversion to negative cultures
- Drug resistance (often multiple drug resistance [MDRTB]) increased by:
  1. Prior treatment
  2. Acquisition of TB in developing countries
  3. Homelessness
  4. AIDS
  5. Prisoners
  6. IV drug addicts
  7. Known contact with MDRTB
- Never add single drug to failing regimen
- Never treat TB with fewer than two to three drugs or two to three new additional drugs
- Monitor for clinical toxicity (especially hepatitis)
  1. Patient and physician awareness that anorexia, nausea, RUQ pain, and unexplained malaise require immediate cessation of treatment
  2. Evaluation of LFTs
     a. Minimal SGOT/SGPT elevations without symptoms generally transient and not clinically significant
- Preventive treatment for PPD conversion only (infection without disease)
  1. Must be certain that chest x-ray examination is negative and patient has no symptoms of TB
  2. INH 300 mg daily for 6 to 12 mo; at least 12 mo if HIV-positive
  3. Most important groups:
     a. HIV-positive
     b. Close contact of active TB
     c. Recent converter
     d. Old TB on chest x-ray examination
     e. IV drug addict
     f. Medical risk factor
     g. High-risk foreign country
     h. Homeless
- Infants generally given prophylaxis immediately if recent contact of active TB (even if infant PPD negative), then retested with PPD in 3 mo (continuing INH if PPD becomes positive and stopping INH if PPD remains negative)
- Chronic, stable PPD (several years) given INH prophylaxis generally only if patient is <35 yr old
  1. INH toxicity may outweigh benefit
  2. Individualize decision
- Preventive therapy for suspected INH-resistant organisms is unclear

■ CHRONIC Rx
- Generally not indicated beyond treatment described previously
- Prolonged treatment, supervised by infectious disease expert, in a few very complicated infections caused by resistant organisms

■ DISPOSITION
- Monthly follow-up by physician experienced in TB treatment
- Confirm sensitivity testing and alter treatment appropriately
- Frequent sputum samples until culture is negative
- Confirm chest x-ray regression at 2 to 3 mo

■ REFERRAL
- To infectious disease expert for:
  1. HIV-positive patient
  2. Patient with suspected drug-resistant TB
  3. Patients previously treated for TB
  4. Patients whose fever has not decreased and sputum has not converted to negative in 2 to 4 wk
  5. Patients with overwhelming pulmonary or extrapulmonary tuberculosis
- To pulmonologist for bronchoscopy or pleural biopsy

☼ PEARLS & CONSIDERATIONS

■ COMMENTS
- All contacts (especially close household contacts and infants) should be properly tested for PPD conversions during 3 mo following exposure.
- Those with positive PPD should be evaluated for active TB and properly treated or given prophylaxis.

REFERENCES

Benator D et al: Rifapentine and isoniazid once a week versus rifampicin and isoniazid twice a week for treatment of drug susceptible pulmonary tuberculosis in HIV-negative patients: a randomized clinical trial, *Lancet* 360(9332):528, 2002.

Espinal MA et al: Infectiousness of *my-cobacterium tuberculosis* in HIV-1-infected patients with tuberculosis: a prospective study, *Lancet* 355(9200):275, 2000.

Kanaya AM, Glidden DV, Chambers HF: Identifying pulmonary tuberculosis in patients with negative sputum smear results, *Chest* 120(2):349, 2001.

Karcic AA et al: An elderly woman with chronic knee pain and abnormal chest radiography, *Postgrad Med* 77(911):600, 2001.

Mulder K: Tuberculosis: a case history, *Lancet* 358(9283):776, 2001.

Salazar GE et al: Pulmonary tuberculosis in children in a developing country, *Pediatrics* 108(2):448, 2001.

Small P, Fujiwara P: Management of tuberculosis in the United States, *N Engl J Med* 345:189, 2001.

Tudo G et al: Detection of unsuspected cases of nosocomial transmission of tuberculosis by use of a molecular typing method, *Clin Infect Dis* 33(4):453, 2001.

Author: **George O. Alonso, M.D.**

BASIC INFORMATION

■ DEFINITION
Tularemia is a Zoonosis caused by small, facultative gram-negative intracellular coccobacillus *Francisella tularensis*. Clinical manifestations range from asymptomatic illness to septic shock and death.

ICD-9CM CODES
021.9 Tularemia

■ EPIDEMIOLOGY & DEMOGRAPHICS
INCIDENCE (IN U.S.): Highest overall incidence in Arkansas, Missouri, and Okalahoma. It also found in Canada, Mexico, and European countries, Turkey, Israel, China and Japan.
PREDOMINANT SEX: Male
PREDOMINANT AGE: Occurs at any age
PEAK INCIDENCE: June through August and in December
PHYSICAL FINDINGS:
- Incubation period is 2-10 days.
- Most common initial signs and symptoms:
  1. Fever
  2. Chills
  3. Headache
  4. Malaise
  5. Anorexia
  6. Fatigue
  7. Cough
  8. Myalgias
  9. Chest discomfort
  10. Vomiting
  11. Abdominal pain
  12. Diarrhea

■ CLINICAL SYNDROME OF TULAREMIA
1. Ulcer glandular and glandular: Account for 75%-80% of cases. Fever and a single erythematous papuloulcerative lesion with a central Escher accompanied by tender lymphadenopathy.
2. Oculoglandular: Accounts for 1%-2% of cases. Painful inflamed conjunctiva with numerous yellowish nodules and pinpoint ulcers. Purulent conjunctivitis with regional lymphadenopathy. Corneal perforation may occur.
3. Oropharyngeal and gastrointestinal: Account for 1%-4% of cases. Acute exudative membranes pharyngitis associated with cervical lymphadenopathy. Ulcerative intestinal lesion associated with mesenteric lymphadepathy, diarrhea, abdominal pain, nausea, vomiting and GI bleeding.

4. Pulmonary tularemia: Occurs often in the elderly and has a higher mortality. Symptoms include nonproductive cough, dysnoea, or pleuritic chest pain.
5. Typhoidal tularemia: 10% of all cases of tularemia. Rare in U.S. Symptoms include high continuous fever, signs of endotoxemia, and severe headache. Mortality can approach 30%.

■ COMPLICATIONS
1. Intravascular coagulation
2. Renal failure
3. Rhabitomyolysis
4. Jaundice
5. Hepatitis
6. Meningitis
7. Encephalitis
8. Percarditis
9. Peritonitis
10. Osteomyelitis
11. Spleenic rupture
12. Thrombophlebitis
13. Myositis and septicemia

■ ETIOLOGY
1. Caused by infection with *F. tularensis*.
2. Two main biovars of *F. tularensis*: Type A and Type B. Type A produces severe disease in humans. Type B produces milder subclinical infection.
3. Transmitted by ticks, tabanid flies, and mosquitoes. Also acquired by inhalation and ingestion.
4. Cases also occur after exposure to animals (wild rabbit, squirrels, birds, sheep, beavers, muskrats, and domestic dogs and cats) or animal products.
5. Laboratory acquisition is possible.
6. Pathogenesis: After inoculation into the skin the organism multiplies locally with in 2-5 days, then it produces erythematous tender or pruritic papule. The papule rapidly enlarges and forms an ulcer with a black base. The bacteria spread to the regional lymph nodes producing lymphadenopathy, and with bacremia may spread to distant organs.

 # DIAGNOSIS

■ DIFFERENTIAL DIAGNOSIS
1. Rickettsial infections
2. Meningococcal infections
3. Cat-scratch disease
4. Infectious mononucleosis
5. Atypical pneumonia
6. Group A strep pharyngitis
7. Typhoid fever
8. Fungal infection—sporotrichosis
9. Anthrax
10. Bacterial skin infections

■ WORKUP
1. CBC
2. Chest x-ray examination
3. Cultures of blood, lymph node, pleural fluid, wounds, sputum, and gastric aspirate
4. Antigen detection in urine
5. PCR
6. Serology

■ LABORATORY TESTS
1. WBC count and ESR normal or elevated
2. Rarely seen on Gram-stained smears or tissue biopsies
3. Antibodies to *F. tularensis* demonstrated by tube agglutination, micro agglutination, heme agglutination, and ELISA; definitive serologic diagnosis requires a fourfold or greater rise in titer between acute and convalescent specimens
4. Polymerase chain reaction (PCR) to facilitate early diagnosis

■ IMAGING STUDIES
Chest x-ray examination to show bilateral patchy infiltrate, lobar parenchymal infiltrate, cavitory lesion, pleural effusion, or emphysema

TREATMENT

■ ACUTE GENERAL Rx
Immediate therapy to limit extent of acute illness and complication
- Streptomycin 10 mg/kg IM q12h (daily dose should not exceed 2 g) or Gentamicin 3-5 mg/kg q8h
- Tetracycline 500 mg PO qid or Doxycycline 100 mg PO bid or Chloramphenicol 25-60 mg/kg q6h (do not exceed 6 g)
- Combination antibiotics required for tularemic meningitis— Chloramphenicol plus Streptomycin Surgical therapies are limited to drainage of abscessed lymph nodes and chest tube drainage of empyemas

■ PROGNOSIS

The mortality rate of severe untreated infection (tularemic pneumonia and typhoidal tularemia) can be as high as 30%. Overall mortality associated with tularemia is 2%-4% with appropriate treatment. Lifelong immunity usually follows tularemia.

■ DISPOSITION

Follow-up as outpatient

■ PREVENTION

1. Educate the public to prevent sick or dead animals.
2. Use insect repellants.
3. Remove ticks promptly.
4. Drink only portable water.
5. Adequately cook wild meats.
6. Tularemia vaccine has been developed but is not commercially available in U.S.; however, it is available from the Centers for Disease Control and Prevention (CDC). Vaccination of high-risk individuals working with large quantities of cultured organism is recommended.
7. Avoid skinning wild animals, especially rabbits; wear gloves while handling animal carcasses.
8. Do not use wells or other water that are contaminated by dead animals.
9. Hospitalized patients with tularemia do not need special isolation. Standard universal precautions for contaminated secretion are adequate when handling drainage from wounds.
10. Laboratory personnel should be notified of potential danger.

■ REFERRAL

For consultation with infectious diseases specialist in suspected cases

☼ PEARLS & CONSIDERATIONS

- Alert the microbiology laboratory to the possibility of tularemia.
- Do not use doxycyclin or tetracyclin in children or pregnant women.
- Because of its highly contagious nature with low inoculums, tularemia is considered an agent that could be used by terrorists. It is classified as a category A critical biologic agent by the CDC.

REFERENCES

Chocarro A, Gonzalez A, Garcia I: Treatment of tularemia with ciprofloxacin, *Clin Infect Dis* 31:623, 2000.

Jensen WA, Kirsch CM: Tularemia, *Semina Respir Infect* 18(3):146, 2003.

Author: **Vasanthi Arumugam, M.D.**

BASIC INFORMATION

■ DEFINITION

Turner's syndrome refers to a pattern of malformation characterized by short stature, ovarian hypofunction, loose nuchal skin, and cubitus valgus as described by Turner in 1938. An associated 45,X chromosome constitution was recognized by Ford et al in 1959.

■ SYNONYMS

All obsolete:
Ullrich-Turner syndrome
Bonnevie-Ullrich-Turner syndrome

ICD-9CM CODES

758.6 Syndrome, Turner's

■ EPIDEMIOLOGY & DEMOGRAPHICS

INCIDENCE: 1 case out of every 2500 to 5000 live births

■ PHYSICAL FINDINGS & CLINICAL PRESENTATION

- Turner's phenotype is recognizable at any point on the developmental spectrum.
- In spontaneous abortuses the most common sex chromosome abnormality detected (45,X chromosome constitution) is found in 75% of affected individuals and accounts for 20% of such cases.
- In fetuses, it is suspected because of such ultrasonographic manifestations as thickening of the nuchal folds, frank nuchal cystic hygromas, or mild shortness of the femora at midtrimester.
- In infants:
  1. At birth may display loose nuchal skin (pterygium colli) and edema on the dorsa of hands and feet
  2. Canthal folds reflecting midface hypoplasia and redundant skin in the periorbital region
  3. Nipples appearing widely spaced
  4. Heart and cardiovascular system: murmur of aortic stenosis or bicuspid aortic valve or diminished femoral pulses suggestive of aortic coarctation
  5. Renal ultrasonography: renal ectopia such as pelvic kidney or horseshoe kidneys
- In older children:
  1. Slow linear growth
  2. Short stature—may be improved with growth hormone therapy (Fig. 1-285)
  3. Delayed or absent menses— secondary sex characteristics possibly normalized with estrogen replacement therapy

4. Intelligence is often normal, but delays in spatial perception or visual motor integration are commonly observed; frank mental retardation is rare

■ ETIOLOGY

- Phenotype caused by absence of the second sex chromosome, whether X or Y
- 45,X chromosome constitution in about 50% of affected individuals
- Other chromosome aberrations (40% of cases): isochromosome Xq (46,X,i[Xq]) or mosaicism (XX/X)
- With deletions involving the short (or "p") arm of the X chromosome: short stature but little ovarian hypofunction
- Deletions involving Xq13-q27: ovarian failure
- Usually a deficiency of paternal contribution of sex chromosome, reflecting paternal nondisjunction

DIAGNOSIS

■ DIFFERENTIAL DIAGNOSIS

- Noonan syndrome, an autosomally dominant inherited disorder also characterized by loose nuchal skin, midface hypoplasia, canthal folds, and stenotic cardiac valvular defects and affecting males and females equally; also have normal chromosome constitutions
- Other conditions in the differential diagnosis of loose skin, whether or not associated with edema:
  1. Fetal hydantoin syndrome (loose nuchal skin, midface hypoplasia, distal digital hypoplasia)
  2. Disorders of chromosome constitution (trisomy 21, tetrasomy 12p mosaicism)
  3. Congenital lymphedema (Milroy edema)

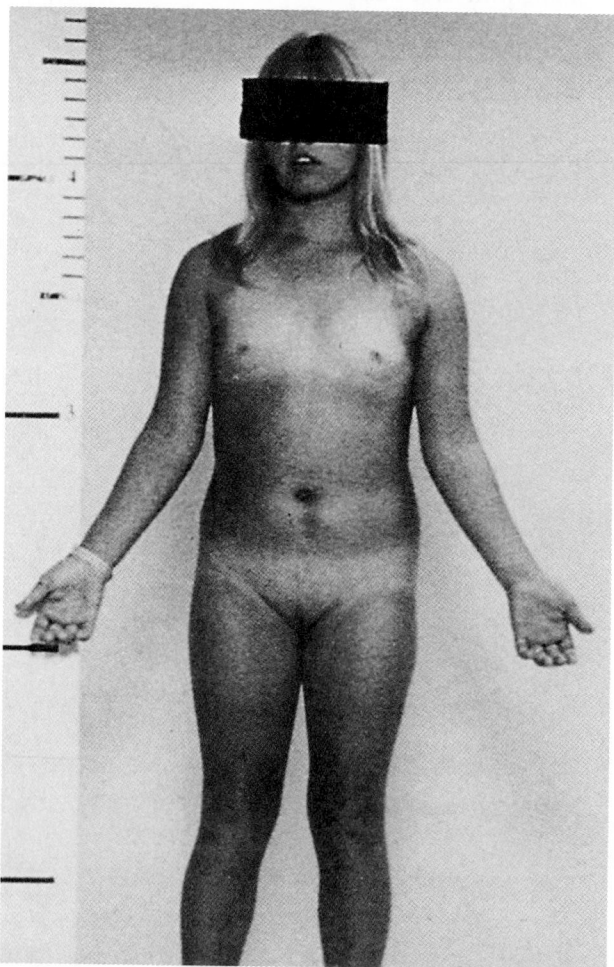

Fig. 1-285 A 17-year-old patient with Turner's syndrome demonstrating short stature, poor sexual development, and increased carrying angles at elbows. Patient also has webbing of the neck. (From Mishell D [ed]: *Comprehensive gynecology,* ed 3, St Louis, 1997, Mosby.)

■ WORKUP

- Giemsa banded karyotype to confirm clinical diagnosis
- Once diagnosis is established: cardiologic consultation for evaluation for cardiac valvular abnormalities or aortic coarctation
- Renal ultrasonography
- Endocrine evaluations in older patients with short stature or amenorrhea
- Psychometrics to document known or suspected learning disabilities

■ LABORATORY TESTS

- As noted, routine Giemsa banded karyotype on peripheral lymphocytes to confirm the clinical impression in all suspected cases of Turner's syndrome
- Recognition of associated medical problems, such as hypergonadotropic hypogonadism or autoimmune thyroiditis prompting periodic evaluation of these potential areas

■ IMAGING STUDIES

- Echocardiogram
- Renal ultrasonography
- Abdominal ultrasonography for evaluation of ovarian and uterine size and morphology
- MRI of brain (especially in cases with known or suspected neurologic impairment)
- Radiographs (for evaluation of carpal/metacarpal abnormalities, radioulnar synostosis)
- Bone age (for evaluation of short stature)

 TREATMENT

Recognition of the multisystem involvement of Turner's syndrome necessitates multiple medical specialists working in concert with the primary care provider to maximize and improve outcome while minimizing unnecessary or redundant testing.

■ NONPHARMACOLOGIC THERAPY

General medical care guided by normal medical standards with special attention paid to identifying such age-related problems as developmental delays, learning disabilities, slow growth, or amenorrhea.

■ ACUTE GENERAL Rx

Specific treatment geared to the specific medical problem (e.g., cardiac or renal dysfunction)

■ CHRONIC Rx

- Estrogen replacement therapy in early adolescence
- Some benefit from recombinant human growth hormone therapy

■ REFERRAL

- To geneticist: clinical diagnosis, differential diagnosis, recurrence risk counseling, cytogenetic tests
- To endocrinologist (pediatric): evaluation of short stature, estrogen or growth hormone replacement therapy
- To cardiologist

⚙ PEARLS & CONSIDERATIONS

■ COMMENTS

- Although newer studies are optimistic regarding outcomes, previous reports suffered from retrospective observations, case reports, and ascertainment bias, contributing to a generally poor interaction between physician and patient.
- Affected individuals and families often benefit from the contemporary experiences and expertise of members of genetic support groups. The Turner Syndrome Association (phone: 612-379-3607 or 800-365-9944; Internet: http://www.turner-syndrome-us.org) and the Alliance of Genetic Support Groups (phone: 800-336-4363; Internet: http://medhelp.org/www/agsg.htm) are valuable resources.

REFERENCES

Conniff C: Turner's syndrome, *Adolesc Med* 13(2):359, 2002.
Elsheikh M et al: Turner's syndrome in adulthood, *Endocr Rev* 23(1):120, 2002.
Author: **Luther K. Robinson, M.D.**

BASIC INFORMATION

■ DEFINITION
Typhoid fever is a systemic infection caused by *Salmonella typhi.*

■ SYNONYMS
Typhoid
Enteric fever

ICD-9CM CODES
002.0 Typhoid fever

■ EPIDEMIOLOGY & DEMOGRAPHICS
INCIDENCE (IN U.S.): Approximately 500 cases of *S. typhi* infections are reported annually.

■ PHYSICAL FINDINGS & CLINICAL PRESENTATION
- Incubation period of a few days to several weeks.
- Usual manifestations:
  1. Prolonged fever
  2. Myalgias
  3. Headache
  4. Cough
  5. Sore throat
  6. Malaise
  7. Anorexia, at times with abdominal pain and hepatosplenomegaly
  8. Diarrhea or constipation may occur early in the course of illness
  9. Rose spots, which are faint, maculopapular, blanching lesions, may sometimes be seen on the chest or abdomen
- In the untreated patient, fever may last 1 to 2 mo. The main complication of untreated disease is GI bleeding as a result of perforation from ulceration of Peyer's patches in the ileum. Mental status changes and shock are rare complications. The relapse rate is approximately 10%.

■ ETIOLOGY
- *Salmonella typhi*
- *S. paratyphi*
- *S. typhi* or *S. paratyphi* found only in humans
- Acquisition of disease by ingestion of food or water contaminated by other humans
- In the U.S. most cases are acquired either during foreign travel or by ingestion of food prepared by chronic carriers, many of whom acquired the organism outside of the U.S.

DIAGNOSIS

■ DIFFERENTIAL DIAGNOSIS
- Malaria
- Tuberculosis
- Brucellosis
- Amebic liver abscess

■ WORKUP
- Blood, stool, and urine cultures are helpful.
- Cultures should be repeated if initially negative.
- Blood cultures are more likely to be positive early in the course of illness.
- Stool and urine cultures are more commonly positive in the second and third weeks of illness.
- Bone marrow biopsy cultures are 90% positive, although this procedure is usually not necessary.
- Serology using Widal test is helpful in retrospect, showing a fourfold increase in convalescent titers.

■ LABORATORY TESTS
- Neutropenia is common.
- Transaminitis is possible.
- Culture:
  1. Blood
  2. Body fluids
  3. Biopsy specimens

TREATMENT

■ ACUTE GENERAL Rx
- Ciprofloxacin 500 mg PO bid or 400 mg IV bid for 14 days
- Ceftriaxone 2 g IV qd for 14 days
- If organism sensitive
  1. SMX/TMP, 1 to 2 DS tabs PO bid *or*
  2. Amoxicillin, 2 g PO q8h to complete 14 days
- Dexamethasone, 3 mg IV initially, followed by 1 mg IV q6h for 8 doses for patients with shock or mental status changes

■ CHRONIC Rx
- Carrier states possible
- More common in age >60 yr and in persons with gallstones
- Usual site of colonization: gallbladder
- Treatment in those with persistently positive stool cultures and in food-handlers
- Suggested regimens for eradication of carrier state
  1. Ciprofloxacin 500 mg PO bid for 4 wk
  2. SMX/TMP 1 to 2 tabs PO bid for 6 wk (if susceptible)
  3. Amoxicillin, 2 g PO q8h for 6 wk (if susceptible)

- Cholecystectomy possibly required in carriers with gallstones who fail medical therapy

■ DISPOSITION
- Treated patients usually respond to therapy, with a small percentage becoming chronic carriers.
- The relapse rate is approximately 10%.
- Untreated patients may have serious complications.

■ REFERRAL
- Failure of therapy
- Chronic carrier

PEARLS & CONSIDERATIONS

■ COMMENTS
- Oral and parenteral vaccines are available for travelers to areas of high risk.
- Vaccines are about 70% effective.
- Immunity wanes after several years.
- Parenteral preparations are accompanied by frequent side effects:
  1. Pain at injection site
  2. Fever
  3. Malaise
  4. Headaches

REFERENCES
Ackers ML et al: Laboratory-based surveillance of *Salmonella* serotype *typhi* infections in the United States: antimicrobial resistance on the rise, *JAMA* 283(20):2668, 2000.

Guerrant RL, Kosek M: Polysaccharide conjugate typhoid vaccine, *N Engl J Med* 344(17):1322, 2001.

Hoffer RJ et al: Emergency department presentations of typhoid fever, *J Emerg Med* 19(4):317, 2000.

Koul PA: A *Salmonella typhi* Vi conjugate vaccine, *N Engl J Med* 345(7):545, 2001.

O'Brien D et al: Fever in returned travelers: review of hospital admissions for a 3-year period, *Clin Infect Dis* 33(50):603, 2001.

Yang HH et al: An outbreak of typhoid fever, Xing-An County, People's Republic of China, 1999: estimation of the field effectiveness of Vi polysaccharide typhoid vaccine, *J Infect Dis* 183(15):1775, 2001.

Author: **Maurice Policar, M.D.**

BASIC INFORMATION

■ DEFINITION

Ulcerative colitis is a chronic inflammatory bowel disease of undetermined etiology.

■ SYNONYMS

Inflammatory bowel disease (IBD)
Idiopathic proctocolitis

ICD-9CM CODES

556.9 Ulcerative colitis

■ EPIDEMIOLOGY & DEMOGRAPHICS

INCIDENCE:
- 50 to 150 cases/100,000 persons; most common between age 14 and 38 yr.
- Appendectomy for an inflammatory condition (appendicitis or lymphadenitis) but not for nonspecific abdominal pain is associated with a low risk of subsequent ulcerative colitis. This inverse relation is limited to patients who undergo surgery before the age of 20 yr.

■ PHYSICAL FINDINGS & CLINICAL PRESENTATION

- Patients with ulcerative colitis often present with bloody diarrhea accompanied by tenesmus, fever, dehydration, weight loss, anorexia, nausea, and abdominal pain.
- Abdominal distention and tenderness
- Bloody diarrhea
- Fever, evidence of dehydration
- Evidence of extraintestinal manifestations may be present: liver disease, sclerosing cholangitis, iritis, uveitis, episcleritis, arthritis, erythema nodosum, pyoderma gangrenosum, aphthous stomatitis

DIAGNOSIS

■ DIFFERENTIAL DIAGNOSIS

- Crohn's disease
- Bacterial infections
  1. Acute: *Campylobacter, Yersinia, Salmonella, Shigella, Chlamydia, Escherichia coli, Clostridium difficile,* gonococcal proctitis
  2. Chronic: Whipple's disease, TB, enterocolitis
- Irritable bowel syndrome
- Protozoal and parasitic infections (amebiasis, giardiasis, cryptosporidiosis)
- Neoplasm (intestinal lymphoma, carcinoma of colon)
- Ischemic bowel disease
- Diverticulitis
- Celiac sprue, collagenous colitis, radiation enteritis, endometriosis, gay bowel syndrome

■ WORKUP

Diagnostic workup includes:
- Comprehensive history, physical examination
- Laboratory and radiographic studies
- Sigmoidoscopy to establish the presence of mucosal inflammation: typical endoscopic findings in ulcerative colitis are friable mucosa, diffuse, uniform erythema replacing the usual mucosal vascular pattern, and pseudopolyps; rectal involvement is invariably present if the disease is active

■ LABORATORY TESTS

- Anemia, high sedimentation rate (in severe colitis) are common.
- Potassium, magnesium, calcium, albumin may be decreased.
- Antineutrophil cytoplasmic antibodies (ANCA) with a perinuclear staining pattern (pANCA) can be found in >45% of patients; there is an increased frequency in treatment-resistant left-sided colitis, suggesting a possible association between these antibodies and a relative resistance to medical therapy in patients with ulcerative colitis.

■ IMAGING STUDIES

Image studies are generally not indicated. Air-contrast barium enema, when used, may reveal continuous involvement (including the rectum), pseudopolyps, decreased mucosal pattern, and fine superficial ulcerations.

TREATMENT

■ NONPHARMACOLOGIC THERAPY

- Correct nutritional deficiencies; TPN with bowel rest may be necessary in severe cases; folate supplementation may reduce the incidence of dysplasia and cancer in chronic ulcerative colitis.
- Avoid oral feedings during acute exacerbation to decrease colonic activity; a low-roughage diet may be helpful in *early* relapse.
- Psychotherapy is useful in most patients. Referral to self-help groups is also important because of the chronicity of the disease and the young age of the patients.

■ ACUTE GENERAL Rx

The therapeutic options vary with the degree of disease (mild, severe, fulminant) and areas of involvement (distal, extensive):
- Mild or moderate disease can be treated with mesalamine (Rowasa). It can be administered as an enema (40 mg once daily at bedtime for 3 to 6 wk) or suppository (500 mg bid)

for patients with distal colonic disease. Oral forms in which the 5-ASA is in a slow-release or pH-dependent matrix (Pentasa 1 g qid, Asacol 800 mg PO tid) can deliver therapeutic concentrations to the more proximal small bowel or distal ileum.
- Olsalazine (Dipentum) is often useful for maintenance of remission of ulcerative colitis in patients intolerant to sulfasalazine. Usual dose is 500 mg bid taken with food.
- Balsalazide (Colazal) is indicated for mild to moderately active ulcerative colitis. Usual dose is three 750 mg capsules tid.
- Severe disease usually responds to oral corticosteroids (e.g., prednisone 40 to 60 mg/day); corticosteroid suppositories or enemas are also useful for distal colitis.
- Fulminant disease generally requires hospital admission and parenteral corticosteroids (e.g., IV hydrocortisone 100 mg q6h); when bowel movements have returned to normal and the patient is able to eat normally, oral prednisone is resumed. IV cyclosporine can also be used in severe refractory cases; renal toxicity is a potential complication.
- Surgery is indicated in patients who fail to respond to intensive medical therapy. Colectomy is usually curative in these patients and also eliminates the high risk of developing adenocarcinoma of the colon (10% to 20% of patients develop it after 10 yr with the disease); newer surgical techniques allow for the preservation of the sphincter.

■ CHRONIC Rx

- Colonoscopic surveillance and multiple biopsies should be instituted approximately 10 yr after diagnosis because of the increased risk of colon carcinoma.
- Erythropoietin is useful in patients with anemia refractory to treatment with iron and vitamins.

■ DISPOSITION

The clinical course is variable; 15% to 20% of patients will eventually require colectomy; >75% of patients treated medically will experience relapse.

■ REFERRAL

- GI consultation for initial diagnostic sigmoidoscopy/colonoscopy in suspected cases
- Surgical referral for patients with severe disease unresponsive to medical therapy

Author: **Fred F. Ferri, M.D.**

BASIC INFORMATION

■ DEFINITION
Urethritis is a well-defined clinical syndrome manifested by dysuria, a urethral discharge, or both.

ICD-9CM CODES
597.80 Urethritis, unspecified
098.20 Gonococcal

■ EPIDEMIOLOGY & DEMOGRAPHICS
- The major single specific etiology of acute urethritis is *Neisseria gonorrhoeae,* producing GCU. Urethritis of all other etiologies is called *nongonococcal urethritis* (NGU).
- NGU is twice as common as GCU in the U.S. NGU is the most common STD syndrome occurring in men, accounting for 6 million office visits annually. NGU is more frequently encountered in higher socioeconomic groups. GCU is more common in homosexual males than heterosexual males with acute urethritis.
- The gonococcus is a gram-negative, kidney-shaped diplococcus with flattened opposed margins. The urethra is the most common site of infection in all men. In heterosexual men, the pharynx is infected in 7%, and in homosexual men, the pharynx is infected in 40% and the rectum in 25%. A single episode of intercourse with an infected partner carries a transmission risk of 20% for males; female partners of an infected male will contract the disease 80% of the time.

■ PHYSICAL FINDINGS & CLINICAL PRESENTATION
SYMPTOMS OF GONOCOCCAL URETHRITIS: Urethral discharge and dysuria are the most common symptoms. There is complaint of urethral itching. Prostatic involvement can cause frequency, urgency, and nocturia. It can involve the epididymis through spreading down the vas deferens, causing acute epididymitis.
INCUBATION PERIOD: 3 to 10 days. Without treatment urethritis persists for 3 to 7 wk, with 95% of men becoming asymptomatic after 3 mo. GCU is asymptomatic in up to 60% of contacts.

SIGNS OF GONOCOCCAL URETHRITIS: Yellow-brown discharge, meatal edema, urethral tenderness to palpation. Rectal bleeding with pus is seen with gonococcal proctitis. Periurethritis leading to urethral stenosis can occur. Disseminated infection can occur. Tenosynovitis and arthritis can occur. Rarely, hepatitis, myocarditis, endocarditis, and meningitis can occur.

DIAGNOSIS

■ DIFFERENTIAL DIAGNOSIS
- NGU
- Herpes simplex virus

■ LABORATORY TESTS
- Calcium alginate or rayon swab on a metal shaft (*not* cotton-tipped swabs, which are bactericidal) of the urethra should be done anywhere from 2 to 4 hr after voiding to prevent bacterial washout with voiding.
- Cultures of the pharynx and rectum when indicated.
- Gram staining should be done. Modified Thayer-Martin media is used.
- On examination of the urethral smear, the presence of small numbers of PMNs provides objective evidence of urethritis. The complete absence of PMNs on a urethral smear argues against urethritis. If in addition to the PMNs there are gram-negative, intracellular diplococci, the diagnosis of gonorrhea is established.

TREATMENT

■ NONPHARMACOLOGIC THERAPY
BEHAVIORAL MANAGEMENT: Avoid intercourse until cure has been attained and sexual partners have been evaluated and treated.

■ ACUTE GENERAL Rx
FOR UNCOMPLICATED URETHRAL, CERVICAL, AND RECTAL GCU:
Ceftriaxone 125 mg IM + doxycycline 100 mg bid × 7 days. Alternative therapy: ciprofloxacin 500 mg PO × 1 day; ofloxacin 400 mg PO × 1 day (all of these to be followed by 7 days of doxycycline 100 mg PO bid).

- In uncomplicated gonococcal infections, single-drug regimens using selected fluoroquinolones, selected cephalosporins, or spectinomycin are highly effective and safe.
- Resistance to penicillins, sulphonamides, and tetracyclines is now widespread.
- Dual treatment for gonococcal and chlamydial infections is based on theory and expert opinion rather than on evidence from clinical trials.
FOR EPIDIDYMITIS: Ceftriaxone 250 mg IM followed by doxycycline 100 mg PO bid × 10 days. Alternative therapy: ofloxacin 300 mg PO bid × 10 days.

■ CHRONIC Rx
POSTGONOCOCCAL URETHRITIS (PGU): Reinfection is the most common cause of recurrence. Repeat swab and culture of the urethra, pharynx, and rectum (where applicable) are mandatory. Persistence of PMNs with the absence of gram-negative intracellular diplococci suggests a diagnosis of postgonococcal urethritis. This occurs when GCU is treated with a regimen that is ineffective against coincident chlamydial infection; it represents NGU following GCU. The syndrome should be treated as NGU. Persistence of *N. gonorrhoeae* by smear or culture requires treatment for *N. gonorrhoeae.*

PEARLS & CONSIDERATIONS

■ COMMENTS
- CAUTION: Tetracyclines and fluoroquinolones are *contraindicated* in pregnancy. *Chlamydia* infection in pregnancy can be treated with amoxicillin 500 mg PO tid for 7 days or with clindamycin 450 mg PO tid for 10 days.
- *Posttreatment cultures are required.*

REFERENCE
Centers for Disease Control and Prevention: 2002 sexually transmitted diseases treatment guidelines, *MMWR Morb Mortal Wkly Rep* 51(RR-6), 2002.
Author: **Philip J. Aliotta, M.D., M.S.H.A.**

BASIC INFORMATION

■ DEFINITION
Nongonococcal urethritis is urethral inflammation caused by any of several organisms.

■ SYNONYMS
NGU

ICD-9CM CODES
099.40 Nongonococcal
099.41 Chlamydial

■ EPIDEMIOLOGY & DEMOGRAPHICS
- Occurrence is 50% in STD clinics.
- NGU most commonly affects men in higher socioeconomic class, affecting heterosexual men more frequently than homosexual men.
- NGU carries a greater morbidity than GCU.

■ ETIOLOGY
- Most common agent is *Chlamydia* spp., an obligate intracellular parasite possessing both DNA and RNA, replicating by binary fission. It causes 20% to 50% of NGU cases. Two species exist:
  1. *Chlamydia psittaci*
  2. *Chlamydia trachomatis* with its 15 serotypes
     a. Serotypes A-C cause hyperendemic blinding trachoma.
     b. Serotypes D-K cause genital tract infection.
     c. Serotypes L1-L3 cause lymphogranuloma venereum.
- Other causes of NGU: *Ureaplasma urealyticum* causing 15% to 30% of the cases of NGU, *Trichomonas vaginalis,* and herpes simplex virus. The cause of 20% of the cases of NGU has not been identified.
- Asymptomatic infection occurs in 28% of the contacts of women with chlamydial cervical infection.

INCUBATION PERIOD: 2 to 35 days
SYMPTOMS: Dysuria, whitish-to-clear urethral discharge, and urethral itching. The onset of symptoms in NGU is less acute than GCU.

SIGNS: Whitish-to-clear urethral discharge, meatal edema, and erythema. Infected women manifest pyuria, and the disease can present as acute urethral syndrome.
COMPLICATIONS: Epididymitis in heterosexual men may be linked to nonbacterial prostatitis, proctitis in homosexual men, and Reiter's syndrome.

DIAGNOSIS

■ DIFFERENTIAL DIAGNOSIS
- GCU
- Herpes simplex virus
- Trichomoniasis

■ LABORATORY TESTS
- Requires demonstration of urethritis and exclusion of infection with *N. gonorrhoeae.*
- The appearance of PMNs on urethral smear confirms the diagnosis of urethritis. Because *Chlamydia* is an intracellular parasite of the columnar epithelium, the best specimen for culture is an endourethral swab taken from an area 2 to 4 cm inside the urethra. The organism can only be grown in tissue culture, which is expensive.
- New techniques have been developed and are useful in making the diagnosis: nucleic acid hybridization, enzyme-linked immunosorbent assay (ELISA), and direct immunofluorescence.
- For culture, a Dacron-tipped swab is used; avoid calcium alginate or cotton swabs.

TREATMENT

Because it is impossible to differentiate among the common etiologies of NGU, the condition is treated syndromically, including in the initial treatment regimen those drugs effective against the common causative agents.
- Recommended: doxycycline 100 mg PO bid for 7 days

- Other drugs: tetracycline 500 mg PO qid for 7 days
- Alternative regimens: azithromycin 1000 mg as a single dose, erythromycin 500 mg PO qid for 7 days, ofloxacin 300 mg PO bid for 7 days

In pregnant women:
- Both amoxicillin and erythromycin are likely effective in achieving microbiologic cure.
- Clindamycin and erythromycin have a similar effect on cure rates.
- A single dose of azithromycin is more effective in achieving microbiologic cure of *C. trachomatis* than a 7-day course of erythromycin.

In men and nonpregnant women:
- Multiple-dose regimens of tetracyclines and macrolides achieve microbiologic cure in at least 95% of patients.
- Erythromycin daily dose of 2 g is likely beneficial.
- Ciprofloxacin is less effective in the treatment of *C. trachomatis* infection when compared with doxycycline.
- A single dose of azithromycin is as successful at curing *C. trachomatis* as a 7-day course of doxycycline.

PEARLS & CONSIDERATIONS

■ COMMENTS
- CAUTION: Tetracyclines and fluoroquinolones are *contraindicated* in pregnancy. *Chlamydia* infection in pregnancy can be treated with amoxicillin 500 mg PO tid for 7 days or with clindamycin 450 mg PO tid for 10 days.
- *Posttreatment cultures are required.*

REFERENCES
Centers for Disease Control and Prevention: 2002 sexually transmitted diseases treatment guidelines, *MMWR Morb Mortal Wkly Rep* 51(RR-6), 2002.
Gaydos CA et al: *Chlamydia trachomatis* infections in female military recruits, *N Engl J Med* 339:739, 1998.
Author: Philip J. Aliotta, M.D., M.S.H.A.

BASIC INFORMATION

■ DEFINITION

Urinary tract infection (UTI) is a term that encompasses a broad range of clinical entities that have in common a positive urine culture. A conventional threshold is growth of >100,000 colony-forming units per ml from a midstream-catch urine sample. In symptomatic patients, a smaller number of bacteria (between 100 and 10,000 colony-forming units per ml of midstream urine) is recognized as an infection.

■ SYNONYMS

UTI

ICD-9CM CODES

595.0 Acute cystitis
595.3 Trigonitis
595.2 Chronic cystitis
590.1 Acute pyelonephritis
590.0 Chronic pyelonephritis
590.8 Nonspecific pyelonephritis

■ CLASSIFICATION

FIRST INFECTION: The first documented UTI; tends to be uncomplicated and is easily treated.
UNRESOLVED BACTERIURIA: UTI in which the urinary tract is not sterilized during therapy. Main causes are bacterial resistance, patient noncompliance with medication, resistance, mixed bacterial infection, rapid reinfection, azotemia, infected stones, Munchausen's, and papillary necrosis.
BACTERIAL PERSISTENCE: UTI in which the urine cultures become sterile during therapy, but a persistent source of infection from a site within the urinary tract that was excluded from the high urinary concentrations gives rise to reinfection by the same organism. Causes: infected stone, chronic bacterial prostatitis, atrophic infected kidney, vesicovaginal or enterovesical fistulas, obstructive uropathy, infected pyelocalyceal diverticula, infected ureteral stump following nephrectomy, infected necrotic papillae from papillary necrosis, infected urachal cysts, infected medullary sponge kidney, urethral diverticula, and foreign bodies.
REINFECTION: UTI in which a new infection occurs with new pathogens at variable intervals after a previous infection has been eradicated.
Relapse: The less common form of recurrent infection; occurs within 2 wk of treatment when the same organism reappears in the same site as the previous infection. Relapsing infections of the urinary tract most commonly occur in pyelonephritis, kidney obstruction from a stone, and prostatitis.

■ EPIDEMIOLOGY & DEMOGRAPHICS

INCIDENCE:
In Neonates: More common in boys as a result of anatomic abnormalities.
In Preschool Children: More common in girls (4.5% vs. 0.5% for boys).
In Adulthood: More common in women, with a 1% to 3% prevalence in nonpregnant women. In pregnancy at 12 wk, the incidence of asymptomatic bacteriuria is similar to nonpregnant women, at 2% to 10%. However, 70% to 80% of women with asymptomatic bacteriuria develop acute pyelonephritis, especially in the second and third trimesters, and suffer a pyelonephritic recurrence rate of 10%. In adults, 65 yr and older, at least 10% of men and 20% of women have bacteriuria.
PATHOGENESIS:
• Four major pathways:
  1. Ascending from the urethra
  2. Lymphatic
  3. Hematogenous
  4. Direct extension from another organ system
• Other risk factors: neurologic diseases, renal failure, diabetes; anatomic abnormalities: bladder outlet obstruction, urethral stricture, vesicoureteral reflux, fistula, urinary diversion, megacystis, and infected stones; age; pregnancy; instrumentation, poor patient compliance, poor hygiene, infrequent voider, diaphragm contraceptives, tampon use, douches, and catheters
Catheters: All patients who require a long-term Foley catheter eventually develop significant levels of bacteriuria. Treatment is reserved for those individuals who become symptomatic (i.e., leukocytosis, fever, chills, malaise, loss of appetite, etc.) Using prophylactic antibiotics to treat patients who have chronic catheters is to be discouraged because of the risk of acquiring bacteria that are resistant to antibiotic therapy.
• Once bacteria reach the urinary tract, three factors determine whether the infection occurs (Box 1-24):
  1. Virulence of the microorganism
  2. Inoculum size
  3. Adequacy of the host defense mechanisms
• These factors also determine the anatomic level of the UTI.
Urinary Pathogens: In >95% of UTIs the infecting organism is a member of the Enterobacteriaceae, *Pseudomonas aeruginosa,* enterococci, or, in young women, *Staphylococcus saprophyticus.* In contrast, the organisms that commonly colonize the distal urethra and skin of both men and women and the vagina of women are *Staphylococcus epidermidis,* diphtheroids, lactobacilli, *Gardnerella vaginalis,* and a variety of anaerobes that rarely cause UTI. Generally, the isolation of two or more bacterial species from a urine culture signifies a contaminated specimen, unless the patient is being managed with an indwelling catheter or urinary diversion or has a chronic complicated infection.
Defense Mechanisms Against Cystitis: Low pH and high osmolarity, mucopolysaccharide glycosaminoglycan protective layer, normal bladder that empties completely and has no incontinence, and the presence of estrogen

■ PHYSICAL FINDINGS

• UTI presentation is inconsistent and cannot be relied upon to diagnose UTI accurately or to localize the site of infection. Patients complain of:
  1. Urinary frequency, urgency
  2. Dysuria

BOX 1-24 Bacterial Factors

1. The size of the inoculum
2. The virulence of the infecting organism:
   a. Virulence factors:
      i. P-fimbriae facilitate the adherence of bacteria to biologic surfaces.
      ii. K-antigens facilitate adherence and protect the organisms from the host-immune response.
      iii. O-antigens are an important source of the systemic reactions, such as fever and shock, that occur with bacterial infections.
      iv. H antigens are associated with flagella and are related to bacterial locomotion.
      v. Hemolysin may potentiate tissue damage and facilitate local bacterial growth.
      vi. Urease alkalinizes the urine and facilitates stone formation, thus potentiating infection.
   b. Biofilms harbor bacteria on prosthetic devices and may be a source of recurrent infections.
   c. The presence of sialosyl galactosyl globoside (SGG) on the surface of kidney cells. This compound is a highly powerful receptor for *E. coli* bacteria.
   d. Women with a deficiency in human beta-defensin-1 (HBD-1) are at greater risk for urinary tract infection.
3. Adequacy of host defense mechanisms

3. Urge incontinence
4. Suprapubic pain
5. Gross or microscopic hematuria
- When negative cultures are associated with significant pyuria, vaginal discharge, or hematuria, infections with *Chlamydia trachomatis, Neisseria gonorrhoeae,* and *Trichomonas vaginalis* should be considered.
- Acute pyelonephritis (PN) presents with fever, flank or abdominal pain, chills, malaise, vomiting, and diarrhea. It is these systemic symptoms that distinguish pyelonephritis from cystitis. Complications of acute pyelonephritis are renal abscess, perinephric abscess, emphysematous pyelonephritis, and pyonephrosis.

🔬 DIAGNOSIS

■ DIFFERENTIAL DIAGNOSIS
- Interstitial cystitis
- Vaginitis
- Urethritis (gonococcal, nongonococcal, *Trichomonas*)
- Frequency-urgency syndrome, prostatitis (acute and chronic)
- Obstructive uropathy
- Infected stones
- Fistulas
- Papillary necrosis
- Vesicoureteral reflux

■ LABORATORY TESTS
- Urinalysis with microscopic evaluation of clean-catch urine for bacteria and pyuria
- Urine C&S
- CBC with differential (shows leukocytosis)
- Antibody-coated bacteria are seen with pyelonephritis

■ IMAGING STUDIES
- Warranted only if renal infection or genitourinary abnormality is suspected
- KUB, VCUG, renal sonogram, IVP, CT scan, and nuclear scan
- Specialty examination: cystoscopy with occasional retrograde pyelography to rule out obstructive uropathy; stenting the obstruction possibly required

℞ TREATMENT

■ NONPHARMACOLOGIC THERAPY
- Hot sitz baths, anticholinergics, urinary analgesics
- For pyelonephritis: bed rest, analgesics, antipyretics, and IV hydration

■ ACUTE GENERAL Rx
- Conventional therapy of 7 days; short-term therapy of 1, 3, or 5 days.
- Agents of choice: amoxicillin/clavulanate, cephalosporins, fluoro-

quinolones, nitrofurantoin, and trimethoprim with sulfonamide.
- For pyelonephritis: hospitalization until afebrile and stable, then at home via home care agency with IV antibiotic composed of aminoglycoside plus cephalosporin × 1 wk followed by oral agents (based on sensitivity) for 2 wk. Moderate forms of pyelonephritis have been successfully treated with fluoroquinolone therapy for 21 days, without requiring hospitalization. Most important, complicating factors such as obstructive uropathy or infected stones must be identified and treated.
- Section III, Fig. 3-187 describes an approach to the management of UTI.

☼ PEARLS & CONSIDERATIONS

■ COMMENTS
- *Asymptomatic bacteriuria:* occurs in both anatomically normal and abnormal urinary tracts. This can clear spontaneously, persist, or lead to symptomatic kidney infection. Treatment is recommended in patients with vesicoureteral reflux, stones, obstructive uropathy, parenchymal renal disease, diabetes mellitus, and pregnant or immunocompromised patients.
- *Pregnancy:* 20% to 40% of pregnant women with untreated bacteriuria develop pyelonephritis. This is associated with prematurity and low-birth-weight infants. Confirmed significant bacteriuria should be treated with an aminopenicillin and cephalosporin.
- *Recurrent UTI:* caused by an unresolved infection, vaginal colonization of the originally infecting organism, or reinfection with a new strain. Management of recurrent UTI includes continuous antibiotic prophylaxis, intermittent self-treatment, and postcoital prophylaxis. Prophylaxis is recommended for women who experience two or more symptomatic UTIs over a 6-mo period or three or more episodes over a 12-mo period.
  1. Changes after menopause: lower levels of lactobacilli, decreased estrogen, senile atrophy of the genitalia, and loss of bladder elasticity (compliance).
  2. Biologic factors altering defense systems: the presence of sialosyl galactosyl globoside (SGG) on the surface of the kidney acts as a powerful receptor for *E. coli* and increases the risk for UTI; the presence of the blood group P1 causes increased binding of *E. coli* that is resistant to normal infection-fighting mechanisms in the body and it is believed that some individuals are deficient in a compound called *human beta-*

defensin-1 (HBD-1), a naturally occurring antibiotic that fights *E. coli* within the urinary tract.
Resistance:
- Because of the overuse of antibiotics, organisms once sensitive to a number of agents are now increasingly more resistant, making effective management of UTI and pyelonephritis more difficult and potentially more dangerous. Most important has been the increasing resistance to TMP-SMX, the current primary care provider drug of choice for acute uncomplicated UTI in women.
- Facts about bacterial resistance:
  1. Given enough antibiotic and time, resistance will develop
  2. Organisms that are resistant to one antibiotic will likely become resistant to others
  3. Resistance is progressive, moving from low to intermediate to high levels
  4. Once selected, drug resistance will not disappear; because of poorly reversible genetic and environmental factors, it may decline slowly
  5. When antibiotics are used by any patient, this use affects other people by changing the immediate and extended environment
  6. No counterselective steps against resistant bacteria now exist
- When choosing a treatment regimen physicians should consider such factors as:
  1. In-vitro susceptibility
  2. Adverse effects
  3. Cost effectiveness
  4. Resistance rates in the respective communities

REFERENCES

Bent S et al: Does this woman have an acute uncomplicated urinary tract infection? *JAMA* 287:2701, 2002.

Gomolin IH et al: Efficacy and safety of ciprofloxacin oral suspension versus trimethoprim-sulfamethoxazole oral suspension for treatment of older women with acute urinary tract infection, *J Am Geriatr Soc* 49:1606, 2001.

Gupta K et al: Increasing antimicrobial resistance and the management of uncomplicated community-acquired urinary tract infections, *Ann Int Med* 135:41, 2001.

Levy SB: Multidrug resistance—a sign of the times, *N Engl J Med* 338:1376, 1998 [editorial].

McIsaac WJ et al: The impact of empirical management of acute cystitis on unnecessary antibiotic use, *Arch Int Med* 161:600, 2002.

Saint S et al: The effectiveness of a clinical practical guideline for the management of presumed uncomplicated UTI in women, *Am J Med* 106:636, 1999.

Author: **Philip J. Aliotta, M.D., M.S.H.A.**

BASIC INFORMATION

■ DEFINITION

Urolithiasis is the presence of calculi within the urinary tract. The five major types of urinary stones are calcium oxalate (>50%), calcium phosphate (10% to 20%), uric acid (8%), struvite (15%), and cystine (3%).

■ SYNONYMS

Nephrolithiasis
Renal colic

ICD-9CM CODES
592.9 Urinary calculus

■ EPIDEMIOLOGY & DEMOGRAPHICS

- Urinary stone disease afflicts 250,000 to 750,000 Americans/yr.
- Male:female ratio is 4:1. After the sixth decade, the ratio is 1.5:1.
- Incidence of symptomatic nephrolithiasis is greatest during the summer (resulting from increased humidity and temperatures with increased risk of dehydration and concentrated urine).
- Calcium oxalate or mixed calcium oxalate/calcium phosphate stones account for 70% of urolithiasis.

■ PHYSICAL FINDINGS & CLINICAL PRESENTATION

Stones may be asymptomatic or may cause the following signs and symptoms from obstruction:
- Sudden onset of flank tenderness
- Nausea and vomiting
- Patient in constant movement, attempting to lessen the pain (patients with an acute abdomen are usually still because movement exacerbates the pain)
- Pain may be referred to the testes or labium (progression of stone down the urinary ureter)

- Fever and chills accompanying the acute colic if there is superimposed infection
- Pain may radiate anteriorly over to the abdomen and result in intestinal ileus

■ ETIOLOGY

- Increased absorption of calcium in the small bowel: type I absorptive hypercalciuria (independent of calcium intake)
- Idiopathic hypercalciuria nephrolithiasis is the most common diagnosis for patients with calcium stones; the diagnosis is made only if there is no hypercalcemia and no known cause for hypercalciuria
- Increased vitamin D synthesis (e.g., secondary to renal phosphate loss: type III absorptive hypercalciuria)
- Renal tubular malfunction with inadequate reabsorption of calcium and resulting hypercalciuria
- Heterozygous mutations in the NPT2a gene result in hypophosphatemia and urinary phosphate loss
- Hyperparathyroidism with resulting hypercalcemia
- Elevated uric acid level (metabolic defects, dietary excess)
- Chronic diarrhea (e.g., inflammatory bowel disease) with increased oxalate absorption
- Type I (distal tubule) renal tubular acidosis (<1% of calcium stones)
- Chronic hydrochlorothiazide treatment
- Chronic infections with urease-producing organisms (e.g., *Proteus, Providencia, Pseudomonas, Klebsiella*). Struvite, or magnesium ammonium phosphate crystals, are produced when the urinary tract is colonized by bacteria, producing elevated concentrations of ammonia
- Abnormal excretion of cystine
- Chemotherapy for malignancies

DIAGNOSIS

■ DIFFERENTIAL DIAGNOSIS

- Urinary tract infection
- Pyelonephritis
- Diverticulitis
- PID
- Ovarian pathology
- Factitious (drug addicts)
- Appendicitis
- Small bowel obstruction
- Ectopic pregnancy
- The differential diagnosis of obstructive uropathy is described in Section II

■ WORKUP

- Laboratory and imaging studies. Stone analysis should be performed on recovered stones.
- A clinical algorithm for evaluation of nephrolithiasis is described in Section III.
- Box 1-25 describes past medical history significant for urolithiasis.

■ LABORATORY TESTS

- Urinalysis: hematuria may be present; however, its absence does not exclude urinary stones. Evaluation of urinary pH is of value in identification of type of stone (pH >7.5 is associated with struvite stones, whereas pH <5 generally is seen with uric acid or with cystine stones).
- Urine C&S should be obtained for all patients.
- Serum chemistries should include calcium, electrolytes, phosphate, and uric acid.
- Additional tests: 24-hr urine collection for calcium, uric acid, phosphate, oxalate, and citrate excretion is generally reserved for patients with recurrent stones.

BOX 1-25   Past Medical History Significant for Urolithiasis

Diseases associated with disturbances of calcium metabolism: primary hyperparathyroidism, Wilson's disease, medullary sponge kidney, osteoporosis, immobilization, sarcoidosis, osteolytic metastases, plasmacytoma, neuroendocrine tumors, Paget's disease
    Dietary history: purine gluttony, calcium excess, milk alkali, oxalate excess, sodium excess, low citrus fruit intake
    Medications: uricosurics, diuretics, analgesics, vitamins C and D, antacids (especially phosphorus-binding agents), acetazolamide, calcium channel blockers, triamterene, theophylline, protease inhibitors (indinavir), sulfonamides
Diseases associated with disturbances of oxalate metabolism: primary hyperoxaluria types I and II, Crohn's disease, ulcerative colitis, intestinal bypass surgery (especially jejunoileal bypass), ileal resection
Diseases associated with disturbances of purine metabolism
    Intrinsic metabolic disorders—anemia, neoplastic disorders (especially leukemias), intoxication, myocardial infarction, irradiation, cytotoxic chemotherapy
    Enzyme deficiency—primary gout, Lesch-Nyhan syndrome
    Altered excretion—renal insufficiency, metabolic acidosis
    Infectious history: organisms (particularly *Proteus* and *Klebsiella*), febrile upper tract involvement and dates if hospitalized.

From Nseyo UO (ed): *Urology for primary care physicians*, Philadelphia, 1999, WB Saunders.

■ IMAGING STUDIES

- Plain films of the abdomen can identify radioopaque stones (calcium, uric acid stones).
- Renal sonogram may be helpful.
- IVP demonstrates the size and location of the stone, as well as degree of obstruction.
- Unenhanced (noncontrast) helical CT scan does not require contrast media and can visualize the calculus (identified by the "rim sign" or "halo" representing the edematous ureteral wall around the stone). It is fast, accurate (sensitivity 15% to 100%, specificity 94% to 96%), and readily identifies all stone types in all locations. This modality is being used increasingly in the initial assessment of renal colic.

■ TREATMENT

■ NONPHARMACOLOGIC THERAPY

- Increase in water or other fluid intake (doubling of previous fluid intake unless patient has a history of CHF or fluid overload)
- Normal dietary calcium intake. If one does not consume enough calcium, less is available to bind to dietary oxalate; as a result, more oxalate reaches the colon, is absorbed into the bloodstream, and is excreted as calcium oxalate, setting the stage for calcium urolithiasis.
- Sodium restriction (to decrease calcium excretion), decreased protein intake to 1 g/kg/day (to decrease uric acid, calcium, and oxalate excretion)
- Increase in bran (may decrease bowel transit time with increased binding of calcium and subsequent decrease in urinary calcium)

■ ACUTE GENERAL Rx

- Pain control (use of narcotics is generally indicated because of the severity of pain)
- Specific therapy tailored to the stone type:
  1. Uric acid calculi: control of hyperuricosuria with allopurinol 100 to 300 mg/day; increase urinary pH with potassium citrate, 10-mEq tablets tid
  2. Calcium stones:
     a. HCTZ 25 to 50 mg qd in patients with type I absorptive hypercalciuria

---

b. Decrease bowel absorption of calcium with cellulose phosphate 10 g/day in patients with type I absorptive hypercalciuria
c. Orthophosphates to inhibit vitamin B synthesis in patients with type III absorptive hypercalciuria
d. Potassium citrate supplementation in patients with hypocitraturic calcium nephrolithiasis
e. Purine dietary restrictions or allopurinol in patients with hyperuricosuric calcium nephrolithiasis

3. Struvite stones:
   a. Most of the stones are large and cause obstruction and bleeding.
   b. ESWL and percutaneous nephrolithotomy are generally necessary.
   c. Prolonged use of antibiotics directed against the predominant urinary tract organism may be beneficial to prevent recurrence.
4. Cystine stones: Hydration and alkalization of the urine to pH >6.5, penicillamine, and tiopronin can also be used to reduce the formation of cystine; captopril is also beneficial and causes fewer side effects

- Surgical treatment in patients with severe pain unresponsive to medication and patients with persistent fever or nausea or significant impediment of urine flow:
  a. Ureteroscopic stone extraction
  b. Extracorporeal shock wave lithotripsy (ESWL) for most renal stones
- In 1997 the American Urological Association issued the following guidelines for the treatment of ureteral stones:
  1. Proximal ureteral stones <1 cm in diameter: options are ESWL, percutaneous nephroureterolithotomy, and ureteroscopy
  2. Proximal ureteral stones >1 cm in diameter: options are ESWL, percutaneous nephroureterolithotomy, and ureteroscopy. Placement of a ureteral stent should be considered if the stone is causing high-grade obstruction
  3. Distal ureteral stones <1 cm in diameter: most of these pass spontaneously. ESWL and ureteroscopy are two accepted modes of therapy

---

4. Distal ureteral stones >1 cm in diameter: watchful waiting, ESWL, ureteroscopy (following stone fragmentation)

- Section III describes an approach to the management of ureteral calculi.

■ CHRONIC Rx

Maintenance of proper hydration and dietary restrictions (see "Acute General Rx")

■ DISPOSITION

- >50% of patients will pass the stone within 48 hr.
- Stones will recur in approximately 50% of patients within 5 yr if no medical treatment is provided.

■ REFERRAL

Urology referral in complicated or recurrent urolithiasis; most patients with small uncomplicated ureteral or renal calculi can be followed as outpatient, whereas patients with persistent vomiting, suspected UTI, pain unresponsive to oral analgesics, or obstructing calculus associated with solitary kidney should be admitted

☼ PEARLS & CONSIDERATIONS

■ COMMENTS

- Early identification and aggressive treatment of urinary tract infections is indicated in all patients with struvite stones.
- Alkalinization of urine (pH >7.5 with penicillamine) is useful in patients with recurrent cystine stones.
- An algorithmic approach to the management of ureteral calculi is described in Section III.

REFERENCES

Borghi L et al: Comparison of two diets for the prevention of recurrent stones in idiopathic hypercalciuria, *N Engl J Med* 346:77, 2002.

Prie D et al: Nephrolithiasis and osteoporosis associated with hypophosphatemia caused by mutations in the type 2a sodium-phosphate cotransporter, *N Engl J Med* 347:983, 2002.

Worster A et al: The accuracy of noncontrast helical computed tomography versus intravenous pyelography in the diagnosis of suspected acute urolithiasis: a meta-analysis, *Ann Intern Med* 40:280, 2002.

Author: **Fred F. Ferri, M.D.**

BASIC INFORMATION

DEFINITION

Urticaria is a pruritic rash involving the epidermis and the upper portions of the dermis, resulting from localized capillary vasodilation and followed by transudation of protein-rich fluid in the surrounding tissue and manifesting clinically with the presence of hives.

SYNONYMS

Hives
Wheals

ICD-9CM CODES

708.8 Other unspecified urticaria

EPIDEMIOLOGY & DEMOGRAPHICS

- At least 20% of the population will have one episode of hives during their lifetime.
- Incidence is increased in atopic patients.
- The etiology of chronic urticaria (hives lasting longer than 6 wk) is determined in only 5% to 20% of cases.

PHYSICAL FINDINGS & CLINICAL PRESENTATION

- Presence of elevated, erythematous, or white nonpitting plaques that change in size and shape over time; they generally last a few hours and disappear without a trace.
- Annular configuration with central pallor (Fig. 1-286).

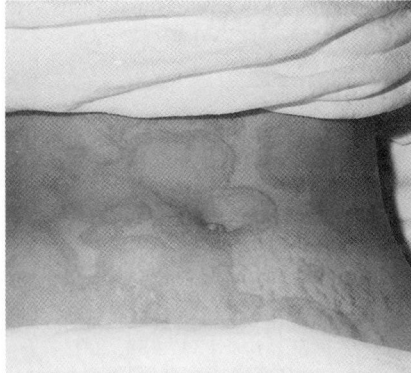

Fig. 1-286   Wheal (urticaria). Note central cleaning, giving annular configuration. (From Noble J et al: *Textbook of primary care medicine*, ed 3, St Louis, 2001, Mosby.)

ETIOLOGY

- Foods (e.g., shellfish, eggs, strawberries, nuts)
- Drugs (e.g., penicillin, aspirin, sulfonamides)
- Systemic diseases (e.g., SLE, serum sickness, autoimmune thyroid disease, polycythemia vera)
- Food additives (e.g., salicylates, benzoates, sulfites)
- Infections (viral infections, fungal infections, chronic bacterial infections)
- Physical stimuli (e.g., pressure urticaria, exercise-induced, solar urticaria, cold urticaria)
- Inhalants (e.g., mold spores, animal danders, pollens)
- Contact (nonimmunologic) urticaria (e.g., caterpillars, plants)
- Other: hereditary angioedema, urticaria pigmentosa, pregnancy, cold urticaria, hair bleaches, chemicals, saliva, cosmetics, perfumes, pemphigoid, emotional stress

DIAGNOSIS

DIFFERENTIAL DIAGNOSIS

- Erythema multiforme
- Erythema marginatum
- Erythema infectiosum
- Urticarial vasculitis
- Herpes gestationis
- Drug eruption
- Multiple insect bites
- Bullous pemphigoid

WORKUP

- It is useful to determine whether hives are acute or chronic; a medical history focused on various etiologic factors is necessary before embarking on extensive laboratory testing.
- A diagnostic approach to chronic urticaria is described in Section III, Fig. 3-188.

LABORATORY TESTS

- CBC with differential
- Stool for ova and parasites in patients with suspected parasitic infestations
- ANA, ESR, TSH, LFTs, eosinophil count are indicated only in selected patients
- Measurement of C_4 in patients who present with angioedema alone
- Skin biopsy is helpful in patients with fever, arthralgias, and elevated ESR

TREATMENT

NONPHARMACOLOGIC THERAPY

- Remove suspected etiologic agents (e.g., stop aspirin and all nonessential drugs), restrict diet (e.g., elimination of tomatoes, nuts, eggs, shellfish).
- Elimination of yeast should be attempted in patients with chronic urticaria (*Candida albicans* sensitivity may be a factor in patients with chronic urticaria).

ACUTE GENERAL Rx

- Oral antihistamines: use of nonsedating antihistamines (e.g., loratadine [Claritin] 10 mg qd or cetirizine [Zyrtec] 10 mg qd) is preferred over first-generation antihistamines (e.g., hydroxyzine, diphenhydramine).
- Doxepin (a tricyclic antidepressant) that blocks both H_1 and H_2 receptors 25 to 75 mg qhs may be effective in patients with chronic urticaria.
- Oral corticosteroids should be reserved for refractory cases (e.g., prednisone 20 mg qd or 20 mg bid).
- H_2 receptor antagonists (cimetidine, ranitidine, famotidine) can be added to H_1 antagonists in refractory cases.

CHRONIC Rx

- Use of nonsedating antihistamines, doxepin, and/or oral corticosteroids (see "Acute General Rx")
- Low dose of the immunosuppressant cyclosporine (2.5 to 3 mg/kg body weight/day) has been shown to be effective and corticosteroid sparing in chronic urticaria
- There is insufficient data to support use of leukotriene antagonists (zafirlukast, montelukast) in patients with chronic urticaria

DISPOSITION

- Most cases of urticaria resolve within 6 wk.
- Only 25% of patients with a history of chronic urticaria are completely cured after 5 yr.

PEARLS & CONSIDERATIONS

COMMENTS

Local treatment (e.g., starch baths or Aveeno baths) may be helpful in selected patients; however, local treatment is generally not rewarding.

REFERENCE

Kaplan AP: Chronic urticaria and angioedema, *N Engl J Med* 346:157, 2002.
Author: **Fred F. Ferri, M.D.**

BASIC INFORMATION

■ DEFINITION
Uterine malignancy includes tumors from the endometrium (discussed elsewhere in this text) and sarcomas. Uterine sarcoma is an abnormal proliferation of cells originating from the mesenchymal, or connective tissue, elements of the uterine wall.

■ SYNONYMS
Leiomyosarcomas
Endometrial stromal sarcoma
Malignant mixed mullerian tumors
Adenosarcomas

ICD-9CM CODES
182.0 Malignant neoplasm of body of uterus (corpus uteri), except isthmus
182.1 Malignant neoplasm of body of uterus, isthmus
182.8 Malignant neoplasm of body of uterus, other specified sites of body of uterus

■ EPIDEMIOLOGY & DEMOGRAPHICS
PREVALENCE: Uterine sarcoma accounts for 4.3% of all cancers of the uterine corpus and is the most lethal gynecologic malignancy.
INCIDENCE: 17.1 cases/1 million females
MEAN AGE AT DIAGNOSIS: The age at diagnosis is variable. Mean age at diagnosis is 52 yr.
RISK FACTORS: Similar to endometrial carcinoma

■ PHYSICAL FINDINGS & CLINICAL PRESENTATION
• Abnormal vaginal bleeding is the most common symptom
• May also present as pelvic pain or pressure and pelvic mass on examination
• May appear as tumor protruding through the cervix
• Vaginal discharge may also be a presenting symptom
• Rapidly enlarging uterus

■ ETIOLOGY
• The exact etiology is unknown.
• Prior pelvic radiation is a risk factor for sarcoma.
• Black women may be at higher risk.

DIAGNOSIS

■ DIFFERENTIAL DIAGNOSIS
Leiomyoma

■ WORKUP
Diagnosis is made histologically by biopsy for abnormal bleeding.

■ LABORATORY TESTS
Chest radiography, CT scans, and MRI are used to evaluate spread.

■ IMAGING STUDIES
• Chest radiography is usually done as routine preoperative testing.
• CT scans and MRI are good for assessing tumor spread once diagnosis is made.

TREATMENT

■ NONPHARMACOLOGIC THERAPY
• Surgery excision is the mainstay of treatment.
• Grade and stage of tumor affect prognosis (Fig. 1-287).
• Adjuvant radiotherapy may improve pelvic disease control, but it does not improve survival.
• Chemotherapeutic agents have produced only partial and short-term responses.

■ DISPOSITION
• Survival varies with each type of sarcoma but is generally very poor.

• Five-year survival for leiomyosarcoma ranges from 48% for stage I to 0% for stage IV.
• Five-year survival for malignant mixed mesodermal tumor ranges from 36% for stage I to 6% for stage IV.

■ REFERRAL
Uterine sarcoma should be managed by a gynecologic oncologist and radiation oncologist.

REFERENCES
Elima Y et al: Para-aortic lymph node metastasis in relation to serum CA 125 levels and nuclear grade in endometrial carcinoma, *Acta Obstet Gynecol Scond* 81(5):458, 2002.
Pitsm G et al: Stage II endometrial carcinoma: prognostic factors and risk classification in 170 patients, *Intern J Radiat Oncol Biol Physics* 53(4):862, 2002.
Author: **Gil Farkash**, M.D.

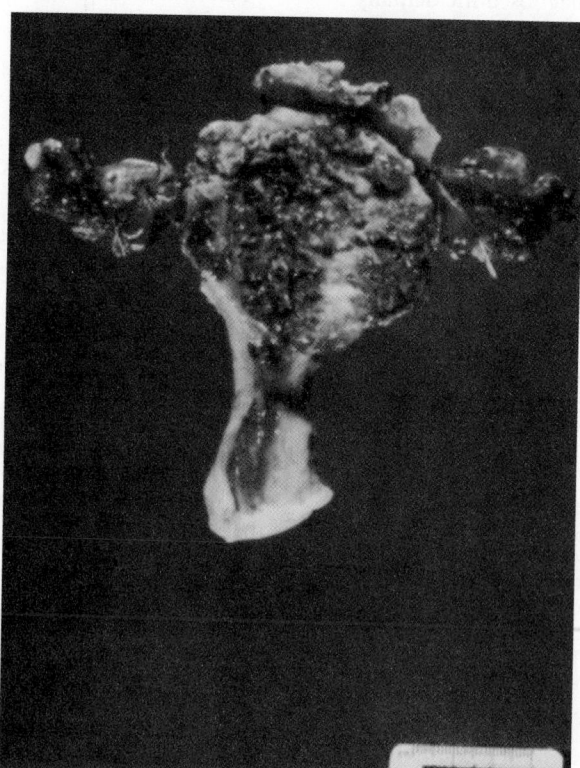

Fig. 1-287 This grade 3 adenocarcinoma demonstrates extensive myometrial invasion. The tumor has penetrated the uterine serosa and extends onto the fundus and into the upper left broad ligament. (From Copeland LJ: *Textbook of gynecology*, ed 2, Philadelphia, 2000, WB Saunders.)

BASIC INFORMATION

■ DEFINITION
Uterine myomas are discrete nodular tumors that vary in size and number and that may be found subserosal, intramucosal, or submucosal within the uterus or may be found in the cervix or broad ligament or on a pedicle.

■ SYNONYMS
Leiomyomas, fibroids

ICD-9CM CODES
218.9 Leiomyomas, fibroids

■ EPIDEMIOLOGY & DEMOGRAPHICS
- Estimated presence in at least 20% of all reproductive age women
- The most common benign uterine tumor
- More common in black than in white women
- Asymptomatic fibroids may be present in 40% to 50% of women >40 yr of age
- May occur singly but are often multiple
- Fewer than half of all fibroids are estimated to produce symptoms
- Frequently diagnosed incidentally on pelvic examination
- There is increased familial incidence
- Potential to enlarge during pregnancy, as well as to regress after menopause
- Infrequent primary cause of infertility in <3% of infertile patients

■ PHYSICAL FINDINGS & CLINICAL PRESENTATION
- Enlarged, irregular uterus on pelvic examination.
- Presenting symptoms:
  1. Menorrhagia (most common)
  2. Chronic pelvic pain (dysmenorrhea, dyspareunia, pelvic pressure)
  3. Acute pain (torsion of pedunculated myoma, infarction, and degeneration)
  4. Urinary symptoms (frequency from bladder pressure, partial ureteral obstruction, complete ureteral obstruction)
  5. Rectosigmoid compression with constipation or intestinal obstruction
  6. Prolapse through cervix of pedunculated submucosal tumor
  7. Venous stasis of lower extremities
  8. Polycythemia
  9. Ascites

■ ETIOLOGY
Unknown. It is suggested that myomas arise from a single neoplastic smooth muscle cell in the myometrium. Malignant degeneration of preexisting leiomyoma is extremely uncommon (<0.5%).

DIAGNOSIS

■ DIFFERENTIAL DIAGNOSIS
Leiomyosarcoma, ovarian mass (neoplastic, nonneoplastic, endometrioma), inflammatory mass, pregnancy

■ WORKUP
- Complete pelvic examination, rectovaginal examination, Pap test
- Estimation of size of mass in centimeters
- Endometrial sampling may be indicated (biopsy or D&C) when abnormal bleeding and pelvic mass are present
- If urinary symptoms are prominent, cystometry, cystoscopy to rule out bladder lesions, IVP to rule out impingement on urinary system

■ LABORATORY TESTS
- Pregnancy test
- Pap smear
- CBC, ESR
- Fecal occult blood

■ IMAGING STUDIES
- Pelvic ultrasound (transvaginal may have higher diagnostic accuracy) is useful.
- CT scan is helpful in planning treatment if malignancy is strongly suspected.
- Hysteroscopy may provide direct evidence of intrauterine pathology or submucosal leiomyoma that distorts uterine cavity.

TREATMENT

Management should be based on primary symptoms and may include observation with close follow-up, temporizing surgical therapies, medical management, or definitive surgical procedures.

■ NONSURGICAL Rx
- Patient observation and follow-up with periodic repeat pelvic examinations to ensure that tumors are not growing rapidly.
- GnRH agonist use results in 40% to 60% reduction in uterine volume. Hypoestrogenism, reversible bone loss, hot flushes associated with use. Limit to short-term use and consider low-dose hormonal replacement to minimize hypoestrogenic effects.
- Regrowth occurs in about 50% of women treated a few months after cessation.
- Indications for GnRH:
  1. Fertility preservation in women with large myomas before attempting conception or preoperative myectomy treatment
  2. Anemia treatment to normalize hemoglobin before surgery
  3. Women approaching menopause to avoid surgery
  4. Preoperative for large myomas to make vaginal hysterectomy, hysteroscopic resection/ablation, or laparoscopic destruction more feasible
  5. Women with medical contraindications for surgery
  6. Personal or medical indications for delaying surgery
- Progestational agents may also result in decrease in uterine size and amenorrhea, allowing iron therapy to treat anemia with limited success.

■ SURGICAL Rx
- Indications
  1. Abnormal uterine bleeding with anemia, refractory to hormonal therapy
  2. Chronic pain with severe dysmenorrhea, dyspareunia, or lower abdominal pressure/pain
  3. Acute pain, torsion, or prolapsing submucosal fibroid
  4. Urinary symptoms or signs such as hydronephrosis
  5. Rapid uterine enlargement premenopausal or any postmenopausal increase in size
  6. Infertility with leiomyoma as only finding
  7. Enlarged uterus with compression symptoms or discomfort
- Procedures
  1. Hysterectomy (definitive procedure)
  2. Abdominal myomectomy (to preserve fertility)
  3. Vaginal myomectomy for prolapsed pedunculated submucous fibroid
  4. Hysteroscopic resection
  5. Laparoscopic myomectomy
  6. Uterine fibroid embolization

■ REFERRAL
Consultation with gynecologic oncologist if suspicion of malignancy

REFERENCE
DeWaay DJ et al: Natural history of uterine polyps and leiomyomata, *Obstet Gynecol* 100:3, 2002.
Author: **Eugene J. Louie-Ng, M.D.**

BASIC INFORMATION

■ DEFINITION

Uterine prolapse refers to the protrusion of the uterus into or out of the vaginal canal. In a *first-degree uterine prolapse,* the cervix is visible when the perineum is depressed. In a *second-degree uterine prolapse,* the uterine cervix has prolapsed through the vaginal introitus, with the fundus remaining within the pelvis proper. In a *third-degree uterine prolapse* (i.e., *complete uterine prolapse, uterine procidentia*), the entire uterus is outside the introitus.

■ SYNONYMS

Genital prolapse
Uterine descensus
Pelvic organ prolapse

ICD-9CM CODES

618.8 Genital prolapse
618.1 Uterine descensus
618.8 Pelvic organ prolapse

■ EPIDEMIOLOGY & DEMOGRAPHICS

Most prevalent in postmenopausal multiparous women.
RISK FACTORS:
• Pregnancy
• Labor
• Vaginal childbirth
• Obesity
• Chronic coughing
• Constipation
• Pelvic tumors
• Ascites
• Strenuous physical exertion
• Caucasian race
GENETICS: Increased incidence in women with spina bifida occulta.

■ PHYSICAL FINDINGS & CLINICAL PRESENTATION

• Pelvic pressure
• Bearing-down sensation
• Bilateral groin pain
• Sacral backache
• Coital difficulty
• Protrusion from vagina
• Spotting
• Ulceration
• Bleeding
• Examination of patient in lithotomy, sitting, and standing positions and before, during, and after a maximum Valsalva effort
• Erosion or ulceration of the cervix possible in the most dependent area of the protrusion

■ ETIOLOGY

• Vaginal childbirth and chronic increases in intraabdominal pressure leading to detachments, lacerations, and denervations of the vaginal support system
• Further weakening of pelvic support system by hypoestrogenic atrophy
• Some cases from congenital or inherited weaknesses within the pelvic support system
• Neonatal uterine prolapse mostly coexistent with congenital spinal defects

DIAGNOSIS

■ DIFFERENTIAL DIAGNOSIS

Occasionally, elongated cervix; body of the uterus remains undescended

■ WORKUP

• Diagnosis is based on history and physical examination.
• If erosion or ulceration of the cervix is present, a Pap smear followed by a cervical biopsy should be performed if indicated.
• If urinary symptoms are significant, further urodynamic workup is indicated, looking for concurrent cystourethrocele, cystocele, enterocele, or rectocele.

■ LABORATORY TESTS

Urine culture

■ IMAGING STUDIES

Ultrasound if concurrent fibroids need further evaluation

TREATMENT

■ NONPHARMACOLOGIC THERAPY

• Prophylactic measures
  1. Diagnosis and treatment of chronic respiratory and metabolic disorders
  2. Correction of constipation
  3. Weight control, nutrition, and smoking cessation counseling
  4. Teaching of pelvic muscle exercises
• Supportive pessary therapy
  1. Ring-type pessary useful for first- or second-degree prolapse
  2. Gellhorn pessary preferred for more advanced prolapse
  3. Use of pessaries in conjunction with continuous hormone replacement therapy, unless contraindicated
  4. Perineorrhaphy under local anesthesia possibly needed to support the pessary if the vaginal outlet is very relaxed

■ ACUTE GENERAL Rx

• Patients who are only infrequently symptomatic: insertion of a tampon or diaphragm for temporary relief when prolonged standing is anticipated
• Neonatal uterine prolapse: simple digital reduction or the use of a small pessary

■ CHRONIC Rx

• Hormone replacement therapy at the time of menopause helps preserve tissue strength, maintain elasticity of the vagina, and promote the durability of surgical repairs.
• Gold standard for therapy is vaginal hysterectomy.
• Vaginal apex should be well suspended, but a prophylactic sacrospinous ligament fixation is not routinely required.
• If occult enterocele present, McCall culdoplasty is performed.
• If vaginal approach to hysterectomy is contraindicated, abdominal hysterectomy is performed; vaginal apex likewise well supported.
• Colpocleisis is considered for the elderly patient who is sexually inactive and is a high-risk patient from a surgical point of view; can be done rapidly under local anesthesia with mild sedation if necessary.
• For symptomatic women who desire childbearing: management with pessaries or pelvic muscle exercises is recommended; if surgical correction is required, transvaginal sacrospinous fixation is the preferred method.
• Other surgical options are sling operations and sacral cervicopexy.

■ DISPOSITION

If untreated, uterine prolapse progressively worsens.

■ REFERRAL

To a gynecologist if pessary fitting or surgical intervention is needed

PEARLS & CONSIDERATIONS

■ COMMENTS

Surgery contraindicated in mild or asymptomatic uterine prolapse because the patient will seldom benefit from the operation although exposed to its risks.

REFERENCES

Glass RH, Curtis MG, Hopkins MP: *Glass' office gynecology,* ed 5, Baltimore, 1999, Lippincott Williams & Wilkins.
Thaker R: Management of uterine prolapse, *BMJ* 324:1258, 2002.
Author: **Wan J. Kim, M.D.**

BASIC INFORMATION

■ DEFINITION
Uveitis is inflammation of the uveal tract, including the iris, ciliary body, and choroid. It may also involve other closed structures such as the sclera, retina, and vitreous humor.

■ SYNONYMS
Anterior uveitis
Posterior uveitis
Acute or chronic uveitis
Granulomatous or nongranulomatous uveitis

ICD-9CM CODES
364.3 Unspecified iridocyclitis, uveitis

■ EPIDEMIOLOGY & DEMOGRAPHICS
INCIDENCE (IN U.S.): Common; busy ophthalmologist will see two or more cases per week
PREVALENCE (IN U.S.): 17 cases/100,000 persons
PREDOMINANT SEX: None
PREDOMINANT AGE: 38 yr
PEAK INCIDENCE: Middle age or older

■ PHYSICAL FINDINGS & CLINICAL PRESENTATION
- Photophobia
- Blurred visual acuity
- Irregular pupil
- Hazy cornea
- Abnormal cells and flare in anterior chamber or vitreous humor
- Retinal hemorrhage, vascular sheathing (Fig. 1-288)
- Conjunctival injection
- Ciliary flush
- Keratitic precipitates (precipitates on the cornea)
- Hazy vitreous
- Retinal inflammation
- Iris nodules
- Glaucoma

DIAGNOSIS

■ DIFFERENTIAL DIAGNOSIS
- Glaucoma
- Conjunctivitis
- Retinal detachment
- Retinopathy
- Keratitis
- Scleritis
- Episcleritis

■ WORKUP
- Associated with arthritis, syphilis, tuberculosis, granulomatous disease, collagen-vascular disease, allergies, AIDS, sarcoid, Behçet's disease, histoplasmosis, and toxoplasmosis
- Slit lamp examination, indirect ophthalmoscopy

■ LABORATORY TESTS
- CBC
- Laboratory tests for specific inflammatory causes cited previously in "Workup" (e.g., ANA, ESR, VDRL, HLA-B27 PPD, Lyme titer)

■ IMAGING STUDIES
- Chest x-ray examination in suspected sarcoidosis, TB, histoplasmosis
- Sacroiliac x-ray examination in suspected ankylosing spondylitis

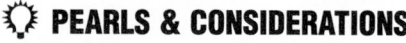 TREATMENT

■ NONPHARMACOLOGIC THERAPY
Treat the underlying disease.

■ ACUTE GENERAL Rx
- Cycloplegic drops (cyclopentolate [Cyclogyl]) or cycloplegic agents (homatropine hydrobromide [Optic] 1gtt q3-4h while awake) and topical steroids (prednisone acetate 1% 1 gtt qh during day, prn at night until favorable response, then q4-6h); avoid topical corticosteroids in infectious uveitis
- Antibiotics when infection is suspected
- Systemic steroids if appropriate for the underlying disease

■ CHRONIC Rx
Topical steroids and cycloplegics

■ DISPOSITION
Urgent referral to ophthalmologist

■ REFERRAL
- Eye problem should be followed early on by an ophthalmologist.
- Underlying medical disease should be treated by the primary care physician.

PEARLS & CONSIDERATIONS

■ COMMENTS
- In 90% of cases, the condition is idiopathic.
- Associated causes are found approximately 10% of the time, usually chronic and recurrent.

REFERENCE
Gardiner AM et al: Correlation between visual function and visual ability in patients with uveitis, *Br J Ophthmol* 86(9):993, 2002.
Author: **Melvyn Koby, M.D.**

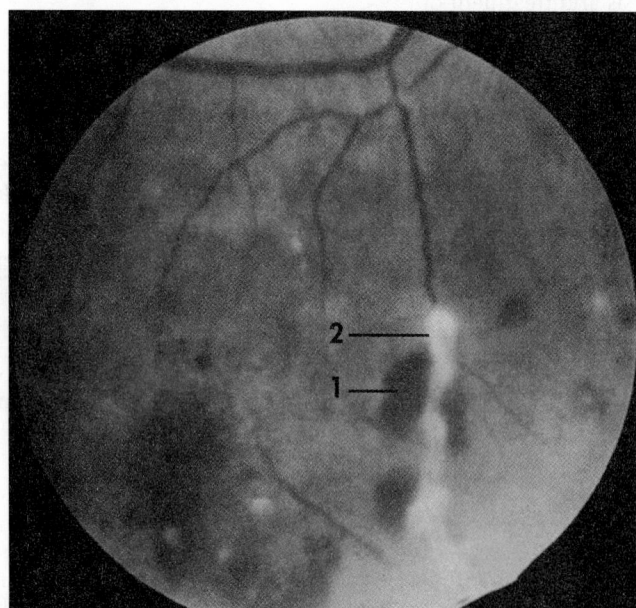

Fig. 1-288   Sarcoid posterior uveitis showing retinal hemorrhage (*1*) and vascular sheating (*2*). (Palay D [ed]: *Ophthalmology for the primary care physician,* St Louis, 1997, Mosby.)

BASIC INFORMATION

■ DEFINITION
Bleeding per vagina at any time during pregnancy must be regarded as abnormal and is associated with an increased likelihood of pregnancy complications.

■ SYNONYMS
Hemorrhage

ICD-9CM CODES
634.9 Spontaneous abortion
633.9 Ectopic pregnancy
630/631 Molar pregnancy
622.7 Cervical polyps
180.9/180.0/180.8 Cervical dysplasia/cancer
616.0 Cervicitis
616.10 Vulvovaginitis
184.0 Vaginal cancer
644.2 Premature labor term labor
641.1 Placenta previa
641.2 Placental abruption

■ EPIDEMIOLOGY & DEMOGRAPHICS
- Common in U.S.; 20% to 25% of patients have vaginal spotting/bleeding in first trimester; of those, miscarriage occurs in 50%.
- Occurs in women of childbearing age.
- Between 1% and 2% of all pregnancies in the U.S. are ectopic.
- After one ectopic pregnancy, the chance of another is 7% to 15%.
- Ectopic pregnancy is the leading cause of maternal mortality in the first trimester.
- Average reported frequency for placental abruption is about 1 in 150 deliveries (0.3%).
- Incidence of placenta previa is <1 in 200 deliveries (0.5%).

■ PHYSICAL FINDINGS & CLINICAL PRESENTATION
- Bleeding: ranges from scant to life-threatening with hemodynamic instability
- Color: brown to bright red
- Can be painless or painful (cramps, back pain, severe abdominal pain)
- Fetal compromise: ranges from none to fetal demise

■ ETIOLOGY
- Influenced by gestational age
- Vaginal
- Cervical
- Uterine

DIAGNOSIS

■ DIFFERENTIAL DIAGNOSIS
- Any gestational age:
  1. Cervical lesions: polyps, decidual reaction, neoplasia
  2. Vaginal trauma
  3. Cervicitis/vulvovaginitis
  4. Postcoital trauma
  5. Bleeding dyscrasias
- Gestation <20 wk:
  1. Spontaneous abortion
  2. Presence of intrauterine device
  3. Ectopic pregnancy
  4. Molar pregnancy
  5. Implantation bleeding
  6. Low-lying placenta
- Gestation >20 wk:
  1. Molar pregnancy
  2. Placenta previa
  3. Placental abruption
  4. Vasa previa
  5. Marginal separation of the placenta
  6. Bloody show at term
  7. Preterm labor
- Section II describes the differential diagnosis of vaginal bleeding in pregnancy.

■ WORKUP
- Gestation <20 wk (Section III, Fig. 3-29 describes a clinical algorithm for evaluation of vaginal bleeding in early pregnancy.)
  1. Pelvic examination
  2. Culdocentesis
  3. Laparoscopy
  4. Laparotomy
- Gestation >20 wk:
  1. Ultrasound to locate placenta before pelvic examination
  2. If placenta previa, no speculum or bimanual examination
  3. If preterm labor, appropriate evaluation done

■ LABORATORY TESTS
- Urine pregnancy test: if positive, get quantitative β human chorionic gonadotropin (hCG)
  1. Early pregnancy: follow serially every 48 hr
  2. Normal pregnancy: hCG doubles approximately every 48 hr
  3. Spontaneous abortion: hCG levels will fall
  4. Ectopic pregnancy: hCG level will rise inappropriately
  5. Molar pregnancy: hCG level is extremely high

- CBC
- Blood type and screen (Rh-negative patients need RhoGAM)
- Coagulation profile (useful in missed abortion and abruption)
- Cervical cultures/wet mount
- Pap smear for cervical malignancy; caution with biopsy, because cervix can bleed extensively

■ IMAGING STUDIES
Ultrasound:
- 5 to 6 wk: gestational sac (transvaginally); hCG >2500 mIU/ml (third IS) or >1000 mIU/ml (second IS)
- 8 to 9 wk: fetal cardiac activity
- Molar pregnancy: characteristic cluster of cysts
- Location of placenta
- Degree of placental separation: difficult to assess

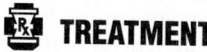

TREATMENT

■ NONPHARMACOLOGIC THERAPY
- Pelvic rest: no coitus, douching, or tampons
- Bed rest, if >20 wk
- Counseling: genetic, bereavement

■ ACUTE GENERAL Rx
- Hemodynamic stabilization
- Emergency D&C, laparotomy, or cesarean section as necessary

■ CHRONIC Rx
Depends on diagnosis

■ DISPOSITION
Depends on diagnosis

■ REFERRAL
- If patient is unstable and needs emergency ob/gyn management and/or surgery
- If patient has diagnosis of ectopic or molar pregnancy, because immediate surgical treatment is indicated
- Perinatal consultation for high-risk pregnancy

REFERENCES
Alexander JD, Schneider FD: Vaginal bleeding associated with pregnancy primary care; clinic in office, *Practice* 27(1):137, 2000.
Coppola PT, Coppola M: Vaginal bleeding in the first 20 weeks of pregnancy, *Emerg Med Clin North Am* 21(3):667, 2003.
Author: George T. Danakas, M.D.

BASIC INFORMATION

DEFINITION
Vaginal malignancy is an abnormal proliferation of vaginal epithelium demonstrating malignant cells below the basement membrane.

SYNONYMS
Squamous cell carcinoma of the vagina
Adenocarcinoma of the vagina
Melanoma of the vagina
Sarcoma of the vagina
Endodermal sinus tumor

ICD-9CM CODES
184.0 Vagina, vaginal neoplasm

EPIDEMIOLOGY & DEMOGRAPHICS
PREVALENCE: Vaginal cancer is the second rarest gynecologic cancer. It comprises 2% of malignancies of the female genital tract.
INCIDENCE: 0.42 cases/100,000 persons
MEAN AGE AT DIAGNOSIS: Predominantly a disease of menopause. Mean age at diagnosis is 60 yr old.

PHYSICAL FINDINGS & CLINICAL PRESENTATION
- Majority of cases are asymptomatic
- Postmenopausal vaginal bleeding and/or vaginal discharge are the most common symptoms
- May also present as pelvic pain or pressure, dyspareunia, dysuria, malodor, or postcoital bleeding
- May present as a vaginal lesion or abnormal Pap smear

ETIOLOGY
- The exact etiology is unknown.
- Vaginal intraepithelial neoplasia is thought to be a precursor for squamous cell carcinoma of the vagina.
- Chronic pessary use has been associated with vaginal malignancy.
- Prior pelvic radiation may be a risk factor.
- Clear-cell adenocarcinoma is related to in utero diethylstilbestrol exposure.

 DIAGNOSIS

DIFFERENTIAL DIAGNOSIS
- Extension from other primary carcinoma; more common than primary vaginal cancer
- Vaginitis

WORKUP
- Diagnosis is made histologically by biopsy.
- Colposcopy and biopsy should follow suspicious Pap smear.
- Cystoscopy, proctosigmoidoscopy, chest radiography, IV urography, and barium enema may be used for clinical staging.
- CT scan and MRI are being used to evaluate spread.
- Staging I-IV (Fig. 1-289).

IMAGING STUDIES
- Chest radiography, IV urography, and barium enema are used for staging.
- CT scan and MRI are good for assessing tumor spread.

TREATMENT

NONPHARMACOLOGIC THERAPY
- Radiation therapy is the mainstay of treatment.
- Stage I tumors that are small and confined to the posterior, upper third of the vagina may be treated with radical surgery.
- Other stages require a whole-pelvis, interstitial, and/or intracavitary radiation therapy.
- Chemotherapy is used in conjunction with radiotherapy in rare select cases.

DISPOSITION
Five-year survival ranges from 80% for stage I to 17% for stage IV.

REFERRAL
Vaginal cancer should be managed by a gynecologic oncologist and radiation oncologist.

REFERENCES
Kim H et al: Case report: magnetic resonance imaging of vaginal malignant melanoma, *J Comput Assist Tomogr* 27(3):357, 2003.
Stryker JA: Radiotherapy for vaginal carcinoma: a 23-year review, *Br J Radiol* 73 (875):1200, 2000.
Author: **Gil Farkash, M.D.**

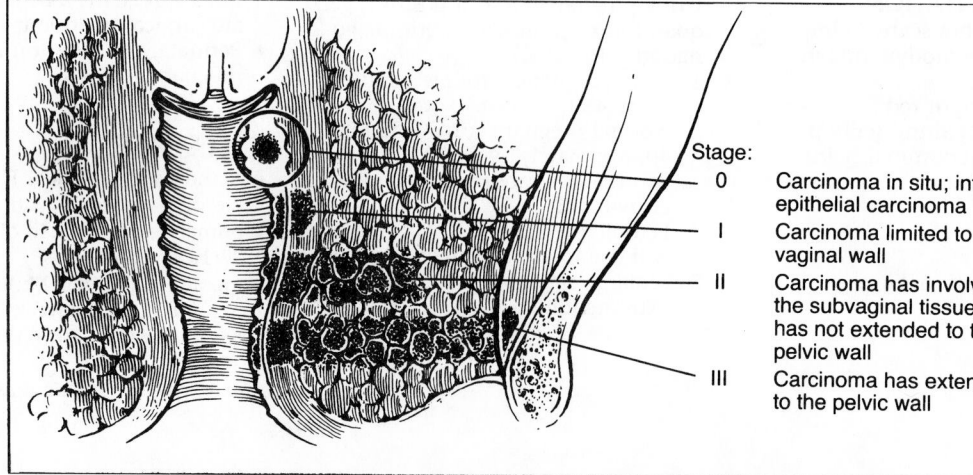

Fig. 1-289 **Staging system for vaginal cancer.** Metastatic disease that involves the bladder or rectum is stage IV-a. Metastatic disease beyond the pelvis is stage IV-b. (From Copeland LJ: *Textbook of gynecology,* ed 2, Philadelphia, 2000, WB Saunders.)

BASIC INFORMATION

■ DEFINITION
Vaginismus refers to the involuntary spasm of the vaginal, introital, and/or levator ani muscles, preventing penetration or causing painful intercourse.

ICD-9CM CODES
300.11 Hysterical vaginismus
306.51 Psychogenic or functional vaginismus
625.1 Reflex vaginismus

■ EPIDEMIOLOGY & DEMOGRAPHICS
PREVALENCE: Affects approximately 1:200 women
INCIDENCE: Estimated at about 11.7% to 42% of women presenting to sexual dysfunction clinics
RISK FACTORS: Any previous sexual trauma, including incest or rape
PREDOMINANT SEX: Affects only females

■ PHYSICAL FINDINGS & CLINICAL PRESENTATION
- Fear of pain with coitus
- Dyspareunia
- Orgasmic dysfunction

■ ETIOLOGY
- Learned conditioned response to real or imagined painful vaginal experience (e.g., traumatic speculum examination, incest, rape)
- Vaginitis
- PID
- Endometriosis
- Anatomic anomalies
- Atrophic vaginitis
- Mucosal tears
- Inadequate lubrication
- Focal vulvitis
- Painful hymenal tags
- Scarring secondary to episiotomy
- Skin disorders
- Topical allergies
- Postherpetic neuralgia

DIAGNOSIS

■ WORKUP
- Thorough history (including sexual history)
- Careful pelvic examination
- Behavioral therapy

TREATMENT

■ NONPHARMACOLOGIC THERAPY
- Deconditioning the response by systematic self-administered progressive dilation techniques using fingers or dilators
- Behavioral and/or psychosexual therapy

■ ACUTE GENERAL Rx
- Botulinum toxin therapy given locally has been shown to relieve the perineal muscle spasms associated with vaginismus, allowing resumption of intercourse.
  1. Acts by preventing neuromuscular transmission, causing muscle weakness
  2. Considered experimental treatment for vaginismus at this time
- Cause should be determined by history and explained to the patient so that she understands the mechanics of the muscle spasms.
- Patient must be motivated to desire painless vaginal insertion for such reasons as pleasurable coitus, tampon insertion, or gynecologic examination.
- Patient (and her partner) must be willing to patiently undergo the process of systematic desensitization and counseling.

■ DISPOSITION
A high percentage of successfully treated patients

■ REFERRAL
To a gynecologist or sex therapist

PEARLS & CONSIDERATIONS

■ COMMENTS
- May uncover early sexual abuse or an aversion to sexuality in general.
- To American Association of Sex Educators, Counselors and Therapists, 11 Dupont Circle, NW, Washington, DC, 20036.
- To Sex Information and Education Council of the U.S. (SIECUS), 85th Avenue, New York, NY 10022.

REFERENCES
Brin MF, Vapnek JM: Treatment of vaginismus with botulinum toxin injections, *Lancet* 349:252, 1997.

Heim LJ: Evaluation and differential diagnosis of dyspareunia, *Am Fam Physician* 63(8):1535, 2001.

McGuire H, Hawton K: Interventions for vaginismus. [update of Cochrane Database Syst Rev. 2001;(2):CD001760; PMID:11406006]. Cochrane Database of Systematic Reveiws (1):CD001760, 2003.

Phillips NA: Female sexual dysfunction evaluation and treatment, *Am Fam Physician* 62(1):127, 2000.

Author: **Beth J. Wutz, M.D.**

BASIC INFORMATION

■ DEFINITION

Bacterial vaginosis (BV) is a thin, gray, homogenous, malodorous vaginal discharge that results from a shift in the vaginal flora from a predominance of lactobacilli to high concentrations of anaerobic bacteria.

■ PREVIOUS NAMES

Before 1955: nonspecific vaginitis
1955: *Haemophilus vaginalis* vaginitis
1963: *Corynebacterium vaginalis* vaginitis
1980: *Gardnerella vaginalis* vaginitis
1990: Bacterial vaginosis

ICD-9CM CODES

616.10 Vaginitis, bacterial

■ EPIDEMIOLOGY & DEMOGRAPHICS

- Most common vaginal infection
- Studies by Thomason et al report that BV is present in:
  1. 16% of private patients
  2. 10% to 25% of obstetric clinic patients
  3. 38% to 64% of STD clinic patients
- *Gardnerella, Mycoplasma,* and *Mobiluncus* are harbored in the urethra of male partners; however,
  1. Male partners are asymptomatic.
  2. There is no improved cure rate or lower reinfection rate if the infected patient's male partner is treated.
  3. Abstinence from intercourse or condom use while the patient completes her treatment regimen may improve cure rates and lessen recurrences.

■ PHYSICAL FINDINGS & CLINICAL PRESENTATION

- 50% of patients are asymptomatic
- A thin, dark, or dull gray homogenous discharge that adheres to the vaginal walls
- An offensive, "fishy" odor that is accentuated after intercourse or menses
- Pruritus (only in 13%)

■ ETIOLOGY & PATHOGENESIS

- *Gardnerella vaginalis* is detected in 40% to 50% of vaginal secretions.
  1. Increase in vaginal pH caused by decrease in hydrogen peroxide–producing lactobacilli
  2. Anaerobes predominate and produce amines
- Amines, when alkalinized by semen, menstrual blood, the use of alkaline douches, or the addition of 10% KOH, volatilize and cause the unpleasant "fishy" odor.

- In BV:
  1. *Bacteroides* (anaerobes) species are increased 1000× the usual concentration.
  2. *G. vaginalis* are 100× normal.
  3. *Peptostreptococcus* are 10× normal.
  4. *Mycoplasma hominis* and Enterobacteriacea members are present in increased concentrations.

■ ASSOCIATIONS WITH OTHER DISORDERS

Bacterial vaginosis has been associated with PID, cystitis, posthysterectomy vaginal cuff cellulitis, postabortal infection, preterm delivery, premature rupture of membranes (PROM), amnionitis, chorioamnionitis, and postpartum endometritis.

DIAGNOSIS

Detecting three of the four following signs will diagnose 90% correctly, with <10% false positives:
  1. Thin, gray, homogenous, malodorous discharge that adheres to the vaginal walls
  2. Elevated pH >4.5
  3. Positive KOH whiff test
  4. Clue cells present on wet mount
- Cultures are unnecessary.
- Pap smear will not identify *G. vaginalis.*
- Gram stain of vaginal secretions will reveal clue cells and abnormal mixed bacteria (Fig. 1-290).

TREATMENT

■ RECOMMENDED REGIMENS

1. Metronidazole 500 mg PO bid for 7 days
2. 0.75% metronidazole gel in vagina bid for 5 days
3. 2% clindamycin cream qd for 7 days

■ ALTERNATE REGIMENS (LOWER EFFICACY FOR BV)

1. Clindamycin ovules 100 g intravaginally qhs for 3 days
2. Clindamycin 300 mg PO bid for 7 days (increased incidence of diarrhea)
3. Metronidazole ER 750 mg PO qd for 7 days
4. Metronidazole 2 g PO single dose (higher relapse rate)

Patients should be advised to avoid alcohol while taking metronidazole and for 24 hr thereafter.

■ TREATMENT IN PREGNANCY

All pregnant patients proven to have BV should be treated because of its association with preterm labor, chorioamnionitis, and PROM.

■ RECOMMENDED REGIMENS

1. Metronidazole 250 mg PO tid for 7 days
2. Clindamycin 300 mg PO bid for 7 days
- Existing data do not support the use of topical agents during pregnancy.
- Multiple studies and meta-analysis have not demonstrated associations between metronidazole use during pregnancy and teratogenic effects in newborns.

Author: **Tiffany B. Genewick, M.D.**

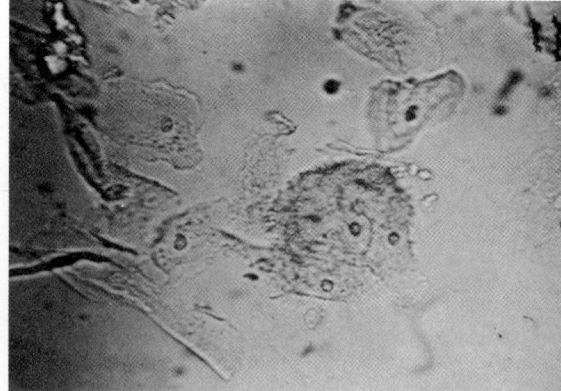

Fig. 1-290 Clue cells characteristic of bacterial vaginosis, squamous epithelial cells whose borders are obscured by bacteria. (From Carlson K [ed]: *Primary care of women,* St Louis, 1995, Mosby.)

BASIC INFORMATION

■ DEFINITION
Varicose veins are dilated networks of the subcutaneous venous system that result from valvular incompetence.

■ SYNONYMS
Chronic venous insufficiency
Stasis skin changes

ICD-9CM CODES
454.9 Varicose veins

■ EPIDEMIOLOGY & DEMOGRAPHICS
PREVALENCE:
- Approximately 30% of adults, with increasing incidence with age
- Increased incidence during pregnancy, especially with advanced maternal age

GENETICS:
- Familial tendency
- Evidence for dominant, recessive, and multifactorial types of inheritance

PREDOMINANT SEX: Female > male

RISK FACTORS:
- Advancing age
- Prolonged standing
- Pregnancy
- Obesity
- Use of oral contraceptives

■ PHYSICAL FINDINGS & CLINICAL PRESENTATION
- Dull ache, burning, or cramping in leg muscles
- Worsening discomfort with standing, warm temperatures, or menses
- Tortuous dilation of superficial veins
- Edema
- Varicose ulcer, sometimes with superficial infection
- Dermatitis pigmentation

■ ETIOLOGY
- Normally, blood flow directed from the superficial venous system to the deep venous system via communication of perforating vessels
- Best thought of as "venous hypertension"
- Valvular incompetence in perforator veins of lower extremity leading to reverse flow of fluid from high-pressure deep venous system to low-pressure superficial venous system, resulting in dilation of superficial veins, leg edema, and pain
- Rarely associated with deep vein thrombophlebitis
- Exacerbated by restrictive clothing

■ DIAGNOSIS

■ DIFFERENTIAL DIAGNOSIS
Conditions that can lead to superficial venous stasis other than primary valvular insufficiency include:
- Arterial occlusive disease
- Diabetes
- Deep vein thrombophlebitis
- Peripheral neuropathies
- Unusual infections
- Carcinoma

■ WORKUP
- Mainly a clinical diagnosis
- Arterial studies to rule out arterial insufficiency before initiating therapy for venous insufficiency

■ LABORATORY TESTS
Not useful

■ IMAGING STUDIES
Duplex ultrasound
- Gold standard for evaluation of varicose veins
- Quantitation of flow through venous valves under direct visualization
- Allows precise anatomic identification of source of venous reflux

■ TREATMENT

■ NONPHARMACOLOGIC THERAPY
- Leg elevation and rest
- Graded compression stockings: used early in morning before edema accumulates and removed before going to bed
- Weight loss
- Avoidance of occlusive clothing

■ ACUTE GENERAL Rx
- For associated stasis dermatitis: topical corticosteroids
- Treatment of secondary infection with appropriate antibiotics

■ CHRONIC Rx
- Sclerotherapy: injection of 1% to 3% solution of sodium tetradecyl sulfate
- Surgery: indications include the following:
  1. Persistent varicosities with conservative treatment
  2. Failed sclerotherapy
  3. Previous or impending bleeding from ulcerated varicosities
  4. Disabling pain
  5. Cosmetic concerns
- Surgical methods include (must be combined with compressive therapy):
  1. Saphenous vein ligation
  2. Ligation of incompetent perforating veins
  3. Saphenous vein stripping with or without avulsion of varicosities
  4. Ambulatory "miniphlebectomies": avulsion of superficial varicosities with saphenous vein stripping

■ DISPOSITION
A chronic condition in which a combination of compressive and surgical therapy can adequately control varicosities

■ REFERRAL
- To dermatologist for dermatitis complications
- To surgeon for failed conservative management

REFERENCES
Bradbury A et al: What are the symptoms of varicose veins? Edinburgh Vein Study cross sectional population survey, *BMJ* 318:353, 1999.

Hagen MD, Johnson ED: What treatments are effective for varicose veins? *J Fam Pract* 52(4):329, 2003.

Author: **Matthew L. Withiam-Leitch, M.D., Ph.D.**

BASIC INFORMATION

■ DEFINITION
- Ventricular septal defect (VSD) refers to an abnormal hole or opening in the septum separating the right and left ventricles.
- VSDs may be large or small, single or multiple.
- VSDs are located at various anatomic regions of the septum and classified as:
  1. Membranous (75% to 80%): Most common defect that can extend into the vascular septum.
  2. Canal or inlet defects (8%): Commonly lie beneath the septal leaflet of the tricuspid valve and often seen in patients with Down syndrome.
  3. Muscular or trabecular defects (5% to 20%): Can be single or multiple, small or large.
  4. Subarterial defect (5% to 7%): Least common and also called outlet, infundibular, or supracristal defect. Commonly found beneath the aortic valve, leading to aortic valve prolapse and regurgitation.

■ SYNONYMS
VSD

ICD-9CM CODES
745.4 Ventricular septal defect

■ EPIDEMIOLOGY & DEMOGRAPHICS
- Isolated VSD is the most common congenital heart abnormality found at birth (excluding bicuspid aortic valve and mitral valve prolapse) and accounts for 30% of all congenital cardiac defects.
- Prevalence is 1.17 per 1000 live births and at 0.5 per 1000 adults.
- Found equally in males and females.
- Approximately 25% of all congenital heart defects found in children are VSDs.
- Approximately 10% of all congenital heart defects found in adults are VSDs.
- VSDs may be associated with:
  1. Coarctation of the aorta (17%)
  2. Patent ductus arteriosus (22%)
  3. Subvalvular aortic stenosis (4%)
  4. Subpulmonic stenosis
  5. Atrial septal defect (35%)
- Multiple VSDs are more prevalent in patients with tetralogy of Fallot and double outlet right ventricular defects.

■ PHYSICAL FINDINGS & CLINICAL PRESENTATION
- Clinical presentation is dictated by the direction and volume of the VSD shunt along with the ratio of the pulmonary to systemic vascular resistance.
- Infants at birth may be asymptomatic because of elevated pulmonary artery pressure and resistance. Over the next few weeks, pulmonary arterial resistance decreases, allowing more blood shunting through the VSD into the right ventricle, with subsequent increased flow into the lungs, left atrium, and left ventricle, causing LV volume overload. Tachypnea, failure to thrive, and congestive heart failure ensue.
- In adults with VSD, the shunt is left to right in the absence of pulmonary stenosis and pulmonary hypertension, and patients typically manifest with symptoms of heart failure (e.g., shortness of breath, orthopnea, and dyspnea on exertion).
- A spectrum of physical findings may be seen including:
  1. Holosystolic murmur heard best along the left sternal border
  2. Systolic thrill
  3. Mid-diastolic rumble heard at the apex
  4. S_3
  5. Rales
- With the development of pulmonary hypertension:
  1. Augmented pulmonic component of S_2
  2. Cyanosis and clubbing (seen in Eisenmenger's complex with reversal of the shunt in a right to left direction)

■ ETIOLOGY
Usually congenital (focus of our review), but may occur postmyocardial infarction

DIAGNOSIS

The diagnosis of VSD is suspected by physical examination. Imaging studies, particularly transthoracic echocardiography, establishes the diagnosis.

■ DIFFERENTIAL DIAGNOSIS
Based on physical examination, the diagnosis of VSD may be confused with other causes of systolic murmurs such as mitral regurgitation, aortic stenosis, asymmetric septal hypertrophy, and pulmonary stenosis.

■ WORKUP
Any person that is suspected of having a VSD should have an ECG, a chest x-ray, and an echocardiogram and be considered for a cardiac catheterization and angiography.

■ LABORATORY TESTS
- Laboratory tests are not specific but may offer insight into the severity of the disease
- CBC may show polycythemia, especially in patients with Eisenmenger's complex
- Arterial blood gases showing hypoxemia

■ IMAGING STUDIES
- Chest x-ray findings in patients with VSD include: Cardiomegaly resulting from volume overload directly related to the magnitude of the shunt.
- Enlargement of the proximal pulmonary arteries along with redistribution and pruning of the distal pulmonary vessels resulting from sustained pulmonary hypertension (Fig. 1-291, A).
- ECG findings vary according to the size of the VSD and whether pulmonary hypertension is present or not. In large VSDs with pulmonary hypertension, right axis deviation is seen along with evidence of right ventricular hypertrophy.
- Echocardiography is the noninvasive procedure of choice in the diagnosis of VSD.
  1. Two-dimensional echo and color Doppler displays the size and location of the VSD (Fig. 1-291, B).
  2. Continuous wave Doppler not only approximates the gradient between the left and right ventricle but also estimates the pulmonary artery pressure.
- Cardiac catheterization measures right heart pressures and detects and estimates the size of the shunt by the calculation of the pulmonary to systemic flow ratio.
- Angiography also locates the VSD.

TREATMENT

The decision to treat a VSD depends on its type, size, shunt severity, pulmonary vascular resistance, functional capacity, and associated valvular abnormalities.

■ NONPHARMACOLOGIC THERAPY
- In young children, small asymptomatic VSDs with a pulmonary to systemic blood flow ratio of ≤1.5:1 and no evidence of pulmonary hypertension can be observed.
- Oxygen and low-salt diet is recommended in patients with congestive heart failure.

■ ACUTE GENERAL Rx

Surgery is indicated in:
- Infants with congestive heart failure
- Children between the ages of 1 to 6 with persistent VSD and a pulmonary to systemic blood flow ratios >2:1
- Adults with VSD and flow ratios >1.5:1

Percutaneous transcatheter closure by umbrella or clamshell occluder devices are currently under investigation with anecdotal success.

■ CHRONIC Rx

See "Acute General Rx."

■ DISPOSITION

- The natural history of isolated VSD depends on the type of defect, its size, and associated abnormalities.
- Approximately 75% to 80% of small VSDs close spontaneously by age 10 yr.
- In patients with large VSDs, only 10% to 15% will close spontaneously.
- Large VSDs left untreated may lead to arrhythmias, congestive heart failure, pulmonary hypertension, and Eisenmenger's complex.

- Eisenmenger's complex carries a poor prognosis, with most patients dying before the age of 40 yr.

■ REFERRAL

All infants and children diagnosed with VSD should be referred to a pediatric cardiologist. Adults with VSD should be referred to a cardiologist. Cardiothoracic surgeons experienced in congenital heart disease surgery should be consulted if surgery is indicated.

☼ PEARLS & CONSIDERATIONS

■ COMMENTS

- Ventricular septal defect was first described by Dalrymple in 1847.
- Risk of patients with VSD developing infective endocarditis is 4%. The risk is higher if aortic insufficiency is present.
- Bacterial endocarditis prophylaxis is recommended in all patients with VSD.
- Postoperatively, if no shunt remains, endocarditis prophylaxis is not indicated after 6 mo.

REFERENCES

Ammash NM, Warnes CA: Ventricular septal defects in adults, *Ann Intern Med* 135:812, 2001.

Braunwald: *Heart disease: a textbook of cardiovascular medicine,* ed 6, Philadelphia, 2001, WB Saunders.

Congenital heart disease and vascular interventions, *Am J Cardiol* 88(Suppl 5A):118G, 2001.

Interventional approaches to septal defects, valve disease, and hypertrophic cardiomyopathy, *Am J Cardiol* 92(6A): 160L, 2003.

McDaniel NL: Ventricular and atrial septal defects, *Pediatr Rev* 22(8):265, 2001.

Merrick AF et al: Management of ventricular septal defect: a survey of practice in the United Kingdom, *Ann Thorac Surg* 68(3):983, 1999.

Turner SW, Hunter S, Wyllie JP: The natural history of ventricular septal defects, *Arch Dis Child* 81(5):413, 1999.

Authors: **Wen-Chih Wu, M.D., and Peter Petropoulos, M.D.**

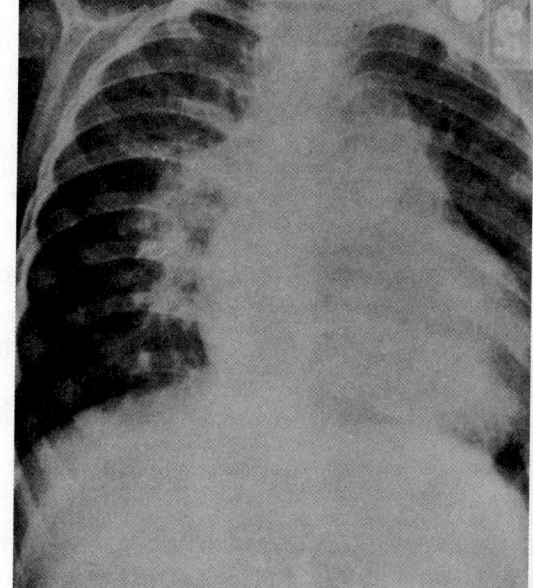
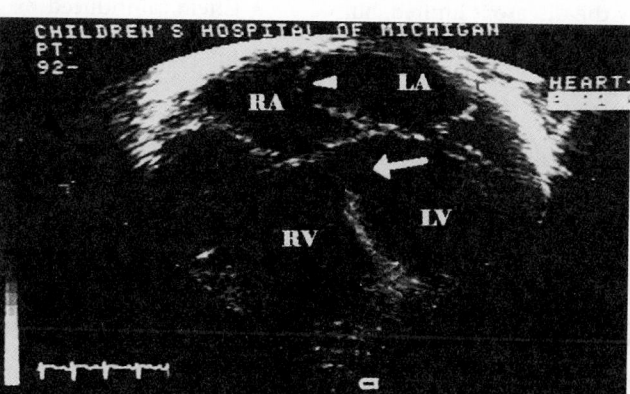

Fig. 1-291 **A,** Chest roentgenogram of a child with a large VSD, large pulmonary blood flow, and pulmonary hypertension, but only mild elevation of PVR. This is reflected in the evidence of left and right ventricular enlargement, enlargement of the main pulmonary artery, and marked increase in pulmonary blood flow. **B,** Apical four-chamber echocardiographic view of ventricular septal defect *(large arrow).* Small arrow points to interatrial septum. *RA,* Right atrium; *LA,* left atrium; *RV,* right ventricle; *LV,* left ventricle. (**A** From Pacifico AD, Kirklin JW, Kirklin JK: Surgical treatment of ventricular septal defect. In Sabiston DC, Jr, spencer FC [eds]: *Surgery of the chest,* ed 5, Philadelphia, 1990, WB Saunders. **B** Courtesty Richard Humes, M.D., Associate Professor of Pediatrics, Director of Echocardiography Laboratory, Children's Hospital of Michigan, Detroit.)

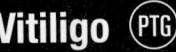

 BASIC INFORMATION

■ **DEFINITION**

Vitiligo is the acquired loss of epidermal pigmentation characterized histologically by the absence of epidermal melanocytes.

ICD-9CM CODES
709.1 Vitiligo

■ **EPIDEMIOLOGY & DEMOGRAPHICS**

- Prevalence: 1% of the population
- Positive family history in 25% to 30%
- Can begin at any age, but age at onset is under 20 yr for half the patients

■ **CLINICAL PRESENTATION & PHYSICAL FINDINGS**

- Hypopigmented and depigmented lesions (Fig. 1-292) favor sun-exposed regions, intertriginous areas, genitalia, and sites over bony prominences (type A vitiligo).
- Areas around body orifices are also frequently involved.
- The lesions tend to be symmetric.
- Occasionally the lesions are linear or pseudodermatomal (type B vitiligo).
- Vitiligo lesions may occur at trauma sites (Koebner's phenomenon).
- The hair in affected areas may be white.
- The margins of the lesions are usually well demarcated, and when a ring of hyperpigmentation is seen, the term *trichrome vitiligo* is used.
- The term *marginal inflammatory vitiligo* is used to describe lesions with raised borders.
- Initially the disease is limited, but the lesions tend to become more extensive over the years.

- Type B vitiligo is more common in children.
- Vitiligo may begin around pigmented nevi, producing a halo (Sutton's nevus); in such cases the central nevus often regresses and disappears over time.

■ **ETIOLOGY & PATHOGENESIS**

Three pathophysiologic theories:
- Autoimmune theory (autoantibodies against melanocytes)
- Neural theory (neurochemical mediator selectively destroys melanocytes)
- Self-destructive process whereby melanocytes fail to protect themselves against cytotoxic melanin precursors

Although vitiligo is considered to be an acquired disease, 25% to 30% is familial; the mode of transmission is unknown (polygenic or autosomal dominant with incomplete penetrance and variable expression).

Associated disorders:
- Alopecia areata
- Type 1 diabetes mellitus
- Adrenal insufficiency
- Hyper- and hypothyroidism
- Mucocutaneous candidiasis
- Pernicious anemia
- Polyglandular autoimmune syndromes
- Melanoma

DIAGNOSIS

■ **DIFFERENTIAL DIAGNOSIS (OTHER HYPOPIGMENTATION DISORDERS)**

Acquired:
- Chemical-induced
- Halo nevus
- Idiopathic guttate hypomelanosis

- Leprosy
- Leukoderma associated with melanoma
- Pityriasis alba
- Postinflammatory hypopigmentation
- Tinea versicolor
- Vogt-Koyanagi syndrome (vitiligo, uveitis, and deafness)

Congenital:
- Albinism, partial (piebaldism)
- Albinism, total
- Nevus anemicus
- Nevus depigmentosus
- Tuberous sclerosis

■ **WORKUP**

- Physical examination
- Wood's light examination may enhance lesions in light-skinned individuals

TREATMENT

- Treatment indicated primarily for cosmetic purposes when depigmentation causes emotional or social distress. Depigmentation is more noticeable in darker complexions.
- Cosmetic masking agents (Dermablend, Covermark) or stains (Dy-O-Derm, Vita-Dye).
- Sunless tanning lotions (dihydroxyacetone).
- Repigmentation (achieved by activation and migration of melanocytes from hair follicles; therefore skin with little or no hair responds poorly to treatment).
- PUVA (psoralen phototherapy): oral or topical psoralen administration followed by phototherapy with UVA (150 to 200 treatments required over 1 to 2 yr).
- Psoralens and sunlight (Puvasol).
- Topical midpotency steroids (e.g., triamcinolone 0.1% or desonide 0.05% cream qd for 3 to 4 mo).
- Intralesional steroid injection.
- Systemic steroids (betamethasone 5 mg qd on two consecutive days per wk for 2 to 4 mo).
- Total depigmentation (in cases of extensive vitiligo) with 20% monobenzyl ether or hydroquinone. This is a permanent procedure, and patients will require lifelong protection from sun exposure.

REFERENCE

Habif TP: Vitiligo. In Habif TP (ed): *Clinical dermatology,* ed 3, St Louis, 1996, Mosby.

Author: **Tom J. Wachtel, M.D.**

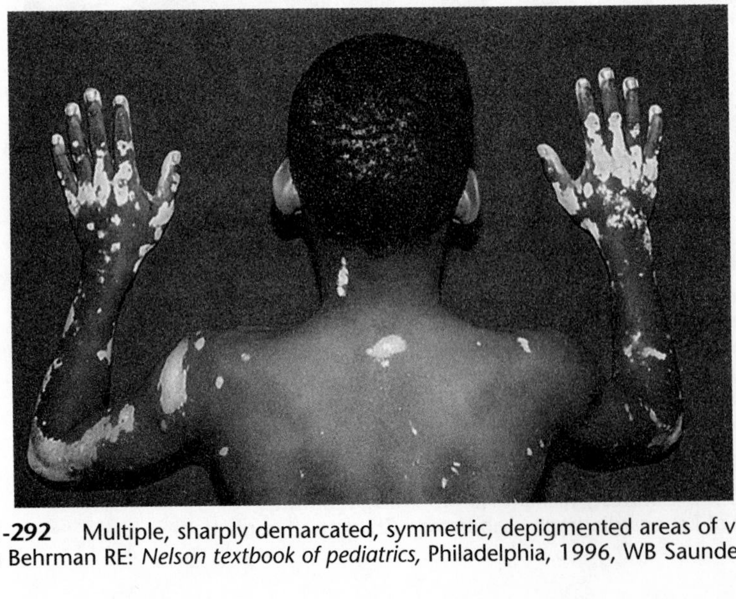

Fig. 1-292 Multiple, sharply demarcated, symmetric, depigmented areas of vitiligo. (From Behrman RE: *Nelson textbook of pediatrics,* Philadelphia, 1996, WB Saunders.)

BASIC INFORMATION

■ DEFINITION
Von Hippel-Lindau disease (VHL) is an autosomal dominant inherited disease characterized by the formation of hemangioblastomas, cysts, and malignancies involving multiple organs and systems.

■ SYNONYMS
Hippel-Lindau syndrome
Cerebelloretinal hemangioblastomatosis
Retinocerebellar angiomatosis

ICD-9CM CODE
759.6 von Hippel-Lindau disease

■ EPIDEMIOLOGY & DEMOGRAPHICS
- The incidence of VHL is 1 case/36,000 people.
- Age of onset varies but usually presents between the ages of 25 to 40 yr.
- In the U.S. approximately 7000 people are affected.
- Affected individuals are at risk of developing renal cell carcinoma, pheochromocytoma, pancreatic islet cell tumor, endolymphatic sac tumor, and hemangioblastomas of the cerebellum and retina.

■ PHYSICAL FINDINGS & CLINICAL PRESENTATION
The most common manifestations of VHL disease are:
- Retinal angiomas (59%)
  1. Most common presentation usually occurs by age 25
  2. Multiple angiomas
  3. Detached retina
  4. Glaucoma
  5. Blindness
- CNS hemangioblastomas (59%)
  1. Cerebellum is the most common site followed by the spine and medulla
  2. Usually multiple and occurs by the age of 30
  3. Headache, ataxia, slurred speech, nystagmus, vertigo, nausea, and vomiting
- Renal cysts (~60%) and clear cell renal cell carcinoma (25% to 45%)
  1. Usually occurs by the age of 40
  2. May be asymptomatic or cause abdominal and flank pain
  3. Renal cell carcinoma is bilateral in 75% of patients
- Pancreatic cysts
  1. Usually asymptomatic
  2. Large cysts can cause biliary obstructive symptoms
  3. Diarrhea and diabetes may develop if enough of the pancreas is replaced by cysts
- Pheochromocytoma (7% to 18%)
  1. Bilateral in 50% to 80% of cases
  2. Hypertension, palpitations, sweating, and headache
  3. Commonly occurs with pancreatic islet cell tumors
- Papillary cystadenoma of the epididymis (10% to 25% of men with VHL)
  1. Palpable scrotal mass
  2. May be unilateral or bilateral
- Endolymphatic sac tumors
  1. Ataxia
  2. Loss of hearing
  3. Facial paralysis

■ ETIOLOGY
VHL disease is primarily caused by a mutation of the von Hippel-Lindau gene located on chromosome 3. The VHL disease gene codes for a cytoplasmic protein that functions in tumor suppression.

DIAGNOSIS

- The diagnosis of VHL disease is established if in the presence of a positive family history, a single retinal or cerebellar hemangioblastoma is noted or a visceral lesion is found (e.g., renal cell carcinoma, pheochromocytoma, pancreatic cysts or tumor).
- If no clear family history is present, two or more hemangioblastomas or one hemangioblastoma with a visceral lesion are required to make the diagnosis.
- Screening family members is essential in the early detection of VHL disease.

■ WORKUP
All patients with VHL disease or patients at risk for the disease should have screening laboratory, ophthalmoscopic, and imaging studies performed to look for sites of involvement.

■ LABORATORY TESTS
- CBC may reveal erythrocytosis requiring periodic phlebotomies
- Electrolytes, BUN, and creatinine
- Urine for norepinephrine, epinephrine, and vanillylmandelic acid looking for pheochromocytoma

■ IMAGING STUDIES
- Indirect and direct ophthalmoscopy, fluorescein angioscopy, and tonometry are studies used in screening for retinal angiomas and glaucoma.
- CT scan of the abdomen is used in the screening, detection, and monitoring of patients with renal cysts renal tumors, pheochromocytomas, pancreatic cysts, and tumors (Fig. 1-293).
  1. Renal cysts grow on average 0.5 cm/yr.
  2. Renal tumors grow on average 1.5 cm/yr.
  3. CT scans are done every 6 mo for the first 2 yr and every year for life in patients who have had surgery for renal cell carcinoma.
- MRI with gadolinium is used for screening and evaluation of CNS and spinal hemangioblastomas, endolymphatic sac tumors, and pheochromocytomas.
- Angiography may be done before CNS surgery.

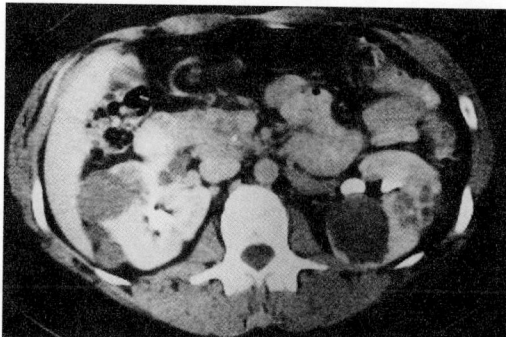

Fig. 1-293   Von Hippel-Lindau syndrome. Contrast CT demonstrates cystic and solid renal masses bilaterally. (From Barbaric ZL: *Principles of genitourinary radiology*, ed 2, New York, 1994, Thieme Medical.)

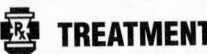 **TREATMENT**

■ NONPHARMACOLOGIC THERAPY
Genetic counseling is essential in patients diagnosed with VHL and in family members at risk.

■ ACUTE GENERAL Rx
- Laser photocoagulation and cryotherapy is used in patients with retinal angiomas to prevent blindness.
- For cerebellar hemangioblastomas the treatment is surgical removal. External-beam radiation and stereotaxic radiosurgery can also be done.
- For renal tumors, surgery is delayed until one of the renal tumors reaches 3 cm in diameter. Nephron-sparing surgery is the preferred surgical approach.
- Nephrectomy is indicated in patients with end-stage renal disease requiring dialysis because of the malignant potential of the disease.
- Pancreatic islet cell tumors usually require surgical removal.
- Adrenalectomy for pheochromocytoma.

■ CHRONIC Rx
- Dialysis has been delayed in many patients because of nephron-sparing surgery.
- Renal transplantation is usually delayed for 1 yr after bilateral nephrectomy for renal tumors so as to ensure that no metastases occur.

■ DISPOSITION
- Median life expectancy is 49 yr of age.
- The most common cause of death in VHL disease is from renal cell carcinoma.

■ REFERRAL
- A coordinated team of physicians is needed in the management of patients with VHL disease including: geneticist, neurosurgeon, urologist, nephrologist, ophthalmologist, otolaryngologist, neurologist, endocrinologist, and radiation oncologist.
- Patients, family members, and physicians interested in learning more about VHL disease can contact: von Hippel-Lindau Family Alliance (171 Clinton Road, Brookline, MA 02146. Tel: 1-800-767-4VHL).

☼ PEARLS & CONSIDERATIONS

■ COMMENTS
- VHL disease is named after the German ophthalmologist, Eugen von Hippel, who described patients with retinal angiomas in 1904, and Arvid Lindau, a Swedish pathologist who associated the hereditary nature of patients with cerebellar hemangioblastomas and angiomas in 1927.
- Latif et al were the first to discover the VHL gene in 1993.
- Genetic testing is available but should be done under the guidance and expertise of a geneticist.

REFERENCES
Couch V et al: von Hippel-Lindau Disease, *Mayo Clin Proc* 75:265, 2000.

Zbar B et al: Third International meeting on von Hippel-Lindau disease, *Cancer Res* 59:2251, 1999.

Author: **Peter Petropoulos, M.D.**

BASIC INFORMATION

■ DEFINITION

Von Willebrand's disease is a congenital disorder of hemostasis characterized by defective or deficient von Willebrand factor (vWF). There are several subtypes of von Willebrand's disease. The most common type (80% of cases) is type I, which is caused by a quantitative decrease in von Willebrand factor; type IIA and type IIB are results of qualitative protein abnormalities; type III is a rare autosomal recessive disorder characterized by a near complete quantitative deficiency of vWF. Acquired von Willebrand's disease (AvWD) is a rare disorder that usually occurs in elderly patients and usually presents with mucocutaneous bleeding abnormalities and no clinically meaningful family history. It is often accompanied by a hematoproliferative or autoimmune disorder. Successful treatment of the associated illness can reverse the clinical and laboratory manifestations.

■ SYNONYMS

Pseudohemophilia

ICD-9CM CODES

286.4 von Willebrand's disease

■ EPIDEMIOLOGY & DEMOGRAPHICS

- Autosomal dominant disorder
- Most common inherited bleeding disorder
- Occurs in >100/1 million persons

■ PHYSICAL FINDINGS & CLINICAL PRESENTATION

- Generally normal physical examination
- Mucosal bleeding (gingival bleeding, epistaxis) and GI bleeding may occur
- Easy bruising
- Postpartum bleeding, bleeding after surgery or dental extraction, menorrhagia

■ ETIOLOGY

Quantitative or qualitative deficiency of vWF (see "Definition")

DIAGNOSIS

■ DIFFERENTIAL DIAGNOSIS

Platelet function disorders, clotting factor deficiencies

■ WORKUP

- Laboratory evaluation (see "Laboratory Tests")
- Initial testing includes PTT (increased), platelet count (normal), and bleeding time (prolonged)
- Subsequent tests include vWF level (decreased), factor VIII:C (decreased), and ristocetin agglutination (increased in type II B) (Table 1-60)

■ LABORATORY TESTS

- Normal platelet number and morphology
- Prolonged bleeding time
- Decreased factor VIII coagulant activity
- Decreased von Willebrand factor antigen or ristocetin cofactor
- Normal platelet aggregation studies
- Type II A von Willebrand can be distinguished from type I by absence of ristocetin cofactor activity and abnormal multimer
- Type IIB von Willebrand is distinguished from type I by abnormal multimer

TREATMENT

■ NONPHARMACOLOGIC THERAPY

- Avoidance of aspirin and other NSAIDs
- Evaluation for likelihood of bleeding (with measurement of bleeding time) before surgical procedures

■ GENERAL Rx

- Desmopressin acetate (DDAVP) is useful to release stored vWF from endothelial cells. It is used to cover minor procedures and traumatic bleeding in mild type I von Willebrand's disease. Dose is 0.3 µg/kg in 100 ml of normal saline solution IV infused >20 min. DDAVP is also available as a nasal spray (dose of 150 µg spray administered to each nostril) as a preparation for minor surgery and management of minor bleeding episodes. DDAVP is not effective in type IIA von Willebrand's disease and is potentially dangerous in type IIB (increased risk of bleeding and thrombocytopenia).
- In patients with severe disease, replacement therapy in the form of cryoprecipitate is the method of choice. The standard dose is 1 bag of cryoprecipitate per 10 kg of body weight.
- Factor VIII concentrate rich in vWF (Humate-P, Armour) is useful to correct bleeding abnormalities.
- Life-threatening hemorrhage unresponsive to therapy with cryoprecipitate or factor VIII concentrate may require transfusion of normal platelets.

■ DISPOSITION

Prognosis is very good; most patients have minor bleeding complications and are able to lead a normal life.

REFERENCE

Kumar S et al: Acquired von Willebrand disease, *Mayo Clin Proc* 77:181, 2002.
Author: **Fred F. Ferri, M.D.**

TABLE 1-60   **Genetic and Laboratory Findings in von Willebrand's Disease**

TYPE	BT	VIII-C	vW-Ag	R-Cof	RIPA	MULTIMER STRUCTURE	MODE OF INHERITANCE
				PARAMETER			
I (classic)	P	R	R	R	R	N	AD
II							
A	P	N/R	N/R	R	R	Abn	AD
B	P	N/R	N/R	N/R	I	Abn	AD
III	P	R	R	R	R	Variable	AR

From Behrman RE: *Nelson textbook of pediatrics*, ed 15, Philadelphia, 1996, WB Saunders.
Abn, Abnormal; *AD,* autosomal dominant; *AR,* autosomal recessive; *BT,* bleeding time; *I,* increased; *N,* normal; *N/R,* normal or reduced; *P,* prolonged; *R,* reduced; *R-Cof,* ristocetin cofactor; *RIPA,* ristocetin-induced platelet aggregation (agglutination); *vW-Aq,* von Willebrand antigen (protein); *VIII-C,* factor VIII coagulant activity.

BASIC INFORMATION

■ DEFINITION
Vulvar cancer is an abnormal cell proliferation arising on the vulva and exhibiting malignant potential. The majority are of squamous cell origin; however, other types include adenocarcinoma, basal cell carcinoma, sarcoma, and melanoma (Fig. 1-294).

■ SYNONYMS
Squamous cell carcinoma of the vulva (90%)
Basal cell carcinoma of the vulva
Adenocarcinoma of the vulva
Melanoma of the vulva
Bartholin gland carcinoma
Verrucous carcinoma of the vulva
Vulvar sarcoma

ICD-9CM CODES
184.4 Vulvar neoplasm

■ EPIDEMIOLOGY & DEMOGRAPHICS
PREVALENCE: Vulvar cancer is uncommon. It comprises 4% of malignancies of the female genital tract. It is the fourth most common gynecologic malignancy.
INCIDENCE: 1.8 cases/100,000 persons

MEAN AGE AT DIAGNOSIS:
Predominantly a disease of menopause. Mean age at diagnosis is 65 yr.

■ PHYSICAL FINDINGS & CLINICAL PRESENTATION
• Vulvar pruritus or pain is present.
• May produce a malodor or discharge or present as bleeding.
• Raised lesion, may have fleshy, ulcerated, leukoplakic, or warty appearance; may have multifocal lesions.
• Lesions are usually located on labia majora, but may be seen on labia minora, clitoris, and perineum.
• The lymph nodes of groin may be palpable.

■ ETIOLOGY
• The exact etiology is unknown.
• Vulvar intraepithelial neoplasia has been reported in 20% to 30% of invasive squamous cell carcinoma of the vulva, but the malignant potential is unknown.
• Human papillomavirus is found in 30% to 50% of vulvar carcinoma, but its exact role is unclear.
• Chronic pruritus, wetness, industrial wastes, arsenicals, hygienic agents, and vulvar dystrophies have been implicated as causative agents.

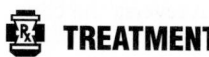

DIAGNOSIS

■ DIFFERENTIAL DIAGNOSIS
• Lymphogranuloma inguinale
• Tuberculosis
• Vulvar dystrophies
• Vulvar atrophy
• Paget's disease

■ WORKUP
• Diagnosis is made histologically by biopsy
• Thorough examination of the lesion and assessment of spread
• Possible colposcopy of adjacent areas
• Cytologic smear of vagina and cervix
• Cystoscopy and proctosigmoidoscopy may be necessary

■ IMAGING STUDIES
• Chest radiography
• CT scan and MRI for assessing local tumor spread

TREATMENT

■ NONPHARMACOLOGIC THERAPY
• Treatment is individualized depending on the stage of the tumor.
• Stage I tumors with <1 mm stromal invasion are treated with complete local excision without groin node dissection.
• Stage I tumors with >1 mm stromal invasion are treated with complete local excision with groin node dissection.
• Stage II tumors require radical vulvectomy with bilateral groin node dissection.
• Advanced-stage disease may require the addition of radiation and chemotherapy to the surgical regimen.
• Section III, Fig. 3-192 describes a treatment algorithm for management of vulvar cancer.

■ DISPOSITION
Five-year survival ranges from 90% for stage I to 15% for stage IV.

■ REFERRAL
Vulvar cancer should be managed by a gynecologic oncologist and radiation oncologist.

REFERENCES
Canavan TP, Cohen D: Vulvar cancer, *Am Fam Physician* 66(7):1269, 2002.
Coleman RL, Santoso JT: Vulvar carcinoma, *Curr Treat Opt Oncol* 1(2):177, 2000.
Grandys EC Jr, Aroris JV: Innovations in the management of vulvar carcinoma, *Curr Opin Obstet Gynecol* 12(1):15, 2000.
Author: **Gil Farkash, M.D.**

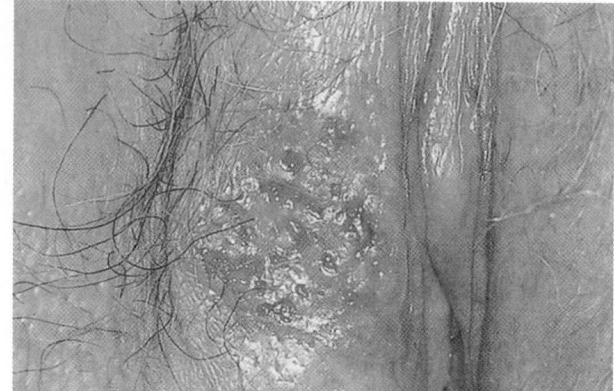

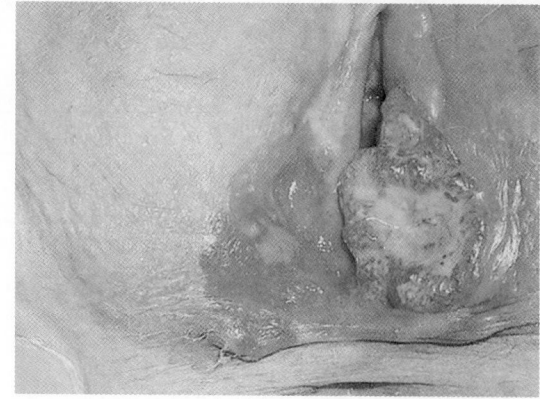

Fig. 1-294 **A,** Basal cell carcinoma of the vulva. **B,** Ulcerative squamous cell carcinoma of the vulva. (From Symonds EM, Macpherson MBA: *Color atlas of obstetrics and gynecology,* St Louis, 1994, Mosby.)

BASIC INFORMATION

■ DEFINITION
Bacterial vulvovaginitis is inflammation affecting the vagina, only rarely affecting the vulva, caused by anaerobic and aerobic bacteria.

■ SYNONYMS
Bacterial vaginosis
Gardnerella vaginalis
Haemophilus vaginalis
Corynebacterium vaginalis

ICD-9CM CODES
616.10 Vulvovaginitis

■ EPIDEMIOLOGY & DEMOGRAPHICS
- Most prevalent form of vaginal infection of reproductive age women in the U.S.
- 32% to 64% in patients visiting STD clinics
- 12% to 25% in other clinic populations
- 10% to 26% in patients visiting obstetric clinics
- May be associated with adverse pregnancy outcomes: premature rupture of membranes, preterm labor, preterm birth
- Organisms frequently found in postpartum or postcesarean endometritis

■ PHYSICAL FINDINGS & CLINICAL PRESENTATION
- >50% of all women may be without symptoms.
- Unpleasant, fishy, or musty vaginal odor in about 50% to 70% of all patients. Odor exacerbated immediately after intercourse or during menstruation.
- Vaginal discharge is increased.
- Vaginal itching and irritation occur.

■ ETIOLOGY
- Synergistic polymicrobial infection characterized by an overgrowth of bacteria normally found in the vagina

- Anaerobics: *Bacteroides* spp., *Peptostreptococcus* spp., *Mobiluncus* spp.
- Facultative anaerobes: *G. vaginalis, Mycoplasma hominis*
- Concentration of anaerobic bacteria increased to 100 to 1000 times normal
- Lactobacilli are absent or greatly reduced

DIAGNOSIS

■ DIFFERENTIAL DIAGNOSIS
- Fungal vaginitis
- *Trichomonas* vaginitis
- Atrophic vaginitis
- Cervicitis

■ WORKUP
- Pelvic examination
- Speculum examination
- Normal saline and 10% KOH slide of discharge
- Amsel criteria for diagnosis (three of four should be present):
  1. pH >4.5
  2. Clue cells (epithelial cells covered with bacteria) on saline solution slide
  3. Positive whiff test on 10% KOH
  4. Homogeneous, white, adherent discharge
- Section III, Fig. 3-189 describes the evaluation of vaginal discharge.

TREATMENT

■ ACUTE GENERAL Rx
- Metronidazole 500 mg PO bid × 7 days, >90% cure rate
- Metronidazole 2 g PO × 1 day, 67% to 92% cure rate
- Metronidazole gel 5 g, intravaginal bid × 5 days
- Clindamycin 2% cream 5 g, intravaginal qd × 7 days

- Clindamycin 300 mg PO bid × 7 days in pregnancy

■ CHRONIC Rx
Clindamycin 300 mg PO bid × 7 days; cure rate similar to those achieved with metronidazole
Related to adverse pregnancy outcomes
- Metronidazole 250 mg PO bid × 7 days
- Metronidazole zympoxidase
- Clindamycin 300 mg PO bid × 7 days
- Good hygiene: avoidance of douching, harsh shower gels, bubble baths; cotton underwear

■ DISPOSITION
- Reevaluate if not cured with treatment
- Recurrence fairly common

■ REFERRAL
Refer to obstetrician/gynecologist for recurrence or pregnant patient with bacterial vaginosis

PEARLS & CONSIDERATIONS

■ COMMENTS
Treating sexual partners has failed to demonstrate a benefit.

REFERENCES
Centers for Disease Control and Prevention: 2002 Guidelines for treatment of sexually transmitted diseases, *MMWR, Morb Mortal Wkly Rep*, 51 (RR-6), 2002.
Mead P, Hager WD, Faro S: *Protocols for infectious diseases in obstetrics and gynecology*, ed 2, New York, 2000, Blackwell Science.
Author: **Julie Anne Szumigala, M.D.**

BASIC INFORMATION

■ DEFINITION
Estrogen-deficient vulvovaginitis is the irritation and/or inflammation of the vulva and vagina because of progressive thinning and atrophic changes secondary to estrogen deficiency (Fig. 1-295).

■ SYNONYMS
Atrophic vaginitis

ICD-9CM CODES
616.10 Vulvovaginitis

■ EPIDEMIOLOGY & DEMOGRAPHICS
- Seen most often in postmenopausal women
- Average age of menopause is 52 yr
- In 1990, there were 36 million women 50 yr of age or older

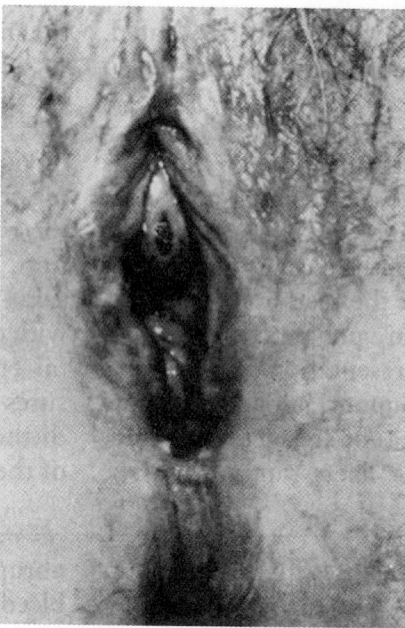

Fig. 1-295 Advanced postmenopausal atrophy of the vulva in a 72-year-old woman. (From Symonds EM, Macpherson MBA: *Color atlas of obstetrics and gynecology,* St Louis, 1994, Mosby.)

■ PHYSICAL FINDINGS & CLINICAL PRESENTATION
- Thinning of pubic hair, labia minora and majora
- Decreased secretions from the vestibular glands, with vaginal dryness
- Regression of subcutaneous fat
- Vulvar and vaginal itching
- Dyspareunia
- Dysuria and urinary frequency
- Vaginal spotting

■ ETIOLOGY
Estrogen deficiency

DIAGNOSIS

■ DIFFERENTIAL DIAGNOSIS
- Infectious vulvovaginitis
- Squamous cell hyperplasia
- Lichen sclerosus
- Vulva malignancy
- Vaginal malignancy
- Cervical and endometrial malignancy

■ WORKUP
- Pelvic examination
- Speculum examination
- Pap smear
- Possible endometrial biopsy if bleeding

■ LABORATORY TESTS
FSH and estradiol: generally after menopause, estradiol <15 pg and FSH >40 mIU/ml

TREATMENT

■ ACUTE GENERAL Rx
- Premarin 0.625 mg PO qd
- Estraderm patch 0.05 mg × 2 per week
- If uterus present:
  1. Estrogen + 2.5 mg PO Provera qd *or*
  2. Estrogen + 10 mg PO Provera × 10 days each mo
- Conjugated estrogen vaginal cream intravaginally. Estradiol vaginal cream 0.01%
  2 to 4 g/day × 2 wk then
  1 to 2 g/day × 2 wk then
  1 to 2 g × 3 days/wk
- Vagifen (estradial vaginal tablets) 25 mg inserted intravaginally daily for 2 wk then twice weekly. May take up to 12 wk to feel the full benefits of the medication.
- Conjugated estrogen vaginal cream: 2-4 g qd (3 wk on, 1 wk off) for 3-5 mo.

■ CHRONIC Rx
See "Acute General Rx." May discontinue vaginal estrogen cream once symptoms alleviate.

■ DISPOSITION
The symptoms should be improved with the therapy. Caution for vaginal bleeding if uterus present

■ REFERRAL
To obstetrician/gynecologist if vaginal bleeding

REFERENCE
Bornstein J et al: The classic approach to diagnosis of vulvovaginitis: a critical analysis, *Infect Dis Obstet Gynecol* 9(2):105, 2001.
Author: **Julie Anne Szumigala, M.D.**

BASIC INFORMATION

■ DEFINITION

Fungal vulvovaginitis is the inflammation of vulva and vagina caused by *Candida* spp.

■ SYNONYMS

Monilial vulvovaginitis

ICD-9CM CODES

112.1 Vulvovaginitis, monilial

■ EPIDEMIOLOGY & DEMOGRAPHICS

- Second most common cause of vaginal infection.
- Approximately 13 million people were affected in 1990.
- 75% of women will have at least one episode during their childbearing years, and approximately 40% to 50% of these will experience a second attack.
- No symptoms in 20% to 40% of women who have positive cultures.

■ PHYSICAL FINDINGS & CLINICAL PRESENTATION

- Intense vulvar and vaginal pruritus
- Edema and erythema of vulva
- Thick, curdlike vaginal discharge
- Adherent, dry, white, curdy patches attached to vaginal mucosa

■ ETIOLOGY

- *Candida albicans* is responsible for 80% to 95% of vaginal fungal infections.
- *Candida tropicalis* and *Torulopsis glabrata (Candida glabrata)* are the most common nonalbicans *Candida* species that can induce vaginitis.

■ PREDISPOSING HOST FACTORS

- Pregnancy
- Oral contraceptives (high-estrogen)
- Diabetes mellitus
- Antibiotics
- Immunosuppression
- Tight, poorly ventilated, nylon underclothing, with increased local perineal moisture and temperature

DIAGNOSIS

■ DIFFERENTIAL DIAGNOSIS

- Bacterial vaginosis
- *Trichomonas* vaginitis
- Atrophic vaginitis
- Section II describes the differential diagnosis of vaginal discharges and infections

■ WORKUP

- Pelvic examination
- Speculum examination
- Hyphae or budding spores on 10% KOH preparation (positive in 50% to 70% of individuals with yeast infection)
- Section III, Fig. 3-189 describes the evaluation of vaginal discharge

■ LABORATORY TESTS

Culture, especially recurrence for identification

TREATMENT

■ ACUTE GENERAL Rx

- Cure rate of the various azole derivatives 85% to 90%; little evidence of superiority of one azole agent over another
- No significant differences in persistent symptoms with oral or vaginal treatment
- Fluconazole (oral) associated with increased frequency of mild nausea, headache, abdominal pain
- Cure rate of polyene (Nystatin) cream and suppositories, 75% to 80%
- Miconazole 200-mg suppository (Monistat 3), one suppository × 3 or 2% vaginal cream (Monistat 7), one applicator full intravaginally qhs × 7
- Clotrimazole 200-mg vaginal tablet, one tablet intravaginally qhs × 3 or 100-mg vaginal tablet (Gyne-Lotrimin, Mycelex-G) one tablet intravaginally qhs × 7, or 1% vaginal cream intravaginally qhs × 7
- Butoconazole 2% cream (Femstat) one applicator intravaginally qhs × 3
- Terconazole 80-mg suppository or 0.8% vaginal cream (Terazol 3), one suppository or one applicator intravaginally qhs × 3 or 0.4% vaginal cream (Terazol 7), one applicator intravaginally qhs × 7
- Gynecazole-1 vaginal cream one applicator intravaginally × 1
- Tioconazole 6.5% ointment (Vagistat), one applicator intravaginally × 1
- Fluconazole (Diflucan) 150 mg PO × 1

■ CHRONIC Rx (FOUR OR MORE SYMPTOMATIC EPISODES/YR)

- Resistance or recurrence
  1. 14- to 21-day course of 7-day regimens mentioned in "Acute General Rx"
  2. Fluconazole (Diflucan) 150 mg PO × 1

  3. Ketoconazole (Nizoral) 200 mg PO bid × 5 to 14 days
  4. Itraconazole (Sporanox) 200 mg PO qd × 3 days
  5. Boric acid 600-mg capsule intravaginally bid × 14 days
- Prophylactic regimens
  1. Clotrimazole one 500-mg vaginal tablet each month
  2. Ketoconazole 200 mg PO bid × 5 days each month
  3. Fluconazole 150 mg PO × 1 each month
  4. Miconazole 100-mg vaginal tablet × 2 weekly

■ DISPOSITION

- Approximately 40% of adult women experience more than one lifetime episode of fungal vulvovaginitis.
- If symptoms do not resolve completely with treatment, or if they recur within a 2- to 3-mo period, further evaluation is indicated.
- Reexamination and possibly culture are necessary.
- Positive culture in absence of symptoms should not lead to treatment. Approximately 30% of women harbor *Candida* spp. and other species in the vagina.

■ REFERRAL

To obstetrician/gynecologist for recurrence

PEARLS & CONSIDERATIONS

■ COMMENTS

- Treatment of sexual partner is not recommended.
- No evidence that treating a woman's male sexual partner significantly improves woman's infection or reduced their rate of relapse.

REFERENCES

Marazzo J: Vulvovaginal candidiasis, *Clin Concise* 7:346, 2002.

Nyirjesy P: Chronic vulvovaginal candidiasis, *Am Fam Physician* 63:687, 2001.

Spinius A et al: Effect of antibiotic use on the prevalence of symptomatic vulvovaginal candidiasis, *Am J Obstet Gynecol* 180:14, 1999.

Author: **Julie Anne Szumigala, M.D.**

BASIC INFORMATION

■ DEFINITION
Prepubescent vulvovaginitis is an inflammatory condition of vulva and vagina.

■ ICD-9CM CODES
616.10 Vulvovaginitis

■ EPIDEMIOLOGY & DEMOGRAPHICS
- Most common gynecologic problem of the premenarcheal female.
- Prepubertal girl is susceptible to irritation and trauma because of the absence of protective hair and labial fat pads and the lack of estrogenization with atrophic vaginal mucosa.
- Symptoms of vulvovaginitis and introital irritation and discharge account for 80% to 90% of gynecologic visits.
- Nonspecific etiology in approximately 75% of children with vulvovaginitis.
- Majority of vulvovaginitis in children involves a primary irritation of the vulva with secondary involvement of the lower one third of the vagina.

■ PHYSICAL FINDINGS & CLINICAL PRESENTATION
- Vulvar pain, dysuria, pruritus
  1. Discharge is not a primary symptom.
  2. If present, vaginal discharge may be foul smelling or bloody.

■ ETIOLOGY
- Infections
  1. Bacterial
  2. Protozoal
  3. Mycotic
  4. Viral
- Endocrine disorders
- Labial adhesions
- Poor hygiene
- Sexual abuse
- Allergic substance
- Trauma
- Foreign body
- Masturbation
- Constipation
- Section II describes the differential diagnosis of vaginal discharge in prepubertal girls.

DIAGNOSIS

■ DIFFERENTIAL DIAGNOSIS
- Physiologic leukorrhea
- Foreign body
- Bacterial vaginosis
- Gonorrhea
- Fungal vulvovaginitis
- *Trichomonas* vulvovaginitis
- Sexual abuse
- Pinworms

■ WORKUP
- Pelvic, genital examination
- Speculum examination
- Rectal examination
- KOH and normal saline preparation of discharge
- Section III, Fig. 3-189 describes the evaluation of vaginal discharge

■ LABORATORY TESTS
- Urinalysis to rule out UTI and diabetes
- Cultures including STDs

TREATMENT

■ NONPHARMACOLOGIC THERAPY
- Avoid tight clothing
- Perineal hygiene
- Avoid irritant chemicals
- Reassurance

■ ACUTE GENERAL Rx
- Group A β *Streptococcus* and *Streptococcus pneumoniae*: penicillin V potassium 125 to 250 mg PO qid × 10 days
- *Chlamydia trachomatis*: erythromycin 50 mg/kg/day PO × 10 days
  1. Children >8 yr of age, doxycycline 100 mg bid PO × 7 days
- *Neisseria gonorrhoeae*: ceftriaxone 125 mg IM × 1 day
  1. Children >8 yr of age should also be given doxycycline 100 mg bid PO × 7 days
- *Staphylococcus aureus*: amoxicillin-clavulanate 20 to 40 mg/kg/day PO × 7 to 10 days
- *Haemophilus influenzae*: amoxicillin 20 to 40 mg/kg/day PO × 7 days
- *Trichomonas*: metronidazole 125 mg (15 mg/kg/day) tid PO × 7 to 10 days
- Pinworms: mebendazole 100-mg tablet chewable, repeat in 2 wk
- Labial agglutination: spontaneous resolution or topical estrogen cream for 7-10 days

■ CHRONIC Rx
See "Referral."

■ DISPOSITION
Further education:
- Young child: hygiene
- Adolescent: pregnancy prevention and "safe sex"

■ REFERRAL
- To obstetrician/gynecologist
- To pediatrician

REFERENCE
Van Neer PA, Korver CR: Constipation presenting as recurrent vulvovaginitis in prepubertal children, *J Am Acad Dermatol* 43(4):718, 2000.
Author: **Julie Anne Szumigala, M.D.**

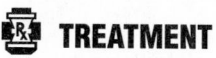
 BASIC INFORMATION

DEFINITION
Trichomonas vulvovaginitis is the inflammation of vulva and vagina caused by *Trichomonas* spp.

■ SYNONYMS
Trichomonas *vaginalis*

ICD-9CM CODES
131.01 Vulvovaginitis, trichomonal

■ EPIDEMIOLOGY & DEMOGRAPHICS
- Acquired through sexual contact
- Diagnosed in:
  1. 50% to 75% of prostitutes
  2. 5% to 15% of women visiting gynecology clinics
  3. 7% to 32% of women in STD clinics
  4. 5% of women in family planning clinics

■ PHYSICAL FINDINGS & CLINICAL PRESENTATION
- Profuse, yellow, malodorous vaginal discharge and severe vaginal itching
- Vulvar itching
- Dysuria
- Dyspareunia
- Intense erythema of the vaginal mucosa
- Cervical petechiae ("strawberry cervix")
- Asymptomatic in approximately 50% of women and 90% of men

■ ETIOLOGY
Single-cell parasite known as *trichomonad*

■ RISK FACTORS
- Multiple sexual partners
- History of previous STDs

🔬 DIAGNOSIS

■ DIFFERENTIAL DIAGNOSIS (TABLE 1-61)
- Bacterial vaginosis
- Fungal vulvovaginitis
- Cervicitis
- Atrophic vulvovaginitis

■ WORKUP
- Pelvic examination
- Speculum examination
- Mobile trichomonads seen on normal saline preparation: 70% sensitivity
- Elevated pH (>5) of vaginal discharge
- Culture is most sensitive commercially available method
- A large number of inflammatory cells on normal saline preparation
- Section III, Fig. 3-189 describes the evaluation of vaginal discharge

■ LABORATORY TESTS
- Culture (modified Diamond media): 90% sensitivity
- Direct enzyme immunoassay
- Fluorescein-conjugated monoclonal antibody test
- Pap test 40% detected

℞ TREATMENT

■ NONPHARMACOLOGIC THERAPY
Condom use

■ ACUTE GENERAL Rx
Metronidazole (Flagyl) 2 g PO × 1 or 500 mg PO bid × 7 days

■ CHRONIC Rx
- Metronidazole gel: less likely to achieve therapeutic levels; therefore not recommended
- Metronidazole (retreat): 500 mg PO bid × 7 days
- Treatment of future recurrences: Metronidazole 2 g PO qd × 3 to 5 days
- Allergy, intolerance, or adverse reactions: Alternatives to metronidazole are not available. Patients who are allergic to metronidazole can be managed by desensitization
- Pregnancy
  1. Associated with adverse outcomes (i.e., PROM)
  2. Metronidazole 2 g PO × 1 day

■ DISPOSITION
Trichomonas infection is considered an STD; therefore treatment of the sexual partner is necessary.

■ REFERRAL
To obstetrician/gynecologist for recurrence and pregnancy

REFERENCE
Workowski KA, Levine WC: Sexually transmitted diseases treatment guidelines, *MMWR Recomm Rep* 51:1, 2002.
Author: **Julie Anne Szumigala, M.D.**

TABLE 1-61   Differential Diagnosis of Vaginitis

CHARACTERISTICS OF VAGINAL DISCHARGE	C. ALBICANS VAGINITIS	T. VAGINALIS VAGINITIS	BACTERIAL VAGINOSIS
pH	4.5	>5.0	>5.0
White curd	Usually	No	No
Odor with KOH	No	Yes	Yes
Clue cells	No	No	Usually
Motile trichomonads	No	Usually	No
Yeast cells3	Yes	No	No

From Goldman L, Ausiello D (eds): *Cecil textbook of medicine*, ed 22, Philadelphia, 2004, WB Saunders.

BASIC INFORMATION

■ DEFINITION

Waldenström's macroglobulinemia (WM) is a plasma cell dyscrasia characterized by the presence of IgM monoclonal macroglobulins.

■ SYNONYMS

WM
Monoclonal macroglobulinemia

ICD-9CM CODES

273.3 Waldenström's macroglobulinemia

■ EPIDEMIOLOGY & DEMOGRAPHICS

- Accounts for 2% of all hematologic cancers
- 1500 people diagnosed each year in the U.S.
- Incidence: 0.61/100,00 in men; 0.36/100,000 in women
- Usually occurs in people over age 65 but can occur in younger people
- More common among men than women and among whites than blacks

■ PHYSICAL FINDINGS & CLINICAL PRESENTATION

- Weakness
- Fatigue
- Weight loss
- Headache, dizziness, vertigo, deafness, and seizures (hyperviscosity syndrome)
- Easy bleeding (e.g., epistaxis)
- Retinal vein link sausage shaped
- Lymphadenopathy (15%)
- Hepatomegaly (20%)
- Splenomegaly (15%)
- Purpura
- Peripheral neuropathy (5%)

■ ETIOLOGY

- The exact cause of WM is not known.
- Genetic predisposition, radiation exposure, occupational chemicals, and chronic inflammatory stimulation have been suggested but there is insufficient evidence to substantiate these hypotheses.

DIAGNOSIS

The diagnosis of WM is usually established by laboratory blood tests and by bone marrow biopsy.

■ DIFFERENTIAL DIAGNOSIS

- Monoclonal gammopathy of unknown significance (MGUS)
- Multiple myeloma
- Chronic lymphocytic leukemia
- Hairy-cell leukemia
- Lymphoma

■ WORKUP

In any patient suspected of having WM, specific blood tests (CBC, ESR, SPEP, IPEP, UPEP, IgM level, serum viscosity) and bone marrow biopsy will confirm the diagnosis.

■ LABORATORY TESTS

- CBC with differential:
  1. Anemia is a common finding, with a median hemoglobin value of approximately 10 g/dl. WBC count is usually normal; thrombocytopenia can occur.
  2. Peripheral smear may reveal malignant lymphoid cells in terminal patients.
- Elevated ESR
- Serum protein electrophoresis (SPEP): homogeneous M spike
- Immunoelectrophoresis: proves IgM
- Urine immunoelectrophoresis: monoclonal light chain usually kappa chains. Bence Jones protein can be seen but is not the typical finding in WM
- IgM levels are high, generally >3 g/dl
- Serum viscosity: symptoms usually occur when the serum viscosity is four times the viscosity of normal serum
- Cryoglobulins, rheumatoid factor, or cold agglutinins may be present
- Bone marrow biopsy: characteristically reveals lymphoplasmacytoid cells that have infiltrated the bone marrow

■ IMAGING STUDIES

Chest x-ray can be obtained to rule out pulmonary involvement.

TREATMENT

■ NONPHARMACOLOGIC THERAPY

Asymptomatic patients do not require treatment, and these patients should be monitored periodically for the onset of symptoms or changes in blood tests (e.g., worsening anemia, thrombocytopenia, rising IgM, and serum viscosity).

■ ACUTE GENERAL Rx

Symptomatic patients with WM usually receive chemotherapy.
- Chlorambucil and prednisone are given daily for 10 days and repeated at 6-wk intervals until a response is seen in the IgM concentration. Approximately 60% of patients respond to chemotherapy as defined by a 75% reduction in IgM concentration.
- Combination melphalan, cyclophosphamide, and prednisone chemotherapy given for 7 days at 4- to 6-wk intervals for 12 courses followed by continuous therapy with chlorambucil and prednisone until relapse has shown promising results.

■ CHRONIC Rx

- Refractory patients can be tried on fludarabine or 2-CdA (2-chlorodeoxyadenosine).
- New investigational treatment includes administration of rituximab, a monoclonal anti-CD 20 antibody.

■ DISPOSITION

- The onset of WM is slow and insidious. Most patients die from progression of the disease with hyperviscosity, hemorrhage, and infection, or from congestive heart failure.
- Some patients develop acute myelogenous leukemia, immunoblastic sarcoma, or chronic myelogenous leukemia as a preterminal event.
- Median survival in patients with WM is about 4 yr.
- Approximately 10% of patients will achieve complete remission with prognosis being more favorable (median survival 11 yr).

■ REFERRAL

If WM is suspected, a hematology consultation is helpful in guiding future workup, treatment, and monitoring.

☀ PEARLS & CONSIDERATIONS

■ COMMENTS

- Waldenström's macroglobulinemia was first described in 1944 by the Swedish physician Jan Gosta Waldenström.
- Patients with MGUS carry a higher risk of developing WM.
- Amyloidosis is rare, occurring in 5% of patients with WM.

REFERENCES

Dimopoulos MA, Galani E, Matsouka C: Waldenström's macroglobulinemia, *Hematol Oncol Clin North Am* 13(6):1351, 1999.
Gertz MA, Fonseca R, Rajkuma SV: Waldenstrom's macroglobulinemia, *Oncologist* 5(1):63, 2000.
Owen RG, Johnson SA, Morgan GJ: Waldenström's macroglobulinemia: laboratory diagnosis and treatment, *Hematol Oncol* 18(2):41, 2000.
Author: **Peter Petropoulos, M.D.**

BASIC INFORMATION

■ DEFINITION
Warts are benign epidermal neoplasms caused by human papillomavirus (HPV).

■ SYNONYMS
Verruca vulgaris (common warts)
Verruca plana (flat warts)
Condyloma acuminatum (venereal warts)
Verruca plantaris (plantar warts)
Mosaic warts (cluster of many warts)

ICD-9CM CODES
0.78.10 Viral warts
0.79.19 Venereal wart (external genital organs)

■ EPIDEMIOLOGY & DEMOGRAPHICS
- Common warts occur most frequently in children and young adults.
- Anogenital warts are most common in young, sexually active patients. Genital warts are the most common viral STD in the U.S., with up to 24 million Americans carrying the virus that causes them.
- Common warts are longer lasting and more frequent in immunocompromised patients (e.g., lymphoma, AIDS, immunosuppressive drugs).
- Plantar warts occur most frequently at points of maximal pressure (over the heads of the metatarsal bones or on the heels).

■ PHYSICAL FINDINGS & CLINICAL PRESENTATION
- Common warts (Fig. 1-296) have an initial appearance of a flesh-colored papule with a rough surface; they subsequently develop a hyperkeratotic appearance with black dots on the surface (thrombosed capillaries); they may be single or multiple and are most common on the hands.
- Warts obscure normal skin lines (important diagnostic feature). Cylindrical projections from the wart may become fused, forming a mosaic pattern.
- Flat warts generally are pink or light yellow, slightly elevated, and often found on the forehead, back of hands, mouth, and beard area; they often occur in lines corresponding to trauma (e.g., a scratch); are often misdiagnosed (particularly when present on the face) and inappropriately treated with topical corticosteroids.
- Filiform warts have a fingerlike appearance with various projections; they are generally found near the mouth, beard, or periorbital and paranasal regions.

- Plantar warts are slightly raised and have a roughened surface; they may cause pain when walking; as they involute, small hemorrhages (caused by thrombosed capillaries) may be noted.
- Genital warts are generally pale pink with several projections and a broad base. They may coalesce in the perineal area to form masses with a cauliflower-like appearance.
- Genital warts on the cervical epithelium can produce subclinical changes that may be noted on Pap smear or colposcopy.

■ ETIOLOGY
- Human papillomavirus (HPV) infection; >60 types of viral DNA have been identified. Transmission of warts is by direct contact.
- Genital warts are usually caused by HPV types 6 or 11.

DIAGNOSIS

■ DIFFERENTIAL DIAGNOSIS
- Molluscum contagiosum
- Condyloma latum
- Acrochordon (skin tags) or seborrheic keratosis
- Epidermal nevi
- Hypertrophic actinic keratosis
- Squamous cell carcinomas
- Acquired digital fibrokeratoma
- Varicella zoster virus in patients with AIDS

- Recurrent infantile digital fibroma
- Plantar corns (may be mistaken for plantar warts)

■ WORKUP
- Diagnosis is generally based on clinical findings.
- Suspect lesions should be biopsied.

■ LABORATORY TESTS
Colposcopy with biopsy of patients with cervical squamous cell changes

TREATMENT

■ NONPHARMACOLOGIC THERAPY
- Importance of use of condoms to reduce transmission of genital warts should be emphasized.
- Watchful waiting is an acceptable option in the treatment of warts, because many warts will disappear without intervention over time.
- Plantar warts that are not painful do not need treatment.

■ GENERAL Rx
- Common warts:
  1. Application of topical salicylic acid 17% (e.g., Duofilm). Soak area for 5 min in warm water and dry. Apply thin layer once or twice daily for up to 12 wk, avoiding normal skin. Bandage.
  2. Liquid nitrogen, electrocautery are also common methods of removal.

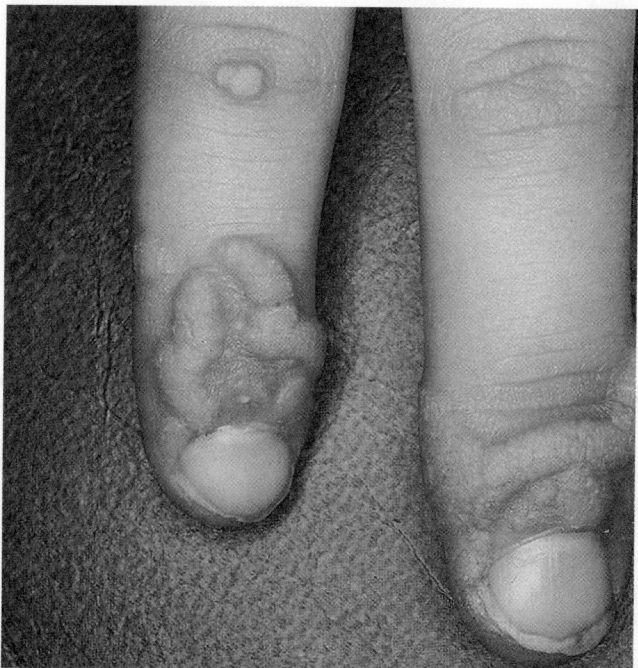

Fig. 1-296   Verruca vulgaris or common viral warts. These papules often have verrucous surface changes. (From Callen JP: *Color atlas of dermatology*, ed 2, Philadelphia, 2000, WB Saunders.)

3. Blunt dissection can be used in large lesions or resistant lesions.
4. Duct tape occlusion is also effective for treating common warts. It is cut to cover warts and left in place for 6 days. It is removed after 6 days and the warts are soaked in water and then filed with pumice stones. New tape is applied 12 hr later. This treatment can be repeated until warts resolve.
- Filiform warts: surgical removal is necessary.
- Flat warts: generally more difficult to treat.
  1. Tretinoin cream applied at hs over the involved area for several weeks may be effective
  2. Application of liquid nitrogen
  3. Electrocautery
  4. 5-Fluorouracil cream (Efudex 5%) applied once or twice a day for 3 to 5 wk is also effective. Persistent hyperpigmentation may occur following Efudex use
- Plantar warts:
  1. Salicylic acid therapy (e.g., Occlusal-HP). Soak wart in warm water for 5 min, remove loose tissue, dry. Apply to area, allow to dry, reapply. Use once or twice daily; maximum 12 wk. Use of 40% salicylic acid plasters (Mediplast) is also a safe, nonscarring treatment; it is particularly useful in treating mosaic warts covering a large area.
  2. Blunt dissection is also a fast and effective treatment modality.
  3. Laser therapy can be used for plantar warts and recurrent warts; however, it leaves open wounds that require 4 to 6 wk to fill with granulation tissue.
  4. Interlesional bleomycin is also effective but generally used when all other treatments fail.

- Genital warts:
  1. Can be effectively treated with 20% podophyllin resin in compound tincture of benzoin applied with a cotton tip applicator by the treating physician and allowed to air dry. The treatment can be repeated weekly if necessary.
  2. Podofilox (Condylox 0.5% gel) is now available for application by the patient. Local adverse effects include pain, burning, and inflammation at the site.
  3. Cryosurgery with liquid nitrogen delivered with a probe or as a spray is effective for treating smaller genital warts.
  4. Carbon dioxide laser can also be used for treating primary or recurrent genital warts (cure rate >90%).
  5. Imiquimod (Aldara) cream, 5% is a patient-applied immune response modifier effective in the treatment of external genital and perianal warts (complete clearing of genital warts in >70% of females and >30% of males in 4 to 16 wk). Sexual contact should be avoided while the cream is on the skin. It is applied three times/wk before normal sleeping hours and is left on the skin for 6-10 hr.
- Application of trichloroacetic acid (TCA) or bichloracetic acid (BCA) 80% to 90% is also effective for external genital warts. A small amount should be applied only to warts and allowed to dry, at which time a white "frosting" develops. This treatment can be repeated weekly if necessary.

■ DISPOSITION
- Warts can be effectively treated with the previous modalities, with complete resolution in the majority of patients; however, recurrence rate is high.
- Cervical carcinomas and precancerous lesions in women are associated with genital papillomavirus infection.
- Squamous cell anal cancer is also associated with a history of genital warts.

■ REFERRAL
- Dermatology referral for warts resistant to conservative therapy
- Surgical referral in selected cases
- STD counseling for patients with anogenital warts

☼ PEARLS & CONSIDERATIONS

■ COMMENTS
- Subungual and periungual warts are generally more resistant to treatment. Dermatology referral for cryosurgery is recommended in resistant cases.
- Examination of sex partners is not necessary for the management of genital warts because no data indicate that reinfection plays a role.

REFERENCES

Focht DR III et al: The efficacy of duct tape vs cryotherapy in the treatment of verruca vulgaris, *Arch Pediatr Adolesc Med* 156:971, 2002.
Gibbs S et al: Local treatment for cutaneous warts: systematic review, *BMJ* 325:461, 2002.

Author: **Fred F. Ferri, M.D.**

BASIC INFORMATION

■ DEFINITION

Wegener's granulomatosis is a multisystem disease generally consisting of the classic triad of:
1. Necrotizing granulomatous lesions in the upper or lower respiratory tractis
2. Generalized focal necrotizing vasculitis involving both arteries and veins
3. Focal glomerulonephritis of the kidneys

"Limited forms" of the disease can also occur and may evolve into the classic triad; Wegener's granulomatosis can be classified using the "ELK" classification, which identifies the three major sites of involvement: *E*, ears, nose, and throat or respiratory tract; *L*, lungs; *K*, kidneys.

ICD-9CM CODES

446.4 Wegener's granulomatosis

■ EPIDEMIOLOGY & DEMOGRAPHICS

• The incidence of Wegener's granulomatosis is 0.5/100,000 persons.
• Mean age at onset is 40 yr.

■ PHYSICAL FINDINGS & CLINICAL PRESENTATION

• Clinical manifestations often vary with the stage of the disease and degree of organ involvement.
• Frequent manifestations are:
  1. Upper respiratory tract: chronic sinusitis, chronic otitis media, mastoiditis, nasal crusting, obstruction and epistaxis, nasal septal perforation, nasal lacrimal duct stenosis, saddle nose deformities (resulting from cartilage destruction)
  2. Lung: hemoptysis, multiple nodules, diffuse alveolar pattern
  3. Kidney: renal insufficiency, glomerulonephritis
  4. Skin: necrotizing skin lesions
  5. Nervous system: mononeuritis multiplex, cranial nerve involvement

  6. Joints: monarthritis or polyarthritis (nondeforming), usually affecting large joints
  7. Mouth: chronic ulcerative lesions of the oral mucosa, "mulberry" gingivitis
  8. Eye: proptosis, uveitis, episcleritis, retinal and optic nerve vasculitis

■ ETIOLOGY

Unknown

DIAGNOSIS

■ DIFFERENTIAL DIAGNOSIS

• Other granulomatous lung diseases (e.g., lymphomatoid granulomatosis, Churg-Strauss syndrome, necrotizing sarcoid granulomatosis, bronchocentric granulomatosis, sarcoidosis); the differential diagnosis of granulomatous lung disease is described in Section II
• Neoplasms
• Goodpasture's syndrome
• Bacterial or fungal sinusitis
• Midline granuloma
• Viral infections

■ WORKUP

Chest x-ray examination, laboratory evaluation, PFTs, and tissue biopsy

■ LABORATORY TESTS

• Positive test for cytoplasmic pattern of ANCA (c-ANCA)
• Anemia, leukocytosis
• Urinalysis: may reveal hematuria, RBC casts, and proteinuria
• Elevated serum creatinine, decreased creatinine clearance
• Increased ESR, positive rheumatoid factor, and elevated C-reactive protein may be found.

■ IMAGING STUDIES

• Chest x-ray: may reveal bilateral multiple nodules, cavitated mass lesions, pleural effusion (20%).
• PFTs: useful in detecting stenosis of the airways.

• Biopsy of one or more affected organs should be attempted; the most reliable source for tissue diagnosis is the lung. Lesions in the nasopharynx (if present) can be easily biopsied.

TREATMENT

■ NONPHARMACOLOGIC THERAPY

• Ensure proper airway drainage.
• Give nutritional counseling.

■ ACUTE GENERAL Rx

• Prednisone 60 to 80 mg/day and cyclophosphamide 2 mg/kg are generally effective and are used to control clinical manifestations; once the disease comes under control, prednisone is tapered and cyclophosphamide is continued.
• TMP-SMX therapy may represent a useful alternative in patients with lesions limited to the upper and/or lower respiratory tracts in absence of vasculitis or nephritis. Treatment with TMP-SMX (160 mg/800 mg bid) also reduces the incidence of relapses in patients with Wegener's granulomatosis in remission.

■ DISPOSITION

Five-year survival with aggressive treatment is approximately 80%; without treatment 2-yr survival is <20%.

■ REFERRAL

Surgical referral for biopsy

PEARLS & CONSIDERATIONS

■ COMMENTS

• Methotrexate (20 mg/wk) represents an alternative to cyclophosphamide in patients who do not have immediately life-threatening disease.
• C-ANCA levels should not dictate changes in therapy, because they correlate erratically with disease activity.

Author: **Fred F. Ferri, M.D.**

BASIC INFORMATION

■ DEFINITION
Wernicke's encephalopathy is the acute onset of extraocular muscle dysfunction, associated with confusion and ataxia, resulting from thiamine deficiency.

■ SYNONYMS
Korsakoff's syndrome
Wernicke-Korsakoff syndrome
Alcoholic polyneuritic psychosis

ICD-9CM CODES
265.1 Wernicke's encephalopathy, disease, or syndrome

■ EPIDEMIOLOGY & DEMOGRAPHICS
- Most commonly seen in alcoholics
- Slightly more common in males
- Age of onset evenly distributed between age 30 and 70

■ PHYSICAL FINDINGS & CLINICAL PRESENTATION
- Disturbance of extraocular motility, including nystagmus, abducens nerve palsy, and disorders of conjugate gaze
- Encephalopathy
- Ataxia of gait
- Peripheral neuropathy may be seen in addition to the typical findings described previously

■ ETIOLOGY
Thiamine deficiency from alcohol abuse or other malnourished state

DIAGNOSIS

■ DIFFERENTIAL DIAGNOSIS
Diagnosis is directed toward the underlying cause of thiamine deficiency.

■ WORKUP
When suspected, treat immediately.

■ LABORATORY TESTS
- CBC
- Serum chemistries
- Serum pyruvate is elevated
- Whole-blood or erythrocyte transketolase are decreased; rapid resolution to normal in 24 hr with thiamine repletion

■ IMAGING STUDIES
- MRI may show diencephalic and mesencephalic lesions acutely, but there is no definitive radiologic study for diagnosis.
- CT scan may show cerebral atrophy from chronic alcoholism.

TREATMENT

■ NONPHARMACOLOGIC THERAPY
Alcoholics Anonymous

■ ACUTE GENERAL Rx
- 100 mg thiamine IV or IM immediately
- Avoid dextrose containing fluids until thiamine repleted

- Prophylactic treatment for delirium tremens if alcoholic

■ CHRONIC Rx
- Attempt to treat alcoholism or underlying malnourished state.
- Inadequately treated disease may progress to Korsakoff's psychosis (see relevant entry).

■ DISPOSITION
Enter substance abuse program after acute phase.

■ REFERRAL
Referral to a neurologist if symptoms do not resolve after thiamine therapy.

PEARLS & CONSIDERATIONS

■ COMMENTS
- Give thiamine if the disease is even suspected.
- A preventable cause is prolonged dextrose-containing IV fluids without supplemental thiamine.

REFERENCES
Lishman WA: Alcohol and the brain, *Br J Psychiatry* 157:454, 1990.
Zubaran C, Fernandes JG, Rodnight R: Wernicke-Korsakoff syndrome, *Postgrad Med J* 73(855):27, 1997.
Author: **Daniel Mattson, M.D., M.Sc.(Med.)**

BASIC INFORMATION

■ DEFINITION
West Nile virus infection is an illness affecting the central nervous system (CNS) caused by the mosquito-borne West Nile virus.

ICD-9CM CODES
066.4 West Nile virus infection

■ EPIDEMIOLOGY & DEMOGRAPHICS
- Before 1999, West Nile virus infection was confined to areas in the Middle East, with occasional outbreaks in Europe. For the past 4 yr, the infection has been diagnosed for the first time in the Western hemisphere. First seen in the northeast and mid-Atlantic states, West Nile virus infection has spread steadily, each year, to new regions of the U.S. In the year 2002, a record number of cases were reported from the U.S. through November 2002, 3949 proven cases, 254 of which were fatal, were reported from 40 states. Hardest hit were Illinois, Ohio, Michigan, and Louisiana, each reporting more than 300 cases.
- The virus is carried by a number of species of birds, as well as horses and several other animals. It is transmitted to humans through the bite of an infected mosquito. For this reason, West Nile virus infection is seen primarily from mid-summer to mid-autumn, the period of maximum mosquito intensity.
- The majority of severe cases have been reported among individuals >50 yr of age. There is no gender predilection.

■ PHYSICAL FINDINGS & CLINICAL PRESENTATION
- Only 20% of infected individuals develop symptomatic disease. The initial phase of illness is nonspecific, with abrupt onset of fever accompanied by malaise, eye pain, anorexia, headache, and, occasionally, rash and lymphadenopathy. Less commonly, myocarditis, hepatitis, or pancreatitis may occur.

- In approximately 1 in 150 cases, especially among elderly patients, severe neurologic sequelae will occur. Most common among these are ataxia, cranial nerve palsies, optic neuritis, seizures, myelitis, and polyradiculitis.

■ ETIOLOGY
The West Nile virus is a member of the flavivirus group, along with the yellow fever, dengue, St. Louis, and Japanese encephalitis viruses. It has a large reservoir in nature, infecting many species of birds, as well as certain mammals, and is thought to be spread to humans exclusively by various species of mosquito. Neurologic disease is caused by direct invasion of the CNS.

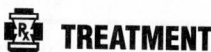

DIAGNOSIS

■ DIFFERENTIAL DIAGNOSIS
- Meningitis or encephalitis caused by more common viruses (e.g., enteroviruses, Herpes simplex)
- Bacterial meningitis
- Vasculitis
- Fungal meningitis (e.g., cryptococcal infection)
- Tuberculous meningitis

■ LABORATORY TESTS
- CBC, electrolytes (hyponatremia common)
- Spinal tap and CSF examination: typically demonstrates lymphocytic pleocytosis with normal level of glucose and elevated level of protein
- CSF West Nile virus IgM antibody level: rare false-positive results in persons recently vaccinated to Japanese encephalitis or yellow fever viruses

■ IMAGING STUDIES
CT or MRI studies of the brain to exclude mass lesions; cerebral edema

TREATMENT

■ NONPHARMACOLOGIC THERAPY
Hospitalization, intravenous hydration, ventilator support may be necessary.

■ ACUTE GENERAL Rx
No specific therapy has been established in clinical trials. Ribavirin and interferon alpha-2b have been shown to have in vitro activity against the virus.

■ CHRONIC Rx
Chronic rehabilitation therapy usually necessary for patients with severe neurologic impairment.

■ DISPOSITION
Chronic rehabilitation as needed following recovery from acute infection

■ REFERRAL
- Infectious disease consultant
- Public health authorities

PEARLS & CONSIDERATIONS

■ COMMENTS
- Diagnosis requires a high index of suspicion, because disease course may be nonspecific and may mimic other, more common disorders.
- Specific laboratory diagnostic studies are available only through public health laboratories.
- Best means of prevention is reduction in mosquito population by draining of stagnant water deposits and, if necessary, insecticide spraying.
- Individuals may reduce risk by covering arms and legs in areas where mosquitoes are likely to be found and using insect repellent.

REFERENCES
Centers for Disease Control and Prevention: www.cdc.gov/ncidod/dvbid/westnile/surv&control.htm.

Kahler SC: APHIS: West Nile virus vaccine safe for use, *J Am Vet Med Assoc* 223(4):416, 2003.

Petersen LR, Marfin AA: West Nile virus: a primer for the clinician, *Ann Intern Med* 137:173, 2002.

Author: **Joseph R. Masci, M.D.**

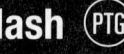

 BASIC INFORMATION

■ **DEFINITION**
Whiplash refers to a hyperextension injury to the neck, often the result of being struck from behind by a fast-moving vehicle. It is an acceleration-deceleration injury to the neck.

■ **SYNONYMS**
• Cervical strain
• Soft tissue cervical hyperextension injury
• Acceleration flexion-extension neck injury

ICD-9CM CODES
847.0 Whiplash injury or syndrome

■ **EPIDEMIOLOGY & DEMOGRAPHICS**
• Whiplash occurs in more than 1 million people each year.
• Most injuries (40%) are the result of rear-end motor vehicle accidents.
• Whiplash occurs at all ages, in both sexes, and at all socioeconomic levels.
• Incidence is 4 per 1000 persons and is higher in women than men.
• Nearly 50% of patients with whiplash seek legal advice.
• Whiplash is also seen in shaken baby syndrome.

■ **PHYSICAL FINDINGS & CLINICAL PRESENTATION**
• Most present with a history of being involved in a motor vehicle accident and rear-ended by another vehicle
• Pain not present initially but usually develops hours to a few days later
• Neck tightness and stiffness
• Occipital headache
• Shoulder, arm, and back pain
• Numbness in the arms
• Tinnitus
• TMJ pain
• Dysphagia (retropharyngeal hematoma)
• Decreased range of motion of the neck

■ **ETIOLOGY**
• The mechanism of injury is due to the sudden acceleration of the body forward, forcing the neck to hyperextend backward, causing injury to ligaments, muscles, bone, and/or intervertebral disk. At the end of the accident the head is thrust forward in a flexion position, sometimes causing injury to C5-C6-C7.
• Motor vehicle accidents, trauma from falls, contact sports, physical abuse, and altercations are all possible causes of whiplash.

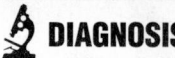 **DIAGNOSIS**

The clinical presentation and physical examination determine both the diagnosis and clinical classification of whiplash-associated disorders (Table 1-62).

■ **DIFFERENTIAL DIAGNOSIS**
The differential diagnosis of cervical strain is:
• Osteoarthritis
• Cervical disk disease
• Fibrositis
• Neuritis
• Torticollis
• Spinal cord tumor
• TMJ syndrome
• Tension headache
• Migraine headache

■ **WORKUP**
Any patient who presents with symptoms of whiplash and musculoskeletal or neurologic signs merits a workup to exclude cervical spine fractures or herniated disk disease.

■ **LABORATORY TESTS**
Laboratory studies are not helpful in the diagnosis of whiplash or in excluding complications of acute neck injuries.

■ **IMAGING STUDIES**
• Plain C-spine films (AP, lateral, and odontoid views) to exclude cervical spine fractures
• Flexion/extension x-rays looking for C-spine instability
• CT scan to exclude fracture if suspected by plain films
• MRI to look for cervical disk bulging or herniation

■ **TREATMENT**

■ **NONPHARMACOLOGIC THERAPY**
• Bed rest
• Soft cervical collar for no longer than 72 hr
• Moist heat 15 to 20 min four to six times per day

■ **ACUTE GENERAL Rx**
• Analgesics
  1. Ibuprofen 800 mg PO tid
  2. Naproxen 500 mg PO bid
  3. Acetaminophen 1 g PO qid
• Muscle relaxants (short-term use)
  1. Cyclobenzaprine 10 mg PO tid
  2. Methocarbamol 1 g PO qid
  3. Carisoprodol 350 mg PO qid

■ **CHRONIC Rx**
• NSAIDs as described previously can be used long term.
• Intraarticular corticosteroids have been tried in the past; however, recently they were found not to be effective for pain relief in patients with chronic whiplash syndrome.

■ **DISPOSITION**
• Most patients recover from the acute whiplash injury within weeks.
• 20% to 40% may develop chronic whiplash syndrome (symptoms of headache, neck pain, and psychiatric complaints that persist for 6 mo).

■ **REFERRAL**
If symptoms are not relieved with conservative nonpharmacologic and acute treatments within 1 to 2 mo, a referral to orthopedic or rheumatology may be helpful.

TABLE 1-62 Proposed Clinical Classification of Whiplash-Associated Disorders

GRADE	CLINICAL PRESENTATION
0	No complaint about the neck No physical sign(s)
I	Neck complaint of pain, stiffness, or tenderness only No physical sign(s)
II	Neck complaint and musculoskeletal sign(s)*
III	Neck complaint and neurologic sign(s)†
IV	Neck complaint and fracture or dislocation

From the Scientific Monograph of the Quebec Task Force on Whiplash Associated Disorders: *Spine* 20(8S):1S, 1995.
*Musculoskeletal signs include decreased range of motion and point tenderness.
†Neurologic signs include decreased or absent deep tendon reflexes, weakness, and sensory deficits.
Symptoms and disorders that can be manifest in all grades include deafness, dizziness, tinnitus, headache, memory loss, dysphagia, and temporomandibular joint pain.

☼ PEARLS & CONSIDERATIONS

■ COMMENTS

- The entity of chronic whiplash syndrome remains elusive. Some authorities argue that financial motivation is a factor leading to persistent neck symptoms. Other studies do not substantiate this, countering a true chronic injury to the soft tissues of the neck.
- Nearly one third of all personal injury cases involve cervical injuries.

REFERENCES

Barnsley L et al: Lack of effect of intraarticular corticosteroids for chronic pain in the cervical-zygapophyseal joints, *N Engl J Med* 330(15):1047, 1994.

Eck JC, Hodges SD, Humphreys SC: Whiplash: a review of a commonly misunderstood injury, *Am J Med* 110(8):651, 2001.

Livingston M: Whiplash injury, *J Rheumatol* 26(5):1206, 1999.

Sptizer WO et al: Scientific monograph of the Quebec Task Force on whiplash-associated disorders, *Spine* 208S:1S, 1995.

Young WF: The enigma of whiplash injury: current management strategies and controversies, *Postgrad Med* 93(10):526, 2000.

Author: **Peter Petropoulos, M.D.**

BASIC INFORMATION

■ DEFINITION

Whipple's disease is a multisystem illness characterized by malabsorption and its consequences, lymphadenopathy, arthritis, cardiac involvement, ocular symptoms and neurologic problems, caused by the gram-positive bacillus *Tropheryma whippelii*.

■ SYNONYMS

Intestinal lipodystrophy (name used by Dr. Whipple in 1907)

ICD-9CM CODES
040.2 Whipple's disease

■ EPIDEMIOLOGY & DEMOGRAPHICS
• Uncommon illness
• Peak age: 30 to 60 yr of age
• More frequent in men than women

■ PHYSICAL FINDINGS & CLINICAL PRESENTATION
PRESENTATION: The disease may present with extraintestinal symptoms (e.g., arthralgia), but few clinicians will suspect the diagnosis unless or until GI symptoms are present.
The GI manifestations are those seen in malabsorption of any cause:
• Diarrhea: 5 to 10 semiformed, malodorous steatorrheic stools per day
• Abdominal bloating and cramps
• Anorexia
Extraintestinal manifestations of malabsorption:
• Weight loss, fatigue
• Anemia
• Bleeding diathesis
• Edema and ascites
• Osteomalacia
Extraintestinal involvement:
• Arthritis (intermittent, migratory, affecting small, large, and axial joints)
• Pleuritic chest pain and cough
• Pericarditis, endocarditis
• Dementia, ophthalmoplegia, myoclonus, and many other symptoms, because any portion of the central nervous system may be a disease site
• Fever
PHYSICAL FINDINGS:
• Abdominal distention, sometimes with tenderness and less commonly fullness or mass, which represents enlarged mesenteric lymph nodes

• Signs of weight loss, cachexia
• Clubbing
• Lymphadenopathy
• Inflamed joints
• Heart murmur or rub
• Sensory loss or motor weakness related to peripheral neuropathy
• Abnormal mental status examination
• Pallor

■ ETIOLOGY & PATHOGENESIS
• Infectious disease caused by *Tropheryma whippelii,* an actinobacter.
• The bacillus has never been cultured, nor has direct transmission from patient to patient ever been documented; however, the agent can be seen in tissue samples by electron microscopy and identified by polymerase chain reaction (PCR).
• Predictable response to appropriate antibiotic therapy confirms the pathogenic role of the infection.
• Tissue infiltration by macrophages is believed to be the mechanism of specific organ dysfunction and symptoms.

DIAGNOSIS

■ DIFFERENTIAL DIAGNOSIS
Malabsorption/maldigestion:
• Celiac disease
• *Mycobacterium avium-intracellulare* intestinal infection in patients with AIDS
• Intestinal lymphoma
• Abetalipoproteinemia
• Amyloidosis
• Systemic mastocytosis
• Radiation enteritis
• Crohn's disease
• Short bowel syndrome
• Pancreatic insufficiency
• Intestinal bacterial overgrowth
• Lactose deficiency
• Postgastrectomy syndrome
• Other cause of diarrhea (see Section III Figs. 3-60 and 3-61)
Seronegative inflammatory arthritis (see Section II for differential diagnosis)
Pericarditis and pleuritis
Lymphadenitis
Neurologic disorders

■ WORKUP
Laboratory tests and imaging studies

■ LABORATORY TESTS
• Anemia (iron, folate, and/or vitamin B_{12} deficiency)
• Hypokalemia
• Hypocalcemia
• Hypomagnesemia
• Hypoalbuminemia
• Prolonged prothrombin time
• Low serum carotene
• Low cholesterol
• Leukocytosis
• Steatorrhea demonstrated by a Sudan fecal fat stain
• 72-Hr stool collection demonstrating more than 7 g/24 hr of fat in the stool is impractical to perform, especially in ambulatory patients
• Defective D-xylose absorption

■ IMAGING STUDIES
Small bowel x-rays after barium ingestion often show thickening of mucosal folds.

■ BIOPSY
Infiltration of the intestinal lamina propria by PAS-positive macrophages containing gram-positive, acid-fast negative bacilli, associated with lymphatic dilation (diagnostic); PCR of the involved tissue in uncertain cases

TREATMENT

• Antibiotics: TMP/SMX DS bid for 6 to 12 mo
• Alternative antibiotics: penicillin alone, penicillin plus streptomycin, ampicillin, tetracycline, chloramphenicol, ceftriaxone
• Treat specific vitamin, mineral, and nutrient deficiencies

REFERENCES

Malwald M et al: *Tropheryma whippelii* DNA is rare in the intestinal mucosa of patients without other evidence of Whipple disease, *Ann Intern Med* 136:115, 2001.

Trier JS: Whipple's disease. In Feldman M, Scharschmidt BF, Sleisenger MH (eds): *Sleisenger and Fordtran's gastrointestinal and liver disease,* ed 6, Philadelphia, 1998, WB Saunders.

Author: **Tom J. Wachtel, M.D.**

BASIC INFORMATION

■ DEFINITION

Wilson's disease is a disorder of copper transport with inadequate biliary copper excretion, leading to an accumulation of the metal in liver, brain, kidneys, and corneas.

ICD-9CM CODES

275.1 Wilson's disease

■ EPIDEMIOLOGY & DEMOGRAPHICS

- Prevalence: 1 in 30,000
- Affects men and women equally (autosomal recessive gene)
- Onset of symptoms: 3 to 40 yr of age

■ CLINICAL PRESENTATION & PHYSICAL FINDINGS

Hepatic presentation:
- Acute hepatitis with malaise, anorexia, nausea, jaundice, elevated transaminase, prolonged prothrombin time; rarely fulminant hepatic failure
- Chronic active (or autoimmune) hepatitis with fatigue, malaise, rashes, arthralgia, elevated transaminase, elevated serum IgG, positive ANA and anti–smooth muscle antibody
- Chronic liver disease/cirrhosis with hepatosplenomegaly, ascites, low serum albumin, prolonged prothrombin time, portal hypertension

Neurologic presentation:
- Movement disorder: tremors, ataxia
- Spastic dystonia: masklike facies, rigidity, gait disturbance, dysarthria, drooling, dysphagia

Psychiatric presentation:
- Depression, obsessive-compulsive disorder, psychopathic behaviors

Other organs:
- Hemolytic anemia
- Renal disease (i.e., Fanconi's syndrome with hematuria, phosphaturia, renal tubular acidosis, vitamin D–resistant rickets)
- Cardiomyopathy
- Arthritis
- Hypoparathyroidism
- Hypogonadism

PHYSICAL FINDINGS:
- Ocular: the Kayser-Fleischer ring is a gold-yellow ring seen at the periphery of the iris (Fig. 1-297)
- Stigmata of acute or chronic liver disease
- Neurologic abnormalities: see previous

■ ETIOLOGY & PATHOGENESIS

- Dietary copper is transported from the intestine to the liver where normally it is metabolized into ceruloplasmin. In Wilson's disease, defective incorporation of copper into ceruloplasmin and a decrease of biliary copper excretion lead to accumulation of this mineral.
- The gene for Wilson's disease is located in chromosome 13.

DIAGNOSIS

■ DIFFERENTIAL DIAGNOSIS

- Hereditary hypoceruloplasminemia
- Menkes' disease
- Consider the diagnosis of Wilson's disease in all cases of acute or chronic liver disease where another cause has not been established
- Consider Wilson's disease in patients with movement disorders or dystonia even without symptomatic liver disease

■ LABORATORY TESTS

- Abnormal LFTs (note that AST may be higher than ALT)
- Low serum ceruloplasmin level (<200 mg/L)
- Low serum copper (<65 μg/L)
- 24-hr urinary copper excretion greater than 100 μg (normal <30 μg); increases to greater than 1200 μg/24 hr after 500 mg of d-penicillamine (normal <500 μg/24 hr)
- Low serum uric acid and phosphorus
- Abnormal urinalysis (hematuria)

■ BIOPSY

- Early:
  Steatosis, focal necrosis, glycogenated hepatocyte nuclei
  May reveal inflammation and piecemeal necrosis
- Late: cirrhosis
- Hepatic copper content (>250 μg/g of dry weight) (normal is 20 to 50 μg)

TREATMENT

- Penicillamine: (chelator therapy) 0.75 to 1.5 g/day divided bid (with pyridoxine 25 mg/day)
  Monitor CBC and urinalysis weekly
- Trientine: (triethylene tetramine) (chelator therapy)
  1 to 2 g/day divided tid
  Monitor CBC
- Zinc: (inhibits intestinal copper absorption)
  50 mg tid
  Monitor zinc level
- Ammonium tetrathiomolybdate for neurologic symptoms
- Antioxidants
- Liver transplant (for severe hepatic failure unresponsive to chelation)

■ PROGNOSIS

Good with early chelation treatment

■ REFERRAL

To gastroenterologist

REFERENCES

Cox DW, Roberts EA: Wilson's disease. In Feldman M, Scharschmidt BF, Sleisenger MH (eds): *Sleisenger & Fordtran's gastrointestinal and liver disease,* ed 6, Philadelphia, 1998, WB Saunders.

El-Youssef M: Wilson's disease, *Mayo Clin Proc* 78:1126, 2003.

Author: **Tom J. Wachtel, M.D.**

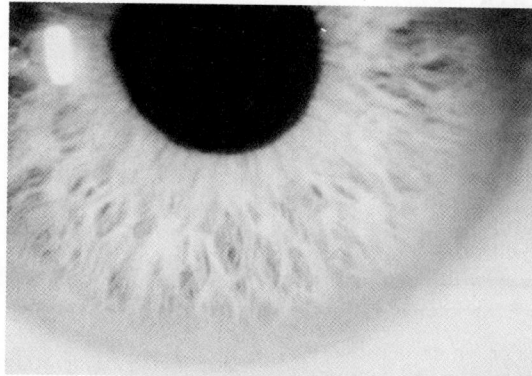

Fig. 1-297 Wilson's disease. A Kayser-Fleisher ring, which is a gold-yellow ring, extends to the limbus without a clear interval. (From Palay D [ed]: *Ophthalmology for the primary care physician,* St Louis, 1997, Mosby.)

BASIC INFORMATION

■ DEFINITION

Wolff-Parkinson-White syndrome is an electrocardiographic abnormality associated with earlier than normal ventricular depolarization following the atrial impulse and predisposing the affected person to tachyarrhythmias.

■ SYNONYMS

Preexcitation syndrome

ICD-9CM CODES

426.7 Wolff-Parkinson-White syndrome
426.81 Lown-Ganong-Levine syndrome

■ EPIDEMIOLOGY & DEMOGRAPHICS

- Prevalence: 1.5 cases/1000 persons
- Prevalence higher in males and decreases with age
- Most patients with WPW syndrome have normal hearts, but associations with mitral valve prolapse, cardiomyopathies, and Ebstein's anomaly have been reported

■ PHYSICAL FINDINGS & CLINICAL PRESENTATION

Paroxysmal tachycardias
- 10% of WPW patients aged 20 to 40 yr
- 35% of WPW patients aged over 60 yr

The type of tachycardia is:
- Reciprocating tachycardia at 150 to 250 beats per minute (80%)
- Atrial fibrillation (15%)
- Atrial flutter (5%)
- Ventricular tachycardia: rare
- Sudden death is rare (<1/1000 cases)

■ PATHOPHYSIOLOGY

- Existence of accessory pathways (Kent bundles)
- If the accessory pathway is capable of anterograde conduction, two parallel routes of AV conduction are possible, one subject to delay through the AV mode, the other without delay through the accessory pathway. The resulting QRS complex is a fusion beat with the "delta" wave representing ventricular activation through the accessory pathway (Fig. 1-298).
- Tachycardias occur when, because of different refractory periods, conduction is anterograde in one pathway (usually the normal AV pathway) and retrograde in the other (usually the accessory pathway). Some patients (5% to 10%) with WPW syndrome have multiple accessory pathways.

DIAGNOSIS

Three basic features characterize the ECG abnormalities in WPW syndrome (Fig. 1-299):
- PR interval <120 msec
- QRS complex >120 msec with a slurred, slowly rising onset of QRS in some lead (delta wave)
- ST-T wave changes

Variants
- Lown-Ganong-Levine syndrome: atriohisian pathway with short PR interval and normal QRS complex on ECG (no delta wave)
- Atriofascicular accessory pathways: duplication of the AV node, with normal baseline ECG

TREATMENT

- No treatment in the absence of tachyarrhythmias.
- Symptomatic tachyarrhythmias.
- Acute episode: adenosine, verapamil, or diltiazem can be used to terminate an episode of reciprocal tachycardia.
- Digitalis should not be used because it can reduce refractoriness in the accessory pathway and accelerate the tachycardia. Cardioversion should be used in the presence of hemodynamic impairment.

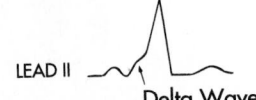

Fig. 1-298 With Wolff-Parkinson-White syndrome an abnormal accessory conduction pathway called a bypass tract (BT) connects the atria and ventricles. (From Goldberger AL [ed]: *Clinical electrocardiography: a simplified approach*, ed 6, St Louis, 1999, Mosby.)

- Prevention:
Empiric trials or serial electrophysiologic drug testing of:
  1. Quinidine and propranolol
  2. Procainamide and verapamil
  3. Amiodarone
  4. Sotalol

Electrical or surgical ablation of the accessory pathway

REFERENCES

Gollob MH et al: Identification of a gene responsible for familial Wolff-Parkinson-White syndrome, *N Engl J Med* 366:1823, 2001.

Olgin JE, Zipes DP: Preexcitation syndrome. In Braunwald E (ed): *Heart disease: a textbook of cardiovascular medicine*, ed 6, vol 2, Philadelphia, 2001, WB Saunders.

Author: **Tom J. Wachtel, M.D.**

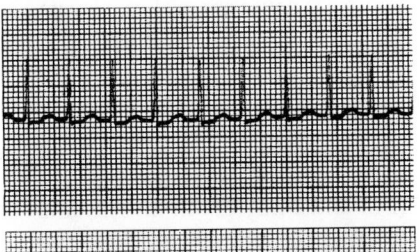

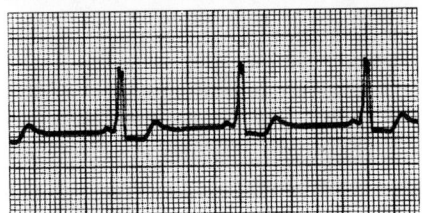

Fig. 1-299 **A,** SVT in a child with Wolff-Parkinson-White (WPW) syndrome. Note the normal QRS complexes during the tachycardia. **B,** Later the typical features of WPW syndrome are apparent (short P-R interval, delta wave, and wide QRS). (From Behrman RE: *Nelson textbook of pediatrics*, ed 16, Philadelphia, 2000, WB Saunders.)

BASIC INFORMATION

■ DEFINITION

Yellow fever is an infection, primarily of the liver, with systemic manifestations caused by the yellow fever virus (YFV).

ICD-9CM CODES
060.9 Yellow fever

■ EPIDEMIOLOGY & DEMOGRAPHICS

INCIDENCE (IN U.S.):
- None
- Approximate attack rates of 3% in Africa and Amazon

PREVALENCE (IN U.S.):
- None
- Endemic areas: 20% of population

PREDOMINANT SEX: In Africa and Amazon, male agricultural workers

PREDOMINANT AGE: 20 to 40 yr

PEAK INCIDENCE: Variable with outbreaks

■ PHYSICAL FINDINGS & CLINICAL PRESENTATION

- Clinical illness with jaundice in about 5% to 20% of infections
- Most subclinical
- Onset sudden after incubation period of 3 to 6 days
- Viremic (early) phase
  1. Fever, chills
  2. Severe headache
  3. Lumbosacral pain
  4. Myalgias
  5. Nausea
  6. Severe malaise
  7. Conjunctivitis
  8. Relative bradycardia
- After brief recovery, toxic phase:
  1. Jaundice
  2. Oliguria
  3. Albuminuria
  4. Hemorrhage (especially hematemesis)
  5. Encephalopathy
  6. Shock
  7. Acidosis

■ ETIOLOGY

- Yellow fever virus (*L. flavus*)
  1. Prototype flavivirus
  2. Infects primarily hepatic cells
  3. Replication
     a. Exclusively intracellular and intracytoplasmic
     b. Primarily in the endoplasmic reticulum
  4. Late in infection, cytopathic effects (antibody- and cell-mediated) produce pathology
- Vector
  1. *Aedes aegypti* (urban)
  2. *Aedes* spp., *Haemagogus* (especially in Amazon) mosquitos (sylvan)
  3. Primary hosts humans and simian species
  4. Virus maintained in mosquito ova during dry season
  5. Sylvan cycle interrupted by humans: agriculture, forest clearing

- Geographic distribution
  1. South American and Africa, in countries between +15 and −15 degrees latitude
  2. Not in Asia
- Recent increase in epidemics in Africa (especially Nigeria)
  1. Several hundred thousand cases between 1987 and 1991
  2. Fatality rate approximately 20% in jaundiced patients
  3. Death between days 7 and 10
- Pathogenesis
  1. Unclear
  2. Probably involves Kupffer cell, followed by hepatocyte infection
  3. Renal failure accompanied by viral antigen in glomeruli
  4. Shock and lactic acidosis accompanied by release of vasoactive mediators from liver, nodes, spleen
  5. Myocarditis contributes to shock and collapse
  6. Hemorrhage
     a. Decreased synthesis of clotting factors
     b. DIC
  7. Encephalopathy secondary to cerebral edema

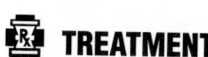 **DIAGNOSIS**

■ DIFFERENTIAL DIAGNOSIS

- Viral hepatitis
- Leptospirosis
- Malaria
- Typhoid fever
- Hemorrhagic fevers (HF) with jaundice
  1. Dengue (HF)
  2. Rift Valley fever
  3. Crimean-Congo (HF)

■ WORKUP

- CBC
- Liver function tests
- Serum for serology (YFV, viral isolation)
- Coagulation studies
  1. Prothrombin time
  2. Fibrinogen
  3. Fibrin split products
- Liver biopsy contraindicated (death from bleeding)

■ LABORATORY TESTS

- CBC
  1. Generally nonspecific
  2. Mild leukopenia
  3. Thrombocytopenia
  4. Anemia
- LFTs
  1. Mildly to severely abnormal ALT, AST, and bilirubin
- Elevated creatinine and BUN
- Coagulation studies
  1. Normal *or*
  2. Demonstrate abnormal prothrombin time *or*
  3. Reveal DIC
- Terminal hypoglycemia

- Specific diagnosis confirmed by viral isolation from blood
- Serologic diagnosis
  1. Viral antigen in serum (ELISA)
  2. Viral RNA by PCR
  3. IgM by:
     a. Antibody-capture ELISA
     b. Hemagglutination inhibition
     c. Complement fixation
     d. Neutralization assays
  4. Appear within 5 to 7 days
     a. IgM
     b. HI
     c. N Ab
  5. Appear within 7 to 14 days
     a. CF Ab
  6. Rising Ab confirmed by paired sera
  7. CF persists up to 1 yr

TREATMENT

■ ACUTE GENERAL Rx

- Treatment symptomatic
- Acetaminophen (headache and fever)
- Antacids, cimetidine (GI bleeding)
- Blood transfusion, volume replacement for hemorrhage and shock
- Dialysis for renal failure
- No clearly useful antiviral agents

■ DISPOSITION

Follow-up until hepatic, renal, CNS disease resolved

■ REFERRAL

To infectious diseases expert for accurate diagnosis and management

PEARLS & CONSIDERATIONS

■ COMMENTS

- Yellow fever is preventable.
- Recovery from yellow fever confers lasting immunity.
- Live, attenuated yellow fever vaccine provides protective immunity in 95% of vaccinees within 10 days of vaccination.
- Reimmunization at 10-yr intervals is required for travel.
- Vaccine contraindicated in:
  1. Infants <6 mo (postvaccinal encephalitis)
  2. Immunosuppressed patients
  3. Pregnant women (congenital infection may result, although generally without adverse effects on the fetus)
  4. Patients with egg hypersensitivity
- Cases of multiple organ system failure have been associated with recent administration of yellow fever vaccine. More data are needed to clearly define a causal association. Health care providers should provide vaccine only to persons planning to travel to areas reporting yellow fever activity or areas in the yellow fever endemic zone.

Author: **Marilyn Fabbri, M.D.**

■ BASIC INFORMATION

■ DEFINITION
Zenker's (hypopharyngeal) diverticulum refers to the acquired physiologic obstruction of the esophageal introitus that results from mucosal herniation (false diverticulum) posteriorly between the cricopharyngeus muscle and the inferior pharyngeal constrictor muscle (Fig. 1-300).

■ SYNONYMS
- Pharyngoesophageal diverticulum
- Pulsion diverticulum

ICD-9CM CODES
530.6 Zenker's diverticulum (esophagus)

■ EPIDEMIOLOGY & DEMOGRAPHICS
- Rare disease: <1% of all barium swallows
- Commonly seen in people over 50 yr of age (most common in women and elderly)
- Peak incidence is seventh to ninth decades
- Associated with GERD and hiatal hernia

■ PHYSICAL FINDINGS & CLINICAL PRESENTATION
Small Zenker's diverticulum may be asymptomatic. As they become larger, symptoms include:
- Dysphagia to solids and liquids
- Regurgitation of undigested food
- Sensation of globus or fullness in the neck
- Cough
- Halitosis
- Aspiration pneumonia
- Weight loss
- Voice changes

■ ETIOLOGY
The specific cause of Zenker's diverticulum is not known; however, the leading hypothesis suggests the following:
- During swallowing there is raised intraluminal pressure secondary to the incomplete opening of the cricopharyngeus muscle (improperly timed relaxation) before the bolus of food can be driven forward into the stomach.
- Discordination of the swallowing mechanism leads to increased pressure on the mucosa of the hypopharynx resulting in the slow progressive distention of the mucosa in the weakest area of the esophagus, namely being the posterior wall. The end result being the formation of a false diverticulum where food elements and secretions may be lodged, causing the symptoms listed previously.

🔬 DIAGNOSIS

Clinical presentation and barium swallow typically make the diagnosis of Zenker's diverticulum.

■ DIFFERENTIAL DIAGNOSIS
The differential diagnosis is similar to anyone presenting with dysphagia:
- Achalasia
- Esophageal spasm
- Esophageal carcinoma
- Esophageal webs
- Peptic stricture
- Lower esophageal (Schatzki) ring
- Foreign bodies
- CNS disorders (stroke, Parkinson's disease, ALS, multiple sclerosis, myasthenia gravis, muscular dystrophies)
- Dermatomyositis
- Infection

■ WORKUP
The workup for suspected Zenker's diverticulum should include a barium swallow. Upper endoscopy runs the risk of perforation. Manometry motility studies are usually not indicated because they will not change the course of treatment.

■ LABORATORY TESTS
There are no specific laboratory tests to diagnose Zenker's diverticulum.

■ IMAGING STUDIES
- Barium swallow is the diagnostic procedure of choice. Radiographically Zenker's diverticulum is easily demonstrated with a barium contrast study (Fig. 1-301).
- Endoscopy is indicated if barium studies show mucosal irregularities to rule out neoplasia.
- Barium swallow characteristically demonstrates a herniated sac with a narrow diverticular neck that typically originates just proximal to the cricopharyngeus at the level of C5-C6.
- A chest x-ray is performed in cases of suspected aspiration pneumonia.

℞ TREATMENT

■ NONPHARMACOLOGIC THERAPY
- Soft mechanical diet can be tried in patients with symptoms of dysphagia.
- Avoid seeds, skins, and nuts.

■ ACUTE GENERAL Rx
- Endoscopic techniques (esophagodiverticulostomy) have largely replaced conventional treatment by open surgery.
- Surgery is the recommended treatment for symptomatic patients with Zenker's diverticulum.
- Surgical treatment relieves symptoms (dysphagia, cough, aspiration) in nearly all patients with Zenker's diverticulum.
- Surgical procedures include:
  1. Cervical diverticulectomy with cricopharyngeal myotomy (most common approach)

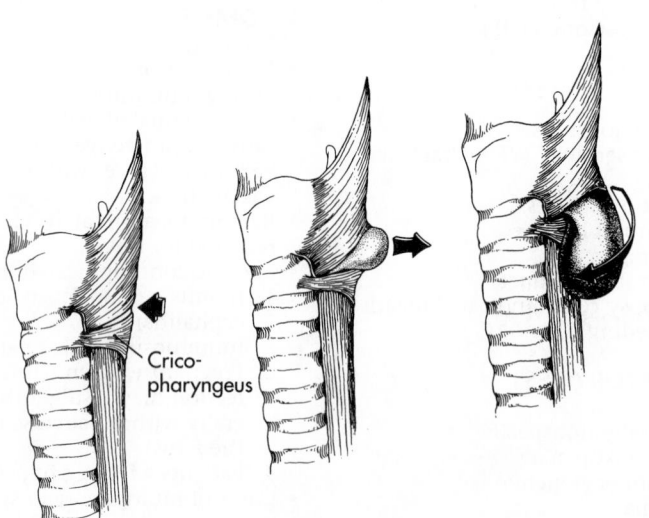
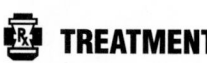

Fig. 1-300 Formation of pharyngoesophageal (Zenker's) diverticulum. *Left,* Herniation of the pharyngeal mucosa and submucosa occurs at the point of transition *(arrow)* between the oblique fibers of the thyropharyngeus muscle and the more horizontal fibers of the cricopharyngeus muscle. *Center and right,* As the diverticulum enlarges, it dissects toward the left side and downward into the superior mediastinum in the prevertebral space. (From Sabiston D: *Textbook of surgery,* ed 15, Philadelphia, 1997, WB Saunders.)

2. Diverticulopexy or diverticular inversion with cricopharyngeal myotomy
3. Diverticulectomy alone
4. Cricopharyngeal myotomy alone
- Surgical mortality <1.5%.

■ CHRONIC Rx

In patients not having surgery, treatment is directed toward any complications that may occur:
- Antibiotics for aspiration pneumonia
- H_2 antagonists for ulcerations that can develop within the diverticulum
- Botulinum toxin is considered for temporary relief of dysphagia

■ DISPOSITION
- The natural history of Zenker's diverticulum if left untreated is one of progressive enlargement of the diverticulum.
- As the diverticulum enlarges, the risk of complications, including aspiration pneumonia, increases.
- Recurrence of Zenker's diverticulum (4%) postoperatively can occur; however, patients are usually not symptomatic.

■ REFERRAL

Any patient with dysphagia requires a gastroenterology consultation. A thoracic surgical, ENT, or head and neck surgeon may be consulted if surgery is considered for Zenker's diverticulum.

☼ PEARLS & CONSIDERATIONS

■ COMMENTS
- The association of cancer with Zenker's diverticulum is rare (0.4%).
- Zenker's diverticulum forms in "Killian's triangle," the point between the oblique fibers of the inferior pharyngeal muscle and the horizontal fibers of the cricopharyngeus muscle.

REFERENCES

Achkar E: Zenker's diverticulum, *Dig Dis* 16(3):144, 1998.

Blitzer A, Brin MF: Use of botulinum toxin for diagnosis and management of cricopharyngeal achalasia, *Otolaryngol Head Neck Surg* 116(3):328, 1997.

Bremner CG: Zenker's diverticulum, *Arch Surg* 133(10):1131, 1998.

Bremmer CG, DeMeester TR: Endoscopic treatment of Zenker's diverticulum, *Gastrointestl Endosc* 49(1):126, 1999.

Richtsmeire WJ: Endoscopic management of Zenker diverticulum: a staple assisted approach, *Am J Med* 3A:175S, 2003.

Siddiq MA, Sood S, Strachan D: Pharyngeal pouch (Zenker's diculum), *Postgrad Med J* 77(910):506, 2001.

Authors: **Hemchand Ramberan, M.D., and Peter Petropoulos, M.D.**

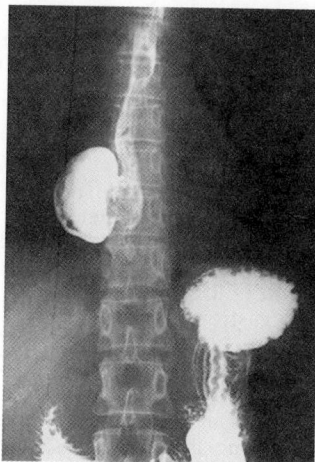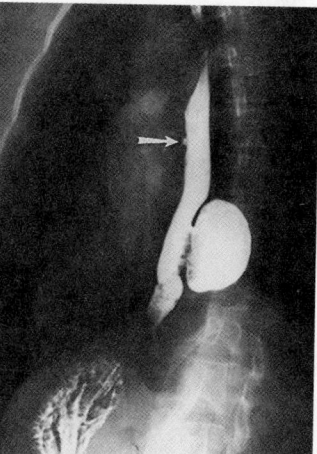

Fig. 1-301   Posteroanterior *(left)* and oblique *(right)* views from barium esophagogram showing both a typical diverticulum of the junction of the mid- and distal esophagus and a small traction diverticulum *(arrow)* of the mid-esophagus. (From Sabiston D: *Textbook of surgery,* ed 15, Philadelphia, 1997, Saunders.)

BASIC INFORMATION

■ DEFINITION

Zollinger-Ellison (ZE) syndrome is a hypergastrinemic state caused by a pancreatic or extrapancreatic non–beta islet cell tumor (gastrinoma) and resulting in peptic acid disease.

■ SYNONYMS

Gastrinoma

ICD-9CM CODES

251.5 Zollinger-Ellison syndrome

■ EPIDEMIOLOGY & DEMOGRAPHICS

- Incidence is unknown, but 0.1% of all duodenal ulcers are believed to be caused by ZE.
- Occurs in both genders and at any age (most common in 30 to 50 yr of age).
- Two thirds of gastrinomas are sporadic, and one third are associated with multiple endocrine neoplasia type 1 (MEN-1), an autosomal dominant genetic disorder that also includes hyperparathyroidism and pituitary tumors.
- About 60% of gastrinomas are malignant.

■ PHYSICAL FINDINGS & CLINICAL PRESENTATION

- The vast majority of patients (95%) present with symptoms of peptic ulcer (see Section I).
- 60% of patients have symptoms related to gastroesophageal reflux disease (see Section I).
- One third of patients with ZE have diarrhea and, less commonly, steatorrhea.

The following circumstances warrant suspicion of ZE syndrome:
- Ulcers distal to the first portion of the duodenum
- Multiple peptic ulcers
- Ineffective treatment for peptic ulcer disease with the usual drug doses and schedules
- Peptic ulcer and diarrhea
- Familial history of peptic ulcer
- Patients with a personal or family history suggesting parathyroid or pituitary tumors of dysfunction
- Peptic ulcer and urinary tract calculi
- Patients with peptic ulcer who are negative for *H. pylori* and do not have a history of NSAID use

■ ETIOLOGY

- The pathophysiologic manifestations of ZE syndrome are related to the effects of hypergastrinemia. Gastrin stimulates gastric acid secretion, which in turn is responsible for the development of duodenal ulcers and diarrhea. Gastrin also promotes gastric mucosal epithelial cell growth and resulting parietal cell hyperplasia.
- Gastrinomas are usually small (0.1 to 2 cm) but sometimes large (>20 cm) tumors.
- 60% of gastrinomas are malignant, with liver and regional lymph nodes the most common site of metastases. Histology is not a good predictor of the biology of gastrinomas.
- 60% of patients with MEN-1 have gastrinomas.
- 10% of patients with ZE syndrome have islet cell hyperplasia rather than gastrinomas; in 10% to 20% of patients with gastrinoma the tumors cannot be located because of small size.

DIAGNOSIS

■ DIFFERENTIAL DIAGNOSIS

- Peptic ulcer disease (see Section I)
- Gastroesophageal reflux disease (see Section I)

Diarrhea (see Section III, Figs. 3-60 and 3-61)

■ WORKUP

- Diagnosis of peptic ulcer
  UGI series (may also show prominent gastric rugal folds)
  Endoscopy
- Gastric acid secretion
- Serum gastrin level (fasting) >150 pg/ml (causes of false-positive: pernicious anemia, renal failure, retained gastric antrum syndrome, diabetes mellitus, rheumatoid arthritis)
- Provocative gastrin level tests
  Secretin stimulation
  Calcium stimulation
  Standard test meal stimulation
- Gastrinoma localization
  Arteriography (Fig. 1-302)
  Abdominal sonography
  Abdominal CT scan
  Abdominal MRI
  Selective portal vein branch gastrin level
  Octreotide scan

TREATMENT

- Surgical resection of the gastrinoma (NOTE: 90% of gastrinomas can be located, resulting in a 40% overall cure rate)
- Total gastrectomy or vagotomy (palliative in some patients)
- Medical treatment
  Proton pump inhibitors (e.g., omeprazole or lansoprazole)
  Somatostatin or octreotide
  Chemotherapy for metastatic gastrinoma with streptozotocin, 5-FU, and doxorubicin

■ PROGNOSIS

Five-year survival:
- Two thirds of all patients
- 20% with liver metastases
- 90% without liver metastases

■ REFERRAL

To gastroenterologist

REFERENCES

McGuigan JE: Zollinger-Ellison syndrome. In Feldman M, Scharschmidt BF, Sleisenger MH (eds): *Sleisenger & Fordtran's gastrointestinal and liver disease,* ed 6, St Louis, 1998, WB Saunders.

Norten JA et al: Surgery to cure Zollinger-Ellison syndrome, *N Engl J Med* 341:635, 1999.

Author: **Tom J. Wachtel, M.D.**

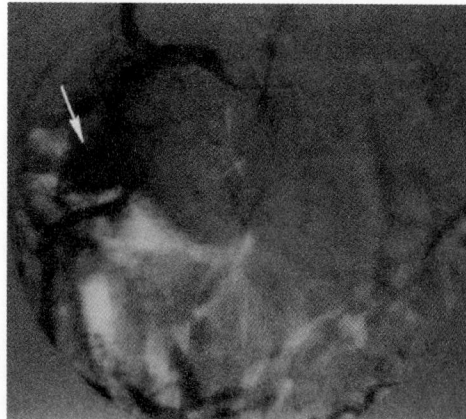

Fig. 1-302   Selective celiac arteriogram in a patient with Zollinger-Ellison syndrome. The hepatic artery injection fills the gastroduodenal artery, which reveals a tumor blush *(arrow)* in the region of the duodenum or head of the pancreas. At exploration, a 2-cm benign duodenal gastrinoma was identified and locally resected. (From Sabiston D: *Textbook of surgery,* ed 15, Philadelphia, 1997, WB Saunders.)

Differential Diagnosis

ABDOMINAL DISTENTION

ICD-9CM # 787.3

■ **NONMECHANICAL OBSTRUCTION**
Excessive intraluminal gas.
Intraabdominal infection.
Trauma.
Retroperitoneal irritation (renal colic, neoplasms, infections, hemorrhage).
Vascular insufficiency (thrombosis, embolism).
Mechanical ventilation.
Extraabdominal infection (sepsis, pneumonia, empyema, osteomyelitis of spine).
Metabolic/toxic abnormalities (hypokalemia, uremia, lead poisoning).
Chemical irritation (perforated ulcer, bile, pancreatitis).
Peritoneal inflammation.
Severe pain, pain medications.

■ **MECHANICAL OBSTRUCTION**
Neoplasm (intraluminal, extraluminal).
Adhesions, endometriosis.
Infection (intraabdominal abscess, diverticulitis).
Gallstones.
Foreign body, bezoars.
Pregnancy.
Hernias.
Volvulus.
Stenosis at surgical anastomosis, radiation stenosis.
Fecaliths.
Inflammatory bowel disease.
Gastric outlet obstruction
Hematoma.
Other: parasites, superior mesenteric artery (SMA) syndrome, pneumatosis intestinalis, annular pancreas, Hirschsprung's disease, intussusception, meconium.

ABDOMINAL PAIN, DIFFUSE

ICD-9CM # 789.67

Early appendicitis.
Aortic aneurysm.
Gastroenteritis.
Intestinal obstruction.
Diverticulitis.
Peritonitis.
Mesenteric insufficiency or infarction.
Pancreatitis.
Inflammatory bowel disease.
Irritable bowel.
Mesenteric adenitis.
Metabolic: toxins, lead poisoning, uremia, drug overdose, diabetic ketoacidosis (DKA), heavy metal poisoning.
Sickle cell crisis.
Pneumonia (rare).
Trauma.
Urinary tract infection, pelvic inflammatory disease (PID).
Other: acute intermittent porphyria, tabes dorsalis, periarteritis nodosa, Henoch-Schönlein purpura, adrenal insufficiency.

ABDOMINAL PAIN, EPIGASTRIC

ICD-9CM # 789.66

Gastric: peptic ulcer disease (PUD), gastric outlet obstruction, gastric ulcer.
Duodenal: PUD, duodenitis.

Biliary: cholecystitis, cholangitis.
Hepatic: hepatitis.
Pancreatic: pancreatitis.
Intestinal: high small bowel obstruction, early appendicitis.
Cardiac: angina, MI, pericarditis.
Pulmonary: pneumonia, pleurisy, pneumothorax.
Subphrenic abscess.
Vascular: dissecting aneurysm, mesenteric ischemia.

ABDOMINAL PAIN, SUPRAPUBIC

ICD-9CM # 789.85

Intestinal: colon obstruction or gangrene, diverticulitis, appendicitis.
Reproductive system: ectopic pregnancy, mittelschmerz, torsion of ovarian cyst, PID, salpingitis, endometriosis, rupture of endometrioma.
Cystitis, rupture of urinary bladder.

ABDOMINAL PAIN, RIGHT UPPER QUADRANT

ICD-9CM # 789.61

Biliary: calculi, infection, inflammation, neoplasm.
Hepatic: hepatitis, abscess, hepatic congestion, neoplasm, trauma.
Gastric: PUD, pyloric stenosis, neoplasm, alcoholic gastritis, hiatal hernia.
Pancreatic: pancreatitis, neoplasm, stone in pancreatic duct or ampulla.
Renal: calculi, infection, inflammation, neoplasm, rupture of kidney.
Pulmonary: pneumonia, pulmonary infarction, right-sided pleurisy.
Intestinal: retrocecal appendicitis, intestinal obstruction, high fecal impaction, diverticulitis.
Cardiac: myocardial ischemia (particularly involving the inferior wall), pericarditis.
Cutaneous: herpes zoster.
Trauma.
Fitz-Hugh-Curtis syndrome (perihepatitis).

ABDOMINAL PAIN, LEFT LOWER QUADRANT

ICD-9CM # 789.64

Gastric: PUD, gastritis, pyloric stenosis, hiatal hernia.
Pancreatic: pancreatitis, neoplasm, stone in pancreatic duct or ampulla.
Cardiac: MI, angina pectoris.
Splenic: splenomegaly, ruptured spleen, splenic abscess, splenic infarction.
Renal: calculi, pyelonephritis, neoplasm.
Pulmonary: pneumonia, empyema, pulmonary infarction.
Vascular: ruptured aortic aneurysm.
Cutaneous: herpes zoster.
Trauma.
Intestinal: high fecal impaction, perforated colon, diverticulitis.

ABDOMINAL PAIN, PERIUMBILICAL

ICD-9CM # 789.65

Intestinal: small bowel obstruction or gangrene, early appendicitis.
Vascular: mesenteric thrombosis, dissecting aortic aneurysm.

Pancreatic: pancreatitis.
Metabolic: uremia, DKA.
Trauma.

ABDOMINAL PAIN, RIGHT LOWER QUADRANT

ICD-9CM # 789.63

Intestinal: acute appendicitis, regional enteritis, incarcerated hernia, cecal diverticulitis, intestinal obstruction, perforated ulcer, perforated cecum, Meckel's diverticulitis.
Reproductive: ectopic pregnancy, ovarian cyst, torsion of ovarian cyst, salpingitis, tuboovarian abscess, mittelschmerz, endometriosis, seminal vesiculitis.
Renal: renal and ureteral calculi, neoplasms, pyelonephritis.
Vascular: leaking aortic aneurysm.
Psoas abscess.
Trauma.
Cholecystitis.

ABDOMINAL PAIN, LEFT LOWER QUADRANT

ICD-9CM # 789.64

Intestinal: diverticulitis, intestinal obstruction, perforated ulcer, inflammatory bowel disease, perforated descending colon, inguinal hernia, neoplasm, appendicitis.
Reproductive: ectopic pregnancy, ovarian cyst, torsion of ovarian cyst, tuboovarian abscess, mittelschmerz, endometriosis, seminal vesiculitis.
Renal: renal or ureteral calculi, pyelonephritis, neoplasm.
Vascular: leaking aortic aneurysm.
Psoas abscess.
Trauma.

ABDOMINAL PAIN, INFANCY[23]

ICD-9CM # 789.67

Acute gastroenteritis.
Appendicitis.
Intussusception.
Volvulus.
Meckel's diverticulum.
Other:
　Colic.
　Trauma.

ABDOMINAL PAIN, CHILDHOOD[23]

ICD-9CM # 789.67

Acute gastroenteritis.
Appendicitis.
Constipation.
Cholecystitis, acute.
Intestinal obstruction.
Pancreatitis.
Neoplasm.
Inflammatory bowel disease.
Other:
　Functional abdominal pain.
　Pyelonephritis.
　Pneumonia.
　Diabetic ketoacidosis.
　Heavy metal poisoning.
　Sickle cell crisis.
　Trauma.

ABDOMINAL PAIN, ADOLESCENCE[23]

ICD-9CM # 789.67

Acute gastroenteritis.
Appendicitis.
Inflammatory bowel disease.
Peptic ulcer disease.
Cholecystitis.
Neoplasm.
Other.
Functional abdominal pain.
Pelvic inflammatory disease.
Pregnancy.
Pyelonephritis.
Renal stone.
Trauma.

ABDOMINAL PAIN, POORLY LOCALIZED[23]

ICD-9CM # 789.60

■ EXTRAABDOMINAL
Metabolic
DKA, acute intermittent porphyria, hyperthyroidism, hypothyroidism, hypercalcemia, hypokalemia, uremia, hyperlipidemia, hyperparathyroidism.
Hematologic
Sickle cell crisis, leukemia or lymphoma, Henoch-Schönlein purpura.
Infectious
Infectious mononucleosis, Rocky Mountain spotted fever, acquired immunodeficiency syndrome (AIDS), streptococcal pharyngitis (in children), herpes zoster.
Drugs and toxins
Heavy metal poisoning, black widow spider bites, withdrawal syndromes, mushroom ingestion.
Referred pain
Pulmonary: pneumonia, pulmonary embolism, pneumothorax.
Cardiac: angina, myocardial infarction, pericarditis, myocarditis.
Genitourinary: prostatitis, epididymitis, orchitis, testicular torsion.
Musculoskeletal: rectus sheath hematoma.
Functional
Somatization disorder, malingering, hypochondriasis, Munchausen syndrome.

■ INTRAABDOMINAL
Early appendicitis, gastroenteritis, peritonitis, pancreatitis, abdominal aortic aneurysm, mesenteric insufficiency or infarction, intestinal obstruction, volvulus, ulcerative colitis.

ABDOMINAL PAIN, PREGNANCY[23]

ICD-9CM # 789.67

■ GYNECOLOGIC (GESTATIONAL AGE IN PARENTHESES)

Miscarriage	(<20 wk; 80% <12 wk)
Septic abortion	(<20 wk)
Ectopic pregnancy	(<14 wk)
Corpus luteum cyst rupture	(<12 wk)
Ovarian torsion	(Especially <24 wk)
Pelvic inflammatory disease	(<12 wk)
Chorioamnionitis	(>16 wk)
Abruptio placentae	(>16 wk)

■ NONGYNECOLOGIC

Appendicitis	(Throughout)
Cholecystitis	(Throughout)
Hepatitis	(Throughout)
Pyelonephritis	(Throughout)
Preeclampsia	(>20 wk)

ABORTION, RECURRENT

ICD-9CM # 761.8

Congenital anatomic abnormalities.
Adhesions (uterine synechiae).
Uterine fibroids.
Endometriosis.
Endocrine abnormalities (luteal phase insufficiency, hypothyroidism, uncontrolled diabetes mellitus).
Parenteral chromosome abnormalities.
Maternal infections (cervical mycoplasma, ureaplasma, chlamydia).
DES exposure, heavy metal exposure.
Thrombocytosis.
Allogenic immunity, autoimmunity, lupus anticoagulant.

ACHES AND PAINS, DIFFUSE[21]

ICD-9CM # 719.49

Postviral arthralgias/myalgias.
Bilateral soft tissue rheumatism.
Overuse syndromes.
Fibrositis.
Hypothyroidism.
Metabolic bone disease.
Paraneoplastic syndrome.
Myopathy (polymyositis, dermatomyositis).
RA.
Sjögren's syndrome.
Polymyalgia rheumatica.
Hypermobility.
Benign arthralgias/myalgias.
Chronic fatigue syndrome.
Hypophosphatemia.

ACIDOSIS, LACTIC

ICD-9CM # 276.2

■ TISSUE HYPOXIA

Shock (hypovolemic, cardiogenic, endotoxic).
Respiratory failure (asphyxia).
Severe CHF.
Severe anemia.
Carbon monoxide or cyanide poisoning.

■ ASSOCIATED WITH SYSTEMIC DISORDERS

Neoplastic diseases (e.g., leukemia, lymphoma).
Liver or renal failure.
Sepsis.
Diabetes mellitus.
Seizure activity.
Abnormal intestinal flora.
Alkalosis.
HIV.

■ SECONDARY TO DRUGS OR TOXINS

Salicylates.
Ethanol, methanol, ethylene glycol.
Fructose or sorbitol.

Biguanides (phenformin, metformin [usually occurring in patients with renal insufficiency]).
Isoniazid.
Streptozocin.
Nucleoside reverse transcriptase inhibitors (zidovudine, didanosine, stavudine).

■ HEREDITARY DISORDERS

G6PD deficiency and others.

ACIDOSIS, METABOLIC

ICD-9CM # 276.2

■ METABOLIC ACIDOSIS WITH INCREASED AG (AG ACIDOSIS)

Lactic acidosis.
Ketoacidosis (diabetes mellitus, alcoholic ketoacidosis).
Uremia (chronic renal failure).
Ingestion of toxins (paraldehyde, methanol, salicylate, ethylene glycol).
High-fat diet (mild acidosis).

■ METABOLIC ACIDOSIS WITH NORMAL AG (HYPERCHLOREMIC ACIDOSIS)

Renal tubular acidosis (including acidosis of aldosterone deficiency).
Intestinal loss of HCO_3^- (diarrhea, pancreatic fistula).
Carbonic anhydrase inhibitors (e.g., acetazolamide).
Dilutional acidosis (as a result of rapid infusion of bicarbonate-free isotonic saline).
Ingestion of exogenous acids (ammonium chloride, methionine, cystine, calcium chloride).
Ileostomy.
Ureterosigmoidostomy.
Drugs: amiloride, triamterene, spironolactone, β-blockers.

ACIDOSIS RESPIRATORY

ICD-9CM # 276.2

Pulmonary disease (COPD, severe pneumonia, pulmonary edema, interstitial fibrosis).
Airway obstruction (foreign body, severe bronchospasm, laryngospasm).
Thoracic cage disorders (pneumothorax, flail chest, kyphoscoliosis).
Defects in muscles of respiration (myasthenia gravis, hypokalemia, muscular dystrophy).
Defects in peripheral nervous system (amyotrophic lateral sclerosis, poliomyelitis, Guillain-Barré syndrome, botulism, tetanus, organophosphate poisoning, spinal cord injury).
Depression of respiratory center (anesthesia, narcotics, sedatives, vertebral artery embolism or thrombosis, increased intracranial pressure).
Failure of mechanical ventilator.

ACUTE SCROTUM

ICD-9CM # 608.9

Testicular torsion.
Epididymitis.
Testicular neoplasm.
Orchitis.

ADNEXAL MASS[23]

ICD-9CM # VARIES WITH SPECIFIC DISORDER

Ovary (neoplasm, endometriosis, functional cyst).
Fallopian tube (ectopic pregnancy, neoplasm, tuboovarian abscess, hydrosalpinx, paratubal cyst).
Uterus (fibroid, neoplasm).
Retroperitoneum (neoplasm, abdominal wall hematoma or abscess).
Urinary tract (pelvic kidney, distended bladder, urachal cyst).
Inflammatory bowel disease.
GI tract neoplasm.
Diverticular disease.
Appendicitis.
Bowel loop with feces.

ADRENAL MASSES[33]

ICD-9CM # 194.0 ADRENOCORTICAL CARCINOMA
255.8 ADRENAL HYPERPLASIA

■ **UNILATERAL ADRENAL MASS**
Functional lesions
Adrenal adenoma.
Adrenal carcinoma.
Pheochromocytoma.
Primary aldosteronism, adenomatous type.
Nonfunctional lesions
Incidentaloma of adrenal.
Ganglioneuroma.
Myelolipoma.
Hematoma.
Adenolipoma.
Metastasis.

■ **BILATERAL ADRENAL MASS**
Functional lesions:
ACTH-dependent Cushing's syndrome.
Congenital adrenal hyperplasia.
Pheochromocytoma.
Conn's syndrome, hyperplastic variety.
Micronodular adrenal disease.
Idiopathic bilateral adrenal hypertrophy.
Nonfunctional lesions:
Infection (tuberculosis, fungi).
Infiltration (leukemia, lymphoma).
Replacement (amyloidosis).
Hemorrhage.
Bilateral metastases.

ADYNAMIC ILEUS[23]

ICD-9CM # 560.1

Abdominal trauma.
Infection (retroperitoneal, pelvic, intrathoracic).
Laparotomy.
Metabolic disease (hypokalemia).
Renal colic.
Skeletal injury (rib fracture, vertebral fracture).
Medications (e.g., narcotics).

AEROPHAGIA (BELCHING, ERUCTATION)

ICD-9CM # 787.3

Anxiety disorders.
Rapid food ingestion.
Carbonated beverages.
Nursing infants (especially when nursing in horizontal position).
Eating or drinking in supine position.
Gum chewing.
Poorly fitting dentures, orthodontic appliances.
Hiatal hernia, gastritis, nonulcer dyspepsia.
Cholelithiasis, cholecystitis.
Ingestion of legumes, onions, peppers.

AIRWAY OBSTRUCTION, PEDIATRIC AGE[17]

ICD-9CM # 496 OBSTRUCTION DUE TO
BRONCHOSPASM
934.9 OBSTRUCTION DUE TO FOREIGN
BODY
478.75 OBSTRUCTION DUE TO
LARYNGOSPASM
506.9 OBSTRUCTION DUE TO INHALATION
OF FUMES OR VAPORS

■ **CONGENITAL CAUSES**
Craniofacial dysmorphism.
Hemangioma.
Laryngeal cleft/web.
Laryngoceles, cysts.
Laryngomalacia.
Macroglossia.
Tracheal stenosis.
Vascular ring.
Vocal cord paralysis.

■ **ACQUIRED INFECTIOUS CAUSES**
Acute laryngotracheobronchitis.
Epiglottitis.
Laryngeal papillomatosis.
Membranous croup (bacterial tracheitis).
Mononucleosis.
Retropharyngeal abscess.
Spasmodic croup.
Diphtheria.

■ **ACQUIRED NONINFECTIOUS CAUSES**
Anaphylaxis.
Foreign body aspiration.
Supraglottic hypotonia.
Thermal/chemical burn.
Trauma.
Vocal cord paralysis.
Angioneurotic edema.

AKINETIC/RIGID SYNDROME[1]

ICD-9CM # NOT AVAILABLE

Parkinsonism (idiopathic, drug-induced).
Catatonia (psychosis).
Progressive supranuclear palsy.
Multisystem atrophy (Shy-Drager syndrome, olivopontocerebellar atrophy).
Diffuse Lewy-body disease.
Toxins (MPTP, manganese, carbon monoxide).
Huntington's disease and other hereditary neurodegenerative disorders.

ALKALOSIS, METABOLIC

ICD-9CM # 276.3

■ CHLORIDE-RESPONSIVE
Vomiting.
Nasogastric (NG) suction.
Diuretics.
Posthypercapnic alkalosis.
Stool losses (laxative abuse, cystic fibrosis, villous adenoma).
Massive blood transfusion.
Exogenous alkali administration.

■ CHLORIDE-RESISTANT
Hyperadrenocorticoid states (Cushing's syndrome, primary hyperaldosteronism, secondary mineralocorticoidism [licorice, chewing tobacco]).
Hypomagnesemia.
Hypokalemia.
Bartter's syndrome.

ALKALOSIS, RESPIRATORY

ICD-9CM # 276.3

Hypoxemia (pneumonia, pulmonary embolism, atelectasis, high-altitude living).
Drugs (salicylates, xanthenes, progesterone, epinephrine, thyroxine, nicotine).
Central nervous system (CNS) disorders (tumor, cerebrovascular accident [CVA], trauma, infections).
Psychogenic hyperventilation (anxiety, hysteria).
Hepatic encephalopathy.
Gram-negative sepsis.
Hyponatremia.
Sudden recovery from metabolic acidosis.
Assisted ventilation.

ALOPECIA[12,25]

ICD-9CM # 704.00 ALOPECIA NOS
          704.01 ALOPECIA, ANDROGENIC
          704.01 ALOPECIA AREATA
          757.4 ALOPECIA, CONGENITAL
          316 ALOPECIA, PSYCHOGENIC

■ SCARRING ALOPECIA
Congenital (aplasia cutis).
Tinea capitis with inflammation (kerion).
Bacterial folliculitis.
Discoid lupus erythematosus.
Lichen planopilaris.
Folliculitis decalvans.
Neoplasm.
Trauma.

■ NONSCARRING ALOPECIA
Cosmetic treatment.
Tinea capitis.
Structural hair shaft disease.
Trichotillomania (hair pulling).
Anagen arrest.
Telogen arrest.
Alopecia areata.
Androgenetic alopecia.

ALVEOLAR CONSOLIDATION

ICD-9CM # 514

Infection.
Neoplasm (Bronchoalveolar carcinoma, lymphoma).
Aspiration.
Trauma.
Hemorrhage (Wegener's Goodpasture, bleeding diathesis).
ARDS.
CHF.
Renal failure.
Eosinophilic pneumonia.
Bronchiolitis obliterans.
Pulmonary alveolar proteinosis.

ALVEOLAR HEMORRHAGE[25]

ICD-9CM # 770.3

Hematologic disorders (coagulopathies, thrombocytopenia).
Goodpasture syndrome (Antibasement-membrane antibody disease).
Wegener's vasculitis.
Immune complex-mediated vasculitis.
Idiopathic pulmonary hemosiderosis.
Drugs (penicillamine).
Lymphangiogram contrast.
Mitral stenosis.

AMENORRHEA

ICD-9CM # 626.0

■ PREGNANCY

■ EARLY MENOPAUSE
HYPOTHALAMIC DYSFUNCTION: defective synthesis or release of LHRH, anorexia nervosa, stress, exercise.
PITUITARY DYSFUNCTION: neoplasm, postpartum hemorrhage, surgery, radiotherapy.
OVARIAN DYSFUNCTION: gonadal dysgenesis, 17-α-hydroxylase deficiency, premature ovarian failure, polycystic ovarian disease, gonadal stromal tumors.

■ UTEROVAGINAL ABNORMALITIES
Congenital: imperforate hymen, imperforate cervix, imperforate or absent vagina, müllerian agenesis.
Acquired: destruction of endometrium with curettage (Asherman's syndrome), closure of cervix or vagina caused by traumatic injury, hysterectomy.

■ OTHER
metabolic diseases (liver, kidney), malnutrition, rapid weight loss, exogenous obesity, endocrine abnormalities (Cushing's syndrome, Graves' disease, hypothyroidism).

AMNESIA

ICD-9CM # 292.83 DRUG INDUCED
          300.12 HYSTERICAL
          780.9 RETROGRADE
          437.7 TRANSIENT GLOBAL

Degenerative diseases (e.g., Alzheimer's, Huntington's disease).
CVA (especially when involving thalamus, basal forebrain, and hippocampus).
Head trauma.

Postsurgical (e.g., mammillary body surgery, bilateral temporal lobectomy).
Infections (herpes simplex encephalitis, meningitis).
Wernicke-Korsakoff syndrome.
Cerebral hypoxia.
Hypoglycemia.
CNS neoplasms.
Creutzfeldt-Jakob disease.
Medications (e.g., midazolam and other benzodiazepines).
Psychosis.
Malingering.

ANAL INCONTINENCE[23]

ICD-9CM # 787.6

■ TRAUMATIC
Nerve injured in surgery.
Spinal cord injury.
Obstetric trauma.
Sphincter injury.

■ NEUROLOGIC
Spinal cord lesions.
Dementia.
Autonomic neuropathy (e.g., diabetes mellitus).
Obstetrics: pudendal nerve stretched during surgery.
Hirschsprung's disease.

■ MASS EFFECT
Carcinoma of anal canal.
Carcinoma of rectum.
Foreign body.
Fecal impaction.
Hemorrhoids.

■ MEDICAL
Procidentia.
Inflammatory disease.
Diarrhea.
Laxative abuse.

■ PEDIATRIC
Congenital.
Meningocele.
Myelomeningocele.
Spina bifida.
After corrective surgery for imperforate anus.
Sexual abuse.
Encopresis.

ANAPHYLAXIS[18]

ICD-9CM # 995.0

■ PULMONARY
Laryngeal edema.
Epiglottitis.
Foreign body aspiration.
Pulmonary embolus.
Asphyxiation.
Hyperventilation.

■ CARDIOVASCULAR
Myocardial infarction.
Arrhythmia.
Hypovolemic shock.
Cardiac arrest.

■ CNS
Vasovagal reaction.
CVA.
Seizure disorder.
Drug overdose.

■ ENDOCRINE
Hypoglycemia.
Pheochromocytoma.
Carcinoid syndrome.
Catamenial (progesterone-induced anaphylaxis).

■ PSYCHIATRIC
Vocal cord dysfunction syndrome.
Munchausen's disease.
Panic attack/globus hystericus.

■ OTHER
Hereditary angioedema.
Cord urticaria.
Idiopathic urticaria.
Mastocytosis.
Serum sickness.
Idiopathic capillary leak syndrome.
Sulfite exposure.
Scombroid poisoning (tuna, blue fish, mackerel).

ANEMIA, DRUG-INDUCED[15]

ICD-9CM # 283.0

■ DRUGS THAT MAY INTERFERE WITH RED CELL PRODUCTION BY INDUCING MARROW SUPPRESSION OR APLASIA
Alcohol.
Antineoplastic drugs.
Antithyroid drugs.
Antibiotics.
Oral hypoglycemic agents.
Phenylbutazone.
Azidothymidine (AZT).

■ DRUGS THAT INTERFERE WITH VITAMIN B$_{12}$, FOLATE, OR IRON ABSORPTION OR UTILIZATION
Nitrous oxide.
Anticonvulsant drugs.
Antineoplastic drugs.
Isoniazid, cycloserine A.

■ DRUGS CAPABLE OF PROMOTING HEMOLYSIS
Immune Mediated
Penicillins.
Quinine.
Alpha-methyldopa.
Procainamide.
Mitomycin C.
Oxidative Stress
Antimalarials.
Sulfonamide drugs.
Nalidixic acid.

■ DRUGS THAT MAY PRODUCE OR PROMOTE BLOOD LOSS
Aspirin.
Alcohol.
Nonsteroidal antiinflammatory agents.
Corticosteroids.
Anticoagulants.

ANEMIA, LOW RETICYLOCYTE COUNT[1]

ICD-9CM # 285.9

■ MICROCYTIC ANEMIA (MCV <80)
Iron deficiency.
Thalassemia minor.
Sideroblastic anemia.
Lead poisoning.

■ MACROCYTIC ANEMIA (MCV >100)
Megaloblastic anemias.
Folate deficiency.
Vitamin B_{12} deficiency.
Drug-induced megaloblastic anemia.
Nonmegaloblastic macrocytosis.
Liver disease.
Hypothyroidism.

■ NORMOCYTIC ANEMIA (MCV 80-100)
Early iron deficiency.
Aplastic anemia.
Myelophthisic disorders.
Endocrinopathies.
Anemia of chronic disease.
Uremia.
Mixed nutritional deficiency.

ANEMIA, MEGALOBLASTIC[33]

ICD-9CM # 281.0 PERNICIOUS ANEMIA
    281.1 B_{12} DEFICIENCY
    281.2 FOLATE DEFICIENCY
    281.3 B_{12} WITH FOLATE DEFICIENCY
    281.4 PROTEIN OR AMINO ACID
        DEFICIENCY
    281.8 NUTRITIONAL
    281.9 NOS

■ COBALAMIN (CBL) DEFICIENCY
Nutritional Cbl deficiency (insufficient Cbl intake): vegetarians, vegans, breast-fed infants of mothers with pernicious anemia.

Abnormal intragastric events (inadequate proteolysis of food Cbl): atrophic gastritis, partial gastrectomy with hypochlorhydria

Loss/atrophy of gastric oxyntic mucosa (deficient IF molecules): total or partial gastrectomy, pernicious anemia (PA), caustic destruction (lye).

Abnormal events in small bowel lumen:
Inadequate pancreatic protease (R-Cbl not degraded, Cbl not transferred to IF).
- Insufficiency of pancreatic protease—pancreatic insufficiency.
- Inactivation of pancreatic protease—Zollinger-Ellison syndrome.
Usurping of luminal Cbl (inadequate Cbl binding to IF).
- By bacteria—stasis syndromes (blind loops, pouches of diverticulosis, strictures, fistulas, anastomoses); impaired bowel motility (scleroderma, pseudoobstruction), hypogammaglobulinemia.
- By *Diphyllobothrium latum.*

Disorders of ileal mucosa/IF receptors (IF-Cbl not bound to IF receptors):
Diminished or absent IF receptors—ileal bypass/resection/fistula.
Abnormal mucosal architecture/function—tropical/nontropical sprue, Crohn's disease, TB ileitis, infiltration by lymphomas, amyloidosis.

IF-/post IF-receptor defects—Imerslund-Graesbeck syndrome, TC II deficiency.
Drug-induced effects (slow K, biguanides, cholestyramine, colchicine, neomycin, PAS).

DISORDERS OF PLASMA CBL TRANSPORT (TC II-CBL NOT DELIVERED TO TC II RECEPTORS)
Congenital TC II deficiency, defective binding of TC II-Cbl to TC II receptors (rare).

METABOLIC DISORDERS (CBL NOT UTILIZED BY CELL)
Inborn enzyme errors (rare).
Acquired disorders: (Cbl oxidized to cob[III]alamin)—N_2O inhalation.

■ FOLATE DEFICIENCY
Nutritional causes
Decreased dietary intake—poverty and famine (associated with kwashiorkor, marasmus), institutionalized individuals (psychiatric/nursing homes), chronic debilitating disease/goats' milk (low in folate), special diets (slimming), cultural/ethnic cooking techniques (food folate destroyed) or habits (folate-rich foods not consumed)
Decreased diet and increased requirements:
- Physiologic: pregnancy and lactation, prematurity, infancy
- Pathologic: intrinsic hematologic disease (autoimmune hemolytic disease), drugs, malaria; hemoglobinopathies (SS, thalassemia), RBC membrane defects (hereditary spherocytosis, paroxysmal nocturnal hemoglobinopathy); abnormal hematopoiesis (leukemia/lymphoma, myelodysplastic syndrome, agnogenic myeloid metaplasia with myelofibrosis); infiltration with malignant disease; dermatologic (psoriasis)
Folate malabsorption
With normal intestinal mucosa:
- Some drugs (controversial).
- Congenital folate malabsorption (rare).
With mucosal abnormalities—tropical and nontropical sprue, regional enteritis.
Defective cellular folate uptake—familial aplastic anemia (rare)
Inadequate cellular utilization
Folate antagonists (methotrexate).
Hereditary enzyme deficiencies involving folate.
Drugs (multiple effects on folate metabolism)
alcohol, sulfasalazine, triamterine, pyrimethamine, trimethoprim-sulfamethoxazole, diphenylhydantoin, barbiturates.

■ MISCELLANEOUS MEGALOBLASTIC ANEMIAS (NOT CAUSED BY CBL OR FOLATE DEFICIENCY)
Congenital disorders of DNA synthesis (rare)
Orotic aciduria, Lesch-Nyhan syndrome, congenital dyserythropoietic anemia.
Acquired disorders of DNA synthesis
Thiamine-responsive megaloblastosis (rare).
Malignancy—erythroleukemia—refractory sideroblastic anemias—all antineoplastic drugs that inhibit DNA synthesis.
Toxic—alcohol.

ANERGY, CUTANEOUS[33]

ICD-9CM # 279.9

■ IMMUNOLOGIC
Acquired (AIDS, acute leukemia, carcinoma, CLL, Hodgkin's lymphoma, NHL).
Congenital (ataxia-telangiectasia, Di George's syndrome, severe combined immunodeficiency, Wiskott-Aldrich syndrome).

■ INFECTIONS

Bacterial (bacterial pneumonia, brucellosis).
Disseminated mycotic infections.
Mycobacterial (lepromatous leprosy, TB).
Viral (varicella, hepatitis, influenza, mononucleosis, measles, mumps).

■ IMMUNOSUPPRESSIVE MEDICATIONS

Systemic corticosteroids.
Methotrexate, cyclophosphamide.
Rifampin.

■ OTHER

Alcoholic cirrhosis, biliary cirrhosis, sarcoidosis, rheumatic disease.
Diabetes, Crohn's disease, uremia.
Anemia, pyridoxine deficiency, sickle cell anemia.
Burns, malnutrition, pregnancy, old age, surgery.

ANEURYSMS, THORACIC AORTA

ICD-9CM # 441.2

Trauma.
Infection.
Inflammatory (Syphilis, Takayasu disease).
Collagen vascular disease (rheumatoid arthritis, ankylosing spondylitis).
Annuloaortic ectasia (Marfan's syndrome, Ehlers-Danlos syndrome).
Congenital.
Coarctation.
Cystic medial necrosis.

ANISOCORIA

ICD-9CM # 379.41

Mydriatic or miotic drugs.
Prosthetic eye.
Inflammation (keratitis, iridocyclitis).
Infections (herpes zoster, syphilis, meningitis, encephalitis, TB, diphtheria, botulism).
Subdural hemorrhage.
Cavernous sinus thrombosis.
Intracranial neoplasm.
Cerebral aneurysm.
Glaucoma.
CNS degenerative diseases.
Internal carotid ischemia.
Toxic polyneuritis (alcohol, lead).
Adie's syndrome.
Horner's syndrome.
Diabetes mellitus (DM).
Trauma.
Congenital.

APPETITE LOSS IN INFANTS AND CHILDREN[17]

ICD-9CM # 783.0 APPETITE LOSS
307.59 APPETITE LOSS, PSYCHOGENIC
ORIGIN

■ ORGANIC DISEASE

Infection (acute or chronic)
Neurologic
Congenital degenerative disease.
Hypothalamic lesion.
Increased intracranial pressure (including a brain tumor).
Swallowing disorders (neuromuscular).
Gastrointestinal
Oral lesions (e.g., thrush or herpes simplex).
Gastroesophageal reflux.
Obstruction (especially with gastric or intestinal distention).
Inflammatory bowel disease.
Celiac disease.
Constipation.
Cardiac
Congestive heart failure (especially associated with cyanotic lesions).
Metabolic
Renal failure and/or renal tubule acidosis.
Liver failure.
Congenital metabolic disease.
Lead poisoning.
Nutritional
Marasmus.
Iron deficiency.
Zinc deficiency.
Fever
Rheumatoid arthritis.
Rheumatic fever.
Drugs
Morphine.
Digitalis.
Antimetabolites.
Methylphenidate.
Amphetamines.
Miscellaneous
Prolonged restriction of oral feedings, beginning in the neonatal period.
Systemic lupus erythematosus.
Tumor.

■ PSYCHOLOGIC FACTORS

Anxiety, fear, depression, mania (limbic influence on the hypothalamus).
Avoidance of symptoms associated with meals (abdominal pain, diarrhea, bloating, urgency, dumping syndrome).
Anorexia nervosa.
Excessive weight loss and food aversion in athletes, simulating anorexia nervosa.

ARTERIAL OCCLUSION[13]

ICD-9CM # 444.22 ARTERIAL OCCLUSION, LOWER
EXTREMITIES
444.21 ARTERIAL OCCLUSION, UPPER
EXTREMITIES

Thromboembolism (post-MI, mitral stenosis, rheumatic valve disease, atrial fibrillation, atrial myxoma, marantic endocarditis, bacterial endocarditis, Libman-Sacks endocarditis).
Atheroembolism (microemboli composed of cholesterol, calcium, and platelets from proximal atherosclerotic plaques).
Arterial thrombosis (endothelial injury, altered arterial blood flow, trauma, severe atherosclerosis, acute vasculitis).
Vasospasm.
Trauma.
Hypercoagulable states
Miscellaneous (irradiation, drugs, infections, necrotizing).

ARTHRITIS AND EYE LESIONS[6]

ICD-9CM # CODE VARIES WITH SPECIFIC DIAGNOSIS

SLE.
Sjögren's syndrome.
Behçet's syndrome.
Sarcoidosis.
SBE.
Lyme disease.
Wegener's granulomatosis.
Giant cell arteritis.
Takayasu arteritis.
Rheumatoid arthritis, JRA.
Scleroderma.
Inflammatory bowel disease.
Whipple's disease.
Ankylosing spondylitis.
Reactive arthritis.
Psoriatic arthritis.

ARTHRITIS AND HEART MURMUR[6]

ICD-9CM # CODE VARIES WITH SPECIFIC DIAGNOSIS

Subacute bacterial endocarditis (SBE).
Cardiac myxoma.
Ankylosing spondylitis.
Reactive arthritis.
Acute rheumatic fever.
Rheumatoid arthritis (RA).
SLE with Libman-Sacks endocarditis.
Relapsing polychondritis.

ARTHRITIS AND MUSCLE WEAKNESS[8]

ICD-9CM # CODE VARIES WITH SPECIFIC DIAGNOSIS

RA.
Ankylosing spondylitis.
Polymyositis.
Dermatomyositis.
SLE, scleroderma, mixed connective tissue disease.
Sarcoidosis.
HIV-associated arthritis.
Whipple's disease.

ARTHRITIS AND RASH[6]

ICD-9CM # CODE VARIES WITH SPECIFIC DIAGNOSIS

Chronic urticaria.
Vasculitic urticaria.
SLE.
Dermatomyositis.
Polymyositis.
Psoriatic arthritis.
Reactive arthritis.
Chronic sarcoidosis.
Serum sickness.
Sweet's syndrome.
Leprosy.

ARTHRITIS AND SUBCUTANEOUS NODULES[6]

ICD-9CM # CODE VARIES WITH SPECIFIC DIAGNOSIS

RA.
Gout.
Pseudogout (rare).
Sarcoidosis.
Light chain (LA) amyloidosis (primary, multiple myeloma).
Acute rheumatic fever (ARF).
Hemochromatosis.
Whipple's disease.
Multicentric reticulohistiocytosis.

ARTHRITIS AND WEIGHT LOSS[6]

ICD-9CM # CODE VARIES WITH SPECIFIC DIAGNOSIS

Severe RA.
RA with vasculitis.
Reactive arthritis.
RA or psoriatic arthritis or ankylosing spondylitis with amyloidosis.
Cancer.
Enteropathic arthritis (Crohn's, ulcerative colitis).
HIV infection.
Whipple's disease.
Blind loop syndrome.
Scleroderma with intestinal bacterial overgrowth.

ARTHRITIS, AXIAL SKELETON

**ICD-9CM # 720.0 ARTHRITIS, RHEUMATOID, SPINE
696.0 ARTHRITIS, PSORIATIC
715.9 ARTHRITIS, DEGENERATIVE, NOS
720.0 ANKYLOSING SPONDYLITIS**

RA.
Psoriatic arthritis.
Reiter's syndrome.
Ankylosing spondylitis.
Juvenile RA.
Degenerative disease of the nucleus pulposus.
Spondylosis deformans.
Diffuse idiopathic skeletal hyperostosis (DISH).
Alkaptonuria.
Infection.

ARTHRITIS, FEVER, AND RASH[6]

ICD-9CM # CODE VARIES WITH SPECIFIC DIAGNOSIS

Rubella, parvovirus B-19.
Gonococcemia, meningococcemia.
Secondary syphilis, Lyme borreliosis.
Adult acute rheumatic fever, adult Still's disease, adult Kawasaki disease.
Vasculitic urticaria.
Acute sarcoidosis.
Familial Mediterranean fever.
Hyperimmunoglobulinemia D and periodic fever syndrome.

ARTHRITIS, MONOARTICULAR AND OLIGOARTICULAR[2]

> ICD-9CM # 715.3 OSTEOARTHRITIS, LOCALIZED
> 711.9 INFECTIOUS ARTHRITIS
> 716.6 MONOARTICULAR ARTHRITIS
> 5TH DIGIT TO BE ADDED TO THE ABOVE
> DEPENDING ON SITE OF ARTHRITIS
> 0. SITE UNSPECIFIED
> 1. SHOULDER REGION
> 1. UPPER ARM
> 1. FOREARM
> 1. HAND
> 1. PELVIC REGION AND THIGH
> 1. LOWER LEG
> 1. ANKLE AND/OR FOOT
> 1. OTHER SPECIFIED EXCEPT SPINE

Septic arthritis (*S. aureus, Neisseria gonorrhea, Meningococci, Streptococci, S. pneumoniae, enteric gram-neg bacilli*).
Crystalline-induced arthritis (gout, pseudogout, calcium oxalate, hydroxyapatite and other basic calcium/phosphate crystals).
Traumatic joint injury.
Hemarthrosis.
Monoarticular or oligoarticular flare of an inflammatory polyarticular rheumatic disease (RA, psoriatic arthritis, Reiter's syndrome, SLE).

ARTHRITIS, PEDIATRIC AGE[17]

> ICD-9CM # 711.9 INFECTIOUS ARTHRITIS
> 714.30 JUVENILE CHRONIC OR
> UNSPECIFIED
> 714.31 JUVENILE RHEUMATOID
> POLYARTICULAR ACUTE
> 714.32 JUVENILE RHEUMATOID
> PAUCIARTICULAR
> 714.33 JUVENILE RHEUMATOID
> MONOARTICULAR

■ RHEUMATIC DISEASES OF CHILDHOOD
Acute rheumatic fever.
Systemic lupus erythematosus.
Juvenile ankylosing spondylitis.
Polymyositis and dermatomyositis.
Vasculitis.
Scleroderma.
Psoriatic arthritis.
Mixed connective tissue disease and overlap syndromes.
Kawasaki disease.
Behçet's syndrome.
Familial Mediterranean fever.
Reiter's syndrome.
Reflex sympathetic dystrophy.
Fibromyalgia (fibrositis).

■ INFECTIOUS DISEASES
Bacterial arthritis.
Viral or postviral arthritis.
Fungal arthritis.
Osteomyelitis.
Reactive arthritis.

■ NEOPLASTIC DISEASES
Leukemia.
Lymphoma.
Neuroblastoma.
Primary bone tumors.

■ NONINFLAMMATORY DISORDERS
Trauma.
Avascular necrosis syndromes.
Osteochondroses.
Slipped capital femoral epiphysis.
Diskitis.
Patellofemoral dysfunction (chondromalacia patellae).
Toxic synovitis of the hip.
Overuse syndromes.

■ GENETIC OR CONGENITAL SYNDROMES

■ HEMATOLOGIC DISORDERS
Sickle cell disease.
Hemophilia.

■ INFLAMMATORY BOWEL DISEASE

■ MISCELLANEOUS
Growing pains.
Psychogenic arthralgias (conversion reactions).
Hypermobility syndrome.
Villonodular synovitis.
Foreign body arthritis.

2.26 ARTHRITIS, POLYARTICULAR

> ICD-9CM # 715.09 GENERALIZED OSTEOARTHRITIS,
> MULTIPLE SITES
> 716.89 ARTHRITIS, MULTIPLE SITES
> 714.31 JUVENILE RHEUMATOID,
> POLYARTICULAR, ACUTE

RA, juvenile (rheumatoid) polyarthritis.
SLE, other connective tissue diseases, erythema nodosum, palindromic rheumatism, relapsing polychondritis.
Psoriatic arthritis, ankylosing spondylitis.
Sarcoidosis.
Lyme arthritis, bacterial endocarditis, *Neisseria gonorrhoeae* infection, rheumatic fever, Reiter's disease.
Crystal deposition disease.
Hypersensitivity to serum or drugs.
Hepatitis B, HIV, rubella, mumps
Other: serum sickness, leukemias, lymphomas, enteropathic arthropathy, Whipple's disease, Behçet's syndrome, Henoch-Schönlein purpura, familial Mediterranean fever, hypertrophic pulmonary osteoarthropathy.

2.27 ASCITES

> ICD-9CM # 789.5 ASCITES NOS
> 197.6 ASCITES, CANCEROUS
> (MALIGNANT)
> 457.8 ASCITES, CHYLOUS

Hypoalbuminemia: nephrotic syndrome, protein-losing gastroenteropathy, starvation.
Cirrhosis.
Hepatic congestion: CHF, constrictive pericarditis, tricuspid insufficiency, hepatic vein obstruction (Budd-Chiari syndrome), inferior vena cava or portal vein obstruction.
Peritoneal infections: TB and other bacterial infections, fungal diseases, parasites.
Neoplasms: primary hepatic neoplasms, metastases to liver or peritoneum, lymphomas, leukemias, myeloid metaplasia.
Lymphatic obstruction: mediastinal tumors, trauma to the thoracic duct, filariasis.
Ovarian disease: Meigs' syndrome, struma ovarii.

Chronic pancreatitis or pseudocyst: pancreatic ascites.
Leakage of bile: bile ascites.
Urinary obstruction or trauma: urine ascites.
Myxedema.
Chylous ascites.

ASTHMA, CHILDHOOD[4]

ICD-9CM # 493.0 USE 5TH DIGIT
0. WITHOUT MENTION OF STATUS ASTHMATICUS
1. WITH STATUS ASTHMATICUS

■ INFECTIONS
Bronchiolitis (RSV).
Pneumonia.
Croup.
Tuberculosis, histoplasmosis.
Bronchiectasis.
Bronchiolitis obliterans.
Bronchitis.
Sinusitis.

■ ANATOMIC, CONGENITAL
Cystic fibrosis.
Vascular rings.
Ciliary dyskinesia.
B lymphocyte immune defect.
Congestive heart failure.
Laryngotracheomalacia.
Tumor, lymphoma.
H-type tracheoesophageal fistula.
Repaired tracheoesophageal fistula.
Gastroesophageal reflux.

■ VASCULITIS, HYPERSENSITIVITY
Allergic bronchopulmonary aspergillosis.
Allergic alveolitis, hypersensitivity pneumonitis.
Churg-Strauss syndrome.
Periarteritis nodosa.

■ OTHER
Foreign body aspiration.
Pulmonary thromboembolism.
Psychogenic cough.
Sarcoidosis.
Bronchopulmonary dysplasia.
Vocal cord dysfunction.

ATAXIA

ICD-9CM # 781.3 ATAXIA NOS
303.0 ALCOHOLIC, ACUTE
303.9 ALCOHOLIC, CHRONIC
334.3 CEREBELLAR
331.89 CEREBRAL
334.0 FRIEDREICH'S
300.11 HYSTERICAL

Vertebral-basilar artery ischemia.
Diabetic neuropathy.
Tabes dorsalis.
Vitamin B_{12} deficiency.
Multiple sclerosis and other demyelinating diseases.
Meningomyelopathy.
Cerebellar neoplasms, hemorrhage, abscess, infarct.
Nutritional (Wernicke's encephalopathy).
Paraneoplastic syndromes.
Parainfectious: Guillain-Barré syndrome, acute ataxia of childhood and young adults.

Toxins: phenytoin, alcohol, sedatives, organophosphates.
Wilson's disease (hepatolenticular degeneration).
Hypothyroidism.
Myopathy.
Cerebellar and spinocerebellar degeneration: ataxia/telangiectasia, Friedreich's ataxia.
Frontal lobe lesions: tumors, thrombosis of anterior cerebral artery, hydrocephalus.
Labyrinthine destruction: neoplasm, injury, inflammation, compression.
Hysteria.
AIDS.

ATELECTASIS

ICD-9CM # 518.0

Lung neoplasm (primary or metastatic).
Infection (pneumonia, TB, fungal, histoplasmosis).
Postoperative (lower lobes).
Sarcoidosis.
Mucoid impaction.
Foreign body.
Postinflammatory (middle lobe syndrome).
Pneumothorax.
Pleural effusion.
Pneumoconiosis.
Interstitial fibrosis.
Bulla.
Mediastinal or adjacent mass.

AV NODAL BLOCK[13]

ICD-9CM # 426.10 AV BLOCK (INCOMPLETE, PARTIAL)
426.0 AV BLOCK, COMPLETE

Idiopathic fibrosis (Lenegre's disease).
Sclerodegenerative processes (e.g., Lev's disease with calcification of the mitral and aortic annuli).
AV node radiofrequency ablation procedure.
Medications (e.g., digoxin, beta blockers, calcium channel blockers, class III antiarrhythmics).
Acute inferior wall MI.
Myocarditis.
Infections (endocarditis, Lyme disease).
Infiltrative diseases (e.g., hemochromatosis, sarcoidosis, amyloidosis).
Trauma (including cardiac surgical procedures).
Collagen vascular diseases.
Aortic root diseases (e.g., spondylitis).
Electrolyte abnormalities (e.g., hyperkalemia).

BACK PAIN

ICD-9CM # 724.5 BACK PAIN (POSTURAL)
724.2 LOW BACK PAIN
307.89 BACK PAIN PSYCHOGENIC
724.8 STIFF BACK
847.9 BACK STRAIN
724.6 BACKACHE, SACROILIAC

Trauma: injury to bone, joint, or ligament.
Mechanical: pregnancy, obesity, fatigue, scoliosis.
Degenerative: osteoarthritis.
Infections: osteomyelitis, subarachnoid or spinal abscess, TB, meningitis, basilar pneumonia.
Metabolic: osteoporosis, osteomalacia.
Vascular: leaking aortic aneurysm, subarachnoid or spinal hemorrhage/infarction.

II

Neoplastic: myeloma, Hodgkin's disease, carcinoma of pancreas, metastatic neoplasm from breast, prostate, lung.
GI: penetrating ulcer, pancreatitis, cholelithiasis, inflammatory bowel disease.
Renal: hydronephrosis, calculus, neoplasm, renal infarction, pyelonephritis.
Hematologic: sickle cell crisis, acute hemolysis.
Gynecologic: neoplasm of uterus or ovary, dysmenorrhea, salpingitis, uterine prolapse.
Inflammatory: ankylosing spondylitis, psoriatic arthritis, Reiter's syndrome.
Lumbosacral strain.
Psychogenic: malingering, hysteria, anxiety.
Endocrine: adrenal hemorrhage or infarction.

BLEEDING, LOWER GI

ICD-9CM # 578.9

■ (ORIGINATING BELOW THE LIGAMENT OF TREITZ)
Small Intestine
Ischemic bowel disease (mesenteric thrombosis, embolism, vasculitis, trauma).
Small bowel neoplasm: leiomyomas, carcinoids.
Hereditary hemorrhagic telangiectasia (Rendu-Osler-Weber syndrome).
Meckel's diverticulum and other small intestine diverticula.
Aortoenteric fistula.
Intestinal hemangiomas: blue rubber-bleb nevi, intestinal hemangiomas, cutaneous vascular nevi.
Hamartomatous polyps: Peutz-Jeghers syndrome (intestinal polyps, mucocutaneous pigmentation).
Infections of small bowel: tuberculous enteritis, enteritis necroticans.
Volvulus.
Intussusception.
Lymphoma of small bowel, sarcoma, Kaposi's sarcoma.
Irradiation ileitis.
AV malformation of small intestine.
Inflammatory bowel disease.
Polyarteritis nodosa.
Other: pancreatoenteric fistulas, Henoch-Schönlein purpura, Ehlers-Danlos syndrome, systemic lupus erythematosus, amyloidosis, metastatic melanoma.
Colon
Carcinoma (particularly left colon).
Diverticular disease.
Inflammatory bowel disease.
Ischemic colitis.
Colonic polyps.
Vascular abnormalities: angiodysplasia, vascular ectasia.
Radiation colitis.
Infectious colitis.
Uremic colitis.
Aortoenteric fistula.
Lymphoma of large bowel.
Hemorrhoids.
Anal fissure.
Trauma, foreign body.
Solitary rectal/cecal ulcers.
Long-distance running.

BLEEDING, LOWER GI, PEDIATRIC[2]

ICD-9CM # 578.9

■ <3 MONTHS
Swallowed maternal blood.
Infectious colitis.

Milk allergy.
Bleeding diathesis.
Intussusception.
Midgut volvulus.
Meckel's diverticulum.
Necrotizing enterocolitis.

■ <2 YEARS OLD
Anal fissure.
Infectious colitis.
Milk allergy.
Colitis.
Intussusception.
Meckel's diverticulum.
Polyp.
Duplication.
Hemolytic uremic syndrome.
Inflammatory bowel disease.
Pseudomembranous enterocolitis.

■ <5 YEARS OLD
Infectious colitis.
Anal fissure.
Polyp.
Intussusception.
Meckel's diverticulum.
Henoch-Schönlein purpura.
Hemolytic uremic syndrome.
Inflammatory bowel disease.
Pseudomembranous enterocolitis.

■ 5-18 YEARS
Infectious colitis.
Inflammatory bowel disease.
Pseudomembranous enterocolitis.
Polyp.
Hemolytic-uremic syndrome.
Hemorrhoid.

BLEEDING, UPPER GI

ICD-9CM # 578.9

■ (ORIGINATING ABOVE THE LIGAMENT OF TREITZ)
Oral or pharyngeal lesions: swallowed blood from nose or oropharynx.
Swallowed hemoptysis
Esophageal: varices, ulceration, esophagitis, Mallory-Weiss tear, carcinoma, trauma.
Gastric: peptic ulcer (including Cushing and Curling's ulcers), gastritis, angiodysplasia, gastric neoplasms, hiatal hernia, gastric diverticulum, pseudoxanthoma elasticum, Rendu-Osler-Weber syndrome.
Duodenal: peptic ulcer, duodenitis, angiodysplasia, aortoduodenal fistula, duodenal diverticulum, duodenal tumors, carcinoma of ampulla of Vater, parasites (e.g., hookworm), Crohn's disease.
Biliary: hematobilia (e.g., penetrating injury to liver, hepatobiliary malignancy, endoscopic papillotomy).

BLEEDING, UPPER GI, PEDIATRIC[2]

ICD-9CM # 578.9

■ <3 MONTHS OLD
Swallowed maternal blood.
Gastritis.
Ulcer, stress.

Bleeding diathesis.
Foreign body (NG tube).
Vascular malformation.
Duplication.

■ <2 YEARS OLD
Esophagitis.
Gastritis.
Ulcer.
Pyloric stenosis.
Mallory-Weiss syndrome.
Vascular malformation.
Duplication.

■ <5 YEARS OLD
Esophagitis.
Gastritis.
Ulcer.
Esophageal varices.
Foreign body.
Mallory-Weiss syndrome.
Hemophilia.
Vascular malformations.

■ 5-18 YEARS OLD
Esophagitis.
Gastritis.
Ulcer.
Esophageal varices.
Mallory-Weiss syndrome.
Inflammatory bowel disease.
Hemophilia.
Vascular malformation.

BLINDNESS, PEDIATRIC AGE[20]

ICD-9CM # VARIES WITH SPECIFIC DISORDER

■ CONGENITAL
Optic nerve hypoplasia or aplasia.
Optic coloboma.
Congenital hydrocephalus.
Hydranencephaly.
Porencephaly.
Micrencephaly.
Encephalocele, particularly occipital type.
Morning glory disc.
Aniridia.
Anterior microphthalmia.
Peter's anomaly.
Persistent pupillary membrane.
Glaucoma.
Cataracts.
Persistent hyperplastic primary vitreous.

■ PHAKOMATOSES
Tuberous sclerosis.
Neurofibromatosis (special association with optic glioma).
Sturge-Weber syndrome.
von Hippel–Lindau disease.

■ TUMORS
Retinoblastoma.
Optic glioma.
Perioptic meningioma.
Craniopharyngioma.
Cerebral glioma.
Posterior and intraventricular tumors when complicated by hydrocephalus.
Pseudotumor cerebri.

■ NEURODEGENERATIVE DISEASES
Cerebral storage disease.
Gangliosidoses, particularly Tay-Sachs disease (infantile amaurotic familial idiocy), Sandhoff's variant, generalized gangliosidosis.
Other lipidoses and ceroid lipofuscinoses, particularly the late-onset amaurotic familial idiocies such as those of Jansky-Bielschowsky and of Batten-Mayou-Spielmeyer-Vogt.
Mucopolysaccharidoses, particularly Hurler's syndrome and Hunter's syndrome.
Leukodystrophies (dysmyelination disorders), particularly metachromatic leukodystrophy and Canavan's disease.
Demyelinating sclerosis (myelinoclastic diseases), especially Schilder's disease and Devic's neuromyelitis optica.
Special types: Dawson's disease, Leigh's disease, Bassen-Kornzweig syndrome, Refsum's disease.
Retinal degenerations: retinitis pigmentosa and its variants, Leber's congenital type.
Optic atrophies: congenital autosomal recessive type, infantile and congenital autosomal dominant types, Leber's disease, and atrophies associated with hereditary ataxias—the types of Behr, of Marie, and of Sanger-Brown.

■ INFECTIOUS PROCESSES
Encephalitis, especially in the prenatal infection syndromes caused by Toxoplasma gondii, cytomegalovirus, rubella virus, *Treponema pallidum,* herpes simplex.
Meningitis; arachnoiditis.
Chorioretinitis.
Endophthalmitis.
Keratitis.

■ HEMATOLOGIC DISORDERS
Leukemia with central nervous system involvement.

■ VASCULAR AND CIRCULATORY DISORDERS
Collagen vascular diseases.
Arteriovenous malformations—intracerebral hemorrhage, subarachnoid hemorrhage.
Central retinal occlusion.

■ TRAUMA
Contusion or avulsion of optic nerves, chiasm, globe, cornea.
Cerebral contusion or laceration.
Intracerebral, subarachnoid, or subdural hemorrhage.

■ DRUGS AND TOXINS
OTHER
Retinopathy of prematurity.
Sclerocornea.
Conversion reaction.
Optic neuritis.
Osteopetrosis.

BLISTERS, SUBEPIDERMAL

ICD-9CM # 919.2

Burns.
Porphyria cutanea tarda.
Bullous pemphigoid.
Bullous drug reaction.
Arthropod bite reaction.
Toxic epidermal necrosis.
Dermatitis herpetiformis.
Polymorphous light eruption.
Variegate porphyria.
Lupus erythematosus.

Epidermolysis bullosa.
Pseudoporphyria.
Acute graft-versus host reaction.
Linear IgA disease.
Leukocytoclastic vasculitis.
Pressure necrosis.
Urticaria pigmentosa.
Amyloidosis.

BONE LESIONS, PREFERENTIAL SITE OF ORIGIN[32]

ICD-9CM # 170.0 SKULL AND FACE
170.1 MANDIBLE
170.2 VERTEBRAL COLUMN
170.3 RIBS, STERNUM, CLAVICLE
170.4 SCAPULA, LONG BONES UPPER LIMB
170.5 SHORT BONES AND UPPER LIMB
170.6 PELVIC BONES, SACRUM COCCYX
170.7 LONG BONES LOWER LIMB
170.8 SHORT BONES LOWER LIMB
170.9 BONE CANCER NOS
198.5 BONE CANCER, METASTATIC

■ EPIPHYSIS
Chondroblastoma.
Giant-cell tumor—after fusion of growth plate.
Langerhans' cell histiocytosis.
Clear cell chondrosarcoma.
Osteosarcoma.

■ METAPHYSIS
Parosteal sarcoma.
Chondrosarcoma.
Fibrosarcoma.
Nonossifying fibroma.
Giant-cell tumor—before fusion of growth plate.
Unicameral bone cyst.
Aneurysmal bone cyst.

■ DIAPHYSIS
Myeloma.
Ewing's tumor.
Reticulum cell sarcoma.

■ METADIAPHYSEAL
Fibrosarcoma.
Fibrous dysplasia.
Enchondroma.
Osteoid osteoma.
Chondromyofibroma.

BONE PAIN

ICD-9CM # NOT AVAILABLE

Trauma.
Neoplasm (primary or metastatic).
Osteoporosis with compression fracture.
Paget's disease of bone.
Infection (osteomyelitis, septic arthritis).
Osteomalacia.
Viral syndrome.
Sickle cell disease.
Anxiety.

BONE RESORPTION[32]

ICD-9CM # 733.90 BONE DISORDER

■ DISTAL CLAVICLE
Hyperparathyroidism.
Rheumatoid arthritis.
Scleroderma.
Posttraumatic osteolysis.
Progeria.
Pycnodysostosis.
Cleidocranial dysplasia.

■ INFERIOR ASPECT OF RIBS
Vascular impression, associated with but not limited to
coarctation of the aorta.
Hyperparathyroidism.
Neurofibromatosis.

■ TERMINAL PHALANGEAL TUFTS
Scleroderma.
Raynaud's phenomenon.
Vascular disease.
Frostbite, electrical burns.
Psoriasis.
Tabes dorsalis.
Hyperparathyroidism.

■ GENERALIZED RESORPTION
Paraplegia.
Myositis ossificans.
Osteoporosis.

BRADYCARDIA, SINUS[13]

ICD-9CM # 427.89

Idiopathic.
Degenerative processes (e.g., Lev's disease, Lenegre's disease).
Medications
Beta blockers.
Some calcium channel blockers (diltiazem, verapamil).
Digoxin (when vagal tone is high).
Class I antiarrhythmic agents (e.g., procainamide).
Class III antiarrhythmic agents (amiodarone, sotalol).
Clonidine.
Lithium carbonate.
Acute myocardial ischemia and infarction
Right or left circumflex coronary artery occlusion or spasm.
High vagal tone (e.g., athletes).

BREAST INFLAMMATORY LESION[10]

ICD-9CM # 611.0 ACUTE MASTITIS
610.1 CHRONIC CYSTIC MASTITIS
771.5 NEONATAL INFECTIVE MASTITIS
778.7 NEONATAL NONINFECTIVE
MASTITIS

Mastitis (*S. aureus, Beta-hemolytic Strep*).
Trauma.
Foreign body (sutures, breast implants).
Granuloma (TB, fungal).
Fat necrosis post biopsy.
Necrosis or infarction (anticoagulant therapy, pregnancy).
Breast malignancy.

BREAST MASS

ICD-9CM # 611.72

Fibrocystic breasts.
Benign tumors (fibroadenoma, papilloma).
Mastitis (acute bacterial mastitis, chronic mastitis).
Malignant neoplasm.
Fat necrosis.
Hematoma.
Duct ectasia.
Mammary adenosis.

BREATH ODOR[31]

ICD-9CM # 784.9 HALITOSIS

Sweet, fruity: DKA, starvation ketosis.
Fishy, stale: uremia (trimethylamines).
Ammonia-like: uremia (ammonia).
Musty fish, clover: fetor hepaticus (hepatic failure).
Foul, feculent: intestinal obstruction/diverticulum.
Foul, putrid: nasal/sinus pathology (infection, foreign body, cancer), respiratory infections (empyema, lung abscess, bronchiectasis).
Halitosis: tonsillitis, gingivitis, respiratory infections, Vincent's angina, gastroesophageal reflux, achalasia.
Cinnamon: pulmonary TB.

BREATHING, NOISY[31]

ICD-9CM # 786.09 BREATHING LABORED,
789.09 SNORING, WHEEZING
786.1 STRIDOR

Infection: upper respiratory infection, peritonsillar abscess, retropharyngeal abscess, epiglottitis, laryngitis, tracheitis, bronchitis, bronchiolitis.
Irritants and allergens: hyperactive airway, asthma (reactive airway disease), rhinitis, angioneurotic edema.
Compression from outside of the airway: esophageal cysts or foreign body, neoplasms, lymphadenopathy.
Congenital malformation and abnormality: vascular rings, laryngeal webs, laryngomalacia, tracheomalacia, hemangiomas within the upper airway, stenoses within the upper airway, cystic fibrosis.
Acquired abnormality (at every level of the airway): nasal polyps, hypertrophied adenoids and/or tonsils, foreign body, intraluminal tumors, bronchiectasis.
Neurogenic disorder: vocal cord paralysis.

BULLOUS DISEASES

ICD-9CM # 694.9 BULLOUS DERMATOSES
694.5 BULLOUS PEMPHIGOID
694.4 PEMPHIGUS VULGARIS
694.4 PEMPHIGUS FOLIACEUS

Bullous pemphigoid.
Pemphigus vulgaris.
Pemphigus foliaceus.
Paraneoplastic pemphigus.
Cicatricial pemphigoid.
Erythema multiforme.
Dermatitis herpetiformis.
Herpes gestationis.
Impetigo.
Erosive lichen planus.

Linear IgA bullous dermatosis.
Epidermolysis bullosa acquisita.

CALCIFICATION ON CHEST X-RAY

ICD-9CM # 722.92

Lung neoplasm (primary or metastatic).
Silicosis.
Idiopathic pulmonary fibrosis.
Tuberculosis.
Histoplasmosis.
Disseminated varicella infection.
Mitral stenosis (end-stage).
Secondary hyperparathyroidism.

CARDIAC ARREST, NONTRAUMATIC[23]

ICD-9CM # 427.5 CARDIAC ARREST NOS

Cardiac (coronary artery disease, cardiomyopathies, structural abnormalities, valve dysfunction, arrhythmias).
Respiratory (upper airway obstruction, hypoventilation, pulmonary embolism, asthma, COPD exacerbation, pulmonary edema).
Circulatory (tension pneumothorax, pericardial tamponade, PE, hemorrhage, sepsis).
Electrolyte abnormalities (hypokalemia or hyperkalemia, hypomagnesemia or hypermagnesemia, hypocalcemia).
Medications (tricyclic antidepressants, digoxin, theophylline, calcium channel blockers).
Drugs abuse (cocaine, heroin, amphetamines).
Toxins (carbon monoxide, cyanide).
Environmental (drowning/near-drowning, electrocution, lightning, hypothermia or hyperthermia, venomous snakes).

CARDIAC ENLARGEMENT[13]

ICD-9CM # 429.3 CARDIOMEGALY, IDIOPATHIC
746.89 CARDIOMEGALY, CONGENITAL
402.0 CARDIOMEGALY, MALIGNANT
402.1 CARDIOMEGALY, BENIGN

■ CARDIAC CHAMBER ENLARGEMENT
Chronic volume overload
Mitral or aortic regurgitation.
Left-to-right shunt (PDA, VSD, AV fistula).
Cardiomyopathy
Ischemic.
Nonischemic.
Decompensated pressure overload
Aortic stenosis.
Hypertension.
High-output states
Severe anemia.
Thyrotoxicosis.
Bradycardia
Severe sinus bradycardia.
Complete heart block.

■ LEFT ATRIUM
LV failure of any cause.
Mitral valve disease.
Myxoma.

■ RIGHT VENTRICLE
Chronic volume overload.
   Tricuspid or pulmonic regurgitation.
   Left-to-right shunt (ASD).
Decompensated pressure overload.
   Pulmonic stenosis.
   Pulmonary artery hypertension.
     Primary.
     Secondary (PE, COPD).
   Pulmonary venoocclusive disease.

■ RIGHT ATRIUM
RV failure of any cause.
Tricuspid valve disease.
Myxoma.
Ebstein's anomaly.

■ MULTICHAMBER ENLARGEMENT
Hypertrophic cardiomyopathy.
Acromegaly.
Severe obesity.

■ PERICARDIAL DISEASE
Pericardial effusion with or without tamponade.
Effusive constrictive disease.
Pericardial cyst, loculated effusion.

■ PSEUDOCARDIOMEGALY
Epicardial fat.
Chest wall deformity (pectus excavatum, straight back syndrome).
Low lung volumes.
AP chest x-ray.
Mediastinal tumor, cyst.

CARDIAC MURMURS

ICD-9CM # CODE VARIES WITH SPECIFIC DISORDER

■ SYSTOLIC
Mitral regurgitation (MR).
Tricuspid regurgitation (TR).
Ventricular septal defect (VSD).
Aortic stenosis (AS).
Idiopathic hypertrophic subaortic stenosis (IHSS).
Pulmonic stenosis (PS).
Innocent murmur of childhood.
Coarctation of aorta.
Mitral valve prolapse (MVP).

■ DIASTOLIC
Aortic regurgitation (AR).
Atrial myxoma.
Mitral stenosis (MS).
Pulmonary artery branch stenosis.
Tricuspid stenosis (TS).
Graham Steell murmur (diastolic decrescendo murmur heard in severe pulmonary hypertension).
Pulmonic regurgitation (PR).
Severe mitral regurgitation (MR).
Austin Flint murmur (diastolic rumble heard in severe AR).
Severe VSD and patent ductus arteriosus.

■ CONTINUOUS
Patent ductus arteriosus.
Pulmonary AV fistula.

CAVITARY LESION ON CHEST X-RAY[14]

ICD-9CM # 793.1 CHEST X-RAY LUNG SHADOW

■ NECROTIZING INFECTIONS
Bacteria: anaerobes, *Staphylococcus aureus*, enteric gram-negative bacteria, *Pseudomonas aeruginosa*, *Legionella* species, *Haemophilus influenzae*, *Streptococcus pyogenes*, *Streptococcus pneumoniae* (?), *Rhodococcus*, *Actinomyces*.
Mycobacteria: *Mycobacterium tuberculosis*, *Mycobacterium kansasii*, MAI.
Bacteria-like: *Nocardia* species.
Fungi: *Coccidioides immitis*, *Histoplasma capsulatum*, *Blastomyces hominis*, *Aspergillus* species, *Mucor* species.
Parasitic: *Entamoeba histolytica*, *Echinococcus*, *Paragonimus westermani*.

■ CAVITARY INFARCTION
Bland infarction (with or without superimposed infection).
Lung contusion.

■ SEPTIC EMBOLISM
S. aureus, anaerobes, others.

■ VASCULITIS
Wegener's granulomatosis, periarteritis.

■ NEOPLASMS
Bronchogenic carcinoma, metastatic carcinoma, lymphoma.

■ MISCELLANEOUS LESIONS
Cysts, blebs, bullae, or pneumatocele with or without fluid collections.
Sequestration.
Empyema with air-fluid level.
Bronchiectasis.

CEREBROVASCULAR DISEASE, ISCHEMIC[35]

ICD-9CM # 437.9

■ VASCULAR DISORDERS
Large-vessel atherothrombotic disease.
Lacunar disease.
Arterial-to-arterial embolization.
Carotid or vertebral artery dissection.
Fibromuscular dysplasia.
Migraine.
Venous thrombosis.
Radiation.
Complications of arteriography.
Multiple, progressive intracranial arterial occlusions.

■ INFLAMMATORY DISORDERS
Giant cell arteritis.
Polyarteritis nodosa.
Systemic lupus erythematosus.
Granulomatous angiitis.
Takayasu's disease.
Arteritis associated with amphetamine, cocaine, or phenylpropanolamine.
Syphilis, mucormycosis.
Sjögren syndrome.
Behçet's syndrome.

■ CARDIAC DISORDERS
Rheumatic heart disease.
Mural thrombus.
Arrhythmias.

Mitral valve prolapse.
Prosthetic heart valve.
Endocarditis.
Myxoma.
Paradoxical embolus.

■ **HEMATOLOGIC DISORDERS**
Thrombotic thrombocytopenic purpura.
Sickle cell disease.
Hypercoagulable states.
Polycythemia.
Thrombocytosis.
Leukocytosis.
Lupus anticoagulant.

CHEST PAIN, CHILDREN[4]

| ICD-9CM # 786.50 CHEST PAIN NOS |
| 786.59 CHEST PRESSURE |
| 786.52 CHEST PAIN, PLEURITIC |

■ **MUSCULOSKELETAL (COMMON)**
Trauma (accidental, abuse).
Exercise, overuse injury (strain, bursitis).
Costochondritis (Tietze's syndrome).
Herpes zoster (cutaneous).
Pleurodynia.
Fibrositis.
Slipping rib.
Sickle cell anemia vaso-occlusive crisis.
Osteomyelitis (rare).
Primary or metastatic tumor (rare).

■ **PULMONARY (COMMON)**
Pneumonia.
Pleurisy.
Asthma.
Chronic cough.
Pneumothorax.
Infarction (sickle cell anemia).
Foreign body.
Embolism (rare).
Pulmonary hypertension (rare).
Tumor (rare).

■ **GASTROINTESTINAL (LESS COMMON)**
Esophagitis (gastroesophageal reflux).
Esophageal foreign body.
Esophageal spasm.
Cholecystitis.
Subdiaphragmatic abscess.
Perihepatitis (Fitz-Hugh-Curtis syndrome).
Peptic ulcer disease.

■ **CARDIAC (LESS COMMON)**
Pericarditis.
Postpericardiotomy syndrome.
Endocarditis.
Mitral valve prolapse.
Aortic or subaortic stenosis.
Arrhythmias.
Marfan's syndrome (dissecting aortic aneurysm).
Anomalous coronary artery.
Kawasaki disease.
Cocaine, sympathomimetic ingestion.
Angina (familial hypercholesterolemia).

■ **IDIOPATHIC (COMMON)**
Anxiety, hyperventilation.
Panic disorder.

■ **OTHER (LESS COMMON)**
Spinal cord or nerve root compression.
Breast-related pathologic condition.
Castleman's disease (lymph node neoplasm).

CHEST PAIN (NONPLEURITIC)[8]

| ICD-9CM # 786.50 CHEST PAIN NOS |
| 786.59 CHEST DISCOMFORT |

Cardiac: myocardial ischemia/infarction, myocarditis.
Esophageal: spasm, esophagitis, ulceration, neoplasm, achalasia, diverticula, foreign body.
Referred pain from subdiaphragmatic GI structures.
Gastric and duodenal: hiatal hernia, neoplasm, PUD.
Gallbladder and biliary: cholecystitis, cholelithiasis, impacted stone, neoplasm.
Pancreatic: pancreatitis, neoplasm.
Dissecting aortic aneurysm.
Pain originating from skin, breasts, and musculoskeletal structures: herpes zoster, mastitis, cervical spondylosis.
Mediastinal tumors: lymphoma, thymoma.
Pulmonary: neoplasm, pneumonia, pulmonary embolism/infarction.
Psychoneurosis.
Chest pain associated with mitral valve prolapse.

CHEST PAIN (PLEURITIC)

| ICD-9CM #786.52 CHEST PAIN, PLEURITIC |

Cardiac: pericarditis, postpericardiotomy/Dressler's syndrome.
Pulmonary: pneumothorax, hemothorax, embolism/infarction, pneumonia, empyema, neoplasm, bronchiectasis, pneumomediastinum, TB, carcinomatous effusion.
GI: liver abscess, pancreatitis, esophageal rupture, Whipple's disease with associated pericarditis or pleuritis.
Subdiaphragmatic abscess.
Pain originating from skin and musculoskeletal tissues: costochondritis, chest wall trauma, fractured rib, interstitial fibrositis, myositis, strain of pectoralis muscle, herpes zoster, soft tissue and bone tumors.
Collagen vascular diseases with pleuritis.
Psychoneurosis.
Familial Mediterranean fever.

CHOREOATHETOSIS[25]

| ICD-9CM # 275.1 CHOREOATHETOSIS-AGITANS |
| SYNDROME |
| 33.5 CHOREOATHETOSIS PAROXYSMAL |

■ **SYSTEMIC DISEASES**
Systemic lupus erythematosus.
Polycythemia.
Thyrotoxicosis.
Rheumatic fever.
Cirrhosis of the liver (acquired hepatocerebral degeneration).
Diabetes mellitus.
Wilson's disease.

■ PRIMARY DEGENERATIVE BRAIN DISEASES

Huntington's chorea.
Olivopontocerebellar atrophies.
Neuroacanthocytosis.

■ FOCAL BRAIN DISEASES

Hemichorea.
Stroke.
Tumor.
Arteriovenous malformation.

■ DRUG-INDUCED CHOREOATHETOSIS

Parkinson's disease drugs
Levodopa.
Epilepsy drugs
Phenytoin.
Carbamazepine.
Phenobarbital.
Gabapentin.
Valproate.
Psychostimulant drugs
Cocaine.
Amphetamine.
Methamphetamine.
Dextroamphetamine.
Methylphenidate.
Pemoline.
Psychotropic drugs
Lithium.
Tricyclic antidepressant drugs.
Oral contraceptive drugs
Cimetidine.

CLUBBING

ICD-9CM # 781.5 CLUBBING FINGER

Pulmonary neoplasm (lung, pleura).
Other neoplasm (GI, liver, Hodgkin's, thymus, osteogenic sarcoma).
Pulmonary infectious process (empyema, abscess, bronchiectasis, TB, chronic pneumonitis).
Extrapulmonary infectious process (subacute bacterial endocarditis, intestinal TB, bacterial or amebic dysentery, arterial graft sepsis).
Pneumoconiosis.
Cystic fibrosis.
Sarcoidosis.
Cyanotic congenital heart disease.
Endocrine (Graves' disease, hyperparathyroidism).
Inflammatory bowel disease.
Celiac disease.
Chronic liver disease, cirrhosis (particularly biliary and juvenile).
Pulmonary AV malformations.
Idiopathic.
Thyroid acropachy
Hereditary (pachydermoperiostosis).
Chronic trauma (jackhammer operators, machine workers).

COLOR CHANGES, CUTANEOUS[31]

ICD-9CM # 709.00 PIGMENTATION ANOMALY

■ BROWN

Generalized: pituitary, adrenal, liver disease, ACTH-producing tumor (e.g., oat cell lung carcinoma)
Localized: nevi, neurofibromatosis.

■ WHITE

Generalized: albinism.
Localized: vitiligo, Raynaud's syndrome.

■ RED (ERYTHEMA)

Generalized: fever, polycythemia, urticaria, viral exanthems.
Localized: inflammation, infection, Raynaud's syndrome.

■ YELLOW

Generalized: liver disease, chronic renal disease, anemia.
Generalized (except sclera): hypothyroidism, increased intake of vegetables containing carotene.
Localized: resolving hematoma, infection, peripheral vascular insufficiency.

■ BLUE

Lips, mouth, nail beds: cardiovascular and pulmonary diseases, Raynaud's.

COMA

ICD-9CM # 780.01

Vascular: hemorrhage, thrombosis, embolism.
CNS infections: meningitis, encephalitis, cerebral abscess.
Cerebral neoplasms with herniation.
Head injury: subdural hematoma, cerebral concussion, cerebral contusion.
Drugs: narcotics, sedatives, hypnotics.
Ingestion or inhalation of toxins: CO, alcohol, lead.
Metabolic disturbances.
Hypoxia.
Acid-base disorders.
Hypoglycemia, hyperglycemia.
Hepatic failure.
Electrolyte disorders.
Uremia.
Hypothyroidism.
Hypothermia, hyperthermia.
Hypotension, malignant hypertension.
Postictal.

COMA, NORMAL COMPUTED TOMOGRAPHY[1]

ICD-9CM # 780.01

■ MENINGEAL DISORDERS

Subarachnoid hemorrhage (uncommon).
Bacterial meningitis.
Encephalitis.
Subdural empyema.

■ EXOGENOUS TOXINS

Sedative drugs and barbiturates.
Anesthetics and γ-hydroxybutyrate.[*]
Alcohols.
Stimulants:
    Phencyclidine.[†]
    Cocaine and amphetamine.[‡]
Psychotropic drugs:
    Cyclic antidepressants.
    Phenothiazines.
    Lithium.
Anticonvulsants.
Opioids.
Clonidine.[§]
Penicillins.
Salicylates.
Anticholinergics.
Carbon monoxide, cyanide, and methemoglobinemia.

■ ENDOGENOUS TOXINS/DEFICIENCIES/DERANGEMENTS
Hypoxia and ischemia.
Hypoglycemia.
Hypercalcemia.
Osmolar:
  Hyperglycemia.
  Hyponatremia.
  Hypernatremia.
Organ system failure.
  Hepatic encephalopathy.
  Uremic encephalopathy.
  Pulmonary insufficiency (carbon dioxide narcosis).

■ SEIZURES
Prolonged postictal state.
Spike-wave stupor.

■ HYPOTHERMIA OR HYPERTHERMIA
Brainstem ischemia
Basilar artery stroke
Brainstem or cerebellar hemorrhage
Conversion or malingering

---

*General anesthetic, similar to γ-aminobutyric acid; recreational drug and body building aid. Rapid onset, rapid recovery often with myoclonic jerking and confusion. Deep coma (2-3 hr; Glasgow Coma Scale = 3) with maintenance of vital signs.
† Coma associated with cholinergic signs: lacrimation, salivation, bronchorrhea, and hyperthermia.
‡ Coma after seizures or status (i.e., a prolonged postictal state).
§ An antihypertensive agent active through the opiate receptor system; frequent overdose when used to treat narcotic withdrawal.

COMA, PEDIATRIC POPULATION[28]

ICD-9CM # 780.01

■ ANOXIA
Birth asphyxia.
Carbon monoxide poisoning.
Croup/epiglottitis.
Meconium aspiration.

■ INFECTION
Hemolysis.
Blood loss.
Hydrops fetalis.
Infection.
Meningoencephalitis.
Sepsis.
Postimmunization encephalitis.

■ INCREASED INTRACRANIAL PRESSURE
Anoxia.
Inborn metabolic errors.
Toxic encephalopathy.
Reye's syndrome.
Head trauma/intracranial bleed.
Hydrocephalus.
Posterior fossa tumors.

■ HYPERTENSIVE ENCEPHALOPATHY
Coarctation of aorta.
Nephritis.
Vasculitis.

Pheochromocytoma.

■ ISCHEMIA
Hypoplastic left heart.
Shunting lesions.
Aortic stenosis.
Cardiovascular collapse (any cause).

■ PURPURIC CAUSES
Disseminated intravascular coagulation.
Hemolytic-uremic syndrome.
Leukemia.
Thrombotic purpura.

■ HYPERCAPNIA
Cystic fibrosis.
Bronchopulmonary dysplasia.
Congenital lung anomalies.

■ NEOPLASM
Medulloblastoma.
Glioma of brainstem.
Posterior fossa tumors.

■ DRUGS/TOXINS
Maternal sedation.
Alcohol.
Any drug.
Lead.
Salicylism.
Arsenic.
Pesticides.

■ ELECTROLYTE ABNORMALITIES
Hypernatremia (diarrhea, dehydration, salt poisoning).
Hyponatremia (SIADH, androgenital syndrome, gastroenteritis).
Hyperkalemia (renal failure, salicylism, androgenitalism).
Hypokalemia (diarrhea, hyperaldosteronism, salicylism, DKA).
Hypocalcemia (vitamin D deficiency, hyperparathyroidism).
Severe acidosis (sepsis, cold injury, salicylism, DKA).

■ HYPOGLYCEMIA
Birth injury or stress.
Diabetes.
Alcohol.
Salicylism.
Hyperinsulinemia.
Iatrogenic.

■ POSTSEIZURE
Renal causes
Nephritis.
Hypoplastic kidneys.
Hepatic causes
Acute hepatitis.
Fulminant hepatic failure.
Inborn metabolic errors.
Bile duct atresia.

CONSTIPATION

ICD-9CM # 564.0

Intestinal obstruction:
Fecal impaction.
Diverticular disease.
GI neoplasm.
Strangulated femoral hernia.
Gallstone ileus.
Tuberculous stricture.

Adhesions.
Ameboma.
Volvulus.
Intussusception.
Inflammatory bowel disease.
Hematoma of bowel wall, secondary to trauma or anticoagulants.
Poor dietary habits: insufficient bulk in diet, inadequate fluid intake.
Change from daily routine: travel, hospital admission, physical inactivity.
Acute abdominal conditions: renal colic, salpingitis, biliary colic, appendicitis, ischemia.
Hypercalcemia or hypokalemia, uremia.
Irritable bowel syndrome, pregnancy, anorexia nervosa, depression.
Painful anal conditions: hemorrhoids, fissure, stricture.
Decreased intestinal peristalsis: old age, spinal cord injuries, myxedema, diabetes, multiple sclerosis, parkinsonism and other neurologic diseases.
Drugs: codeine, morphine, antacids with aluminum, verapamil, anticonvulsants, anticholinergics, disopyramide, cholestyramine, alosetron, iron supplements.
Hirschsprung's disease, meconium ileus, congenital atresia in infants.

COUGH

ICD-9CM # 786.2

Infectious process (viral, bacterial).
Postinfectious.
"Smoker's cough."
Rhinitis (allergic, vasomotor, postinfectious).
Asthma.
Exposure to irritants (noxious fumes, smoke, cold air).
Drug-induced (especially ACE inhibitors, β-blockers).
GERD.
Interstitial lung disease.
Lung neoplasms.
Lymphomas, mediastinal neoplasms.
Bronchiectasis.
Cardiac (CHF, pulmonary edema, mitral stenosis, pericardial inflammation).
Recurrent aspiration.
Inflammation of larynx, pleura, diaphragm, mediastinum.
Cystic fibrosis.
Anxiety.
Other: pulmonary embolism, foreign body inhalation, aortic aneurysm, Zenker's diverticulum, osteophytes, substernal thyroid, thyroiditis, PMR.

CYANOSIS

ICD-9CM # 782.5 CYANOSIS NOS
770.8 CYANOSIS, NEWBORN

Congenital heart disease with right-to-left shunt.
Pulmonary embolism.
Hypoxia.
Pulmonary edema.
Pulmonary disease (oxygen diffusion and alveolar ventilation abnormalities).
Hemoglobinopathies.
Decreased cardiac output.
Vasospasm.
Arterial obstruction.
Pulmonary AV fistulas.
Elevated hemidiaphragm.

Neoplasm (bronchogenic carcinoma, mediastinal neoplasm, intrahepatic lesion).
Substernal thyroid.
Infectious process (pneumonia, empyema, TB, subphrenic abscess, hepatic abscess).
Atelectasis.
Idiopathic.
Eventration.
Phrenic nerve dysfunction (myelitis, myotonia, herpes zoster).
Trauma to phrenic nerve or diaphragm (e.g., surgery).
Aortic aneurysm.
Intraabdominal mass.
Pulmonary infarction.
Pleurisy.
Radiation therapy.
Rib fracture.
Superior vena cava syndrome.

DELIRIUM[23]

ICD-9CM # 780.09 DELIRIUM NOS
293.0 ACUTE DELIRIUM

■ PHARMACOLOGIC AGENTS
Anxiolytics (benzodiazepines).
Antidepressants (e.g., amitriptyline, doxepin, imipramine).
Cardiovascular agents (e.g., methyldopa, digitalis, reserpine, propranolol, procainamide, captopril, disopyramide).
Antihistamine.
Cimetidine.
Corticosteroids.
Antineoplastics.
Drugs of abuse (alcohol, cannabis, amphetamines, cocaine, hallucinogens, opioids, sedative-hypnotics, phencyclidine).

■ METABOLIC DISORDERS
Hypercalcemia.
Hypercarbia.
Hypoglycemia.
Hyponatremia.
Hypoxia.

■ INFLAMMATORY DISORDERS
Sarcoidosis.
SLE.
Giant cell arteritis.

■ ORGAN FAILURE
Hepatic encephalopathy.
Uremia.

■ NEUROLOGIC DISORDERS
Alzheimer's disease.
CVA.
Encephalitis (including HIV).
Encephalopathies.
Epilepsy.
Huntington's disease.
Multiple sclerosis.
Neoplasms.
Normal pressure hydrocephalus.
Parkinson's disease.
Pick's disease.
Wilson's disease.

■ ENDOCRINE DISORDERS
Addison's disease.
Cushing's disease.

Panhypopituitarism.
Parathyroid disease.
Postpartum psychosis.
Recurrent menstrual psychosis.
Sydenham's chorea.
Thyroid disease.

■ DEFICIENCY STATES
Niacin.
Thiamine, Vitamin B$_{12}$, and folate

DELIRIUM, DIALYSIS PATIENT[23]

ICD-9CM # 293.0 ACUTE DELIRIUM
293.9 ENCEPHALOPATHY FROM DIALYSIS

■ STRUCTURAL
Cerebrovascular accident (particularly hemorrhage).
Subdural hematoma.
Intracerebral abscess.
Brain tumor.

■ METABOLIC
Disequilibrium syndrome.
Uremia.
Drug effects.
Meningitis.
Hypertensive encephalopathy.
Hypotension.
Postictal state.
Hypernatremia or hyponatremia.
Hypercalcemia.
Hypermagnesemia.
Hypoglycemia.
Severe hyperglycemia.
Hypoxemia.
Dialysis dementia.

DEMYELINATING DISEASES[35]

ICD-9CM # 341.9

■ MULTIPLE SCLEROSIS
Relapsing and chronic progressive forms.
Acute multiple sclerosis.
Neuromyelitis optica (Devic's disease).

■ DIFFUSE CEREBRAL SCLEROSIS
Schilder's encephalitis periaxialis diffusa.
Baló's concentric sclerosis.

■ ACUTE DISSEMINATED ENCEPHALOMYELITIS
After measles, chickenpox, rubella, influenza, mumps.
After rabies or smallpox vaccination.

■ NECROTIZING HEMORRHAGIC ENCEPHALITIS
Hemorrhagic leukoencephalitis.

■ LEUKODYSTROPHIES
Krabbe's globoid leukodystrophy.
Metachromatic leukodystrophy.
Adrenoleukodystrophy.
Adrenomyeloneuropathy.
Pelizaeus-Merzbacher leukodystrophy.
Canavan's disease.
Alexander's disease.

DIPLOPIA, BINOCULAR

ICD-9CM # 368.2

Cranial nerve palsy (3rd, 4th, 6th).
Thyroid eye disease.
Myasthenia gravis.
Decompensated strabismus.
Orbital trauma with blow-out fracture.
Orbital pseudotumor.
Cavernous sinus thrombosis

DYSPAREUNIA[10]

ICD-9CM # 625.0 DYSPAREUNIA
608.89 DYSPAREUNIA, MALE
302.76 DYSPAREUNIA, PSYCHOGENIC

■ INTROITAL
Vaginismus.
Intact or rigid hymen.
Clitoral problems.
Vulvovaginitis.
Vaginal atrophy: hypoestrogen.
Vulvar dystrophy.
Bartholin or Skene gland infection.
Inadequate lubrication.
Operative scarring.

■ MIDVAGINAL
Urethritis.
Trigonitis.
Cystitis.
Short vagina.
Operative scarring.
Inadequate lubrication.

■ DEEP
Endometriosis.
Pelvic infection.
Uterine retroversion.
Ovarian pathology.
Gastrointestinal.
Orthopedic.
Abnormal penile size or shape.

DYSPHAGIA

ICD-9CM # 787.2

Esophageal obstruction: neoplasm, foreign body, achalasia, stricture, spasm, esophageal web, diverticulum, Schatzki's ring.
Peptic esophagitis with stricture, Barrett's stricture.
External esophageal compression: neoplasms (thyroid neoplasm, lymphoma, mediastinal tumors), thyroid enlargement, aortic aneurysm, vertebral spurs, aberrant right subclavian artery (dysphagia lusoria).
Hiatal hernia, GERD.
Oropharyngeal lesions: pharyngitis, glossitis, stomatitis, neoplasms.
Hysteria: globus hystericus.
Neurologic and/or neuromuscular disturbances: bulbar paralysis, myasthenia gravis, ALS, multiple sclerosis, parkinsonism, CVA, diabetic neuropathy.
Toxins: poisoning, botulism, tetanus, postdiphtheritic dysphagia.
Systemic diseases: scleroderma, amyloidosis, dermatomyositis.
Candida and herpes esophagitis.
Presbyesophagus.

DYSPNEA

ICD-9CM # 786.00

Upper airway obstruction: trauma, neoplasm, epiglottitis, laryngeal edema, tongue retraction, laryngospasm, abductor paralysis of vocal cords, aspiration of foreign body.

Lower airway obstruction: neoplasm, COPD, asthma, aspiration of foreign body.

Pulmonary infection: pneumonia, abscess, empyema, TB, bronchiectasis.

Pulmonary hypertension.

Pulmonary embolism/infarction.

Parenchymal lung disease.

Pulmonary vascular congestion.

Cardiac disease: ASHD, valvular lesions, cardiac dysrhythmias, cardiomyopathy, pericardial effusion, cardiac shunts.

Space-occupying lesions: neoplasm, large hiatal hernia, pleural effusions.

Disease of chest wall: severe kyphoscoliosis, fractured ribs, sternal compression, morbid obesity.

Neurologic dysfunction: Guillain-Barré syndrome, botulism, polio, spinal cord injury.

Interstitial pulmonary disease: sarcoidosis, collagen vascular diseases, DIP, Hamman-Rich pneumonitis, etc.

Pneumoconioses: silicosis, berylliosis, etc.

Mesothelioma.

Pneumothorax, hemothorax, pleural effusion.

Inhalation of toxins.

Cholinergic drug intoxication.

Carcinoid syndrome.

Hematologic: anemia, polycythemia, hemoglobinopathies.

Thyrotoxicosis, myxedema.

Diaphragmatic compression caused by abdominal distention, subphrenic abscess, ascites.

Lung resection.

Metabolic abnormalities: uremia, hepatic coma, DKA.

Sepsis.

Atelectasis.

Psychoneurosis.

Diaphragmatic paralysis.

Pregnancy.

DYSURIA

ICD-9CM # 788.1 DYSURIA
306.53 DYSURIA, PSYCHOGENIC

Urinary tract infection.

Estrogen deficiency (in postmenopausal female).

Vaginitis.

Genital infection (e.g., herpes, condyloma).

Interstitial cystitis.

Chemical irritation (e.g., deodorant aerosols, douches).

Meatal stenosis or stricture.

Reiter's syndrome.

Bladder neoplasm.

GI etiology (diverticulitis, Crohn's disease).

Impaired bladder or sphincter action.

Urethral carbuncle.

Chronic fibrosis posttrauma.

Radiation therapy.

Prostatitis.

Urethritis (gonococcal, *Chlamydiae*).

Behçet's syndrome.

Stevens-Johnson syndrome.

EARACHE[30]

ICD-9CM # 388.70 EARACHE
388.72 EAR PAIN, REFERRED

Otitis media.

Serous otitis media.

Eustachitis.

Otitis externa.

Otitic barotrauma.

Mastoiditis.

Foreign body.

Impacted cerumen.

Referred otalgia, as with TMJ dysfunction, dental problems, and tumors.

EDEMA, CHILDREN[17]

ICD-9CM # 782.3 EDEMA NOS

■ **CARDIOVASCULAR**

Congestive heart failure.

Acute thrombi or emboli.

Vasculitis of many types.

■ **RENAL**

Nephrotic syndrome.

Glomerulonephritis of many types.

End-stage renal failure.

■ **ENDOCRINE OR METABOLIC**

Thyroid disease.

Starvation.

Hereditary angioedema.

■ **IATROGENIC**

Drugs (diuretics and steroids).

Water or salt overload.

■ **HEMATOLOGIC**

Hemolytic disease of the newborn.

■ **GASTROINTESTINAL**

Hepatic cirrhosis.

Protein-losing enteritis.

Lymphangiectasis.

Cystic fibrosis.

Celiac disease.

Enteritis of many types.

■ **LYMPHATIC ABNORMALITIES**

Congenital (gonadal dysgenesis).

Acquired.

EDEMA, GENERALIZED

ICD-9CM # 782.3 EDEMA NOS

Congestive heart failure (CHF).

Cirrhosis.

Nephrotic syndrome.

Pregnancy.

Idiopathic.

Acute nephritic syndrome.

Myxedema.

Medications (NSAIDs, estrogens, vasodilators).

EDEMA, LEG, UNILATERAL[23]

ICD-9CM # 782.3

■ WITH PAIN
DVT.
Postphlebitic syndrome.
Popliteal cyst rupture.
Gastrocnemius rupture.
Cellulitis.
Psoas or other abscess.

■ WITHOUT PAIN
DVT.
Postphlebitic syndrome.
Other venous insufficiency (after saphenous vein harvest, varicosities).
Lymphatic obstruction/lymphedema (carcinoma, lymphoma, sarcoidosis, filariasis, retroperitoneal fibrosis).

EDEMA OF LOWER EXTREMITIES

ICD-9CM # 782.3

CHF (right-sided).
Hepatic cirrhosis.
Nephrosis.
Myxedema.
Lymphedema.
Pregnancy.
Abdominal mass: neoplasm, cyst.
Venous compression from abdominal aneurysm.
Varicose veins.
Bilateral cellulitis.
Bilateral thrombophlebitis.
Vena cava thrombosis, venous thrombosis.
Retroperitoneal fibrosis.

ELEVATED HEMIDIAPHRAGM

ICD-9CM # 519.4 DIAPHRAGM DISORDER
519.4 DIAPHRAGM PARALYSIS
756.6 DIAPHRAGM EVENTRATION, CONGENITAL

Neoplasm (bronchogenic carcinoma, mediastinal neoplasm, intrahepatic lesion).
Substernal thyroid.
Infectious process (pneumonia, empyema, TB, subphrenic abscess, hepatic abscess).
Atelectasis.
Idiopathic.
Eventration.
Phrenic nerve dysfunction (myelitis, myotonia, herpes zoster).
Trauma to phrenic nerve or diaphragm (e.g., surgery).
Aortic aneurysm.
Intraabdominal mass.
Pulmonary infarction.
Pleurisy.
Radiation therapy.
Rib fracture.

EMBOLI, ARTERIAL[23]

ICD-9CM # 444.22 EMBOLISM, ARTERY, LOWER EXTREMITY
444.21 EMBOLISM, ARTERY, UPPER EXTREMITY

Myocardial infarction with mural thrombi.
Atrial fibrillation.
Cardiomyopathies.
Prosthetic heart valves.
CHF.
Endocarditis.
Left ventricular aneurysm.
Left atrial myxoma.
Sick sinus syndrome.
Paradoxical embolus from venous thrombosis.
Aneurysms of large blood vessels.
Atheromatous ulcers of large blood vessels.

EMESIS, PEDIATRIC AGE[17]

ICD-9CM # 787.03

■ INFANCY
Gastrointestinal tract
Congenital:
Regurgitation—chalasia, gastroesophageal reflux.
Atresia—stenosis (tracheoesophageal fistula, prepyloric diaphragm, intestinal atresia).
Duplication.
Volvulus (errors in rotation and fixation, Meckel's diverticulum).
Congenital bands.
Hirschsprung's disease.
Meconium ileus (cystic fibrosis), meconium plug.
Acquired:
Acute infectious gastroenteritis, food poisoning (staphylococcal, clostridial).
Pyloric stenosis.
Gastritis, duodenitis.
Intussusception.
Incarcerated hernia—inguinal, internal secondary to old adhesions.
Cow's milk protein intolerance, food allergy, eosinophilic gastroenteritis.
Disaccharidase deficiency.
Celiac disease—presents after introduction of gluten in diet; inherited risk.
Adynamic ileus—the mediator for many nongastrointestinal causes.
Neonatal necrotizing enterocolitis.
Chronic granulomatous disease with gastric outlet obstruction.
Nongastrointestinal tract
Infectious—otitis, urinary tract infection, pneumonia, upper respiratory tract infection, sepsis, meningitis.
Metabolic—aminoaciduria and organic aciduria, galactosemia, fructosemia, adrenogenital syndrome, renal tubular acidosis, diabetic ketoacidosis, Reye's syndrome.
Central nervous system—trauma, tumor, infection, diencephalic syndrome, rumination, autonomic responses (pain, shock).
Medications—anticholinergics, aspirin, alcohol, idiosyncratic reaction (e.g., codeine).

■ CHILDHOOD
Gastrointestinal tract
Peptic ulcer—vomiting is a common presentation in children younger than 6 yr old.

Trauma—duodenal hematoma, traumatic pancreatitis, perforated bowel.
Pancreatitis—mumps, trauma, cystic fibrosis, hyperparathyroidism, hyperlipidemia, organic acidemias.
Crohn's disease.
Idiopathic intestinal pseudoobstruction.
Superior mesenteric artery syndrome.
Nongastrointestinal tract
Central nervous system—cyclic vomiting, migraine, anorexia nervosa, bulimia.

ENCEPHALOPATHY, METABOLIC[33]

> **ICD-9CM # 291.2 ALCOHOLIC ENCEPHALOPATHY**
> **572.2 HEPATIC ENCEPHALOPATHY**
> **251.2 HYPOGLYCEMIC ENCEPHALOPATHY**
> **349.82 TOXIC ENCEPHALOPATHY**
> **984.9 LEAD ENCEPHALOPATHY**
> **293.9 ENCEPHALOPATHY**

Substrate deficiency: hypoxia/ischemia, carbon monoxide poisoning, hypoglycemia.
Cofactor deficiency: thiamine, Vitamin B_{12}, pyridoxine (INH administration).
Electrolyte disorders: hyponatremia, hypercalcemia, carbon dioxide narcosis, dialysis, hypermagnesemia, disequilibrium syndrome.
Endocrinopathies: DKA, hyperosmolar coma, hypothyroidism, hyperadrenocorticism, hyperparathyroidism.
Endogenous toxins: liver disease, uremia, porphyria.
Exogenous toxins: drug overdose (sedative/hypnotics, ethanol, narcotics, salicylates, tricyclic antidepressants), drug withdrawal, toxicity of therapeutic medications, industrial toxins (e.g., organophosphates, heavy metals), sepsis.
Heat stroke.
Epilepsy (postictal).

ENTHESOPATHY

> **ICD-9CM # CODE NOT AVAILABLE**

Viremia or bacteremia.
Ankylosing spondylitis.
Psoriatic arthritis.
Drug-induced (quinolones, etretinate).
Reactive arthritis.
Disseminated idiopathic skeletal hyperostosis (DISH).
Reiter's syndrome.

EPILEPSY

> **ICD-9CM # 345.9 EPILEPSY NOS**

Psychogenic spells.
Transient ischemic attack.
Hypoglycemia.
Syncope.
Narcolepsy.
Migraine.
Paroxysmal vertigo.
Arrhythmias.
Drug reaction.

EPISTAXIS

> **ICD-9CM # 784.7**

Trauma.
Medications (nasal sprays, NSAIDs, anticoagulants, antiplatelets).
Nasal polyps.
Cocaine use.
Coagulopathy (hemophilia, liver disease, DIC, thrombocytopenia).
Systemic disorders (hypertension, uremia).
Infections.
Anatomic malformations.
Rhinitis.
Nasal polyps.
Local neoplasms (benign and malignant).
Desiccation.
Foreign body.

ERECTILE DYSFUNCTION, ORGANIC[28]

> **ICD-9CM # 607.84**

Neurogenic abnormalities: Somatic nerve neuropathy, central nervous system abnormalities.
Psychogenic causes: Depression, performance anxiety, marital conflict.
Endocrine causes: Hyperprolactinemia, hypogonadotropic hypogonadism, testicular failure, estrogen excess.
Trauma: Pelvic fracture, prostate surgery, penile fracture.
Systemic disease: Diabetes mellitus, renal failure, hepatic cirrhosis.
Medications: Diuretics, antidepressants, H_2 blockers, exogenous hormones, alcohol, antihypertensives, nicotine abuse, finasteride, etc.
Structural abnormalities: Peyronie's disease.

ESOPHAGEAL PERFORATION[23]

> **ICD-9CM # 530.4 PERFORATION, NONTRAUMATIC**
> **862.22 INJURY, TRAUMATIC**

Trauma.
Caustic burns.
Iatrogenic.
Foreign bodies.
Spontaneous rupture (Boerhaave's syndrome).
Postoperative breakdown of anastomosis.

EXANTHEMS[25]

> **ICD-9CM # 782.1**

Measles.
Rubella.
Erythema infectiosum (fifth disease).
Roseola exanthema.
Varicella.
Enterovirus.
Adenovirus.
Epstein-Barr virus.
Kawasaki disease.
Staphylococcal scalded skin.
Scarlet fever.
Meningococcemia.
Rocky Mountain spotted fever.

EYE PAIN

ICD-9CM # 379.91

Foreign body.
Herpes zoster.
Trauma.
Conjunctivitis.
Iritis.
Iridocyclitis.
Uveitis.
Blepharitis.
Ingrown lashes.
Orbital or periorbital cellulitis/abscess.
Sinusitis.
Headache.
Glaucoma.
Inflammation of lacrimal gland.
Tic douloureux.
Cerebral aneurysm.
Cerebral neoplasm.
Entropion.
Retrobulbar neuritis.
UV light.
Dry eyes.
Irritation or inflammation from eye drops, dust, cosmetics, etc.

FACIAL PAIN

ICD-9CM # 784.0

Infection, abscess.
Postherpetic neuralgia.
Trauma, posttraumatic neuralgia.
Tic douloureux.
Cluster headache, "lower-half headache."
Geniculate neuralgia.
Anxiety, somatization syndrome.
Glossopharyngeal neuralgia.
Carotidynia.

FACIAL PARALYSIS[25]

ICD-9CM # 351.0 FACIAL (7TH NERVE) PALSY

■ INFECTION
Bacterial: otitis media, mastoiditis, meningitis, Lyme disease.
Viral: herpes zoster, mononucleosis, varicella, rubella, mumps, Bell's palsy
Mycobacterial: TB, meningitis, leprosy.
Miscellaneous: syphilis, malaria.

■ TRAUMA
Temporal bone fracture, facial laceration.
Surgery.

■ NEOPLASM
Malignant: squamous cell carcinoma, basal cell and adenocystic tumors, leukemia, parotid neoplasms, metastic tumors.
Benign: facial nerve neuroma, vestibular schwannoma, congenital cholesteatoma.

■ IMMUNOLOGIC
Guillain-Barré syndrome, periarteritis nodosa.
Reaction to tetanus antiserum.

■ METABOLIC
Pregnancy.
Hypothyroidism.
DM.

FAILURE TO THRIVE

ICD-9CM # 783.4

■ MALABSORPTION
Cow's milk protein allergy.
Cystic fibrosis.
Celiac disease.
Biliary atresia.

■ INSUFFICIENT CALORIC INTAKE
Parental neglect.
Feeding difficulties (CNS lesion, severe reflux, oromotor abnormalities).
Use of diluted formula preparation.
Food shortage (poverty).

■ INCREASED NEEDS
Hyperthyroidism.
Congenital heart defects.
Malignancy.
Renal or hepatic disease.
HIV.

■ IMPROPER UTILIZATION
Storage disorders.
Amino acid disorders.
Trisomy 13, 21, 18.

FATIGUE

ICD-9CM # 780.7 FATIGUE NOS
300.5 FATIGUE PSYCHOGENIC
780.7 CHRONIC FATIGUE SYNDROME

Depression.
Anxiety, emotional stress.
Inadequate sleep.
Prolonged physical activity.
Pregnancy and postpartum period.
Anemia.
Hypothyroidism.
Medications (beta-blockers, anxiolytics, antidepressants, sedating antihistamines, clonidine, methyldopa).
Viral or bacterial infections.
Sleep apnea syndrome.
Dieting.
Renal failure, CHF, COPD, liver disease.

FATTY LIVER

ICD-9CM # 571.8

Obesity.
Alcohol abuse.
Diabetes mellitus.
Acute fatty liver of pregnancy.
Medications (tetracycline, valproic acidglucocorticoids, amiodarone, estrogen, methotrexate).
Reye's syndrome.
Wilson's disease.
Nonalcoholic steatosis.

FEVER AND JAUNDICE

ICD-9CM # 789.6 FEVER
782.4 JAUNDICE

Cholecystitis.
Hepatic abscess (pyogenic, amebic).
Ascending cholangitis.
Pancreatitis.
Malaria.
Neoplasm (hepatic pancreatic, biliary tract, metastatic).
Mononucleosis.
Viral hepatitis.
Sepsis.
Babesiosis.
HIV (cryptosporidium).
Biliary ascariasis.
Toxic shock syndrome.
Yersinia infection, leptospirosis, Yellow fever, Dengue fever, relapsing fever.

FEVER AND RASH

ICD-9CM # 782.1 EXANTHEM
57.9 EXANTHEM VIRAL
789.6 FEVER

Drug hypersensitivity: penicillin, sulfonamides, thiazides, anticonvulsants, allopurinol.
Viral infection: measles, rubella, varicella, erythema infectiosum, roseola, enterovirus infection, viral hepatitis, infectious mononucleosis, acute HIV.
Other infections: meningococcemia, staphylococcemia, scarlet fever, typhoid fever, Pseudomonas bacteremia, Rocky Mountain spotted fever, Lyme disease, secondary syphilis, bacterial endocarditis, babesiosis, brucellosis, listeriosis.
Serum sickness.
Erythema multiforme.
Erythema marginatum.
Erythema nodosum.
SLE.
Dermatomyositis.
Allergic vasculitis.
Pityriasis rosea.
Herpes zoster.

FEVER IN RETURNING TRAVELERS AND IMMIGRANTS[25]

ICD-9CM # CODE VARIES WITH SPECIFIC DISORDER

Differential Diagnosis of Some Selected Systemic Febrile Illnesses to Consider in Returned Travelers and Immigrants.*

■ COMMON

Acute respiratory tract infection (worldwide).
Gastroenteritis (worldwide) [foodborne, waterborne, fecal-oral].
Enteric fever, including typhoid (worldwide) [food, water].
Urinary tract infection (worldwide) [sexual contact].
Drug reactions [antibiotics, prophylactic agents, other] {rash frequent}.
Malaria (tropics, limited areas of temperate zones) [mosquitoes].
Arboviruses (Africa; tropics) [mosquitoes, ticks, mites].
Dengue (Asia, Caribbean, Africa) [mosquitoes].
Viral hepatitis (worldwide).

Hepatitis A (worldwide) [food, fecal-oral].
Hepatitis B (worldwide, especially Asia, sub-Saharan Africa) [sexual contact] {long incubation period}.
Hepatitis C (worldwide) [blood or sexual contact].
Hepatitis E (Asia, North Africa, Mexico, ?others) [food, water].
Tuberculosis (worldwide) [airborne, milk] {long period to symptomatic infection}.
Sexually transmitted diseases (worldwide) [sexual contact].

■ LESS COMMON

Filariasis (Asia, Africa, South America) [biting insects] {long incubation period, eosinophilia}.
Measles (developing world) [airborne] {in susceptible individual}.
Amebic abscess (worldwide) [food].
Brucellosis (worldwide) [milk, cheese, food, animal contact].
Listeriosis (worldwide) [foodborne] {meningitis}.
Leptospirosis (worldwide) [animal contact, open fresh water] {jaundice, meningitis}.
Strongyloidiasis (warm and tropical areas) [soil contact] {eosinophilia}.
Toxoplasmosis (worldwide) [undercooked meat].

■ RARE

Relapsing fever (western Americas, Asia, northern Africa) [ticks lice].
Hemorrhagic fevers (worldwide) [arthropod and nonarthropod transmitted].
Yellow fever (tropics) [mosquitoes] {hepatitis}.
Hemorrhagic fever with renal syndrome (Europe, Asia, North America) [rodent urine] {renal impairment}.
Hantavirus pulmonary syndrome (western North America, ?other) [rodent urine] {respiratory distress syndrome}.
Lassa fever (Africa) [rodent excreta, person to person] {high mortality rate}.
Other—chikungunya, Rift Valley, Ebola-Marburg, etc. (various) [insect bites, rodent excreta, aerosols, person to person] {often severe}.
Rickettsial infections {Rashes and eschars}.
Leishmaniasis, visceral (Middle East, Mediterranean, Africa, Asia, South America) [biting flies] {long incubation period}.
Acute schistosomiasis (Africa, Asia, South America, Caribbean) [fresh water].
Chagas' disease (South and Central America) [reduviid bug bites] {often asymptomatic}.
African trypanosomiasis (Africa) [tsetse fly bite] {neurologic syndromes, sleeping sickness}.
Bartonellosis (South America) [sandfly bite; cb] {skin nodules}.
HIV infection/AIDS (worldwide) [sexual and blood contact].
Trichinosis (worldwide) [undercooked meat] {eosinophilia}.
Plague (temperate and tropical plains) [animal exposures and fleas].
Tularemia (worldwide) [animal contact, fleas, aerosols] {ulcers, lymph nodes}.
Anthrax (worldwide) [animal, animal product contact] {ulcers}.
Lyme disease (North America, Europe) [tick bites] {arthritis, meningitis, cardiac abnormalities}.

---

*Diagnoses for which particular symptoms are indicative are in italics. Exposure to regions of the world that are most likely to be significant to the diagnosis are presented in (parentheses). Vectors, risk behaviors, and sources associated with acquisition are presented in [brackets]. Special clinical characteristics are listed within {braces}.

FLATULENCE AND BLOATING[30]

ICD-9CM # 787.3

Ingestion of nonabsorbable carbohydrates.
Ingestion of carbonated beverages.
Malabsorption: pancreatic insufficiency, biliary disease, celiac disease, bacterial overgrowth in small intestine.
Lactase deficiency.
Irritable bowel syndrome.
Anxiety disorders.
Food poisoning, giardiasis.

FLUSHING[24]

ICD-9CM # 782.62

Physiologic flushing: menopause, ingestion of monosodium glutamate (Chinese restaurant syndrome), ingestion of hot drinks.
Drugs: alcohol (with or without disulfiram, metronidazole, or chlorpropamide), nicotinic acid, diltiazem, nifedipine, levodopa, bromocriptine, vancomycin, amyl nitrate.
Neoplastic disorders: carcinoid syndrome, Vipoma syndrome, medullary carcinoma of thyroid, systemic mastocytosis, basophilic chronic myelocytic leukemia, renal cell carcinoma.
Anxiety.
Agnogenic flushing.

FOOT PAIN

ICD-9CM # CODE VARIES WITH SPECIFIC DIAGNOSIS

Trauma (fractures, musculoskeletal and ligamentous strain).
Inflammation (Plantar fasciitis, Achilles tendonitis or bursitis, calcaneal apophysitis).
Arterial insufficiency, Raynaud's phenomenon, thromboangiitis obliterans.
Gout, pseudogout.
Calcaneal spur.
Infection (cellulitis, abscess, lymphangitis, gangrene).
Decubitus ulcer.
Paronychia, ingrown toenail.
Thrombophlebitis, postphlebitic syndrome.

FOREARM AND HAND PAIN

ICD-9CM # 959.3 FOREARM INJURY
959.4 HAND INJURY

Epicondylitis.
Tenosynovitis.
Osteoarthritis.
Cubital tunnel syndrome.
Carpal tunnel syndrome.
Trauma.
Herpes zoster.
Peripheral vascular insufficiency.
Infection (cellulitis, abscess).

GAIT ABNORMALITY

ICD-9CM # 781.2 GAIT ABNORMALITY

Parkinsonism.
Degenerative joint disease (hips, back, knees).
Multiple sclerosis.
Trauma, foot pain.
CVA.

Cerebellar lesions.
Infections (tabes, encephalitis, meningitis).
Sensory ataxia.
Dystonia, cerebral palsy, neuromuscular disorders.
Metabolic abnormalities.

GALACTORRHEA[25]

ICD-9CM # 611.6

Prolonged suckling.
Drugs (INH, phenothiazines, reserpine derivatives, amphetamines, spironolactone and tricyclic antidepressants).
Major stressors (surgery, trauma).
Hypothyroidism.
Pituitary tumors.

GASTRIC EMPTYING, DELAYED[1]

ICD-9CM # 536.8 GASTRIC MOTILITY DISORDER

■ **MECHANICAL OBSTRUCTION**
Duodenal or pyloric channel ulcer.
Pyloric stricture.
Tumor of the distal stomach.

■ **FUNCTIONAL OBSTRUCTION (GASTROPARESIS)**
Drugs: anticholinergics, beta-adrenergics, opiates.
Electrolyte imbalance: hypokalemia, hypocalcemia, hypomagnesemia.
Metabolic disorders: DM, hypoparathyroidism, hypothyroidism, pregnancy.
Vagotomy.
Viral infections.
Neuromuscular disorders (myotonic dystrophy, autonomic neuropathy, scleroderma, polymyositis).
Gastric pacemaker (i.e., tachygastria).
Brainstem tumors.
GERD.
Psychiatric disorders: anorexia nervosa, psychogenic vomiting.
Idiopathic.

GASTRIC EMPTYING, RAPID

ICD-9CM # 536.8 GASTRIC MOTILITY DISORDER

Pancreatic insufficiency.
Dumping syndrome.
Peptic ulcer.
Celiac disease.
Promotility agents.
Zollinger-Ellison disease.

GENITAL DISCHARGE, FEMALE[10]

ICD-9CM # 629.9

Physiologic discharge: cervical mucus, vaginal transudation, bacteria, squamous epithelial cells.
Individual variation.
Pregnancy.
Sexual response.
Menstrual cycle variation.
Infection.
Foreign body: tampon, cervical cap, other.
Neoplasm.
Fistula.
IUD.

Cervical ectropion.
Spermicide.
Nongenital causes: urinary incontinence, urinary tract fistula, Crohn's disease, rectovaginal fistula.

GENITAL SORES[1]

```
ICD-9CM # 054.10 GENITAL HERPES
          91.0 GENITAL SYPHILIS
          078.11 CONDYLOMA ACUMINATUM
          099.0 CHANCROID
          099.2 GRANULOMA INGUINALE
          099.1 LYMPHOGRANULOMA VENEREUM
          629.8 ULCER, GENITAL SITE, FEMALE
          608.89 ULCER, GENITAL SITE, MALE
```

Herpes genitalis.
Syphilis.
Chancroid.
Lymphogranuloma venereum.
Granuloma inguinale.
Condyloma acuminatum.
Neoplastic lesion.
Trauma.

GOITER

```
ICD-9CM # 240.9 GOITER, UNSPECIFIED
          241.9 GOITER, ADENOMATOUS
          246.1 GOITER, CONGENITAL
          240.9 GOITER, NONTOXIC DIFFUSE
          241.1 GOITER, NONTOXIC
                MULTINODULAR
          240.0 SIMPLE GOITER
          242.1 THYROTOXIC GOITER
```

Thyroiditis.
Toxic multinodular goiter.
Graves' disease.
Medications (PTU, methimazole, sulfonamides, sulfonylureas, ethionamide, amiodarone, lithium, etc.).
Iodine deficiency.
Sarcoidosis, amyloidosis.
Defective thyroid hormone synthesis.
Resistance to thyroid hormone.

GRANULOMATOUS DISORDERS[29]

```
ICD-9CM # 446.4 GRANULOMATOSIS
          288.1 GRANULOMATOUS DISEASE
```

■ INFECTIONS

Fungi
Histoplasma.
Coccidioides.
Blastomyces.
Sporothrix.
Aspergillus.
Cryptococcus.
Protozoa
Toxoplasma.
Leishmania.
Metazoa
Toxocara.
Schistosoma.
Spirochetes
Treponema pallidum.
T. pertenue.
T. carateum.

Mycobacteria
M. tuberculosis.
M. leprae.
M. kansasii.
M. marinum.
M. avian.
Bacille Calmette-Guérin (BCG) vaccine.
Bacteria
Brucella.
Yersinia.
Other Infections
Cat scratch.
Lymphogranuloma.

■ NEOPLASIA

Carcinoma.
Reticulosis.
Pinealoma.
Dysgerminoma.
Seminoma.
Reticulum cell sarcoma.
Malignant nasal granuloma.

■ CHEMICALS

Beryllium.
Zirconium.
Silica.
Starch.

■ IMMUNOLOGIC ABERRATIONS

Sarcoidosis.
Crohn's disease.
Primary biliary cirrhosis.
Wegener's granulomatosis.
Giant-cell arteritis.
Peyronie's disease.
Hypogammaglobulinemia.
Systemic lupus erythematosus.
Lymphomatoid granulomatosis.
Histiocytosis X.
Hepatic granulomatous disease.
Immune complex disease.
Rosenthal-Melkersson syndrome.
Churg-Strauss allergic granulomatosis.

■ LEUKOCYTE OXIDASE DEFECT

Chronic granulomatous disease of childhood.

■ EXTRINSIC ALLERGIC ALVEOLITIS

Farmer's lung.
Bird fancier's.
Mushroom worker's.
Suberosis (cork dust).
Bagassosis.
Maple bark stripper's.
Paprika splitter's.
Coffee bean.
Spatlese lung.

■ OTHER DISORDERS

Whipple's disease.
Pyrexia of unknown origin.
Radiotherapy.
Cancer chemotherapy.
Panniculitis.
Chalazion.
Sebaceous cyst.
Dermoid.
Sea urchin spine injury.

GROIN PAIN, ACTIVE PATIENT[34]

**ICD-9CM # 959.1 GROIN INJURY
848.8 GROIN PAIN**

■ MUSCULOSKELETAL

Avascular necrosis of the femoral head.
Avulsion fracture (lesser trochanter, anterior superior iliac spine, anterior inferior iliac spine).
Bursitis (iliopectineal, trochanteric).
Entrapment of the ilioinguinal or iliofemoral nerve.
Gracilis syndrome.
Muscle tear (adductors, iliopsoas, rectus abdominis, gracilis, sartorius, rectus femoris).
Myositis ossificans of the hip muscles.
Osteitis pubis.
Osteoarthritis of the femoral head.
Slipped capital femoral epiphysis.
Stress fracture of the femoral head or neck and pubis.
Synovitis.

■ HERNIA-RELATED

Avulsion of the internal oblique muscle in the conjoined tendon.
Defect at the insertion of the rectus abdominis muscle.
Direct inguinal hernia.
Femoral ring hernia.
Indirect inguinal hernia.
Inguinal canal weakness.

■ UROLOGIC

Epididymitis.
Fracture of the testis.
Hydrocele.
Kidney stone.
Posterior urethritis.
Prostatis.
Testicular cancer.
Torsion of the testis.
Urinary tract infection.
Varicocele.

■ GYNECOLOGIC

Ectopic pregnancy.
Ovarian cyst.
Pelvic inflammatory disease.
Torsion of the ovary.
Vaginitis.

■ LYMPHATIC ENLARGEMENT IN GROIN

GYNECOMASTIA

ICD-9CM # 611.1 GYNECOMASTIA, NONPUERPERAL

Physiologic (puberty, newborns, aging).
Drugs (estrogen and estrogen precursors, digitalis, testosterone and exogenous androgens, clomiphene, cimetidine, spironolactone, ketoconazole, amiodarone, ACE inhibitors, isoniazid, phenytoin, methyldopa, metoclopramide, phenothiazine).
Increased prolactin level (prolactinoma).
Liver disease.
Adrenal disease.
Thyrotoxicosis.
Increased estrogen production (hCG-producing tumor, testicular tumor, bronchogenic carcinoma).
Secondary hypogonadism.
Primary gonadal failure (trauma, castration, viral orchitis, granulomatous disease).
Defects in androgen synthesis.

Testosterone deficiency.
Klinefelter's syndrome.

HALITOSIS

ICD-9CM # 784.9

Tobacco use.
Alcohol use.
Dry mouth (mouth breathing, inadequate fluid intake).
Foods (onion, garlic, meats, nuts).
Disease of mouth or nose (infections, cancer, inflammation).
Medications (antihistamines, antidepressants).
Systemic disorders (diabetes, uremia).
GI disorders (esophageal diverticula, hiatal hernia, GERD, achalasia).
Sinusitis.
Pulmonary disorders (bronchiectasis, pneumonia, neoplasms, TB).

HAND PAIN AND SWELLING[6]

ICD-9CM # CODE VARIES WITH SPECIFIC DIAGNOSIS

Trauma.
Gout.
Pseudogout.
Cellulitis.
Lymphangitis.
DVT of upper extremity.
Thrombophlebitis.
Rheumatoid arthritis.
Remitting seronegative symmetrical synovitis with pitting edema (RS3PE).
Polymyalgia rheumatica.
Mixed connective tissue disease.
Scleroderma.
Rupture of the olecranon bursa.
Metzger's syndrome (neoplasia).
The puffy hand of drug addiction.
Reflex sympathetic dystrophy.
Eosinophilic fasciitis.
Sickle cell (hand-foot syndrome).
Leprosy.
Factitial (the rubber band syndrome).

HEADACHE[11]

**ICD-9CM # 784.0 HEADACHE NOS
307.81 HEADACHE, TENSION
346.2 HEADACHE, CLUSTER
346.9 HEADACHE, MIGRAINE
784.0 HEADACHE, VASCULAR**

Vascular: migraine, cluster headaches, temporal arteritis, hypertension, cavernous sinus thrombosis.
Musculoskeletal: neck and shoulder muscle contraction, strain of extraocular and/or intraocular muscles, cervical spondylosis, temporomandibular arthritis.
Infections: meningitis, encephalitis, brain abscess, sepsis, sinusitis, osteomyelitis, parotitis, mastoiditis.
Cerebral neoplasm.
Subdural hematoma.
Cerebral hemorrhage/infarct.
Pseudotumor cerebri.
Normal pressure hydrocephalus (NPH).
Postlumbar puncture.
Cerebral aneurysm, arteriovenous malformations.
Posttrauma.

Dental problems: abscess, periodontitis, poorly fitting dentures.
Trigeminal neuralgia, glossopharyngeal neuralgia.
Otitis and other ear diseases.
Glaucoma and other eye diseases.
Metabolic: uremia, carbon monoxide inhalation, hypoxia.
Pheochromocytoma, hypoglycemia, hypothyroidism.
Effort induced: benign exertional headache, cough, headache, coital cephalalgia.
Drugs: alcohol, nitrates, histamine antagonists.
Paget's disease of the skull.
Emotional, psychiatric.

HEADACHE AND FACIAL PAIN[33]

**ICD-9CM # 784.0 HEADACHE NOS
784.0 FACIAL PAIN**

■ VASCULAR HEADACHES
Migraine
Migraine with headaches and inconspicuous neurologic features:
  - Migraine without aura ("common migraine").
Migraine with headaches and conspicuous neurologic features:
  -With transient neurologic symptoms:
    Migraine with typical aura ("classic migraine").
    Sensory, basilar, and *hemiplegic migraine.*
  -With prolonged or permanent neurologic features ("complicated migraine"):
    Ophthalmoplegic migraine.
    Migrainous infarction.
Migraine without headaches but with conspicuous neurologic features ("migraine equivalents"):
  -Abdominal migraine.
  - Benign paroxysmal vertigo of childhood.
  - Migraine aura without headache ("isolated auras," transient migrainous accompaniments).
Cluster headaches
Episodic cluster headache ("cyclic cluster headaches").
Chronic cluster headaches.
Chronic paroxysmal hemicrania.
Other vascular headaches
Headaches of reactive vasodilation (fever, drug-induced, postictal, hypoglycemia, hypoxia, hypercarbia, hyperthyroidism).
Headaches associated with arterial hypertension:
  -Chronic severe hypertension (diastolic >120 mm Hg).
  -Paroxysmal severe hypertension (pheochromocytoma, some coital headaches).
Headaches caused by cranial arteritis:
  -Giant cell arteritis ("temporal arteritis").
  -Other vasculitides.

■ HEADACHES ASSOCIATED WITH DEMONSTRABLE MUSCLE SPASM
Headache caused by posturally induced or perilesional muscle spasm:
  -Headaches of sustained or impaired posture (e.g., prolonged close work, driving).
  -Headaches associated with cervical spondylosis and other diseases of cervical spine.
  -Myofascial pain dysfunction syndrome (headache or facial pain associated with disorders of teeth, jaws, and related structures, or "TMJ syndrome").
Headaches caused by psychophysiologic muscular contraction ("muscle contraction headaches," or tension-type headache associated with disorder of pericranial muscles).

■ HEADACHES AND FACIAL PAIN WITHOUT DEMONSTRABLE PHYSICAL SUBSTRATE
Headaches of uncertain etiology:
  -"Tension headaches" (tension-type headache unassociated with disorder of pericranial muscles).
  -Some forms of posttraumatic headache.
Psychogenic headaches (e.g., hypochondriacal, conversional, delusional, malingered).
Facial pain of uncertain etiology ("atypical facial pain").

■ COMBINED TENSION-MIGRAINE HEADACHES
Episodic migraine superimposed on chronic tension headaches.
Chronic daily headaches:
  -Associated with analgesic and/or ergotamine overuse ("rebound headaches").
  -Not associated with drug overuse.

■ HEADACHES AND HEAD PAINS CAUSED BY DISEASES OF EYES, EARS, NOSE, SINUSES, TEETH, OR SKULL

■ HEADACHES CAUSED BY MENINGEAL INFLAMMATION
Subarachnoid hemorrhage.
Meningitis and meningoencephalitis.
Others (e.g., meningeal carcinomatosis).

■ HEADACHES ASSOCIATED WITH ALTERED INTRACRANIAL PRESSURE ("TRACTION HEADACHES")
Increased intracranial pressure
Intracranial mass lesions (neoplasm, hematoma, abscess, etc.).
Hydrocephalus.
Benign intracranial hypertension.
Venous sinus thrombosis.
Decreased intracranial pressure
Post–lumbar puncture headaches.
Spontaneous hypoliquorrheic headaches.

■ HEADACHES AND HEAD PAINS CAUSED BY CRANIAL NEURALGIAS
Presumed irritation of superficial nerves
Occipital neuralgia.
Supraorbital neuralgia.
Presumed irritation of intracranial nerves
Trigeminal neuralgia ("tic douloureux").
Glossopharyngeal neuralgia.

HEARING LOSS, ACUTE[23]

ICD-9CM # 388.2

Infectious: mumps, measles, influenza, herpes simplex, herpes zoster, CMV, mononucleosis, syphilis.
Vascular: macroglobulinemia, sickle cell disease, Berger's disease, leukemia, polycythemia, fat emboli, hypercoagulable states.
Metabolic: diabetes, pregnancy, hyperlipoproteinemia.
Conductive: cerumen impaction, foreign bodies, otitis media, otitis externa, barotrauma, trauma.
Medications: aminoglycosides, loop diuretics, antineoplastics, salicylates, vancomycin.
Neoplasm: acoustic neuroma, metastatic neoplasm.

HEARTBURN AND INDIGESTION[30]

> ICD-9CM # 787.1 HEARTBURN
> 536.8 INDIGESTION

Reflux esophagitis.
Gastritis.
Nonulcer dyspepsia.
Functional GI disorder (anxiety disorder, social/environmental stresses).
Excessive intestinal gas (ingestion of flatulogenic foods, GI stasis, constipation).
Gas entrapment (hepatitis or splenic flexure syndrome).
Neoplasm (adenocarcinoma of stomach or esophagus, lymphoma).
Gallbladder disease.

HEEL PAIN, PLANTAR[21]

> ICD-9CM # 729.5

■ SKIN
Keratoses.
Verruca.
Ulcer.
Fissure.

■ CONNECTIVE TISSUE
Fat
Atrophy.
Panniculitis.
Dense Connective Tissue
Inflammatory fasciitis.
Fibromatosis.
Enthesopathy.
Bursitis.
Bone (Calcaneus)
Stress fracture.
Paget's disease.
Benign bone cyst/tumor.
Malignant bone tumor.
Metabolic bone disease (osteopenia).
Nerve
Tarsal tunnel.
Plantar nerve entrapment.
S1 nerve root radiculopathy.
Painful peripheral neuropathy.

■ INFECTION
Dermatomycoses.
Acute osteomyelitis.
Plantar abscess.

■ MISCELLANEOUS
Foreign body.
Nonunion calcaneus fracture.
Psychogenic.
Idiopathic.

HEMARTHROSIS

> ICD-9CM # 848.9 HEMARTHROSIS (SPRAIN) NOS

Trauma.
Anticoagulant therapy.
Thrombocytopenia, thrombocytosis.
Bleeding disorders (e.g., von Willebrand's disease).
Charcot's joint.
Idiopathic.

Other: pigmented villonodular synovitis, hemangioma, synovioma, AV fistula, ruptured aneurysm.

HEMATURIA

> ICD-9CM # 599.7 HEMATURIA, BENIGN (ESSENTIAL)

Use the mnemonic TICS:
T (trauma): blow to kidney, insertion of Foley catheter or foreign body in urethra, prolonged and severe exercise, very rapid emptying of overdistended bladder.
(tumor): hypernephroma, Wilms' tumor, papillary carcinoma of the bladder, prostatic and urethral neoplasms.
(toxins): turpentine, phenols, sulfonamides and other antibiotics, cyclophosphamide, NSAIDs.
I (infections): glomerulonephritis, TB, cystitis, prostatitis, urethritis, Schistosoma haematobium, yellow fever, blackwater fever.
(inflammatory processes): Goodpasture's syndrome, periarteritis, postirradiation.
C (calculi): renal, ureteral, bladder, urethra.
(cysts): simple cysts, polycystic disease.
(congenital anomalies): hemangiomas, aneurysms, AVM.
S (surgery): invasive procedures, prostatic resection, cystoscopy.
(sickle cell disease and other hematologic disturbances): hemophilia, thrombocytopenia, anticoagulants.
(somewhere else): bleeding genitals, factitious (drug addicts).

HEMATURIA, CAUSE BY AGE AND SEX

> ICD-9CM # 599.7 HEMATURIA BENIGN (ESSENTIAL)
> OTHER CODES FOR HEMATURIA VARY
> WITH CAUSE OF HEMATURIA

■ 0-20 YR
Acute urinary tract infections.
Acute glomerulonephritis.
Congenital urinary tract anomalies with obstruction.
Trauma to genitals.

■ 20-40 YR
Acute urinary tract infection.
Trauma to genitals.
Urolithiasis.
Bladder cancer.

■ 40-60 YR (WOMEN)
Acute urinary tract infection.
Bladder cancer.
Urolithiasis.

■ 40-60 YR (MEN)
Acute urinary tract infection.
Bladder cancer.
Urolithiasis.

■ 60 YR AND OLDER (WOMEN)
Acute urinary tract infection.
Bladder cancer.
Vaginal trauma or irritation.
Urolithiasis.

■ 60 YR AND OLDER (MEN)
Acute urinary tract infection.
Benign prostatic hyperplasia.
Bladder cancer.
Urolithiasis.
Trauma.

HEMIPARESIS/HEMIPLEGIA

> **ICD-9CM # 436.0 ACQUIRED DUE TO ACUTE CVA, FLACCID**
> **436.1 ACQUIRED DUE TO CVA, ACUTE, SPASTIC**

CVA.
Transient ischemic attack.
Cerebral neoplasm.
Multiple sclerosis or other demyelinating disorder.
CNS infection.
Migraine.
Hypoglycemia
Subdural hematoma.
Vasculitis.
Todd's paralysis.
Epidural hematoma.
Metabolic (hyperosmolar state, electrolyte imbalance).
Psychiatric disorders.
Congenital disorders.
Leukodystrophies.

HEMOLYSIS AND HEMOGLOBINURIA

> **ICD-9CM # 773.2 HEMOLYSIS**
> **791.2 HEMOGLOBINURIA**

Erythrocyte trauma (prosthetic cardiac valves, marching and severe trauma, extensive burns).
Infections (malaria, *Bartonella, Clostridium Welchii*).
Brown recluse spider bite.
Incompatible blood transfusions.
Hemolytic uremic syndrome.
Thrombotic thrombocytopenic purpura (TTP).
Paroxysmal nocturnal hemoglobinuria (PNH).
Drugs (penicillins, quinidine, methyldopa, sulfonamides, nitrofurantoin).
Erythrocyte enzyme deficiencies (e.g., exposure to fava beans in patients with glucose-6-phosphate dehydrogenase deficiency).

HEMOLYSIS, INTRAVASCULAR

> **ICD-9CM # 283.2**

Infections.
Exertional hemolysis (e.g., prolonged march).
Valve hemolysis.
Microangiopathic hemolytic anemia.
Osmotic and chemical agents.
Thermal injury.
Cold agglutinins.
Venoms (snakes, spiders).
Paroxysmal nocturnal hemoglobinuria (PNH).

HEMOPTYSIS

> **ICD-9CM # 786.3**

■ CARDIOVASCULAR
Pulmonary embolism/infarction.
Left ventricular failure.
Mitral stenosis.
AV fistula.
Severe hypertension.
Erosion of aortic aneurysm.

■ PULMONARY
Neoplasm (primary or metastatic).
Infection.
Pneumonia: *Streptococcus pneumoniae, Klebsiella pneumoniae, Staphylococcus aureus, Legionella* pneumophila.
Bronchiectasis.
Abscess.
TB.
Bronchitis.
Fungal infections (aspergillosis, coccidioidomycosis).
Parasitic infections (amebiasis, ascariasis, paragonimiasis).
Vasculitis: Wegener's granulomatosis, Churg-Strauss syndrome, Henoch-Schönlein purpura.
Goodpasture's syndrome.
Trauma (needle biopsy, foreign body, right-sided heart catheterization, prolonged and severe cough).
Cystic fibrosis, bullous emphysema.
Pulmonary sequestration.
Pulmonary AV fistula.
SLE.
Idiopathic pulmonary hemosiderosis.
Drugs: aspirin, anticoagulants, penicillamine.
Pulmonary hypertension.
Mediastinal fibrosis.

■ OTHER
Epistaxis, trauma.
Laryngeal bleeding (laryngitis, laryngeal neoplasm).
Hematologic disorders (clotting abnormalities, DIC, thrombocytopenia).

HEPATIC CYSTS[33]

> **ICD-9CM # 751.62 HEPATIC CYST, CONGENITAL**
> **122.8 ECHINOCOCCUS INFECTION, LIVER**

■ CONGENITAL HEPATIC CYSTS
Parenchymal: solitary cyst, polycystic disease.
Ductal: localized dilatation, multiple cystic dilatations of intrahepatic ducts (Caroli's disease).

■ ACQUIRED HEPATIC CYSTS
Inflammatory cysts: retention cysts, echinococcal cyst, amebic cyst.
Neoplastic cyst.
Peliosis hepatis.

HEPATIC GRANULOMAS[1]

> **ICD-9CM # 572.8**

■ INFECTIONS
Bacterial, spirochetal: TB and atypical mycobacterial infections, tularemia, brucellosis, leprosy, syphilis, Whipple's disease, listeriosis.
Viral: mononucleosis, CMV.
Rickettsial: Q fever.
Fungal: coccidioidomycosis, histoplasmosis, cryptococcal infections, actinomycosis, aspergillosis, nocardiosis.
Parasitic: schistosomiasis, clonorchiasis, toxocariasis, ascariasis, toxoplasmosis, amebiasis.

■ HEPATOBILIARY DISORDERS
Primary biliary cirrhosis, granulomatous hepatitis, jejunoileal bypass.

■ SYSTEMIC DISORDERS
Sarcoidosis, Wegener's granulomatosis, inflammatory bowel disease, Hodgkin's disease, lymphoma.

■ DRUGS/TOXINS

Beryllium, parenteral foreign material (starch, talc, silicone, etc.), phenylbutazone, α-methyldopa, procainamide, allopurinol, phenytoin, nitrofurantoin, hydralazine.

HEPATITIS, CHRONIC[22]

ICD-9CM # 571.40 HEPATITIS, NONINFECTIOUS, CHRONIC
072.22 HEPATITIS B, CHRONIC
070.44 HEPATITIS C, CHRONIC

Chronic viral hepatitis:
    Hepatitis B.
    Hepatitis C.
    Hepatitis D.
Autoimmune hepatitis and variant syndromes.
Hereditary hemochromatosis.
Wilson's disease.
α-Antitrypsin deficiency.
Fatty liver and nonalcoholic steatohepatitis.
Alcoholic liver disease.
Drug-induced liver disease.
Hepatic granulomas:
    Infectious.
    Drug induced.
    Neoplastic.
    Idiopathic.

HEPATOMEGALY

ICD-9CM # 789.1

■ FREQUENT JAUNDICE

Infectious hepatitis.
Toxic hepatitis.
Carcinoma: liver, pancreas, bile ducts, metastatic neoplasm to liver.
Cirrhosis.
Obstruction of common bile duct.
Alcoholic hepatitis.
Biliary cirrhosis.
Cholangitis.
Hemochromatosis with cirrhosis.

■ INFREQUENT JAUNDICE

CHF.
Amyloidosis.
Liver abscess.
Sarcoidosis.
Infectious mononucleosis.
Alcoholic fatty infiltration.
Nonalcoholic steatohepatitis
Lymphoma.
Leukemia.
Budd-Chiari syndrome.
Myelofibrosis with myeloid metaplasia.
Familial hyperlipoproteinemia type 1.
Other: amebiasis, hydatid disease of liver, schistosomiasis, kala-azar *(Leishmania donovani)*, Hurler's syndrome, Gaucher's disease, kwashiorkor.

HERMAPHRODITISM[4]

ICD-9CM # 752.7 HERMAPHRODITISM, CONGENITAL

■ FEMALE PSEUDOHERMAPHRODITISM

Androgen exposure:
    Fetal source:
        21-Hydroxylase (P450 c21) deficiency.
        11β-Hydroxylase (P450 c11) deficiency.
        3β-Hydroxysteroid dehydrogenase II (3β-HSD II) deficiency.
        Aromatase (P450$_{arom}$) deficiency.
    Maternal source.
    Virilizing ovarian tumor.
    Virilizing adrenal tumor.
    Androgenic drugs.
Undetermined origin:
    Associated with genitourinary and gastrointestinal tract defects.

■ MALE PSEUDOHERMAPHRODITISM

Defects in testicular differentiation:
    Denys-Drash syndrome (mutation in WT1 gene).
    WAGR syndrome (*W*ilms tumor, *a*niridia, *g*enitourinary malformation, *r*etardation).
    Deletion of 11p13.
    Camptomelic syndrome (autosomal gene at 17q24.3-q25.1) and SOX 9 mutation.
    XY pure gonadal dysgenesis (Swyer syndrome).
        Mutation in SRY gene.
        Unknown cause.
    XY gonadal agenesis.
Deficiency of testicular hormones:
    Leydig cell aplasia.
    Mutation in LH receptor.
    Lipoid adrenal hyperplasia (P450 scc) deficiency; mutation in StAR (steroidogenic acute regulatory protein).
    3β-HSDII deficiency.
    17-Hydroxylase/17, 20-lyase (P450 c17) deficiency.
    Persistent müllerian duct syndrome.
        Gene mutations, müllerian-inhibiting substance (MIS).
        Receptor defects for MIS.
Defect in androgen action:
    5α-Reductase II mutations.
    Androgen receptor defects:
        Complete androgen insensitivity syndrome.
        Partial androgen insensitivity syndrome.
        (Reifenstein and other syndromes).
        Smith-Lemli-Opitz syndrome.
           Defect in conversion of 7-dehydrocholesterol to cholesterol.

■ TRUE HERMAPHRODITISM

XX.
XY.
XX/XY chimeras.

HICCUPS[18]

ICD-9CM # 786.8

■ TRANSIENT HICCUPS

Sudden excitement, emotion.
Gastric distention.
Esophageal obstruction.
Alcohol ingestion.
Sudden change in temperature.

■ PERSISTENT OR CHRONIC HICCUPS

Toxic/metabolic: uremia, DM, hyperventilation, hypocalcemia, hypokalemia, hyponatremia, gout, fever.

Drugs: benzodiazepines, steroids, α-methyldopa, barbiturates.

Surgery/general anesthesia.

Thoracic/diaphragmatic disorders: pneumonia, lung cancer, asthma, pleuritis, pericarditis, myocardial infarction, aortic aneurysm, esophagitis, esophageal obstruction, diaphragmatic hernia or irritation.

Abdominal disorders: gastric ulcer or cancer, hepatobiliary or pancreatic disease, IBD, bowel obstruction, intraabdominal or subphrenic abscess, prostatic infection or cancer.

Central nervous system disorders: traumatic, infectious, vascular, structural.

Ear, nose, and throat disorders: pharyngitis, laryngitis, tumor, irritation of auditory canal.

Psychogenic disorders.

Idiopathic disorders.

HIP PAIN, CHILDREN[23]

> ICD-9CM # 959.6 HIP INJURY
> 719.95 HIP JOINT DISORDER
> 843.9 HIP STRAIN

■ TRAUMA

Hip or pelvis fractures.
Overuse injuries.

■ INFECTION

Septic arthritis.
Osteomyelitis.

■ INFLAMMATION

Transient synovitis.
Juvenile rheumatoid arthritis.
Rheumatic fever.

■ NEOPLASM

Leukemia.
Osteogenic or Ewing's sarcoma.
Metastatic disease.

■ HEMATOLOGIC DISORDERS

Hemophilia.
Sickle cell anemia.

■ MISCELLANEOUS

Legg-Calvé-Perthes disease.
Slipped capital femoral epiphysis.

HIRSUTISM

> ICD-9CM # 704.1

Idiopathic: familial, possibly increased sensitivity to androgens.

Menopause.

Polycystic ovarian syndrome.

Drugs: androgens, anabolic steroids, methyltestosterone, minoxidil, diazoxide, phenytoin, glucocorticoids, cyclosporine.

Congenital adrenal hyperplasia.

Adrenal virilizing tumor.

Ovarian virilizing tumor: arrhenoblastoma, hilus cell tumor.

Pituitary adenoma.

Cushing's syndrome.

Hypothyroidism (congenital and juvenile).

Acromegaly.

Testicular feminization.

HIV INFECTION, ANORECTAL LESIONS[23]

> ICD-9CM # 042 HIV INFECTION, SYMPTOMATIC
> V08 HIV INFECTION, ASYMPTOMATIC

■ COMMON CONDITIONS

Anal fissure.
Abscess and fistula.
Hemorrhoids.
Pruritus ani.
Pilonidal disease.

■ COMMON STDs

Gonorrhea.
Chlamydia.
Herpes.
Chancroid.
Syphilis.
Condylomata acuminata.

■ ATYPICAL CONDITIONS

Infectious: TB, CMV, actinomycosis, cryptococcus.
Neoplastic: lymphoma, Kaposi's sarcoma, squamous cell carcinoma.
Other: idiopathic and ulcer.

HIV INFECTION, CHEST RADIOGRAPHIC ABNORMALITIES[23]

> ICD-9CM # 042 HIV INFECTION, SYMPTOMATIC
> V08 HIV INFECTION, ASYMPTOMATIC

■ DIFFUSE INTERSTITIAL INFILTRATION

Pneumocystis carinii.
Cytomegalovirus.
Mycobacterium tuberculosis.
Mycobacterium avium complex.
Histoplasmosis.
Coccidioidomycosis.
Lymphoid interstitial pneumonitis.

■ FOCAL CONSOLIDATION

Bacterial pneumonia.
Mycoplasma pneumoniae.
Pneumocystis carinii.
Mycobacterium tuberculosis.
Mycobacterium avium complex.

■ NODULAR LESIONS

Kaposi's sarcoma.
Mycobacterium tuberculosis.
Mycobacterium avium complex.
Fungal lesions.
Toxoplasmosis.

■ CAVITARY LESIONS

Pneumocystis carinii.
Mycobacterium tuberculosis.
Bacterial infection.

■ PLEURAL EFFUSION

Kaposi's sarcoma.
(Small effusion may be associated with any infection).

■ **ADENOPATHY**

Kaposi's sarcoma.
Lymphoma.
Mycobacterium tuberculosis.
Cryptococcus.

■ **PNEUMOTHORAX**

Kaposi's sarcoma.

HIV INFECTION, COGNITIVE IMPAIRMENT[22]

ICD-9CM # 042 HIV INFECTION, SYMPTOMATIC

■ **EARLY TO MID-STAGE HIV DISEASE**

Depression.
Alcohol and substance abuse.
Medication-induced cognitive impairment.
Metabolic encephalopathies.
HIV-related cognitive impairment.

■ **ADVANCED HIV DISEASE (CD4⁺ <100/mm³)**

Opportunistic infection of CNS.
Neurosyphilis.
CNS lymphoma.
Progressive multifocal leukoencephalopathy.
Depression.
Metabolic encephalopathies.
Medication-induced cognitive impairment.
Stroke.
HIV dementia.

HIV INFECTION, CUTANEOUS MANIFESTATIONS[18]

ICD-9CM # 042 HIV INFECTION, SYMPTOMATIC
V08 HIV INFECTION, ASYMPTOMATIC

■ **BACTERIAL INFECTION**

Bacillary angiomatosis: Numerous angiomatous nodules associated with fever, chills, weight loss.
Staphylococcus aureus: Folliculitis, ecthyma, impetigo, bullous impetigo, furuncles, carbuncles.
Syphilis: May occur in different forms (primary, secondary, tertiary); chancre may become painful because of secondary infection.

■ **FUNGAL INFECTION**

Candidiasis: Mucous membranes (oral, vulvovaginal), less commonly candida intertrigo or paronychia.
Cryptococcoses: Papules or nodules that strongly resemble molluscum contagiosum; other forms include pustules, purpuric papules, and vegetating plaques.
Seborrheic dermatitis: Scaling and erythema in the hair-bearing areas (eyebrows, scalp, chest, and pubic area).

■ **ARTHROPOD INFESTATIONS**

Scabies: Pruritus with or without rash, usually generalized but can be limited to a single digit.

■ **VIRAL INFECTION**

Herpes simplex: Vesicular lesion in clusters; perianal, genital, orofacial, or digital; can be disseminated.
Herpes zoster: Painful dermatomal vesicles that may ulcerate or disseminate.
HIV: Discrete erythematous macules and papules on the upper trunk, palms, and soles are the most characteristic cutaneous finding of acute HIV infection.
Human papillomavirus: Genital warts (may become unusually extensive).

Kaposi's sarcoma (herpesvirus): Erythematous macules or papules; enlarge at varying rates; violaceous nodules or plaques; occasionally painful.
Molluscum contagiosum: Discrete umbilicated papules commonly on the face, neck, and intertriginous sites (axilla, groin, or buttocks).

■ **NONINFECTIOUS**

Drug reactions: More frequent and severe in HIV patients.
Nutritional deficiencies: Mainly seen in children and patients with chronic diarrhea; diffuse skin manifestations, depending upon the deficiency.
Psoriasis: Scaly lesions; diffuse or localized; can be associated with arthritis.
Vasculitis: Palpable purpuric eruption (can resemble septic emboli).

HIV INFECTION, ESOPHAGEAL DISEASE

ICD-9CM # CODE VARIES WITH SPECIFIC DIAGNOSIS

Candida infection.
Cytomegalovirus infection.
Aphthous ulcer.
Herpes simplex.

HIV INFECTION, HEPATIC DISEASE[22]

ICD-9CM # 042 HIV INFECTION, SYMPTOMATIC

■ **VIRUSES**

Hepatitis A.
Hepatitis B.
Hepatitis C.
Hepatitis D (with HBV).
Epstein-Barr virus.
Cytomegalovirus.
Herpes simplex virus.
Adenovirus.
Varicella-zoster virus.

■ **MYCOBACTERIA**

Mycobacterium avium complex.
Mycobacterium tuberculosis.

■ **FUNGI**

Histoplasma capsulatum.
Cryptococcus neoformans.
Coccidioides immitis.
Candida albicans.
Pneumocystis carinii.
Penicillium marneffei.

■ **PROTOZOA**

Toxoplasma gondii.
Cryptosporidium parvum.
Microsporida spp.
Schistosoma.

■ **BACTERIA**

Bartonella henselae (peliosis hepatis).

■ **MALIGNANCY**

Kaposi's sarcoma (HHV-8).
Non-Hodgkin's lymphoma.
Hepatocellular carcinoma.

■ **MEDICATIONS**

Zidovudine.
Didanosine.

Ritonavir.
Other HIV-1 protease inhibitors.
Fluconazole.
Macrolide antibiotics.
Isoniazid.
Rifampin.
Trimethoprim-sulfamethoxazole.

HIV INFECTION, LOWER GI TRACT DISEASE[22]

ICD-9CM # 042 HIV INFECTION, SYMPTOMATIC

■ CAUSES OF ENTEROCOLITIS
Bacteria
Campylobacter jejuni and other spp.
Salmonella spp.
Shigella flexneri.
Aeromonas hydrophila.
Plesiomonas shigelloides.
Yersinia enterocolitica.
Vibrio spp.
Mycobacterium avium complex.
Mycobacterium tuberculosis.
Escherichia coli (enterotoxigenic, enteroadherent).
Bacterial overgrowth.
Clostridium difficile (toxin).
Parasites
Cryptosporidium parvum.
Microsporida *(Enterocytozoon bieneusi, Septata intestinalis).*
Isospora belli.
Entamoeba histolytica.
Giardia lamblia.
Cyclospora cayetanensis.
Viruses
Cytomegalovirus.
Adenovirus.
Calicivirus.
Astrovirus.
Picobirnavirus.
Human immunodeficiency virus.
Fungi
Histoplasma capsulatum.

■ CAUSES OF PROCTITIS
Bacteria
Chlamydia trachomatis.
Neisseria gonorrhoeae.
Treponema pallidum.
Viruses
Herpes simplex.
Cytomegalovirus.

HIV INFECTION, OCULAR MANIFESTATIONS[33]

ICD-9CM # 042 HIV INFECTION, SYMPTOMATIC
V08 HIV INFECTION, ASYMPTOMATIC

■ EYELIDS
Molluscum contagiosum.
Kaposi's sarcoma.

■ CORNEA/CONJUNCTIVA
Keratoconjunctivitis sicca.
Bacterial/fungal ulcerative keratitis.
Herpes simplex.
Herpes zoster ophthalmicus.
Conjunctival microvasculopathy.
Kaposi's sarcoma.

■ RETINA, CHOROID, AND VITREOUS
Microvasculopathy.
Endophthalmitis.
Cytomegalovirus retinitis.
Acute retinal necrosis.
Syphilis.
Toxoplasmosis.
Pneumocystis choroidopathy.
Cryptococcosis.
Mycobacterial infection.
Intraocular lymphoma.
Candidiasis.
Histoplasmosis.

■ DRUGS ASSOCIATED WITH OCULAR TOXICITY
Rifabutin.
Didanosine.

■ NEUROOPHTHALMIC
Disc edema.
Primary or secondary optic neuropathy.
Cranial nerve palsies.

■ ORBITAL
Lymphoma.
Infection.
Pseudotumor.

HIV INFECTION, PULMONARY DISEASE[22]

ICD-9CM # 042 HIV INFECTION, SYMPTOMATIC

■ MYCOBACTERIAL
M. tuberculosis.
M. kansasii.
M. avium complex.
Other nontuberculous mycobacteria.

■ OTHER BACTERIAL
Streptococcus pneumoniae.
Staphylococcus aureus.
Haemophilus influenzae.
Enterobacteriaceae.
Pseudomonas aeruginosa.
Moraxella catarrhalis.
Group A *Streptococcus.*
Nocardia species.
Rhodococcus equi.
Chlamydia pneumoniae.

■ FUNGAL
Pneumocystis carinii.
Cryptococcus neoformans.
Histoplasma capsulatum.
Coccidioides immitis.
Aspergillus species.
Blastomyces dermatitidis.
Penicillium marneffei.

■ VIRAL
Cytomegalovirus.
Herpes simplex virus.
Adenovirus.
Respiratory syncytial virus.
Influenza viruses.
Parainfluenza virus.

■ OTHER
Toxoplasma gondii.
Strongyloides stercoralis.

Kaposi's sarcoma.
Lymphoma.
Lung cancer.
Lymphocytic interstitial pneumonitis.
Nonspecific interstitial pneumonitis.
Bronchiolitis obliterans with organizing pneumonia.
Pulmonary hypertension.
Emphysema-like or bullous disease.
Pneumothorax.
Congestive heart failure.
Diffuse alveolar damage.
Pulmonary embolus.

HOARSENESS

ICD-9CM # 784.49

Allergic rhinitis.
Infections (laryngitis, epiglottitis, tracheitis, croup).
Vocal cord polyps.
Voice strain.
Irritants (tobacco smoke).
Vocal cord trauma (intubation, surgery).
Neoplastic involvement of vocal cord (primary or metastatic).
Neurologic abnormalities (multiple sclerosis, ALS, parkinsonism).
Endocrine abnormalities (puberty, menopause, hypothyroidism).
Other (laryngeal webs or cysts, psychogenic, muscle tension abnormalities).

HYPERCALCEMIA

ICD-9CM # 275.42 HYPERCALCEMIA DISORDER

Malignancy: increased bone resorption via osteoclast-activating factors, secretion of PTH-like substances, prostaglandin E_2, direct erosion by tumor cells, transforming growth factors, colony-stimulating activity.
Hypercalcemia is common in the following neoplasms:
Solid tumors: breast, lung, pancreas, kidneys, ovary.
Hematologic cancers: myeloma, lymphosarcoma, adult T-cell lymphoma, Burkitt's lymphoma.
Hyperparathyroidism: increased bone resorption, GI absorption, and renal absorption; etiology:
Parathyroid hyperplasia, adenoma.
Hyperparathyroidism or renal failure with secondary hyperparathyroidism.
    Granulomatous disorders: increased GI absorption (e.g., sarcoidosis).
    Paget's disease: increased bone resorption, seen only during periods of immobilization.
    Vitamin D intoxication, milk-alkali syndrome; increased GI absorption.
    Thiazides: increased renal absorption.
Other causes: familial hypocalciuric hypercalcemia, thyrotoxicosis, adrenal insufficiency, prolonged immobilization, vitamin A intoxication, recovery from acute renal failure, lithium administration, pheochromocytoma, disseminated SLE.

HYPERCAPNIA, PERSISTENT[33]

ICD-9CM # 786.09

Hypercapnia with normal lungs: CNS disturbances (CVA, parkinsonism, encephalitis), metabolic alkalosis, myxedema, primary alveolar hypoventilation, spinal cord lesions.

Diseases of the chest wall (e.g., kyphoscoliosis, ankylosing spondylitis).
Neuromuscular disorders (e.g., myasthenia gravis, Guillain-Barré syndrome, amyotrophic lateral sclerosis, muscular dystrophy, poliomyelitis).
COPD.

HYPERHIDROSIS[4]

ICD-9CM # 780.8 HYPERHIDROSIS

■ CORTICAL
Emotional.
Familial dysautonomia.
Congenital ichthyosiform erythroderma.
Epidermolysis bullosa.
Nail-patella syndrome.
Jadassohn-Lewandowsky syndrome.
Pachyonychia congenita.
Palmoplantar keratoderma.

■ HYPOTHALAMIC
Drugs
Antipyretics.
Emetics.
Insulin.
Meperidine.
Exercise
Infection
Defervescence.
Chronic illness.
Metabolic
Debility.
Diabetes mellitus.
Hyperpituitarism.
Hyperthyroidism.
Hypoglycemia.
Obesity.
Porphyria.
Pregnancy.
Rickets.
Infantile scurvy.
Cardiovascular
Heart failure.
Shock.
Vasomotor
Cold injury.
Raynaud phenomenon.
Rheumatoid arthritis.
Neurologic
Abscess.
Familial dysautonomia.
Postencephalitic.
Tumor.
Miscellaneous
Chédiak-Higashi syndrome.
Compensatory.
Phenylketonuria.
Pheochromocytoma.
Vitiligo.
Medullary
Physiologic gustatory sweating.
Encephalitis.
Granulosis rubra nasi.
Syringomyelia.
Thoracic sympathetic trunk injury.
Spinal
Cord transection.
Syringomyelia.

Changes in blood flow
Mallucci syndrome.
Arteriovenous fistula.
Klippel-Trenaunay syndrome.
Glomus tumor.
Blue rubber bleb nevus syndrome.

HYPERKALEMIA

ICD-9CM # 276.7

Pseudohyperkalemia.
  Hemolyzed specimen.
  Severe thrombocytosis (platelet count >10^6 ml).
  Severe leukocytosis (white blood cell count >10^5 ml).
  Fist clenching during phlebotomy.
Excessive potassium intake (often in setting of impaired excretion).
  Potassium replacement therapy.
  High-potassium diet.
  Salt substitutes with potassium.
  Potassium salts of antibiotics.
Decreased renal excretion.
  Potassium-sparing diuretics (e.g., spironolactone, triamterene, amiloride).
  Renal insufficiency.
  Mineralocorticoid deficiency.
  Hyporeninemic hypoaldosteronism (DM).
  Tubular unresponsiveness to aldosterone (e.g., SLE, multiple myeloma, sickle cell disease).
  Type 4 RTA.
  ACE inhibitors.
  Heparin administration.
  NSAIDs.
  Trimethoprim-sulfamethoxazole.
  β-Blockers.
  Pentamidine.
Redistribution (excessive cellular release).
  Acidemia (each 0.1 decrease in pH increases the serum potassium by 0.4 to 0.6 mEq/L). Lactic acidosis and ketoacidosis cause minimal redistribution.
  Insulin deficiency.
  Drugs (e.g., succinylcholine, markedly increased digitalis level, arginine, β-adrenergic blockers).
  Hypertonicity.
  Hemolysis.
  Tissue necrosis, rhabdomyolysis, burns.
  Hyperkalemic periodic paralysis

HYPERKINETIC MOVEMENT DISORDERS[27]

ICD-9CM # 314.8 HYPERKINETIC SYNDROME
          275.1 CHOREOATHETOSIS
          335.5 HEMIBALLISM
          333.7 DYSTONIA DUE TO DRUGS
          333.6 DYSTONIA, IDIOPATHIC

Chorea, choreoathetosis: drug-induced, Huntington's chorea, Sydenham's chorea.
Tardive dyskinesia (e.g., phenothiazines).
Hemiballismus (lacunar CVA near subthalamic nuclei in basal ganglia, metastatic lesions, toxoplasmosis [in AIDS]).
Dystonia (idiopathic, familial, drug-induced [prochlorperazine, metoclopramide]), Wilson's disease.
Liver failure.
Thyrotoxicosis.
SLE, polycythemia.

HYPERMAGNESEMIA

ICD-9CM # 275.2

Renal failure (decreased GFR).
Decreased renal excretion secondary to salt depletion.
Abuse of antacids and laxatives containing magnesium in patients with renal insufficiency.
Endocrinopathies (deficiency of mineralocorticoid or thyroid hormone).
Increased tissue breakdown (rhabdomyolysis).
Redistribution: acute DKA, pheochromocytoma.
Other: lithium, volume depletion, familial hypocalciuric hypercalcemia.

HYPERPHOSPHATEMIA

ICD-9CM # 275.3

Excessive phosphate administration.
Excessive oral intake or IV administration.
Laxatives containing phosphate (phosphate tablets, phosphate enemas).
Decreased renal phosphate excretion.
Acute or chronic renal failure.
Hypoparathyroidism or pseudohypoparathyroidism.
Acromegaly, thyrotoxicosis.
Biphosphonate therapy.
Tumor calcinosis.
Sickle cell anemia.
Transcellular shift out of cells.
Chemotherapy of lymphoma or leukemia, tumor lysis syndrome, hemolysis.
Acidosis.
Rhabdomyolysis, malignant hyperthermia.
Artifact: in vitro hemolysis.
Pseudohyperphosphatemia: hyperlipidemia, paraproteinemia, hyperbilirubinemia.

HYPERPIGMENTATION[5]

ICD-9CM # 709.00

Addison's disease.*
Arsenic ingestion.
ACTH or MSH producing tumors (e.g., oat cell carcinoma of the lung).*
Drug induced (i.e., antimalarials, some cytotoxic agents).
Hemochromatosis ("bronze" diabetes).
Malabsorption syndrome (Whipple's disease and celiac sprue).
Melanoma.
Melanotropic hormone injection.*
Pheochromocytoma.
Porphyrias (porphyria cutanea tarda and variegate porphyria).
Pregnancy.
Progressive systemic sclerosis and related conditions.
PUVA therapy (psoralen administration) for psoriasis and vitiligo.*

(*ACTH*, Adrenocorticotropic hormone; *MSH*, melanocyte-stimulating hormone; *PUVA*, psoralen plus ultraviolet A.)
*Accentuation on sun-exposed surfaces.

HYPERTRICHOSIS[7]

ICD-9CM # 704.1 HYPERTRICHOSIS NOS
757.4 HYPERTRICHOSIS, CONGENITAL

■ DRUGS
Dilantin.
Streptomycin.
Hexachlorobenzene.
Penicillamine.
Diazoxide.
Minoxidil.
Cyclosporine.

■ SYSTEMIC ILLNESS
Hypothyroidism.
Anorexia nervosa.
Malnutrition.
Porphyria.
Dermatomyositis.

■ IDIOPATHIC

HYPERVENTILATION, PERSISTENT[33]

ICD-9CM # 786.01

Fibrotic lung disease.
Metabolic acidosis (e.g., diabetes, uremia).
CNS disorders (midbrain and pontine lesions).
Hepatic coma.
Salicylate intoxication.
Fever.
Sepsis.
Psychogenic (e.g., anxiety).

HYPOCALCEMIA

ICD-9CM # 275.41

Renal insufficiency: hypocalcemia caused by:
  Increased calcium deposits in bone and soft tissue secondary to increased serum PO_4^-3 level.
  Decreased production of 1,25-dihydroxyvitamin D.
  Excessive loss of 25-OHD (nephrotic syndrome).
Hypoalbuminemia: each decrease in serum albumin (g/L) will decrease serum calcium by 0.8 mg/dl but will not change free (ionized) calcium.
Vitamin D deficiency:
  Malabsorption (most common cause).
  Inadequate intake.
  Decreased production of 1,25-dihydroxyvitamin D (vitamin D dependent rickets, renal failure).
  Decreased production of 25-OHD (parenchymal liver disease).
  Accelerated 25-OHD catabolism (phenytoin, phenobarbital).
  End-organ resistance to 1,25-dihydroxyvitamin D.
Hypomagnesemia: hypocalcemia caused by:
  Decreased PTH secretion.
  Inhibition of PTH effect on bone.
Pancreatitis, hyperphosphatemia, osteoblastic metastases: hypocalcemia is secondary to increased calcium deposits (bone, abdomen).
Pseudohypoparathyroidism (PHP): autosomal recessive disorder characterized by short stature, shortening of metacarpal bones, obesity, and mental retardation; the hypocalcemia is secondary to congenital end-organ resistance to PTH.

Idiopathic hypoparathyroidism, surgical removal of parathyroids (e.g., neck surgery).
"Hungry bones syndrome": rapid transfer of calcium from plasma into bones after removal of a parathyroid tumor.
Sepsis.
Massive blood transfusion (as a result of EDTA in blood).

HYPOCAPNIA

ICD-9CM # 786.01

Hyperventilation.
Pneumonia, pneumonitis.
Fever, sepsis.
Medications (salicylates, β-adrenergic agonists, progesterone, methylxanthines).
Pulmonary disease (asthma, interstitial fibrosis).
Pulmonary embolism.
Hepatic failure.
Metabolic acidosis.
High altitude.
CHF.
Pregnancy.
Pain.
CNS lesions.

HYPOGONADISM

ICD-9CM # 256.3 FEMALE
257.2 MALE
256.3 OVARIAN
253.4 PITUITARY
257.2 TESTICULAR

■ HYPERGONADOTROPIC HYPOGONADISM
Hormone resistance (androgen, LH insensitivity).
Gonadal defects (e.g., Klinefelter's syndrome, myotonic dystrophy).
Drug induced (e.g., spironolactone, cytotoxins).
Alcoholism, radiation-induced.
Mumps orchitis.
Anatomic defects, castration.

■ HYPOGONADOTROPIC HYPOGONADISM
Pituitary lesions (neoplasms, granulomas, infarction, hemochromatosis, vasculitis).
Drug-induced (e.g., glucocorticoids).
Hyperprolactinemia.
Genetic disorders (Laurence-Moon-Biedl syndrome, Prader-Willi).
Delayed puberty.
Other: chronic disease, nutritional deficiency, Kallmann's syndrome, idiopathic isolated LH or FSH deficiency.

HYPOKALEMIA

ICD-9CM # 276.8

Cellular shift (redistribution) and undetermined mechanisms.
Alkalosis (each 0.1 increase in pH decreases serum potassium by 0.4 to 0.6 mEq/L).
Insulin administration.
Vitamin B_{12} therapy for megaloblastic anemias, acute leukemias.
Hypokalemic periodic paralysis: rare familial disorder manifested by recurrent attacks of flaccid paralysis and hypokalemia.

β-Adrenergic agonists (e.g., terbutaline), decongestants, bronchodilators, theophylline, caffeine.
Barium poisoning, toluene intoxication, verapamil intoxication, chloroquine intoxication.
Correction of digoxin intoxication with digoxin antibody fragments (Digibind).
Increased renal excretion.
  Drugs:
    Diuretics, including carbonic anhydrase inhibitors (e.g., acetazolamide).
    Amphotericin B.
    High-dose sodium penicillin, nafcillin, ampicillin, or carbenicillin.
    Cisplatin.
    Aminoglycosides.
    Corticosteroids, mineralocorticoids.
    Foscarnet sodium.
  RTA: distal (type 1) or proximal (type 2).
    Diabetic ketoacidosis (DKA), ureteroenterostomy.
    Magnesium deficiency.
    Postobstruction diuresis, diuretic phase of ATN.
    Osmotic diuresis (e.g., mannitol).
    Bartter's syndrome: hyperplasia of juxtaglomerular cells leading to increased renin and aldosterone, metabolic alkalosis, hypokalemia, muscle weakness, and tetany (seen in young adults).
    Increased mineralocorticoid activity (primary or secondary aldosteronism), Cushing's syndrome.
    Chronic metabolic alkalosis from loss of gastric fluid (increased renal potassium secretion).
GI loss.
  Vomiting, nasogastric suction.
    Diarrhea.
    Laxative abuse.
    Villous adenoma.
    Fistulas.
    Inadequate dietary intake (e.g., anorexia nervosa).
    Cutaneous loss (excessive sweating).
    High dietary sodium intake, excessive use of licorice.

HYPOMAGNESEMIA

ICD-9CM # 275.2

GI and nutritional
Defective GI absorption (malabsorption).
Inadequate dietary intake (e.g., alcoholics).
Parenteral therapy without magnesium.
Chronic diarrhea, villous adenoma, prolonged nasogastric suction, fistulas (small bowel, biliary).
Excessive renal losses
Diuretics.
RTA.
Diuretic phase of ATN.
Endocrine disturbances (DKA, hyperaldosteronism, hyperthyroidism, hyperparathyroidism), SIADH, Bartter's syndrome, hypercalciuria, hypokalemia.
Cisplatin, alcohol, cyclosporine, digoxin, pentamidine, mannitol, amphotericin B, foscarnet, methotrexate.
Antibiotics (gentamicin, ticarcillin, carbenicillin).
Redistribution: hypoalbuminemia, cirrhosis, administration of insulin and glucose, theophylline, epinephrine, acute pancreatitis, cardiopulmonary bypass.
Miscellaneous: sweating, burns, prolonged exercise, lactation, "hungry-bones" syndrome.

HYPOPHOSPHATEMIA

ICD-9CM # 275.3

Decreased intake (prolonged starvation [alcoholics], hyperalimentation, or IV infusion without phosphate
Malabsorption.
Phosphate-binding antacids.
Renal loss:
  RTA.
  Fanconi syndrome, vitamin D-resistant rickets.
  ATN (diuretic phase).
  Hyperparathyroidism (primary or secondary).
  Familial hypophosphatemia.
  Hypokalemia, hypomagnesemia.
  Acute volume expansion.
  Glycosuria, idiopathic hypercalciuria.
  Acetazolamide.
Transcellular shift into cells:
  Alcohol withdrawal.
  DKA (recovery phase).
  Glucose-insulin or catecholamine infusion.
  Anabolic steroids.
  Total parenteral nutrition.
  Theophylline overdose.
  Severe hyperthermia; recovery from hypothermia.
  "Hungry bones" syndrome.

HYPOTENSION, POSTURAL

ICD-9CM # 458.0

Antihypertensive medications (especially α-blockers, diuretics, ACE inhibitors).
Volume depletion (hemorrhage, dehydration).
Impaired cardiac output (constrictive pericarditis, aortic stenosis).
Peripheral autonomic dysfunction (DM, Guillain Barré).
Idiopathic orthostatic hypotension.
Central autonomic dysfunction (Shy-Grager syndrome).
Peripheral venous disease.
Adrenal insufficiency.

IMPOTENCE[24]

ICD-9CM # 302.72 PSYCHOSEXUAL
607.84 ORGANIC
997.99 ORGANIC POSTPROSTATECTOMY

Psychogenic.
Endocrine: hyperprolactinemia, DM, Cushing's syndrome, hypothyroidism or hyperthyroidism, abnormality of hypothalamic-pituitary-testicular axis.
Vascular: arterial insufficiency, venous leakage, AV malformation, local trauma.
Medications.
Neurogenic: autonomic or sensory neuropathy, spinal cord trauma or tumor, CVA, multiple sclerosis, temporal lobe epilepsy.
Systemic illness: renal failure, COPD, cirrhosis of liver, myotonic dystrophy.
Peyronie's disease.
Prostatectomy.

INSOMNIA[30]

ICD-9CM # 780.52 INSOMNIA NOS
307.42 INSOMNIA, CHRONIC ASSOCIATED WITH ANXIETY OR DEPRESSION
780.51 INSOMNIA WITH SLEEP APNEA

Anxiety disorder, psychophysiologic insomnia.
Depression.
Drugs (e.g., caffeine, amphetamines, cocaine), hypnotic-dependent sleep disorder.
Pain, fibromyalgia.
Inadequate sleep hygiene.
Restless leg syndrome.
Obstructive sleep apnea.
Sleep bruxism.
Medical illness (e.g., GERD, sleep-related asthma, parkinsonism and movement disorders).
Narcolepsy.
Other: periodic leg movement of sleep, central sleep apnea, REM behavioral disorder.

INTESTINAL PSEUDOOBSTRUCTION[33]

ICD-9CM # 560.1 ADYNAMIC INTESTINAL OBSTRUCTION
564.9 INTESTINAL DISORDER, FUNCTIONAL

■ "PRIMARY" (IDIOPATHIC INTESTINAL PSEUDOOBSTRUCTION)
Hollow visceral myopathy:
  Familial.
  Sporadic.
Neuropathic:
  Abnormal myenteric plexus.
  Normal myenteric plexus.

■ SECONDARY
Scleroderma.
Myxedema.
Amyloidosis.
Muscular dystrophy.
Hypokalemia.
Chronic renal failure.
Diabetes mellitus.
Drug toxicity caused by:
  Anticholinergics.
  Opiate narcotics.
Ogilvie's syndrome.

IRON OVERLOAD

ICD-9CM # 790.6 IRON, ABNORMAL BLOOD LEVEL
275, IRON, METABOLISM DISORDER

Hereditary hemochromatosis.
Chronic iron supplementation (PO, IM, transfusions).
Nonalcoholic steatohepatitis.
Chronic viral hepatitis.
Alcoholic liver disease.
Chronic anemias (e.g., sideroblastic anemia, thalassemia major).
Porphyria cutanea tarda.

ISCHEMIC COLITIS, NONOCCLUSIVE[18]

ICD-9CM # 557.1

■ ACUTE DIMINUTION OF COLONIC INTRAMURAL BLOOD FLOW
Small vessel obstruction
Collagen-vascular disease.
Vasculitis, diabetes.
Oral contraceptives.
Nonocclusive hypoperfusion
Hemorrhage.
CHF, MI, Arrhythmias.
Sepsis.
Vasoconstricting agents: vasopressin, ergot.
Increased viscosity: polycythemia, sickle cell disease, thrombocytosis.

■ INCREASED DEMAND ON MARGINAL BLOOD FLOW
Increased motility
Mass lesion, stricture.
Constipation.
Increased intraluminal pressure
Bowel obstruction.
Colonoscopy.
Barium enema.

JAUNDICE

ICD-9CM # 782.4 JAUNDICE NOS
576.8 JAUNDICE, OBSTRUCTIVE
277.4 BILIRUBIN EXCRETION DISORDERS

■ PREDOMINANCE OF DIRECT (CONJUGATED) BILIRUBIN
Extrahepatic obstruction.
Common duct abnormalities: calculi, neoplasm, stricture, cyst, sclerosing cholangitis.
Metastatic carcinoma.
Pancreatic carcinoma, pseudocyst.
Ampullary carcinoma.
Hepatocellular disease: hepatitis, cirrhosis.
Drugs: estrogens, phenothiazines, captopril, methyltestosterone, labetalol.
Cholestatic jaundice of pregnancy.
Hereditary disorders: Dubin-Johnson syndrome, Rotor's syndrome.
Recurrent benign intrahepatic cholestasis.

■ PREDOMINANCE OF INDIRECT (UNCONJUGATED) BILIRUBIN
Hemolysis: hereditary and acquired hemolytic anemias.
Inefficient marrow production.
Impaired hepatic conjugation: chloramphenicol.
Neonatal jaundice.
Hereditary disorders: Gilbert's syndrome, Crigler-Najjar syndrome.

II

JOINT PAIN, ANTERIOR HIP, MEDIAL THIGH, KNEE[25]

ICD-9CM # 719.4 ADD 5TH DIGIT
    0 SITE NOS
    1 SHOULDER REGION
    2 UPPER ARM (ELBOW, HUMERUS)
    3 FOREARM (RADIUS, WRIST, ULNA)
    4 HAND
    5 PELVIC REGION AND THIGH
    6 LOWER LEG (FIBULA, PATELLA, TIBIA)
    7 ANKLE AND/OR FOOT

■ ACUTE
Acute rheumatic fever.
Adductor muscle strain.
Avascular necrosis.
Crystal arthritis.
Femoral artery (pseudo) aneurysm.
Fracture (femoral neck or intertrochanteric).
Hemarthrosis.
Hernia.
Herpes zoster.
Iliopectineal bursitis.
Iliopsoas tendinitis.
Inguinal lymphadenitis.
Osteomalacia.
Painful transient osteoporosis of hip.
Septic arthritis.

■ SUBACUTE AND CHRONIC
Adductory muscle strain.
Amyloidosis.
Acute rheumatic fever.
Femoral artery aneurysm.
Hernia (inguinal or femoral).
Iliopectineal bursitis.
Iliopsoas tendinitis.
Inguinal lymphadenopathy.
Osteochondromatosis.
Osteomyelitis.
Osteitis deformans (Paget's disease).
Osteomalacia (pseudofracture).
Postherpetic neuralgia.
Sterile synovitis (e.g., rheumatoid arthritis, psoriatic, systemic lupus erythematosus).

JOINT PAIN, HIP, LATERAL THIGH[25]

ICD-9CM # 959.6 HIP INJURY
    719.95 HIP JOINT DISORDER
    843.9 HIP STRAIN

■ ACUTE
Herpes zoster.
Iliotibial tendinitis.
Impacted fracture of femoral neck.
Lateral femoral cutaneous neuropathy (meralgia paresthetica).
Radiculopathy: L4-5.
Trochanteric avulsion fracture (greater trochanter).
Trochanteric bursitis.
Trochanteric fracture.

■ SUBACUTE AND CHRONIC
Lateral femoral cutaneous neuropathy (meralgia paresthetica).
Osteomyelitis.
Postherpetic neuralgia.
Radiculopathy: L4-5.
Tumors.

JOINT PAIN, POSTERIOR HIPS, THIGH, BUTTOCKS[25]

ICD-9CM # 719.4 ADD 5TH DIGIT
    0 SITE NOS
    1 SHOULDER REGION
    2 UPPER ARM (ELBOW, HUMERUS)
    3 FOREARM (RADIUS, WRIST, ULNA)
    4 HAND
    5 PELVIC REGION AND THIGH
    6 LOWER LEG (FIBULA, PATELLA, TIBIA)
    7 ANKLE AND/OR FOOT

■ ACUTE
Gluteal muscle strain.
Herpes zoster.
Ischial bursitis.
Ischial or sacral fracture.
Osteomalacia (pseudofracture).
Sciatic neuropathy.
Radiculopathy: L5-S1.

■ SUBACUTE AND CHRONIC
Gluteal muscle strain.
Ischial bursitis.
Lumbar spinal stenosis.
Osteoarthritis of hip.
Osteitis deformans (Paget's disease).
Osteomyelitis.
Osteochondromatosis.
Osteomalacia (pseudofracture).
Postherpetic neuralgia.
Radiculopathy: L5-S1.
Tumors.

JOINT SWELLING

ICD-9CM # 719.0 ADD 5TH DIGIT
    0 SITE NOS
    1 SHOULDER REGION
    2 UPPER ARM (ELBOW, HUMERUS)
    3 FOREARM (RADIUS, WRIST, ULNA)
    4 HAND
    5 PELVIC REGION AND THIGH
    6 LOWER LEG (FIBULA, PATELLA, TIBIA)
    7 ANKLE AND/OR FOOT

Trauma.
Osteoarthritis.
Gout.
Pyogenic arthritis.
Pseudogout.
Rheumatoid arthritis.
Viral syndrome.

JUGULAR VENOUS DISTENTION

ICD-9CM # 459.89 INCREASED VENOUS PRESSURE

Right-sided heart failure.
Cardiac tamponade.
Constrictive pericarditis.
Goiter.
Tension pneumothorax.
Pulmonary hypertension.
Cardiomyopathy (restrictive).
Superior vena cava syndrome.
Valsalva maneuver.
Right atrial myxoma.
COPD.

KNEE PAIN[25]

ICD-9CM # 844.1 COLLATERAL LIGAMENT SPRAIN,
MEDIAL
844.2 CRUCIATE LIGAMENT SPRAIN
716.96 KNEE INFLAMMATION
959.7 KNEE INJURY
718.86 KNEE INSTABILITY
836.1 LATERAL MENISCUS TEAR
836.0 MEDIAL MENISCUS TEAR
844.8 PATELLAR SPRAIN
719.56 KNEE STIFFNESS
719.06 KNEE SWELLING

■ DIFFUSE

Articular.
Anterior.
Prepatellar bursitis.
Patellar tendon enthesopathy.
Chondromalacia patellae.
Patellofemoral osteoarthritis.
Cruciate ligament injury.
Medial plica syndrome.

■ MEDIAL

Anserine bursitis.
Spontaneous osteonecrosis.
Osteoarthritis.
Medial meniscal tear.
Medial collateral ligament bursitis.
Referred pain from hip and L3.
Fibromyalgia.

■ LATERAL

Iliotibial band syndrome.
Meniscal cyst.
Lateral meniscal tear.
Collateral ligament.
Peroneal tenosynovitis.

■ POSTERIOR

Popliteal cyst (Baker's cyst).
Tendinitis.
Aneurysms, ganglions, sarcoma.

LEFT AXIS DEVIATION[19]

ICD-9CM # 426.3 LEFT BUNDLE BRANCH BLOCK
426.2 LEFT BUNDLE BRANCH HEMIBLOCK
429.3 LEFT VENTRICULAR HYPERTROPHY

Normal variation.
Left anterior fascicular block (hemiblock).
Left bundle branch block.
Left ventricular hypertrophy.
Mechanical shifts causing a horizontal heart, high diaphragm, pregnancy, ascites.
Some forms of ventricular tachycardia.
Endocardial cushion defects and other congenital heart disease.

LEG CRAMPS, NOCTURNAL

ICD-9CM # 729.82 MUSCLE CRAMPS

Diabetic neuropathy.
Medications.
Electrolyte abnormalities (hypokalemia, hyponatremia, hypocalcemia, hyperkalemia, hypophosphatemia).

Respiratory alkalosis.
Uremia.
Hemodialysis.
Peripheral nerve injury.
ALS.
Alcohol use.
Heat cramps.
Vitamin B_{12} deficiency.
Hyperthyroidism.
Contractures.
DVT.
Hypoglycemia.
Peripheral vascular insufficiency.
Baker cyst

LEG LENGTH DISCREPANCIES[20]

ICD-9CM # 736.81 LEG LENGTH DISCREPANCY,
ACQUIRED
755.30 LEG LENGTH DISCREPANCY,
CONGENITAL

■ CONGENITAL

Proximal femoral local deficiency.
Coxa vara.
Hemiatrophy-hemihypertrophy (anisomelia).
Development dysplasia of the hip.

■ DEVELOPMENTAL

Legg-Calvé-Perthes disease.

■ NEUROMUSCULAR

Polio.
Cerebral palsy (hemiplegia).

■ INFECTIOUS

Pyogenic osteomyelitis with physeal damage.

■ TRAUMA

Physeal injury with premature closure.
Overgrowth.
Malunion (shortening).

■ TUMOR

Physeal destruction.
Radiation-induced physeal injury.
Overgrowth.

LEG PAIN WITH EXERCISE

ICD-9CM # 729.82 MUSCLE CRAMPS

Shin splints.
Arteriosclerosis obliterans.
Neurogenic (spinal cord compression or ischemia).
Venous claudication.
Popliteal cyst.
DVT.
Thromboangiitis obliterans.
Adventitial cysts.
Popliteal artery entrapment syndrome.
McArdle syndrome.

LEG ULCERS[25]

ICD-9CM # 440.23 LOWER LIMB, ARTERIOSCLEROTIC
707.1 LOWER LIMB, CHRONIC
707.1 LOWER LIMB, NEUROGENIC
250.70 LOWER LIMB, CHRONIC DIABETES MELLITUS TYPE II
250.71 LOWER LIMB, CHRONIC, DIABETES MELLITUS TYPE I

■ VASCULAR
Arterial: arteriosclerosis, thromboangiitis obliterans, AV malformation, cholesterol emboli.
Venous: superficial varicosities, incompetent perforators, DVT, lymphatic abnormalities.

■ VASCULITIS HEMATOLOGIC
Sickle cell anemia, thalassemia, polycythemia vera, leukemia, cold agglutinin disease.
Macroglobulinemia, protein C and protein S deficiency, cryoglobulinemia, lupus anticoagulant, antiphospholipid syndrome.

■ INFECTIOUS
Fungus: Blastomycosis, coccidioidomycosis, histoplasmosis, sporotrichosis.
Bacterial: Furuncle, ecthyma, septic emboli.
Protozoal: leishmaniasis.

■ METABOLIC
Necrobiosis lipoidica diabeticorum.
Localized bullous pemphigoid.
Gout, calcinosis cutis, Gaucher's disease.

■ TUMORS
Basal cell carcinoma, squamous cell carcinoma, melanoma.
Mycosis fungoides, Kaposi's sarcoma, metastatic neoplasms.

■ TRAUMA
Burns, cold injury, radiation dermatitis.
Insect bites.
Factitial, excessive pressure.

■ NEUROPATHIC
Diabetic trophic ulcers.
Tabes dorsalis, syringomyelia.

■ DRUGS
Warfarin, IV colchicine extravasation, methotrexate, halogens, ergotism, hydroxyurea.

■ PANNICULITIS
Weber-Christian disease.
Pancreatic fat necrosis, alpha-antitrypsinase deficiency.

LIMP

ICD-9CM # 781.2 GAIT ABNORMALITY
719.75 GAIT DISORDER DUE TO JOINT ABNORMALITY IN HIP, BUTTOCK, OR FEMUR
719.76 GAIT DISORDER DUE TO JOINT ABNORMALITY IN LOWER LEG
719.77 GAIT DISORDER DUE TO JOINT ABNORMALITY IN ANKLE AND/OR FOOT
300.11 HYSTERICAL GAIT DISORDER

Degenerative joint disease, osteochondritis dissecans, chondromalacia patellae.

Trauma to extremities, vertebral disc, hips.
Poorly fitting shoes, foreign body in shoe, unequal leg length.
Splinter in foot.
Joint infection (septic arthritis, osteomyelitis), viral arthritis.
Abdominal pain (e.g., appendicitis, incarcerated hernia), testicular torsion.
Polio, neuromuscular disorders, Guillain-Barré syndrome, multiple sclerosis.
Osgood-Schlatter disease.
Legg-Calvé-Perthes disease.
Factitious, somatization syndrome.
Neoplasm (local or metastatic).
Other: diskitis, periostitis, sickle cell disease, hemophilia.

LIMPING, PEDIATRIC AGE[20]

ICD-9CM # 781.2 GAIT ABNORMALITY

■ TODDLER (1-3 YR)
Infection:
  Septic arthritis:
    -Hip.
    -Knee.
  Osteomyelitis.
  Diskitis.
Occult trauma:
  Toddler's fracture.
Neoplasia.

■ CHILDHOOD (4-10 YR)
Infection:
  Septic arthritis:
    -Hip.
    -Knee.
  Osteomyelitis.
  Diskitis.
  Transient synovitis, hip.
LCPD.
Tarsal coalition.
Rheumatologic disorder:
  JRA.
Trauma.
Neoplasia.

■ ADOLESCENCE (11+ YR)
SCFE.
Rheumatologic disorder:
  JRA.
Trauma.
Tarsal coalition.
Hip dislocation (DDH).
Neoplasia.

LIVEDO RETICULITIS

ICD-9CM # CODE NOT AVAILABLE

Emboli (SBE, left atrial myxoma, cholesterol emboli).
Thrombocythemia or polycythemia.
Antiphospholipid antibody syndrome.
Cryoglobulinemia, cryofibrinogenemia.
Leukocytoclastic vasculitis.
SLE, rheumatoid arthritis, dermatomyositis.
Pancreatitis.

DDH, Developmental dysplasia of the hip; *JRA*, juvenile rheumatoid arthritis; *LCPD*, Legg-Calvé-Perthes disease; *SCFE*, slipped capital femoral epiphysis.

Drugs (quinine, quinidine, amantadine, catecholamines).
Physiologic (cutis marmorata).
Congenital.

LYMPHADENOPATHY[12]

ICD-9CM # 785.6

■ GENERALIZED
AIDS.
Lymphoma: Hodgkin's disease, non-Hodgkin's lymphoma.
Leukemias, reticuloendotheliosis.
Infectious mononucleosis, CMV, and other viral infections.
Diffuse skin infection: generalized furunculosis, multiple tick bites.
Parasitic infections: toxoplasmosis, filariasis, leishmaniasis, Chagas' disease.
Serum sickness.
Collagen vascular diseases (RA, SLE).
Dengue (arbovirus infection).
Sarcoidosis and other granulomatous diseases.
Drugs: INH, hydantoin derivatives, antithyroid and antileprosy drugs.
Secondary syphilis.
Hyperthyroidism, lipid-storage diseases.

■ LOCALIZED
Cervical nodes
Infections of the head, neck, ears, sinuses, scalp, pharynx.
Mononucleosis.
Lymphoma.
TB.
Malignancy of head and neck.
Rubella.
Scalene/supraclavicular nodes
Lymphoma.
Lung neoplasm.
Bacterial or fungal infection of thorax or retroperitoneum.
GI malignancy.
Axillary nodes
Infections of hands and arms.
Cat-scratch disease.
Neoplasm (lymphoma, melanoma, breast carcinoma).
Brucellosis.
Epitrochlear nodes
Infections of the hand.
Lymphoma.
Tularemia.
Sarcoidosis, secondary syphilis (usually bilateral).
Inguinal nodes
Infections of leg or foot, folliculitis (pubic hair).
LGV, syphilis.
Lymphoma.
Pelvic malignancy.
Pasteurella pestis.
Hilar nodes
Sarcoidosis.
TB.
Lung carcinoma.
Fungal infections, systemic.
Mediastinal nodes
Sarcoidosis.
Lymphoma.
Lung neoplasm.
TB.
Mononucleosis.
Histoplasmosis.
Abdominal/retroperitoneal nodes
Lymphoma.
TB.
Neoplasm (ovary, testes, prostate and other malignancies).

MEDIASTINAL MASSES OR WIDENING ON CHEST X-RAY

ICD-9CM # 785.6 ADENOPATHY
519.3 DISEASE NEC
793.2 SHIFT (CXR)

Lymphoma: Hodgkin's disease and non-Hodgkin's lymphoma.
Sarcoidosis.
Vascular: aortic aneurysm, ectasia or tortuosity of aorta or bronchocephalic vessels.
Carcinoma: lungs, esophagus.
Esophageal diverticula.
Hiatal hernia.
Achalasia.
Prominent pulmonary outflow tract: pulmonary hypertension, pulmonary embolism, right-to-left shunts.
Trauma: mediastinal hemorrhage.
Pneumomediastinum.
Lymphadenopathy caused by silicosis and other pneumoconioses.
Leukemias.
Infections: TB, viral (rare), Mycoplasma (rare), fungal, tularemia.
Substernal thyroid.
Thymoma.
Teratoma.
Bronchogenic cyst.
Pericardial cyst.
Neurofibroma, neurosarcoma, ganglioneuroma.

MENINGITIS, CHRONIC[23]

ICD-9CM # 322.2

TB.
Fungal CNS infection.
Tertiary syphilis.
CNS neoplasm.
Metabolic encephalopathies.
Multiple sclerosis.
Chronic subdural hematoma.
SLE cerebritis.
Encephalitides.
Sarcoidosis.
NSAIDs.
Behçet's syndrome.
Anatomic defects (traumatic, congenital, postoperative).
Granulomatous angiitis.

MESENTERIC ISCHEMIA, NONOCCLUSIVE[23]

ICD-9CM # 557.0 MESENTERIC ARTERY EMBOLISM OR INFARCTION
557.1 MESENTERIC ARTERY INSUFFICIENCY, CHRONIC
902.39 MESENTERIC VEIN INJURY

Cardiovascular disease resulting in low-flow states (CHF, cardiogenic shock, post cardiopulmonary bypass, dysrhythmias).
Septic shock.
Drug induced (cocaine, vasopressors, ergot alkaloid poisoning).

MESENTERIC VENOUS THROMBOSIS[23]

ICD-9CM # 557.0

Hypercoagulable states (protein C or S deficiency, antithrombin III deficiency, Factor V Leyden, malignancy, P. Vera, Sickle cell disease, homocystinemia, lupus anticoagulant, cardiolipin antibody).
Trauma (operative venous injury, abdominal trauma, postsplenectomy).
Inflammatory conditions (pancreatitis, diverticulitis, appendicitis, cholangitis).
Other: CHF, renal failure, portal hypertension, decompression sickness.

METASTATIC NEOPLASMS

ICD-9CM # 198.5 BONE AND BONE MARROW
198.3 BRAIN AND SPINAL CORD
197.7 LIVER
197.0 LUNG

To: Bone	To: Brain	To: Liver	To: Lung
Breast	Lung	Colon	Breast
Lung	Breast	Stomach	Colon
Prostate	Melanoma	Pancreas	Kidney
Thyroid	GU tract	Breast	Testis
Kidney	Colon	Lymphomas	Stomach
Bladder	Sinuses	Bronchus	Thyroid
Endometrium	Sarcoma	Lung	Melanoma
Cervix	Skin	Sarcoma	
Melanoma	Thyroid	Choriocarcinoma	
		Kidney	

MICROCEPHALY[4]

ICD-9CM # 742.1 MICROCEPHALUS

■ **PRIMARY (GENETIC)**
Familial (autosomal recessive).
Autosomal dominant.
Syndromes:
Down (21-trisomy).
Edward (18-trisomy).
Cri-du-chat (5 p-).
Cornelia de Lange.
Rubinstein-Taybi.
Smith-Lemli-Opitz.

■ **SECONDARY (NONGENETIC)**
Radiation.
Congenital infections:
Cytomegalovirus.
Rubella.
Toxoplasmosis.
Drugs:
Fetal alcohol.
Fetal hydantoin.
Meningitis/encephalitis.
Malnutrition.
Metabolic.
Hyperthermia.
Hypoxic-ischemic encephalopathy.

MICROPENIS[24]

ICD-9CM # 752.69 PENILE AGENESIS OR ATRESIA
607.89 PENILE ATROPHY
752.64 MICROPENIS (CONGENITAL)

■ **HYPOGONADOTROPIC HYPOGONADISM (HYPOTHALAMIC OR PITUITARY DEFICIENCIES)**
Kallmann's syndrome: autosomal dominant; associated with hyposmia.
Prader-Willi syndrome: hypotonia, mental retardation, obesity, small hands and feet.
Rud syndrome: hyposomia, ichthyosis, mental retardation.
De Morsier's syndrome (septooptic dysplasia): hypopituitarism, hypoplastic optic discs, absent septum pellucidum.

■ **HYPERGONADOTROPIC HYPOGONADISM**
Primary testicular defect: disorders of testicular differentiation or inborn errors of testosterone synthesis.
Klinefelter syndrome.
Other X polysomies (i.e., XXXXY, XXXY).
Robinow's syndrome: brachymesomelic dwarfism, dysmorphic facies.

■ **PARTIAL ANDROGEN INSENSITIVITY**

■ **IDIOPATHIC**
Defective morphogenesis of the penis.

MIOSIS

ICD-9CM # 379.42 MIOSIS PERSISTENT NOT DUE TO MIOTICS

Medications (e.g., morphine, pilocarpine).
Neurosyphilis.
Congenital.
Iritis.
CNS pontine lesion.
CNS infections.
Cavernous sinus thrombosis.
Inflammation/irritation of cornea or conjunctiva.

MONONEUROPATHY

ICD-9CM # 355.9

Herpes zoster.
Herpes simplex.
Vasculitis.
Trauma, compression.
Diabetes.
Postinfectious or inflammatory.

MUSCLE WEAKNESS

ICD-9CM # 728.9

Physical deconditioning.
Impaired cardiac output (e.g., mitral stenosis, mitral regurgitation).
Uremia, liver failure.
Electrolyte abnormalities (hypokalemia, hyperkalemia, hypophosphatemia, hypercalcemia), hypoglycemia.
Drug-induced (e.g., statin myopathy).
Muscular dystrophies.
Steroid myopathy.
Alcoholic myopathy.

Myasthenia gravis, Lambert-Eaton syndrome.
Infections (polio, botulism, HIV, hepatitis, diphtheria, tick paralysis, neurosyphilis, brucellosis, TB, trichinosis).
Pernicious anemia, other anemias, beriberi.
Psychiatric illness (depression, somatization syndrome).
Organophosphate or arsenic poisoning.
Inflammatory myopathies (e.g., collagen vascular disease, RA, sarcoidosis).
Endocrinopathies (e.g., adrenal insufficiency, hypothyroidism), diabetic neuropathy.
Other: motor neuron disease, mitochondrial myopathy, L-tryptophan (eosinophilia-myalgia), rhabdomyolysis, glycogen storage disease, lipid storage disease.

MUSCLE WEAKNESS, LOWER MOTOR NEURON VERSUS UPPER MOTOR NEURON[35]

ICD-9CM # 728.9

■ LOWER MOTOR NEURON
Weakness, usually severe.
Marked muscle atrophy.
Fasciculations.
Decreased muscle stretch reflexes.
Clonus not present.
Flaccidity.
No Babinski sign.
Asymmetric and may involve one limb only in the beginning to become generalized as the disease progresses.

■ UPPER MOTOR NEURON
Weakness, usually less severe.
Minimal disuse muscle atrophy.
No fasciculations.
Increased muscle stretch reflexes.
Clonus may be present.
Spasticity.
Babinski sign.
Often initial impairment of only skilled movements.
In the limbs the following muscles may be the only ones weak or weaker than the others: triceps; wrist and finger extensors; interossei; iliopsoas; hamstrings; and foot dorsiflexors, inverters and extroverters.

MYDRIASIS

ICD-9CM # 379.43 MYDRIASIS PERSISTENT NOT DUE TO MYDRIATICS

Coma.
Medications (cocaine, atropine, epinephrine, etc.).
Glaucoma.
Cerebral aneurysm.
Ocular trauma.
Head trauma.
Optic atrophy.
Cerebral neoplasm.
Iridocyclitis

MYELOPATHY AND MYELITIS[33]

ICD-9CM # 722.70 MYELOPATHY, DISCOGENIC INTERVERTEBRAL NOS
336.9 MYELOPATHY, NONDISCOGENIC UNSPECIFIED

■ INFLAMMATORY
Infectious: spirochetal TB, zoster, rabies, HIV, polio, rickettsial, fungal, parasitic.

Noninfectious: idiopathic transverse myelitis, multiple sclerosis.

■ TOXIC/METABOLIC
DM, pernicious anemia, chronic liver disease, pellagra, arsenic.

■ TRAUMA COMPRESSION
Spinal neoplasm, cervical spondylosis, epidural abscess, epidural hematoma.

■ VASCULAR
AV malformation, SLE, periarteritis nodosa, dissecting aortic aneurysm.

■ PHYSICAL AGENTS
Electrical injury, irradiation.

■ NEOPLASTIC
Spinal cord tumors, paraneoplastic myelopathy.

MYOCARDIAL ISCHEMIA[33]

ICD-9CM # 414.8 ISCHEMIA (CHRONIC)
411.89 ISCHEMIA, ACUTE WITHOUT MI

Atherosclerotic obstructive coronary artery disease.
Nonatherosclerotic coronary artery disease:
  Coronary artery spasm.
  Congenital coronary artery anomalies:
    -Anomalous origin of coronary artery from pulmonary artery.
    -Aberrant origin of coronary artery from aorta or another coronary artery.
    -Coronary arteriovenous fistula.
    -Coronary artery aneurysm.
Acquired disorders of coronary arteries:
  Coronary artery embolism.
  Dissection:
    -Surgica.
    -During percutaneous coronary angioplasty.
    -Aortic dissection.
    -Spontaneous (e.g., during pregnancy).
  Extrinsic compression:
    -Tumors.
    -Granulomas.
    -Amyloidosis.
  Collagen-vascular disease:
    -Polyarteritis nodosa.
    -Temporal arteritis.
    -Rheumatoid arthritis.
    -Systemic lupus erythematosus.
    -Scleroderma.
  Miscellaneous disorders:
    -Irradiation.
    -Trauma.
    -Kawasaki disease.
  Syphilis.
Hereditary disorders:
  Pseudoxanthoma elasticum.
  Gargoylism.
  Progeria.
  Homocystinuria.
  Primary oxaluria.
"Functional" causes of myocardial ischemia in absence of anatomic coronary artery disease:
Syndrome X.
Hypertrophic cardiomyopathy.
Dilated cardiomyopathy.
Muscle bridge.
Hypertensive heart disease.

Pulmonary hypertension.
Valvular heart disease; aortic stenosis, aortic regurgitation.

MYOPATHIES, INFECTIOUS

ICD-9CM # 359.8

HIV.
Viral myositis.
Trichinosis
Toxoplasmosis.
Cysticercosis.

MYOPATHIES, INFLAMMATORY

ICD-9CM # 359.9

SLE, rheumatoid arthritis.
Sarcoidosis.
Paraneoplastic syndrome.
Polymyositis, dermatomyositis.
Polyarteritis nodosa.
Myxed connective tissue disease.
Scleroderma.
Inclusion body myositis.
Sjögren's syndrome.
Cimetidine, D-penicillamine.

MYOPATHIES, TOXIC[1]

ICD-9CM # 359.4

Inflammatory: cimetidine, D-penicillamine.
Noninflammatory necrotizing or vacuolar: cholesterol-lowering agents, chloroquine, colchicine.
Acute muscle necrosis and myoglobinuria: cholesterol-lowering drugs, alcohol, cocaine.
Malignant hyperthermia: halothane, ethylene, others; succinylcholine.
Mitochondrial: zidovudine.
Myosin loss: nondepolarizing neuromuscular blocking agents; glucocorticoids.

MYOSITIS, INFLAMMATORY[1]

ICD-9CM # 729.1

■ INFECTIOUS
Viral myositis:
   Retroviruses (HIV, HTLV-I).
   Enteroviruses (echovirus, Coxsackievirus).
   Other viruses (influenza, hepatitis A and B, Epstein-Barr virus).
Bacterial: pyomyositis.
Parasites: trichinosis, cysticercosis.
Fungi: candidiasis.

■ IDIOPATHIC
Granulomatous myositis (sarcoid, giant cell).
Eosinophilic myositis.
Eosinophilia-myalgia syndrome.

■ ENDOCRINE/METABOLIC DISORDERS
Hypothyroidism.
Hyperthyroidism.
Hypercortisolism.
Hyperparathyroidism.

Hypoparathyroidism.
Hypocalcemia.
Hypokalemia.

■ METABOLIC MYOPATHIES
Myophosphorylase deficiency (McArdle's disease).
Phosphofructokinase deficiency.
Myoadenylate deaminase deficiency.
Acid maltase deficiency.
Lipid storage diseases.
Acute rhabdomyolysis.

■ DRUG-INDUCED MYOPATHIES
Alcohol.
D-Penicillamine.
Zidovudine.
Colchicine.
Chloroquine, hydroxychloroquine.
Lipid-lowering agents.
Cyclosporine.
Cocaine, heroin, barbiturates.
Corticosteroids.

■ NEUROLOGIC DISORDERS
Muscular dystrophies.
Congenital myopathies.
Motor neuron disease.
Guillain-Barré syndrome.
Myasthenia gravis.

NAUSEA AND VOMITING

ICD-9CM # 787.01

Infections (viral, bacterial).
Intestinal obstruction.
Metabolic (uremia, electrolyte abnormalities, DKA, acidosis, etc.).
Severe pain.
Anxiety, fear.
Psychiatric disorders (bulimia, anorexia nervosa).
Pregnancy.
Medications (NSAIDs, erythromycin, morphine, codeine, aminophylline, chemotherapeutic agents, etc.).
Withdrawal from substance abuse (drugs, alcohol).
Head trauma.
Vestibular or middle ear disease.
Migraine headache.
CNS neoplasms.
Radiation sickness.
PUD.
Carcinoma of GI tract.
Reye's syndrome.
Eye disorders.
Abdominal trauma.

NECK AND ARM PAIN

ICD-9CM # 723.1 NECK PAIN
847.0 NECK STRAIN
959.09 NECK INJURY
959.2 ARM INJURY
840.9 ARM STRAIN

Cervical disc syndrome.
Trauma, musculoskeletal strain.
Rotator cuff syndrome.
Bicipital tendonitis.
Glenohumeral arthritis.
Acromioclavicular arthritis.

Thoracic outlet syndrome.
Pancoast tumor.
Infection (cellulitis, abscess).
Angina pectoris.

NECK MASS[25]

ICD-9CM # 784.2

■ CONGENITAL ANOMALIES
Thyroglossal duct cyst.
Bronchial apparatus anomalies.
Teratomas.
Ranula.
Dermoid cysts.
Hemangioma.
Laryngoceles.
Cystic hygroma.

■ NONNEOPLASTIC INFLAMMATORY ETIOLOGIES
Folliculitis.
Adenopathy secondary to peritonsillar abscess.
Retropharyngeal or parapharyngeal abscess.
Salivary gland infections.
Viral infections (mononucleosis, HIV, CMV).
TB.
Cat-scratch disease.
Toxoplasmosis.
Actinomyces.
Atypical mycobacterium.
Jugular vein thrombus.

■ NEOPLASM (PRIMARY OR METASTATIC)
Lipoma

NECK PAIN[25]

ICD-9CM # 723.1 NECK PAIN (NONDISCOGENIC)
959.09 NECK INJURY

■ INFLAMMATORY DISEASES
Rheumatoid arthritis (RA).
Spondyloarthropathies.
Juvenile RA.

■ NONINFLAMMATORY DISEASE
Cervical osteoarthritis.
Diskogenic neck pain.
Diffuse idiopathic skeletal hyperostosis.
Fibromyalgia or myofascial pain.

■ INFECTIOUS CAUSES
Meningitis.
Osteomyelitis.
Infectious diskitis.

■ NEOPLASMS
Primary.
Metastatic.

■ REFERRED PAIN
Temporomandibular joint pain.
Cardiac pain.
Diaphragmatic irritation.
Gastrointestinal sources (gastric ulcer, gallbladder, pancreas).

NEPHRITIC SYNDROME, ACUTE[1]

ICD-9CM # 580.89

■ LOW SERUM COMPLEMENT LEVEL
Acute postinfectious glomerulonephritis.
Membranoproliferative glomerulonephritis.
SLE.
Subacute bacterial endocarditis.
Visceral abscess "shunt" nephritis.
Cryoglobulinemia.

■ NORMAL SERUM COMPLEMENT LEVEL
IgA nephropathy.
Idiopathic rapidly progressive glomerulonephritis.
Antiglomerular basement membrane disease.
Polyarteritis nodosa.
Wegener's glomerulonephritis.
Henoch-Schönlein purpura.
Goodpasture syndrome.

NEUROGENIC BLADDER[26]

ICD-9CM # 396.54

■ SUPRATENTORIAL
CVA.
Parkinson's disease.
Alzheimer's disease.
Cerebral palsy.

■ SPINAL CORD
Spinal cord injury.
Spinal stenosis.
Central cord syndrome.
ALS.
Multiple sclerosis.
Myelodysplasia.

■ PERIPHERAL NEUROPATHY
Diabetes.
Alcohol.
Shingles.
Syphilis.

NEUROLOGIC DEFICIT, FOCAL[23]

ICD-9CM # 436 CVA
435.9 TIA

■ TRAUMATIC: INTRACRANIAL, INTRASPINAL
Subdural hematoma.
Intraparenchymal hemorrhage.
Epidural hematoma.
Traumatic hemorrhagic necrosis.

■ INFECTIOUS
Brain abscess.
Epidural and subdural abscesses.
Meningitis.

■ NEOPLASTIC
Primary central nervous system tumors.
Metastatic tumors.
Syringomyelia.
Vascular.
Thrombosis.
Embolism.

II

Spontaneous hemorrhage: arteriovenous malformation, aneurysm, hypertensive.

■ METABOLIC
Hypoglycemia.
B_{12} deficiency.
Postseizure.
Hyperosmolar nonketotic.

■ OTHER
Migraine.
Bell's palsy.
Psychogenic.

NEUROLOGIC DEFICIT, MULTIFOCAL[23]

> **ICD-9CM # 436 CVA**
> **435.9 TIA**

Acute disseminated encephalomyelitis: Postviral or postimmunization.
Infectious encephalomyelitis: Poliovirus, enteroviruses, arbovirus, herpes zoster, Epstein-Barr virus.
Granulomatous encephalomyelitis: Sarcoid.
Autoimmune: Systemic lupus erythematosus.
Other: Familial spinocerebellar degenerations.

NEUROPATHIES, PAINFUL[35]

> **ICD-9CM # 355.9 NEUROPATHY NOS**
> **357.5 ALCOHOLIC**
> **357.8 CHRONIC PROGRESSIVE OR RELAPSING**
> **356.2 CONGENITAL SENSORY**
> **356.0 DEJERINE-SOTTAS**
> **356.60 DIABETIC POLYNEUROPATHY, TYPE II**
> **356.61 DIABETIC POLYNEUROPATHY TYPE I**

■ MONONEUROPATHIES
Compressive neuropathy (carpal tunnel, meralgia paresthetica).
Trigeminal neuralgia.
Ischemic neuropathy.
Polyarteritis nodosa.
Diabetic mononeuropathy.
Herpes zoster.
Idiopathic and familial brachial plexopathy.

■ POLYNEUROPATHIES
Diabetes mellitus.
Paraneoplastic sensory neuropathy.
Nutritional neuropathy.
Multiple myeloma.
Amyloid.
Dominantly inherited sensory neuropathy.
Toxic (arsenic, thallium, metronidazole).
AIDS-associated neuropathy.
Tangier disease.
Fabry disease.

NYSTAGMUS

> **ICD-9CM # 379.50 NYSTAGMUS NOS**
> **386.11 BENIGN POSITIONAL**
> **386.2 CENTRAL POSITIONAL**
> **379.59 CONGENITAL**

Medications (meperidine, barbiturates, phenytoin, phenothiazines, etc.).
Multiple sclerosis.
Congenital.
Neoplasm (cerebellar, brainstem, cerebral).
Labyrinthine or vestibular lesions.
CNS infections.
Optic atrophy.
Other: Arnold-Chiari malformation, syringobulbia, chorioretinitis, meningeal cysts.

OPHTHALMOPLEGIA[1]

> **ICD-9CM # 378.9 OPHTHALMOPLEGIA NOS**
> **378.52 CEREBELLAR ATAXIA SYNDROME**
> **376.22 EXOPHTHALMIC**

■ BILATERAL
Botulism.
Myasthenia gravis.
Wernicke's encephalopathy.
Acute cranial polyneuropathy.
Brainstem stroke.

■ UNILATERAL
Carotid-posterior (3rd cranial nerve, pupil involved communicating aneurysm).
Diabetic-idiopathic (3rd or 6th cranial nerve, pupil spared).
Myasthenia gravis.
Brainstem stroke.

ORAL MUCOSA, ERYTHEMATOUS LESIONS[8]

> **ICD-9CM # 528.3 ORAL ABSCESS**
> **528.9 ORAL DISEASE (SOFT TISSUE)**
> **528.8 HYPERPLASIA (TONGUE)**

Allergy.
Erythroplakia.
Candidiasis.
Geographic tongue.
Stomatitis areata migrans.
Plasma cell gingivitis.
Pemphigus vulgaris.

ORAL MUCOSA, PIGMENTED LESIONS[8]

> **ICD-9CM # 528.3 ORAL ABSCESS**
> **528.9 ORAL DISEASE (SOFT TISSUE)**
> **528.8 HYPERPLASIA (TONGUE)**

Racial pigmentation.
Oral melanotic macule.
Peutz-Jeghers syndrome.
Neurofibromatosis.
Albright's syndrome.
Addison's disease.
Chloasma.
Drug reaction: quinacrine, Minocin, chlorpromazine, Myleran.
Amalgam tattoo.
Lead line.

Smoker's melanosis.
Nevi.
Melanoma.

ORAL MUCOSA, PUNCTATE EROSIVE LESIONS[8]

ICD-9CM # 528.3 ORAL ABSCESS
528.9 ORAL DISEASE (SOFT TISSUE)
528.8 HYPERPLASIA (TONGUE)

Viral lesion: Herpes simplex, coxsackievirus (A, B, A16), herpes zoster.
Aphthous stomatitis.
Sutton's disease (giant aphthae).
Behçet's syndrome.
Reiter's syndrome.
Neutropenia.
Acute necrotizing ulcerative gingivostomatitis (ANUG).
Drug reaction.
Inflammatory bowel disease.
Contact allergy.

ORAL MUCOSA, WHITE LESIONS[8]

ICD-9CM # 528.3 ORAL ABSCESS
528.9 ORAL DISEASE (SOFT TISSUE)
528.8 HYPERPLASIA (TONGUE)

Leukoplakia.
White, hairy leukoplakia.
Squamous cell carcinoma.
Lichen planus.
Stomatitis nicotinica.
Benign intraepithelial dyskeratosis.
White spongy nevus.
Leukoedema.
Darier-White disease.
Pachyonychia congenital.
Candidiasis.
Allergy.
SLE.

ORAL VESICLES AND ULCERS[1]

ICD-9CM # 528.9

Aphthous stomatitis.
Primary herpes simplex infection.
Vincent's stomatitis.
Syphilis.
Coxsackievirus A (herpangina).
Fungi (histoplasmosis).
Behçet's syndrome.
Systemic lupus erythematosus.
Reiter's syndrome.
Crohn's disease.
Erythema multiforme.
Pemphigus.
Pemphigoid.

ORGASM DYSFUNCTION[10]

ICD-9CM # 302.73 ORGASM INHIBITED FEMALE
PSYCHOSEXUAL
302.74 ORGASM INHIBITED MALE
PSYCHOSEXUAL

Anorgasmia: inadequate stimulation or learning.
Spinal cord lesion or injury.

Multiple sclerosis.
Alcoholic neuropathy.
Amyotrophic lateral sclerosis.
Spinal cord accident.
Spinal cord trauma.
Peripheral nerve damage.
Radical pelvic surgery.
Herniated lumbar disk.
Hypothyroidism.
Addison's disease.
Cushing's disease.
Acromegaly.
Hypopituitarism.
Pharmacologic agents (e.g., SSRIs, β-blockers).
Psychogenic.

OVULATORY DYSFUNCTION[18]

ICD-9CM # 628.0 ANOVULATORY CYCLE
626.5 OVULATION PAIN

■ HYPERANDROGENIC ANOVULATION
Polycystic ovarian syndrome.
Late-onset congenital adrenal hyperplasias.
Ovarian hyperthecosis.
Androgen-producing ovarian tumors.
Androgen-producing adrenal tumors.
Cushing's syndrome.

■ HYPOESTROGENIC ANOVULATION (HYPOTHALAMIC OR PITUITARY ETIOLOGY)
Hypogonadotropic hypoestrogenic states
Reversible:
Functional hypothalamic amenorrheas:
　Eating disorders (anorexia nervosa, excessive weight loss).
　Excessive athletic training.
Neoplastic:
　Craniopharyngioma.
　Pituitary stalk compression.
Infiltrative diseases:
　Histiocytosis-X.
　Sarcoidosis.
Hypophysitis.
Pituitary adenomas:
　Hyperprolactinemia.
　Euprolactinemic galactorrhea.
Endocrinopathies:
　Hypothyroidism/hyperthyroidism.
　Cushing's disease.
Irreversible:
　Kallmann's syndrome.
　Isolated gonadotropin deficiency (hypothalamic or pituitary origin).
　Panhypopituitarism/pituitary insufficiency:
　　-Sheehan's syndrome, pituitary apoplexy.
　　-Pituitary irradiation or ablation.
Hypergonadotropic hypoestrogenic states
Physiologic states:
　Menopause.
　Perimenopause.
Premature ovarian failure.
Immune-related:
　Radiation/chemotherapy-induced.
Ovarian dysgenesis.
Turner's syndrome.
46XX with mutations of X.
Androgen insensitivity syndrome.

■ **MISCELLANEOUS**
Endometriosis.
Luteal phase defect.

PALINDROMIC RHEUMATISM[6]

> ICD-9CM # 719.3 USE 5TH DIGIT
>   0. SITE UNSPECIFIED
>   1. SHOULDER REGION
>   2. UPPER ARM (ELBOW, HUMERUS)
>   3. FOREARM (RADIUS, WRIST, ULNA)
>   4. HAND (CARPAL, METACARPAL,
>   FINGERS)
>   5. PELVIC REGION AND THIGH
>   6. LOWER LEG
>   7. ANKLE AND FOOT
>   8. OTHER
>   9. MULTIPLE

Palindromic rheumatoid arthritis.
Essential palindromic rheumatism.
Crystal synovitis (gout, CPPD, pseudogout, calcific peri-
    arthritis).
Lyme borreliosis, stages 2 and 3.
Sarcoidosis.
Whipple's disease.
Acute rheumatic fever.
Reactive arthritis (rare).

PALPITATIONS[30]

> ICD-9CM # 785.1 PALPITATIONS

Anxiety.
Electrolyte abnormalities (hypokalemia, hypomagnesemia).
Exercise.
Hyperthyroidism.
Ischemic heart disease.
Ingestion of stimulant drugs (cocaine, amphetamines, caf-
    feine).
Medications (digoxin, beta blockers, calcium channel antag-
    onists, hydralazines, diuretics, minoxidil).
Hypoglycemia in type 1 DM.
Mitral valve prolapse.
Wolff-Parkinson-White (WPW) syndrome.
Sick sinus syndrome.

PANCYTOPENIA[33]

> ICD-9CM # 284.8

■ **PANCYTOPENIA WITH HYPOCELLULAR BONE MARROW**
Acquired aplastic anemia.
Constitutional aplastic anemia.
Exposure to chemical or physical agents, including ionizing
    irradiation and chemotherapeutic agents.
Some hematologic malignancies, including myelodysplasia
    and aleukemic leukemia.

■ **PANCYTOPENIA WITH NORMAL OR INCREASED CELLULARITY OF HEMATOPOIETIC ORIGIN**
Some hematologic malignancies, including myelodysplasia,
    and some leukemias, lymphomas, and myelomas.
Paroxysmal nocturnal hemoglobinuria.
Hypersplenism.
Vitamin B_{12}, folate deficiencies.
Overwhelming infection.

■ **PANCYTOPENIA WITH BONE MARROW REPLACEMENT**
Tumor metastatic to marrow.
Metabolic storage diseases
Osteopetrosis.
Myelofibrosis.

PAPILLEDEMA

> ICD-9CM # 377.00 PAPILLEDEMA NOS
>   377.02 WITH DECREASED OCULAR
>   PRESSURE
>   377.01 WITH INCREASED INTRACRANIAL
>   PRESSURE
>   377.03 WITH RETINAL DISORDER

CNS infections (viral, bacterial, fungal).
Medications (lithium, cisplatin, corticosteroids, tetracycline,
    etc.).
Head trauma.
CNS neoplasm (primary or metastatic).
Pseudotumor cerebri.
Cavernous sinus thrombosis.
SLE.
Sarcoidosis.
Subarachnoid hemorrhage.
Carbon dioxide retention.
Arnold-Chiari malformation and other developmental or
    congenital malformations.
Orbital lesions.
Central retinal vein occlusion.
Hypertensive encephalopathy.
Metabolic abnormalities.

PARANEOPLASTIC SYNDROMES, ENDOCRINE[33]

> ICD-9CM # CODE VARIES WITH SPECIFIC DISORDER

Hypercalcemia.
Syndrome of inappropriate secretion of antidiuretic hor-
    mone.
Hypoglycemia.
Zollinger-Ellison syndrome.
Ectopic secretion of human chorionic gonadotropin.
Cushing's syndrome.

PARANEOPLASTIC SYNDROMES, NONENDOCRINE[33]

> ICD-9CM # CODE VARIES WITH SPECIFIC DISORDER

■ **CUTANEOUS**
Dermatomyositis.
Acanthosis nigricans.
Sweet's syndrome.
Erythema gyratum repens.
Systemic nodular panniculitis (Weber-Christian disease).

■ **RENAL**
Nephrotic syndrome.
Nephrogenic diabetes insipidus.

■ **NEUROLOGIC**
Subacute cerebellar degeneration.
Progressive multifocal leukoencephalopathy.
Subacute motor neuropathy.
Sensory neuropathy.
Ascending acute polyneuropathy (Guillain-Barré syndrome).
Myasthenic syndrome (Eaton-Lambert syndrome).

■ HEMATOLOGIC

Microangiopathic hemolytic anemia.
Migratory thrombophlebitis (Trousseau's syndrome).
Anemia of chronic disease.

■ RHEUMATOLOGIC

Polymyalgia rheumatica.
Hypertrophic pulmonary osteoarthropathy.

PARAPLEGIA

ICD-9CM # 344.1 PARAPLEGIA, ACQUIRED
343.0 PARAPLEGIA, CONGENITAL
438.50 PARAPLEGIA, LATE EFFECT OF CVA

Trauma: penetrating wounds to motor cortex, fracture-dislocation of vertebral column with compression of spinal cord or cauda equina, prolapsed disk, electrical injuries.
Neoplasm: parasagittal region, vertebrae, meninges, spinal cord, cauda equina, Hodgkin's disease, NHL, leukemic deposits, pelvic neoplasms.
Multiple sclerosis and other demyelinating disorders.
Mechanical compression of spinal cord, cauda equina, or lumbosacral plexus: Paget's disease, kyphoscoliosis, herniation of intervertebral disk, spondylosis, ankylosing spondylitis, RA, aortic aneurysm.
Infections: spinal abscess, syphilis, TB, poliomyelitis, leprosy.
Thrombosis of superior sagittal sinus.
Polyneuritis: Guillain-Barré syndrome, diabetes, alcohol, beriberi, heavy metals.
Heredofamilial muscular dystrophies.
ALS.
Congenital and familial conditions: syringomyelia, myelomeningocele, myelodysplasia.
Hysteria.

PARESTHESIAS

ICD-9CM # 782.0

Multiple sclerosis.
Nutritional deficiencies (thiamin, vitamin B$_{12}$, folic acid).
Compression of spinal cord or peripheral nerves.
Medications (e.g., INH, lithium, nitrofurantoin, gold, cisplatin, hydralazine, amitriptyline, sulfonamides, amiodarone, metronidazole, dapsone, disulfiram, chloramphenicol).
Toxic chemicals (e.g., lead, arsenic, cyanide, mercury, organophosphates).
DM.
Myxedema.
Alcohol.
Sarcoidosis.
Neoplasms.
Infections (HIV, Lyme disease, herpes zoster, leprosy, diphtheria).
Charcot-Marie-Tooth syndrome and other hereditary neuropathies.
Guillain-Barré neuropathy.

PAROTID SWELLING[3]

ICD-9CM # 527.2 ALLERGIC PAROTITIS
72.9 INFECTIOUS PAROTITIS
527.8 SALIVARY GLAND OBSTRUCTION
527.5 SALIVARY GLAND OBSTRUCTION
WITH CALCULUS
527.8 SALIVARY GLAND STRICTURE
527.3 SALIVARY GLAND ABSCESS
235.1 SALIVARY GLAND NEOPLASM

■ INFECTIOUS

Mumps.
Parainfluenza.
Influenza.
Cytomegalovirus infection.
Coxsackievirus infection.
Lymphocytic choriomeningitis.
Echovirus infection.
Suppuration (bacterial).
Actinomyces infection.
Mycobacterial infection.
Cat-scratch disease.

■ NONINFECTIOUS

Drug hypersensitivity (thiouracil, phenothiazines, thiocyanate, iodides, copper, isoprenaline, lead, mercury, phenylbutazone).
Sarcoidosis.
Tumors, mixed.
Hemangioma, lymphangioma.
Sialectasis.
Sjögren syndrome.
Mikulicz syndrome (scleroderma, mixed connective tissue disease, systemic lupus erythematosus).
Recurrent idiopathic parotitis.
Pneumoparotitis.
Trauma.
Sialolithiasis.
Foreign body.
Cystic fibrosis.
Malnutrition (marasmus, alcohol cirrhosis).
Dehydration.
Diabetes mellitus.
Waldenström macroglobulinemia.
Reiter syndrome.
Amyloidosis.

■ NONPAROTID SWELLING

Hypertrophy of masseter muscle.
Lymphadenopathy.
Rheumatoid mandibular joint swelling.
Tumors of jaw.
Infantile cortical hyperostosis.

PELVIC MASS

ICD-9CM # 789.39

Hemorrhagic ovarian cyst.
Simple ovarian cyst (follicle or corpus luteum).
Ovarian carcinoma, carcinoma of fallopian tube, colorectal carcinoma, metastatic carcinoma, prostate carcinoma, bladder carcinoma, lymphoma, Hodgkin's disease.
Cystadenoma, teratoma, endometrioma.
Leiomyoma.
Leiomyosarcoma.
Diverticulitis, diverticular abscess.
Appendiceal abscess, tuboovarian abscess.
Ectopic pregnancy, intrauterine pregnancy.
Paraovarian cyst.
Hydrosalpinx.

PELVIC PAIN, CHRONIC[7]

ICD-9CM # 625.9 PELVIC PAIN, FEMALE
789.09 PELVIC PAIN, MALE

■ GYNECOLOGIC DISORDERS
Primary dysmenorrhea.
Endometriosis.
Adenomyosis.
Adhesions.
Fibroids.
Retained ovary syndrome after hysterectomy.
Previous tubal ligation.
Chronic pelvic infection.

■ MUSCULOSKELETAL DISORDERS
Myofascial pain syndrome.

■ GASTROINTESTINAL DISORDERS
Irritable bowel syndrome.
Inflammatory bowel disease.

■ URINARY TRACT DISORDERS
Interstitial cystitis.
Nonbacterial urethritis.

PELVIC PAIN, GENITAL ORIGIN[23]

ICD-9CM # 625.9 PELVIC PAIN, FEMALE
789.09 PELVIC PAIN, MALE

■ PERITONEAL IRRITATION
Ruptured ectopic pregnancy.
Ovarian cyst rupture.
Ruptured tuboovarian abscess.
Uterine perforation.

■ TORSION
Ovarian cyst or tumor.
Pedunculated fibroid.

■ INTRATUMOR HEMORRHAGE OR INFARCTION
Ovarian cyst.
Solid ovarian tumor.
Uterine leiomyoma.

■ INFECTION
Endometritis.
Pelvic inflammatory disease.
Trichomonas cervicitis or vaginitis.
Tuboovarian abscess.

■ PREGNANCY-RELATED
First Trimester
Ectopic pregnancy.
Abortion.
Corpus luteum hematoma.
Late Pregnancy
Placental problems.
Preeclampsia.
Premature labor.

■ MISCELLANEOUS
Endometriosis.
Foreign objects.
Pelvic adhesions.
Pelvic neoplasm.
Primary dysmenorrhea.

PERICARDIAL EFFUSION

ICD-9CM # 420.90

Pericarditis.
Uremia.
Myxedema.
Neoplasm (leukemia, lymphoma, metastatic).
Hemorrhage (trauma, leakage of thoracic aneurysm).
SLE, Rheumatoid disease.
Myocardial infarction.

PERITONEAL EFFUSION[16]

ICD-9CM # 792.9

■ TRANSUDATES
Increased hydrostatic pressure or decreased plasma oncotic
    pressure.
Congestive heart failure.
Hepatic cirrhosis.
Hypoproteinemia.

■ EXUDATES
Increased capillary permeability or decreased lymphatic re-
    sorption.
Infections (TB, spontaneous bacterial peritonitis, secondary
    bacterial peritonitis).
Neoplasms (hepatoma, metastatic carcinoma, lymphoma,
    mesothelioma).
Trauma.
Pancreatitis.
Bile peritonitis (e.g., ruptured gallbladder).

■ CHYLOUS EFFUSION
Damage or obstruction to thoracic duct.
Trauma.
Lymphoma.
Carcinoma.
Tuberculosis.
Parasitic infection.

PHOTOSENSITIVITY

ICD-9CM # 692.72

Solar urticaria.
Photoallergic reaction.
Phototoxic reaction.
Polymorphous light eruption.
Porphyria cutanea tarda.
SLE.
Drug-induced (e.g., tetracyclines).

PLEURAL EFFUSIONS

ICD-9CM # 511.9 PLEURAL EFFUSION, UNSPECIFIED

■ EXUDATIVE
Neoplasm: bronchogenic carcinoma, breast carcinoma,
    mesothelioma, lymphoma, ovarian carcinoma, multiple
    myeloma, leukemia, Meigs' syndrome.
Infections: viral pneumonia, bacterial pneumonia,
    Mycoplasma, TB, fungal and parasitic diseases, extension
    from subphrenic abscess.
Trauma.
Collagen vascular diseases: SLE, RA, scleroderma, polyarteri-
    tis, Wegener's granulomatosis.
Pulmonary infarction.

Pancreatitis.
Postcardiotomy/Dressler's syndrome.
Drug-induced lupus erythematosus (hydralazine, procainamide).
Postabdominal surgery.
Ruptured esophagus.
Chronic effusion secondary to congestive failure.

■ TRANSUDATIVE
CHF.
Hepatic cirrhosis.
Nephrotic syndrome.
Hypoproteinemia from any cause.
Meigs' syndrome.

PNEUMONIA, RECURRENT

> ICD-9CM # 482.9 BACTERIAL PNEUMONIA
> 480.9 VIRAL PNEUMONIA
> 484.1 FUNGAL PNEUMONIA
> 485 SEGMENTAL PNEUMONIA

Mechanical obstruction from neoplasm.
Chronic aspiration (tube feeding, alcoholism, CVA, neuromuscular disorders, seizure disorder, inability to cough).
Bronchiectasis.
Kyphoscoliosis.
COPD, CHF, asthma, silicosis, pulmonary fibrosis, cystic fibrosis.
Pulmonary TB, chronic sinusitis.
Immunosuppression (HIV, corticosteroids, leukemia, chemotherapy, splenectomy).

POLYNEUROPATHY[35]

> ICD-9CM # 357.9

■ PREDOMINANTLY MOTOR
Guillain-Barré syndrome.
Porphyria.
Diphtheria.
Lead.
Hereditary sensorimotor neuropathy, types I and II.
Paraneoplastic neuropathy.

■ PREDOMINANTLY SENSORY
Diabetes.
Amyloidosis.
Leprosy.
Lyme disease.
Paraneoplastic neuropathy.
Vitamin B_{12} deficiency.
Hereditary sensory neuropathy, types I-IV.

■ PREDOMINANTLY AUTONOMIC
Diabetes.
Amyloidosis.
Alcoholic neuropathy.
Familial dysautonomias.

■ MIXED SENSORIMOTOR
Systemic diseases: Renal failure, hypothyroidism, acromegaly, rheumatoid arthritis, periarteritis nodosa, systemic lupus erythematosus, multiple myeloma, macroglobulinemia, remote effect of malignancy.
Medications: Isoniazid, nitrofurantoin, ethambutol, chloramphenicol, chloroquine, vincristine, vinblastine, dapsone, disulfiram, diphenylhydantoin, cisplatin, 1-tryptophan.

Environmental toxins: N-hexane, methyl N-butyl ketone, acrylamide, carbon disulfide, carbon monoxide, hexachlorophene, organophosphates.
Deficiency disorders: Malabsorption, alcoholism, vitamin B_1 deficiency, Refsum's disease, metachromatic leukodystrophy.

POLYNEUROPATHY, DRUG-INDUCED[35]

> ICD-9CM # 357.6

■ DRUGS IN ONCOLOGY
Vincristine.
Procarbazine.
Cisplatin.
Misonidazole.
Metronidazole (Flagyl).
Taxol.

■ DRUGS IN INFECTIOUS DISEASES
Isoniazid.
Nitrofurantoin.
Dapsone.
ddC (dideoxycytidine).
ddI (dideoxyinosine).

■ DRUGS IN CARDIOLOGY
Hydralazine.
Perhexiline maleate.
Procainamide.
Disopyramide.

■ DRUGS IN RHEUMATOLOGY
Gold salts.
Chloroquine.

■ DRUGS IN NEUROLOGY AND PSYCHIATRY
Diphenylhydantoin.
Glutethimide.
Methaqualone.

■ MISCELLANEOUS
Disulfiram (Antabuse).
Vitamin: pyridoxine (megadoses).

POLYNEUROPATHY, SYMMETRIC[35]

> ICD-9CM # 357.9

■ ACQUIRED NEUROPATHIES
Toxic:
  Drugs.
  Industrial toxins.
  Heavy metals.
  Abused substances.
Metabolic/endocrine:
  Diabetes.
  Chronic renal failure.
  Hypothyroidism.
  Polyneuropathy of critical illness.
Nutritional deficiency:
  Vitamin B_{12} deficiency.
  Alcoholism.
  Vitamin E deficiency.
Paraneoplastic:
  Carcinoma.
  Lymphoma.
Plasma cell dyscrasia:
  Myeloma, typical, atypical, and solitary forms.
  Primary systemic amyloidosis.

Idiopathic chronic inflammatory demyelinating polyneuropathies.
Polyneuropathies associated with peripheral nerve autoantibodies.
Acquired immunodeficiency syndrome.

■ INHERITED NEUROPATHIES
Neuropathies with biochemical markers
Refsum's disease.
Bassen-Kornzweig disease.
Tangier disease.
Metachromatic leukodystrophy.
Krabbe's disease.
Adrenomyeloneuropathy.
Fabry's disease.
Neuropathies without biochemical markers or systemic involvement
Hereditary motor neuropathy.
Hereditary sensory neuropathy.
Hereditary sensorimotor neuropathy.

POLYURIA

ICD-9CM # 788.42

DM.
Diabetes insipidus.
Primary polydipsia (compulsive water drinking).
Hypercalcemia.
Hypokalemia.
Postobstructive uropathy.
Diuretic phase of renal failure.
Drugs: diuretics, caffeine, alcohol, lithium.
Sickle cell trait or disease, chronic pyelonephritis (failure to concentrate urine).
Anxiety, cold weather.

POPLITEAL SWELLING

ICD-9CM # 459.2 VENOUS OBSTRUCTION
747.4 VEIN ANOMALY, LOWER LIMB VESSEL
442.3 ARTERY ANEURYSM
904.41 ARTERY INJURY
447.8 ENTRAPMENT SYNDROME
727.51 BAKER'S CYST
451.2 PHLEBITIS, LOWER EXTREMITY
727.67 RUPTURE OF ACHILLES TENDON

Phlebitis (superficial).
Lymphadenitis.
Trauma: fractured tibia or fibula, contusion, traumatic neuroma.
DVT.
Ruptured varicose vein.
Baker's cyst.
Popliteal abscess.
Osteomyelitis.
Ruptured tendon.
Aneurysm of popliteal artery.
Neoplasm: lipoma, osteogenic sarcoma, neurofibroma, fibrosarcoma.

PORTAL HYPERTENSION[1]

ICD-9CM # 572.3

■ INCREASED RESISTANCE TO FLOW
Presinusoidal
Portal or splenic vein occlusion (thrombosis, tumor).
Schistosomiasis.
Congenital hepatic fibrosis.
Sarcoidosis.
Sinusoidal
Cirrhosis (all causes).
Alcoholic hepatitis.
Postsinusoidal
Venoocclusive disease.
Budd-Chiari syndrome.
Constrictive pericarditis.

■ INCREASED PORTAL BLOOD FLOW
Splenomegaly not caused by liver disease.
Arterioportal fistula.

PROPTOSIS[27]

ICD-9CM # 376.30

Thyrotoxicosis.
Orbital pseudotumor.
Optic nerve tumor.
Cavernous sinus AV fistula, cavernous sinus thrombosis.
Cellulitis.
Metastatic tumor to orbit

PROTEINURIA

ICD-9CM # 791.0

Nephrotic syndrome as a result of primary renal diseases.
Malignant hypertension.
Malignancies: multiple myeloma, leukemias, Hodgkin's disease.
CHF.
DM.
SLE, RA.
Sickle cell disease.
Goodpasture's syndrome.
Malaria.
Amyloidosis, sarcoidosis.
Tubular lesions: cystinosis.
Functional (after heavy exercise).
Pyelonephritis.
Pregnancy.
Constrictive pericarditis.
Renal vein thrombosis.
Toxic nephropathies: heavy metals, drugs.
Radiation nephritis.
Orthostatic (postural) proteinuria.
Benign proteinuria: fever, heat, or cold exposure.

PRURITUS

ICD-9CM # 698.9 PRURITUS NOS
697.0 PRURITUS ANI
698.1 PRURITUS, GENITAL ORGANS

Dry skin.
Drug-induced eruption, fiberglass exposure.
Scabies.
Skin diseases.

Myeloproliferative disorders: mycosis fungoides, Hodgkin's lymphoma, multiple myeloma, polycythemia vera.
Cholestatic liver disease.
Endocrine disorders: DM, thyroid disease, carcinoid, pregnancy.
Carcinoma: breast, lung, gastric.
Chronic renal failure.
Iron deficiency.
AIDS.
Neurosis.
Sjögren's syndrome.

PRURITUS ANI[23]

ICD-9CM # 697.0

■ FECAL IRRITATION
Poor hygiene.
Anorectal conditions (fissure, fistula, hemorrhoids, skin tags, perianal clefts).
Spicy foods, citrus foods, caffeine, colchicine, quinidine.

■ CONTACT DERMATITIS
Anesthetic agents, topical corticosteroids, perfumed soap.

■ DERMATOLOGIC DISORDERS
Psoriasis, seborrhea, lichen simplex or sclerosus.

■ SYSTEMIC DISORDERS
Chronic renal failure, myxedema, DM, thyrotoxicosis, polycythemia vera, Hodgkin's disease.

■ SEXUALLY TRANSMITTED DISEASES
Syphilis, herpes simplex virus, human papillomavirus.

■ OTHER INFECTIOUS AGENTS
Pinworms.
Scabies.
Bacterial infection, viral infection.

PSEUDOINFARCTION[19]

ICD-9CM # CODE NOT AVAILABLE

Cardiac tumors, primary and secondary.
Cardiomyopathy (particularly hypertrophic and dilated).
Chagas disease.
Chest deformity.
COPD (particularly emphysema).
HIV infection.
Hyperkalemia.
Left anterior fascicular block.
Left bundle branch block.
Left ventricular hypertrophy.
Myocarditis and pericarditis.
Normal variant.
Pneumothorax.
Poor R wave progression, rotational changes, and lead placement.
Pulmonary embolism.
Trauma to chest (nonpenetrating).
Wolff-Parkinson-White syndrome.
Rare causes: pancreatitis, amyloidosis, sarcoidosis, scleroderma.

PSYCHOSIS[25]

ICD-9CM # 298.9 PSYCHOSIS NOS
298.90 PSYCHOSIS, AFFECTIVE
291.0 PSYCHOSIS, ALCOHOLIC
290.41 PSYCHOSIS, ACUTE
ARTERIOSCLEROTIC

■ PRIMARY
Schizophrenia related.*
Major depression.
Dementia.
Bipolar disorder.

■ SECONDARY
Drug use.†
Drug withdrawal.‡
Drug toxicity.§
Charles Bonnet syndrome.
Infections (pneumonia).
Electrolyte imbalance.
Syphilis.
Congestive heart failure.
Parkinson's disease.
Trauma to temporal lobe.
Postpartum psychosis.
Hypothyroidism/hyperthyroidism.
Hypomagnesemia.
Epilepsy
Meningitis.
Encephalitis.
Brain abscess.
Herpes encephalopathy.
Hypoxia.
Hypercarbia.
Hypoglycemia.
Thiamine deficiency.
Postoperative states.

---

*Includes schizophrenia, schizophreniaform disorder, brief reactive psychosis.
†Includes hypnotics, glucocorticoids, marijuana, phencyclidine, atropine, dopaminergic agents (e.g., amantadine, bromocriptine, L-dopa), immunosuppressants.
‡Includes alcohol, barbiturates, benzodiazepines.
§Includes digitalis, theophylline, cimetidine, anticholinergics, glucocorticoids, catecholaminergic agents.

PTOSIS

ICD-9CM # 374.30 PTOSIS NOS
743.61 CONGENITAL
374.33 MECHANICAL
374.32 MYOGENIC
374.31 PARALYTIC

Third nerve palsy.
Myasthenia gravis.
Horner's syndrome.
Senile ptosis.

PUBERTY, DELAYED[24]

ICD-9CM # 259.0

■ NORMAL OR LOW SERUM GONADOTROPIN LEVELS
Constitutional delay in growth and development.

Hypothalamic and/or pituitary disorders:
Isolated deficiency of growth hormone.
Isolated deficiency on Gn-RH.
Isolated deficiency of LH and/or FSH.
Multiple anterior pituitary hormone deficiencies.
Associated with congenital anomalies: Kallmann's syndrome; Prader-Willi syndrome; Laurence-Moon-Biedl syndrome; Friedreich's ataxia.
Trauma.
Postinfection.
Hyperprolactinemia.
Postirradiation.
Infiltrative disease (histiocytosis).
Tumor.
Autoimmune hypophysitis.
Idiopathic.
Functional:
Chronic endocrinologic or systemic disorders.
Emotional disorders.
Drugs: cannabis.

■ **INCREASED SERUM GONADOTROPIN LEVELS**
Gonadal abnormalities:
Congenital:
Gonadal dysgenesis.
Klinefelter's syndrome.
Bilateral anorchism.
Resistant ovary syndrome.
Myotonic dystrophy in males.
17-Hydroxylase deficiency in females.
Galactosemia.
Acquired:
Bilateral gonadal failure resulting from trauma or infection or after surgery, irradiation, or chemotherapy.
Oophoritis: isolated or with other autoimmune disorders.
Uterine or vaginal disorders:
Absence of uterus and/or vagina.
Testicular feminization: complete or incomplete androgen insensitivity.
(*FSH*, Follicle-stimulating hormone; *Gn-RH*, gonadotropin-releasing hormone; *LH*, luteinizing hormone.)

PULMONARY CRACKLES

ICD-9CM # NOT AVAILABLE

Pneumonia.
Left ventricular failure.
Asbestosis, silicosis, interstitial lung disease.
Chronic bronchitis.
Alveolitis (allergic, fibrosing).
Neoplasm.

PULMONARY LESIONS

ICD-9CM # 518.3 PULMONARY INFILTRATE
518.89 PULMONARY NODULE
508.9 PULMONARY DISORDER DUE TO
UNSPECIFIED EXTERNAL AGENT
861.20 PULMONARY INJURY NOS

TB.
Legionella pneumonia.
Mycoplasma pneumonia.
Viral pneumonia.
Pneumocystis carinii.
Hypersensitivity pneumonitis.
Aspiration pneumonia.
Fungal disease (aspergillosis, histoplasmosis).

ARDS associated with pneumonia.
Psittacosis.
Sarcoidosis.
Septic emboli.
Metastatic cancer.
Multiple pulmonary emboli.
Rheumatoid nodules.

PULMONARY NODULE, SOLITARY

ICD-9CM # 518.89

Bronchogenic carcinoma.
Granuloma from histoplasmosis.
TB granuloma.
Granuloma from coccidioidomycosis.
Metastatic carcinoma.
Bronchial adenoma.
Bronchogenic cyst.
Hamartoma.
AV malformation.
Other: fibroma, intrapulmonary lymph node, sclerosing hemangioma, bronchopulmonary sequestration.

PULSELESS ELECTRICAL ACTIVITY

ICD-9CM # CODE NOT AVAILABLE

Hypovolemia.
Hypoxia.
Hyperkalemia.
Acidosis.
Cardiac tamponade.
Tension pneumothorax.
Pulmonary embolus.
Drug overdose.
Hypothermia

PURPURA

ICD-9CM # 287.2 PURPURA NOS
287.0 AUTOIMMUNE
287.0 HENOCH-SCHÖNLEIN
287.3 IDIOPATHIC THROMBOCYTOPENIC
446.6 THROMBOCYTOPENIC
THROMBOTIC

Trauma.
Septic emboli, atheromatous emboli.
DIC.
Thrombocytopenia.
Meningococcemia.
Rocky Mountain spotted fever.
Hemolytic-uremic syndrome.
Viral infection: echo, coxsackie.
Scurvy.
Other: left atrial myxoma, cryoglobulinemia, vasculitis, hyperglobulinemic purpura.

QT INTERVAL PROLONGATION[19]

ICD-9CM # 794.31

Drugs:
Class I antiarrhythmics (e.g., disopyramide, procainamide, quinidine).
Class III antiarrhythmics.
Tricyclic antidepressants.
Phenothiazines.

Astemizole.
Terfenadine.
Adenosine.
Antibiotics (e.g., erythromycin and other macrolides).
Antifungal agents.
Pentamidine, chloroquine.
Ischemic heart disease.
Cerebrovascular disease.
Rheumatic fever.
Myocarditis.
Mitral valve prolapse.
Electrolyte abnormalities.
Hypocalcemia.
Hypothyroidism.
Liquid protein diets.
Organophosphate insecticides.
Congenital prolonged QT syndrome.

RECTAL PAIN

ICD-9CM # 569.42

Anal fissure.
Thrombosed hemorrhoid.
Anorectal abscess.
Foreign bodies.
Fecal impaction.
Endometriosis.
Neoplasms (primary or metastatic).
Pelvic inflammatory disease.
Inflammation of sacral nerves.
Compression of sacral nerves.
Prostatitis.
Other: proctalgia fugax, uterine abnormalities, myopathies, coccygodynia.

RED EYE

ICD-9CM # 379.93

Infectious conjunctivitis (bacterial, viral).
Allergic conjunctivitis.
Acute glaucoma.
Keratitis (bacterial, viral).
Iritis.
Trauma.

RENAL FAILURE, INTRINSIC OR PARENCHYMAL CAUSES[33]

ICD-9CM # 584. ACUTE, USE 4TH DIGIT
   5. WITH ACUTE TUBULAR NECROSIS
   6. WITH CORTICAL NECROSIS
   7. WITH MEDULLARY NECROSIS
   8. WITH OTHER UNSPECIFIED
     PATHOLOGIC CONDITION IN KIDNEY
   9. RENAL FAILURE UNSPECIFIED
   585 RENAL FAILURE, CHRONIC

■ ABNORMALITIES OF THE VASCULATURE
Renal arteries: atherosclerosis, thromboembolism, arteritis.
Renal veins: thrombosis.
Microvasculature: vasculitis, thrombotic microangiopathy.

■ ABNORMALITIES OF GLOMERULI (ACUTE GLOMERULONEPHRITIS)
Antiglomerular membrane disease (Goodpasture syndrome).
Immune complex glomerulonephritis: SLE, postinfectious, idiopathic, membranoproliferative.

■ ABNORMALITIES OF INTERSTITIUM (ACUTE INTERSTITIAL NEPHRITIS)
Drugs (e.g., antibiotics, NSAIDs, diuretics, anticonvulsants, allopurinol).
Infectious pyelonephritis.
Infiltrative: lymphoma, leukemia, sarcoidosis.

■ ABNORMALITIES OF TUBULES
Physical obstruction (uric acid, oxalate, light chains).
Acute tubular necrosis:
  Ischemic.
  Toxic (antibiotics, chemotherapy, immunosuppressives, radiocontrast dyes, heavy metals, myoglobin, hemolysed RBCs.

RENAL FAILURE, PRERENAL CAUSES[33]

ICD-9CM # 584. ACUTE, USE 4TH DIGIT
   5. WITH ACUTE TUBULAR NECROSIS
   6. WITH CORTICAL NECROSIS
   7. WITH MEDULLARY NECROSIS
   8. WITH OTHER UNSPECIFIED
     PATHOLOGIC CONDITION IN KIDNEY
   9. RENAL FAILURE UNSPECIFIED
   585 RENAL FAILURE, CHRONIC

■ DECREASED CARDIAC OUTPUT
CHF.
Arrhythmias.
Pericardial constriction or tamponade.
Pulmonary embolism.

■ HYPOVOLEMIA
GI tract loss (vomiting, diarrhea, nasogastric suction).
Blood losses (trauma, GI tract surgery).
Renal losses (diuretics, mineralocorticoid deficiency, postobstructive diuresis).
Skin losses (burns).

■ VOLUME REDISTRIBUTION (DECREASE IN EFFECTIVE BLOOD VOLUME)
Hypoalbuminemic states (cirrhosis, nephrosis).
Sequestration of fluid in "third" space (ischemic bowel, peritonitis, pancreatitis).
Peripheral vasodilation (sepsis, vasodilators, anaphylaxis).

■ ALTERED RENAL VASCULAR RESISTANCE
Increase in afferent vascular resistance (NSAIDs, liver disease, sepsis, hypercalcemia, cyclosporine).
Decrease in efferent arteriolar tone (ACE inhibitors).

RENAL FAILURE, POSTRENAL CAUSES[33]

ICD-9CM # 584. ACUTE, USE 4TH DIGIT
   5. WITH ACUTE TUBULAR NECROSIS
   6. WITH CORTICAL NECROSIS
   7. WITH MEDULLARY NECROSIS
   8. WITH OTHER UNSPECIFIED
     PATHOLOGIC CONDITION IN KIDNEY
   9. RENAL FAILURE UNSPECIFIED
   585 RENAL FAILURE, CHRONIC

■ URETER AND RENAL PELVIS
Intrinsic obstruction:
  Blood clots.
  Stones.
  Sloughed papillae: diabetes, sickle cell disease, analgesic nephropathy.
  Inflammatory: fungus ball.

II

Extrinsic obstruction:
  Malignancy.
  Retroperitoneal fibrosis.
  Iatrogenic: inadvertent ligation of ureters.

■ BLADDER
Prostatic hypertrophy or malignancy.
Neuropathic bladder.
Blood clots.
Bladder cancer.
Stones.

■ URETHRAL
Strictures.
Congenital valves.

RESPIRATORY FAILURE, HYPOVENTILATORY[25]

ICD-9CM # 518.81 RESPIRATORY FAILURE

■ ABNORMAL RESPIRATORY CAPACITY (NORMAL RESPIRATORY WORKLOADS)
Acute depression of central nervous system:
  Various causes.
Chronic central hypoventilation syndromes:
  Obesity-hypoventilation syndrome.
  Sleep apnea syndrome.
  Hypothyroidism.
  Shy-Drager syndrome (multisystem atrophy syndrome).
Acute toxic paralysis syndromes:
  Botulism.
  Tetanus.
  Toxic ingestion or bites.
  Organophosphate poisoning.
Neuromuscular disorders (acute and chronic):
  Myasthenia gravis.
  Guillain-Barré syndrome.
  Drugs.
  Amyotrophic lateral sclerosis.
  Muscular dystrophies.
  Polymyositis.
  Spinal cord injury.
  Traumatic phrenic nerve paralysis.

■ ABNORMAL PULMONARY WORKLOADS
Chronic obstructive pulmonary disease:
  Chronic bronchitis.
  Asthmatic bronchitis.
  Emphysema.
Asthma and acute bronchial hyperreactivity syndromes.
Upper airway obstruction.
Interstitial lung diseases.

■ ABNORMAL EXTRAPULMONARY WORKLOADS
Chronic thoracic cage disorders:
  Severe kyphoscoliosis.
  After thoracoplasty.
  After thoracic cage injury.
Acute thoracic cage trauma and burns.
Pneumothorax.
Pleural fibrosis and effusions.
Abdominal processes.

RIGHT AXIS DEVIATION[19]

ICD-9CM # CODE VARIES WITH SPECIFIC DIAGNOSIS

Normal variation.
Right ventricular hypertrophy.
Left posterior fascicular block.

Lateral myocardial infarction.
Pulmonary embolism.
Dextrocardia.
Mechanical shifts or emphysema causing a vertical heart.

SCROTAL PAIN[25]

ICD-9CM # 878.2 SCROTAL INJURY, TRAUMATIC
  608.9 SCROTAL DISORDER NOS
  608.4 SCROTAL CELLULITIS
  608.83 SCROTAL HEMORRHAGE, NONTRAUMATIC
  608.4 SCROTAL NODULE, INFLAMMATORY

Torsion:
  Appendages.
  Spermatic cord.
Infection:
  Orchidis.
  Abscess.
  Epididymitis.
Neoplasia:
  Benign.
  Malignant.
Incarcerated hernia.
Trauma.
Hydrocele.
Spermatocele.
Varicocele.

SCROTAL SWELLING

ICD-9CM # 608.86

Hydrocele.
Varicocele.
Neoplasm.
Acute epididymitis.
Orchitis.
Trauma.
Hernia.
Torsion of spermatic cord.
Torsion of epididymis.
Torsion of testis.
Insect bite.
Folliculitis.
Sebaceous cyst.
Thrombosis of spermatic vein.
Other: lymphedema, dermatitis, fat necrosis, Henoch-Schönlein purpura, idiopathic scrotal edema.

SEIZURE

ICD-9CM # 780.39

Syncope.
Alcohol abuse/withdrawal.
TIA.
Hemiparetic migraine.
Psychiatric disorders.
Carotid sinus hypersensitivity.
Hyperventilation, prolonged breath holding.
Hypoglycemia.
Narcolepsy.
Movement disorders (tics, hemiballismus).
Hyponatremia.
Brain tumor (primary or metastatic).
Tetanus.
Strychnine, phencyclidine poisoning.

SEIZURE, PEDIATRIC[2]

ICD-9CM # 780.39 INFANTILE SEIZURES
779.0 SEIZURES, NEWBORN

■ FIRST MONTH OF LIFE

First Day
Hypoxia.
Drugs.
Trauma.
Infection.
Hyperglycemia.
Hypoglycemia.
Pyridoxine deficiency.
Day 2-3
Infection.
Drug withdrawal.
Hypoglycemia.
Hypocalcemia.
Developmental malformation.
Intracranial hemorrhage.
Inborn error of metabolism.
Hyponatremia or hypernatremia.
Day >4
Infection.
Hypocalcemia.
Hyperphosphatemia.
Hyponatremia.
Developmental malformation.
Drug withdrawal.
Inborn error of metabolism.

■ 1 TO 6 MONTHS
As above.

■ 6 MONTHS TO 3 YEARS
Febrile seizures.
Birth injury.
Infection.
Toxin.
Trauma.
Metabolic disorder.
Cerebral degenerative disease.

■ >3 YEARS
Idiopathic.
Infection.
Trauma.
Cerebral degenerative disease

SEXUAL PRECOCITY[36]

ICD-9CM # 259.1

■ TRUE PRECOCIOUS PUBERTY
Premature reactivation of LHRH pulse generator.

■ INCOMPLETE SEXUAL PRECOCITY
(Pituitary Gonadotropin Independent).
Males
Chorionic gonadotropin-secreting tumor.
Leydig cell tumor.
Familial testotoxicosis.
Virilizing congenital adrenal hyperplasia.
Virilizing adrenal tumor.
Premature adrenarche.
Females
Granulosa cell tumor (follicular cysts may be manifested similarly).
Follicular cyst.

Feminizing adrenal tumor.
Premature thelarche.
Premature adrenarche.
Late-onset virilizing congenital adrenal hyperplasia.
In both sexes
McCune-Albright syndrome.
Primary hypothyroidism.

SEXUALLY TRANSMITTED DISEASES, ANORECTAL REGION[23]

ICD-9CM # 569.49 INFECTION AND REGION

■ ULCERATIVE
Lymphogranuloma venereum.
Herpes simplex virus.
Early (primary) syphilis.
Chancroid (Haemophilus ducreyi).
Cytomegalovirus.
Idiopathic (usually HIV positive).

■ NONULCERATIVE
Condyloma acuminatum.
Gonorrhea.
Chlamydia (Chlamydia trachomitis).
Syphilis.

SHOULDER PAIN

ICD-9CM # 952.2 SHOULDER INJURY
718.81 SHOULDER INSTABILITY
726.19 SHOULDER LIGAMENT OR MUSCLE INSTABILITY
840.9 SHOULDER STRAIN, SITE UNSPECIFIED

■ WITH LOCAL FINDINGS IN SHOULDER
Trauma: contusion, fracture, muscle strain, trauma to spinal cord.
Arthrosis, arthritis, RA, ankylosing spondylitis.
Bursitis, synovitis, tendinitis, tenosynovitis.
Aseptic (avascular) necrosis.
Local infection: septic arthritis, osteomyelitis, abscess, herpes zoster, TB.

■ WITHOUT LOCAL FINDINGS IN SHOULDER
Cardiovascular disorders: ischemic heart disease, pericarditis, aortic aneurysm.
Subdiaphragmatic abscess, liver abscess.
Cholelithiasis, cholecystitis.
Pulmonary lesions: apical bronchial carcinoma, pleurisy, pneumothorax, pneumonia.
GI lesions: PUD, gastric neoplasm, peptic esophagitis.
Pancreatic lesions: carcinoma, calculi, pancreatitis.
CNS abnormalities: neoplasm, vascular abnormalities.
Multiple sclerosis.
Syringomyelia.
Polymyositis/dermatomyositis.
Psychogenic.
Polymyalgia rheumatica.
Ectopic pregnancy.

SHOULDER PAIN BY LOCATION

> **ICD-9CM # 952.2 SHOULDER INJURY**
> **726.19 SHOULDER LIGAMENT OR MUSCLE INSTABILITY**
> **840.8 SHOULDER SEPARATION**

■ TOP OF SHOULDER (C4)
Cervical source.
Acromioclavicular.
Sternoclavicular.
Diaphragmatic.

■ SUPEROLATERAL (C5)
Rotator cuff tendinitis.
Impingement.
Adhesive capsulitis.
Glenohumeral arthritis.

■ ANTERIOR
Bicipital tendinitis and rupture.
Glenoid labral tear.
Adhesive capsulitis.
Glenohumeral arthritis.
Osteonecrosis.

■ AXILLARY
Neoplasm (Pancoast's, mediastinal).
Herpes zoster.

SMALL BOWEL OBSTRUCTION[23]

> **ICD-9CM # 751.1 SMALL INTESTINE OBSTRUCTION, CONGENITAL**
> **560.81 SMALL INTESTINE OBSTRUCTION DUE TO ADHESION**

■ INTRINSIC
Congenital (artesia, stenosis).
Inflammatory (Crohn's, radiation enteritis).
Neoplasms (metastatic or primary).
Intussusception.
Traumatic (hematoma).

■ EXTRINSIC
Hernias (internal and external).
Adhesions.
Volvulus.
Compressing masses (tumors, abscesses, hematomas).

■ INTRALUMINAL
Foreign body.
Gallstones.
Bezoars.
Barium.
Ascaris infestation.

SORE THROAT[30]

> **ICD-9CM # 426 PHARYNGITIS**
> **075 MONONUCLEOSIS**
> **472.1 CHRONIC PHARYNGITIS**
> **487.1 PHARYNGITIS, INFLUENZAL**
> **074.0 COXSACKIE VIRUS PHARYNGITIS**

■ WITHOUT PHARYNGEAL ULCERS
Viral pharyngitis.
Allergic pharyngitis.
Infectious mononucleosis.
Streptococcal pharyngitis.
Gonococcal pharyngitis.
Sinusitis with postnasal drip.

■ WITH PHARYNGEAL ULCERS
Herpangina.
Herpes simplex.
Candidiasis.
Fusospirochetal infection (Vincent's angina).

SPINAL CORD DYSFUNCTION

> **ICD-9CM # 336.9 SPINAL CORD COMPRESSION**
> **336.9 SPINAL CORD DISEASE NOS**
> **742.9 SPINAL CORD DISEASE, CONGENITAL**
> **281.1 SPINAL CORD DEGENERATION, B_{12} DEFICIENCY ANEMIA**
> **336.8 SPINAL CORD ATROPHY, ACUTE**
> **336.10 SPINAL CORD ATROPHY, ADULT**

Trauma.
Multiple sclerosis.
Transverse myelitis.
Neoplasm (primary, metastatic).
Syringomyelia.
Spinal epidural abscess.
HIV myelopathy.
Diskitis.
Spinal epidural hematoma.
Spinal cord infarction.
Spinal AV malformation.
Subarachnoid hemorrhage.

SPLENOMEGALY

> **ICD-9CM # 789.2 SPLENOMEGALY UNSPECIFIED**
> **289.51 CHRONIC CONGESTIVE**
> **759.0 CONGENITAL**
> **789.2 UNKNOWN ORIGIN**

Hepatic cirrhosis.
Neoplastic involvement: CML, CLL, lymphoma, multiple myeloma.
Bacterial infections: TB, infectious endocarditis, typhoid fever, splenic abscess.
Viral infections: infectious mononucleosis, viral hepatitis, HIV.
Gaucher's disease and other lipid storage diseases.
Sarcoidosis.
Parasitic infections (malaria, kala-azar, histoplasmosis).
Hereditary and acquired hemolytic anemias.
Idiopathic thrombocytopenic purpura (ITP).
Collagen vascular disorders: SLE, RA (Felty's syndrome), polyarteritis nodosa.
Serum sickness, drug hypersensitivity reaction.
Splenic cysts and benign tumors: hemangioma, lymphangioma.
Thrombosis of splenic or portal vein.
Polycythemia vera, myeloid metaplasia.

STEATOHEPATITIS

> **ICD-9CM # 571.8**

Alcohol abuse.
Obesity.
Diabetes mellitus.
Parenteral nutrition.

Medications (high-dose estrogen, amiodarone, cortico-
steroids, methotrexate, nifedipine).
Jejunoileal bypass.
Abetalipoproteinemia.
Wilson's disease, Weber-Christian disease.

STOMATITIS, BULLOUS

ICD-9CM # 528.0

Erythema multiforme.
Erosive lichen planus.
Bullous pemphigoid.
SLE.
Pemphigus vulgaris.
Mucous membrane pemphigoid.

STRIDOR, PEDIATRIC AGE[4]

**ICD-9CM # 786.1 STRIDOR
748.3 STRIDOR LARYNGEAL CONGENITAL**

■ RECURRENT
Allergic (spasmodic) croup.
Respiratory infections in a child with otherwise asympto-
matic anatomic narrowing of the large airways.
Laryngomalacia.

■ PERSISTENT
Laryngeal obstruction:
   Laryngomalacia.
   Papillomas, other tumors.
   Cysts and laryngoceles.
   Laryngeal webs.
   Bilateral abductor paralysis of the cords.
   Foreign body.
Tracheobronchial disease:
   Tracheomalacia.
   Subglottic tracheal webs.
Endotracheal, endobronchial tumors.
Subglottic tracheal stenosis.
Congenital.
Acquired.
Extrinsic masses.
Mediastinal masses.
Vascular ring.
Lobar emphysema.
Bronchogenic cysts.
Thyroid enlargement.
Esophageal foreign body.
Tracheoesophageal fistulas.
Other.
Gastroesophageal reflux.
Macroglossia, Pierre Robin syndrome.
Cri du chat syndrome.
Hysterical stridor.
Hypocalcemia.

STROKE[33]

ICD-9CM # 436 ACUTE STROKE

Hypoglycemia.
Drug overdose or intoxication.
Hysterical conversion reaction.
Hyperventilation.
Metabolic encephalopathy.
Migraine.
Syncope.

Transient global amnesia.
Seizures.
Vestibular vertigo.

STROKE, PEDIATRIC AGE[20]

ICD-9CM # 436 STROKE, ACUTE

■ CARDIAC DISEASE
Congenital:
   Aortic stenosis.
   Mitral stenosis; mitral prolapse.
   Ventricular septal defects.
   Patent ductus arteriosus.
   Cyanotic congenital heart disease involving right-to-left
   shunt.
Acquired:
   Endocarditis (bacterial, SLE).
   Kawasaki disease.
   Cardiomyopathy.
   Atrial myxoma.
   Arrhythmia.
   Paradoxical emboli through patent foramen ovale.
   Rheumatic fever.
   Prosthetic heart valve.

■ HEMATOLOGIC ABNORMALITIES
Hemoglobinopathies:
   Sickle cell (SS) disease.
   Sickle (SC) disease.
Polycythemia.
Leukemia/lymphoma.
Thrombocytopenia.
Thrombocytosis.
Disorders of coagulation:
   Protein C deficiency.
   Protein S deficiency.
   Factor V Leiden.
   Antithrombin III deficiency.
   Lupus anticoagulant.
      Oral contraceptive pill use.
      Pregnancy and the postpartum state.
      Disseminated intravascular coagulation.
      Paroxysmal nocturnal hemoglobinuria.
      Inflammatory bowel disease (thrombosis).

■ INFLAMMATORY DISORDERS
Meningitis:
   Viral.
   Bacterial.
   Tuberculosis.
Systemic infection:
   Viremia.
   Bacteremia.
   Local head and neck infections.
Drug-induced inflammation:
   Amphetamine.
   Cocaine.
Autoimmune disease:
   Systemic lupus erythematosus.
   Juvenile rheumatoid arthritis.
   Takayasu arteritis.
   Mixed connective tissue disease.
   Polyarteritis nodosum.
   Primary CNS vasculitis.
   Sarcoidosis.
   Behçet's syndrome.
   Wegener granulomatosis.

II

■ METABOLIC DISEASE ASSOCIATED WITH STROKE

Homocystinuria.
Pseudoxanthoma elasticum.
Fabry disease.
Sulfite oxidase deficiency.
Mitochondrial disorders:
   MELAS.
   Leigh syndrome.
Ornithine transcarbamylase deficiency.

■ INTRACEREBRAL VASCULAR PROCESSES

Ruptured aneurysm.
Arteriovenous malformation.
Fibromuscular dysplasia.
Moyamoya disease.
Migraine headache.
Postsubarachnoid hemorrhage vasospasm.
Hereditary hemorrhagic telangiectasia.
Sturge-Weber syndrome.
Carotid artery dissection.
Post varicella.

■ TRAUMA AND OTHER EXTERNAL CAUSES

Child abuse.
Head trauma/neck trauma.
Oral trauma.
Placental embolism.
ECMO therapy.
(*CNS*, Central nervous system; *ECMO*, extracorporeal membrane oxygenation; *MELAS*, mitochondrial encephalomyopathy, lactic acidosis, and stroke.)

STROKE, YOUNG ADULT, CAUSES[1]

ICD-9CM # 436

Cardiac factors (ASD, MVP, patent foramen ovale).
Inflammatory factors (SLE, polyarteritis nodosa).
Infections (endocarditis, neurosyphilis).
Drugs (cocaine, heroin, oral contraceptives, decongestants).
Arterial dissection.
Hematolic factors (DIC, TTP, deficiency of protein S, protein C, antithrombin III).
Migraine.
Postpartum angiopathy.
Others: premature atherosclerosis, fibromuscular dysplasia.

SUDDEN DEATH, YOUNG ATHLETE

ICD-9CM # CODE VARIES WITH SPECIFIC DIAGNOSIS

Hyperthrophic cardiomyopathy.
Coronary artery anomalies.
Myocarditis.
Ruptured aortic aneurysm (Marfan's syndrome).
Arrhythmias.
Aortic valve stenosis.
Asthma.
Trauma (cerebral, cardiac).
Drug and alcohol abuse.
Heat stroke.
Cardiac sarcoidosis.
Atherosclerotic coronary artery disease.
Dilated cardiomyopathy.

SUDDEN DEATH, PEDIATRIC AGE[4]

ICD-9CM # CODE VARIES WITH SPECIFIC DISORDER

■ SIDS AND SIDS "MIMICS"

SIDS.
Long Q-T syndromes.
Inborn errors of metabolism.
Child abuse.
Myocarditis.
Duct-dependent congenital heart disease.

■ CORRECTED OR UNOPERATED CONGENITAL HEART DISEASE

Aortic stenosis.
Tetralogy of Fallot.
Transposition of great vessels (postoperative atrial switch).
Mitral valve prolapse.
Hypoplastic left heart syndrome.
Eisenmenger's syndrome.

■ CORONARY ARTERIAL DISEASE

Anomalous origin.
Anomalous tract.
Kawasaki disease.
Periarteritis.
Arterial dissection.
Marfan's syndrome.
Myocardial infarction.

■ MYOCARDIAL DISEASE

Myocarditis.
Hypertrophic cardiomyopathy.
Dilated cardiomyopathy.
Arrhythmogenic right ventricular dysplasia.

■ CONDUCTION SYSTEM ABNORMALITY/ARRHYTHMIA

Long Q-T syndromes.
Proarrhythmic drugs.
Preexcitation syndromes.
Heart block.
Commotio cordis.
Idiopathic ventricular fibrillation.
Heart tumor.

■ MISCELLANEOUS

Pulmonary hypertension.
Pulmonary embolism.
Heat stroke.
Cocaine.
Anorexia nervosa.
Electrolyte disturbances.
SIDS, Sudden infant death syndrome.

SWOLLEN LIMB

ICD-9CM # 729.81 SWOLLEN ARM OR HAND
729.81 SWOLLEN LEG OR FOOT

Trauma.
Insect bite.
Abscess.
Lymphedema.
Thrombophlebitis.
Lipoma.
Neurofibroma.
Postphlebitic syndrome.
Myositis ossificans.
Nephrosis, cirrhosis, CHF.

Hypoalbuminemia.
Varicose veins.

TALL STATURE[24]

ICD-9CM # 253.0 GROWTH HORMONE OVERPRODUCTION, GIGANTISM

■ CONSTITUTIONAL (FAMILIAL OR GENETIC)—MOST COMMON CAUSE

■ ENDOCRINE CAUSES

Growth hormone excess—gigantism.
Sexual precocity (tall as children, short as adults):
  True sexual precocity.
  Pseudosexual precocity.
Androgen deficiency:
  Klinefelter's syndrome.
  Bilateral anorchism.

■ GENETIC CAUSES

Klinefelter's syndrome.
Syndromes of XYY, XXYY.

■ MISCELLANEOUS SYNDROMES AND DISORDERS

Cerebral gigantism or Sotos' syndrome: prominent forehead, hypertelorism, high arched palate, dolichocephaly, mental retardation, large hands and feet, and premature eruption of teeth. Large at birth, with most rapid growth in first 4 years of life.
Marfan's syndrome: disorder of mesodermal tissues, subluxation of the lenses, arachnodactyly, and aortic aneurysm.
Homocystinuria: same phenotype as Marfan's syndrome.
Obesity: tall as infants, children, and adolescents.
Total lipodystrophy: large hands and feet, generalized loss of subcutaneous fat, insulin-resistant diabetes mellitus, and hepatomegaly.
Beckwith-Wiedemann syndrome: neonatal tallness, omphalocele, macroglossia, and neonatal hypoglycemia.
Weaver-Smith syndrome: excessive intrauterine growth, mental retardation, megalocephaly, widened bifrontal diameter, hypertelorism, large ears, micrognathia, camptodactyly, broad thumbs, and limited extension of elbows and knees.
Marshall-Smith syndrome: excessive intrauterine growth, mental retardation, blue sclerae, failure to thrive, and early death.

TARDIVE DYSKINESIA[11]

ICD-9CM # 781.3 DYSKINESIA
300.11 HYSTERICAL DYSKINESIA
333.82 OROFACIAL DYSKINESIA
307.9 PSYCHOGENIC DYSKINESIA

■ DIFFERENTIAL DIAGNOSIS:

Medications (antidepressants, anticholinergics, amphetamines, lithium, L-Dopa, phenytoin).
Brain neoplasms.
Ill-fitting dentures.
Huntington's disease.
Idiopathic dystonias (tics, blepharospasm, aging).
Wilson's disease.
Extrapyramidal syndrome (postanoxic or postencephalitic).
Torsion dystonia.

TASTE AND SMELL LOSS[1]

ICD-9CM # 781.1 SMELL AND TASTE DISTURBANCE OF SENSATION

■ TASTE

Local: radiation therapy.
Systemic: cancer, renal failure, hepatic failure, nutritional deficiency (vitamin B_{12}, zinc), Cushing's syndrome, hypothyroidism, DM, infection (influenza), drugs (antirheumatic and antiproliferative).
Neurologic: Bell's palsy, familial dysautonomia, multiple sclerosis.

■ SMELL

Local: allergic rhinitis, sinusitis, nasal polyposis, bronchial asthma.
Systemic: renal failure, hepatic failure, nutritional deficiency (vitamin B_{12}), Cushing's syndrome, hypothyroidism, DM, infection (viral hepatitis, influenza), drugs (nasal sprays, antibiotics).
Neurologic: head trauma, multiple sclerosis, Parkinson's disease, frontal brain tumor.

TELANGIECTASIA

ICD-9CM # 448.9

Oral contraceptive agents.
Pregnancy.
Rosacea.
Varicose veins.
Trauma.
Drug induced (corticosteroids, systemic or topical).
Spider telangiectases.
Hepatic cirrhosis.
Mastocytosis.
SLE, dermatomyositis, systemic sclerosis.

TENDINOPATHY[23]

ICD-9CM # 727.9

■ INTRINSIC FACTORS
Anatomic factors
Malalignment.
Muscle weakness or imbalance.
Muscle inflexibility.
Decreased vascularity.
Systemic factors
Inflammatory conditions (e.g., SLE).
Pregnancy.
Quinolone-induced tendinopathy.
Age-related factors
Tendon degeneration.
Increased tendon stiffness.
Tendon calcification.
Decreased vascularity.

■ EXTRINSIC FACTORS
Repetitive mechanical load
Excessive duration.
Excessive frequency.
Excessive intensity.
Poor technique.
Workplace factors.
Equipment problems
Footwear.
Athletic field surface.
Equipment factors (e.g., racquet size).
Protective gear.

II

TESTICULAR FAILURE[9]

ICD-9CM # 257.1 TESTICULAR FAILURE

■ PRIMARY
Klinefelter's syndrome (XXY).
XYY.
Vanishing testes syndrome (in utero or early postnatal torsion).
Noonan's syndrome.
Varicocele.
Myotonic dystrophy.
Orchitis (mumps, gonorrhea).
Cryptorchidism.
Chemical exposure.
Irradiation to testes.
Spinal cord injury.
Polyglandular failure.
Idiopathic oligospermia or azoospermia.
Germinal cell aplasia (Sertoli cell–only syndrome).
Idiopathic testicular failure.
Testicular torsion.
Testicular trauma.
Diethylstilbestrol (maternal use during pregnancy resulting in in utero estrogen exposure).
Testicular tumor with subsequent irradiation therapy, chemotherapy, or surgery (retroperitoneal lymph node dissection or orchiectomy).

■ SECONDARY
Delayed puberty.
Kallmann's syndrome.
Isolated gonadotropin deficiency.
Prader-Labhart-Willi syndrome.
Lawrence-Moon-Biedl syndrome.
Central nervous system irradiation.
Prepubertal panhypopituitarism.
Postpubertal panhypopituitarism.
Hypogonadism secondary to hyperprolactinemia.
Adrenogenital syndrome.
Chronic liver disease.
Chronic renal failure/uremia.
Hemochromatosis.
Cushing's syndrome.
Malnutrition.
Massive obesity.
Sickle cell anemia.
Hyper/hypothyroidism.
Anabolic steroid use.

TESTICULAR PAIN

ICD-9CM # 608.9

Testicular torsion.
Trauma.
Epididymitis.
Orchitis.
Neoplasm.
Urolithiasis.
Inguinal hernia.
Infection (cellulitis, abscess, folliculitis).
Anxiety.

TESTICULAR SIZE VARIATIONS[9]

ICD-9CM # 608.3 TESTICULAR ATROPHY
608.89 TESTICULAR MASS
257.2 HYPOGONADISM

■ SMALL TESTES
Hypothalamic-pituitary dysfunction.
Gonadotropin deficiency.
Growth hormone deficiency.
Normal variant.
Primary hypogonadism.
Autoimmune destruction, chemotherapy, cryptorchidism, irradiation, Klinefelter's syndrome, orchiditis, testicular regression syndrome, torsion, trauma.

■ LARGE TESTES
Adrenal rest tissue.
Compensatory.
Fragile X syndrome.
Idiopathic.
Tumor.

TETANUS[23]

ICD-9CM # 037

Acute abdomen.
Black widow spider bite.
Dental abscess.
Dislocated mandible.
Dystonic reaction.
Encephalitis.
Head trauma.
Hyperventilation syndrome.
Hypocalcemia.
Meningitis.
Peritonsillar abscess.
Progressive fluctuating muscular rigidity (stiff-man syndrome).
Psychogenic.
Rabies.
Sepsis.
Subarachnoid hemorrhage.
Status epilepticus.
Strychnine poisoning.
Temporomandibular joint syndrome.

THROMBOCYTOPENIA

ICD-9CM # 287.3 CONGENITAL OR PRIMARY
287.4 SECONDARY
287.5 THROMBOCYTOPENIA NOS

■ INCREASED DESTRUCTION
Immunologic
Drugs: quinine, quinidine, digitalis, procainamide, thiazide diuretics, sulfonamides, phenytoin, aspirin, penicillin, heparin, gold, meprobamate, sulfa drugs, phenylbutazone, nonsteroidal antiinflammatory drugs (NSAIDs), methyldopa, cimetidine, furosemide, INH, cephalosporins, chlorpropamide, organic arsenicals, chloroquine, platelet glycoprotein IIb/IIIa receptor inhibitors, ranitidine, indomethacin, carboplatin, ticlopidine, clopidogrel.
Idiopathic thrombocytopenic purpura (ITP).
Transfusion reaction: transfusion of platelets with plasminogen activator (PLA) in recipients without PLA-1.
Fetal/maternal incompatibility.

Collagen vascular diseases (e.g., systemic lupus erythematosus [SLE]).
Autoimmune hemolytic anemia.
Lymphoreticular disorders (e.g., CLL).
Nonimmunologic
Prosthetic heart valves.
Thrombotic thrombocytopenic purpura (TTP).
Sepsis.
DIC.
Hemolytic-uremic syndrome (HUS).
Giant cavernous hemangioma.

■ DECREASED PRODUCTION
(1) Abnormal marrow.
(2) Marrow infiltration (e.g., leukemia, lymphoma, fibrosis).
(3) Marrow suppression (e.g., chemotherapy, alcohol, radiation).
(4) Hereditary disorders.
(5) Wiskott-Aldrich syndrome: X-linked disorder characterized by thrombocytopenia, eczema, and repeated infections.
(6) May-Hegglin anomaly: increased megakaryocytes but ineffective thrombopoiesis.
(7) Vitamin deficiencies (e.g., vitamin B_{12}, folic acid).

■ SPLENIC SEQUESTRATION, HYPERSPLENISM

■ DILUTIONAL, AS A RESULT OF MASSIVE TRANSFUSION

THROMBOCYTOSIS

ICD-9CM # 289.9 THROMBOCYTOSIS, ESSENTIAL

Iron deficiency.
Posthemorrhage.
Neoplasms (GI tract).
CML.
Polycythemia vera.
Myelofibrosis with myeloid metaplasia.
Infections.
After splenectomy.
Postpartum.
Hemophilia.
Pancreatitis.
Cirrhosis.
Idiopathic.

TICK-RELATED INFECTIONS

ICD-9CM # 082.0 ROCKY MOUNTAIN SPOTTED FEVER
066.1 COLORADO TICK FEVER
088.82 BABESIOSIS
082.8 EHRLICHIOSIS
088.81 LYME DISEASE

Lyme disease.
Rocky Mountain spotted fever.
Babesiosis.
Tularemia.
Q Fever.
Colorado tick fever.
Ehrlichiosis.
Relapsing fever.

TORSADES DE POINTES[19]

ICD-9CM # CODE NOT AVAILABLE

Antiarrhythmics known to increase the QT interval (e.g., quinidine, procainamide, amiodarone, disopyramide, sotalol).
Tricyclic antidepressants and phenothiazines.
Histamine (H1) antagonists (e.g., astemizole, terfenadine).
Antiviral and antifungal agents and antibiotics.
Hypokinemia.
Hypomagnesemia.
Insecticide poisoning.
Bradyarrhythmias.
Congenital long QT syndrome.
Subarachnoid hemorrhage.
Chloroquinine, pentamidine.
Cocaine abuse.

TREMOR

ICD-9CM # 781.0 TREMOR NOS
333.1 BENIGN ESSENTIAL TREMOR
333.1 FAMILIAL TREMOR

■ TREMOR PRESENT AT REST
Parkinsonism.
CNS neoplasms.
Tardive dyskinesia.

■ POSTURAL TREMOR (PRESENT DURING MAINTENANCE OF A POSTURE)
Essential senile tremor.

■ ACTION TREMOR (PRESENT WITH MOVEMENT)
Anxiety.
Medications (bronchodilators, caffeine, corticosteroids, lithium, etc.).
Endocrine disorders (hyperthyroidism, pheochromocytoma, carcinoid).
Withdrawal from substance abuse.

URETHRAL DISCHARGE AND DYSURIA

ICD-9CM # 788.7 URETHRAL DISCHARGE
599.9 URETHRAL DISCHARGE BLOODY
788.1 DYSURIA

Urethritis (gonococcal, chlamydial, trichomonal).
Cystitis.
Prostatitis.
Vaginitis (candidiasis, chemical).
Meatal stenosis.
Interstitial cystitis.
Trauma (foreign body, masturbation, horseback or bike riding).

URINARY RETENTION, ACUTE

ICD-9CM # 788.20

Mechanical obstruction: urethral stone, foreign body, urethral stricture, BPH, prostate carcinoma, prostatitis, trauma with hematoma formation).
Neurogenic bladder.
Neurologic disease (MS, parkinsonism, tabes dorsalis, CVA).
Spinal cord injury.
CNS neoplasm (primary or metastatic).
Spinal anesthesia.

II

Lower urinary tract instrumentation.
Medications (antihistamines, antidepressants, narcotics, anticholinergics).
Abdominal or pelvic surgery.
Alcohol toxicity.
Pregnancy.
Anxiety.
Encephalitis.
Postoperative pain.
Encephalitis.
Spina bifida occulta.

URINE, RED[26]

ICD-9CM # CODE VARIES WITH SPECIFIC DIAGNOSIS

■ WITH A POSITIVE DIPSTICK
Hematuria.
Hemoglobinuria: negative urinalysis.
Myoglobinuria: negative urinalysis.

■ WITH A NEGATIVE DIPSTICK
Drugs
Aminosalicylic acid.
Deferoxamine mesylate.
Ibuprofen.
Phenacetin.
Phenolphthalein.
Phensuximide.
Rifampin.
Anthraquinone laxatives.
Doxorubicin.
Methyldopa.
Phenazopyridine.
Phenothiazine.
Phenytoin.
Dyes
Azo dyes.
Eosin.
Foods
Beets, berries, maize.
Rhodamine B.
Metabolic
Porphyrins.
Serratia marcescens (red diaper syndrome).
Urate crystalluria.

UROPATHY, OBSTRUCTIVE[33]

ICD-9CM # 599.6

■ INTRINSIC CAUSES
Intraluminal
Intratubular deposition of crystals (uric acid, sulfas).
Stones.
Papillary tissue.
Blood clots.
Intramural
Functional.
Ureter (ureteropelvic or ureterovesical dysfunction).
Bladder (neurogenic): spinal cord defect or trauma, diabetes, multiple sclerosis, Parkinson's disease, cerebrovascular accidents.
Bladder neck dysfunction.
Anatomic
Tumors.
Infection, granuloma.
Strictures.

■ EXTRINSIC CAUSES
Originating in the reproductive system
Prostate: benign hypertrophy or cancer.
Uterus: pregnancy, tumors, prolapse, endometriosis.
Ovary: abscess, tumor, cysts.
Originating in the vascular system
Aneurysms (aorta, iliac vessels).
Aberrant arteries (ureteropelvic junction).
Venous (ovarian veins, retrocaval ureter).
Originating in the gastrointestinal tract: Crohn's disease, pancreatitis, appendicitis, tumors
Originating in the retroperitoneal space
Inflammations.
Fibrosis.
Tumor, hematomas.

UTERINE BLEEDING, ABNORMAL[10]

ICD-9CM # 626.9

■ PREGNANCY
Threatened abortion.
Incomplete abortion.
Complete abortion.
Molar pregnancy.
Ectopic pregnancy.
Retained products of conception.

■ OVULATORY
Vulva: infection, laceration, tumor.
Vagina: infection, laceration, tumor, foreign body.
Cervix: polyps, cervical erosion, cervicitis, carcinoma.
Uterus: fibroids (submucous fibroids most likely to cause abnormal bleeding), polyps, adenomyosis, endometritis, intrauterine device, atrophic endometrium.
Pregnancy complications: ectopic pregnancy; threatened, incomplete, complete abortion; retained products of conception.
Abnormality of clotting system.
Midcycle bleeding.
Halban's disease (persistent corpus luteum).
Menorrhagia.
Pelvic inflammatory disease.

■ ANOVULATORY
Physiologic causes:
    Puberty.
    Perimenopausal.
Pathologic causes:
    Ovarian failure (FSH over 40 IU/ml).
    Hyperandrogenism.
    Hyperprolactinemia.
    Obesity.
    Hypothalamic dysfunction (polycystic ovaries); LH/FSH ratio greater than 2 to 1.
    Hyperplasia.
    Endometrial carcinoma.
    Estrogen-producing tumors.
    Hypothyroidism.

VAGINAL BLEEDING, PREGNANCY[7]

ICD-9CM # 626.6 IRREGULAR VAGINAL BLEEDING

■ FIRST TRIMESTER
Implantation bleeding.
Abortion.
Threatened.
Complete.

Incomplete.
Missed.
Ectopic pregnancy.
Neoplasia.
Hydatidiform mole.
Cervix.

■ THIRD TRIMESTER
Placenta previa.
Placental abruption.
Premature labor.
Choriocarcinoma.

VAGINAL DISCHARGE, PREPUBERTAL GIRLS[17]

ICD-9CM # 623.5 VAGINAL DISCHARGE

Irritative (bubble baths, sand).
Poor perineal hygiene.
Foreign body.
Associated systemic illness (group A streptococci, chicken-
   pox).
Infections.
Escherichia coli with foreign body.
Shigella organisms.
Yersinia organisms.
Infections (consider sexual abuse).
Chlamydia trachomatis.
Neisseria gonorrhoeae.
Trichomonas vaginalis.
Tumor (rare).

VASCULITIS, CLASSIFICATION[23]

ICD-9CM # 447.6

■ LARGE VESSEL DISEASE
Arteritis
Giant cell arteritis.
Takayasu's arteritis.
Arteritis associated with Reiter's syndrome, ankylosing
   spondylitis.

■ MEDIUM AND SMALL VESSEL DISEASE
Polyarteritis nodosa
Primary (idiopathic).
Associated with viruses (Hepatitis B or C, CMV, HIV, herpes
   zoster).
Associated with malignancy (hairy cell leukemia).
Familial Mediterranean fever.
Granulomatous vasculitis
Wegener's granulomatosis.
Lymphomatoid granulomatosis.
Behçet's disease
Kawasaki disease (mucocutaneous lymph node syndrome)

■ PREDOMINANTLY SMALL VESSEL DISEASE
Hypersensitivity vasculitis (leukocytoclastic vasculitis)
Henoch-Schönlein purpura.
Mixed cryoglobulinemia.
Serum sickness.
Vasculitis associated with connective tissue diseases (SLE,
   Sjögren's syndrome).
Vasculitis associated with specific syndromes:
   Primary biliary cirrhosis.
   Lyme disease.
   Chronic active hepatitis.
   Drug-induced vasculitis.

Churg-Strauss syndrome
Goodpasture syndrome
Erythema nodosum
Panniculitis
Buerger's disease (thrombophlebitis obliterans)

VASCULITIS[25]

DISEASES THAT MIMIC VASCULITIS

ICD-9CM # VARIES WITH SPECIFIC DISEASE

■ EMBOLIC DISEASE
Infectious or marantic endocarditis.
Cardiac mural thrombus.
Atrial myxoma.
Cholesterol embolization syndrome.

■ NONINFLAMMATORY VESSEL WALL DISRUPTION
Atherosclerosis.
Arterial fibromuscular dysplasia.
Drug effects (vasoconstrictors, anticoagulants).
Radiation.
Genetic disease (neurofibromatosis, Ehlers-Danlos syn-
   drome).
Amyloidosis.
Intravascular malignant lymphoma.

■ DIFFUSE COAGULATION
Disseminated intravascular coagulation.
Thrombotic thrombocytopenic purpura.
Hemolytic-uremic syndrome.
Protein C and S deficiencies, factor V/Leiden mutation.
Antiphospholipid syndrome.

VENTRICULAR FAILURE

ICD-9CM # 429.9 VENTRICULAR DYSFUNCTION

■ LEFT VENTRICULAR FAILURE
Systemic hypertension.
Valvular heart disease (AS, AR, MR).
Cardiomyopathy, myocarditis.
Bacterial endocarditis.
Myocardial infarction.
Idiopathic hypertrophic subaortic stenosis.

■ RIGHT VENTRICULAR FAILURE
Valvular heart disease (mitral stenosis).
Pulmonary hypertension.
Bacterial endocarditis (right-sided).
Right ventricular infarction.

■ BIVENTRICULAR FAILURE
Left ventricular failure.
Cardiomyopathy.
Myocarditis
Arrhythmias.
Anemia.
Thyrotoxicosis.
Arteriovenous fistula.
Paget's disease.
Beri-beri.

VERTIGO

> ICD-9CM # 780.4 VERTIGO NOS
> 386.11 BENIGN PAROXYSMAL POSITIONAL
> 386.2 CENTRAL ORIGIN
> 386.10 PERIPHERAL
> 386.12 VESTIBULAR (NEURONITIS)

■ PERIPHERAL
Otitis media.
Acute labyrinthitis.
Vestibular neuronitis.
Benign positional vertigo.
Meniere's disease.
Ototoxic drugs: streptomycin, gentamicin.
Lesions of the eighth nerve: acoustic neuroma, meningioma, mononeuropathy, metastatic carcinoma.
Mastoiditis.

■ CNS OR SYSTEMIC
Vertebrobasilar artery insufficiency.
Posterior fossa tumor or other brain tumors.
Infarction/hemorrhage of cerebral cortex, cerebellum, or brainstem.
Basilar migraine.
Metabolic: drugs, hypoxia, anemia, fever.
Hypotension/severe hypertension.
Multiple sclerosis.
CNS infections: viral, bacterial.
Temporal lobe epilepsy.
Arnold-Chiari malformation, syringobulbia.
Psychogenic: ventilation, hysteria.

VISION LOSS, ACUTE, PAINFUL

> ICD-9CM # 368.11 VISION LOSS, SUDDEN

Acute angle-closure glaucoma.
Corneal ulcer.
Uveitis.
Endophthalmitis.
Factitious.
Somatization syndrome.
Trauma.

VISION LOSS, ACUTE, PAINLESS

> ICD-9CM # 368.11 VISION LOSS, SUDDEN

Retinal artery occlusion.
Optic neuritis.
Retinal vein occlusion.
Vitreous hemorrhage.
Retinal detachment.
Exudative macular degeneration.
CVA.
Ischemic optic neuropathy.
Factitious.
Somatization syndrome, anxiety reaction.

VISION LOSS, CHRONIC, PROGRESSIVE

> ICD-9CM # 369.9 VISION LOSS NOS

Cataract.
Macular degeneration.
Cerebral neoplasm.
Refractive error.
Open-angle glaucoma.

VOCAL CORD PARALYSIS

> ICD-9CM # 478.30 UNSPECIFIED
> 478.31 UNILATERAL PARTIAL
> 478.32 UNILATERAL COMPLETE
> 478.33 BILATERAL PARTIAL
> 478.34 BILATERAL COMPLETE

Neoplasm: primary or metastatic (e.g,. lung, thyroid, parathyroid, mediastinum).
Neck surgery (parathyroid, thyroid, carotid endarterectomy, cervical spine).
Idiopathic.
Viral, bacterial, or fungal infection.
Trauma (intubation, penetrating neck injury).
Cardiac surgery.
Rheumatoid arthritis.
Multiple sclerosis.
Parkinsonism.
Toxic neuropathy.
CVA.
CNS abnormalities: hydrocephalus, Arnold-Chiari malformation, meningomyelocele.

VOLUME DEPLETION[1]

> ICD-9CM # 276.5

Gastrointestinal losses:
  Upper: bleeding, nasogastric suction, vomiting.
  Lower: bleeding, diarrhea, enteric or pancreatic fistula, tube drainage.
Renal losses:
  Salt and water: diuretics, osmotic diuresis, postobstructive diuresis, acute tubular necrosis (recovery phase), salt-losing nephropathy, adrenal insufficiency, renal tubular acidosis.
Water loss: diabetes insipidus.
Skin and respiratory losses:
  Sweat, burns, insensible losses.
Sequestration without external fluid loss:
  Intestinal obstruction, peritonitis, pancreatitis, rhabdomyolysis, internal bleeding.

VOLUME EXCESS[1]

> ICD-9CM # CODE VARIES WITH SPECIFIC DIAGNOSIS

■ PRIMARY RENAL SODIUM RETENTION (INCREASED EFFECTIVE CIRCULATING VOLUME)
Renal failure, nephritic syndrome, acute glomerulonephritis.
Primary hyperaldosteronism.
Cushing syndrome.
Liver disease.

■ SECONDARY RENAL SODIUM RETENTION (DECREASED EFFECTIVE CIRCULATING VOLUME)
Heart failure.
Liver disease.
Nephrotic syndrome (minimal change disease).
Pregnancy.

VOMITING

> ICD-9CM # 787.03

GI disturbances:
Obstruction: esophageal, pyloric, intestinal.

Infections: viral or bacterial enteritis, viral hepatitis, food poisoning, gastroenteritis

Pancreatitis.

Appendicitis.

Biliary colic.

Peritonitis.

Perforated bowel.

Diabetic gastroparesis.

Other: gastritis, PUD, IBD, GI tract neoplasms.

Drugs: morphine, digitalis, cytotoxic agents, bromocriptine.

Severe pain: MI, renal colic.

Metabolic disorders: uremia, acidosis/alkalosis, hyperglycemia, DKA, thyrotoxicosis.

Trauma: blows to the testicles, epigastrium.

Vertigo.

Reye's syndrome.

Increased intracranial pressure.

CNS disturbances: trauma, hemorrhage, infarction, neoplasm, infection, hypertensive encephalopathy, migraine.

Radiation sickness.

Nausea and vomiting of pregnancy, hyperemesis gravidarum

Motion sickness.

Bulimia, anorexia nervosa.

Psychogenic: emotional disturbances, offensive sights or smells.

Severe coughing.

Pyelonephritis.

Boerhaave's syndrome

Carbon monoxide poisoning

VULVAR LESIONS[10]

ICD-9CM #		
625.8	VULVAR MASS
098.0	VULVAR ULCER, GONOCOCCAL
091.0	VULVAR ULCER, SYPHILITIC
616.51	BEHÇET'S
624.0	LEUKOPLAKIA
624.8	DYSPLASIA
233.3	CARCINOMA
616.9	INFLAMMATORY LESION
624.4	VULVAR SCAR (OLD)
624.1	VULVAR ATROPHY

■ RED LESION

Infection/infestation

Fungal infection:

Candida.

Tinea cruris.

Intertrigo.

Pityriasis versicolor.

Sarcoptes scabiei.

Erythrasma: *Corynebacterium minutissimum.*

Granuloma inguinale: *Calymmatobacterium granulomatis.*

Folliculitis: *Staphylococcus aureus.*

Hidradenitis suppurativa.

Behçet's syndrome.

Inflammation

Reactive vulvitis.

Chemical irritation:

Detergent.

Dyes.

Perfume.

Spermicide.

Lubricants.

Hygiene sprays.

Podophyllum.

Topical 5-FU.

Saliva.

Gentian violet.

Semen.

Mechanical trauma: scratching.

Vestibular adenitis.

Essential vulvodynia.

Psoriasis.

Seborrheic dermatitis.

Neoplasm

Vulvar intraepithelial neoplasia (VIN):

Mild dysplasia.

Moderate dysplasia.

Severe dysplasia.

Carcinoma-in-situ.

Vulvar dystrophy.

Bowen's disease.

Invasive cancer:

Squamous cell carcinoma.

Malignant melanoma.

Sarcoma.

Basal cell carcinoma.

Adenocarcinoma.

Paget's disease.

Undifferentiated.

■ WHITE LESION

Vulvar dystrophy:

Lichen sclerosus.

Vulvar dystrophy.

Vulvar hyperplasia.

Mixed dystrophy.

VIN.

Vitiligo.

Partial albinism.

Intertrigo.

Radiation treatment.

■ DARK LESION

Lentigo.

Nevi (mole).

Neoplasm (see Neoplasm, Vulvar, below).

Reactive hyperpigmentation.

Seborrheic keratosis.

Pubic lice.

■ ULCERATIVE LESION

Infection

Herpes simplex.

Vaccinia.

Treponema pallidum.

Granuloma inguinale.

Pyoderma.

Tuberculosis.

Noninfection

Behçet's disease.

Crohn's disease.

Pemphigus.

Pemphigoid.

Hidradenitis suppurativa (see Neoplasm, Vulvar, below).

Neoplasm

Basal cell carcinoma.

Squamous cell carcinoma.

Vulvar tumor <1 cm:

Condyloma acuminatum.

Molluscum contagiosum.

Epidermal inclusion.

Vestibular cyst.

Mesenephric duct.

VIN.

Hemangioma.

Hidradenoma.

Neurofibroma.

Syringoma.

Accessory breast tissue.

Acrochordon.
Endometriosis.
Fox-Fordyce disease.
Pilonidal sinus.
Vulvar tumor >1 cm:
  Bartholin cyst or abscess.
  Lymphogranuloma venereum.
  Fibroma.
  Lipoma.
  Verrucous carcinoma.
  Squamous cell carcinoma.
  Hernia.
  Edema.
  Hematoma.
  Acrochordon.
  Epidermal cysts.
  Neurofibromatosis.
  Accessory breast tissue.

WEAKNESS, ACUTE, EMERGENT[23]

ICD-9CM # 780.7

Demyelinating disorders (Guillain-Barré, chronic inflammatory demyelinating polyneuropathy [CIDP]).
Myasthenia gravis.
Infectious (poliomyelitis, diphtheria).
Toxic (botulism, tick paralysis, paralytic shellfish toxin, puffer fish, newts).
Metabolic (acquired or familial hypokalemia, hypophosphatemia, hypermagnesemia).
Metals poisoning (arsenic, thallium).
Porphyria.

WEIGHT GAIN

ICD-9CM # 783.1 ABNORMAL WEIGHT GAIN
278.00 OBESITY

Sedentary lifestyle.
Fluid overload.
Discontinuation of tobacco abuse.
Endocrine disorders (hypothyroidism, hyperinsulinism associated with maturity-onset DM, Cushing's syndrome, hypogonadism, insulinoma, hyperprolactinemia, acromegaly).
Medications (nutritional supplements, oral contraceptives, glucocorticoids, etc.).
Anxiety disorders with compulsive eating.
Laurence-Moon-Biedl syndrome, Prader-Willi syndrome, other congenital diseases.
Hypothalamic injury (rare; <100 cases reported in medical literature).

WEIGHT LOSS

ICD-9CM # 783.2 ABNORMAL WEIGHT LOSS

Malignancy.
Psychiatric disorders (depression, anorexia nervosa).
New-onset DM.
Malabsorption.
COPD.
AIDS.
Uremia, liver disease.
Thyrotoxicosis, pheochromocytoma, carcinoid syndrome.
Addison's disease.
Intestinal parasites.
Peptic ulcer disease.
Inflammatory bowel disease.
Food faddism.
Postgastrectomy syndrome.

WHEEZING

ICD-9CM # 786.09

Asthma.
COPD.
Interstitial lung disease.
Infections (pneumonia, bronchitis, bronchiolitis, epiglottitis).
Cardiac asthma.
GERD with aspiration.
Foreign body aspiration.
Pulmonary embolism.
Anaphylaxis.
Obstruction airway (neoplasm, goiter, edema or hemorrhage from trauma, aneurysm, congenital abnormalities, strictures, spasm).
Carcinoid syndrome.

WHEEZING, PEDIATRIC AGE[4]

ICD-9CM # 786.09 WHEEZING

Reactive airways disease.
Atopic asthma.
Infection-associated airway reactivity.
Exercise-induced asthma.
Salicylate-induced asthma and nasal polyposis.
Asthmatic bronchitis.
Other hypersensitivity reactions:
  Hypersensitivity pneumonitis.
  Tropical eosinophilia.
  Visceral larva migrans.
  Allergic bronchopulmonary aspergillosis.
Aspiration:
  Foreign body.
  Food, saliva, gastric contents.
  Laryngotracheoesophageal cleft.
  Tracheoesophageal fistula, H-type.
  Pharyngeal incoordination or neuromuscular weakness.
Cystic fibrosis.
Primary ciliary dyskinesia.
Cardiac failure.
Bronchiolitis obliterans.
Extrinsic compression of airways:
  Vascular ring.
  Enlarged lymph node.
  Mediastinal tumor.
  Lung cysts.
Tracheobronchomalacia.
Endobronchial masses.
Gastroesophageal reflux.
Pulmonary hemosiderosis.
Sequelae of bronchopulmonary dysplasia.
"Hysterical" glottic closure.
Cigarette smoke, other environmental insults.

XEROPHTHALMIA[25]

ICD-9CM # 372.53 XEROPHTHALMIA

Medications
Tricyclic antidepressants: amitriptyline (Elavil), doxepin (Sinequan).
Antihistamines: diphenhydramine (Benadryl), chlorpheniramine (Chlor-Trimeton), promethazine (Phenergan), and many cold and decongestant preparations.

Anticholinergic agents: antiemetics such as scopolamine, antispasmodic agents such as oxybutynin chloride (Ditropan).

Abnormalities of eyelid function
Neuromuscular disorders.
Aging.
Thyrotoxicosis.

Abnormalities of tear production
Hypovitaminosis A.
Stevens-Johnson syndrome.
Familial diseases affecting sebaceous secretions.

Abnormalities of corneal surfaces
Scarring from past injuries and herpes simplex infection.

XEROSTOMIA[25]

ICD-9CM # 527.7

Medications
Tricyclic antidepressants: amitriptyline (Elavil), doxepin (Sinequan).
Antihistamines: diphenhydramine (Benadryl), chlorpheniramine (Chlor-Trimeton), promethazine (Phenergan), and many cold and decongestant preparations.
Anticholinergic agents: antiemetics such as scopolamine, antispasmodic agents such as oxybutynin chloride (Ditropan).

Dehydration
Debility.
Fever.

Polyuria
Alcohol intake.
Arrhythmia.
Diabetes.

Previous head and neck irradiation

Systemic diseases
Sjögren's syndrome.
Sarcoidosis.
Amyloidosis.
Human immunodeficiency virus (HIV) infection.
Graft-vs.-host disease.

REFERENCES

1. Andreoli TE, editor: *Cecil essentials of medicine,* ed 5, Philadelphia, 2001, WB Saunders.
2. Barkin RM, Rosen P: *Emergency pediatrics: a guide to ambulatory care,* ed 5, St Louis, 1998, Mosby.
3. Baude AI: *Infectious diseases and medical microbiology,* ed 2, Philadelphia, 1986, WB Saunders.
4. Behrman RE: *Nelson textbook of pediatrics,* ed 16, Philadelphia, 2000, WB Saunders.
5. Callen JP: *Color atlas of dermatology,* ed 2, Philadelphia, 2000, WB Saunders.
6. Canoso J: *Rheumatology in primary care,* Philadelphia, 1997, WB Saunders.
7. Carlson KJ: *Primary care of women,* ed 2, St Louis, 2000, Mosby.
8. Conn R: *Current diagnosis,* ed 9, Philadelphia, 1997, WB Saunders.
9. Copeland LJ: *Textbook of gynecology,* ed 2, Philadelphia, 2000, WB Saunders.
10. Danakas G, editor: *Practical guide to the care of the gynecologic/obstetric patient,* St Louis, 1997, Mosby.
11. Goldberg RJ: *The care of the psychiatric patient,* ed 2, St Louis, 1998, Mosby.
12. Goldman L, Bennet JC: *Cecil textbook of medicine,* ed 21, Philadelphia, 2000, WB Saunders.
13. Goldman L, Braunwauld E, editors: *Primary cardiology,* Philadelphia, 1998, WB Saunders.
14. Gorbach SL: *Infectious diseases,* ed 2, Philadelphia, 1998, WB Saunders.
15. Harrington J: *Consultation in internal medicine,* ed 2, St Louis, 1997, Mosby.
16. Henry JB: *Clinical diagnosis and management by laboratory methods,* ed 20, Philadelphia, 2001, WB Saunders.
17. Hoekelman R: *Primary pediatric care,* ed 3, St Louis, 1997, Mosby.
18. Kassirer J, editor: *Current therapy in adult medicine,* ed 4, St Louis, 1998, Mosby.
19. Khan MG: *Rapid ECG interpretation,* Philadelphia, 2003, WB Saunders.
20. Kliegman R: *Practical strategies in pediatric diagnosis and therapy,* Philadelphia, 1996, WB Saunders.
21. Klippel J, editor: *Practical rheumatology,* London, 1995, Mosby.
22. Mandell GL: *Mandell, Douglas, and Bennett's principles and practice of infectious diseases,* ed 5, New York, 2000, Churchill Livingstone.
23. Marx J, editor: *Rosen's emergency medicine: concepts and clinical practice,* ed. 5, St Louis, 2002, Mosby.
24. Moore WT, Eastman RC: *Diagnostic endocrinology,* ed 2, St Louis, 1996, Mosby.
25. Noble J, editor: *Primary care medicine,* ed 3, St Louis, 2001, Mosby.
26. Nseyo UO: *Urology for primary care physicians,* Philadelphia, 1999, WB Saunders.
27. Palay D, editor: *Ophthalmology for the primary care physician,* St Louis, 1997, Mosby.
28. Rakel RE: *Principles of family practice,* ed 6, Philadelphia, 2002, WB Saunders.
29. Schwarz MI: *Interstitial lung disease,* ed 2, St Louis, 1993, Mosby.
30. Seller RH: *Differential diagnosis of common complaints,* ed 4, Philadelphia, 2000, WB Saunders.
31. Siedel HM, editor: *Mosby's guide to physical examination,* ed 4, St Louis, 1999, Mosby.
32. Specht N: *Practical guide to diagnostic imaging,* St Louis, 1998, Mosby.
33. Stein JH, editor: *Internal medicine,* ed 5, St Louis, 1998, Mosby.
34. Swain R, Snodgrass: *Phys Sportmed* 23:56, 1995.
35. Wiederholt WC: *Neurology for non-neurologists,* ed 4, Philadelphia, 2000, WB Saunders.
36. Wilson JD: *Williams textbook of endocrinology,* ed 9, Philadelphia, 1998, WB Saunders.

II

Clinical Algorithms

PLEASE NOTE: These algorithms are designed to assist clinicians in the evaluation and treatment of patients. They may not apply to all patients with a particular condition and are not intended to replace a clinician's individual judgment.

ABUSE, CHILD

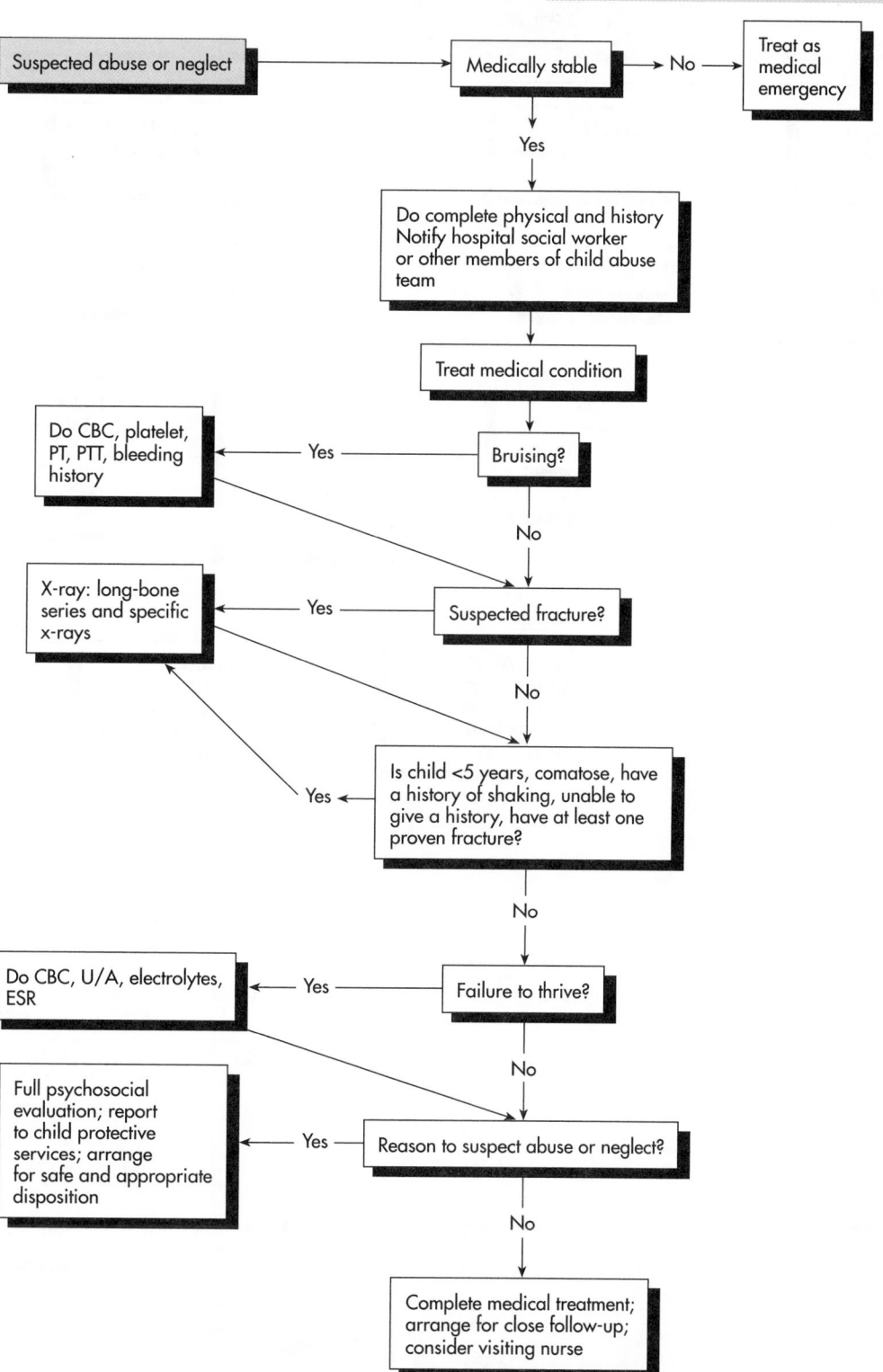

Fig. 3-1   Management of suspected child abuse. *CBC,* Complete blood count; *ESR,* erythrocyte sedimentation rate; *PT,* prothrombin time; *PTT,* partial thromboplastin time; *U/A,* urinalysis. (From Marx J [ed]: *Rosen's emergency medicine,* ed 5, St Louis, 2002, Mosby.)

ACETAMINOPHEN INGESTION

Acetaminophen ingestion
ICD-9CM # 965.4 Acetaminophen poisoning

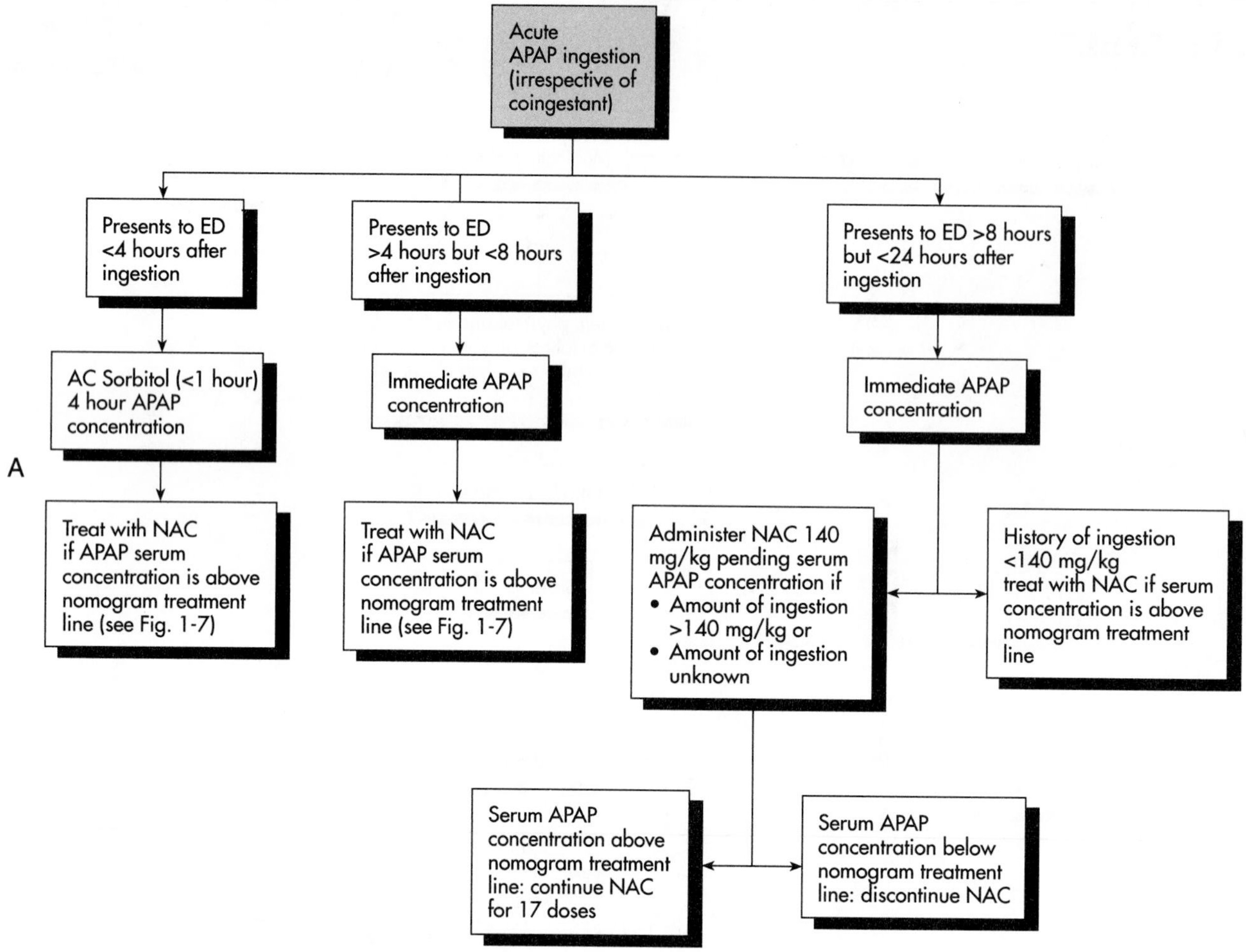

Acute APAP ingestion (irrespective of coingestant)
Presents to ED <4 hours after ingestion
Presents to ED >4 hours but <8 hours after ingestion
Presents to ED >8 hours but <24 hours after ingestion
AC Sorbitol (<1 hour) 4 hour APAP concentration
Immediate APAP concentration
Immediate APAP concentration
A
Treat with NAC if APAP serum concentration is above nomogram treatment line (see Fig. 1-7)
Treat with NAC if APAP serum concentration is above nomogram treatment line (see Fig. 1-7)
Administer NAC 140 mg/kg pending serum APAP concentration if
• Amount of ingestion >140 mg/kg or
• Amount of ingestion unknown
History of ingestion <140 mg/kg treat with NAC if serum concentration is above nomogram treatment line
Serum APAP concentration above nomogram treatment line: continue NAC for 17 doses
Serum APAP concentration below nomogram treatment line: discontinue NAC

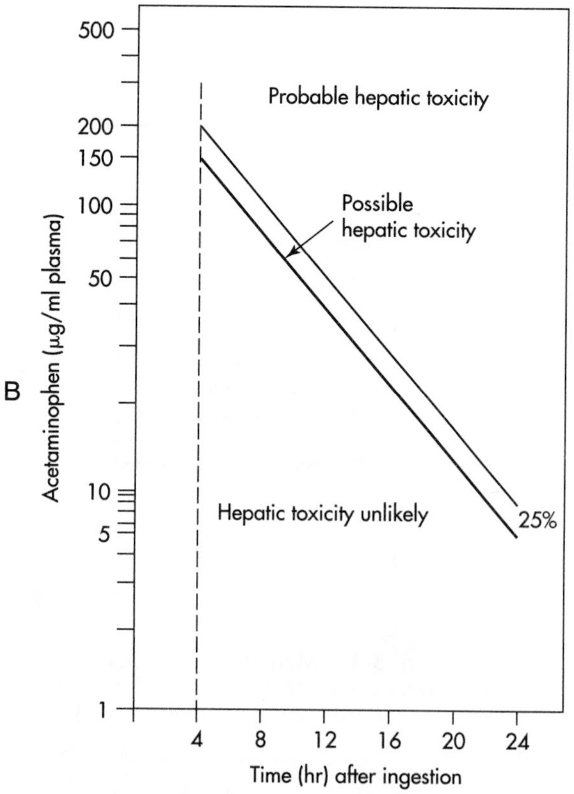

B
500
200
150
100
50
10
5
1
Acetaminophen (μg/ml plasma)
Probable hepatic toxicity
Possible hepatic toxicity
Hepatic toxicity unlikely
25%
4
8
12
16
20
24
Time (hr) after ingestion

Fig. 3-2 A, Treatment of acetaminophen ingestion. *APAP,* Acetaminophen; *ED,* emergency department; *NAC, N*-acetylcysteine. (From Marx J [ed]: *Rosen's emergency medicine,* ed 5, St Louis, 2002, Mosby.)
B, Rumack-Matthew nomogram for acetaminophen poisoning. (From Rumack BH, Matthew H: *Pediatrics* 55:871, 1975. In Marx J [ed]: *Rosen's emergency medicine,* ed 5, St Louis, 2002, Mosby.)

ACID-BASE HOMEOSTASIS

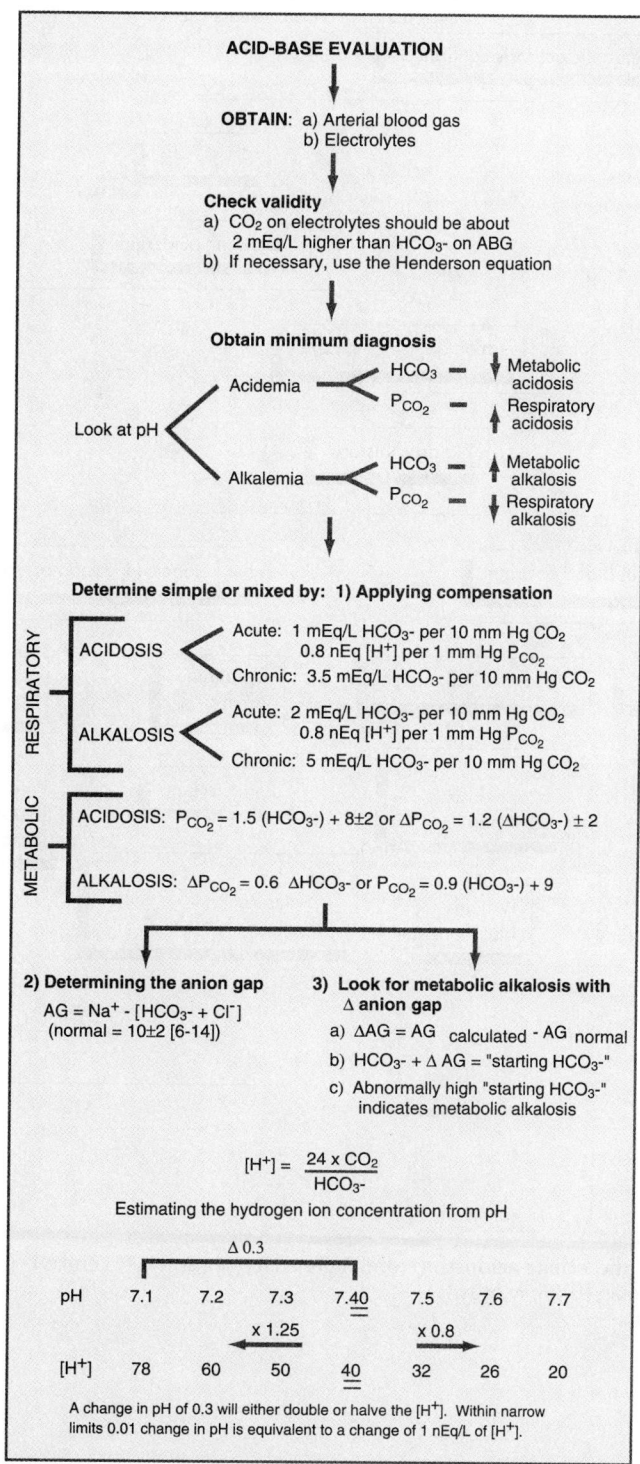

Fig. 3-3   Scheme for assessing acid-base homeostasis. (From Andreoli TE [ed]: *Cecil essentials of medicine,* ed 4, Philadelphia, 1997, WB Saunders.)

ACIDOSIS, METABOLIC

Acidosis, metabolic
ICD-9CM # 276.2

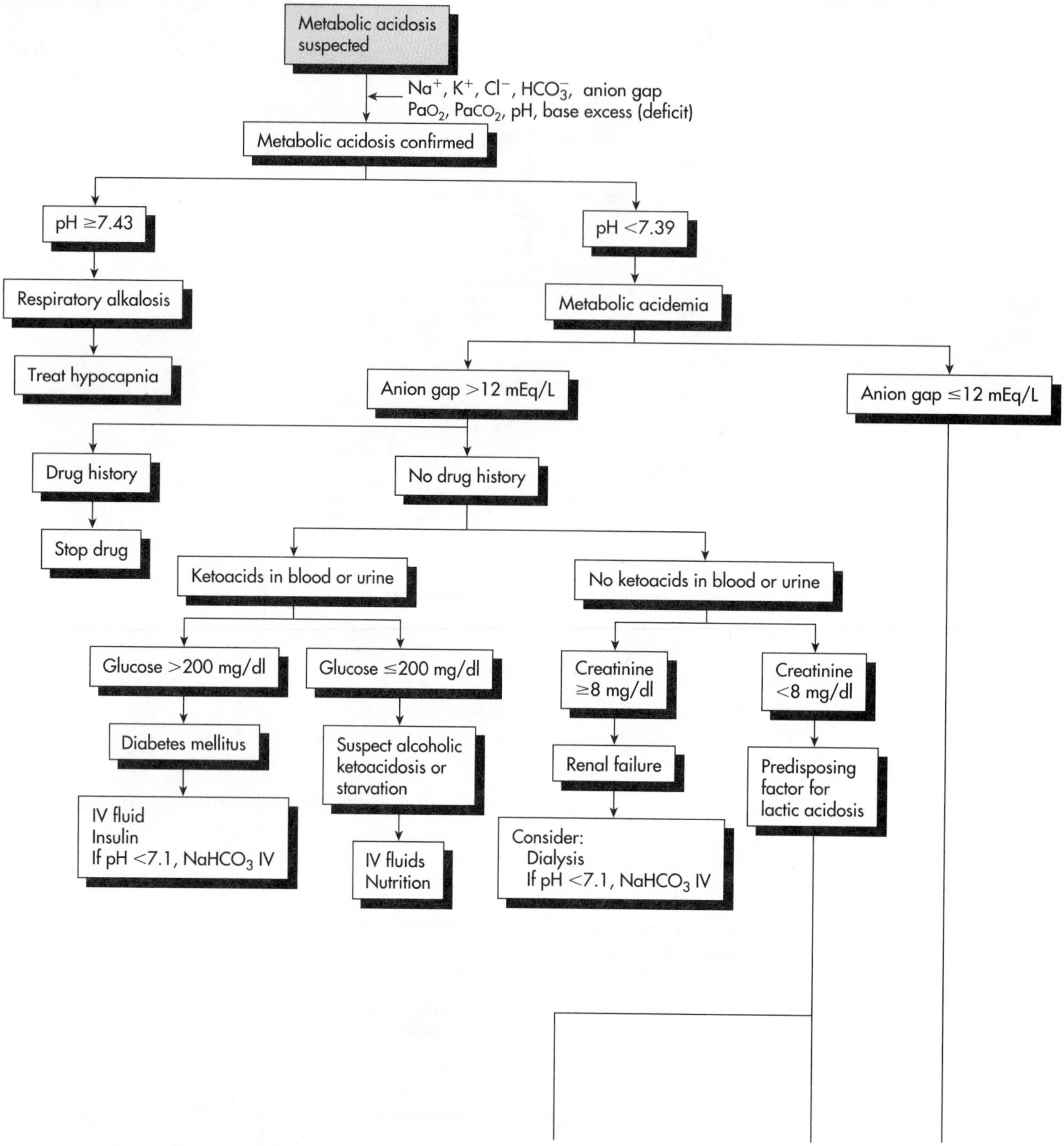

Fig. 3-4 Suspected metabolic acidosis. (From Greene HL, Johnson WP, Lemke D [eds]: *Decision making in medicine,* ed 2, St Louis, 1998, Mosby.)

Continued

ACIDOSIS, METABOLIC—cont'd

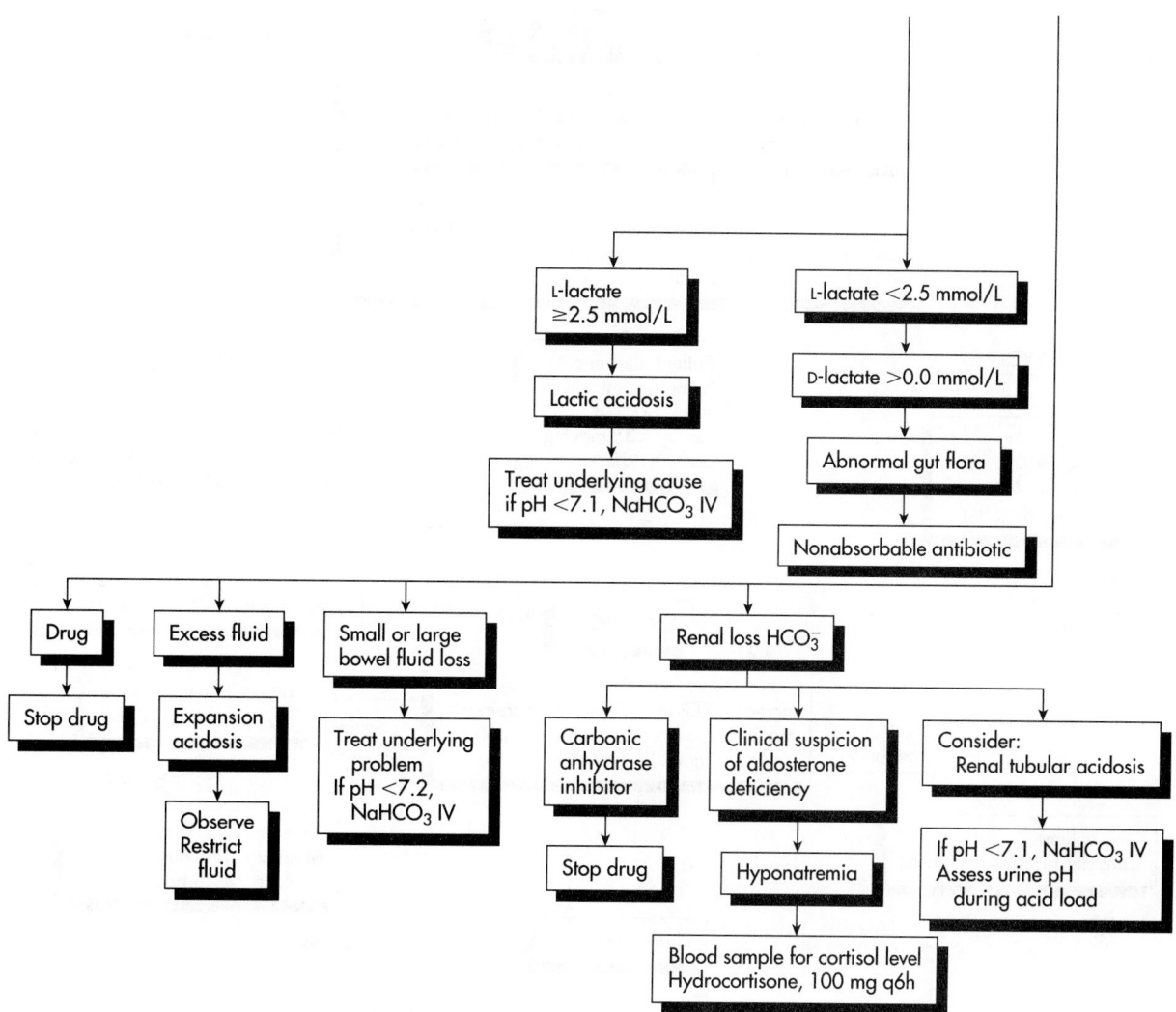

Fig. 3-4, cont'd **Suspected metabolic acidosis.** (From Greene HL, Johnson WP, Lemke D [eds]: *Decision making in medicine,* ed 2, St Louis, 1998, Mosby.)

ACUTE RESPIRATORY DISTRESS SYNDROME

**Acute respiratory distress syndrome
ICD-9CM # 518.82**

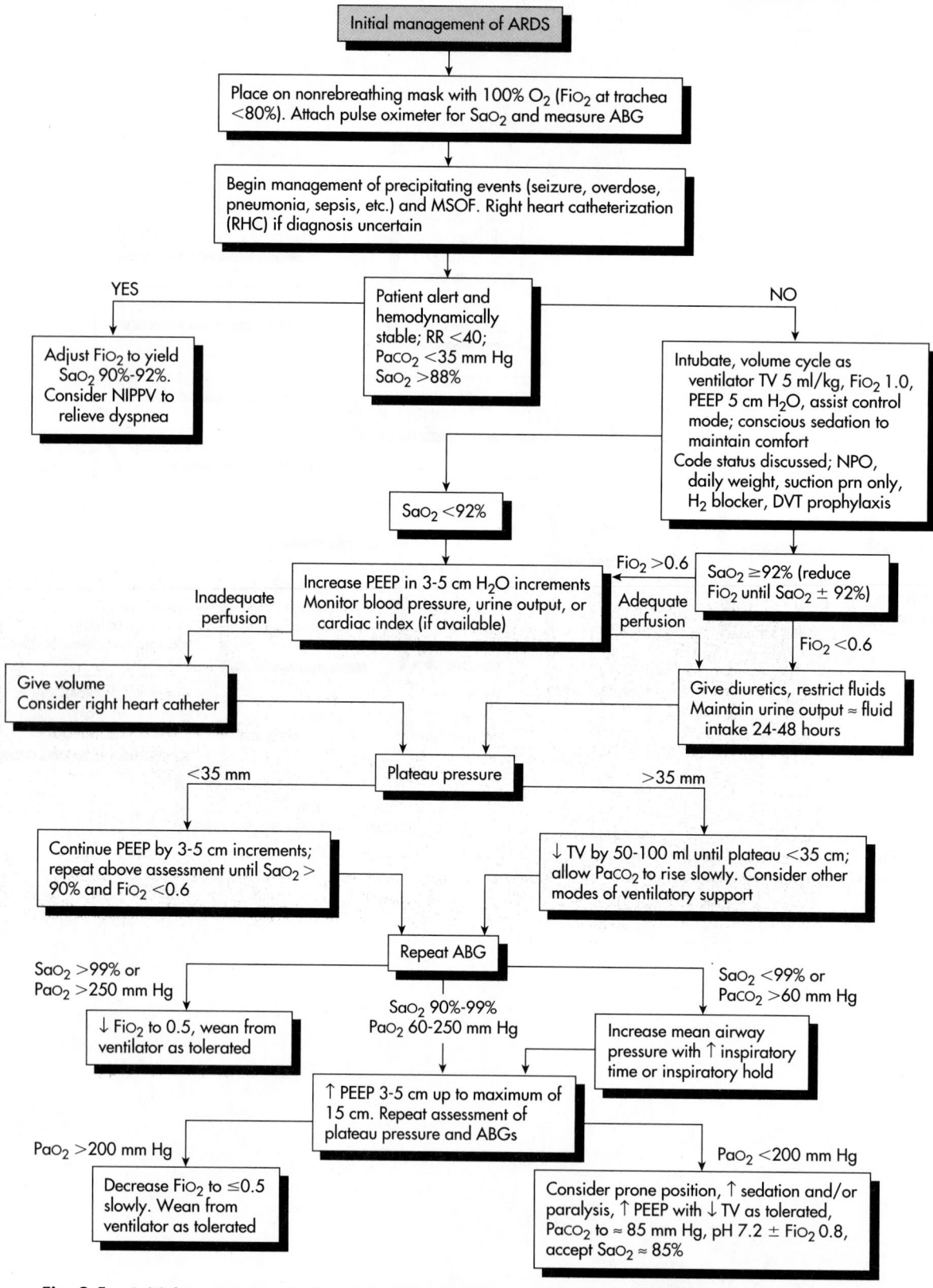

Fig. 3-5   Initial management of acute respiratory distress syndrome (ARDS). *ABG,* Arterial blood gas analysis; *CO₂,* carbon dioxide; *DVT,* deep venous thrombosis; *Fio₂,* inspired oxygen concentration; *MSOF,* multisystem organ failure; *NIPPV,* noninvasive intermittent positive-pressure ventilation; *O₂,* oxygen; *Paco₂,* arterial partial pressure of carbon dioxide; *Pao₂,* arterial partial pressure of oxygen; *PEEP,* positive end-expiratory pressure; *RR,* respiratory rate; *Sao₂,* arterial oxygen saturation; *V_T,* tidal volume. (From Goldman L, Ausiello D [eds]: *Cecil textbook of medicine,* ed 22, Philadelphia, 2004, WB Saunders.)

ADRENAL INCIDENTALOMA

Adrenal incidentaloma
ICD-9CM # 255.9

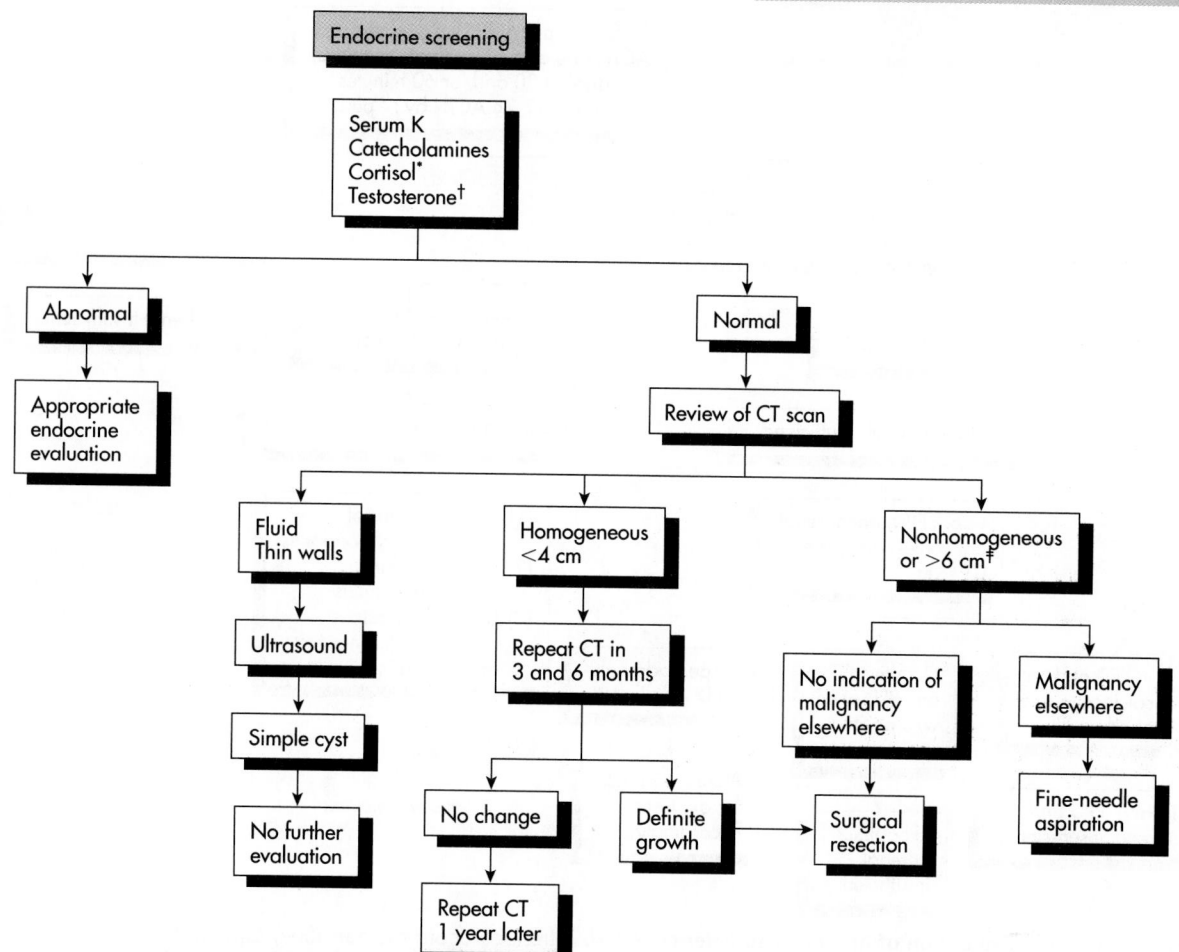

Fig. 3-6   Algorithm for evaluation of an adrenal incidentaloma. *CT,* Computed tomography.
*Only if there are clinical indications of excess cortisol. †Only in women with hirsutism. ‡Measure dehy-droepiandrosterone sulfate, a marker of primary adrenal carcinoma. (From Nseyo UO [ed]: *Urology for primary care physicians,* Philadelphia, 1999, WB Saunders.)

ADRENAL INSUFFICIENCY

Adrenal insufficiency
ICD-9CM # 255.4 Addison's disease

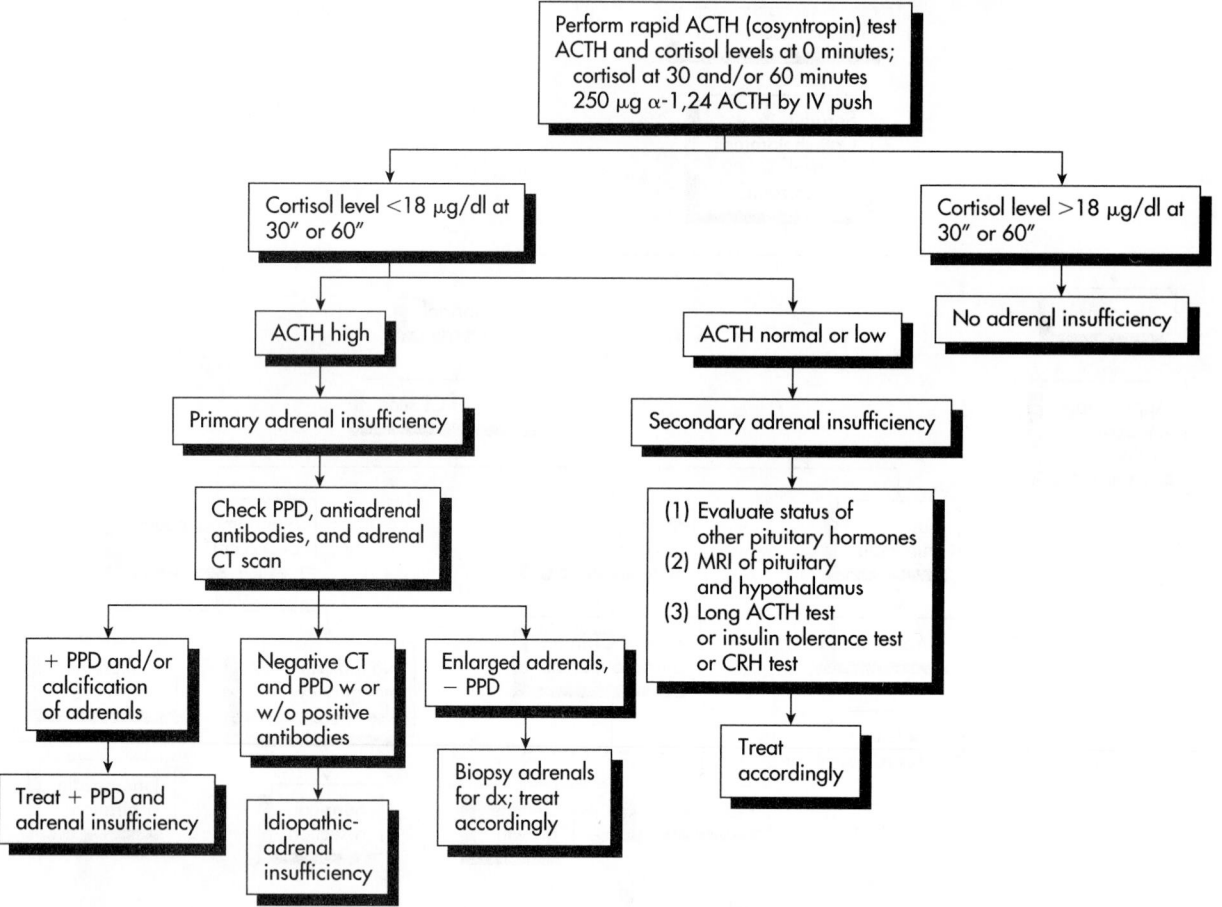

Fig. 3-7   Evaluation of adrenal insufficiency. *ACTH,* Adrenocorticotropic hormone; *CRH,* corticotropin-releasing hormone; *CT,* computed tomography; *MRI,* magnetic resonance imaging; *PPD,* purified protein derivative. (From Noble J: *Primary care medicine,* ed 3, St Louis, 2001, Mosby.)

ADRENAL MASS

Adrenal mass
ICD-9CM # 194.0 Adrenal cortical carcinoma
site NOS M8370/3
255.8 Adrenal hyperplasia

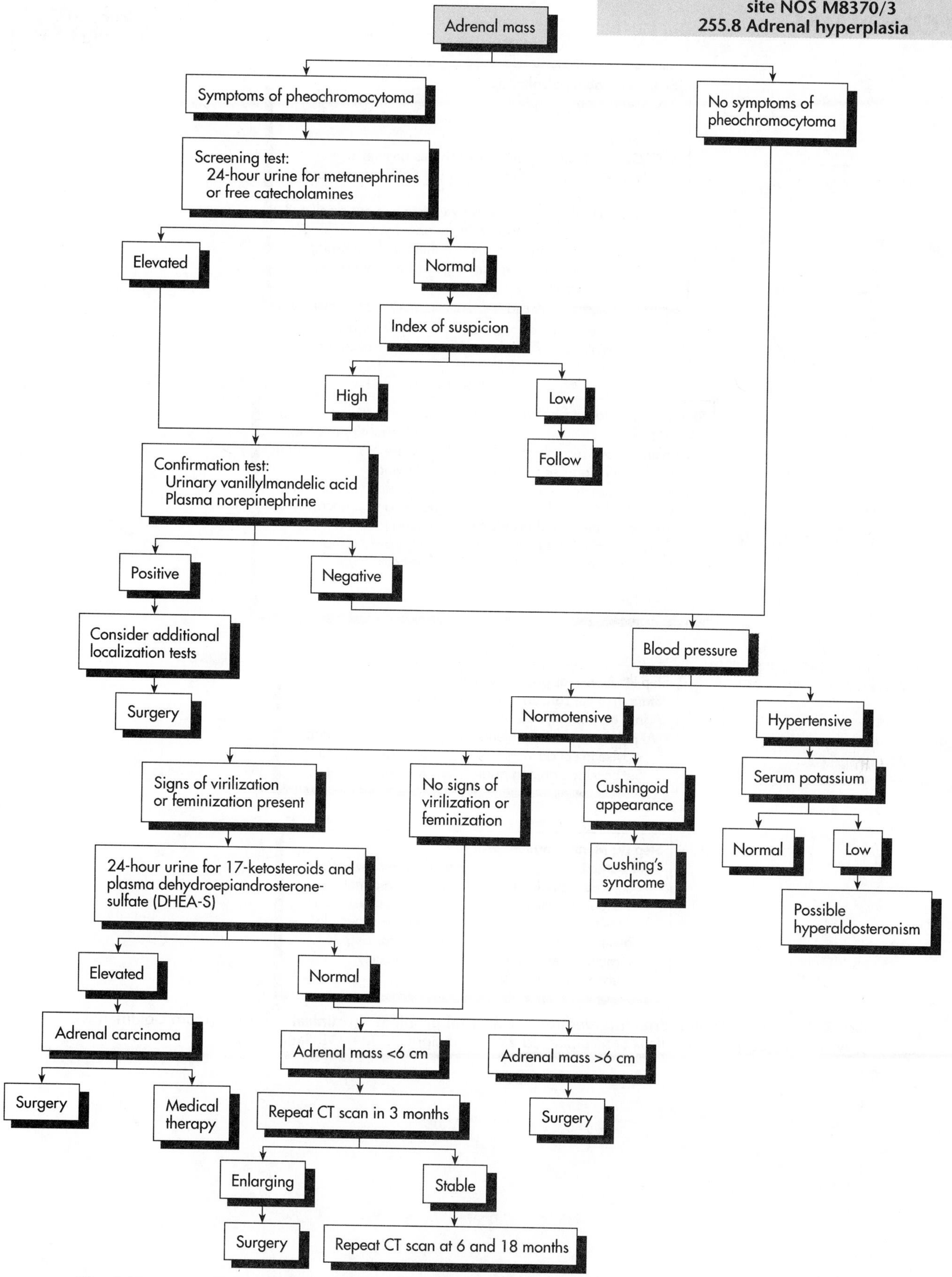

Fig. 3-8 **Evaluation of adrenal mass.** *CT,* Computed tomography. (From Greene HL, Johnson WP, Lemcke D [eds]: *Decision making in medicine,* ed 2, St Louis, 1998, Mosby.)

ALCOHOLISM

**Alcoholism
ICD-9CM # 303.9**

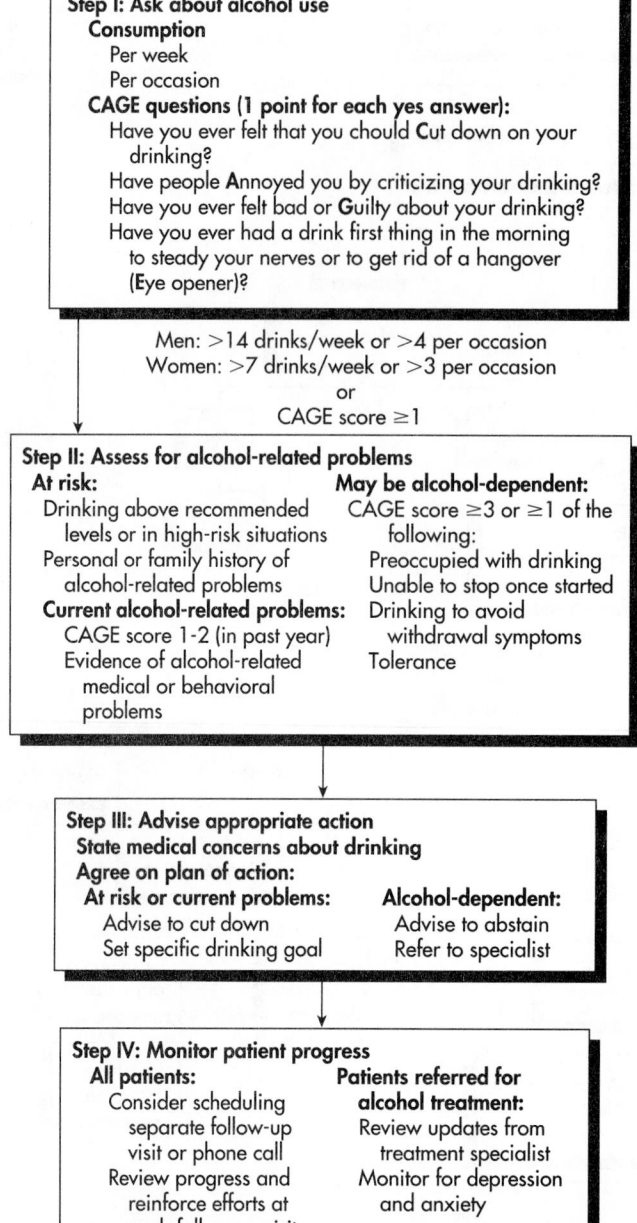

Step I: Ask about alcohol use
Consumption
Per week
Per occasion
CAGE questions (1 point for each yes answer):
Have you ever felt that you chould **C**ut down on your
drinking?
Have people **A**nnoyed you by criticizing your drinking?
Have you ever felt bad or **G**uilty about your drinking?
Have you ever had a drink first thing in the morning
to steady your nerves or to get rid of a hangover
(**E**ye opener)?

Men: >14 drinks/week or >4 per occasion
Women: >7 drinks/week or >3 per occasion
or
CAGE score ≥1

Step II: Assess for alcohol-related problems
At risk:
Drinking above recommended
levels or in high-risk situations
Personal or family history of
alcohol-related problems
Current alcohol-related problems:
CAGE score 1-2 (in past year)
Evidence of alcohol-related
medical or behavioral
problems

May be alcohol-dependent:
CAGE score ≥3 or ≥1 of the
following:
Preoccupied with drinking
Unable to stop once started
Drinking to avoid
withdrawal symptoms
Tolerance

Step III: Advise appropriate action
State medical concerns about drinking
Agree on plan of action:
At risk or current problems:
Advise to cut down
Set specific drinking goal

Alcohol-dependent:
Advise to abstain
Refer to specialist

Step IV: Monitor patient progress
All patients:
Consider scheduling
separate follow-up
visit or phone call
Review progress and
reinforce efforts at
each follow-up visit

**Patients referred for
alcohol treatment:**
Review updates from
treatment specialist
Monitor for depression
and anxiety

Fig. 3-9   Screening and brief intervention for alcohol problems in clinical practice. (From Goldman
L, Ausiello D [eds]: *Cecil textbook of medicine,* ed 22, Philadelphia, 2004, WB Saunders.)

ALKALOSIS, METABOLIC

Alkalosis, metabolic
ICD-9CM # 273.6

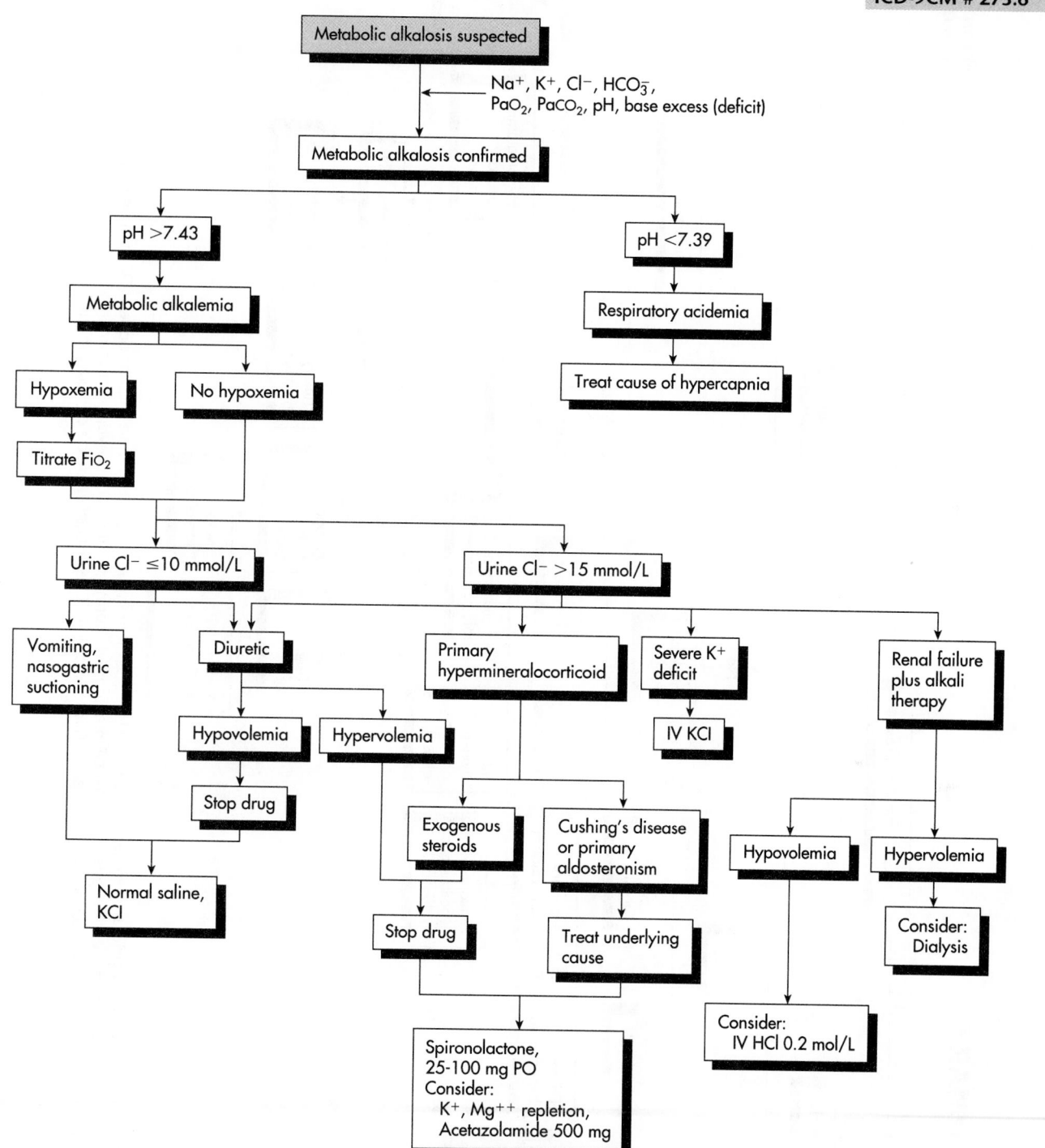

Fig. 3-10 Suspected metabolic alkalosis. (From Greene HL, Johnson WP, Lemke D [eds]: *Decision making in medicine,* ed 2, St Louis, 1998, Mosby.)

AMENORRHEA, PRIMARY

Amenorrhea, primary
ICD-9CM # 626.0

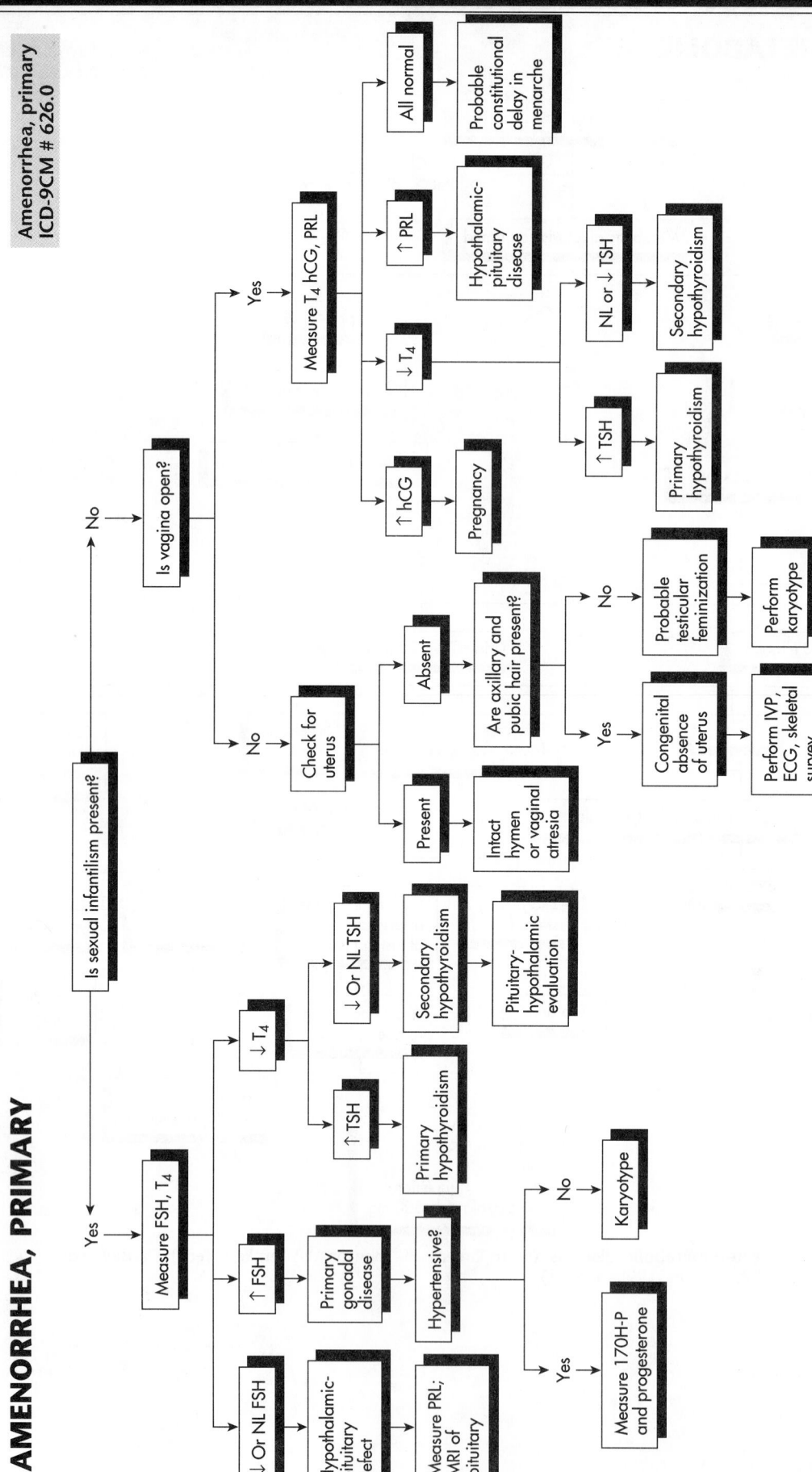

Fig. 3-11 **Diagnostic evaluation of primary amenorrhea.** *ECG,* Electrocardiogram; *FSH,* follicle-stimulating hormone; *hCG,* human chorionic gonadotropin; *IVP,* intravenous pyelogram; *MRI,* magnetic resonance imaging; *NL,* normal; *170H-P,* 17 α-hydroxyprogesterone; *T₄,* thyroxine; *TSH,* thyroid-stimulating hormone; ↓, decreased; ↑, increased. (From Andreoli TE [ed]: *Cecil essentials of medicine,* ed 5, Philadelphia, 2001, WB Saunders.)

AMENORRHEA, SECONDARY

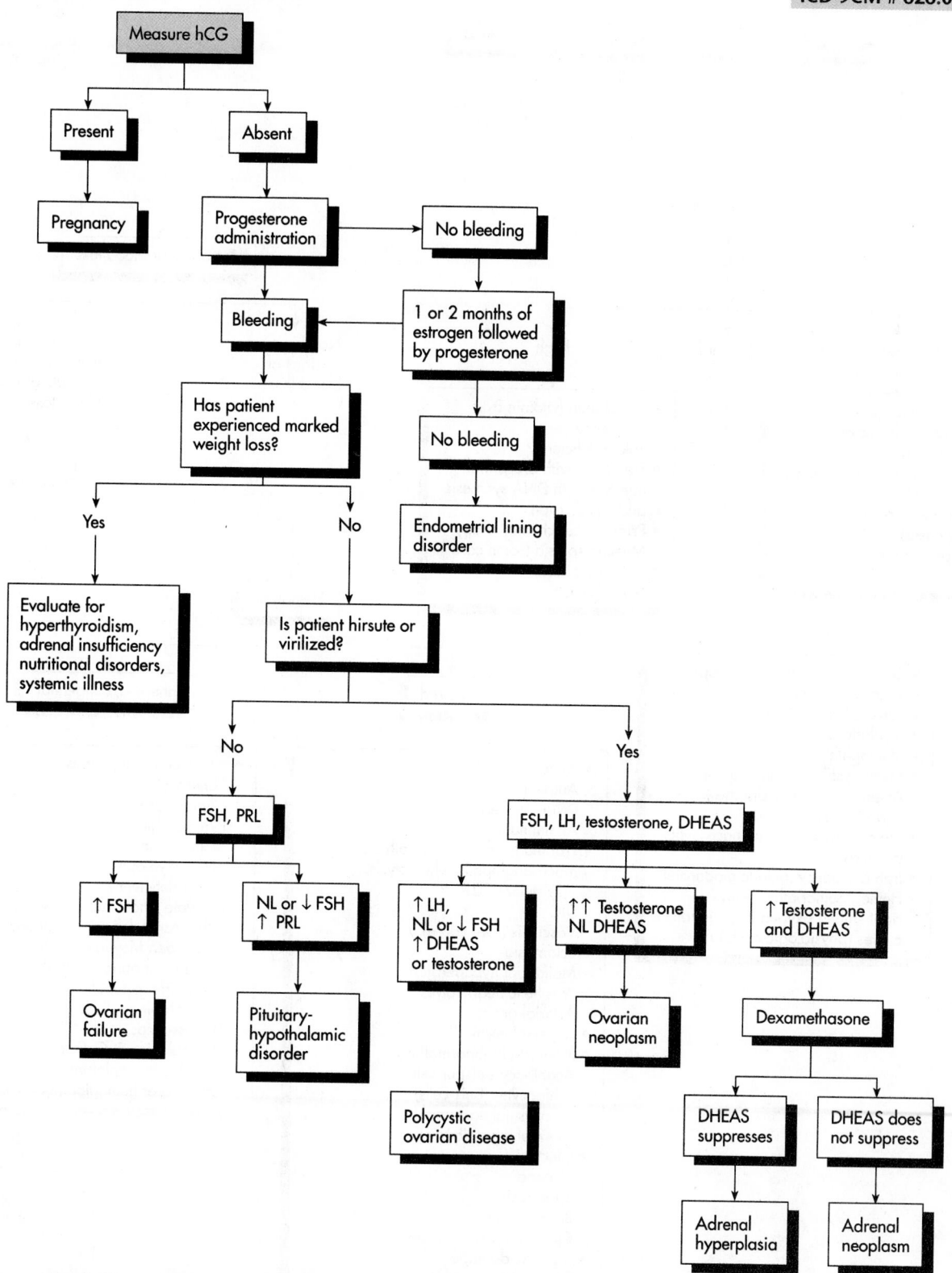

Fig. 3-12   Evaluation of secondary amenorrhea. *DHEAS,* Dehydroepiandrosterone-sulfate; *FSH,* follicle-stimulating hormone; *hCG,* human chorionic gonadotropin; *LH,* luteinizing hormone; *NL,* normal; *PRL,* prolactin; ↑, increased; ↑↑, markedly increased; ↓, decreased. (From Andreoli TE [ed]: *Cecil essentials of medicine,* ed 5, Philadelphia, 2001, WB Saunders.)

ANEMIA

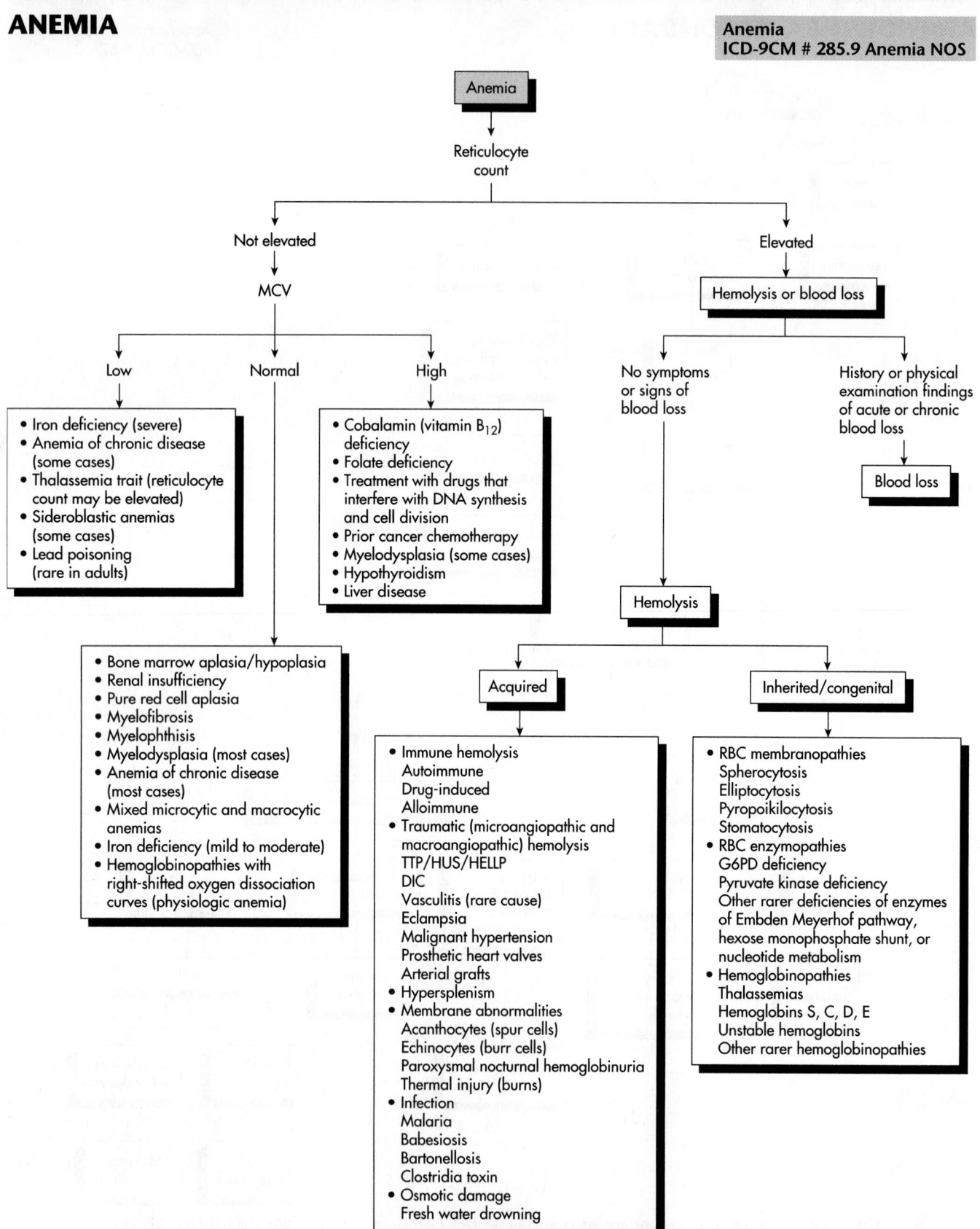

Fig. 3-13   Algorithm for diagnosis of anemias. *DIC,* Disseminated intravascular coagulation; *HELLP, h*epatomegaly-*e*levated *l*iver (function tests)-*l*ow *p*latelets; *HUS,* hemolytic-uremic syndrome; *MCV,* mean corpuscular volume; *RBC,* red blood cell; *TTP,* thrombotic thrombocytopenic purpura. (From Goldman L, Ausiello D [eds]: *Cecil textbook of medicine,* ed 22, Philadelphia, 2004, WB Saunders.)

ANEMIA, MACROCYTIC

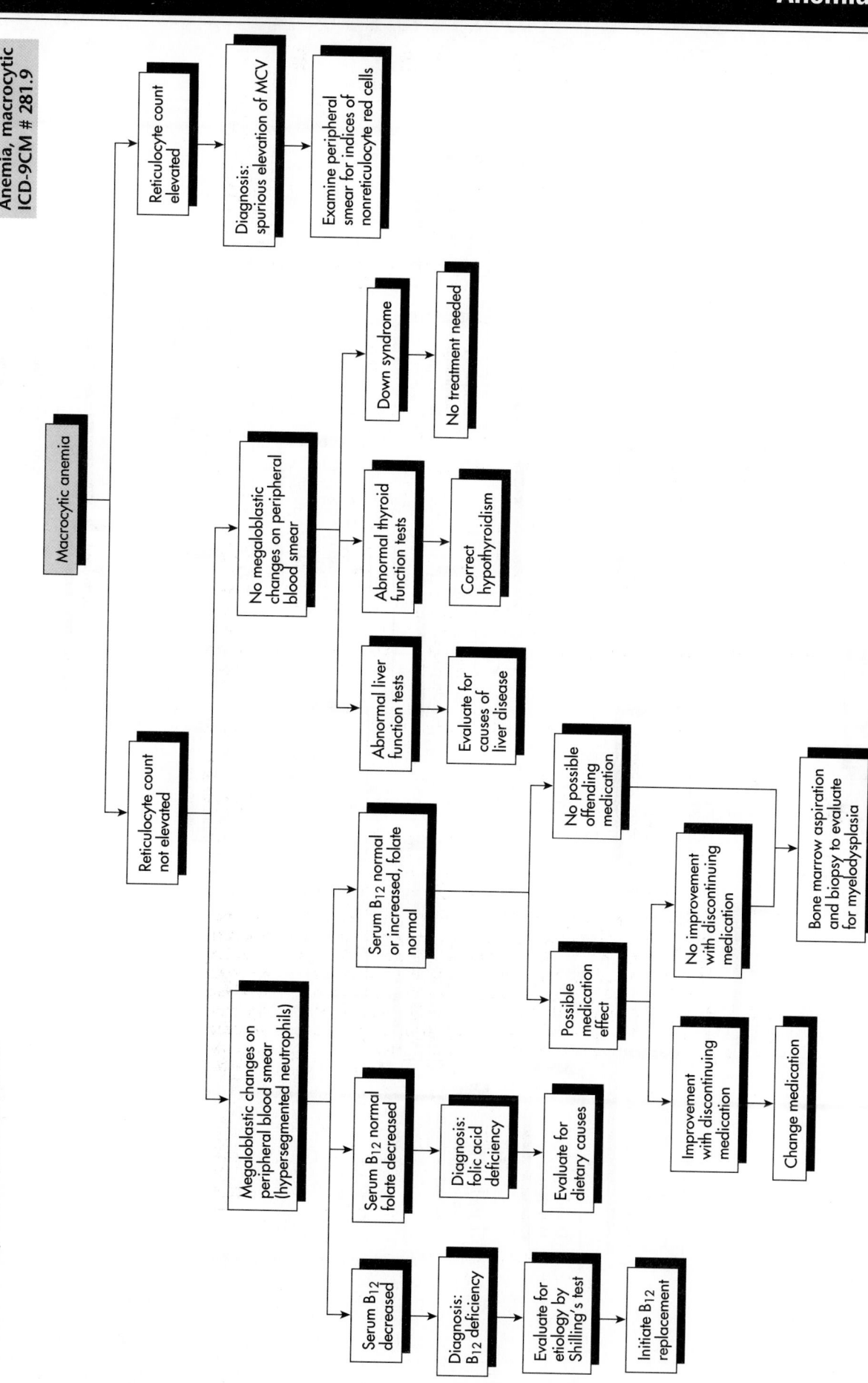

Fig. 3-14 Differential diagnosis of macrocytic anemia. (From Rakel RE [ed]: *Principles of family practice,* ed 6, Philadelphia, 2002, WB Saunders.)

ANEMIA, MICROCYTIC

Anemia, microcytic
ICD-9CM # 282.4

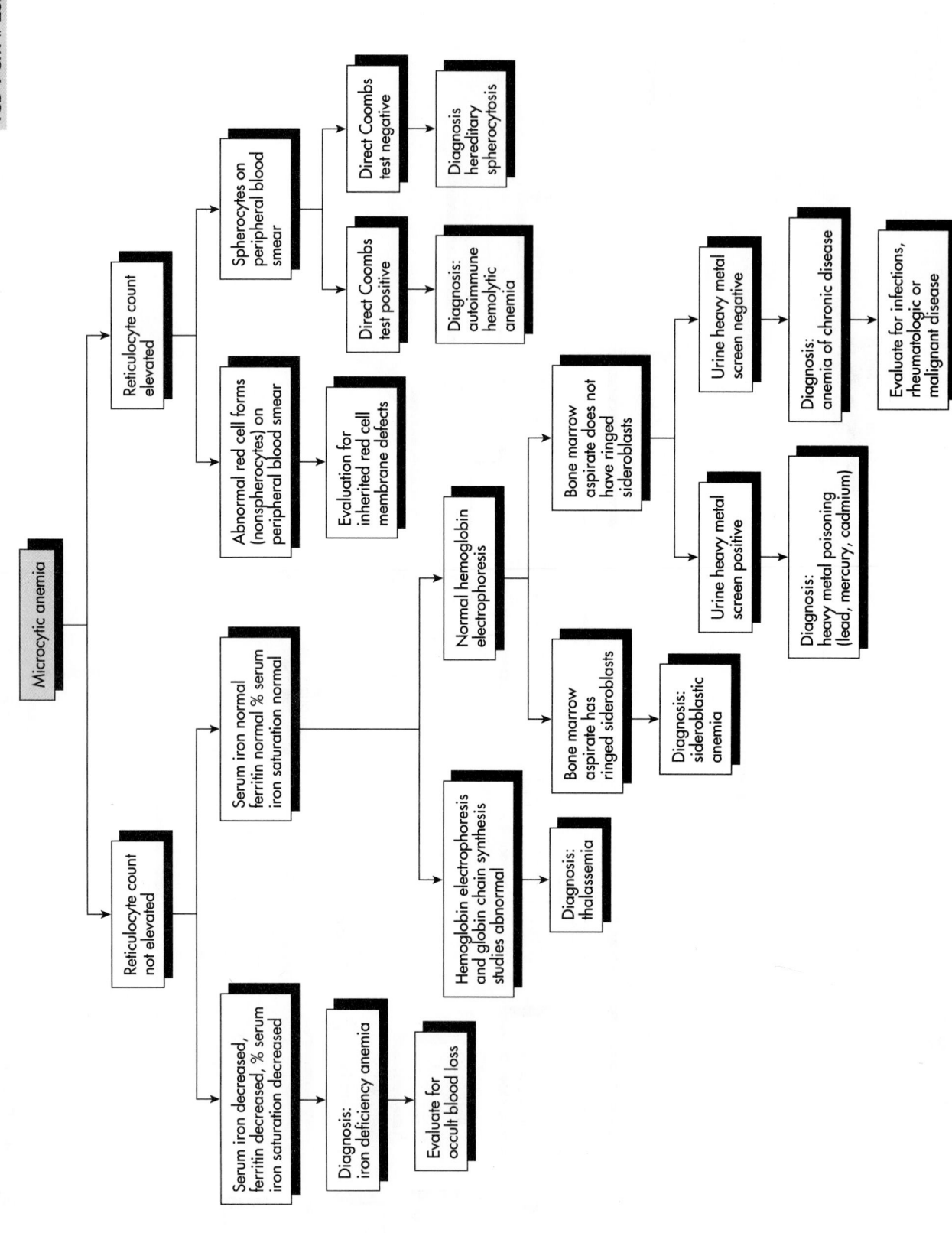

Fig. 3-15   Differential diagnosis of microcytic anemia. (From Rakel RE [ed]: *Principles of family practice*, ed 6, Philadelphia, 2002, WB Saunders.)

ANEMIA, WITH RETICULOCYTOSIS

Anemia with reticulocytosis
ICD-9CM # 790.99

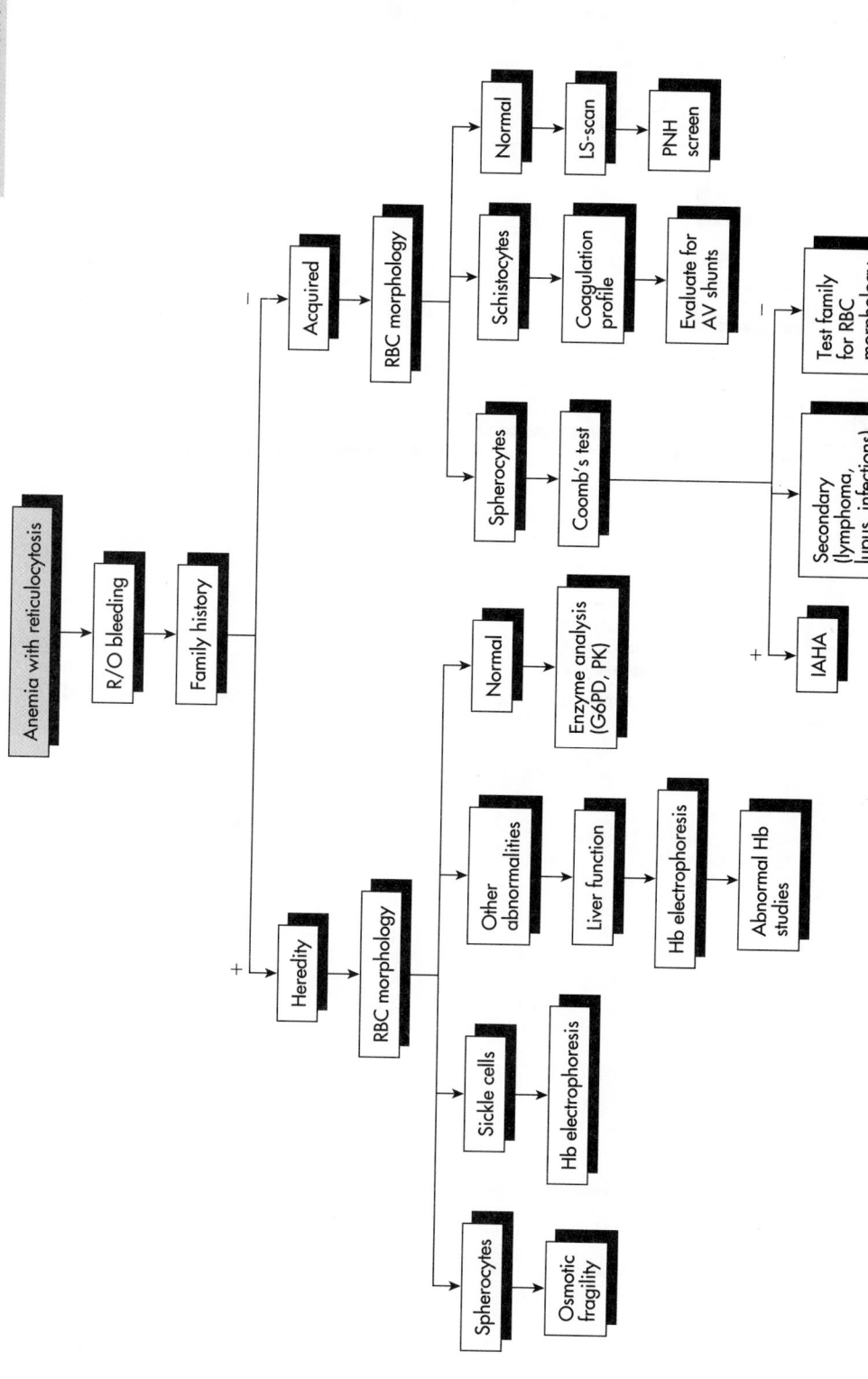

Fig. 3-16   Evaluations of patients with hemolytic anemia. *AV,* Arteriovenous; *Hb,* hemoglobin; *IAHA,* idiopathic autoimmune hemolytic anemia; *LS,* liver spleen; *PK,* pyruvate kinase; *PNH,* paroxysmal nocturnal hemoglobinuria; *RBC,* red blood cell. (From Stein JH: *Internal medicine,* ed 5, St Louis, 1997, Mosby.)

III

ANISOCORIA

**Anisocoria
ICD-9CM # 379.41**

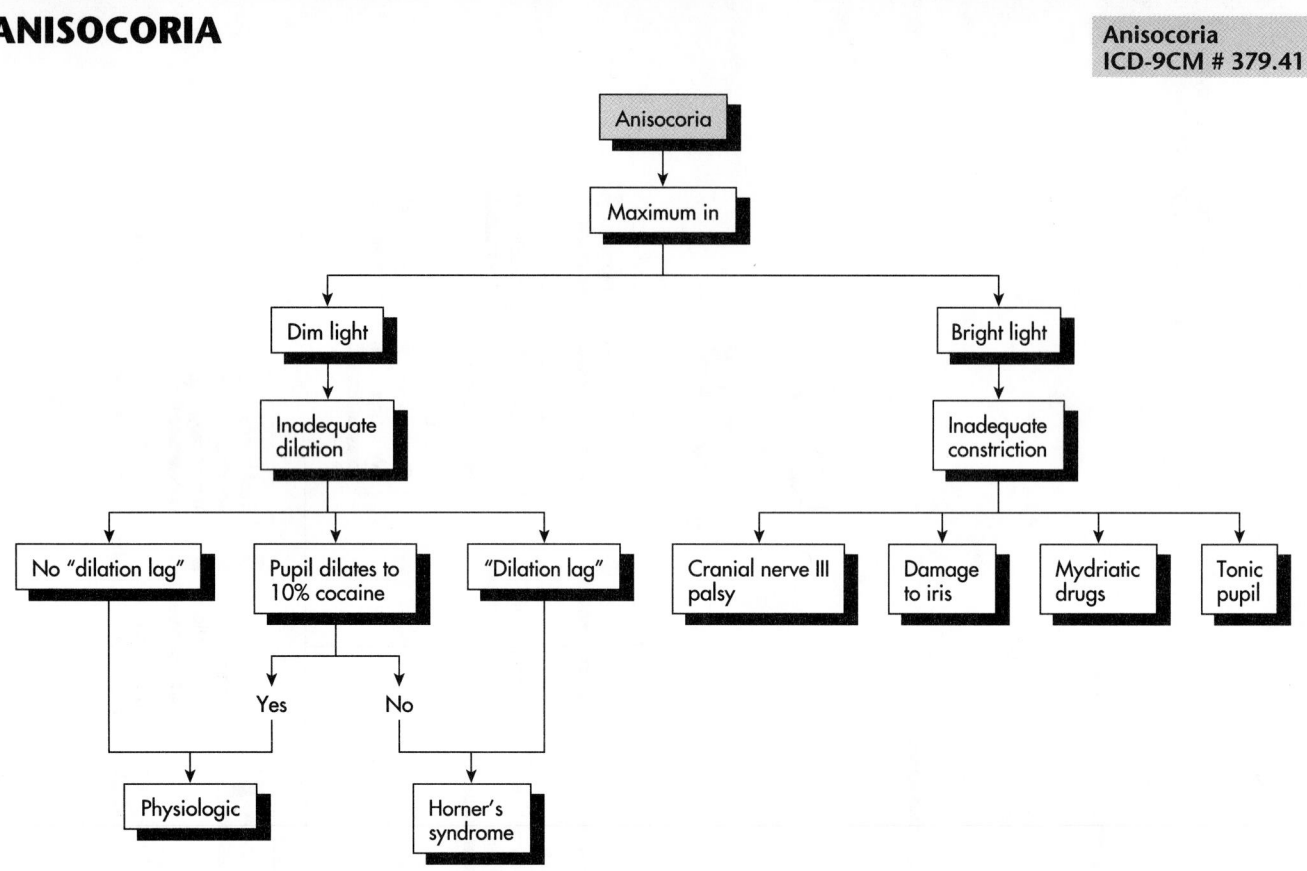

Fig. 3-17   Algorithm for the approach to unequal pupils (anisocoria). (From Andreoli TE [ed]: *Cecil essentials of medicine,* ed 5, Philadelphia, 2001, WB Saunders.)

ANOREXIA

Patient with anorexia

History
Physical examination

Diagnostic tests
Chemistry panel
CBC
ESR
Urinalysis
Thyroid function tests
Fasting plasma cortisol level
ECG

Medical disease

Nonmedical etiology

Eating disorders

Social factors

Psychologic disorders

Age-related conditions

Consider:
Depression
Dementia
Alcoholism
Drug abuse
Psychosis
Anxiety
Bereavement

Consider:
Decreased olfactory sense
Hypogeusia
Visual disorders
Hearing disorders
Dental disorders

Medications

CNS disease

Endocrine disorders

GI disorders

Other medical diseases

Consider:
Sedatives and psychotropics
Digoxin
Laxatives
Appetite suppressants
Thiazide diuretics
Levodopa
Narcotics
Antibiotics
Miscellaneous

Consider:
Thyroid disease
Adrenal insufficiency
Diabetes
Hyperparathyroidism
Hypercalcemia

Consider:
Malabsorption syndromes
PUD
Biliary disease
Hepatitis
Gastroesophageal reflux disease
Esophageal motility disease
Oral cavity problems
GI malignancy

Consider:
Chronic infection
Malignancy
Cardiopulmonary disease
Cerebrovascular disease
Abdominal ischemia

Diagnostic tests:
Stool for blood, fat, parasites
Flexible sigmoidoscopy
Upper GI with small bowel follow-through

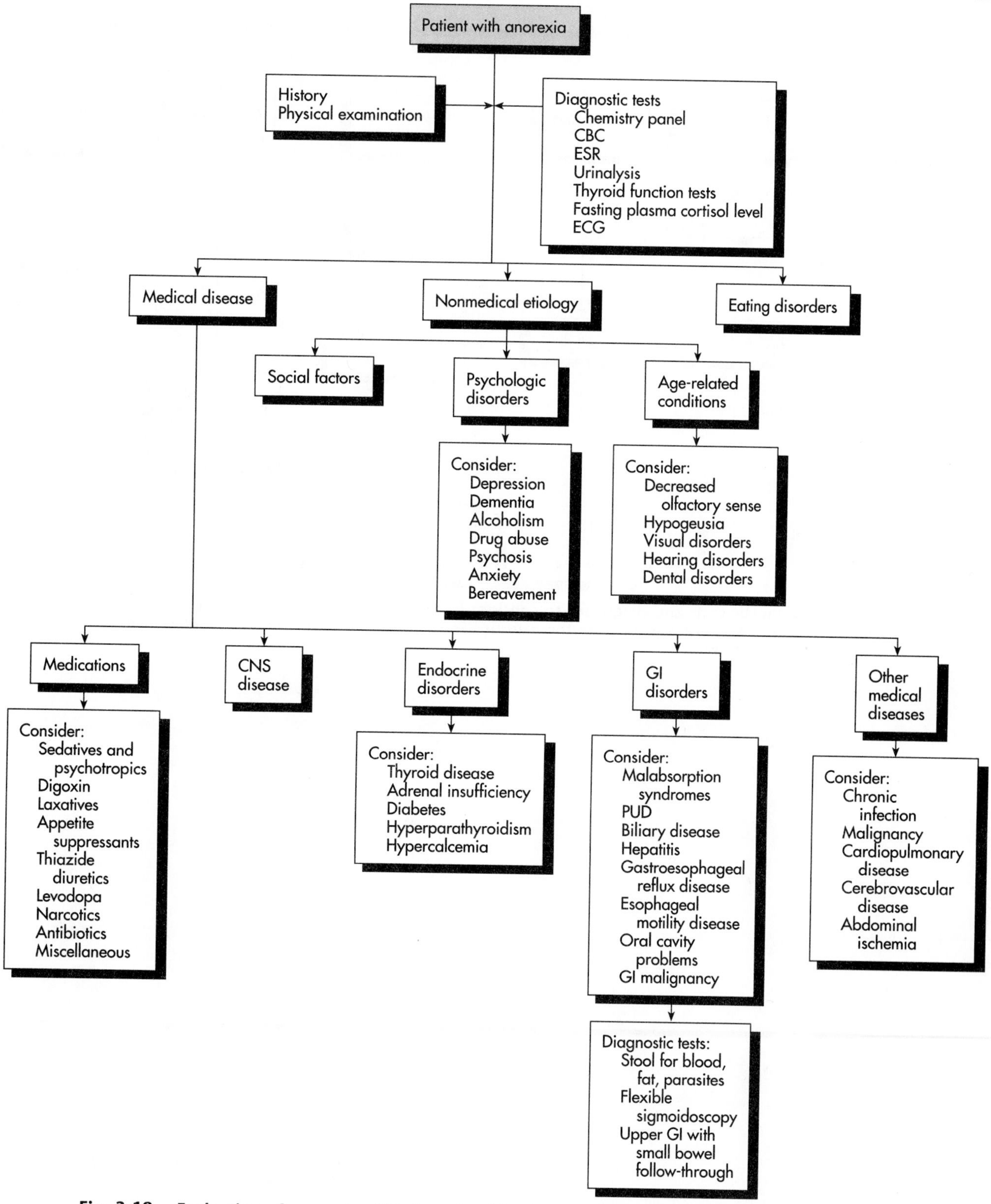

Fig. 3-18 **Evaluation of anorexia.** *CBC,* Complete blood count; *CNS,* central nervous system; *ECG,* electrocardiogram; *ESR,* erythrocyte sedimentation rate; *GI,* gastrointestinal; *PUD,* peptic ulcer disease. (From Greene HL, Johnson WP, Lemcke D [eds]: *Decision making in medicine,* ed 2, St Louis, 1998, Mosby.)

ANTINUCLEAR ANTIBODY TESTING

Antinuclear antibody testing
ICD-9CM # 795.79

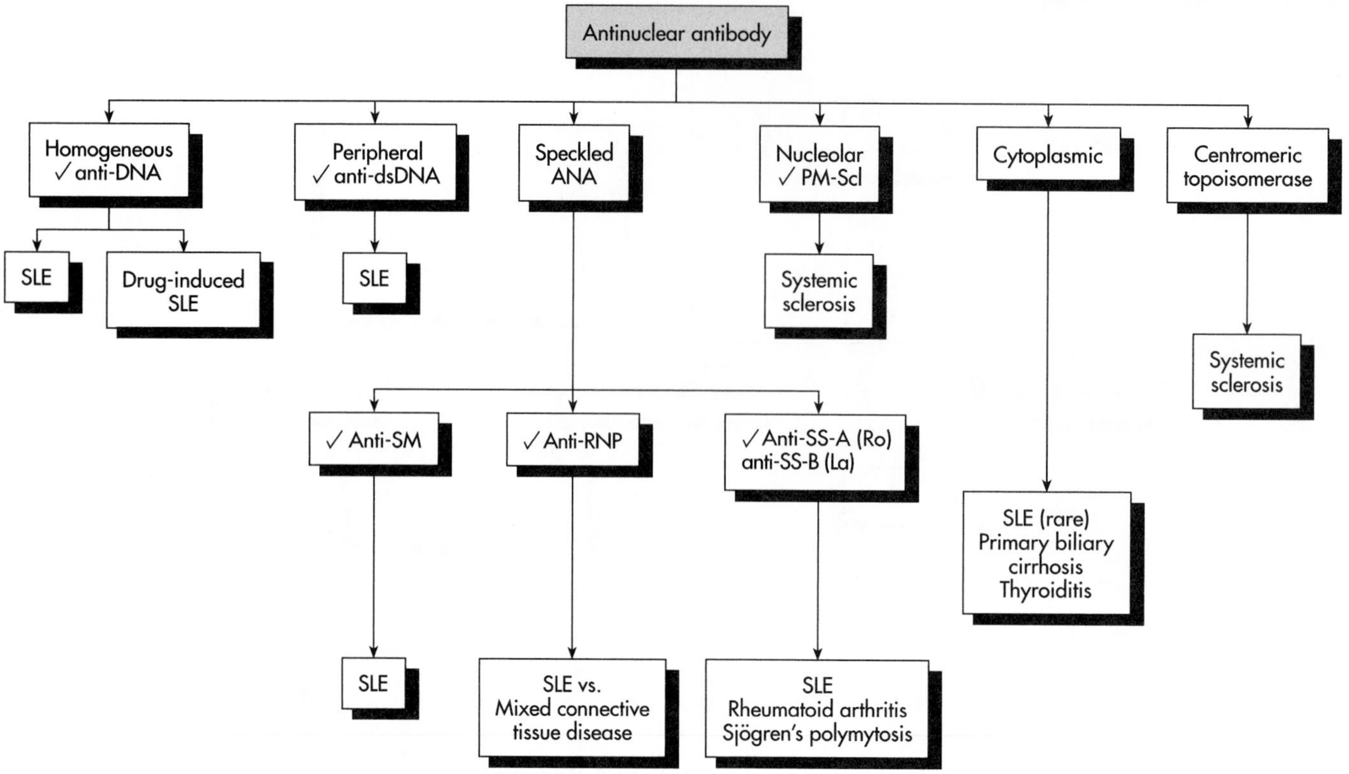

Fig. 3-19 Diagnostic tests and diagnoses to consider from antinuclear antibody pattern. *ANA,* Antinuclear antibody; *SLE,* systemic lupus erythematosus. (From Carlson KJ et al: *Primary care of women,* ed 2, St Louis, 2002, Mosby.)

ARTHRALGIA LIMITED TO ONE OR FEW JOINTS

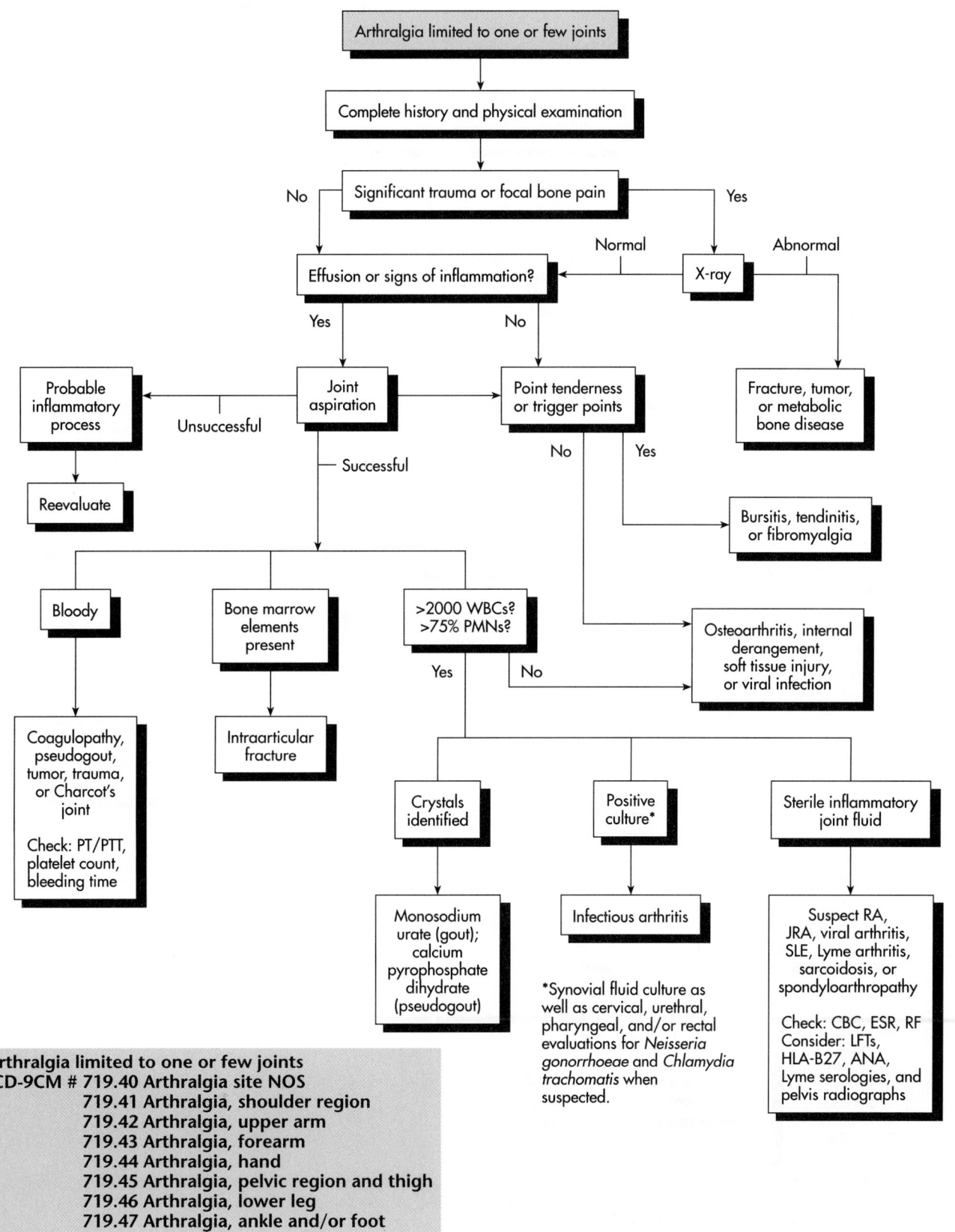

Arthralgia limited to one or few joints
ICD-9CM # 719.40 Arthralgia site NOS
719.41 Arthralgia, shoulder region
719.42 Arthralgia, upper arm
719.43 Arthralgia, forearm
719.44 Arthralgia, hand
719.45 Arthralgia, pelvic region and thigh
719.46 Arthralgia, lower leg
719.47 Arthralgia, ankle and/or foot

Fig. 3-20   A diagnostic approach to arthralgia in a few joints. *ANA,* Antinuclear antibodies; *CBC,* complete blood count; *ESR,* erythrocyte sedimentation rate; *JRA,* juvenile rheumatoid arthritis; *LFTs,* liver function tests; *PMNs,* polymorphonuclear neutrophils; *PT,* prothrombin time; *PTT,* partial thromboplastin time; *RA,* rheumatoid arthritis; *RF,* rheumatoid factor; *SLE,* systemic lupus erythematosus; *WBCs,* white blood cells. (Modified from American College of Rheumatology Ad Hoc Committee on Clinical Guidelines: *Arthritis Rheum* 39:1, 1996.)

ASCITES

Ascites
ICD-9CM # 789.5 Ascites NOS
            197.6 Ascites, cancerous
                  (malignant) M8000/6
            457.8 Chylous
            014.0 Tuberculous

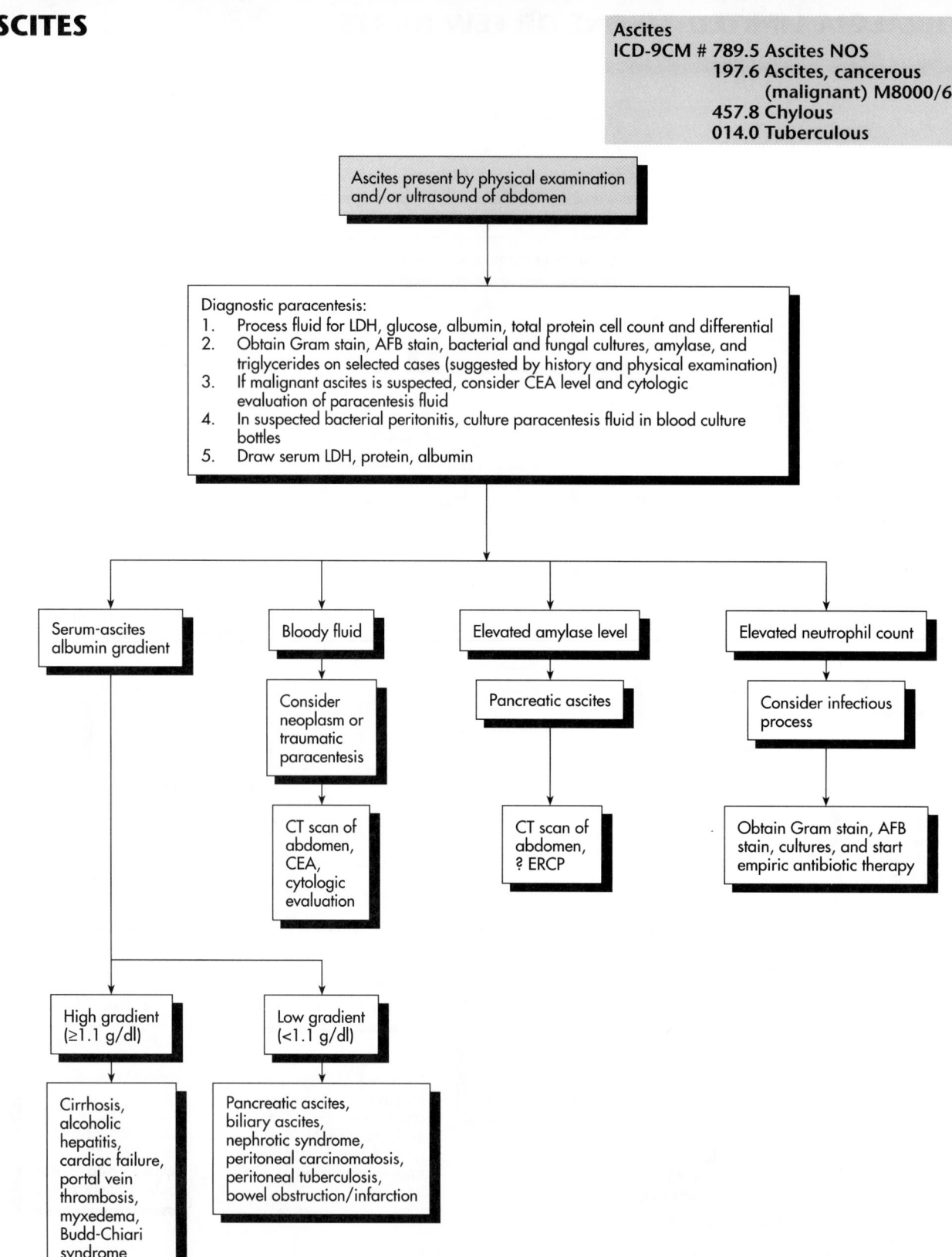

Fig. 3-21   Evaluation of ascites. *AFB,* Acid-fast bacillus; *CEA,* carcinoembryonic antigen; *CT,* computed tomography; *ERCP,* endoscopic retrograde cholangiopancreatography; *LDH,* lactate dehydrogenase.

ASPIRATION, GASTRIC CONTENTS

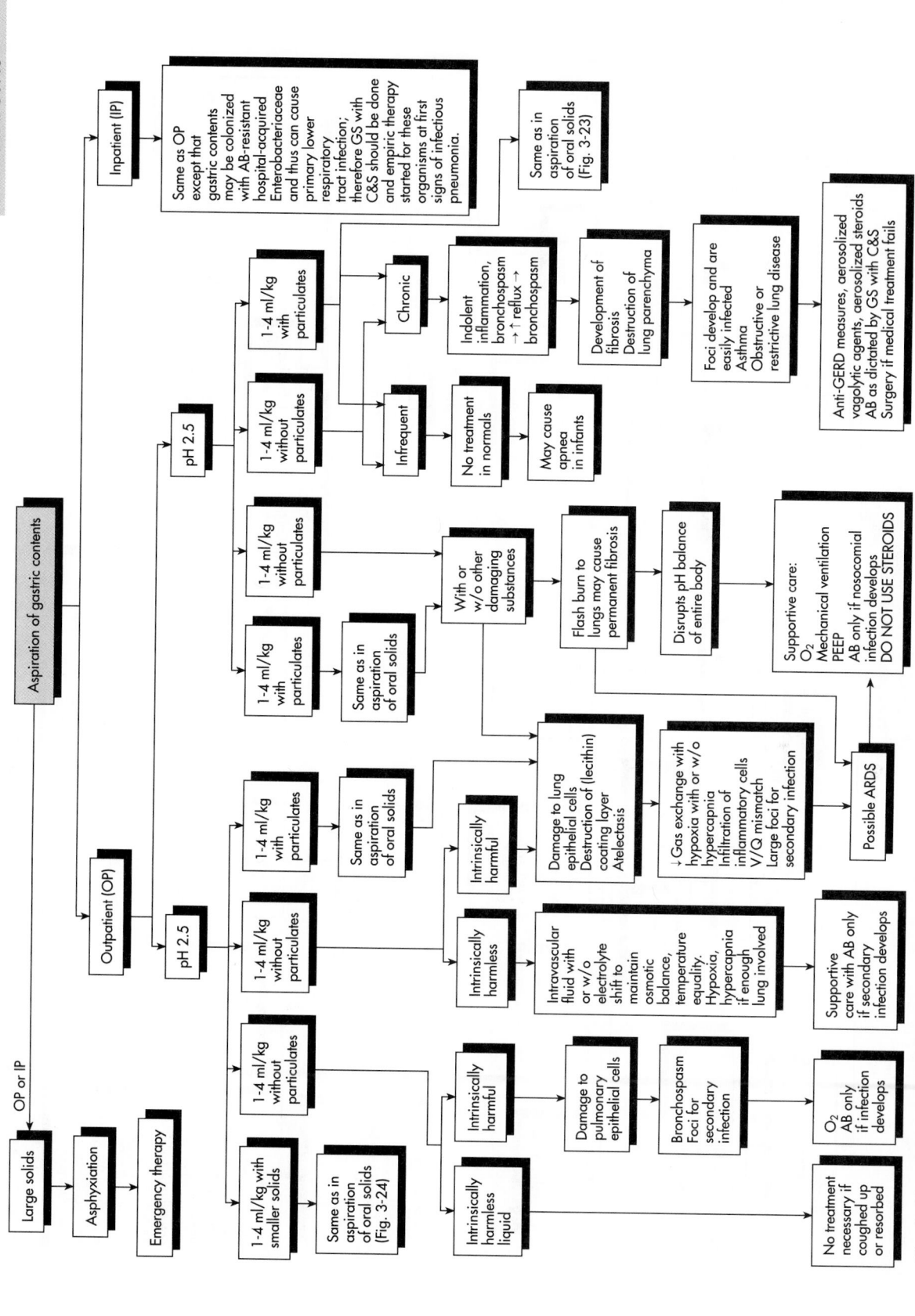

Fig. 3-22 **Management of aspiration of gastric contents.** *AB,* Antibiotics; *ARDS,* acute respiratory distress syndrome; *C&S,* culture and sensitivity; *GERD,* gastroesophageal reflux disease; *GS,* Gram's stain; *PEEP,* positive end-expiratory pressure; *V/Q,* ventilation-perfusion. (From Kassirer J [ed]: *Current therapy in adult medicine,* ed 4, St Louis, 1998, Mosby.)

ASPIRATION, ORAL CONTENTS

Aspiration, oral contents
ICD-9CM # 507.0

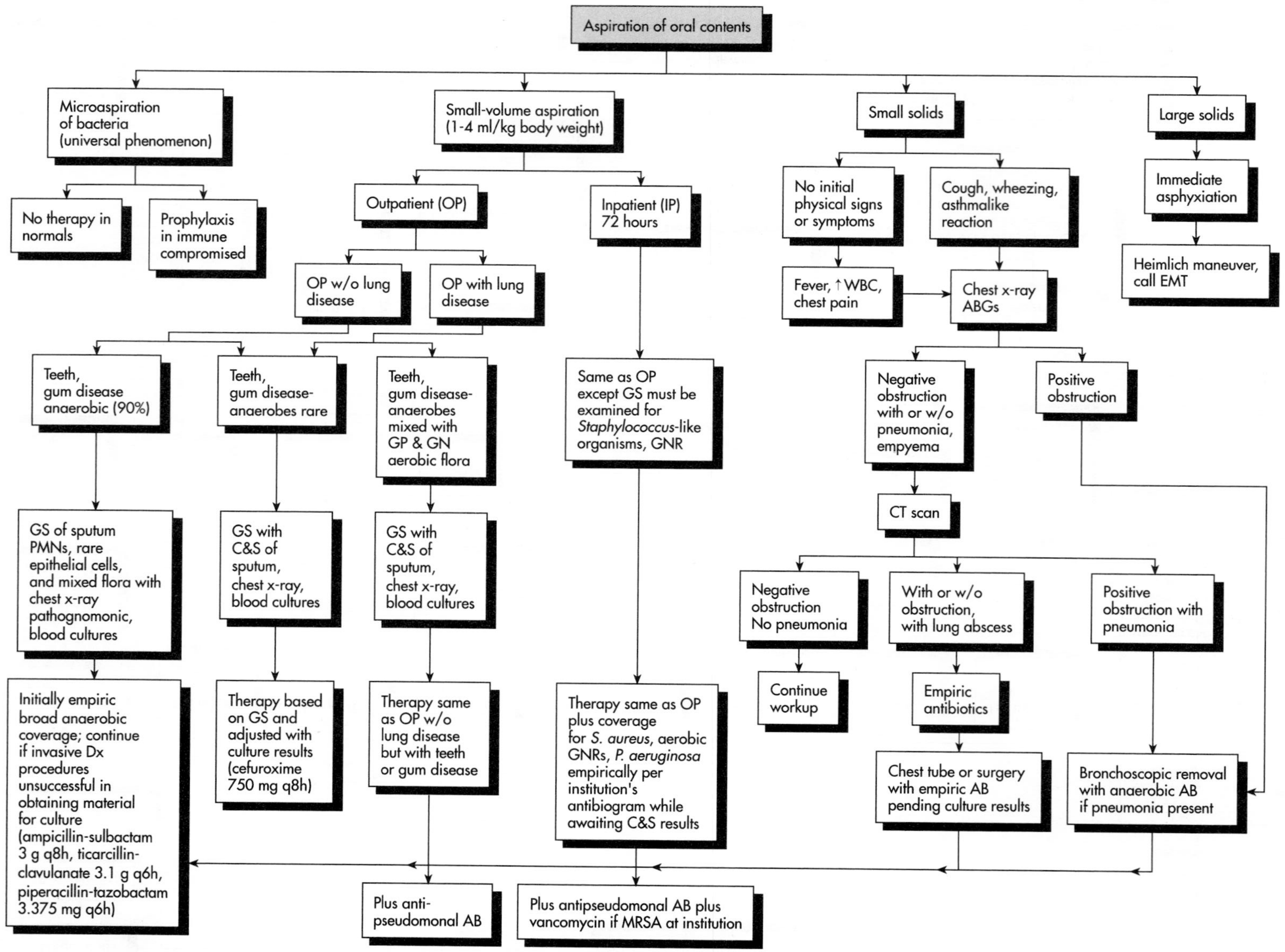

Fig. 3-23   Management of aspiration of oral contents. *AB,* Antibiotics; *ABG,* arterial blood gases; *C&S,* culture and sensitivity; *CT,* computed tomography; *Dx,* diagnostic; *EMT,* emergency medical technician; *GN,* gram-negative; *GNRs,* gram-negative rods; *GP,* gram-positive; *GS,* Gram stain; *MRSA,* methicillin-resistant *Staphylococcus aureus; PMNs,* polymorphonuclear leukocytes; *WBC,* white blood cells. (From Kassirer J [ed]: *Current therapy in adult medicine,* ed 4, St Louis, 1998, Mosby.)

ASTHMA, EMERGENCY DEPARTMENT AND HOSPITAL-BASED CARE

Asthma, emergency department and hospital-based care
ICD-9CM # 493.9 Asthma, unspecified
493.1 Intrinsic asthma
493.0 Extrinsic asthma

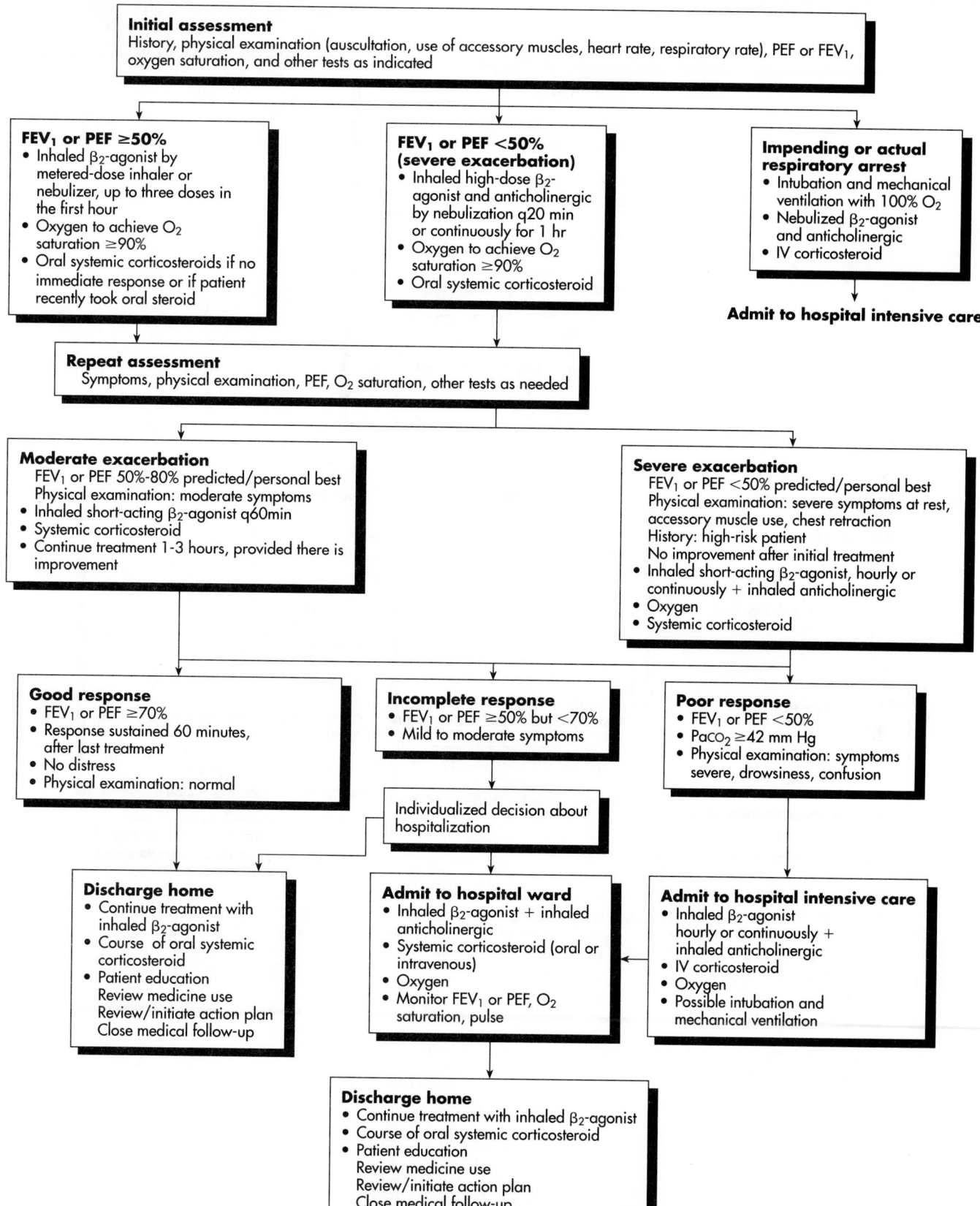

Fig. 3-24 **Management of asthma exacerbations: emergency department and hospital-based care.** *FEV₁,* Forced expiratory volume in 1 second; *PEF,* peak expiratory flow. (From National Asthma Education and Prevention Program: *Guidelines for the diagnosis and management of asthma,* NIH Pub No 97-4051A, Bethesda, Md, 1997, National Institutes of Health, National Heart, Lung, and Blood Institute.)

ASTHMA, HOME MANAGEMENT

Asthma, home management
ICD-9CM # 493.9 Asthma, unspecified
        493.1 Intrinsic asthma
        493.0 Extrinsic asthma

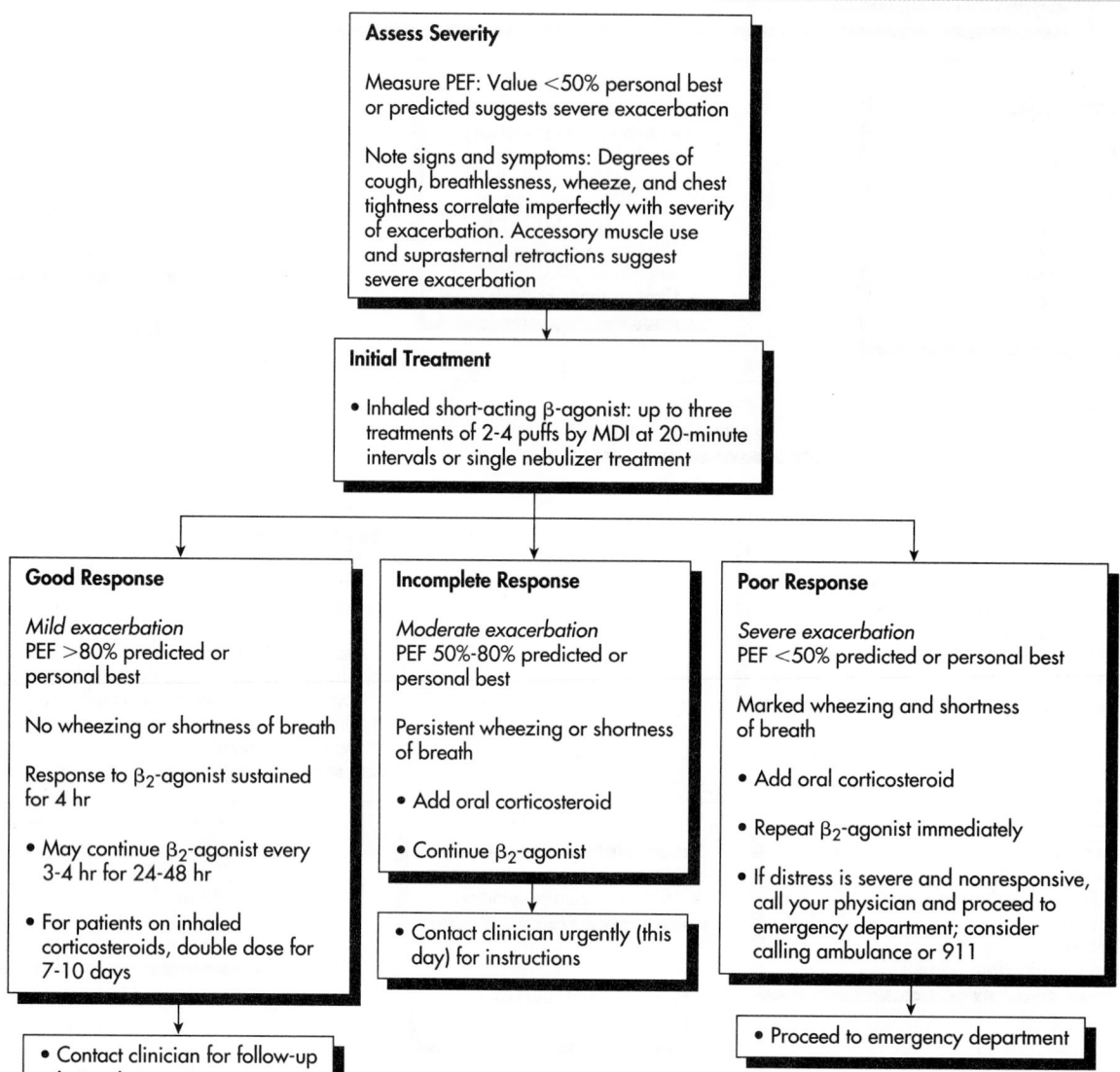

Assess Severity

Measure PEF: Value <50% personal best or predicted suggests severe exacerbation

Note signs and symptoms: Degrees of cough, breathlessness, wheeze, and chest tightness correlate imperfectly with severity of exacerbation. Accessory muscle use and suprasternal retractions suggest severe exacerbation

Initial Treatment

• Inhaled short-acting β-agonist: up to three treatments of 2-4 puffs by MDI at 20-minute intervals or single nebulizer treatment

Good Response

Mild exacerbation
PEF >80% predicted or personal best

No wheezing or shortness of breath

Response to β₂-agonist sustained for 4 hr

• May continue β₂-agonist every 3-4 hr for 24-48 hr

• For patients on inhaled corticosteroids, double dose for 7-10 days

• Contact clinician for follow-up instructions

Incomplete Response

Moderate exacerbation
PEF 50%-80% predicted or personal best

Persistent wheezing or shortness of breath

• Add oral corticosteroid

• Continue β₂-agonist

• Contact clinician urgently (this day) for instructions

Poor Response

Severe exacerbation
PEF <50% predicted or personal best

Marked wheezing and shortness of breath

• Add oral corticosteroid

• Repeat β₂-agonist immediately

• If distress is severe and nonresponsive, call your physician and proceed to emergency department; consider calling ambulance or 911

• Proceed to emergency department

Fig. 3-25   Home management of acute asthma. *MDI,* Metered-dose inhaler; *PEF,* peak expiratory flow rate. (Modified from National Asthma Education and Prevention Program, National Heart, Lung, and Blood Institute, Expert Panel Report 2: *Guidelines for the diagnosis and management of asthma,* NIH Pub No 97-4051, July 1997.)

BACK PAIN

Back pain
ICD-9CM # 847.9

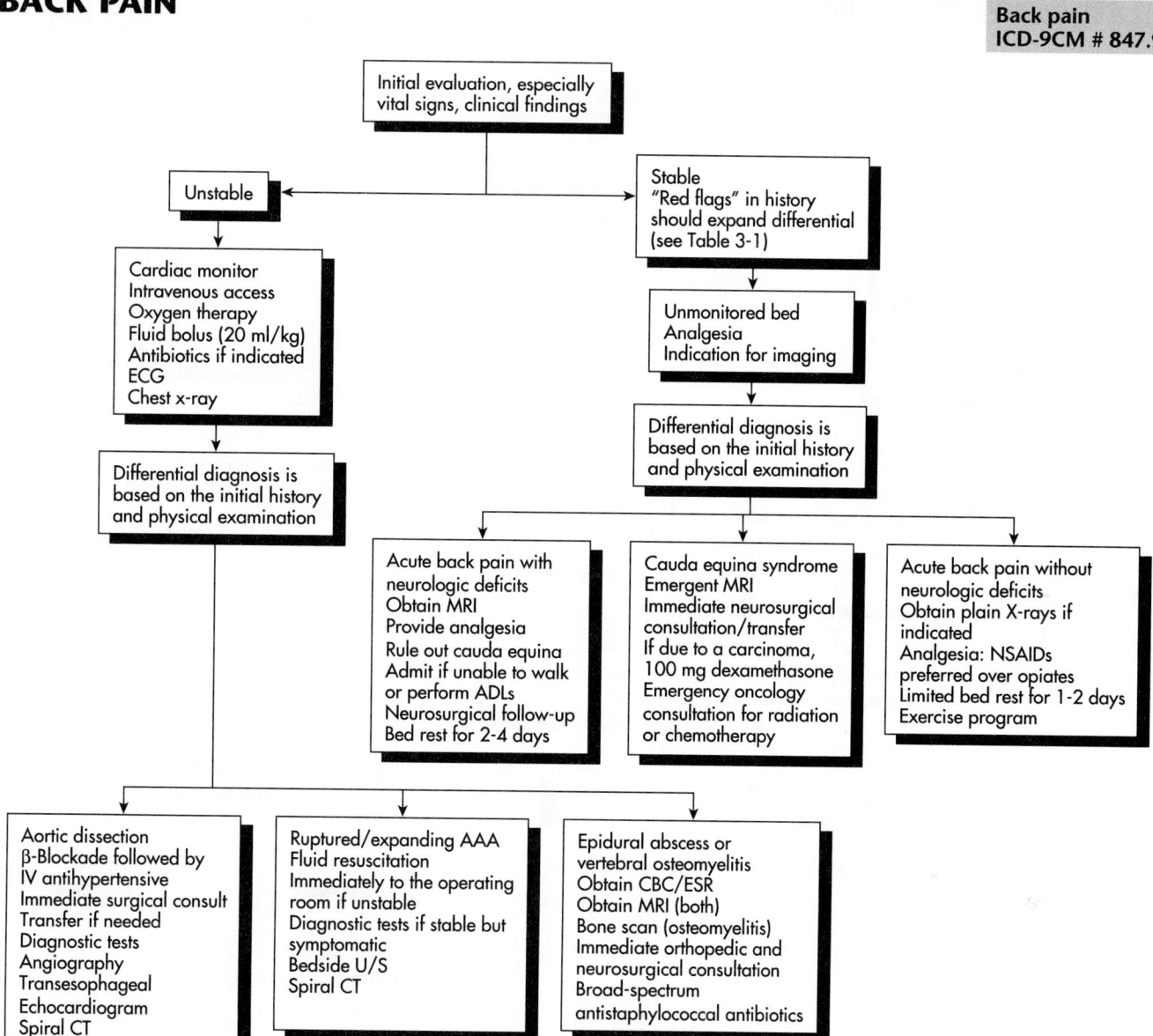

Fig. 3-26 **Management of acute low back pain.** *AAA,* Abdominal aortic aneurysm; *ADL,* activities of daily living; *CBC,* complete blood count; *CT,* computed tomography; *ECG,* electrocardiogram; *ESR,* erythrocyte sedimentation rate; *IV,* intravenous; *NSAIDs,* nonsteroidal antiinflammatory drugs. (From Marx JA [ed]: *Rosen's emergency medicine,* ed 5, St Louis 2002, Mosby.

III

TABLE 3-1 Red Flags for Potentially Serious Conditions

POSSIBLE FRACTURE	POSSIBLE TUMOR OR INFECTION	POSSIBLE CAUDA EQUINA SYNDROME
From Medical History		
Major trauma, such as vehicle accident or fall from height	Age over 50 or under 20 yr	Saddle anesthesia
Minor trauma or even strenuous lifting (in older or potentially osteoporotic patient)	History of cancer	Recent onset of bladder dysfunction, such as urinary retention, increased frequency, or overflow incontinence
	Constitutional symptoms, such as recent fever or chills or unexplained weight loss	
	Risk factors for spinal infection: recent bacterial infection (e.g., urinary tract infection); intravenous drug abuse; or immune suppression (from steroids, transplant, or human immunodeficiency virus)	Severe or progressive neurologic deficit in the lower extremity
	Pain that worsens when supine; severe nighttime pain	

BILIRUBIN ELEVATION

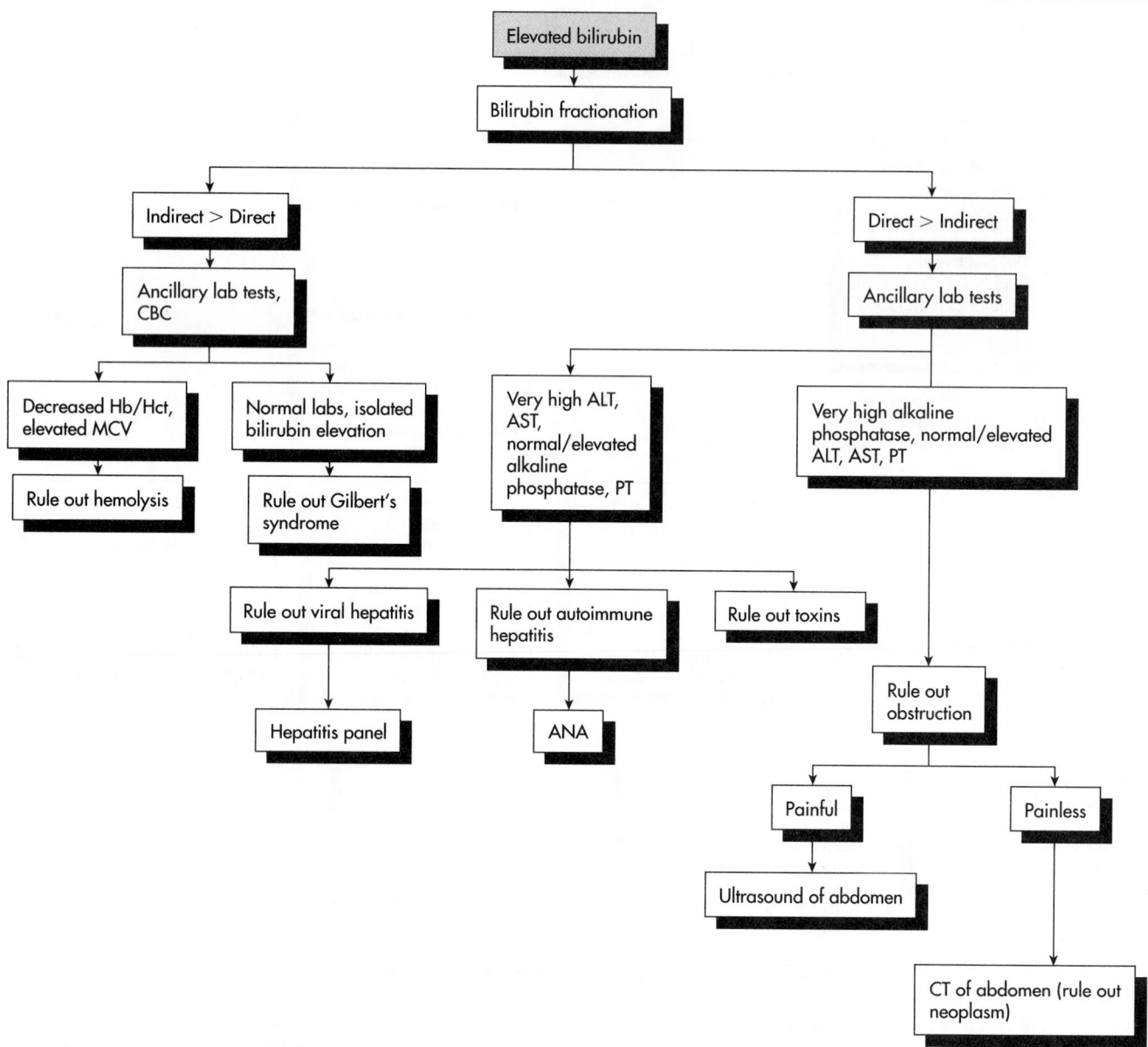

Fig. 3-27   Bilirubin elevation. *ALT,* Alanine aminotransferase; *ANA,* antinuclear antibody; *AST,* aspartate aminotransferase; *CBC,* complete blood count; *CT,* computed tomography; *MCV,* mean corpuscular volume; *PT,* prothrombin time.

BLEEDING, CONGENITAL DISORDER

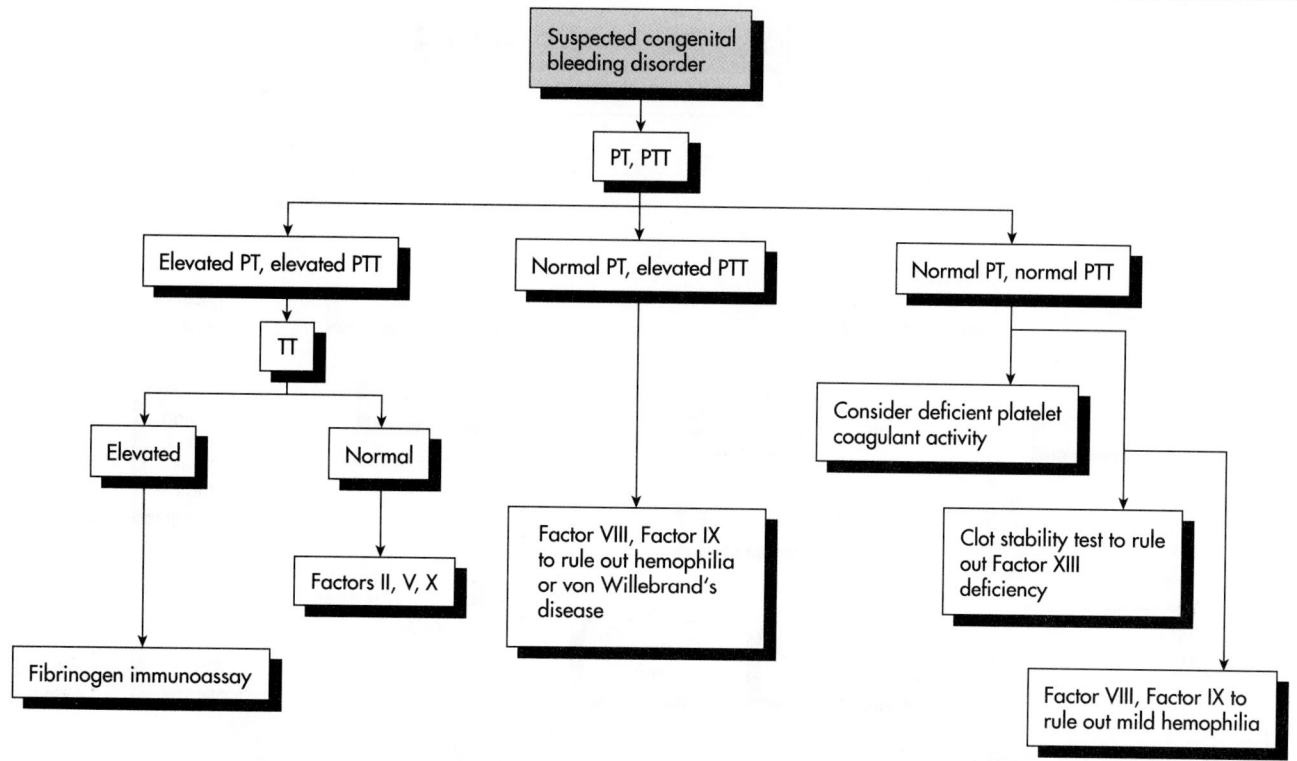

Fig. 3-28   Bleeding, congenital disorder. *PT,* Prothrombin time; *PTT,* partial thromboplastin time; *TT,* thrombin time.

III

BLEEDING, EARLY PREGNANCY

Bleeding, early pregnancy
ICD-9CM # 641.9 Vaginal bleeding NOS in pregnancy

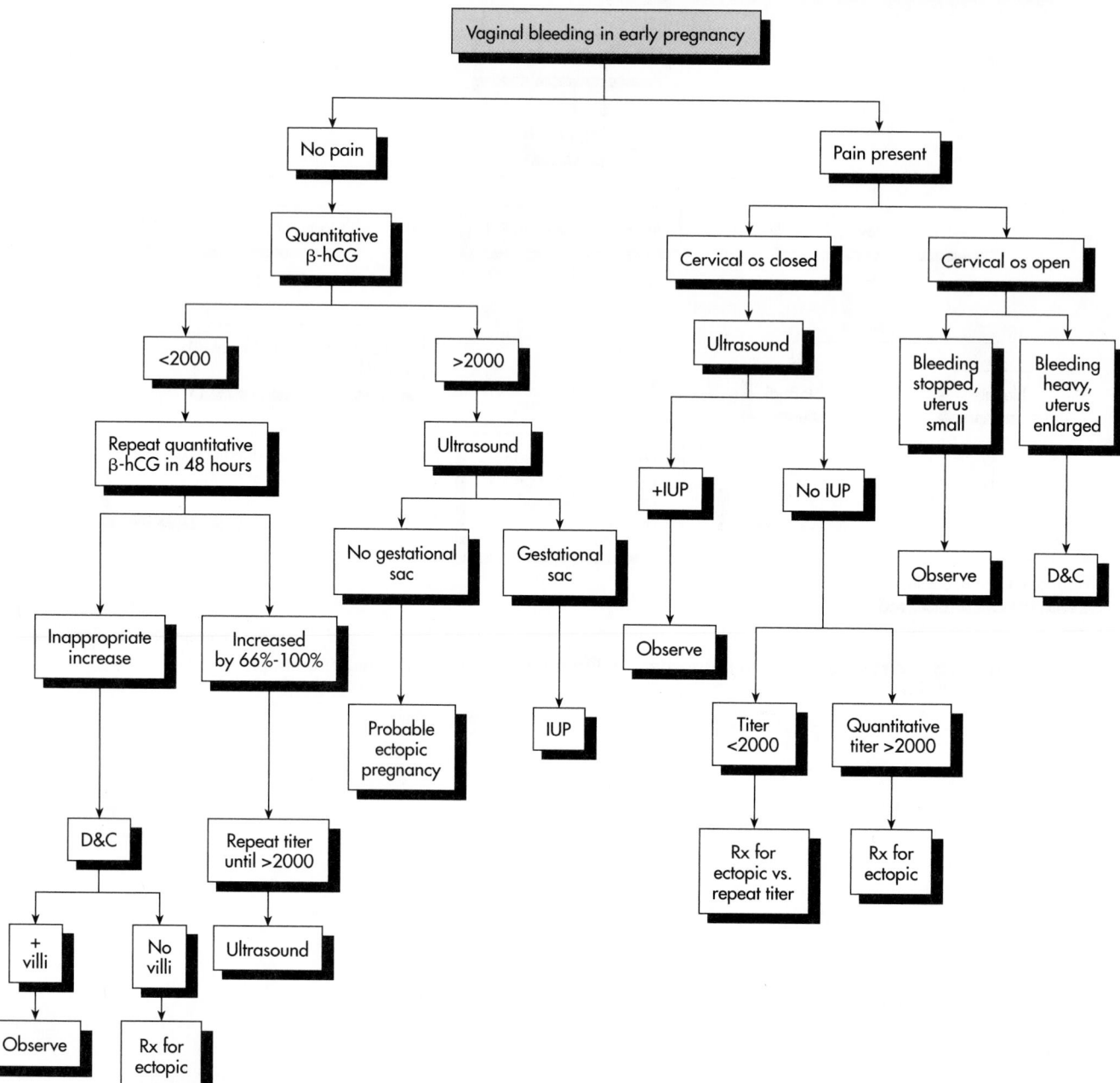

Fig. 3-29 **Diagnosis of vaginal bleeding in early pregnancy.** *D&C,* Dilation and curettage; β-*hCG,* β-human chorionic gonadotropin; *IUP,* intrauterine pregnancy. (From Carlson KJ et al: *Primary care of women,* ed 2, St Louis, 2002, Mosby.)

BLEEDING, GASTROINTESTINAL

Bleeding, gastrointestinal
ICD-9CM # 578.9

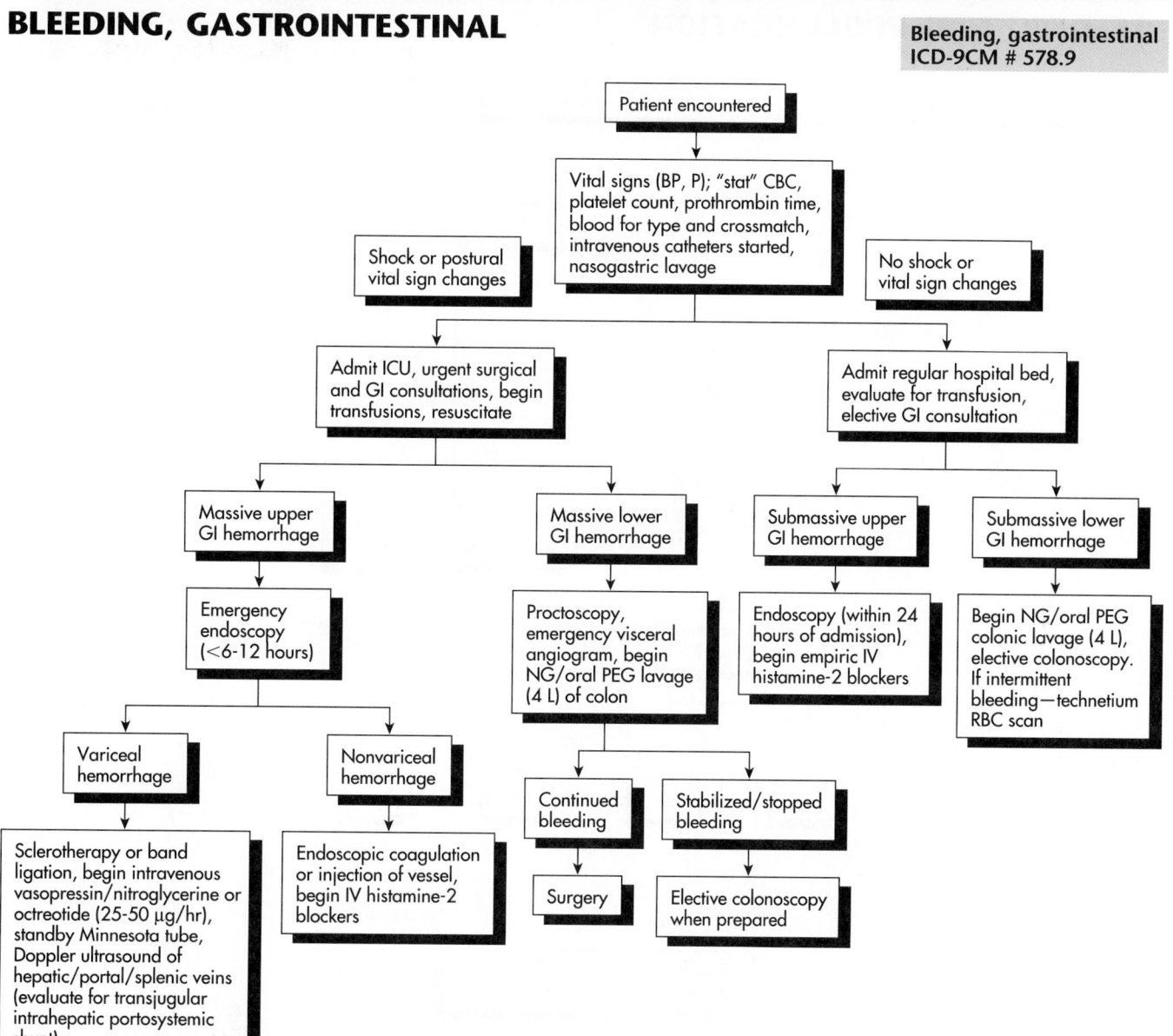

Fig. 3-30   Approach to the patient with gastrointestinal hemorrhage. *BP,* Blood pressure; *CBC,* complete blood count; *GI,* gastrointestinal; *ICU,* intensive care unit; *IV,* intravenous; *NG,* nasogastric; *P,* weight; *PEG,* percutaneous endoscopic gastrostomy; *RBC,* red blood cell. From Goldman L, Ausiello D [eds]: *Cecil textbook of medicine,* ed 22, Philadelphia, 2004, WB Saunders.)

BLEEDING TIME PROLONGATION

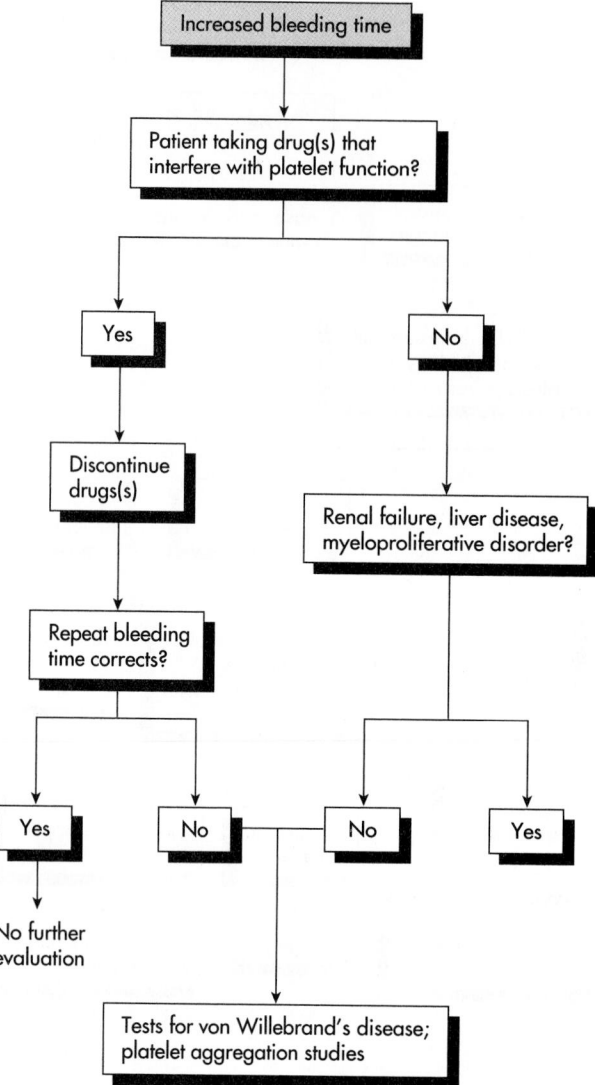

Fig. 3-31 An algorithm for diagnostic decisions in evaluating patients with a prolonged bleeding time. The scheme assumes that the platelet count is normal, because thrombocytopenia itself can prolong the bleeding time. (From Goldman L, Ausiello D [eds]: *Cecil textbook of medicine,* ed 22, Philadelphia, 2004, WB Saunders.)

BLEEDING, VAGINAL

Bleeding, vaginal
ICD-9CM # 623.8 Vaginal bleeding NOS

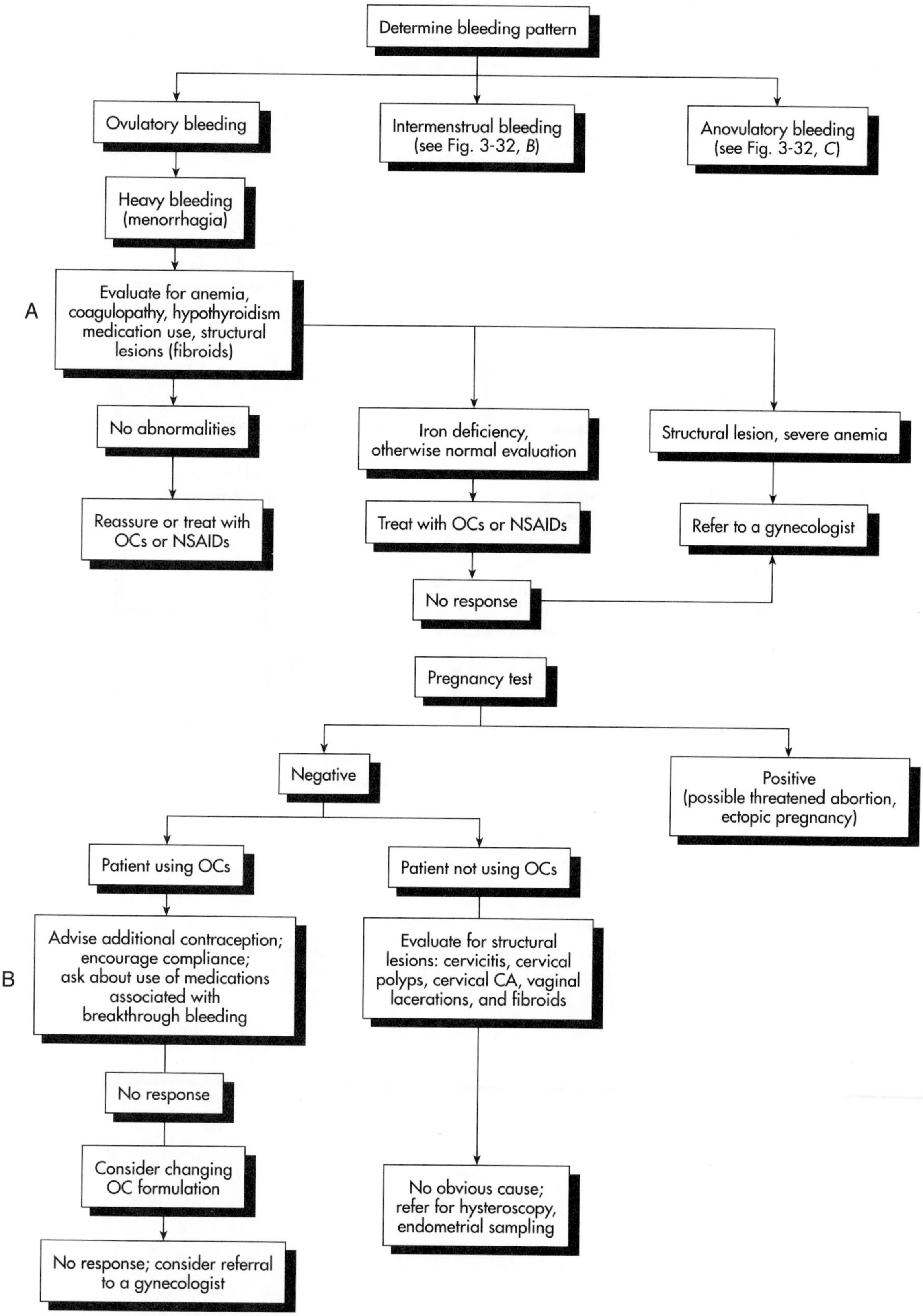

Fig. 3-32   A, Evaluation of ovulatory bleeding. B, Evaluation of intermenstrual bleeding. *NSAIDs,* Nonsteroidal antiinflammatory drugs; *OCs,* oral contraceptives. (From Appleby J, Henderson M, Wathen PI: *Intern Med* Sept:17, 1996.)

BLEEDING, VAGINAL—cont'd

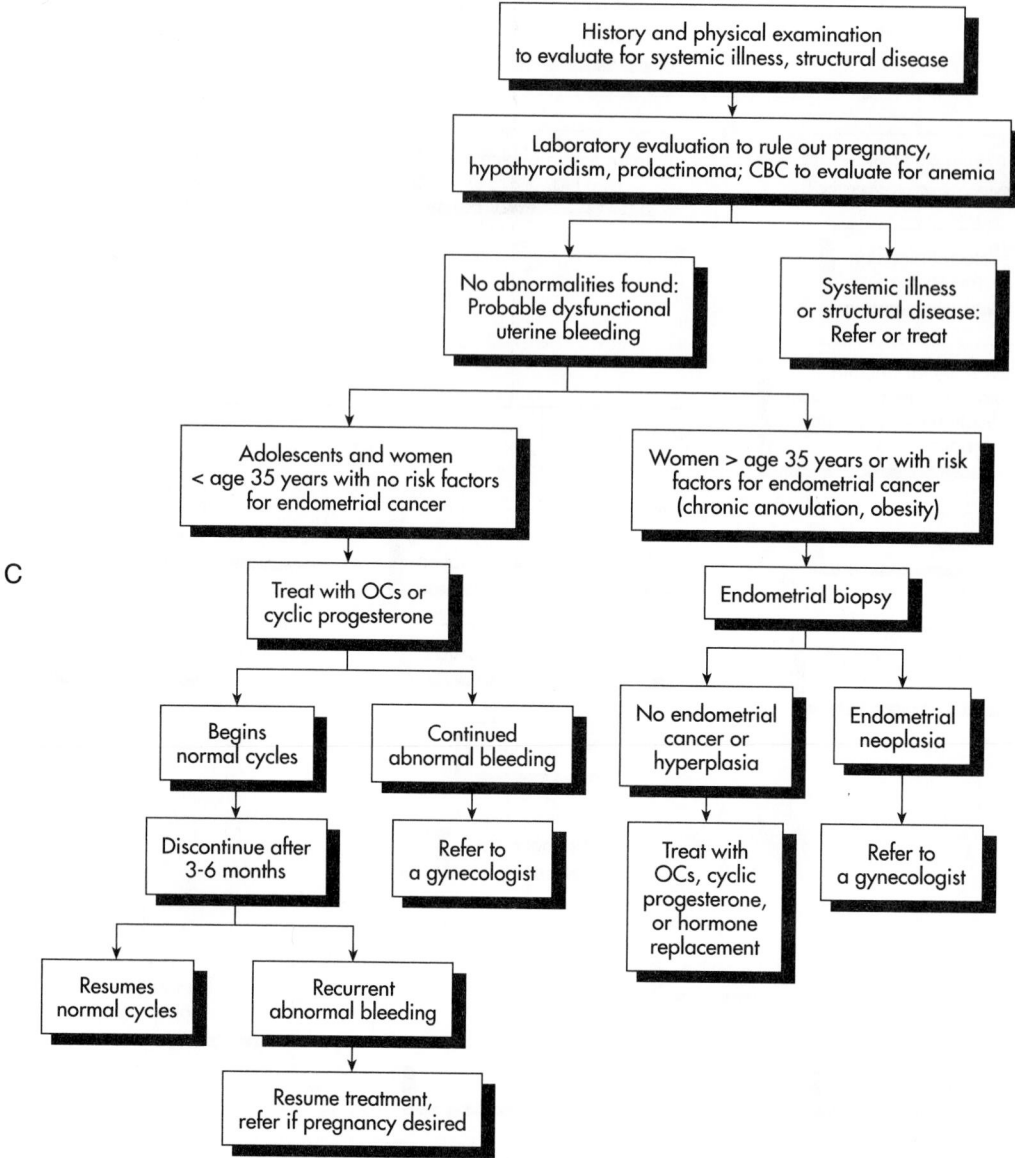

Fig. 3-32, cont'd   C, Evaluation of anovulatory bleeding. *CBC,* Complete blood count; *OCs,* oral contraceptives. (From Appleby J, Henderson M, Wathen PI: *Intern Med* Sept:17, 1996.)

BLEEDING VARICEAL

Bleeding, variceal
ICD-9CM # 456.0

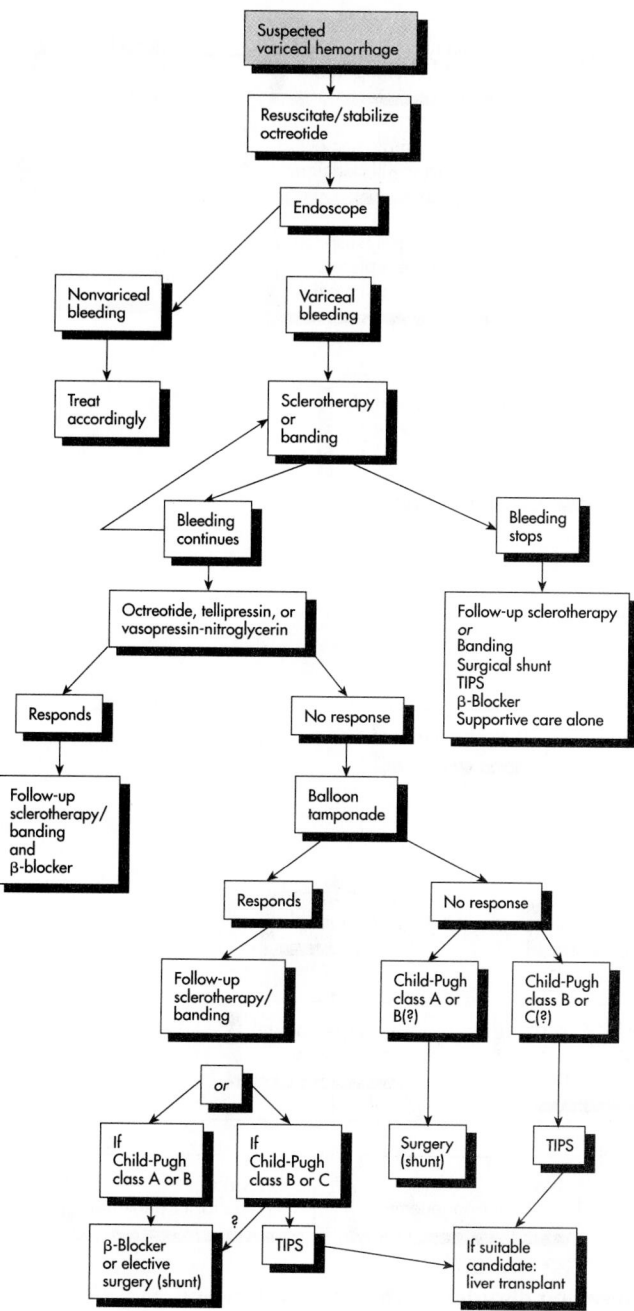

Fig. 3-33 **Management of bleeding varices.** Practice may vary according to local resources, personnel, expertise, and preference. Where hepatic transplant is available, candidates may undergo placement of transjugular intrahepatic portosystemic shunt (TIPS) sooner, especially if sclerotherapy or banding for esophageal varices fails (gastric varices are generally not readily amenable to these procedures). Those who are not transplant candidates may benefit from portacaval shunt (side-to-side if ascites is present) to stop active bleeding or from distal splenorenal shunt if the patient is not actively bleeding and without ascites. (From Stein J [ed]: *Internal medicine,* ed 5, St Louis, 1998, Mosby.)

TABLE 3-2 **Child-Pugh Classes**

PROGNOSTIC VARIABLES	CHILD-PUGH SCORE* POINTS		
	1	2	3
Bilirubin (mg/dl)	>1.1-2.0	>2.0-3.0	>3.0
Albumin (g/dl)		2.8-3.5	<2.8
Prothrombin time (seconds above control)	1-3	4-6	>6
Encephalopathy		Grade 1-2	Grade 3-4
Ascites		Mild	Moderate
Age (years)			
Edema (± diuretics)			
Splenomegaly			
Histologic stage			

From Stein J (ed): *Internal medicine,* ed 5, St Louis, 1998, Mosby.
*Child-Pugh classes: A, score 1-6; B, score 7-9; C, score 10-15.

III

BLEEDING DISORDER, CONGENITAL

Bleeding disorder, congenital
ICD-9CM # 286.9

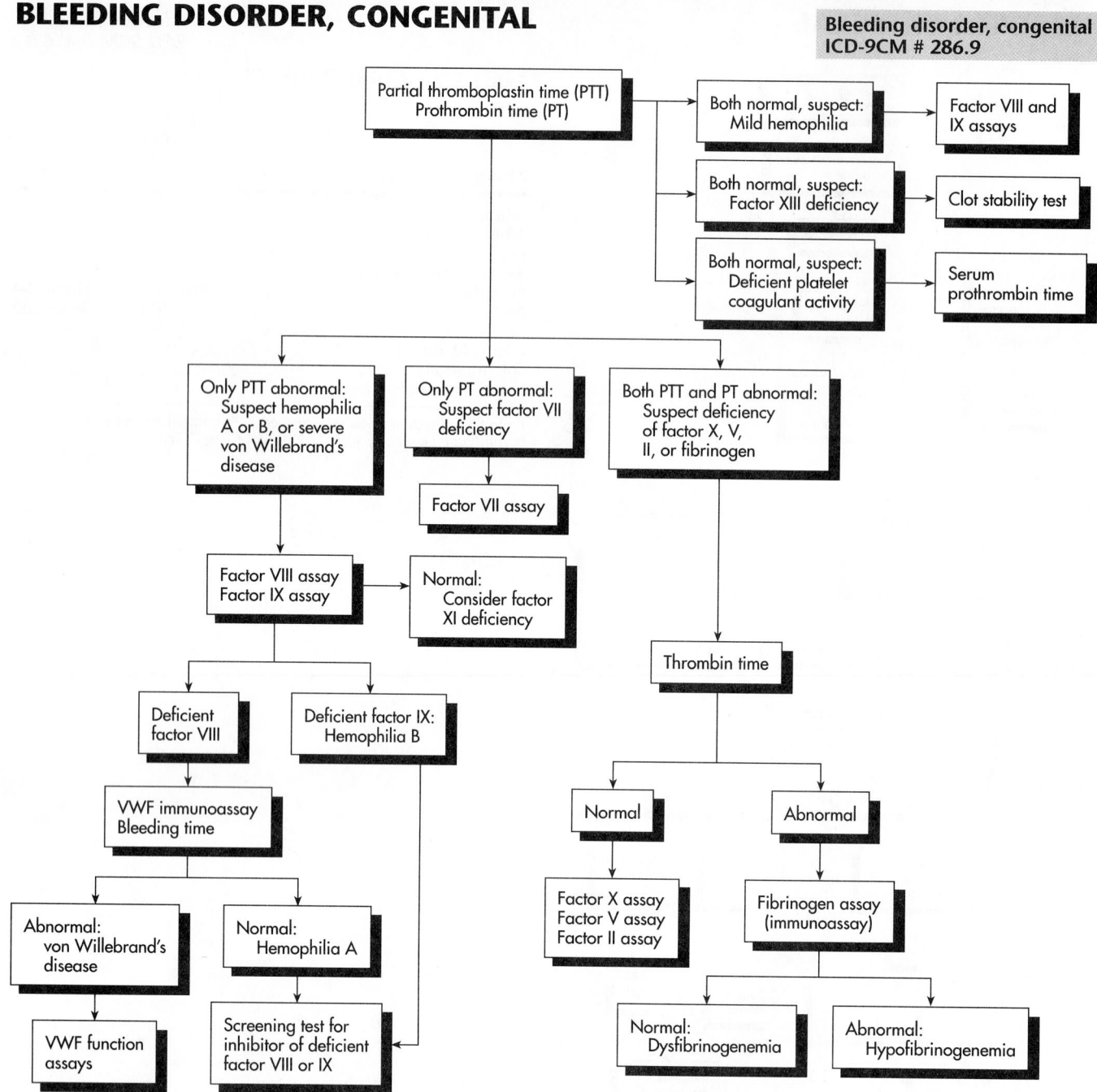

Fig. 3-34 Laboratory evaluation of a patient with a bleeding disorder in whom the history and physical examination suggest a congenital coagulation disorder. *VWF,* von Willebrand factor. (From Stein JH [ed]: *Internal medicine,* ed 5, St Louis, 1998, Mosby.)

BRADYCARDIA

ICD-9CM # 427.89 Unspecified bradycardia
427.81 Chronic bradycardia
770.8 Newborn bradycardia
427.89 Postoperative bradycardia
337 Reflex bradycardia
427.89 Sinus bradycardia

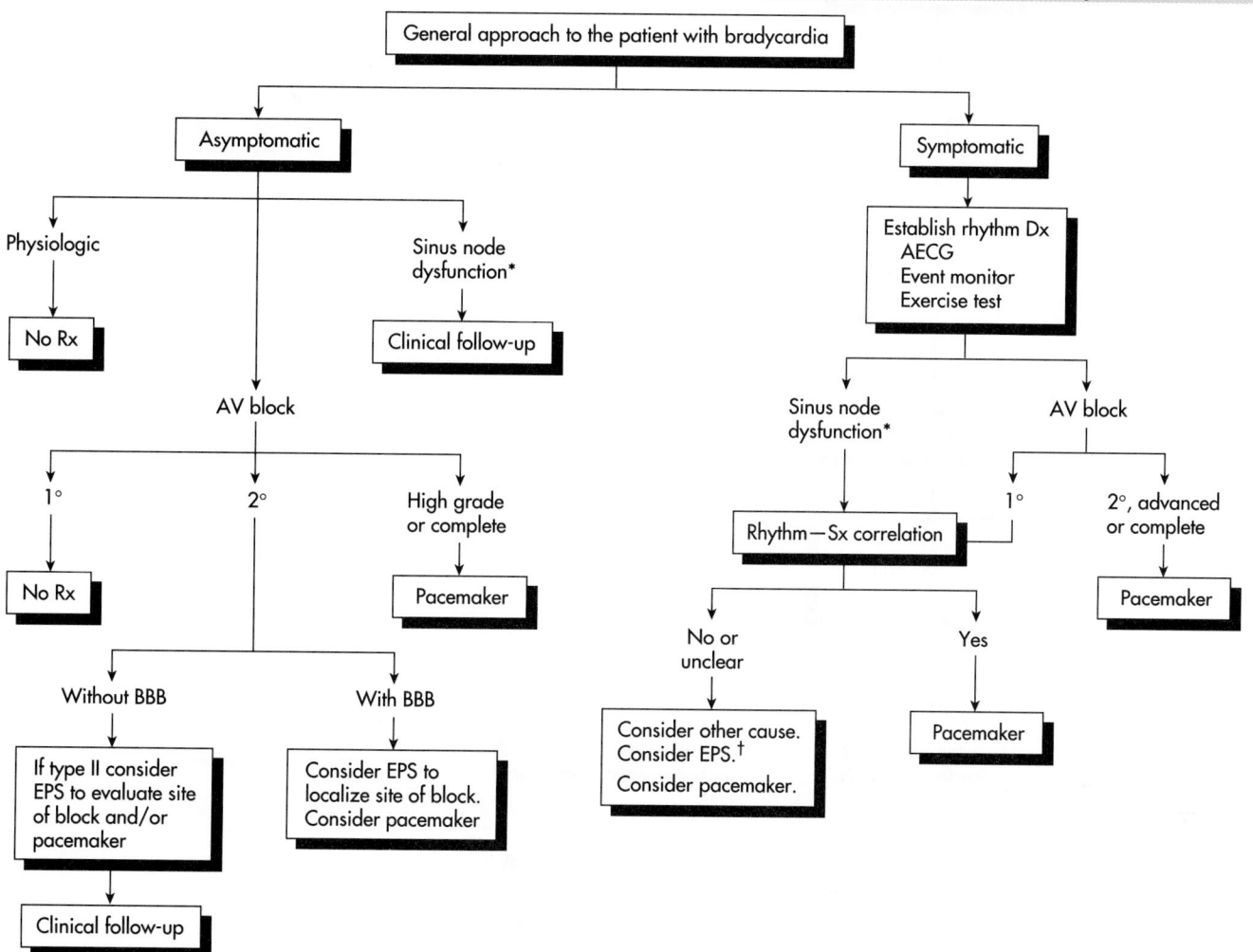

*Includes bradycardia-tachycardia syndrome.
†EPS includes sinus node function and ventricular arrhythmia induction studies.

Fig. 3-35   General approach to the patient with bradycardia. *AECG,* Ambulatory electrocardiography; *AV,* atrioventricular; *BBB,* bundle branch block; *Dx,* diagnostic; *EPS,* electrophysiologic study; *Rx,* treatment; *Sx,* symptoms; 1°, first-degree; 2°, second-degree. (From Goldman L, Braunwald E [eds]: *Primary cardiology,* Philadelphia, 1998, WB Saunders.)

BREAST, NIPPLE DISCHARGE EVALUATION*

Breast, nipple discharge evaluation
ICD-9CM # 611.79

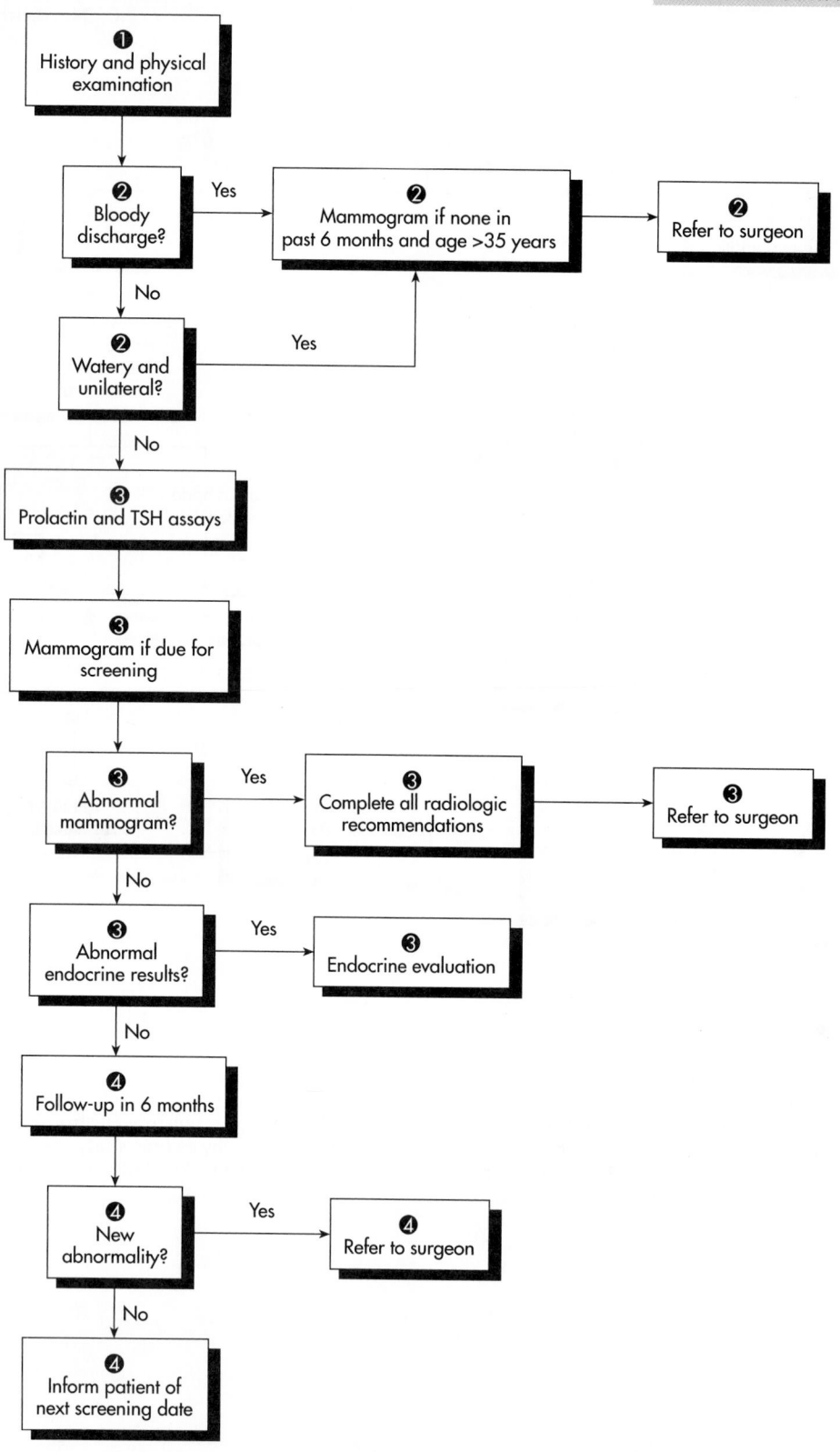

*Without palpable mass.

Fig. 3-36   Breast cancer screening and evaluation. (From Institute for Clinical Systems Integration, Minneapolis: *Postgrad Med* 100:182, 1996.)

Fig. 3-36, cont'd

1. **History and physical examination.*** Patients who present with a complaint of nipple discharge should be evaluated with breast-related history taking and a physical examination. History taking is aimed at uncovering and characterizing any other breast-related symptom. A risk assessment should also be undertaken for identified risk factors, including patient age over 50 years, any past personal history of breast cancer, history of hyperplasia on previous breast biopsies, and family history of breast cancer in first-degree relatives (mother, sister, daughter). Physical examination should include inspection of the breast for any evidence of ulceration or contour changes and inspection of the nipple for Paget's disease. Palpation should be performed with the patient in both the upright and the supine positions to determine the presence of any palpable mass.

2. **Bloody discharge?** If the discharge appears frankly bloody, the patient should be referred to a surgeon for evaluation. At the time of referral, a mammogram of the involved breast should be obtained if the patient is over 35 years of age and has not had a mammogram within the preceding 6 months. Similarly, patients with a watery, unilateral discharge should be referred to a surgeon for evaluation and possible biopsy.

3. **Endocrine tests. Mammogram.** If the discharge appears frankly milky or is bilateral, serum prolactin and serum thyroid-stimulating hormone (TSH) assays should be performed to rule out the presence of an endocrinologic basis for the symptoms. At the time of that visit, a mammogram should also be performed if the patient is due for routine mammographic screening according to the recommended intervals. A patient with an abnormal mammogram should be further evaluated radiologically to better characterize the lesion and then be referred to a surgeon if appropriate. Make certain that all recommended additional views, ultrasound examinations, and follow-up studies have been obtained before referral to a surgeon. Should the mammogram appear normal, results of the assays for TSH and prolactin should be reviewed. If the results are abnormal the patient should undergo appropriate evaluation for etiology, either by a primary care physician or by an endocrinologist.

4. **Six-month follow-up results.** If results of the mammogram and the endocrinologic screening studies are normal, the patient should return for a follow-up visit in 6 months to ensure that there has been no specific change in the character of the discharge, such as development of frank bleeding or Paget's disease, that would warrant surgical evaluation. If the evaluation at that follow-up visit fails to reveal any palpable or visible abnormalities, the patient should be returned to the routine screening process with studies performed at the recommended intervals.

---

*ICSI healthcare guidelines are designed to assist clinicians by providing an analytic framework for the evaluation and treatment of patients. They are not intended either to replace a clinician's judgment or to establish a protocol for all patients with a particular condition. A guideline will rarely establish the only approach to a problem. In addition, guidelines are "living documents" that are expected to be imperfect and are subject to annual review and revision.

ICSI is a nonprofit organization that provides healthcare quality improvement services to 20 medical groups affiliated with HealthPartners in central and southern Minnesota and western Wisconsin. The guidelines are developed through a process that involves physicians, nurses, and other healthcare professionals from beginning to end, and healthcare purchasers are included in decision making. To order any of the more than 40 guidelines ICSI has developed, contact the ICSI Publications Fulfillment Center, in care of the ARDEL Group, 6518 Walker St., Suite 150, Minneapolis, MN 55426; 612-927-6707.

III

BREAST, RADIOLOGIC EVALUATION

Breast, radiologic evaluation
ICD-9CM # V76.10

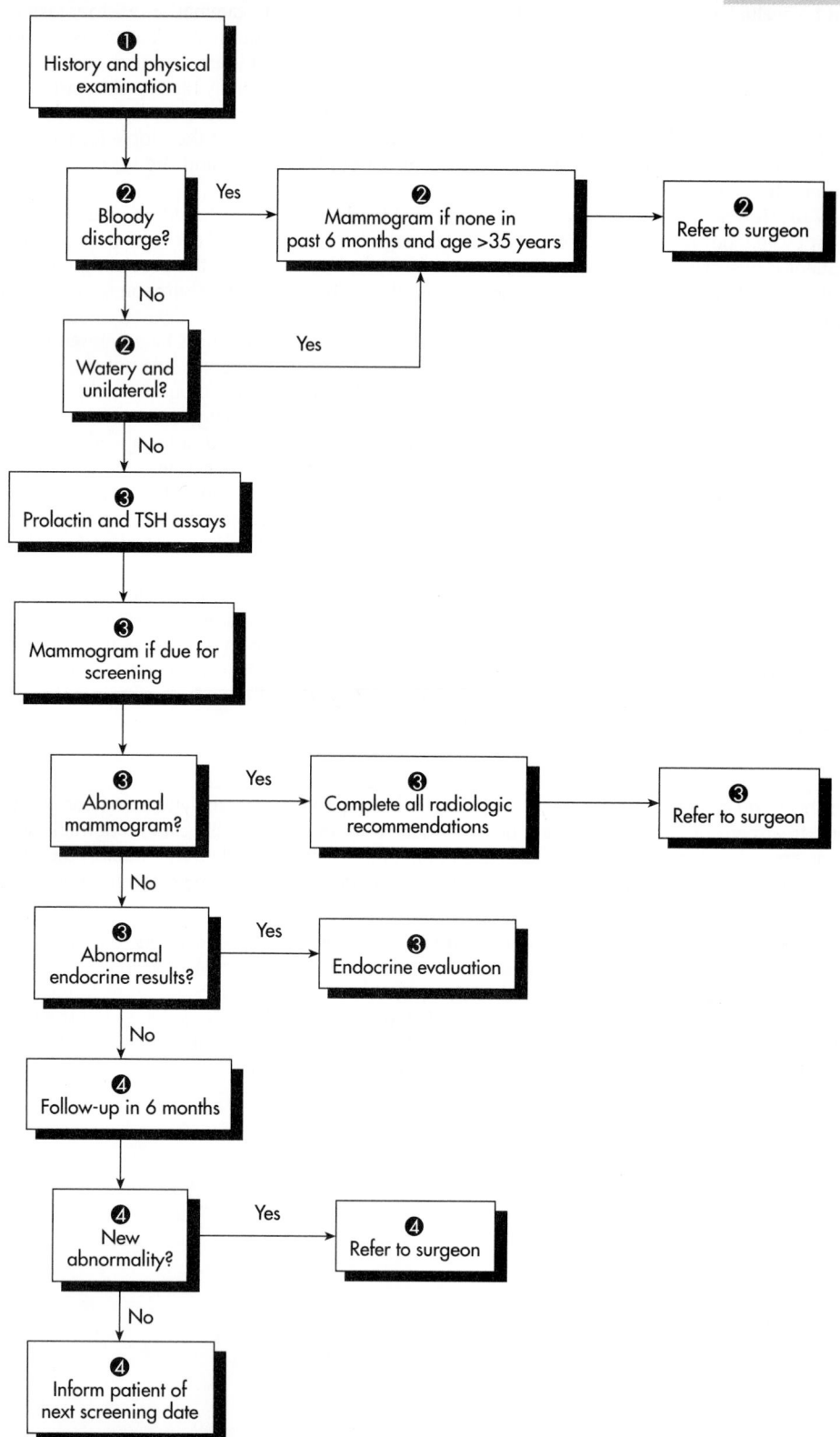

Fig. 3-37 Breast cancer screening and evaluation. (From Institute for Clinical Systems Integration, Minneapolis: *Postgrad Med* 100:182-187, 1996.)

Fig. 3-37, cont'd

1. **Screening mammogram.*** Patients are most commonly referred to a radiologist for screening mammography. Occasionally, however, patients are referred for diagnostic mammography based on symptoms or findings on breast exam. In the event of an abnormal finding on the mammogram, complete evaluation under the direction of a radiologist is recommended. It is the responsibility of the radiologist to complete the radiologic assessment so that the best possible characterization of the abnormality can be provided in an expeditious fashion to the primary care physician who ordered the original study. Any recommendations for referral to a surgeon for possible biopsy should be made directly to the primary care physician. The ultimate responsibility to make the referral will rest with the primary care physician.

2. **Abnormal mammogram. Sorting abnormalities. Suspicious for cancer?** On obtaining an abnormal finding on a mammogram, the radiologist determines whether further mammographic images are required for completion of the evaluation process. This may include a repeated image of the involved breast at 6 months to document stability of a low-risk, probably benign lesion. Alternatively, spot compression, magnification, or both may be necessary to obtain further characterization of indeterminate breast lesions. These additional studies should be done with the radiologist present to reduce the risk of patient recall for further studies necessary to evaluate the same lesion.

   On completion of these views, each and every abnormality uncovered for each independent lesion of the breast studied should be sorted according to the nature of the abnormality. The radiologist should classify the lesion as representing either suspicious microcalcifications, architectural distortion, or a soft-tissue mass. For any lesions identified as demonstrating microcalcifications that suggest cancer, biopsy will be recommended. It is up to the primary care physician to make the referral to a surgeon for biopsy. If a soft-tissue mass is identified on the mammogram, it should be studied further to determine its relative risk for malignancy. Any suspect lesions identified as having associated microcalcifications, architectural distortion, or interval growth when compared with the previous mammogram should likewise be referred to a surgeon for possible biopsy.

3. **Ultrasound results.** When the mass is not immediately suggestive of cancer, an ultrasound should be performed to determine whether the lesion is solid. A solid mass should be further characterized for its level of benignity according to three criteria:
   - Size less than 15 mm
   - Three or fewer lobulations
   - More than 50% of the margin of the lesion appearing well circumscribed in any view

   Patients who have lesions that fit all three criteria may be observed and then evaluated with a 6-month follow-up study. Any lesion that does not fit all three criteria for benignity should be characterized as indeterminate, and biopsy should be considered. Likewise, any solid mass that is palpable should be referred to a surgeon for possible open biopsy. Finally, any lesion that appears to be new since the last screening mammogram should be considered for biopsy.

4. **Aspiration and results.** If the ultrasound of the soft-tissue mass demonstrates that it is a cystic lesion, the cyst should be further categorized by the criteria listed in the algorithm: irregular wall, as seen on ultrasonography; internal echoes; complex, septated appearance; and palpability within the region of the ultrasound-proven cyst. A positive finding for any of these criteria would be an indication for ultrasound-directed aspiration of the cyst. Aspiration should also be offered if the patient requests it.

   After cyst aspiration, a single-view mammogram should be obtained to demonstrate complete resolution of the lesion. If the lesion is sufficiently complex, a cyst pneumogram may be performed. Should any residual mass be present or if the cyst pneumogram findings are abnormal, biopsy should be recommended. If, on the other hand, the mass is a simple cyst that does not fit any of the previously listed criteria, the patient should be returned to the screening process, and completion of this evaluation should be reported to the ordering health care provider.

---

*ICSI healthcare guidelines are designed to assist clinicians by providing an analytic framework for the evaluation and treatment of patients. They are not intended either to replace a clinician's judgment or to establish a protocol for all patients with a particular condition. A guideline will rarely establish the only approach to a problem. In addition, guidelines are "living documents" that are expected to be imperfect and are subject to annual review and revision.

ICSI is a nonprofit organization that provides healthcare quality improvement services to 20 medical groups affiliated with HealthPartners in central and southern Minnesota and western Wisconsin. The guidelines are developed through a process that involves physicians, nurses, and other healthcare professionals from beginning to end, and healthcare purchasers are included in decision making. To order any of the more than 40 guidelines ICSI has developed, contact the ICSI Publications Fulfillment Center, in care of the ARDEL Group, 6518 Walker St., Suite 150, Minneapolis, MN 55426; 612-927-6707.

III

BREAST, ROUTINE SCREEN OR PALPABLE MASS EVALUATION

Breast, routine screen or palpable mass evaluation
ICD-9CM # 611.72 Breast mass or lump, nonpuerperal

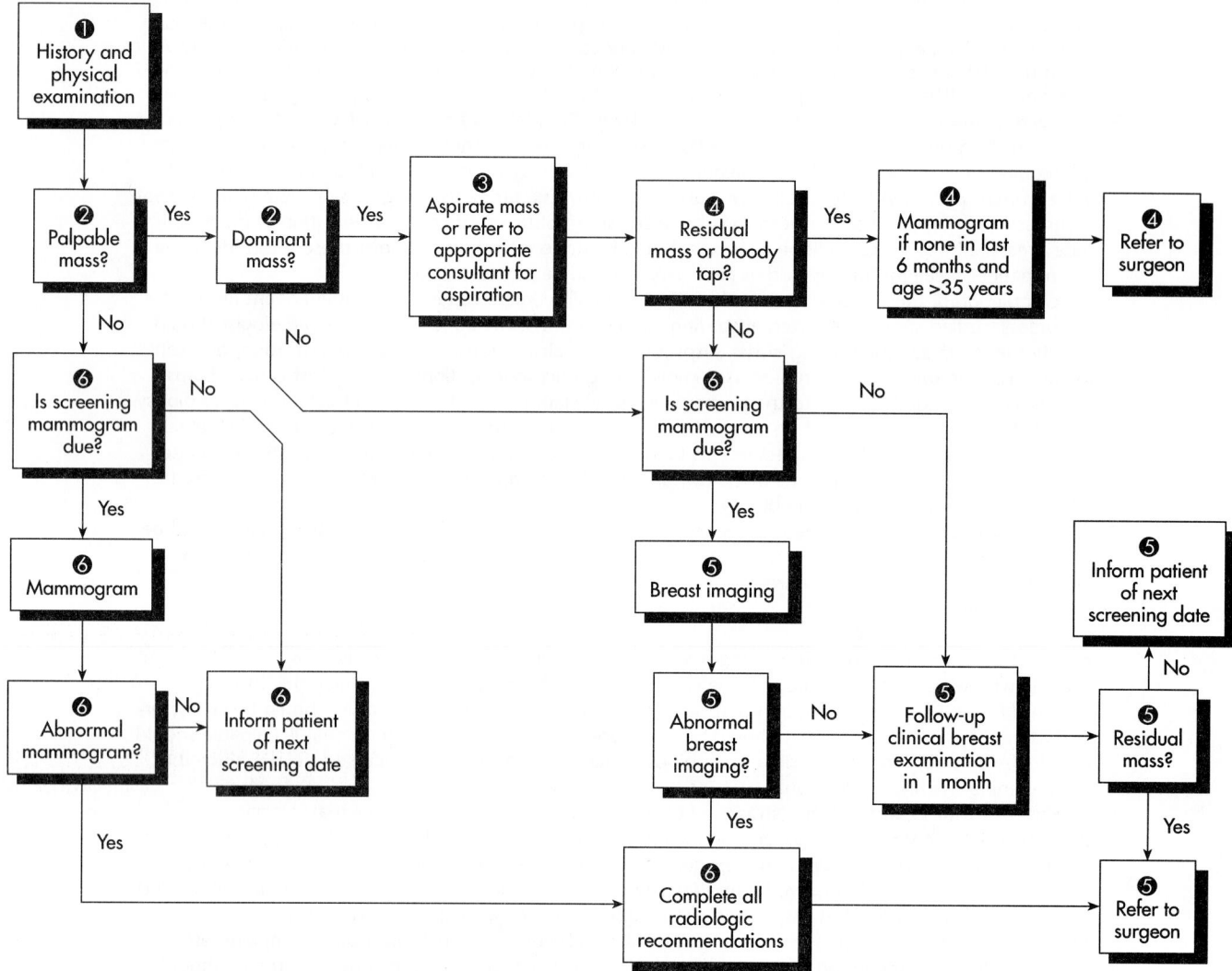

Fig. 3-38   Breast cancer screening and evaluation. (From Institute for Clinical Systems Integration, Minneapolis: *Postgrad Med* 100:182, 1996.)

1. **History and physical examination.*** Primary care evaluation is initiated with history taking aimed at uncovering and characterizing any breast-related symptom. A risk assessment should also be undertaken for identified risk factors, including patient age over 50 years, any past personal history of breast cancer, history of hyperplasia on previous breast biopsies, and family history of breast cancer in first-degree relatives (mother, sister, daughter). Physical examination should include inspection of the breast for any evidence of ulceration or contour changes and inspection of the nipple for Paget's disease. Palpation should be performed with the patient in both the upright and supine positions to determine the presence of any palpable mass.

2. **Palpable mass? Dominant mass?** A dominant mass is a palpable finding that is discrete and clearly different from the surrounding parenchyma. If a palpable mass is identified, it should be determined whether it represents a dominant (i.e., discrete) mass, which requires immediate evaluation. The primary care physician or appropriate consultant should attempt to aspirate any dominant mass because a simple cyst may be uncovered, in which case aspiration completes the evaluation process.

3. **Aspirate mass or refer for aspiration.** Aspiration of a dominant palpable mass should be performed by the primary care physician or by the appropriate consultant. The breast skin is prepped with alcohol. Then, with the lesion immobilized by the nonoperating hand, an 18- to 25-gauge needle mounted on a 10-ml syringe is directed to the central portion of the mass for a single attempt at aspiration. Successful aspiration of a simple cyst would yield a nonbloody fluid with complete resolution of the dominant mass. Typical watery fluid may be discarded. However, cyst fluid that is bloody or unusually tenacious should be examined cytologically.

Fig. 3-38, cont'd

4. **Residual mass or bloody tap? Mammogram if none in past 6 months. Refer to surgeon.** Should the mass remain after the attempt at aspiration or should frank blood be aspirated during the process, the presence of a malignant process cannot be ruled out. Patients with a residual mass or bloody tap should be referred to a surgeon for possible biopsy. Before the referral, a mammogram should be obtained for any patient over age 35 years who has not had a mammogram within the preceding 6 months. In patients 35 years and under, obtaining any other breast-imaging studies should be left to the discretion of the surgeon or radiologist.

5. **Is screening mammogram due? Breast imaging. Follow-up clinical breast examination. Refer to surgeon.** Should physical examination demonstrate a palpable mass that is not clearly a discrete and dominant mass, its size, location, and character should be documented in anticipation of a follow-up examination. A screening mammogram should be obtained if one has not been done within the recommended interval. If no mammogram is required or if a required mammogram demonstrates no abnormality, a follow-up examination in 1 month is indicated. Should any residual mass be identified, the patient should be referred to a surgeon for possible biopsy. Patients with a persisting nondominant palpable mass that does not resolve within 1 month and those with any recurring cystic mass should be referred for surgical evaluation. If no mass is apparent at the time of the follow-up examination, the patient should then be informed of the appropriate date for her next screening examination, according to the recommended intervals.

6. **Screening mammogram and results.** After completion of the physical examination, the appropriateness of a routine screening mammogram should be determined. If a mammogram is done, the radiologist should provide the results to the primary care physician for reporting to the patient. Should any abnormalities be uncovered, it will be the responsibility of the radiologist to complete any additional imaging studies required for the complete radiographic characterization of the lesion. The radiologist should make certain that all recommended additional views, follow-up studies, and ultrasound examinations have been completed before referral to a surgeon. However, it is important that the primary care physician who ordered the mammogram review the results of these studies to understand fully the opinion of the radiologist and to ensure that all recommendations of the radiologist have been completed. Should the radiologist recommend that surgical consultation is warranted, it will be the responsibility of the primary care physician to establish this referral.

NOTE: *The importance of communication between the surgical consultant and the primary care physician cannot be overstated. Biopsy results should be reported both to the surgeon and to the primary care physician. More important, patients who do not require biopsy after surgical consultation should be returned to the routine screening process. This process is under the supervision of the primary care physician. Therefore it is absolutely necessary for the primary care physician to know when the patient reenters the routine screening population. In the event that new symptoms arise during the screening interval, the patient should be evaluated by the primary care physician using the primary care evaluation process of this guideline.*

*ICSI healthcare guidelines are designed to assist clinicians by providing an analytic framework for the evaluation and treatment of patients. They are not intended either to replace a clinician's judgment or to establish a protocol for all patients with a particular condition. A guideline will rarely establish the only approach to a problem. In addition, guidelines are "living documents" that are expected to be imperfect and are subject to annual review and revision.

ICSI is a nonprofit organization that provides healthcare quality improvement services to 20 medical groups affiliated with HealthPartners in central and southern Minnesota and western Wisconsin. The guidelines are developed through a process that involves physicians, nurses, and other healthcare professionals from beginning to end, and healthcare purchasers are included in decision making. To order any of the more than 40 guidelines ICSI has developed, contact the ICSI Publications Fulfillment Center, in care of the ARDEL Group, 6518 Walker St., Suite 150, Minneapolis, MN 55426; 612-927-6707.

III

BREASTFEEDING DIFFICULTIES

Breastfeeding difficulties
ICD-9CM # 676.8

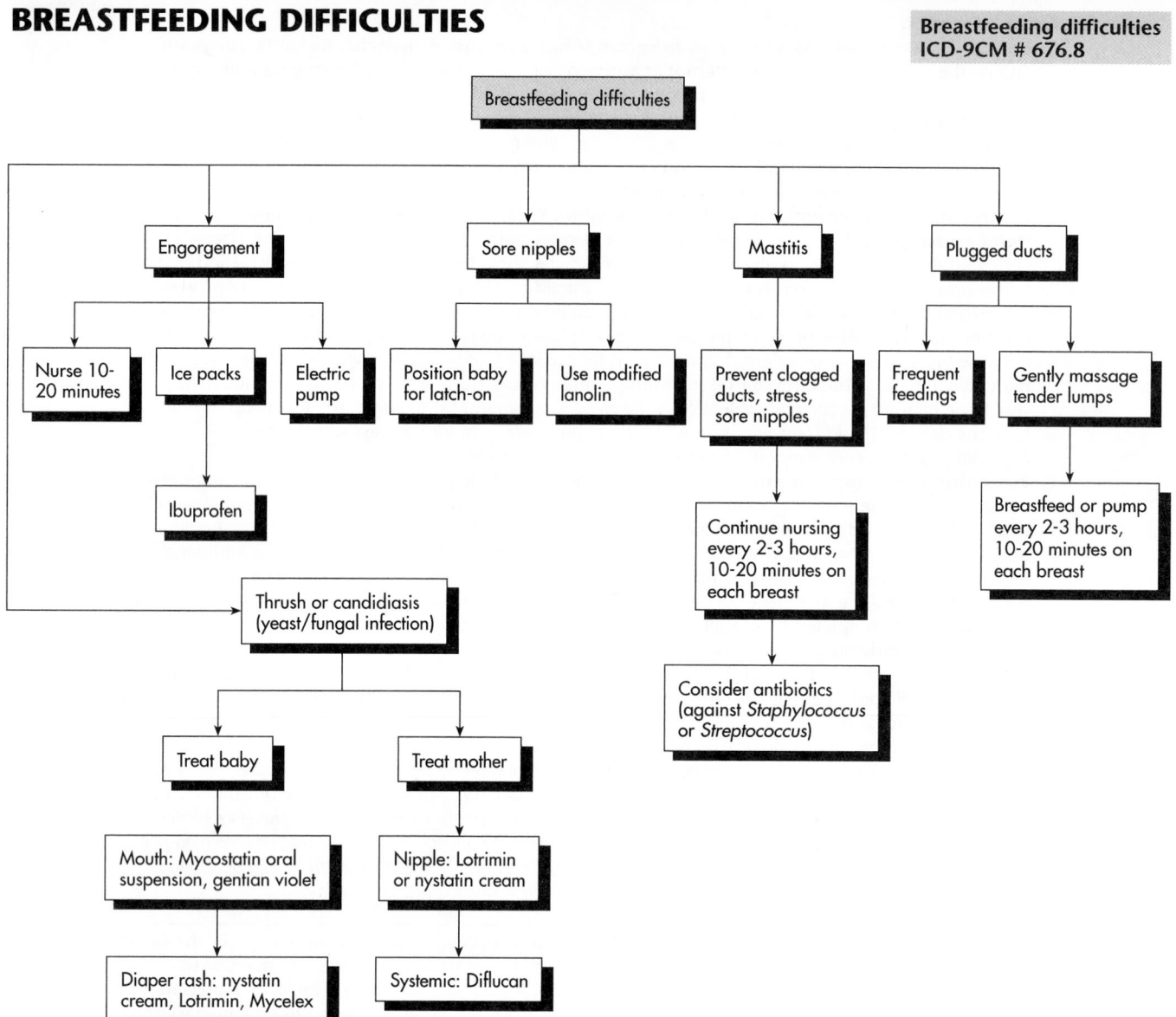

Fig. 3-39   Management of breastfeeding difficulties. (From Zuspan FP [ed]: *Handbook of obstetrics, gynecology, and primary care,* St Louis, 1998, Mosby.)

CARCINOID TUMORS

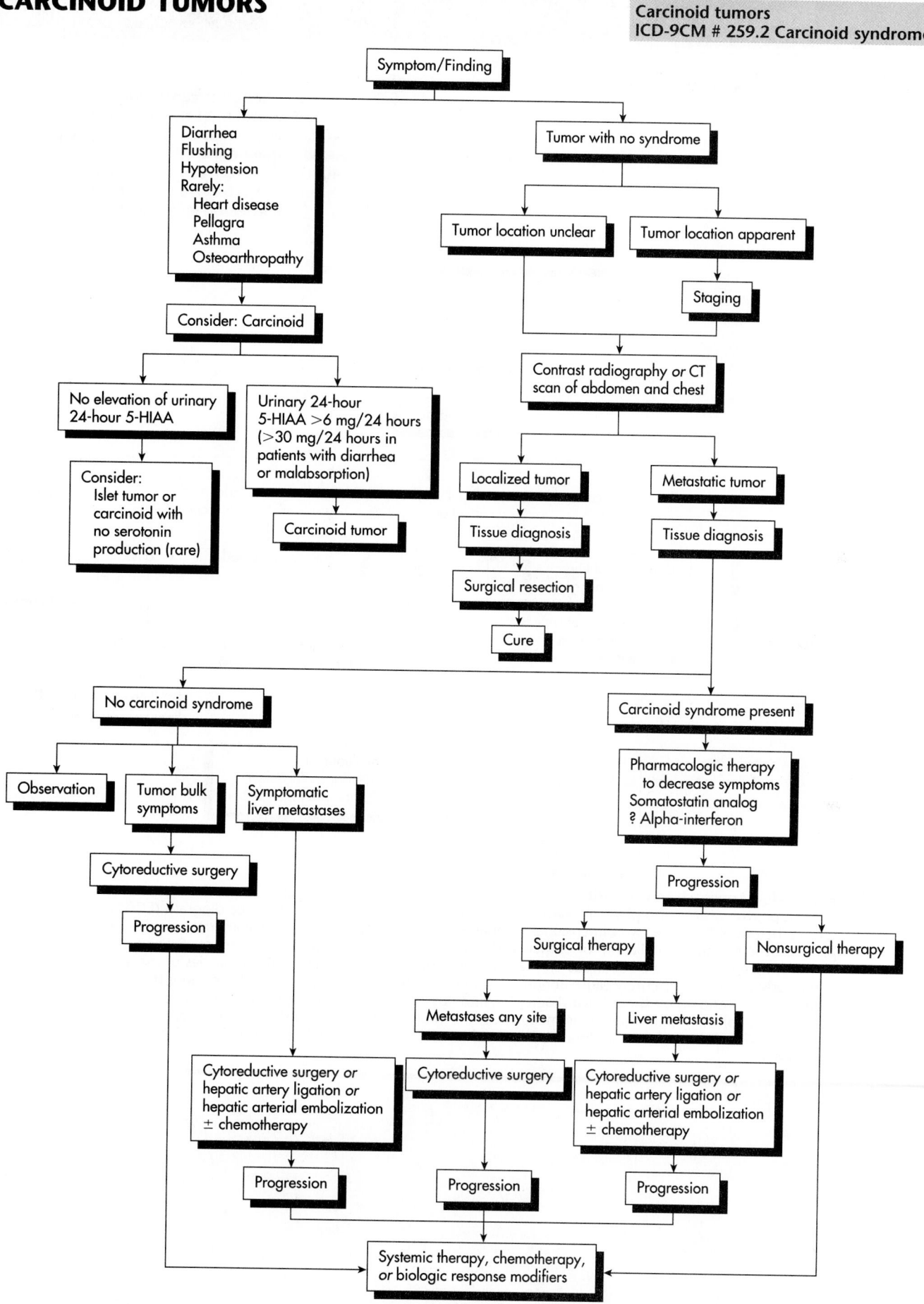

Fig. 3-40 Diagnosis and treatment of carcinoid tumors. *5-HIAA,* 5-Hydroxyindoleacetic acid. (From Abeloff MD: *Clinical oncology,* ed 2, New York, 2000, Churchill Livingstone.)

CARDIOMEGALY ON CHEST X-RAY

Cardiomegaly
ICD-9CM # 429.3 Idiopathic cardiomegaly
746.89 Congenital cardiomegaly
402.0 Hypertensive cardiomegaly, malignant
402.1 Hypertensive cardiomegaly, benign
402.11 Hypertensive cardiomegaly with congestive heart failure

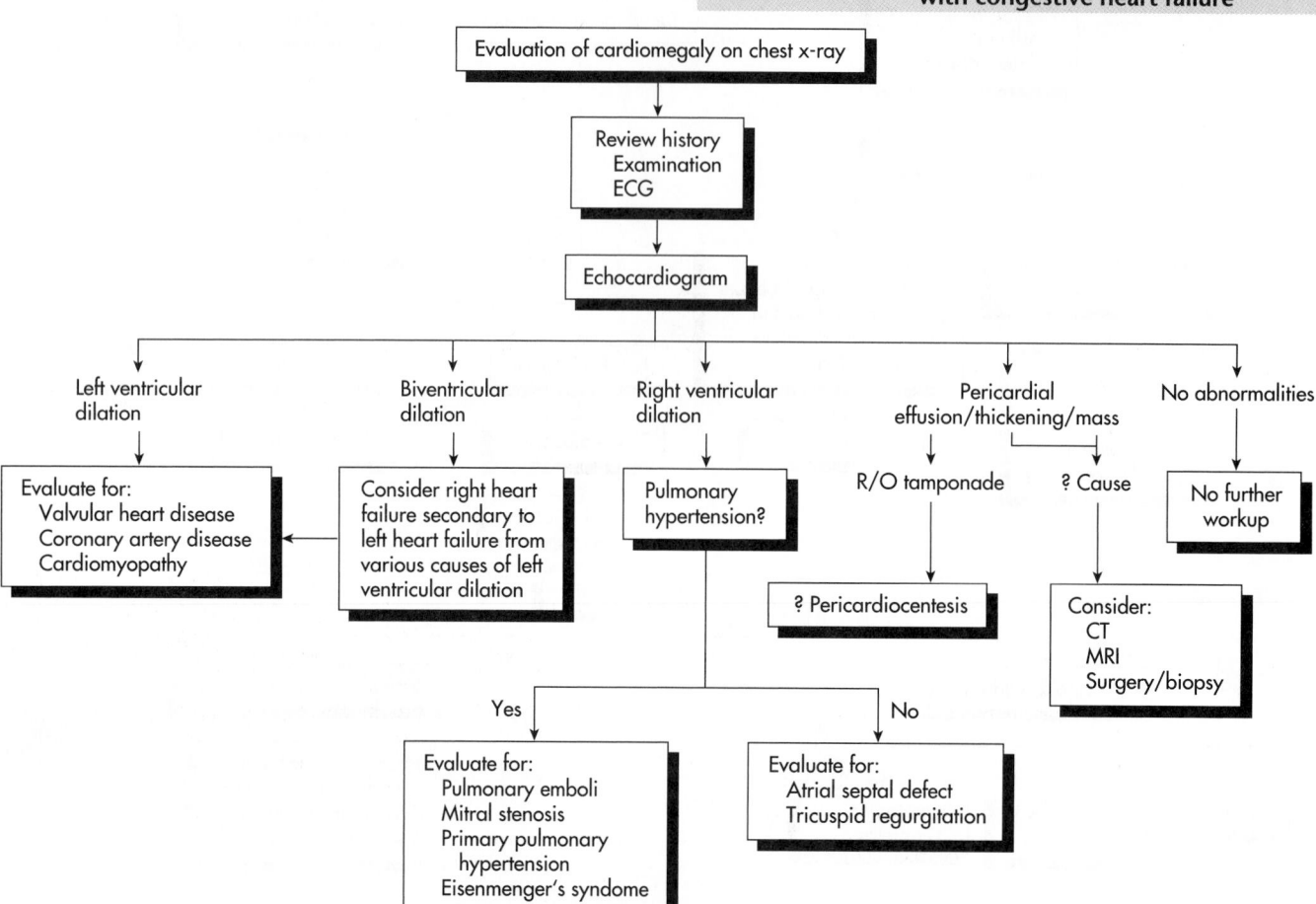

Fig. 3-41 Approach to the patient with cardiomegaly. When cardiomegaly is found on the chest radiograph, the history and physical examination should be reviewed and an electrocardiogram (ECG) performed before obtaining a two-dimensional Doppler echocardiographic study. Cardiomegaly may be explained by left ventricular dilation, biventricular dilation, right ventricular dilation, or pericardial abnormalities, or it may be found to be spurious on the echocardiogram. Rarely, isolated abnormalities of the atrium, particularly the left atrium, may cause abnormalities on the chest radiograph but will not cause true cardiomegaly. Depending on the echocardiographic findings, further tests can help elucidate the cause of echocardiographically confirmed cardiomegaly. *CT,* Computer tomography; *MRI,* magnetic resonance imaging; *R/O,* rule out. (From Goldman L, Branwald E [eds]: *Primary cardiology,* Philadelphia, 1998, WB Saunders.)

CEREBRAL ISCHEMIA

Cerebral ischemia
ICD-9CM # 437.1 Cerebral ischemia (chronic)
435.9 Cerebral ischemia
intermittent (transient)

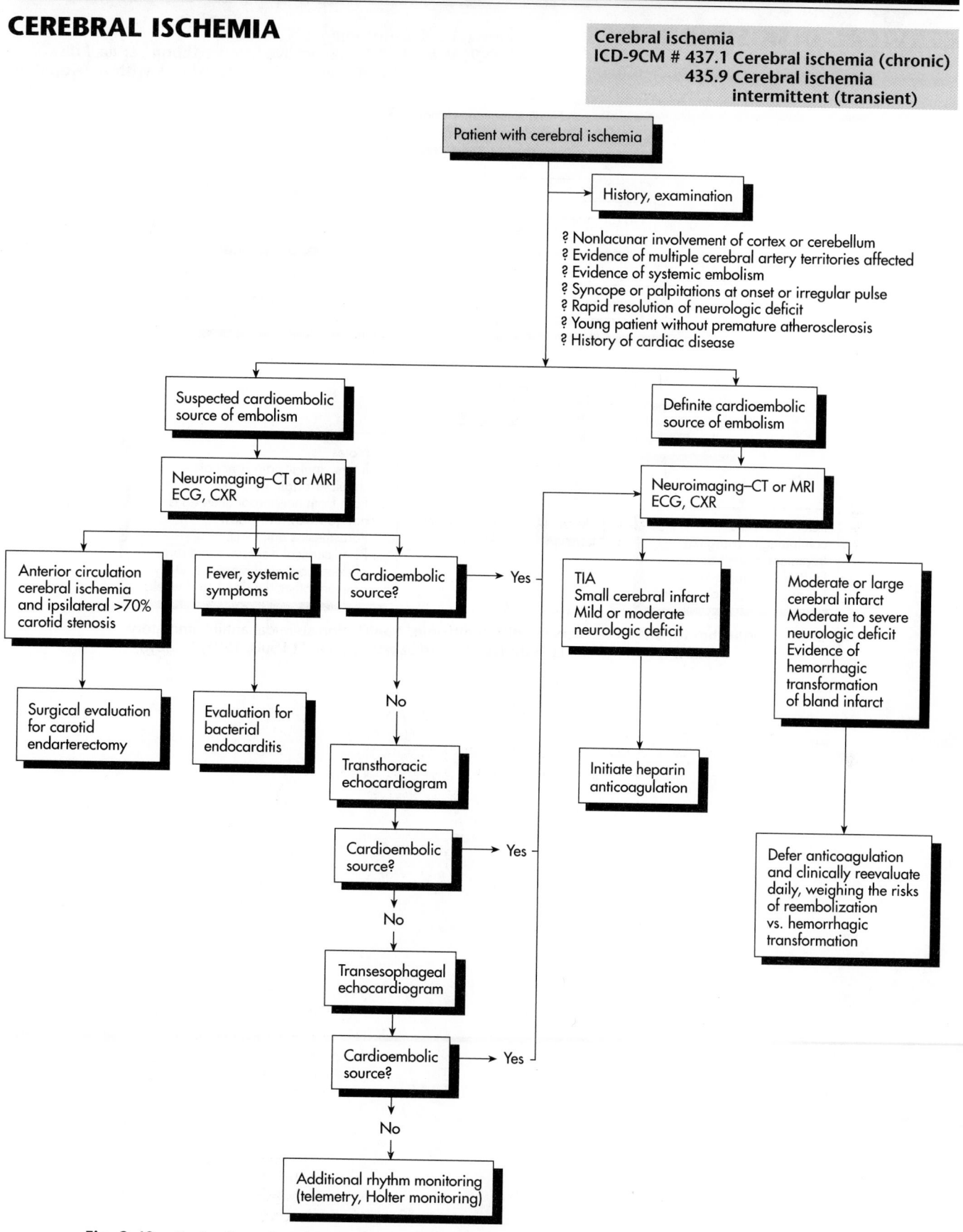

Fig. 3-42   Evaluation of patients with cerebral ischemia for a cardioembolic source. *CT,* computed tomography; *CXR,* chest radiograph; *ECG,* electrocardiogram; *MRI,* magnetic resonance imaging; *TIA,* transient ischemic attack. (From Johnson R [ed]: *Current therapy in neurologic disease,* ed 5, St Louis, 1997, Mosby.)

CERVICAL DISK SYNDROME

Cervical disk syndrome
ICD-9CM # 722.4 Degenerative intervertebral cervical disk
722.71 Degenerative cervical disk with myelopathy

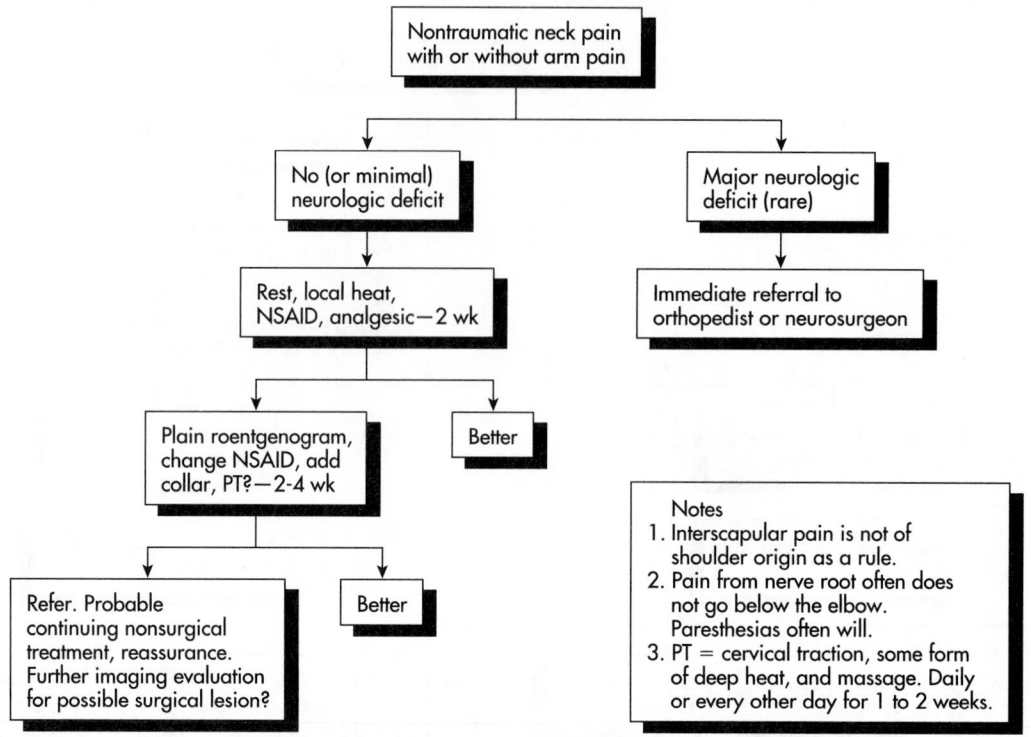

Fig. 3-43   **Algorithm for suspected cervical disk syndrome.** *NSAID,* Non-steroidal antiinflammatory drug; *PT,* physical therapy. (From Mercier LR [ed]: *Practical orthopaedics,* ed 4, St Louis, 1995, Mosby.)

CHRONIC OBSTRUCTIVE PULMONARY DISEASE

Chronic obstructive pulmonary disease
ICD-9CM # 496   COPD
                 492.8 Emphysema

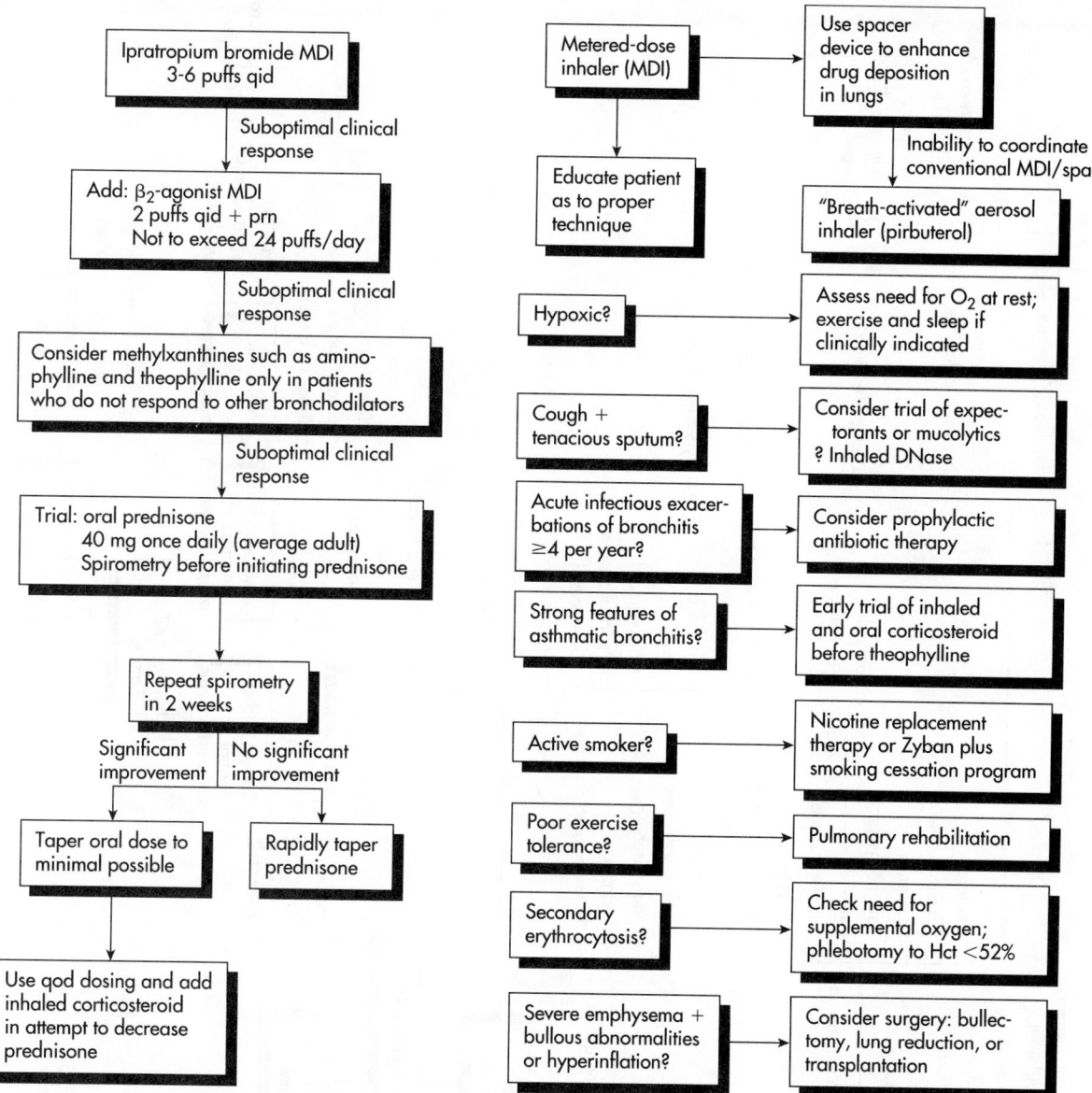

Fig. 3-44   Managed care guide: pharmacotherapy and general management approaches for chronic obstructive pulmonary disease (COPD). *DNase,* Deoxyribonuclease; *Hct,* hematocrit; *prn,* as needed; *qid,* four times a day; *qod,* every other day. (Modified from Noble J: *Primary care medicine,* ed 3, St Louis, 2001, Mosby.)

III

CONSTIPATION

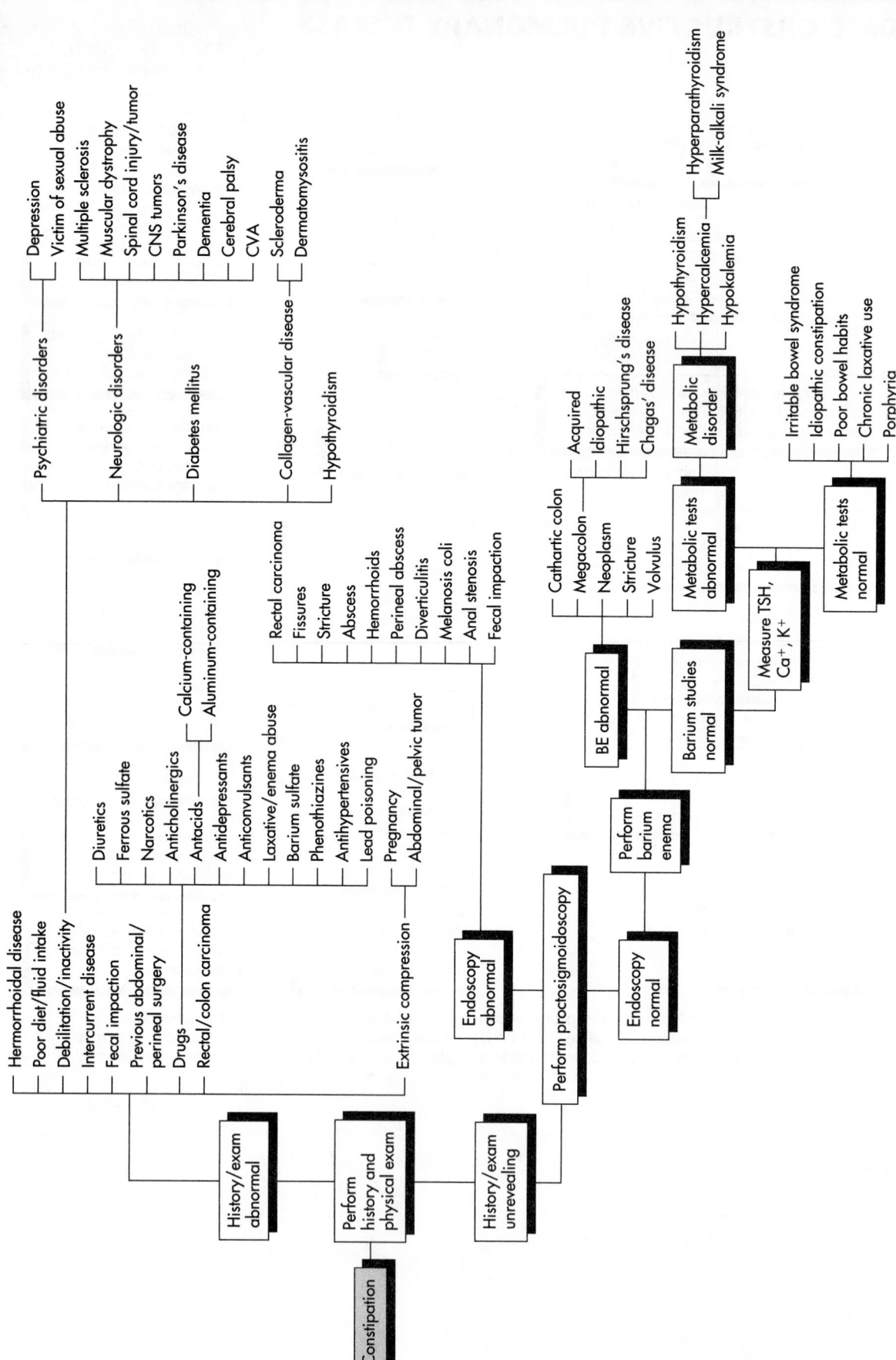

Fig. 3-45   Constipation. *BE*, Barium enema; *CNS*, central nervous system; *CVA*, cerebral vascular accident; *TSH*, thyroid-stimulating hormone. (From Healey PM: *Common medical diagnosis: an algorithmic approach*, ed 3, Philadelphia, 2000, WB Saunders.)

CONTRACEPTIVE METHOD SELECTION

Contraceptive method selection
ICD-9CM # V25.09

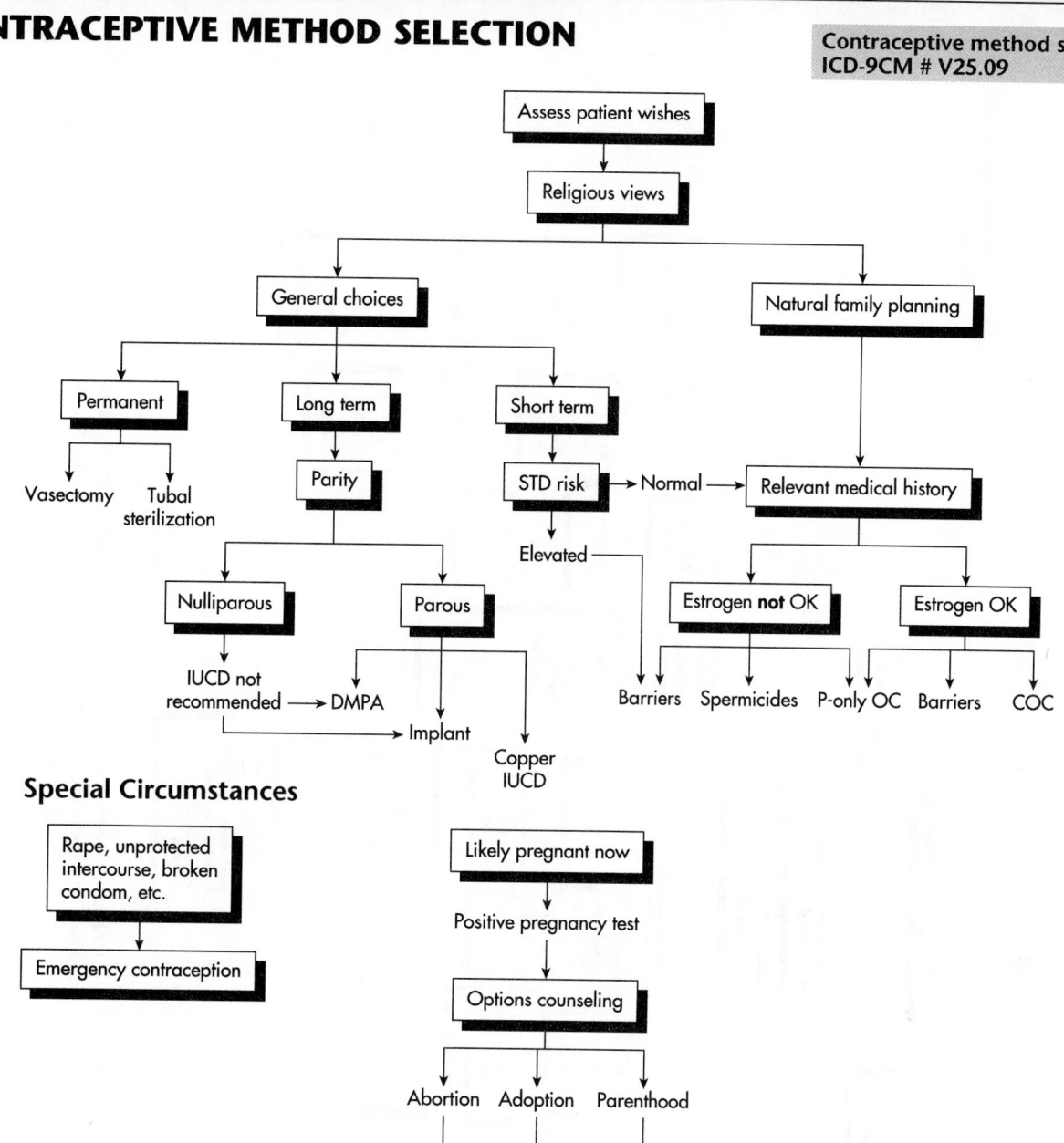

Special Circumstances

Fig. 3-46   Helping couples select a contraceptive method. *COC,* Combination estrogen-progestin oral contraceptive; *DMPA,* depot medroxyprogesterone acetate; *IUCD,* intrauterine contraceptive device; *P-only OC,* progestin-only oral contraceptive; *STD,* sexually transmitted disease. (From Copeland LJ: *Textbook of gynecology,* ed 2, Philadelphia, 2000, WB Saunders.)

CONTRACEPTIVE USE, ORAL

Contraceptive use, oral
ICD-9CM # V25.01 Prescription or use, oral
contraceptive

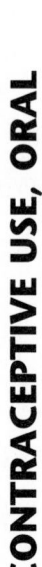

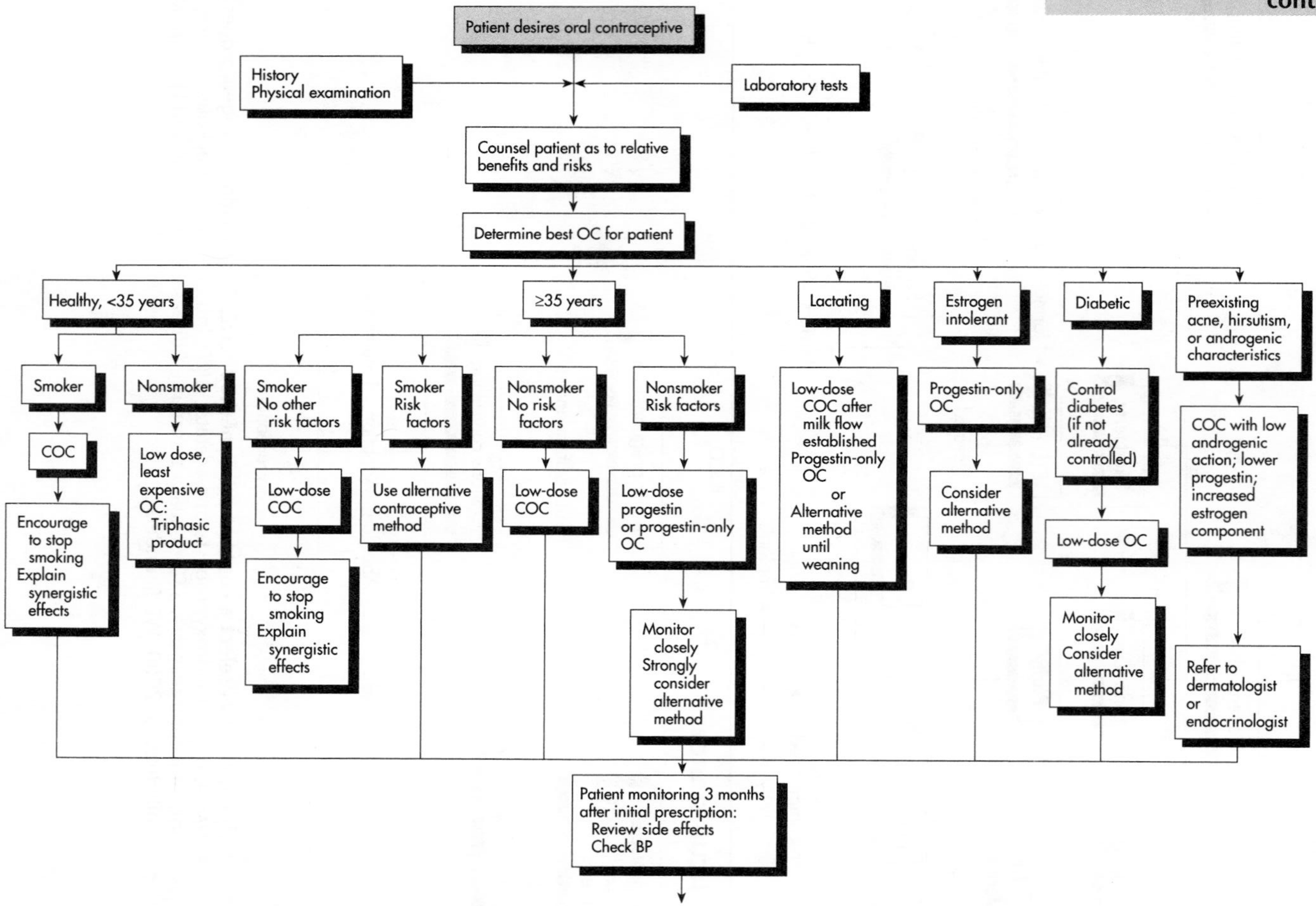

Fig. 3-47 **Contraceptive use.** *BP,* Blood pressure; *BTB,* breakthrough bleeding; *COC,* combination oral contraceptives; *CVA,* cerebrovascular accident; *OC,* oral contraceptive. (From Robles TA: Use of oral contraceptives. In Greene HL, Johnson WP, Lemcke D [eds]: *Decision making in medicine,* ed 2, St Louis, 1998, Mosby.)

Continued

CONTRACEPTIVE USE, ORAL—cont'd

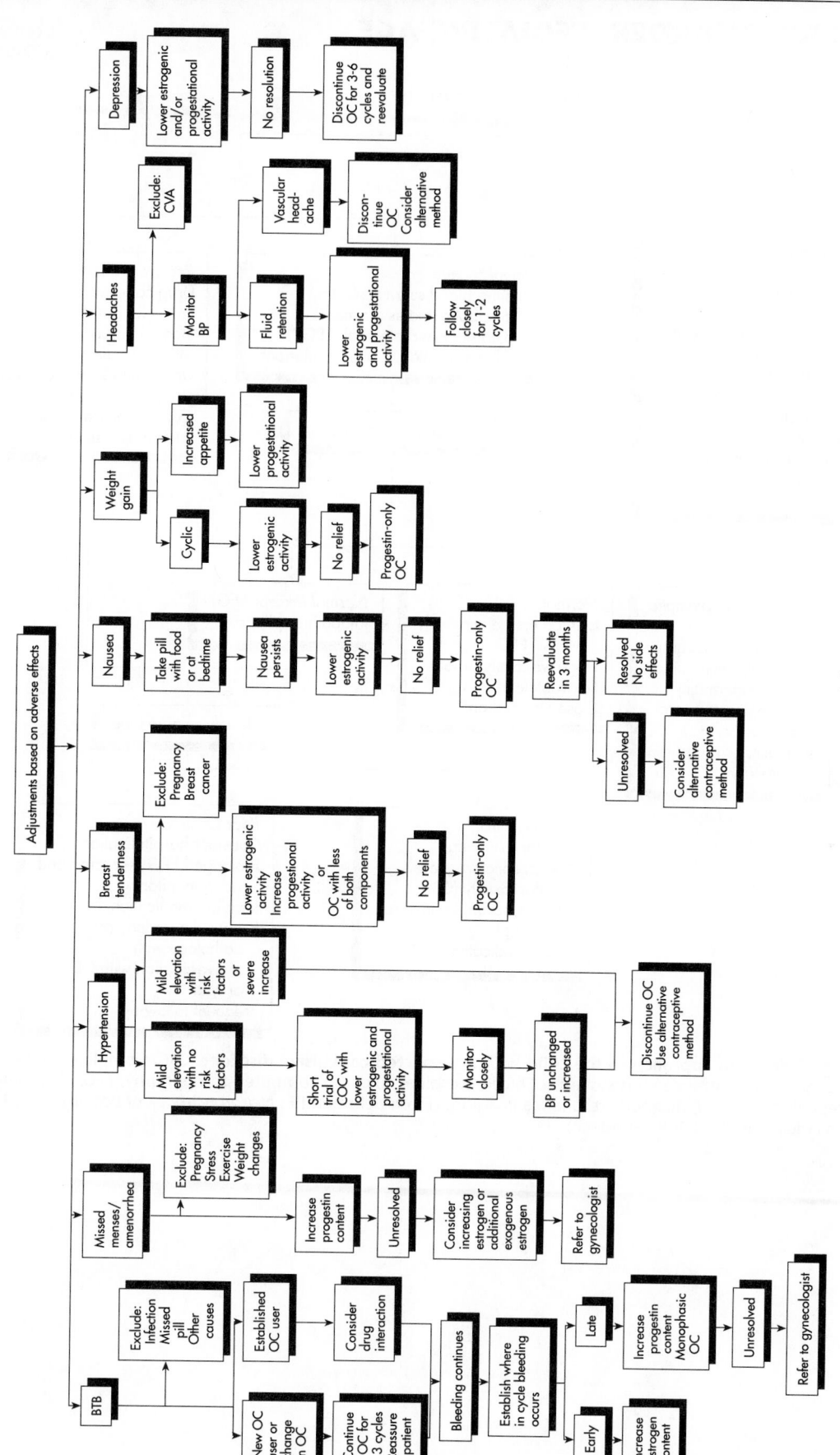

Fig. 3-47, cont'd

CONVULSIVE DISORDER, PEDIATRIC AGE

Convulsive disorder
ICD-9CM # 780.39

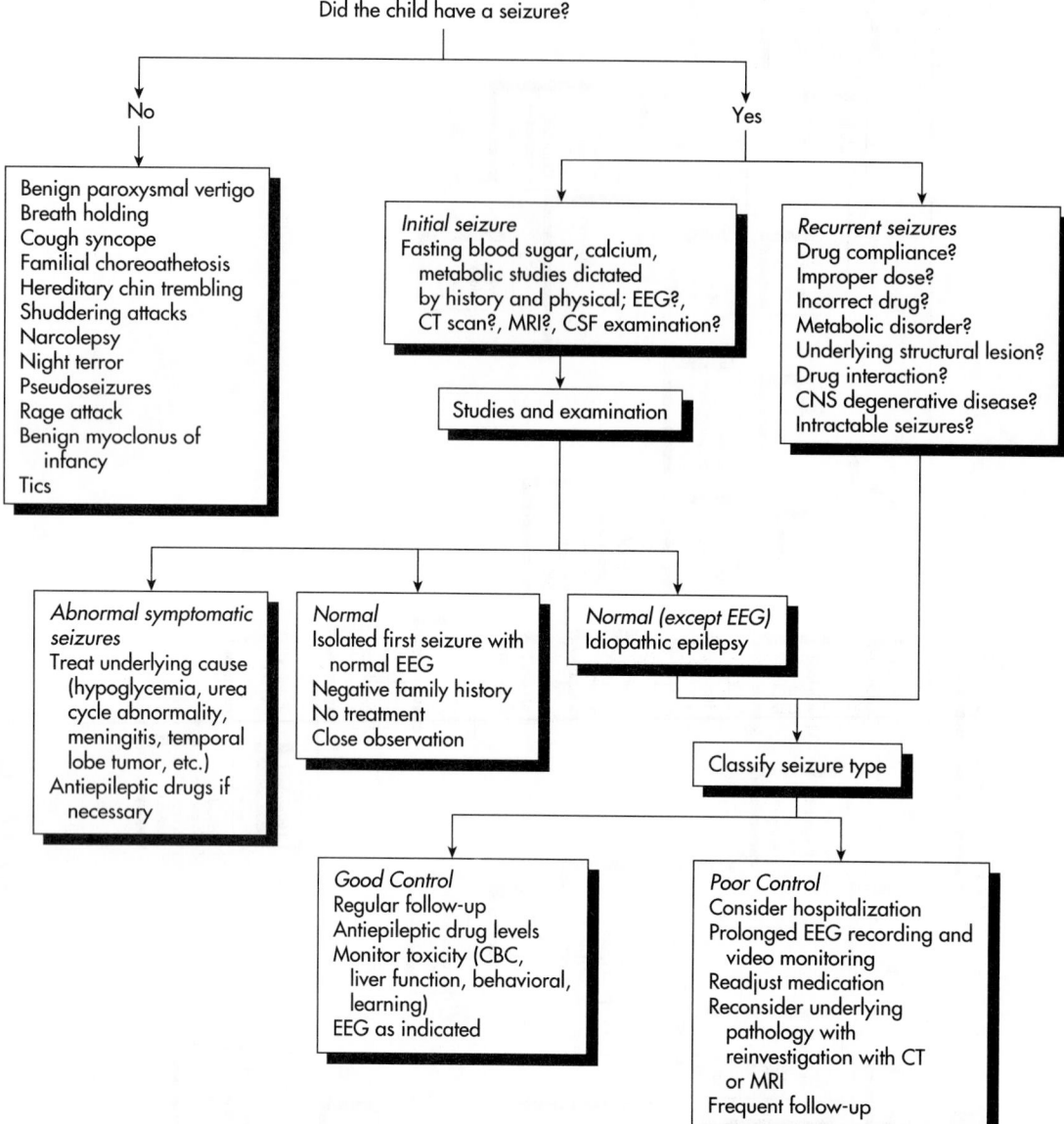

Fig. 3-48 **An approach to the child with a suspected convulsive disorder.** *CBC,* Complete blood count; *CNS,* central nervous system; *CSF,* cerebrospinal fluid; *CT,* computed tomography; *EEG,* electroencephalogram; *MRI,* magnetic resonance imaging. (From Behrman RE: *Nelson textbook of pediatrics,* ed 16, Philadelphia, 2000, WB Saunders.)

CORNEAL DISORDERS

Corneal disorders
**ICD-9CM # 918.1 Corneal abrasion
743.9 Corneal anomalies NOS**

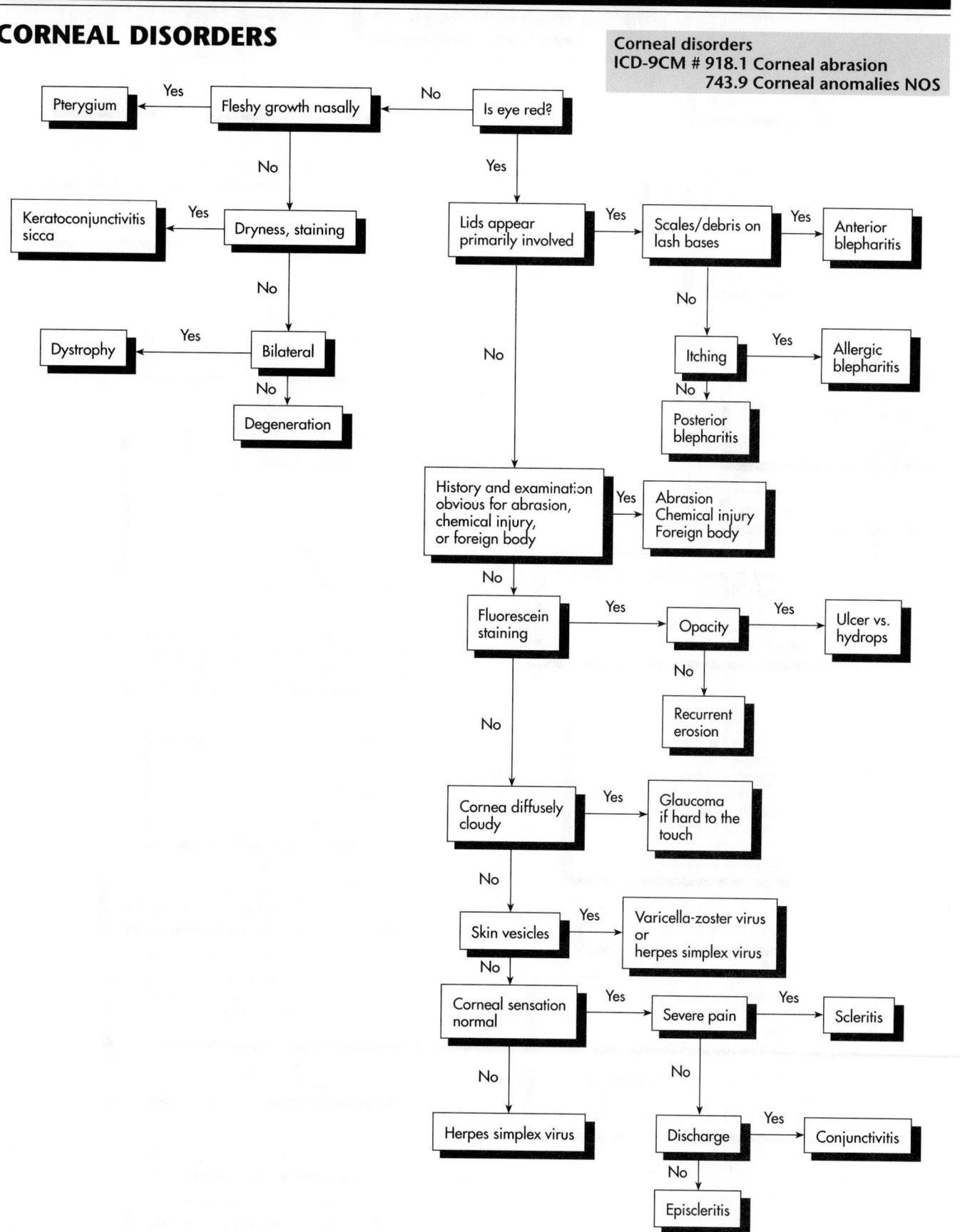

Fig. 3-49 **Approach to the patient with corneal disorders.** (From Noble J [ed]: *Primary care medicine,* ed 3, St Louis, 2001, Mosby.)

COUGH

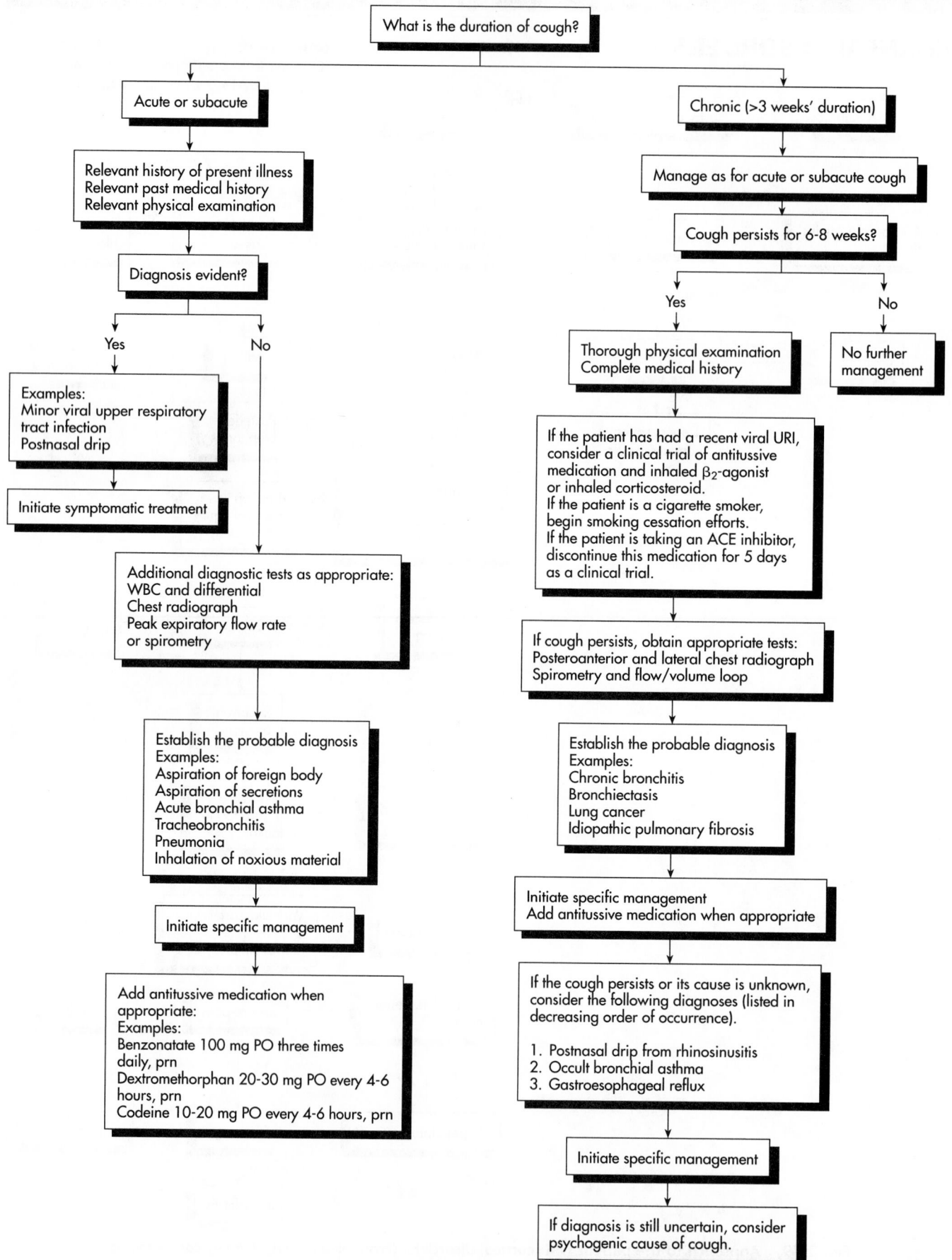

Fig. 3-50   Evaluation and treatment of the patient with cough. *ACE,* Angiotensin-converting enzyme; *URI,* upper respiratory infection; *WBC,* white blood count. (From Stein J [ed]: *Internal medicine,* ed 5, St Louis, 1998, Mosby.)

CREATINE KINASE ELEVATION

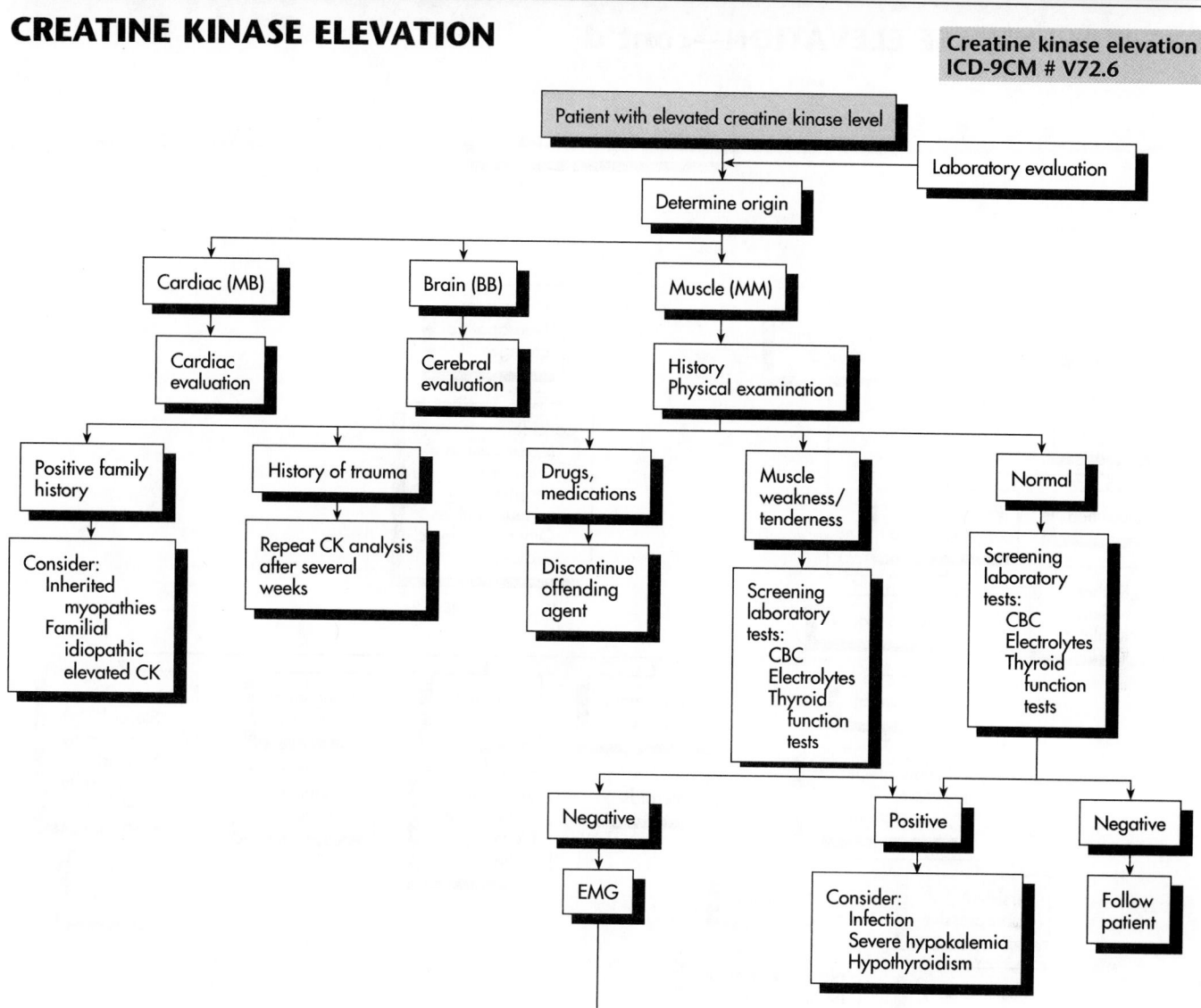

Fig. 3-51 **Evaluation of creatine kinase elevation.** *CBC,* Complete blood count; *CK,* creatine kinase; *EMG,* electromyography. (From Greene HL, Johnson WP, Lemcke D [eds]: *Decision making in medicine,* ed 2, St Louis, 1998, Mosby.)

III

CREATINE KINASE ELEVATION—cont'd

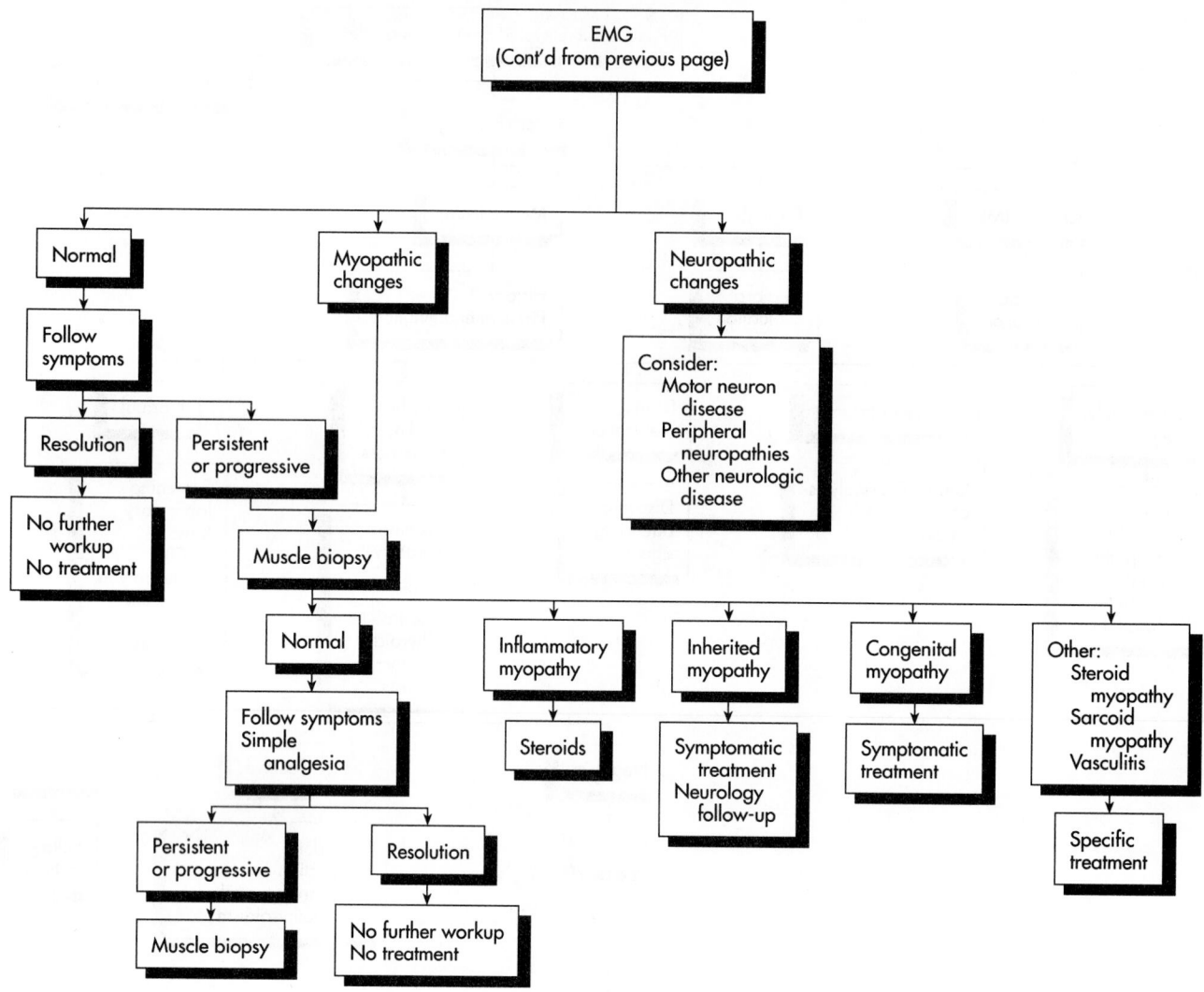

Fig. 3-51, cont'd

CUSHING'S SYNDROME

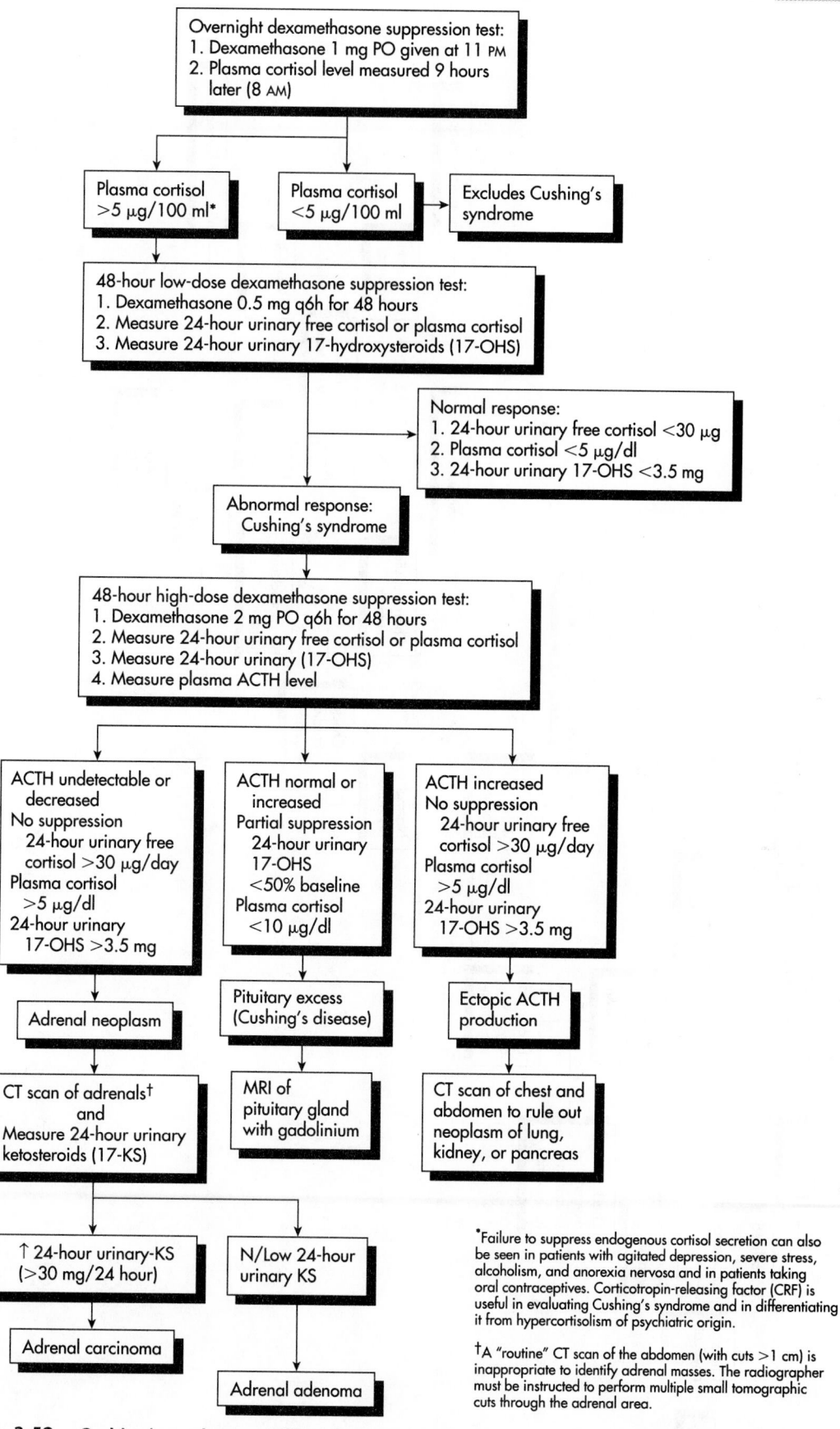

Fig. 3-52   Cushing's syndrome. *ACTH,* Adrenocorticotropic hormone; *CT,* computed tomography; *MRI,* magnetic resonance imaging; *PO,* by mouth. (From Ferri F: *Practical guide to the care of the medical patient,* ed 6, St Louis, 2004, Mosby.)

CYANOSIS

Cyanosis
ICD-9CM # 782.5 Cyanosis NOS

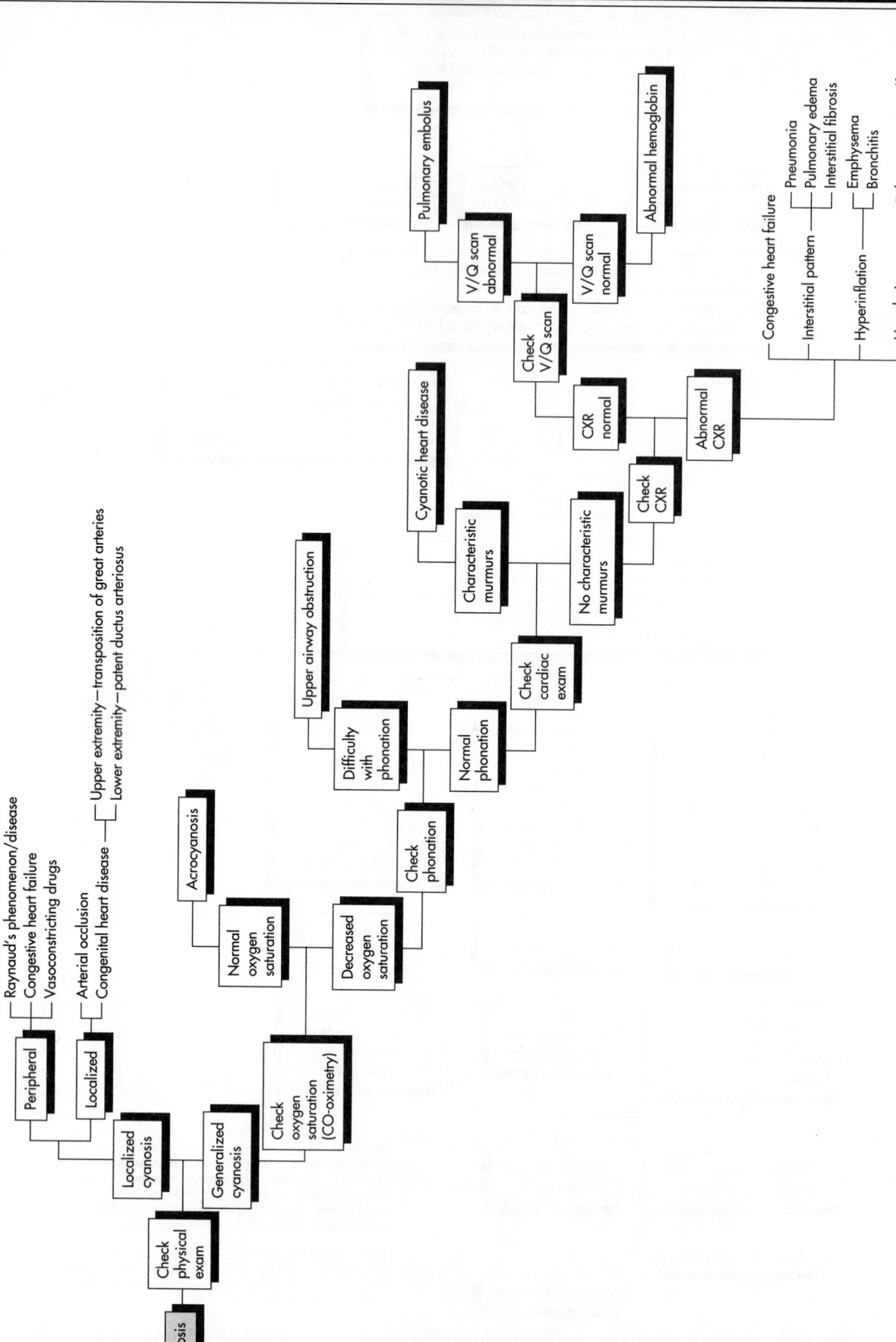

Fig. 3-53 Cyanosis. *A-V,* Arteriovenous; *CXR,* chest x-ray; *V/Q,* ventilation-perfusion. (From Healey PM: *Common medical diagnosis: an algorithmic approach,* ed 3, Philadelphia, 2000, WB Saunders.)

DELIRIUM

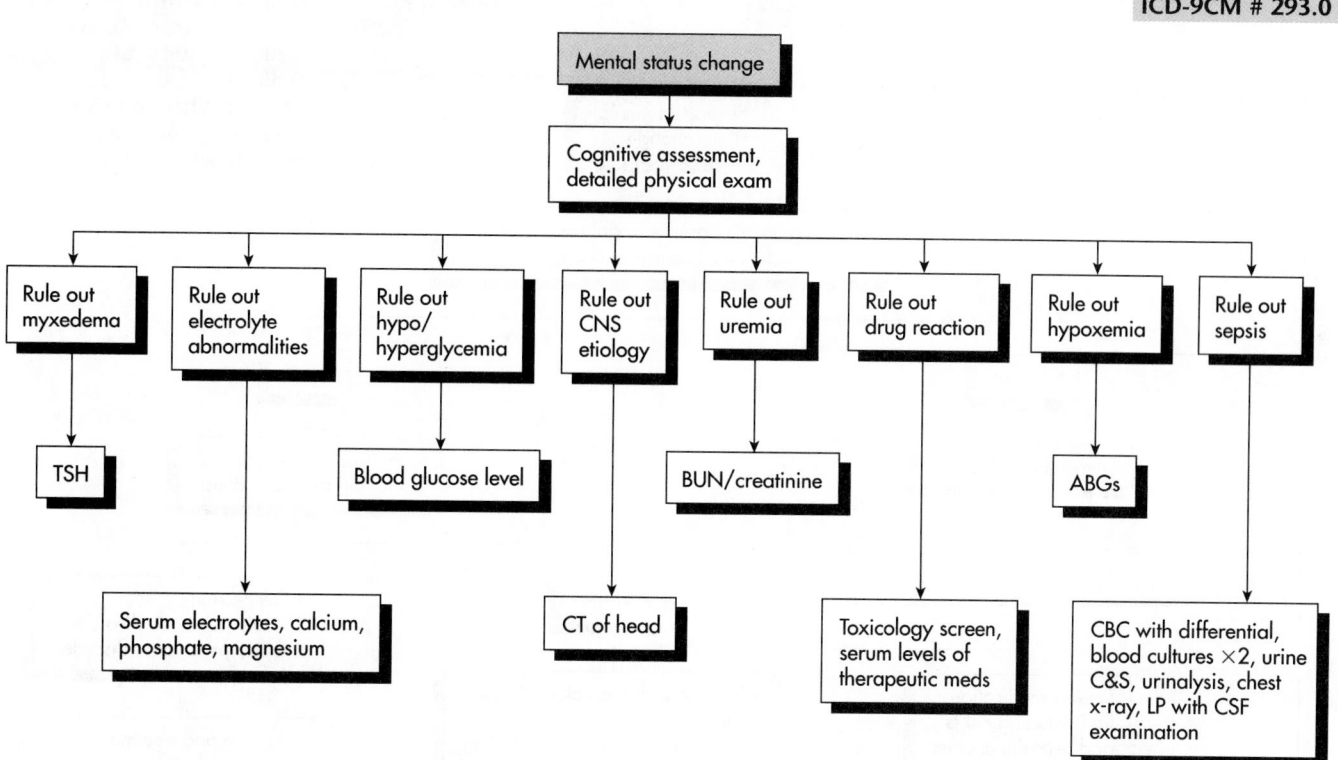

Fig. 3-54 **Delirium.** *ABG,* Arterial blood gas; *BUN,* blood urea nitrogen; *CBC,* complete blood count; *CNS,* central nervous system; *C&S,* culture and sensitivity; *CSF,* cerebrospinal fluid; *CT,* computed tomography; *TSH,* thyroid-stimulating hormone.

III

DELIRIUM, GERIATRIC PATIENT

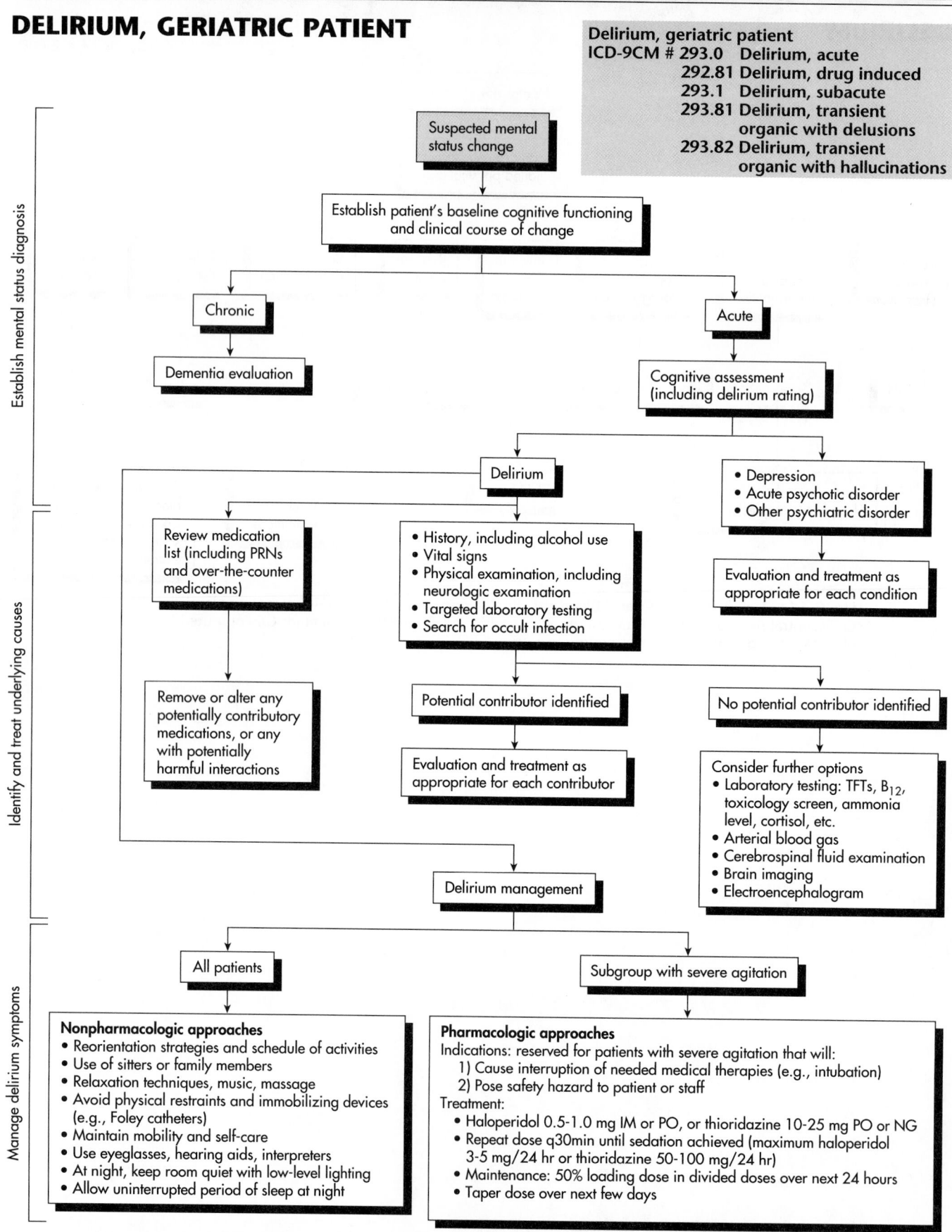

Delirium, geriatric patient
ICD-9CM # 293.0 Delirium, acute
292.81 Delirium, drug induced
293.1 Delirium, subacute
293.81 Delirium, transient organic with delusions
293.82 Delirium, transient organic with hallucinations

Establish mental status diagnosis

Suspected mental status change

Establish patient's baseline cognitive functioning and clinical course of change

Chronic

Dementia evaluation

Acute

Cognitive assessment (including delirium rating)

Delirium

- Depression
- Acute psychotic disorder
- Other psychiatric disorder

Evaluation and treatment as appropriate for each condition

Identify and treat underlying causes

Review medication list (including PRNs and over-the-counter medications)

- History, including alcohol use
- Vital signs
- Physical examination, including neurologic examination
- Targeted laboratory testing
- Search for occult infection

Remove or alter any potentially contributory medications, or any with potentially harmful interactions

Potential contributor identified

Evaluation and treatment as appropriate for each contributor

No potential contributor identified

Consider further options
- Laboratory testing: TFTs, B$_{12}$, toxicology screen, ammonia level, cortisol, etc.
- Arterial blood gas
- Cerebrospinal fluid examination
- Brain imaging
- Electroencephalogram

Delirium management

Manage delirium symptoms

All patients

Subgroup with severe agitation

Nonpharmacologic approaches
- Reorientation strategies and schedule of activities
- Use of sitters or family members
- Relaxation techniques, music, massage
- Avoid physical restraints and immobilizing devices (e.g., Foley catheters)
- Maintain mobility and self-care
- Use eyeglasses, hearing aids, interpreters
- At night, keep room quiet with low-level lighting
- Allow uninterrupted period of sleep at night

Pharmacologic approaches
Indications: reserved for patients with severe agitation that will:
1) Cause interruption of needed medical therapies (e.g., intubation)
2) Pose safety hazard to patient or staff
Treatment:
- Haloperidol 0.5-1.0 mg IM or PO, or thioridazine 10-25 mg PO or NG
- Repeat dose q30min until sedation achieved (maximum haloperidol 3-5 mg/24 hr or thioridazine 50-100 mg/24 hr)
- Maintenance: 50% loading dose in divided doses over next 24 hours
- Taper dose over next few days

Fig. 3-55 **Algorithm for evaluation of suspected mental status change in an older patient.** *IM,* Intramuscular; *NG,* nasogastric; *PO,* by mouth; *PRNs,* as needed; *TFTs,* thyroid function tests. (From Goldman L, Ausiello D [eds]: *Cecil textbook of medicine,* ed 22, Philadelphia, 2004, WB Saunders.)

DEMENTIA

Dementia
ICD-9CM # 290.10 Dementia, presenile
290.0 Dementia, senile
437.0 Dementia, arteriosclerotic

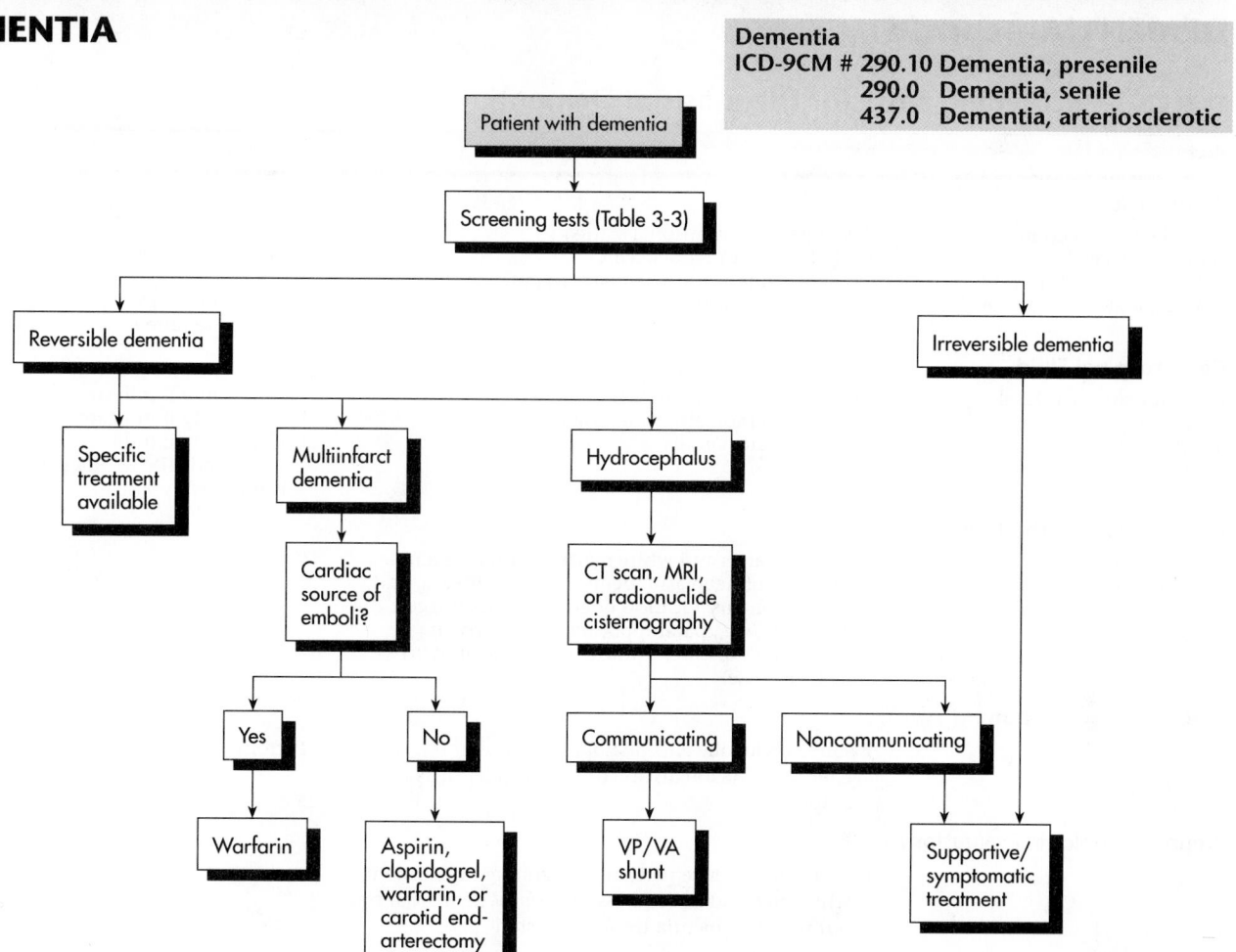

Fig. 3-56 **Management of dementia.** *VA,* Ventriculoatrial; *VP,* ventriculoperitoneal.

III

DEMENTIA—cont'd

TABLE 3-3 Screening Tests for Diagnosis of Dementia

TEST	RATIONALE	REMARKS
Blood Test		
Complete blood count	Assess general nutritional status	
Serum B_{12} level	Exclude vitamin B_{12} deficiency	Consider Schilling's test if B_{12} level is low
TSH + free T_4 *or* TSH + FTI	Exclude primary and secondary hypothyroidism	
HIV serology	Exclude HIV infection	Perform only if indicated; consent from patient required
Cerebrospinal Fluid		
Cell count/protein level	Exclude chronic meningitis	Perform only if indicated
Cytology	Exclude carcinomatous meningitis	Perform only if indicated
VDRL	Exclude neurosyphilis	Perform only if indicated; check serum TPHA and HIV serology if CSF VDRL is positive
CT Scan/MRI of the Brain		
	Identify infarcts and white matter changes; exclude presence of neoplasm, demyelinating disease, and hydrocephalus; location of atrophy may suggest the diagnosis (e.g., parahippocampal atrophy in Alzheimer's disease, frontotemporal atrophy in Pick's disease)	
Electroencephalogram		
	Exclude metabolic encephalopathies; useful if Creutzfeldt-Jakob disease or status epilepticus is suspected	Perform only if indicated
Neuropsychologic Evaluation		
	Help to characterize pattern of cognitive impairment, which may aid in the classification of dementia; rule out pseudodementia from depression	

From Johnson RT, Griffin JW: Current therapy in neurologic disease, ed 5, St Louis, 1997, Mosby.
CSF, Cerebrospinal fluid; *CT,* computed tomography; *FTI,* free thyroxine index; *HIV,* human immunodeficiency virus; *MRI,* magnetic resonance imaging; T_4, thyroxine; *TPHA, Treponema pallidum* hemagglutination assay; *TSH,* thyroid-stimulating hormone; *VDRL,* Venereal Disease Research Laboratory test.

DEPRESSION

Depression
ICD-9CM # 296.2 Major depressive disorder, single episode

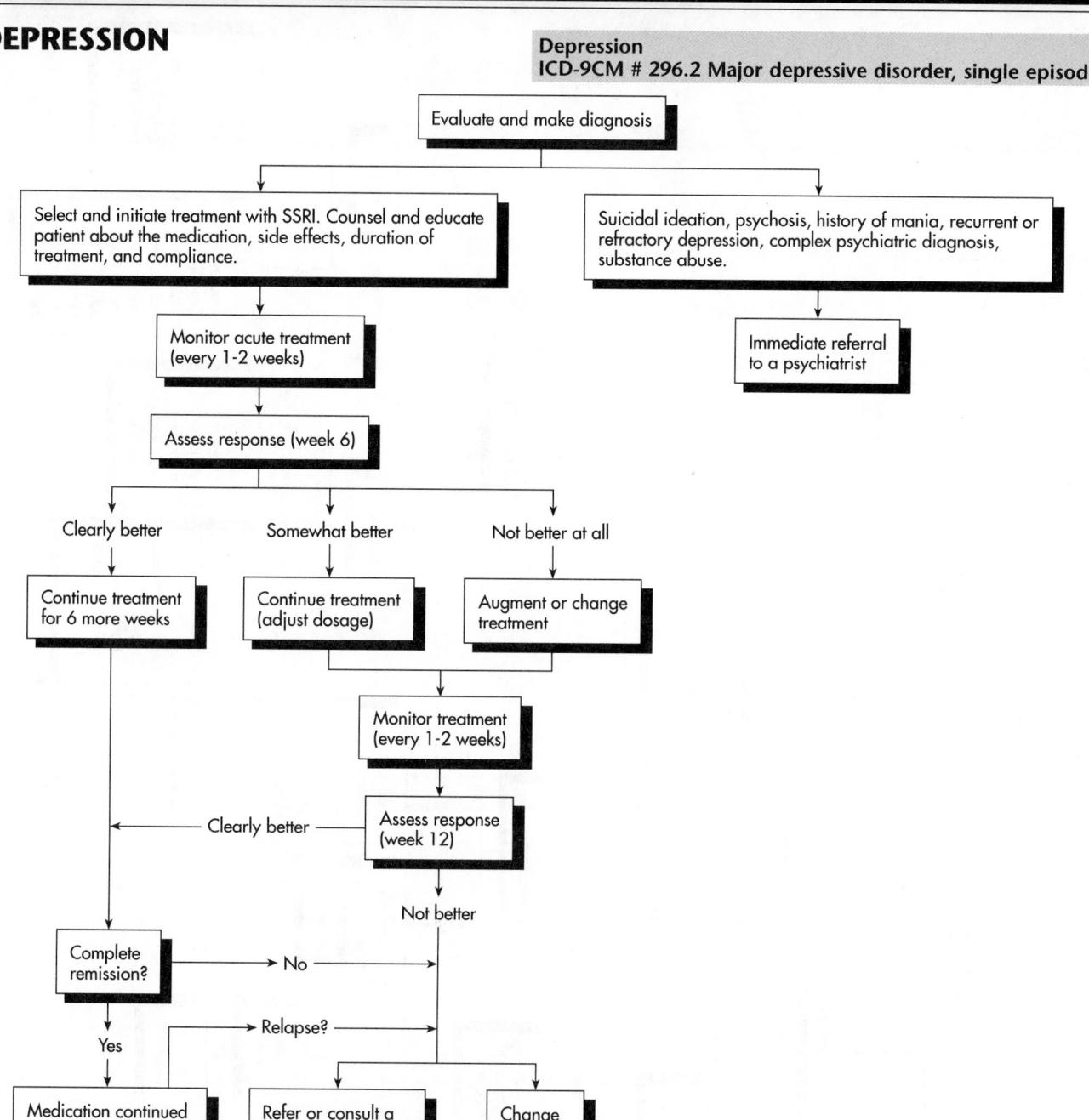

Fig. 3-57   Guidelines for the treatment of depression in the primary care setting. *SSRI,* Selective serotonin reuptake inhibitor. NOTE: Time of assessment (weeks 6 and 12) rests on very modest data. It may be necessary to revise the treatment plan earlier for patients who fail to respond. (From AHCPR Quick Reference Guide of Clinicians, No. 5: Depression in primary care: *Detection, diagnosis and treatment,* 1993; and American Psychiatric Association: *Diagnostic and statistical manual of mental disorders,* ed 4, Washington, DC, 1994, American Psychiatric Association.)

DEVELOPMENTAL DELAY

Developmental delay
ICD-9CM # 783.4 Developmental delay, physiological

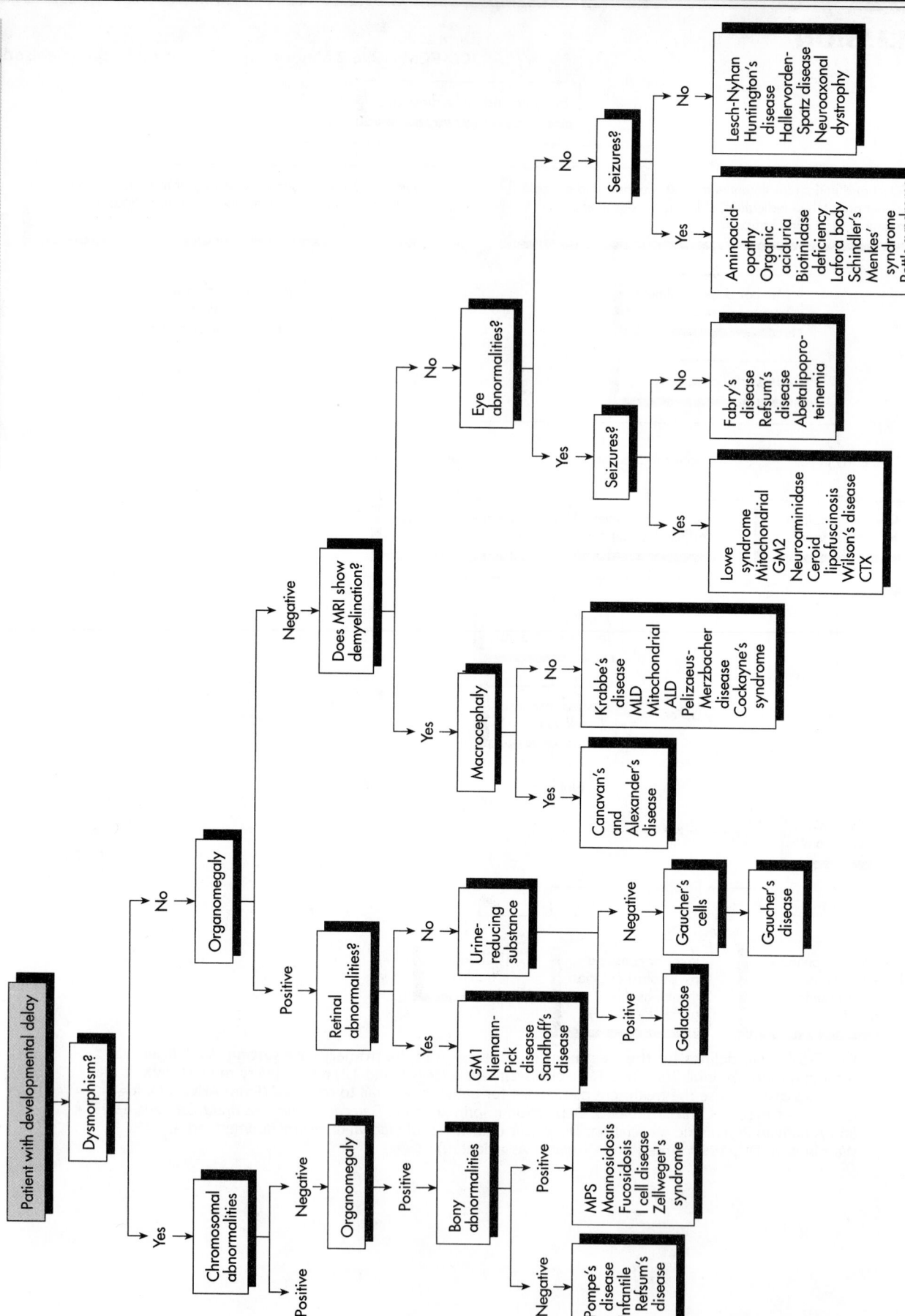

Fig. 3-58 **Workup for developmental delay.** *ALD,* Adrenoleukodystrophy; *CTX,* cerebrotendinous xanthomatosis; *MLD,* metachromatic leukodystrophy; *MPS,* mucopolysaccharidosis; *MRI,* magnetic resonance imaging. (From Johnson RT, Griffin JW: *Current therapy in neurologic disease,* ed 5, St Louis, 1997, Mosby.)

DIABETES INSIPIDUS

Diabetes insipidus
ICD-9CM # 253.5

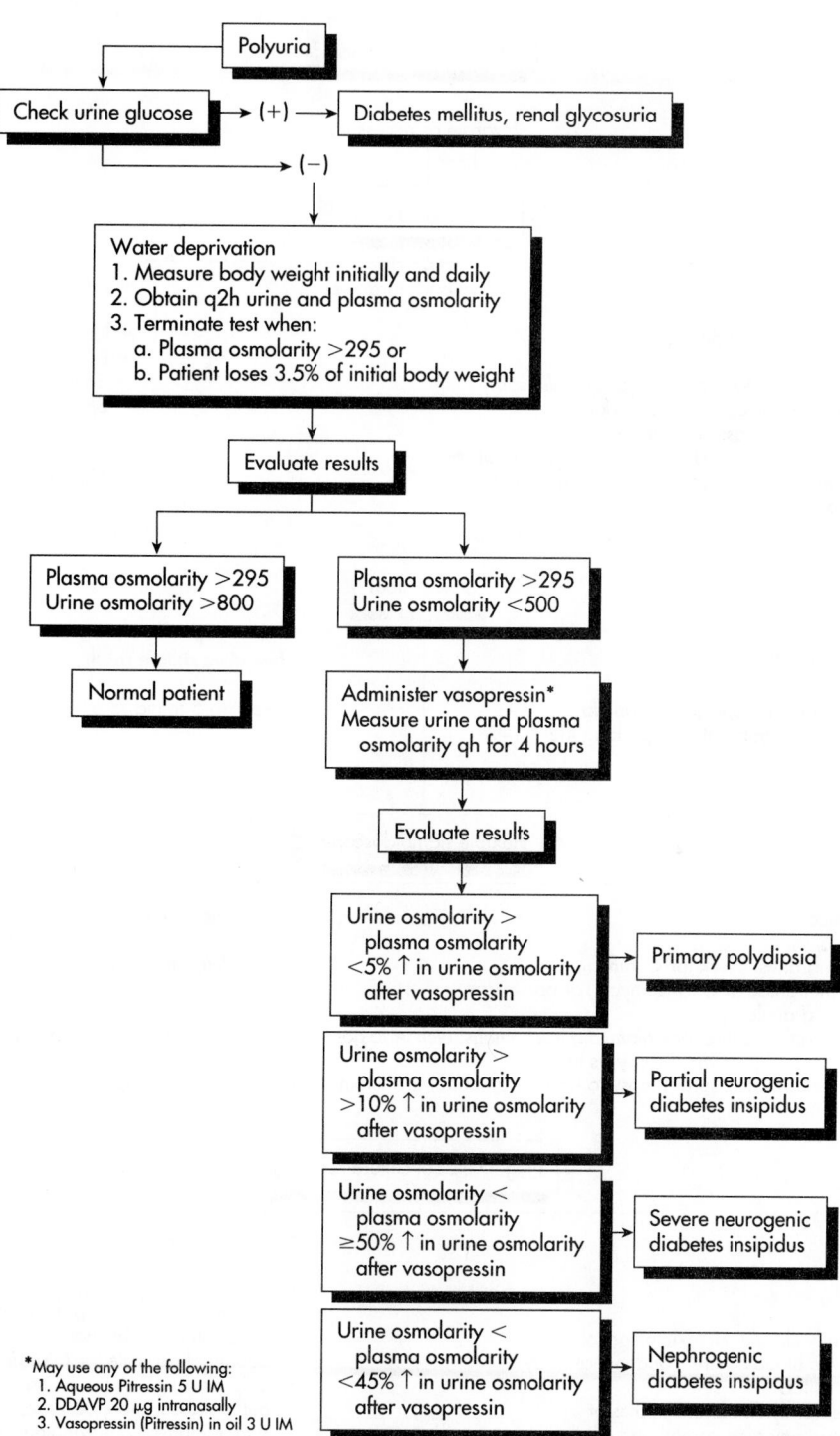

Fig. 3-59 **Diagnostic flowchart for diabetes insipidus.** (From Ferri F: *Practical guide to the care of the medical patient,* ed 6, St Louis, 2004, Mosby.)

DIARRHEA, ACUTE

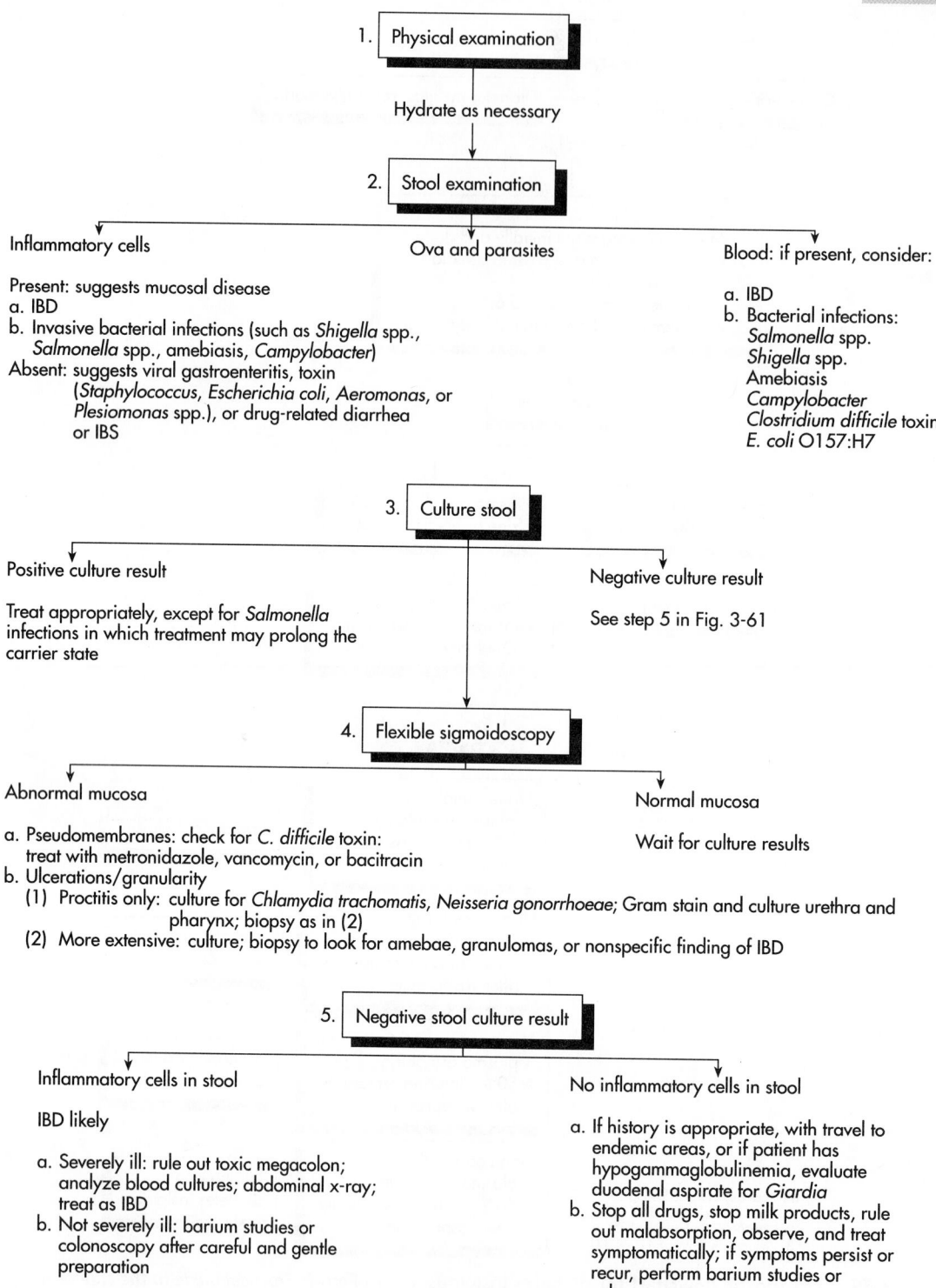

1. Physical examination

Hydrate as necessary

2. Stool examination

Inflammatory cells

Present: suggests mucosal disease
a. IBD
b. Invasive bacterial infections (such as *Shigella* spp.,
   Salmonella spp., amebiasis, *Campylobacter*)
Absent: suggests viral gastroenteritis, toxin
   (*Staphylococcus, Escherichia coli, Aeromonas,* or
   Plesiomonas spp.), or drug-related diarrhea
   or IBS

Ova and parasites

Blood: if present, consider:

a. IBD
b. Bacterial infections:
   Salmonella spp.
   Shigella spp.
   Amebiasis
   Campylobacter
   Clostridium difficile toxin
   E. coli O157:H7

3. Culture stool

Positive culture result

Treat appropriately, except for *Salmonella*
infections in which treatment may prolong the
carrier state

Negative culture result

See step 5 in Fig. 3-61

4. Flexible sigmoidoscopy

Abnormal mucosa

a. Pseudomembranes: check for *C. difficile* toxin:
   treat with metronidazole, vancomycin, or bacitracin
b. Ulcerations/granularity
   (1) Proctitis only: culture for *Chlamydia trachomatis, Neisseria gonorrhoeae*; Gram stain and culture urethra and
       pharynx; biopsy as in (2)
   (2) More extensive: culture; biopsy to look for amebae, granulomas, or nonspecific finding of IBD

Normal mucosa

Wait for culture results

5. Negative stool culture result

Inflammatory cells in stool

IBD likely

a. Severely ill: rule out toxic megacolon;
   analyze blood cultures; abdominal x-ray;
   treat as IBD
b. Not severely ill: barium studies or
   colonoscopy after careful and gentle
   preparation

No inflammatory cells in stool

a. If history is appropriate, with travel to
   endemic areas, or if patient has
   hypogammaglobulinemia, evaluate
   duodenal aspirate for *Giardia*
b. Stop all drugs, stop milk products, rule
   out malabsorption, observe, and treat
   symptomatically; if symptoms persist or
   recur, perform barium studies or
   colonoscopy

Fig. 3-60   Diagnostic steps in the assessment of acute diarrhea. *IBD,* Inflammatory bowel disease; *IBS,*
irritable bowel syndrome. (From Stein JH [ed]: *Internal medicine,* ed 5, St Louis, 1998, Mosby.)

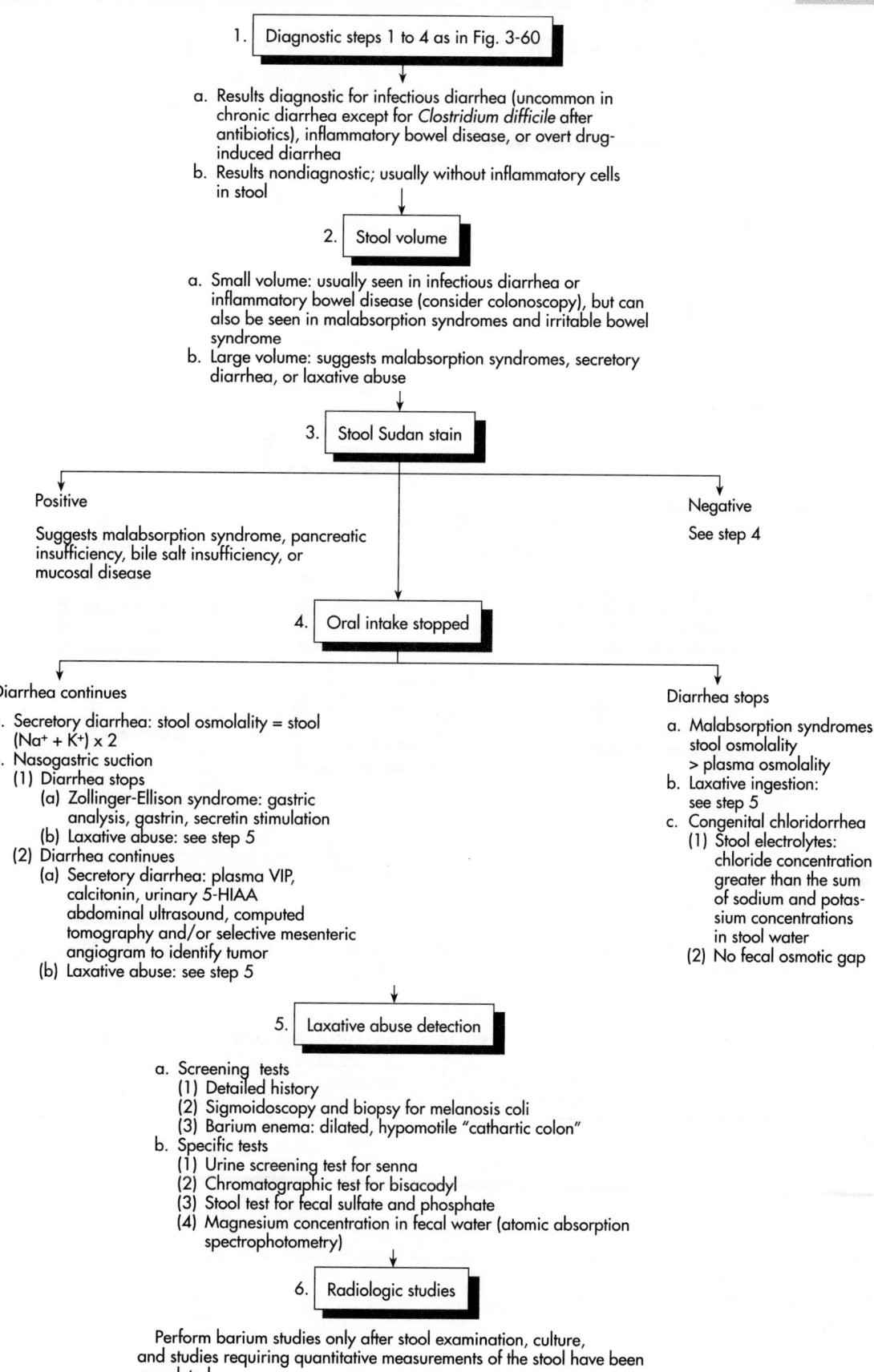

1. Diagnostic steps 1 to 4 as in Fig. 3-60

   a. Results diagnostic for infectious diarrhea (uncommon in chronic diarrhea except for *Clostridium difficile* after antibiotics), inflammatory bowel disease, or overt drug-induced diarrhea
   b. Results nondiagnostic; usually without inflammatory cells in stool

2. Stool volume

   a. Small volume: usually seen in infectious diarrhea or inflammatory bowel disease (consider colonoscopy), but can also be seen in malabsorption syndromes and irritable bowel syndrome
   b. Large volume: suggests malabsorption syndromes, secretory diarrhea, or laxative abuse

3. Stool Sudan stain

Positive

Suggests malabsorption syndrome, pancreatic insufficiency, bile salt insufficiency, or mucosal disease

Negative

See step 4

4. Oral intake stopped

Diarrhea continues

   a. Secretory diarrhea: stool osmolality = stool $(Na^+ + K^+) \times 2$
   b. Nasogastric suction
     (1) Diarrhea stops
       (a) Zollinger-Ellison syndrome: gastric analysis, gastrin, secretin stimulation
       (b) Laxative abuse: see step 5
     (2) Diarrhea continues
       (a) Secretory diarrhea: plasma VIP, calcitonin, urinary 5-HIAA abdominal ultrasound, computed tomography and/or selective mesenteric angiogram to identify tumor
       (b) Laxative abuse: see step 5

Diarrhea stops

   a. Malabsorption syndromes: stool osmolality > plasma osmolality
   b. Laxative ingestion: see step 5
   c. Congenital chloridorrhea
     (1) Stool electrolytes: chloride concentration greater than the sum of sodium and potassium concentrations in stool water
     (2) No fecal osmotic gap

5. Laxative abuse detection

   a. Screening tests
     (1) Detailed history
     (2) Sigmoidoscopy and biopsy for melanosis coli
     (3) Barium enema: dilated, hypomotile "cathartic colon"
   b. Specific tests
     (1) Urine screening test for senna
     (2) Chromatographic test for bisacodyl
     (3) Stool test for fecal sulfate and phosphate
     (4) Magnesium concentration in fecal water (atomic absorption spectrophotometry)

6. Radiologic studies

Perform barium studies only after stool examination, culture, and studies requiring quantitative measurements of the stool have been completed.

Fig. 3-61 **Diagnostic approach to the patient with chronic diarrhea.** *5-HIAA,* 5-Hydroxyindoleacetic acid; *VIP,* vasoactive intestinal polypeptide. (Modified from Stein JH [ed]: *Internal medicine,* ed 5, St Louis, 1998, Mosby.)

III

DIARRHEA, CHRONIC, IN PATIENTS WITH HIV INFECTION

Diarrhea, chronic, in patients with HIV infection
ICD-9CM # 787.1 Diarrhea, chronic

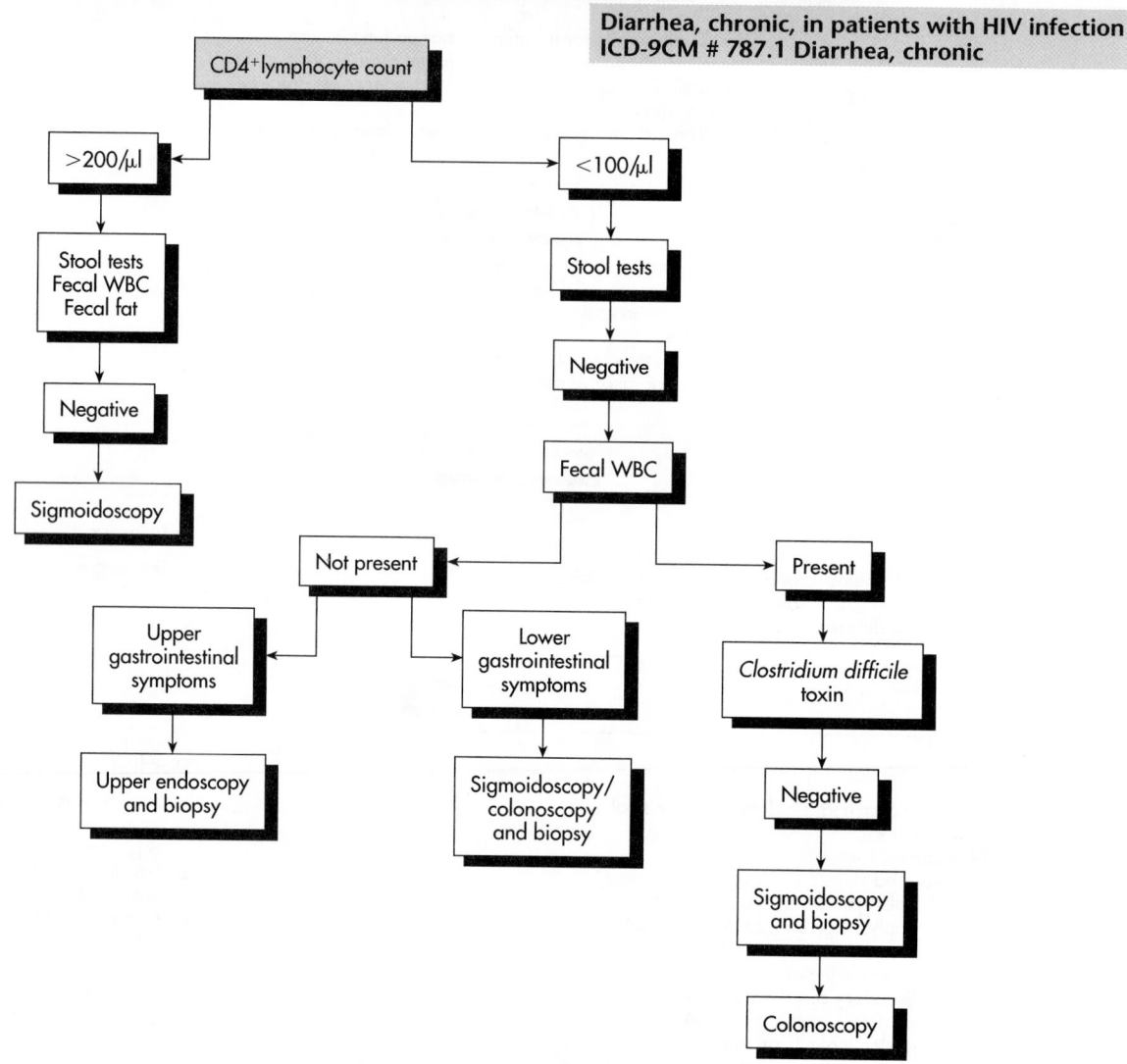

Fig. 3-62 Approach to evaluating chronic diarrhea in patients with HIV infection. *WBC,* White blood cell count. (From Wilcox CM: *Gastrointest Dis Today* 5:9, 1996.)

TABLE 3-4 Common Gastrointestinal Pathogens Associated with HIV Infection

PATHOGEN	CD4+ CELLS/μl	STOOL VOLUME AND FREQUENCY	ABDOMINAL PAIN	WEIGHT LOSS	FEVER	FECAL LEUKOCYTES
Cytomegalovirus*	<100	Mild to moderate	++	++	++	+
Cryptosporidiosis	<100	Moderate to severe	−	++	−	−
Microsporidiosis	<100	Mild to moderate	−	+	−	−
Mycobacterium avium complex†	<100	Mild to moderate	+	+++	+++	−

From Wilcox CM: *Gastrointest Dis Today* 5:9, 1996.
*Can have proctitis symptoms when involving the distal colon.
†Typical presentation is fever and wasting; diarrhea is usually secondary.
+++, Very common; ++, frequent; +, can occur; −, absent.

DILATED PUPIL

Dilated pupil
ICD9-CM # 379.43 Pupil dilation

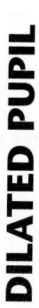

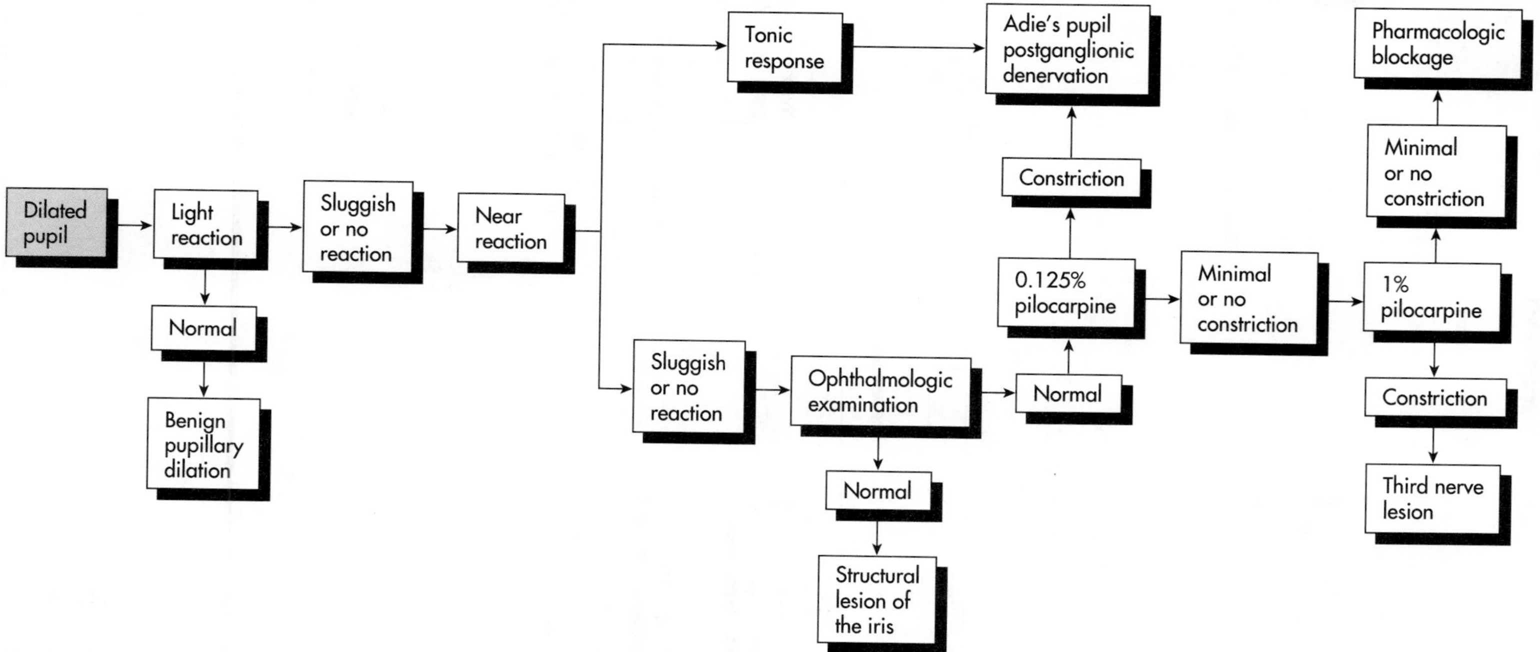

Fig. 3-63   Use of pilocarpine to help differentiate between different causes of a dilated pupil. (From Goldman L, Ausiello D [eds]: *Cecil textbook of medicine*, ed 22, Philadephia, 2004, WB Saunders.)

III

DYSPEPSIA

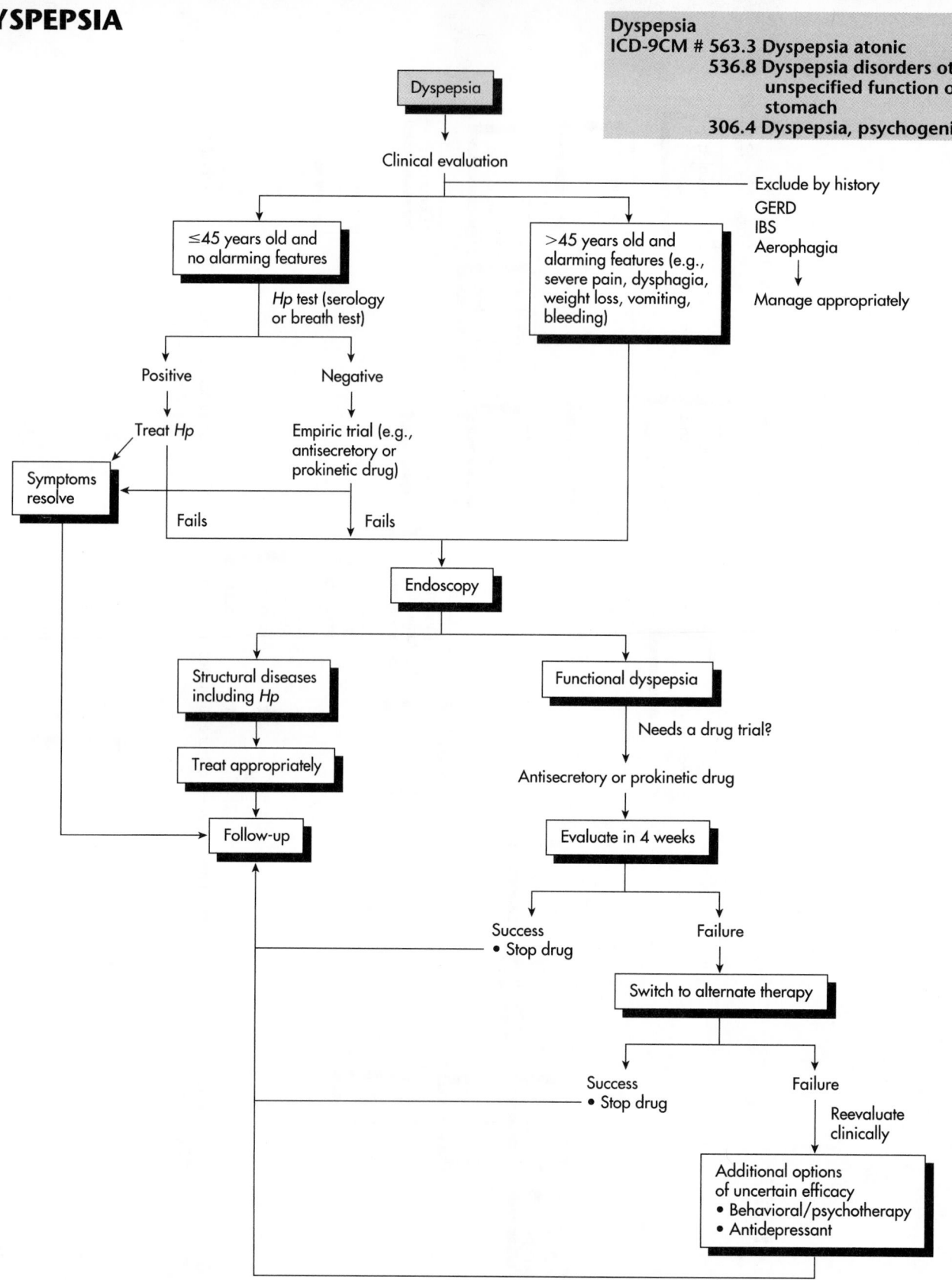

Fig. 3-64 Algorithm for the evaluation of dyspepsia. *GERD,* Symptomatic gastroesophageal reflux disease; *Hp, Helicobacter pylori; IBS,* irritable bowel syndrome. (From Goldman L, Ausiello D [eds]: *Cecil textbook of medicine,* ed 22, Philadelphia, 2004, WB Saunders.)

DYSPHAGIA

Dysphagia
ICD-9CM # 787.2

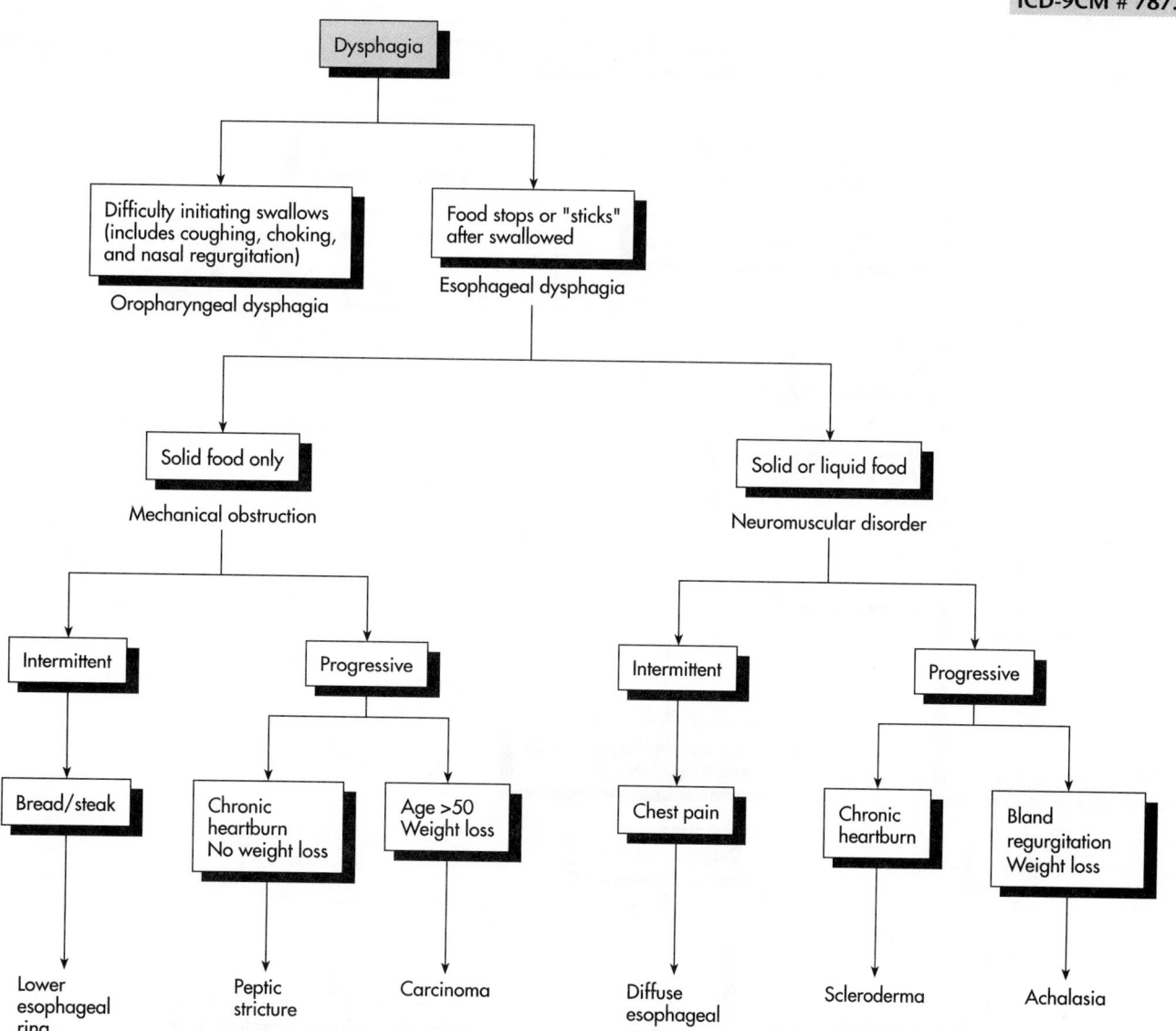

Fig. 3-65   Differential diagnosis of dysphagia. (From Andreoli TE [ed]: *Cecil essentials of medicine,* ed 5, Philadelphia, 2001, WB Saunders.)

DYSPNEA, ACUTE

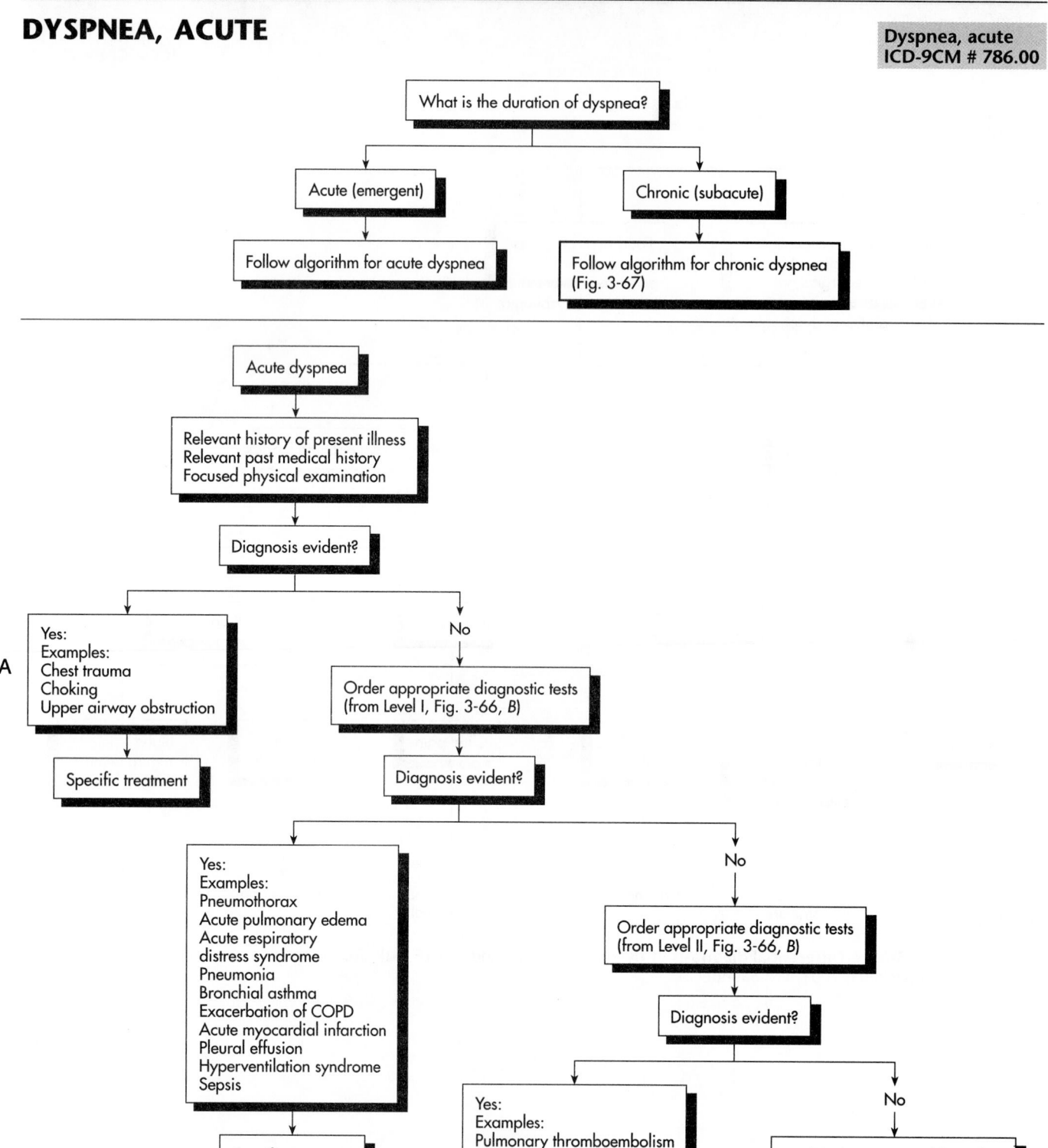

Fig. 3-66   A, Evaluation of the patient with dyspnea. *COPD,* Chronic obstructive pulmonary disease.
(From Stein J [ed]: *Internal medicine,* ed 5, St Louis, 1998, Mosby.)

DYSPNEA, ACUTE—cont'd

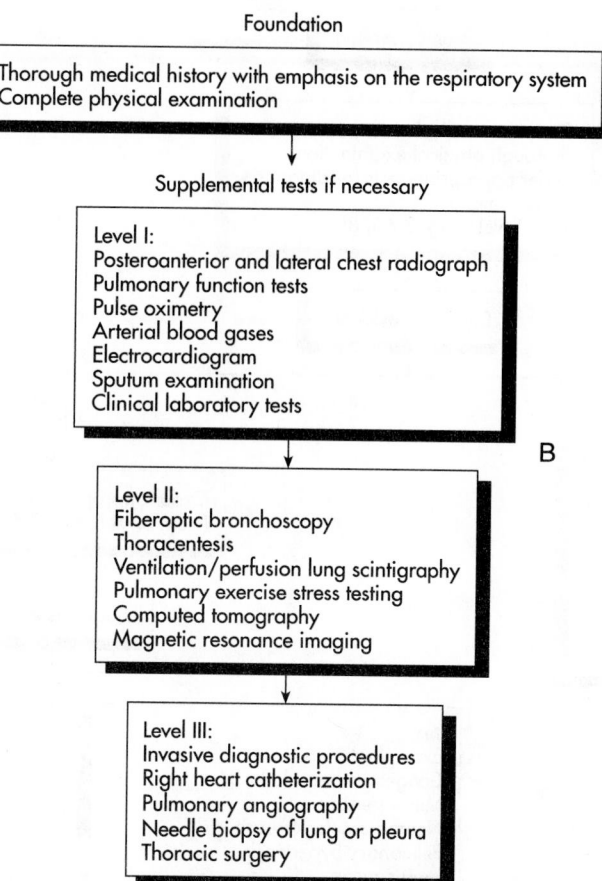

Foundation

Thorough medical history with emphasis on the respiratory system
Complete physical examination

Supplemental tests if necessary

Level I:
Posteroanterior and lateral chest radiograph
Pulmonary function tests
Pulse oximetry
Arterial blood gases
Electrocardiogram
Sputum examination
Clinical laboratory tests

B

Level II:
Fiberoptic bronchoscopy
Thoracentesis
Ventilation/perfusion lung scintigraphy
Pulmonary exercise stress testing
Computed tomography
Magnetic resonance imaging

Level III:
Invasive diagnostic procedures
Right heart catheterization
Pulmonary angiography
Needle biopsy of lung or pleura
Thoracic surgery

Fig. 3-66, cont'd **B, Medical history and physical examination are the foundation for the diagnosis of respiratory system disease.** Diagnostic tests of increasing levels of complexity and invasiveness are performed if necessary to supplement the initial history and physical examination. (From Stein J [ed]: *Internal medicine,* ed 5, St Louis, 1998, Mosby.)

III

DYSPNEA, CHRONIC

Dyspnea, chronic
ICD-9CM # 786.00

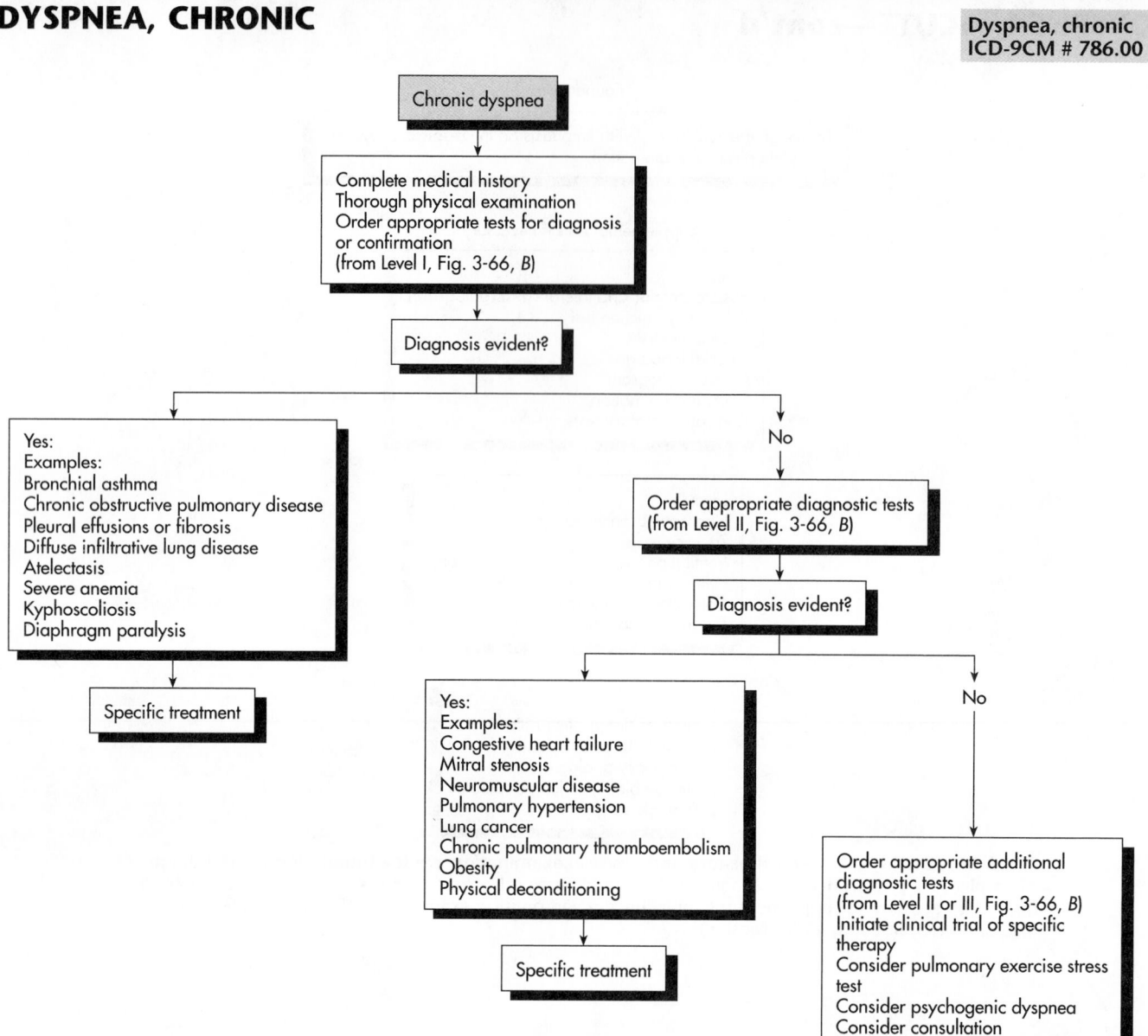

Fig. 3-67 **Chronic dyspnea.** (From Stein J [ed]: *Internal medicine,* ed 5, St Louis, 1998, Mosby.)

DYSURIA AND/OR URETHRAL/VAGINAL DISCHARGE

Dysuria and/or urethral/vaginal discharge
ICD-9CM # 788.1 Dysuria
           788.7 Urethral discharge
           623.5 Vaginal discharge

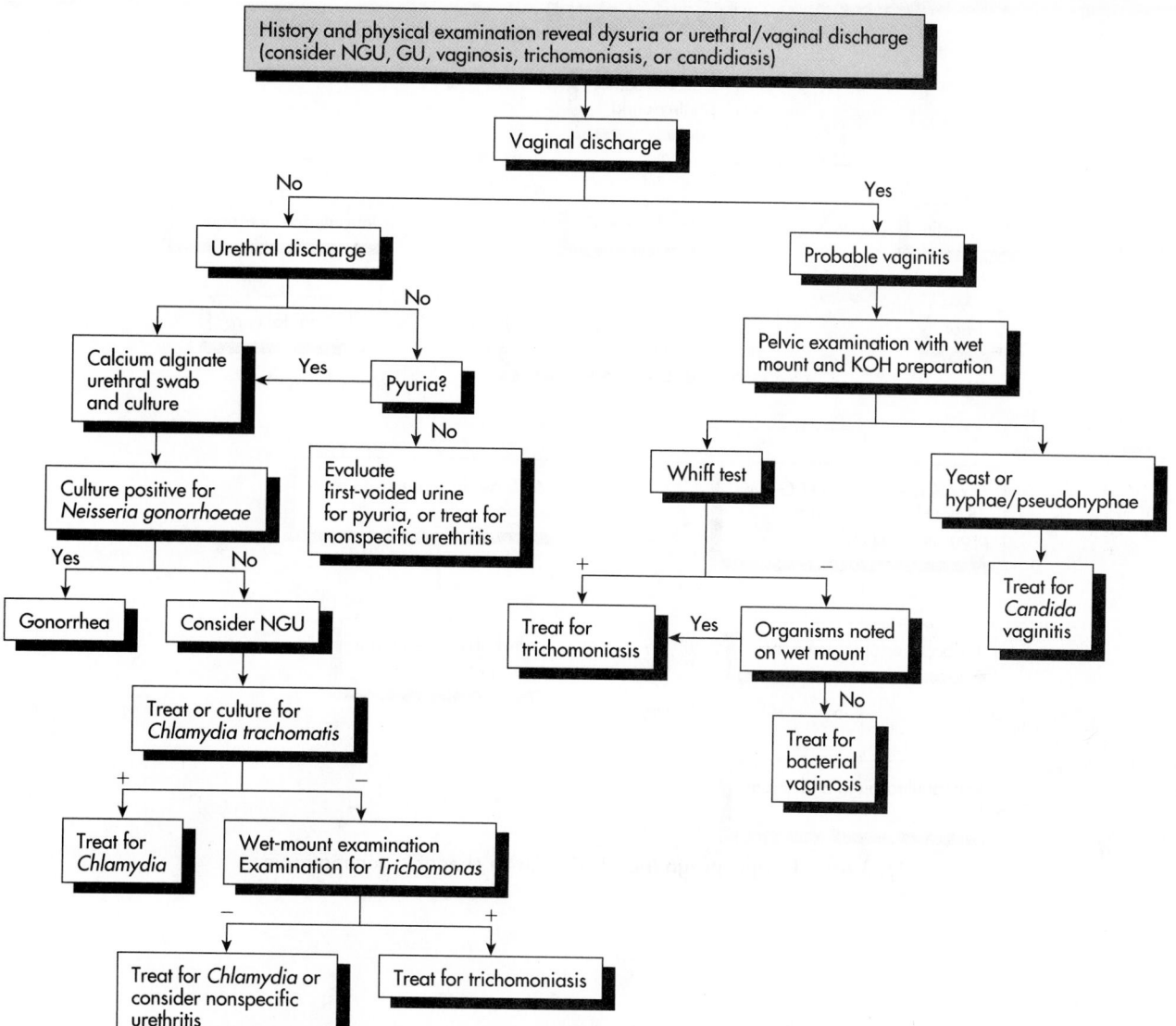

Fig. 3-68   **Evaluation of patients with dysuria and/or urethral/vaginal discharge.** *GU,* Gonococcal urethritis; *KOH,* potassium hydroxide; *NGU,* nongonococcal urethritis. (From Nseyo UO [ed]: *Urology for primary care physicians,* Philadelphia, 1999, WB Saunders.)

ECTOPIC PREGNANCY

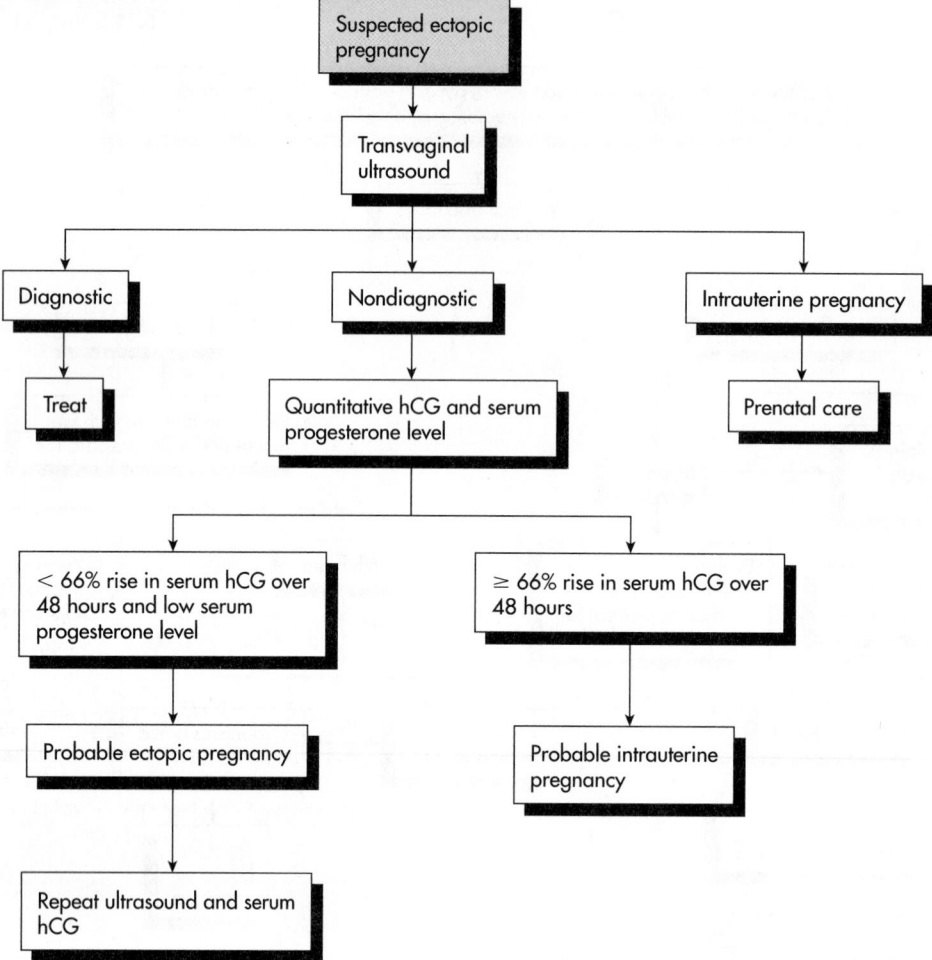

Fig. 3-69 **Ectopic pregnancy.** *hCG,* Human chorionic gonadotropin.

EDEMA, GENERALIZED

Edema, generalized
ICD-9CM # 782.3 Edema NOS
782.3 Edema, lower extremities

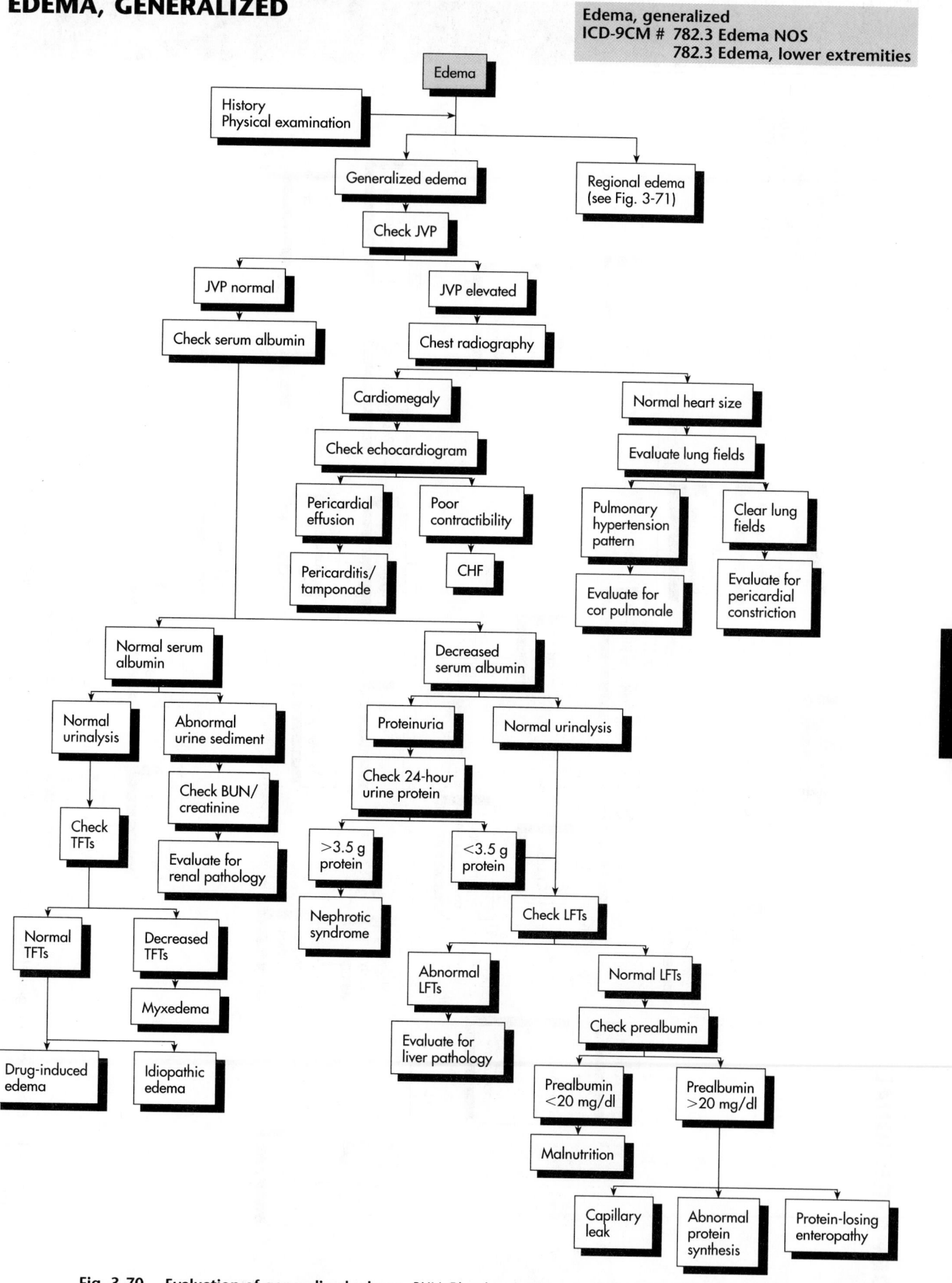

Fig. 3-70 **Evaluation of generalized edema.** *BUN,* Blood urea nitrogen; *CHF,* congestive heart failure; *JVP,* jugular venous pressure; *LFT,* liver function tests; *TFT,* thyroid function tests. (From Greene HL, Johnson WP, Lemcke D [eds]: *Decision making in medicine,* ed 2, St Louis, 1998, Mosby.)

EDEMA, REGIONAL

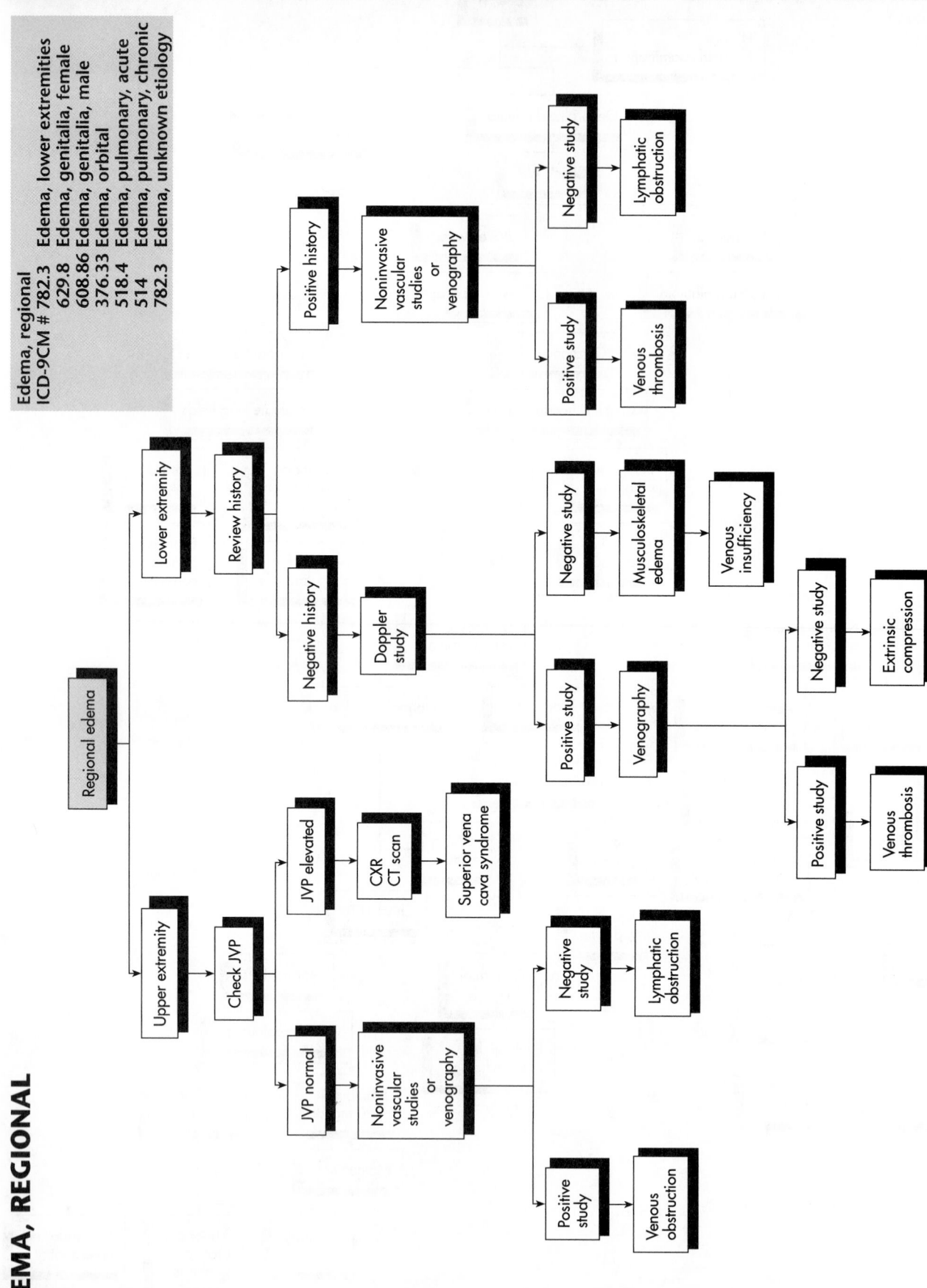

Edema, regional
ICD-9CM # 782.3   Edema, lower extremities
629.8   Edema, genitalia, female
608.86   Edema, genitalia, male
376.33   Edema, orbital
518.4   Edema, pulmonary, acute
514   Edema, pulmonary, chronic
782.3   Edema, unknown etiology

Fig. 3-71   Evaluation of regional edema. *CT,* Computed tomography; *CXR,* chest x-ray examination; *JVP,* jugular venous pressure. (From Greene HL, Johnson WP, Lemcke D [eds]: *Decision making in medicine,* ed 2, St Louis, 1998, Mosby.)

ENURESIS AND VOIDING DYSFUNCTION, PEDIATRIC

Enuresis and voiding dysfunction, pediatric
ICD-9CM # 788.30

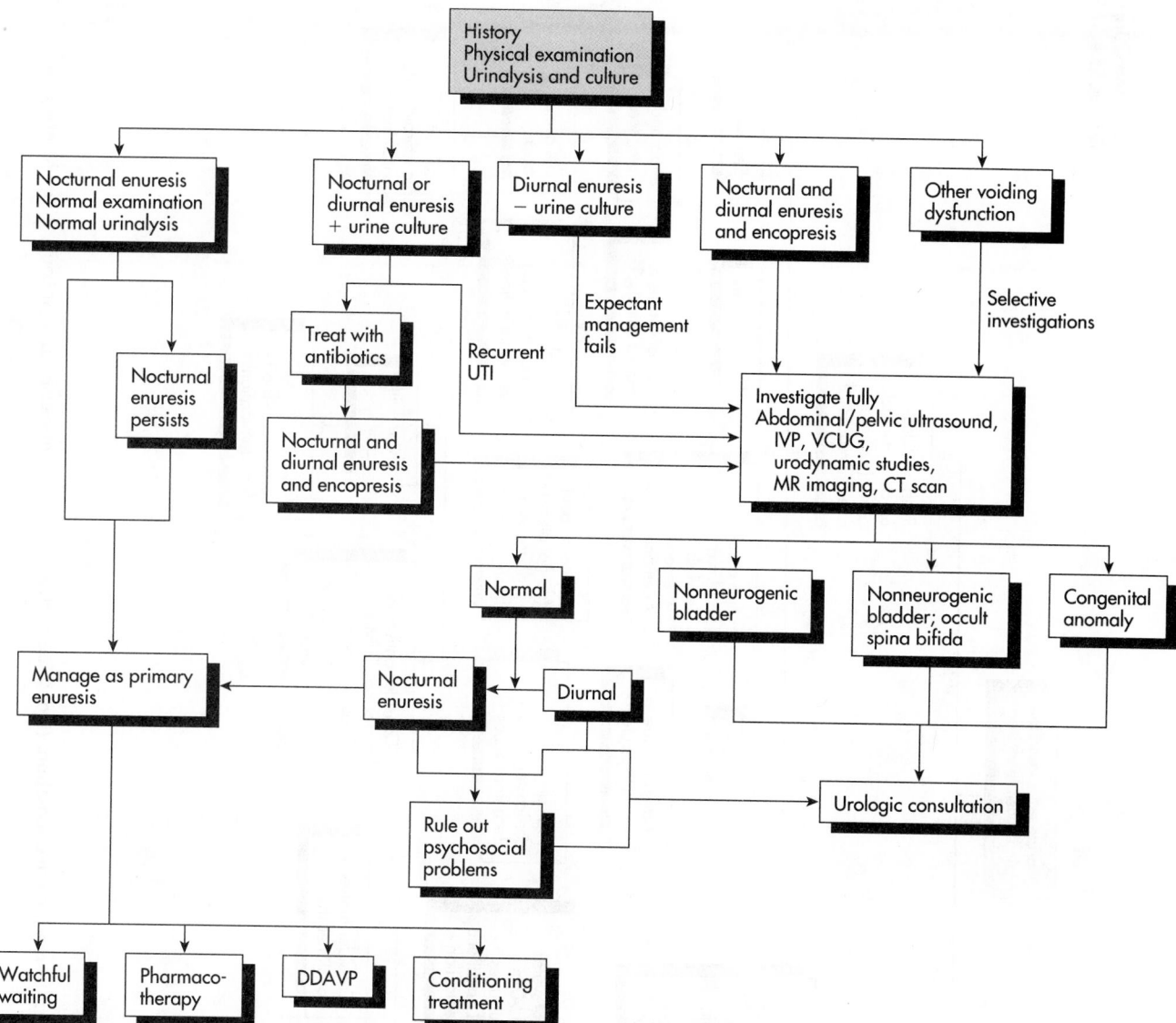

Fig. 3-72 Algorithm of management of pediatric enuresis and voiding dysfunction. *CT,* Computed tomography; *DDAVP,* desmopressin acetate; *IVP,* intravenous pyelogram; *MR,* magnetic resonance; *UTI,* urinary tract infection; *VCUG,* voiding cystourethrogram. (From Nseyo UO [ed]: *Urology for primary care physicians,* Philadelphia, 1999, WB Saunders.)

ENVENOMATION, MARINE

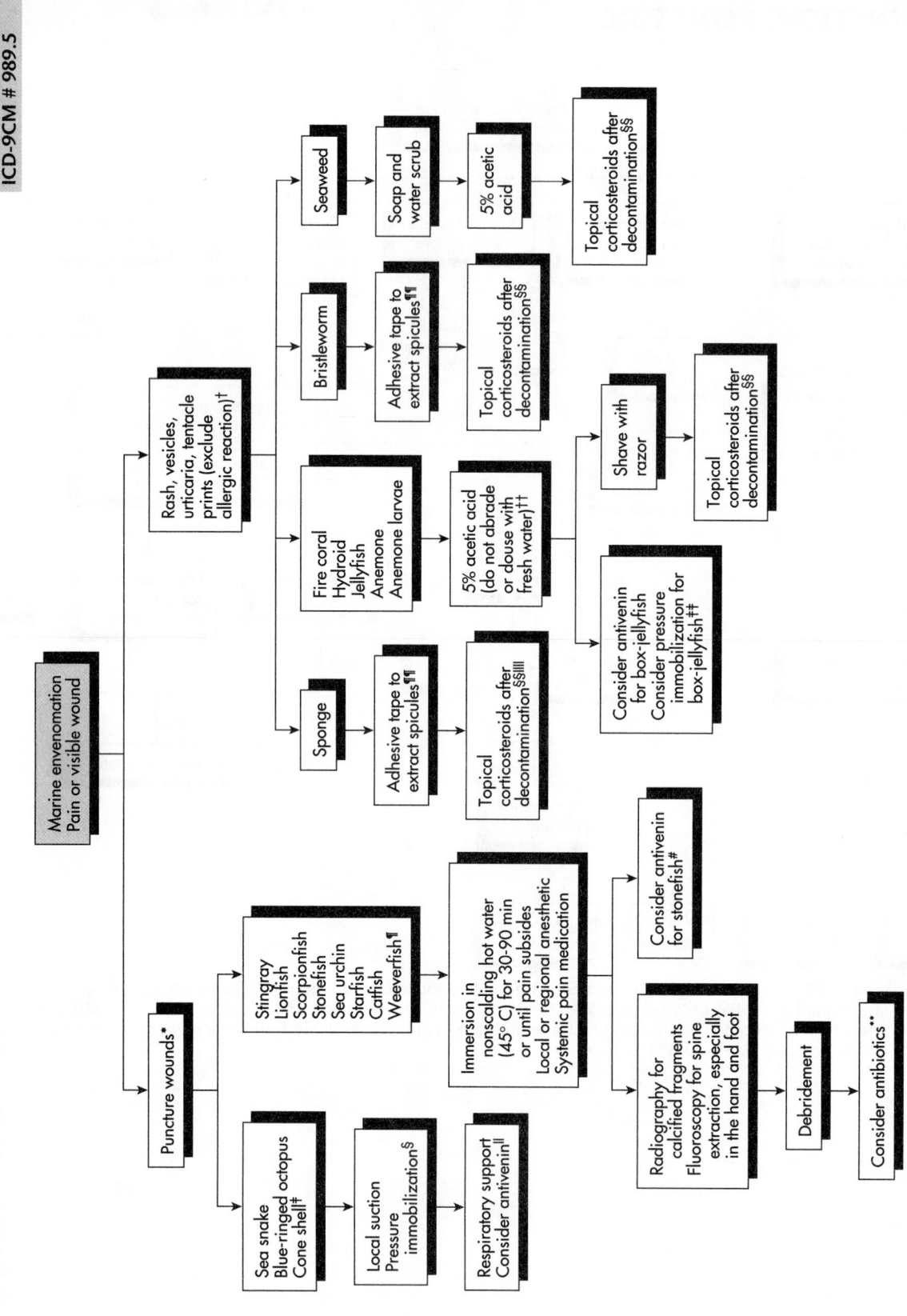

Fig. 3-73 Algorithmic approach to marine envenomation. (From Auerbach PS: *Wilderness medicine*, ed 4, St Louis, 2001, Mosby.)

Continued

*A gaping laceration, particularly of the lower extremity, with cyanotic edges suggests a stingray wound. Multiple punctures in an erratic pattern with or without purple discoloration or retained fragments are typical of a sea urchin sting. One to eight (usually two) fang marks are usually present after a sea snake bite. A single ischemic puncture wound with an erythematous halo and rapid swelling suggests scorpionfish envenomation. Blisters often accompany a lionfish sting. Painless punctures with paralysis suggest the bite of a blue-ringed octopus; the site of a cone shell sting is punctate, painful, and ischemic in appearance.

†Wheal and flare reactions are nonspecific. Rapid (within 24 hours) onset of skin necrosis suggests an anemone sting. "Tentacle prints" with cross-hatching or a frosted appearance are pathognomonic for box-jellyfish (*Chironex fleckeri*) envenomation. Ocular or intraoral lesions may be caused by fragmented hydroids or coelenterate tentacles. An allergic reaction must be treated promptly.

‡Sea snake venom causes weakness, respiratory paralysis, myoglobinuria, myalgias, blurred vision, vomiting, and dysphagia. The blue-ringed octopus injects tetrodotoxin, which causes rapid neuromuscular paralysis.

§If *immediately* available (which is rarely the case), local suction can be applied without incision using a plunger device, such as The Extractor (Sawyer Products, Safety Harbor, Fla.). As soon as possible, venom should be sequestered locally with a proximal venous-lymphatic occlusive band of constriction or (preferably) the pressure immobilization technique, in which a cloth pad is compressed directly over the wound by an elastic wrap that should encompass the entire extremity at a pressure of 9.33 kPa (70 mm Hg) or less. Incision and suction are not recommended.

‖Early ventilatory support has the greatest influence on outcome. The minimal initial dose of sea snake antivenin is 1 to 3 vials; up to 10 vials may be required.

¶The wounds range from large lacerations (stingrays) to minute punctures (stonefish). Persistent pain after immersion in hot water suggests a stonefish sting or a retained fragment of spine. The puncture site can be identified by forcefully injecting 1% to 2% lidocaine or another local anesthetic agent without epinephrine near the wound and observing the egress of fluid. Do not attempt to crush the spines of sea urchins if they are present in the wound. Spine dye from already-extracted sea urchin spines will disappear (be absorbed) in 24 to 36 hours.

#The initial dose of stonefish antivenin is one vial per two puncture wounds.

**The antibiotics chosen should cover *Staphylococcus*, *Streptococcus*, and microbes of marine origin, such as *Vibrio*.

††Acetic acid 5% (vinegar) is a good all-purpose decontaminant and is mandated for the sting from a box-jellyfish. Alternatives, depending on the geographic region and indigenous jellyfish species, include isopropyl alcohol, bicarbonate (baking soda), ammonia, papain, and preparations containing these agents.

‡‡The initial dose of box-jellyfish antivenin is one ampule intravenously or three ampules intramuscularly.

§§If inflammation is severe, steroids should be given systematically (beginning with at least 60 to 100 mg of prednisone or its equivalent) and the dose tapered over a period of 10 to 14 days.

‖‖An alternative is to apply and remove commercial facial peel materials.

¶¶An alternative is to apply and remove commercial facial peel materials followed by topical soaks of 30 ml of 5% acetic acid (vinegar) diluted in 1 L of water for 15 to 30 minutes several times a day until the lesions begin to resolve. Anticipate surface desquamation in 3 to 6 weeks.

III

EPIGLOTTITIS

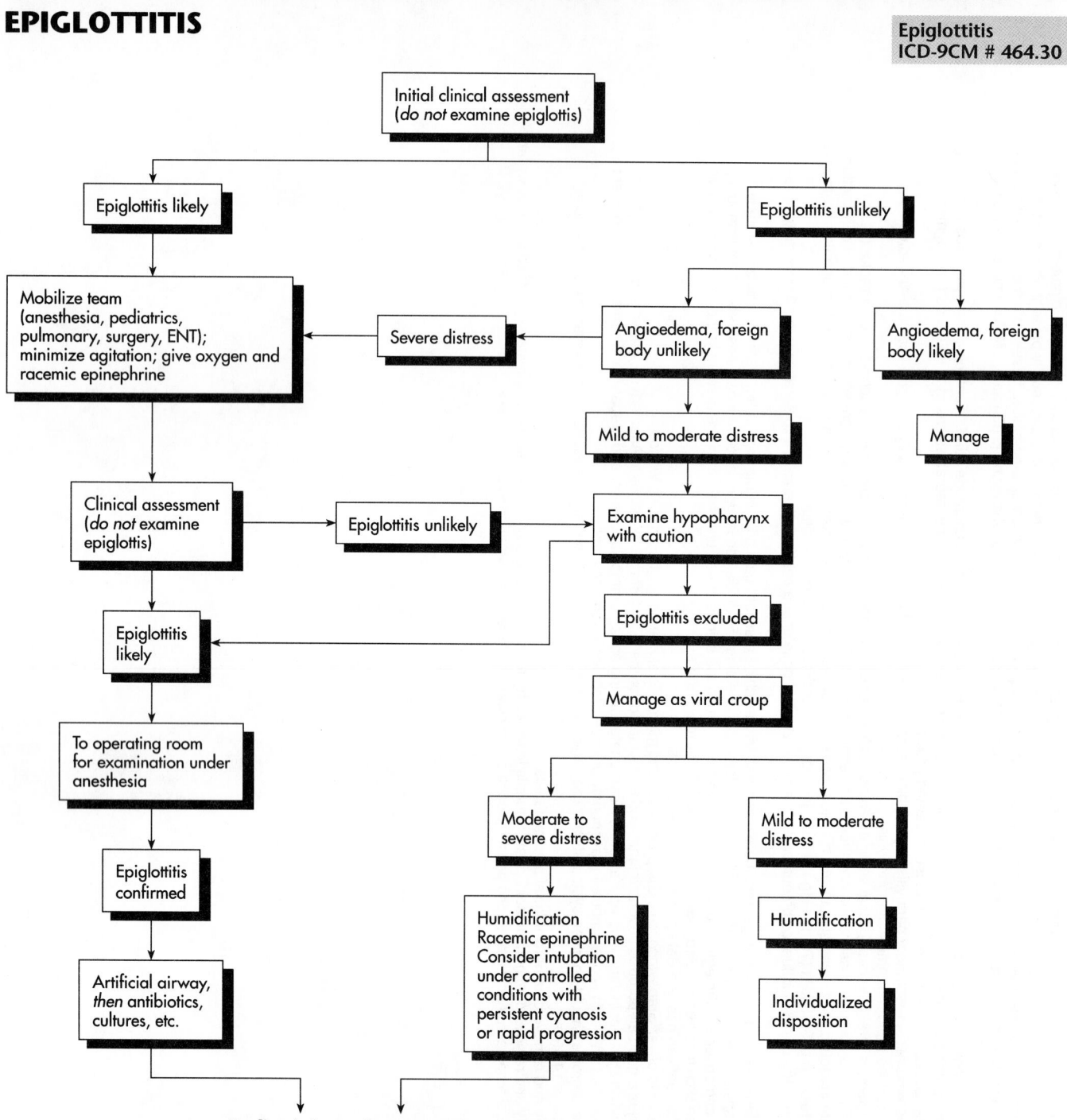

Pediatric intensive care unit

Fig. 3-74 **Optimal assessment and management of upper airway obstruction caused by epiglottitis or severe croup. Care must be individualized to reflect resources and logistic issues within a given institution.** *ENT,* Ear, nose, throat. (From Barkin RM, Rosen P: *Emergency pediatrics,* St Louis, 1999, Mosby.)

ERYTHROCYTOSIS, ACQUIRED

Erythrocytosis, acquired
ICD-9CM # 289.0 Polycythemia, acquired

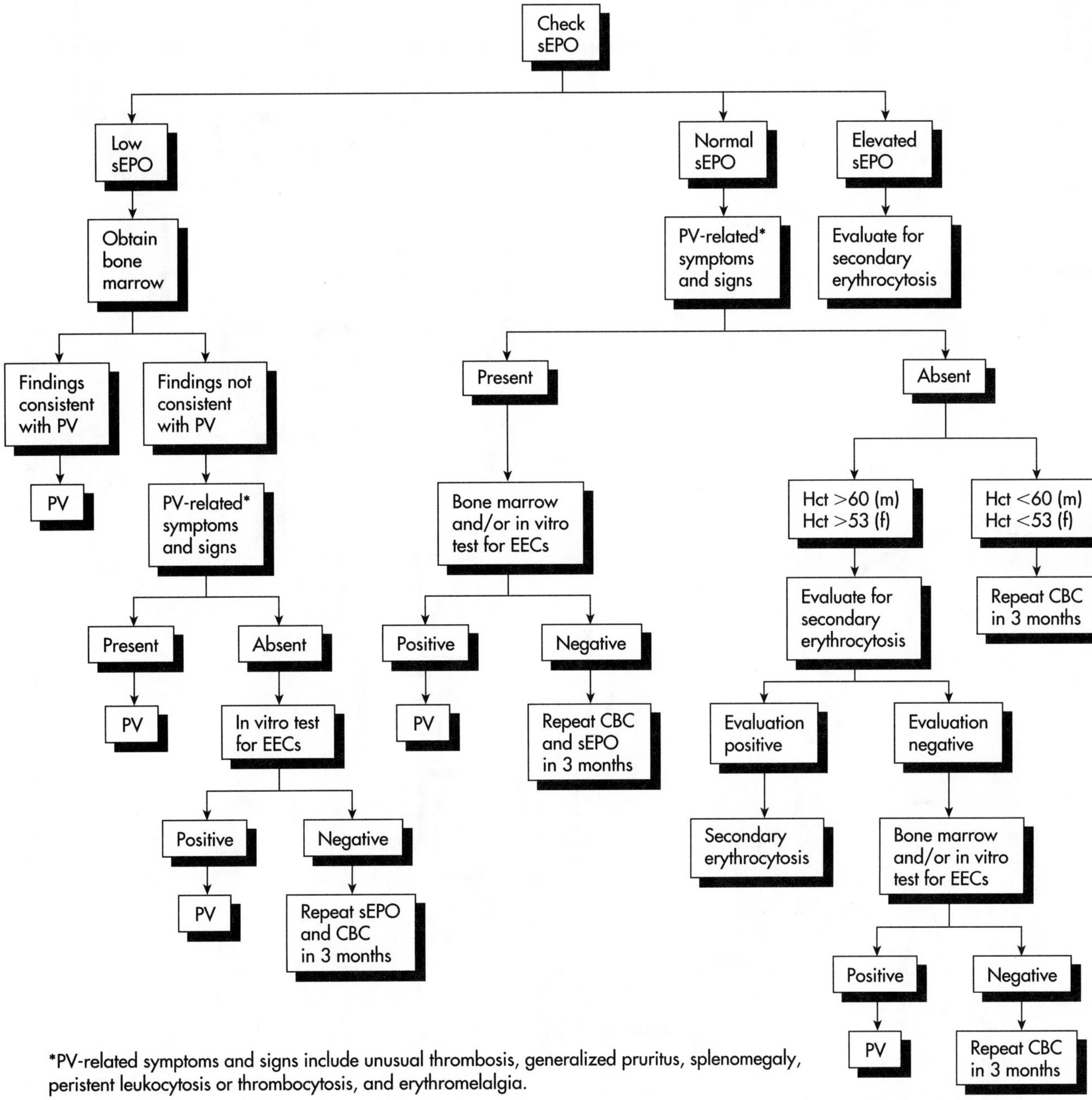

*PV-related symptoms and signs include unusual thrombosis, generalized pruritus, splenomegaly, peristent leukocytosis or thrombocytosis, and erythromelalgia.

Fig. 3-75   A diagnostic approach to acquired erythrocytosis. *CBC,* Complete blood cell count; *EEC,* endogenous (spontaneous) erythroid colonies; *f,* female; *Hct,* hematocrit; *m,* male; *PV,* polycythemia vera; *sEPO,* serum erythropoietin level. (From Goldman L, Ausiello D [eds]: *Cecil textbook of medicine,* ed 22, Philadelphia, 2004, WB Saunders.)

FATIGUE

Fatigue
ICD-9CM # 780.7 Fatigue, general

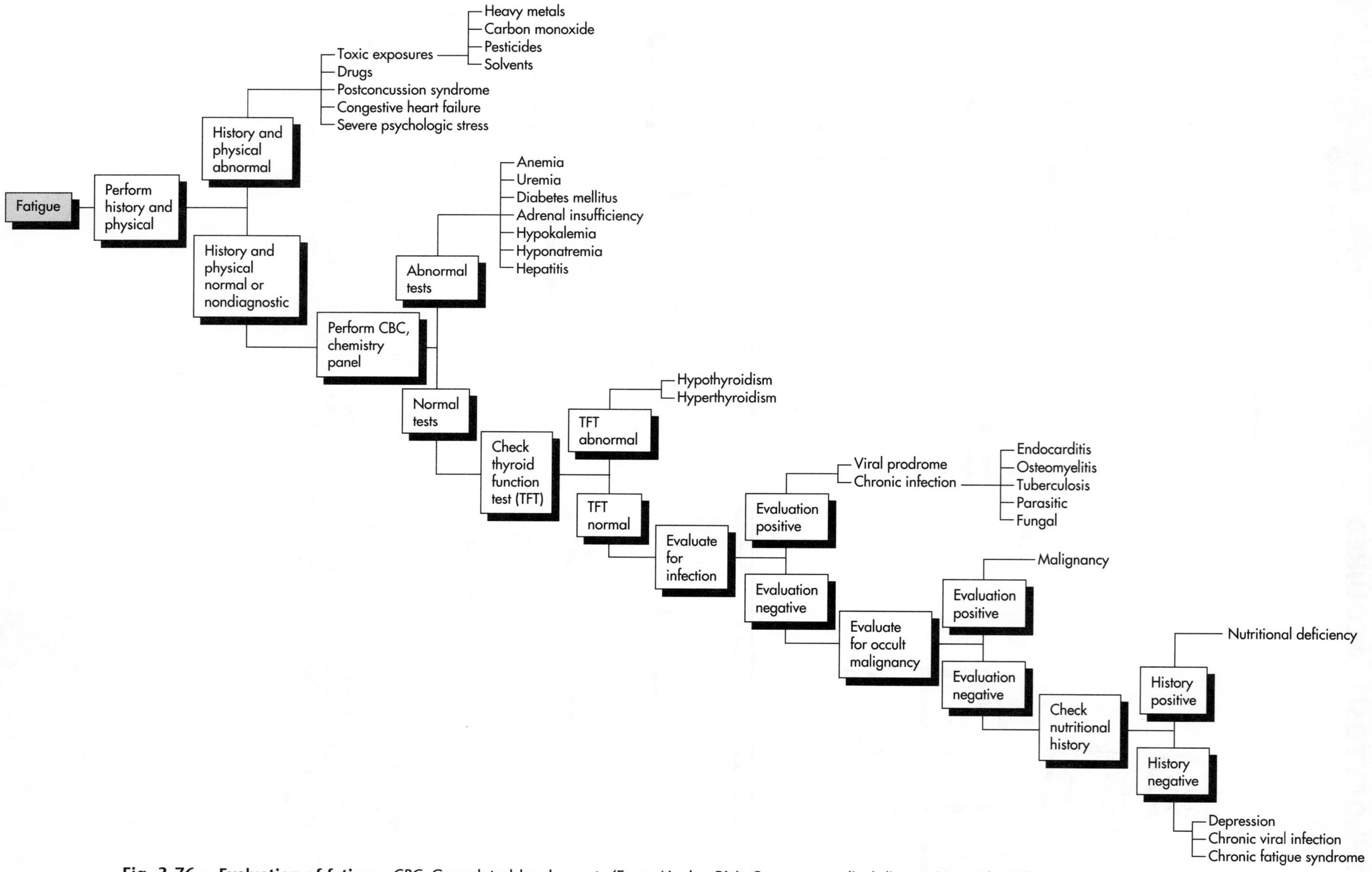

Fatigue
↓
Perform history and physical
├─ History and physical abnormal
│   └─ Toxic exposures
│   ├─ Heavy metals
│   ├─ Carbon monoxide
│   ├─ Pesticides
│   └─ Solvents
│   ├─ Drugs
│   ├─ Postconcussion syndrome
│   ├─ Congestive heart failure
│   └─ Severe psychologic stress
│
└─ History and physical normal or nondiagnostic
    └─ Perform CBC, chemistry panel
        ├─ Abnormal tests
        │   ├─ Anemia
        │   ├─ Uremia
        │   ├─ Diabetes mellitus
        │   ├─ Adrenal insufficiency
        │   ├─ Hypokalemia
        │   ├─ Hyponatremia
        │   └─ Hepatitis
        └─ Normal tests
            └─ Check thyroid function test (TFT)
                ├─ TFT abnormal
                │   ├─ Hypothyroidism
                │   └─ Hyperthyroidism
                └─ TFT normal
                    └─ Evaluate for infection
                        ├─ Evaluation positive
                        │   ├─ Viral prodrome
                        │   └─ Chronic infection
                        │   ├─ Endocarditis
                        │   ├─ Osteomyelitis
                        │   ├─ Tuberculosis
                        │   ├─ Parasitic
                        │   └─ Fungal
                        └─ Evaluation negative
                            └─ Evaluate for occult malignancy
                                ├─ Evaluation positive
                                │   └─ Malignancy
                                └─ Evaluation negative
                                    └─ Check nutritional history
                                        ├─ History positive
                                        │   └─ Nutritional deficiency
                                        └─ History negative
                                            ├─ Depression
                                            ├─ Chronic viral infection
                                            └─ Chronic fatigue syndrome

Fig. 3-76 Evaluation of fatigue. *CBC,* Complete blood count. (From Healey PM: *Common medical diagnosis: an algorithmic approach,* ed 3, Philadelphia, 2000, WB Saunders.)

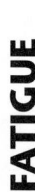

FEVER OF UNDETERMINED ORIGIN

Fever of undetermined origin
ICD-9CM #

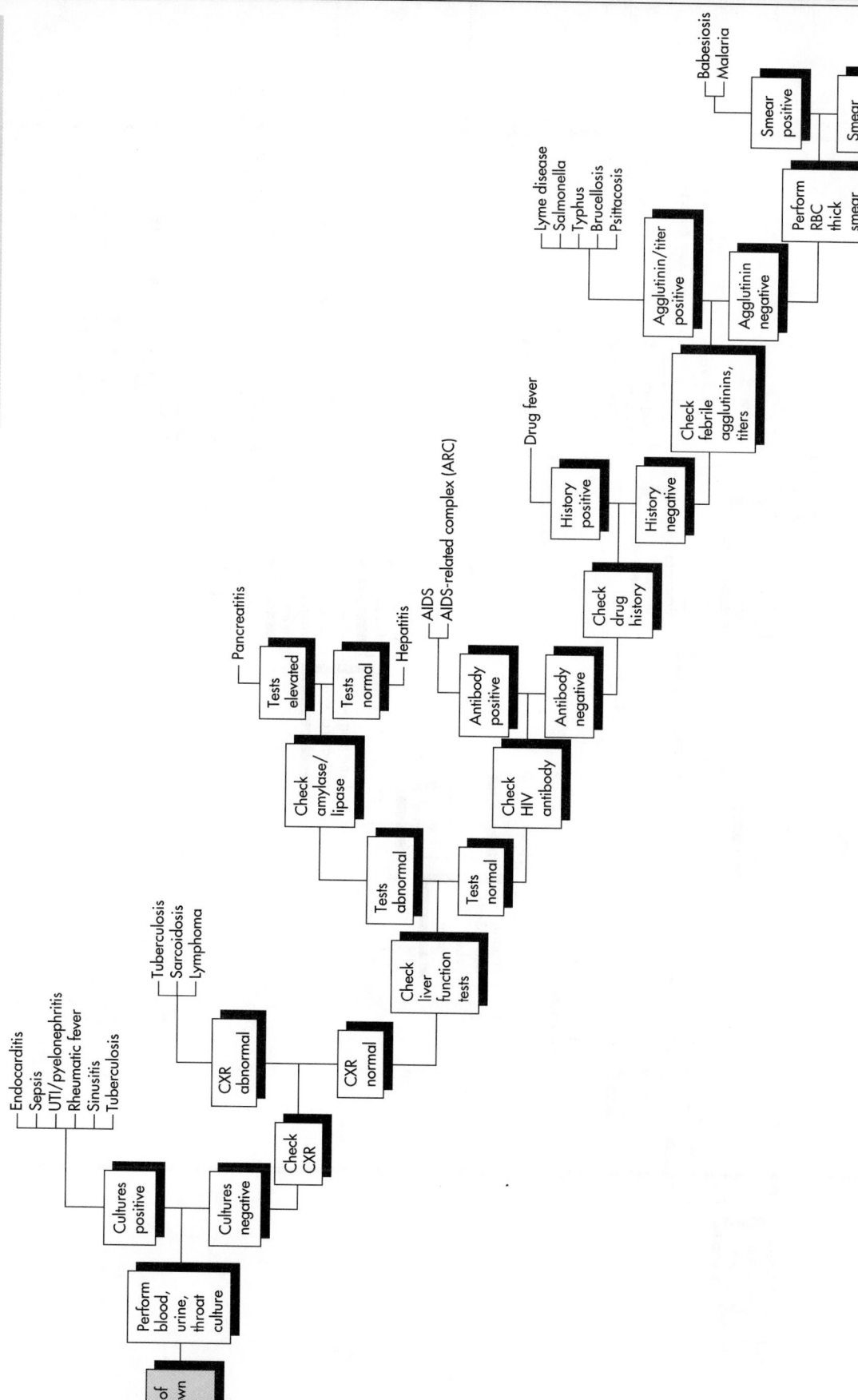

Fig. 3-77   Approach to the patient with fever of undetermined origin. *AIDS*, Acquired immunodeficiency syndrome; *ANA*, antinuclear antibody; *CT*, computed tomography; *CSR*, chest x-ray; *ESR*, erythrocyte sedimentation rate; *GI*, gastrointestinal; *HIV*, human immunodeficiency virus; *RBC*, red blood cell; *UTI*, urinary tract infection. (From Healey PM: *Common medical diagnosis: an algorithmic approach*, ed 3, Philadelphia, 2000, WB Saunders.)

FEVER OF UNDETERMINED ORIGIN—cont'd

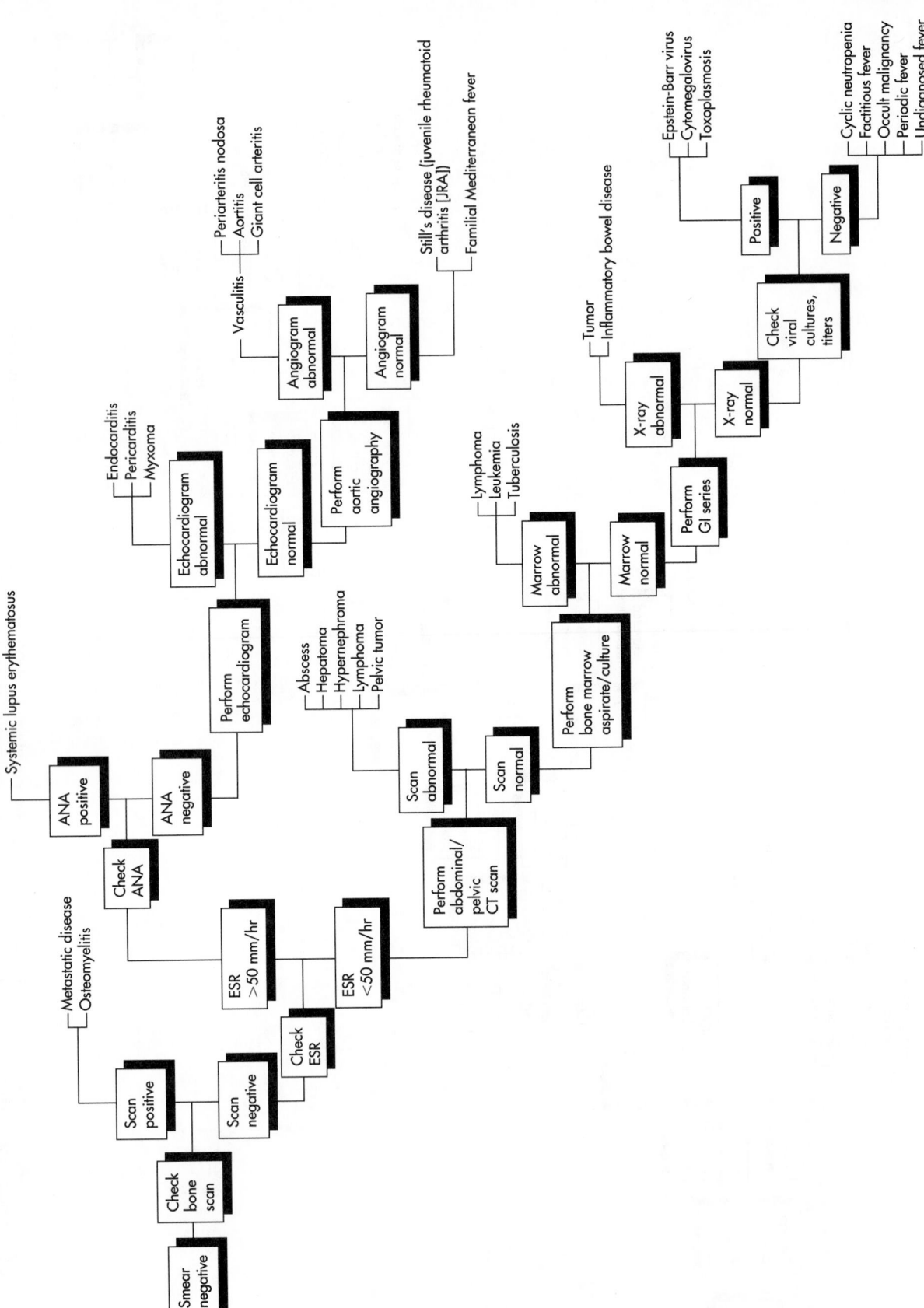

Fig. 3-77, cont'd *AIDS,* Acquired immunodeficiency syndrome; *ANA,* antinuclear antibody; *CT,* computed tomography; *CSR,* chest x-ray; *ESR,* erythrocyte sedimentation rate; *GI,* gastrointestinal; *HIV,* human immunodeficiency virus; *RBC,* red blood cell; *UTI,* urinary tract infection. (From Healey PM: *Common medical diagnosis: an algorithmic approach,* ed 3, Philadelphia, 2000, WB Saunders.)

FRACTURE, BONE

Fracture, bone
ICD-9CM # 829.0 Fracture bone(s) NOS closed
           829.1 Fracture bone(s) NOS open

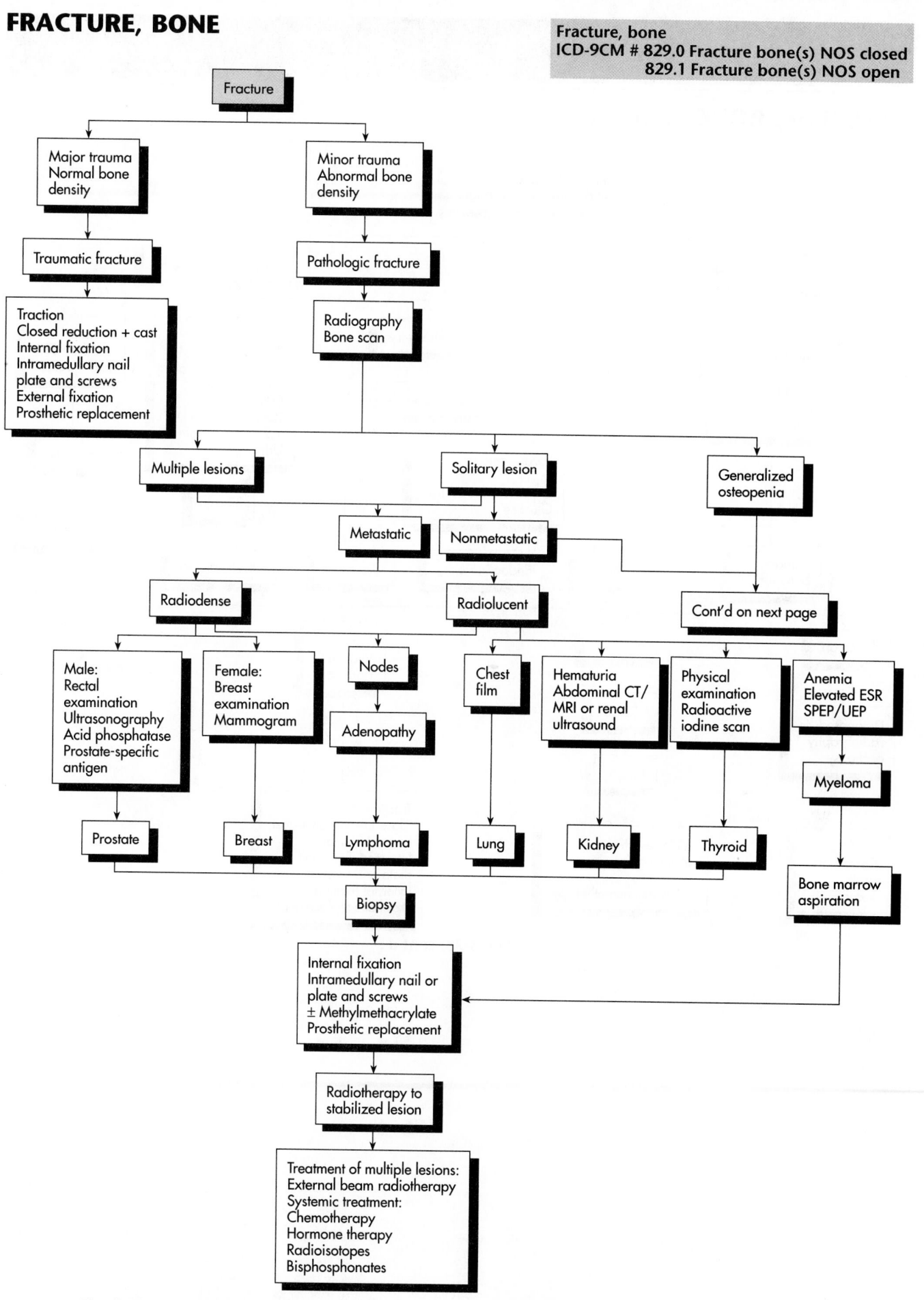

Fig. 3-78   Bone fracture. *CT,* Computed tomography; *ESR,* erythrocyte sedimentation rate; *MRI,* magnetic resonance imaging; *SPEP,* serum protein electrophoresis; *UEP,* urine electrophoresis. (From Greene HL, Johnson WP, Lemcke D [eds]: *Decision making in medicine,* ed 2, St Louis, 1998, Mosby.)

FRACTURE, BONE—cont'd

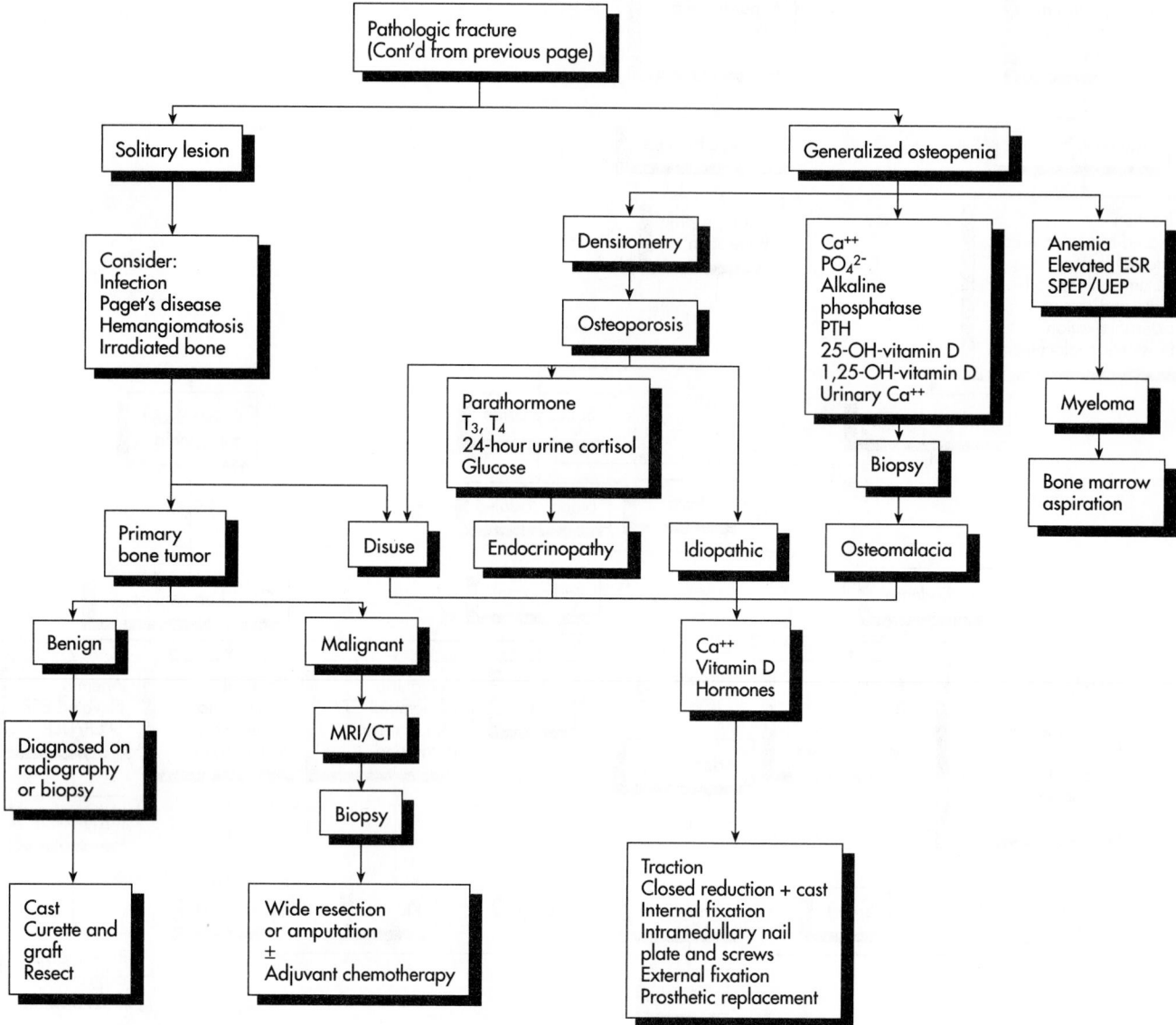

Fig. 3-78, cont'd

GENITAL LESIONS OR ULCERS

Genital sores
ICD-9CM # 054.10 Genital herpes
           91.0   Genital syphilis
        078.11 Condyloma acuminatum
        099.0 Chancroid
        099.2 Granuloma inguinale
        099.1 Lymphogranuloma venereum
        629.8 Ulcer, genital site, female
        608.89 Ulcer, genital site, male

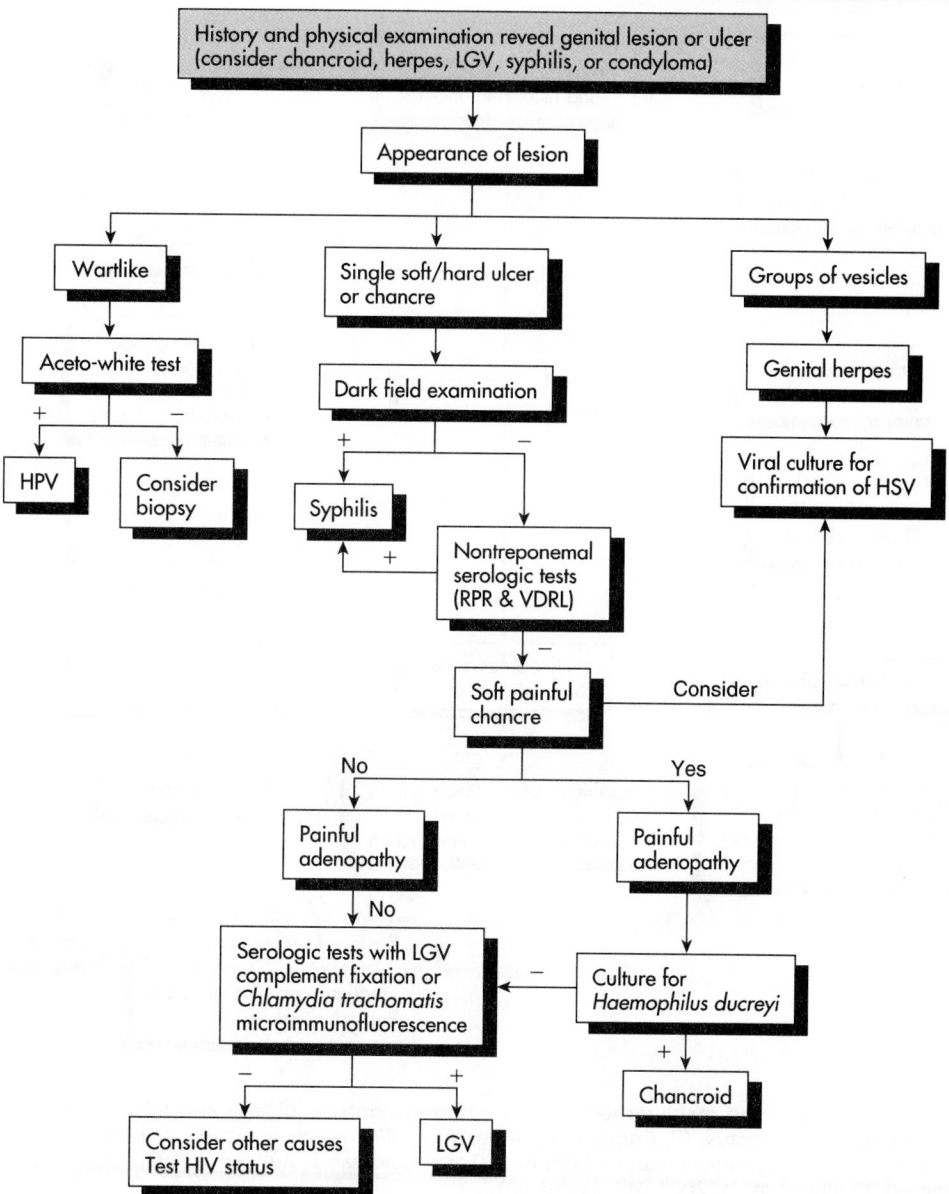

Fig. 3-79   **Evaluation of patients with genital lesions or ulcers.** *HIV,* Human immunodeficiency virus; *HPV,* human papillomavirus; *HSV,* herpes simplex virus; *LGV,* lymphogranuloma venereum; *RPR,* rapid plasma reagin; *VDRL,* Venereal Disease Research Laboratory. (From Nseyo UO [ed]: *Urology for primary care physicians,* Philadelphia, 1999, WB Saunders.)

GOITER EVALUATION AND MANAGEMENT

Goiter evaluation and management
ICD-9CM # 240.9 Goiter, unspecified
240.0 Goiter, simple
241.9 Goiter, adenomatous
246.1 Goiter, congenital
242.1 Goiter, uninodular with thyrotoxicosos
242.2 Goiter, multinodular with thyrotoxicosos

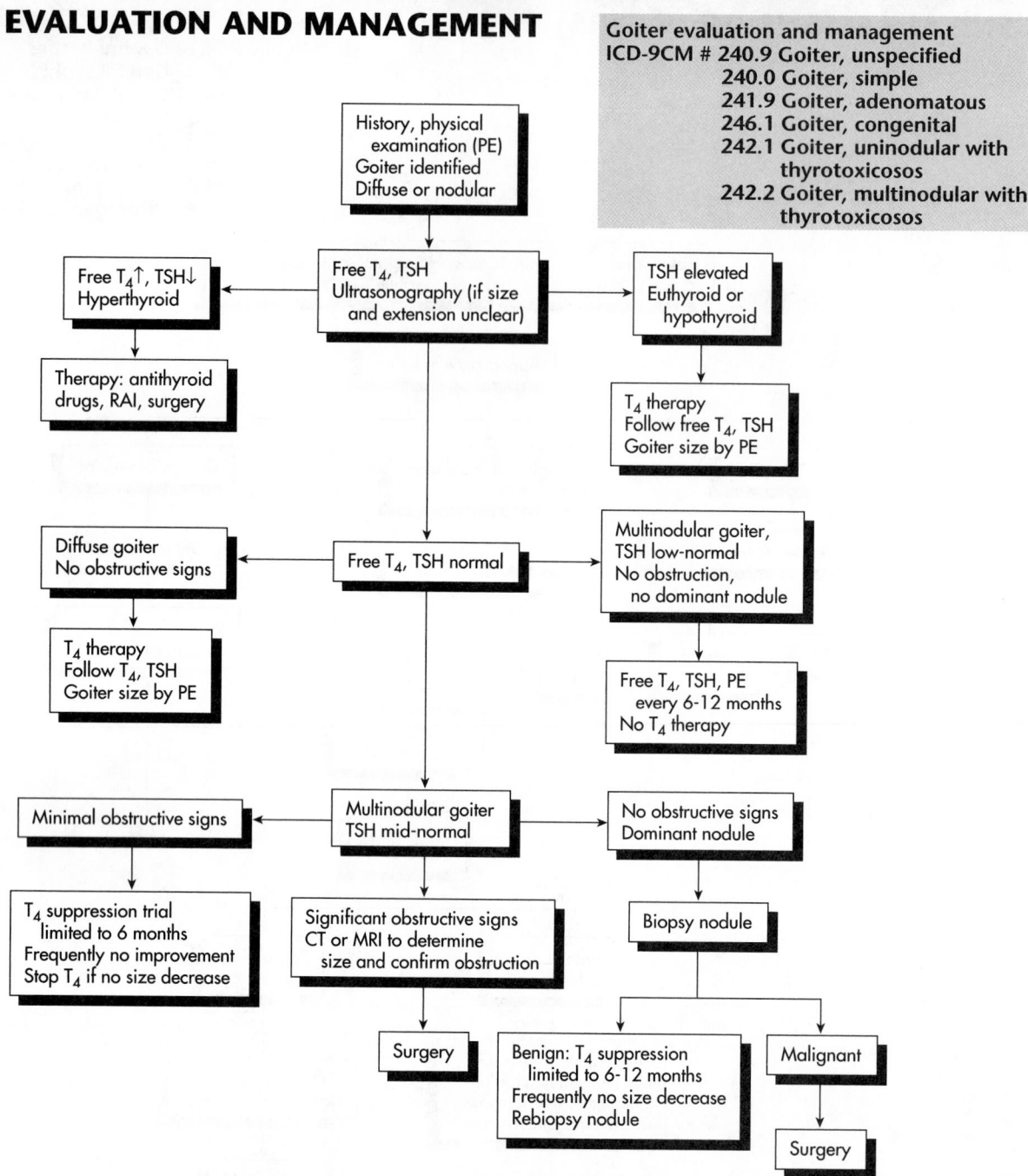

Fig. 3-80 **Evaluation and management of patients with nontoxic diffuse and nodular goiter and undetermined thyroid status.** *CT,* Computed tomography; *MRI,* magnetic resonance imaging; *RAI,* radioactive iodine; *TSH,* thyroid-stimulating hormone. (From Goldman L, Ausiello D [eds]: *Cecil textbook of medicine,* ed 22, Philadelphia, 2004, WB Saunders.)

GYNECOMASTIA

Gynecomastia
ICD-9CM # 611.1 Gynecomastia nonpuerperal

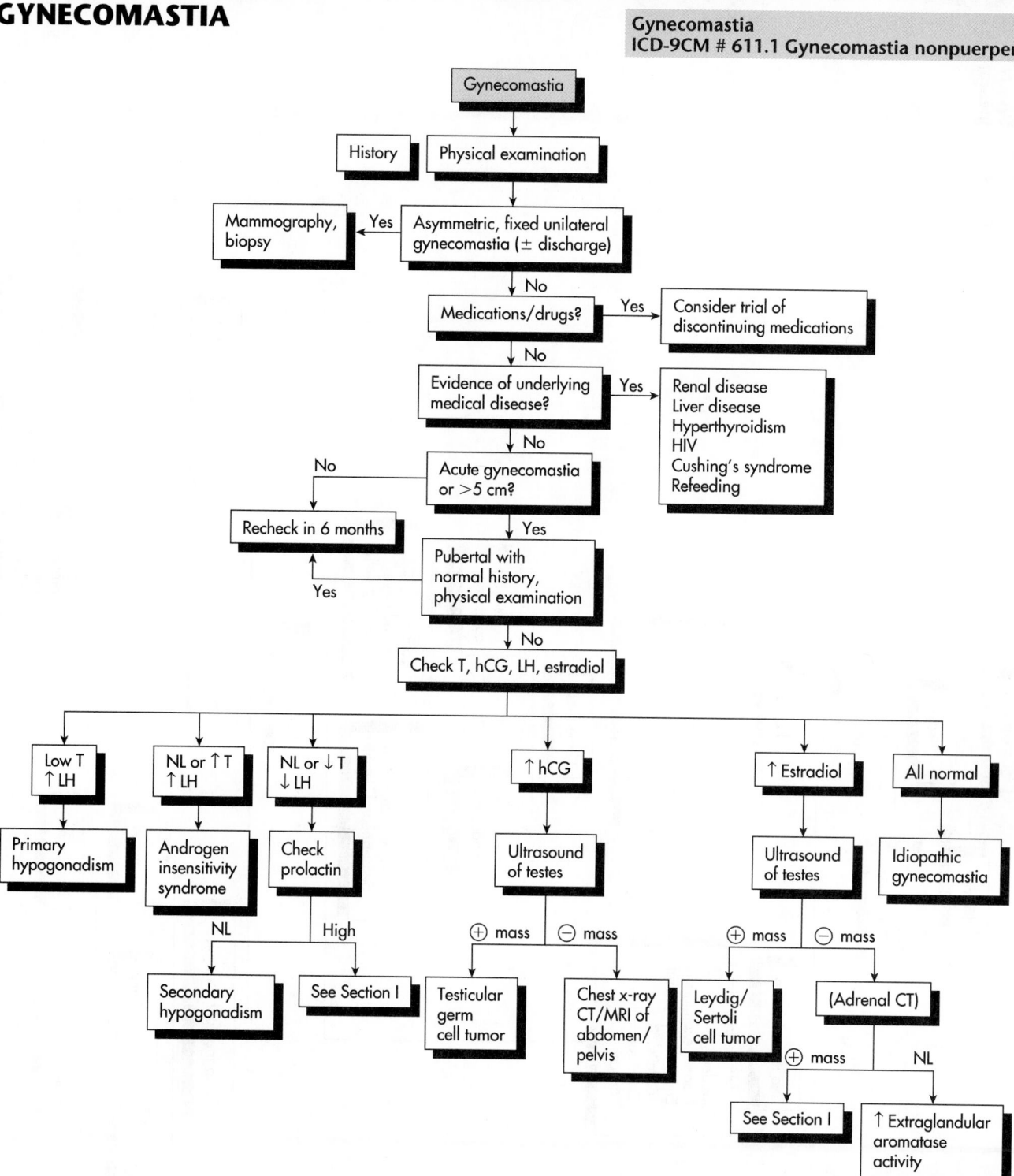

Fig. 3-81   Evaluation of gynecomastia. *CT,* Computed tomography; *hCG,* human chorionic gonadotropin; *HIV,* human immunodeficiency syndrome; *LH,* luteinizing hormone; *MRI,* magnetic resonance
imaging; *NL,* normal limits; *T,* testosterone. (From Noble J: *Primary care medicine,* ed 3, St Louis, 2001,
Mosby.)

III

HEARING LOSS

Hearing loss
ICD-9CM # 389.00 Conductive NOS
389.10 Sensorineural NOS

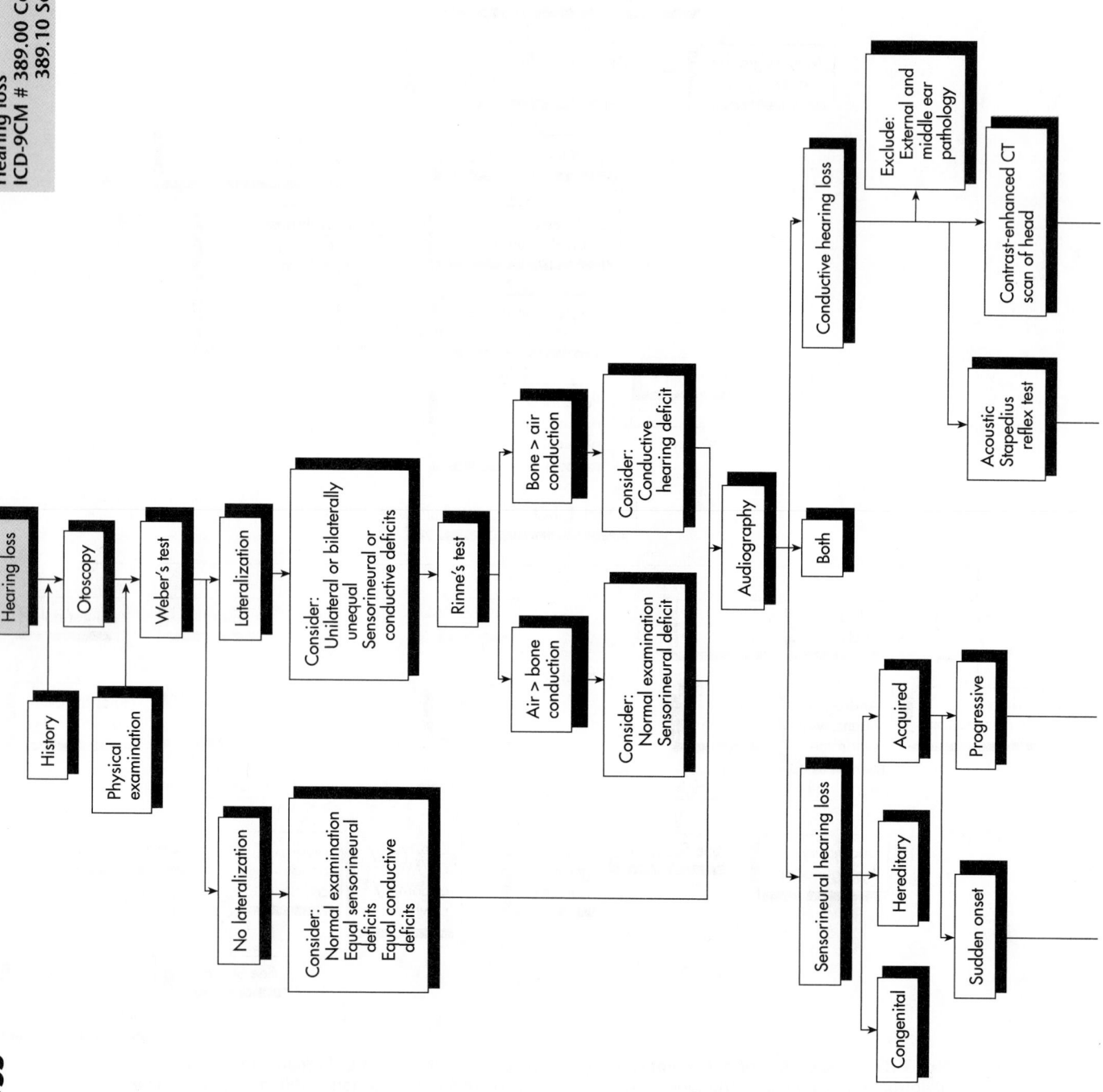

Hearing loss

History

Physical examination

Otoscopy

Weber's test

Lateralization

No lateralization

Consider:
Unilateral or bilaterally unequal
Sensorineural or conductive deficits

Consider:
Normal examination
Equal sensorineural deficits
Equal conductive deficits

Rinne's test

Bone > air conduction

Air > bone conduction

Consider:
Conductive hearing deficit

Consider:
Normal examination
Sensorineural deficit

Audiography

Both

Conductive hearing loss

Sensorineural hearing loss

Exclude:
External and middle ear pathology

Acoustic Stapedius reflex test

Contrast-enhanced CT scan of head

Congenital

Hereditary

Acquired

Sudden onset

Progressive

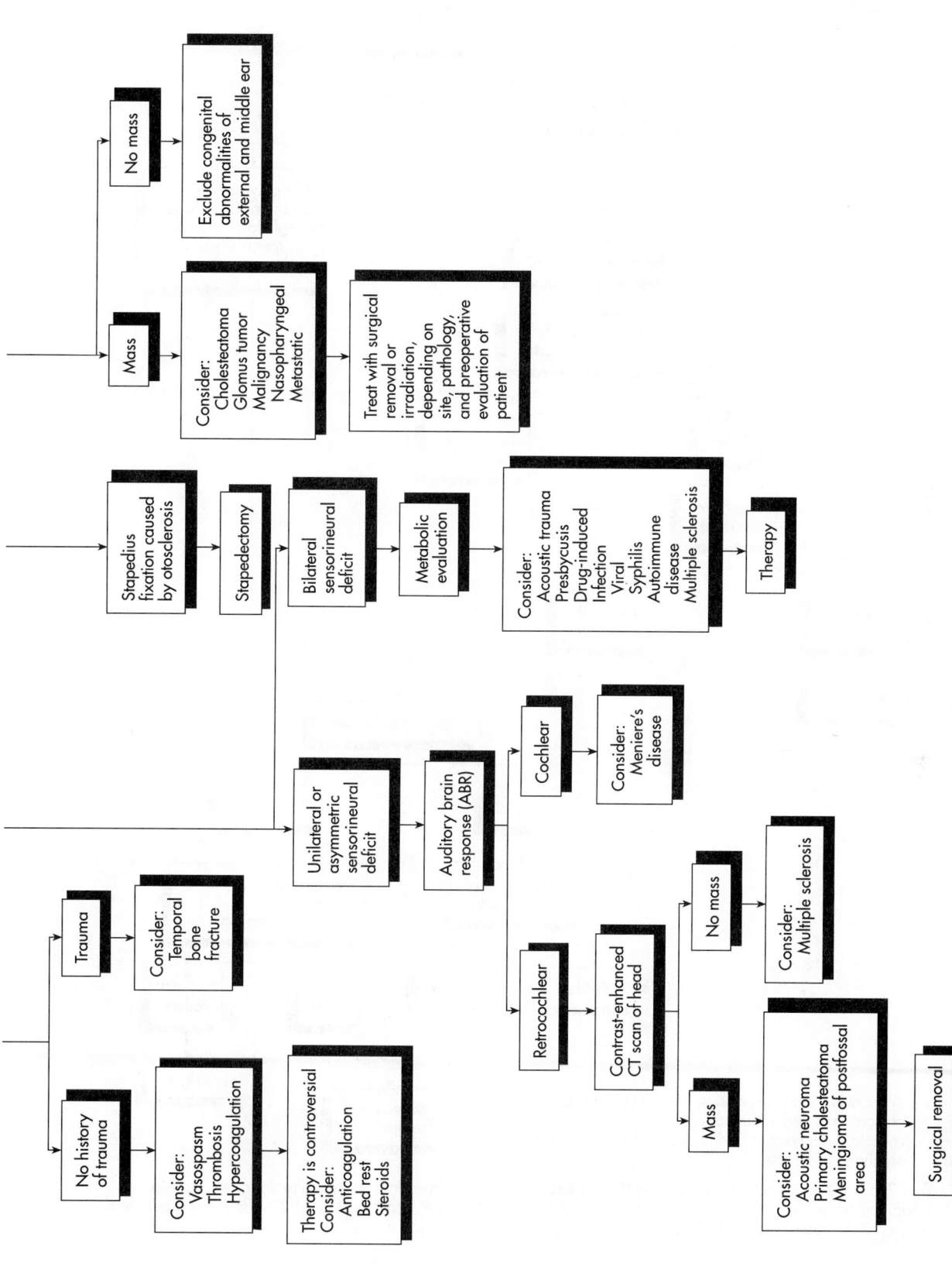

Fig. 3-82 **Evaluation of hearing loss.** *CT,* Computed tomography. (From Greene HL, Johnson WP, Lemcke D [eds]: *Decision making in medicine,* ed 2, St Louis, 1998, Mosby.)

HEARTBURN

Heartburn
ICD-9CM # 787.1

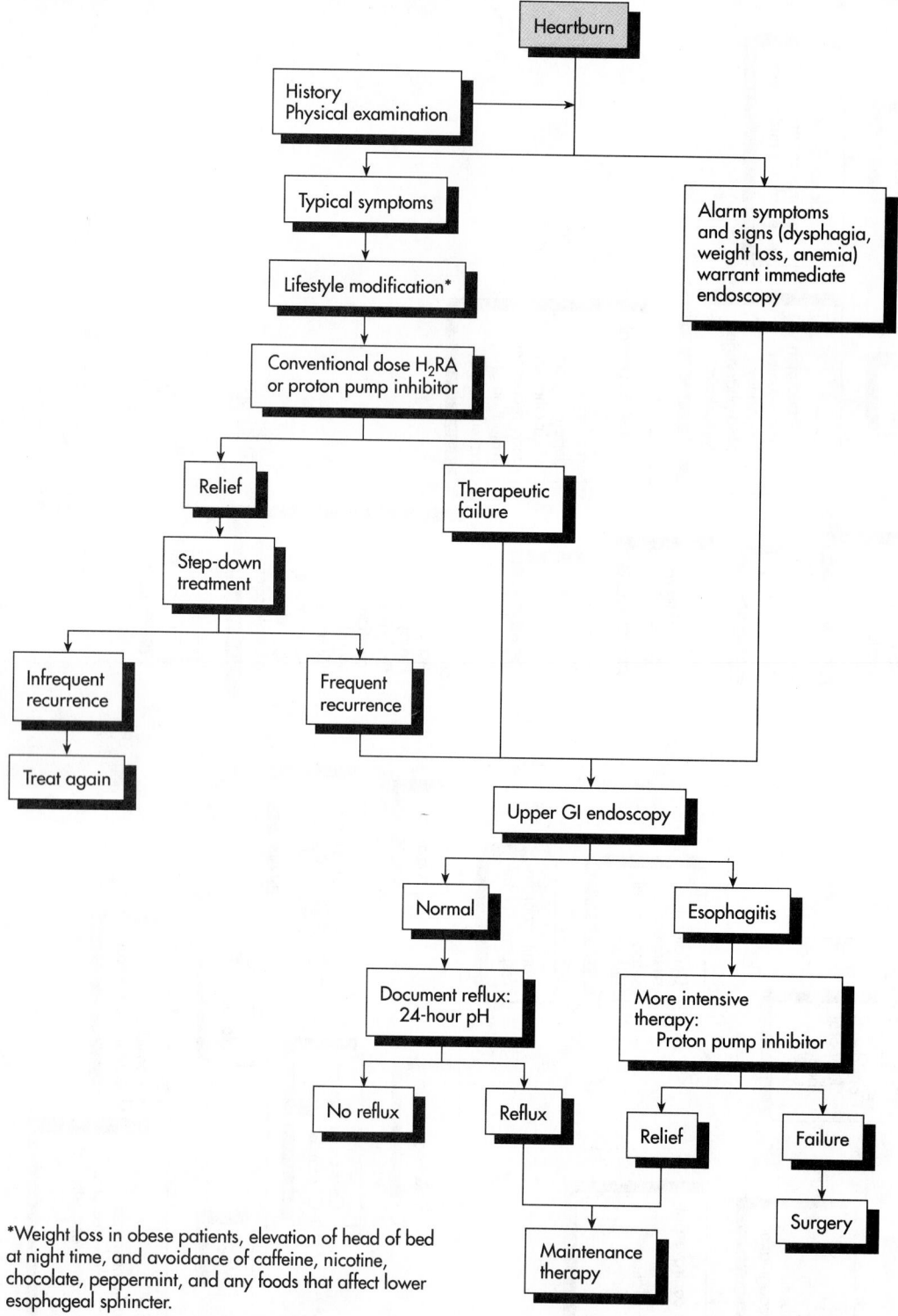

*Weight loss in obese patients, elevation of head of bed at night time, and avoidance of caffeine, nicotine, chocolate, peppermint, and any foods that affect lower esophageal sphincter.

Fig. 3-83   **Treatment of a patient with heartburn.** *GI,* Gastrointestinal; *H₂RA,* H₂ receptor antagonist. (Modified from Sampliner RE: Heartburn. In Greene HL, Johnson WP, Lemcke D [eds]: *Decision making in medicine,* ed 2, St Louis, 1998, Mosby.)

HEMATURIA, ASYMPTOMATIC

Hematuria, asymptomatic
ICD-9CM # 599.7

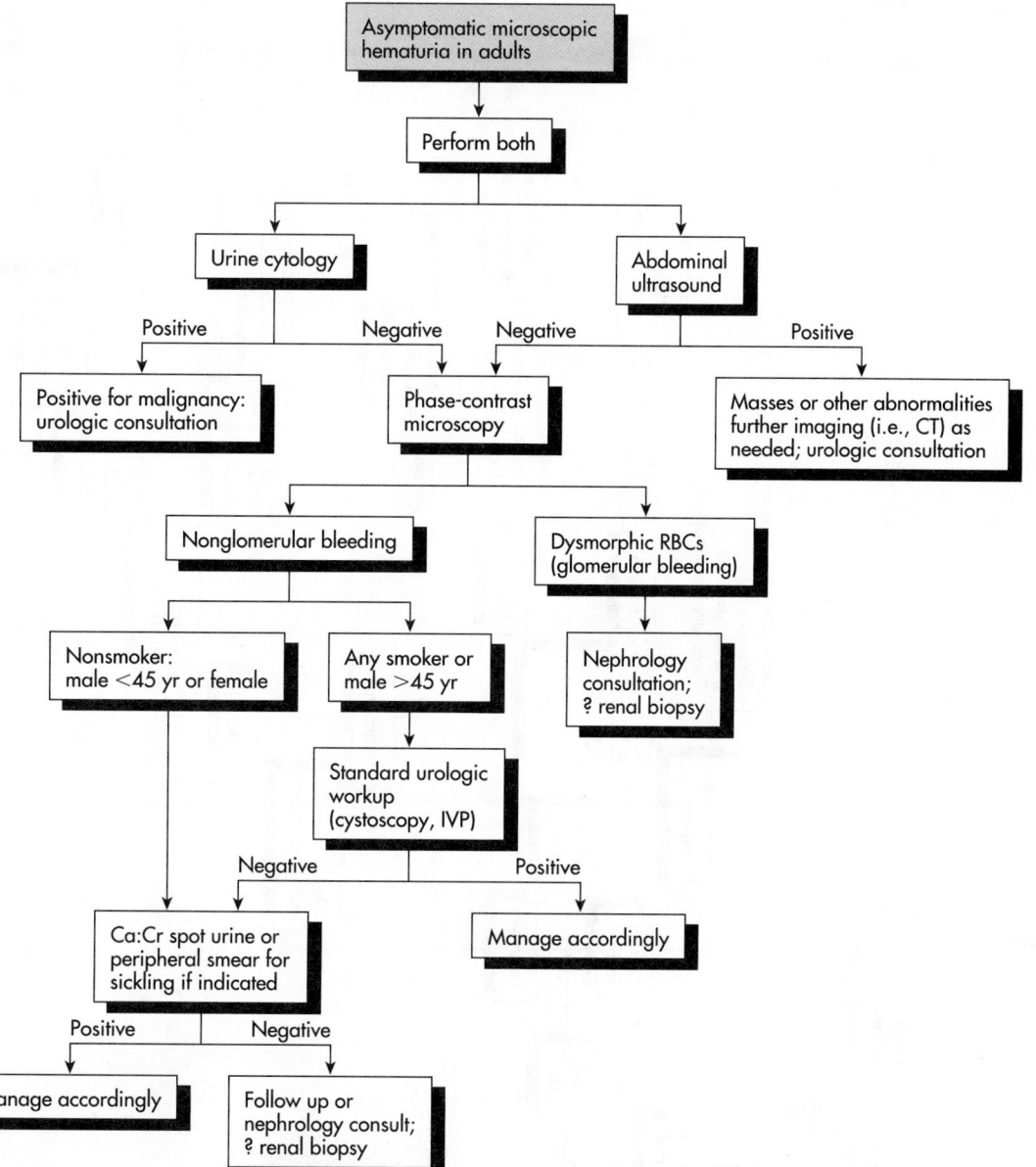

Fig. 3-84   Suggested algorithm for the evaluation of adult asymptomatic microscopic hematuria.
These patients must have no symptoms referable to the hematuria and a negative urinalysis except for red blood cells (RBCs). Adults with gross hematuria require a full urologic evaluation. *Ca:Cr,* Calcium:creatinine ratio; *IVP,* intravenous pyelogram. (From Nseyo UO [ed]: *Urology for primary care physicians,* Philadelphia, 1999, WB Saunders.)

HEMOPTYSIS

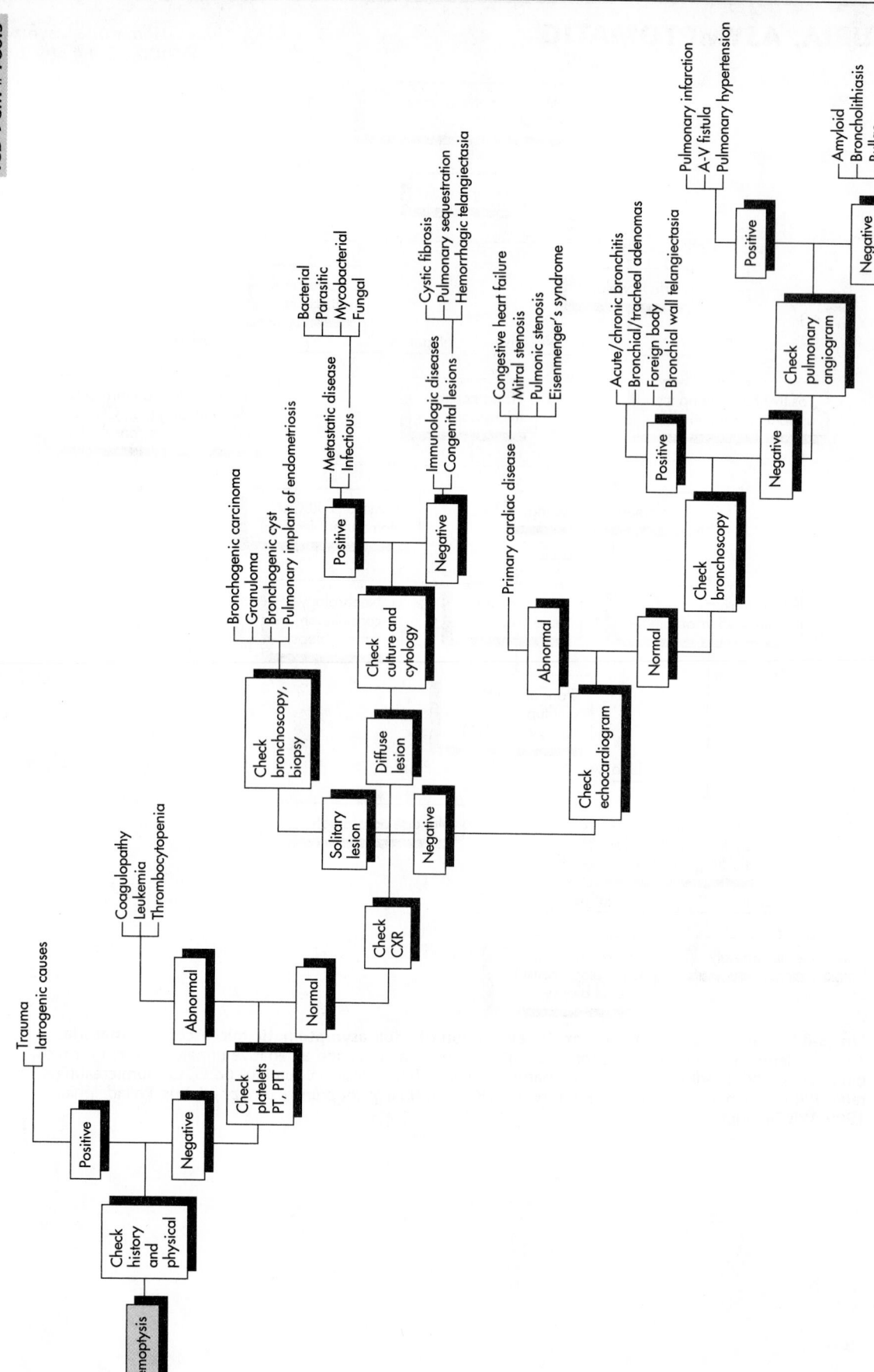

Fig. 3-85 **Evaluation of hemoptysis.** *A-V,* Arteriovenous; *CXR,* chest x-ray; *PT,* prothrombin time; *PTT,* partial thromboplastin time. (From Healey PM: *Common medical diagnosis: an algorithmic approach,* ed 3, Philadelphia, 2000, WB Saunders.)

HEPATITIS, VIRAL

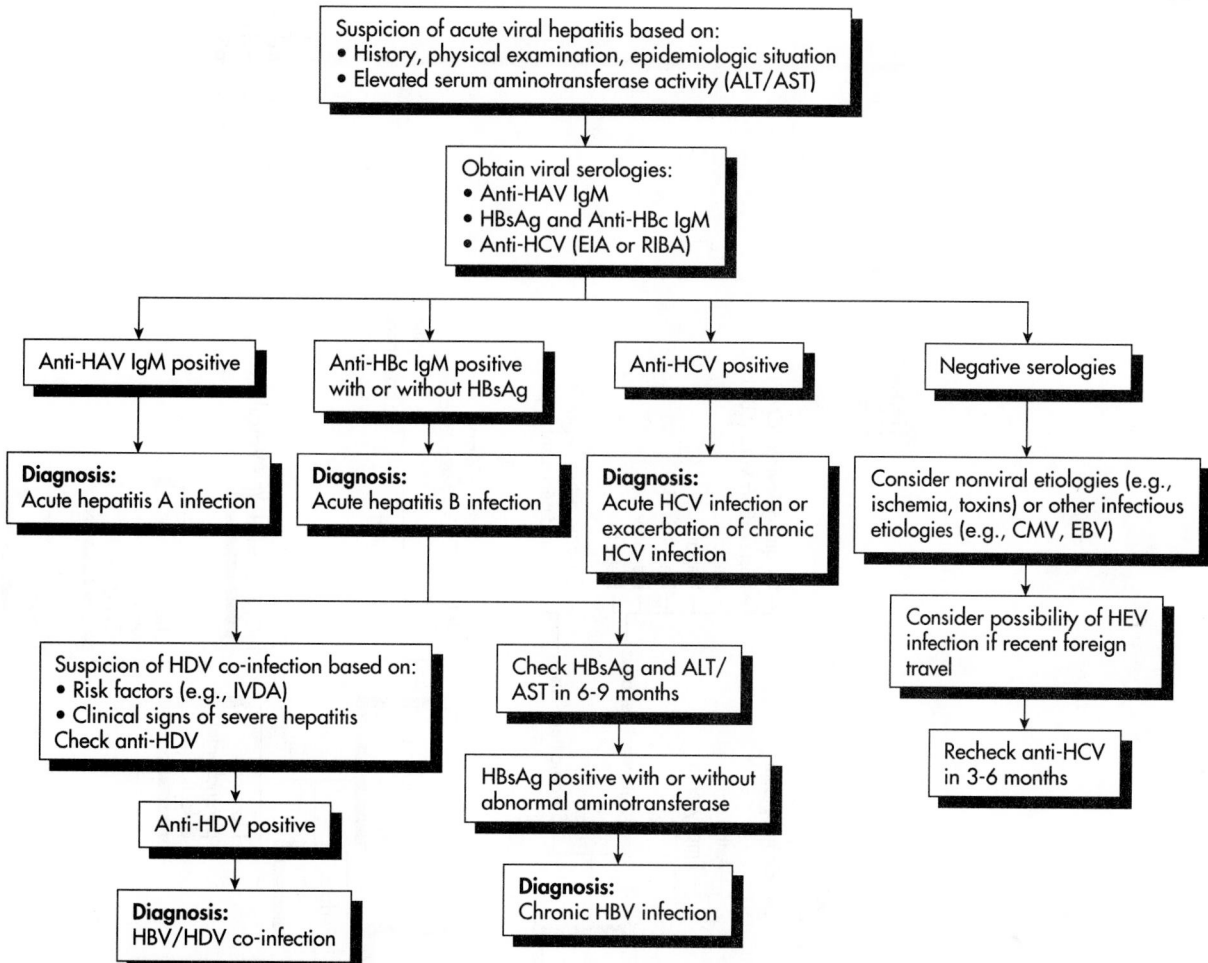

Fig. 3-86 A flow diagram showing the use of specific serologic tests for the diagnosis of acute viral hepatitis in relation to the clinical and epidemiologic setting. Co-infections and superinfections of chronic hepatitis B or C patients should always be considered in cases that do not fit well with the clinical or serologic picture. *CMV*, Cytomegalovirus; *EBV*, Epstein-Barr virus; *EIA*, enzyme immunoassay; *HBV*, hepatitis B virus; *HCV*, hepatitis C virus; *HDV*, hepatitis D virus; *HEV*, hepato-encephalomyelitis virus; *IVDA*, intravenous drug abuse; *RIBA*, recombinant immunoblot assay. (From Mandell GL: *Mandell, Douglas, and Bennett's principles and practice of infectious diseases*, ed 5, New York, 2000, Churchill Livingstone.)

III

HEPATOMEGALY

Hepatomegaly
ICD-9CM # 789.1

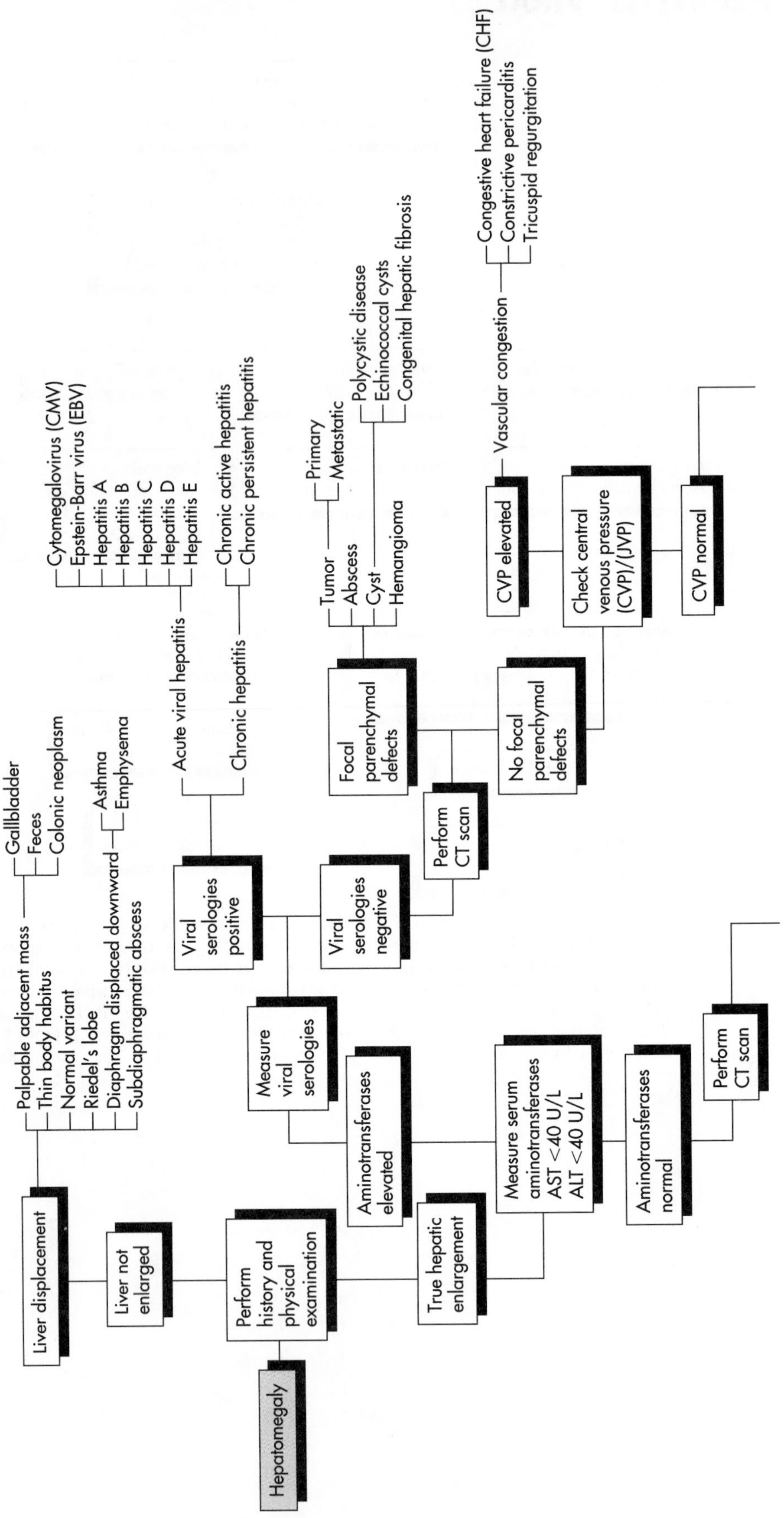

Hepatomegaly

→ Perform history and physical examination

→ Liver displacement
  - Palpable adjacent mass
    - Gallbladder
    - Feces
    - Colonic neoplasm
  - Thin body habitus
  - Normal variant
  - Riedel's lobe
  - Diaphragm displaced downward
    - Asthma
    - Emphysema
  - Subdiaphragmatic abscess

→ Liver not enlarged

→ True hepatic enlargement
  → Measure serum aminotransferases AST <40 U/L ALT <40 U/L
    → Aminotransferases elevated
      → Measure viral serologies
        → Viral serologies positive
          → Acute viral hepatitis
            - Cytomegalovirus (CMV)
            - Epstein-Barr virus (EBV)
            - Hepatitis A
            - Hepatitis B
            - Hepatitis C
            - Hepatitis D
            - Hepatitis E
          → Chronic hepatitis
            - Chronic active hepatitis
            - Chronic persistent hepatitis
        → Viral serologies negative
          → Perform CT scan
            → Focal parenchymal defects
              - Tumor
                - Primary
                - Metastatic
              - Abscess
              - Cyst
                - Polycystic disease
                - Echinococcal cysts
                - Congenital hepatic fibrosis
              - Hemangioma
            → No focal parenchymal defects
              → Check central venous pressure (CVP)/(JVP)
                → CVP elevated
                  - Vascular congestion
                    - Congestive heart failure (CHF)
                    - Constrictive pericarditis
                    - Tricuspid regurgitation
                → CVP normal
    → Aminotransferases normal
      → Perform CT scan

HEPATOMEGALY—cont'd

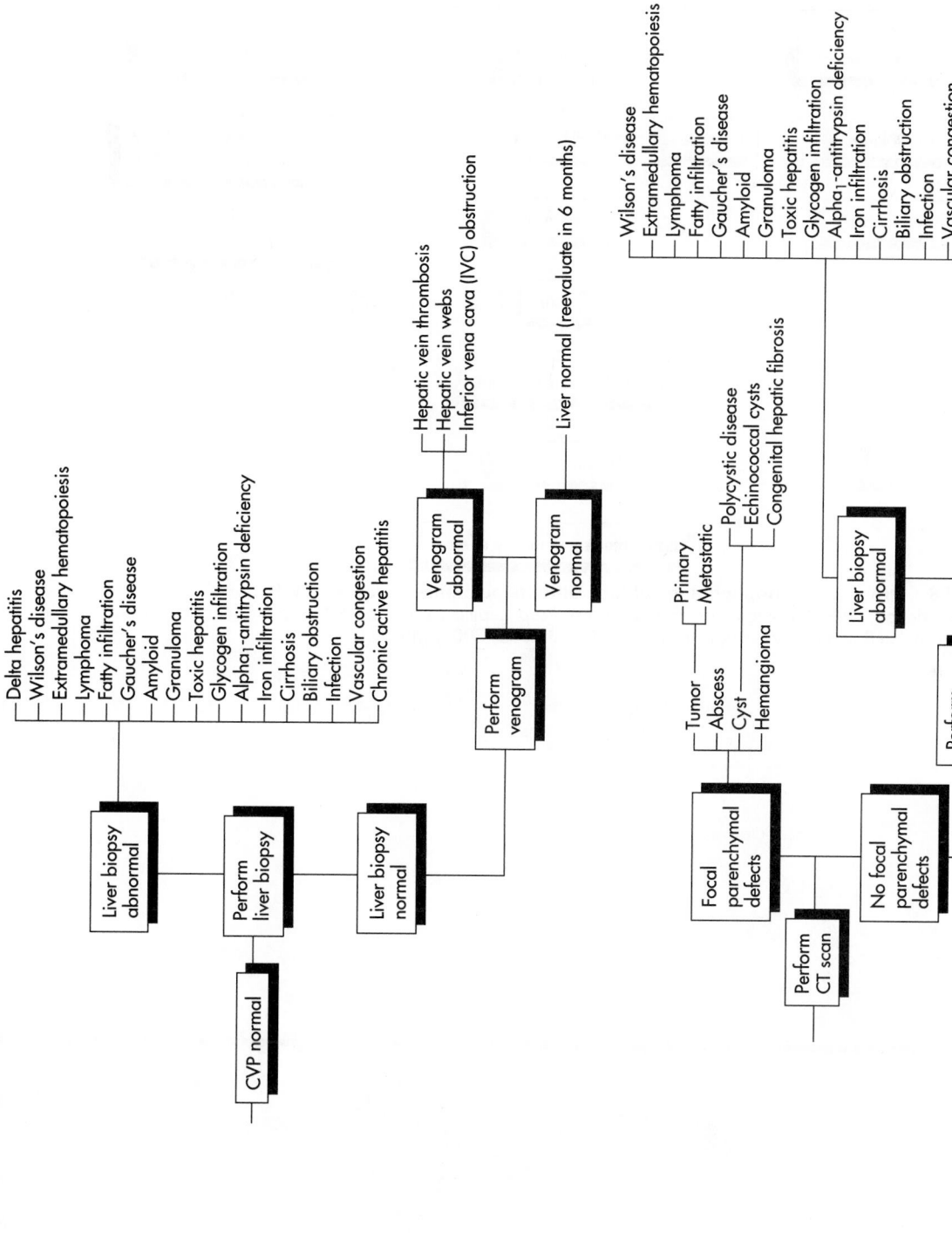

Fig. 3-87 Hepatomegaly. *ALT,* Alanine aminotransferase; *AST,* aspartate aminotransferase; *CT,* computed tomography; *JVP,* jugular venous pressure. (From Healey PM: *Common medical diagnosis: an algorithmic approach,* ed 3, Philadelphia, 2000, WB Saunders.)

HIGH-ALTITUDE PULMONARY EDEMA

High-altitude pulmonary edema
ICD-9CM # 289   Mountain sickness, acute
993.2 High altitude, effects

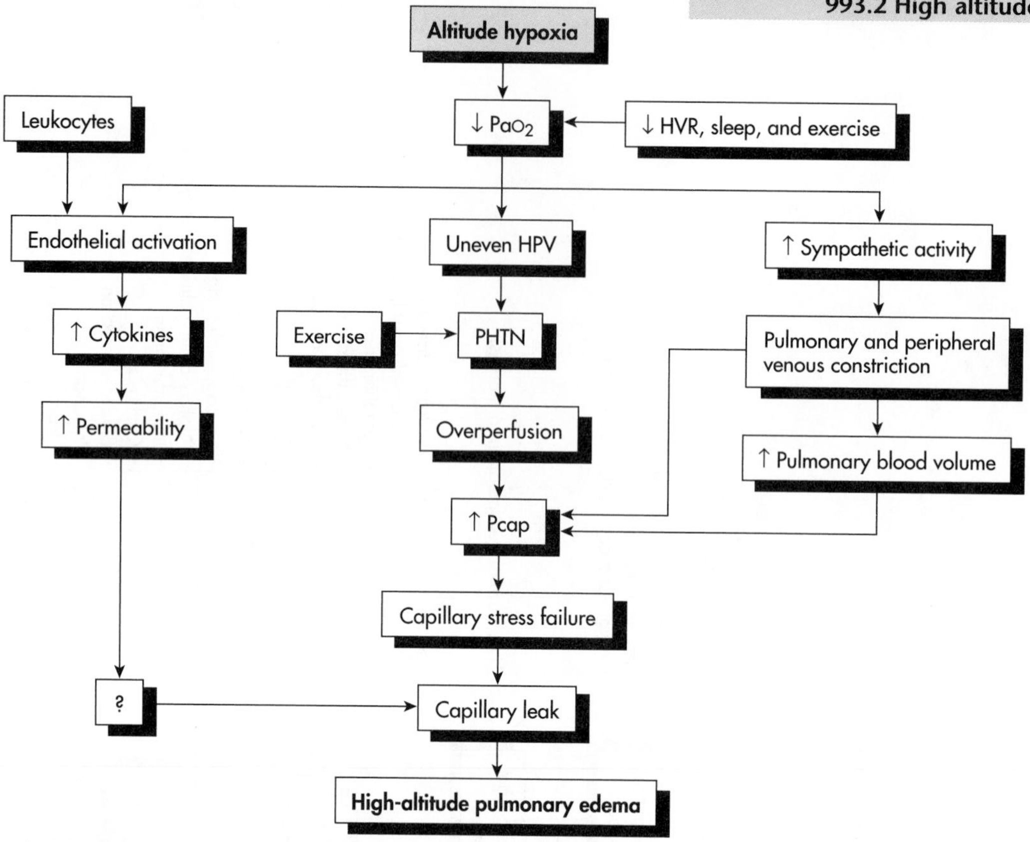

Fig. 3-88   Proposed pathophysiology of high-altitude pulmonary edema. *HPV,* Hypoxic pulmonary vasoconstriction; *HVR,* hypoxic ventilatory response; *Pcap,* capillary pressure; *PHTN,* pulmonary hypertension. (From Auerbach PS: *Wilderness medicine,* ed 4, St Louis, 2001, Mosby.)

HIRSUTISM

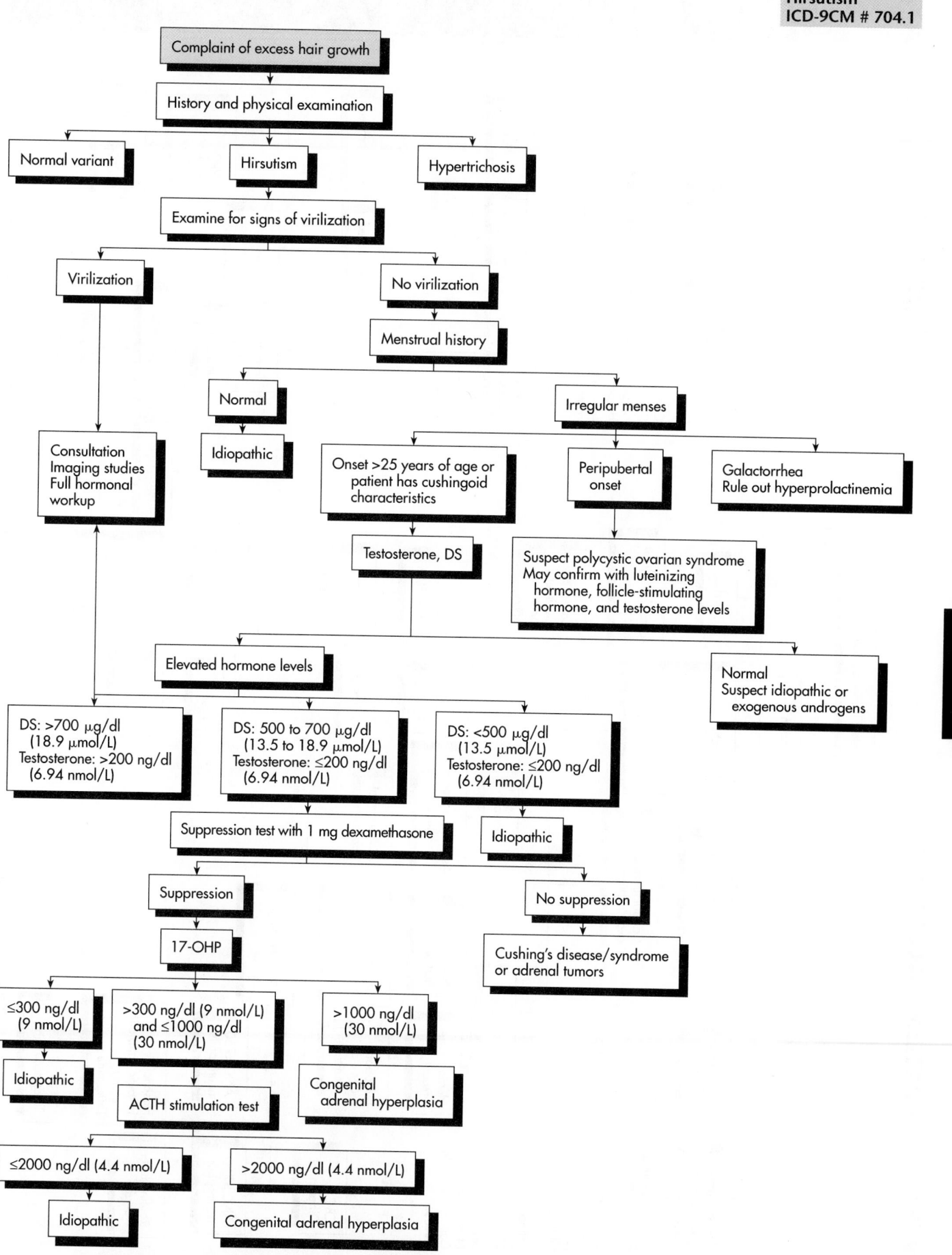

Fig. 3-89 Algorithm showing the evaluation and treatment of hirsutism. *ACTH*, Adrenocorticotropic hormone; *DS*, dehydroepiandrosterone; *17-OHP*, 17-hydroxyprogesterone. (From Gilchrist VJ, Hecht BR: *Am Fam Physician* 52:1837, 1995.)

HIV-INFECTED PATIENT, ACUTELY ILL

HIV-infected patient, acutely ill
ICD-9CM # 042 HIV infection, symptomatic

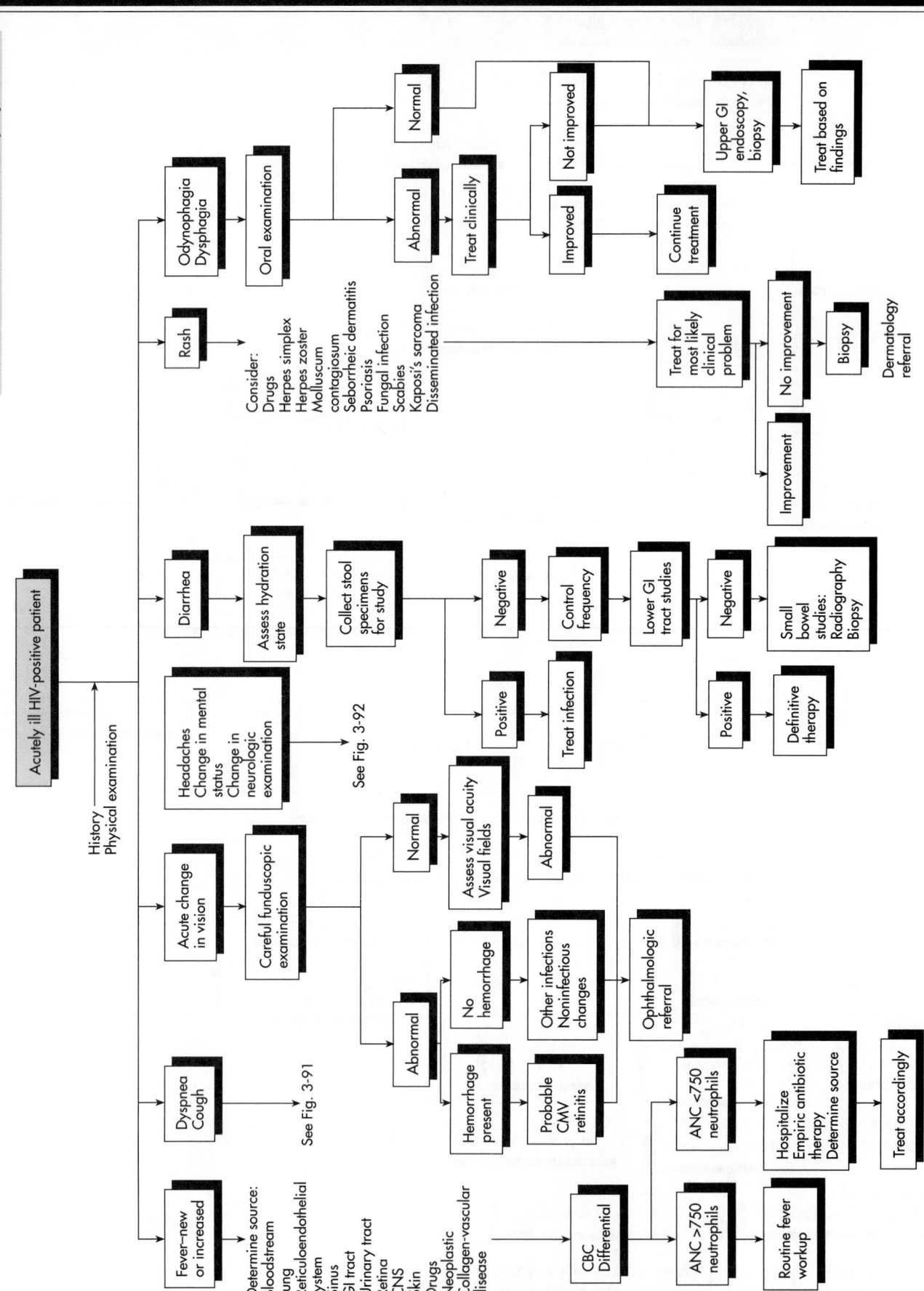

Fig. 3-90   Acutely ill HIV-positive patient. *ANC*, Absolute neutrophil count; *CBC*, complete blood count; *CMV*, cytomegalovirus; *CNS*, central nervous system; *GI*, gastrointestinal. (From Greene HL, Johnson WP, Lemcke D [eds]: *Decision making in medicine*, ed 2, St Louis, 1998, Mosby.)

HIV-INFECTED PATIENT WITH RESPIRATORY COMPLAINTS

HIV-infected patient with respiratory complaints
ICD-9CM # 042 HIV infection, symptomatic

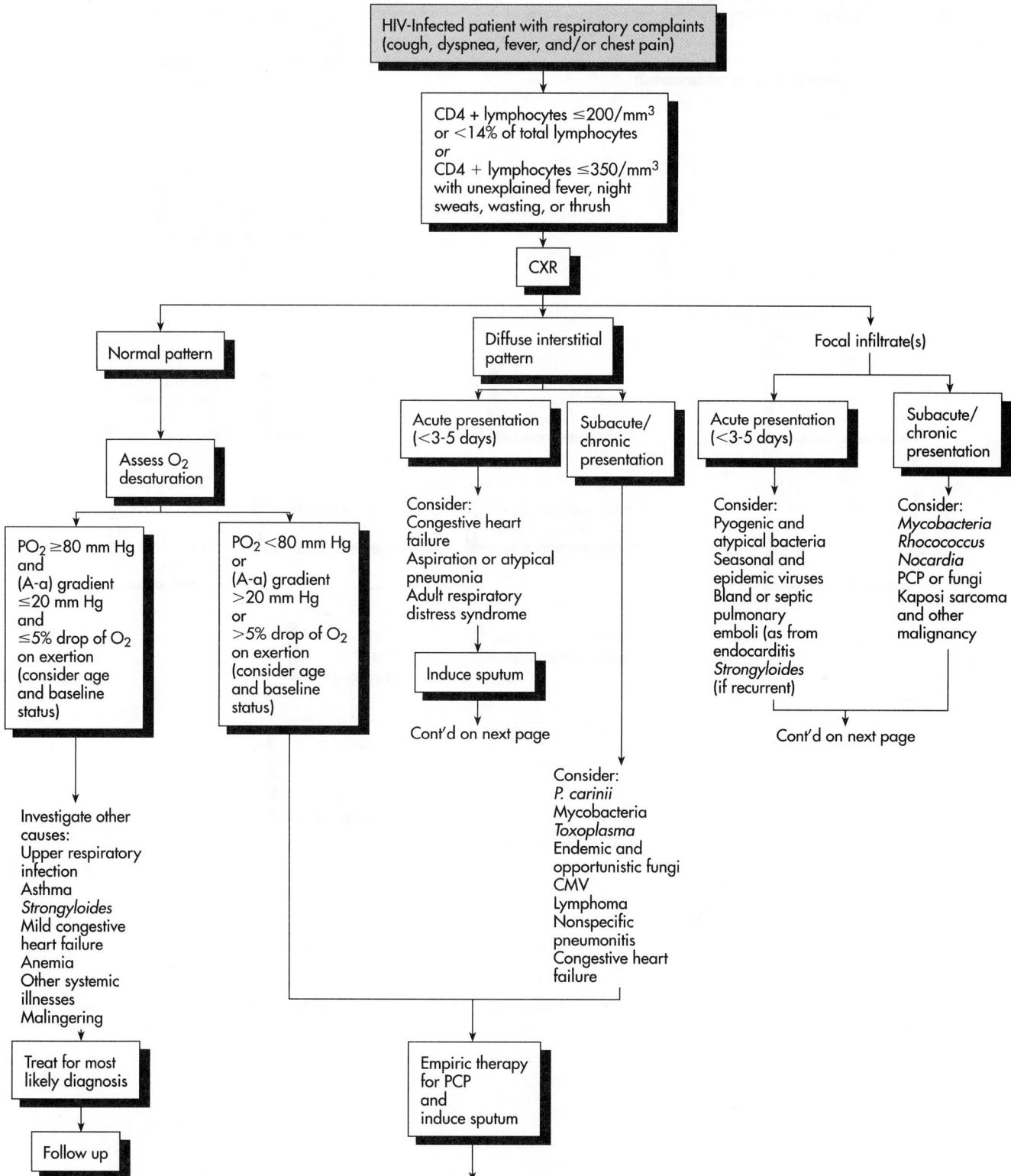

Fig. 3-91   HIV-infected patient with respiratory complaints. *BAL,* Bronchoalveolar lavage; *CMV,* cytomegalovirus; *CXR,* chest x-ray examination; *PCP, Pneumocystis carinii* pneumonia; *TBB,* transbronchial biopsy. (From Greene HL, Johnson WP, Lemcke D [eds]: *Decision making in medicine,* 2, St Louis, 1998, Mosby.)

HIV-INFECTED PATIENT WITH
RESPIRATORY COMPLAINTS—cont'd

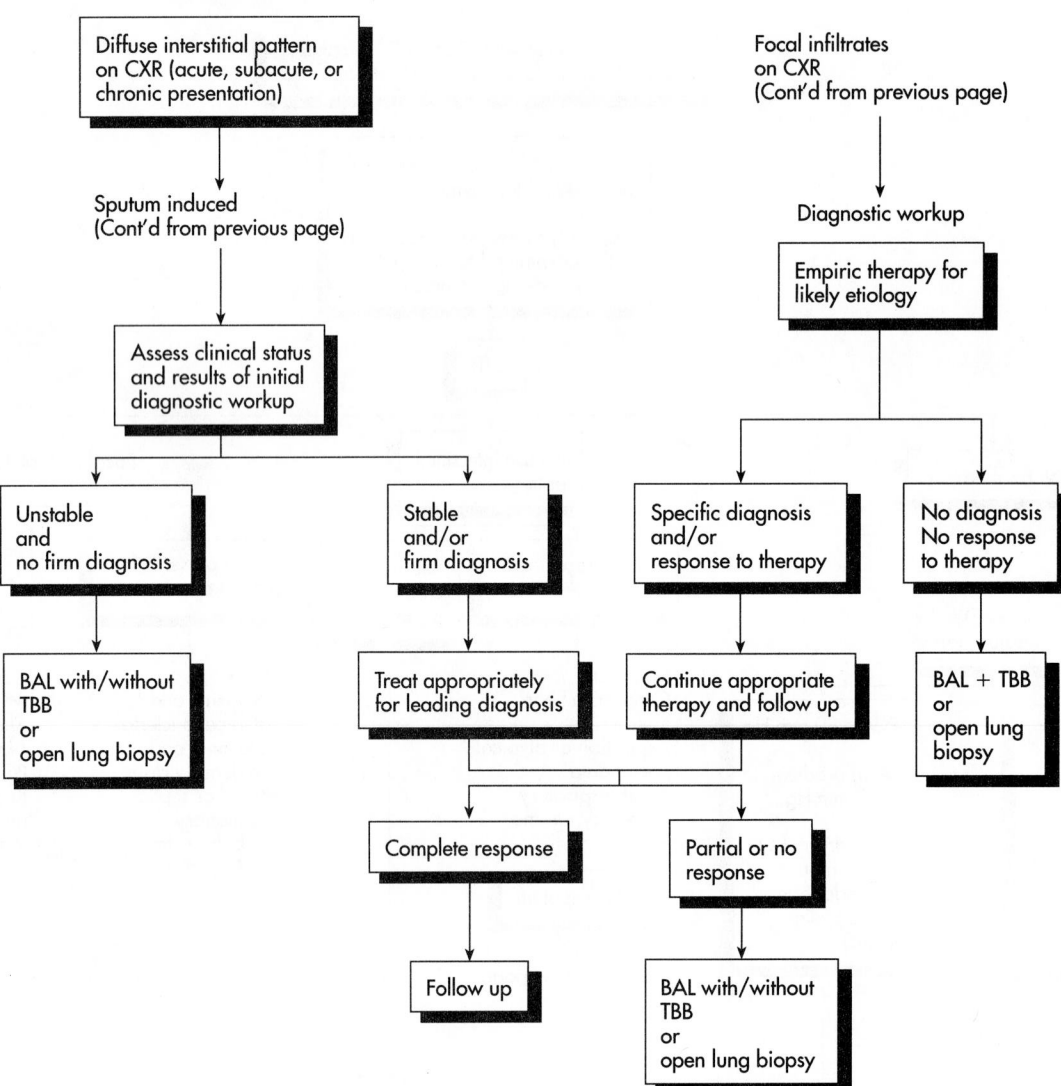

Fig. 3-91, cont'd

HIV-INFECTED PATIENT WITH SUSPECTED CENTRAL NERVOUS SYSTEM INFECTION

HIV-infected patient with suspected CNS infection
ICD-9CM # 042 HIV infection, symptomatic

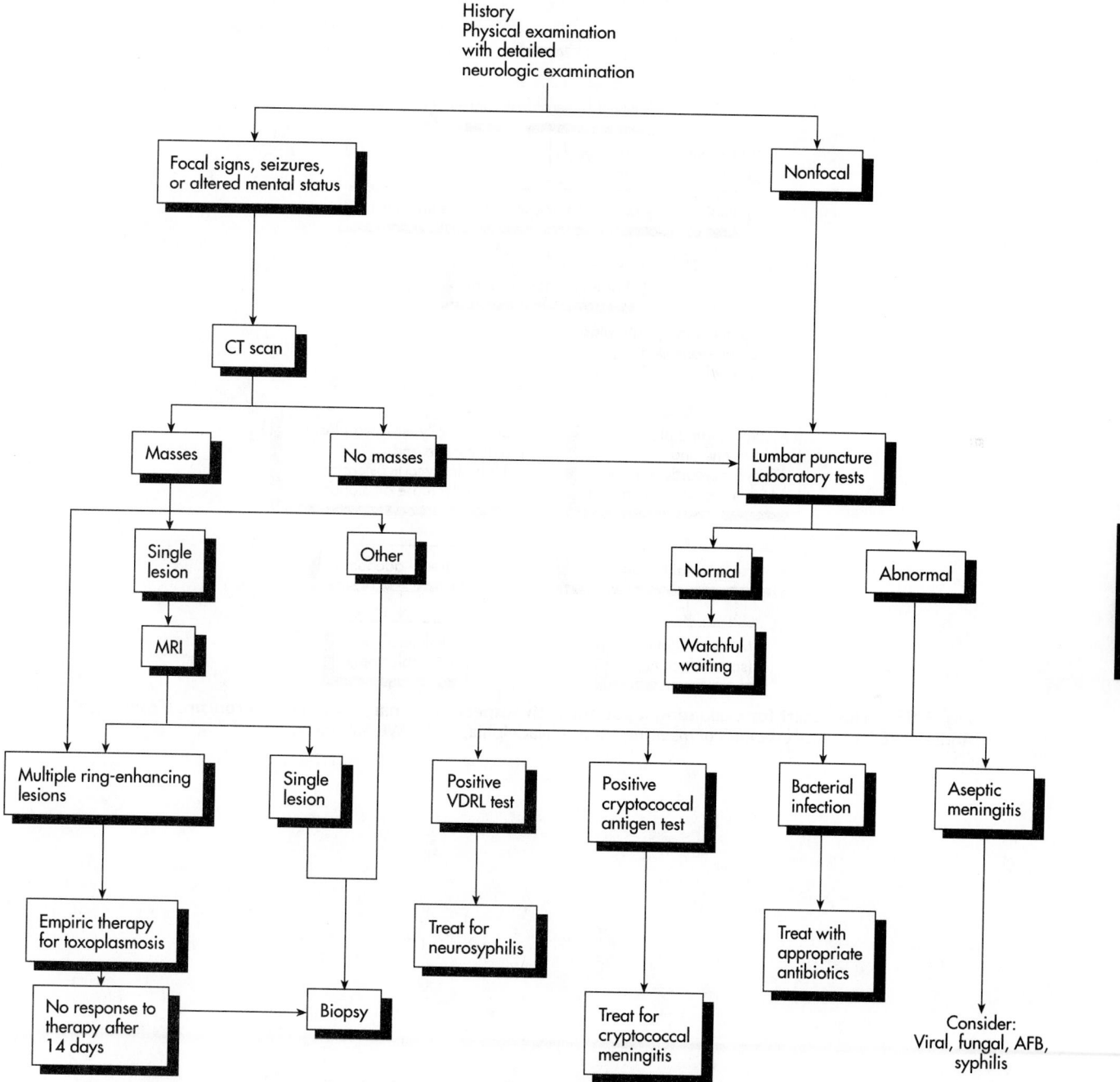

Fig. 3-92 HIV-positive patient with suspected central nervous system infection. *AFB,* Acid-fast bacilli; *CNS,* central nervous system; *CT,* computed tomography; *MRI,* magnetic resonance imaging; *VDRL,* Venereal Disease Research Laboratory. (From Greene HL, Johnson WP, Lemcke D [eds]: *Decision making in medicine,* ed 2, St Louis, 1998, Mosby.)

HYPERALDOSTERONISM

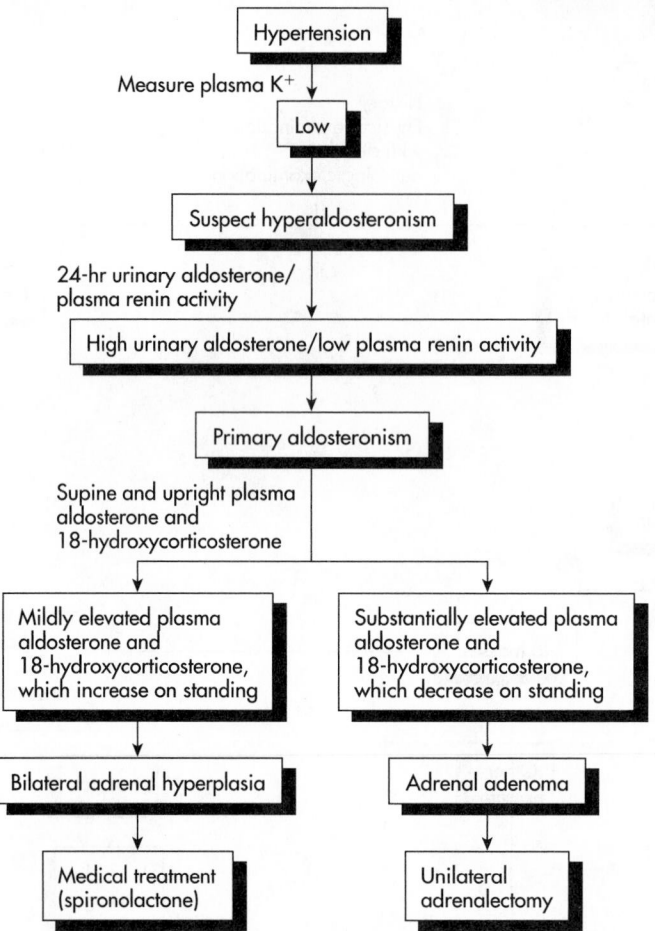

Fig. 3-93   Flow chart for evaluating a patient with suspected primary hyperaldosteronism. (From Andreoli TE [ed]: *Cecil essentials of medicine,* ed 5, Philadelphia, 2001, WB Saunders.)

HYPERCALCEMIA

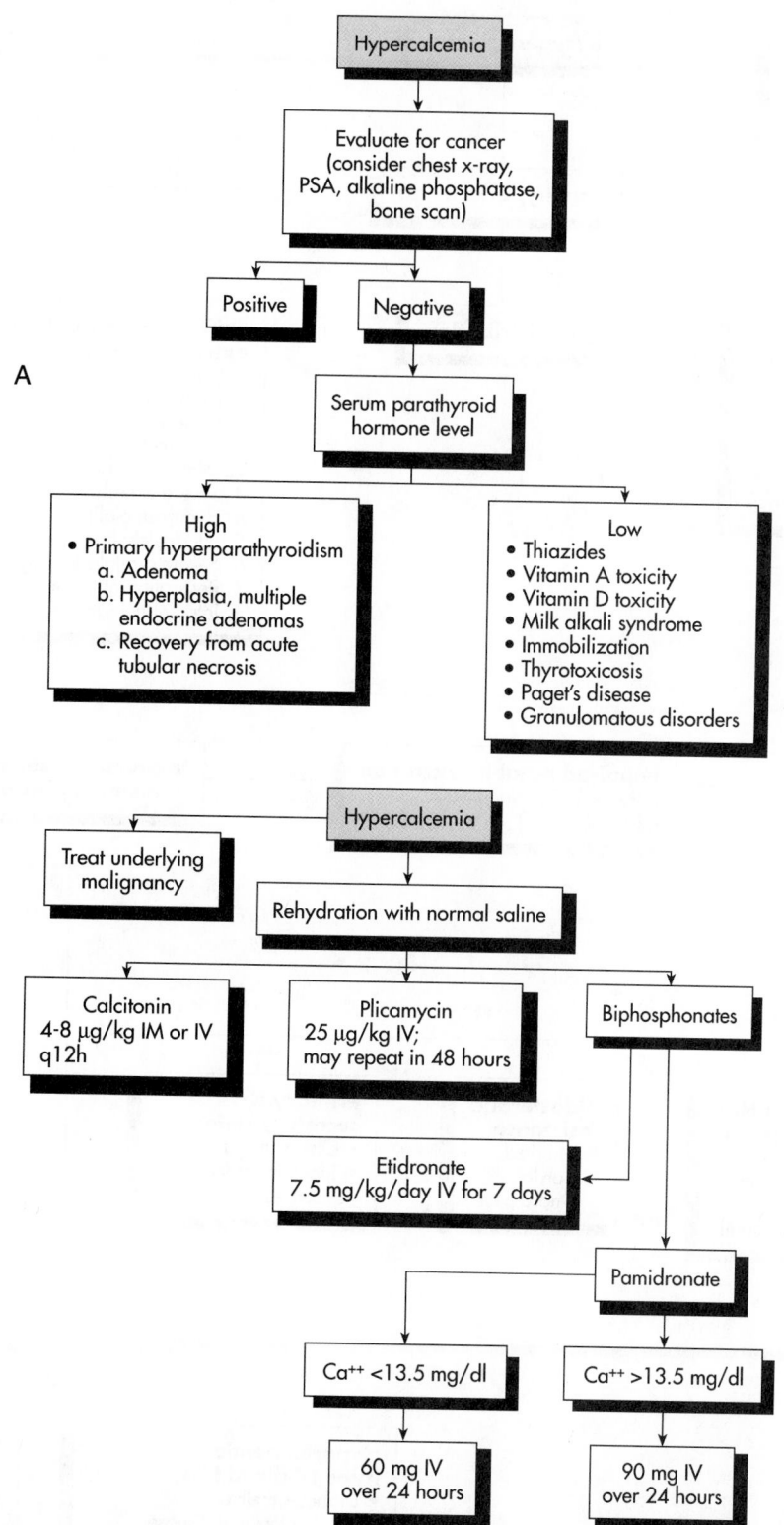

Fig. 3-94   A, Evaluation of hypercalcemia. *PSA,* Prostate-specific antigen. **B, Therapy for hypercalcemia.** *IM,* Intramuscularly; *IV,* intravenously. (From Noble J [ed]: *Primary care medicine,* ed 3, St Louis, 2001, Mosby.) (From Wachtel TJ, Stein MD: *Practical guide to the care of the ambulatory patient,* ed 2, St Louis, 2000, Mosby.)

III

HYPERKALEMIA, DIAGNOSTIC APPROACH

Hyperkalemia
ICD-9CM # 276.7

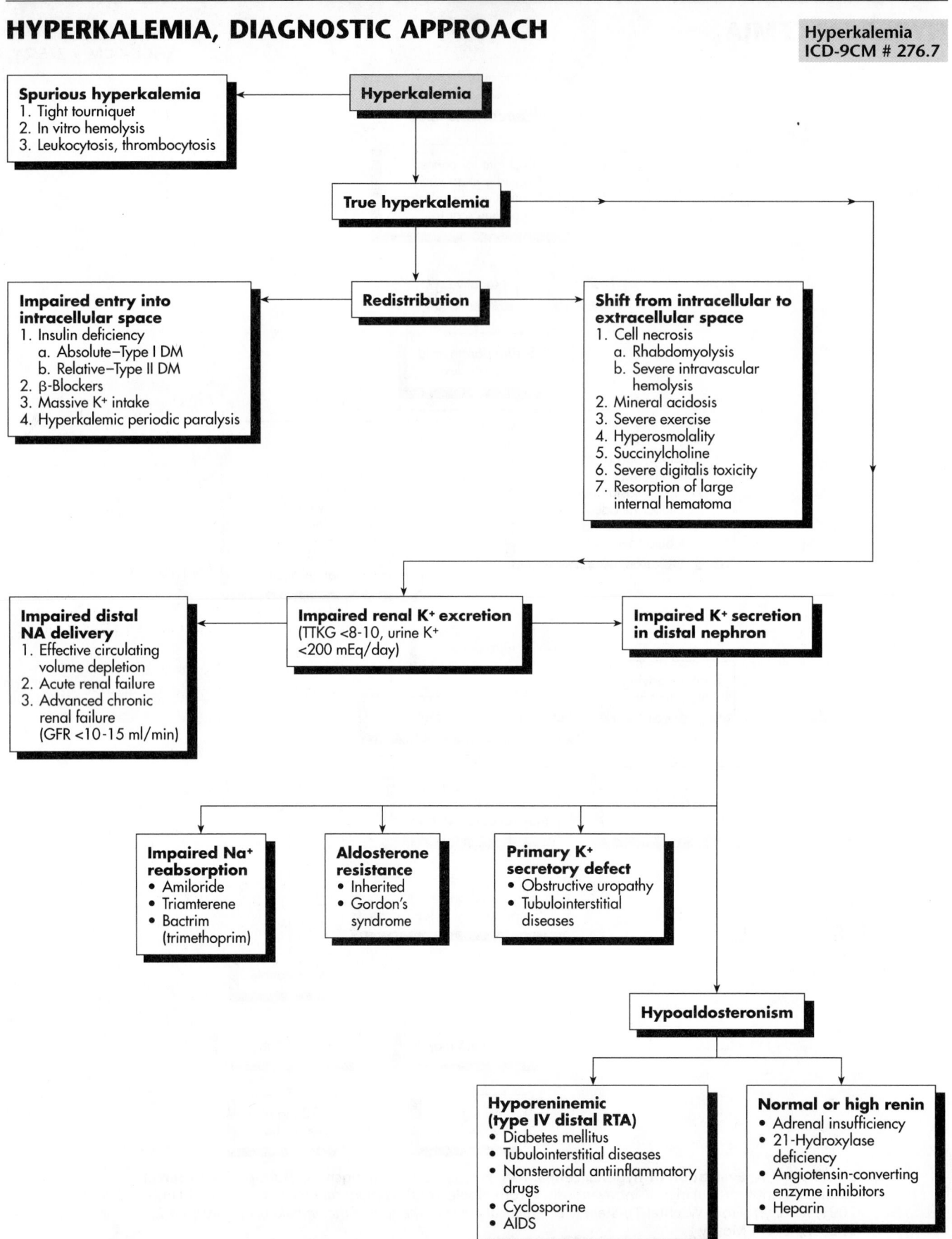

Fig. 3-95 Diagnostic approach to hyperkalemia. *AIDS,* Acquired immunodeficiency syndrome; *DM,* diabetes mellitus; *GFR,* glomerular filtration rate; *RTA,* renal tubular acidosis; *TTKG,* transtubular potassium gradient. (From Andreoli TE [ed]: *Cecil essentials of medicine,* ed 4, Philadelphia, 1997, WB Saunders.)

HYPERKALEMIA, EVALUATION AND TREATMENT

Hyperkalemia, evaluation and treatment
ICD-9CM # 276.7

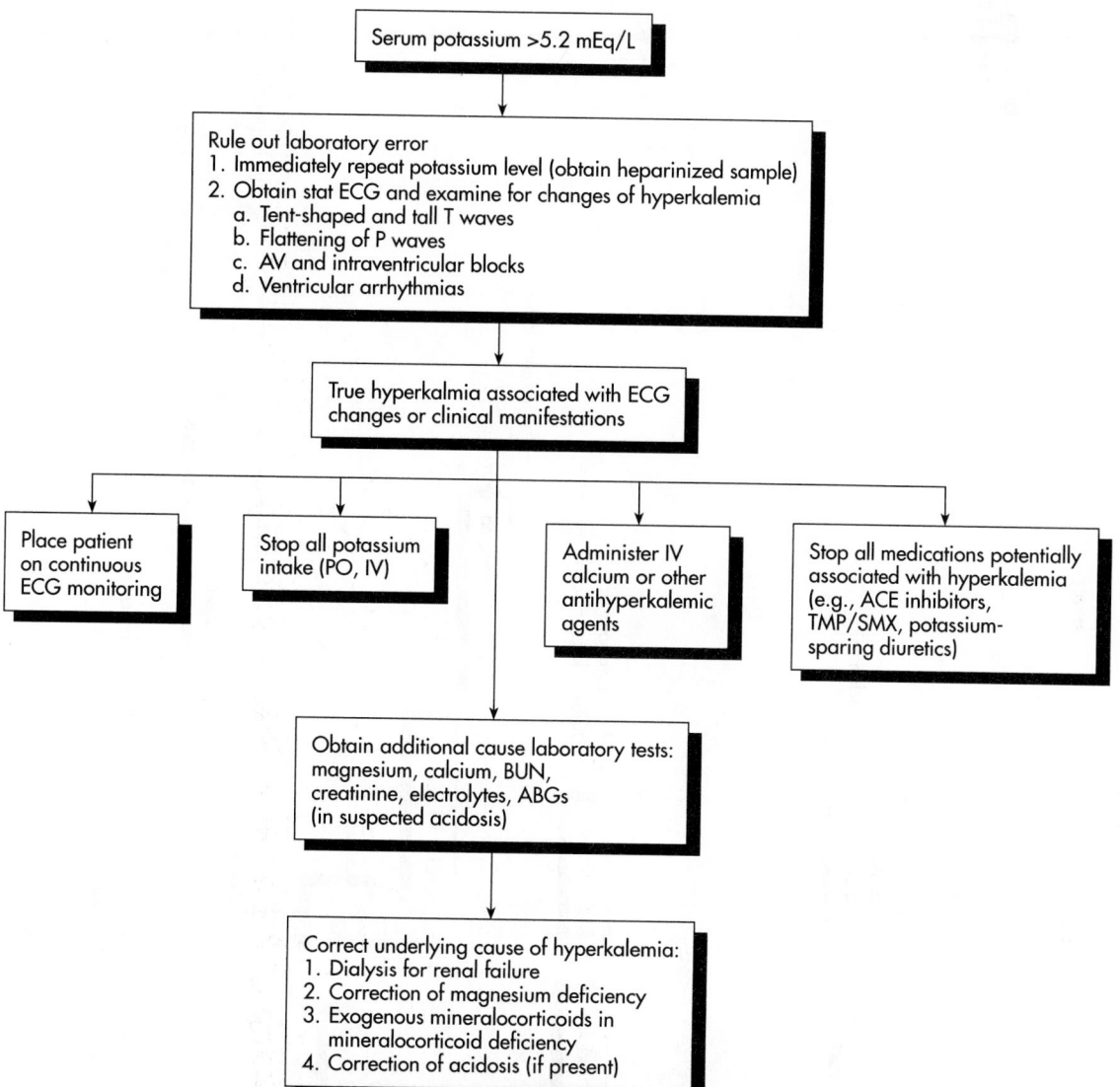

Fig. 3-96   Evaluation and treatment of hyperkalemia. *ABGs,* Arterial blood gases; *ACE,* angiotensin-converting enzyme; *AV,* atrioventricular; *BUN,* blood urea nitrogen; *ECG,* electrocardiogram; *IV,* intravenous; *PO,* oral; *TMP/SMX,* trimethoprim-sulfamethoxazole. (From Ferri F: *Practical guide to the care of the medical patient,* ed 6, St Louis, 2004, Mosby.)

HYPERMAGNESEMIA

Hypermagnesemia
ICD-9CM # 275.2

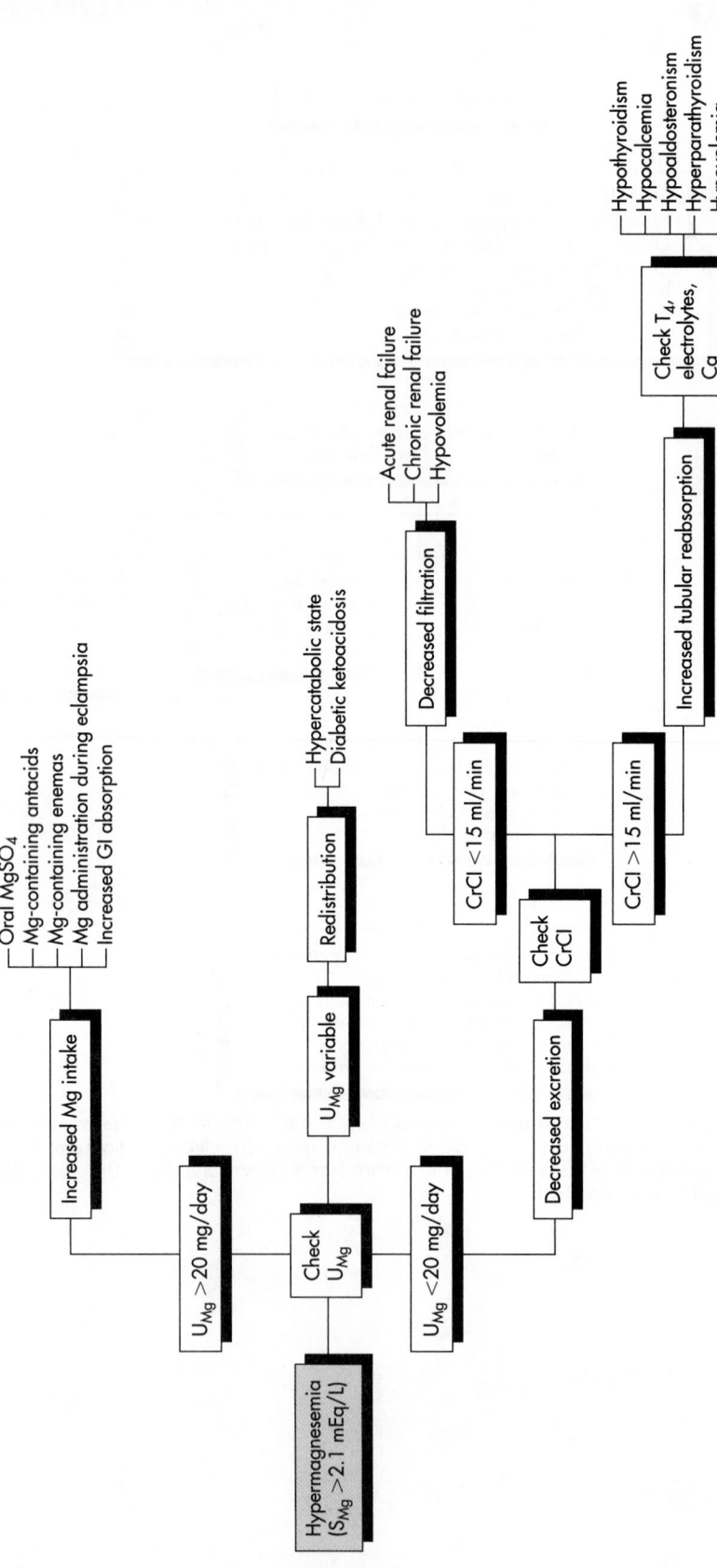

Fig. 3-97 Hypermagnesemia. *CrCl,* Creatinine clearance; *GI,* gastrointestinal; *MgSO₄,* magnesium sulfate. (From Healey PM: *Common medical diagnosis: an algorithmic approach,* ed 3, Philadelphia, 2000, WB Saunders.)

HYPERNATREMIA

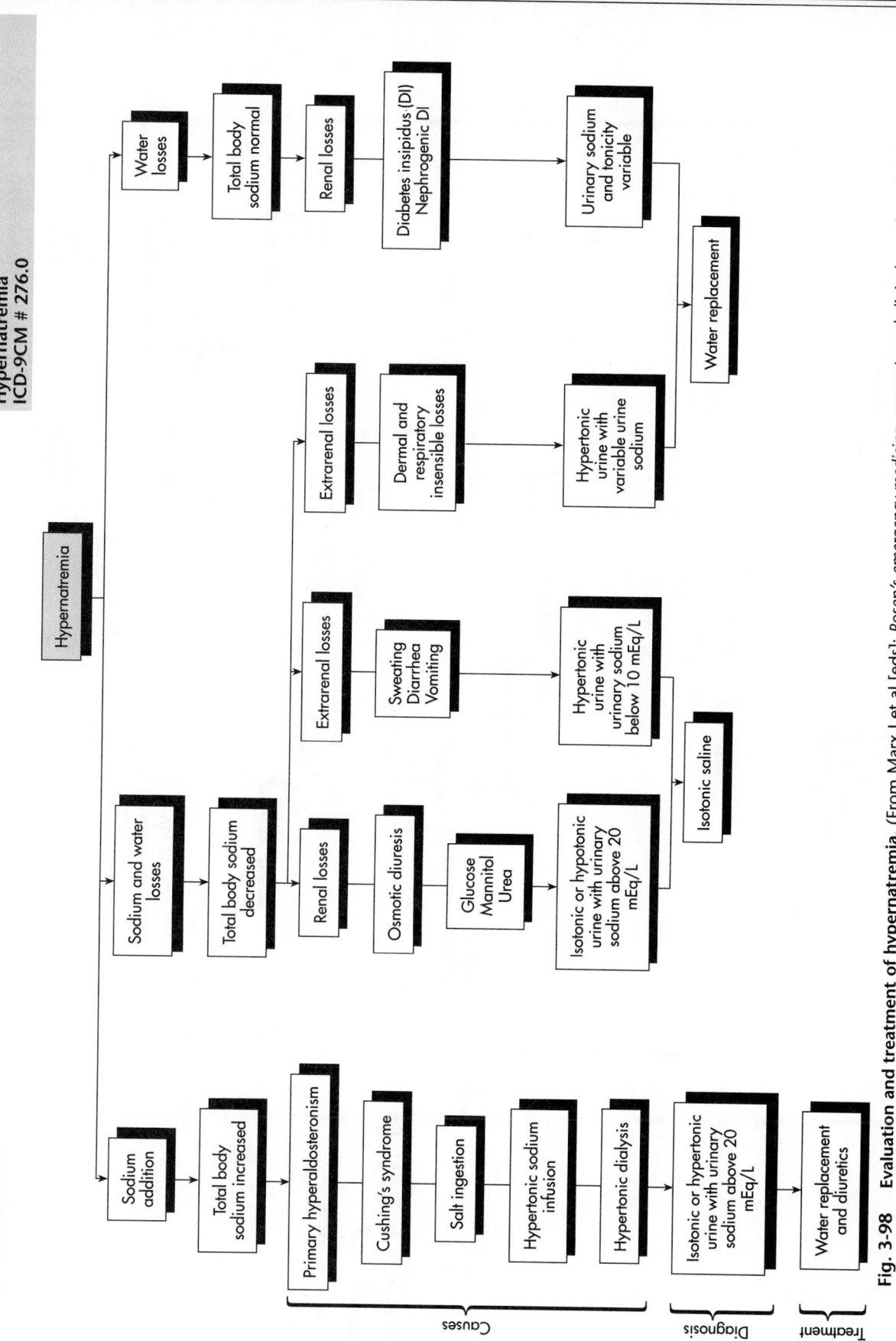

Fig. 3-98   Evaluation and treatment of hypernatremia. (From Marx J et al [eds]: *Rosen's emergency medicine: concepts and clinical practice*, ed 6, St Louis, 2004, Mosby.)

HYPERPHOSPHATEMIA

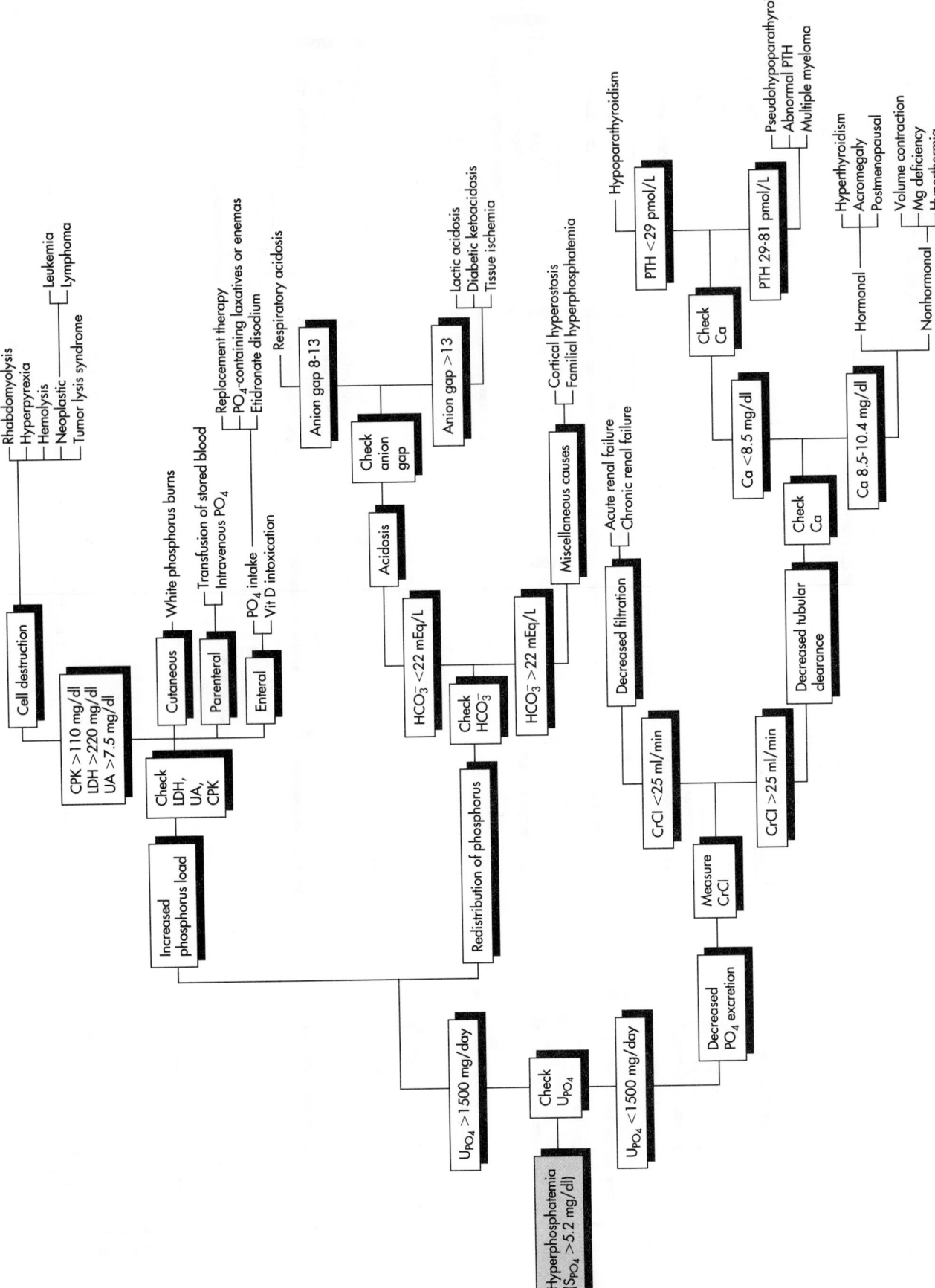

Fig. 3-99 **Approach to hyperphosphatemia.** *CT,* Computerized tomography; *MRI,* magnetic resonance imaging; *T₄,* thyroxine; *TSH,* thyroid-stimulating hormone. (From Healey PM: *Common medical diagnosis: An algorithmic approach,* ed 3, Philadelphia, 2000, WB Saunders.)

HYPERPROLACTINEMIA

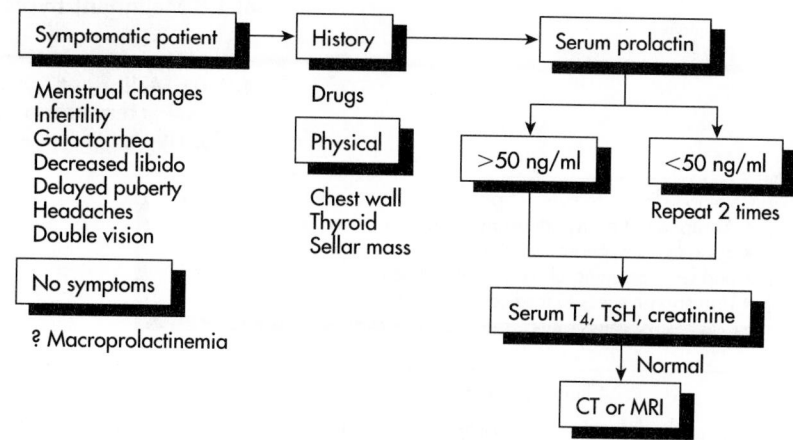

Fig. 3-100   Approach to hyperprolactinemia. *CT,* Computed tomography; *MRI,* magnetic resonance imaging; *T₄,* thyroxine; *TSH,* thyroid-stimulating hormone. (From Copeland LJ: *Textbook of gynecology,* ed 2, Philadelphia, 2000, WB Saunders.)

HYPERTENSION, SECONDARY CAUSES

Hypertension, secondary causes
ICD-9CM # 401.1 Essential hypertension
401.0 Malignant hypertension due to renal artery stenosis
642   Hypertension complicating pregnancy
405.01 Malignant hypertension secondary to renal artery stenosis
437.2 Hypertensive encephalopathy

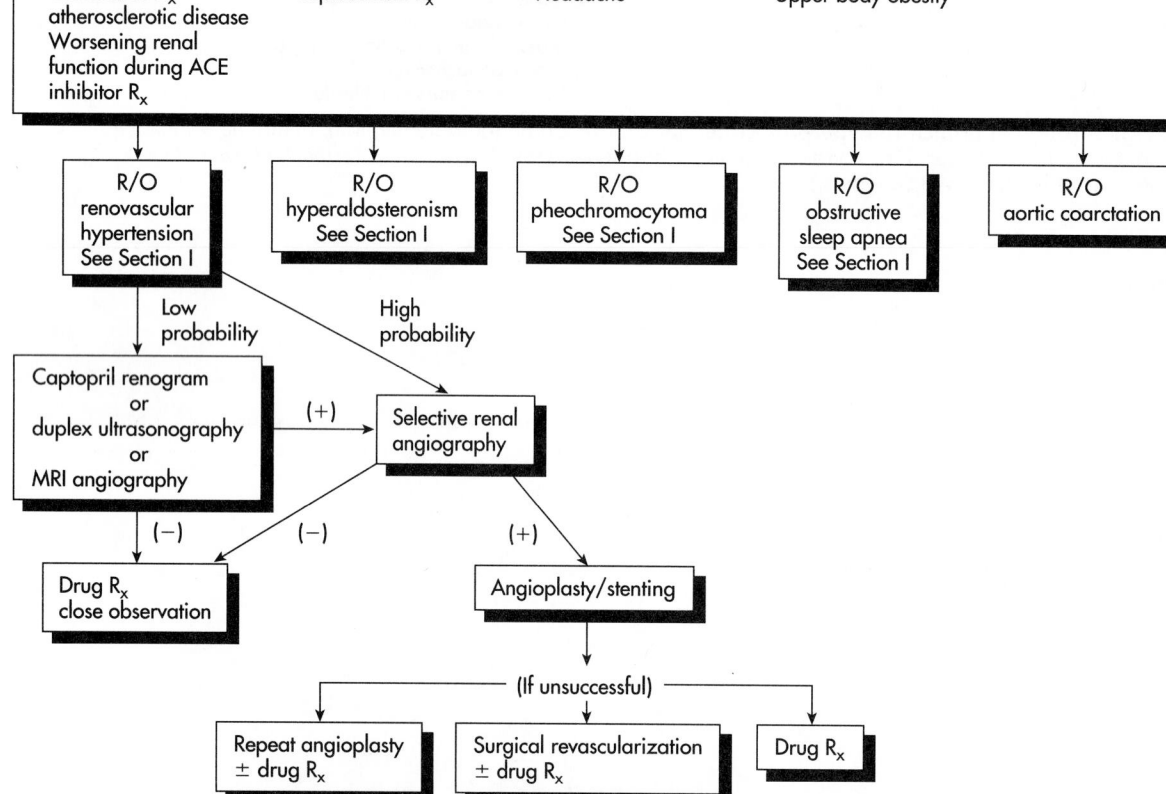

Fig. 3-101   Algorithm for identifying patients for evaluation of secondary causes of hypertension.
ACE, Angiotension-converting enzyme; *Hx,* history; *K+,* potassium; *R/O,* rule out. (From Goldman L, Ausiello D [eds]: *Cecil textbook of medicine,* ed 22, Philadelphia, 2004, WB Saunders.)

HYPERTHYROIDISM

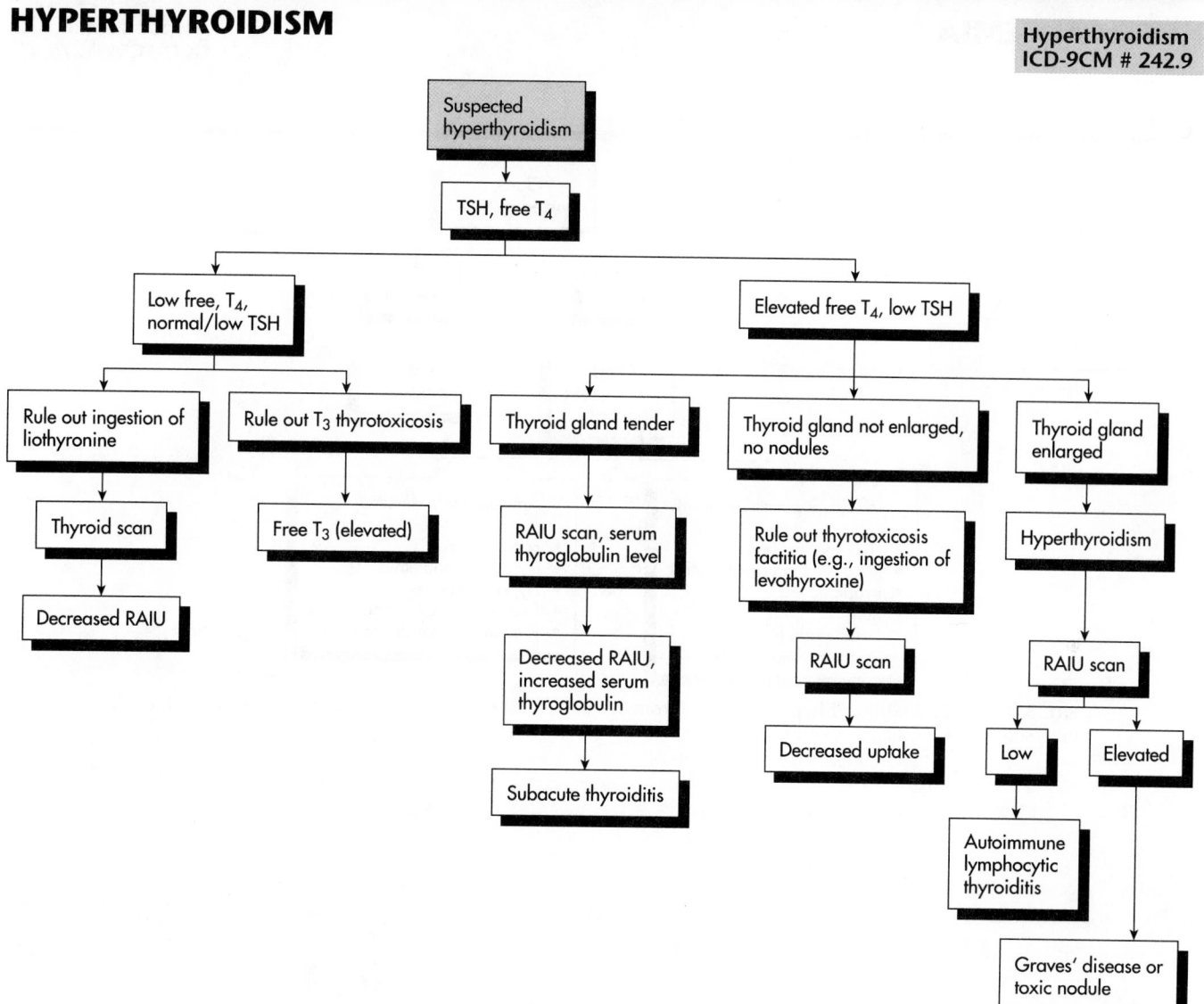

Fig. 3-102   Hyperthyroidism. *RAIU,* Radioactive iodine uptake; *TSH,* thyroid-stimulating hormone.

III

HYPOCALCEMIA

Hypocalcemia
ICD-9CM # 275.41

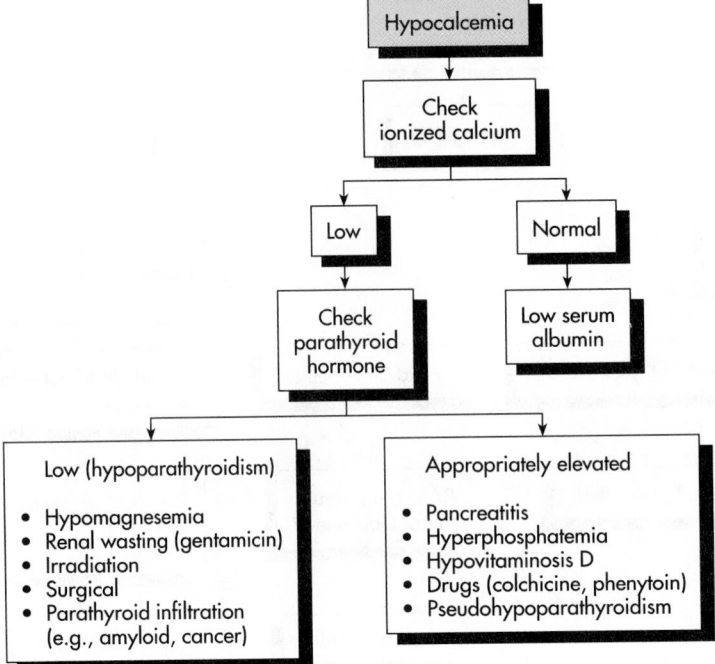

Fig. 3-103 **Evaluation of hypocalcemia.** (From Wachtel TJ, Stein MD: *Practical guide to the care of the ambulatory patient,* ed 2, St Louis, 2000, Mosby.)

HYPOGLYCEMIA

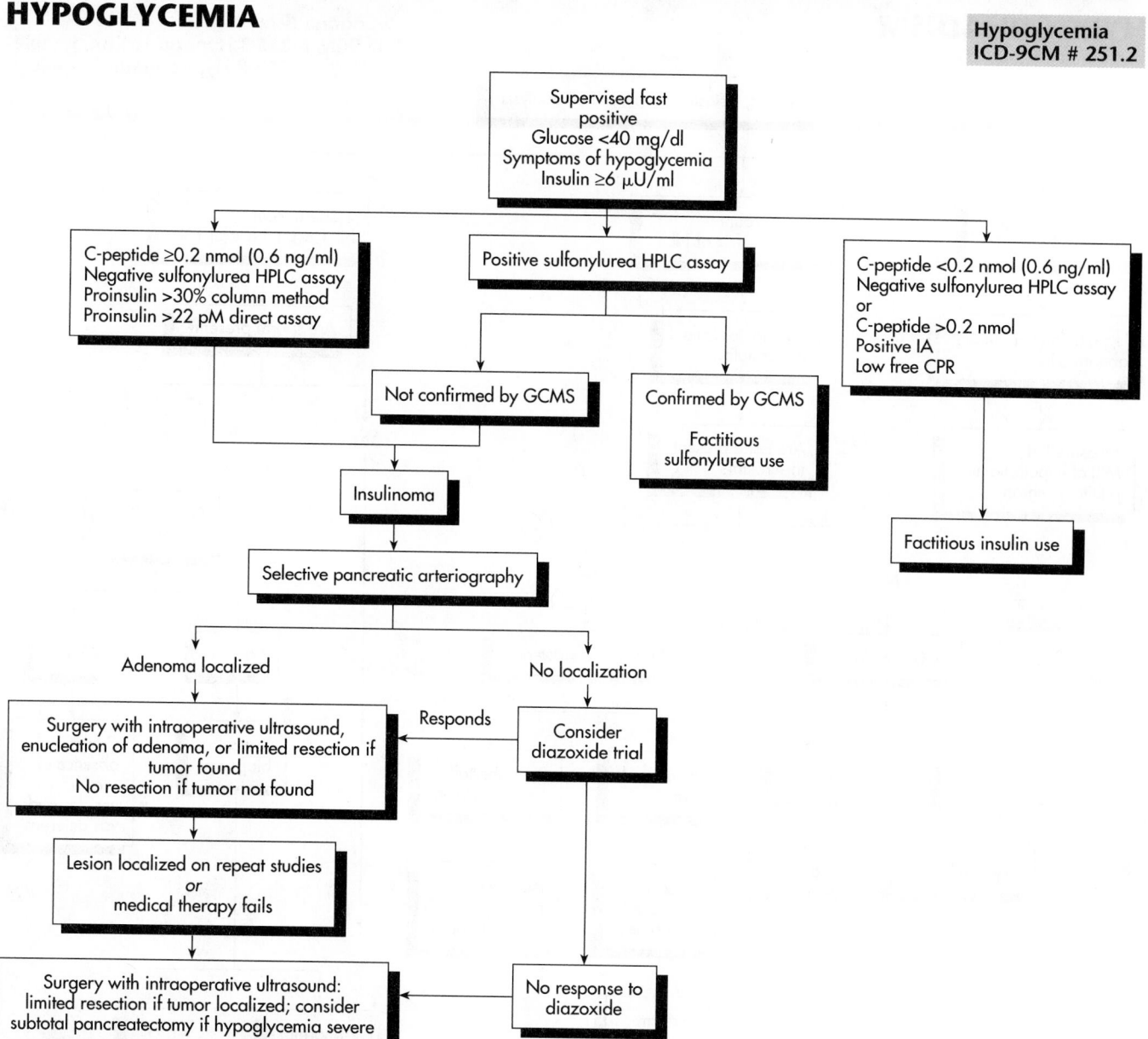

Fig. 3-104   Diagnostic evaluation of patients with documented hypoglycemia and elevated insulin.
CPR, C-peptide immunoreactivity; *GCMS,* gas chromatography mass spectrometry; *HPLC,* high-pressure liquid chromatography; *IA,* insulin antibodies. (From Moore WT, Eastman RC: *Diagnostic endocrinology,* ed 2, St Louis, 1996, Mosby.)

III

HYPOGONADISM

Hypogonadism
ICD-9CM # 256.3 Hypogonadism, female
257.2 Hypogonadism, male

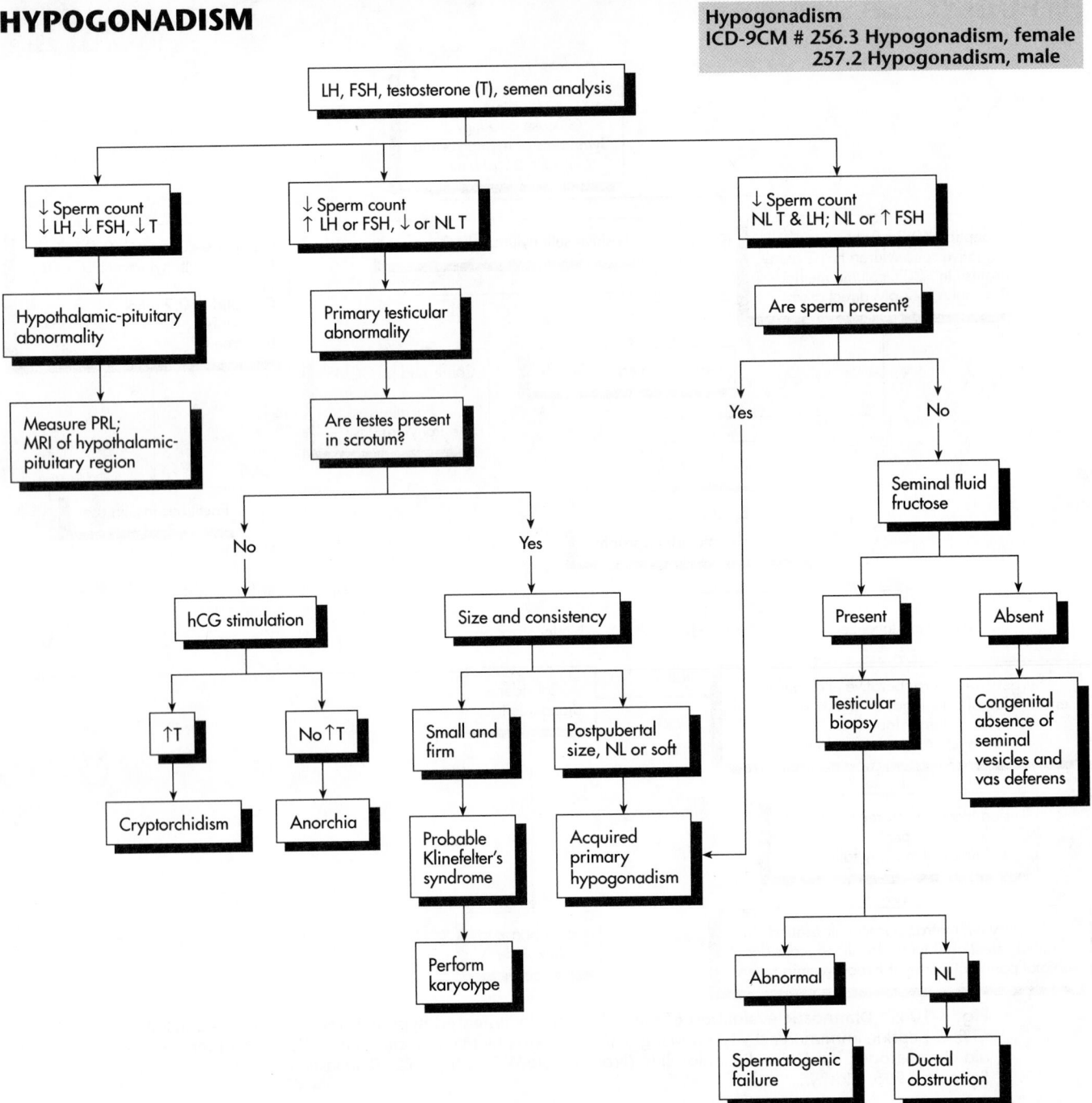

Fig. 3-105 **Laboratory evaluation of hypogonadism.** *FSH,* Follicle-stimulating hormone; *hCG,* human chorionic gonadotropin; *LH,* luteinizing hormone; *MRI,* magnetic resonance imaging; *NL,* normal; *PRL,* prolactin; ↑, elevated; ↓, decreased or low. (From Andreoli TE [ed]: *Cecil essentials of medicine,* ed 5, Philadelphia, 2001, WB Saunders.)

HYPOKALEMIA

Hypokalemia
ICD-9CM # 276.8

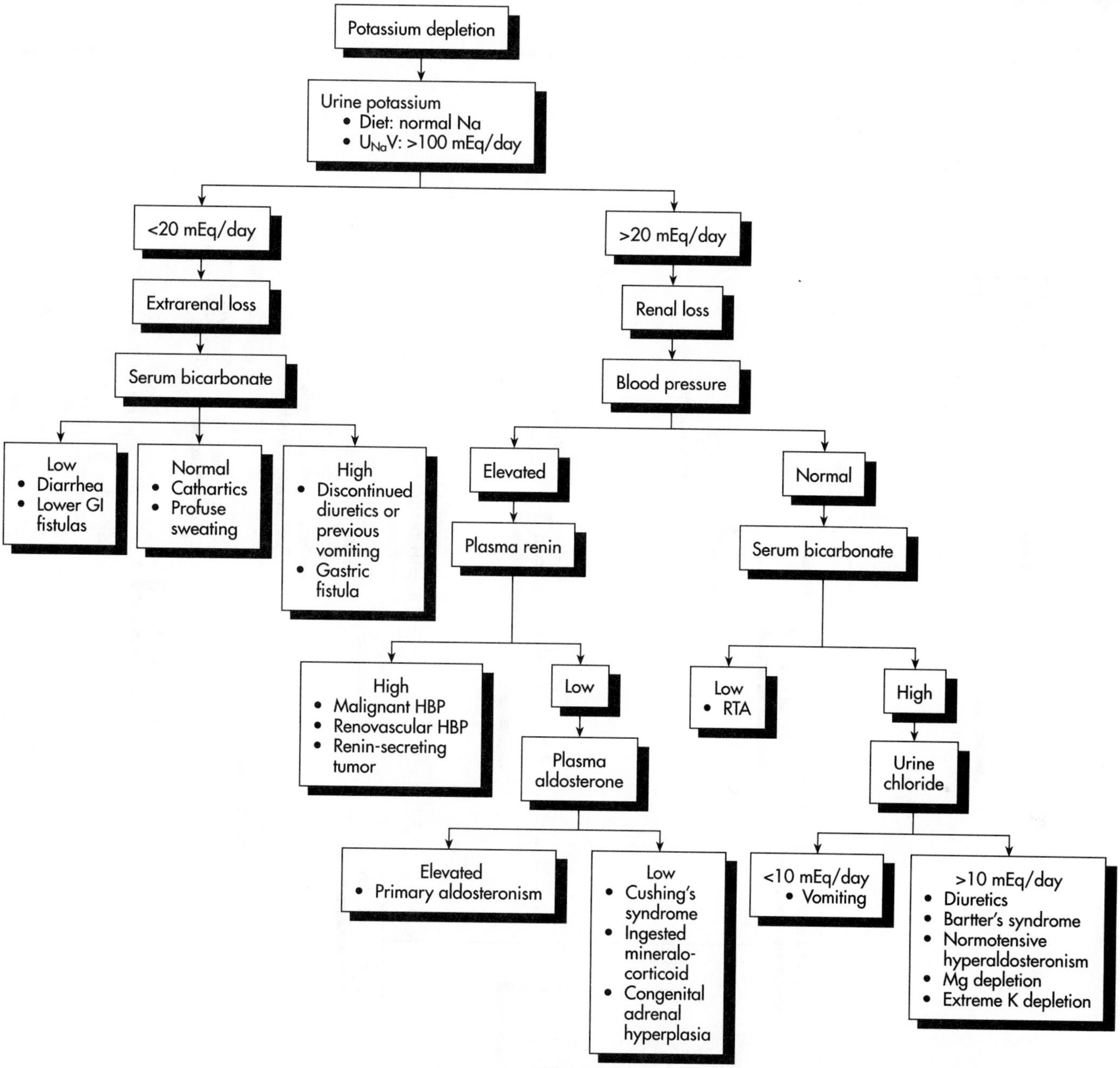

Fig. 3-106   Diagnostic approach to hypokalemia. Because renal potassium wasting may improve during sodium restriction, diminished potassium excretion is indicative of extrarenal loss only when the diet (and therefore the urine) is rich in sodium. *GI,* Gastrointestinal; *HBP,* high blood pressure; *RTA,* renal tubular acidosis; $U_{Na}V$, urinary sodium volume. (From Stein JH [ed]: *Internal medicine,* ed 5, St Louis, 1998, Mosby.)

HYPOMAGNESEMIA

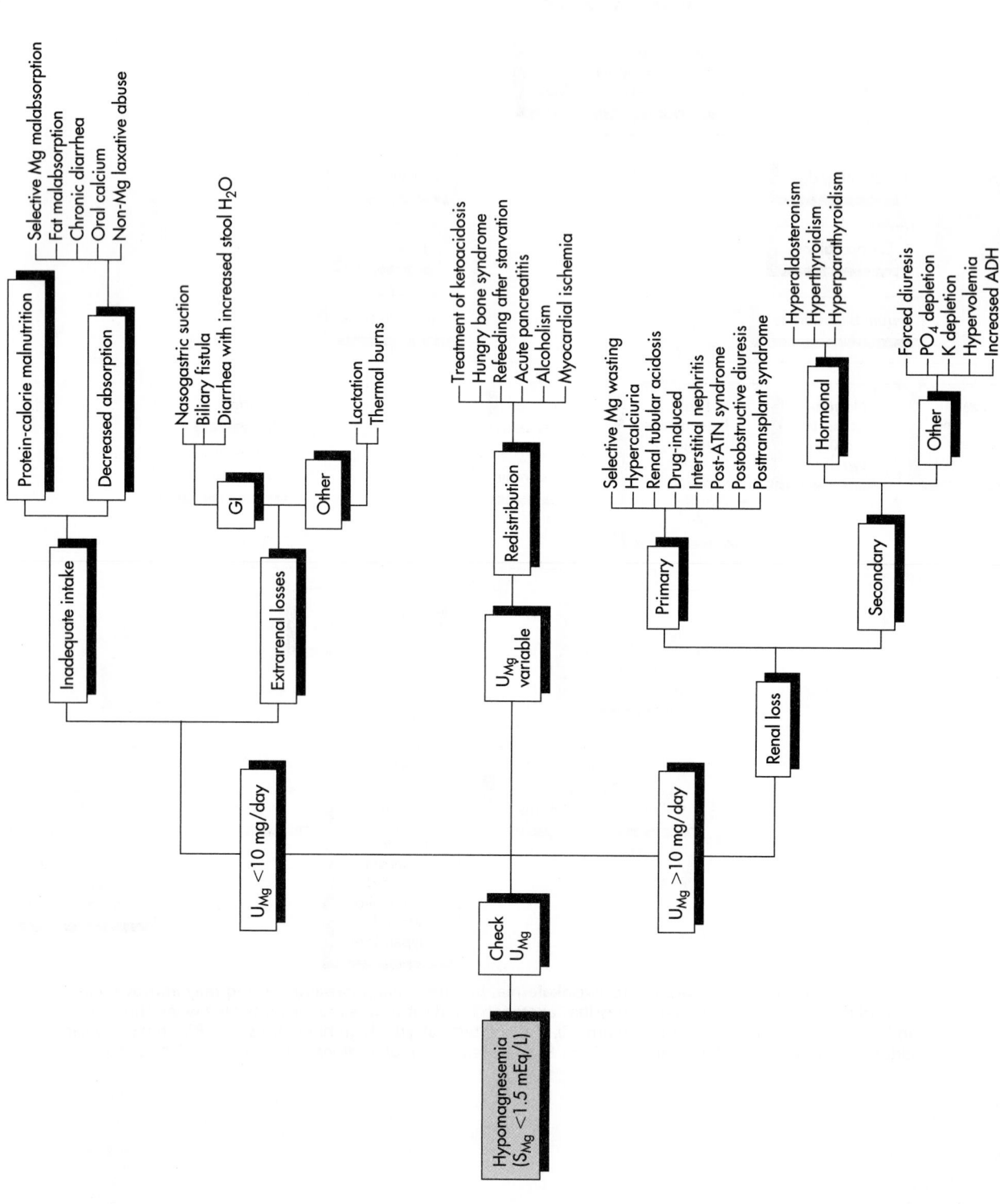

Fig. 3-107   Hypomagnesemia. *ADH,* Antidiuretic hormone; *GI,* gastrointestinal; *post-ATN,* post acute tubular necrosis. (From Healy PM: *Common medical diagnosis: an algorithmic approach,* ed 3, Philadelphia, 2000, WB Saunders.)

HYPONATREMIA

Hyponatremia
ICD-9CM # 276.1

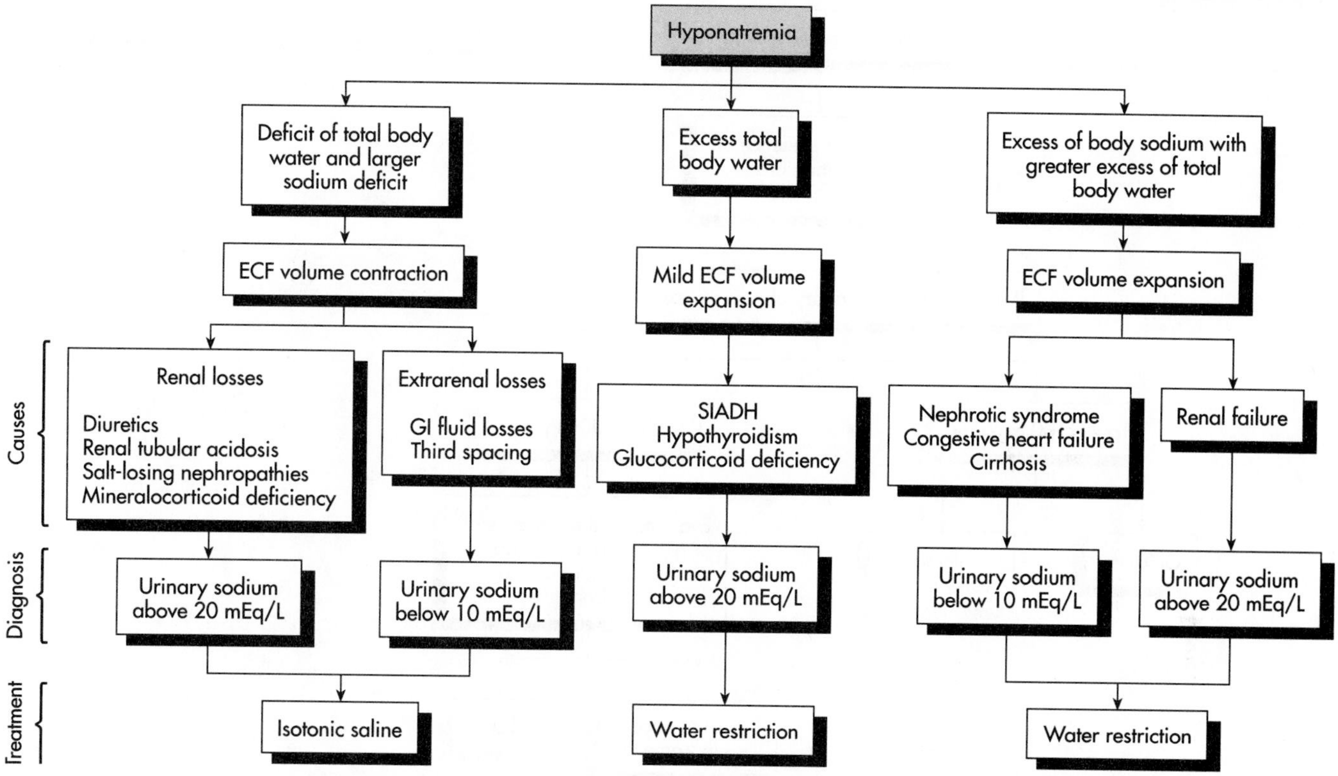

Fig. 3-108 Evaluation and treatment of asymptomatic, mild hyponatremia. *ECF,* Extracellular fluid; *GI,* gastrointestinal; *SIADH,* syndrome of inappropriate secretion of antidiuretic hormone. (From Marx J et al [eds]: *Rosen's emergency medicine: concepts and clinical practice,* ed 5, St Louis, 2002, Mosby.)

HYPOPHOSPHATEMIA

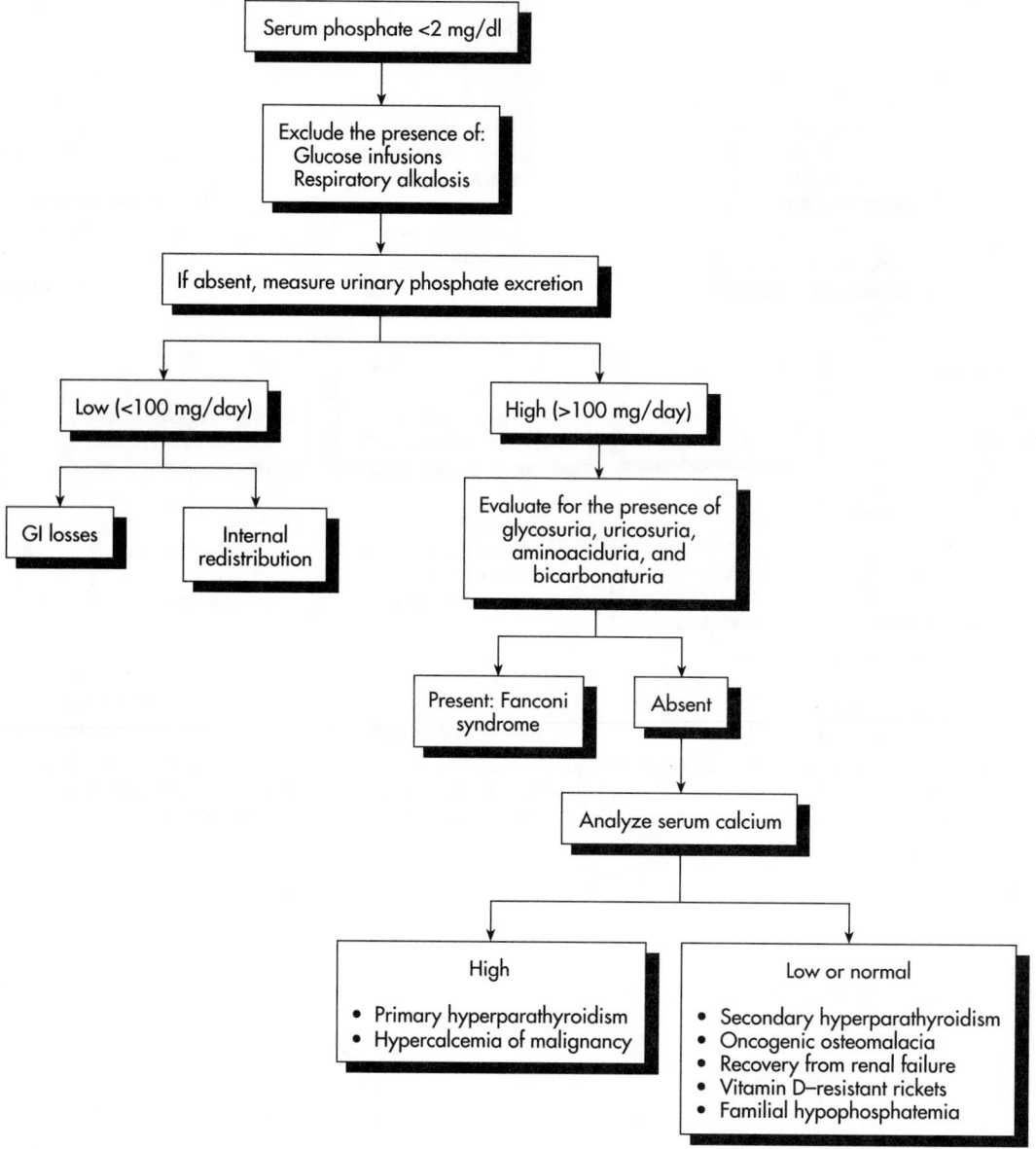

Fig. 3-109 **Diagnostic workup of hypophosphatemia.** *GI,* Gastrointestinal. (From Stein JH [ed]: *Internal medicine,* ed 5, St Louis, 1998, Mosby.)

HYPOTENSION

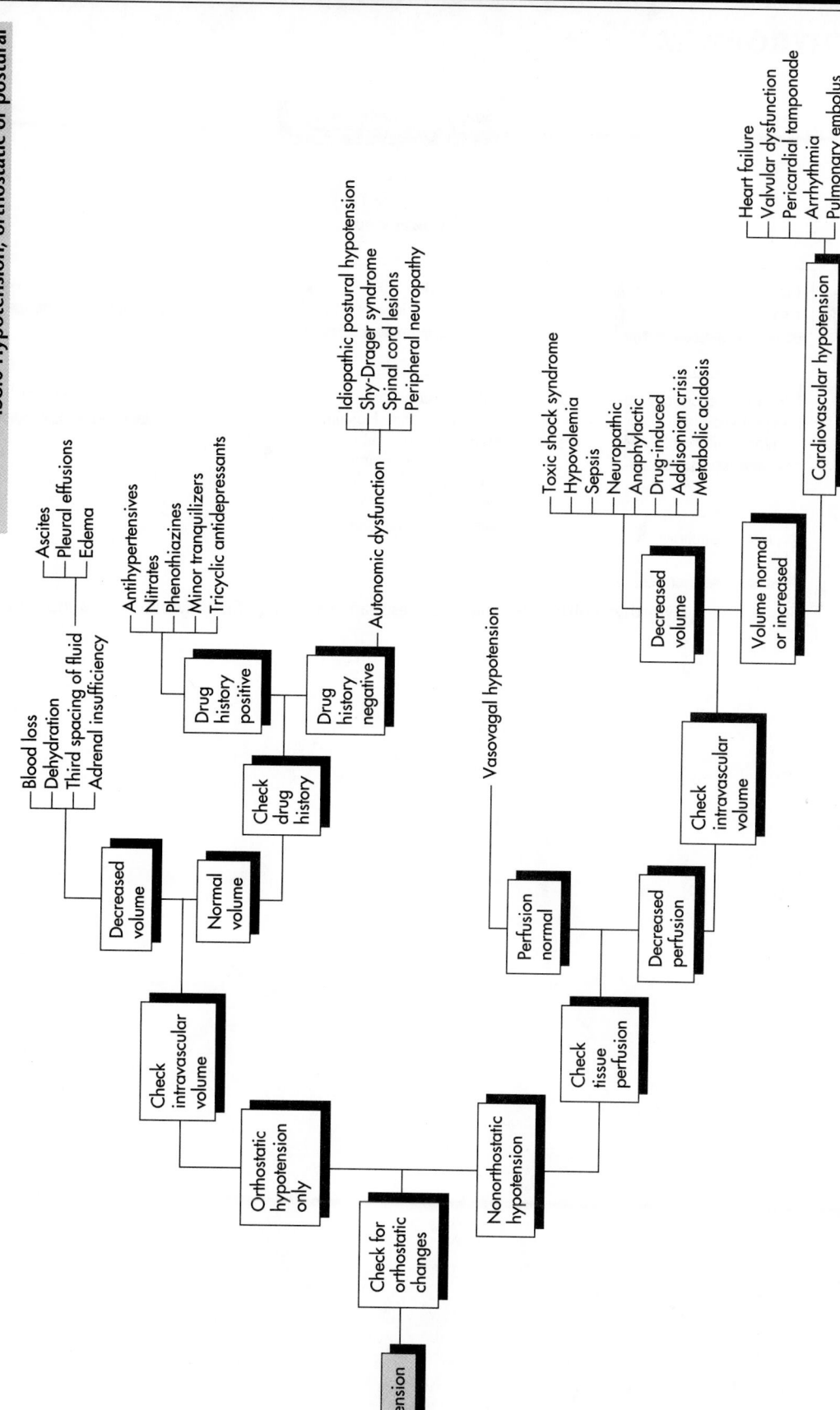

Hypotension
ICD-9CM # 458.9 Hypotension, NOS
458.1 Hypotension, chronic
458.2 Hypotension, iatrogenic
458.0 Hypotension, orthostatic or postural

Fig. 3-110   **Hypotension.** (From Healey PM: *Common medical diagnosis: an algorithmic approach*, ed 3, Philadelphia, 2000, WB Saunders.)

HYPOTHYROIDISM

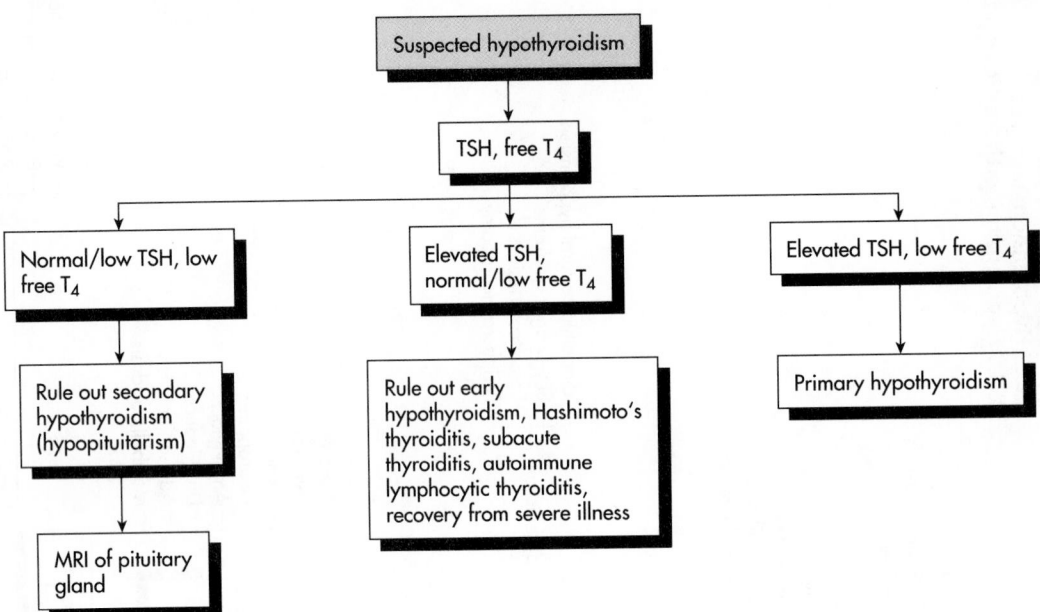

Fig. 3-111 **Hypothyroidism.** *MRI,* Magnetic resonance imaging; *TSH,* thyroid-stimulating hormone.

INFERTILITY

Infertility
ICD-9CM # 628.9 Infertility, female, unspecified
          606.9 Infertility, male, unspecified

A

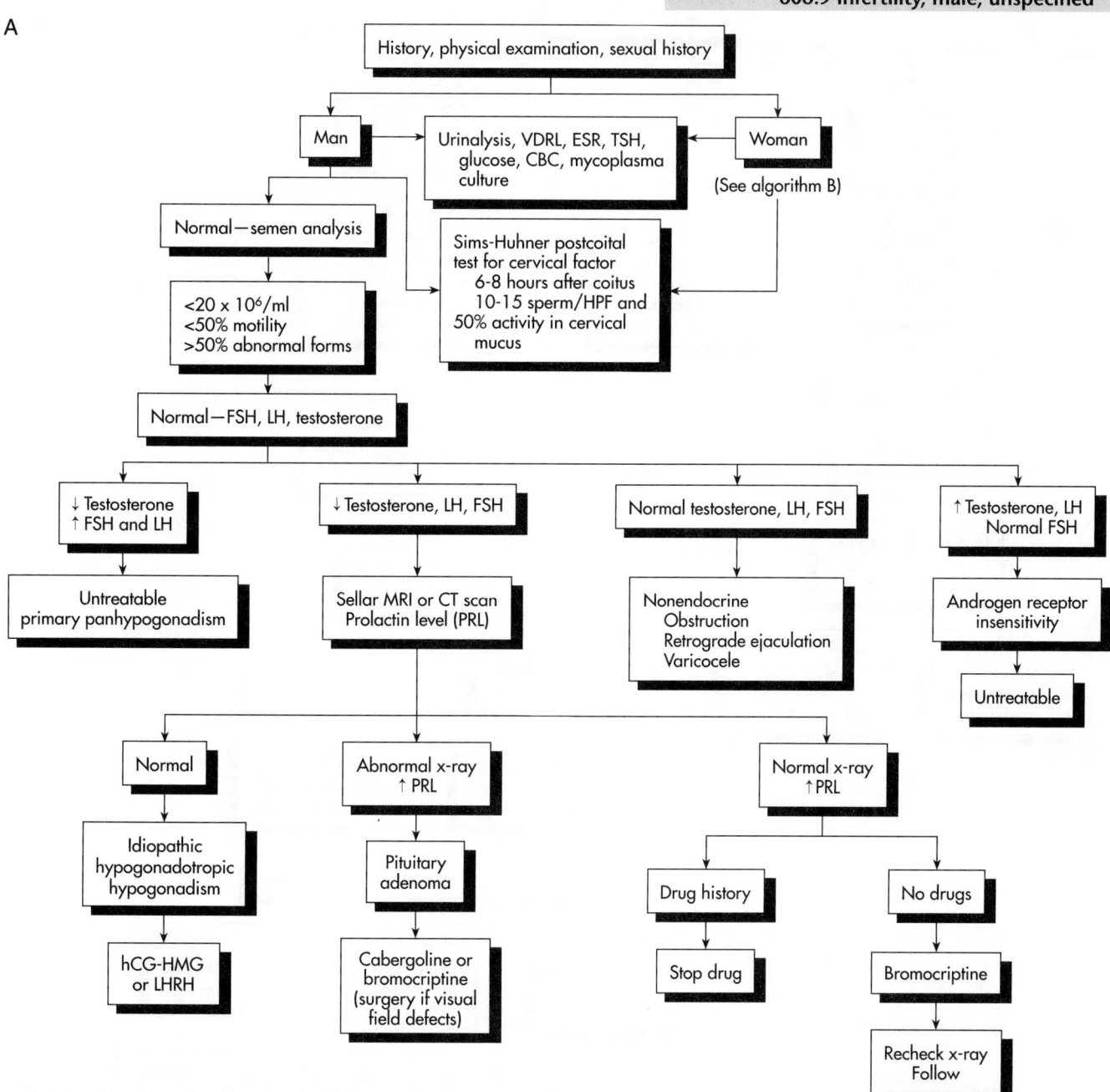

Fig. 3-112   A, Evaluating infertility in the man. *CBC,* Complete blood count; *CT,* computed tomography; *ESR,* erythrocyte sedimentation rate; *FSH,* follicle-stimulating hormone; *hCG-HMG,* human chorionic gonadotropin/human menopausal gonadotropin; *HPF,* high-power field; *LH,* luteinizing hormone; *LHRH,* luteinizing hormone–reducing hormone; *PRL,* prolactin level; *TSH,* thyroid-stimulating hormone; *VDRL,* Venereal Disease Research Laboratory. (Modified from Driscoll CE et al: *The family practice desk reference,* ed 3, St Louis, 1996, Mosby.)

Continued

B

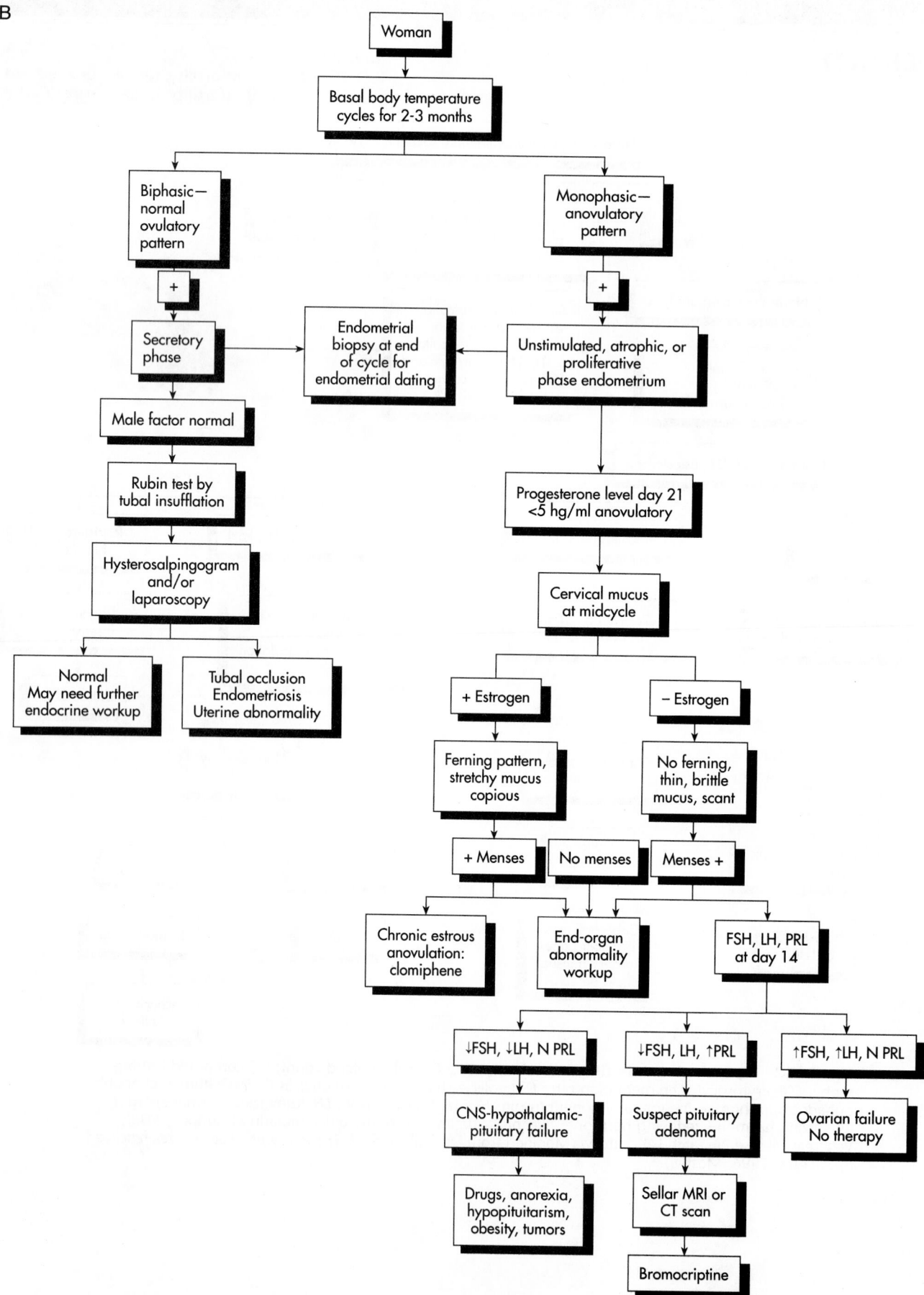

Fig. 3-112, cont'd   B, Evaluating infertility in the woman. *CNS,* Central nervous system; *CT,* computed tomography; *FSH,* follicle-stimulating hormone; *LH,* luteinizing hormone; *N,* normal; *PRL,* prolactin level. (Modified from Driscoll CE et al: *The family practice desk reference,* ed 3, St Louis, 1996, Mosby.)

JAUNDICE AND HEPATOBILIARY DISEASE

Jaundice and hepatobiliary disease
ICD-9CM # 782.4 Jaundice NOS
277.4 Bilirubin excretion disorders
576.8 Jaundice, obstructive

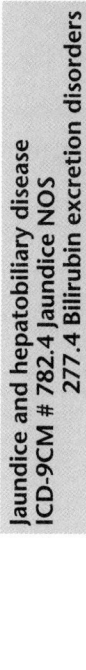

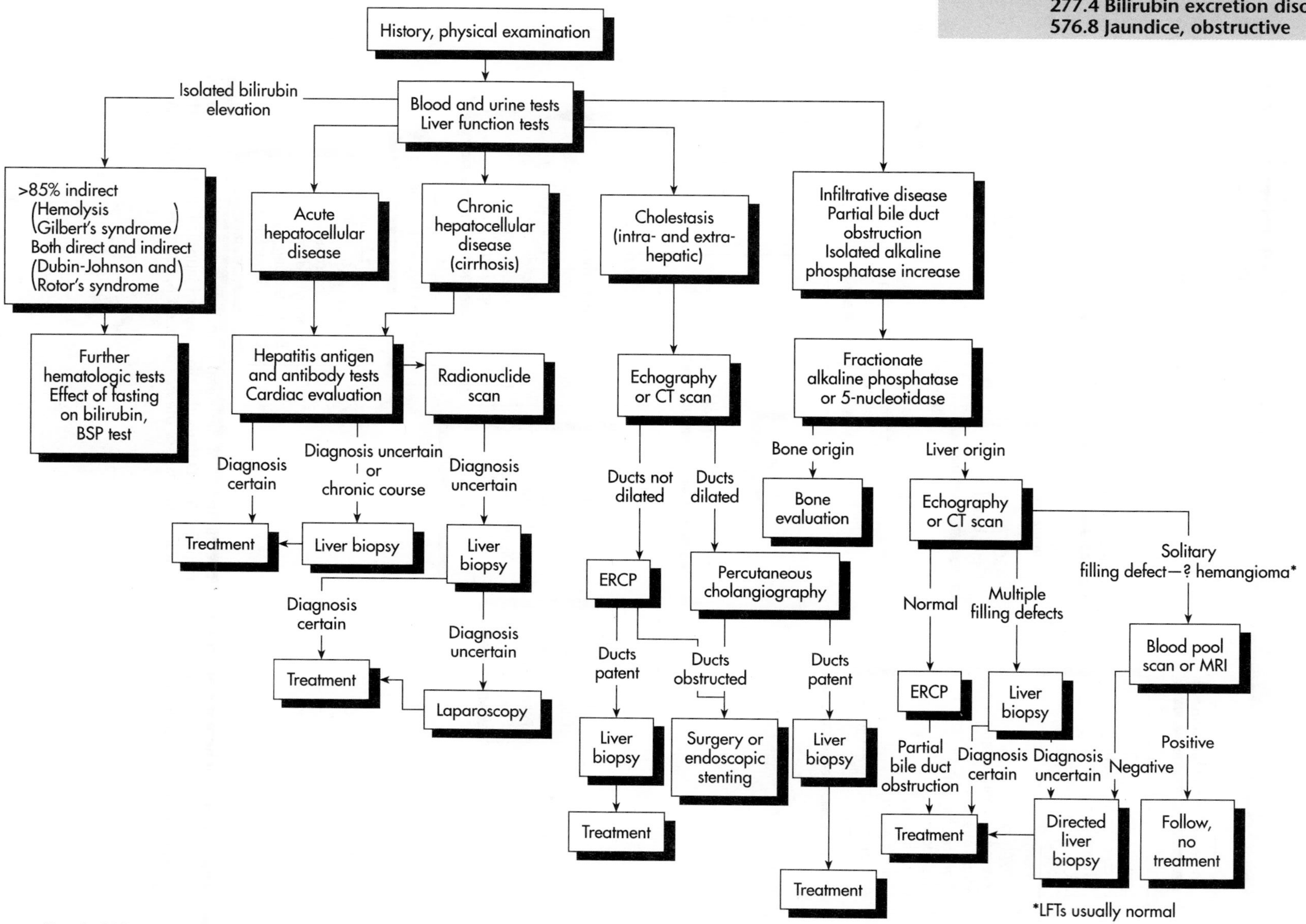

Fig. 3-113   Evaluation of jaundice and hepatobiliary disease. *BSP,* Bromsulphalein; *CT,* computed tomography; *ERCP,* endoscopic retrograde cholangiopancreatography; *LFTs,* liver function tests; *MRI,* magnetic resonance imaging. (From Stein JH [ed]: *Internal medicine,* ed 5, St Louis, 1998, Mosby.)

III

JAUNDICE, NEONATAL

Jaundice, neonatal
ICD-9CM # 774.6 Jaundice neonatal, NOS
            773.1 ABO reaction perinatal
            774.1 Hemolytic perinatal
            773.0 RH reaction perinatal
            751.61 Bile duct obstruction, congenital

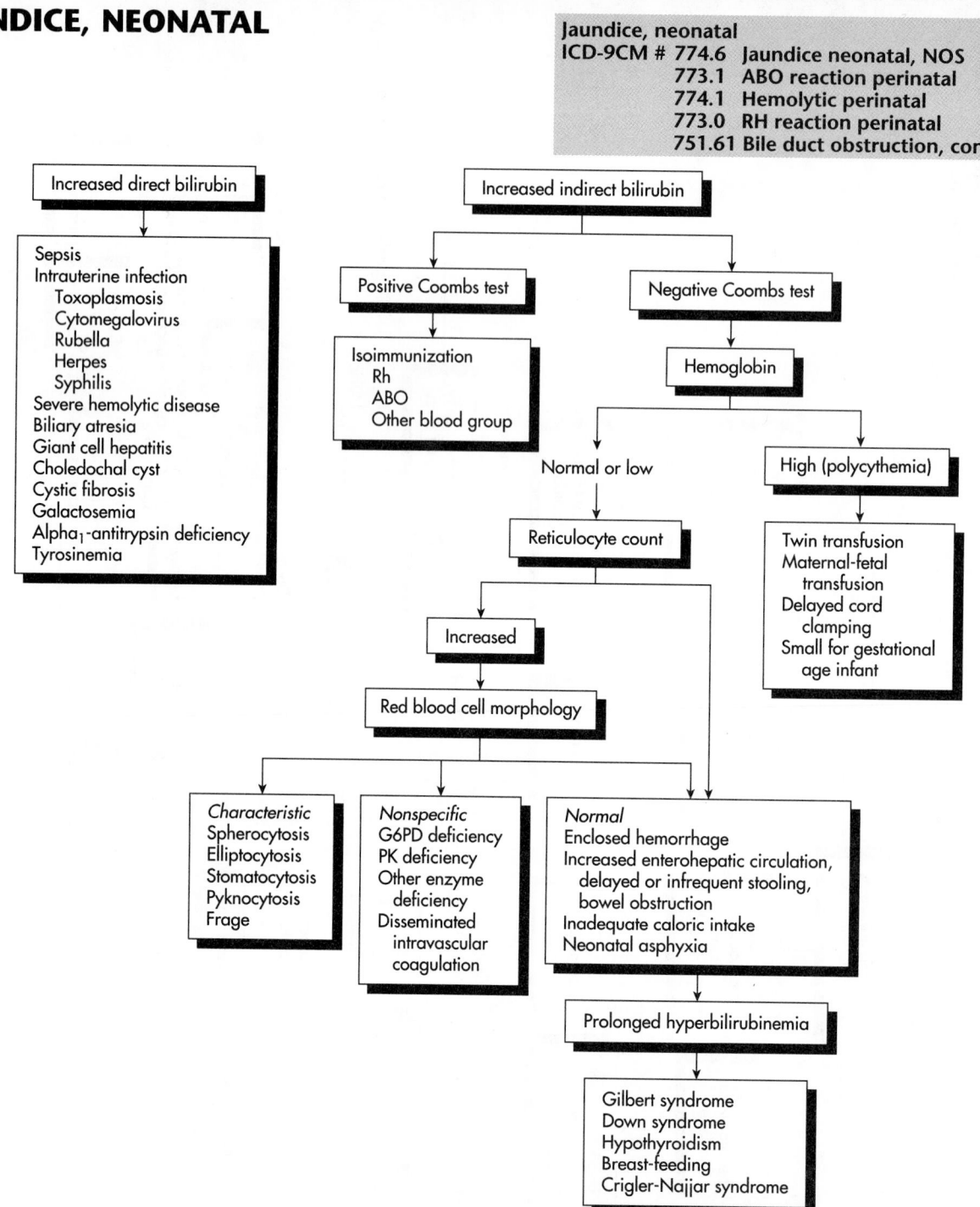

Fig. 3-114   Schematic approach to the diagnosis of neonatal jaundice. *G6PD,* Glucose-6-phosphate dehydrogenase; *PK,* pyruvate kinase. (From Oski FA: Differential diagnosis of jaundice. In Taeusch HW, Ballard RA, Avery MA [eds]: *Schaffer and Avery's diseases of the newborn,* ed 6, Philadelphia, 1991, WB Saunders.)

JOINT EFFUSION

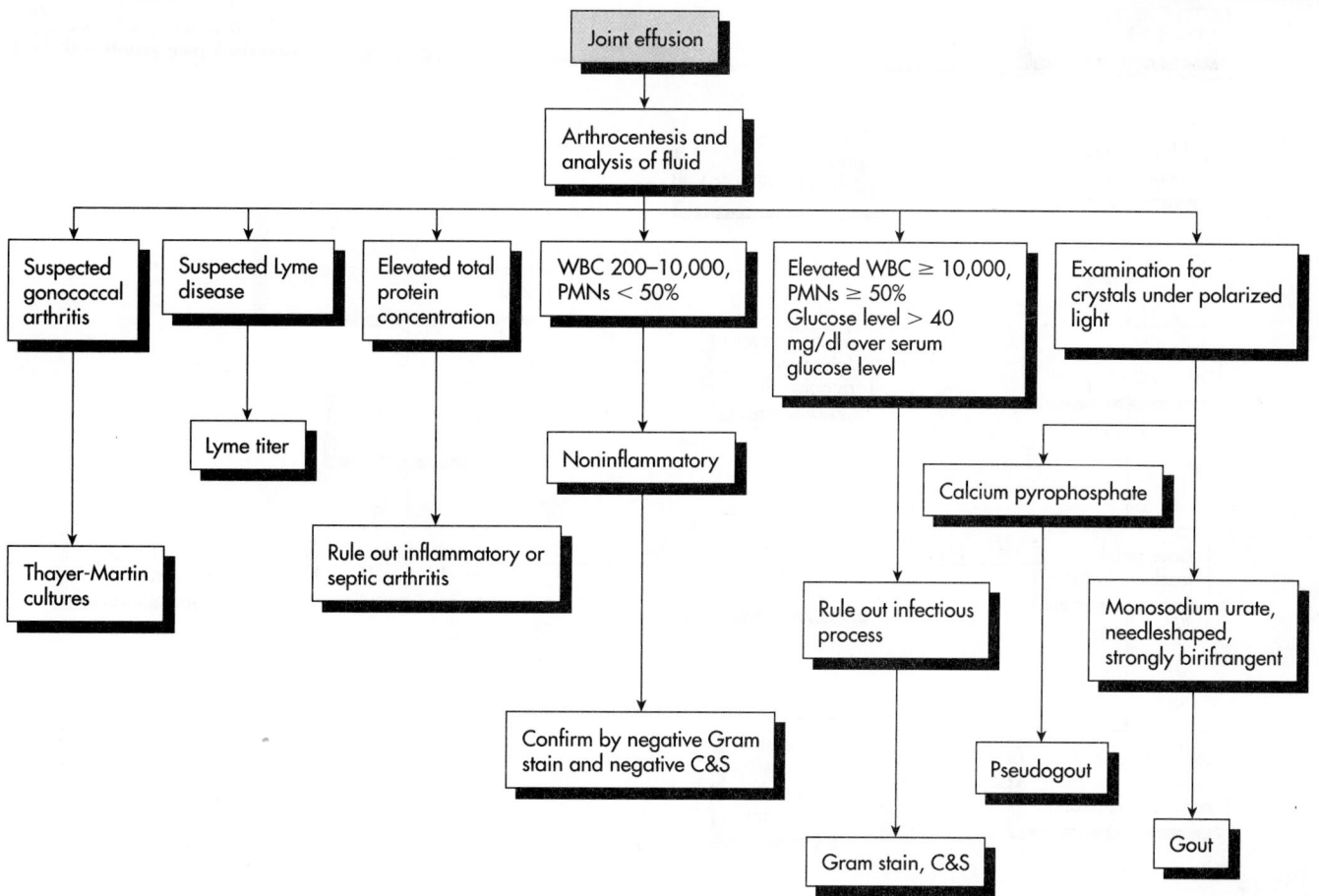

Fig. 3-115   **Joint effusion.** *C&S,* Culture and sensitivity; *WBC,* white blood cell count.

KNEE PAIN, ANTERIOR

Knee pain, anterior
ICD-9CM # 716.96 Knee inflammation
959.7 Knee injury
719.56 Knee stiffness
719.06 Knee swelling

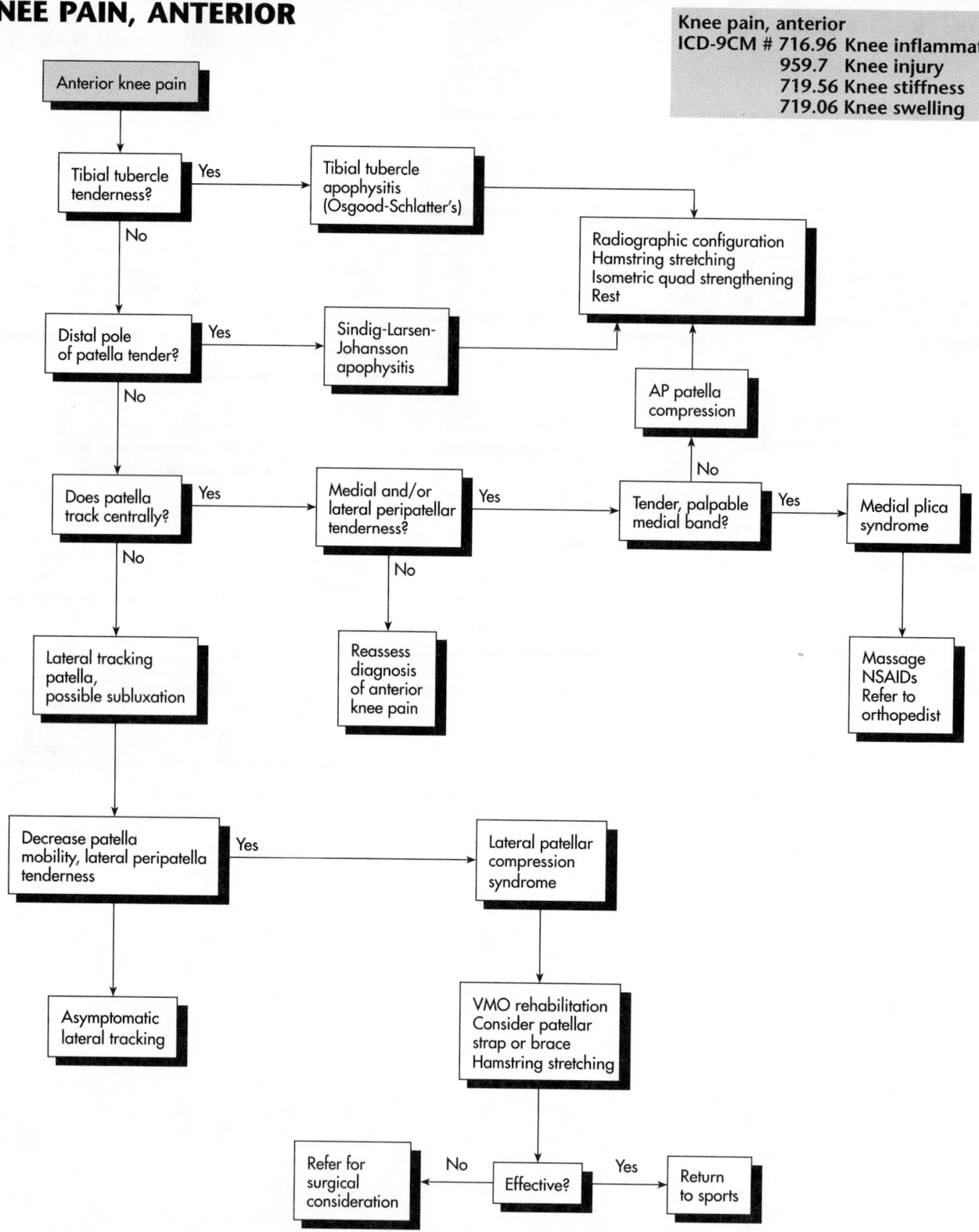

Fig. 3-116   Evaluation and management of knee extensor mechanism pain. Focused treatment based on specific etiology will prevent recurrence. *AP,* Anteroposterior; *NSAIDs,* nonsteroidal antiinflammatory drugs; *VMO,* vastus medialis obliquus muscle. (From Scudieri G [ed]: *Sports medicine, principles of primary care,* St Louis, 1997, Mosby.)

LEG ULCER

Leg ulcer
ICD-9CM # 440.23 Ulcer, lower limb, arteriosclerotic
707.1 Ulcer, lower limb, chronic
707.1 Ulcer, lower limb, neurogenic
707.9 Ulcer, non-healing
707.0 Pressure ulcer

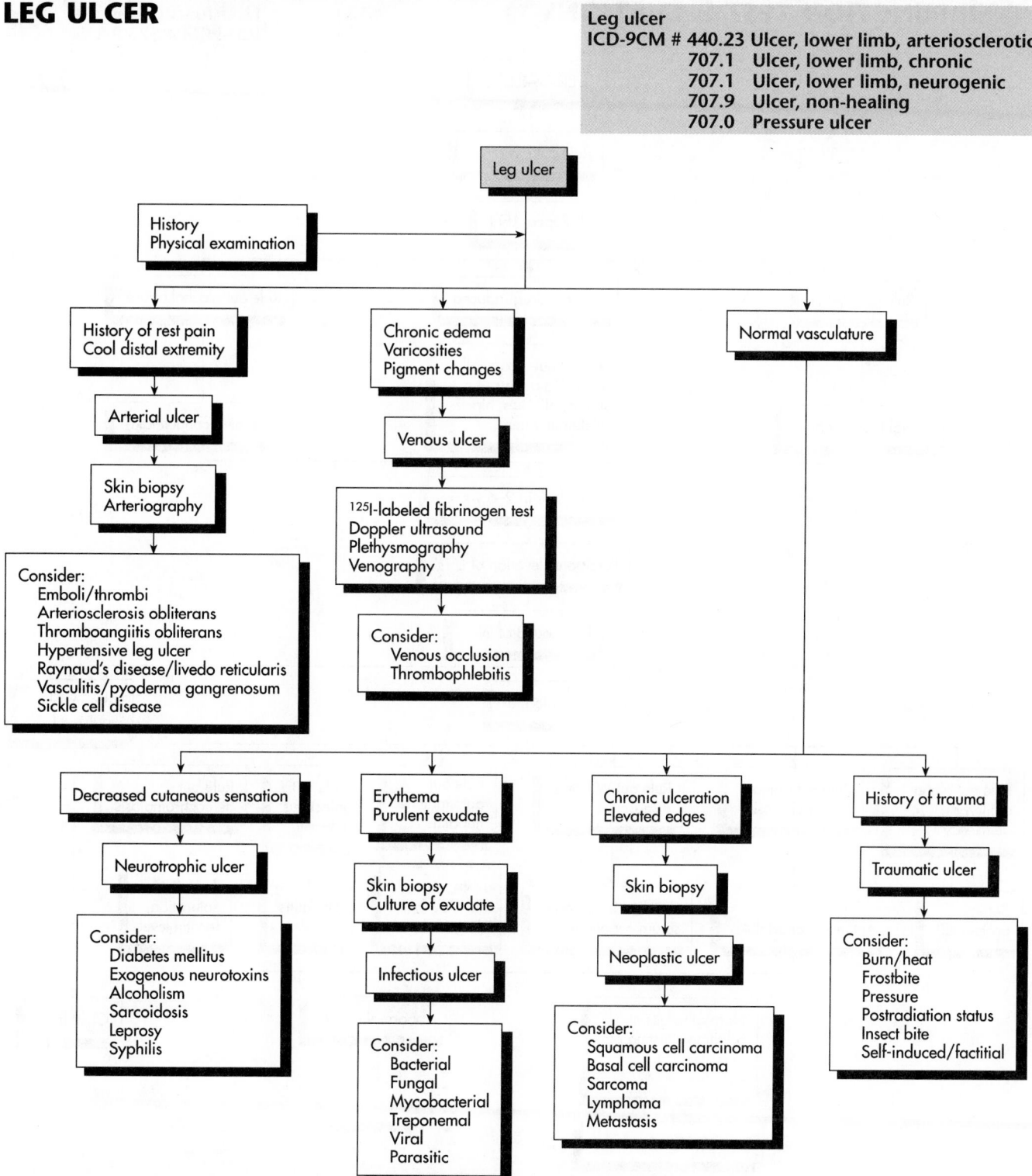

Fig. 3-117 **Leg ulcer.** (From Greene HL, Johnson WP, Lemcke D [eds]: *Decision making in medicine*, ed 2, St Louis, 1998, Mosby.)

LIVER FUNCTION TEST ELEVATIONS

Liver function test elevations
ICD-9CM # 573.9

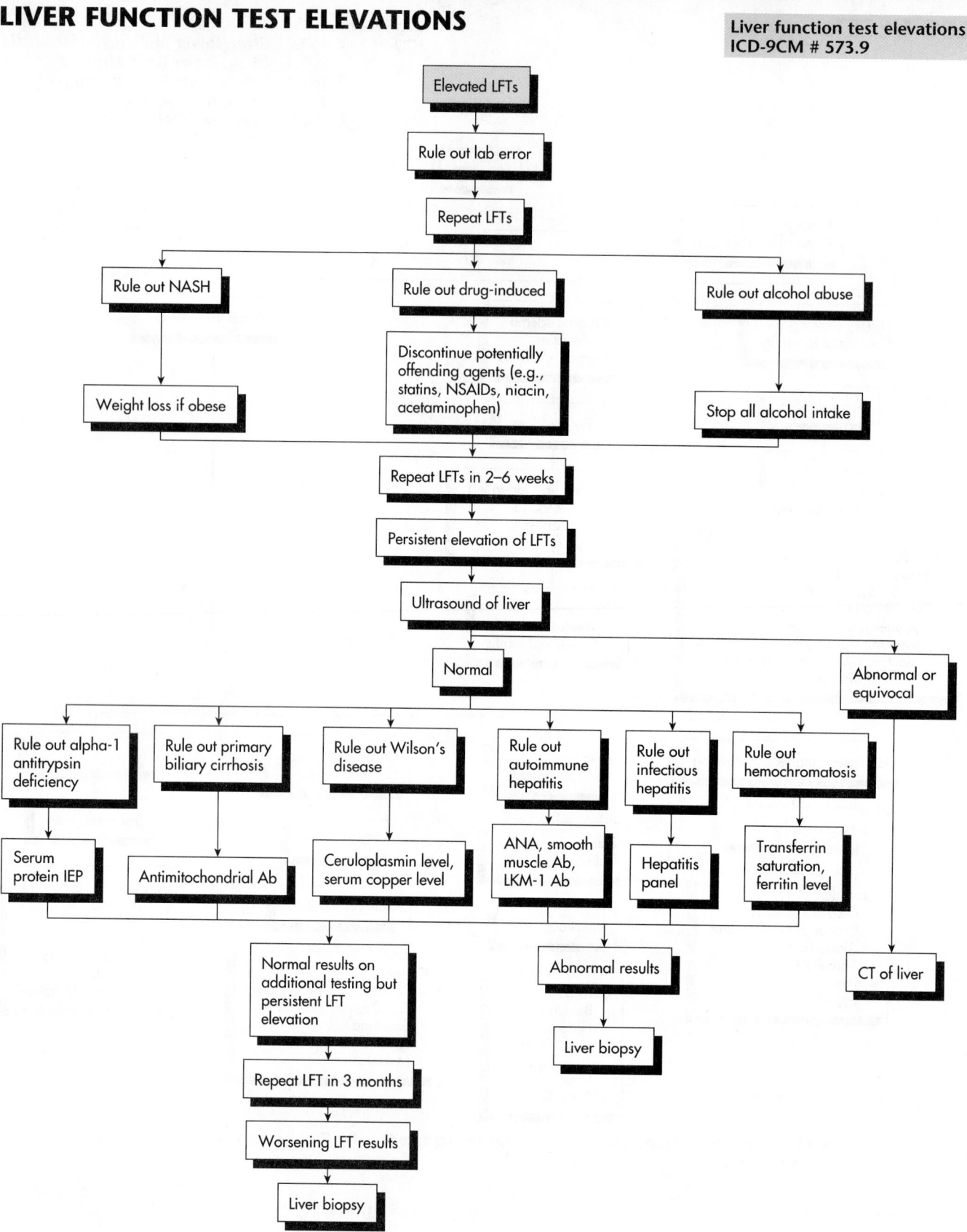

Fig. 3-118   Liver function test elevations. *Ab,* Antibody; *ANA,* antibody to nuclear antigens; *CT,* computed tomography; *IEP,* immuno-electrophoresis; *LFT,* liver function test; *LKM,* liver-kidney microsome; *NSAIDs,* nonsteroidal antiinflammatory drugs.

LYMPHADENOPATHY, AXILLARY

Lymphadenopathy, axillary
ICD-9CM # 785.6

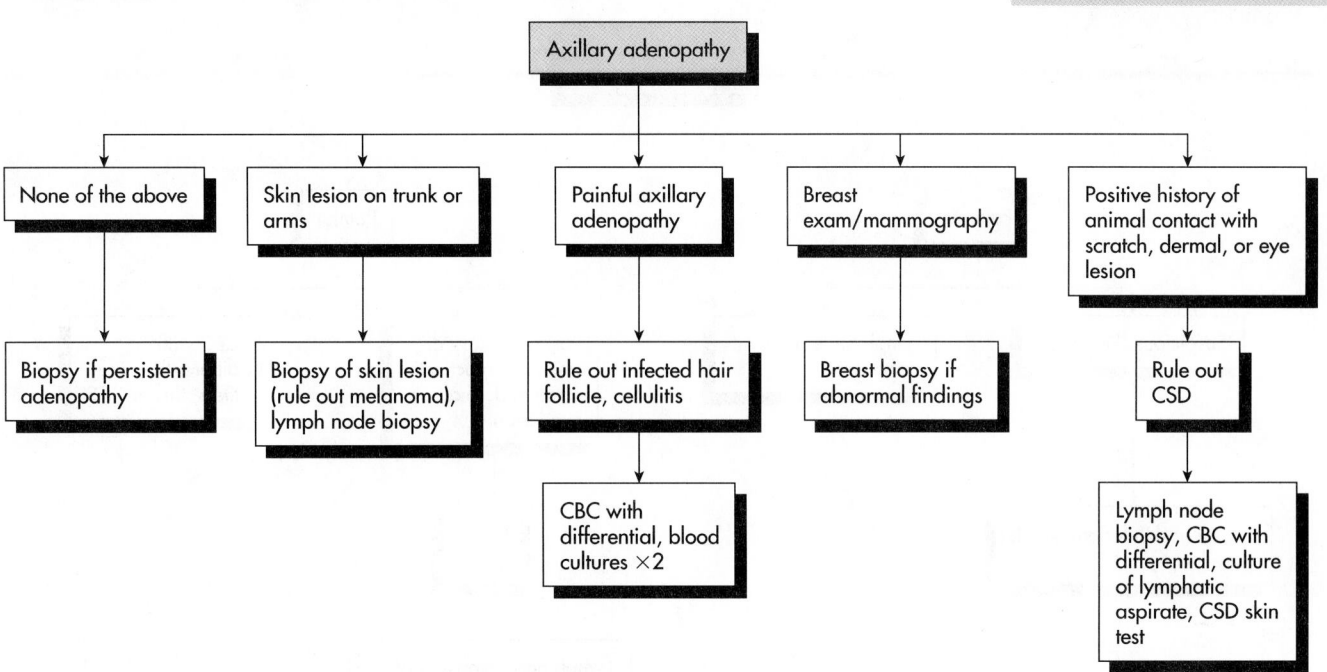

Fig. 3-119 **Lymphadenopathy, axillary.** *CBC,* Complete blood count; *CSD,* cat-scratch disease.

III

LYMPHADENOPATHY, CERVICAL

Lymphadenopathy, cervical
ICD-9CM # 785.6

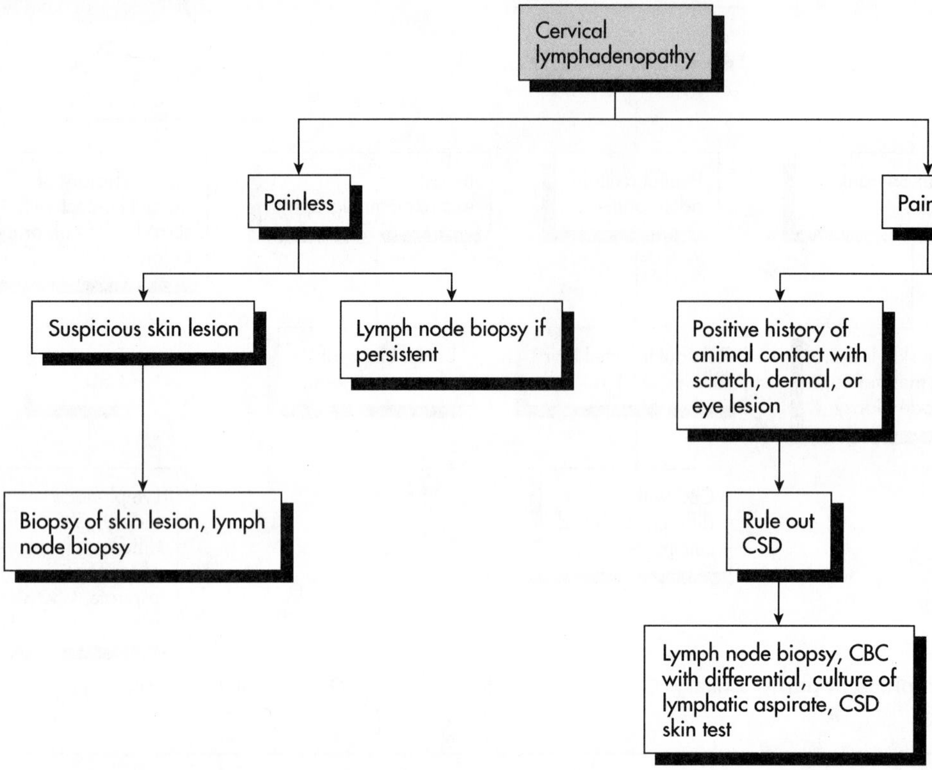
Cervical lymphadenopathy
Painless
Painful
Suspicious skin lesion
Lymph node biopsy if persistent
Positive history of animal contact with scratch, dermal, or eye lesion
CBC with differential, viral titers, throat C&S
Biopsy of skin lesion, lymph node biopsy
Rule out CSD
Lymph node biopsy, CBC with differential, culture of lymphatic aspirate, CSD skin test

Fig. 3-120 Lymphadenopathy, cervical. *CBC,* Complete blood count; *C&S,* culture and sensitivity; *CSD,* cat-scratch disease.

LYMPHADENOPATHY, EPITROCHLEAR

Lymphadenopathy, epitrochlear
ICD-9CM # 785.6

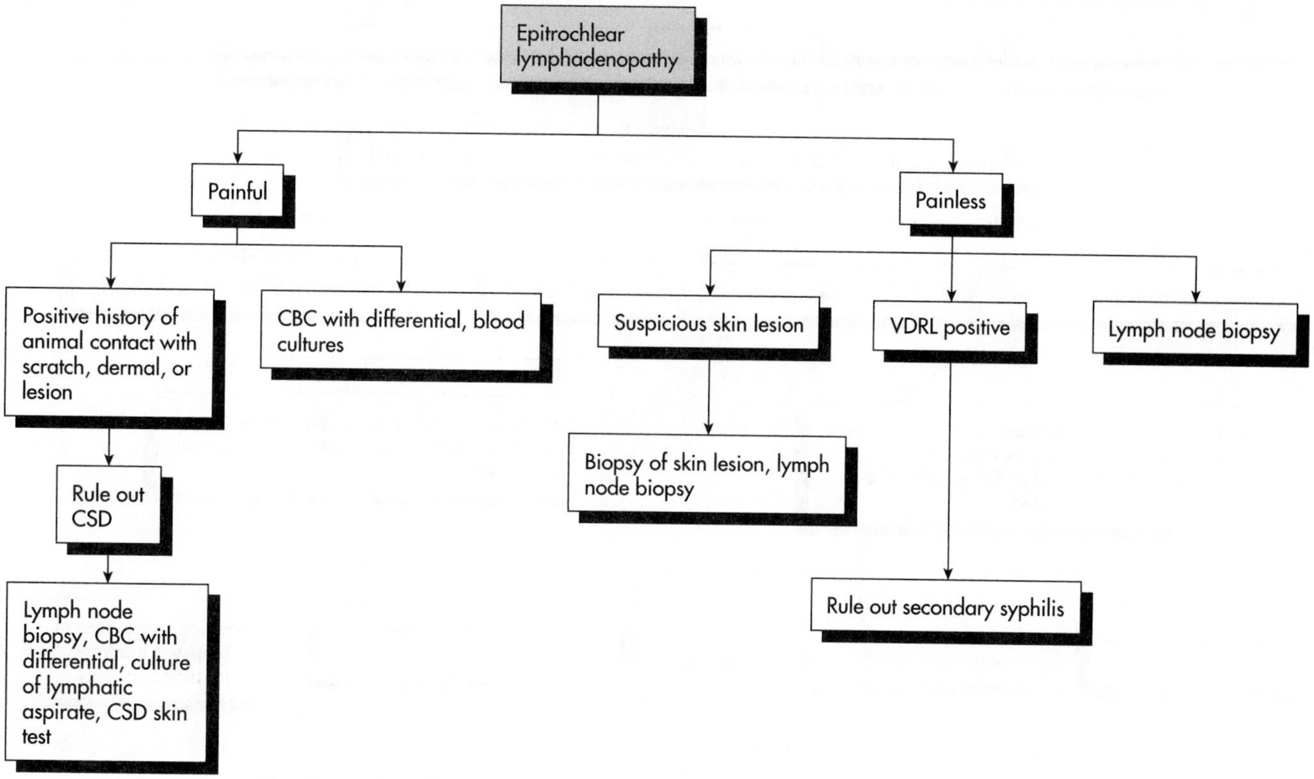

Fig. 3-121 **Lymphadenopathy, epitrochlear.** *CBC,* Complete blood count; *CSD,* cat-scratch disease; *VDRL,* Venereal Disease Research Laboratory.

III

LYMPHADENOPATHY, GENERALIZED

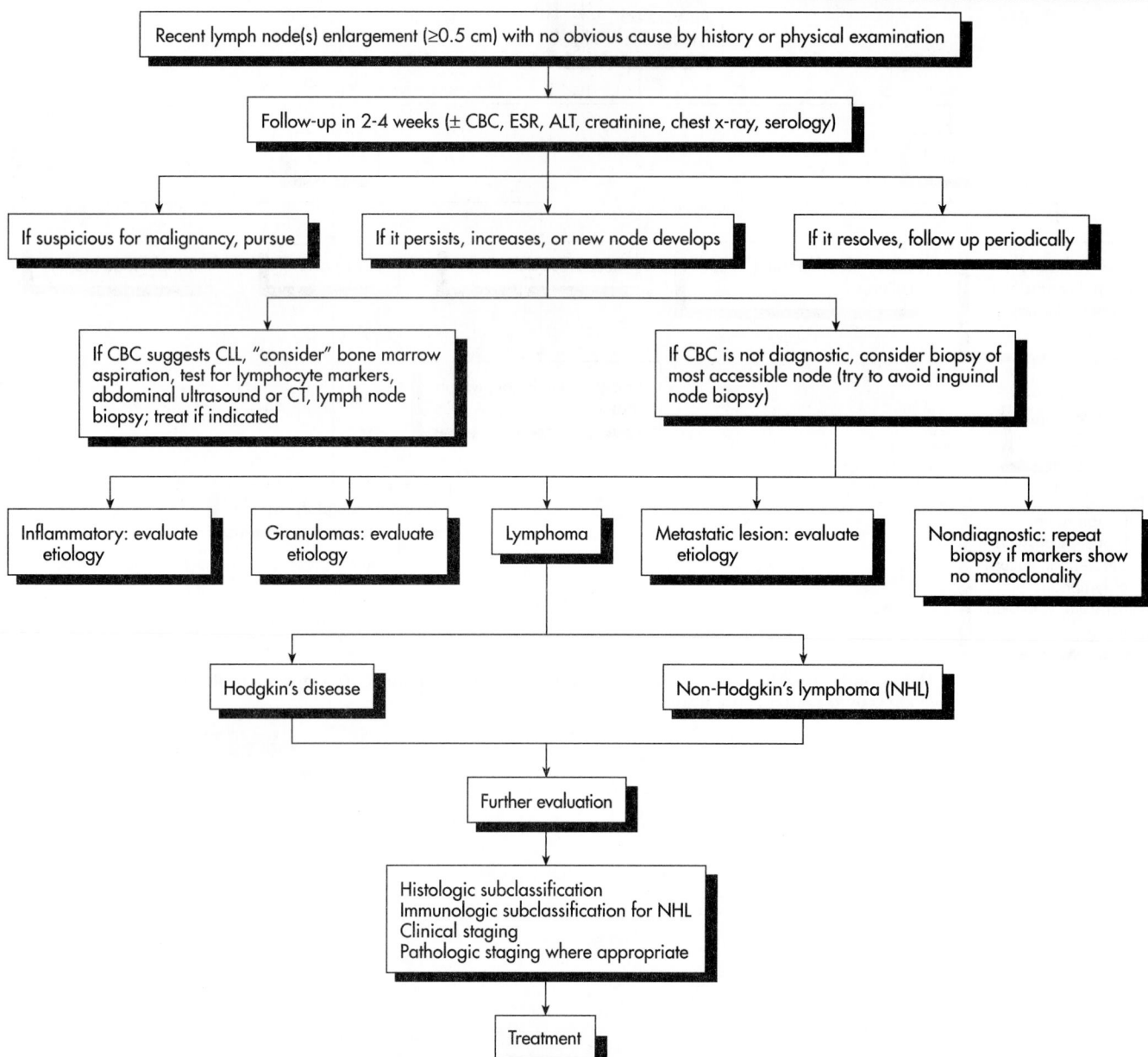

Fig. 3-122 Workup of lymphadenopathy. *ALT,* Alanine aminotransferase; *CBC,* complete blood count; *CLL,* chronic lymphocytic leukemia; *CT,* computed tomography; *ESR,* erythrocyte sedimentation rate. (Modified from Noble J [ed]: *Primary care medicine,* ed 3, St Louis, 2001, Mosby.)

LYMPHADENOPATHY, INGUINAL

Lymphadenopathy, inguinal
ICD-9CM # 785.6

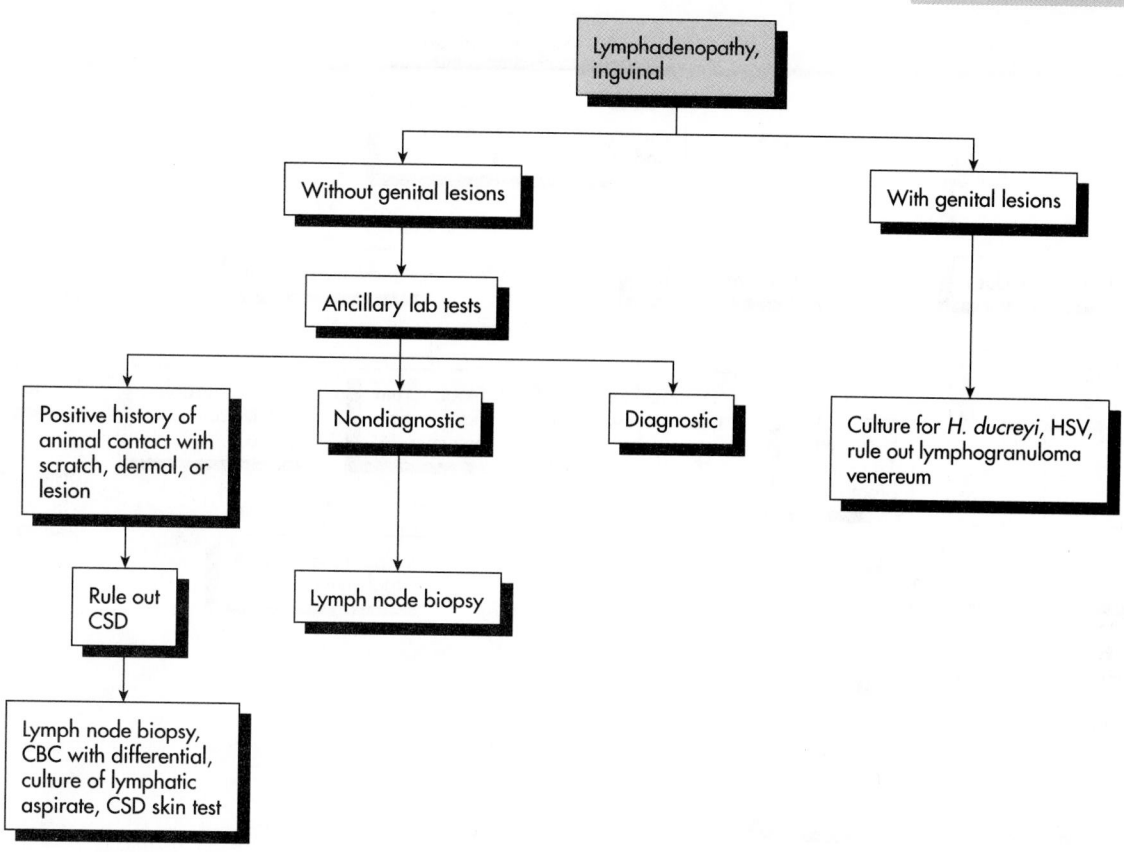

Fig. 3-123   Lymphadenopathy, inguinal. *CBC,* Complete blood count; *CSD,* cat-scratch disease; *HSV,* herpes simplex virus.

MALABSORPTION, SUSPECTED

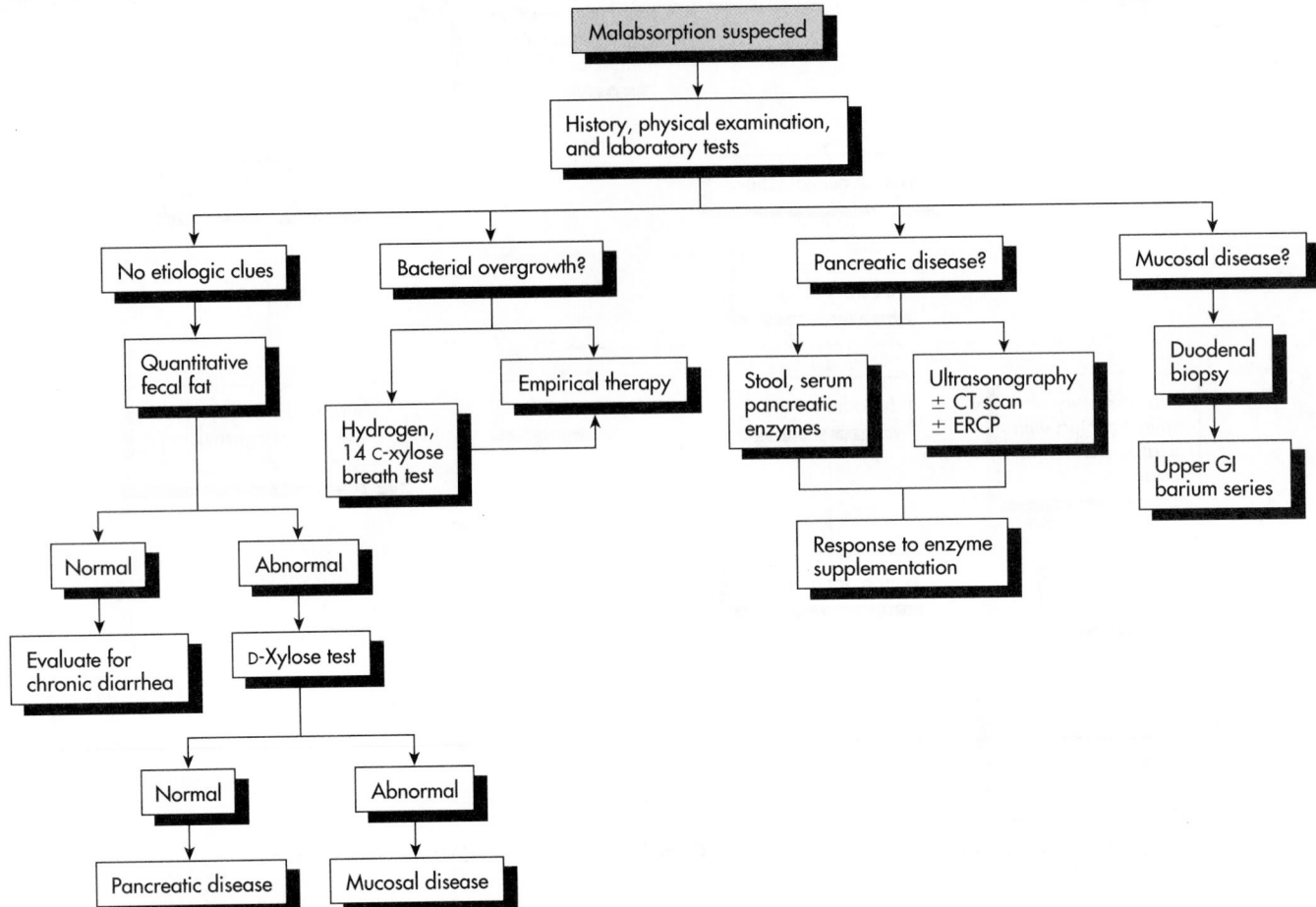

Fig. 3-124   Approach to the patient with suspected malabsorption. *CT,* Computed tomography; *ERCP,* endoscopic retrograde cholangiopancreatography; *GI,* gastrointestinal. (Adapted from Riley SA, Marsh MN: Maldigestion and malabsorption. In Feldman M, Scharschmidt BF, Sleisenger MH [eds]: *Sleisenger and Fordtran's gastrointestinal and liver diseases: pathophysiology/diagnosis/management,* ed 6, Philadelphia, 1998, WB Saunders.)

MENINGITIS

Meningitis
ICD-9CM # 320   Bacterial meningitis
             047.8 Meningitis, aseptic

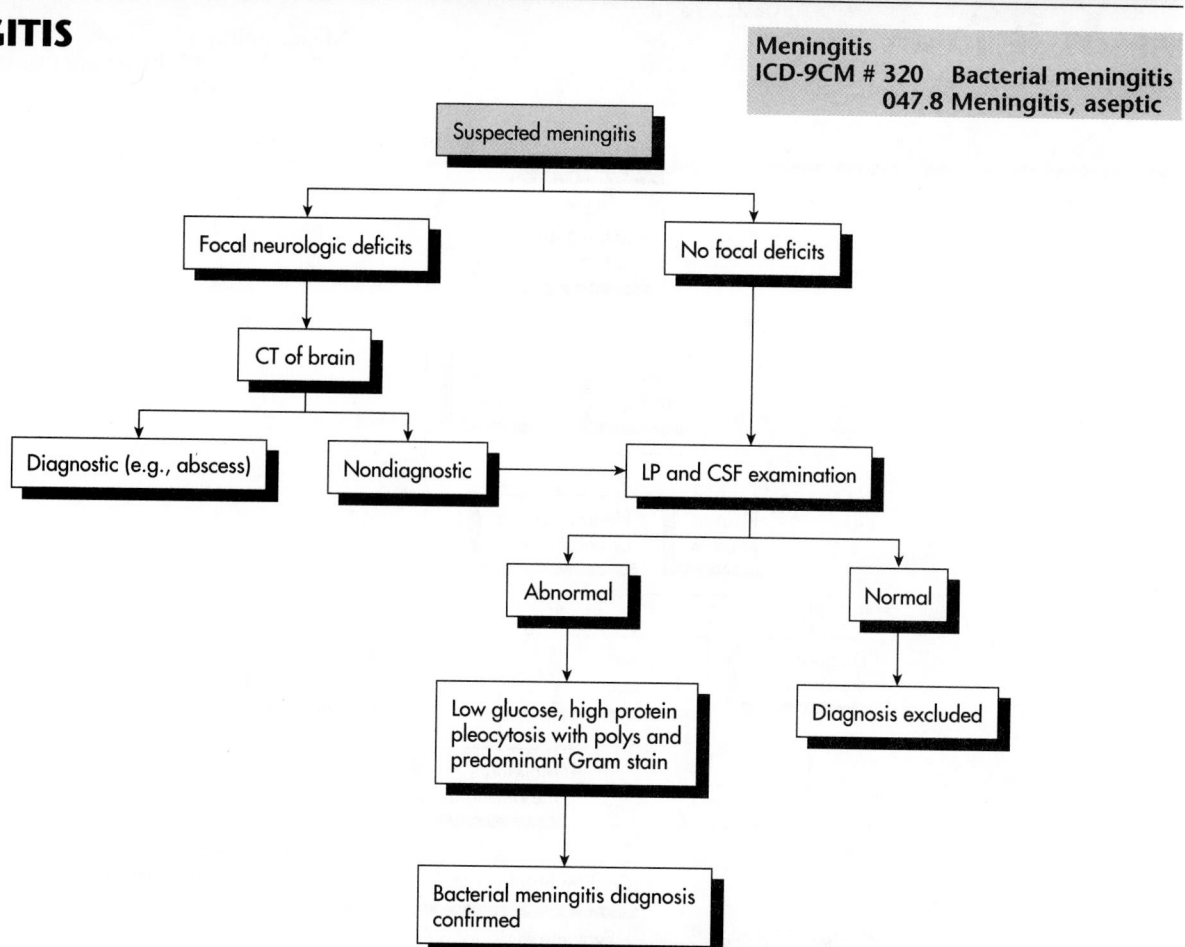

Fig. 3-125   Meningitis. *CSF,* Cat-scratch fever; *CT,* computed tomography; *LP,* lumbar puncture.

MESOTHELIOMA

Mesothelioma
ICD-9CM # 199.1 Malignant mesothelioma,
site Nos

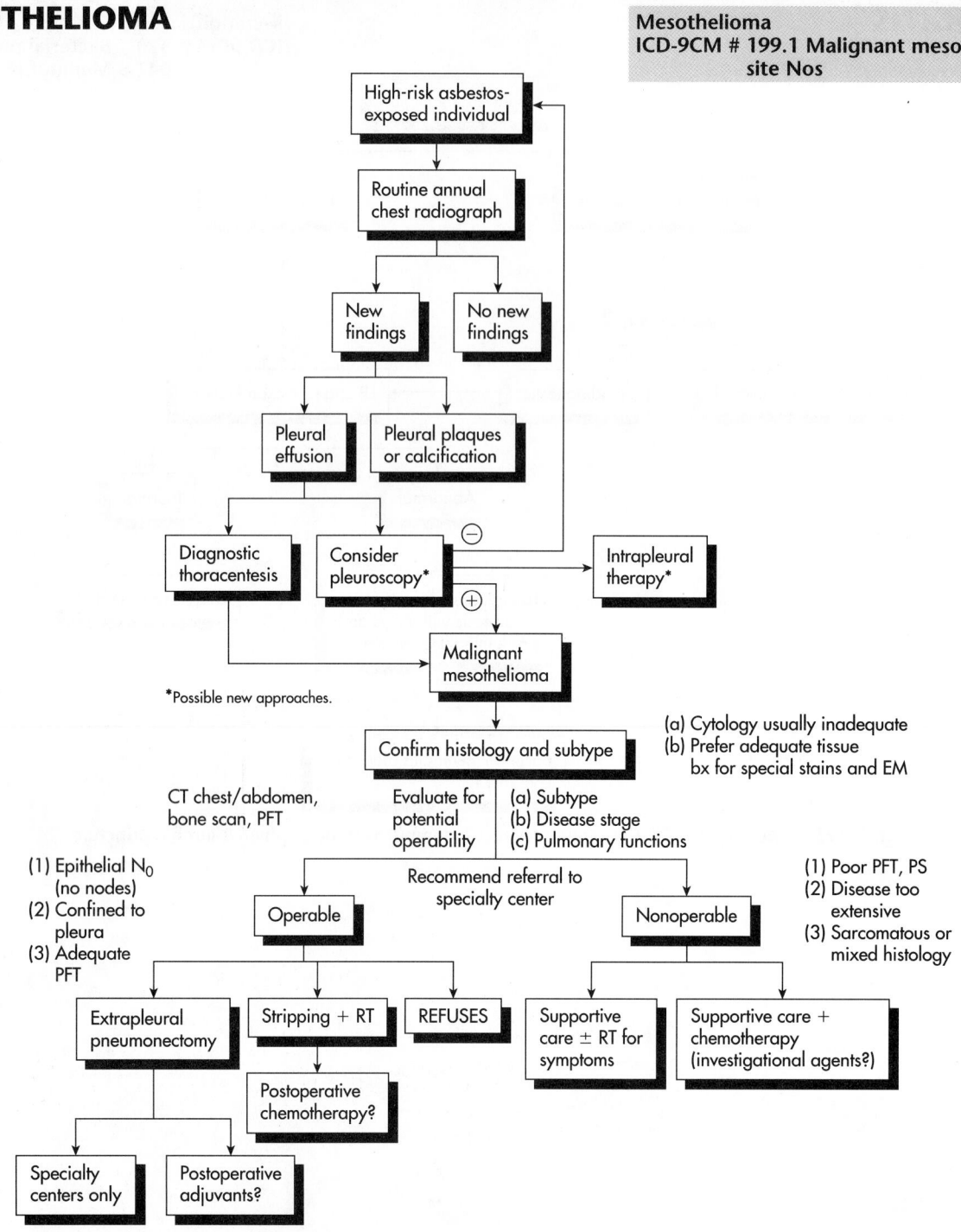

Fig. 3-126   Evaluation and treatment of mesothelioma. *bx,* Biopsy; *CT,* computed tomography; *EM,* electron microscopy; *PFT,* pulmonary function test; *PS,* pleural sclerosis; *RT,* respiratory therapy. (From Abeloff MD: *Clinical oncology,* ed 2, New York, 2000, Churchill Livingstone.)

MULTIPLE MYELOMA

Multiple myeloma
ICD-9CM # 203.0

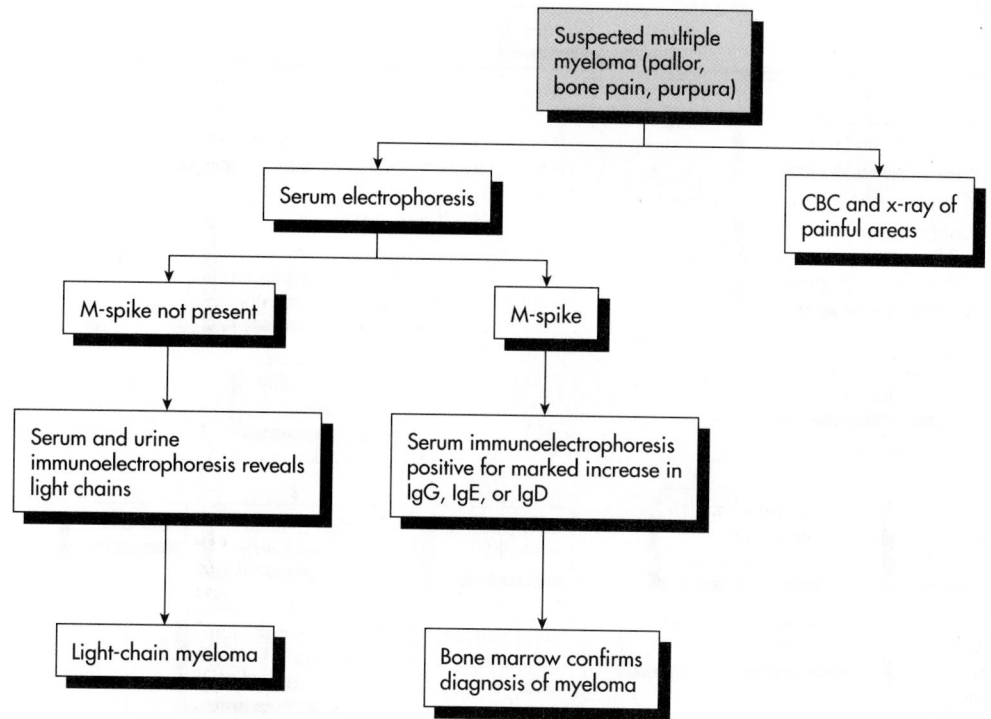

Fig. 3-127   **Multiple myeloma.** *CBC,* Complete blood count; *Ig,* immunoglobulin.

III

MURMUR, DIASTOLIC

Murmur, diastolic
ICD-9CM # 785.2 Murmur heart

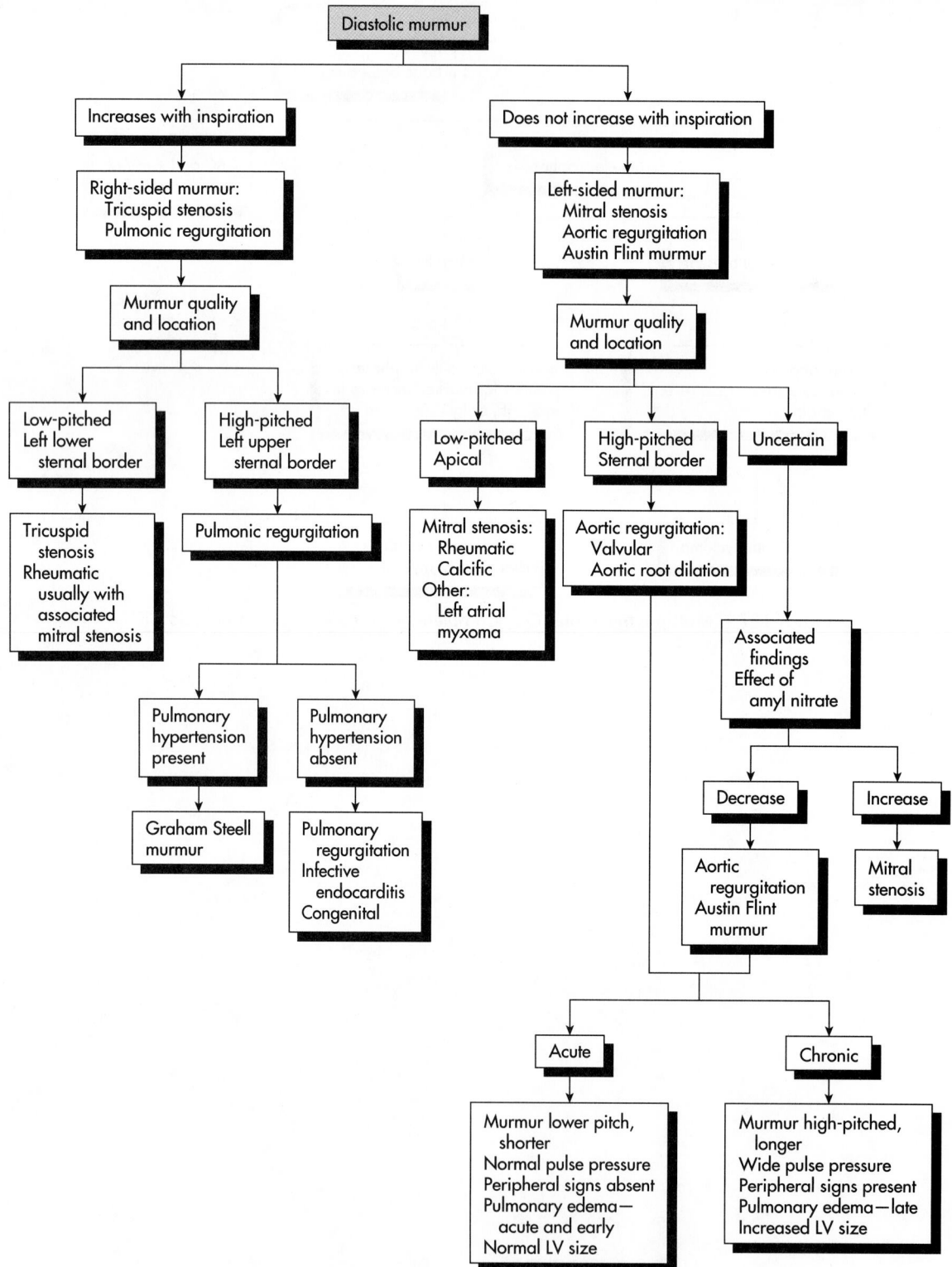

Fig. 3-128 **Diastolic murmur.** *LV,* Left ventricle. (From Greene HL, Johnson WP, Lemke D [eds]: *Decision making in medicine,* ed 2, St Louis, 1998, Mosby.)

MURMUR, SYSTOLIC

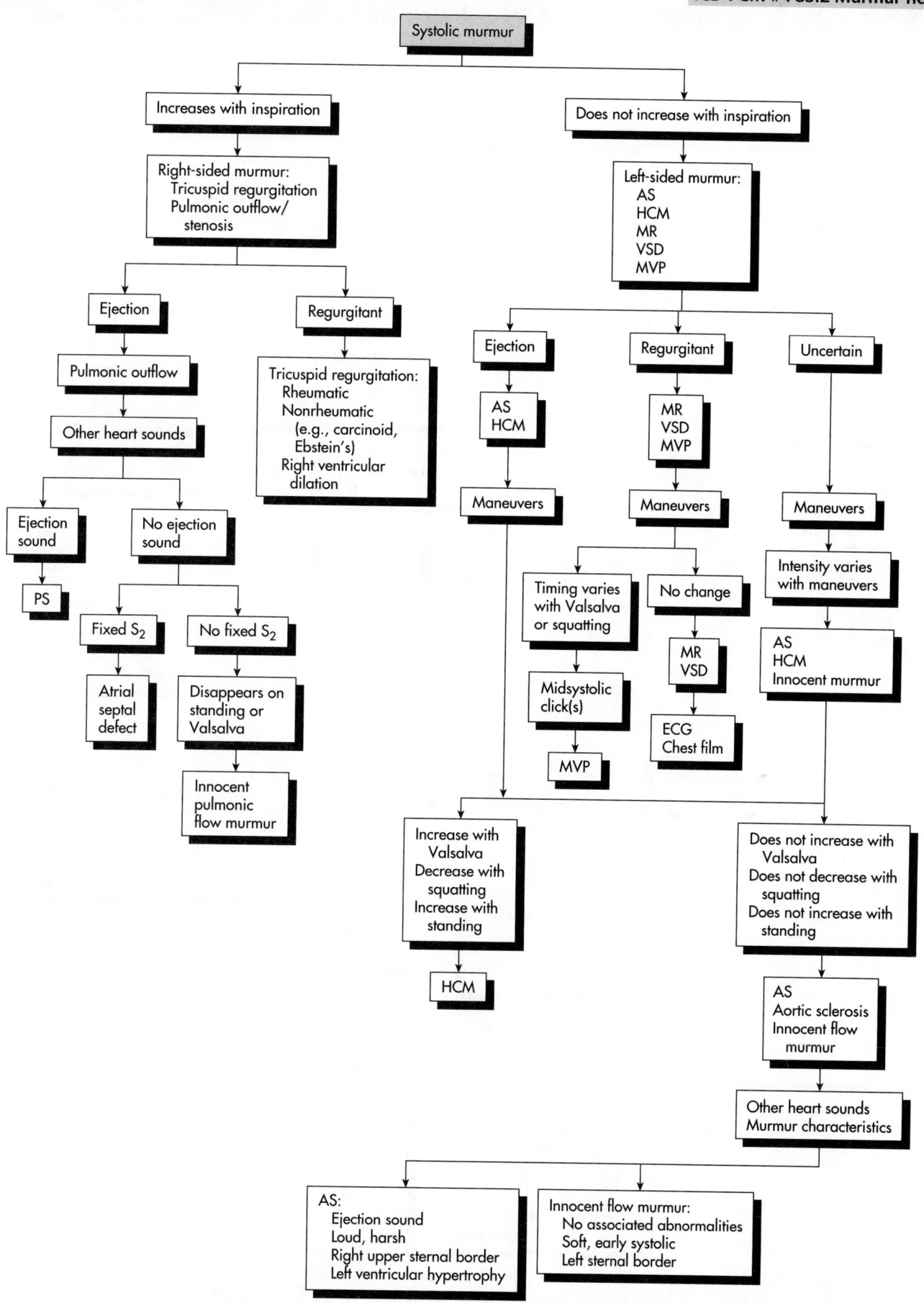

Fig. 3-129   Systolic murmur. *AS,* Aortic stenosis; *ECG,* electrocardiogram; *HCM,* hypertrophic cardiomyopathy; *MR,* mitral regurgitation; *MVP,* mitral valve prolapse; *PS,* pulmonary stenosis; *VSD,* ventricular septal defect. (From Greene HL, Johnson WP, Lemke D [eds]: *Decision making in medicine,* ed 2, St Louis, 1998, Mosby.)

MUSCLE CRAMPS AND ACHES

Muscle cramps and aches
ICD-9CM # 729.82

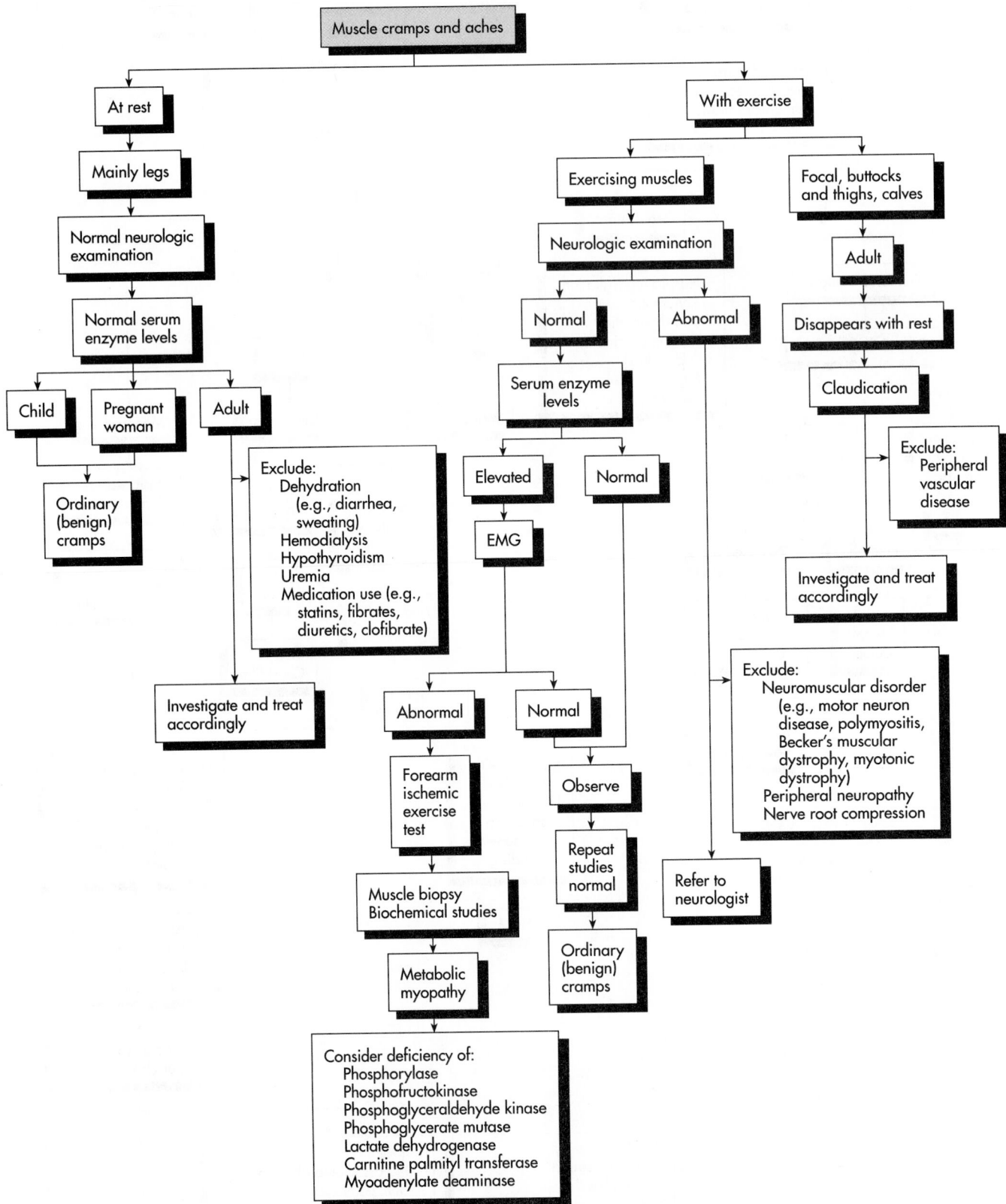

Fig. 3-130   Evaluation of muscle cramps and aches. *EMG,* Electromyography. (From Greene HL, Johnson WP, Lemcke D [eds]: *Decision making in medicine,* ed 2, St Louis, 1998, Mosby.)

MUSCLE WEAKNESS

Muscle weakness
ICD-9CM # 728.9

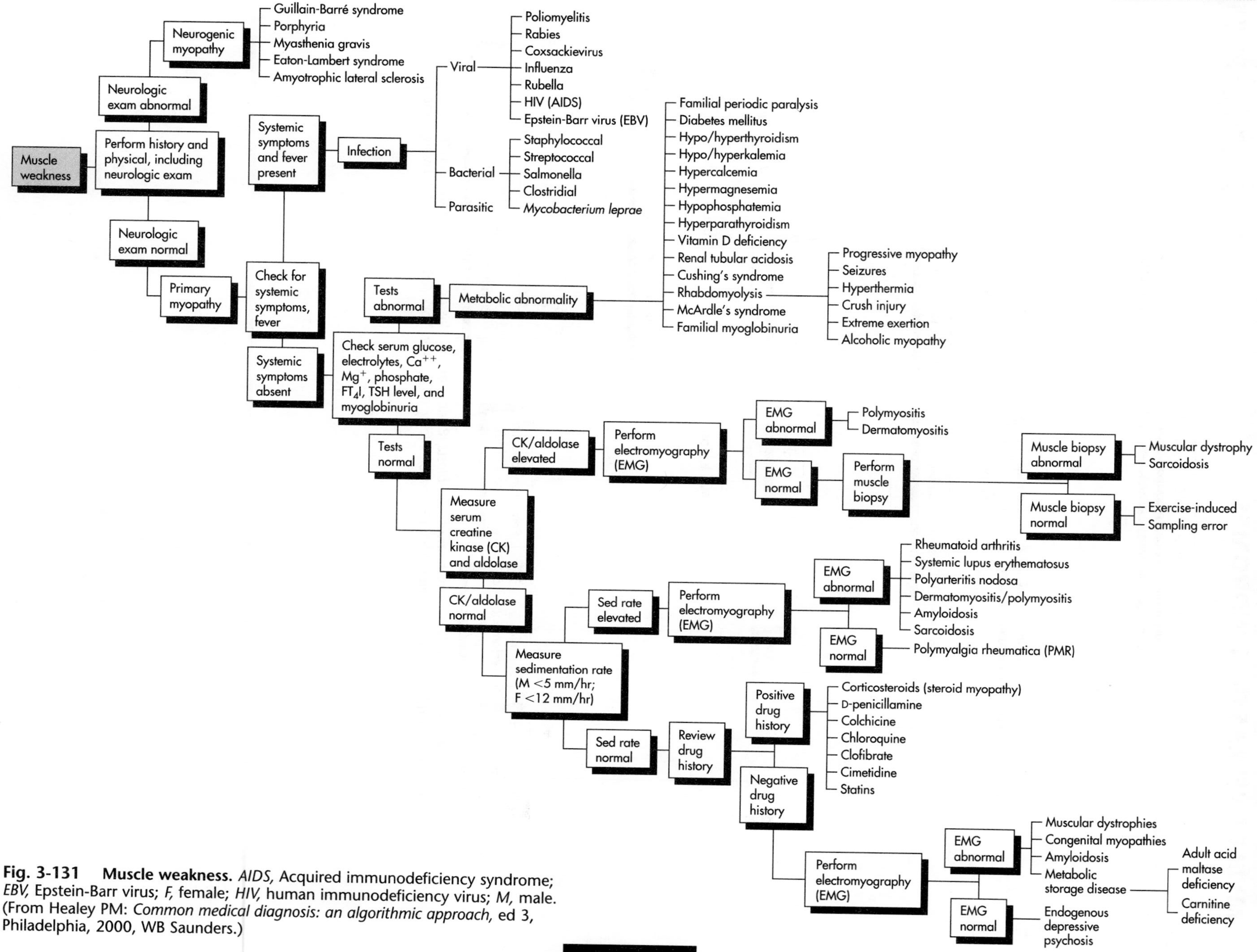

Fig. 3-131   Muscle weakness. *AIDS,* Acquired immunodeficiency syndrome; *EBV,* Epstein-Barr virus; *F,* female; *HIV,* human immunodeficiency virus; *M,* male. (From Healey PM: *Common medical diagnosis: an algorithmic approach,* ed 3, Philadelphia, 2000, WB Saunders.)

MYELODYSPLASTIC SYNDROMES

Myelodysplastic syndrome
ICD-9CM # 238.7

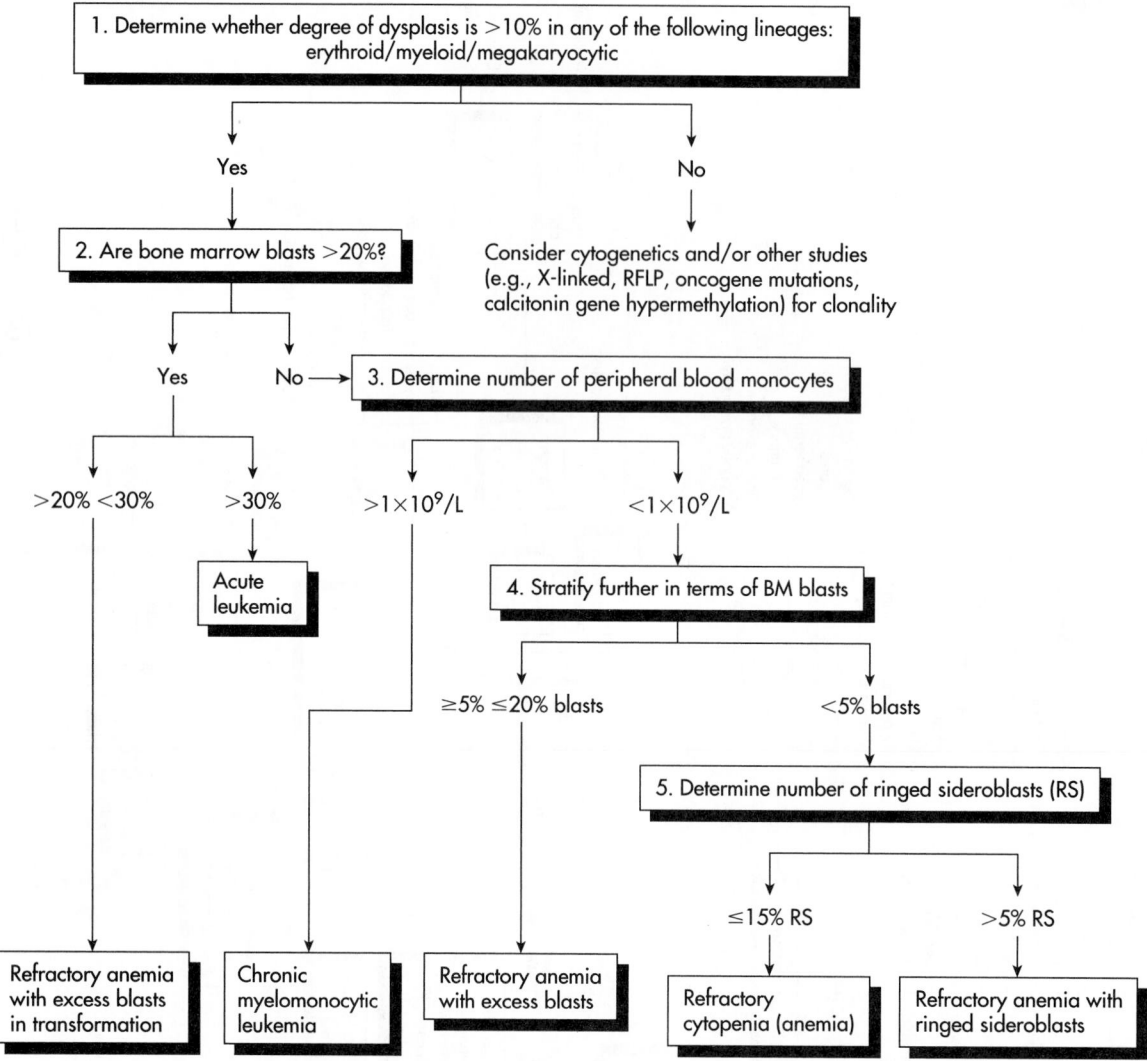

Fig. 3-132   Myelodysplastic syndromes. *BM blasts,* Bone marrow blastocyst; *RFLP,* restriction fragment length polymorphism. (From Abeloff MD: *Clinical oncology,* ed 2, New York, 2000, Churchill Livingstone.)

MYOCARDIAL ISCHEMIA, SUSPECTED

Dementia
ICD-9CM # 290.10 Dementia, presenile
                290.0 Dementia, senile
                437.0 Dementia, arteriosclerotic

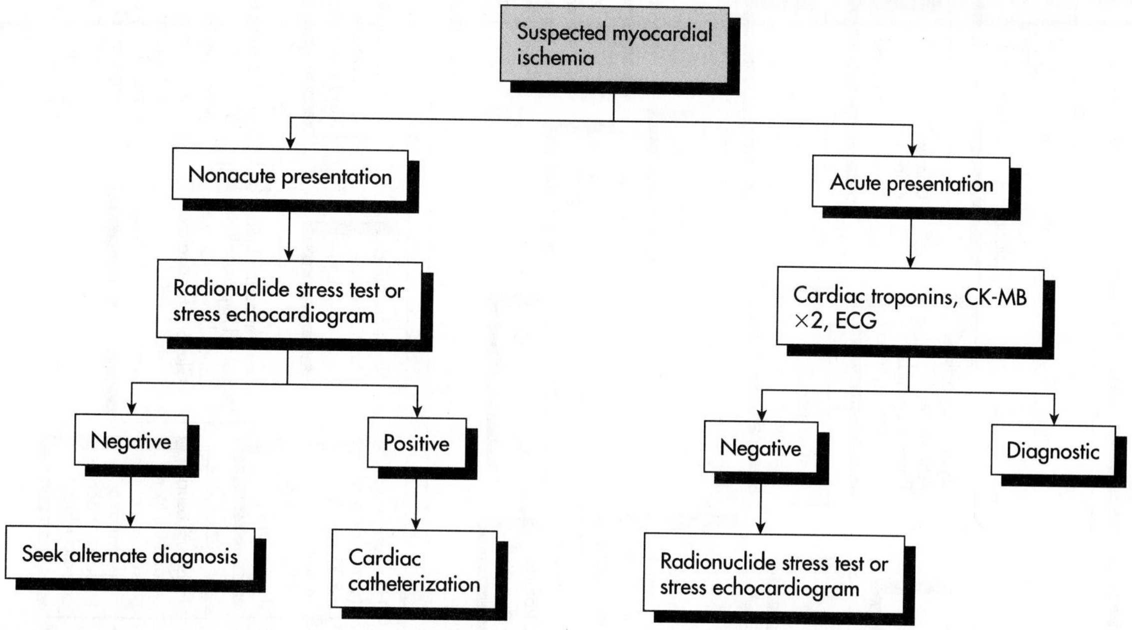

Fig. 3-133 **Myocardial ischemia, suspected.** *CK-MB,* Myocardial muscle creatine kinase isoenzyme; *ECG,* electrocardiogram.

III

NEPHROLITHIASIS

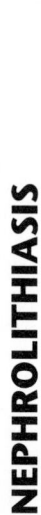

Nephrolithiasis
ICD-9CM # 592.9 Urinary calculus

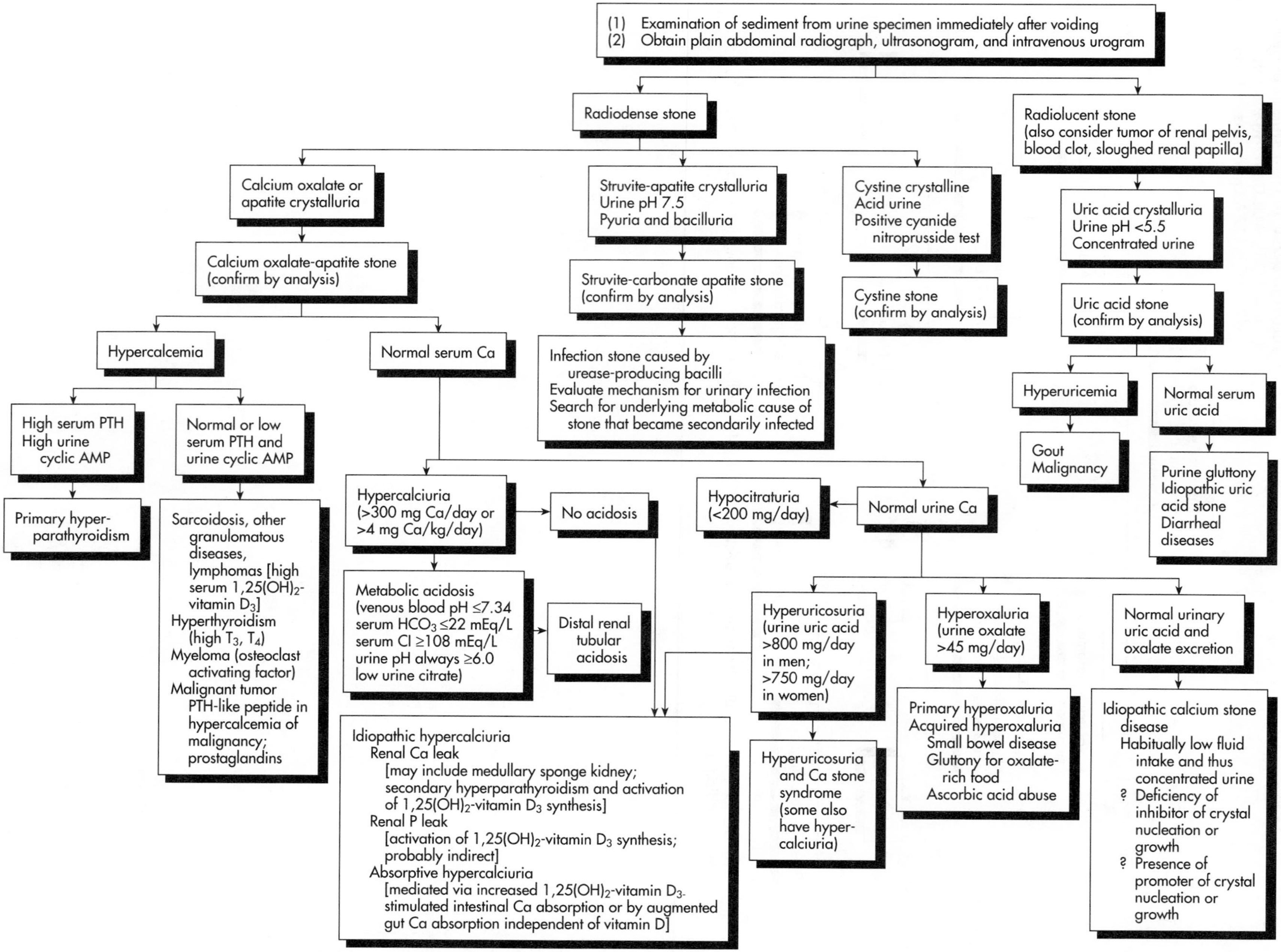

(1) Examination of sediment from urine specimen immediately after voiding
(2) Obtain plain abdominal radiograph, ultrasonogram, and intravenous urogram

Radiolucent stone (also consider tumor of renal pelvis, blood clot, sloughed renal papilla)

Uric acid crystalluria
Urine pH <5.5
Concentrated urine

Uric acid stone (confirm by analysis)

Normal serum uric acid

Purine gluttony
Idiopathic uric acid stone
Diarrheal diseases

Hyperuricemia

Gout
Malignancy

Normal urinary uric acid and oxalate excretion

Idiopathic calcium stone disease
Habitually low fluid intake and thus concentrated urine
? Deficiency of inhibitor of crystal nucleation or growth
? Presence of promoter of crystal nucleation or growth

Radiodense stone

Cystine crystalline
Acid urine
Positive cyanide nitroprusside test

Cystine stone (confirm by analysis)

Struvite-apatite crystalluria
Urine pH 7.5
Pyuria and bacilluria

Struvite-carbonate apatite stone (confirm by analysis)

Infection stone caused by urease-producing bacilli
Evaluate mechanism for urinary infection
Search for underlying metabolic cause of stone that became secondarily infected

Normal urine Ca

Hyperoxaluria (urine oxalate >45 mg/day)

Primary hyperoxaluria
Acquired hyperoxaluria
Small bowel disease
Gluttony for oxalate-rich food
Ascorbic acid abuse

Hypocitraturia (<200 mg/day)

Hyperuricosuria (urine uric acid >800 mg/day in men; >750 mg/day in women)

Hyperuricosuria and Ca stone syndrome (some also have hypercalciuria)

Calcium oxalate or apatite crystalluria

Calcium oxalate-apatite stone (confirm by analysis)

Normal serum Ca

No acidosis

Distal renal tubular acidosis

Idiopathic hypercalciuria
Renal Ca leak [may include medullary sponge kidney; secondary hyperparathyroidism and activation of 1,25(OH)₂-vitamin D₃ synthesis]
Renal P leak [activation of 1,25(OH)₂-vitamin D₃ synthesis; probably indirect]
Absorptive hypercalciuria [mediated via increased 1,25(OH)₂-vitamin D₃-stimulated intestinal Ca absorption or by augmented gut Ca absorption independent of vitamin D]

Hypercalciuria (>300 mg Ca/day or >4 mg Ca/kg/day)

Metabolic acidosis (venous blood pH ≤7.34 serum HCO₃ ≤22 mEq/L serum Cl ≥108 mEq/L urine pH always ≥6.0 low urine citrate)

Hypercalcemia

Normal or low serum PTH and urine cyclic AMP

Sarcoidosis, other granulomatous diseases, lymphomas [high serum 1,25(OH)₂-vitamin D₃]
Hyperthyroidism (high T₃, T₄)
Myeloma (osteoclast activating factor)
Malignant tumor
PTH-like peptide in hypercalcemia of malignancy; prostaglandins

High serum PTH
High urine cyclic AMP

Primary hyper-parathyroidism

Fig. 3-134 **Evaluation of patients with suspected nephrolithiasis (flank pain, ureteral colic, hematuria, fever).** *AMP,* Adenosine monophosphate; *PTH,* parathyroid hormone. (From Stein JH [ed]: *Internal medicine,* ed 5, St Louis, 1998, Mosby.)

NEUTROPENIA

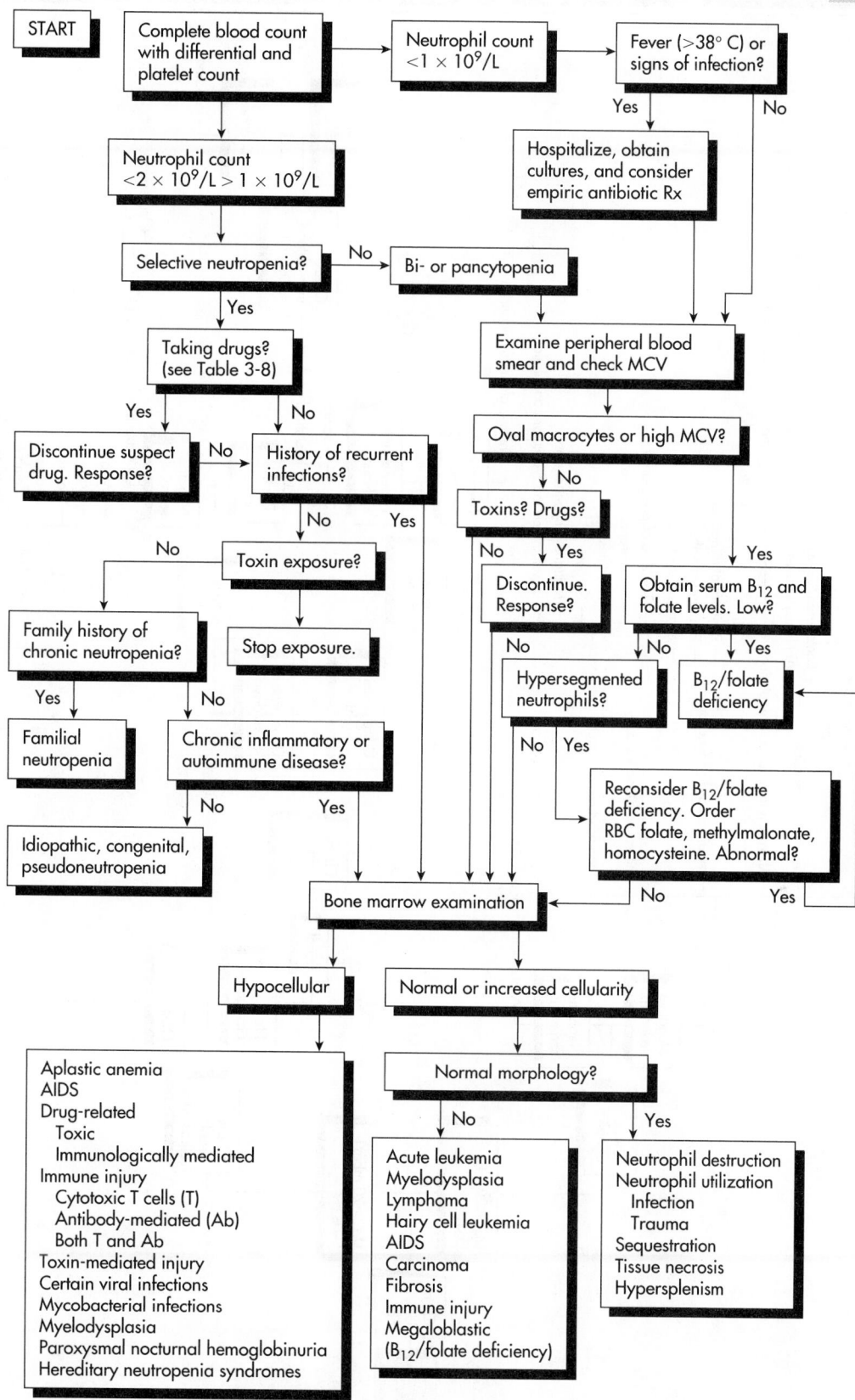

Fig. 3-135   A practical algorithm for the evaluation of patients with neutropenia. The fundamental diagnostic principle is that for patients with severe neutropenia or for those with bicytopenia or pancytopenia, bone marrow examination will likely be necessary unless the following diagnoses are made: (1) a nutritional (folate or vitamin B_{12}) deficiency or (2) drug- or toxin-induced neutropenia in a patient whose neutropenia resolves after discontinuation of the offending agent. *AIDS,* Acquired immunodeficiency syndrome; *MCV,* mean corpuscular volume; *RBC,* red blood cell. (From Goldman L, Ausiello D [eds]: *Cecil textbook of medicine,* ed 22, Philadelphia, 2004, WB Saunders.)

OLIGURIA

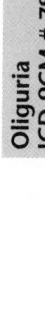

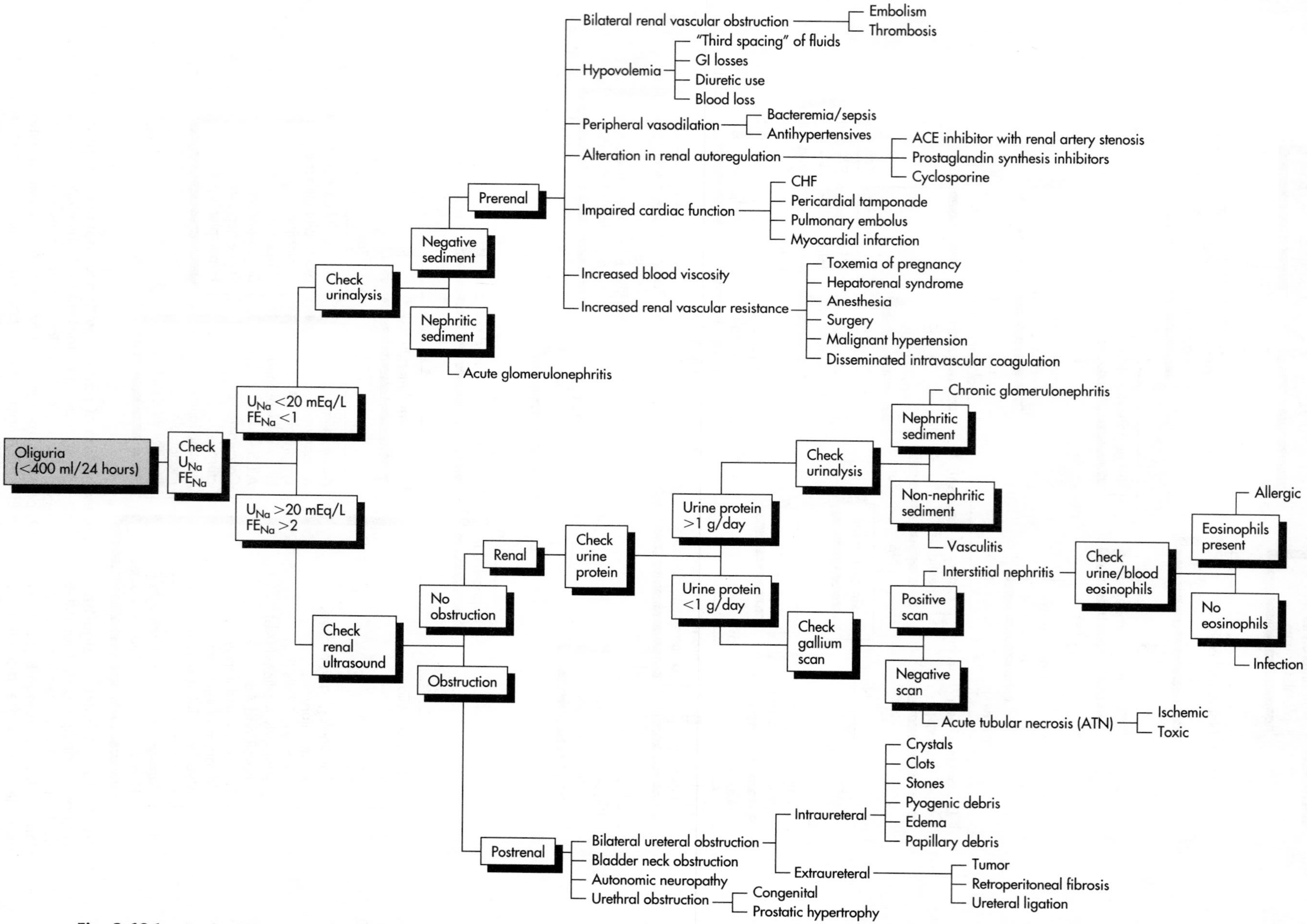

Oliguria (<400 ml/24 hours)

Check U_{Na} FE_{Na}

- U_{Na} <20 mEq/L FE_{Na} <1
- U_{Na} >20 mEq/L FE_{Na} >2

U_{Na} <20 mEq/L, FE_{Na} <1 → Check urinalysis

- Negative sediment → **Prerenal**
  - Bilateral renal vascular obstruction
    - Embolism
    - Thrombosis
  - Hypovolemia
    - "Third spacing" of fluids
    - GI losses
    - Diuretic use
    - Blood loss
  - Peripheral vasodilation
    - Bacteremia/sepsis
    - Antihypertensives
  - Alteration in renal autoregulation
    - ACE inhibitor with renal artery stenosis
    - Prostaglandin synthesis inhibitors
    - Cyclosporine
  - Impaired cardiac function
    - CHF
    - Pericardial tamponade
    - Pulmonary embolus
    - Myocardial infarction
  - Increased blood viscosity
  - Increased renal vascular resistance
    - Toxemia of pregnancy
    - Hepatorenal syndrome
    - Anesthesia
    - Surgery
    - Malignant hypertension
    - Disseminated intravascular coagulation
- Nephritic sediment → Acute glomerulonephritis

U_{Na} >20 mEq/L, FE_{Na} >2 → Check renal ultrasound

- No obstruction → **Renal** → Check urine protein
  - Urine protein >1 g/day → Check urinalysis
    - Nephritic sediment → Chronic glomerulonephritis
    - Non-nephritic sediment → Vasculitis
  - Urine protein <1 g/day → Check gallium scan
    - Positive scan → Interstitial nephritis → Check urine/blood eosinophils
      - Eosinophils present → Allergic
      - No eosinophils → Infection
    - Negative scan → Acute tubular necrosis (ATN)
      - Ischemic
      - Toxic
- Obstruction → **Postrenal**
  - Bilateral ureteral obstruction
    - Intraureteral
      - Crystals
      - Clots
      - Stones
      - Pyogenic debris
      - Edema
      - Papillary debris
    - Extraureteral
      - Tumor
      - Retroperitoneal fibrosis
      - Ureteral ligation
  - Bladder neck obstruction
    - Congenital
    - Prostatic hypertrophy
  - Autonomic neuropathy
  - Urethral obstruction

Fig. 3-136 Evaluation of oliguria. *ACE*, Angiotensin-converting enzyme; *CHF*, congestive heart failure; *GI*, gastrointestinal. (From Healey PM: *Common medical diagnosis: an algorithmic approach*, ed 3, Philadelphia, 2000, WB Saunders.)

PANCREATIC ISLET CELL TUMORS

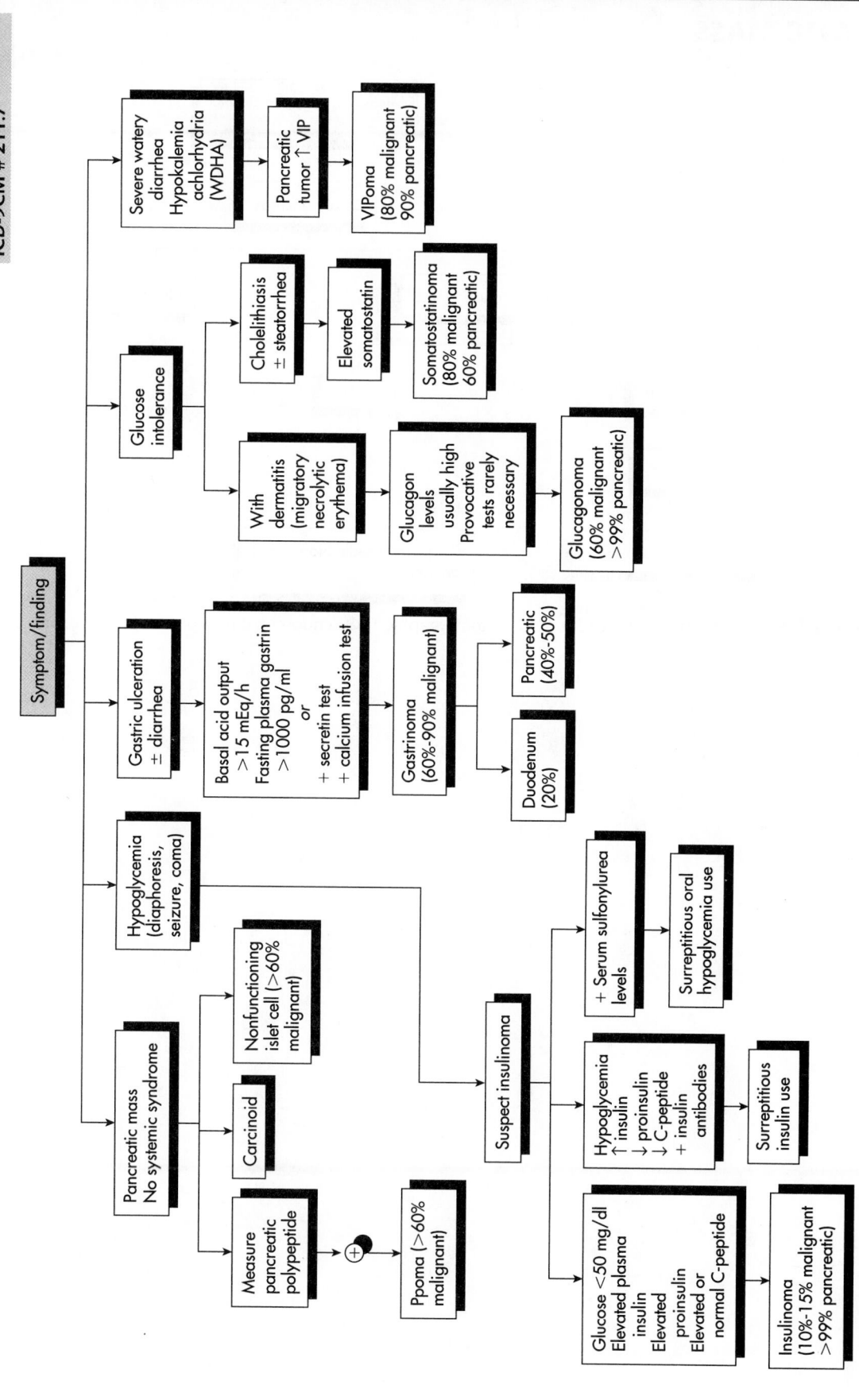

Fig. 3-137   Diagnosis of pancreatic islet cell tumors. *Ppoma,* Islet cell tumor secreting pancreatic polypeptide; *VIP,* vasoactive intestinal peptide; *VIPoma,* islet cell tumor secreting vasoactive intestinal peptide. (From Abeloff MD: *Clinical oncology,* ed 2, New York, 2000, Churchill Livingstone.)

PANCREATIC MASS

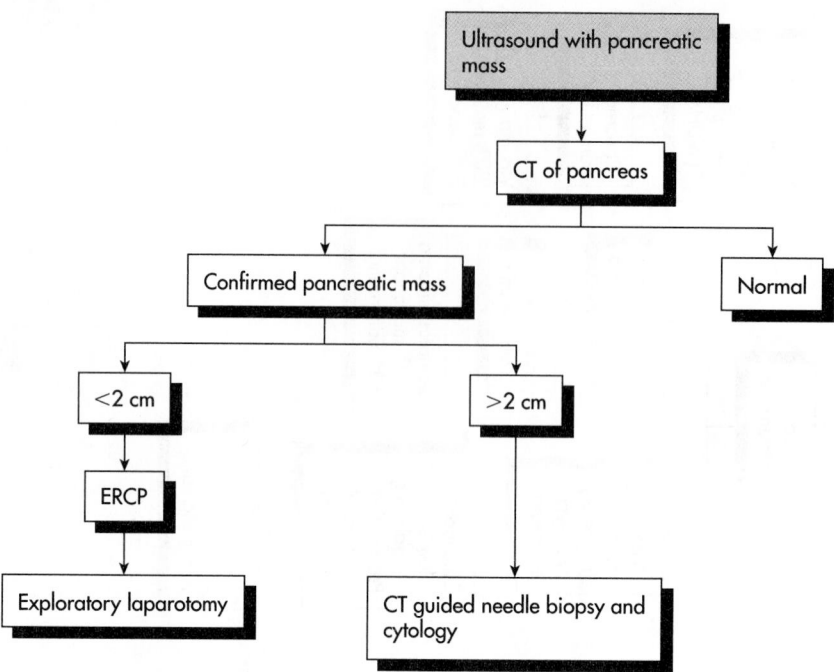

Fig. 3-138   **Pancreatic mass.** *CT,* Computed tomography; *ERCP,* endoscopic retrograde cholangiopancreatography.

PATIENT WITH ILL-DEFINED PHYSICAL COMPLAINTS

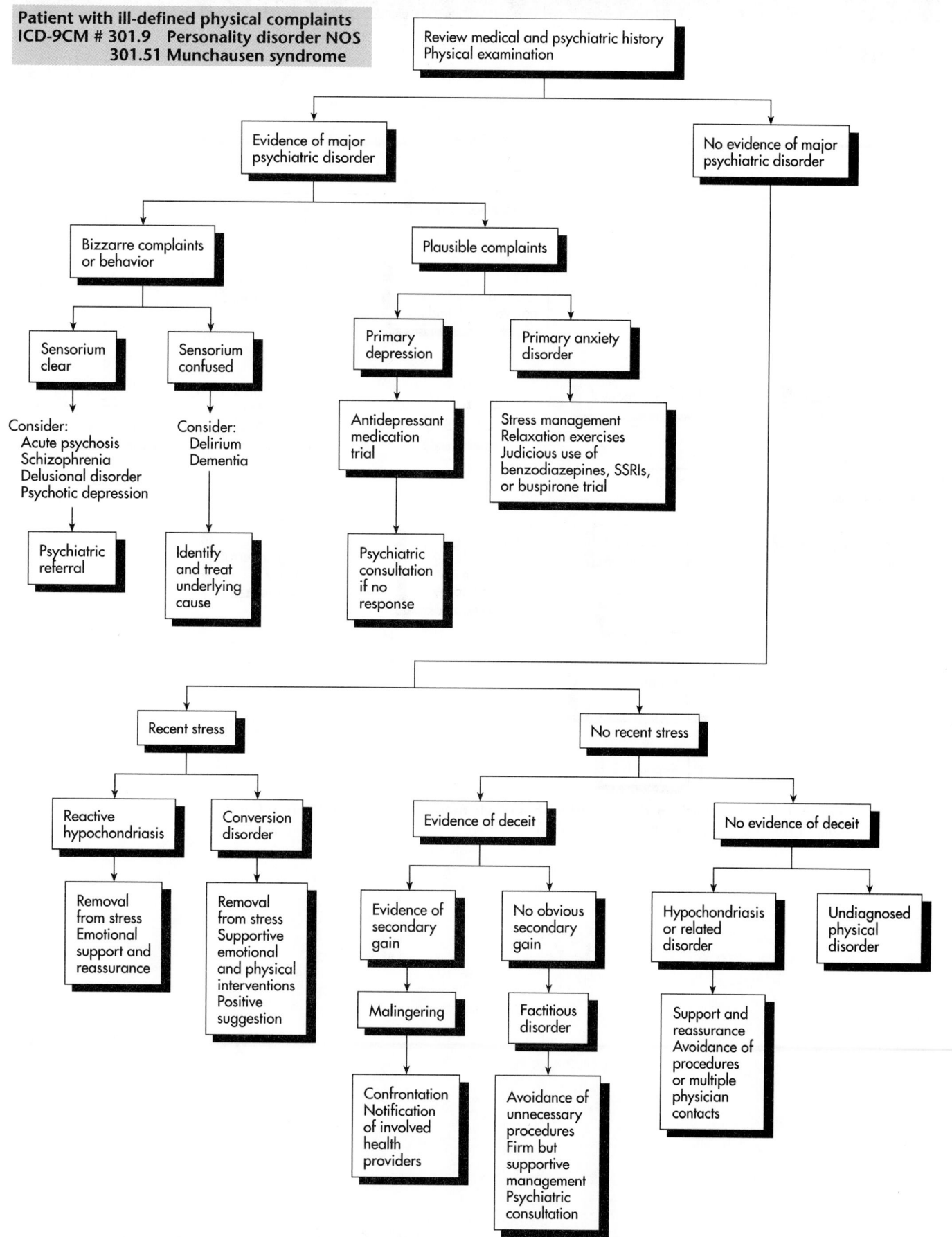

Patient with ill-defined physical complaints
ICD-9CM # 301.9   Personality disorder NOS
301.51 Munchausen syndrome

Review medical and psychiatric history
Physical examination

Evidence of major psychiatric disorder

No evidence of major psychiatric disorder

Bizzarre complaints or behavior

Plausible complaints

Sensorium clear

Sensorium confused

Primary depression

Primary anxiety disorder

Consider:
Acute psychosis
Schizophrenia
Delusional disorder
Psychotic depression

Consider:
Delirium
Dementia

Antidepressant medication trial

Stress management
Relaxation exercises
Judicious use of benzodiazepines, SSRIs, or buspirone trial

Psychiatric referral

Identify and treat underlying cause

Psychiatric consultation if no response

Recent stress

No recent stress

Reactive hypochondriasis

Conversion disorder

Evidence of deceit

No evidence of deceit

Removal from stress
Emotional support and reassurance

Removal from stress
Supportive emotional and physical interventions
Positive suggestion

Evidence of secondary gain

No obvious secondary gain

Hypochondriasis or related disorder

Undiagnosed physical disorder

Malingering

Factitious disorder

Support and reassurance
Avoidance of procedures or multiple physician contacts

Confrontation
Notification of involved health providers

Avoidance of unnecessary procedures
Firm but supportive management
Psychiatric consultation

Fig. 3-139   Patient with ill-defined physical complaints. Previous or recent evaluations are noncontributory. *SSRIs,* Selective serotonin reuptake inhibitors. (From Greene H, Johnson WP, Lemcke D [eds]: *Decision making in medicine,* ed 2, St Louis, 1998, Mosby.)

PELVIC MASS

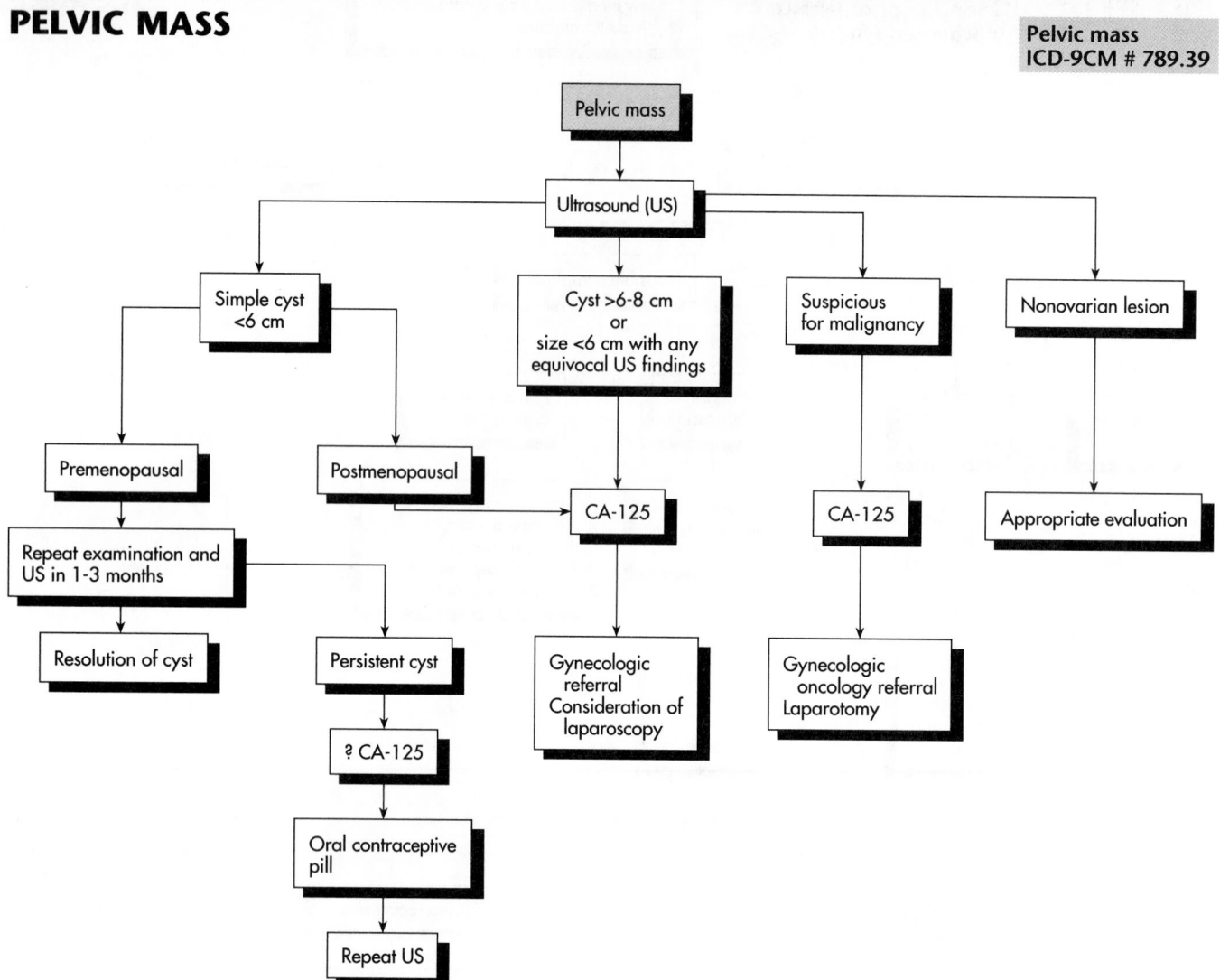

Fig. 3-140 **Approach to the patient with a pelvic mass.** *US,* Ultrasound. (From Carlson KJ et al: *Primary care of women,* ed 2, St Louis, 2002, Mosby.)

PELVIC PAIN, REPRODUCTIVE-AGE WOMAN

Pelvic pain, reproductive-age woman
ICD-9CM # 625.9

1. Rapid history and external abdominal examination

- **If surgical abdomen**: consider early ob/gyn/surgery consultation
  - Rupture (ectopic, cyst, abscess)
  - Torsion (adnexal, fibroid)
  - Perforation (uterine)
  - Appendicitis

2. Vital signs

- **If unstable**: Establish venous access and administer fluid bolus
  Spin Hct, type and crossmatch blood as needed
  Consider early ob/gyn/surgery consult without ultrasound
  - Rupture (ectopic, cyst)
  - Septic (abortion, abscess)
  - Placental (previa, abruptio)

3. Complete history and physical examination, and perform pelvic examination

- **If obvious abortion**: consult obstetrician and consider ultrasound
  - Abortion (incomplete, septic)

- **If late pregnancy**: forego pelvic exam
  Check for fetal heart tones
  Consider ultrasound followed by ob/gyn consultation
  - Placenta previa or abruptio
  - Premature labor contractions

4. Laboratory diagnostic workup (pregnancy test, CBC, UA/micro)

- **If pregnant**: consider ultrasound followed by ob/gyn consultation
  - R/I viable intrauterine gestation
  - R/O ectopic pregnancy, abortion, placental problems
  - R/O free intraperitoneal fluid, abscess formation

- **If not pregnant**: consider ultrasound and ob/gyn/surgery consultation
  - R/O gynecologic surgical problems
  - Ovarian cyst rupture, hemorrhage
  - Tubo-ovarian abscess rupture
  - Adnexal or fibroid torsion
  - Uterine perforation

  - Consider nonsurgical gynecologic problems
  - PID, pelvic adhesions, endometriosis, neoplasm, menstrual

  - R/O general surgery problems
  - Appendicitis and complications
  - Other, GI, GU, vascular, orthopedic surgery problems

  - Consider nonsurgical nongynecologic problems
  - Systemic illnesses

Fig. 3-141   Evaluation and management of reproductive-age women with acute pelvic pain. *CBC,* Complete blood count; *GI,* gastrointestinal; *GU,* genitourinary; *Hct,* hematocrit; *PID,* pelvic inflammatory disease; *UA/micro,* urinalysis with microscopy. (From Marx JA (ed): *Rosen's emergency medicine,* ed 5, St Louis, 2002, Mosby.)

PERIPHERAL NEUROPATHY

Peripheral neuropathy
ICD-9CM # 356.9 Peripheral nerve neuropathy
355.10 Lower extremity neuropathy
354.11 Upper extremity neuropathy

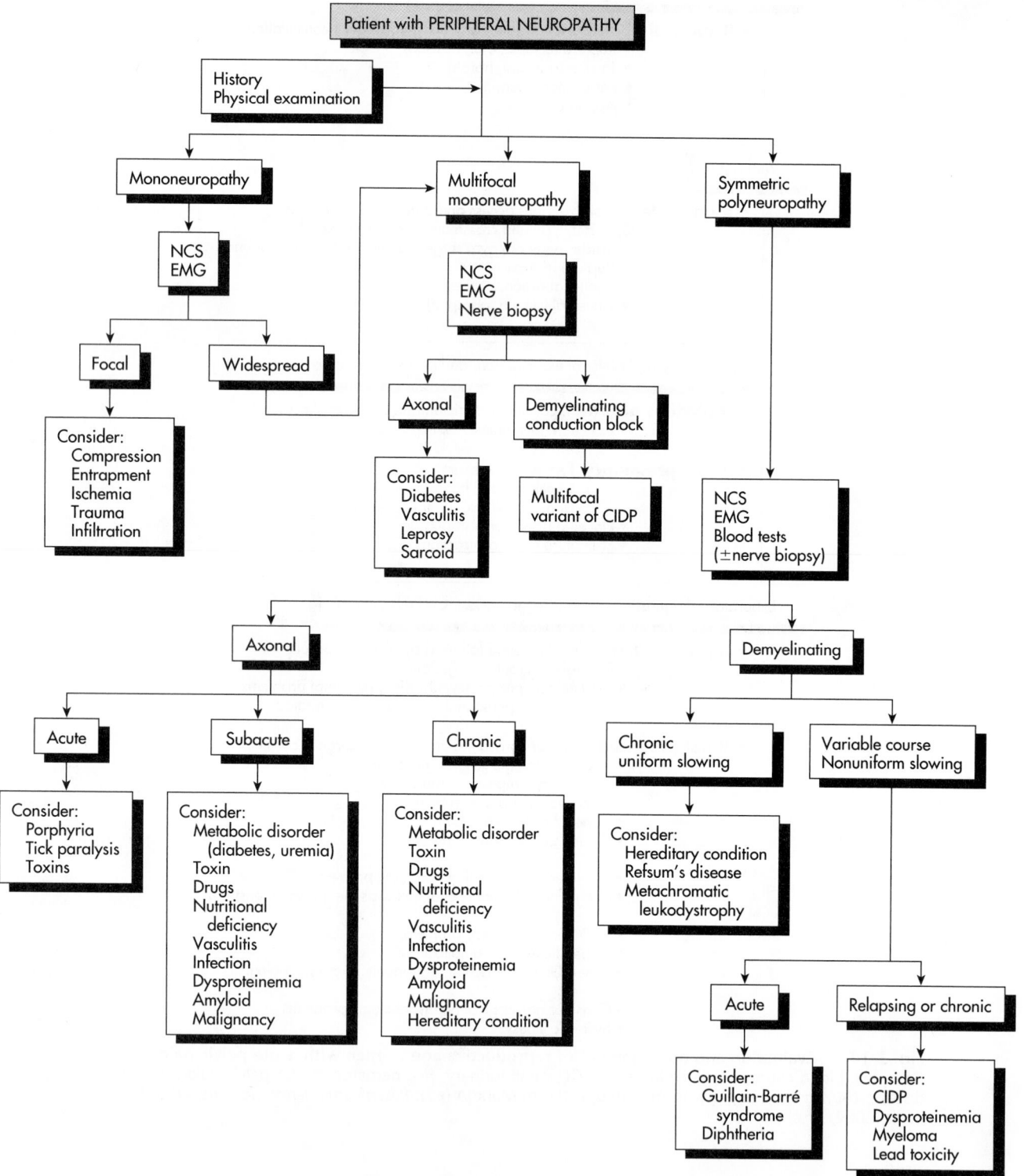

Fig. 3-142   Approach to the patient with peripheral neuropathy. *CIDP,* Chronic inflammatory demyelinating polyradioneuropathy; *EMG,* electromyogram; *NCS,* nerve conduction studies. (From Greene HL, Johnson WP, Lemcke DL: *Decision making in medicine,* ed 2, St Louis, 1988, Mosby.)

PHEOCHROMOCYTOMA

Pheochromocytoma
ICD-9CM # 194.0

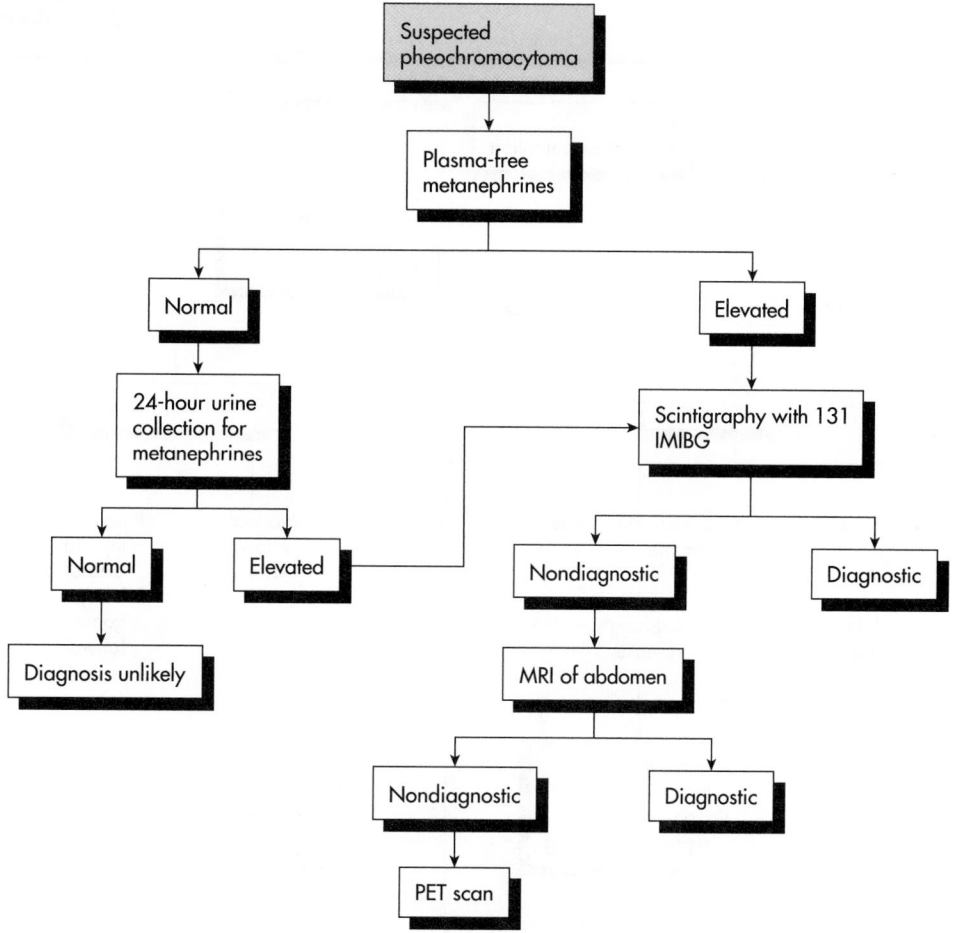

Fig. 3-143   Pheochromocytoma. *IMIBG,* Iodine metaiodobenzyl guanidine; *MRI,* magnetic resonance imaging; *PET,* positron emission tomography.

III

PITUITARY TUMOR

Pituitary tumor
ICD-9CM # 253   **Pituitary adenoma**
          253.0 **Acromegaly**
          253.1 **Prolactinoma**

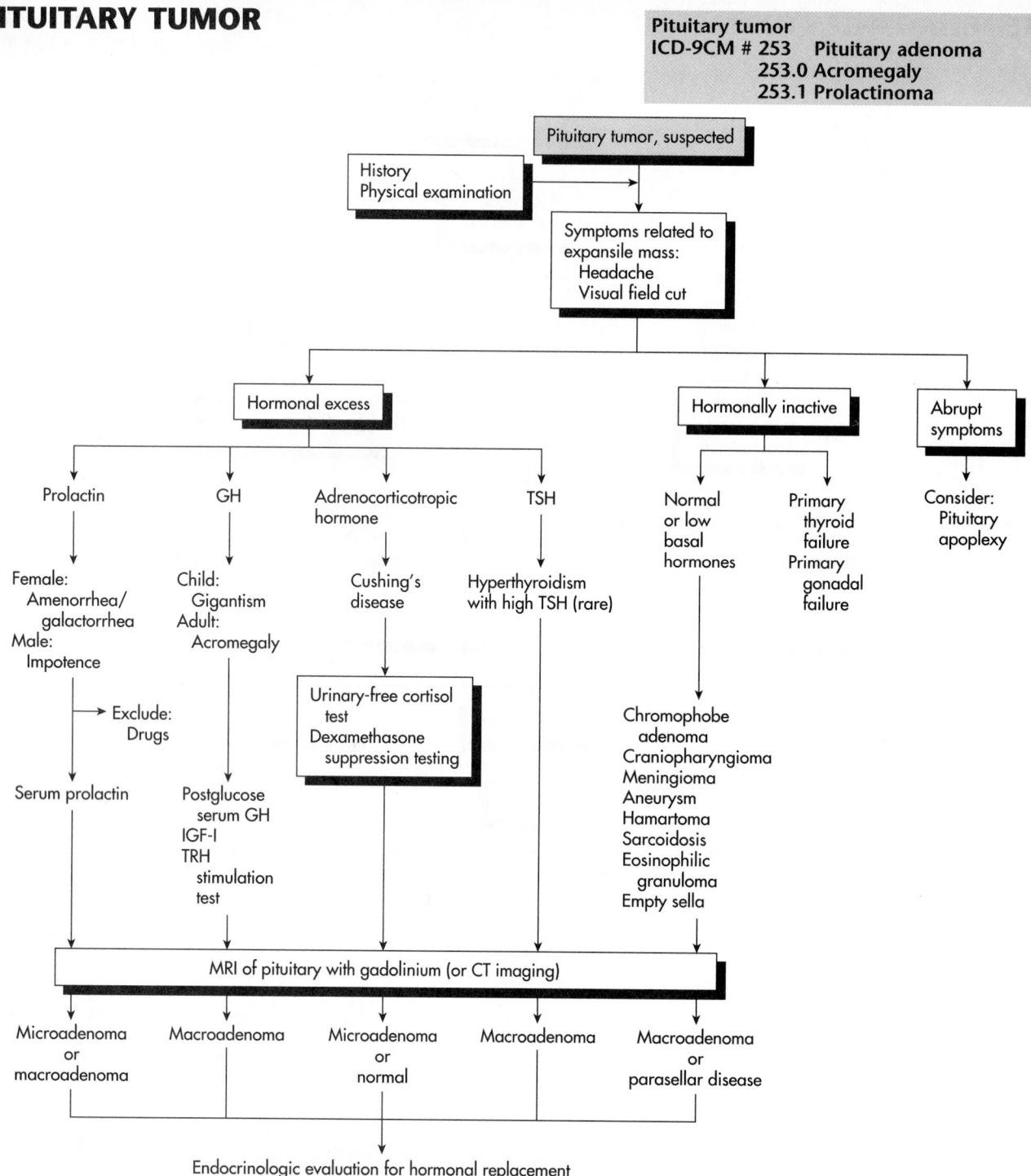

Fig. 3-144   **Evaluation of suspected pituitary tumor.** *CT,* Computed tomography; *GH,* growth hormone; *IGF-I,* one of the insulin-like growth factors; *MRI,* magnetic resonance imaging; *TRH,* thyrotropin-releasing hormone; *TSH,* thyroid-stimulating hormone. (From Greene HL, Johnson WP, Lemcke D: *Decision making in medicine,* ed 2, St Louis, 1998, Mosby.)

PLEURAL SPACE FLUID

Pleural space fluid
ICD-9CM # 511.9 Pleural effusion, unspecified

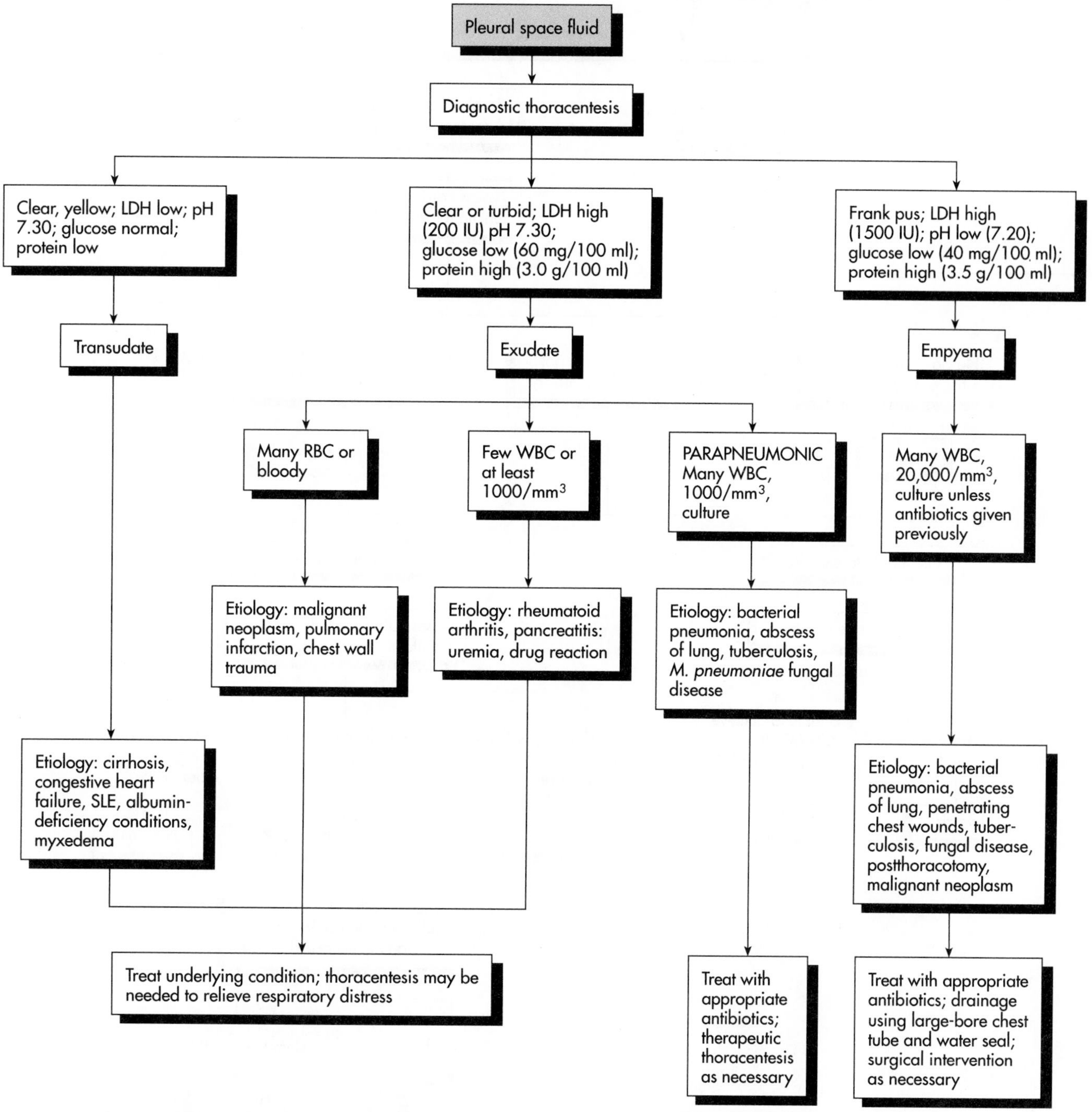

Pleural space fluid

↓

Diagnostic thoracentesis

Clear, yellow; LDH low; pH 7.30; glucose normal; protein low

→ Transudate

Clear or turbid; LDH high (200 IU) pH 7.30; glucose low (60 mg/100 ml); protein high (3.0 g/100 ml)

→ Exudate

Frank pus; LDH high (1500 IU); pH low (7.20); glucose low (40 mg/100 ml); protein high (3.5 g/100 ml)

→ Empyema

Many RBC or bloody

Few WBC or at least 1000/mm^3

PARAPNEUMONIC Many WBC, 1000/mm^3, culture

Many WBC, 20,000/mm^3, culture unless antibiotics given previously

Etiology: malignant neoplasm, pulmonary infarction, chest wall trauma

Etiology: rheumatoid arthritis, pancreatitis; uremia, drug reaction

Etiology: bacterial pneumonia, abscess of lung, tuberculosis, *M. pneumoniae* fungal disease

Etiology: cirrhosis, congestive heart failure, SLE, albumin-deficiency conditions, myxedema

Etiology: bacterial pneumonia, abscess of lung, penetrating chest wounds, tuber-culosis, fungal disease, postthoracotomy, malignant neoplasm

Treat underlying condition; thoracentesis may be needed to relieve respiratory distress

Treat with appropriate antibiotics; therapeutic thoracentesis as necessary

Treat with appropriate antibiotics; drainage using large-bore chest tube and water seal; surgical intervention as necessary

Fig. 3-145   Evaluation, common etiologies, and management of pleural effusion and empyema. *LDH,* Lactate dehydrogenase; *RBC,* red blood cells; *SLE,* systemic lupus erythematosus; *WBC,* white blood cells. (From Kassirer J [ed]: *Current therapy in adult medicine,* ed 4, St Louis, 1998, Mosby.)

PREOPERATIVE EVALUATION, PATIENT WITH CORONARY HEART DISEASE

Preoperative evaluation, patient with coronary heart disease
ICD-9CM # 411.89 Coronary insufficiency, acute
411.8 Coronary insufficiency, chronic
411.1 Coronary insufficiency or intermediate syndrome

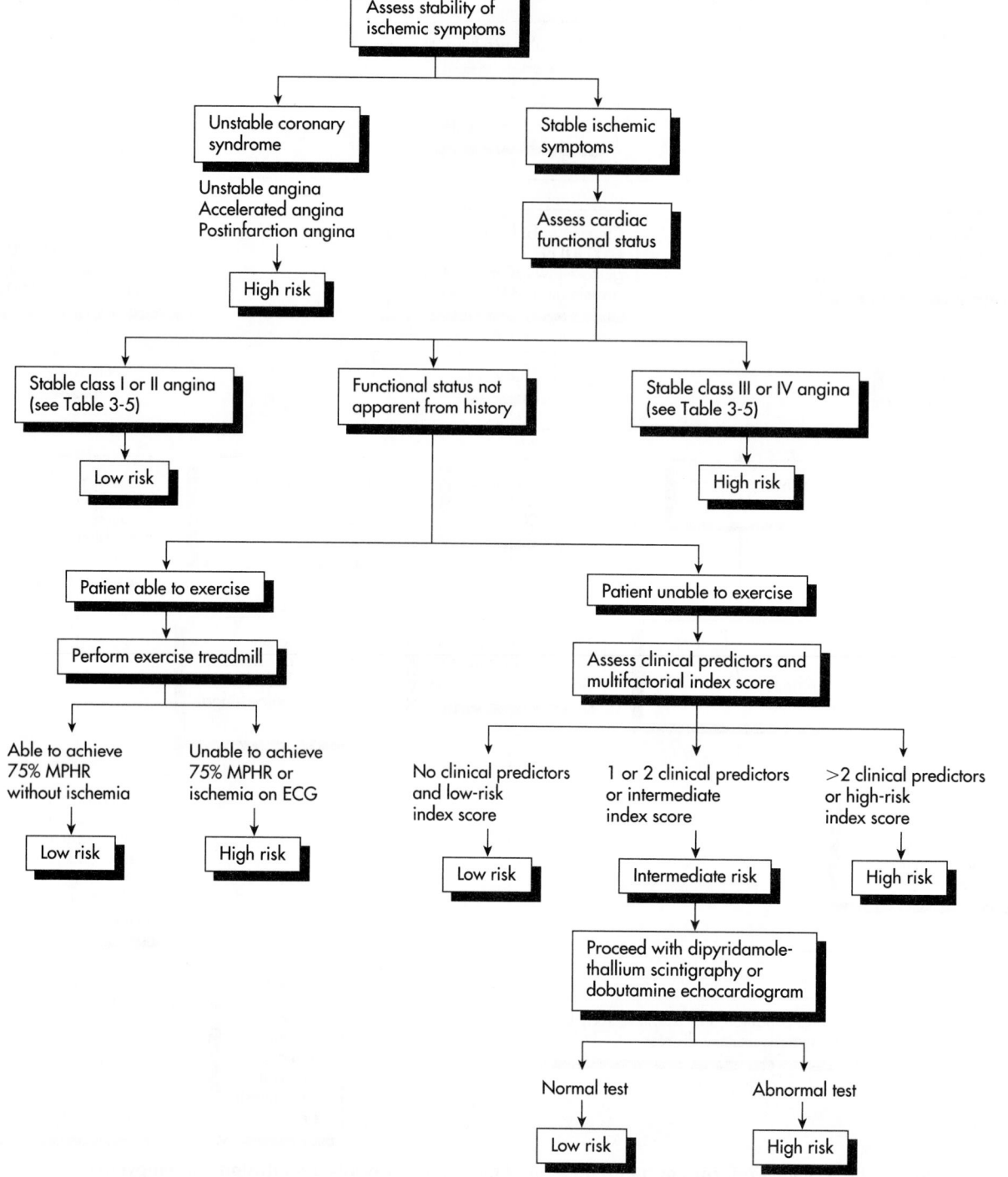

Fig. 3-146 Preoperative evaluation of patients with known or suspected coronary artery disease. (From Goldman L, Braunwald E [eds]: *Primary cardiology*, Philadelphia, 1998, WB Saunders.)

TABLE 3-5 New York Heart Association Functional Classification

Class I	No limitation	Ordinary physical activity does not cause symptoms
Class II	Slight limitation	Comfortable at rest Ordinary physical activity causes symptoms
Class III	Marked limitation	Comfortable at rest Less than ordinary activity causes symptoms
Class IV	Inability to carry on any physical activity	Symptoms present at rest

PROSTATIC HYPERPLASIA, BENIGN

Prostatic hyperplasia, benign
ICD-9CM # 600 Benign prostatic hyperplasia

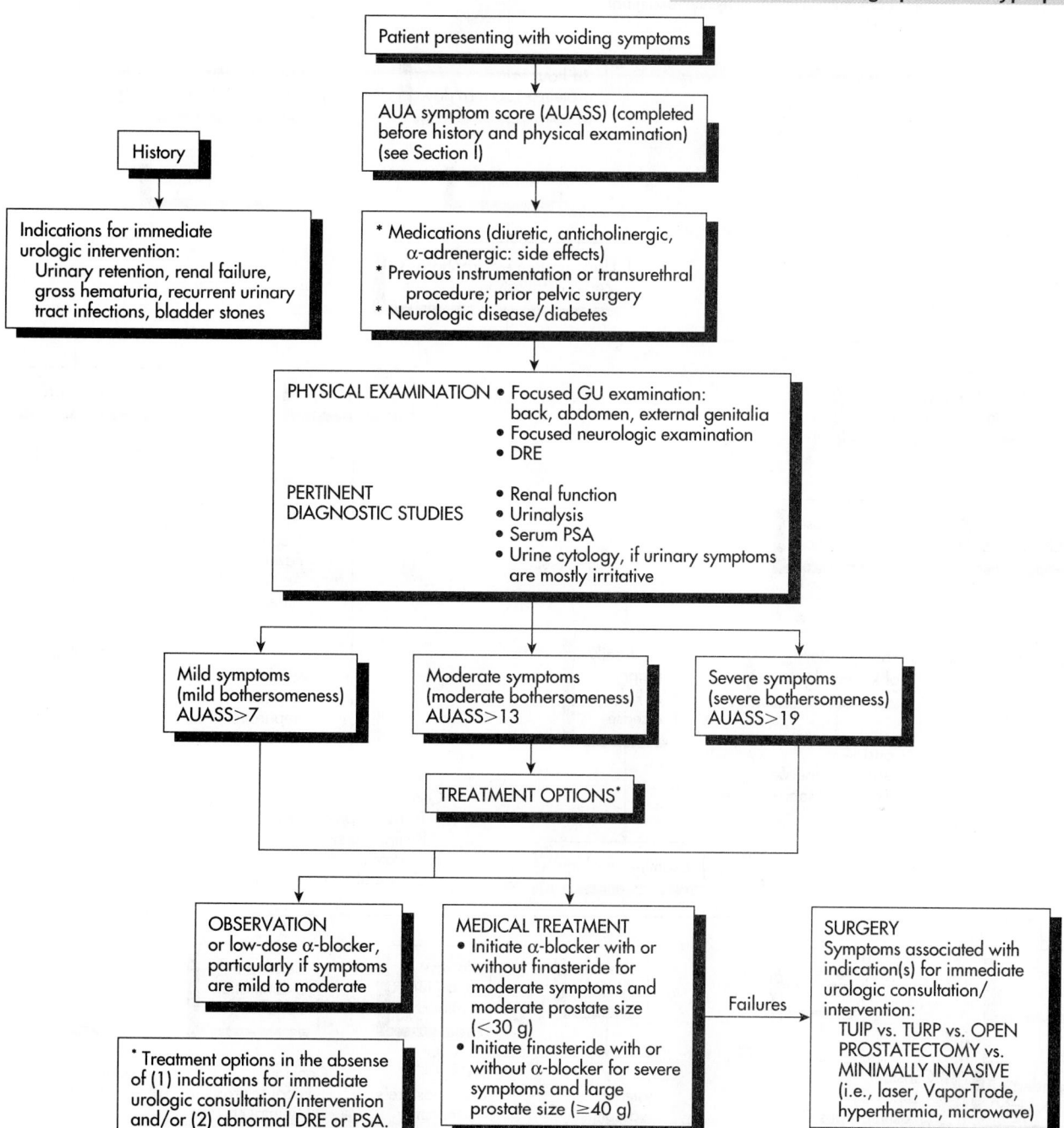

Patient presenting with voiding symptoms

AUA symptom score (AUASS) (completed before history and physical examination) (see Section I)

History

Indications for immediate urologic intervention:
Urinary retention, renal failure, gross hematuria, recurrent urinary tract infections, bladder stones

* Medications (diuretic, anticholinergic, α-adrenergic: side effects)
* Previous instrumentation or transurethral procedure; prior pelvic surgery
* Neurologic disease/diabetes

PHYSICAL EXAMINATION
• Focused GU examination: back, abdomen, external genitalia
• Focused neurologic examination
• DRE

PERTINENT DIAGNOSTIC STUDIES
• Renal function
• Urinalysis
• Serum PSA
• Urine cytology, if urinary symptoms are mostly irritative

Mild symptoms (mild bothersomeness) AUASS>7

Moderate symptoms (moderate bothersomeness) AUASS>13

Severe symptoms (severe bothersomeness) AUASS>19

TREATMENT OPTIONS*

OBSERVATION
or low-dose α-blocker, particularly if symptoms are mild to moderate

* Treatment options in the absense of (1) indications for immediate urologic consultation/intervention and/or (2) abnormal DRE or PSA.

MEDICAL TREATMENT
• Initiate α-blocker with or without finasteride for moderate symptoms and moderate prostate size (<30 g)
• Initiate finasteride with or without α-blocker for severe symptoms and large prostate size (≥40 g)

Failures

SURGERY
Symptoms associated with indication(s) for immediate urologic consultation/ intervention:
TUIP vs. TURP vs. OPEN PROSTATECTOMY vs. MINIMALLY INVASIVE (i.e., laser, VaporTrode, hyperthermia, microwave)

Fig. 3-147   Critical pathway for patients with benign prostatic hypertrophy. *AUA,* American Urological Association; *DRE,* digital rectal examination; *GU,* genitourinary; *PSA,* prostate-specific antigen; *TUIP,* transurethral incision of the prostate; *TURP,* transurethral resection of the prostate. (From Nseyo UO [ed]: *Urology for primary care physicians,* Philadelphia, 1999, WB Saunders.)

III

PROTEINURIA

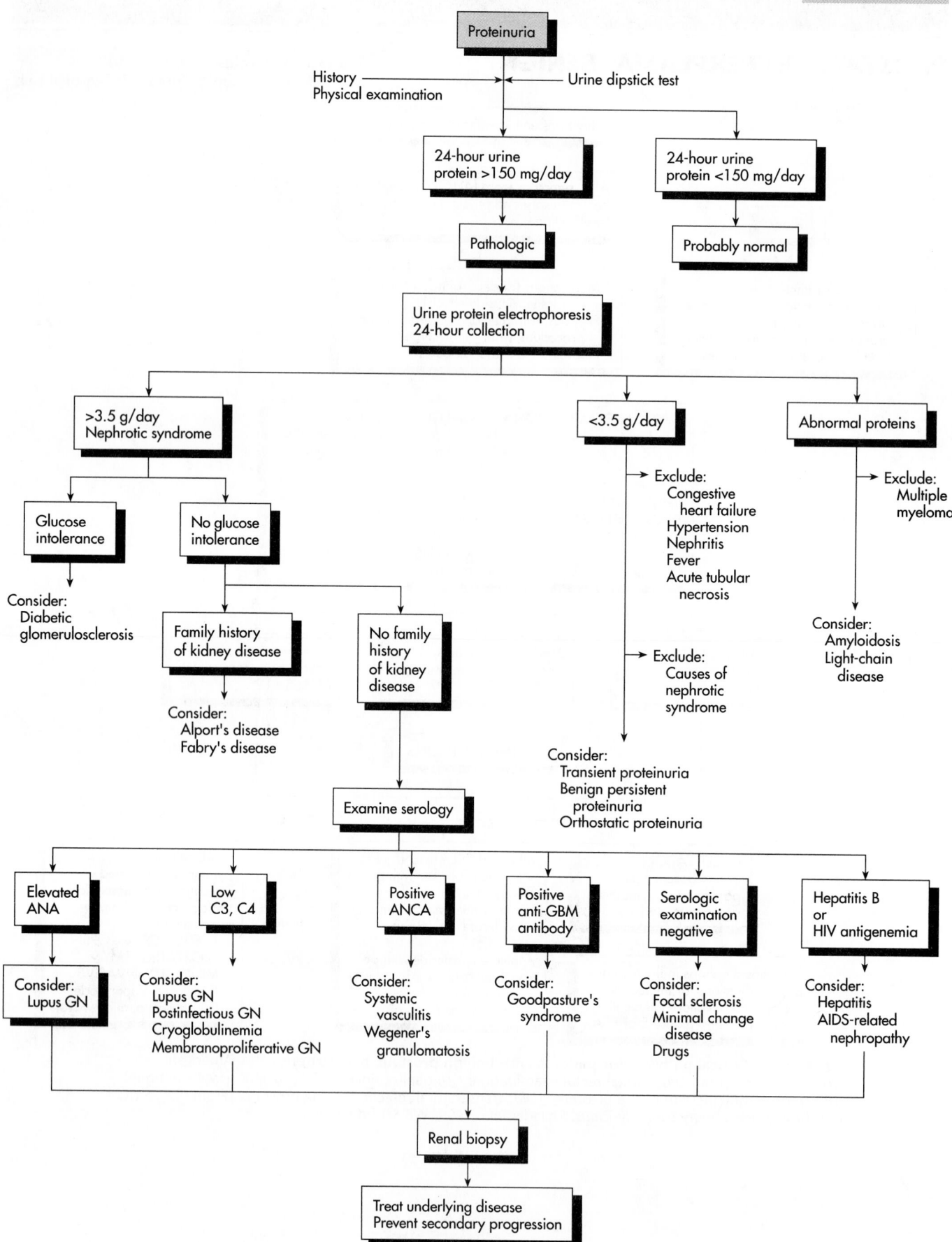

Fig. 3-148 **Proteinuria.** *AIDS,* Acquired immunodeficiency syndrome; *ANA,* antinuclear antibody; *ANCA,* antineutrophil cytoplasmic autoantibody; *anti-GBM,* anti–glomerular basement membrane; *GN,* glomeru-lonephritis. (From Greene HL, Johnson WP, Lemcke D [eds]: *Decision making in medicine,* ed 2, St Louis, 1998, Mosby.)

PRURITUS, GENERALIZED

Pruritus, generalized
ICD-9CM # 698.9 Pruritus NOS

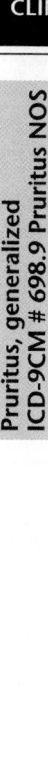

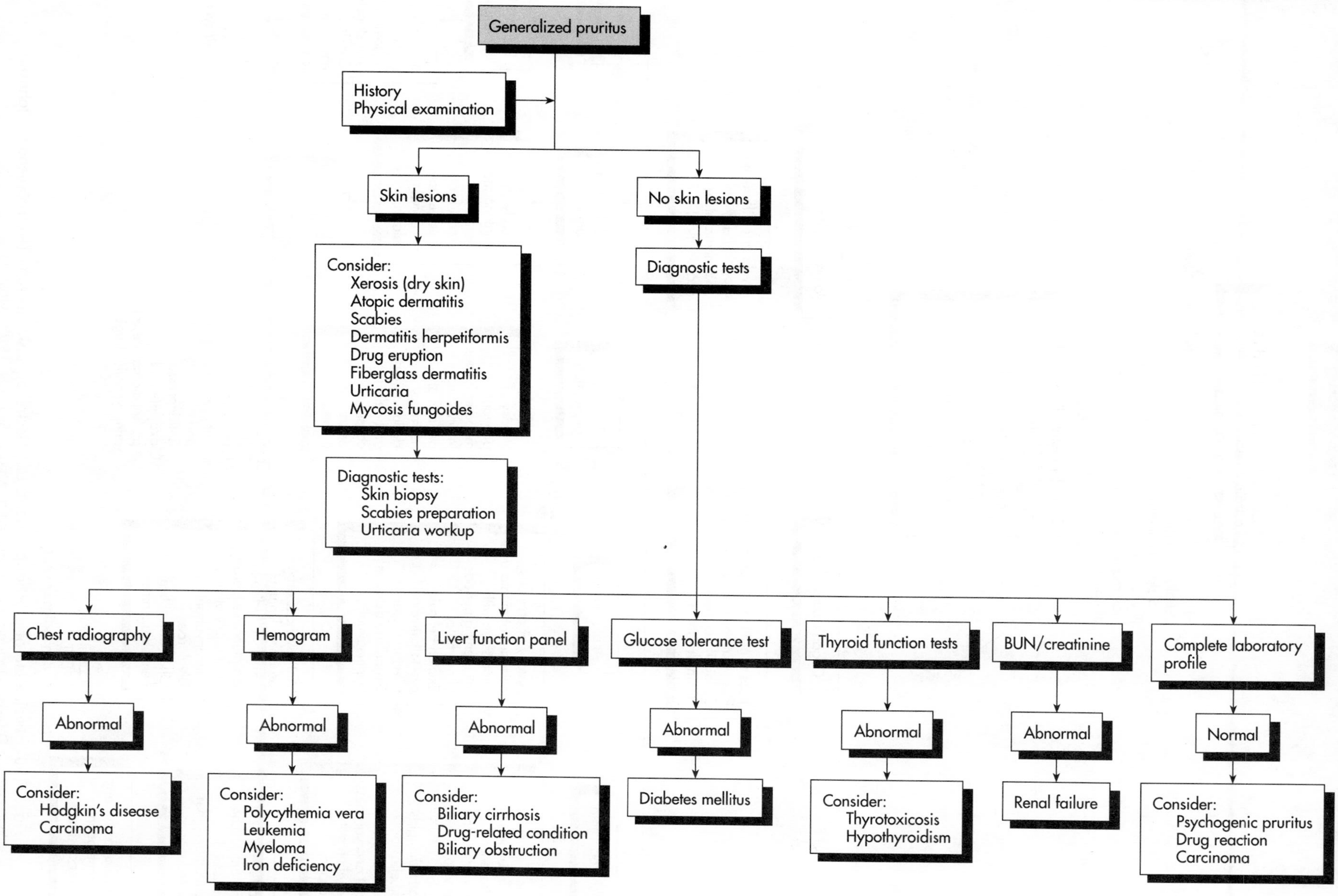

Generalized pruritus

History
Physical examination

Skin lesions

Consider:
Xerosis (dry skin)
Atopic dermatitis
Scabies
Dermatitis herpetiformis
Drug eruption
Fiberglass dermatitis
Urticaria
Mycosis fungoides

Diagnostic tests:
Skin biopsy
Scabies preparation
Urticaria workup

No skin lesions

Diagnostic tests

Chest radiography → Abnormal → Consider: Hodgkin's disease Carcinoma

Hemogram → Abnormal → Consider: Polycythemia vera Leukemia Myeloma Iron deficiency

Liver function panel → Abnormal → Consider: Biliary cirrhosis Drug-related condition Biliary obstruction

Glucose tolerance test → Abnormal → Diabetes mellitus

Thyroid function tests → Abnormal → Consider: Thyrotoxicosis Hypothyroidism

BUN/creatinine → Abnormal → Renal failure

Complete laboratory profile → Normal → Consider: Psychogenic pruritus Drug reaction Carcinoma

Fig. 3-149 **Evaluation of generalized pruritus.** *BUN,* Blood urea nitrogen. (From Greene HL, Johnson WP, Lemcke D [eds]: *Decision making in medicine,* ed 2, St Louis, 1998, Mosby.)

PSYCHOTIC PATIENT

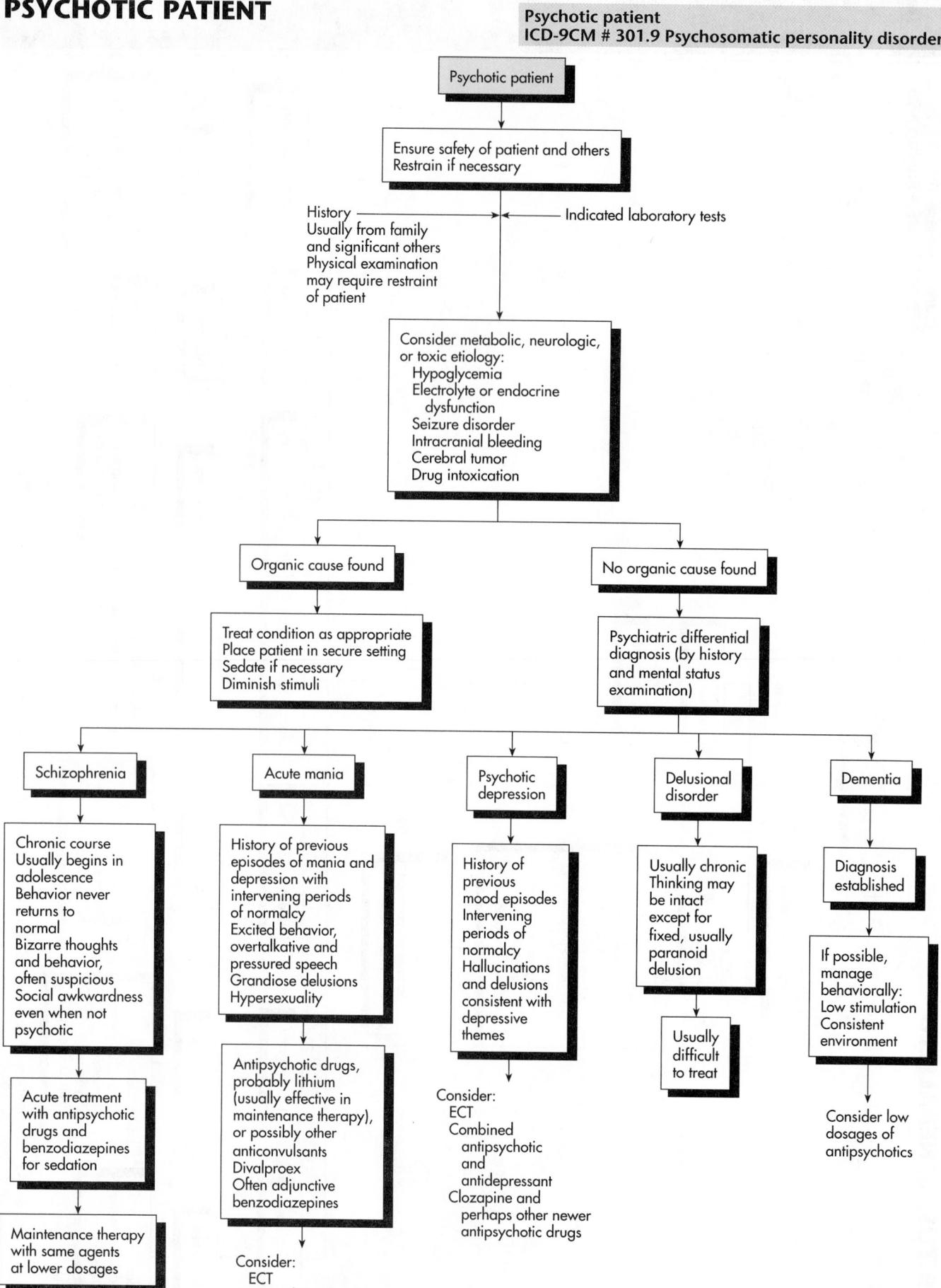

Fig. 3-150   Evaluation of psychotic patient. *ECT,* Electroconvulsive therapy. (From Greene HL, Johnson WP, Lemcke D [eds]: *Decision making in medicine,* ed 2, St Louis, 1998, Mosby.)

PUBERTY, DELAYED

Puberty, delayed
ICD-9CM # 259.0

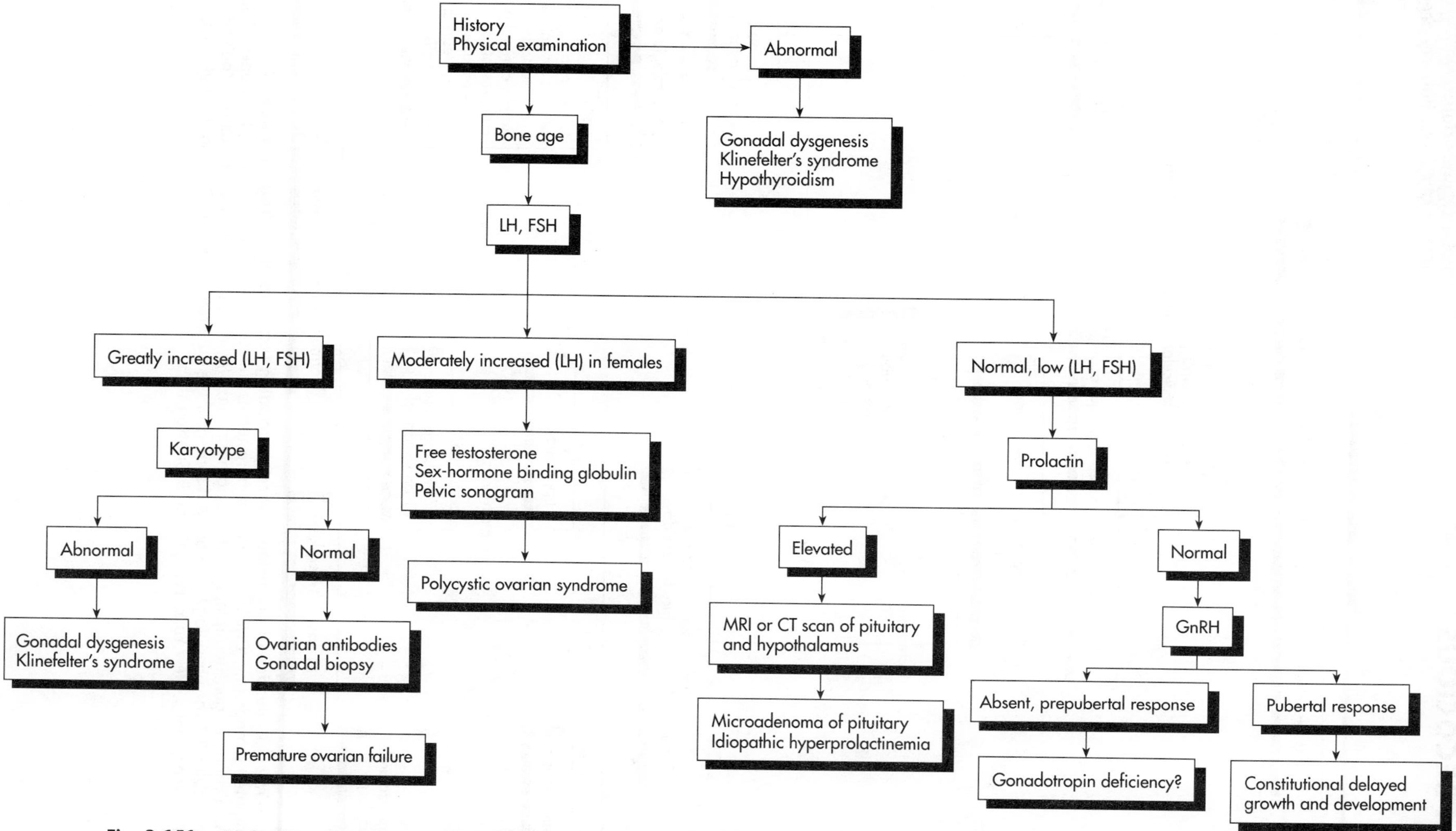

History
Physical examination

Bone age

LH, FSH

Abnormal
→ Gonadal dysgenesis
Klinefelter's syndrome
Hypothyroidism

Greatly increased (LH, FSH)

Karyotype

Normal
→ Ovarian antibodies
Gonadal biopsy
→ Premature ovarian failure

Abnormal
→ Gonadal dysgenesis
Klinefelter's syndrome

Moderately increased (LH) in females

Free testosterone
Sex-hormone binding globulin
Pelvic sonogram
→ Polycystic ovarian syndrome

Normal, low (LH, FSH)

Prolactin

Elevated
→ MRI or CT scan of pituitary and hypothalamus
→ Microadenoma of pituitary
Idiopathic hyperprolactinemia

Normal

GnRH

Pubertal response
→ Constitutional delayed growth and development

Absent, prepubertal response
→ Gonadotropin deficiency?

Fig. 3-151 **Evaluation of patient with delayed puberty.** *CT,* Computed tomography; *FSH,* follicle-stimulating hormone; *GnRH,* gonadotropin-releasing hormone; *LH,* luteinizing hormone; *MRI,* magnetic resonance imaging. (From Moore WT, Eastman RC: *Diagnostic endocrinology,* ed 2, St Louis, 1996, Mosby.)

III

PUBERTY, PRECOCIOUS

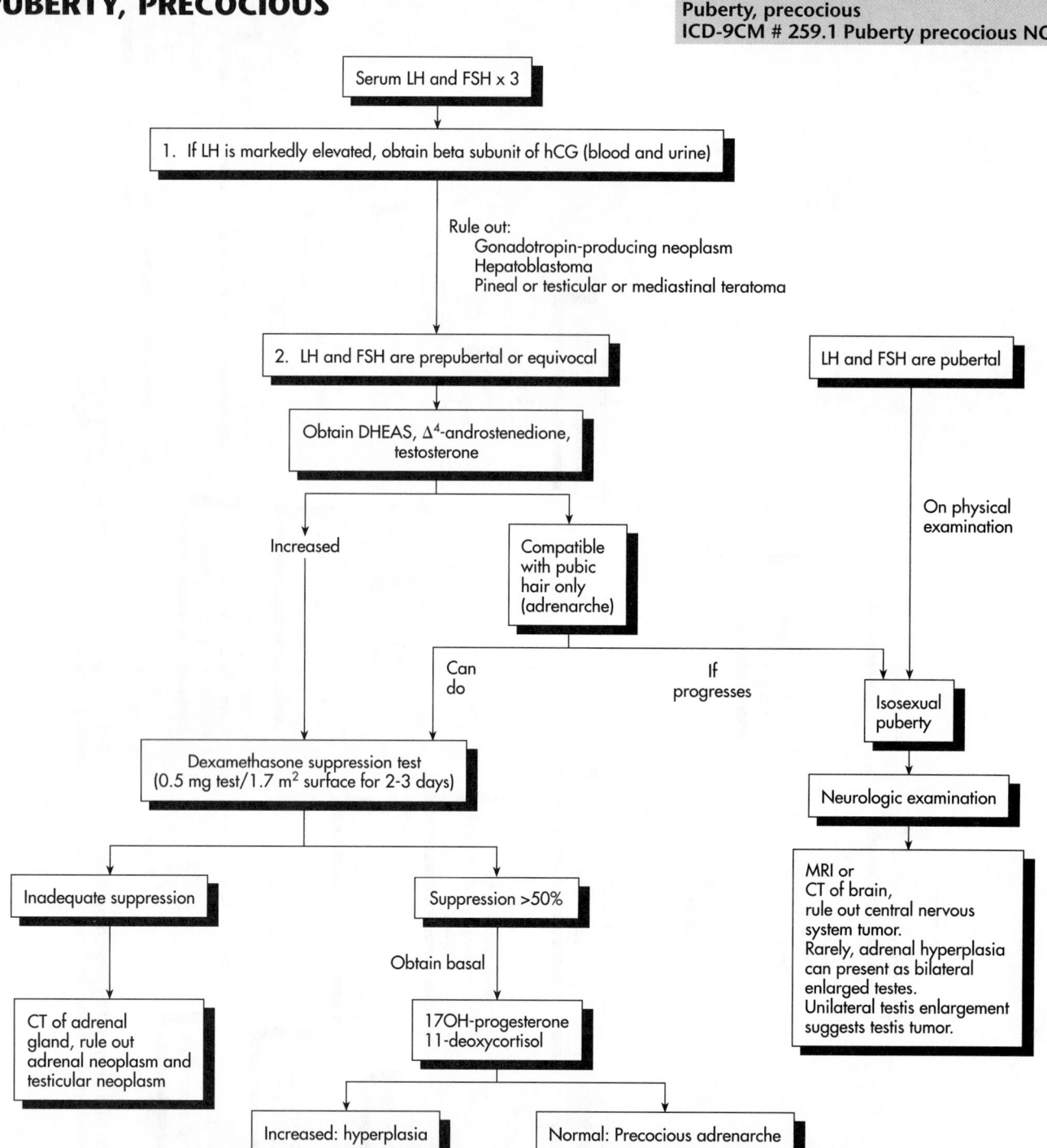

Fig. 3-152 **Evaluation of precocious puberty, excluding factitious and iatrogenic causes.** *CT,* Computed tomography; *DHEAS,* dehydroepiandrosterone sulfate; *FSH,* follicle-stimulating hormone; *hCG,* human chorionic gonadotropin; *LH,* luteinizing hormone; *MRI,* magnetic resonance imaging. (Modified from Odell WD: The physiology of puberty: disorders of the pubertal process. In DeGroot LJ et al [eds]: *Endocrinology,* vol 3, New York, 1979, Grune & Stratton.)

PULMONARY EMBOLISM

Pulmonary embolism
ICD-9CM # 415.1

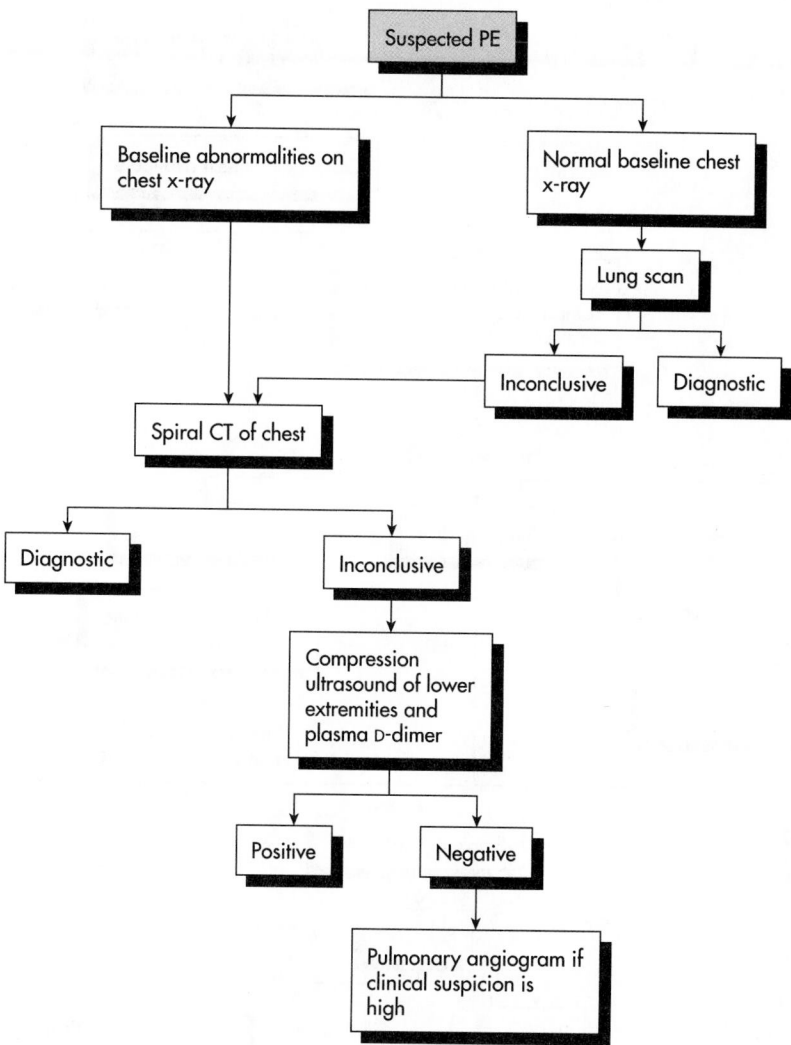

Fig. 3-153   Pulmonary embolism. *CT,* Computed tomography; *PE,* pulmonary embolism.

PULMONARY NODULE

**Pulmonary nodule
ICD-9CM # 518.89**

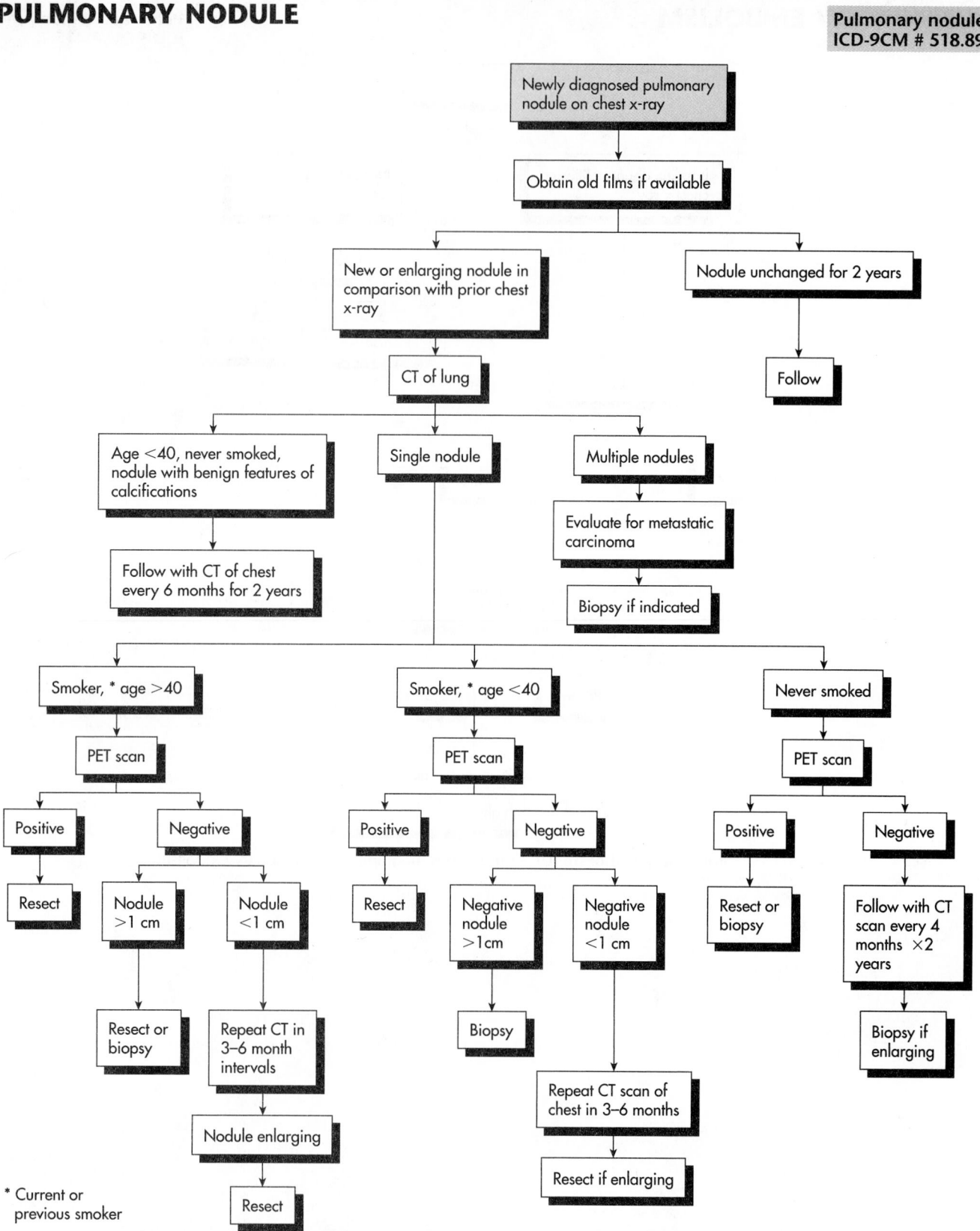

Fig. 3-154   Pulmonary nodule. *CT,* Computed tomography; *PET,* positron emission tomography.

PURPURA, PALPABLE

Purpura, palpable
ICD-9CM # 287.2 Purpura, NOS

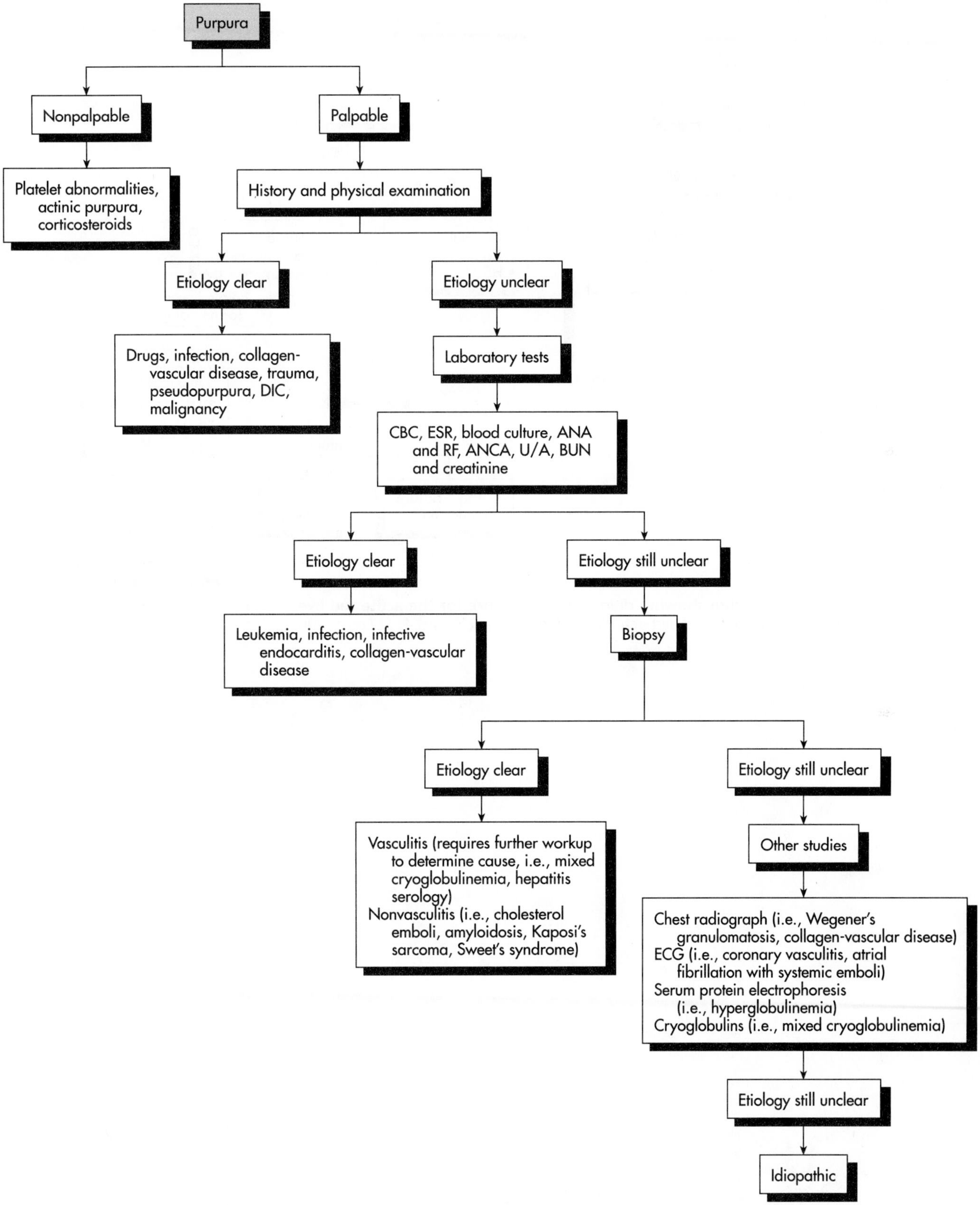

Fig. 3-155 **Diagnostic algorithm for palpable purpura.** *AIDS, Acquired immunodeficiency syndrome; ANA,* antinuclear antibody; *ANCA,* antineutrophil cytoplasmic antibody test; *BUN,* blood urea nitrogen; *CBC,* complete blood cell count; *DIC,* disseminated intravascular coagulation; *ECG,* electrocardiogram; *ESR,* erythrocyte sedimentation rate; *MCV,* mean corpuscular volume; *RF,* rheumatoid factor; *U/A,* urinalysis. (From Stevens GL, Adelman HM, Wallach PM: *Am Fam Physician* 52:1355, 1995.)

RED EYE, ACUTE

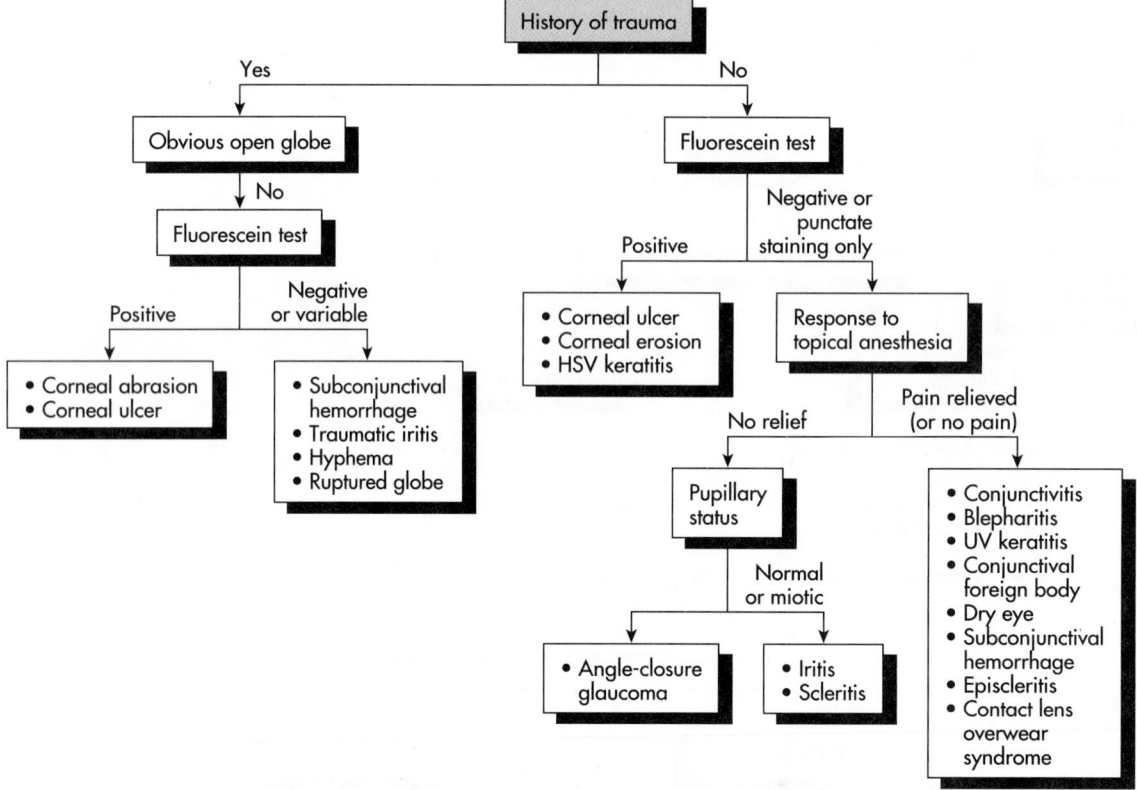

Fig. 3-156 Algorithm showing diagnostic procedure for the acute red eye. *HSV,* Herpes simplex virus; *UV,* ultraviolet. (From Auerbach PS: *Wilderness medicine,* ed 4, St Louis, 2001, Mosby.)

RENAL FAILURE, ACUTE

Renal failure, acute
ICD-9CM # 584.9 Acute renal failure, unspecified

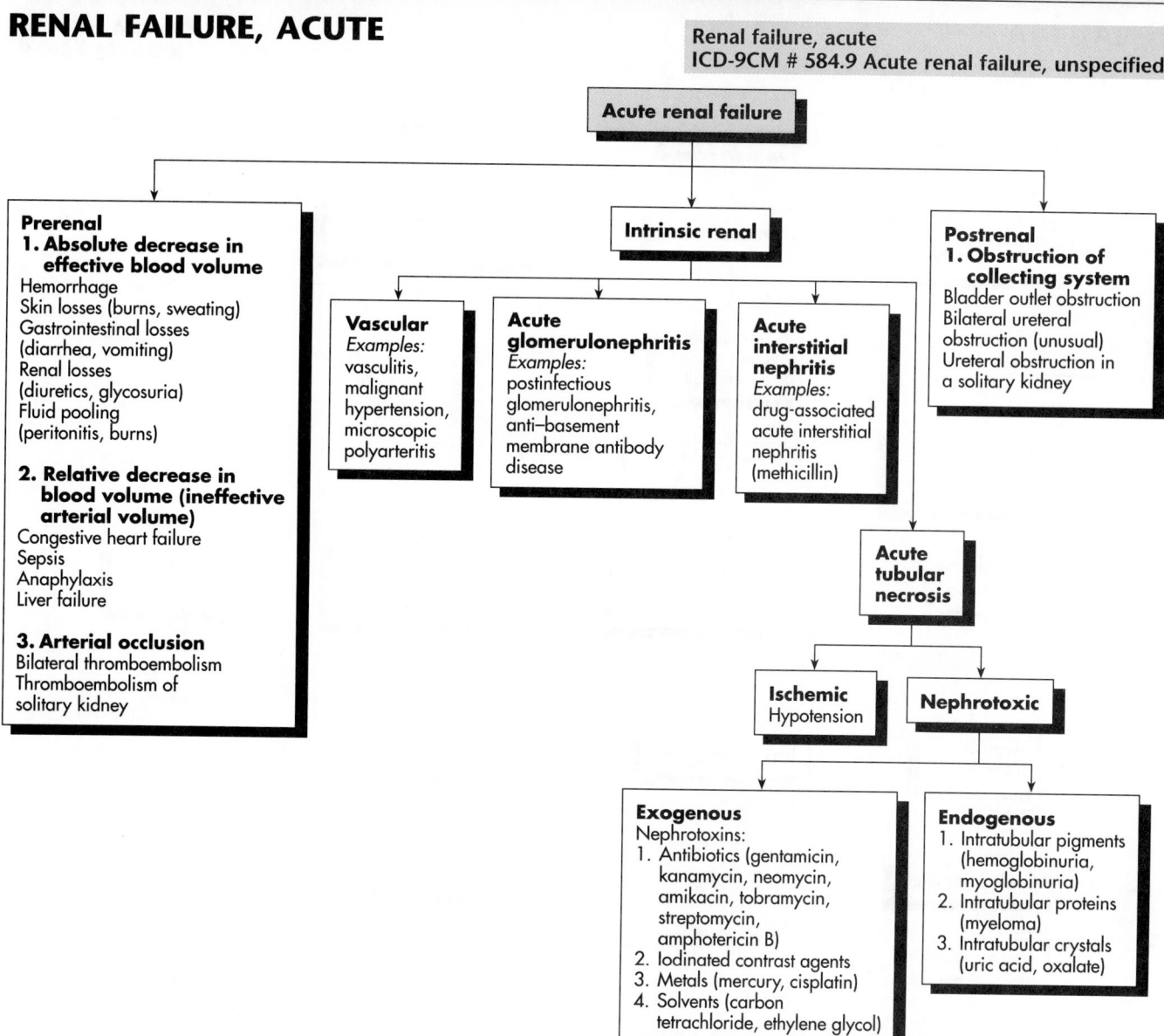

Acute renal failure

Prerenal
**1. Absolute decrease in
   effective blood volume**
Hemorrhage
Skin losses (burns, sweating)
Gastrointestinal losses
(diarrhea, vomiting)
Renal losses
(diuretics, glycosuria)
Fluid pooling
(peritonitis, burns)

**2. Relative decrease in
   blood volume (ineffective
   arterial volume)**
Congestive heart failure
Sepsis
Anaphylaxis
Liver failure

3. Arterial occlusion
Bilateral thromboembolism
Thromboembolism of
solitary kidney

Intrinsic renal

Vascular
Examples:
vasculitis,
malignant
hypertension,
microscopic
polyarteritis

**Acute
glomerulonephritis**
Examples:
postinfectious
glomerulonephritis,
anti–basement
membrane antibody
disease

**Acute
interstitial
nephritis**
Examples:
drug-associated
acute interstitial
nephritis
(methicillin)

Postrenal
**1. Obstruction of
   collecting system**
Bladder outlet obstruction
Bilateral ureteral
obstruction (unusual)
Ureteral obstruction in
a solitary kidney

**Acute
tubular
necrosis**

Ischemic
Hypotension

Nephrotoxic

Exogenous
Nephrotoxins:
1. Antibiotics (gentamicin,
   kanamycin, neomycin,
   amikacin, tobramycin,
   streptomycin,
   amphotericin B)
2. Iodinated contrast agents
3. Metals (mercury, cisplatin)
4. Solvents (carbon
   tetrachloride, ethylene glycol)

Endogenous
1. Intratubular pigments
   (hemoglobinuria,
   myoglobinuria)
2. Intratubular proteins
   (myeloma)
3. Intratubular crystals
   (uric acid, oxalate)

III

Fig. 3-157 **Causes of acute renal failure.** (From Andreoli TE [ed]: *Cecil essentials of medicine,* ed 4, Philadelphia, 1997, WB Saunders.)

RENAL MASS

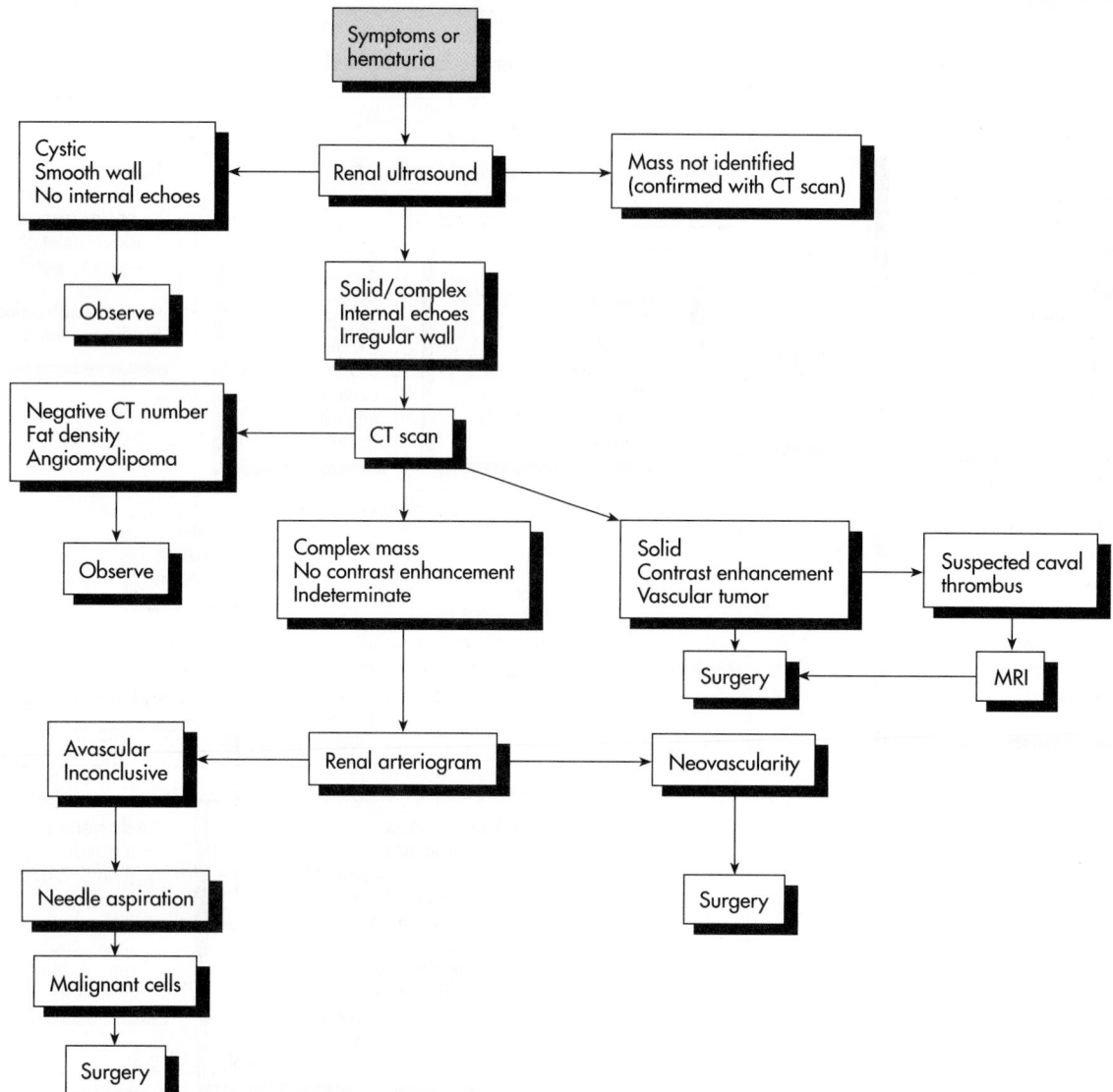

Fig. 3-158   Evaluation of a patient with a renal mass. *CT,* Computed tomography; *MRI,* magnetic resonance imaging. (Modified from Williams RD: Tumors of the kidney, ureter, and bladder. In Goldman L, Ausiello D [eds]: *Cecil textbook of medicine,* ed 22, Philadelphia, 2004, WB Saunders.)

RESPIRATORY DISTRESS

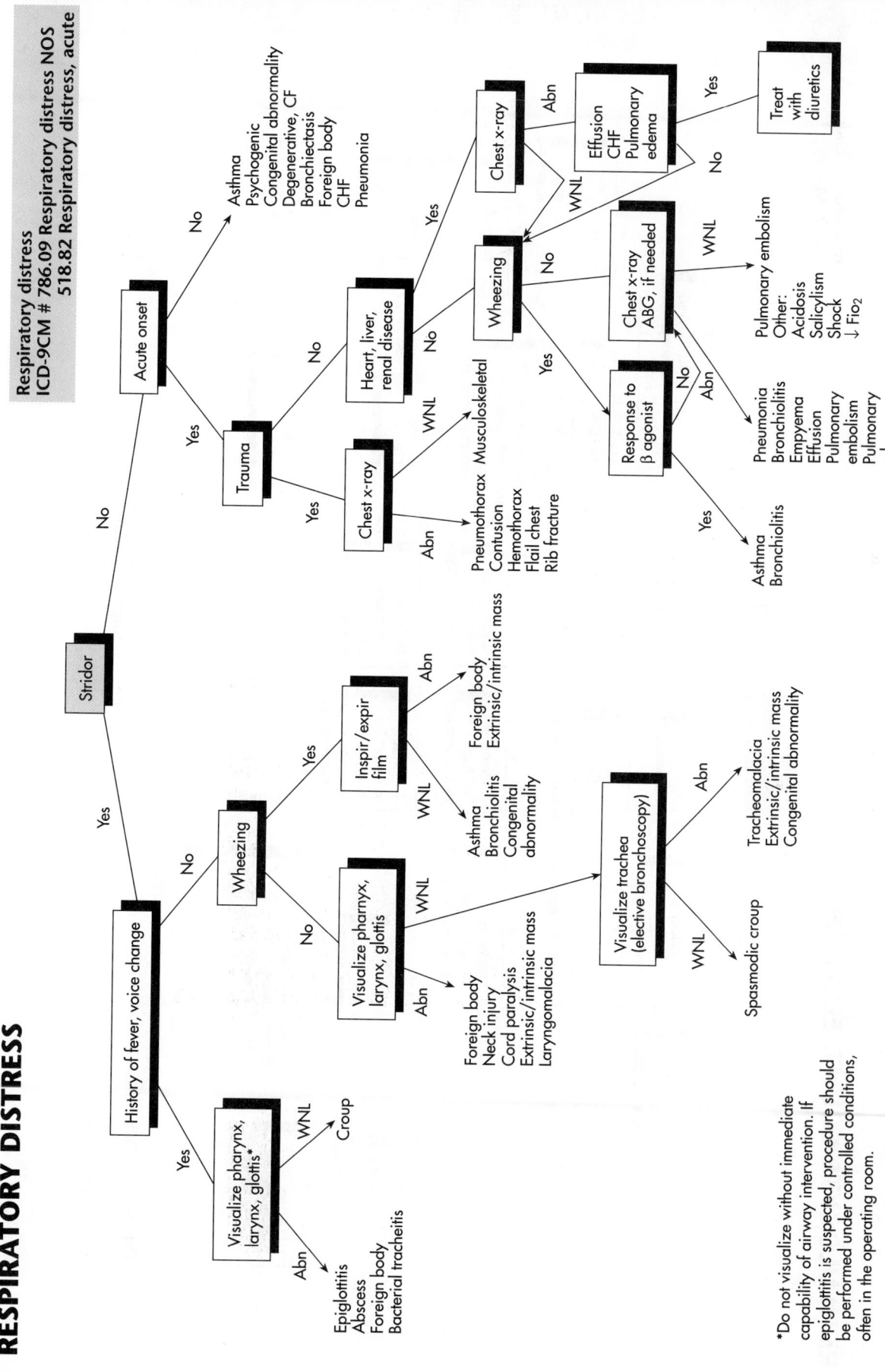

Fig. 3-159   Respiratory distress. *ABG,* Arterial blood gas; *Abn,* abnormal; *CF,* cystic fibrosis; *CHF,* congestive heart failure; *WNL,* within normal limits. (From Barkin RM, Rosen P: *Emergency pediatrics,* St Louis, 1999, Mosby.)

Respiratory distress
ICD-9CM # 786.09 Respiratory distress NOS
518.82 Respiratory distress, acute

*Do not visualize without immediate capability of airway intervention. If epiglottitis is suspected, procedure should be performed under controlled conditions, often in the operating room.

RETICULOCYTE COUNT, ELEVATED

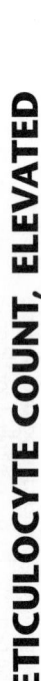

Reticulocyte count, elevated
ICD-9CM # 790.99

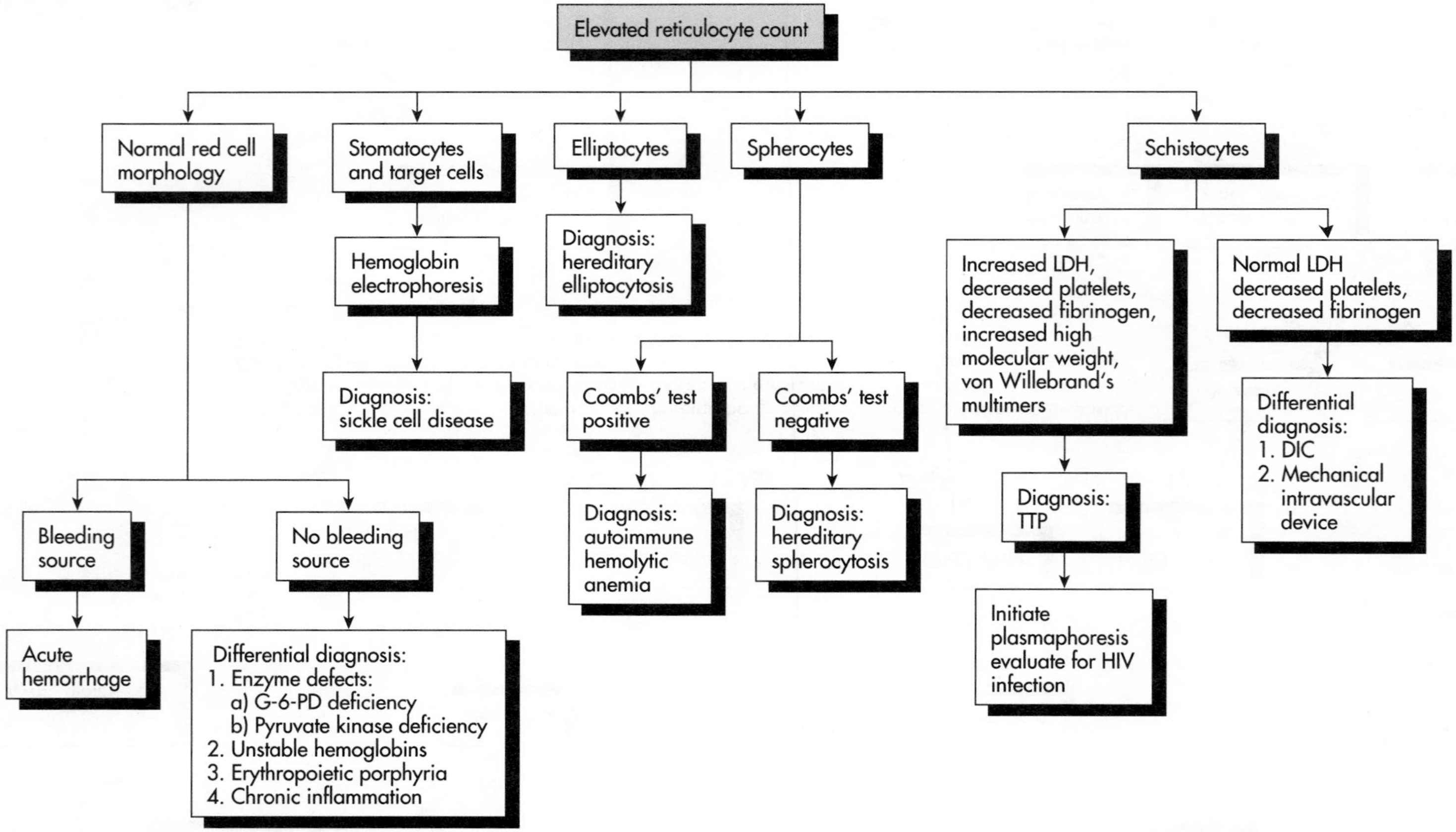

Elevated reticulocyte count

Schistocytes

Normal LDH, decreased platelets, decreased fibrinogen

Differential diagnosis:
1. DIC
2. Mechanical intravascular device

Increased LDH, decreased platelets, decreased fibrinogen, increased high molecular weight, von Willebrand's multimers

Diagnosis: TTP

Initiate plasmaphoresis evaluate for HIV infection

Spherocytes

Coombs' test negative

Diagnosis: hereditary spherocytosis

Elliptocytes

Diagnosis: hereditary elliptocytosis

Coombs' test positive

Diagnosis: autoimmune hemolytic anemia

Stomatocytes and target cells

Hemoglobin electrophoresis

Diagnosis: sickle cell disease

Normal red cell morphology

No bleeding source

Differential diagnosis:
1. Enzyme defects:
  a) G-6-PD deficiency
  b) Pyruvate kinase deficiency
2. Unstable hemoglobins
3. Erythropoietic porphyria
4. Chronic inflammation

Bleeding source

Acute hemorrhage

Fig. 3-160 **Differential diagnosis of elevated reticulocyte count.** *DIC*, Disseminated intravascular coagulation; *G6PD*, glucose-6-phosphate dehydrogenase; *HIV*, human immunodeficiency virus; *LDH*, lactic dehydrogenase; *TTP*, thrombotic thrombocytopenic purpura. (From Rakel RE [ed]: *Principles of family practice*, ed 6, Philadelphia, 2002, WB Saunders.)

RHINORRHEA

Rhinorrhea
ICD-9CM # 478.1

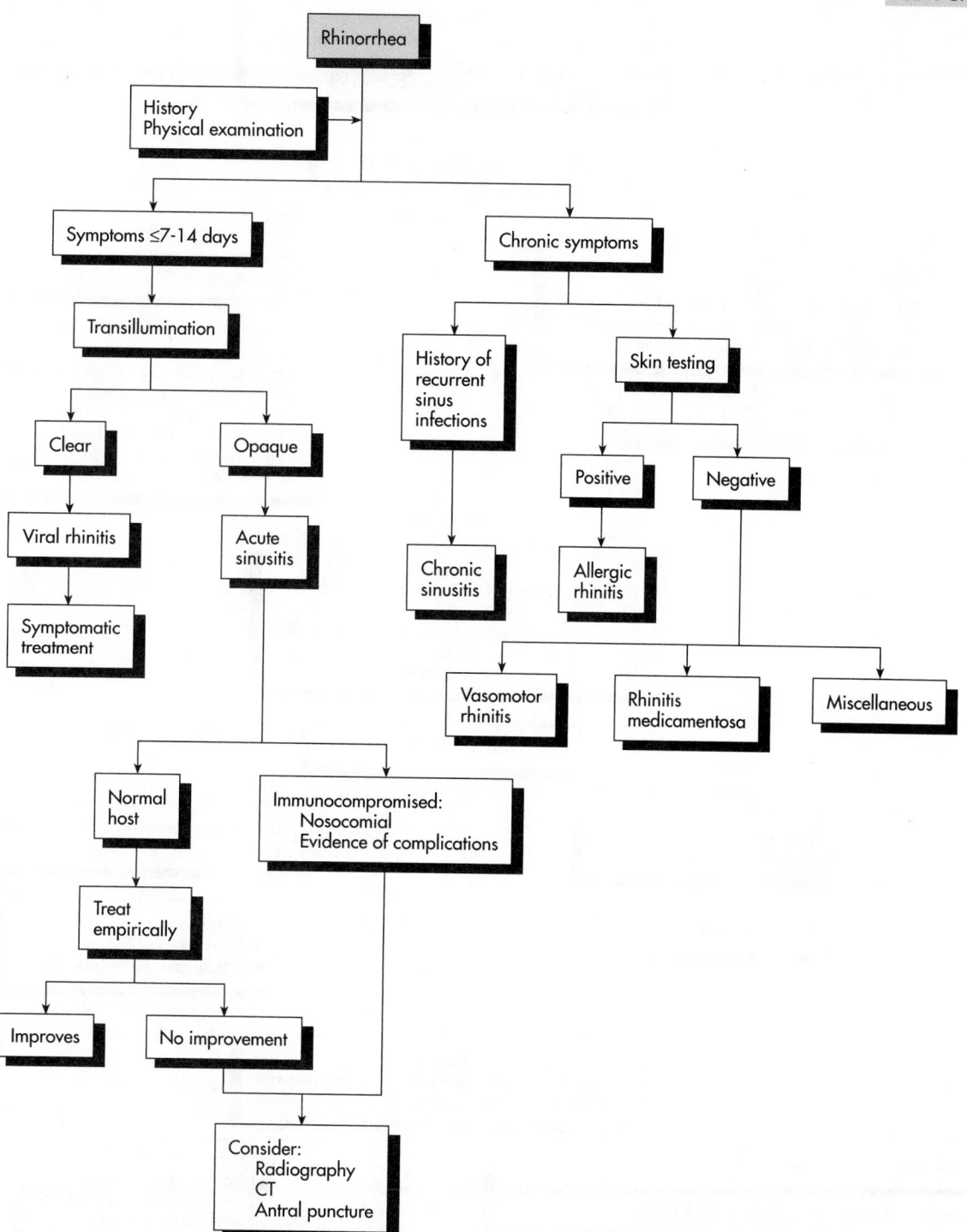

Fig. 3-161   Approach to a patient with rhinorrhea. *CT,* Computed tomography. (From Noble J [ed]: *Primary care medicine,* ed 3, St Louis, 2001, Mosby.)

III

SCHILLING TEST

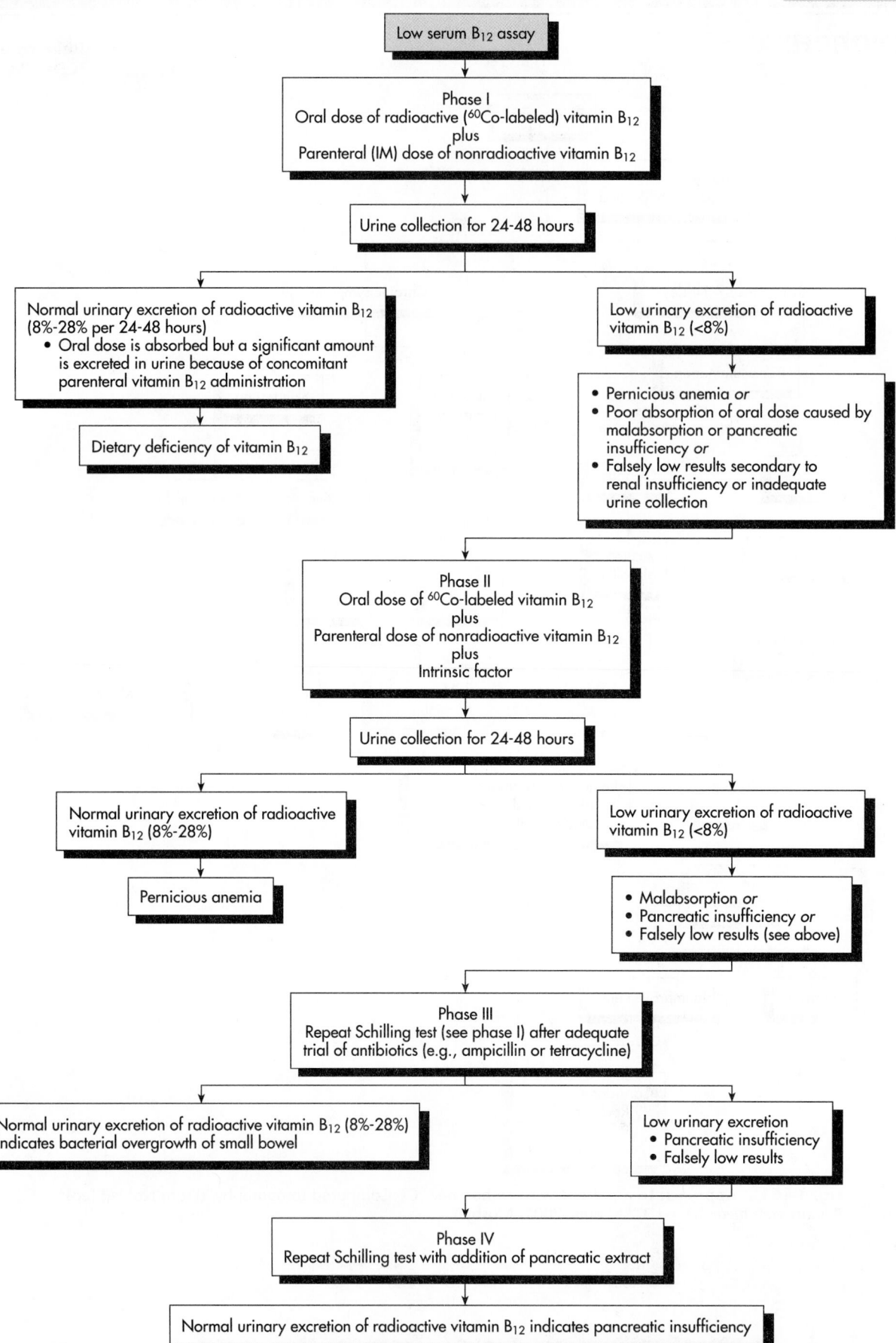

Fig. 3-162   Schilling test. *IM,* Intramuscular. (From Ferri FF: *Practical guide to the care of the medical patient,* ed 6, St Louis, 2004, Mosby.)

SCOLIOSIS

Scoliosis
ICD-9CM # 737.30 Idiopathic scoliosis
737.39 Paralytic scoliosis
754.2 Congenital scoliosis
724.3 Sciatic scoliosis
737.43 Associated with neurofibromatosis

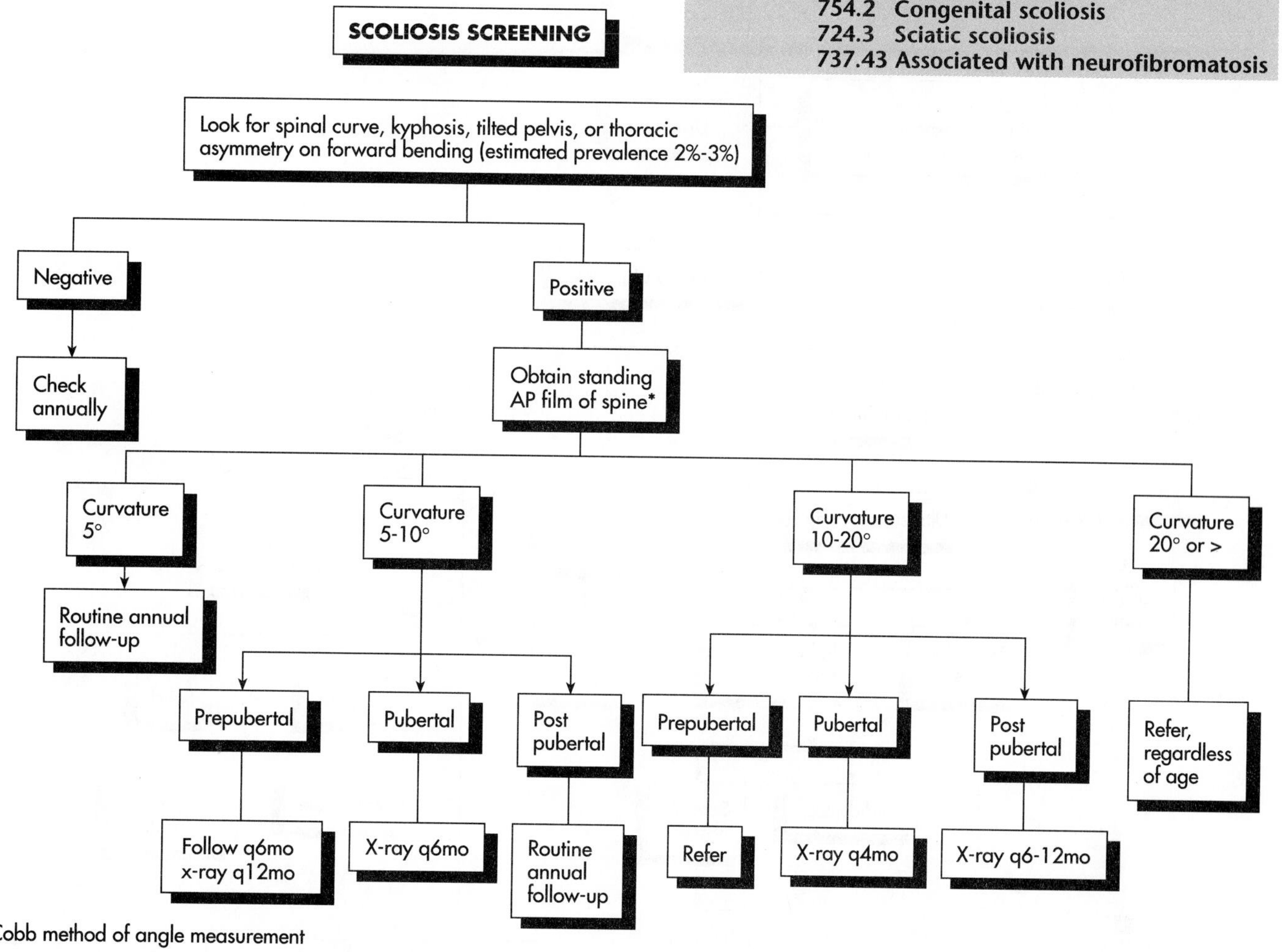

SCOLIOSIS SCREENING

Look for spinal curve, kyphosis, tilted pelvis, or thoracic asymmetry on forward bending (estimated prevalence 2%-3%)

Negative

Check annually

Positive

Obtain standing AP film of spine*

Curvature 5°

Routine annual follow-up

Curvature 5-10°

Curvature 10-20°

Curvature 20° or >

Prepubertal

Follow q6mo x-ray q12mo

Pubertal

X-ray q6mo

Post pubertal

Routine annual follow-up

Prepubertal

Refer

Pubertal

X-ray q4mo

Post pubertal

X-ray q6-12mo

Refer, regardless of age

*Cobb method of angle measurement

1. Find the lowest vertebra whose bottom tilts toward concavity of curve.
2. Erect a perpendicular line from extension of bottom surface.
3. Find highest vertebra as in #1 and erect perpendicular from extension of top surface.
4. Measure intersecting angle = angle of scoliosis.

Fig. 3-163   **Scoliosis screening and follow-up.** *AP,* Anteroposterior. (From Driscoll C [ed]: *The family practice desk reference,* ed 3, St Louis, 1996, Mosby.)

SCROTAL MASS

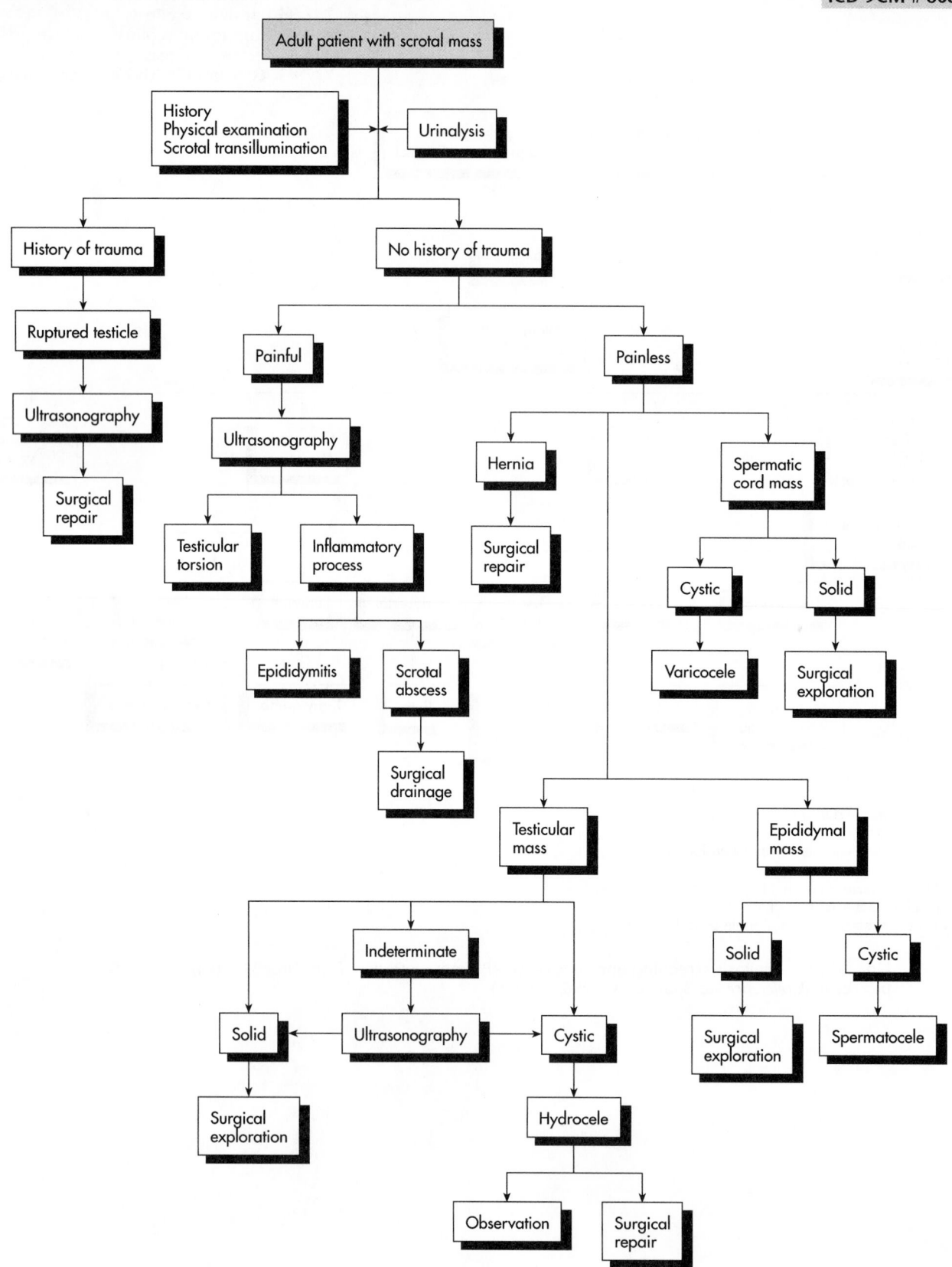

Fig. 3-164 **Evaluation of scrotal mass.** (From Greene HL, Johnson WP, Lemcke D [eds]: *Decision making in medicine*, ed 2, St Louis, 1998, Mosby.)

SEXUAL DYSFUNCTION

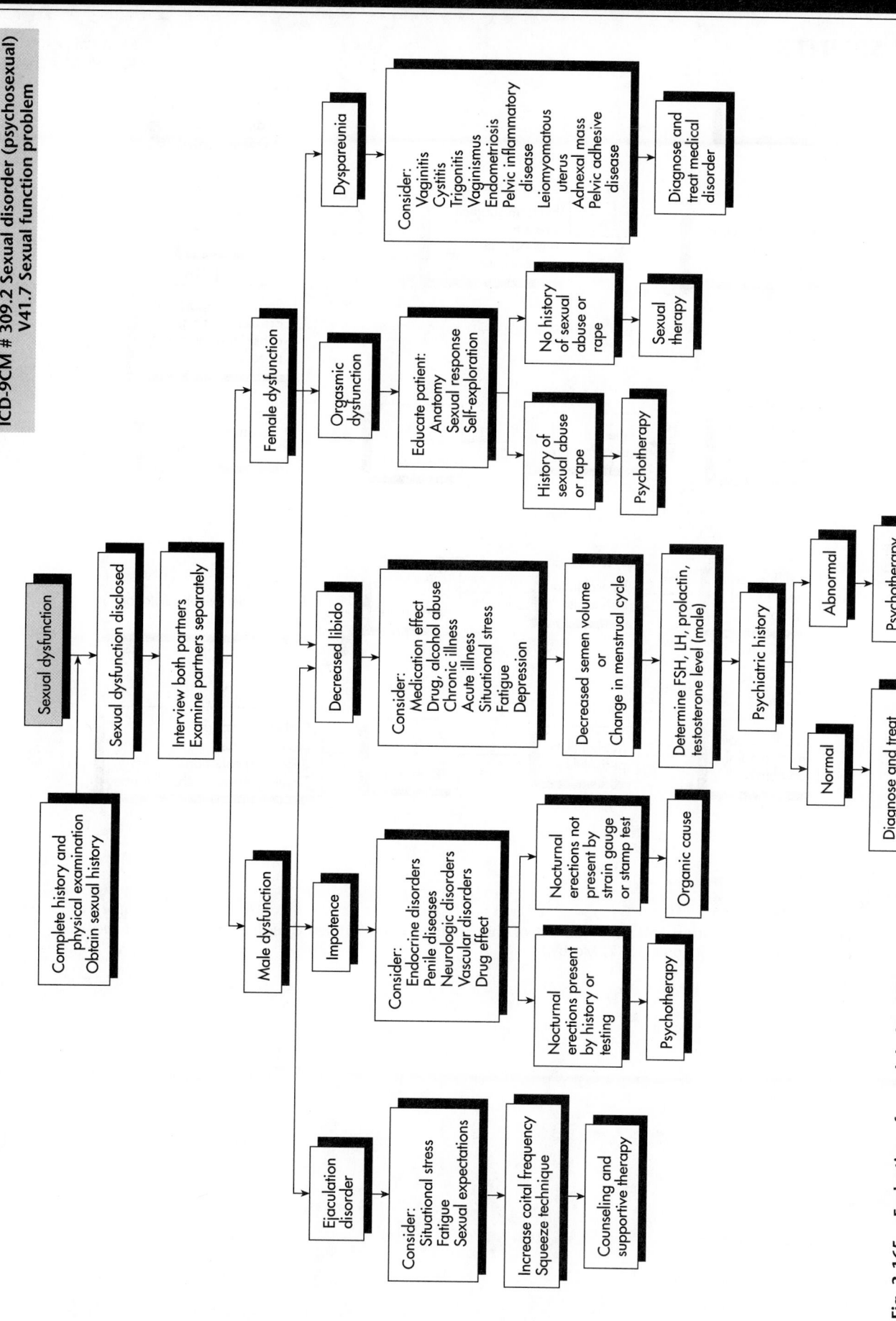

Fig. 3-165 **Evaluation of sexual dysfunction.** *FSH,* Follicle-stimulating hormone; *LH,* luteinizing hormone. (From Greene HL, Johnson WP, Lemcke D [eds]: *Decision making in medicine,* ed 2, St Louis, 1998, Mosby.)

SHIN SPLINTS

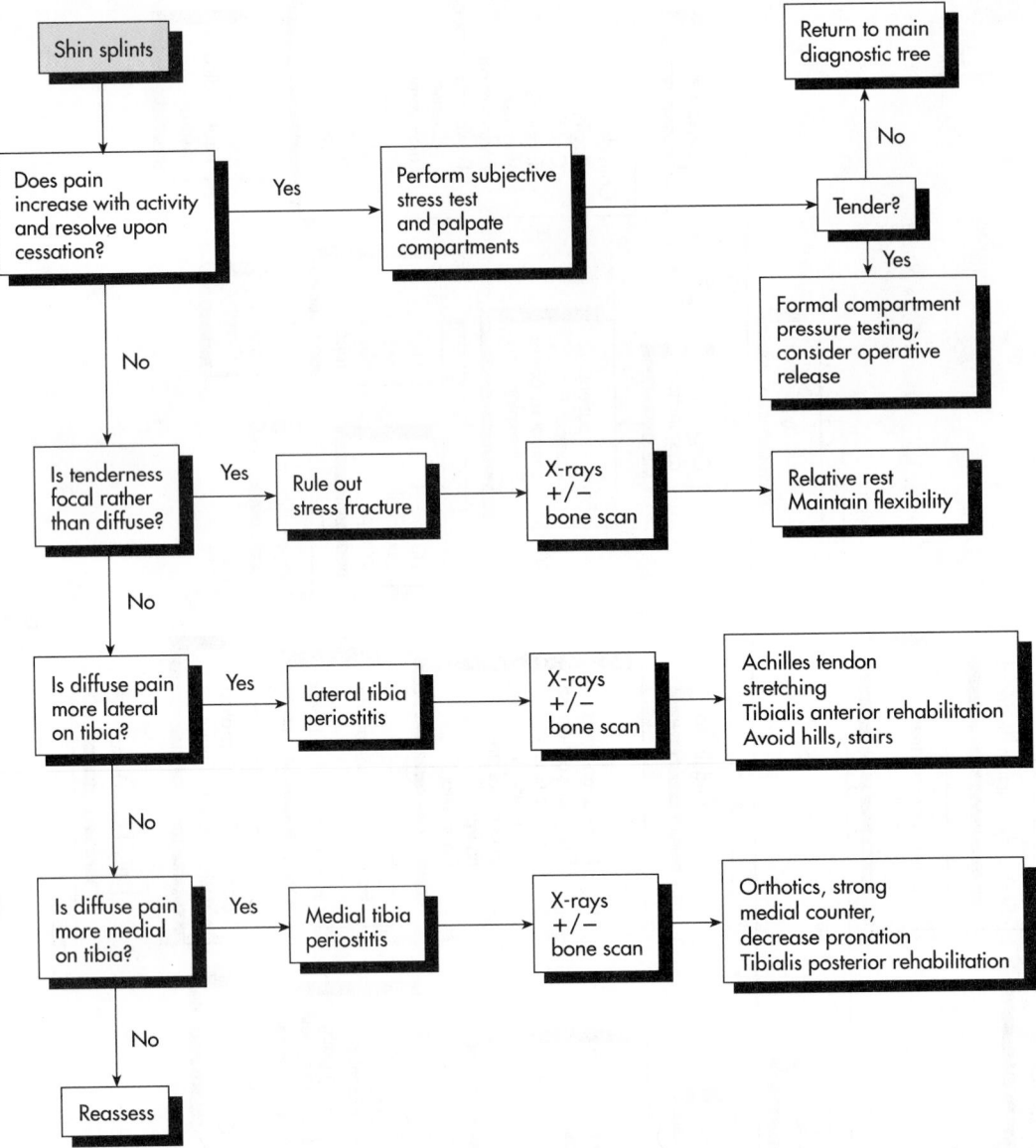

Fig. 3-166   Evaluation and management of shin splints. (From Scudieri G [ed]: *Sports medicine, principles of primary care,* St Louis, 1997, Mosby.)

SHOCK

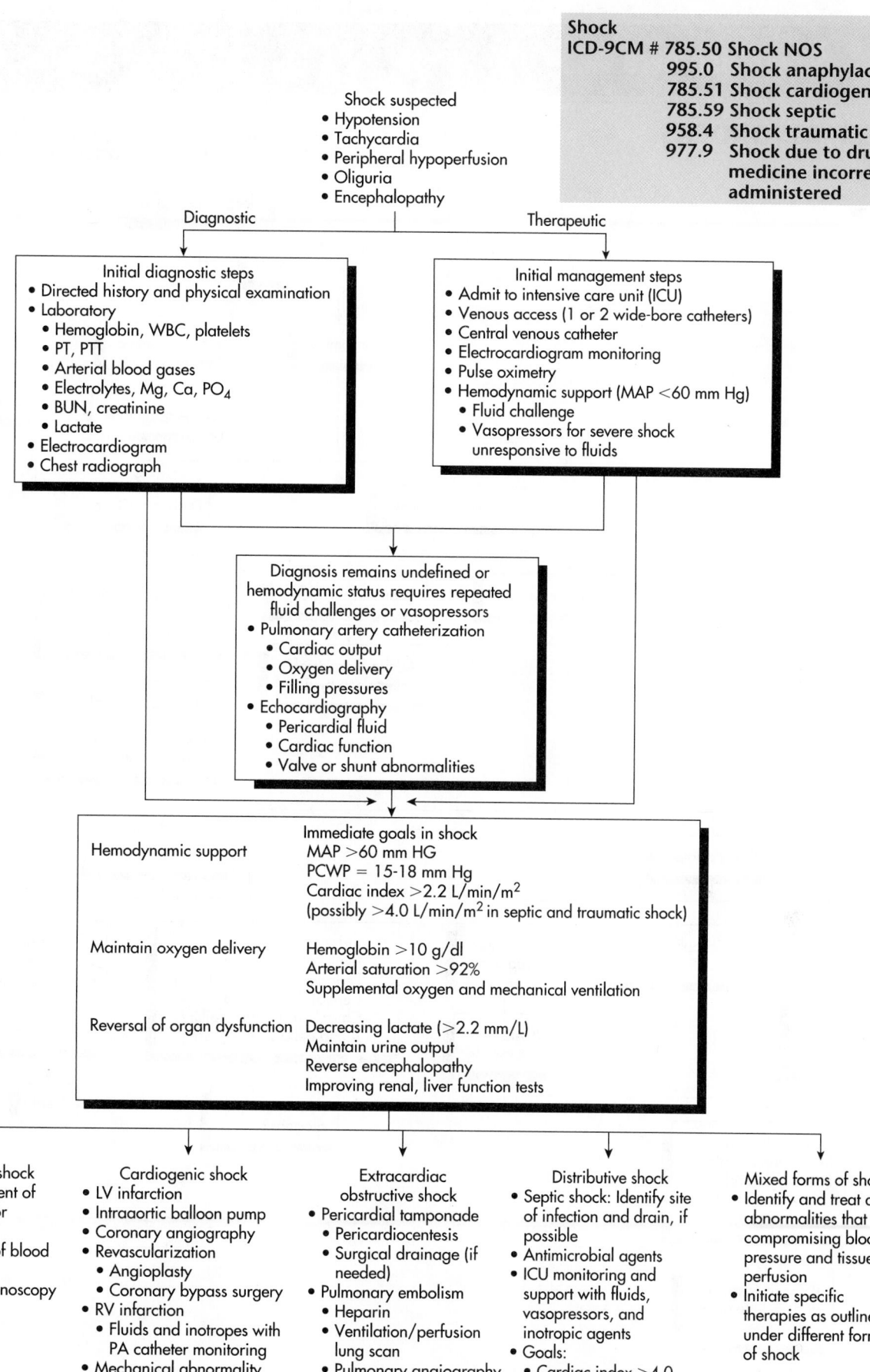

Fig. 3-167   An approach to the diagnosis and treatment of shock. *BUN,* Blood urea nitrogen; *CT,* computed tomography; *LV,* left ventricular; *MAP,* mean arterial pressure; *MRI,* magnetic resonance imaging; *PA,* pulmonary arterial; *PCWP,* pulmonary capillary wedge pressure, *PT,* prothrombin time; *PTT,* partial thromboplastin time; *RV,* right ventricular; *WBC,* white blood cell count. (From Goldman L, Ausiello D [eds]: *Cecil textbook of medicine,* ed 22, Philadelphia, 2004, WB Saunders.)

SLEEP DISORDERS

A

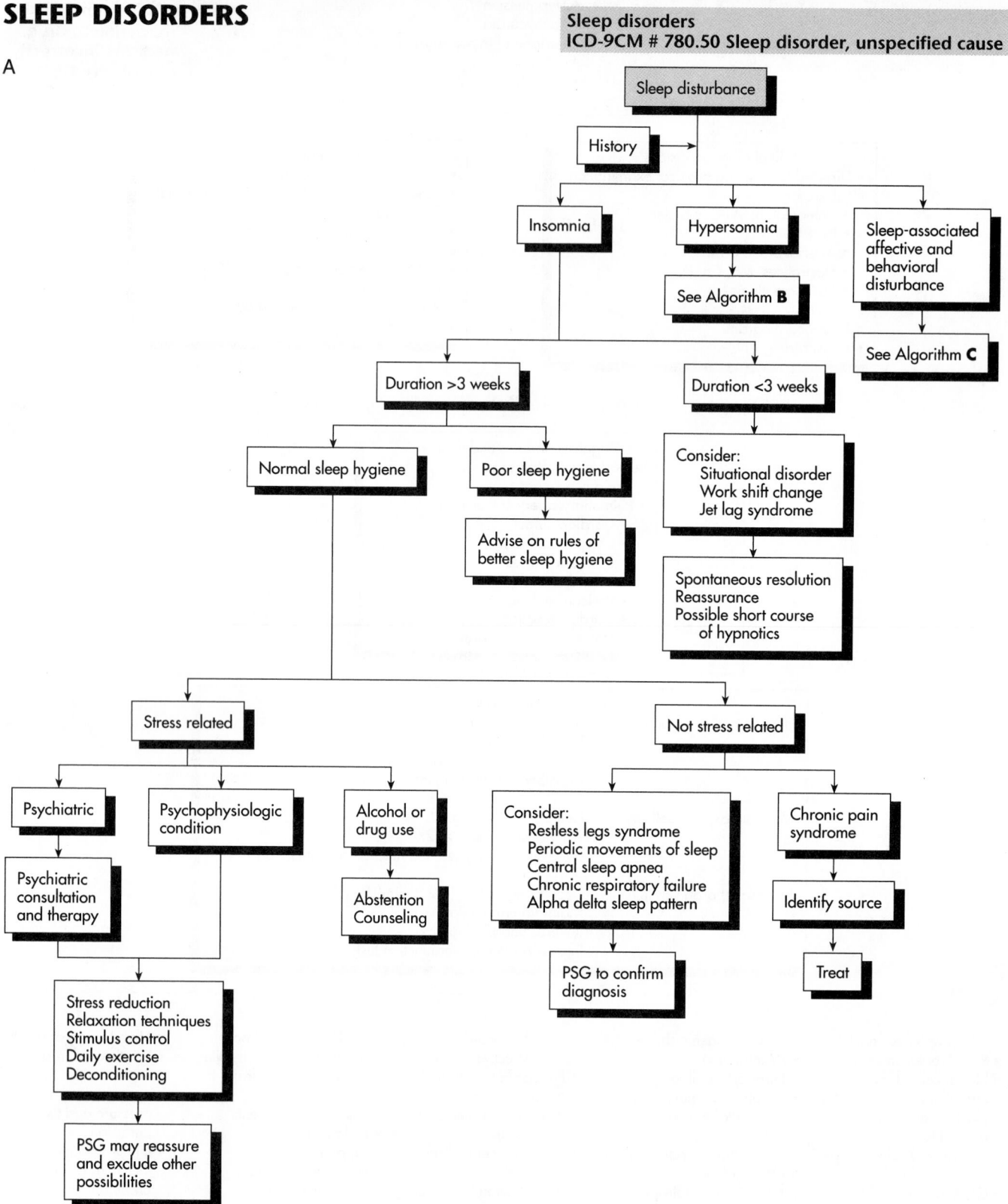

Fig. 3-168 A, Patient with sleep disturbance. *MSLT,* Multiple sleep latency tests; *PSG,* polysomnography. (From Greene HL, Johnson WP, Lemcke D [eds]: *Decision making in medicine,* ed 2, St Louis, 1998, Mosby.)

Continued

SLEEP DISORDERS—cont'd

B

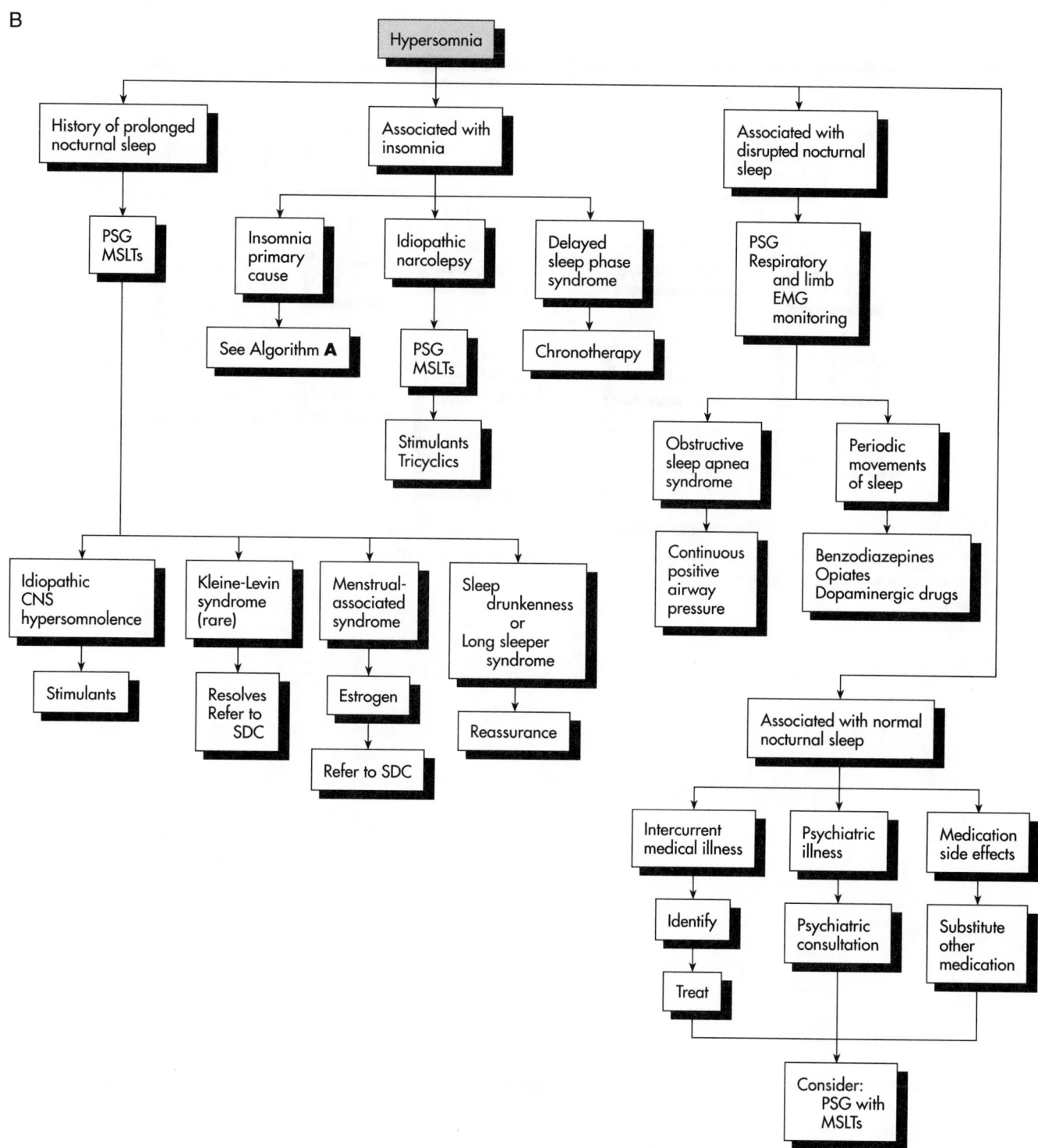

Fig. 3-168, cont'd   B, Hypersomnia. *CNS,* Central nervous system; *EMG,* electromyelogram; *MSLTs,* multiple sleep latency tests; *PSG,* polysomnography; *SDC,* sleep disorders clinic.

SLEEP DISORDERS—cont'd

C

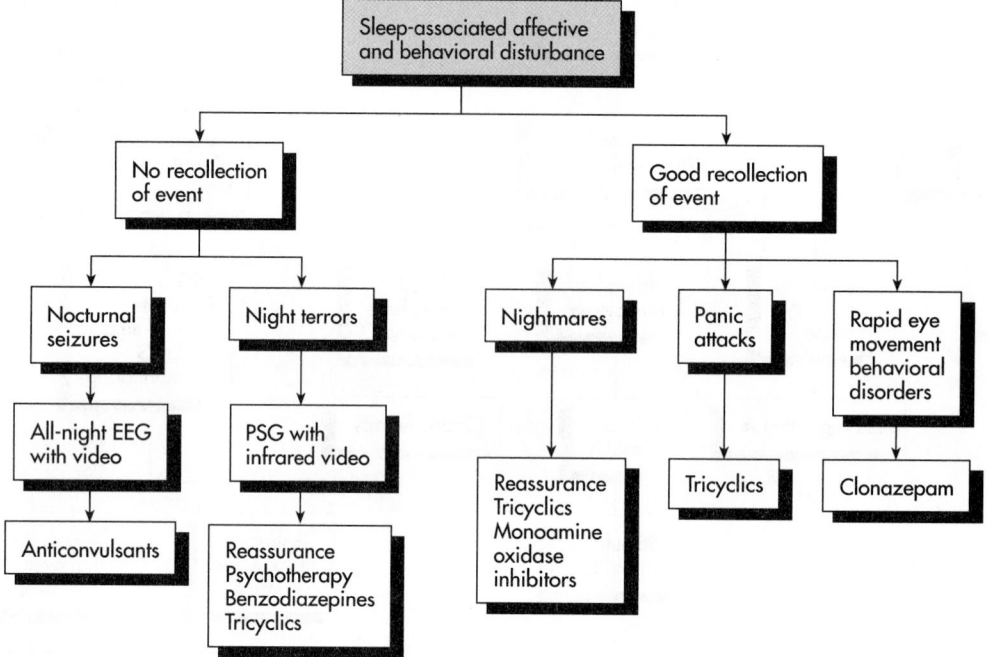

Fig. 3-168, cont'd   C, Sleep-associated affective and behavioral disturbance. *EEG,* Electroencephalogram; *PSG,* polysomnography.

SPLENOMEGALY

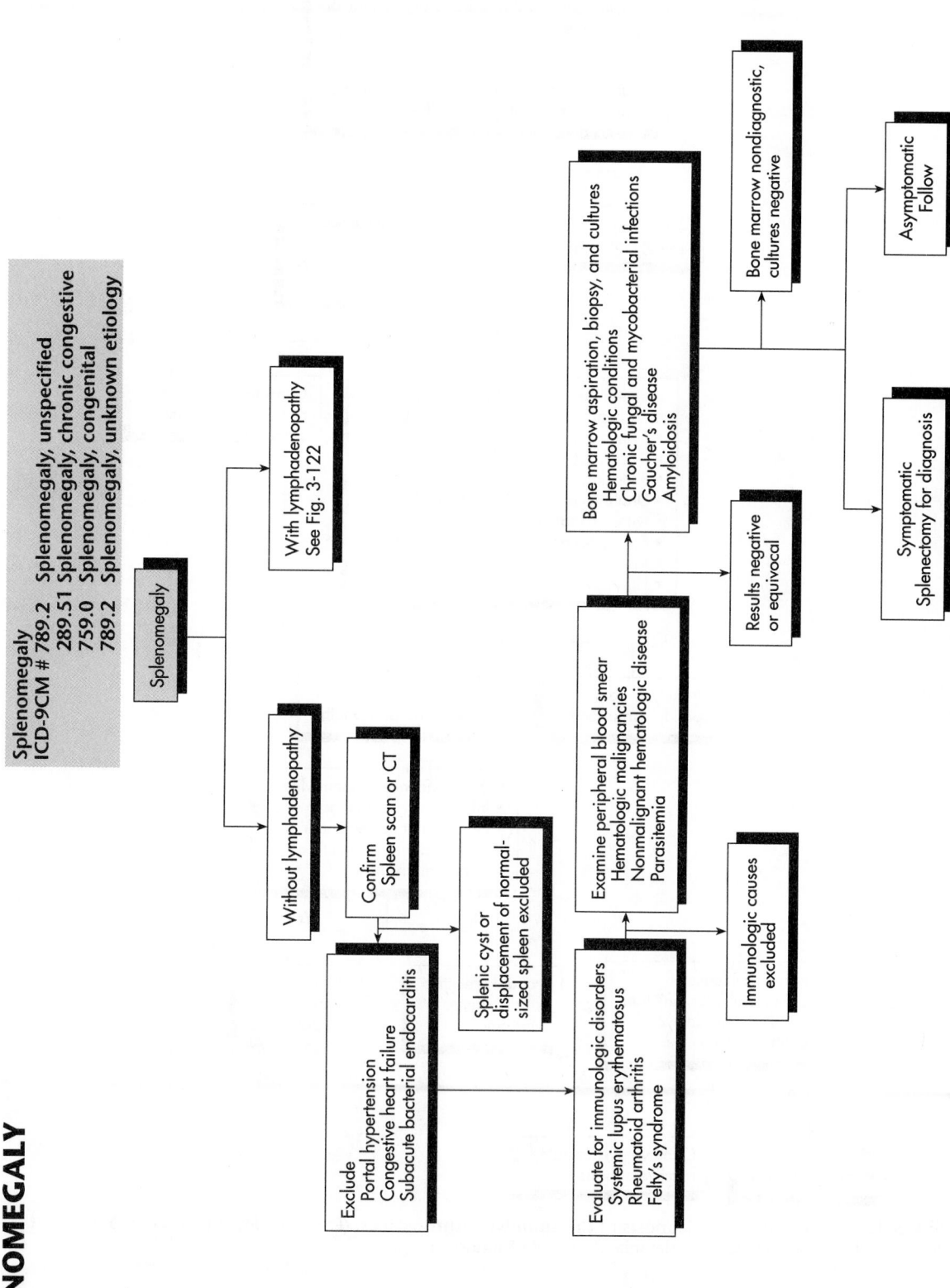

Fig. 3-169 Clinical approach to patient with splenomegaly. *CT,* Computed tomography. (From Stein JH [ed]: *Internal medicine,* ed 5, St Louis, 1998, Mosby.)

SPONDYLOARTHROPATHY, DIAGNOSIS

Spondyloarthropathy, diagnosis
ICD-9CM # 720.7

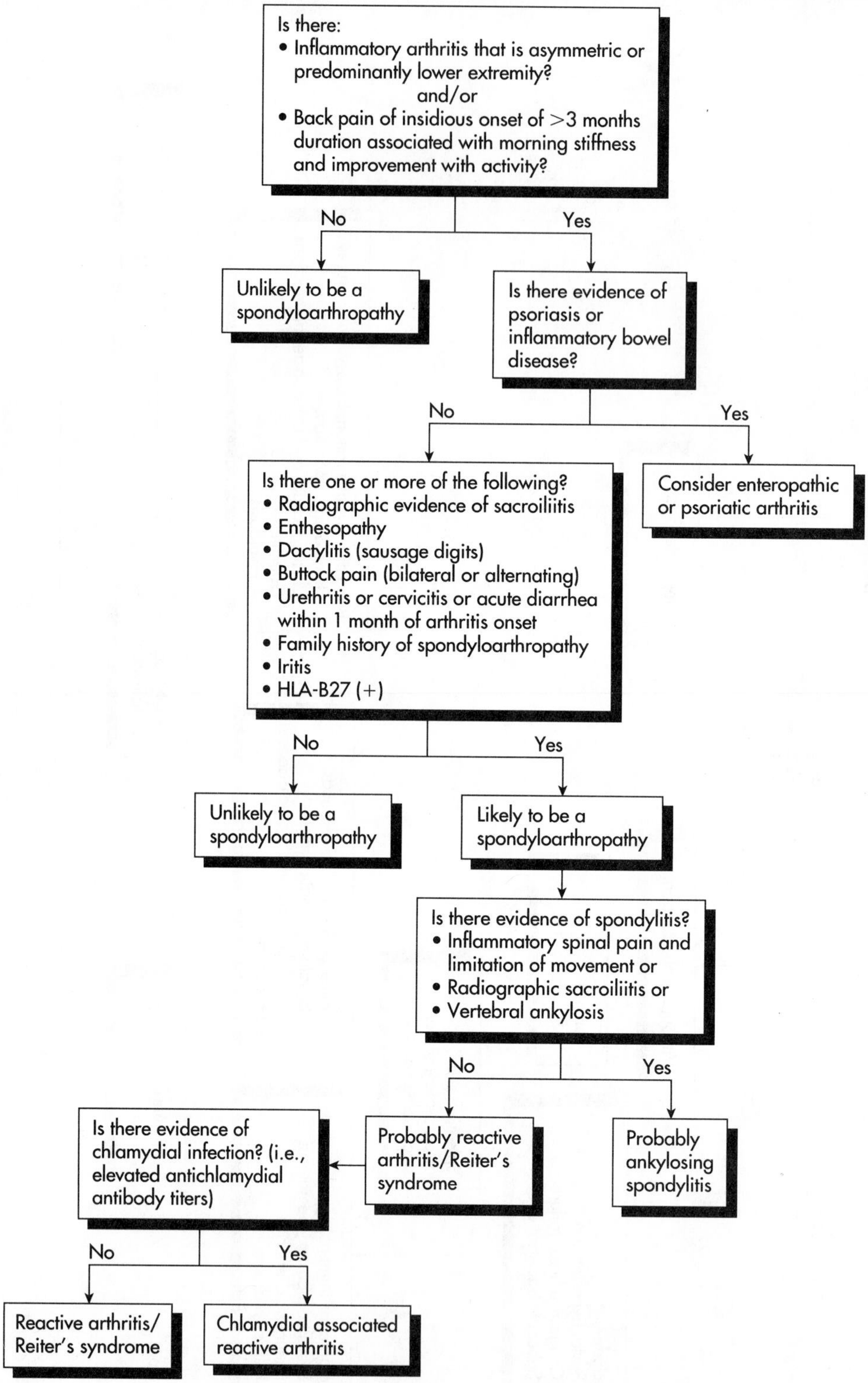

Is there:
- Inflammatory arthritis that is asymmetric or predominantly lower extremity?
  and/or
- Back pain of insidious onset of >3 months duration associated with morning stiffness and improvement with activity?

No → Unlikely to be a spondyloarthropathy

Yes → Is there evidence of psoriasis or inflammatory bowel disease?

No → Is there one or more of the following?
- Radiographic evidence of sacroiliitis
- Enthesopathy
- Dactylitis (sausage digits)
- Buttock pain (bilateral or alternating)
- Urethritis or cervicitis or acute diarrhea within 1 month of arthritis onset
- Family history of spondyloarthropathy
- Iritis
- HLA-B27 (+)

Yes → Consider enteropathic or psoriatic arthritis

No → Unlikely to be a spondyloarthropathy

Yes → Likely to be a spondyloarthropathy

Is there evidence of spondylitis?
- Inflammatory spinal pain and limitation of movement or
- Radiographic sacroiliitis or
- Vertebral ankylosis

No → Probably reactive arthritis/Reiter's syndrome

Yes → Probably ankylosing spondylitis

Is there evidence of chlamydial infection? (i.e., elevated antichlamydial antibody titers)

No → Reactive arthritis/Reiter's syndrome

Yes → Chlamydial associated reactive arthritis

Fig. 3-170   Algorithm for diagnosis of the spondyloarthropathies. (From Goldman L, Ausiello D: *Cecil textbook of medicine,* ed 22, Philadelphia, 2004, WB Saunders.)

SPONDYLOARTHROPATHY, TREATMENT

Spondyloarthropathy, treatment
ICD-9CM # 720.7

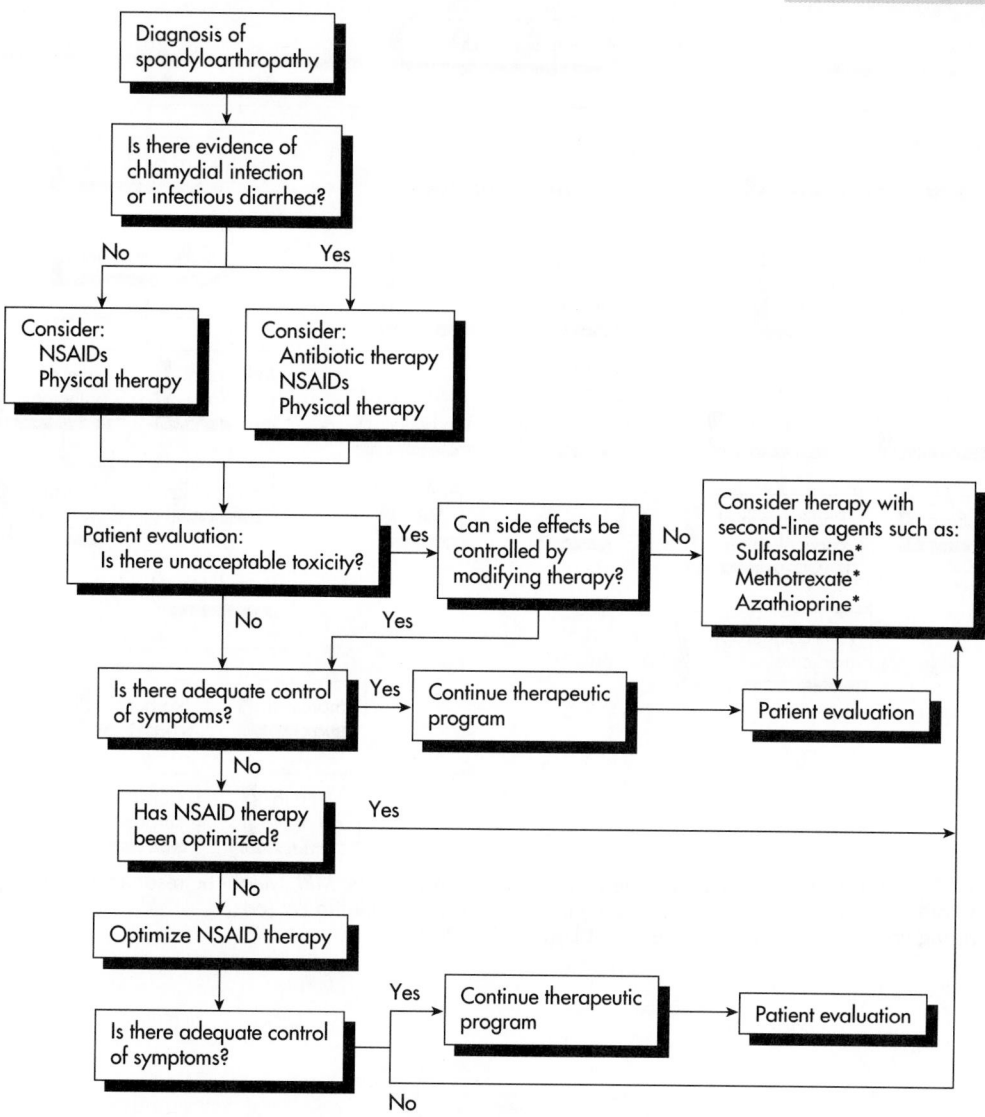

*Not approved by the FDA for treatment of spondyloarthropathies.

Fig. 3-171   Treatment algorithm for patients with a spondyloarthropathy. *FDA,* Food and Drug Administration; *NSAID,* nonsteroidal antiinflammatory drug. (From Goldman L, Ausiello D: *Cecil textbook of medicine,* ed 22, Philadelphia, 2004, WB Saunders.)

SPONDYLOSIS, CERVICAL

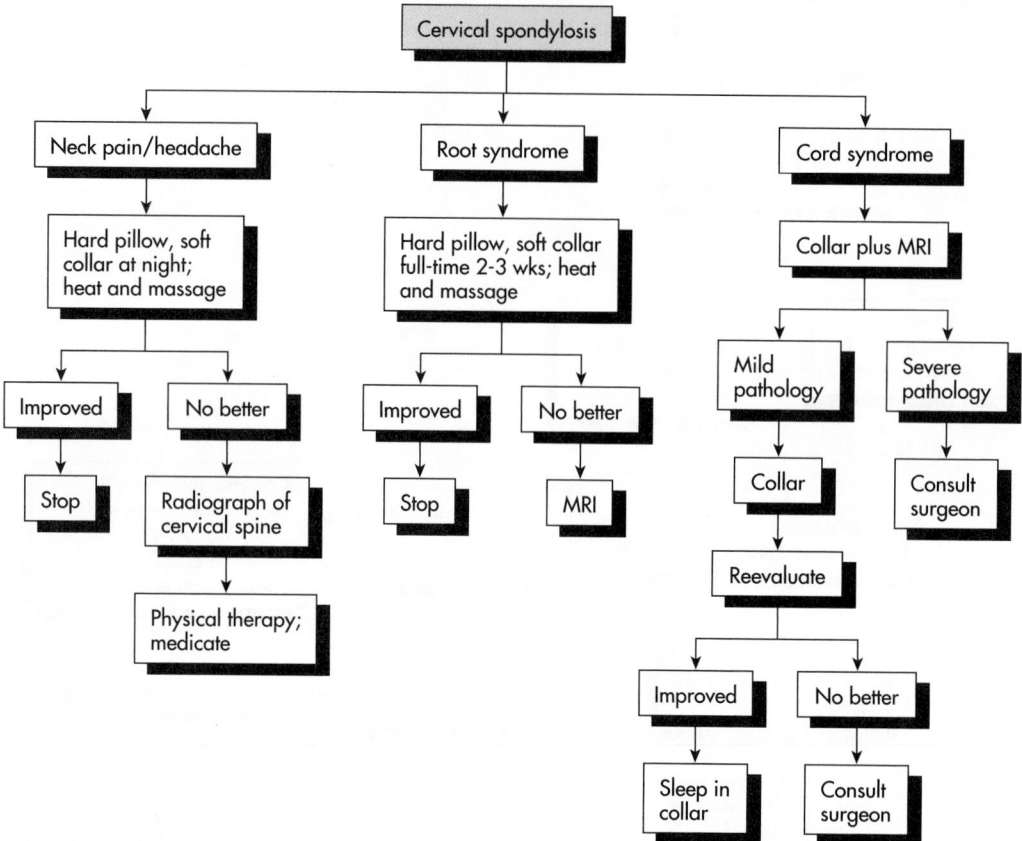

Fig. 3-172 Algorithm for the treatment of cervical spondylosis. *MRI,* Magnetic resonance imaging. (From Ronthal M, Rachlin JR: Cervical spondylosis. In Johnson RT, Griffin JW [eds]: *Current therapy in neurologic disease,* ed 5, St Louis, 1997, Mosby.)

SYNCOPE

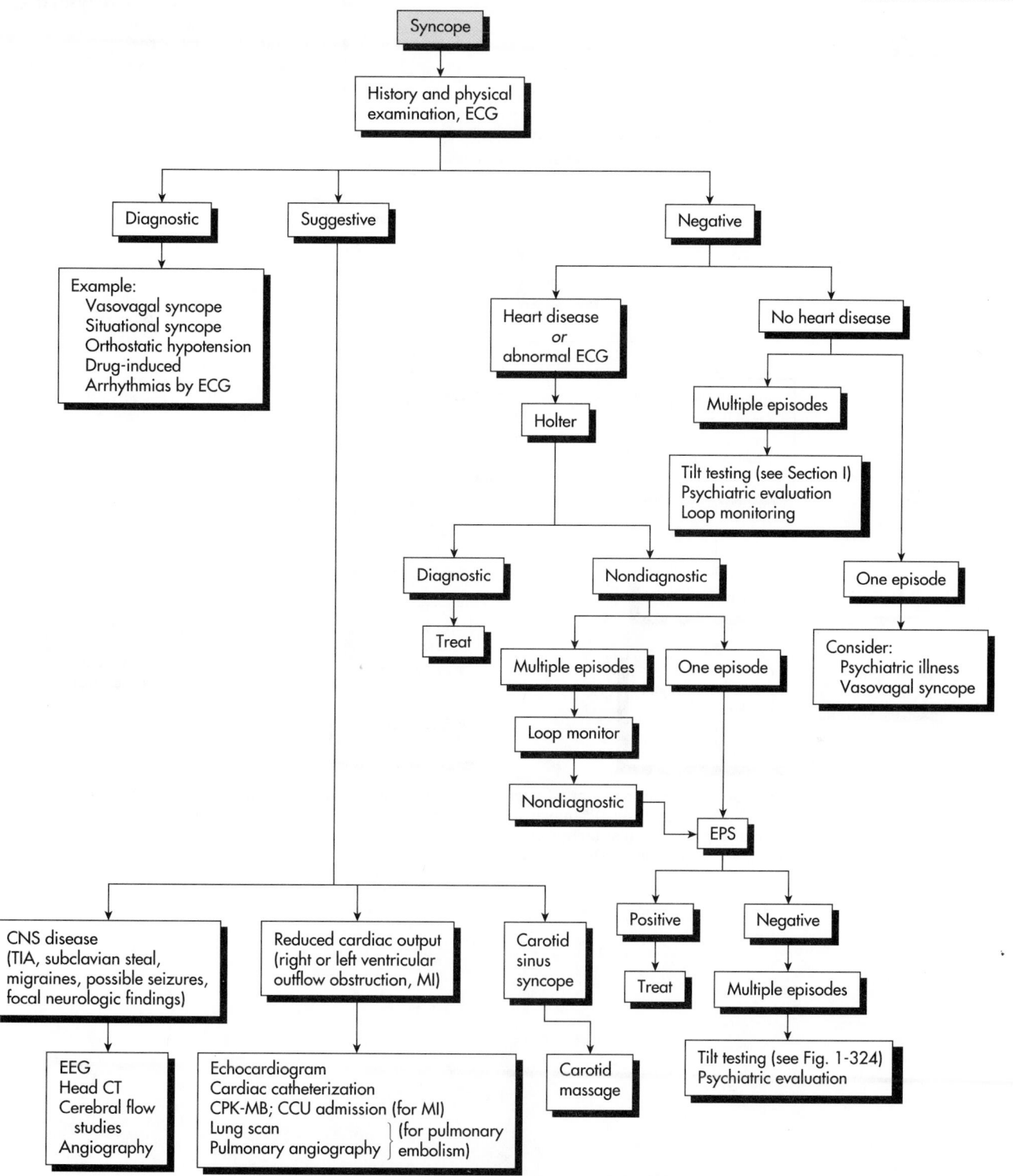

Fig. 3-173   Algorithm summarizing the diagnostic approach to syncope. *CCU,* Critical care unit; *CNS,* central nervous system; *CPK-MB,* isoenzyme of creatine kinase containing M and B subunits; *CT,* computed tomography; *ECG,* electrocardiogram; *EEG,* electroencephalogram; *EPS,* electrophysiologic studies; *MI,* myocardial infarction; *TIA,* transient ischemic attack. (From Noble J: *Primary care medicine,* ed 3, St Louis, 2001, Mosby.)

TACHYCARDIA, NARROW COMPLEX

Tachycardia, narrow complex
ICD-9CM # 427.2   Paroxysmal tachycardia
      427.0   Supraventricular paroxysmal
         tachycardia
      427.42 Ventricular flutter
      427.1   Ventricular paroxysmal tachycardia
      427.89 Atrial tachycardia

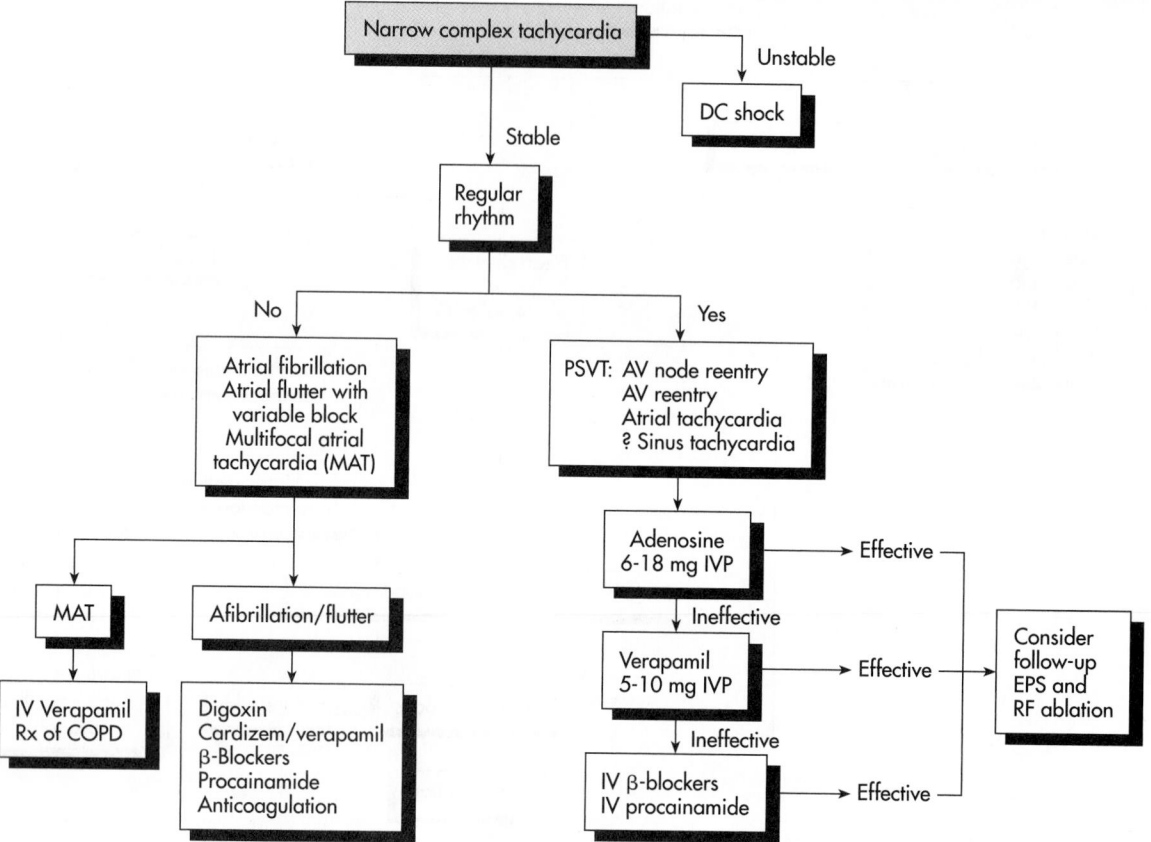

Fig. 3-174   Evaluation and management of narrow complex tachycardia. *AV,* Atrioventricular; *COPD,* chronic obstructive pulmonary disease; *EPS,* electrophysiologic studies; *IV,* intravenous; *IVP,* intravenous push; *PSVT,* paroxysmal supraventricular tachycardia; *RF,* radiofrequency. (From Driscoll CE et al: *The family practice desk reference,* ed 3, St Louis, 1996, Mosby.)

TACHYCARDIA, WIDE COMPLEX

Tachycardia, wide complex
ICD-9CM # 427.2   Paroxysmal tachycardia
           427.0   Supraventricular paroxysmal
                   tachycardia
           427.42 Ventricular flutter
           427.1   Ventricular paroxysmal tachycardia
           427.89 Atrial tachycardia

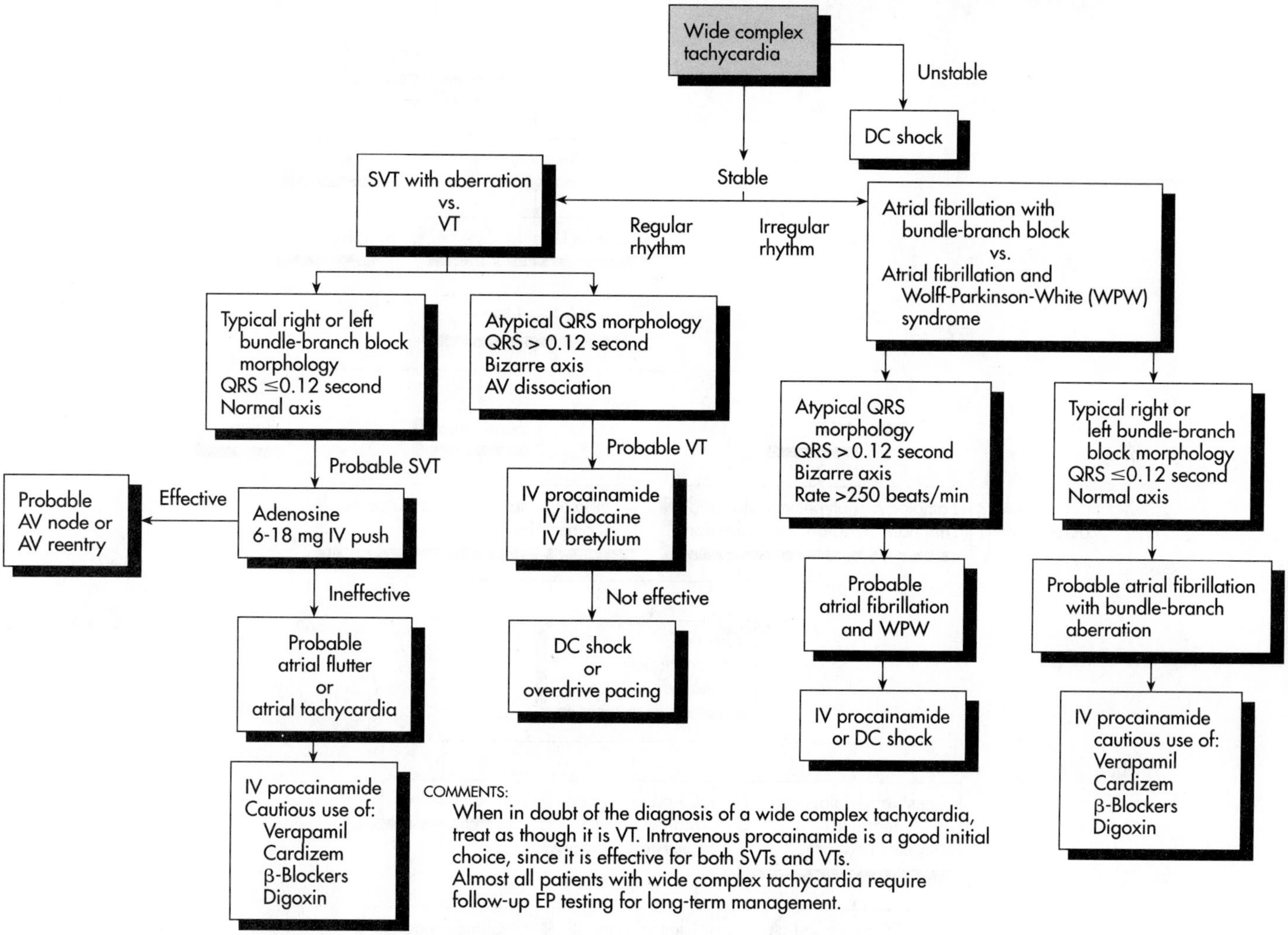

Fig. 3-175   Evaluation and management of wide complex tachycardia. *AV,* Atrioventricular; *EP,* electrophysiologic; *IV,* intravenous; *SVT,* supraventricular tachycardia; *VT,* ventricular tachycardia. (From Driscoll CE et al: *The family practice desk reference,* ed 3, St Louis, 1996, Mosby.)

COMMENTS:
When in doubt of the diagnosis of a wide complex tachycardia, treat as though it is VT. Intravenous procainamide is a good initial choice, since it is effective for both SVTs and VTs.
Almost all patients with wide complex tachycardia require follow-up EP testing for long-term management.

TESTICULAR MASS

Testicular mass
ICD-9CM # 186.9 Testicular neoplasm
        M906/3 (seminoma)
        M9101/3 (embryonal carcinoma or teratoma)
        M9100/3 (choriocarcinoma)

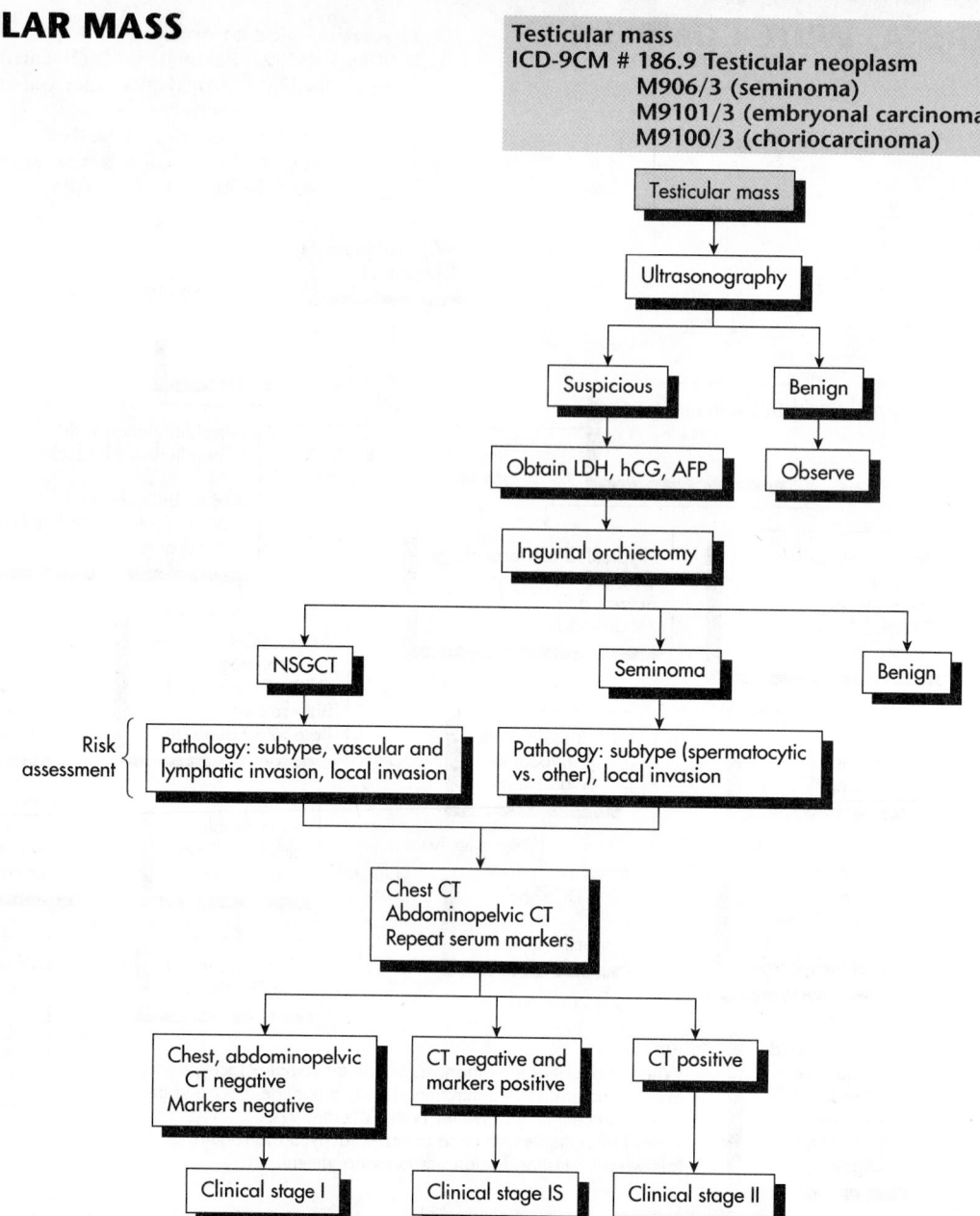

Fig. 3-176 **Diagnosis, staging, and risk assessment of patients with testicular germ cell tumor.** *AFP,* Alpha-fetoprotein; *CT,* computed tomography; *hCG,* human chorionic gonadotropin; *LDH,* lactic dehydrogenase; *NSGCT,* nonseminoma germ cell tumor. (From Abeloff MD: *Clinical oncology,* ed 2, New York, 2000, Churchill Livingstone.)

THORACIC OUTLET SYNDROME

Thoracic outlet syndrome
ICD-9CM # 353.0

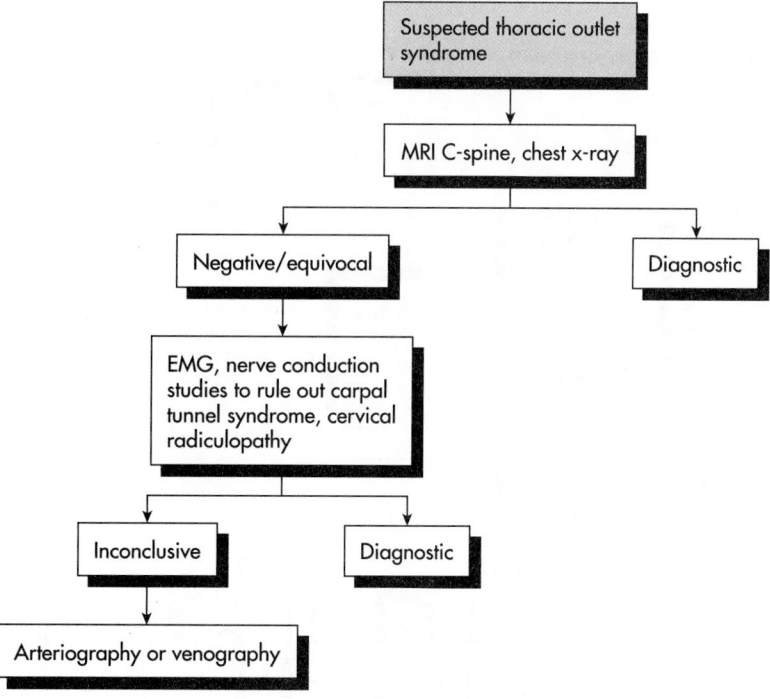

Fig. 3-177   Thoracic outlet syndrome. *EMG,* Electromyogram; *MRI,* magnetic resonance imaging.

III

THROMBOCYTOPENIA

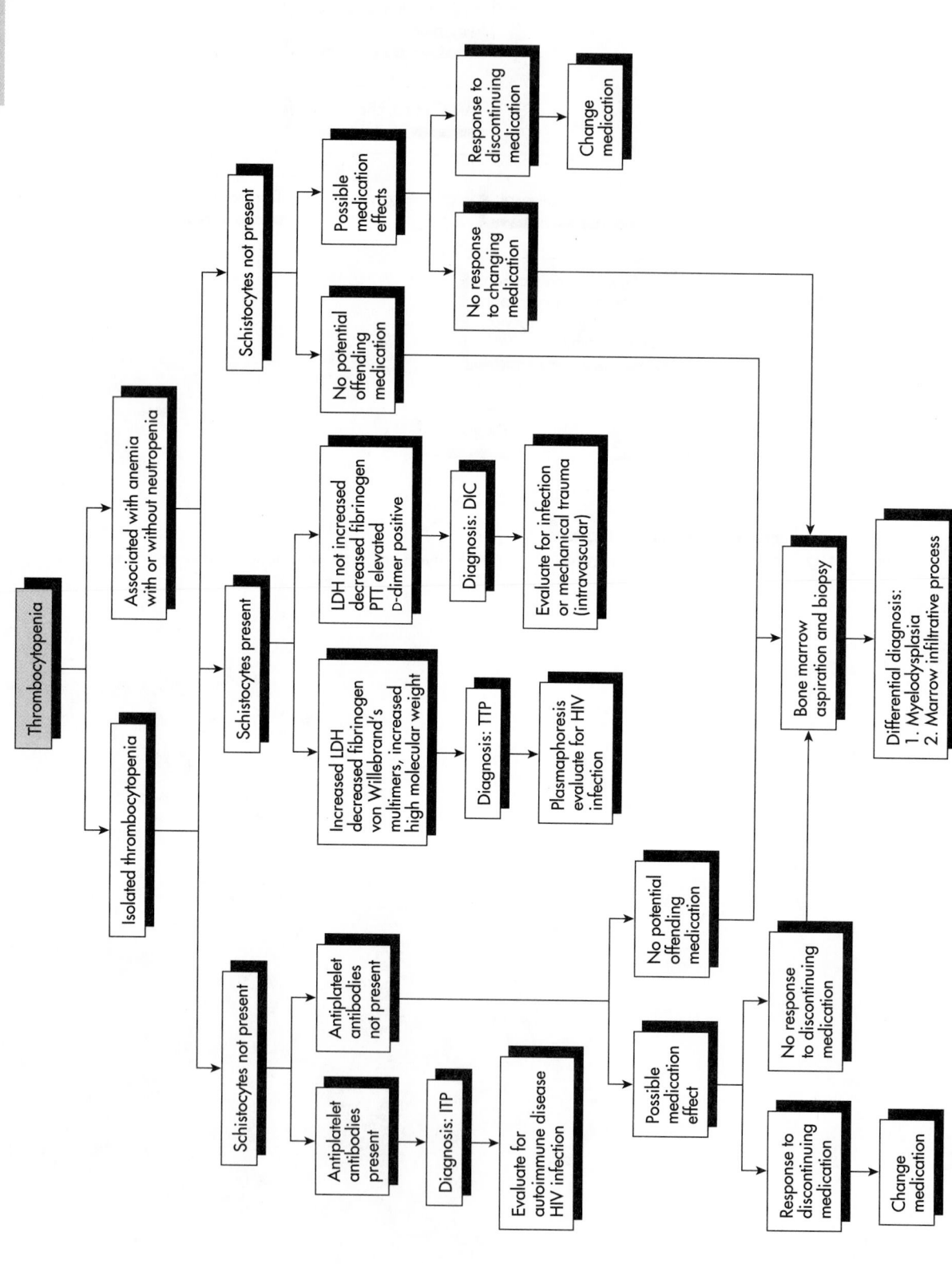

Fig. 3-178 **Differential diagnosis of thrombocytopenia.** *DIC,* Disseminated intravascular coagulation; *HIV,* human immunodeficiency virus; *ITP,* idiopathic thrombocytopenic purpura; *LDH,* lactic dehydrogenase; *PTT,* partial thromboplastin time; *TTP,* thrombotic thrombocytopenic purpura. (From Rakel RE [ed]: *Principles of family practice,* ed 6, Philadelphia, 2002, WB Saunders.)

THROMBOCYTOSIS

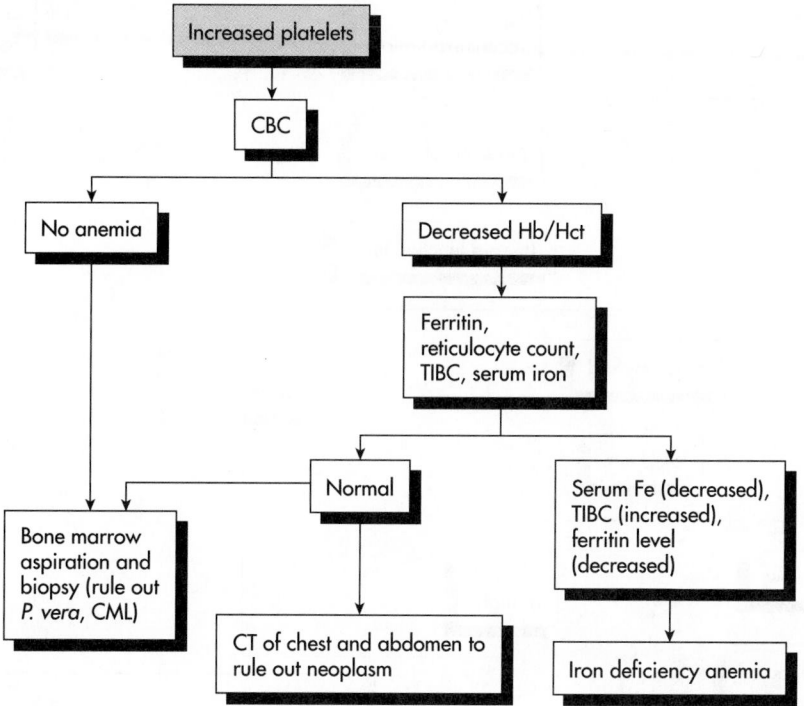

Fig. 3-179   Thrombocytosis. *CBC,* Complete blood count; *CML,* chronic myelogenous leukemia; *CT,* computed tomography; *Fe,* iron; *Hb/Hct,* hemoglobin/hematocrit; *TIBC,* total iron-binding capacity.

III

THYROID, PAINFUL

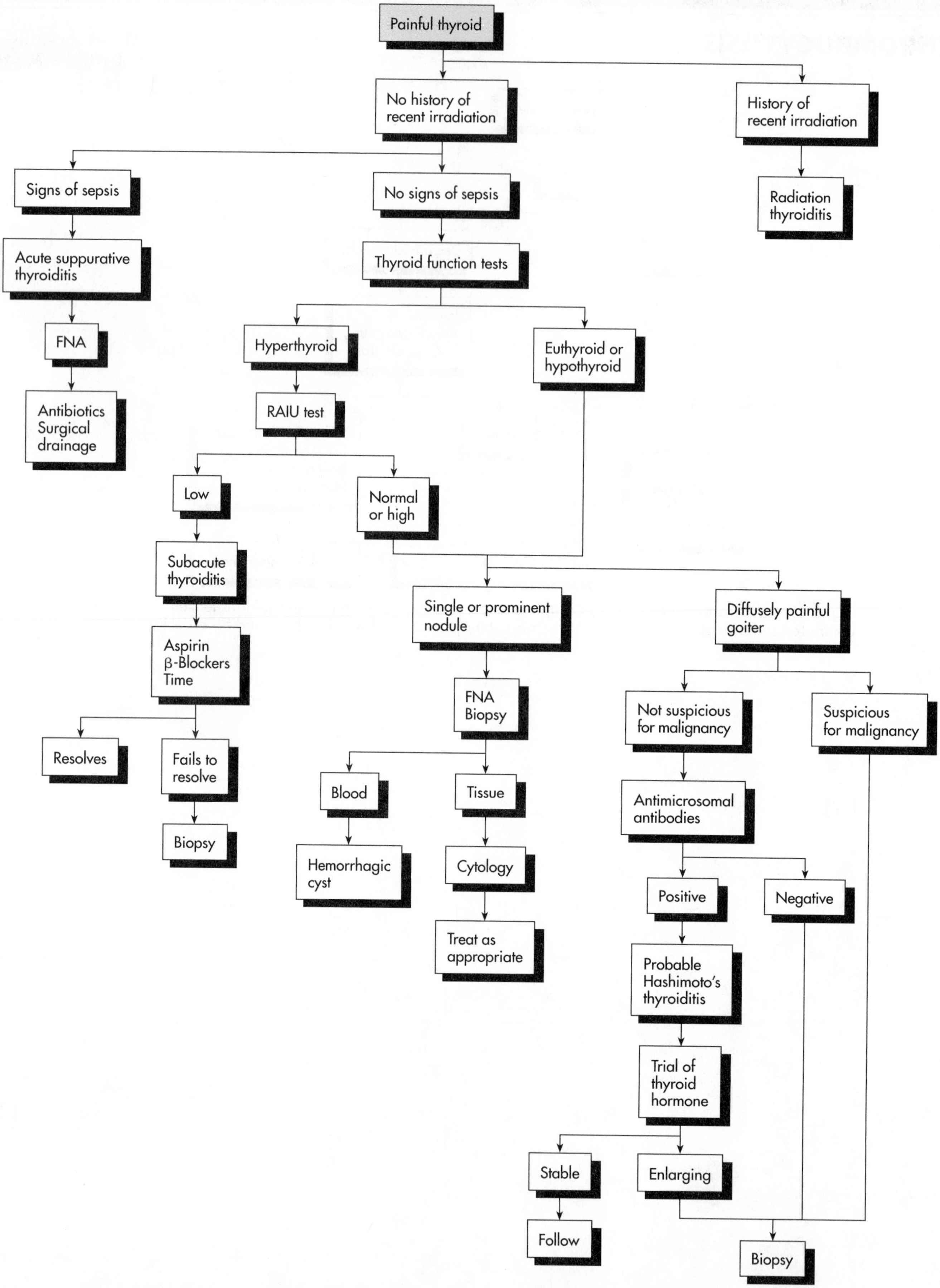

Fig. 3-180   Painful thyroid. *FNA,* Fine-needle aspiration; *RAIU,* radioactive iodine uptake. (From Greene HL, Johnson WP, Lemcke D [eds]: *Decision making in medicine,* ed 2, St Louis, 1998, Mosby.)

THYROID NODULE

Thyroid nodule
ICD-9CM # 241.0 Nodule, thyroid

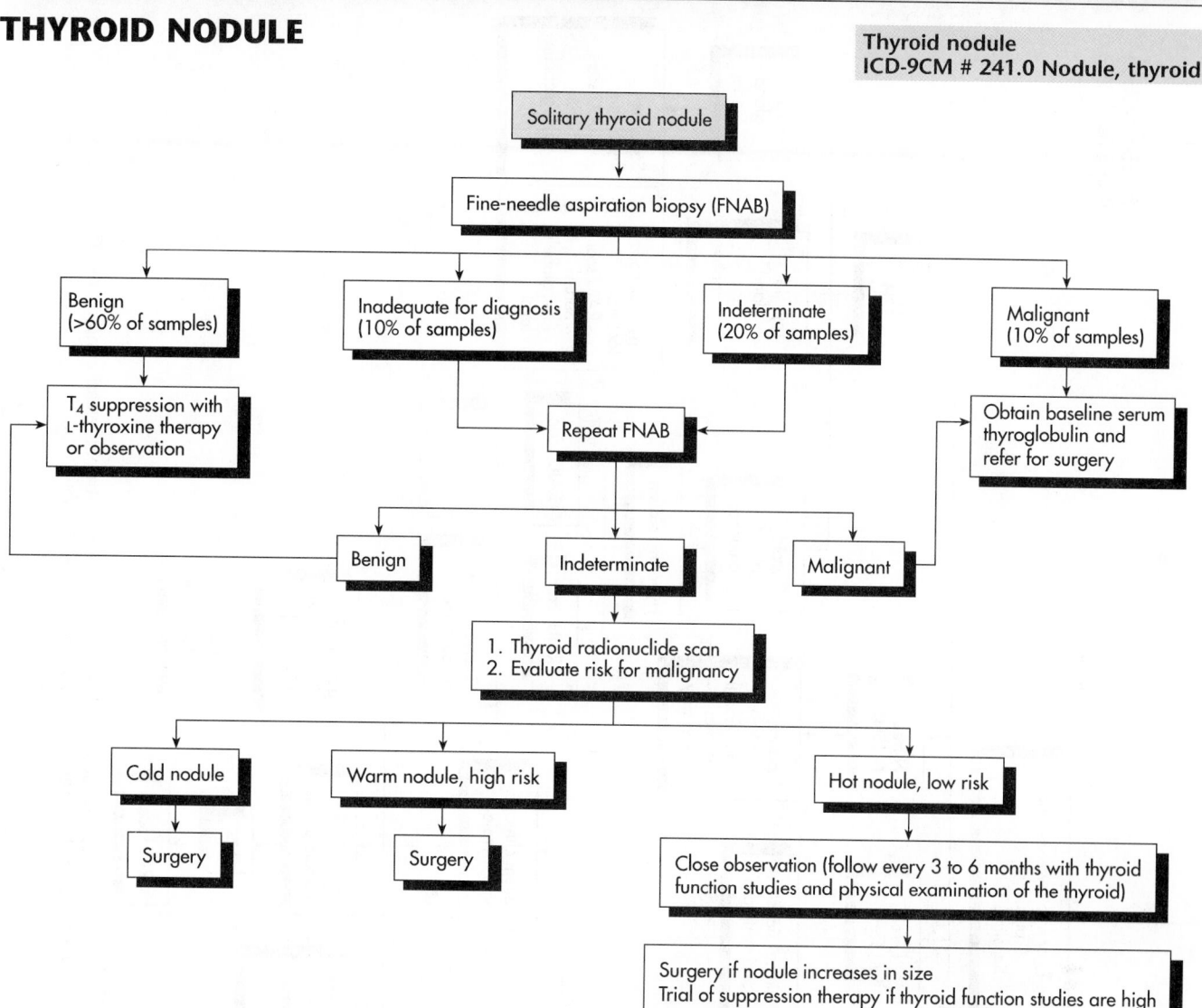

Fig. 3-181   Diagnostic evaluation of solitary thyroid nodule. High risk for malignancy: nodule >2 cm, age <40 yr, male sex, regional lymphadenopathy, fixation to adjacent tissues, history of prior head and neck irradiation. (From Ferri F: *Practical guide to the care of the medical patient,* ed 6, St Louis, 2004, Mosby.)

III

THYROID TESTING

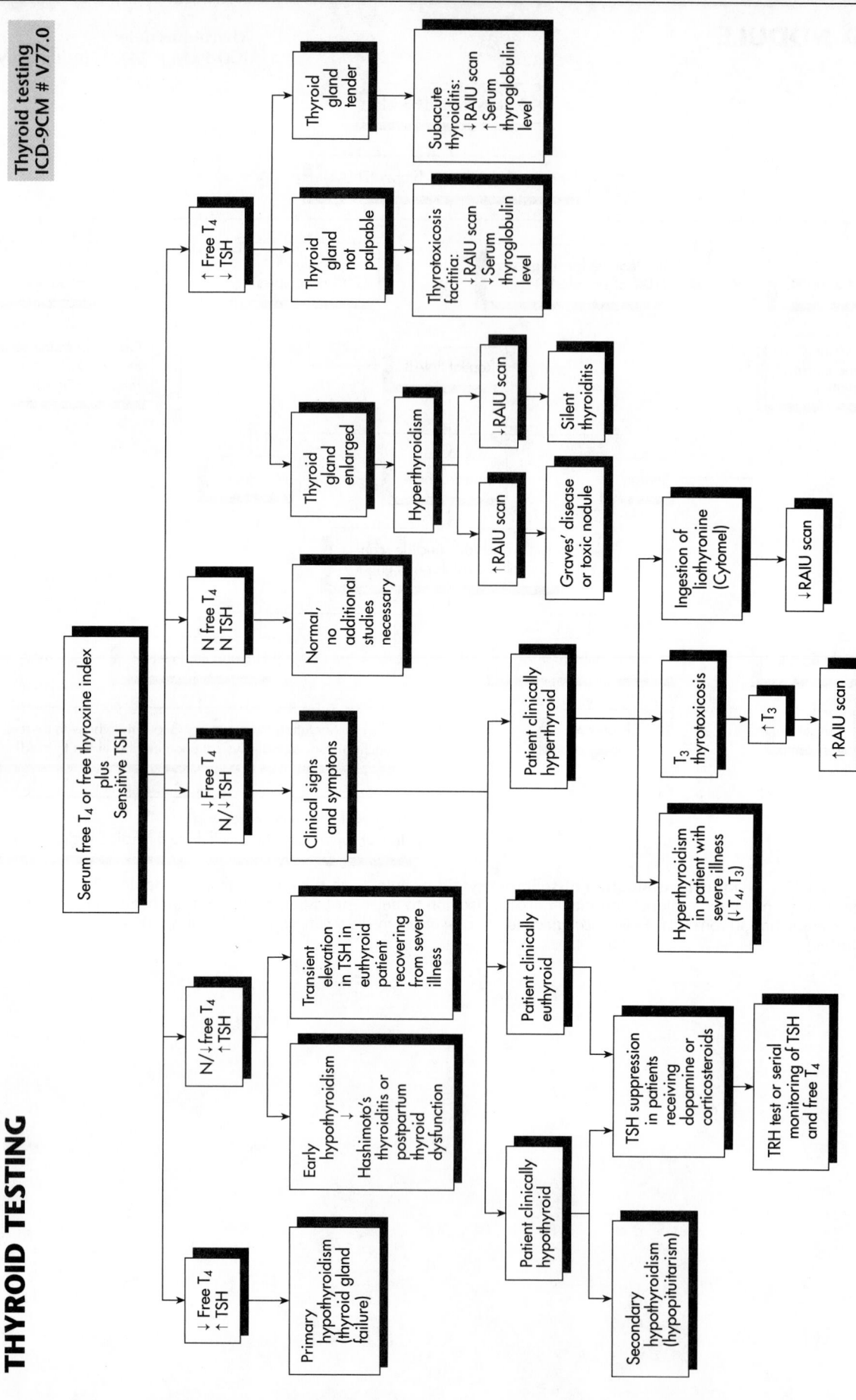

Fig. 3-182   Diagnostic approach to thyroid testing. *N,* Normal; *RAIU,* radioactive iodine uptake; *TRH,* thyrotropin-releasing hormone; *TSH,* thyroid-stimulating hormone. (From Ferri FF: *Practical guide to the care of the medical patient,* ed 6, St Louis, 2004, Mosby.)

TRANSIENT ISCHEMIC ATTACKS

Transient ischemic attacks
ICD-9CM # 435.9 Unspecified transient
cerebral ischemia

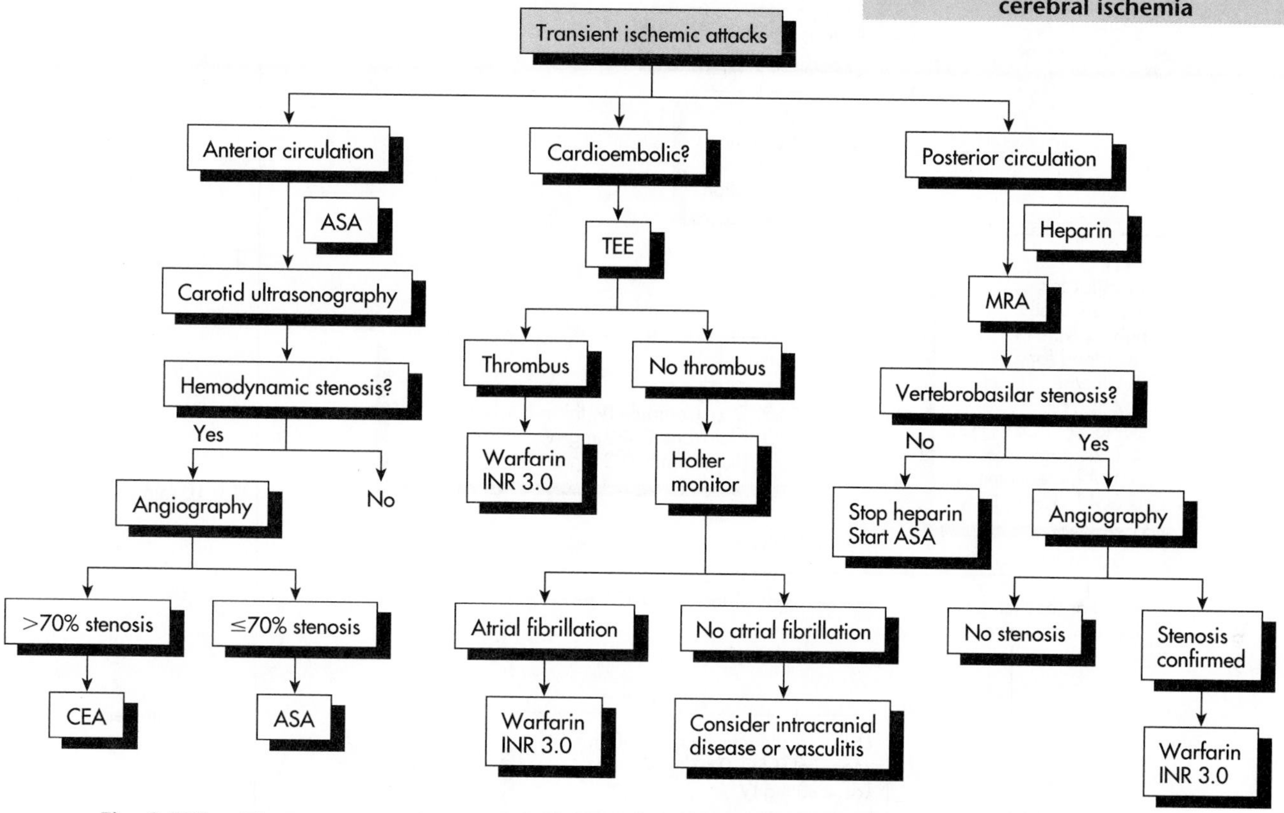

Transient ischemic attacks

Anterior circulation

ASA

Carotid ultrasonography

Hemodynamic stenosis?

Yes

No

Angiography

>70% stenosis

≤70% stenosis

CEA

ASA

Cardioembolic?

TEE

Thrombus

No thrombus

Warfarin
INR 3.0

Holter
monitor

Atrial fibrillation

No atrial fibrillation

Warfarin
INR 3.0

Consider intracranial
disease or vasculitis

Posterior circulation

Heparin

MRA

Vertebrobasilar stenosis?

No

Yes

Stop heparin
Start ASA

Angiography

No stenosis

Stenosis
confirmed

Warfarin
INR 3.0

Fig. 3-183 **The treatment of transient ischemic attacks (TIAs).** *ASA,* Aspirin; *CEA,* carotid endarterectomy; *INR,* International Normalized Ratio; *MRA,* magnetic resonance angiography; *TEE,* transesophageal echocardiography. (Modified from Morgenstern LB, Grotta JC: Transient ischemic attacks. In Johnson RT, Griffin JW [eds]: *Current therapy in neurologic disease,* ed 5, St Louis, 1997, Mosby.)

III

UNCONSCIOUS PATIENT

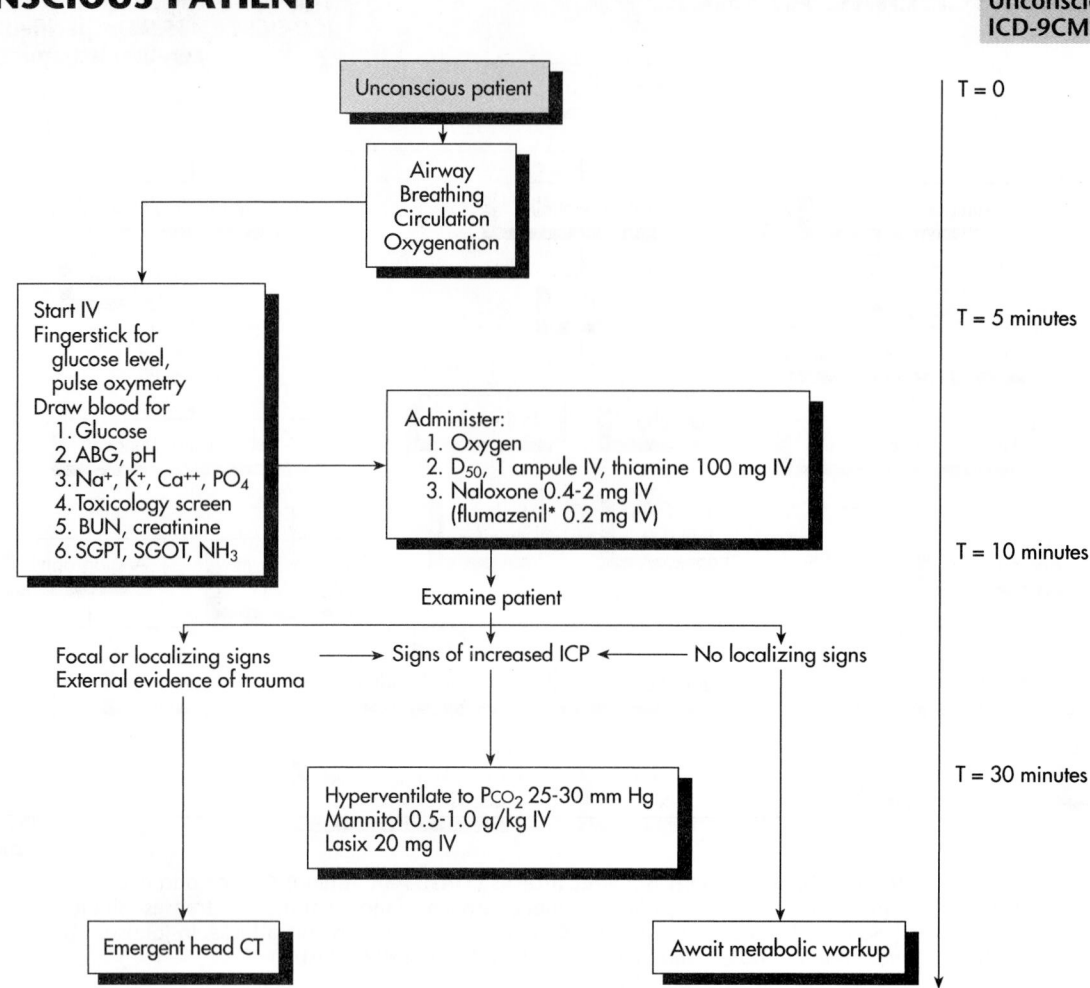

* Use of flumazenil should not be considered routine because
it can precipitate seizures in certain subsets of patients.

Fig. 3-184 **Approach to the unconscious patient.** *ABG,* Arterial blood gas; *BUN,* blood urea nitrogen; *CT,* computed tomography; *ICP,* intracranial pressure; *SGOT,* serum glutamic oxaloacetic transaminase; *SGPT,* serum glutamic pyruvic transaminase. (Modified from Johnson RT, Griffin JW: *Current therapy in neurologic disease,* ed 5, St Louis, 1997, Mosby.)

URETERAL CALCULI

Ureteral calculi
ICD-9CM # 592.9 Urinary calculus

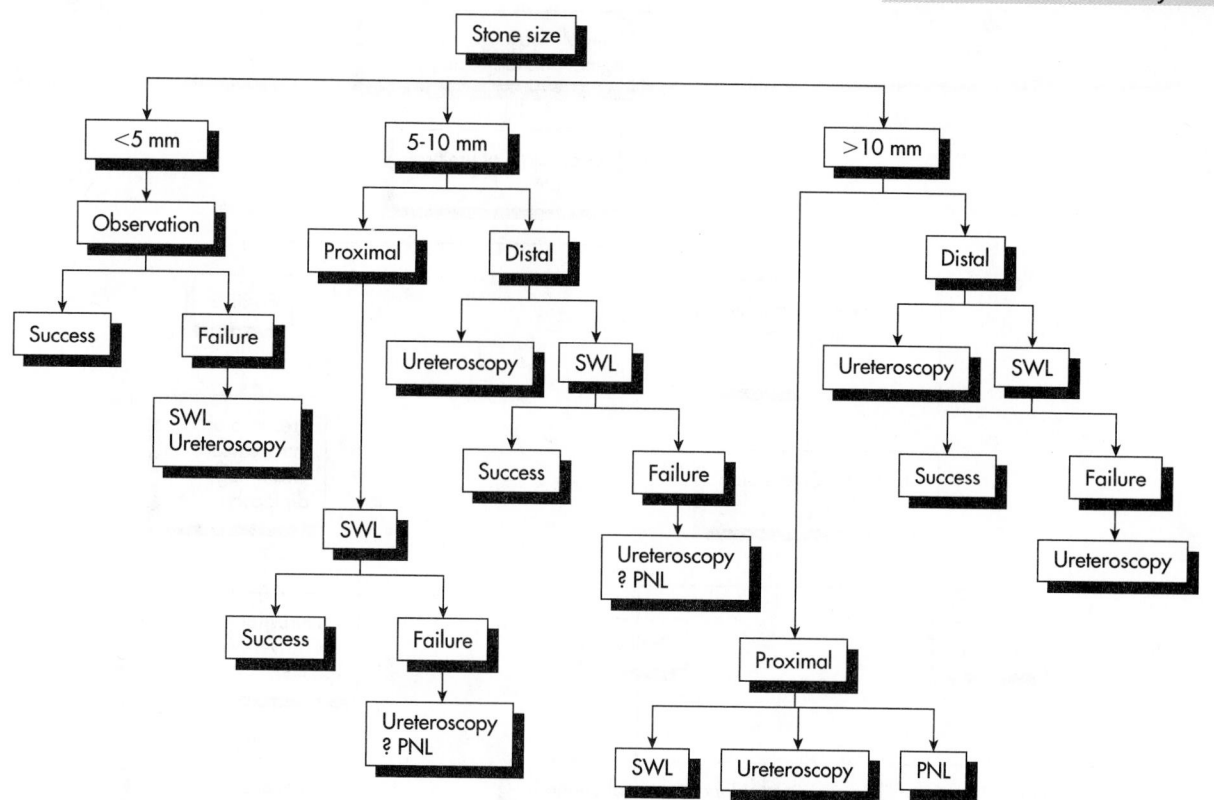

Fig. 3-185   Management of ureteral calculi. *PNL,* Percutaneous nephrostolithotomy; *SWL,* shock wave lithotripsy. (From Noble J: *Primary care medicine,* ed 3, St Louis, 2001, Mosby.)

III

URETHRAL DISCHARGE

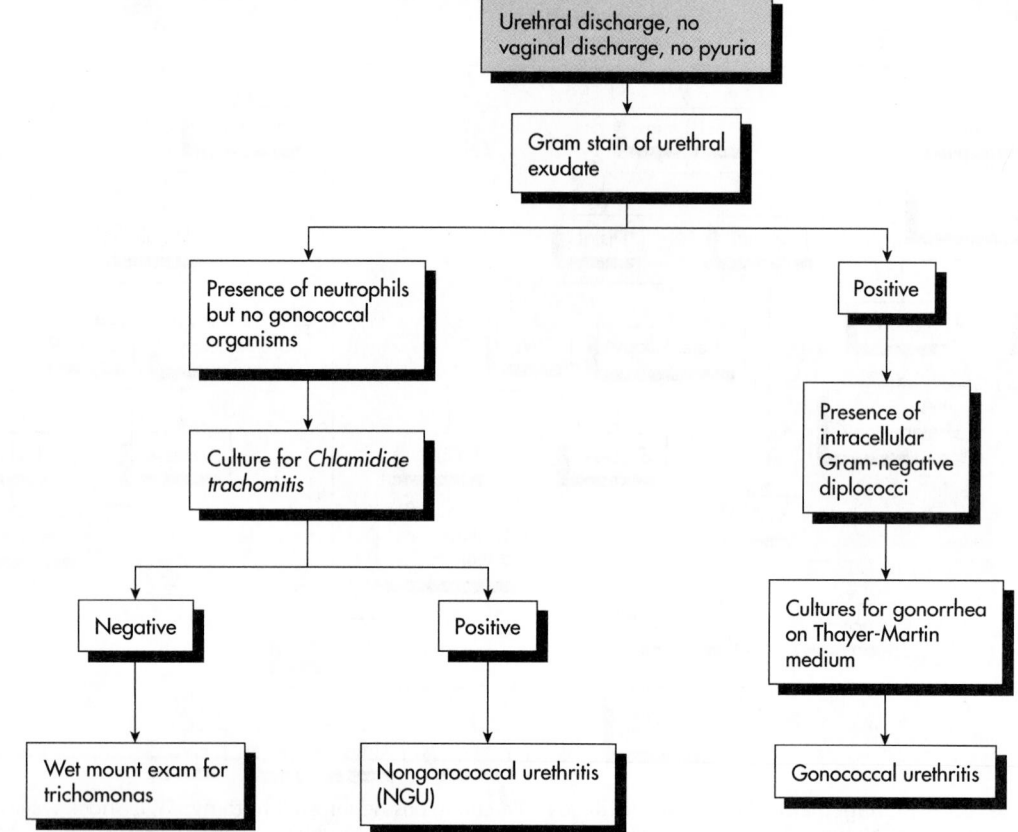

Fig. 3-186   Urethral discharge.

URINARY TRACT INFECTION

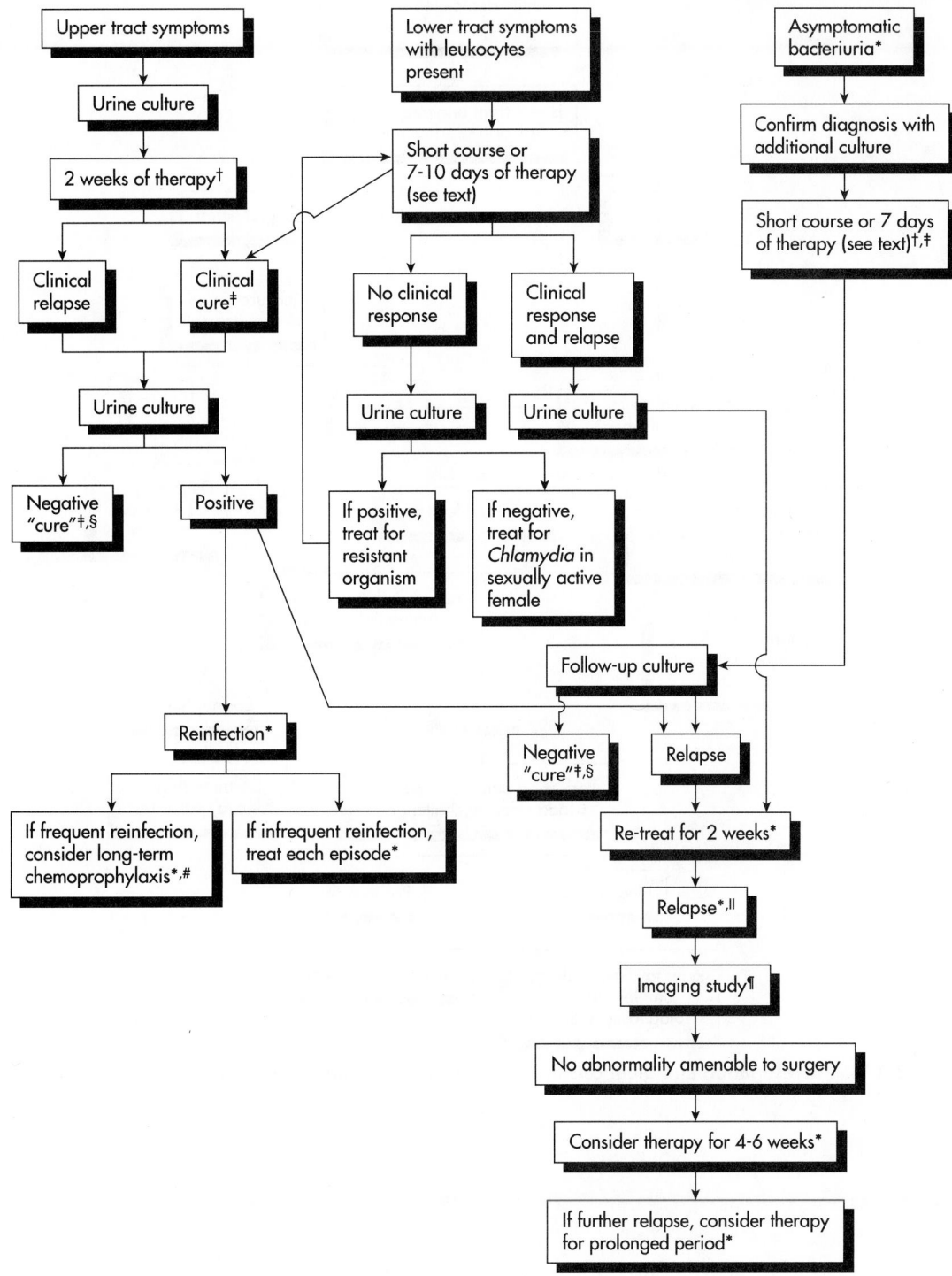

III

* Consider no therapy in nonpregnant adults without obstructive uropathy or symptoms of urinary tract infection.
† Consider imaging studies in all children and men with correction of significant lesions.
‡ Follow-up culture is required only in pregnancy, in children, and in adults with obstructive uropathy.
§ Obtain follow-up cultures monthly in pregnant women and at 6 weeks and 6 months in children.
‖ Evaluate men for chronic bacterial prostatitis.
¶ Delay 2 months postpartum in pregnant women.
# Consider imaging studies after three to four reinfections in women.

Fig. 3-187   Approach to the management of urinary tract infection. (From Mandell GL: *Mandell, Douglas, and Bennett's principles and practice of infectious diseases,* ed 5, New York, 2000, Churchill Livingstone.)

URTICARIA

Urticaria
ICD-9CM # 708.8 Other unspecified urticaria

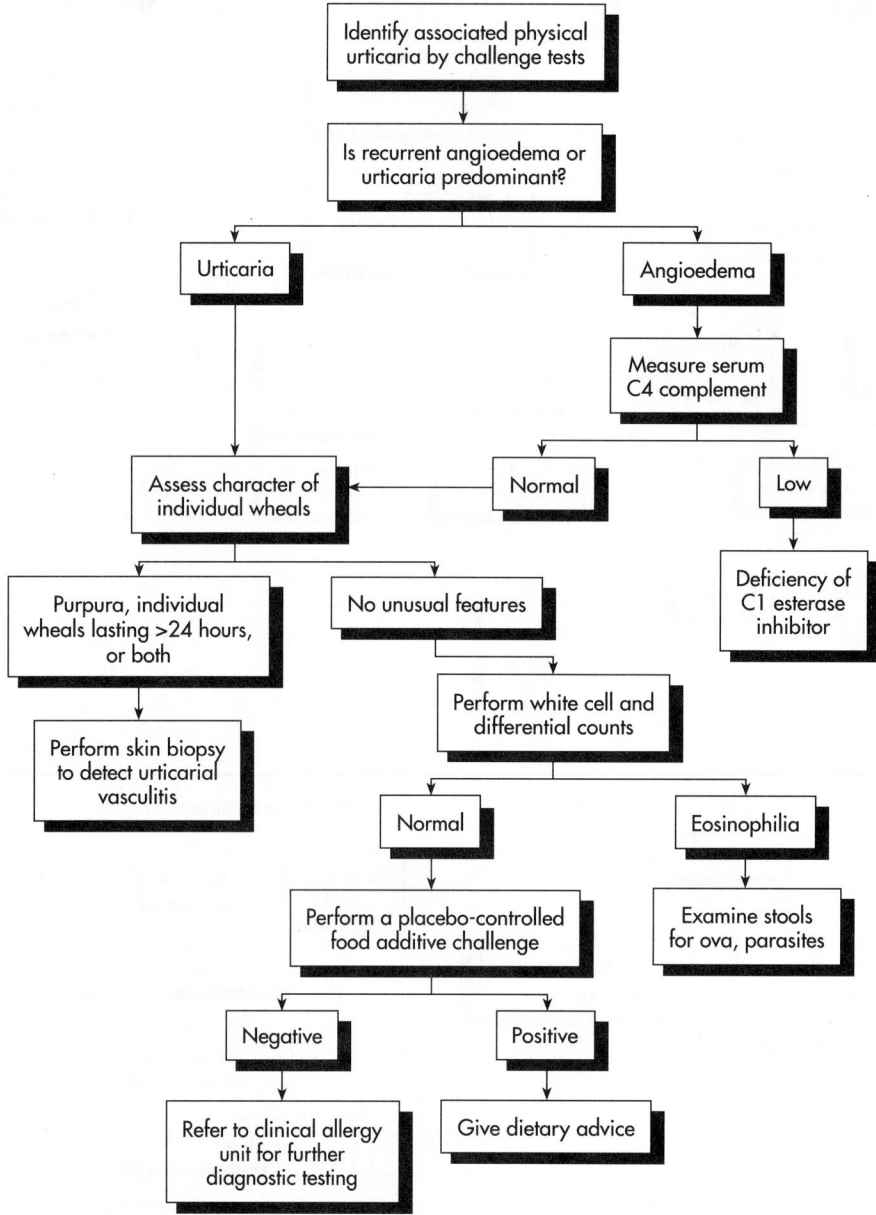

Fig. 3-188   Investigation and diagnosis of chronic urticaria. (From Greaves MW: *N Engl J Med* 332:1767, 1995.)

VAGINAL DISCHARGE

Vaginal discharge
ICD-9CM # 623.5

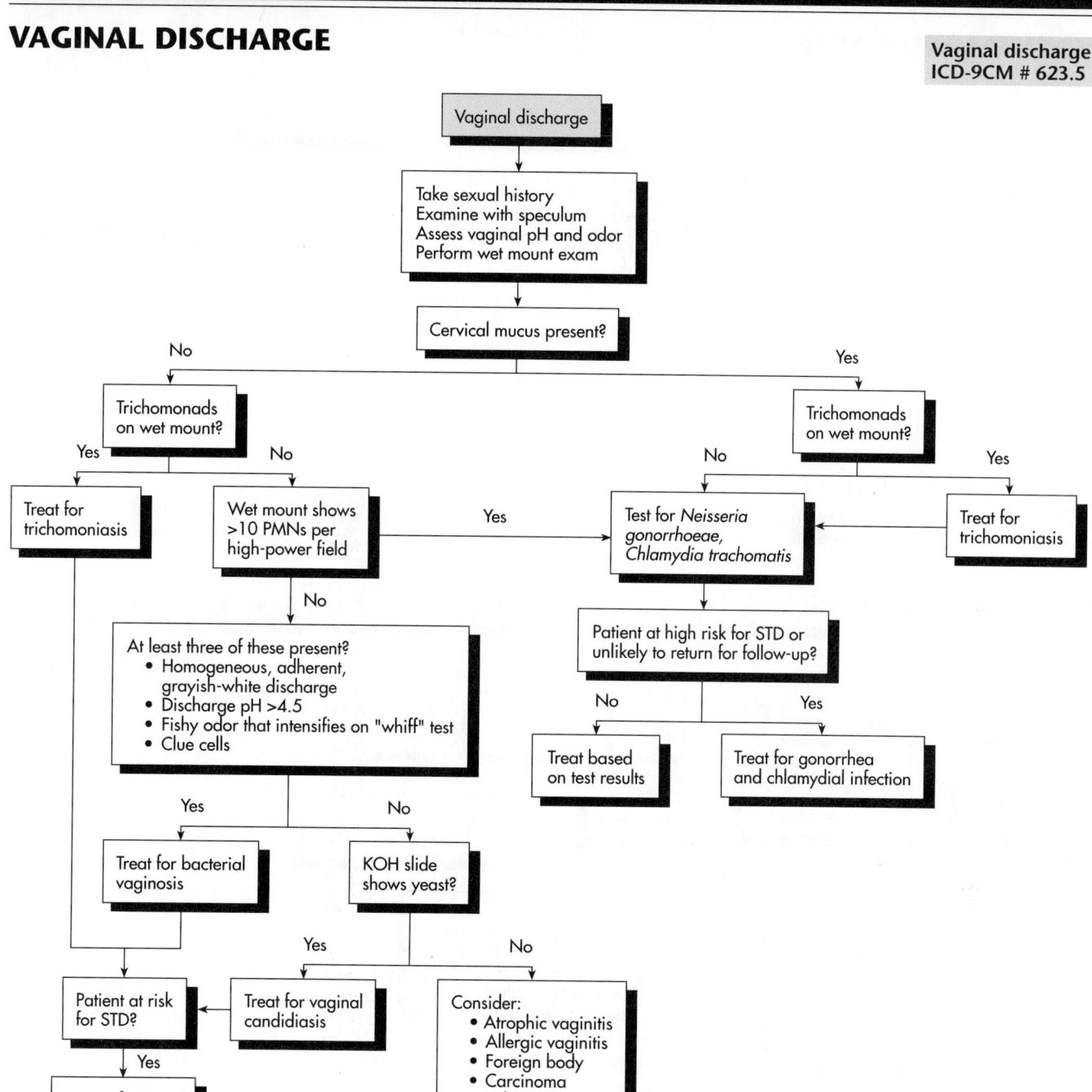

Fig. 3-189   Evaluation of vaginal discharge. *KOH,* Potassium hydroxide; *PMN,* polymorphonuclear leukocyte; *STD,* sexually transmitted disease. (From Fox KK, Behets FMT: *Postgrad Med* 98:87, 1995.)

VAGINAL PROLAPSE

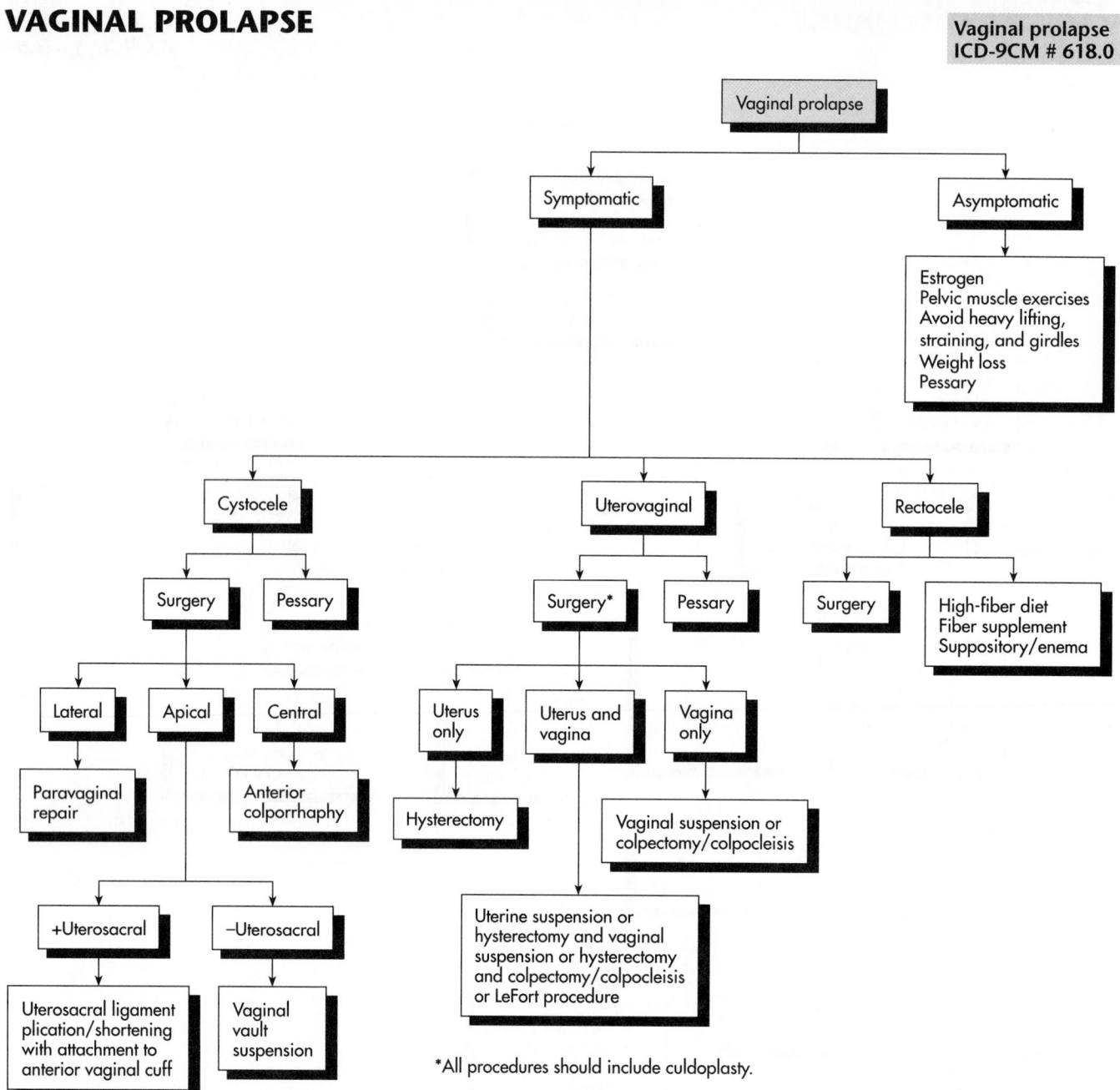

Fig. 3-190 **Management of vaginal prolapse.** (From Zuspan FP [ed]: *Handbook of obstetrics, gynecology, and primary care,* St Louis, 1998, Mosby.)

VERTIGO

Vertigo
ICD-9CM # 780.4 Vertigo NOS
386.11 Benign paroxysmal positional
386.2 Vertigo, central origin
386.10 Vertigo, peripheral

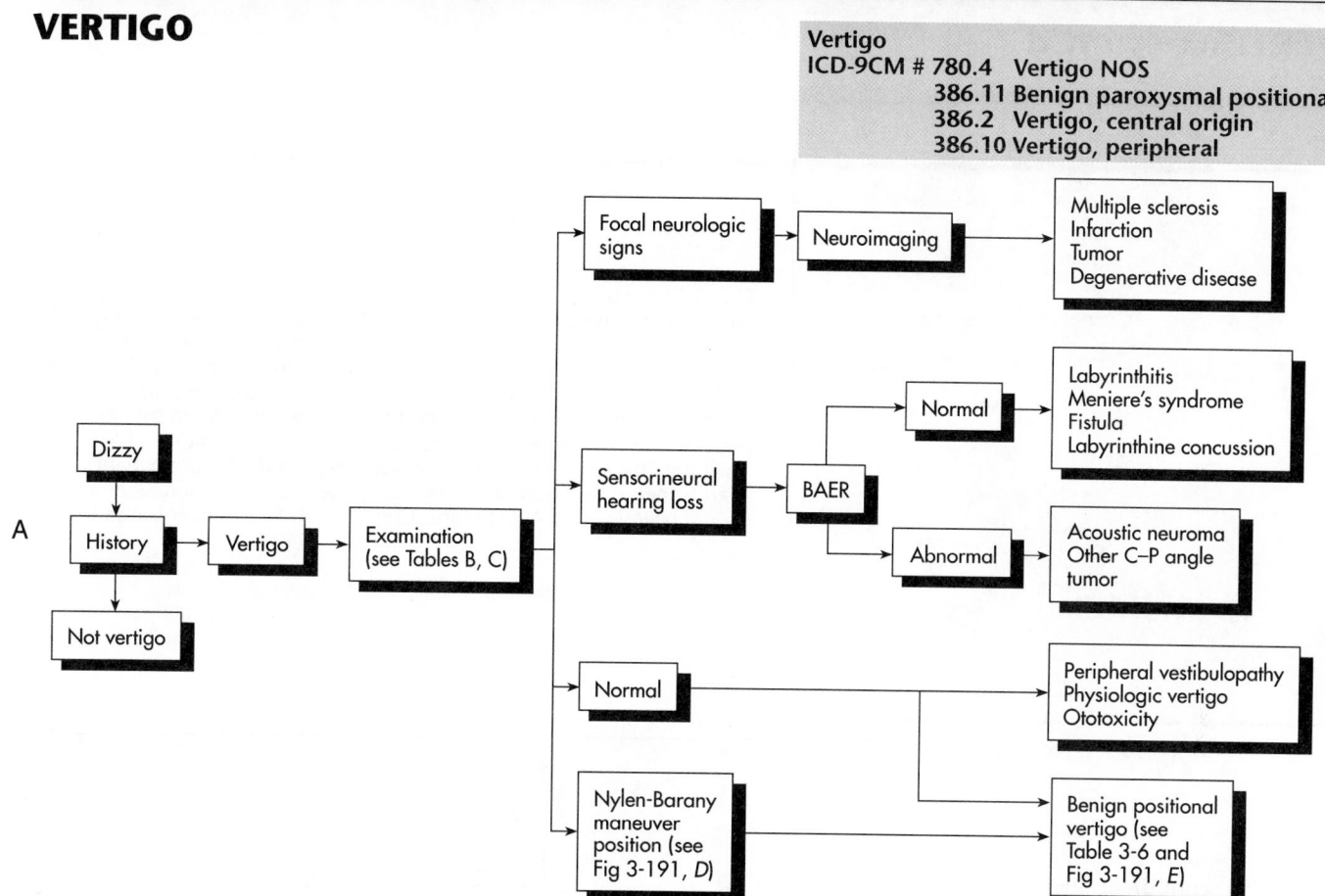

Fig. 3-191   A, Evaluation of vertigo. *BAER,* Brainstem auditory evoked response. (Modified from Baloh RW: Hearing and equilibrium. In Andreoli TE [ed]: *Cecil essentials of medicine,* ed 4, Philadelphia, 1997, WB Saunders.)

SYMPTOM OR SIGN	PERIPHERAL	CENTRAL
Severity	4+	1-4+
Onset	Sudden	Nonparoxysmal
Nausea and vomiting	Common	Uncommon
Nystagmus	*Always* present	Present or absent
Tinnitus and hearing loss	Often present	Very rare
Visual fixation	Inhibits	No effect

Fig. 3-191   B, Symptoms suggestive of central versus peripheral vertigo. (From Andreoli TE [ed]: *Cecil essentials of medicine,* ed 5, Philadelphia, 2001, WB Saunders.)

CHARACTERISTIC	PERIPHERAL	CENTRAL
Direction	Usually horizontal, may have rotary component	Any direction (pure vertical is always central)
Symmetry between eyes	Always symmetric	Dissociation between eyes possible
Lesion side	Fast component away from injured labyrinth	No relation between direction and lesion location
Duration of problem	Minutes to weeks	Days to years
Visual fixation	Decreases	No effect

Fig. 3-191   C, Characteristics of central versus peripheral nystagmus. (From Andreoli TE [ed]: *Cecil essentials of medicine,* ed 5, Philadelphia, 2001, WB Saunders.)

III

VERTIGO—cont'd

D

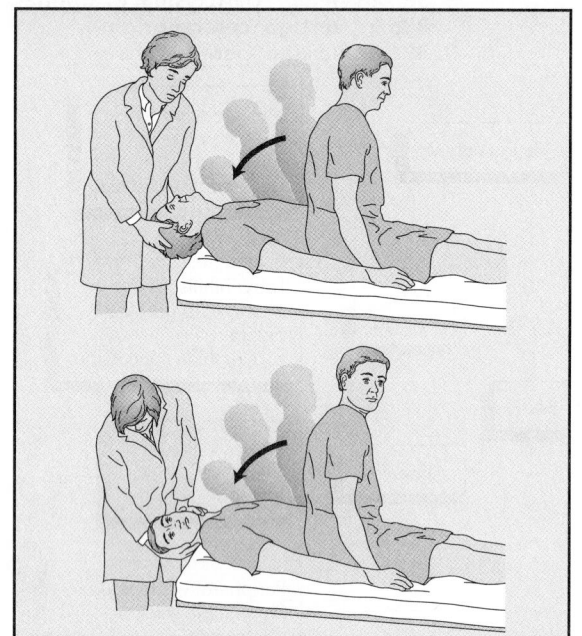

Fig. 3-191, cont'd **D,** Nylen Bárány or Dix-Hallpike maneuver to test for position nystagmus. *Top,* The patient is seated on an examining table with head and eyes directed forward and is then quickly lowered to the supine position with the head over the table edge, 45 degrees below the horizontal. The patient is instructed to keep eyes open; nystagmus is observed for, and the patient is asked to report vertigo. When the test is positive, the affected ear is down; the fast phase of nystagmus beats toward the affected ear. *Bottom,* The test is repeated with the patient's head turned to the right and again to the left. (From Simon RP et al: *Clinical neurology,* ed 4, Stamford, Conn, 1999, Appleton & Lange.)

E

Fig. 3-191, cont'd **E,** Repositioning treatment for benign positional vertigo designed to move endolymphatic debris out of the posterior semicircular canal (PSC) of the right ear and into the utricle (UT). The patient is seated, and the head is turned 45 degrees to the right **(A).** The head is lowered rapidly to below the horizontal **(B).** The examiner shifts hand positions **(C),** and the patient's head is rotated rapidly 90 degrees in the opposite direction, so it now points 45 degrees to the left, where it remains for 30 seconds **(D).** The patient then rolls onto the left side without turning the head in relation to the body and maintains this position for another 30 seconds **(E)** before sitting up. The treatment is repeated until nystagmus is abolished. The procedure is reversed for treating the left ear. The patient must avoid the supine position for 2 days. (Modified from Foster CA, Baloh RW: Episodic vertigo. In Rakel RE [ed]: *Conn's current therapy,* Philadelphia, 1995, WB Saunders.)

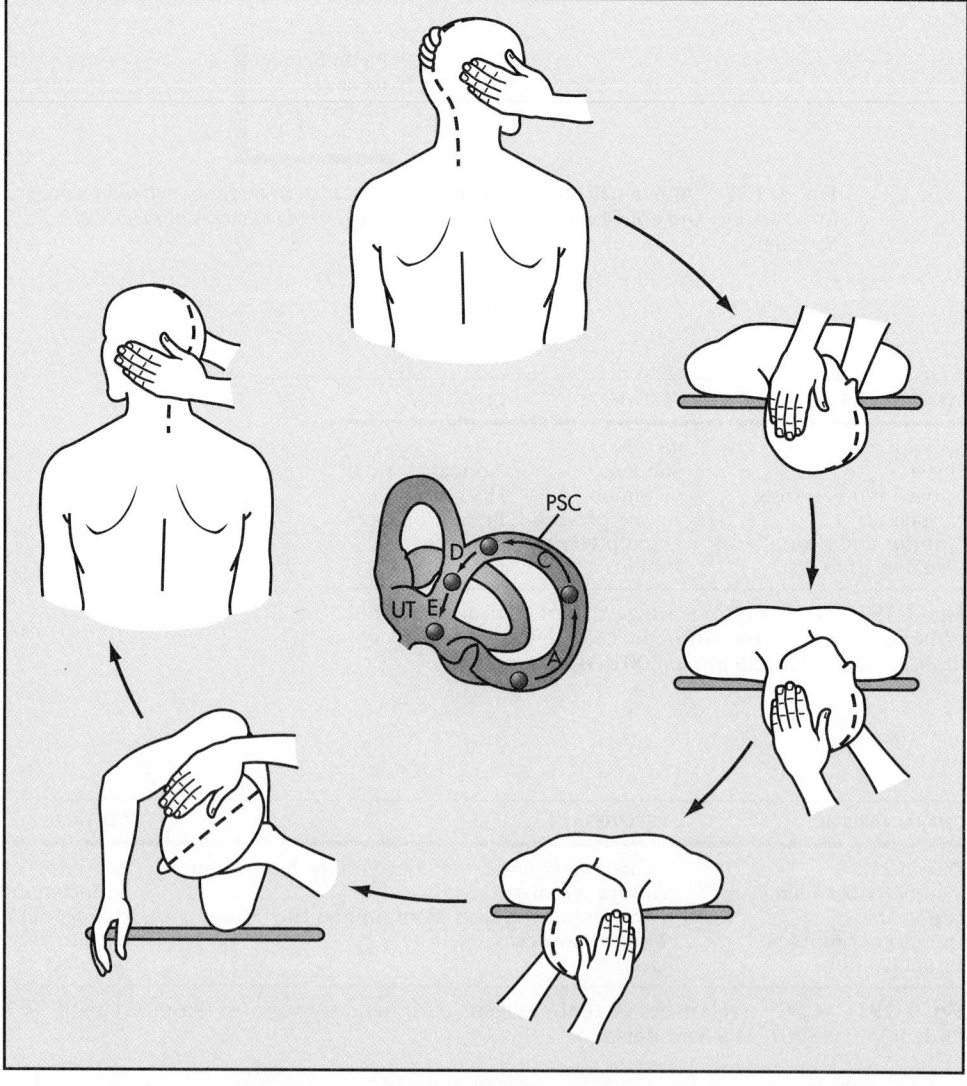

VERTIGO—cont'd

TABLE 3-6 Exercises for Benign Positional Vertigo

Eyes

Look up and down, slowly at first, then quickly, 20 times.
Look from side to side, slowly at first, then quickly, 20 times.
Focus on one's finger at arm's length. Move the finger to the side about 1 foot and then back 20 times.

Head

With eyes open, bend head forward and backward. Move slowly at first and more quickly later. Do this 20 times.
Turn head side to side 20 times
When the dizziness improves, try the head exercises with eyes closed.

Sitting

Shrug shoulders 20 times.
Turn shoulders right and left 20 times.
Bend forward to pick up an object and then sit up 20 times.

Standing

Sit and stand 20 times with eyes open.
Sit and stand 20 times with eyes closed.
Toss a ball from hand to hand above eye level 20 times.
Toss a ball from hand to hand under one knee 20 times.

Moving

Walk across the room with eyes open 10 times.
Walk across the room with eyes closed 10 times.
Walk up and down the steps with eyes open 10 times.
Walk up and down the steps with eyes closed 10 times.

From Rakel RE (ed): *Principles of family practice,* ed 6, Philadelphia, 2002, WB Saunders.
These exercises should be performed twice daily. Initially, the exercises should be performed for 15 minutes. Each exercise session should gradually increase to 30 minutes.
These exercises may need to be modified for elderly patients, especially if they have existing motor, sensory, or cognitive impairments.

III

VULVAR CANCER

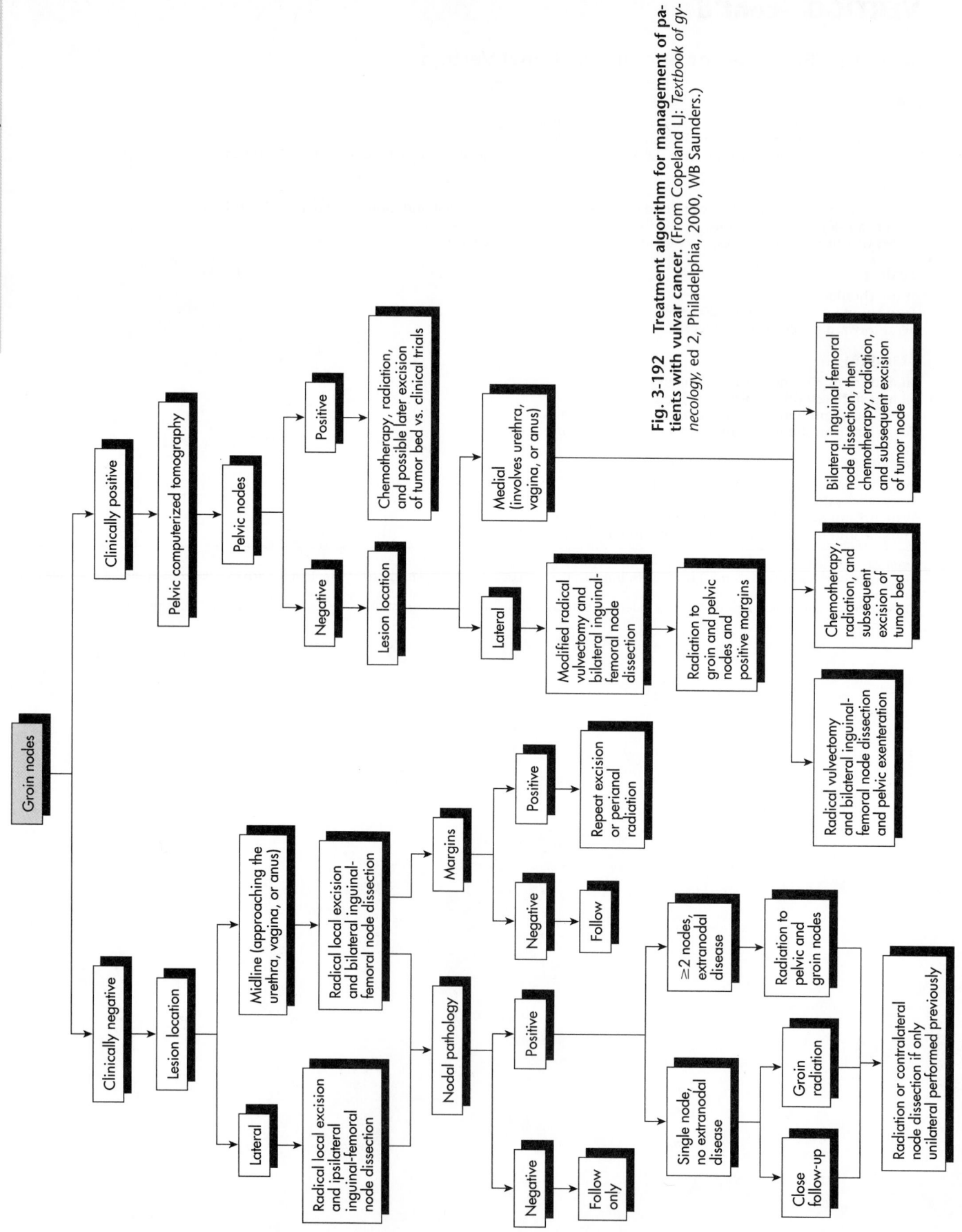

Fig. 3-192 Treatment algorithm for management of patients with vulvar cancer. (From Copeland LJ: *Textbook of gynecology*, ed 2, Philadelphia, 2000, WB Saunders.)

WEIGHT GAIN

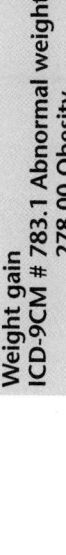

Weight gain
ICD-9CM # 783.1 Abnormal weight gain
278.00 Obesity

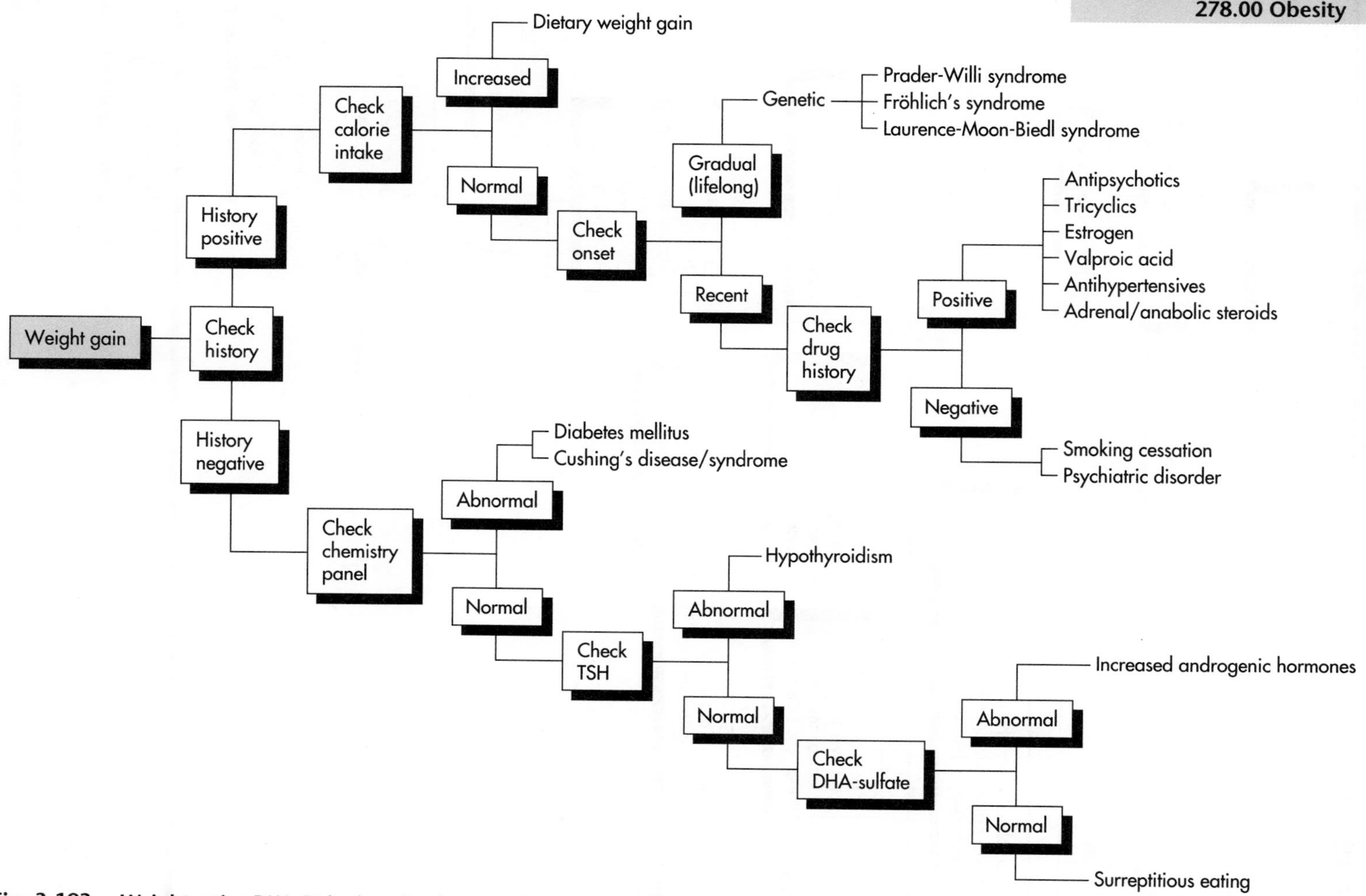

Fig. 3-193   Weight gain. *DHA,* Dehydroepiandrosterone; *TSH,* thyroid-stimulating hormone. (From Healey PM: *Common medical diagnosis: an algorithmic approach,* ed 3, Philadelphia, 2000, WB Saunders.)

WEIGHT LOSS, INVOLUNTARY

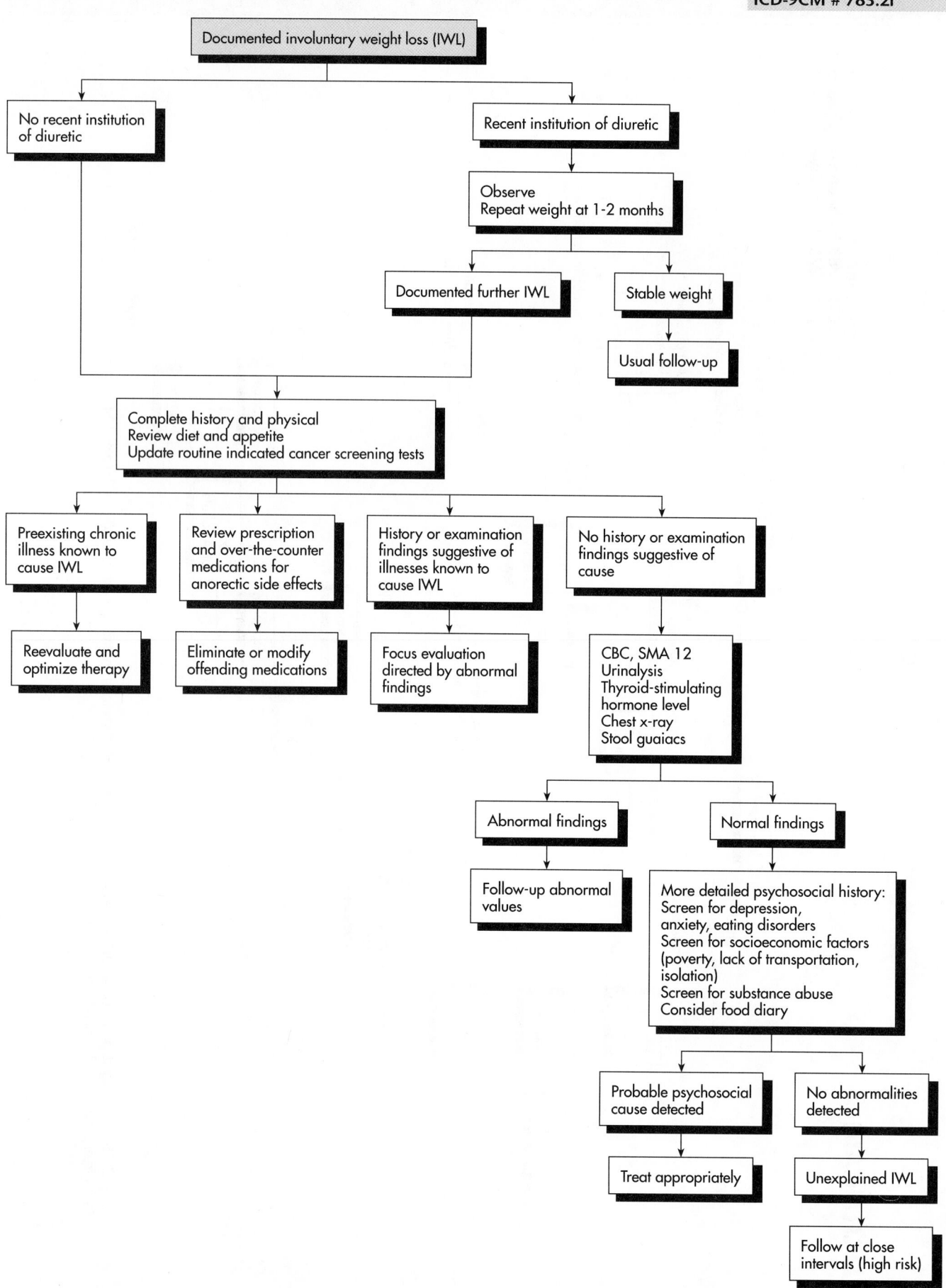

Fig. 3-194 Involuntary weight loss. *CBC,* Complete blood count. (From Greene HL, Johnson WP, Lemcke D [eds]: *Decision making in medicine,* ed 2, St Louis, 1998, Mosby.)

Laboratory Tests and Interpretation of Results

This section contains more than 200 commonly performed laboratory tests. In general, the tests are approached with the following format:

1. Laboratory test
2. Normal range in adult patients
3. Common abnormalities, such as positive test, increased or decreased value
4. Causes of abnormal result

The normal ranges may differ slightly, depending on the laboratory. The reader should be aware of the "normal range" of the particular laboratory performing the test. Every attempt has been made to present current laboratory test data, with emphasis on practical considerations.

■ **ACE LEVEL;** *see* ANGIOTENSIN-CONVERTING ENZYME

■ **ACETONE** (serum or plasma)
Normal: Negative
Elevated in: DKA, starvation, isopropanol ingestion

■ **ACETYLCHOLINE RECEPTOR (ACHR) ANTIBODY**
Normal: <0.03 nmol/L
Elevated in: Myasthenia gravis. Changes in AChR concentration correlate with the clinical severity of myasthenia gravis following therapy and during therapy with prednisone and immunosuppressants. False-positive AChR antibody results may be found in patients with Eaton-Lambert syndrome.

■ **ACID-BASE REFERENCE VALUES;** *see* Tables 4-1 and 4-2.

TABLE 4-1 Commonly Used Acid-Base Reference Values for Arterial and Venous Plasma or Serum (Averaged from Various Sources)

	ARTERIAL		VENOUS	
	CONVENTIONAL UNITS	SI UNITS*	CONVENTIONAL UNITS	SI UNITS*
pH	7.40 (7.35-7.45)	7.40 (7.35-7.45)	7.37 (7.32-7.42)	7.37 (7.32-7.42)
P_{CO_2} (35-45)	40 mm Hg (4.67-6.10)	5.33 kPa (45-50)	45 mm Hg (5.33-6.67)	6.10 kPa
P_{O_2}	80-100 mm Hg	10.66-13.33 kPa (37-43)	40 mm Hg (4.93-5.73)	5.33 kPa
HCO_3 (CO_2 combining power)	24 mEq/L (20-28)	24 mmol/L (20-28)	26 mEq/L (22-30)	26 mmol/L (22-30)
CO_2 content	25 mEq/L (22-28)	25 mmol/L (22-28)	27 mEq/L (24-30)	27 mmol/L (24-30)

From Ravel R: *Clinical laboratory medicine,* ed 6, St Louis, 1995, Mosby.
*International system.

TABLE 4-2 Summary of Laboratory Findings in Primary Uncomplicated Respiratory and Metabolic Acid-Base Disorders*

DISORDER	P_{CO_2}	pH	BASE EXCESS
Acute primary respiratory hypoactivity (respiratory acidosis)	Increase	Decrease	Normal/positive
Acute primary respiratory hyperactivity (respiratory alkalosis)	Decrease	Increase	Normal/negative
Uncompensated metabolic acidosis	Normal	Decrease	Negative
Uncompensated metabolic alkalosis	Normal	Increase	Positive
Partially compensated metabolic acidosis	Decrease	Decrease	Negative
Partially compensated metabolic alkalosis	Increase	Increase	Positive
Chronic primary respiratory hypoactivity (compensated respiratory acidosis)	Increase	Normal	Positive
Fully compensated metabolic alkalosis	Increase	Normal	Positive
Chronic primary respiratory hyperactivity (compensated respiratory alkalosis)	Decrease	Normal	Negative
Fully compensated metabolic acidosis	Decrease	Normal	Negative

From Ravel R: *Clinical laboratory medicine,* ed 6, St Louis, 1995, Mosby.
*Base excess results refer to negative (−) values more than −2 and positive (+) values more than +2.

IV

■ **ACID PHOSPHATASE** (serum)
Normal range: 0-5.5 U/L
Elevated in: Carcinoma of prostate, other neoplasms (breast, bone), Paget's disease, osteogenesis imperfecta, malignant invasion of bone, Gaucher's disease, multiple myeloma, myeloproliferative disorders, benign prostatic hypertrophy, prostatic palpation or surgery, hyperparathyroidism, liver disease, chronic renal failure, idiopathic thrombocytopenic purpura, bronchitis

■ **ACID SERUM TEST;** *see* HAM TEST

■ **ACTIVATED PARTIAL THROMBOPLASTIN TIME (APTT, APTT);** *see* PARTIAL THROMBOPLASTIN TIME

■ **ALANINE AMINOTRANSFERASE (ALT, SGPT)**
Normal range: 0-35 U/L
Elevated in: Liver disease (hepatitis, cirrhosis, Reye's syndrome), hepatic congestion, infectious mononucleosis, myocardial infarction, myocarditis, severe muscle trauma, dermatomyositis/polymyositis, muscular dystrophy, drugs (antibiotics, narcotics, antihypertensive agents, heparin, labetalol, statins, NSAIDs, amiodarone, chlorpromazine, phenytoin), malignancy, renal and pulmonary infarction, convulsions, eclampsia, shock liver

■ **ALBUMIN** (serum)
Normal range: 4-6 g/dl
Elevated in: Dehydration (relative increase)
Decreased in: Liver disease, nephrotic syndrome, poor nutritional status, rapid IV hydration, protein-losing enteropathies (inflammatory bowel disease), severe burns, neoplasia, chronic inflammatory diseases, pregnancy, oral contraceptives, prolonged immobilization, lymphomas, hypervitaminosis A, chronic glomerulonephritis

■ **ALDOLASE** (serum)
Normal range: 0-6 U/L
Elevated in: Muscular dystrophy, rhabdomyolysis, dermatomyositis/polymyositis, trichinosis, acute hepatitis and other liver diseases, myocardial infarction, prostatic carcinoma, hemorrhagic pancreatitis, gangrene, delirium tremens, burns
Decreased in: Loss of muscle mass, late stages of muscular dystrophy

■ **ALDOSTERONE**
Normal range: Recumbent: 50-150 ng/L
Upright: 150-300 ng/L
(Highest levels in neonates, decreasing over time to adult levels)
Elevated in: Primary aldosteronism, secondary aldosteronism, pseudoprimary aldosteronism
Decreased in: Patient with hypertension: diabetes mellitus, Turner's syndrome, acute alcohol intoxication, excess secretion of deoxycorticosterone, corticosterone, and 18-hydroxycorticosterone
Patient without hypertension: Addison's disease, hypoaldosteronism resulting from renin deficiency, isolated aldosterone deficiency

■ **ALKALINE PHOSPHATASE** (serum)
Normal range: 30-120 U/L
Elevated in:
LIVER AND BILIARY TRACT ORIGIN
Extrahepatic bile duct obstruction
Intrahepatic biliary obstruction
Liver cell acute injury
Liver passive congestion
Drug-induced liver cell dysfunction
Space-occupying lesions
Primary biliary cirrhosis
Sepsis
BONE ORIGIN (OSTEOBLAST HYPERACTIVITY)
Physiologic (rapid) bone growth (childhood and adolescent)
Metastatic tumor with osteoblastic reaction
Fracture healing
Paget's disease of bone
CAPILLARY ENDOTHELIAL ORIGIN
Granulation tissue formation (active)
PLACENTAL ORIGIN
Pregnancy
Some parenteral albumin preparations
OTHER
Thyrotoxicosis
Benign transient hyperphosphatasemia
Primary hyperparathyroidism
Decreased in: Hypothyroidism, pernicious anemia, hypophosphatemia, hypervitaminosis D, malnutrition

■ **ALPHA-1-FETOPROTEIN** (serum); *see* α-1 FETOPROTEIN

■ **ALT;** *see* ALANINE AMINOTRANSFERASE

■ **ALUMINUM** (serum)
Normal range: 0-6 ng/mL
Elevated in: Chronic renal failure on dialysis, parenteral nutrition, industrial exposure

■ **AMMONIA** (serum)
Normal range: 10-80 µg/dl
Elevated in: Hepatic failure, hepatic encephalopathy, Reye's syndrome, portacaval shunt, drugs (diuretics, polymyxin B, methicillin)
Decreased in: Drugs (neomycin, lactulose, tetracycline), renal failure

■ **AMYLASE** (serum)
Normal range: 0-130 U/L
Elevated in: Acute pancreatitis, pancreatic neoplasm, abscess, pseudocyst, ascites, macroamylasemia, perforated peptic ulcer, intestinal obstruction, intestinal infarction, acute cholecystitis, appendicitis, ruptured ectopic pregnancy, salivary gland inflammation, peritonitis, burns, diabetic ketoacidosis, renal insufficiency, drugs (morphine), carcinomatosis (of lung, esophagus, ovary), acute ethanol ingestion, mumps, prostate tumors, post–endoscopic retrograde cholangiopancreatography, bulimia, anorexia nervosa
Decreased in: Advanced chronic pancreatitis, hepatic necrosis, cystic fibrosis

■ **AMYLASE, URINE;** *see* URINE AMYLASE

■ **ANA;** *see* ANTINUCLEAR ANTIBODY

■ **ANCA;** *see* ANTINEUTROPHIL CYTOPLASMIC ANTIBODY

■ **ANGIOTENSIN-CONVERTING ENZYME** (ACE level)
Normal range: <40 nmol/ml/min
Elevated in: Sarcoidosis, primary biliary cirrhosis, alcoholic liver disease, hyperthyroidism, hyperparathyroidism, diabetes mellitus, amyloidosis, multiple myeloma, lung disease (asbestosis, silicosis, berylliosis, allergic alveolitis, coccidioidomycosis), Gaucher's disease, leprosy

■ **ANION GAP**
Normal range: 9-14 mEq/L
Elevated in: Lactic acidosis, ketoacidosis (diabetes, alcoholic starvation), uremia (chronic renal failure), ingestion of toxins (paraldehyde, methanol, salicylates, ethylene glycol), hyperosmolar nonketotic coma, antibiotics (carbenicillin)
Decreased in: Hypoalbuminemia, severe hypermagnesemia, IgG myeloma, lithium toxicity, laboratory error (falsely decreased sodium or overestimation of bicarbonate or chloride), hypercalcemia of parathyroid origin, antibiotics (e.g., polymyxin)

■ **ANTICARDIOLIPIN ANTIBODY** (ACA)
Normal range: Negative: Test includes detection of IgG, IgM, and IgA antibody to phospholipid, cardiolipin
Present in: Antiphospholipid antibody syndrome, chronic hepatitis C

■ **ANTICOAGULANT;** *see* CIRCULATING ANTICOAGULANT

■ **ANTI-DNA**
Normal range: Absent
Present in: Systemic lupus erythematosus, chronic active hepatitis, infectious mononucleosis, biliary cirrhosis

■ **ANTIGLOMERULAR BASEMENT ANTIBODY;** *see* GLOMERULAR BASEMENT MEMBRANE ANTIBODY

■ **ANTIMITOCHONDRIAL ANTIBODY**
Normal range: <1:20 titer
Elevated in: Primary biliary cirrhosis (85% to 95%), chronic active hepatitis (25% to 30%), cryptogenic cirrhosis (25% to 30%)

■ **ANTINEUTROPHIL CYTOPLASMIC ANTIBODY** (ANCA)
Positive test: Cytoplasmic pattern (cANCA): positive in Wegener's granulomatosis
Perinuclear pattern (pANCA): positive in inflammatory bowel disease, primary biliary cirrhosis, primary sclerosing cholangitis, autoimmune chronic active hepatitis, crescenteric glomerulonephritis

IV

■ **ANTINUCLEAR ANTIBODY** (ANA)

Normal range: <1:20 titer

Positive test: Systemic lupus erythematosus (more significant if titer >1:160), drugs (phenytoin, ethosuximide, primidone, methyldopa, hydralazine, carbamazepine, penicillin, procainamide, chlorpromazine, griseofulvin, thiazides), chronic active hepatitis, age over 60 years (particularly age over 80 years), rheumatoid arthritis, scleroderma, mixed connective tissue disease, necrotizing vasculitis, Sjögren's syndrome, tuberculosis, pulmonary interstitial fibrosis. Table 4-3 describes diseases associated with ANA subtypes. Fig. 4-1 illustrates various fluorescent ANA test patterns.

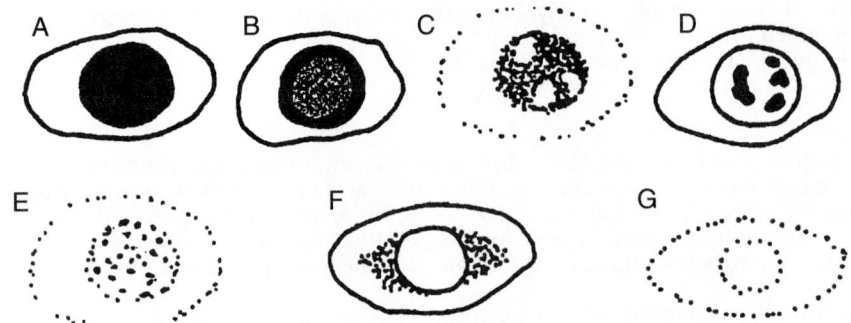

Fig. 4-1   **Fluorescent antinuclear antibody test patterns (HEP-2 cells). A,** Solid (homogeneous). **B,** Peripheral (rim). **C,** Speckled. **D,** Nucleolar. **E,** Anticentromere. **E,** Antimitochondrial. **G,** Normal (nonreactive). (From Ravel R [ed]: *Clinical laboratory medicine,* ed 6, St Louis, 1995, Mosby.)

■ **ANTI-RNP ANTIBODY;** *see* EXTRACTABLE NUCLEAR ANTIGEN

■ **ANTI-SM (ANTI-SMITH) ANTIBODY;** *see* EXTRACTABLE NUCLEAR ANTIGEN

■ **ANTI-SMOOTH MUSCLE ANTIBODY;** *see* SMOOTH MUSCLE ANTIBODY

■ **ANTISTREPTOLYSIN O TITER** (Streptozyme, ASLO titer)

Normal range for adults: <160 Todd units

Elevated in: Streptococcal upper airway infection, acute rheumatic fever, acute glomerulonephritis, increased levels of β-lipoprotein

NOTE: A fourfold increase in titer between acute and convalescent specimens is diagnostic of streptococcal upper airway infection regardless of the initial titer.

■ **ANTITHROMBIN III**

Normal range: 81% to 120% of normal activity; 17-30 mg/dl

Decreased in: Hereditary deficiency of antithrombin III, disseminated intravascular coagulation, pulmonary embolism, cirrhosis, thrombolytic therapy, chronic liver failure, postsurgery, third trimester of pregnancy, oral contraceptives, nephrotic syndrome, IV heparin >3 days, sepsis, acute leukemia, carcinoma, thrombophlebitis

Elevated in: Warfarin drugs, post–myocardial infarction

■ **ARTERIAL BLOOD GASES**

Normal range: Po_2: 75-100 mm Hg

Pco_2: 35-45 mm Hg

HCO_3: 24-28 mEq/L

pH: 7.35-7.45

Abnormal values: Acid-base disturbances (see the following)

METABOLIC ACIDOSIS

Metabolic acidosis with increased AG (AG acidosis)

Lactic acidosis

Ketoacidosis (diabetes mellitus, alcoholic ketoacidosis)

Uremia (chronic renal failure)

Ingestion of toxins (paraldehyde, methanol, salicylate, ethylene glycol)

High-fat diet (mild acidosis)

Metabolic acidosis with normal AG (hyperchloremic acidosis)

Renal tubular acidosis (including acidosis of aldosterone deficiency)

Intestinal loss of HCO_3^- (diarrhea, pancreatic fistula)

Carbonic anhydrase inhibitors (e.g., acetazolamide)

Dilutional acidosis (as a result of rapid infusion of bicarbonate-free isotonic saline)

Ingestion of exogenous acids (ammonium chloride, methionine, cystine, calcium chloride)

Ileostomy

Ureterosigmoidostomy

Drugs: amiloride, triamterene, spironolactone, β-blockers

TABLE 4-3 Disease-Associated ANA Subtypes

NUCLEAR LOCATION	DISEASE(S)
"Native" DNA (dsDNA, or dsDNA/ssDNA complex)	SLE (60%-70%; range, 35%-75%) —also PSS (5%-55%), MCTD (11%-25%), RA (5%-40%), DM (5%-25%), SS (5%)
sNP	SLE (50%) —also other collagen diseases
DNP (DNA-histone complex)	SLE (52%) —also MCTD (8%), RA (3%)
Histones	Drug-induced SLE (95%) —also SLE (30%), RA (15%-24%)
ENA Sm	 SLE (30%-40%; range, 28%-40%) —also MCTD (0%-8%)
RNP (U1-RNP)	MCTD (in high titer without any other ANA subtype present: 95%-100%) —also SLE (26%-50%), PSS (11%-22%), RA (10%), SS (3%)
SS-A (Ro)*	SS without RA (60%-70%) —also SLE (26%-50%), neonatal SLE (over 95%), PSS (30%), MCTD (50%), SS with RA (9%), PBC (15%-19%)
SS-B (La)	SS without RA (40%-60%) —also SLE (5%-15%), SS with RA (5%)
Scl-70*	PSS (15%-43%)
Centromere*	CREST syndrome (70%-90%; range 57%-96%) —also PSS (4%-20%), PBC (12%)
Nucleolar	PSS (scleroderma) (54%-90%) —also SLE (25%-26%), RA (9%)
RAP (RANA)	SS with RA (60%-76%) —also SS without RA (5%)
Jo-1	Polymyositis (30%)
PM-1	Polymyositis or PMS/PSS overlap syndrome (60%-90%) —also DM (17%)
ssDNA	SLE (60%-70%) —also CAH, infectious mononucleosis, RA, chronic GN, chronic infections, PBC

CYTOPLASMIC LOCATION	DISEASE(S)
Mitochondrial	Primary biliary cirrhosis (90%-100%) —also CAH (7%-30%), cryptogenic cirrhosis (30%), acute hepatitis, viral hepatitis (3%), other liver diseases (0%-20%), SLE (5%), SS and PSS (8%)
Microsomal†	Chronic active hepatitis (60%-80%), Hashimoto's thyroiditis (97%)
Ribosomal	SLE (5%-12%)
Smooth muscle‡	Chronic active hepatitis (60%-91%) —also cryptogenic cirrhosis (28%), acute hepatitis, viral hepatitis (5%-87%), infectious mononucleosis (81%), MS (40%-50%), malignancy (67%), PBC (10%-50%)

From Ravel R: *Clinical laboratory medicine,* ed 6, St Louis, 1995, Mosby.
CAH, Chronic active hepatitis; *DM,* dermatomyositis; *GN,* glomerulonephritis; *MS,* multiple sclerosis; *PBC,* primary biliary cirrhosis; *SS,* Sjögren's syndrome.
*Not detected using rat or mouse liver or kidney tissue method.
†Not detected by cultured cell method.
‡Detected by cultured cells but better with rat or mouse tissue.

RESPIRATORY ACIDOSIS
Pulmonary disease (COPD, severe pneumonia, pulmonary edema, interstitial fibrosis)
Airway obstruction (foreign body, severe bronchospasm, laryngospasm)
Thoracic cage disorders (pneumothorax, flail chest, kyphoscoliosis)
Defects in muscles of respiration (myasthenia gravis, hypokalemia, muscular dystrophy)
Defects in peripheral nervous system (amyotrophic lateral sclerosis, poliomyelitis, Guillain-Barré syndrome, botulism, tetanus, organophosphate poisoning, spinal cord injury)
Depression of respiratory center (anesthesia, narcotics, sedatives, vertebral artery embolism or thrombosis, increased intracranial pressure)
Failure of mechanical ventilator
METABOLIC ALKALOSIS
It is divided into chloride-responsive (urinary chloride <15 mEq/L) and chloride-resistant forms (urinary chloride level >15 mEq/L)
Chloride-responsive
Vomiting
Nasogastric (NG) suction
Diuretics

Posthypercapnic alkalosis
Stool losses (laxative abuse, cystic fibrosis, villous adenoma)
Massive blood transfusion
Exogenous alkali administration
Chloride-resistant
Hyperadrenocorticoid states (Cushing's syndrome, primary hyperaldosteronism, secondary mineralocorticoidism [licorice, chewing tobacco])
Hypomagnesemia
Hypokalemia
Bartter's syndrome
RESPIRATORY ALKALOSIS
Hypoxemia (pneumonia, pulmonary embolism, atelectasis, high-altitude living)
Drugs (salicylates, xanthines, progesterone, epinephrine, thyroxine, nicotine)
Central nervous system (CNS) disorders (tumor, cerebrovascular accident [CVA], trauma, infections)
Psychogenic hyperventilation (anxiety, hysteria)
Hepatic encephalopathy
Gram-negative sepsis
Hyponatremia
Sudden recovery from metabolic acidosis
Assisted ventilation

■ **ARTHROCENTESIS FLUID**
Interpretation of results:
1. **Color:** Normally it is clear or pale yellow; cloudiness indicates inflammatory process or presence of crystals, cell debris, fibrin, or triglycerides.
2. **Viscosity:** Normally it has a high viscosity because of hyaluronate; when fluid is placed on a slide, it can be stretched to a string >2 cm in length before separating (low viscosity indicates breakdown of hyaluronate [lysosomal enzymes from leukocytes] or the presence of edema fluid).
3. **Mucin clot:** Add 1 ml of fluid to 5 ml of a 5% acetic acid solution and allow 1 minute for the clot to form; a firm clot (does not fragment on shaking) is normal and indicates the presence of large molecules of hyaluronic acid (this test is nonspecific and infrequently done).
4. **Glucose:** Normally it approximately equals serum glucose level; a difference of more than 40 mg/dl is suggestive of infection.
5. **Protein:** Total protein concentration is <2.5 g/dl in the normal synovial fluid; it is elevated in inflammatory and septic arthritis.
6. Microscopic examination for crystals
   a. Gout: Monosodium urate crystals
   b. Pseudogout: Calcium pyrophosphate dihydrate crystals

■ **ASLO TITER:** *see* ANTISTREPTOLYSIN O TITER

■ **ASPARTATE AMINOTRANSFERASE** (AST, SGOT)
Normal range: 0-35 U/L
Elevated in:
HEART
Acute myocardial infarction
Pericarditis (active: some cases)
LIVER
Hepatitis virus, Epstein-Barr, or cytomegalovirus infection
Active cirrhosis
Liver passive congestion or hypoxia
Alcohol or drug-induced liver dysfunction
Space-occupying lesions (active)
Fatty liver (severe)
Extrahepatic biliary obstruction (early)
Drug-induced
SKELETAL MUSCLE
Acute skeletal muscle injury
Muscle inflammation (infectious or noninfectious)
Muscular dystrophy (active)
Recent surgery
Delirium tremens
KIDNEY
Acute injury or damage
Renal infarct
OTHER
Intestinal infarction
Shock
Cholecystitis
Acute pancreatitis
Hypothyroidism
Heparin therapy (60%-80% of cases)

■ **B-TYPE NATRIURETIC PEPTIDE**
Normal range: Up to 100pg/mL
Elevated in: Heart failure. This test is useful in the emergency department setting to differentiate heart failure patients from those with chronic obstructive pulmonary disease presenting with dyspnea.

■ **BASOPHIL COUNT**
Normal range: 0.4% to 1% of total WBC; 40-100/mm³
Elevated in: Leukemia, inflammatory processes, polycythemia vera, Hodgkin's lymphoma, hemolytic anemia, after splenectomy, myeloid metaplasia, myxedema
Decreased in: Stress, hypersensitivity reaction, steroids, pregnancy, hyperthyroidism, postirradiation

■ **BILE, URINE;** *see* URINE BILE

■ **BILIRUBIN, DIRECT** (conjugated bilirubin)
Normal range: 0-0.2 mg/dl
Elevated in: Hepatocellular disease, biliary obstruction, drug-induced cholestasis, hereditary disorders (Dubin-Johnson syndrome, Rotor's syndrome)

■ **BILIRUBIN, INDIRECT** (unconjugated bilirubin)
Normal range: 0-1.0 mg/dl
Elevated in: A Increased bilirubin production (if normal liver, serum unconjugated bilirubin is usually less than 4 mg/100 ml)
   1. Hemolytic anemia
     a. Acquired
     b. Congenital
   2. Resorption from extravascular sources
     a. Hematomas
     b. Pulmonary infarcts
   3. Excessive ineffective erythropoiesis
     a. Congenital (congenital dyserythropoietic anemias)
     b. Acquired (pernicious anemia, severe lead poisoning; if present, bilirubinemia is usually mild)
B. Defective hepatic unconjugated bilirubin clearance (defective uptake or conjugation)
   1. Severe liver disease
   2. Gilbert's syndrome
   3. Crigler-Najjar type I or II
   4. Drug-induced inhibition
   5. Portacaval shunt
   6. Congestive heart failure
   7. Hyperthyroidism (uncommon)

■ **BILIRUBIN, TOTAL**
Normal range: 0-1.0 mg/dl
Elevated in: Liver disease (hepatitis, cirrhosis, cholangitis, neoplasm, biliary obstruction, infectious mononucleosis), hereditary disorders (Gilbert's disease, Dubin-Johnson syndrome), drugs (steroids, diphenylhydantoin, phenothiazines, penicillin, erythromycin, clindamycin, captopril, amphotericin B, sulfonamides, azathioprine, isoniazid, 5-aminosalicylic acid, allopurinol, methyldopa, indomethacin, halothane, oral contraceptives, procainamide, tolbutamide, labetalol), hemolysis, pulmonary embolism or infarct, hepatic congestion secondary to congestive heart failure

■ **BILIRUBIN, URINE:** *see* URINE BILE

■ **BLEEDING TIME** (modified Ivy method)
Normal range: 2 to 9½ min
Elevated in: Thrombocytopenia, capillary wall abnormalities, platelet abnormalities (Bernard-Soulier disease, Glanzmann's disease), drugs (aspirin, warfarin, antiinflammatory medications, streptokinase, urokinase, dextran, β-lactam antibiotics, moxalactam), disseminated intravascular coagulation, cirrhosis, uremia, myeloproliferative disorders, von Willebrand's disease

■ **BRCA ANALYSIS**
Description of Analysis
Comprehensive BRACAnalysis:
BRCA1: Full sequence determination in both forward and reverse directions of approximately 5500 base pairs comprising 22 coding exons and one noncoding exon (exon 4) and approximately 800 adjacent base pairs in the noncoding intervening sequence (intron). Exon 1, which is noncoding, is not analyzed. The wild-type *BRCA1* gene encodes a protein comprising 1863 amino acids.
BRCA2: Full sequence determination in both forward and reverse directions of approximately 10,200 base pairs comprising 26 coding exons and approximately 900 adjacent base pairs in the noncoding intervening sequence (intron). Exon 1, which is noncoding, is not analyzed. The wild-type *BRCA2* gene encodes a protein comprising 3418 amino acids.

IV

The noncoding intronic regions of *BRCA1* and *BRCA2* that are analyzed do not extend more than 20 base pairs proximal to the 5′ end and 10 base pairs distal to the 3′ end of each exon.

SINGLE-SITE BRACANALYSIS: DNA sequence analysis for a specified mutation in *BRCA1* and/or *BRCA2*.

MULTISITE 3 BRACANALYSIS: DNA sequence analysis of specific portions of *BRCA1* exon 2, *BRCA1* exon 20 and *BRCA2* exon 11 designed to detect only mutations 187delAG and 5385insC in *BRCA1* and 6174delT in *BRCA2*.

Interpretive Criteria

"POSITIVE FOR A DELETERIOUS MUTATION": Includes all mutations (nonsense, insertions, deletions) that prematurely terminate ("truncate") the protein product of *BRCA1* at least 10 amino acids form the C-terminus, or the protein product of *BRCA2* at least 110 amino acids from the C-terminus (based on documentation of deleterious mutations in *BRCA1* and *BRCA2*).

In addition, specific missense mutations and noncoding intervening sequence (IVS) mutations are recognized as deleterious on the basis of data derived from linkage analysis of high-risk families, functional assays, biochemical evidence and/or demonstration of abnormal mRNA transcript processing.

"GENETIC VARIANT, SUSPECTED DELETERIOUS": Includes genetic variants for which the available evidence indicates a likelihood, but not proof, that the mutation is deleterious. The specific evidence supporting such an interpretation will be summarized for individual variants on each such report.

"GENETIC VARIANT, FAVOR POLYMORPHISM": Includes genetic variants for which available evidence indicates that the variant is highly unlikely to contribute substantially to cancer risk. The specific evidence supporting such an interpretation will be summarized for individual variants on each such report.

"GENETIC VARIANT OF UNCERTAIN SIGNIFICANCE": Includes missense mutations and mutations that occur in analyzed intronic regions whose clinical significance has not yet been determined, as well as chain-terminating mutations that truncate *BRCA1* and *BRCA2* distal to amino acid positions 1853 and 3308, respectively.

"NO DELETERIOUS MUTATION DETECTED": Includes nontruncating genetic variants observed at an allele frequency of approximately 1% of a suitable control population (providing that no data suggest clinical significance), as well as all genetic variants for which published data demonstrate absence of substantial clinical significance. Also includes mutations in the protein-coding region that neither alter the amino acid sequence nor are predicted to significantly affect exon splicing, and base pair alterations in noncoding portions of the gene that have been demonstrated to have no deleterious effect on the length or stability of the mRNA transcript.

There may be uncommon genetic abnormalities in *BRCA1* and *BRCA2* that will not be detected by BRACAnalysis. This analysis, however, is believed to rule out the majority of abnormalities in these genes, which are believed responsible for most hereditary susceptibility to breast and ovarian cancer.

"SPECIFIC VARIANT/MUTATION NOT IDENTIFIED": Specific and designated deleterious mutations or variants of uncertain clinical significance are not present in the individual being tested. If one (or rarely two) specific deleterious mutations have been identified in a family member, a negative analysis for the specific mutation(s) indicates that the tested individual is at the general population risk of developing breast or ovarian cancer.

(From Myriad Genetic Laboratories, 320 Wakara Way, Salt Lake City, UT 84108-9930.)

■ **BUN;** *see* UREA NITROGEN

■ **C282Y AND H63D MUTATION ANALYSIS**
PROCEDURE: Detection of the C282Y and H63D mutations is accomplished by amplification of exons 2 and 4 of the HFE gene on chromosome 6 by polymerase chain reaction (PCR) followed by allele-specific hybridization and chemiluminescent detection of hybridized probes. H63D is viewed by some as a polymorphism rather than a mutation because of its prevalence in the population, because 15% of the individuals affected with hereditary hemochromatosis (HH) are compound heterozygotes for C282Y and H63D and about 1% of patients are H63D homozygotes, which suggests that H63D may be causative in the development of the disorder at reduced penetrance. The test is performed by Quest diagnostics pursuant to a license agreement with Roche Molecular systems, Inc.
INTERPRETATION: Homozygosity for the C282Y mutation has been associated with an increased risk of being affected with hereditary hemochromatosis (HH) compared with the general population. The genotype is observed in 60% to 90% of individuals affected with HH and occurs in less than 1% of the general population. However, approximately 25% of asymptomatic individuals with this genotype do not develop the disorder.
C3; *see* COMPLEMENT C3
C4; *see* COMPLEMENT C4

■ **CALCITONIN** (serum)
Normal range: <100 pg/ml
Elevated in: Medullary carcinoma of the thyroid (particularly if level >1500 pg/ml), carcinoma of the breast, apudomas, carcinoids, renal failure, thyroiditis

■ **CALCIUM** (serum)
Normal range: 8.8-10.3 mg/dl
ELEVATED
RELATIVELY COMMON
Neoplasia (noncutaneous)
Bone primary
Myeloma
Acute leukemia
Nonbone solid tumors
Breast
Lung
Squamous nonpulmonary
Kidney
Neoplasm secretion of parathyroid hormone-related protein (PTHrP, "ectopic PTH")
Primary hyperparathyroidism
Thiazide diuretics
Tertiary (renal) hyperparathyroidism
Idiopathic
Spurious (artifactual) hypercalcemia
Dehydration
Serum protein elevation
Laboratory technical problem
RELATIVELY UNCOMMON
Neoplasia (less common tumors)
Sarcoidosis
Hyperthyroidism
Immobilization (mostly seen in children and adolescents)
Diuretic phase of acute renal tubular necrosis
Vitamin D intoxication
Milk-alkali syndrome
Addison's disease
Lithium therapy
Idiopathic hypercalcemia of infancy
Acromegaly
Theophylline toxicity
• Table 4-4 describes the laboratory differential diagnosis of hypercalcemia.

TABLE 4-4 Laboratory Differential Diagnosis of Hypercalcemia

DIAGNOSIS	PLASMA TESTS					URINE TESTS			COMMENTS
	Ca	PO₄	PTH	25(OH)D	1,25(OH)₂D	cAMP	TmP/GFR	Ca	
Primary hyper-parathyroidism	↑	N/↓	↑	N	N/↑	↑	↓	↑	Parathyroid adenoma most common
MEN I									Parathyroid hyperplasia; also includes pituitary and pancreatic neoplasms
MEN IIa									Parathyroid hyperplasia; also includes medullary thyroid carcinoma and pheochromocytoma
MEN IIb									Parathyroid disease uncommon, primarily medullary thyroid carcinoma and pheochromocytoma
FHH	↑	N	N/↑	N	N	N/↑	N/↓	↓↓	Autosomal dominant inheritance; hypercalcemia present within first decade; benign
Malignancy									
Solid tumor—humoral	↑	N/↓	↓	N	N	↑	↓	↑↑	Primarily epidermoid tumors; PTH-related protein(s) is mediator
Solid tumor—osteolytic	↑	N/↑	↓	N	N	↓	↑	↑↑	
Lymphoma	↑	N/↑	↓	N/↓	↑	↓	↑	↑↑	
Granulomatous disease	↑	N/↑	↓	N/↓	↑↑	↓	↑	↑↑	Sarcoid most common etiology
Vitamin D intoxication	↑	N/↑	↓	↑↑	N	↓	↑	↑↑	
Hyperthyroidism	↑	N	↓	N	N	N	N	↑↑	Plasma concentrations of T₄ and/or T₃ are elevated

From Moore WT, Eastman RC: *Diagnostic endocrinology,* ed 2, St Louis, 1996, Mosby.
Ca, Calcium; *cAMP,* cyclic adenosine monophosphate; *FHH,* familial hypocalciuric hypercalcemia; *GFR,* glomerular filtration rate; *MEN,* multiple endocrine neoplasia; *25(OH)D,* 25 hydroxyvitamin D; *PO₄,* phosphate; *PTH,* parathormone; *T₃,* triiodothyronine; *T₄,* thyroxine; *TmP,* renal threshold for phosphorus.

IV

DECREASED
Artifactual
Hypoalbuminemia
Hemodilution
Primary hypoparathyroidism
Pseudohypoparathyroidism
Vitamin D–related
Vitamin D deficiency
Malabsorption
Renal failure
Magnesium deficiency
Sepsis
Chronic alcoholism
Tumor lysis syndrome
Rhabdomyolysis
Alkalosis (respiratory or metabolic)
Acute pancreatitis
Drug-induced hypocalcemia
Large doses of magnesium sulfate
Anticonvulsants
Mithramycin
Gentamicin
Cimetidine
• Table 4-5 describes the laboratory differential diagnosis of hypocalcemia.

■ **CALCIUM, URINE;** *see* URINE CALCIUM

■ **CANCER ANTIGEN 125**
Normal range: Less than 1.4%
The cancer antigen 125 (CA 125) test uses an antibody against antigen from tissue culture of an ovarian tumor cell line. Various published evaluations report sensitivity of about 75%-80% in patients with ovarian carcinoma. There is also an appreciable incidence of elevated values in nonovarian malignancies and in certain benign conditions (see below). Test values may transiently increase during chemotherapy.
MALIGNANT
Epithelial ovarian carcinoma, 75%-80% (range 25%-92%, better in serous than mucinous cystadenocarcinoma)
Endometrial carcinoma, 25%-48% (2%-90%)
Pancreatic carcinoma, 59%
Colorectal carcinoma, 20% (15%-56%)
Endocervical adenocarcinoma, 83%
Squamous cervical or vaginal carcinoma, 7%-14%
Lung carcinoma, 32%
Breast carcinoma, 12%-40%
Lymphoma, 35%
BENIGN
Cirrhosis, 40%-80%
Acute pancreatitis, 38%
Acute peritonitis, 75%
Endometriosis, 88%
Acute pelvic inflammation disease, 33%
Pregnancy first trimester, 2%-24%
During menstruation (occasionally)
Renal failure (?frequency)
Normal persons, 0.6%-1.4%

■ **CARBAMAZEPINE** (tegretol)
Normal therapeutic range: 4-12 mcg/mL

■ **CARBON MONOXIDE;** *see* CARBOXYHEMOGLOBIN

■ **CARBOXYHEMOGLOBIN**
Normal range: Saturation of hemoglobin <2%; smokers <9% (coma: 50%; death: 80%)
Elevated in: Smoking, exposure to smoking, exposure to automobile exhaust fumes, malfunctioning gas-burning appliances

■ **CARCINOEMBRYONIC ANTIGEN** (CEA)
Normal range: Nonsmokers: 0-2.5 ng/ml
Smokers: 0-5 ng/ml
Elevated in: Colorectal carcinomas, pancreatic carcinomas, and metastatic disease (usually produce higher elevations: >20 ng/ml)

TABLE 4-5 Laboratory Differential Diagnosis of Hypocalcemia

DIAGNOSIS	PLASMA TESTS						URINE TESTS				COMMENTS
	Ca	PO$_4$	PTH	25(OH)D	1,25(OH)$_2$D	cAMP	cAMP AFTER PTH	TmP/GFR	TmP/GFR AFTER PTH	Ca	
Hypoparathyroidism	↓	↑	N/↓	N	↓	↓	↑↑	↑	↓↓	N/↓	Deficiency of PTH
Pseudohypoparathyroidism Type I	↓	↑	↑↑	N	↓	↓	NC	↑	↑	N/↓	Resistance to PTH; patients may have Albright's hereditary osteodystrophy and resistance to multiple hormones
Type II	↓	N	↑↑	N	↓	↓	↑	↑	↑	N/↓	Renal resistance to cAMP
Vitamin D deficiency	↓	N/↓	↑↑	↓↓	N/↓	↑	↑	↓	↓	↓↓	Deficient supply (e.g., nutrition) or absorption (e.g., pancreatic insufficiency) of vitamin D
Vitamin D–dependent rickets Type I	↓	N/↓	↑↑	N	↓	↑		↓		↓↓	Deficient activity of renal 25(OH)D-1α-hydroxylase
Type II	↓	N/↓	↑↑	N	↑↑	↑		↓		↓↓	Resistance to 1,25(OH)$_2$D

From Moore WT, Eastman RC: *Diagnostic endocrinology*, ed 2, St Louis, 1996, Mosby.
Ca, Calcium; *cAMP*, cyclic adenosine monophosphate; *FHH*, familial hypocalciuric hypercalcemia; *GFR*, glomerular filtration rate; *MEN*, multiple endocrine neoplasia; *NC*, no change or small increase; *(OH)D*, hydroxycalciferol D; *PO$_4$*, phosphate; *PTH*, parathyroid hormone; *T$_3$*, triiodothyronine; *T$_4$*, thyroxine; *TmP*, renal threshold for phosphorus.

IV

Carcinomas of the esophagus, stomach, small intestine, liver, breast, ovary, lung, and thyroid (usually produce lesser elevations)
Benign conditions (smoking, inflammatory bowel disease, hypothyroidism, cirrhosis, pancreatitis, infections) (usually produce levels <10 ng/ml)

■ **CAROTENE** (serum)
Normal range: 50-250 μg/dl
Elevated in: Carotenemia, chronic nephritis, diabetes mellitus, hypothyroidism, nephrotic syndrome, hyperlipidemia
Decreased in: Fat malabsorption, steatorrhea, pancreatic insufficiency, lack of carotenoids in diet, high fever, liver disease

■ **CATECHOLAMINES, URINE;** *see* URINE CATECHOLAMINES

■ **CBC;** *see* COMPLETE BLOOD COUNT

■ **CD4+ T-LYMPHOCYTE COUNT** (CD4+ T-Cells)
Calculated as total WBC × % lymphocytes × % lymphocytes stained with CD4.
This test is used primarily to evaluate immune dysfunction in HIV infection and should be done every 3-6 months in all HIV-infected persons. It is useful as a prognostic indicator and as a criterion for initiating prophylaxis for several opportunistic infections that are sequelae of HIV infection. Progressive depletion of CD4+ T-lymphocytes is associated with an increased likelihood of clinical complications (Table 4-6). Adolescents and adults with HIV are classified as having AIDS if their CD4+ lymphocyte count is under 200/μL and/or if their CD4+ T-lymphocyte percentage is less than 14%. HIV-infected patients whose CD4+ count is less than 200/μL and who acquire certain infectious diseases or malignancies are also classified as having AIDS. Corticosteroids decrease CD4+ T-cell percentage and absolute number.

TABLE 4-6   Relation of CD4 Lymphocyte Counts to the Onset of Certain, HIV-Associated Infections and Neoplasms in North America

CD4 COUNT (CELLS/MM³)*	OPPORTUNISTIC INFECTION OR NEOPLASM	FREQUENCY (%)†
>500	Herpes zoster, polydermatomal	5-10
200-500	*Mycobacterium tuberculosis* infection, pulmonary and extrapulmonary	2-20
	Oral hairy leukoplakia	40-70
	Candida pharyngitis (thrush)	40-70
	Recurrent *Candida* vaginitis	15-30 (F)
	Kaposi's sarcoma, mucocutaneous	15-30 (M)
	Bacterial pneumonia, recurrent	15-20
	Cervical neoplasia	1-2 (F)
100-200	*Pneumocystis carinii* pneumonia	15-60
	Herpes simplex, chronic, ulcerative	5-10
	Histoplasma capsulatum infection, disseminated	0-20
	Kaposi's sarcoma, visceral	3-8 (M)
	Progressive multifocal leukoencephalopathy	2-3
	Lymphoma, non-Hodgkin's	2-5
<100	*Candida* esophagitis	15-20
	Mycobacterium avium-intracellulare, disseminated	25-40
	Toxoplasma gondii encephalitis	5-25
	Cryptosporidium enteritis	2-10
	Cytomegalovirus (CMV) retinitis	20-35
	Cryptococcus neoformans encephalitis	2-5
	CMV esophagitis or colitis	6-12
	Lymphoma, central nervous system	4-8

From Andreoli TE (ed): *Cecil essentials of medicine,* ed 4, Philadelphia, 1997, WB Saunders.
F, Exclusively in women; *HIV,* human immunodeficiency virus; *M,* almost exclusively in men.
*Table indicates CD4 count at which specific infections or neoplasms generally begin to appear. Each infection may recur or progress during the subsequent course of HIV disease.
†Even within the United States, great regional differences in the incidence of specific opportunistic infections are apparent. For example, disseminated histoplasmosis is common in the Mississippi River drainage area, but very rare in individuals who have lived exclusively on the East or West Coast.

■ **CEA;** *see* CARCINOEMBRYONIC ANTIGEN

■ **CEREBROSPINAL FLUID** (CSF)
Normal range:
Interpretation of results:
1. Appearance of the fluid
   a. Clear: normal.
   b. Yellow color (xanthochromia) in the supernatant of centrifuged CSF within 1 hour or less after collection is usually the result of previous bleeding (subarachnoid hemorrhage); it may also be caused by increased CSF protein, melanin from meningeal melanosarcomas, or carotenoids.
   c. Pinkish color is usually the result of a bloody tap; the color generally clears progressively from tubes 1 to 4 (the supernatant is usually crystal clear in traumatic taps).
   d. Turbidity usually indicates the presence of leukocytes (bleeding introduces approximately 1 WBC/500 RBCs into the CSF).
2. CSF pressure: elevated pressure can be seen with meningitis, meningoencephalitis, pseudotumor cerebri, mass lesions, and intracerebral bleeding.
3. Cell count: in the adult the CSF is normally free of cells (although up to 5 mononuclear cells/mm^3 is considered normal); the presence of granulocytes is never normal.
   a. Neutrophils: seen in bacterial meningitis, early viral meningoencephalitis, and early tuberculosis (TB) meningitis.
   b. Increased lymphocytes: TB meningitis, viral meningoencephalitis, syphilitic meningoencephalitis, fungal meningitis.
4. Protein: serum proteins are generally too large to cross the normal blood-CSF barrier; however, increased CSF protein is seen with meningeal inflammation, traumatic tap, increased CNS synthesis, tissue degeneration, obstruction to CSF circulation, and Guillain-Barré syndrome.
5. Glucose
   a. Decreased glucose is seen with bacterial meningitis, TB meningitis, fungal meningitis, subarachnoid hemorrhage, and some cases of viral meningitis.
   b. A mild increase in CSF glucose can be seen in patients with very elevated serum glucose levels.
Table 4-7, on the following page, describes cerebrospinal fluid findings in central nervous system disorders.

■ **CERULOPLASMIN** (serum)
Normal range: 20-35 mg/dl
Elevated in: Pregnancy, estrogens, oral contraceptives, neoplastic diseases (leukemias, Hodgkin's lymphoma, carcinomas), inflammatory states, systemic lupus erythematosus, primary biliary cirrhosis, rheumatoid arthritis
Decreased in: Wilson's disease (values often <10 mg/dl), nephrotic syndrome, advanced liver disease, malabsorption, total parenteral nutrition, Menkes' syndrome

■ **CHLORIDE** (serum)
Normal range: 95-105 mEq/L
Elevated in: Dehydration, excessive infusion of normal saline solution, cystic fibrosis (sweat test), hyperparathyroidism, renal tubular disease, metabolic acidosis, prolonged diarrhea, drugs (ammonium chloride administration, acetazolamide, boric acid, triamterene)
Decreased in: Congestive heart failure, syndrome of inappropriate antidiuretic hormone secretion, Addison's disease, vomiting, gastric suction, salt-losing nephritis, continuous infusion of D$_5$W, thiazide diuretic administration, diaphoresis, diarrhea, burns, diabetic ketoacidosis

■ **CHLORIDE** (sweat)
Normal: 0-40 mmol/L
Borderline/indeterminate: 41-60 mmol/L
Consistent with cystic fibrosis: > 60 mmol/L
False low results can occur with edema, excessive sweating, and hypoproteinemia.

■ **CHLORIDE, URINE;** *see* URINE CHLORIDE

■ **CHOLESTEROL, HIGH-DENSITY LIPOPROTEIN;** *see* HIGH-DENSITY LIPOPROTEIN CHOLESTEROL

■ **CHOLESTEROL, LOW-DENSITY LIPOPROTEIN;** *see* LOW-DENSITY LIPOPROTEIN CHOLESTEROL

■ **CHOLESTEROL, TOTAL**
Normal range: Varies with age
Generally <200 mg/dl
Elevated in: Primary hypercholesterolemia, biliary obstruction, diabetes mellitus, nephrotic syndrome, hypothyroidism, primary biliary cirrhosis, high-cholesterol diet, pregnancy third trimester, myocardial infarction, drugs (steroids, phenothiazines, oral contraceptives)
Decreased in: Starvation, malabsorption, sideroblastic anemia, thalassemia, abetalipoproteinemia, hyperthyroidism, Cushing's syndrome, hepatic failure, multiple myeloma, polycythemia vera, chronic myelocytic leukemia, myeloid metaplasia, Waldenström's macroglobulinemia, myelofibrosis

IV

TABLE 4-7 Cerebrospinal Fluid Findings in Central Nervous System Disorders

CONDITION	PRESSURE (MM H$_2$O)	LEUKOCYTES (MM^3)	PROTEIN (MG/DL)	GLUCOSE (MG/DL)	COMMENTS
Normal	50-80	<5, ≥75% lymphocytes	20-45	>50 (or 75% serum glucose)	
Common Forms of Meningitis					
Acute bacterial meningitis	Usually elevated (100-300)	100-10,000 or more; usually 300-2000; PMNs predominate	Usually 100-500	Decreased, usually <40 (or <66% serum glucose)	Organisms usually seen on Gram stain and recovered by culture. Latex agglutination of CSF usually positive
Partially treated bacterial meningitis	Normal or elevated	5-10,000; PMNs usual but mononuclear cells may predominate if pretreated for extended period of time	Usually 100-500	Normal or decreased	Organisms may be seen on Gram stain. Latex agglutination CSF may be positive. Pretreatment may render CSF sterile
Viral meningitis or meningoencephalitis	Normal or slightly elevated (80-150)	Rarely >1000 cells. Eastern equine encephalitis and lymphocytic choriomeningitis (LCM) may have cell counts of several thousand. PMNs early but mononuclear cells predominate through most of the course	Usually 50-200	Generally normal; may be decreased to <40 in some viral diseases, particularly mumps (15%-20% of cases)	HSV encephalitis is suggested by focal seizures or by focal findings on CT or MRI scans or EEG. Enteroviruses and HSV infrequently recovered from CSF. HSV and enteroviruses may be detected by PCR of CSF
Uncommon Forms of Meningitis					
Tuberculous meningitis	Usually elevated	10-500; PMNs early, but lymphocytes predominate through most of the course	100-3000; may be higher in presence of block	<50 in most cases; decreases with time if treatment is not provided	Acid-fast organisms almost never seen on smear. Organisms may be recovered in culture of large volumes of CSF. *Mycobacterium tuberculosis* may be detected by PCR of CSF
Fungal meningitis	Usually elevated	5-500; PMNs early but mononuclear cells predominate through most of the course. Cryptococcal meningitis may have no cellular inflammatory response	25-500	<50; decreases with time if treatment is not provided	Budding yeast may be seen. Organisms may be recovered in culture. Cryptococcal antigen (CSF and serum) may be positive in cryptococcal infection
Syphilis (acute) and leptospirosis	Usually elevated	50-500; lymphocytes predominate	50-200	Usually normal	Positive CSF serology. Spirochetes not demonstrable by usual techniques of smear or culture; darkfield examination may be positive
Amebic (*Naegleria*) meningoencephalitis	Elevated	1000-10,000 or more; PMNs predominate	50-500	Normal or slightly decreased	Mobile amebae may be seen by hanging-drop examination of CSF at room temperature

Brain and Parameningeal Abscesses

Condition	Pressure	Cells	Protein	Glucose	Microscopy/Comments
Brain abscess	Usually elevated (100-300)	5-200; CSF rarely acellular; lymphocytes predominate; if abscess ruptures into ventricle, PMNs predominate and cell count may reach >100,000	75-500	Normal unless abscess ruptures into ventricular system	No organisms on smear or culture unless abscess ruptures into ventricular system
Subdural empyema	Usually elevated (100-300)	100-5000; PMNs predominate	100-500	Normal	No organisms on smear or culture of CSF unless meningitis also present; organisms found on tap of subdural fluid
Cerebral epidural abscess	Normal to slightly elevated	10-500; lymphocytes predominate	50-200	Normal	No organisms on smear or culture of CSF
Spinal epidural abscess	Usually low, with spinal block	10-100; lymphocytes predominate	50-400	Normal	No organisms on smear or culture of CSF
Chemical (drugs, dermoid cysts, myelography dye)	Usually elevated	100-1000 or more; PMNs predominate	50-100	Normal or slightly decreased	Epithelial cells may be seen within CSF by use of polarized light in some children with dermoids

Noninfectious Causes

Condition	Pressure	Cells	Protein	Glucose	Microscopy/Comments
Sarcoidosis	Normal or elevated slightly	0-100; mononuclear	40-100	Normal	No specific findings
Systemic lupus erythematosus with CNS involvement	Slightly elevated	0-500; PMNs usually predominate; lymphocytes may be present	100	Normal or slightly decreased	No organisms on smear or culture. LE preparation may be positive. Positive neuronal and ribosomal P protein antibodies in CSF
Tumor, leukemia	Slightly elevated to very high	0-100 or more; mononuclear or blast cells	50-1000	Normal to decreased (20-40)	Cytology may be positive

From Behrman RE: *Nelson textbook of pediatrics*, ed 16, Philadelphia, 2000, WB Saunders.
CSF, Cerebrospinal fluid; EEG, electroencephalogram; HSV, herpes simplex virus; PCR, polymerase chain reaction; PMN, polymorphonuclear neutrophils.

IV

- **CHORIONIC GONADOTROPINS, HUMAN** (serum)
  Normal range, serum: Female, premenopausal: <0.8 IU/L; postmenopausal <3.3 IU/L
  Male: <0.7 IU/L
  Elevated in: Pregnancy, choriocarcinoma, gestational trophoblastic neoplasia (including molar gestations), placental site trophoblastic tumors; human antimouse antibodies (HAMA) can produce false serum assay for hCG.
  The principal use of this test is to diagnose pregnancy. The concentration of hCG increases significantly during the initial 6 weeks of pregnancy. Peak values approaching 100,000 IU/L occur 60-70 days following implantation.
  hCG levels generally double every 1-3 days. In patients with concentration <2000 IU/L, an increase of serum hCG <66% after 2 days is suggestive of spontaneous abortion or ruptured ectopic gestation.

- **CIRCULATING ANTICOAGULANT** (lupus anticoagulant)
  Normal: Negative
  Detected in: Systemic lupus erythematosus, drug-induced lupus, long-term phenothiazine therapy, multiple myeloma, ulcerative colitis, rheumatoid arthritis, postpartum, hemophilia, neoplasms, chronic inflammatory states, AIDS, nephrotic syndrome
  NOTE: The name is a misnomer because these patients are prone to hypercoagulability and thrombosis.

- **CK;** *see* CREATINE KINASE

- **CLOSTRIDIUM DIFFICILE TOXIN ASSAY** (stool)
  Normal: Negative
  Detected in: Antibiotic-associated diarrhea and pseudomembranous colitis

- **CO;** *see* CARBOXYHEMOGLOBIN

- **COAGULATION FACTORS;** *see* Table 4-8 for characteristics of coagulation factors
  Factor reference ranges:
  V: >10%
  VII: >10%
  VIII: 50% to 170%
  IX: 60% to 136%
  X: >10%
  XI: 50% to 150%
  XII: >30%
  • Table 4-9 describes screening laboratory results in coagulation factor deficiencies.

TABLE 4-8   **Characteristics of Coagulation Factors**

FACTOR	DESCRIPTIVE NAME	SOURCE	APPROXIMATE HALF-LIFE (HR)	FUNCTION
I	Fibrinogen	Liver	120	Substrate for fibrin clot (CP)
II	Prothrombin	Liver (VKD)	60	Serine protease (CP)
V	Proaccelerin, labile factor	Liver	12-36	Cofactor (CP)
VII	Serum prothrombin conversion accelerator, proconvertin	Liver (VKD)	6	(?) Serine protease (EP)
VIII	Antihemophilic factor or globulin	Endothelial cells and (?) elsewhere	12	Cofactor (IP)
IX	Plasma thromboplastin component, Christmas factor	Liver (VKD)	24	Serine protease (IP)
X	Stuart-Prower factor	Liver (VKD)	36	Serine protease (CP)
XI	Plasma thromboplastin antecedent	(?) Liver	40-84	Serine protease (IP)
XII	Hageman factor	(?) Liver	50	Serine protease contact activation (IP)
XIII	Fibrin-stabilizing factor	(?) Liver	96-180	Transglutaminase (CP)
Prekallikrein	Fletcher factor	(?) Liver	?	Serine protease contact activation (IP)
High-molecular-weight kininogen	Fitzgerald factor, Flaujeac or Williams factor	(?) Liver	?	Cofactor, contact activation (IP)

From Noble J (ed): *Primary care medicine,* ed 3, St Louis, 2001, Mosby.
CP, Common pathway; *EP,* extrinsic pathway; *IP,* intrinsic pathway; *VKD,* vitamin K dependent.

TABLE 4-9 Screening Laboratory Results in Coagulation Factor Deficiencies

DEFICIENT FACTOR	FREQUENCY	PT	PTT	TT
I (fibrinogen)	Rare	↑	↑	↑
II (prothrombin)	Very rare	↑	↑	↑
V 1:1,000,000		↑	↑	NL
VII	1:500,000	↑	NL	NL
VIII	1:5000 (male)	NL	↑	NL
IX	1:30,000 (male)	NL	↑	NL
X 1:500,000		↑	↑	NL
XI	Rare*	NL	↑	NL
XII† or HMWK† or PK†	Rare	NL	↑	NL
XIII	Rare	NL	NL	NL

From Andreoli TE (ed): *Cecil essentials of medicine,* ed 5, Philadelphia, 2001, WB Saunders.

↑, Increased over normal range; *HMWK,* high-molecular-weight kininogen; *NL,* normal; *PK,* prekallikrein; *PT,* prothrombin time; *PTT,* partial thromboplastin time; *TT,* thrombin time.

*Except in those of Ashkenazi Jewish descent (approximately 4% are heterozygous for factor XI deficiency).

†Not associated with clinical bleeding.

■ **COLD AGGLUTININS TITER**
Normal range: <1:32
Elevated in: Primary atypical pneumonia (mycoplasma pneumonia), infectious mononucleosis, CMV infection
Others: hepatic cirrhosis, acquired hemolytic anemia, frostbite, multiple myeloma, lymphoma, malaria

■ **COMPLEMENT**
Normal range: C3: 70-160 mg/dl
C4: 20-40 mg/dl
Abnormal values:
DECREASED C3: Active SLE, immune complex disease, acute glomerulonephritis, inborn C3 deficiency, membranoproliferative glomerulonephritis, infective endocarditis, serum sickness, autoimmune/chronic active hepatitis
DECREASED C4: Immune complex disease, active SLE, infective endocarditis, inborn C4 deficiency, hereditary angioedema, hypergammaglobulinemic states, cryobulinemic vasculitis
Table 4-10 describes complement deficiency states.

■ **COMPLETE BLOOD COUNT** (CBC)
White blood cells 3200-9800 mm³ (3.2-9.8 × 10⁹/L)
Red blood cells
Male: 4.3-5.9 × 10⁶/mm³ (4.3-5.9 × 10¹²/L)
Female: 3.5-5 × 10⁶/mm³ (3.5-5 × 10¹²/L)
Hemoglobin
Male: 13.6-17.7 g/dl (136-172 g/L)
Female: 12-15 g/dl (120-150 g/L)
Hematocrit
Male: 39% to 49% (0.39-0.49)
Female: 33% to 43% (0.33-0.43)
Mean corpuscular volume (MCV): 76-100 µm³ (76-100 fL)
Mean corpuscular hemoglobin (MCH): 27-33 pg (27-33 pg)
Mean corpuscular hemoglobin concentration (MCHC): 33-37 g/dl (330-370 g/L)
Red blood cell distribution width index (RDW): 11.5% to 14.5%
Platelet count: 130-400 × 10³/mm³ (130-400 × 10⁹/L)
Differential:
2-6 stabs (bands, early mature neutrophils)
60-70 segs (mature neutrophils)
1-4 eosinophils
0-1 basophils
2-8 monocytes
25-40 lymphocytes

■ **CONJUGATED BILIRUBIN;** *see* BILIRUBIN, DIRECT

IV

TABLE 4-10   Complement Deficiency States

COMPONENT	NUMBER OF REPORTED PATIENTS	MODE OF INHERITANCE	FUNCTIONAL DEFECTS	DISEASE ASSOCIATIONS
Classic pathway				
C1qrs	31	ACD	Impaired IC handling, delayed	CVD, 48%; infection (encaps
C4	21	ACD	C´ activation, impaired	bact), 22%; both, 18%;
C2	109	ACD	immune response	healthy, 12%
Alternative pathway				
D	3	ACD	Impaired C´ activation in	Infection (meningococcal), 74%;
P	70	XL	absence of specific antibody	healthy, 26%
Junction of classic and alternative pathways				
C3	19	ACD	Impaired IC handling, opson/phag; granulocytosis, CTX, immune response and absent SBA	CVD, 79%; recurrent infection (encaps bact), 71%
Terminal components				
C5	27	ACD	Impaired CTX; absent SBA	Infection (*Neisseria*, primarily meningococcal), 58%; CVD, 4%
C6	77	ACD	Absent SBA	Both, 1%
C7	73	ACD		Healthy, 25%
C8	73	ACD		
C9	165	ACD	Impaired SBA	Healthy, 91%; infection, 9%
Plasma proteins regulating C´ activation				
C1-INH	Many	AD Acq	Uncontrolled generation of an inflammatory mediator on C´ activation	Hereditary angioedema
H	13	ACD	Uncontrolled AP activation → low C3	CVD, 40%; CVD plus infection (encaps bact), 40%; healthy, 20%
I	14	ACD	Uncontrolled AP activation → low C3	Infection (encaps bact), 100%
Membrane proteins regulating C´ activation				
Decay-accelerating factor Homologous restriction factor CD59	Many	Acq	Impaired regulation of C3b and C8 deposited on host RBC; PMN, platelets → cell lysis	Paroxysmal nocturnal hemoglobinuria
CR3	>20	ACD	Impaired PMN adhesive functions (i.e., margination), CTX, C3bi-mediated opson/phag	Infection (*Staphylococcus aureus*, *Pseudomonas* spp.), 100%
Autoantibodies				
C3 nephritic factors	>59	Acq	Stabilize AP, convertase → low C3	MPGN, 41%; PLD, 25%; infection (encaps bact), 16%; MPGN plus PLD, 10%; PLD plus infection, 5%; MPGN plus PLD plus infection, 3%; MPGN plus infection, 2%
C4 nephritic factor		Acq	Stabilize CP, C3 convertase → low C3	Glomerulonephritis, 50%; CVD, 50%

From Mandell GL: *Mandell, Douglas, and Bennett's principles and practice of infectious diseases*, ed 5, New York, 2000, Churchill Livingstone.
ACD, Autosomal codominant; *Acq*, acquired; *AD*, autosomal dominant; *AP*, alternative pathway; *C´*, complement; *CP*, classic pathway; *CTX*, chemotaxis; *CVD*, collagen-vascular disease; *encaps bact*, encapsulated bacteria; *IC*, immune complex, *MPGN*, membranoproliferative glomerulonephritis; *PLD*, partial lipodystrophy; *PMN*, polymorphonuclear neutrophil; *RBC*, red blood cells; *SBA*, serum bactericidal activity; *XL*, X-linked.

■ **COOMBS, DIRECT**
Normal: Negative
Positive: Autoimmune hemolytic anemia, erythroblastosis fetalis, transfusion reactions, drugs (α-methyldopa, penicillins, tetracycline, sulfonamides, levodopa, cephalosporins, quinidine, insulin)
False positive: May be seen with cold agglutinins

■ **COOMBS, INDIRECT**
Normal: Negative
Positive: Acquired hemolytic anemia, incompatible cross-matched blood, anti-Rh antibodies, drugs (methyldopa, mefenamic acid, levodopa)

- **COPPER** (serum)
  Normal range: 70-140 µg/dl (11-22 µmol/L)
  Decreased in: Wilson's disease, Menkes' syndrome, malabsorption, malnutrition, nephrosis, total parenteral nutrition, acute leukemia in remission
  Elevated in: Aplastic anemia, biliary cirrhosis, systemic lupus erythematosus, hemochromatosis, hyperthyroidism, hypothyroidism, infection, iron deficiency anemia, leukemia, lymphoma, oral contraceptives, pernicious anemia, rheumatoid arthritis

- **COPPER, URINE;** *see* URINE COPPER

- **CORTISOL, PLASMA**
  Normal range: Varies with time of collection (circadian variation):
  8 AM: 4-19 µg/dl (110-520 nmol/L)
  4 PM: 2-15 µg/dl (50-410 nmol/L)
  Elevated in: Ectopic adrenocorticotropic hormone production (i.e., oat cell carcinoma of lung), loss of normal diurnal variation, pregnancy, chronic renal failure iatrogenic, stress, adrenal, or pituitary hyperplasia or adenomas
  Decreased in: Primary adrenocortical insufficiency, anterior pituitary hypofunction, secondary adrenocortical insufficiency, adrenogenital syndromes

- **C-PEPTIDE**
  Elevated in: Insulinoma, sulfonylurea administration
  Decreased in: Insulin-dependent diabetes mellitus, factitious insulin administration

- **CPK;** *see* CREATINE KINASE

- **C-REACTIVE PROTEIN**
  Normal range: 6.8-820 µg/dl (68-8200 µg/L)
  Elevated in: Rheumatoid arthritis, rheumatic fever, inflammatory bowel disease, bacterial infections, myocardial infarction, oral contraceptives, pregnancy third trimester (acute phase reactant), inflammatory and neoplastic diseases

- **C-REACTIVE PROTEIN, HIGH SENSITIVITY** (hs-CRP, Cardio-CRP)
  is a new test used as a cardiac risk marker. It is increased in patients with silent atherosclerosis years before a cardiovascular event and is independent of cholesterol level and other lipoproteins. It can be used to help stratify cardiac risk.
  Interpretation of results:

CARDIO-CRP RESULT (MG/L)	RISK
≤0.6	Lowest risk
0.7-1.1	Low risk
1.2-1.9	Moderate risk
2.0-3.8	High risk
3.9-4.9	Highest risk
≥5.0	Results may be confounded by acute inflammatory disease. If clinically indicated, a repeat test should be performed in 2 or more weeks.

- **CREATINE KINASE** (CK, CPK)
  Normal range: 0-130 U/L
  Elevated in: Myocardial infarction, myocarditis, rhabdomyolysis, myositis, crush injury/trauma, polymyositis, dermatomyositis, vigorous exercise, muscular dystrophy, myxedema, seizures, malignant hyperthermia syndrome, IM injections, cerebrovascular accident, pulmonary embolism and infarction, acute dissection of aorta
  Decreased in: Steroids, decreased muscle mass, connective tissue disorders, alcoholic liver disease, metastatic neoplasms

- **CREATINE KINASE ISOENZYMES**
  CK-BB: Elevated in: cerebrovascular accident, subarachnoid hemorrhage, neoplasms (prostate, gastrointestinal tract, brain, ovary, breast, lung), severe shock, bowel infarction, hypothermia, meningitis
  CK-MB: Elevated in: myocardial infarction (MI), myocarditis, pericarditis, muscular dystrophy, cardiac defibrillation, cardiac surgery, extensive rhabdomyolysis, strenuous exercise (marathon runners), mixed connective tissue disease, cardiomyopathy, hypothermia
  note: CK-MB exists in the blood in two subforms. MB_2 is released from cardiac cells and converted in the blood to MB_1. Rapid assay of CK-MB subforms can detect MI ($CK-MB_2 \geq 1.0$ U/L, with a ratio of $CK-MB_2/CK-MB_1 \geq 1.5$) within 6 hours of onset of symptoms.
  Fig. 4-2 illustrates the time course of CK, AST, troponins, and LDH activity after acute MI.

IV

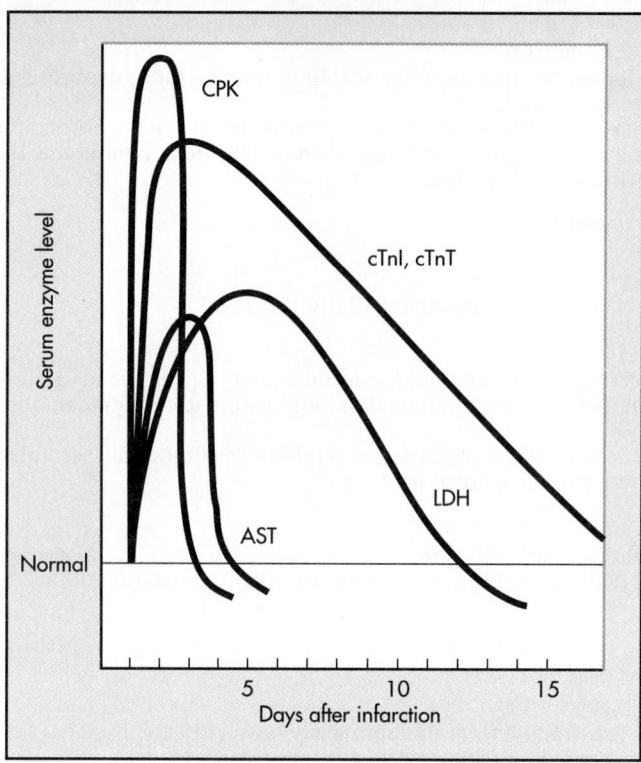

Fig. 4-2   Evaluation of creatine kinase elevation. *CBC,* Complete blood count; *CK,* creatine kinase; *EMG,* electromyography. (From Greene HL, Johnson WP, Lemcke D [eds] : *Decision making in medicine,* ed 2, St Louis, 1998, Mosby.)

CK-MM: Elevated in: crush injury, seizures, malignant hyperthermia syndrome, rhabdomyolysis, myositis, polymyositis, dermatomyositis, vigorous exercise, muscular dystrophy, IM injections, acute dissection of aorta

■ **CREATININE** (serum)
Normal range: 0.6-1.2 mg/dl
Elevated in: Renal insufficiency (acute and chronic), decreased renal perfusion (hypotension, dehydration, congestive heart failure), urinary tract infection, rhabdomyolysis, ketonemia
Drugs (antibiotics [aminoglycosides, cephalosporins], hydantoin, diuretics, methyldopa)
Falsely elevated in: Diabetic ketoacidosis, administration of some cephalosporins (e.g., cefoxitin, cephalothin)
Decreased in: Decreased muscle mass (including amputees and older persons), pregnancy, prolonged debilitation

■ **CREATININE CLEARANCE**
Normal range: 75-124 ml/min Box 4-1 describes a formula for calculation of creatinine clearance. The Cockcroft-Gault formula to calculate creatinine clearance is described in Box 4-2.
Elevated in: Pregnancy, exercise
Decreased in: Renal insufficiency, drugs (cimetidine, procainamide, antibiotics, quinidine)

BOX 4-1   Calculation of the Creatinine Clearance

$C_{cr} = U_{cr} \times V / P_{cr}$
where C_{cr} = clearance of creatinine (ml/min)
        U_{cr} = urine creatinine (mg/dl)
        V = volume of urine (ml/min) (for 24-hr volume: divide by 1440)
        P_{cr} = plasma creatinine (mg/dl)

Normal range: 95 to 105 ml/min/1.75m²

BOX 4-2   Cockroft-Gault Formula to Calculate Creatinine Clearance (C_{cr})

$$C_{cr} = \frac{(140 - \text{age in years}) \times (\text{lean body weight in kg})}{S_{cr} \text{ in mg/dl} \times 72}$$

For women multiply final value by 0.85

Scr, Serum creatinine.

- **CREATININE, URINE;** *see* URINE CREATININE

- **CRYOGLOBULINS** (serum)
  Normal range: Not detectable
  Present in: Collagen-vascular diseases, chronic lymphocytic leukemia, hemolytic anemias, multiple myeloma, Waldenström's macroglobulinemia, chronic active hepatitis, Hodgkin's disease

- **CRYPTOSPORIDIUM ANTIGEN BY EIA** (stool)
  Normal range: Not detected
  Present in: Cryptosporidiosis

- **CSF;** *see* CEREBROSPINAL FLUID

- **D-DIMER**
  Normal range: <0. mcg/mL
  Elevated in: DVT, pulmonary embolism, high levels of rheumatoid factor, activation of coagulation and fibrolytic system from any cause
  D-dimer assay by ELISA assists in the diagnosis of DVT and pulmonary embolism. This test has significant limitations because it can be elevated whenever the coagulation and fibrinolytic systems are activated and can also be falsely elevated with high rheumatoid factor levels.

- **D-XYLOSE ABSORPTION**
  Normal range: 21% to 31% excreted in 5 hr
  Decreased in: Malabsorption syndrome

- **D-XYLOSE ABSORPTION TEST**
  Normal range:
  URINE: ≥ 4 g/5 hours (5-hour urine collection in adults > 12 years (25 g dose)
  SERUM: ≥ 25 mg/dL (adult, I h, 25 g dose, normal renal function)
  Normal results: In patients with malabsorption, normal results suggest pancreatic disease as an etiology of the malabsorption.
  Abnormal results: Celiac disease, Crohn's disease, tropical sprue, surgical bowel resection, AIDS. False-positives can occur with decreased renal function, dehydration/hypovolemia, surgical blind loops, decreased gastric emptying, vomiting.

- **DIGOXIN (LANOXIN)**
  Normal therapeutic range: 0.5-2 ng/mL
  Elevated in: Impaired renal function, excessive dosing, concomitant use of quinidine, amiodarone, verapamil, fluoxetine, nifedipine

- **DILANTIN;** *see* PHENYTOIN

- **DOPAMINE**
  Normal range: 0-175 pg/ml
  Elevated in: Pheochromocytomas, neuroblastomas, stress, vigorous exercise, certain foods (bananas, chocolate, coffee, tea, vanilla)

- **ELECTROLYTES, URINE;** *see* URINE ELECTROLYTES

- **ELECTROPHORESIS, HEMOGLOBIN;** *see* HEMOGLOBIN ELECTROPHORESIS

- **ELECTROPHORESIS, PROTEIN;** *see* PROTEIN ELECTROPHORESIS

- **ENA-COMPLEX;** *see* EXTRACTABLE NUCLEAR ANTIGEN

- **ENDOMYSIAL ANTIBODIES**
  Normal: Not detected
  Present in: Celiac disease, dermatitis herpetiformis

- **EOSINOPHIL COUNT**
  Normal range: 1%-4% eosinophils (0-440/mm^3)
  Elevated in:
  HELMINTHIC PARASITES
  Ascaris lumbricoides (invasive larval stage)
  Hookworms (invasive larval stage)
  Strongyloides stercoralis (initial infection and autoinfection)
  Trichinosis
  Filariasis
  Echinococcus granulosus and *E. multilocularis*
  Toxocara species
  Animal hookworms

IV

Angiostrongylus cantonensis and *A.* costaricensis
Schistosomiasis
Liver flukes
Fasciolopsis buski
Anisakiasis
Capillaria philippinensis
Paragonimus westermani
"Tropical eosinophilia" (unidentified microfilariae)
OTHER INFECTIONS/INFESTATIONS
Pulmonary aspergillosis
Severe scabies
ALLERGIES
Asthma
Hay fever
Drug reactions
Atopic dermatitis
AUTOIMMUNE AND RELATED DISORDERS
Polyarteritis nodosa
Necrotizing vasculitis
Eosinophilic fasciitis
Pemphigus
NEOPLASTIC DISEASES
Hodgkin's disease
Mycosis fungoides
Chronic myelocytic leukemia
Eosinophilic leukemia
Polycythemia vera
Mucin-secreting adenocarcinomas
IMMUNODEFICIENCY STATES
Hyperimmunoglobulin E with recurrent infection
Wiskott-Aldrich syndrome
OTHER
Addison's disease
Inflammatory bowel disease
Dermatitis herpetiformis
Toxic/chemical syndrome
Eosinophilic myalgia syndrome, tryptophan, toxic oil syndrome
Hypereosinophilic syndrome (unknown etiology)

■ **EPINEPHRINE, PLASMA**
Normal range: 0-90 pg/ml
Elevated in: Pheochromocytomas, neuroblastomas, stress, vigorous exercise, certain foods (bananas, chocolate, coffee, tea, vanilla), hypoglycemia

■ **EPSTEIN-BARR VIRUS SEROLOGY**
Normal range: IgG anti VCA <1:10 or negative
Abnormal: IgG anti VCA >1:10 or positive indicates either current or previous infection
IgM anti VCA >1:10 or positive indicates current or recent infection
Anti-EBNA ≥1.5 or positive indicates previous infection
Table 4-11 and Fig. 4-3 describe test interpretation.

TABLE 4-11 Antibody Tests in Epstein-Barr Viral Infection

	APPEARANCE	PEAK	DISAPPEARS
Heterophil Ab	3-5 days after onset of Sx (range, 0-21 days)	During second wk after onset of Sx (1-4 wk)	2-3 mo after onset of Sx (still found at 1 yr in 20% of cases)
VCA-IgM	Beginning of Sx (1 wk before to 1 wk after Sx begins)	During first wk after onset of Sx (0-21 days)	2-3 mo after onset of Sx (1-6 mo)
VCA-IgG	3 days after onset of Sx (0-2 wk)	During second wk after onset of Sx (1-3 wk)	Decline to lower level, then persists for life
EBNA-IgG	3 wk after onset of Sx (1-4 wk)	8 mo after appearance (3-12 mo)	Lifelong
EA-D	5 days after onset of Sx (during first 1-2 wk after onset of Sx)	14-21 days after onset of Sx (1-4 wk)	9 wk after appearance (2-6 mo)
(EBNA-IgM)	(Same as VCA-IgM)	(Same as VCA-IgM)	(Same as VCA-IgM)

From Ravel R: *Clinical laboratory medicine*, ed 6, St Louis, 1995, Mosby.
Ab, Antibody; *EA,* early antigen; *EBNA,* Epstein-Barr virus nuclear antigen; *Sx,* symptoms; *VCA,* viral capsid antigen.

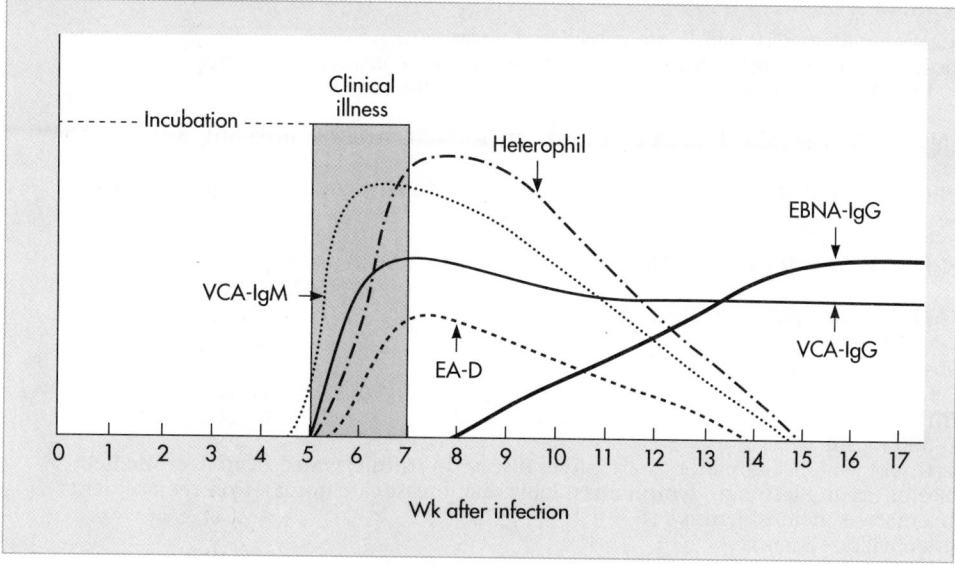

Fig. 4-3 **Tests in Epstein-Barr viral infection.** See Table 4-19 for abbreviations. (From Ravel R: *Clinical laboratory medicine,* ed 6, St Louis, 1995, Mosby.)

■ **ERYTHROCYTE SEDIMENTATION RATE** (ESR; Westergren)
Normal range: Male: 0-15 mm/hr
Female: 0-20 mm/hr
Elevated in: Collagen-vascular diseases, infections, myocardial infarction, neoplasms, inflammatory states (acute phase reactant), hyperthyroidism, hypothyroidism, rouleaux formation
Decreased in: Sickle cell disease, polycythemia, corticosteroids, spherocytosis, anisocytosis, hypofibrinogenemia, increased serum viscosity

■ **ERYTHROPOIETIN** (EP)
Normal: 3.7-16.0 IU/L by radioimmunoassay
Erythropoietin is a glycoprotein secreted by the kidneys that stimulates RBC production by acting on erythroid-committed stem cells.
Increased in: Extremely high: generally seen in patients with severe anemia (Hct <25, <7) such as in cases of aplastic anemia, severe hemolytic anemia, hematologic cancers. Very high: patients with mild to moderate anemia (Hct 25-35, Hb 7-10); high: patients with mild anemia (e.g., AIDS, myelodysplasia).
Erythropoietin can be inappropriately elevated in patients with malignant neoplasms, renal cysts, postrenal transplant, meningioma, hemangioblastoma, and leiomyoma.
Decreased in: Renal failure, polycythemia vera, autonomic neuropathy

■ **ESTRADIOL** (serum)
Normal range: **FEMALE, PREMENOPAUSAL:** 30-400 pg/mL, depending on phase of menstrual cycle
FEMALE, POSTMENOPAUSAL: 0-30 pg/mL
MALE, ADULT: 10-50 pg/mL
Decreased in: Ovarian failure
Elevated in: Tumors of ovary, testis, adrenal, or nonendocrine sites (rare)

■ **ESTROGEN**
Normal range:

Serum:	Males:	20-80 pg/ml
	Females:	Follicular: 60-200 pg/ml
		Luteal: 160-400 pg/ml
		Postmenopausal: <130 pg/ml
Urine:	Males:	4-23 μg/g creatinine
	Females:	Follicular: 7-65 μg/g creatinine
		Midcycle: 32-104 μg/g creatinine
		Luteal: 8-135 μg/g creatinine

Elevated in: Hyperplasia of adrenal cortex, ovarian tumors producing estrogen, granulosa and thecal cell tumors, testicular tumors
Decreased in: Menopause, hypopituitarism, primary ovarian malfunction, anorexia nervosa, hypofunction of adrenal cortex, ovarian agenesis, psychogenic stress, gonadotropin-releasing hormone deficiency

IV

- **ETHANOL** (blood)
  Normal range: Negative (values <10 mg/dL are considered negative)
  Ethanol is metabolized at 10-25 mg/dL/hour. Levels ≥80 mg/dL are considered evidence of impairment for driving. Fatal blood concentration is considered to be >400 mg/dL.

- **EXTRACTABLE NUCLEAR ANTIGEN** (ENA complex, anti-RNP antibody, anti-Sm, anti-Smith)
  Normal: Negative
  Present in: Systemic lupus erythematosus, rheumatoid arthritis, Sjögren's syndrome, mixed connective tissue disease

- **FDP;** *see* FIBRIN DEGRADATION PRODUCT

- **FECAL FAT, QUANTITATIVE** (72-hr collection)
  Normal range: 2-6 g/24 hr
  Elevated in: Malabsorption syndrome

- **FERRITIN** (serum)
  Normal range: 18-300 ng/ml
  Elevated in: Hyperthyroidism, inflammatory states, liver disease (ferritin elevated from necrotic hepatocytes), neoplasms (neuroblastomas, lymphomas, leukemia, breast carcinoma), iron replacement therapy, hemochromatosis, hemosiderosis
  Decreased in: Iron deficiency anemia

- **α-1 FETOPROTEIN**
  Normal range: 0-20 ng/ml
  Elevated in: Hepatocellular carcinoma (usually values >1000 ng/ml), germinal neoplasms (testis, ovary, mediastinum, retroperitoneum), liver disease (alcoholic cirrhosis, acute hepatitis, chronic active hepatitis), fetal anencephaly, spina bifida, basal cell carcinoma, breast carcinoma, pancreatic carcinoma, gastric carcinoma, retinoblastoma, esophageal atresia

- **FIBRIN DEGRADATION PRODUCT** (FDP)
  Normal range: <10 μg/ml
  Elevated in: Disseminated intravascular coagulation, primary fibrinolysis, pulmonary embolism, severe liver disease
  NOTE: The presence of rheumatoid factor may cause falsely elevated FDP.

- **FIBRINOGEN**
  Normal range: 200-400 mg/dl
  Elevated in: Tissue inflammation or damage (acute phase protein reactant), oral contraceptives, pregnancy, acute infection, myocardial infarction
  Decreased in: Disseminated intravascular coagulation, hereditary afibrinogenemia, liver disease, primary or secondary fibrinolysis, cachexia

- **FOLATE** (folic acid)
  Normal range: Plasma: 2-10 ng/ml
  Red blood cells: 140-960 ng/ml
  Decreased in: Folic acid deficiency (inadequate intake, malabsorption), alcoholism, drugs (methotrexate, trimethoprim, phenytoin, oral contraceptives, Azulfidine), vitamin B_{12} deficiency (defective red cell folate absorption), hemolytic anemia
  Elevated in: Folic acid therapy

- **FOLLICLE-STIMULATING HORMONE** (FSH)
  Normal range: 5-20 mIU/mL
  Elevated in: Menopause, primary gonadal failure, alcoholism, castration, Klinefelter's syndrome, gonadotropin-secreting pituitary hormones
  Decreased in: Pregnancy, polycystic ovary disease, anorexia nervosa, anterior pituitary hypofunction

- **FREE T$_4$;** *see* T$_4$, FREE

- **FREE THYROXINE INDEX**
  Normal range: 1.1-4.3
  INCREASED THYROXINE OR FREE THYROXINE VALUES
  Laboratory error
  Primary hyperthyroidism (T_4/T_3 type)
  Severe thyroxine-binding globulin elevation
  Excess therapy of hypothyroidism
  Excessive dose of levothyroxine
  Active thyroiditis (subacute, painless, early active Hashimoto's disease)
  Familial dysalbuminemic hyperthyroxinemia (some FT_4 kits, especially analog types)
  Peripheral resistance to T_4 syndrome
  Amiodarone or propranolol

Postpartum transient toxicosis
Factitious hyperthyroidism
Jod-Basedow (iodine-induced) hyperthyroidism
Severe nonthyroid illness
Acute psychosis (especially paranoid schizophrenia)
T_4 sample drawn 2-4 hr after levothyroxine dose
Struma ovarii
Pituitary thyroid-stimulating hormone–secreting tumor
Certain x-ray contrast media (Telepaque and Oragrafin)
Acute porphyria
Heparin effect (some T_4 and FT_4 kits)
Amphetamine, heroin, methadone, and phencyclidine abuse
Perphenazine or 5-fluorouracil
Antithyroid or anti-IgG heterophil (HAMA) autoantibodies
"T_4" hyperthyroidism
Hyperemesis gravidarum; about 50% of patients
High altitudes
DECREASED THYROXINE OR FREE THYROXINE VALUES
Laboratory error
Primary hypothyroidism
Severe nonthyroid illness*
Lithium therapy
Severe thyroxine-binding globulin decrease (congenital, disease, or drug-induced) or severe albumin decrease*
Dilantin, Depakene, or high-dose salicylate drugs*
Pituitary insufficiency
Large doses of inorganic iodide (e.g., saturated solution of potassium iodide)
Moderate or severe iodine deficiency
Cushing's syndrome
High-dose glucocorticoid drugs
Pregnancy, third trimester (low normal or small decrease)
Addison's disease; some patients (30%)
Heparin effect (a few FT_4 kits)
Desipramine or amiodarone drugs
Acute psychiatric illness

■ **FTA-ABS** (serum)
Normal: Nonreactive
Reactive in: Syphilis, other treponemal diseases (yaws, pinta, bejel), SLE, pregnancy

■ **GAMMA-GLUTAMYL TRANSFERASE** (gGt); *see* γ-GLUTAMYL TRANSFERASE
GASTRIN (serum)
Normal range: 0-180 pg/ml
Elevated in: Zollinger-Ellison syndrome (gastrinoma), pernicious anemia, hyperparathyroidism, retained gastric antrum, chronic renal failure, gastric ulcer, chronic atrophic gastritis, pyloric obstruction, malignant neoplasms of the stomach, H_2-blockers, omeprazole, calcium therapy, ulcerative colitis, rheumatoid arthritis

■ **GLOMERULAR BASEMENT MEMBRANE** (gBm) **ANTIBODY**
Normal: Negative
Present in: Goodpasture's syndrome

■ **GLUCOSE, FASTING**
Normal range: 70-110 mg/dl
Elevated in: Diabetes mellitus, stress, infections, myocardial infarction, cerebrovascular accident, Cushing's syndrome, acromegaly, acute pancreatitis, glucagonoma, hemochromatosis, drugs (glucocorticoids, diuretics [thiazides, loop diuretics]), glucose intolerance
Decreased in: Sulfonylurea therapy, insulin therapy, reactive hypoglycemia (e.g., s/b subtotal gastrectomy), starvation, insulinoma, glycogen storage disorders, severe liver disease or renal disease, ethanol-induced hypoglycemia, mesenchymal tumors that secrete insulin-like hormones

■ **GLUCOSE, POSTPRANDIAL**
Normal range: <140 mg/dl
Elevated in: Diabetes mellitus, glucose intolerance
Decreased in: Postgastrointestinal resection, reactive hypoglycemia, hereditary fructose intolerance, galactosemia, leucine sensitivity

■ **GLUCOSE TOLERANCE TEST**
Normal values above fasting:
30 min: 30-60 mg/dl
60 min: 20-50 mg/dl

IV

120 min: 5-15 mg/dl
180 min: fasting level or below
Abnormal in: Glucose intolerance, diabetes mellitus, Cushing's syndrome, acromegaly, pheochromo-cytoma, gestational diabetes

- **GLUCOSE-6-PHOSPHATE DEHYDROGENASE SCREEN** (blood)
Normal: G_6PD enzyme activity detected
Abnormal: If a deficiency is detected, quantitation of G_6PD is necessary; a G_6PD screen may be falsely interpreted as "normal" after an episode of hemolysis because most G_6PD-deficient cells have been destroyed.

- **γ-GLUTAMYL TRANSFERASE** (GGT)
Normal range: 0-30 U/L
Elevated in: Chronic alcoholic liver disease, neoplasms (hepatoma, metastatic disease to the liver, carcinoma of the pancreas), systemic lupus erythematosus, congestive heart failure, trauma, nephrotic syndrome, sepsis, cholestasis, drugs (phenytoin, barbiturates)

- **GLYCATED (GLYCOSYLATED) HEMOGLOBIN** (HbA_{1C})
Normal range: 4.0% to 6.7%
Elevated in: Uncontrolled diabetes mellitus (glycated hemoglobin levels reflect the level of glucose control over the preceding 120 days), lead toxicity, alcoholism, iron deficiency anemia, hyper-triglyceridemia
Decreased in: Hemolytic anemias, decreased red blood cell survival, pregnancy, acute or chronic blood loss, chronic renal failure, insulinoma, congenital spherocytosis, hemoglobin S, C, and D diseases

- **HAM TEST** (acid serum test)
Normal: Negative
Positive in: Paroxysmal nocturnal hemoglobinuria
False positive in: Hereditary or acquired spherocytosis, recent transfusion with aged red blood cells, aplastic anemia, myeloproliferative syndromes, leukemia, hereditary dyserythropoietic anemia type II

- **HAPTOGLOBIN** (serum)
Normal range: 50-220 mg/dl
Elevated in: Inflammation (acute phase reactant), collagen-vascular diseases, infections (acute phase reactant), drugs (androgens), obstructive liver disease
Decreased in: Hemolysis (intravascular more than extravascular), megaloblastic anemia, severe liver disease, large tissue hematomas, infectious mononucleosis, drugs (oral contraceptives)

- **HDL;** *see* HIGH-DENSITY LIPOPROTEIN CHOLESTEROL

- ***HELICOBACTER PYLORI*** (serology, stool antigen)
Normal range: Not detected
Detected in: H. pylori infection. Positive serology can indicate current or past infection. Positive stool antigen test indicates acute infection (sensitivity and specificity >90%). Stool testing should be delayed at least 4 weeks after eradication therapy.

- **HEMATOCRIT**
Normal range: Male: 39% to 49%
Female: 33% to 43%
Elevated in: Polycythemia vera, smoking, chronic obstructive pulmonary disease, high altitudes, dehydration, hypovolemia
Decreased in: Blood loss (gastrointestinal, genitourinary) anemia

- **HEMOGLOBIN**
Normal range: Male: 13.6-17.7 g/dl
Female: 12.0-15.0 g/dl
Elevated in: Hemoconcentration, dehydration, polycythemia vera, chronic obstructive pulmonary disease, high altitudes, false elevations (hyperlipemic plasma, white blood cells >50,000/mm³), stress
Decreased in: Hemorrhage (gastrointestinal, genitourinary) anemia

- **HEMOGLOBIN A₁c,** *see* GLYCATED HEMOGLOBIN

- **HEMOGLOBIN ELECTROPHORESIS**
Normal range:
HbA_1: 95%-98%
HbA_2: 1.5%-3.5%
HbF: <2%
HbC: absent
HbS: absent

- **HEMOGLOBIN, GLYCATED;** *see* GLYCATED HEMOGLOBIN

- **HEMOGLOBIN, GLYCOSYLATED;** *see* GLYCATED HEMOGLOBIN

- **HEMOGLOBIN, URINE;** *see* URINE HEMOGLOBIN

- **HEMOSIDERIN, URINE;** *see* URINE HEMOGLOBIN

- **HEPATITIS A ANTIBODY**
  Normal: Negative
  Present in: Viral hepatitis A; can be IgM or IgG (if IgM, acute hepatitis A; if IgG, previous infection with hepatitis A)
  See Fig. 4-4 for serologic tests in HAV infection.
  HAV-IGM ANTIBODY
  Appearance
  About the same time as clinical symptoms (3-4 wk after exposure, range 14-60 days), or just before beginning of AST/ALT elevation (range 10 days before–7 days after)
  Peak
  About 3-4 wk after onset of symptoms (1-6 wk)
  Becomes Nondetectable
  3-4 mo after onset of symptoms (1-6 mo). In a few cases HAV-IgM antibody can persist as long as 12-14 mo.
  HAV-TOTAL ANTIBODY
  Appearance
  About 3 wk after IgM becomes detectable (therefore about the middle of clinical symptom period to early convalescence)
  Peak
  About 1-2 mo after onset
  Becomes Nondetectable
  Remains elevated for life, but can slowly fall somewhat

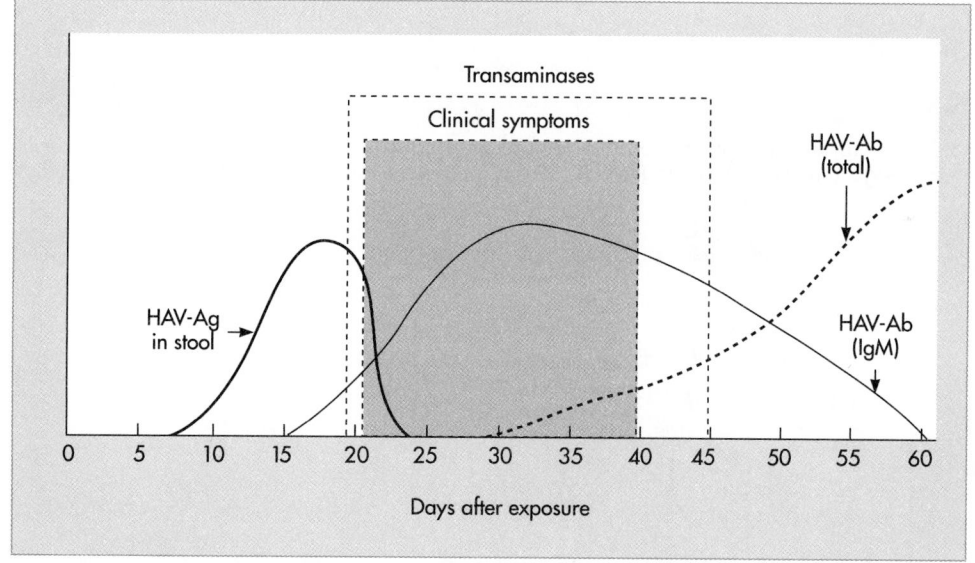

Fig. 4-4   Serologic tests in HAV infection. (From Ravel R: *Clinical laboratory medicine,* ed 6, St Louis, 1995, Mosby.)

- **HEPATITIS A VIRAL INFECTION**
  Best all-purpose test(s) to diagnose acute HAV infection = HAV-Ab (IgM)
  Best all-purpose test(s) to demonstrate past HAV infection/immunity = HAV-Ab (total)

- **HEPATITIS B SURFACE ANTIGEN** (HBSAG)
  Normal: Not detected
  Detected in: Acute viral hepatitis type B, chronic hepatitis B
  Appearance
  2-6 wk after exposure (range 6 days–6 mo); 5%-15% of patients are negative at onset of jaundice
  Peak
  1-2 wk before to 1-2 wk after onset of symptoms
  Becomes Nondetectable
  1-3 mo after peak (range 1 wk-5 mo)

■ HEPATITIS B VIRAL INFECTION

Figs. 4-5, 4-6, and 4-7 illustrate antigens and antibodies in Hepatitis B Infection.

HB$_s$
-Ag

HB$_s$Ag: shows current active HBV infection.

Persistence over 6 mo indicates carrier/chronic HBV infection.

HBV nucleic acid probe: present before and longer than HB$_s$Ag.

More reliable marker for increased infectivity than HB$_s$Ag and/or HB$_e$Ag.

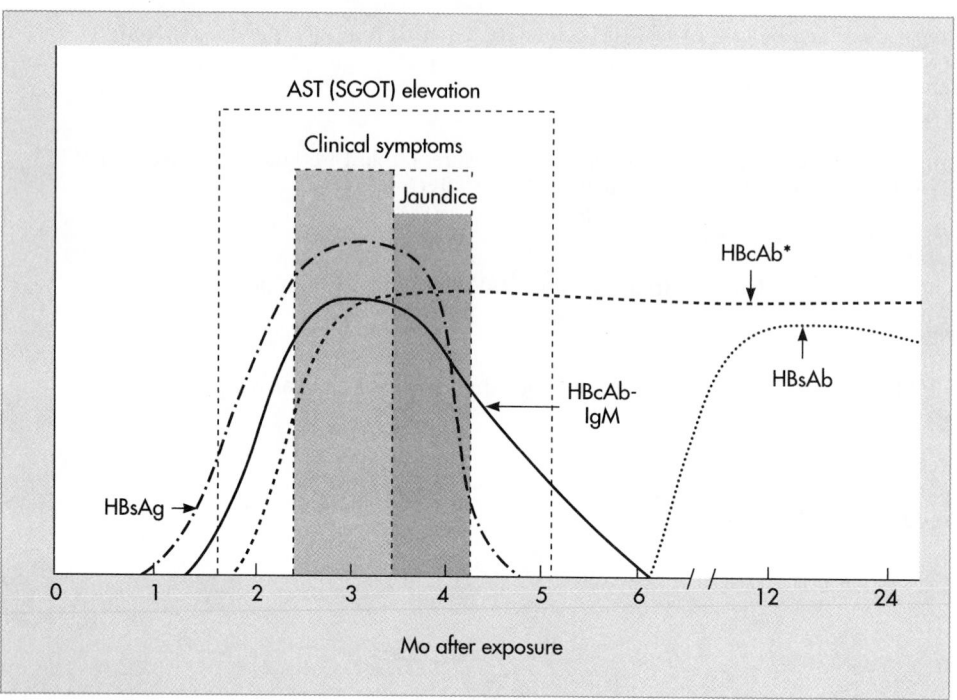

Fig. 4-5   HBV surface antigen-antibody and core antibodies (note "core window"). *HB$_C$Ab = HB$_C$Ab-IgM + HB$_C$Ab-IgG (combined). (From Ravel R: *Clinical laboratory medicine,* ed 6, St Louis, 1995, Mosby.)

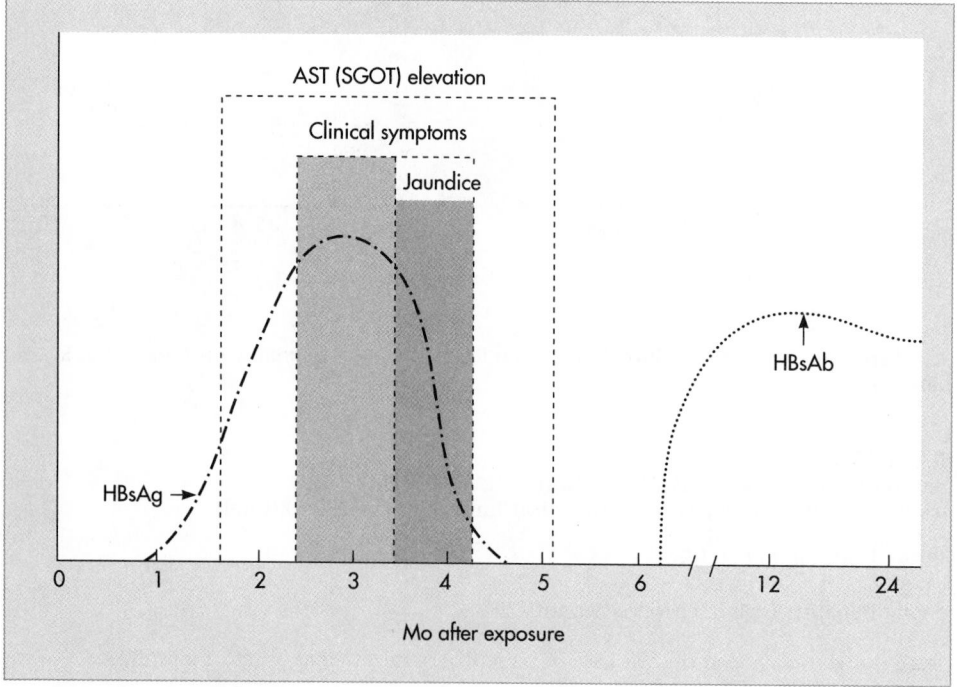

Fig. 4-6   HBV surface antigen and antibody (HB$_s$Ag and HB$_s$Ab-total). (From Ravel R: *Clinical laboratory medicine,* ed 6, St Louis, 1995, Mosby.)

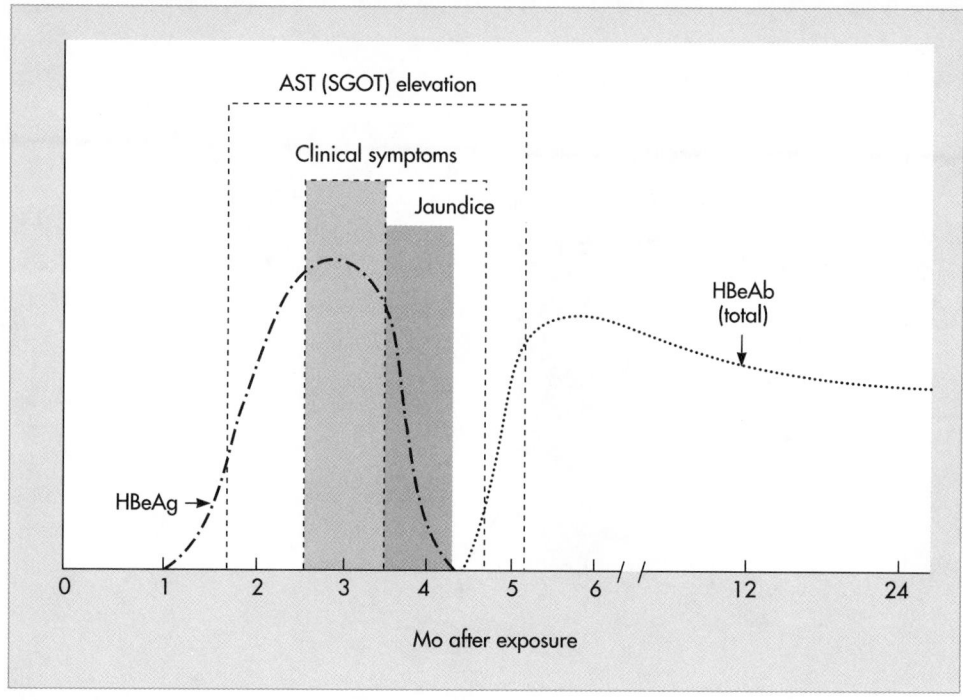

Fig. 4-7 **HBV e antigen and antibody.** (From Ravel R: *Clinical laboratory medicine,* ed 6, St Louis, 1995, Mosby.)

-Ab
HB$_S$Ab-total: shows previous healed HBV infection and evidence of immunity.
HB$_C$
-Ab
HB$_C$Ab-IgM: shows either acute or very recent infection by HBV.
In convalescent phase of acute HBV, may be elevated when HB$_S$Ag has disappeared (core window).
Negative HB$_C$Ab-IgM with positive HB$_S$Ag suggests either very early acute HBV or carrier/chronic HBV.
HB$_C$Ab-total: only useful to show past HBV infection if HB$_S$Ag and HB$_C$Ab-IgM are both negative.
HB$_E$
-Ag
HB$_e$-AbAg: when present, especially without HB$_e$Ab, suggests increased patient infectivity.
HB$_e$Ab-total: when present, suggests less patient infectivity.
I.   HB$_S$Ag positive, HB$_C$Ab negative*
     About 5% (range 0%-17%) of patients with early-stage HBV acute infection (HB$_C$Ab rises later)
II. HB$_S$Ag positive, HB$_C$Ab positive, HB$_S$Ab negative
     a. Most of the clinical symptom stage
     b. Chronic HBV carriers without evidence of liver disease ("asymptomatic carriers")
     c. Chronic HBV hepatitis (chronic persistent type or chronic active type)
III. HB$_S$Ag negative, HB$_C$Ab positive,* HB$_S$Ab negative
     a. Late clinical symptom stage or early convalescence stage (core window)
     b. Chronic HBV infection with HB$_S$Ag below detection levels with current tests
     c. Old previous HBV infection
IV. HB$_S$Ag negative, HB$_C$Ab positive, HB$_S$Ab positive
     a. Late convalescence to complete recovery
     b. Old infection

■ HEPATITIS C VIRAL INFECTION
Fig. 4-8 illustrates antigens and antibodies in Hepatitis C Infection.
HCV
-Ag
HCV nucleic acid probe: shows current infection by HCV (especially using PCR amplification).
-Ab
HCV-Ab (IgG): current, convalescent, or old HCV infection.
HAV
-Ag
HAV-Ag by EM: shows presence of virus in stool early in infection.
-Ab
HAV-Ab (IgM): current or recent HAV infection.
HAV-Ab (total): convalescent or old HAV infection.

IV

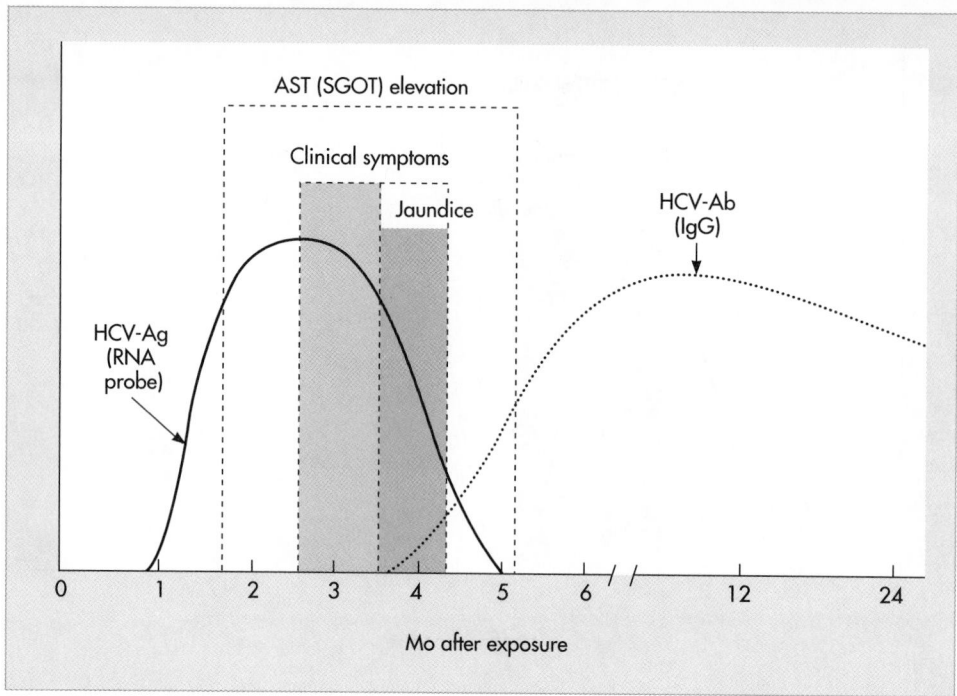

Fig. 4-8   **HCV antigen and antibody.** (From Ravel R: *Clinical laboratory medicine,* ed 6, St Louis, 1995, Mosby.)

■ **HEPATITIS D VIRAL INFECTION**

Fig. 4-9 illustrates antigens and antibodies in Hepatitic D Infection.

Best current all-purpose screening test = ADV-Ab (total)

Best test to differentiate acute from chronic infection = HDV-Ab (IgM)

DELTA HEPATITIS COINFECTION (ACUTE HDV + ACUTE HBV) OR SUPERINFECTION (ACUTE HDV + CHRONIC HBV)

HDV

-Ag

HDV-Ag: shows current infection (acute or chronic) by HDV.

HDV nucleic acid probe: detects antigen before and longer than HDV-Ag by EIA.

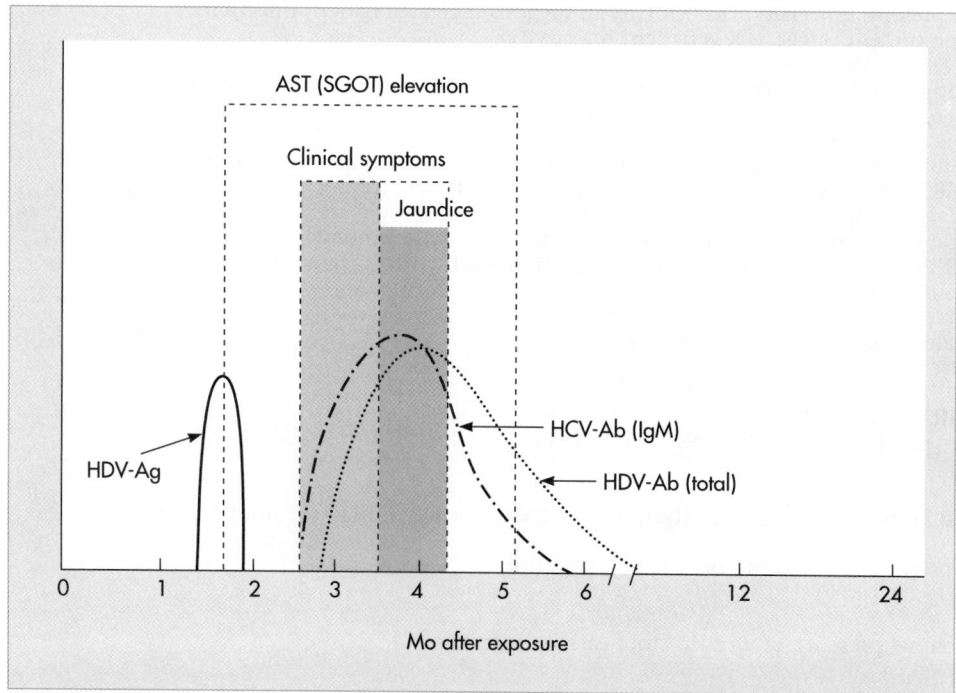

Fig. 4-9   **HDV antigen and antibodies.** (From Ravel R: *Clinical laboratory medicine,* ed 6, St Louis, 1995, Mosby.)

-Ab

HDV-Ab (IgM): high elevation in acute HDV; does not persist.

Low or moderate elevation in convalescent HDV; does not persist.

Low to high persistent elevation in chronic HDV (depends on degree of cell injury and sensitivity of the assay).

HDV-Ab (total): high elevation in acute HDV; does not persist.

High persistent elevation in chronic HDV.

HDV-AG

Detected by DNA probe, less often by immunoassay

Appearance: Prodromal stage (before symptoms); just at or after initial rise in ALT (about a week after appearance of $HB_S Ag$ and about the time $HB_C Ab$-IgM level begins to rise)

Peak: 2-3 days after onset

Becomes nondetectable: 1-4 days (may persist until shortly after symptoms appear)

HDV-AB (IGM)

Appearance: about 10 days after symptoms begin (range 1-28 days)

Peak: about 2 wk after first detection

Becomes nondetectable: about 35 days (range 10-80 days) after first detection (most other IgM antibodies take 3-6 mo to become nondetectable)

HDV-AB (TOTAL)

Appearance: about 50 days after symptoms begin (range 14-80 days); about 5 wk after HDV-Ag (range 3-11 wk)

Peak: About 2 wk after first detection

Becomes nondetectable: about 7 mo after first detection (range 4-14 mo)

■ **HETEROPHIL ANTIBODY**

Normal: Negative

Positive in: Infectious mononucleosis

■ **HIGH-DENSITY LIPOPROTEIN (HDL) CHOLESTEROL**

Normal range:

Male: 45-70 mg/dl

Female: 45-90 mg/dl

Increased in: Use of gemfibrozil, statins, fenofibrate, nicotinic acid, estrogens, regular aerobic exercise, small (1 oz) daily alcohol intake

Decreased in: Deficiency of apoproteins, liver disease, probucol ingestion, Tangier disease

NOTE: A cholesterol/HDL ratio >4.0 is associated with increased risk of coronary artery disease.

■ **HLA ANTIGENS**

Associated disorders: see Table 4-12.

TABLE 4-12 HLA Antigens Associated with Specific Diseases

ANTIGEN	CONDITION	ANTIGEN	CONDITION
HLA-B27	Ankylosing spondylitis	HLA-B8, Dw3	Celiac disease
Reiter's syndrome	HLA-B8, Dw3	Dermatitis herpetiformis	
Psoriatic arthritis	HLA-B8	Myasthenia gravis	
HLA-A10, B18, Dw2	C2 deficiency	HLA-B8	Chronic active hepatitis in children
HLA-A2, B40, Cw3	C4 deficiency	HLA-Drw4	Active chronic hepatitis in adults
HLA-B7, Dw2	Multiple sclerosis	HLA-B13, Bw17	Psoriasis
HLA-A3	Hemochromatosis		

From Cerra FB: *Manual of critical care,* St Louis, 1987, Mosby.

■ **HOMOCYSTEINE, PLASMA**

Normal range:

0-30 years: 4.6-8.1 micromol/L

30-59 years: 6.3-11.2 micromol/L (males), 4-5-7.9 micromol/L (females)

> 59 years: 5.8-11.9 micromol/L

Increased: Thrombophilic states, B_6, B_{12}, folic acid, riboflavin deficiency, pregnancy, homocystinuria

NOTE: An increased homocysteine level is an independent risk factor for atherosclerosis.

■ **HUMAN CHORIONIC GONADOTROPIN** (HCG)

Normal range: Varies with gestational stage

1st week: 5-50 mU/ml

1-2 wk: 50-550 mU/ml

2-3 wk: up to 5000 mU/ml

3-4 wk: up to 10,000 mU/ml

4-5 wk: up to 50,000 mU/ml

2-3 mo: 10,000-100,000 mU/ml

Elevated in: Normal pregnancy, hydatidiform mole, choriocarcinoma, germ cell tumors of testicle, some nontrophoblastic neoplasms (e.g., neoplasms of cervix, gastrointestinal tract, ovary, lung, breast)

IV

■ **HUMAN IMMUNODEFICIENCY VIRUS ANTIBODY, TYPE 1** (HIV-1)

Normal range: Not detected

Abnormal result: HIV antibodies usually appear in the blood 1-4 mo after infection.

Testing sequence:

1. ELISA is the recommended initial screening test. Sensitivity and specificity are >99%. False-positive ELISA may occur with autoimmune disorders, administration of immune globulin manufactured before 1985 within 6 wk of testing, presence of rheumatoid factor, presence of DLA-DR antibodies in multigravida female, administration of influenza vaccine within 3 mo of testing, hemodialysis, positive plasma reagin test, certain medical disorders (hemophilia, hypergammaglobulinemia, alcoholic hepatitis)
2. A positive ELISA is confirmed with Western blot. False-positive Western blot may result from connective tissue disorders, human leukocyte antigen antibodies, polyclonal gammopathies, hyperbilirubinemia, presence of antibody to another human retrovirus, or cross reaction with other non-virus-derived proteins in healthy persons. Undetermined Western blot may occur in AIDS patients with advanced immunodeficiency (caused by loss of antibodies), and in recent HIV infections.
3. Polymerase chain reaction is used to confirm indeterminate Western blot results or negative results in persons with suspected HIV infection.

Fig. 4-10 describes tests in HIV infection.

Indications for plasma HIV RNA testing are described in Table 4-13.

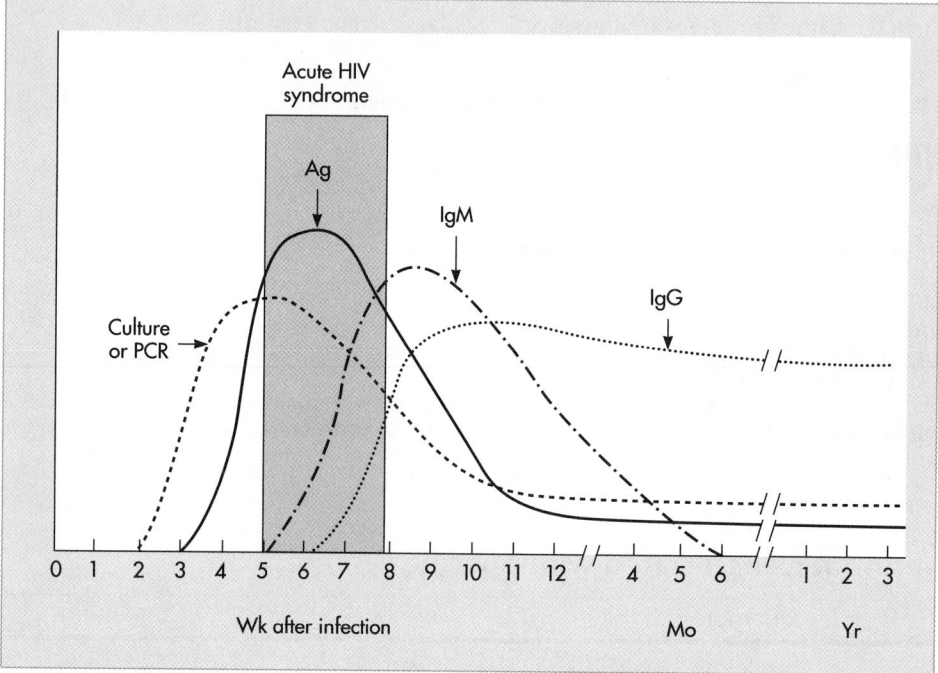

Fig. 4-10   Tests in HIV-1 infection. (From Ravel R: *Clinical laboratory medicine,* ed 6, St Louis, 1995, Mosby.)

TABLE 4-13   Indications for Plasma HIV RNA Testing*

CLINICAL INDICATION	INFORMATION	USE
Syndrome consistent with acute HIV infection	Establishes diagnosis when HIV antibody test is negative or indeterminate	Diagnosis†
Initial evaluation of newly diagnosed HIV infection	Baseline viral load "set point"	Decision to start or defer therapy
Every 3-4 mo in patients not on therapy	Changes in viral load	Decision to start therapy
4-8 wk after initiation of antiretroviral therapy	Initial assessment of drug efficacy	Decision to continue or change therapy
3-4 mo after start of therapy	Maximal effect of therapy	Decision to continue or change therapy
Every 3-4 mo in patients on therapy	Durability of antiretroviral effect	Decision to continue or change therapy
Clinical event or significant decline in CD4+ T cells	Association with changing or stable viral load	Decision to continue, initiate, or change therapy

From *MMWR,* vol 47, no RR-5, Apr 24, 1998.

*Acute illness (e.g., bacterial pneumonia, tuberculosis, HSV, PCP) and immunizations can cause increase in plasma HIV RNA for 2-4 wk; viral load testing should not be performed during this time. Plasma HIV RNA results should usually be verified with a repeat determination before starting or making changes in therapy. HIV RNA should be measured using the same laboratory and the same assay.

†Diagnosis of HIV infection determined by HIV RNA testing should be confirmed by standard methods (e.g., Western blot serology) performed 2-4 mo after the initial indeterminate or negative test.

■ **HUMAN IMMUNODEFICIENCY VIRUS TYPE 1** (HIV-1) **ANTIGEN** (p24), **QUALITATIVE** (p24 antigen)
Normal range: Negative
This test detects uncomplexed HIV-1 p24 antigen. The core protein p24 is the first detectable protein encoded by the group-specific antigen *(gag)* gene. This protein is a marker for viremia. This test should not be used in place of HIV-1 antibody testing as a screen for HIV-1 infection. HIV-1 p24 may be detectable in the first month of acute HIV-1 infection and generally falls to undetectable levels during the asymptomatic stage of HIV-1 infection. A negative result does not exclude the possibility of infection or exposure to HIV-1. It is recommended that a negative result be followed with repeat testing at least 8 weeks after the original test. This test is used primarily for screening of donated blood and plasma and as an aid for the prognosis of HIV-1 infection.

■ **HUMAN IMMUNODEFICIENCY VIRUS TYPE 1** (HIV-1) **VIRAL LOAD**
Normal range: HIV-1 RNA, quant. bDNA 3: less than 50 copies/ml or less than 1.7 log copies/ml
This test should be used only in individuals with documented HIV-1 infection for monitoring the progression of infection, response to antiretroviral therapy, and disease prognosis. It is not indicated for diagnosis of HIV infection.

■ **5-HYDROXYINDOLE-ACETIC ACID, URINE;** *see* URINE 5-HYDROXYINDOLE-ACETIC ACID

■ **IMMUNE COMPLEX ASSAY**
Normal: Negative
Detected in: Collagen-vascular disorders, glomerulonephritis, neoplastic diseases, malaria, primary biliary cirrhosis, chronic acute hepatitis, bacterial endocarditis, vasculitis

■ **IMMUNOGLOBULINS**
Normal range:
IgA: 50-350 mg/dl
IgD: <6 mg/dl
IgE: <25 μg/dl
IgG: 800-1500 mg/dl
IgM: 45-150 mg/dl
Elevated in:
IgA: lymphoproliferative disorders, Berger's nephropathy, chronic infections, autoimmune disorders, liver disease
IgE: allergic disorders, parasitic infections, immunologic disorders, IgE myeloma
IgG: chronic granulomatous infections, infectious diseases, inflammation, myeloma, liver disease
IgM: primary biliary cirrhosis, infectious diseases (brucellosis, malaria), Waldenström's macroglobulinemia, liver disease
Decreased in:
IgA: nephrotic syndrome, protein-losing enteropathy, congenital deficiency, lymphocytic leukemia, ataxia-telangiectasia, chronic sinopulmonary disease
IgE: hypogammaglobulinemia, neoplasma (breast, bronchial, cervical), ataxia-telangiectasia
IgG: congenital or acquired deficiency, lymphocytic leukemia, phenytoin, methylprednisolone, nephrotic syndrome, protein-losing enteropathy
IgM: congenital deficiency, lymphocytic leukemia, nephrotic syndrome

■ **INSULIN-LIKE GROWTH FACTOR-1** (IGF-1), **SERUM**
Normal range:
Age 16-24: 182-780 ng/mL
Age 25-39: 114-492 ng/mL
Age 40-54: 90-360 ng/mL
Age > 55: 71-290 ng/mL
Elevated in: Adolescence, acromegaly, pregnancy, precocious puberty, obesity
Decreased in: Malnutrition, delayed puberty, diabetes mellitus, hypopituitarism, cirrhosis, old age

■ **INTERNATIONAL NORMALIZED RATIO** (INR)
The INR is a comparative rating of prothrombin time (PT) ratios. The INR represents the observed PT ratio adjusted by the International Reference Thromboplastin. It provides a universal result indicative of what the patient's PT result would have been if measured using the primary World Health Organization International Reference reagent. For proper interpretation of INR values, the patient should be on stable anticoagulant therapy.
Recommended INR ranges:
Proximal deep vein thrombosis: 2-3
Pulmonary embolism: 2-3
Transient ischemic attacks: 2-3
Atrial fibrillation: 2-3
Mechanical prosthetic valves: 3-4.5
Recurrent venous thromboembolic disease: 3-4.5

■ **IRON-BINDING CAPACITY, TOTAL** (TIBC)
Normal range: 250-460 μg/dl
Elevated in: Iron deficiency anemia, pregnancy, polycythemia, hepatitis, weight loss

IV

Decreased in: Anemia of chronic disease, hemochromatosis, chronic liver disease, hemolytic anemias, malnutrition (protein depletion)

Table 4-14 describes TIBC and serum iron abnormalities.

TABLE 4-14 Serum Iron and Total Iron-Binding Capacity Patterns

SI↓	TIBC↓	Chronic diseases Uremia
SI↓	TIBC↑	Chronic iron deficiency anemia Pregnancy in third trimester
SI↑	TIBC↓	Hemachromatosis Iron therapy overload (TIBC may be normal) Hemolytic anemia; thalassemia; lead poisoning; megaloblastic anemia; aplastic, pyridoxine deficiency, or other sideroblastic anemias
SI↑	TIBC↑	Oral contraceptives Acute hepatitis (some report TIBC is low normal) Chronic hepatitis (some patients)
SI↑	TIBC NL	B_{12} or folate deficiency
SI↓	TIBC NL	Chronic iron deficiency (some patients) Acute infection, surgery, tissue damage
SI NL	TIBC↑	B_{12}/folate deficiency plus iron deficiency

From Ravel R: *Clinical laboratory medicine,* ed 6, St Louis, 1995, Mosby.
NL, Normal; *SI,* serum iron; *TIBC,* total iron-binding capacity.

■ LACTATE DEHYDROGENASE (LDH)
Normal range: 50-150 U/L
Elevated in: Infarction of myocardium, lung, kidney
Diseases of cardiopulmonary system, liver, collagen, central nervous system
Hemolytic anemias, megaloblastic anemias, transfusions, seizures, muscle trauma, muscular dystrophy, acute pancreatitis, hypotension, shock, infectious mononucleosis, inflammation, neoplasia, intestinal obstruction, hypothyroidism

■ LACTATE DEHYDROGENASE ISOENZYMES
Normal range:
LDH_1: 22% to 36% (cardiac, red blood cell)
LDH_2: 35% to 46% (cardiac, red blood cell)
LDH_3: 13% to 26% (pulmonary)
LDH_4: 3% to 10% (striated muscle, liver)
LDH_5: 2% to 9% (striated muscle, liver)
Normal ratios:
$LDH_1 < LDH_2$
$LDH_5 < LDH_4$
Abnormal values:
$LDH_1 > LDH_2$: myocardial infarction (can also be seen with hemolytic anemias, pernicious anemia, folate deficiency, renal infarct)
$LDH_5 > LDH_4$: liver disease (cirrhosis, hepatitis, hepatic congestion)

■ LAP SCORE; *see* LEUKOCYTE ALKALINE PHOSPHATASE

■ LDH; *see* LACTATE DEHYDROGENASE

■ LDL; *see* LOW-DENSITY LIPOPROTEIN CHOLESTEROL

■ *LEGIONELLA* TITER
Normal:
Negative
Positive in:
Legionnaire's disease (presumptive: ≥1:256 titer; definitive: fourfold titer increase to ≥1:128)

■ LEUKOCYTE ALKALINE PHOSPHATASE
Normal range: 13-100
Elevated in: Leukemoid reactions, neutrophilia secondary to infections (except in sickle cell crisis—no significant increase in LAP score), Hodgkin's disease, polycythemia vera, hairy cell leukemia, aplastic anemia, Down's syndrome, myelofibrosis
Decreased in: Acute and chronic granulocytic leukemia, thrombocytopenic purpura, paroxysmal nocturnal hemoglobinuria, hypophosphatemia, collagen disorders

■ **LEUKOCYTE COUNT;** *see* COMPLETE BLOOD COUNT

■ **LIPASE**
Normal range: 0-160 U/L
Elevated in: Acute pancreatitis, perforated peptic ulcer, carcinoma of pancreas (early stage), pancreatic duct obstruction, bowel infarction, intestinal obstruction

■ **LIPOPROTEIN CHOLESTEROL, HIGH-DENSITY;** *see* HIGH-DENSITY LIPOPROTEIN CHOLESTEROL

■ **LIPOPROTEIN CHOLESTEROL, LOW-DENSITY;** *see* LOW-DENSITY LIPOPROTEIN CHOLESTEROL

■ **LOW-DENSITY LIPOPROTEIN** (LDL) **CHOLESTEROL**
Normal range:
50-130 mg/dl
LDL cholesterol
<100   Optimal
100-129   Near or above optimal
130-159   Borderline high
160-189   High
≥190   Very high

■ **LUPUS ANTICOAGULANT;** *see* CIRCULATING ANTICOAGULANT

■ **LUTEINIZING HORMONE**
Normal range: 5-25 mIU/ml
Elevated in: Postmenopause, pituitary adenoma, primary gonadal dysfunction, polycystic ovary syndrome
Decreased in: Severe illness, anorexia nervosa, malnutrition, pituitary or hypothalamic impairment, severe stress

■ **LYME DISEASE ANTIBODY TITER**
Normal range: Negative
Positive result: Fig. 4-11 illustrates the usual serologic response in Lyme disease.
A serologic test is not necessary or helpful for several days after a tick bite, because it is only 40%-50% sensitive in this stage and a negative test does not rule out the diagnosis.

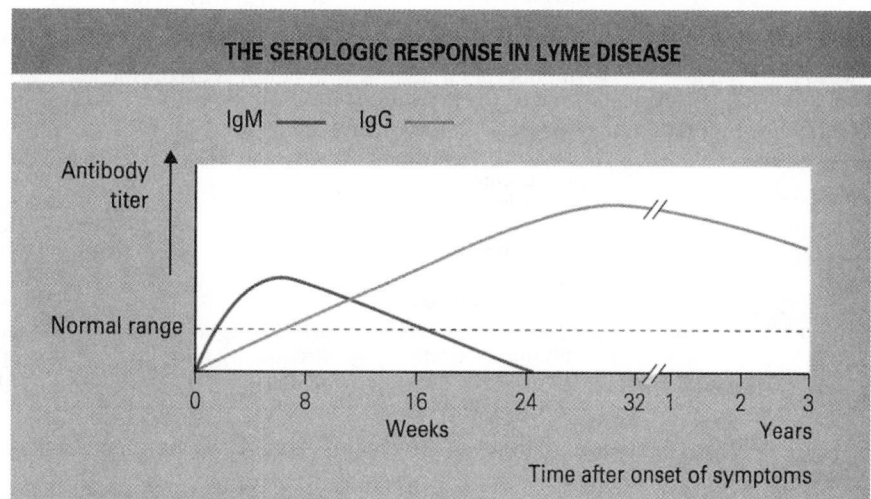

Fig. 4-11   HBV e antigen and antibody. (From Ravel R: *Clinical laboratory medicine,* ed 6, St Louis, 1995, Mosby.)

■ **LYMPHOCYTES**
Normal range:
15% to 40%:   Total lymphocyte count = 800-2600/mm³
              Total T lymphocyte = 800-2200/mm³
              CD4 lymphocytes = ≥400/mm³
              CD8 lymphocytes = 200-800/mm³
              Normal CD4/CD8 ratio is 2.0
Elevated in: Chronic infections, infectious mononucleosis and other viral infections, chronic lymphocytic leukemia, Hodgkin's disease, ulcerative colitis, hypoadrenalism, idiopathic thrombocytopenia

Decreased in: AIDS, bone marrow suppression from chemotherapeutic agents or chemotherapy, aplastic anemia, neoplasms, steroids, adrenocortical hyperfunction, neurologic disorders (multiple sclerosis, myasthenia gravis, Guillain-Barré syndrome)

CD4 lymphocytes are calculated as total white blood cells × % lymphocytes × % lymphocytes stained with CD4. They are decreased in AIDS and other immune dysfunction.

Table 4-15 describes various lymphocyte abnormalities in peripheral blood.

TABLE 4-15 Differential Diagnosis of Abnormal Lymphocytes in Peripheral Blood

LYMPHOCYTE TYPE	USUAL DISEASE ASSOCIATION	CYTOLOGIC FEATURES	LABORATORY FEATURES	CLINICAL FEATURES
Small lymphocyte	Chronic lymphocytic leukemia	B-cell surface markers with low concentration of surface immunoglobulin, CD5 antigen	Hypogammaglobulinemia in 50%; positive direct Coombs' test in 15%; on node biopsy, diffuse, well-differentiated lymphocytic infiltrate	Elderly adults; presentation runs gamut from asymptomatic with lymphocytosis only to bulky disease with adenopathy, splenomegaly, and "packed" bone marrow
Atypical lymphocyte	Infectious mononucleosis, other viral illnesses	Suppressor T-cell markers	Heterophil agglutinin; positive serology for Epstein-Barr virus, cytomegalovirus, toxoplasma, HBsAg	Pharyngitis, fever, adenopathy, rash, splenomegaly, palatal petechiae, jaundice
Plasmacytoid lymphocyte	Waldenström's macroglobulinemia	Cytoplasmic IgM, periodic acid–Schiff (PAS) positivity	IgM paraprotein, rouleaux, cryoglobulins	Adenopathy, splenomegaly, absence of bone lesions, hyperviscosity syndrome, cryopathic phenomena
Lymphoblast	Acute lymphoblastic leukemia (ALL)	Terminal transferase positivity, common ALL antigen, B- or T-precursor markers	Anemia, granulocytopenia, thrombocytopenia, hyperuricemia, diffuse bone marrow infiltration	Peak incidence in childhood, acute onset, bone pain frequent
Lymphosarcoma cell	Lymphocytic lymphoma	B-cell surface markers with high concentration of monoclonal surface immunoglobulin	Nodular or diffuse, poorly differentiated lymphocytic lymphoma on node biopsy, patchy, peritrabecular bone marrow involvement	Middle-aged to older adults, generalized adenopathy, constitutional symptoms
Sézary cell	Cutaneous lymphomas	T-lymphocyte surface markers	Skin biopsy is diagnostic	Exfoliative erythroderma, cutaneous plaques or tumors
Hairy cell	Hairy cell leukemia	B-lymphocyte markers, cytoplasmic projections, tartrate-resistant acid phosphatase, interleukin-2 receptors, CD11 antigen	Pancytopenia	Middle-aged males, moderate to marked splenomegaly without adenopathy
Prolymphocyte	Prolymphocytic leukemia	B-cell surface markers with high concentration of surface immunoglobulin, CD5 negative	Marked lymphocytosis (frequently >100 × 10^9/L)	Elderly adults, massive splenomegaly, minimum adenopathy, poor response to therapy

From Stein JH (ed): *Internal medicine*, ed 5, St Louis, 1998, Mosby.

■ MAGNESIUM (serum)
Normal range: 1.8-3.0 mg/dl
CAUSES OF HYPERMAGNESEMIA

I. Decreased renal excretion
 A. Renal failure—glomerular filtration rate less than 30 ml/min
 B. Hyperparathyroidism
 C. Hypothyroidism
 D. Addison's disease
 E. Lithium intoxication
 F. Familial hypocalciuric hypercalcemia
II. Other causes: usually in association with decrease in glomerular filtration rate
 A. Endogenous loads
  1. Diabetic ketoacidosis
  2. Severe tissue injury—burns

   B. Exogenous loads
     1. Gastrointestinal
       a. Magnesium-containing laxatives and antacids
       b. High-dose vitamin D analogs
     2. Parenteral: management of toxemia of pregnancy
CAUSES OF HYPOMAGNESEMIA
Alcoholic abuse
Diuretic use
Renal losses
Acute and chronic renal failure
Postobstructive diuresis
Acute tubular necrosis
Chronic glomerulonephritis
Chronic pyelonephritis
Interstitial nephropathy
Renal transplantation
Gastrointestinal losses
Chronic diarrhea
Nasogastric suctioning
Short bowel syndrome
Protein calorie malnutrition
Bowel fistula
Total parenteral nutrition
Acute pancreatitis
Endocrine
Diabetes mellitus
Hyperaldosteronism
Hyperthyroidism
Hyperparathyroidism
Acute intermittent porphyria
Pregnancy
Drugs
Aminoglycosides
Amphotericin
β-Agonists
Cisplatin
Cyclosporine
Diuretics
Foscarnet
Pentamidine
Theophylline
Congenital disorders
Familial hypomagnesemia
Maternal diabetes
Maternal hypothyroidism
Maternal hyperparathyroidism

■ **MEAN CORPUSCULAR VOLUME** (MCV)
Normal range: 76-100 μm^3 (76-100 fL)
See Tables 4-16 and 4-17, on the following page, for descriptions of MCV abnormalities.

■ **METANEPHRINES, URINE;** *see* URINE METANEPHRINES

■ **MONOCYTE COUNT**
Normal range: 2% to 8%
Elevated in: Viral diseases, parasites, infections, neoplasms, inflammatory bowel disease, monocytic leukemia, lymphomas, myeloma, sarcoidosis
Decreased in: Aplastic anemia, lymphocytic leukemia, glucocorticoid administration

■ **MYOGLOBIN, URINE;** *see* URINE MYOGLOBIN

■ **NEUTROPHIL COUNT**
Normal range: 50% to 70%
Subsets
Stabs (bands, early mature neutrophils): 2% to 6%
Segs (mature neutrophils): 60% to 70%

IV

TABLE 4-16 Some Causes of Increased Mean Corpuscular Volume (Macrocytosis)

CAUSES	% OF ALL MACROCYTOSIS PATIENTS*	% OF MACROCYTOSIS IN EACH DISEASE†
Common		
Folate or B_{12} deficiency	20-30 (5-50)‡	80-90 (4-100)
Chronic liver disease	15-20 (6-28)	25-30 (8-65)
Chronic alcoholism	10-12 (3-15)	60 (26-90)
Cytotoxic chemotherapy	10-15 (2-20)	30-40 (13-82)
Cardiorespiratory abnormality	8 (7-9.5)	?
Reticulocytosis	6-7 (0-15)	Depends on severity
Myelodysplastic syndromes	Frequent over age 40 yr	>60 in RAEB and RARS
Unexplained	25 (22.5-27)	—
Normal newborn		
Less Common	<4%	
Noncytotoxic drugs		
Zidovudine		
Phenytoin		30 (14-50)
Azathioprine		
Hypothyroidism		20-30 (8-55)
Chronic leukemia/myelofibrosis		
Radiotherapy for malignancy		
Chronic renal disease (occasional patients)		
Distance-runner macrocytosis (some persons)		
Down syndrome		
Artifactual (e.g., cold agglutinins)		

From Ravel R: *Clinical laboratory medicine*, ed 6, St Louis, 1995, Mosby.
RAEB, Refractory anemia with excessive blasts; *RARS*, refractory anemia with ring sideroblasts (formerly called IASA, or idiopathic acquired sideroblastic anemia).
*Percentage of all patients with macrocytosis.
†Percentage of patients with each condition listed who have macrocytosis.
‡Numbers in parentheses are literature range.

TABLE 4-17 Some Causes of Decreased Mean Corpuscular Volume (Microcytosis)

	COMMON	LESS COMMON
	Chronic iron deficiency	Some cases of polycythemia
	α- or β-thalassemia (minor)	Some cases of lead poisoning
	Anemia of chronic disease	Some cases of congenital spherocytosis
	Some cases of sideroblastic anemia	
		Certain abnormal Hbs (Hb E, Hb Lepore)

From Ravel R: *Clinical laboratory medicine*, ed 6, St Louis, 1995, Mosby.

Elevated in: Acute bacterial infections, acute myocardial infarction, stress, neoplasms, myelocytic leukemia
Decreased in: Viral infections, aplastic anemias, immunosuppressive drugs, radiation therapy to bone marrow, agranulocytosis, drugs (antibiotics, antithyroidals, clopidogrel), lymphocytic and monocytic leukemias
• Table 4-18 describes various drugs that can cause neutropenia.

■ **NOREPINEPHRINE**
Normal range: 0-600 pg/ml
Elevated in: Pheochromocytomas, neuroblastomas, stress, vigorous exercise, certain foods (bananas, chocolate, coffee, tea, vanilla)

■ **5′-NUCLEOTIDASE**
Normal range: 2-16 IU/L
Elevated in: Biliary obstruction, metastatic neoplasms to liver, primary biliary cirrhosis, renal failure, pancreatic carcinoma, chronic active hepatitis

■ **OSMOLALITY** (serum)
Normal range: 280-300 mOsm/kg
It can also be estimated by the following formula:
2([Na] + [K]) + glucose/18+ BυN/2.8

TABLE 4-18   Drugs That Cause Neutropenia

Antiarrhythmics
  Tocainide, procainamide, propranolol, quinidine

Antibiotics
  Chloramphenicol, penicillins, sulfonamides, p-aminosalicylic acid (PAS), rifampin, vancomycin, isoniazid, nitrofurantoin

Antimalarials
  Dapsone, quinine, pyrimethamine

Anticonvulsants
  Phenytoin, mephenytoin, trimethadione, ethosuximide, carbamazepine

Hypoglycemic agents
  Tolbutamide, chlorpropamide

Antihistamines
  Cimetidine, brompheniramine, tripelennamine

Antihypertensives
  Methyldopa, captopril

Antiinflammatory agents
  Aminopyrine, phenylbutazone, gold salts, ibuprofen, indomethacin

Antithyroid agents
  Propylthiouracil, methimazole, thiouracil

Diuretics
  Acetazolamide, hydrochlorothiazide, chlorthalidone

Phenothiazines
  Chlorpromazine, promazine, prochlorperazine

Immunosuppressive agents
  Antimetabolites

Cytotoxic agents
  Alkylating agents, antimetabolites, anthracyclines, *Vinca* alkaloids, cisplatin, hydroxyurea, dactinomycin

Other agents
  Recombinant interferons, allopurinol, ethanol, levamisole, penicillamine, zidovudine, streptokinase, carbamazepine, clopidogrel, ticlopidine

Modified from Goldman L, Ausiello D (eds): *Cecil textbook of medicine,* ed 22, Philadelphia, 2004, WB Saunders.

Elevated in: Dehydration, hypernatremia, diabetes insipidus, uremia, hyperglycemia, mannitol therapy, ingestion of toxins (ethylene glycol, methanol, ethanol), hypercalcemia, diuretics
Decreased in: Syndrome of inappropriate diuretic hormone secretion, hyponatremia, overhydration, Addison's disease, hypothyroidism

■ **OSMOLALITY, URINE;** *see* URINE OSMOLALITY

■ **PARACENTESIS FLUID**
  Testing and evaluation of results:
  1. Process the fluid as follows:
     a. Tube 1: LDH, glucose, albumin.
     b. Tube 2: protein, specific gravity.
     c. Tube 3: cell count and differential.
     d. Tube 4: save until further notice.
  2. Draw serum LDH, protein, albumin.
  3. Gram stain, AFB stain, bacterial and fungal cultures, amylase, and triglycerides should be ordered only when clearly indicated; bedside inoculation of blood-culture bottles with ascitic fluid improves sensitivity in detecting bacterial growth.
  4. If malignant ascites is suspected, consider a carcinoembryonic antigen level on the paracentesis fluid and cytologic evaluation.
  5. In suspected spontaneous bacterial peritonitis (SBP) the incidence of positive cultures can be increased by injecting 10 to 20 ml of ascitic fluid into blood culture bottles.
  6. Peritoneal effusion can be subdivided as exudative or transudative based on its characteristics (Section III, Fig 3-21).
  7. The serum-ascites albumin gradient (serum albumin level-ascitic fluid albumin level) correlates directly with portal pressure and can also be used to classify ascite. Patients with gradients ≥1.1 g/dl have portal hypertension, and those with gradients <1.1 g/dl do not; the accuracy of this method is >95%.
  8. For the differential diagnosis of ascites refer to Section III, Fig. 3-21, on page 1004.

IV

9. An ascitic fluid polymorphonuclear leukocyte count >500/μl is suggestive of SBP.
10. A blood-ascitic fluid albumin gradient.

■ **PARTIAL THROMBOPLASTIN TIME** (PTT), **ACTIVATED PARTIAL THROMBOPLASTIN TIME** (APTT)
Normal range: 25-41 sec
Elevated in: Heparin therapy, coagulation factor deficiency (I, II, V, VIII, IX, X, XI, XII), liver disease, vitamin K deficiency, disseminated intravascular coagulation, circulating anticoagulant, warfarin therapy, specific factor inhibition (PCN reaction, rheumatoid arthritis), thrombolytic therapy, nephrotic syndrome
NOTE: Useful to evaluate the intrinsic coagulation system.

■ **PH, BLOOD**
Normal values:
Arterial: 7.35-7.45
Venous: 7.32-7.42
For abnormal values refer to "Arterial Blood Gases."

■ **PH, URINE;** *see* URINE PH

■ **PHENOBARBITAL**
Normal therapeutic range: 15-30 mcg/mL for epilepsy control

■ **PHENYTOIN** (dilantin)
Normal therapeutic range: 10-20 mcg/mL

■ **PHOSPHATASE, ACID;** *see* ACID PHOSPHATASE

■ **PHOSPHATASE, ALKALINE;** *see* ALKALINE PHOSPHATASE

■ **PHOSPHATE** (serum)
Normal range: 2.5-5 mg/dl
DECREASED
Parenteral hyperalimentation
Diabetic acidosis
Alcohol withdrawal
Severe metabolic or respiratory alkalosis
Antacids that bind phosphorus
Malnutrition with refeeding using low-phosphorus nutrients
Renal tubule failure to reabsorb phosphate (Fanconi's syndrome; congenital disorder; vitamin D deficiency)
Glucose administration
Nasogastric suction
Malabsorption
Gram-negative sepsis
Primary hyperthyroidism
Chlorothiazide diuretics
Therapy of acute severe asthma
Acute respiratory failure with mechanical ventilation
INCREASED
Renal failure
Severe muscle injury
Phosphate-containing antacids
Hypoparathyroidism
Tumor lysis syndrome

■ **PLATELET COUNT**
Normal range: 130-400 × 10³/mm³
Elevated in:
REACTIVE THROMBOCYTOSIS
Infections or inflammatory states—vasculitis, allergic reactions, etc.
Surgery and tissue damage—myocardial infarction, pancreatitis, etc.
Postsplenectomy state
Malignancy—solid tumors, lymphoma
Iron deficiency anemia, hemolytic anemia, acute blood loss
Uncertain etiology
Rebound effect after chemotherapy or immune thrombocytopenia
Renal disorders—renal failure, nephrotic syndrome
MYELOPROLIFERATIVE DISORDERS
Chronic myeloid leukemia

Primary thrombocythemia
Polycythemia vera
Idiopathic myelofibrosis
Decreased:
A. Increased destruction
   1. Immunologic
      a. Drugs: quinine, quinidine, digitalis, procainamide, thiazide diuretics, sulfonamides, phenytoin, aspirin, penicillin, heparin, gold, meprobamate, sulfa drugs, phenylbutazone, NSAIDs, methyldopa, cimetidine, furosemide, INH, cephalosporins, chlorpropamide, organic arsenicals, chloroquine
      b. Idiopathic thrombocytopenic purpura
      c. Transfusion reaction: transfusion of platelets with platelet antigen HPA-1a (PL^{A1}) in recipients without PL^{A1}
      d. Fetal/maternal incompatibility
      e. Vasculitis (e.g., systemic lupus erythematosus)
      f. Autoimmune hemolytic anemia
      g. Lymphoreticular disorders (e.g., chronic lymphocytic leukemia)
   2. Nonimmunologic
      a. Prosthetic heart valves
      b. Thrombotic thrombocytopenic purpura
      c. Sepsis
      d. Disseminated intravascular coagulation
      e. Hemolytic-uremic syndrome
      f. Giant cavernous hemangioma
B. Decreased production
   1. Abnormal marrow
      a. Marrow infiltration (e.g., leukemia, lymphoma, fibrosis)
      b. Marrow suppression (e.g., chemotherapy, alcohol, radiation)
   2. Hereditary disorders
      a. Wiskott-Aldrich syndrome: X-linked disorder characterized by thrombocytopenia, eczema, and repeated infections
      b. May-Hegglin anomaly: increased megakaryocytes but ineffective thrombopoiesis
   3. Vitamin deficiencies (e.g., vitamin B$_{12}$, folic acid)
C. Splenic sequestration, hypersplenism
D. Dilutional, secondary to massive transfusion

■ **POTASSIUM** (serum)
Normal range: 3.5-5 mEq/L
CAUSES OF HYPERKALEMIA
I. Pseudohyperkalemia
   A. Hemolysis of sample
   B. Thrombocytosis
   C. Leukocytosis
   D. Laboratory error
II. Increased potassium intake and absorption
   A. Potassium supplements (oral and parenteral)
   B. Dietary—salt substitutes
   C. Stored blood
   D. Potassium-containing medications
III. Impaired renal excretion
   A. Acute renal failure
   B. Chronic renal failure
   C. Tubular defect in potassium secretion
      1. Renal allograft
      2. Analgesic nephropathy
      3. Sickle cell disease
      4. Obstructive uropathy
      5. Interstitial nephritis
      6. Chronic pyelonephritis
      7. Potassium-sparing diuretics
      8. Miscellaneous (lead, systemic lupus erythematosus, pseudohypoaldosteronism)
   D. Hypoaldosteronism
      1. Primary (Addison's disease)
      2. Secondary
         a. Hyporeninemic hypoaldosteronism (type IV RTA)
         b. Congenital adrenal hyperplasia
         c. Drug-induced
            (1) Nonsteroidal antiinflammatory medications
            (2) ACE inhibitors
            (3) Heparin
            (4) Cyclosporine

IV

IV. Transcellular shifts
    A. Acidosis
    B. Hypertonicity
    C. Insulin deficiency
    D. Drugs
        1. β-blockers
        2. Digitalis toxicity
        3. Succinylcholine
    E. Exercise
    F. Hyperkalemic periodic paralysis
V. Cellular injury
    A. Rhabdomyolysis
    B. Severe intravascular hemolysis
    C. Acute tumor lysis syndrome
    D. Burns and crush injuries

CAUSES OF HYPOKALEMIA

I. Decreased intake
    A. Decreased dietary potassium
    B. Impaired absorption of potassium
    C. Clay ingestion
    D. Kayexalate
II. Increased loss
    A. Renal
        1. Hyperaldosteronism
            a. Primary
                1. Conn's syndrome
                2. Adrenal hyperplasia
            b. Secondary
                1. Congestive heart failure
                2. Cirrhosis
                3. Nephrotic syndrome
                4. Dehydration
            c. Bartter's syndrome
        2. Glycyrrhizic acid (licorice, chewing tobacco)
        3. Excessive adrenal corticosteroids
            a. Cushing's syndrome
            b. Steroid therapy
            c. Adrenogenital syndrome
        4. Renal tubular defects
            a. Renal tubular acidosis
            b. Obstructive uropathy
            c. Salt-wasting nephropathy
        5. Drugs
            a. Diuretics
            b. Aminoglycosides
            c. Mannitol
            d. Amphotericin
            e. Cisplatin
            f. Carbenicillin
    B. Gastrointestinal
        1. Vomiting
        2. Nasogastric suction
        3. Diarrhea
        4. Malabsorption
        5. Ileostomy
        6. Villous adenoma
        7. Laxative abuse
    C. Increased losses from the skin
        1. Excessive sweating
        2. Burns
III. Transcellular shifts
    A. Alkalosis
        1. Vomiting
        2. Diuretics
        3. Hyperventilation
        4. Bicarbonate therapy
    B. Insulin
        1. Exogenous
        2. Endogenous response to glucose
    C. β2-Agonists (albuterol, terbutaline, epinephrine)

    D. Hypokalemia periodic paralysis
       1. Familial
       2. Thyrotoxic
  IV. Miscellaneous
    A. Anabolic state
    B. Intravenous hyperalimentation
    C. Treatment of megaloblastic anemia
    D. Acute mountain sickness

■ **POTASSIUM, URINE;** *see* URINE POTASSIUM

■ **PROCAINAMIDE**
Normal therapeutic range: 4-10 mcg/mL

■ **PROLACTIN**
Normal range: <20 ng/ml
Elevated in: Prolactinomas (level >200 highly suggestive), drugs (phenothiazines, cimetidine, tricyclic antidepressants, metoclopramide, estrogens, antihypertensives [methyldopa], verapamil, haloperidol), postpartum, stress, hypoglycemia, hypothyroidism

■ **PROSTATE-SPECIFIC ANTIGEN** (PSA)
Normal range: 0-4 ng/ml
Table 4-19 describes age-specific reference ranges for PSA.
Elevated in: Benign prostatic hypertrophy, carcinoma of prostate, postrectal examination, prostate trauma
Factors affecting serum PSA are described in Table 4-20.
NOTE: Measurement of free PSA is useful to assess the probability of prostate cancer in patients with normal digital rectal examination and total PSA between 4 and 10 ng/ml. In these patients, the global risk of prostate cancer is 25%; however, if the free PSA is >25%, the risk of prostate cancer decreases to 8%, whereas if the free PSA is <10%, the risk of cancer increases to 56%. Free PSA is also useful to evaluate the aggressiveness of prostate cancer. A low free PSA percentage generally indicates a high-grade cancer, whereas a high free PSA percentage is generally associated with a slower growing tumor.

TABLE 4-19 Age-Specific Reference Ranges for PSA

AGE (YR)	SERUM PSA (NG/ML)		
	WHITES	JAPANESE	AFRICAN AMERICAN
40-49	0-2.5	0-2.0	0-2.0
50-59	0-3.5	0-3.0	0-4.0
60-69	0-4.5	0-4.0	0-4.5
70-79	0-6.5	0-5.0	0-5.5

From Nseyo UO (ed): *Urology for primary care physicians,* Philadelphia, 1999, WB Saunders.
PSA, Prostate-specific antigen.

TABLE 4-20 Factors Affecting Serum Prostate-Specific Antigen (PSA)

FACTORS AFFECTING SERUM PSA	DURATION OF EFFECT
Prostate cell number	Not applicable
Prostate size	Not applicable
Recent ejaculation	6-48 hours
Prostate manipulation	
Vigorous massage	1 week
Cystoscopy	1 week
Prostate biopsy	4-6 weeks
Prostatitis	
Acute	3-6 months
Chronic	Unknown
Prostate cancer	Not applicable
Drugs: finasteride (Proscar)*	3-6 months

From Nseyo UO (ed): *Urology for primary care physicians,* Philadelphia, 1999, WB Saunders.
*Lowers PSA for as long as patient is on the medication.

Decreased in: Finasteride therapy, dutasteride therapy, saw palmetto use, bedrest, antiandrogens

■ **PROTEIN** (serum)
Normal range: 6-8 g/dl
Elevated in: Dehydration, multiple myeloma, Waldenström's macroglobulinemia, sarcoidosis, collagen-vascular diseases
Decreased in: Malnutrition, low-protein diet, overhydration, malabsorption, pregnancy, severe burns, neoplasms, chronic diseases, cirrhosis, nephrosis

■ **PROTEIN ELECTROPHORESIS** (serum)
Normal range: Albumin: 60% to 75%
α-1: 1.7% to 5%
α-2: 6.7% to 12.5%
β: 8.3% to 16.3%
γ: 10.7% to 20%

IV

Albumin: 3.6-5.2 g/dl
α-1: 0.1-0.4 g/dl
α-2: 0.4-1 g/dl
β: 0.5-1.2 g/dl
γ: 0.6-1.6 g/dl
Elevated in: Albumin: dehydration
α-1: neoplastic diseases, inflammation
α-2: neoplasms, inflammation, infection, nephrotic syndrome
β: hypothyroidism, biliary cirrhosis, diabetes mellitus
γ: *see* IMMUNOGLOBULINS
Decreased in: Albumin: malnutrition, chronic liver disease, malabsorption, nephrotic syndrome,
burns, systemic lupus erythematosus
α-1: emphysema (α-1 antitrypsin deficiency), nephrosis
α-2: hemolytic anemias (decreased haptoglobin), severe hepatocellular damage
β: hypocholesterolemia, nephrosis
γ: *see* IMMUNOGLOBULINS
Fig. 4-12 describes serum protein electrophoretic patterns.

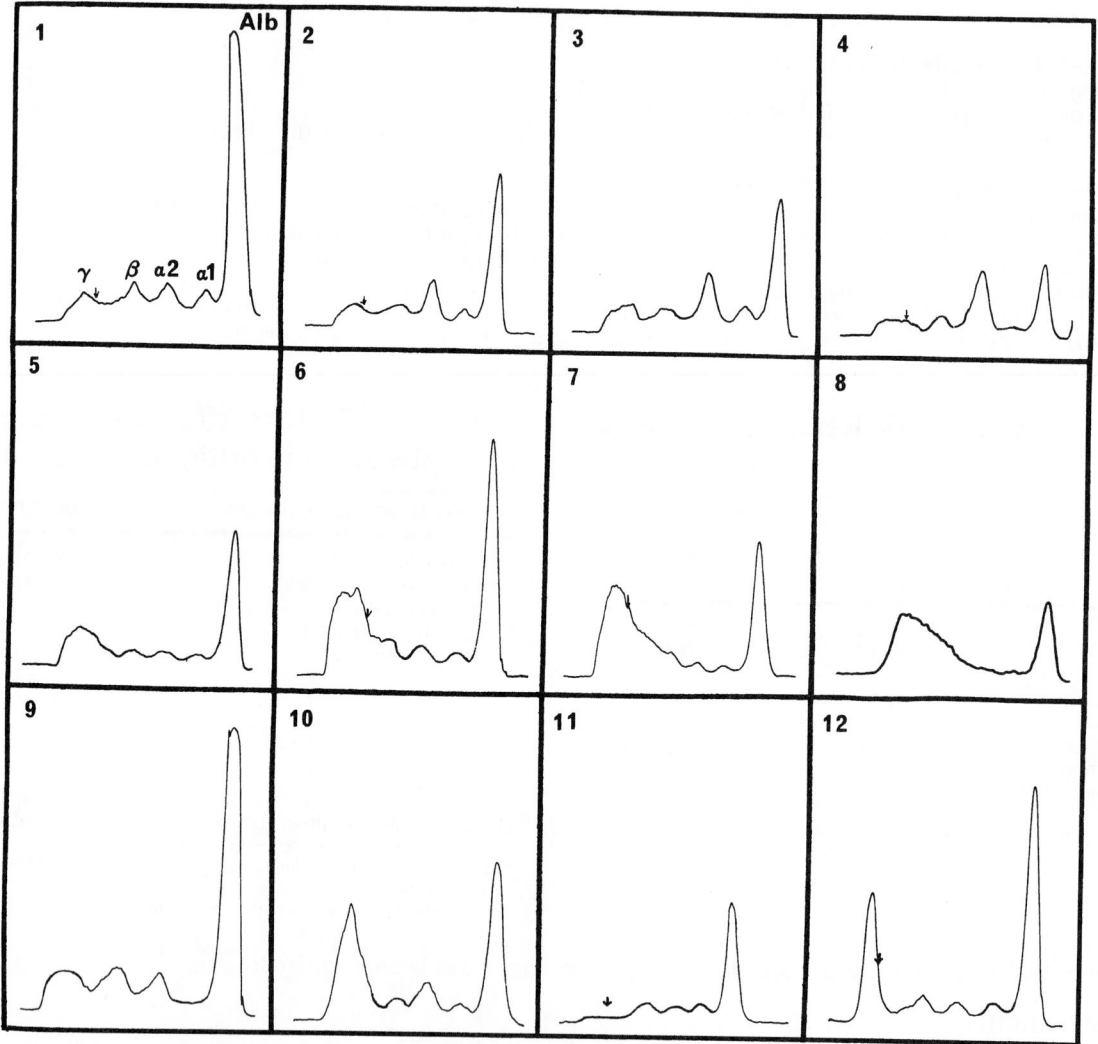

Fig. 4-12   Typical serum protein electrophoretic patterns. *1,* Normal (*arrow* near γ region indicates serum application point). *2,* Acute reaction pattern. *3,* Acute reaction or nephrotic syndrome. *4,* Nephrotic syndrome. *5,* Chronic inflammation, cirrhosis, granulomatous diseases, rheumatoid-collagen group. *6,* Same as *5,* but γ elevation is more pronounced. There is also partial (but not complete) β-γ fusion. *7,* Suggestive of cirrhosis but could be found in the granulomatous diseases or the rheumatoid-collagen group. *8,* Characteristic pattern of cirrhosis. *9,* α-1 Antitrypsin deficiency with mild γ elevation suggesting concurrent chronic disease. *10,* Same as *5,* but the γ elevation is marked. The configuration of the γ peak superficially mimics that of myeloma, but is more broad-based. There are superimposed acute reaction changes. *11,* Hypogammaglobulinemia or light-chain myeloma. *12,* Myeloma, Waldenström's macroglobulinemia, idiopathic or secondary monoclonal gammopathy. (From Ravel R: *Clinical laboratory medicine,* ed 6, St Louis, 1995, Mosby.)

■ **PROTHROMBIN TIME** (PT)
Normal range: 10-12 sec
Elevated in: Liver disease, oral anticoagulants (warfarin), heparin, factor deficiency (I, II, V, VII, X), disseminated intravascular coagulation, vitamin K deficiency, afibrinogenemia, dysfibrinogenemia, drugs (salicylate, chloral hydrate, diphenylhydantoin, estrogens, antacids, phenylbutazone, quinidine, antibiotics, allopurinol, anabolic steroids)
Decreased in: Vitamin K supplementation, thrombophlebitis, drugs (glutethimide, estrogens, griseofulvin, diphenhydramine)

■ **PROTOPORPHYRIN** (free erythrocyte)
Normal range: 16-36 µg/dl of red blood cells
Elevated in: Iron deficiency, lead poisoning, sideroblastic anemias, anemia of chronic disease, hemolytic anemias, erythropoietic protoporphyria

■ **PSA;** *see* PROSTATE-SPECIFIC ANTIGEN

■ **PT;** *see* PROTHROMBIN TIME

■ **PTT;** *see* PARTIAL THROMBOPLASTIN TIME

■ **RDW;** *see* RED BLOOD CELL DISTRIBUTION WIDTH

■ **RED BLOOD CELL** (RBC) **COUNT**
Normal range: Male: $4.3-5.9 \times 10^6/mm^3$ Female: $3.5-5 \times 10^6/mm^3$
Elevated in: Polycythemia vera, smokers, high altitude, cardiovascular disease, renal cell carcinoma and other erythropoietin-producing neoplasms, stress, hemoconcentration/dehydration
Decreased in: Anemias, hemolysis, chronic renal failure, hemorrhage, failure of marrow production

■ **RED BLOOD CELL DISTRIBUTION WIDTH** (RDW)
Measures variability of red cell size (anisocytosis)
Normal range: 11.5-14.5
Normal RDW and:
ELEVATED MEAN CORPUSCULAR VOLUME (MCV): aplastic anemia, preleukemia
NORMAL MCV: normal, anemia of chronic disease, acute blood loss or hemolysis, chronic lymphocytic leukemia (CLL), chronic myelocytic leukemia, nonanemic enzymopathy or hemoglobinopathy
DECREASED MCV: anemia of chronic disease, heterozygous thalassemia
Elevated RDW and:
ELEVATED MCV: vitamin B_{12} deficiency, folate deficiency, immune hemolytic anemia, cold agglutinins, CLL with high count, liver disease
NORMAL MCV: early iron deficiency, early vitamin B_{12} deficiency, early folate deficiency, anemic globinopathy
DECREASED MCV: iron deficiency, red blood cell fragmentation, HbH disease, thalassemia intermedia

■ **RED BLOOD CELL FOLATE;** *see* FOLATE, RED BLOOD CELL

■ **RED BLOOD CELL MASS** (volume)
Normal range:
Male: 20-36 ml/kg of body weight ($1.15-1.21 L/m^2$ body surface area)
Female: 19-31 ml/kg of body weight ($0.95-1.00 L/m^2$ body surface area)
Elevated in: Polycythemia vera, hypoxia (smokers, high altitude, cardiovascular disease), hemoglobinopathies with high oxygen affinity, erythropoietin-producing tumors (renal cell carcinoma)
Decreased in: Hemorrhage, chronic disease, failure of marrow production, anemias, hemolysis

■ **RED BLOOD CELL MORPHOLOGY;** *see* Fig. 4-13

■ **RENIN (SERUM)**
Elevated in: Drugs (thiazides, estrogen, minoxidil), chronic renal failure, Bartter's syndrome, pregnancy (normal), pheochromocytoma, renal hypertension, reduced plasma volume, secondary aldosteronism
Decreased in: Adrenocortical hypertension, increased plasma volume, primary aldosteronism, drugs (propranolol, reserpine, clonidine)
Table 4-21 describes typical renin-aldosterone patterns in various conditions.

IV

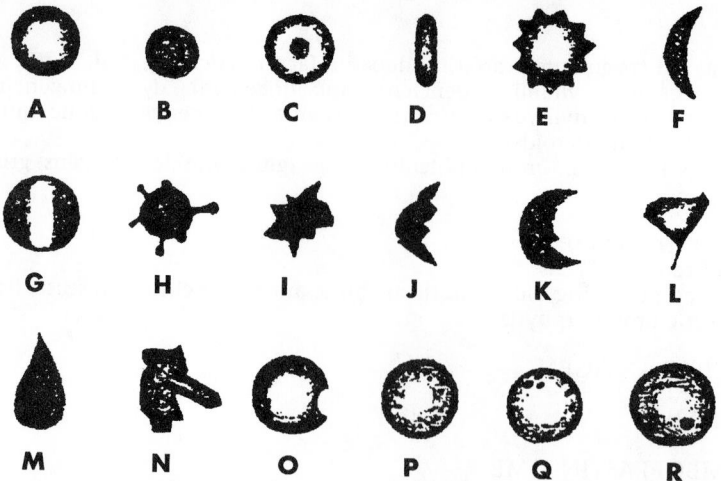

Fig. 4-13   Abnormal red blood cells (RBCs). A, Normal RBC. **B,** Spherocyte. **C,** Target cell. **D,** Elliptocyte. **E,** Echinocyte. **F,** Sickle cell. **G,** Stomatocyte. **H,** Acanthocyte. **I** to **L,** Schistocytes. **M,** Teardrop RBC. **N,** Distorted RBC with Hb C crystal protruding. **O,** Degmacyte. **P,** Basophilic stippling. **Q,** Pappenheimer bodies. **R,** Howell-Jolly body. (From Ravel R: *Clinical laboratory medicine,* ed 6, St Louis, 1995, Mosby.)

TABLE 4-21   Typical Renin-Aldosterone Patterns in Various Conditions

	PLASMA RENIN	ALDOSTERONE
Primary aldosteronism	Low	High
"Low-renin" essential hypertension	Low	Normal
Cushing's syndrome	Low	Low-normal
Licorice ingestion syndrome	Low	Low
High-salt diet	Low	Low
Oral contraceptives	High	Normal
Cirrhosis	High	High
Malignant hypertension	High	High
Unilateral renal disease	High	High
"High-renin" essential hypertension	High	High
Pregnancy	High	High
Diuretic overuse	High	High
Juxtaglomerular tumor (Bartter's syndrome)	High	High
Low-salt diet	High	High
Addison's disease	High	Low
Hypokalemia	High	Low

From Ravel R: *Clinical laboratory medicine,* ed 6, St Louis, 1995, Mosby.

■ RETICULOCYTE COUNT
Normal range: 0.5% to 1.5%
Elevated in: Hemolytic anemia (sickle cell crisis, thalassemia major, autoimmune hemolysis), hemorrhage, postanemia therapy (folic acid, ferrous sulfate, vitamin B_{12}), chronic renal failure
Decreased in: Aplastic anemia, marrow suppression (sepsis, chemotherapeutic agents, radiation), hepatic cirrhosis, blood transfusion, anemias of disordered maturation (iron deficiency anemia, megaloblastic anemia, sideroblastic anemia, anemia of chronic disease)

■ RHEUMATOID FACTOR
Normal: Negative
Present in titer *>1:20*
RHEUMATIC DISEASES
Rheumatoid arthritis
Sjögren's syndrome
Systemic lupus erythematosus
Polymyositis/dermatomyositis
Mixed connective tissue disease
Scleroderma

INFECTIOUS DISEASES
Subacute bacterial endocarditis
Tuberculosis
Infectious mononucleosis
Hepatitis
Syphilis
Leprosy
Influenza
MALIGNANCIES
Lymphoma
Multiple myeloma
Waldenström's macroglobulinemia
Postradiation or postchemotherapy
MISCELLANEOUS
Normal adults, especially the elderly
Sarcoidosis
Chronic pulmonary disease (interstitial fibrosis)
Chronic liver disease (chronic active hepatitis, cirrhosis)
Mixed essential cryoglobulinemia
Hypergammaglobulinemic purpura

■ **RNP;** *see* EXTRACTABLE NUCLEAR ANTIGEN

■ **SEDIMENTATION RATE;** *see* ERYTHROCYTE SEDIMENTATION RATE

■ **SEMEN ANALYSIS**
  • Table 4-22 describes semen analysis reference ranges.

TABLE 4-22   Semen Analysis Reference Ranges

Color	Grayish white
pH	7.3-7.8 (literature range, 7.0-7.8)
Volume	2.0-5.0 ml (literature range, 1.5-6.0 ml)
Sperm count	20-250 million/ml (literature range for upper limit varies from 100-250 million/ml)
Motility	>60% motile <3 hours after specimen is obtained (literature range, >40% to >70%)
% Normal sperm	>60% (literature range, >60% to >70%)
Viscosity	Can be poured from a pipet in droplets rather than a thick strand

From Ravel R (ed): *Clinical laboratory medicine,* ed 6, St Louis, 1995, Mosby.

■ **SGOT;** *see* ASPARTATE AMINOTRANSFERASE

■ **SGPT;** *see* ALANINE AMINOTRANSFERASE

■ **SMOOTH MUSCLE ANTIBODY**
Normal: Negative
Present in: Chronic acute hepatitis (≥1:80), primary biliary cirrhosis (≤1:80), infectious mononucleosis

■ **SODIUM** (serum)
Normal range: 135-147 mEq/L
HYPONATREMIA
A. Sodium and water depletion (deficit hyponatremia)
  1. Loss of gastrointestinal secretions with replacement of fluid but not electrolytes
     a. Vomiting
     b. Diarrhea
     c. Tube drainage
  2. Loss from skin with replacement of fluids but not electrolytes
     a. Excessive sweating
     b. Extensive burns
  3. Loss from kidney
     a. Diuretics
     b. Chronic renal insufficiency (uremia) with acidosis
  4. Metabolic loss
     a. Starvation with acidosis
     b. Diabetic acidosis
  5. Endocrine loss
     a. Addison's disease
     b. Sudden withdrawal of long-term steroid therapy

IV

6. Iatrogenic loss from serous cavities
   a. Paracentesis or thoracentesis
B. Excessive water (dilution hyponatremia)
   1. Excessive water administration
   2. Congestive heart failure
   3. Cirrhosis
   4. Nephrotic syndrome
   5. Hypoalbuminemia (severe)
   6. Acute renal failure with oliguria
C. Inappropriate antidiuretic hormone (IADH) syndrome
D. Intracellular loss (reset osmostat syndrome)
E. False hyponatremia (actually a dilutional effect)
   1. Marked hypertriglyceridemia*
   2. Marked hyperproteinemia*
   3. Severe hyperglycemia

HYPERNATREMIA

Dehydration is the most frequent overall clinical finding in hypernatremia.
1. Deficient water intake (either orally or intravenously)
2. Excess kidney water output (diabetes insipidus, osmotic diuresis)
3. Excess skin water output (excess sweating, loss from burns)
4. Excess gastrointestinal tract output (severe protracted vomiting or diarrhea without fluid therapy)
5. Accidental sodium overdose
6. High-protein tube feedings

■ **STREPTOZYME;** *see* ANTI-STREPTOLYSIN O TITER

■ **SUCROSE HEMOLYSIS TEST** (sugar water test)
Normal: Absence of hemolysis
Positive in: Paroxysmal nocturnal hemoglobinuria
False positive: autoimmune hemolytic anemia, megaloblastic anemias
False negative: may occur with use of heparin or EDTA

■ **SUDAN III STAIN** (qualitative screening for fecal fat)
Normal: Negative. Test should be preceded by diet containing 100-150 g of dietary fat/day for 1 week, avoidance of high-fiber diet, and avoidance of suppositories or oily material before specimen collection.
Positive in: Steatorrhea, use of castor oil or mineral oil droplets

■ **SYNOVIAL FLUID ANALYSIS**
Table 4-23 describes the classification and interpretation of synovial fluid analysis.

TABLE 4-23 Classification and Interpretation of Synovial Fluid Analysis

GROUP	DISEASES	APPEARANCE	VISCOSITY	MUCIN CLOT	WBC/MM³	%PMN	GLUCOSE (MG/DL) (BLOOD–SYNOVIAL FLUID)	PROTEIN (G/DL)
Normal	—	Clear	↑	Firm	<200	<25	<10	<2.5
I (noninflam-matory)	Osteoarthritis, aseptic necrosis, traumatic arthritis, erythema nodosum, osteochondritis dissecans	Clear, yellow (may be xanthochromic if traumatic arthritis)	↑	Firm	↑ Up to 10,000	<25	<10	<2.5
II (inflammatory)	Crystal-induced arthritis, rheumatoid arthritis, Reiter's syndrome, collagen-vascular disease, psoriatic arthritis, serum sickness, rheumatic fever	Clear, yellow, turbid	↓	Friable	↑↑ Up to 100,000	40-90	<40	>2.5
III (septic)	Bacterial (staphylococcal, gonococcal, tuberculosis)	Turbid	↓/↑	Friable	↑↑↑ Up to 5 million	40-100	20-100	>2.5

↑, Elevated; ↑↑, markedly high; ↓, decreased; *PMN*, polymorphonuclear leukocytes. Note that there is considerable overlap in the numbers listed above.

■ **T_3 (triiodothyronine)**
Normal range: 75-220 ng/dl
Abnormal values:
A. Elevated in hyperthyroidism (usually earlier and to a greater extent than serum T_4).
B. Useful in diagnosing:
  1. T_3 hyperthyroidism (thyrotoxicosis): increased T_3, normal FTI.
  2. Toxic nodular goiter: increased T_3, normal or increased T_4.
  3. Iodine deficiency: normal T_3, possibly decreased T_4.
  4. Thyroid replacement therapy with liothyronine (Cytomel): normal T_4, increased T_3 if patient is symptomatically hyperthyroid.
Not ordered routinely but indicated when hyperthyroidism is suspected and serum free T_4 or FTI inconclusive.

■ **T_3 (triiodothyronine)**; *see* Table 4-24 for T_3 abnormalities

TABLE 4-24 Findings in Thyroid Function Tests in Various Clinical Conditions

CONDITION	T_4	FT_4I	T_3	FT_3I	TSH	TSI	TRH STIMULATION
Hyperthyroidism							
Graves' disease	↑	↑	↑	↑	↓	+	↓
Toxic nodular goiter	↑	↑	↑	↑	↓	−	↓
Pituitary TSH-secreting tumors	↑	↑	↑	↑	↑	−	↓
T_3 thyrotoxicosis	N	N	↑	↑	↓	+, −	↓
T_4 thyrotoxicosis	↑	↑	N	N	↓	+, −	↓
Hypothyroidism							
Primary	↓	↓	↓	↓	↑	+, −	↑
Secondary	↓	↓	↓	↓	↓, N	−	↓
Tertiary	↓	↓	↓	↓	↓, N	−	N
Peripheral unresponsiveness	↑, N	↑, N	↑, N	↑	↑, N	−	N, ↑

From Tilton RC, Barrows A: *Clinical laboratory medicine*, St Louis, 1992, Mosby.
N, Normal; ↑, increased; ↓, decreased; +, − variable.

■ **T_3 RESIN UPTAKE (T_3RU)**
Normal range:
25% to 35%
Abnormal values:
Increased in hyperthyroidism. T_3 resin uptake (T_3RU or RT_3U) measures the percentage of free T_4 (not bound to protein); it does not measure serum T_3 concentration; T_3RU and other tests that reflect thyroid hormone binding to plasma protein are also known as *thyroid hormone-binding ratios* (THBR).

■ **T_4, SERUM T_4, AND FREE** (free thyroxine)
Normal range:
0.8-2.8 ng/dl
Abnormal values:
Serum thyroxine (T_4)
Elevated in:
1. Graves' disease
2. Toxic multinodular goiter
3. Toxic adenoma
4. Iatrogenic and factitious
5. Transient hyperthyroidism.
  a. Subacute thyroiditis
  b. Hashimoto's thyroiditis
  c. Silent thyroiditis
6. Rare causes: hypersecretion of TSH (e.g., pituitary neoplasms), struma ovarii, ingestion of large amounts of iodine in a patient with preexisting thyroid hyperplasia or adenoma (Jod-Basedow phenomenon), hydatidiform mole, carcinoma of thyroid, amiodarone therapy of arrhythmias.

Serum thyroxine test measures both circulating thyroxine bound to protein (represents >99% of circulating T_4 and unbound (free) thyroxine. Values vary with protein binding; changes in the concentration of T_4 secondary to changes in thyroxine-binding globulin (TBG) can be caused by the following:

Increased TBG ($\uparrow T_4$)	**Decreased TBG ($\downarrow T_4$)**
Pregnancy	Androgens, glucocorticoids
Estrogens	Nephrotic syndrome, cirrhosis
Acute infectious hepatitis	Acromegaly
Oral contraceptives	Hypoproteinemia
Familial	Familial
Fluorouracil, clofibrate, heroin, methadone	Phenytoin, ASA and other NSAIDs, high-dose penicillin, asparaginase
	Chronic debilitating illness

To eliminate the suspected influence of protein binding on thyroxine values, two additional tests are available: T_3 resin uptake and serum free thyroxine.

■ **T₄, FREE** (free thyroxine)
Normal range: 0.8-2.8 ng/dl
Elevated in: Graves' disease, toxic multinodular goiter, toxic adenoma, iatrogenic and factitious causes, transient hyperthyroidism
Serum free T_4 directly measures unbound thyroxine. Free T_4 can be measured by equilibrium dialysis (gold standard of free T_4 assays) or by immunometric techniques (influenced by serum levels of lipids, proteins, and certain drugs). The free thyroxine index (FTI) can also be easily calculated by multiplying T_4 times T_3RU and dividing the result by 100; the FTI corrects for any abnormal T_4 values secondary to protein binding: $FTI = T_4 \times T_3RU/100$.
Normal values equal 1.1 to 4.3.
Table 4-2, under "Acid-Base Reference Values," describes additional abnormalities of free T_4.

■ **TEGRETOL;** *see* CARBAMAZEPINE; *see* Table 4-24, under "T_3 (triiodothyronine)"

■ **TESTOSTERONE** (total testosterone)
Normal range: (Variable with age and sex)
Serum/plasma: Males: 280-1100 ng/dl
                            Females: 15-70 ng/dl
Urine: Males: 50-135 μg/day
                            Females: 2-12 μg/day
Elevated in: Testicular tumors, ovarian masculinizing tumors
Decreased in: Hypogonadism

■ **THEOPHYLLINE**
Normal therapeutic range: 10-20 mcg/mL

■ **THORACENTESIS FLUID**
Testing and evaluation of results:
1. Pleural effusion fluid should be differentiated in exudate or transudate. The initial laboratory studies should be aimed only at distinguishing an exudate from a transudate.
   a. Tube 1: protein, LDH, albumin.
   b. Tubes 2, 3, 4: save the fluid until further notice. In selected patients with suspected empyema, a pH level may be useful (generally ≤ 7.0). See following for proper procedure to obtain a pH level from pleural fluid.
   NOTE: Do not order further tests until the presence of an exudate is confirmed on the basis of protein and LDH determinations (Section III, Fig. 3-145, on page 1143); however, if the results of protein and LDH determinations cannot be obtained within a reasonable time (resulting in unnecessary delay), additional laboratory tests should be ordered at the time of thoracentesis.
2. A serum/effusion albumin gradient of ≤1.2 g/dl is indicative of exudative effusions, especially in patients with congestive heart failure (CHF) treated with diuretics.
3. Note the appearance of the fluid:
   a. A grossly hemorrhagic effusion can be a result of a traumatic tap, neoplasm, or an embolus with infarction.
   b. A milky appearance indicates either of the following:
      (1) Chylous effusion: caused by trauma or tumor invasion of the thoracic duct; lipoprotein electrophoresis of the effusion reveals chylomicrons and triglyceride levels >115 mg/dl.
      (2) Pseudochylous effusion: often seen with chronic inflammation of the pleural space (e.g., TB, connective tissue diseases).
4. If transudate, consider CHF, cirrhosis, chronic renal failure, and other hypoproteinemic states and perform subsequent workup accordingly.
5. If exudate, consider ordering these tests on the pleural fluid:
   a. Cytologic examination for malignant cells (for suspected neoplasm).
   b. Gram stain, cultures (aerobic and anaerobic), and sensitivities (for suspected infectious process).
   c. AFB stain and cultures (for suspected TB).
   d. pH: a value < 7.0 suggests parapneumonic effusion or empyema; a pleural fluid pH must be drawn anaerobically and iced immediately; the syringe should be prerinsed with 0.2 ml of 1:1000 heparin.
   e. Glucose: a low glucose level suggests parapneumonic effusions and rheumatoid arthritis.

f. Amylase: a high amylase level suggests pancreatitis or ruptured esophagus.

g. Perplexing pleural effusions are often a result of malignancy (e.g., lymphoma, malignant mesothelioma, ovarian carcinoma), TB, subdiaphragmatic processes, prior asbestos exposure, and postcardiac injury syndrome.

■ THROMBIN TIME (TT)
Normal range: 11.3-18.5 sec
Elevated in: Thrombolytic and heparin therapy, disseminated intravascular coagulation, hypofibrinogenemia, dysfibrinogenemia

■ THYROID-STIMULATING HORMONE (TSH)
Normal range: 2-11 µU/ml
CONDITIONS THAT INCREASE SERUM THYROID-STIMULATING HORMONE VALUES
Laboratory error
Primary hypothyroidism
Synthroid therapy with insufficient dose
Lithium or amiodarone; some patients
Hashimoto's thyroiditis in later stage
Large doses of inorganic iodide (e.g., SSKI)
Severe nonthyroid illness in recovery phase
Iodine deficiency (moderate or severe)
Addison's disease
TSH specimen drawn in evening (peak of diurnal variation)
Pituitary TSH-secreting tumor
Therapy of hypothyroidism (3-6 wk after beginning therapy [range, 1-8 wk]; sometimes longer when pretherapy TSH is over 100 µU/ml)
Acute psychiatric illness
Peripheral resistance to T_4 syndrome
Antibodies (e.g., HAMA) interfering with monoclonal sandwich method of TSH assay
Telepaque (iopanoic acid) and Oragrafin (ipodate) x-ray contrast media
Amphetamines
High altitudes
CONDITIONS THAT DECREASE SERUM THYROID-STIMULATING HORMONE VALUES
Laboratory error
T_4/T_3 toxicosis (diffuse or nodular etiology)
Excessive therapy for hypothyroidism
Active thyroiditis (subacute, painless, or early active Hashimoto's disease)
Multinodular goiter containing areas of autonomy
Severe nonthyroid illness (especially acute trauma, dopamine, or glucocorticoid)
T_3 toxicosis
Pituitary insufficiency
Cushing's syndrome (and some patients on high-dose glucocorticoid)
Jod-Basedow (iodine-induced) hyperthyroidism
Thyroid-stimulating hormone drawn 2-4 hr after levothyroxine dose
Postpartum transient toxicosis
Factitious hyperthyroidism
Struma ovarii
Radioimmunoassay, surgery, or antithyroid drug therapy for hyperthyroidism 4-6 wk (range 2 wk–2 yr) after the treatment
Interleukin-2 drugs (3%-6% of cases) or α-interferon therapy (1% of cases)
Hyperemesis gravidarum
Amiodarone therapy

■ THYROXINE (T_4)
Normal range: 4-11 µg/dl

■ TIBC; *see* IRON-BINDING CAPACITY

■ TRANSFERRIN
Normal range: 170-370 mg/dl
Elevated in: Iron deficiency anemia, oral contraceptive administration, viral hepatitis, late pregnancy
Decreased in: Nephrotic syndrome, liver disease, hereditary deficiency, protein malnutrition, neoplasms, chronic inflammatory states, chronic illness, thalassemia, hemochromatosis, hemolytic anemia

■ TRIGLYCERIDES
Normal range: <150 mg/dl
Elevated in: Hyperlipoproteinemias (types I, IIb, III, IV, V), hypothyroidism, pregnancy, estrogens, acute myocardial infarction, pancreatitis, alcohol intake, nephrotic syndrome, diabetes mellitus, glycogen storage disease
Decreased in: Malnutrition, congenital abetalipoproteinemias, drugs (e.g., gemfibrozil, fenofibrate, nicotinic acid, clofibrate)

IV

■ **TRIIODOTHYRONINE;** *see* T$_3$

■ **TROPONINS, SERUM**
Normal range: 0-0.4 ng/ml (negative). If there is clinical suspicion of evolving acute MI or ischemic episode, repeat testing in 5-6 hours is recommended.
Indeterminate: 0.05-0.49 ng/ml. Suggest further tests. In a patient with unstable angina and this troponin I level, there is an increased risk of a cardiac event in the near future.
Strong probability of acute MI: ≥0.05 ng/ml
CARDIAC TROPONIN T (CTNT) is a highly sensitive marker for myocardial injury for the first 48 hours after MI and for up to 5-7 days (see Fig. 4-2, under "Creatine Kinase Isoenzymes"). It may be also elevated in renal failure, chronic muscle disease, and trauma.
CARDIAC TROPONIN I (CTNI) is highly sensitive and specific for myocardial injury (≥CK-MB) in the initial 8 hours, peaks within 24 hours and lasts up to 7 days. With progressively higher levels of cTnI, the risk of mortality increases because the amount of necrosis increases.

■ **TSH;** *see* THYROID-STIMULATING HORMONE

■ **TT;** *see* THROMBIN TIME

■ **TUBERCULIN TEST** (PPD)
Abnormal results: see Boxes 4-3 and 4-4 for interpretation

BOX 4-3   PPD Reaction Size Considered "Positive" (Intracutaneous 5 TU Mantoux Test at 48 hr)

5 mm or More

HIV infection or risk factors for HIV
Close recent contact with active TB case
Persons with chest x-ray consistent with healed TB

10 mm or More

Foreign-born persons from countries with high TB prevalence in Asia, Africa, and Latin America
IV drug users
Medically underserved low-income population groups (including Native Americans, Hispanics, and blacks)

Residents of long-term care facilities (nursing homes, mental institutions)
Medical conditions that increase risk for TB (silicosis, gastrectomy, undernourished, diabetes mellitus, high-dose corticosteroids or immunosuppression Rx, leukemia or lymphoma, other malignancies)
Employees of long-term care facilities, schools, child-care facilities, health care facilities

15 mm or More

All others not already listed

TB, Tuberculosis; *TU,* tuberculin units.

BOX 4-4   Factors Associated with False-Negative Tuberculin Tests

Technical Errors

Improper administration
Inaccurate reading
Loss of potency of antigen

Patient-Related Factors (Anergy)

Age (elderly)
Nutritional status

Medications—corticosteroids, immunosuppressive agents
Severe tuberculosis
Coexisting diseases
  HIV infection
  Viral illness or vaccination
  Lymphoreticular malignancies
  Sarcoidosis
  Solid tumors

Lepromatous leprosy
Sjögren's syndrome
Ataxia telangiectasia
Uremia
Primary biliary cirrhosis
Systemic lupus erythematosus
Severe systemic disease of any etiology

From Stein JH (ed): *Internal medicine,* ed 4, St Louis, 1994, Mosby.

■ **UNCONJUGATED BILIRUBIN;** *see* BILIRUBIN, INDIRECT

■ **UREA NITROGEN, BLOOD** (BUN)
Normal range: 8-18 mg/dl
Box 4-5 describes factors affecting BUN level independent of renal function.
Elevated in: Drugs (aminoglycosides and other antibiotics, diuretics, lithium, corticosteroids), dehydration, gastrointestinal bleeding, decreased renal blood flow (shock, congestive heart failure, myocardial infarction), renal disease (glomerulonephritis, pyelonephritis, diabetic nephropathy), urinary tract obstruction (prostatic hypertrophy)
Decreased in: Liver disease, malnutrition, pregnancy third trimester, overhydration, acromegaly, celiac disease

---

BOX 4-5 PPD Factors Affecting Blood Urea Nitrogen Level Independent of Renal Function

Disproportionate Increase in Blood Urea Nitrogen

Volume depletion "prerenal azotemia"
Gastrointestinal hemorrhage
Corticosteroid or cytotoxic agents
High-protein diet
Obstructive uropathy

Sepsis
Catabolic states tissue breakdown

Disproportionate Decrease in Blood Urea Nitrogen

Low-protein diet
Liver disease

From Andreoli TE (ed): *Cecil essentials of medicine,* ed 5, Philadelphia, 2001, WB Saunders.

■ URIC ACID (serum)

Normal range: 2-7 mg/dl

Elevated in: Renal failure, gout, excessive cell lysis (chemotherapeutic agents, radiation therapy, leukemia, lymphoma, hemolytic anemia), hereditary enzyme deficiency (hypoxanthine-guanine-phosphoribosyl transferase), acidosis, myeloproliferative disorders, diet high in purines or protein, drugs (diuretics, low doses of ASA, ethambutol, nicotinic acid), lead poisoning, hypothyroidism, Addison's disease, nephrogenic diabetes insipidus, active psoriasis, polycystic kidneys

Decreased in: Drugs (allopurinol, high doses of ASA, probenecid, warfarin, corticosteroid), deficiency of xanthine oxidase, syndrome of inappropriate antidiuretic hormone secretion, renal tubular deficits (Fanconi's syndrome), alcoholism, liver disease, diet deficient in protein or purines, Wilson's disease, hemochromatosis

■ URINALYSIS

Normal range:
Color: light straw
Appearance: clear
Ketones: absent
pH: 4.5-8 (average, 6)
Protein: absent
Glucose: absent
Specific gravity: 1.005-1.030
Occult blood absent
Microscopic examination:
Red blood cells: 0-5 (high-power field)
White blood cells: 0-5 (high-power field)
Bacteria (spun specimen): absent
Casts: 0-4 hyaline (low-power field)
Abnormalities in the microscopic examination of urine are described in Table 4-25.

TABLE 4-25 Microscopic Examination of the Urine

FINDING	ASSOCIATIONS
Casts	
Red blood cell	Glomerulonephritis, vasculitis
White blood cell	Interstitial nephritis, pyelonephritis
Epithelial cell	Acute tubular necrosis, interstitial nephritis, glomerulonephritis
Granular	Renal parenchymal disease (nonspecific)
Waxy, broad	Advanced renal failure
Hyaline	Normal finding in concentrated urine
Fatty	Heavy proteinuria
Cells	
Red blood cell	Urinary tract infection, urinary tract inflammation
White blood cell	Urinary tract infection, urinary tract inflammation
Eosinophil	Acute interstitial nephritis
(Squamous) epithelial cell	Contaminants
Crystals	
Uric acid	Acid urine, acute uric acid nephropathy, hyperuricosuria
Calcium phosphate	Alkaline urine
Calcium oxalate	Acid urine, hyperoxaluria, ethylene glycol poisoning
Cystine	Cystinuria
Sulfur	Sulfa-containing antibiotics

From Andreoli TE (ed): *Cecil essentials of medicine,* ed 5, Philadelphia, 2001, WB Saunders.

IV

■ **URINE AMYLASE**
Normal range: 35-260 U Somogyi/hr
Elevated in: Pancreatitis, carcinoma of the pancreas

■ **URINE BILE**
Normal: Absent
Abnormal: Urine bilirubin: hepatitis (viral, toxic, drug-induced), biliary obstruction
Urine urobilinogen: hepatitis (viral, toxic, drug-induced), hemolytic jaundice, liver cell dysfunction (cirrhosis, infection, metastases)

■ **URINE CALCIUM**
Normal range: <250 mg/24 hr
Elevated in: Primary hyperparathyroidism, hypervitaminosis D, bone metastases, multiple myeloma, increased calcium intake, steroids, prolonged immobilization, sarcoidosis, Paget's disease, idiopathic hypercalciuria, renal tubular acidosis
Decreased in: Hypoparathyroidism, pseudohypoparathyroidism, vitamin D deficiency, vitamin D–resistant rickets, diet low in calcium, drugs (thiazide diuretics, oral contraceptives), familial hypocalciuric hypercalcemia, renal osteodystrophy, potassium citrate therapy

■ **URINE CAMP**
Elevated in: Hypercalciuria, familial hypocalciuric hypercalcemia, primary hyperparathyroidism, pseudohypoparathyroidism, rickets
Decreased in: Vitamin D intoxication, sarcoidosis

■ **URINE CATECHOLAMINES**
Normal range:
Norepinephrine: <100 μg/24 hr
Epinephrine: <10 μg/24 hr
Elevated in: Pheochromocytoma, neuroblastoma, severe stress

■ **URINE CHLORIDE**
Normal range: 110-250 mEq/day
Elevated in: Corticosteroids, Bartter's syndrome, diuretics, metabolic acidosis, severe hypokalemia
Decreased in: Chloride depletion (vomiting), colonic villous adenoma, chronic renal failure, renal tubular acidosis

■ **URINE COPPER**
Normal range: <40 μg/24 hr

■ **URINE CORTISOL, FREE**
Normal range: 10-110 μg/24 hr
Elevated: See CORTISOL, plasma

■ **URINE CREATININE** (24 HR)
Normal range:
Male: 0.8-1.8 g/day
Female: 0.6-1.6 g/day
NOTE: Useful test as an indicator of completeness of 24 hr urine collection.

■ **URINE EOSINOPHILS**
Normal:
Absent
Present:
Interstitial nephritis, acute tubular necrosis, urinary tract infection, kidney transplant rejection, hepatorenal syndrome

■ **URINE GLUCOSE** (qualitative)
Normal: Absent
Present in: Diabetes mellitus, renal glycosuria (decreased renal threshold for glucose), glucose intolerance

■ **URINE HEMOGLOBIN, FREE**
Normal: Absent
Present in: Hemolysis (with saturation of serum haptoglobin binding capacity and renal threshold for tubular absorption of hemoglobin)

■ **URINE HEMOSIDERIN**
Normal: Absent
Present in: Paroxysmal nocturnal hemoglobinuria, chronic hemolytic anemia, hemochromatosis, blood transfusion, thalassemias

■ **URINE 5-HYDROXYINDOLE-ACETIC ACID** (urine 5-HIAA)
Normal range: 2-8 mg/24 hr
Elevated in: Carcinoid tumors, after ingestion of certain foods (bananas, plums, tomatoes, avocados, pineapples, eggplant, walnuts), drugs (monoamine oxidase inhibitors, phenacetin, methyldopa, glycerol guaiacolate, acetaminophen, salicylates, phenothiazines, imipramine, methocarbamol, reserpine, methamphetamine)

■ **URINE INDICAN**
Normal: Absent
Present in: Malabsorption secondary to intestinal bacterial overgrowth

■ **URINE KETONES** (semiquantitative)
Normal: Absent
Present in: Diabetic ketoacidosis, alcoholic ketoacidosis, starvation, isopropanol ingestion

■ **URINE METANEPHRINES**
Normal range: 0-2.0 mg/24 hr
Elevated in: Pheochromocytoma, neuroblastoma, drugs (caffeine, phenothiazines, monoamine oxidase inhibitors), stress

■ **URINE MYOGLOBIN**
Normal: Absent
Present in: Severe trauma, hyperthermia, polymyositis/dermatomyositis, carbon monoxide poisoning, drugs (narcotic and amphetamine toxicity), hypothyroidism, muscle ischemia

■ **URINE NITRITE**
Normal: Absent
Present in: Urinary tract infections

■ **URINE OCCULT BLOOD**
Normal: Negative
Positive in: Trauma to urinary tract, renal disease (glomerulonephritis, pyelonephritis), renal or ureteral calculi, bladder lesions (carcinoma, cystitis), prostatitis, prostatic carcinoma, menstrual contamination, hematopoietic disorders (hemophilia, thrombocytopenia), anticoagulants, ASA

■ **URINE OSMOLALITY**
Normal range: 50-1200 mOsm/kg
Elevated in: Syndrome of inappropriate antidiuretic hormone secretion, dehydration, glycosuria, adrenal insufficiency, high-protein diet
Decreased in: Diabetes insipidus, excessive water intake, IV hydration with D_5W, acute renal insufficiency, glomerulonephritis

■ **URINE PH**
Normal range: 4.6-8 (average 6)
Elevated in: Bacteriuria, vegetarian diet, renal failure with inability to form ammonia, drugs (antibiotics, sodium bicarbonate, acetazolamide)
Decreased in: Acidosis (metabolic, respiratory), drugs (ammonium chloride, methenamine mandelate), diabetes mellitus, starvation, diarrhea

■ **URINE PHOSPHATE**
Normal range: 0.8-2.0 g/24 hr
Elevated in: Acute tubular necrosis (diuretic phase), chronic renal disease, uncontrolled diabetes mellitus, hyperparathyroidism, hypomagnesemia, metabolic acidosis, metabolic alkalosis, neurofibromatosis, adult-onset vitamin D–resistant hypophosphatemic osteomalacia
Decreased in: Acromegaly, acute renal failure, decreased dietary intake, hypoparathyroidism, respiratory acidosis

■ **URINE POTASSIUM**
Normal range: 25-100 mEq/24 hr
Elevated in: Aldosteronism (primary, secondary), glucocorticoids, alkalosis, renal tubular acidosis, excessive dietary potassium intake
Decreased in: Acute renal failure, potassium-sparing diuretics, diarrhea, hypokalemia

■ **URINE PROTEIN** (quantitative)
Normal range: <150 mg/24 hr
Elevated in:
Nephrotic syndrome as a result of primary renal diseases
Malignant hypertension
Malignancies: multiple myeloma, leukemias, Hodgkin's disease
Congestive heart failure
Diabetes mellitus

IV

Systemic lupus erythematosus, rheumatoid arthritis
Sickle cell disease
Goodpasture's syndrome
Malaria
Amyloidosis, sarcoidosis
Tubular lesions: cystinosis
Functional (after heavy exercise)
Pyelonephritis
Pregnancy
Constrictive pericarditis
Renal vein thrombosis
Toxic nephropathies: heavy metals, drugs
Radiation nephritis
Orthostatic (postural) proteinuria
Benign proteinuria: fever, heat or cold exposure

■ **URINE SEDIMENT;** *see* Fig. 4-14 for evaluation of common abnormalities

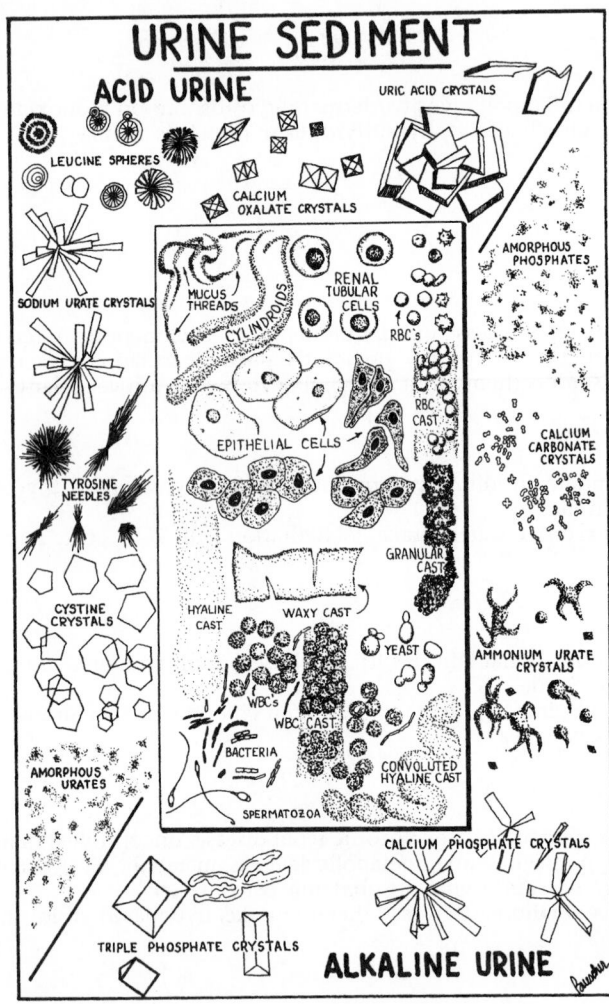

Fig. 4-14 **Microscopic examination of urinary sediment.** (From Grigorian Greene M: *The Harriet Lane handbook: a manual for pediatric house officers,* ed 12, St Louis, 1991, Mosby.)

■ **URINE SODIUM (QUANTITATIVE)**
Normal range: 40-220 mEq/day
Elevated in: Diuretic administration, high sodium intake, salt-losing nephritis, acute tubular necrosis, vomiting, Addison's disease, syndrome of inappropriate antidiuretic hormone secretion, hypothyroidism, congestive heart failure, hepatic failure, chronic renal failure, Bartter's syndrome, glucocorticoid deficiency, interstitial nephritis caused by analgesic abuse, mannitol, dextran, or glycerol therapy, milk-alkali syndrome, decreased renin secretion, postobstructive diuresis
Decreased in: Increased aldosterone, glucocorticoid excess, hyponatremia, prerenal azotemia, decreased salt intake

■ **URINE SPECIFIC GRAVITY**
Normal range: 1.005-1.03
Elevated in: Dehydration, excessive fluid losses (vomiting, diarrhea, fever), x-ray contrast media, diabetes mellitus, congestive heart failure, syndrome of inappropriate antidiuretic hormone secretion, adrenal insufficiency, decreased fluid intake
Decreased in: Diabetes insipidus, renal disease (glomerulonephritis, pyelonephritis), excessive fluid intake or IV hydration

■ **URINE VANILLYLMANDELIC ACID** (VMA)
Normal range: <6.8 mg/24 hr
Elevated in: Pheochromocytoma, neuroblastoma, ganglioblastoma, drugs (isoproterenol, methocarbamol, levodopa, sulfonamides, chlorpromazine), severe stress, after ingestion of bananas, chocolate, vanilla, tea, coffee
Decreased in: Drugs (monoamine oxidase inhibitors, reserpine, guanethidine, methyldopa)

■ **VDRL**
Normal range: Negative
Positive test: Syphilis, other treponemal diseases (yaws, pinta, bejel)
NOTE: A false-positive test may be seen in patients with systemic lupus erythematosus and other autoimmune diseases, infectious mononucleosis, HIV, atypical pneumonia, malaria, leprosy, typhus fever, rat-bite fever, relapsing fever.
NOTE: see Table 4-26 for interpretation of serologic tests for syphilis.

TABLE 4-26 **Interpretation of Serologic Tests for Syphilis***

FINDING		
NONTREPONEMAL TESTS	TREPONEMAL TESTS	INTERPRETATION OF FINDING: IS SYPHILIS PRESENT?*
Nonreactive	Nonreactive	*Early primary syphilis is not ruled out by negative serologic tests.* *Early syphilis* is present in 13%-30% of patients who have a negative microhemagglutination–*Treponema pallidum* test; in about 30% of patients who present with chancre but have a nonreactive reagin test; and in about 10% of patients who have a negative FTA-ABS test. *Late syphilis* is present in a very small fraction of patients. *Adequately treated syphilis in remote past* may produce these results, but treponemal tests usually remain reactive.
	Reactive	Observed in about 10% of patients with chancre. The treponemal tests may turn positive shortly before the reagin tests. Reagin tests repeated after several days are generally positive. *In adequately treated early syphilis,* the reagin test may return to nonreactive within 1-2 yr, whereas the treponemal tests generally do not. *Late syphilis* is not ruled out by a negative reagin test. The sensitivity of the reagin tests is lower than that of treponemal tests in untreated late syphilis. In *secondary syphilis,* rarely, a highly reactive serum appears negative when tested undiluted with a reagin test because flocculation is inhibited by relative antibody excess. Not reported to occur with treponemal tests. Quantitative reagin tests are positive. False-positive treponemal tests occur in 40% of patients with Lyme disease.
Reactive	Nonreactive borderline (FTA-ABS)	Finding is not diagnostic of syphilis but constitutes a classic biologic false-positive reaction. Not diagnostic of syphilis: most patients (90%) with this pattern do not develop clinical or serologic evidence of syphilis. Repeat test is indicated. Chronic borderline results are associated with a variety of conditions other than syphilis.
	Beaded (FTA-ABS)	Not diagnostic of syphilis. Seen with collagen-vascular disease.
	Reactive	Findings diagnostic of syphilis or other treponemal disease. *In adequately treated syphilis,* one would expect (1) a sustained fourfold drop in titer of reagin test, although reagin test may remain positive after adequate therapy; (2) treponemal tests remain positive after adequate therapy. Concurrent false-positive results on both nontreponemal and treponemal tests could occur in rare instances. It may be impossible to rule out syphilis in an individual with this test profile.

From Stein JH (ed): *Internal medicine,* ed 4, St Louis, 1994, Mosby.
FTA-ABS, Fluorescent treponemal antibody, absorbed.
*Serologic data must always be interpreted in the light of a total clinical evaluation. Diagnosis based on serologic criteria alone is fraught with error. Serologic tests apparently in conflict with clinical diagnosis should be confirmed by repetition or possibly referral to a reference laboratory.

IV

■ **VISCOSITY** (serum)
Normal range: 1.4-1.8 relative to water (1.10-1.22 centipoise)
Elevated in: Monoclonal gammopathies (Waldenström's macro-globulinemia, multiple myeloma), hyperfibrinogenemia, systemic lupus erythematosus, rheumatoid arthritis, polycythemia, leukemia

■ **VITAMIN B$_{12}$**
Normal:
190-900 ng/ml
Causes of Vitamin B$_{12}$ deficiency:
1. Pernicious anemia (antibodies against intrinsic factor and gastric parietal cells)
2. Dietary (strict lacto-ovovegetarians, food faddists)
3. Malabsorption (achlorhydria, gastrectomy, ileal resection, pancreatic insufficiency, drugs [omeprazole, cholestyramine])
Falsely low levels occur in patients with severe folate deficiency, in patients using high doses of ascorbic acid, and when cobalamin levels are measured after nuclear medicine studies (radioactivity interferes with cobalamin radioimmunoassay).
Falsely high or normal levels in patients with cobalamin deficiency can occur in severe liver disease and chronic granulocytic leukemia.
The absence of anemia or macrocytosis does not exclude the diagnosis of cobalamin deficiency.

■ **WBC;** *see* COMPLETE BLOOD COUNT

■ **WESTERGREN;** *see* ERYTHROCYTE SEDIMENTATION RATE

■ **WHITE BLOOD COUNT;** *see* COMPLETE BLOOD COUNT

Clinical Preventive Services

*Data modified from US Preventive Services Task Force: *Guide to clinical preventive services: report of the US Preventive Services Task Force*, ed 2, Washington, DC, 1996 (revised 2001), US Department of Health and Human Services. Text downloaded from Internet site: http://text.nlm.nih.gov

THE PERIODIC HEALTH EXAMINATION
Age-Specific Charts

TABLE 5-1   Birth to 10 Years

Interventions considered and recommended for the Periodic Health Examination	Leading causes of death
	Conditions originating in perinatal period
	Congenital anomalies
	Sudden infant death syndrome (SIDS)
	Unintentional injuries (non–motor vehicle)
	Motor vehicle injuries

Interventions for the General Population

Screening

Height and weight

Blood pressure

Vision screen (age 3-4 yr)

Hemoglobinopathy screen (birth)[1]

Phenylalanine level (birth)[2]

T_4 and/or TSH (birth)[3]

Counseling

Injury prevention

Child safety car seats (age <5 yr)

Lap/shoulder belts (age ≥5 yr)

Bicycle helmet; avoid bicycling near traffic

Smoke detector, flame-retardant sleepwear

Hot water heater temperature <120°-130° F

Window/stair guards, pool fence

Safe storage of drugs, toxic substances, firearms, and matches

Syrup of ipecac, poison control phone number

CPR training for parents/caretakers

Diet and exercise

Breast-feeding, iron-enriched formula and foods (infants and toddlers)

Limit fat and cholesterol; maintain caloric balance; emphasize grains, fruits, vegetables (age ≥2 yr)

Regular physical activity*

Substance use

Effects of passive smoking*

Antitobacco message*

Dental health

Regular visits to dental care provider*

Floss, brush with fluoride toothpaste daily*

Advice about baby bottle tooth decay*

Immunizations

Diphtheria-tetanus-pertussis (DTP)[4]

Inactivated poliovirus vaccine (IPV)[5]

Measles-mumps-rubella (MMR)[6]

H. influenzae type b (Hib) conjugate[7]

Hepatitis B[8]

Varicella[9]

Pneumococcal vaccine[10]

Influenza[11]

Chemoprophylaxis

Ocular prophylaxis (birth)

Interventions for High-Risk Populations

Population	Potential Interventions (See detailed high-risk definitions)
Preterm or low birth weight	Hemoglobin/hematocrit (HR1)
Infants of mothers at risk for HIV	HIV testing (HR2)
Low income; immigrants	Hemoglobin/hematocrit (HR1); PPD (HR3)
TB contacts	PPD (HR3)
Native American/Alaska Native	Hemoglobin/hematocrit (HR1); PPD (HR3); hepatitis A vaccine (HR4); pneumococcal vaccine (HR5)
Travelers to developing countries	Hepatitis A vaccine (HR4)
Residents of long-term care facilities	PPD (HR3); hepatitis A vaccine (HR4); influenza vaccine (HR6)
Certain chronic medical conditions	PPD (HR3); pneumococcal vaccine (HR5); influenza vaccine (HR6)
Increased individual or community lead exposure	Blood lead level (HR7)
Inadequate water fluoridation	Daily fluoride supplement (HR8)
Family hx of skin cancer; nevi; fair skin, eyes, hair	Avoid excess/midday sun, use protective clothing* (HR9)

[1]Whether screening should be universal or targeted to high-risk groups will depend on the proportion of high-risk individuals in the screening area, and other considerations. [2]If done during first 24 hr of life, repeat by age 2 wk. [3]Optimally between day 2 and 6, but in all cases before newborn nursery discharge. [4]2, 4, 6, and 12-18 mo; once between ages 4-6 yr (DTaP may be used at 15 mo and older). [5]2, 4, 6-18 mo; once between ages 4-6 yr. [6]12-15 mo and 4-6 yr. [7]2, 4, 6 and 12-15 mo; no dose needed at 6 mo if PRP-OMP vaccine is used for first 2 doses. [8]Birth, 1 mo, 6 mo; or, 0-2 mo, 1-2 mo later, and 6-18 mo. If not done in infancy: current visit, and 1 and 6 mo later. [9]12-18 mo; or any child without hx of chickenpox or previous immunization. Include information on risk in adulthood, duration of immunity, and potential need for booster doses. [10]The 7-Valent conjugate vaccine (PCV) can be administered at the same time as the other childhood vaccines at a separate site. [11]Influenza vaccine is beneficial in children 6 to 23 months of age because they have been shown to be at increased risk for complications associated with influenza vaccination.
*The ability of clinician counseling to influence this behavior is unproven.

HR1 = Infants age 6-12 mo who are living in poverty, black, Native American or Alaska Native, immigrants from developing countries, preterm and low birth weight infants, infants whose principal dietary intake is unfortified cow's milk.

HR2 = Infants born to high-risk mothers whose HIV status is unknown. Women at high risk include past or present injection drug use; persons who exchange sex for money or drugs, and their sex partners; injection drug–using, bisexual, or HIV-positive sex partners currently or in past; persons seeking treatment for STDs; blood transfusion during 1978-1985.

HR3 = Persons infected with HIV, close contacts of persons with known or suspected TB, persons with medical risk factors associated with TB, immigrants from countries with high TB prevalence, medically underserved low-income populations (including homeless), residents of long-term care facilities.

HR4 = Persons ≥2 yr living in or traveling to areas where the disease is endemic and where periodic outbreaks occur (e.g., countries with high or intermediate endemicity; certain Alaska Native, Pacific Island, Native American, and religious communities). Consider for institutionalized children aged ≥2 yr. Clinicians should also consider local epidemiology.

HR5 = Immunocompetent persons ≥2 yr with certain medical conditions, including chronic cardiac or pulmonary disease, dia-betes mellitus, cochlear implant candidates and recipients, and anatomic asplenia. Immunocompetent persons ≥2 yr living in high-risk environments or social settings (e.g., certain Native American and Alaska Native populations).

HR6 = Annual vaccination of children ≥6 mo who are residents of chronic care facilities or who have chronic cardiopulmonary disorders, metabolic diseases (including diabetes mellitus), hemoglobinopathies, immunosuppression, or renal dysfunction.

HR7 = Children about age 12 mo who: (1) live in communities in which the prevalence of lead levels requiring individual intervention, including residental lead hazard control or chelation, is high or undefined; (2) live in or frequently visit a home built before 1950 with dilapidated paint or with recent or ongoing renovation or remodeling; (3) have close contact with a person who has an elevated lead level; (4) live near lead industry or heavy traffic; (5) live with someone whose job or hobby involves lead exposure; (6) use lead-based pottery; or (7) take traditional ethnic remedies that contain lead.

HR8 = Children living in areas with inadequate water fluoridation (<0.6 ppm).

HR9 = Persons with a family history of skin cancer, a large number of moles, atypical moles, poor tanning ability, or light skin, hair, and eye color.

TABLE 5-2   Ages 11-24 Years

Interventions considered and recommended for the Periodic Health Examination	Leading causes of death
	Motor vehicle/other unintentional injuries
	Homicide
	Suicide
	Malignant neoplasms
	Heart diseases

Interventions for the General Population

Screening

Height and weight

Blood pressure[1]

Papanicolaou (Pap) test[2] (females)

Chlamydia screen[3] (females <25 yr)

Lipid panel (in high-risk young adults only)

Rubella serology or vaccination hx[4] (females >12 yr)

Assess for problem drinking

Counseling

Injury prevention
Lap/shoulder belts

Bicycle/motorcycle/ATV helmets*

Smoke detector*

Safe storage/removal of firearms*
Substance use
Avoid tobacco use

Avoid underage drinking and illicit drug use*

Avoid alcohol/drug use while driving, swimming, boating, etc.*

Sexual behavior
STD prevention: abstinence*; avoid high-risk behavior*; condoms/female barrier with spermicide*
Unintended pregnancy: contraception

Diet and exercise
Limit fat and cholesterol; maintain caloric balance; emphasize grains, fruits, vegetables

Adequate calcium intake (females)

Regular physical activity*
Dental health
Regular visits to dental care provider*

Floss, brush with fluoride toothpaste daily

Immunizations

Tetanus-diphtheria (Td) boosters (11-16 yr)

Hepatitis B[5]

MMR (11-12 yr)[6]

Varicella (11-12 yr)[7]

Rubella[4] (females >12 yr)

Chemoprophylaxis

Multivitamin with folic acid (females)

Interventions for High-Risk Populations

Population	*Potential Interventions (See detailed high-risk definitions)*
High-risk sexual behavior	RPR/VDRL (HR1); screen for gonorrhea (female) (HR2), HIV (HR3), chlamydia (female) (HR4); hepatitis A vaccine (HR5)
Injection or street drug use	RPR/VDRL (HR1); HIV screen (HR3); hepatitis A vaccine (HR5); PPD (HR6); advice to reduce infection risk (HR7)
TB contacts; immigrants; low income	PPD (HR6)
Native Americans/Alaska Natives	Hepatitis A vaccine (HR5); PPD (HR6); pneumococcal vaccine (HR8)
Travelers to developing countries	Hepatitis A vaccine (HR5)
Certain chronic medical conditions	PPD (HR6); pneumococcal vaccine (HR8); influenza vaccine (HR9)
Settings where adolescents and young adults congregate	Second MMR (HR10)
Susceptible to varicella, measles, mumps	Varicella vaccine (HR11); MMR (HR12)
Blood transfusion between 1975-1985	HIV screen (HR3)
Institutionalized persons; health care/lab workers	Hepatitis A vaccine (HR5); PPD (HR6); influenza vaccine (HR9)
Family hx of skin cancer; nevi; fair skin, eyes, hair	Avoid excess/midday sun, use protective clothing* (HR13)
Prior pregnancy with neural tube defect	Folic acid 4.0 mg (HR14)
Inadequate water fluoridation	Daily fluoride supplement (HR15)

V

[1]Periodic BP for persons aged ≥21 yr. [2]If sexually active at present or in the past: q ≤3 yr. If sexual history is unreliable, begin Pap tests at age 18 yr. [3]If sexually active. [4]Serologic testing, documented vaccination history, and routine vaccination against rubella (preferably with MMR) are equally acceptable alternatives. [5]If not previously immunized: current visit, 1 and 6 mo later. [6]If no previous second dose of MMR. [7]If susceptible to chickenpox.
*The ability of clinician counseling to influence this behavior is unproven.

HR1 = Persons who exchange sex for money or drugs, and their sex partners; persons with other STDs (including HIV); and sexual contacts of persons with active syphilis. Clinicians should also consider local epidemiology.

HR2 = Females who have two or more sex partners in the last year; a sex partner with multiple sexual contacts; exchanged sex for money or drugs; or a history of repeated episodes of gonorrhea. Clinicians should also consider local epidemiology.

HR3 = Males who had sex with males after 1975; past or present injection drug use; persons who exchange sex for money or drugs, and their sex partners; injection drug–using, bisexual, or HIV-positive sex partner currently or in the past; blood transfusion during 1978-1985; persons seeking treatment for STDs. Clinicians should also consider local epidemiology.

HR4 = Sexually active females with multiple risk factors including history of prior STD; new or multiple sex partners; age under 25; nonuse or inconsistent use of barrier contraceptives; cervical ectopy. Clinicians should consider local epidemiology of the disease in identifying other high-risk groups.

HR5 = Persons living in, traveling to, or working in areas where the disease is endemic and where periodic outbreaks occur (e.g., countries with high or intermediate endemicity; certain Alaska Native, Pacific Island, Native American, and religious communities); men who have sex with men; injection or street drug users. Vaccine may be considered for institutionalized persons and workers in these institutions, military personnel, and day-care, hospital, and laboratory workers. Clinicians should also consider local epidemiology.

HR6 = HIV positive, close contacts of persons with known or suspected TB, health care workers, persons with medical risk factors associated with TB, immigrants from countries with high TB prevalence, medically underserved low-income populations (including homeless), alcoholics, injection drug users, and residents of long-term facilities.

HR7 = Persons who continue to inject drugs.

HR8 = Immunocompetent persons with certain medical conditions, including chronic cardiac or pulmonary disease, diabetes mellitus, cochlear implants candidates and recipients, and anatomic asplenia. Immunocompetent persons who live in high-risk environments or social settings (e.g., certain Native American and Alaska Native populations).

HR9 = Annual vaccination of residents of chronic care facilities; persons with chronic cardiopulmonary disorders, metabolic diseases (including diabetes mellitus), hemoglobinopathies, immunosuppression, or renal dysfunction; and health care providers for high-risk patients.

HR10 = Adolescents and young adults in settings where such individuals congregate (e.g., high schools and colleges), if they have not previously received a second dose.

HR11 = Healthy persons aged ≥13 yr without a history of chickenpox or previous immunization. Consider serologic testing for presumed susceptible persons aged ≥13 yr.

HR12 = Persons born after 1956 who lack evidence of immunity to measles or mumps (e.g., documented receipt of live vaccine on or after the first birthday, laboratory evidence of immunity, or a history of physician-diagnosed measles or mumps).

HR13 = Persons with a family or personal history of skin cancer, a large number of moles, atypical moles, poor tanning ability, or light skin, hair, and eye color.

HR14 = Women with prior pregnancy affected by neural tube defect who are planning pregnancy.

HR15 = Persons aged <17 yr living in areas with inadequate water fluoridation (<0.6 ppm).

TABLE 5-3 Ages 25-64 Years

Interventions considered
and recommended for the
Periodic Health Examination

Leading causes of death
  Malignant neoplasms
  Heart diseases
  Motor vehicle and other unintentional injuries
  Human immunodeficiency virus (HIV) infection
  Suicide and homicide

Interventions for the General Population

Screening

Blood pressure

Height and weight

Lipid panel (men age 35-64, women age 45-64)

Papanicolaou (Pap) test (women)[1]

Fecal occult blood test[2] and/or colonoscopy (≥50 yr)

Mammogram ± clinical breast exam[3] (women 50-69 yr)

Assess for problem drinking

Rubella serology or vaccination hx[4] (women of childbearing age)

Counseling

Substance use
Tobacco cessation

Avoid alcohol/drug use while driving, swimming, boating, etc.*
Diet and exercise
Limit fat and cholesterol; maintain caloric balance; emphasize grains, fruits, vegetables

Adequate calcium intake (women)

Regular physical activity*
Injury prevention
Lap/shoulder belts

Motorcycle/bicycle/ATV helmets*

Smoke detector*

Safe storage/removal of firearms*
Sexual behavior
STD prevention: avoid high-risk behavior*; condoms/female barrier with spermicide*

Unintended pregnancy: contraception
Dental health
Regular visits to dental care provider*

Floss, brush with fluoride toothpaste daily*

Immunizations

Tetanus-diphtheria (Td) boosters

Rubella[4] (women of childbearing age)

Influenza vaccine for people over age 50†

Chemoprophylaxis

Multivitamin with folic acid (women planning or capable of pregnancy)

Discuss hormone prophylaxis (peri- and postmenopausal women)

Interventions for High-Risk Populations

Population	*Potential Interventions (See detailed high-risk definitions)*
High-risk sexual behavior	RPR/VDRL (HR1); screen for gonorrhea (female) (HR2), HIV (HR3), chlamydia (female) (HR4); hepatitis B vaccine (HR5); hepatitis A vaccine (HR6)
Injection or street drug use	RPR/VDRL (HR1); HIV screen (HR3); hepatitis B vaccine (HR5); hepatitis A vaccine (HR6); PPD (HR7); advice to reduce infection risk (HR8)
Low income; TB contacts; immigrants; alcoholics	PPD (HR7)
Native Americans/Alaska Natives	Hepatitis A vaccine (HR6); PPD (HR7); pneumococcal vaccine (HR9)
Travelers to developing countries	Hepatitis B vaccine (HR5); hepatitis A vaccine (HR6)
Certain chronic medical conditions	PPD (HR7); pneumococcal vaccine (HR9); influenza vaccine (HR10)
Blood product recipients	HIV screen (HR3); hepatitis B vaccine (HR5)
Susceptible to measles, mumps, or varicella	MMR (HR11); varicella vaccine (HR12)
Institutionalized persons	Hepatitis A vaccine (HR6); PPD (HR7); pneumococcal vaccine (HR9); influenza vaccine (HR10)
Health care/lab workers	Hepatitis B vaccine (HR5); hepatitis A vaccine (HR6); PPD (HR7); influenza vaccine (HR10)
Family hx of skin cancer; fair skin, eyes, hair	Avoid excess/midday sun, use protective clothing* (HR13)
Previous pregnancy with neural tube defect	Folic acid 4.0 mg (HR14)

[1]Women who are or have been sexually active and who have a cervix: q ≤3 yr. [2]Annually. [3]Mammogram q1-2 yr, or mammogram q1-2 yr with annual clinical breast examination. [4]Serologic testing, documented vaccination history, and routine vaccination (preferably with MMR) are equally acceptable.
*The ability of clinician counseling to influence this behavior is unproven.
†A live attenuated influenza vaccine (LAIV, Flumist) administered intranasally is available for healthy persons 5 to 49 years of age.

V

HR1 = Persons who exchange sex for money or drugs, and their sex partners; persons with other STDs (including HIV); and sexual contacts of persons with active syphilis. Clinicians should also consider local epidemiology.

HR2 = Women who exchange sex for money or drugs, or who have had repeated episodes of gonorrhea. Clinicians should also consider local epidemiology.

HR3 = Men who had sex with men after 1975; past or present injection drug use; persons who exchange sex for money or drugs, and their sex partners; injection drug–using, bisexual, or HIV-positive sex partner currently or in the past; blood transfusion during 1978-1985; persons seeking treatment for STDs. Clinicians should also consider local epidemiology.

HR4 = Sexually active women with multiple risk factors including history of STD; new or multiple sex partners; nonuse or inconsistent use of barrier contraceptives; cervical ectopy. Clinicians should also consider local epidemiology.

HR5 = Blood product recipients (including hemodialysis patients), persons with frequent occupational exposure to blood or blood products, men who have sex with men, injection drug users and their sex partners, persons with multiple recent sex partners, persons with other STDs (including HIV), travelers to countries with endemic hepatitis B.

HR6 = Persons living in, traveling to, or working in areas where the disease is endemic and where periodic outbreaks occur (e.g., countries with high or intermediate endemicity; certain Alaska Native, Pacific Island, Native American, and religious communities); men who have sex with men; injection or street drug users. Consider for institutionalized persons and workers in these institutions, military personnel, and day-care, hospital, and laboratory workers. Clinicians should also consider local epidemiology.

HR7 = HIV positive, close contacts of persons with known or suspected TB, health care workers, persons with medical risk factors associated with TB, immigrants from countries with high TB prevalence, medically underserved low-income populations (including homeless), alcoholics, injection drug users, and residents of long-term care facilities.

HR8 = Persons who continue to inject drugs.

HR9 = Immunocompetent institutionalized persons aged ≥50 yr and immunocompetent persons with certain medical conditions, including chronic cardiac or pulmonary disease, diabetes mellitus, cochlear implants candidates and recipients, and anatomic asplenia. Immunocompetent persons who live in high-risk environments or social settings (e.g., certain Native American and Alaska Native populations).

HR10 = Annual vaccination of residents of chronic care facilities; persons with chronic cardiopulmonary disorders, metabolic diseases (including diabetes mellitus), hemoglobinopathies, immunosuppression or renal dysfunction; and health care providers for high-risk patients.

HR11 = Persons born after 1956 who lack evidence of immunity to measles or mumps (e.g., documented receipt of live vaccine on or after the first birthday, laboratory evidence of immunity, or a history of physician-diagnosed measles or mumps).

HR12 = Healthy adults without a history of chickenpox or previous immunization. Consider serologic testing for presumed susceptible adults.

HR13 = Persons with a family or personal history of skin cancer, a large number of moles, atypical moles, poor tanning ability, or light skin, hair, and eye color.

HR14 = Women with previous pregnancy affected by neural tube who are planning pregnancy.

TABLE 5-4 Age 65 and Older

Interventions considered and recommended for the Periodic Health Examination	Leading causes of death
	Heart diseases
	Malignant neoplasms (lung, colorectal, breast)
	Cerebrovascular disease
	Chronic obstructive pulmonary disease
	Pneumonia and influenza

Interventions for the General Population

Screening

Blood pressure

Height and weight

Fecal occult blood test[1] and/or colonoscopy

Mammogram ± clinical breast exam[2] (women ≤69 yr)

Papanicolaou (Pap) test (women)[3]

Vision screening

Assess for hearing impairment

Assess for problem drinking

Counseling

Substance use

Tobacco cessation

Avoid alcohol/drug use while driving, swimming, boating, etc.*

Diet and exercise

Limit fat and cholesterol; maintain caloric balance; emphasize grains, fruits, vegetables

Adequate calcium intake (women)

Regular physical activity*

Injury prevention

Lap/shoulder belts

Motorcycle and bicycle helmets*

Fall prevention*

Safe storage/removal of firearms*

Smoke detector*

Set hot water heater to <120°-130° F

CPR training for household members

Dental health

Regular visits to dental care provider*

Floss, brush with fluoride toothpaste daily*

Sexual behavior

STD prevention: avoid high-risk sexual behavior*; use condoms

Immunizations

Pneumococcal vaccine

Influenza[1]

Tetanus-diphtheria (Td) boosters

Chemoprophylaxis

Discuss hormone prophylaxis (peri- and postmenopausal women)

Interventions for High-Risk Populations

Population	*Potential Interventions (See detailed high-risk definitions)*
Institutionalized persons	PPD (HR1); hepatitis A vaccine (HR2); amantadine/rimantadine (HR4)
Chronic medical conditions; TB contacts; low income; immigrants; alcoholics	PPD (HR1)
Persons ≥75 yr, or ≥70 yr with risk factors for falls	Fall prevention intervention (HR5)
Cardiovascular disease risk factors	Consider cholesterol screening (HR6)
Family hx of skin cancer; nevi; fair skin, eyes, hair	Avoid excess/midday sun, use protective clothing* (HR7)
Native Americans/Alaska Natives	PPD (HR1); hepatitis A vaccine (HR2)
Travelers to developing countries	Hepatitis A vaccine (HR2); hepatitis B vaccine (HR8)
Blood product recipients	HIV screen (HR3); hepatitis B vaccine (HR8)
High-risk sexual behavior	Hepatitis A vaccine (HR2); HIV screen (HR3); hepatitis B vaccine (HR8); RPR/VDRL (HR9)
Injection or street drug use	PPD (HR1); hepatitis A vaccine (HR2); HIV screen (HR3); hepatitis B vaccine (HR8); RPR/VDRL (HR9); advice to reduce infection risk (HR10)
Health care/lab workers	PPD (HR1); hepatitis A vaccine (HR2); amantadine/rimantadine (HR4); hepatitis B vaccine (HR8)
Persons susceptible to varicella	Varicella vaccine (HR11)

[1]Annually. [2]Mammogram q1-2 yr, or mammogram q1-2 yr with annual clinical breast exam. [3]All women who are or have been sexually active and who have a cervix. Consider discontinuation of testing after age 65 yr if previous regular screening with consistently normal results.
*The ability of clinician counseling to influence this behavior is unproven.

V

HR1 = HIV positive, close contacts of persons with known or suspected TB, health care workers, persons with medical risk factors associated with TB, immigrants from countries with high TB prevalence, medically underserved low-income populations (including homeless), alcoholics, injection drug users, and residents of long-term care facilities.

HR2 = Persons living in, traveling to, or working in areas where the disease is endemic and where periodic outbreaks occur (e.g., countries with high or intermediate endemicity; certain Alaska Native, Pacific Island, Native American, and religious communities); men who have sex with men; injection or street drug users. Consider for institutionalized persons and workers in these institutions, and day-care, hospital, and laboratory workers. Clinicians should also consider local epidemiology.

HR3 = Men who had sex with men after 1975; past or present injection drug use; persons who exchange sex for money or drugs, and their sex partners; injection drug–using, bisexual, or HIV-positive sex partner currently or in the past; blood transfusion during 1978-1985; persons seeking treatment for STDs. Clinicians should also consider local epidemiology.

HR4 = Consider for persons who have not received influenza vaccine or are vaccinated late; when the vaccine may be ineffective due to major antigenic changes in the virus; for unvaccinated persons who provide home care for high-risk persons; to supplement protection provided by vaccine in persons who are expected to have a poor antibody response; and for high-risk persons in whom the vaccine is contraindicated.

HR5 = Persons aged 75 years and older; or aged 70-74 with one or more additional risk factors including use of certain psychoactive and cardiac medications (e.g., benzodiazepines, antihypertensives); use of ≥ 4 prescription medications; impaired cognition, strength, balance, or gait. Intensive individualized home-based multifactorial fall prevention intervention is recommended in settings where adequate resources are available to deliver such services.

HR6 = Although evidence is insufficient to recommend routine screening in elderly persons, clinicians should consider cholesterol screening on a case-by-case basis for persons aged 65-75 with additional risk factors (e.g., smoking, diabetes, or hypertension).

HR7 = Persons with a family or personal history of skin cancer, a large number of moles, atypical moles, poor tanning ability, or light skin, hair, and eye color.

HR8 = Blood product recipients (including hemodialysis patients), persons with frequent occupational exposure to blood or blood products, men who have sex with men, injection drug users and their sex partners, persons with multiple recent sex partners, persons with other STDs (including HIV), travelers to countries with endemic hepatitis B.

HR9 = Persons who exchange sex for money or drugs and their sex partners; persons with other STDs (including HIV); and sexual contacts of persons with active syphilis. Clinicians should also consider local epidemiology.

HR10 = Persons who continue to inject drugs.

HR11 = Healthy adults without a history of chickenpox or previous immunization. Consider serologic testing for presumed susceptible adults.

TABLE 5-5   Pregnant Women*

Interventions considered and recommended for the Periodic Health Examination

Interventions for the General Population

Screening

First visit

Blood pressure

Hemoglobin/hematocrit

Hepatitis B surface antigen (HBsAg)

RPR/VDRL

Chlamydia screen (<25 yr)

Rubella serology or vaccination history

D(Rh) typing, antibody screen

Offer CVS (<13 wk)[1] or amniocentesis (15-18 wk)[1] (age ≥35 yr)

Offer hemoglobinopathy screening

Assess for problem or risk drinking

Offer HIV screening[2]

Follow-up visits

Blood pressure

Urine culture (12-16 wk)

Offer amniocentesis (15-18 wk)[1] (age ≥35 yr)

Offer multiple marker testing[1] (15-18 wk)

Offer serum α-fetoprotein[1] (16-18 wk)

Counseling

Tobacco cessation; effects of passive smoking

Alcohol/other drug use

Nutrition, including adequate calcium intake

Encourage breast-feeding

Lap/shoulder belts

Infant safety car seats

STD prevention: avoid high-risk sexual behavior†; use condoms†

Chemoprophylaxis

Multivitamin with folic acid[3]

Interventions for High-Risk Populations

Population	Potential Interventions (See detailed high-risk definitions)
High-risk sexual behavior	Screen for chlamydia (1st visit) (HR1), gonorrhea (1st visit) (HR2), HIV (1st visit) (HR3); HBsAg (3rd trimester) (HR4); RPR/VDRL (3rd trimester) (HR5)
Blood transfusion 1978-1985	HIV screen (1st visit) (HR3)
Injection drug use	HIV screen (HR3); HBsAg (3rd trimester) (HR4); advice to reduce infection risk (HR6)
Unsensitized D-negative women	D(Rh) antibody testing (24-28 wk) (HR7)
Risk factors for Down syndrome	Offer CVS[1] (1st trimester), amniocentesis[1] (15-18 wk) (HR8)
Prior pregnancy with neural tube defect	Offer amniocentesis[1] (15-18 wk), folic acid 4.0 mg[3] (HR9)

[1]Women with access to counseling and follow-up services, reliable standardized laboratories, skilled high-resolution ultrasound, and, for those receiving serum marker testing, amniocentesis capabilities. [2]Universal screening is recommended for areas (states, counties, or cities) with an increased prevalence of HIV infection among pregnant women. In low-prevalence areas, the choice between universal and tangled screening may depend on other considerations. [3]Beginning at least 1 mo before conception and continuing through the first trimester.
*See Tables 5-2 and 5-3 for other preventive services recommended for women of this age group.
†The ability of clinician counseling to influence this behavior is unproven.

HR1 = Women with history of STD or new or multiple sex partners. Clinicians should also consider local epidemiology. Chlamydia screen should be repeated in 3rd trimester if at continued risk.

HR2 = Women under age 25 with two or more sex partners in the last year, or whose sex partner has multiple sexual contacts; women who exchange sex for money or drugs; and women with a history of repeated episodes of gonorrhea. Clinicians should also consider local epidemiology. Gonorrhea screen should be repeated in the third trimester if at continued risk.

HR3 = In areas where universal screening is not performed due to low prevalence of HIV infection, pregnant women with the following individual risk factors should be screened: past or present injection drug use; women who exchange sex for money or drugs; injection drug–using, bisexual, or HIV-positive sex partner currently or in the past; blood transfusion during 1978-1985; persons seeking treatment for STDs.

HR4 = Women who are initially HBsAg negative who are at high risk due to injection drug use, suspected exposure to hepatitis B during pregnancy, multiple sex partners.

HR5 = Women who exchange sex for money or drugs, women with other STDs (including HIV), and sexual contacts of persons with active syphilis. Clinicians should also consider local epidemiology.

HR6 = Women who continue to inject drugs.

HR7 = Unsensitized D-negative women.

HR8 = Prior pregnancy affected by Down syndrome, advanced maternal age (≥35 yr), known carriage of chromosome rearrangement.

HR9 = Women with previous pregnancy affected by neural tube defect.

V

IMMUNIZATIONS AND CHEMOPROPHYLAXIS
Childhood Immunizations

TABLE 5-6, A Recommended Childhood Immunization Schedule—United States

Recommended childhood immunization schedule—United States

Vaccine ▼ / Age ▶	Birth	1 mo	2 mos	4 mos	6 mos	12 mos	15 mos	18 mos	24 mos	4-6 yrs	11-12 yrs	13-18 yrs
											Preadolescent Assessment	
Hepatitis B[1]	Hep B #1 only if mother HBsAg (−)		Hep B #2			Hep B #3				Hep B series		
Diphtheria, tetanus, pertussis[2]			DTaP	DTaP	DTaP		DTaP			DTaP	Td	
Haemophilus influenzae type b[3]			Hib	Hib	Hib	Hib						
Inactivated polio			IPV	IPV		IPV				IPV		
Measles, mumps, rubella[4]						MMR #1				MMR #2	MMR #2	
Varicella[5]						Varicella				Varicella		
Pneumococcal[6]			PCV	PCV	PCV	PCV				PCV	PCV	
Hepatitis A[7]										Hepatitis A series		
Influenza[8]						Influenza (yearly)						

Range of Recommended Ages — *Catch-Up Vaccination* — *Preadolescent Assessment*

.... Vaccines below this line are for selected populations

This schedule indicates the recommended ages for routine administration of currently licensed childhood vaccines for children through age 18 years. Any dose not given at the recommended age should be given at any subsequent visit when indicated and feasible. ▓ Indicates age groups that warrant special effort to administer those vaccines not previously given. Additional vaccines may be licensed and recommended during the year. Licensed combination vaccines may be used whenever any components of the combination are indicated and the vaccine's other components are not contraindicated. Providers should consult the manufacturers' package inserts for detailed recommendations.

1. Hepatitis B vaccine (Hep B). All infants should receive the first dose of hepatitis B vaccine soon after birth and before hospital discharge; the first dose may also be given by age 2 months if the infant's mother is HBsAg-negative. Only monovalent hepatitis B vaccine can be used for the birth dose. Monovalent or combination vaccine containing Hep B may be used to complete the series. Four doses of vaccine may be administered when a birth dose is given. The second dose should be given at least 4 weeks after the first dose, except for combination vaccines, which cannot be administered before age 6 weeks. The third dose should be given at least 16 weeks after the first dose and at least 8 weeks after the second dose. The last dose in the vaccination series (third or fourth dose) should not be administered before age 6 months.

Infants born to HBsAg-positive mothers should receive hepatitis B vaccine and 0.5 ml hepatitis B immune globulin (HBIG) within 12 hours of birth at separate sites. The second dose is recommended at age 1-2 months. The last dose in the vaccination series should not be administered before age 6 months. These infants should be tested for HBsAg and anti-HBs at 9-15 months of age.

Infants born to mothers whose HBsAg status is unknown should receive the first dose of the hepatitis B vaccine series within 12 hours of birth. Maternal blood should be drawn as soon as possible to determine the mother's HBsAg status; if the HBsAg test is positive, the infant should receive HBIG as soon as possible (no later than age 1 week). The second dose is recommended at age 1-2 months. The last dose in the vaccination series should not be administered before age 6 months.

2. Diphtheria and tetanus toxoids and acellular pertussis vaccine (DTaP). The fourth dose of DTaP may be administered as early as age 12 months, provided 6 months have elapsed since the third dose and the child is unlikely to return at age 15-18 months. **Tetanus and diphtheria toxoids (Td)** is recommended at age 11-12 years if at least 5 years have elapsed since the last dose of tetanus and diphtheria toxoid-containing vaccine. Subsequent routine Td boosters are recommended every 10 years.

3. Haemophilus influenzae type b (Hib) conjugate vaccine. Three Hib conjugate vaccines are licensed for infant use. If PRP-OMP (PedvaxHIB or ComVax [Merck] is administered at ages 2 and 4 months, a dose at age 6 months is not required. DTaP/Hib combination products should not be used for primary immunization in infants at ages 2, 4, or 6 months, but can be used as boosters following any Hib vaccine.

4. Measles, mumps, and rubella vaccine (MMR). The second dose of MMR is recommended routinely at age 4-6 years but may be administered during any visit, provided at least 4 weeks have elapsed since the first dose and that both doses are administered beginning at or after age 12 months. Those who have not previously received the second dose should complete the schedule by the 11- to 12-year-old visit.

5. Varicella vaccine. Varicella vaccine is recommended at any visit at or after age 12 months for susceptible children (i.e., those who lack a reliable history of chickenpox). Susceptible persons aged ≥ 13 years should receive two doses, given at least 4 weeks apart.

6. Pneumococcal vaccine. The heptavalent **pneumococcal conjugate vaccine (PCV)** is recommended for all children age 2-23 months. It is also recommended for certain children age 24-59 months. **Pneumococcal polysaccharide vaccine (PPV)** is recommended in addition to PCV for certain high-risk groups. See MMWR 2000;49(RR-9):1-38.

7. Hepatitis A vaccine. Hepatitis A vaccine is recommended for children and adolescents in selected states and regions, and for certain high-risk groups; consult your local public health authority. Children and adolescents in these states, regions, and high-risk groups who have not been immunized against hepatitis A can begin the hepatitis A vaccination series during any visit. The two doses in the series should be administered at least 6 months apart. See MMWR 1999;48(RR-12):1-37.

8. Influenza vaccine. Influenza vaccine is recommended annually for children age ≥ 6 months. Children aged ≤ 12 years should receive vaccine in a dosage appropriate for their age (0.25 ml if age 6-35 months or 0.5 ml if aged ≥ 3 years). Children aged ≤ 8 years who are receiving influenza vaccine for the first time should receive two doses separated by at least 4 weeks.

For additional information about vaccines, including precautions and contraindications for immunization and vaccine shortages, please visit the National Immunization Program Web site at www.cdc.gov/nip or call the National Immunization Hotline at 800-232-2522 (English) or 800-232-0233 (Spanish).
Approved by the Advisory Committee on Immunization Practices (www.cdc.gov/nip/acip), the American Academy of Pediatrics (www.aap.org), and the American Academy of Family Physicians (www.aafp.org).

TABLE 5-6, B Catch-up Schedule for Children 4 Months Through 6 Years of Age

MINIMUM INTERVAL BETWEEN DOSES

DOSE ONE (MINIMUM AGE)	DOSE ONE TO DOSE TWO	DOSE TWO TO DOSE THREE	DOSE THREE TO DOSE FOUR	DOSE FOUR TO DOSE FIVE
DTaP (6 wk)	4 wk	4 wk	6 mo	6 mo[a]
IPV (6 wk)	4 wk	4 wk	4 wk[b]	
Hep B:[c] (birth)	4 wk	8 wk (and 16 wk after first dose)		
MMR (12 mo)	4 wk[d]			
Varicella (12 mo)				
Hib[e] (6 wk)	4 wk: if first dose given at age <12 mo	4 wk[f]: if current age <12 mo	8 wk (as final dose): this dose only necessary for children aged 12 mo to 5 yr who received three doses before age 12 mo	
	8 wk (as final dose): if first dose given at age 12 to 14 mo	8 wk (as final dose): if current age ≥12 mo and second dose given at age <15 mo		
	No further doses needed: if first dose given at age ≥15 mo	No further doses needed: if previous dose given at age ≥15 mo		
PCV[g] (6 wk)	4 wk: if first dose given at age <12 mo and current age <24 mo	4 wk: if current age <12 months	8 wk (as final dose): this dose only necessary for children aged 12 mo to 5 yr who received three doses before age 12 mo	
	8 wk (as final dose): if first dose given at age ≥12 mo or current age 24 to 59 mo	8 wk (as final dose): if current age ≥12 mo		
	No further doses needed: for healthy children if first dose given at age ≥24 mo	No further doses needed: for healthy children if previous dose given at age ≥24 mo		

Approved by the Advisory Committee on Immunization Practices (www.cdc.gov/nip/acip), the American Academy of Pediatrics (www.aap.org), and the American Academy of Family Physicians (www.aafp.org).
DTaP, Diphtheria and tetanus toxoids and acellular pertussis vaccine; *Hib, Haemophilus influenzae* type b vaccine; *IPV,* inactivated polio vaccine; *MMR,* measles-mumps-rubella vaccine; *PCV,* pneumococcal conjugate vaccine.
[a]DTaP: The fifth dose is not necessary if the fourth dose was given after the fourth birthday.
[b]IPV: For children who received an all-IPV or all-OPV series, a fourth dose is not necessary if third dose was given at age ≥4 years. If OPV and IPV were given as part of a series, a total of four doses should be given, regardless of the child's current age.
[c]Hep B: All children and adolescents who have not been immunized against hepatitis B should begin the hepatitis B vaccination series during any visit. Providers should make special efforts to immunize children who were born in, or whose parents were born in, areas of the world where hepatitis B virus infection is moderately or highly endemic.
[d]MMR: The second dose of MMR is recommended routinely at age 4-6 years, but may be given earlier if desired.
[e]Hib: Vaccine is not generally recommended for children aged ≥5 years.
[f]Hib: If current age <12 months and the first two doses were PRP-OMP (PedvaxHIB or ComVax), the third (and final) dose should be given at age 12-15 months and at least 8 weeks after the second dose.
[g]PCV: Vaccine is not generally recommended for children aged ≥5 years.
NOTE: Report adverse reactions to vaccine through the federal Vaccine Adverse Event Reporting System. For information on reporting reactions following vaccines, please visit www.vaers.org or call the 24-hour national toll-free information line 800-822-7967. Report suspected cases of vaccine-preventable diseases to your state or local health department.

TABLE 5-6, C Catch-up Schedule for Children 7 Through 18 Years of Age

MINIMUM INTERVAL BETWEEN DOSES

DOSE ONE TO DOSE TWO	DOSE TWO TO DOSE THREE	DOSE THREE TO BOOSTER DOSE
Td: 4 wk	Td: 6 mo	Td*:
		6 mo: if first dose given at age <12 mo and current age <11 yr
		5 yr: if first dose given at age ≥12 mo and third dose given at age <7 yr and current age ≥11 yr
		10 yr: if third dose given at age ≥7 yr
IPV†: 4 wk	IPV†: 4 wk	IPV†
Hep B: 4 wk	Hep B: 8 wk (and 16 wk after first dose)	
MMR: 4 wk		
Varicella‡: 4 wk		

Approved by the Advisory Committee on Immunization Practices (www.cdc.gov/nip/acip), the American Academy of Pediatrics (www.aap.org), and the American Academy of Family Physicians (www.aafp.org).
IPV, Inactivated polio vaccine; *MMR,* measles-mumps-rubella vaccine; *Td,* tetanus-diphtheria (toxoid) vaccine.
*Td: For children 7 to 10 years of age, the interval between the third and booster dose is determined by the age when the first dose was given. For adolescents 11 to 18 years of age, the interval is determined by the age when the third dose was given.
†IPV: Vaccine is not generally recommended for persons aged ≥18 years.
‡Varicella: Give two-dose series to all susceptible adolescents aged ≥13 years.
NOTE: Report adverse reactions to vaccines through the federal Vaccine Adverse Event Reporting System. For information on reporting reactions following vaccines, please visit www.vaers.org or call the 24-hour national toll-free information line 800-822-7967. Report suspected cases of vaccine-preventable diseases to your state or local health department.

V

TABLE 5-6, D Minimal Age for Initial Childhood Vaccinations and Minimal Interval Between Vaccine Doses by Type of Vaccine[a]

VACCINE TYPE	MINIMAL AGE FOR DOSE 1	MINIMAL INTERVAL BETWEEN DOSES 1 AND 2	MINIMAL INTERVAL BETWEEN DOSES 2 AND 3	MINIMAL INTERVAL BETWEEN DOSES 3 AND 4
Hepatitis B	Birth	1 mo	2 mo	[b]
DTaP (DT)[c]	6 wk	4 wk	4 wk	6 mo
Combined DTwP–Hib[d]	6 wk	1 mo	1 mo	6 mo
Hib (primary series)				
HbOC	6 wk	1 mo	1 mo	[d]
PRP-T	6 wk	1 mo	1 mo	[d]
PRP-OMP	6 wk	1 mo	[d]	
Inactivated poliovirus	6 wk	4 wk	4 wk[e]	[f]
Pneumococcal conjugate	6 wk	1 mo	1 mo	[d]
MMR	12 mo[g]	1 mo		
Varicella	12 mo	4 wk		

Modified from *Epidemiology and prevention of vaccine-preventable diseases*, ed 6, Atlanta, 2000, Centers for Disease Control and Prevention.

DTaP (DT), Diphtheria and tetanus toxoids and acellular pertussis vaccine (diphtheria and tetanus toxoids vaccine); *DTwP–Hib*, diphtheria and tetanus toxoids and whole-cell pertussis vaccine–*Haemophilus influenzae* type b conjugate vaccine; *HbOC*, oligosaccharides conjugated to diphtheria CRM_{197} toxin protein; *MMR*, measles-mumps-rubella vaccine; *PRP-OMP*, polyribosylribitol phosphate polysaccharide conjugated to a meningococcal outer membrane protein; *PRP-T*, polyribosylribitol phosphate polysaccharide conjugated to tetanus toxoid.

[a]The minimal acceptable ages and intervals may not correspond with the optimal recommended ages and intervals for vaccination. For current recommended routine schedules, see the annual Recommended Childhood Immunization Schedule on the facing page.

[b]This final dose of hepatitis B vaccine is recommended at least 4 months after the first dose and no earlier than 6 months of age.

[c]The total number of doses of diphtheria and tetanus toxoids should not exceed six each before the seventh birthday.

[d]The booster doses of Hib and pneumococcal vaccines that are recommended following the primary vaccination series should be administered no earlier than 12 months of age and at least 2 months after the previous dose.

[e]For unvaccinated adults at increased risk of exposure to poliovirus with less than 3 months but more than 2 months available before protection is needed, 3 doses of IPV should be administered at least 1 month apart.

[f]If the third dose is given after the third birthday, the fourth (booster) dose is not needed.

[g]Although the age for measles vaccination may be as young as 6 months in outbreak areas where cases are occurring in children younger than 1 year, children initially vaccinated before the first birthday should be revaccinated at 12-15 months of age and an additional dose of vaccine should be administered at the time of school entry or according to local policy. Doses of MMR or other measles-containing vaccines should be separated by at least 1 month.

TABLE 5-7 Accelerated Schedule of Routine Childhood Immunizations if Necessary for Travel

VACCINE	ROUTINE SCHEDULE	ACCELERATED SCHEDULE
Diphtheria, tetanus, pertussis	DTaP: 2, 4, 6, 15-18 mo of age	DTaP: 6 wk of age, with 4 wk between 1st, 2nd, and 3rd doses, and 6 mo between 3rd and 4th doses
	DTaP: 4-6 yr of age (booster)	DTaP: 4 yr of age
	dT every 10 yr	dT every 5 yr if at high risk
Poliomyelitis	IPV: at 2 and 4 mo, 6-18 mo, and 4-6 yr	IPV: 6 wk of age, with 1 mo between 1st and 2nd doses and 6 mo between 2nd and 3rd doses
	No additional boosters unless traveling to an endemic area	A single IPV lifetime booster for adolescents and adults who have completed primary immunization
Measles, mumps. rubella	MMR: 12-15 mo of age, with second dose at age 4-6 yr	Two doses at ≥12 mo of age, 4 wk apart
	Not routinely recommended for children <12 mo of age	May give first measles as early as age 6 mo, with additional two doses ≥12 mo of age
Haemophilus influenzae type b	2, 4, 6 (if HbOC or PRP-T), and 12-15 mo	HbOC and PRP-T: 6 wk of age, with 1 mo between the 1st and 2nd and the 2nd and 3rd doses; booster at ≥12 mo of age (≥2 mo from the 3rd dose)
		PRO-OMP: 6 wk of age, with 1 mo between the 1st and 2nd doses; booster at ≥12 mo of age (≥2 mo from the 3rd dose)
Hepatitis B	Birth, 1-2 mo, 6 mo	0, 1, and 4 mo of age
Varicella	12-18 mo of age	12 mo of age (two doses 1 mo apart for persons age ≥13 yr)
Rotavirus	2, 4, 6 mo of age	6 wk of age, with 2nd and 3rd doses each separated by 3 wk

From Behrman RE: *Nelson textbook of pediatrics*, ed 16, Philadelphia, 2000, WB Saunders.

TABLE 5-8 Recommended Immunization Schedule for HIV-Infected Children*

AGE ▶ / VACCINE ▼	BIRTH	1 MO	2 MOS	4 MOS	6 MOS	12 MOS	15 MOS	18 MOS	24 MOS	4-6 YRS	11-12 YRS	14-16 YRS
↪ Recommendations for these vaccines are the same as those for immunocompetent children ↪												
Hepatitis B†	Hep B-1		Hep B-2		Hep B-3						Hep B‡	
Diphtheria, Tetanus, Pertussis¶			DTaP or DTP	DTaP or DTP	DTaP or DTP		DTaP or DTP			DTaP or DTP	Td	
Haemophilus** *influenzae* type b			Hib	Hib	Hib	Hib						
↪ Recommendations for these vaccines differ from those for immunocompetent children ↪												
Polio††			IPV	IPV		IPV			IPV			
Measles, Mumps, Rubella§§						MMR	MMR					
Influenza¶¶						Influenza (a dose is required every year)						
Streptococcus pneumoniae***									Pneumo-coccal			
Varicella						CONTRAINDICATED in all HIV-infected persons						

Modified from *MMWR Morb Mortal Wkly Rep* 46(RR-12), 1997.

NOTE: Modified from the immunization schedule for immunocompetent children. This schedule also applies to children born to HIV-infected mothers whose HIV infection status has not been determined. Once a child is known not to be HIV-infected, the schedule for immunocompetent children applies. This schedule indicates the recommended age for routine administration of currently licensed childhood vaccines. Some combination vaccines are available and may be used whenever administration of all components of the vaccine is indicated. Providers should consult the manufacturers' package inserts for detailed recommendations.

*Vaccines are listed under the routinely recommended ages. Bars indicate range of acceptable ages for vaccination. Shaded bars indicate catch-up vaccination: at 11-12 yrs of age, hepatitis B vaccine should be administered to children not previously vaccinated.

†*Infants born to HBsAg-negative mothers* should receive 2.5 μg of Merck vaccine (Recombivax HB) or 10 μg of SmithKline Beecham (SB) vaccine (Engerix-B). The 2nd dose should be administered >1 mo after the 1st dose.

Infants born to HBsAg-positive mothers should receive 0.5 ml of hepatitis B immune globulin (HBIG) within 12 hr of birth and either 5 μg of Merck vaccine (Recombivax HB) or 10 μg of SB vaccine (Engerix-B) at a separate site. The 2nd dose is recommended at 1-2 mo of age and the 3rd dose at 6 mo of age.

Infants born to mothers whose HBsAg status is unknown should receive either 5 μg of Merck vaccine (Recombivax HB) or 10 μg of SB vaccine (Engerix-B) within 12 hr of birth. The 2nd dose of vaccine is recommended at 1 mo of age and the 3rd dose at 6 mo of age. Blood should be drawn at the time of delivery to determine the mother's HBsAg status; if it is positive, the infant should receive HBIG as soon as possible (no later than 1 wk of age). The dosage and timing of subsequent vaccine doses should be based upon the mother's HBsAg status.

§Children and adolescents who have not been vaccinated against hepatitis B in infancy may begin the series during any childhood visit. Those who have not previously received three doses of hepatitis B vaccine should initiate or complete the series during the 11- to 12-year-old visit. The 2nd dose should be administered at least 1 mo after the 1st dose, and the 3rd dose should be administered at least 4 mo after the 1st dose and at least 2 mo after the 2nd dose.

¶DTaP (diphtheria and tetanus toxoids and acellular pertussis vaccine) is the preferred vaccine for all doses in the vaccination series, including completion of the series in children who have received > one dose of whole-cell DTP vaccine. Whole-cell DTP is an acceptable alternative to DTaP. The 4th dose of DTaP may be administered as early as 12 mo of age, provided 6 mo have elapsed since the 3rd dose, and if the child is considered unlikely to return at 15-18 mo of age. Td (tetanus and diphtheria toxoids, adsorbed, for adult use) is recommended at 11-12 yr of age if at least 5 yr have elapsed since the last dose of DTP, DTaP, or DT. Subsequent routine Td boosters are recommended every 10 yr.

**Three *H. influenzae* type b (Hib) conjugate vaccines are licensed for infant use. If PRP-OMP (PedvaxHIB [Merck]) is administered at 2 and 4 mo of age, a dose at 6 mo is not required. After the primary series has been completed, any Hib conjugate vaccine may be used as a booster.

††Inactivated poliovirus vaccine (IPV) is the only polio vaccine recommended for HIV-infected persons and their household contacts. Although the 3rd dose of IPV is generally administered at 12-18 mo, the 3rd dose of IPV has been approved to be administered as early as 6 mo of age. Oral poliovirus vaccine (OPV) should NOT be administered to HIV-infected persons or their household contacts.

§§MMR should not be administered to severely immunocompromised children. HIV-infected children without severe immunosuppression should routinely receive their first dose of MMR as soon as possible upon reaching the 1st birthday. Consideration should be given to administering the second dose of MMR vaccine as soon as 1 mo (i.e., minimum 28 days) after the 1st dose, rather than waiting until school entry.

¶¶Influenza virus vaccine should be administered to all HIV-infected children >6 mo of age each year. Children aged 6 mo-8 yr who are receiving influenza vaccine for the first time should receive two doses of split virus vaccine separated by at least 1 mo. In subsequent years, a single dose of vaccine (split virus for persons ≤12 yr of age, whole or split virus for persons >12 yr of age) should be administered each year. The dose of vaccine for children aged 6-35 mo is 0.25 ml; the dose for children aged ≥3 yr is 0.5 ml.

***Pneumococcal vaccine should be administered to HIV-infected children at 24 mo of age. Revaccination should generally be offered to HIV-infected children vaccinated 3-5 yr (children aged ≤10 yr) or >5 yr (children aged >10 yr) earlier.

V

TABLE 5-9 **Immunizations for Immunocompromised Infants and Children**

VACCINE	ROUTINE	HIV/AIDS	SEVERE IMMUNO-SUPPRESSION*	ASPLENIA	RENAL FAILURE	DIABETES
Routine Infant Immunizations						
DTaP/DTP (DT/T/Td)	Recommended	Recommended	Recommended	Recommended	Recommended	Recommended
IPV	Recommended	Recommended	Recommended	Use as indicated	Use as indicated	Use as indicated
MMR/MR/M/R	Recommended	Recommended/considered	Contraindicated	Recommended	Recommended	Recommended
Hib	Recommended	Recommended	Recommended	Recommended	Recommended	Recommended
Hepatitis B	Recommended	Recommended	Recommended	Recommended	Recommended	Recommended
Varicella	Recommended	Contraindicated/considered§	Contraindicated	Contraindicated	Use if indicated	Use if indicated
Rotavirus	Recommended	Contraindicated	Contraindicated	Contraindicated	Use if indicated	Use if indicated
Other Childhood Immunizations						
Pneumococcus†	Use if indicated	Recommended	Recommended	Recommended	Recommended	Recommended
Influenza‡	Use if indicated	Recommended	Recommended	Recommended	Recommended	Recommended

Modified from Centers for Disease Control and Prevention: Recommendations of the Advisory Committee on Immunization Practices (ACIP): Use of vaccines and immune globulins in persons with altered immunity, *MMWR* 42 (RR-4):15, 1993.

*Severe immunosuppression can result from congenital immunodeficiency, HIV infection, leukemia, lymphoma, aplastic anemia, generalized malignancy, alkylating agents, antimetabolites, radiation, or large amounts of corticosteroids.

†Recommended for persons ≥2 yr of age.

‡Not recommended for infants <6 mo of age.

§Varicella vaccine should be considered for asymptomatic or mildly symptomatic HIV-infected children in CDC class N1 or A1 with age-specific CD4$^+$ T-lymphocyte percentages of ≥25%. Eligible children should receive two doses of varicella vaccine with a 3-month interval between doses.

TABLE 5-10 Contraindications to and Precautions in Routine Childhood Vaccinations

TRUE CONTRAINDICATIONS AND PRECAUTIONS	NOT CONTRAINDICATIONS (VACCINES MAY BE ADMINISTERED)

GENERAL FOR ALL ROUTINE VACCINES (DTAP/DTP, OPV, IPV, MMR, HIB, HEPATITIS B, VARICELLA, ROTAVIRUS)

Contraindications

Anaphylactic reaction to a vaccine contraindicates further doses of that vaccine

Anaphylactic reaction to a vaccine constituent contraindicates the use of vaccines containing that substance

Moderate or severe illnesses with or without a fever

Not Contraindications

Mild to moderate local reaction (soreness, redness, swelling), after a dose of an injectable antigen

Low-grade or moderate fever after a prior vaccine dose

Mild acute illness with or without low-grade fever

Current antimicrobial therapy

Convalescent phase of illness

Prematurity (same dose and indications as for normal full-term infants)

Recent exposure to an infectious disease

History of penicillin or other nonspecific allergies or fact that relatives have such allergies

Pregnancy of mother or household contact

Unvaccinated household contact

DTaP/DTP

Contraindications

Encephalopathy within 7 days of administration of previous dose of DTaP/DTP

Precautions*

Temperature of ≥40.5° C (105° F) within 48 hr after vaccination with a prior dose of DTaP/DTP and not attributable to another identifiable cause

Collapse or shocklike state (hypotonic-hyporesponsive episode) within 48 hr of receiving a prior dose of DTaP/DTP

Convulsions within 3 days of receiving a prior dose of DTaP/DTP†

Persistent, inconsolable crying lasting ≥3 hr, within 48 hr of receiving a prior dose of DTaP/DTP

Guillain-Barré syndrome within 6 wk after a dose‡

Not Contraindications

Temperature of <40.5° C (105° F) after a previous dose of DTaP/DTP

Family history of convulsions†

Family history of sudden infant death syndrome

Family history of an adverse event after DTaP/DTP administration

OPV

Contraindications

Infection with HIV or a household contact with HIV infection

Known immunodeficiency (hematologic and solid tumors; congenital immunodeficiency; long-term immunosuppressive therapy)

Immunodeficient household contact

Precaution*

Pregnancy

Not Contraindications

Breast-feeding

Current antimicrobial therapy

Mild diarrhea

IPV

Contraindications

Anaphylactic reaction to neomycin, streptomycin, or polymyxin B

Precaution*

Pregnancy

MMR

Contraindications

Anaphylactic reaction to neomycin or gelatin

Pregnancy

Known immunodeficiency (hematologic and solid tumors; congenital immunodeficiency; long-term immunosuppressive therapy; HIV infection with evidence of severe immunosuppression)

Not Contraindications

Tuberculosis or positive PPD test result

Simultaneous tuberculin skin testing§

Breast-feeding

Pregnancy of mother or household contact of vaccine recipient

Immunodeficient family member or household contact

HIV infection without evidence of severe immunosuppression

Allergic reaction to eggs‖

Nonanaphylactic reactions to neomycin

V

Precautions*

Recent (within 3-11 mo, depending on product and dose)
   administration of a blood product or immune globulin
   preparation
Thrombocytopenia*
History of thrombocytopenic purpura¶

HIB

Contraindications
None

Precautions
None

HEPATITIS B

Contraindications
Anaphylactic reaction to common baker's yeast

Precautions
None

Not contraindications
Pregnancy

VARICELLA

Contraindications
Anaphylactic reaction to neomycin or gelatin
Pregnancy
HIV infection with evidence of severe immunosuppression
Known immunodeficiency (hematologic and solid tumors;
   congenital immunodeficiency; long-term immuno-
   suppressive therapy)

Precautions*
Recent (within 3-11 mo, depending on product and dose)
   administration of a blood product or immune globulin
   preparation
Family history of immunodeficiency**

Not Contraindications
Breast-feeding
Immunodeficiency in a household contact
HIV infection in a household contact
Pregnancy of mother or household contact of vaccine recipient

---

ROTAVIRUS

Contraindications
Hypersensitivity to aminoglycosides, amphotericin B, or
   monosodium glutamate
Moderate or severe febrile illness
Known immunodeficiency (hematologic and solid tumors;
   congenital immunodeficiency; long-term immunosuppressive therapy)
Children of HIV-infected mothers, until tests for HIV infection
   in the infant are negative at ≥2 mo of age by PCR or culture

Precautions*
Acute vomiting or diarrhea

Not Contraindications
Breast-feeding
Immunodeficiency in a household contact
HIV infection in a household contact

This information is based on the recommendations of the Advisory Committee on Immunization Practices (ACIP) and of the Committee on Infectious Diseases of the American Academy of Pediatrics (AAP). Some recommendations may vary from those in the manufacturer's product label. For more detailed information, health care providers should consult the published recommendations of the ACIP, AAP, the American Academy of Family Physicians (AAFP), and the manufacturer's product label. These guidelines have been adapted and updated from Centers for Disease Control and Prevention: Update: vaccine side effects, adverse reactions, contraindications, and precautions. Recommendations of the Advisory Committee on Immunization Practices (ACIP), *MMWR* 45(RR-12):1, 1996.
DTaP, Diphtheria and tetanus toxoids plus acellular pertussis vaccine; *DTP*, diphtheria, tetanus, and pertussis vaccine; *IPV*, inactivated poliovirus vaccine; *MMR*, measles, mumps, and rubella vaccine; *OPV*, oral poliovirus vaccine; *PCR*, polymerase chain reaction; *PPd*, purified protein derivative; *VZIG*, varicella-zoster immune globulin.
*The events or conditions listed as precautions, although not contraindications, should be carefully reviewed. The benefits and risks of administering a specific vaccine to an individual under the circumstances should be considered. If the risks are believed to outweigh the benefits, the vaccine should be withheld; if the benefits are believed to outweigh the risks (e.g., during an outbreak or foreign travel), the vaccine should be administered. Whether and when to administer DTaP/DTP to children with proven or suspected underlying neurologic disorders should be decided individually. Avoiding administration of certain vaccines to pregnant women is prudent on theoretic grounds. If immediate protection against poliomyelitis is needed, either OPV or IPV is recommended.
†Acetaminophen administered before DTaP or DTP vaccination and thereafter every 4 hr for 24 hr should be considered for children with a personal or family history of convulsions in siblings or parents.
‡The decision to give additional doses of DTaP or DTP should be based on consideration of the benefit of further vaccination vs the risk of recurrence of Guillain-Barré syndrome. For example, completion of the primary vaccination series in children is justified.
§Measles vaccination may temporarily suppress tuberculin skin test reactivity. MMR vaccine may be administered after or on the same day as Mantoux tuberculin skin testing. If MMR has been given recently, the tuberculin test should be postponed until 4-6 wk after administration of MMR.
‖Recent data suggest that most anaphylactic reactions to measles- and mumps-containing vaccines are not associated with hypersensitivity to egg antigens but to other components of the vaccines, such as gelatin. Because the risk of anaphylactic reactions after administration of measles- or mumps-containing vaccines by persons who are allergic to eggs is extremely low, and skin testing with vaccine is not predictive of allergic reactions to these vaccines, skin testing and desensitization are no longer required before administration of MMR vaccine to persons who are allergic to eggs.
¶The decision to vaccinate should be based on consideration of the benefits of immunity to measles, mumps, and rubella vs the risk of recurrence or exacerbation of thrombocytopenia after vaccination, or from natural infections of measles or rubella. In most instances, the benefits of vaccination are much greater than the potential risks and justify giving MMR, particularly in view of the even greater risk of thrombocytopenia after measles or rubella disease. However, if a prior episode of thrombocytopenia occurred in close temporal proximity to vaccination, avoiding a subsequent dose may be prudent.
**Varicella vaccine should not be administered to a member of a household with a family history of immunodeficiency until the immune status of the recipient and other children in the family is documented.

TABLE 5-11 Vaccines for Children Who Travel

VACCINE	DESCRIPTION	DOSING	COMMENTS/ CONTRAINDICATIONS	LENGTH OF TRAVEL		
				BRIEF (<2 WK)	INTERMEDIATE (2 WK TO 3 MO)	LONG TERM RESIDENTIAL (>3 MO)
Routine						
Polio*	OPV: live attenuated, oral IPV: inactivated, injection	IPV at 2, 4 mo; OPV at 12-18 mo, 4-6 yr; may accelerate to q 4-8 wk × 3 doses	IPV at 2 and 4 mo decreases risk of polio in undiagnosed immunocompromised infants; AAP recommendation may change to IPV only	+	+	+
Diphtheria-tetanus-pertussis*	DPT: D, T toxoid + whole cell P DtaP: DT toxoid + acellular P Td: booster	DtaP recommended at 2, 4, 6, 15-18 mo and 4-6 yr; Td booster at age 12, then q10yr	May accelerate to dose every 4 wk × 3 doses if necessary; decreased incidence of vaccine-related reactions with DTaP	+	+	+
Haemophilus B*	Hib polysaccharide: protein conjugate	0.5 ml IM at 2, 4, 6, 12-15 mo	Typically given as combination with DTaP	+	+	+
Hepatitis B	Recombivax HB: inactivated viral antigen Engerix-B: same	3 doses: 0, 1, 6 mo <11 yr: 0.25 ml IM >11 yr: 0.5 ml IM 3 doses 0, 1, 6 mo <11 yr: 0.5 ml IM >11 yr: 1.0 ml IM	Some protection after just 1 or 2 doses; may accelerate Engerix-B to 0, 1, 2, 12 mo	+	+	+
Measles-mumps-rubella†	Live attenuated viruses	0.25 ml IM at 12-15 mo, then booster at 4-6 or 11-12 yr	May accelerate to 6-12 mo, repeat 1 mo later, then per usual schedule; give at least 2-3 wk before IgG	+	+	+
Varicella	Live attenuated virus	12 mo-12 yr: 0.5 ml SC as single dose >12 yr: 2 doses 4-8 wk apart	Give at least 2-3 wk before IgG; may be given with MMR using different sites; avoid if immunocompromised	+	+	+
Routine for Travel						
Hepatitis A	Havrix: inactive virus (720ELU) Vaqta (24U)	>2 yr: 2 × 0.5 ml doses 6-12 mo apart	Preferred for hepatitis A protection if over age 2 yr Protects in 4 wk after dose 1	+	+	+
Immune globulin (IgG)	Antibodies	<2 yr: 0.02 ml/kg for <3 mo of travel; 0.06 ml/kg q5mo and 3 days before travel	Hepatitis A protection for those under age 2 yr; beware of timing with live virus vaccines			

Consult Centers for Disease Control and Prevention (CDC) for current and specific vaccine recommendations for destination country. From Auerbach PS: *Wilderness medicine*, ed 4, St Louis, 2001, Mosby.
+, Recommended; ±, consider; *AAP*, American Academy of Pediatrics; *DTaP*, diphtheria and tetanus toxoids plus acellular pertussis vaccine; *IM*, intramuscularly; *q*, every; *SC*, subcutaneously.

TABLE 5-11 **Vaccines for Children Who Travel—cont'd**

				LENGTH OF TRAVEL		
VACCINE	DESCRIPTION	DOSING	COMMENTS/ CONTRAINDICATIONS	BRIEF (<2 WK)	INTERMEDIATE (2 WK TO 3 MO)	LONG TERM RESIDENTIAL (>3 MO)
Required or Geographically Indicated						
Yellow fever	Live virus	>9 mo: 0.5 ml SC at least 10 days before departure; booster q10yr	Required for parts of sub-Saharan Africa, of tropical South America; may give at 4-9 mo if traveling to epidemic area; under 9 mo: risk of vaccine-related encephalitis	+	+	+
Typhoid	Heat inactivated	6 mo-2 yr: 2 × 0.25 ml SC 4 wk apart, booster q3yr	Fever, pain with heat killed: significantly fewer side effects with ViCPS and Ty21a; important for Latin America, Asia, Africa; vaccine not a substitute for eating and drinking cleanly	±	+	+
	ViCPS: polysaccharide Ty21a: oral live attenuated	2-6 yr: 0.5 ml IM × 1 booster q2yr >6 yr: 1 capsule q 2 days × 4; booster q 5 yr				
Meningococcal	Serogroups A, C, Y, W-135: polysaccharide	>2 years: 0.5 ml SC; booster in 1 yr if 1st dose after age 4 yr, otherwise in 5 yr	Use for central Africa, Saudi Arabia for the Hajj, Nepal, and epidemic areas; minimal efficacy under age 2 yr	±	±	±
Japanese encephalitis	Inactivated virus	1-3 yr: 0.5 ml SC at 0, 7, 14-30 days >3 years: 1.0 ml SC at 0, 7, 14-30 days Last dose >10 days before travel	Indicated for parts of India and rural Asia if stay >1 mo; no safety data for under age 1 yr; high rate of hypersensitivity	±	±	+
Cholera	Inactivated bacteria	>6 mo: 0.2 ml SC	Vaccine of questionable efficacy; not recommended by CDC or WHO; do not use under 6 mo			
Lyme disease	LYMErix: antigenic protein*	>15 yr: 0.5 ml IM at 0, 1, 12 mo	Indicated for frequent, prolonged exposure to Lyme-endemic area, not brief exposures			
Extended Stay						
Rabies	HDCV: human diploid cell	1 ml IM in deltoid muscle at 0, 7, 21-28 days if >1 mo stay	If exposed and immunized: give vaccine, 1 ml IM at 0, 3 days If exposed and unimmunized: give rabies Ig (RIG), 20 IU/kg half at site and half IM; give vaccine, 1 ml IM at 0, 3, 7, 14, 28 days	±	+	+

*Not readily available.

TABLE 5-12   Schedule for Catch-Up Administration of PCV (Prevnar) in Unvaccinated Infants and Children

AGE AT FIRST DOSE	PRIMARY SERIES	BOOSTER DOSE
2-6 mo	Three doses, 2 mo apart*	One dose at 12-15 mo†
7-11 mo	Two doses, 2 mo apart*	One dose at 12-15 mo†
12-23 mo	Two doses, 2 mo apart	—
24-59 mo		
Healthy children	One dose	—
Children with sickle cell disease, asplenia, HIV infection, chronic illness, or immunocompromising condition‡	Two doses, 2 mo apart	—

Modified from *MMWR Morb Mortal Wkly Rep* 49(RR-9):24, 2000.
HIV, Human immunodeficiency virus; *PCV*, pneumococcal conjugate vaccine.
*For the primary series in children vaccinated before 12 mo of age, the minimum interval between doses is 4 wk.
†The booster dose should be administered at least 8 wk after the primary series is completed.
‡Recommendations do not include children who have undergone bone marrow transplant.

TABLE 5-13   Administration Schedule for PCV (Prevnar) When a Lapse in Immunization Has Occurred

AGE AT PRESENTATION (MONTHS)	PREVIOUS PCV IMMUNIZATION HISTORY	RECOMMENDED REGIMEN
7 to 11	One dose	One dose at 7 to 11 mo followed by a booster at 12 to 15 mo with a minimal interval of 2 mo
	Two doses	One dose at 7 to 11 mo followed by a booster at 12 to 15 mo with a minimal interval of 2 mo
12 to 23	One dose before 12 mo	Two doses at least 2 mo apart
	Two doses before 12 mo	One dose at least 2 mo following the most recent dose
24 to 59	Any incomplete schedule	One dose*

Modified from *MMWR Morb Mortal Wkly Rep* 49(RR-9):24, 2000.
PCV, Pneumococcal conjugate vaccine.
*Children with certain chronic illnesses or immunosuppressing conditions should receive two doses at least 2 mo apart.

TABLE 5-14   Using PPV in High-Risk Children 2 Years and Older Who Have Been Immunized with PCV (Prevnar)

HEALTH STATUS	PPV SCHEDULE	REVACCINATE WITH PPV
Healthy	None	No
Sickle cell disease, anatomic or functional asplenia, HIV-infection, immunocompromising conditions	1 dose PPV given at least 2 mo after PCV	Yes*
Chronic illness	1 dose PPV given at least 2 mo after PCV	No

Modified from *MMWR Morb Mortal Wkly Rep* 49(RR-9):24, 2000.
HIV, Human immunodeficiency virus; *PCV*, pneumococcal conjugate vaccine; *PPV*, pneumococcal polysaccharide vaccine.
* If patient is older than 10 yr, a single revaccination should be given at least 5 yr after previous dose; if patient is 10 yr or younger, revaccinate 3 to 5 yr after previous dose. Regardless of when administered, a second dose of PPV should not be given less than 3 yr following the previous PPV dose.

V

TABLE 5-15, A   Recommended Adult Immunization Schedule—United States

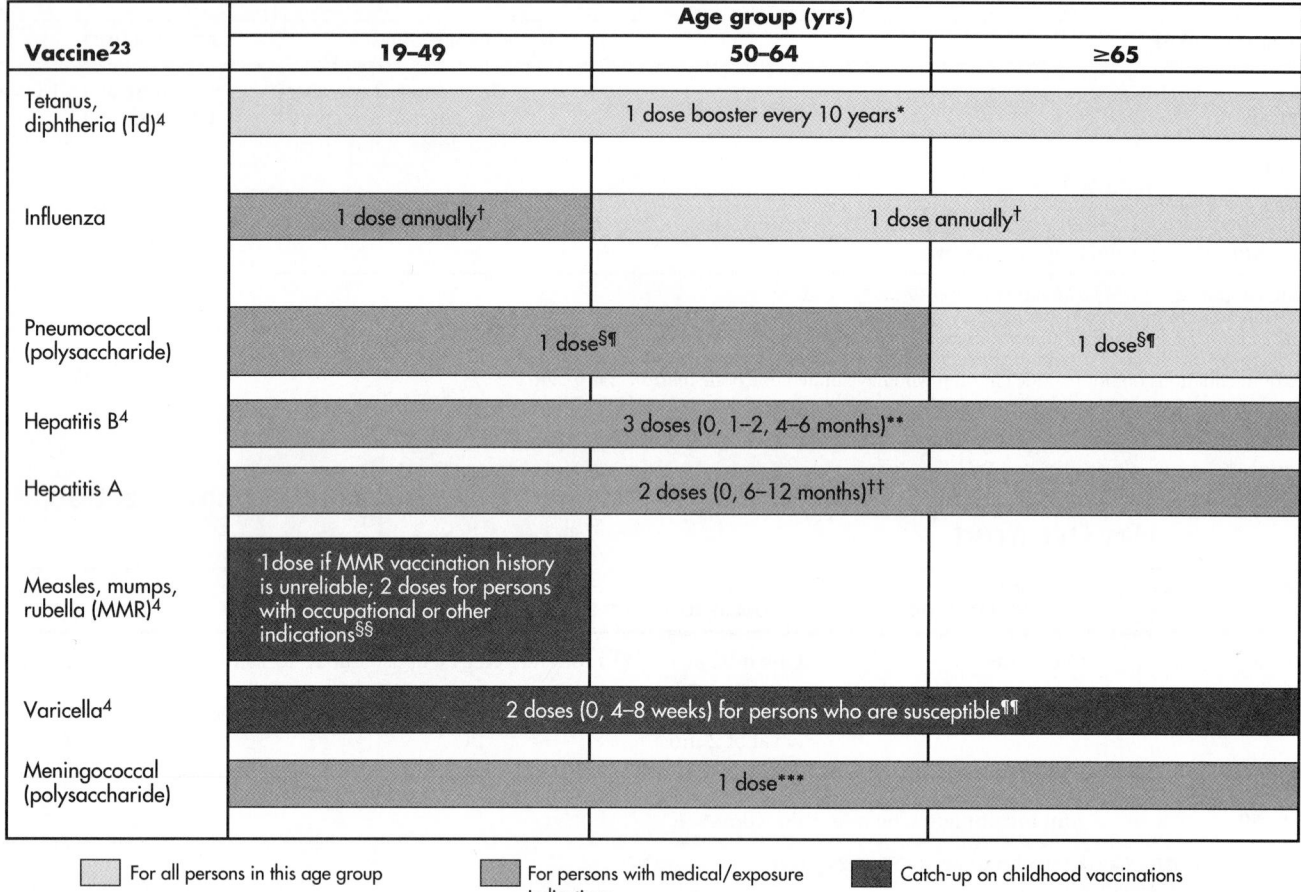

Vaccine[23]	Age group (yrs)		
	19–49	**50–64**	**≥65**
Tetanus, diphtheria (Td)[4]	1 dose booster every 10 years*		
Influenza	1 dose annually†	1 dose annually†	
Pneumococcal (polysaccharide)	1 dose§¶		1 dose§¶
Hepatitis B[4]	3 doses (0, 1–2, 4–6 months)**		
Hepatitis A	2 doses (0, 6–12 months)††		
Measles, mumps, rubella (MMR)[4]	1 dose if MMR vaccination history is unreliable; 2 doses for persons with occupational or other indications§§		
Varicella[4]	2 doses (0, 4–8 weeks) for persons who are susceptible¶¶		
Meningococcal (polysaccharide)	1 dose***		

▢ For all persons in this age group   ▢ For persons with medical/exposure indications   ▢ Catch-up on childhood vaccinations

[1]Approved by the Advisory Committee on Immunization Practices and accepted by the American College of Obstetricians and Gynecologists (ACOG) and the American Academy of Family Physicians (AAFP).

[2]This schedule indicates recommended age groups for routine administration of currently licensed vaccines for persons aged ≥19 years. Licensed combination vaccine may be used whenever any components of the combination are indicated and the vaccine's other components are not contraindicated. Health-care providers should consult manufacturers' package inserts for detailed recommendations.

[3]Additional information regarding these vaccines and contraindications for vaccination is available from the National Immunization Hotline (telephone, 800-232-2522 [English] or 800-232-0233 [Spanish] or at http://www.cdc.gov/nip.

[4]Covered by the Vaccine Injury Compensation Program. Information on how to file a claim is available at http://www.hrsa.gov/osp/vicp or by telephone, 800-338-2382. Vaccine injury claims are filed with U.S. Court of Federal Claims, 717 Madison Place, N.W., Washington, D.C. 20005; telephone, 202-219-9657.

***Tetanus and diphtheria (Td).** Adults, including pregnant women with uncertain histories of a complete primary vaccination series, should receive a primary series of Td. A primary series for adults is 3 doses: the first 2 doses administered at least 4 weeks apart and the third dose, 6–12 months after the second. Administer 1 dose if the person received the primary series and the last vaccination was ≥10 years previously. In addition, information is available regarding administration of Td as prophylaxis in wound management (1). The American College of Physicians Task Force on Adult Immunization supports a second option for Td use in adults: a single Td booster at age 50 years for persons who have completed the full pediatric series, including the teenage/young adult booster.

†**Influenza vaccination.** *Medical indications:* chronic disorders of the cardiovascular or pulmonary systems including asthma; chronic metabolic diseases including diabetes mellitus, renal dysfunction, hemoglobinopathies, or immunosuppression (including immunosuppression caused by medications or by human immunodeficiency virus [HIV]) requiring medical follow-up or hospitalization during the preceding year; women who will be in the second or third trimester of pregnancy during the influenza season. *Occupational indications:* health-care workers (HCWs). *Other indications:* residents of nursing homes and other long-term-care facilities; persons likely to transmit influenza to persons at high risk (e.g., in-home caregivers to persons with medical indications; household contact and out-of-home caregivers for children aged ≤23 months, or children with asthma or other indicator conditions for influenza vaccination; household members and caregivers for elderly and adults with high-risk conditions); and anyone who wishes to be vaccinated. For healthy persons age 5-49 years without high-risk conditions, either the inactivated vaccine or the intranasally administered influenza vaccine (FluMist™) may be administered (2,3).

§**Pneumococcal polysaccharide vaccination.** *Medical indications:* chronic disorders of the pulmonary system, excluding asthma, cardiovascular diseases, diabetes mellitus, chronic liver diseases (including liver disease as a result of alcohol abuse [e.g., cirrhosis]), chronic renal failure or nephrotic syndrome, functional or anatomic asplenia (e.g., sickle cell disease or splenectomy), immunosuppressive conditions (e.g., congenital immunodeficiency, HIV infection, leukemia, lymphoma, multiple myeloma, Hodgkins disease, generalized malignancy, and organ or bone marrow transplantation), chemotherapy with alkylating agents, antimetabolites, or long-term systemic corticosteroids. *Geographic/other indications:* Alaska Natives and certain American Indian populations. *Other indications:* residents of nursing homes and other long-term-care facilities (4).

¶**Revaccination with pneumococcal polysaccharide vaccine.** One-time revaccination after 5 years for persons with chronic renal failure or nephrotic syndrome, functional or anatomic asplenia (e.g., sickle cell disease or splenectomy), immunosuppressive conditions (e.g., congenital immunodeficiency, HIV infection, leukemia, lymphoma, multiple myeloma, Hodgkins disease, generalized malignancy, and organ or bone marrow transplantation), chemotherapy with alkylating agents, antimetabolites, or long-term systemic corticosteroids. For persons aged ≥65 years, one-time revaccination if they were vaccinated ≥5 years previously and were aged <65 years at the time of primary vaccination (4).

**Hepatitis B (HepB) vaccine. *Medical indications:* hemodialysis patients, patients who receive clotting-factor concentrates. *Occupational indications:* HCWs and public-safety workers who have exposure to blood in the workplace, persons in training in schools of medicine, dentistry, nursing, laboratory technology, and other allied health professions. *Behavioral indications:* injection-drug users, persons with more than one sex partner during the previous 6 months, persons with a recently acquired sexually transmitted disease (STD), all clients in STD clinics, men who have sex with men (MSM). *Other indications:* household contacts and sex partners of persons with chronic Hepatitis B virus (HBV) infection, clients and staff of institutions for the developmentally disabled, international travelers to countries with high or intermediate prevalence of chronic HBV infection for >6 months, and inmates of correctional facilities (5).

††Hepatitis A (HepA) vaccine. For the combined HepA-HepB vaccine, use 3 doses (at 0, 1, and 6 months). *Medical indications:* persons with clotting-factor disorders or chronic liver disease. *Behavioral indications:* MSM, users of injecting and noninjecting illegal drugs. *Occupational indications:* persons working with Hepatitis A virus (HAV)-infected primates or with HAV in a research laboratory setting. *Other indications:* persons traveling to or working in countries that have high or intermediate endemicity of HAV (6).

§§Measles, Mumps, Rubella (MMR) vaccination. *Measles component:* adults born before 1957 might be considered immune to measles. Adults born in or after 1957 should receive at least 1 dose of MMR unless they have a medical contraindication, documentation of at least 1 dose, or other acceptable evidence of immunity. A second dose of MMR is recommended for adults who 1) were exposed recently to measles or were in an outbreak setting, 2) were previously vaccinated with killed measles vaccine, 3) were vaccinated with an unknown vaccine during 1963–1967, 4) are students in postsecondary educational institutions, 5) work in health-care facilities, or 6) plan to travel internationally. *Mumps component:* 1 dose of MMR should be adequate for protection. *Rubella component:* Administer 1 dose of MMR to women whose rubella vaccination history is unreliable and counsel women to avoid becoming pregnant for 4 weeks after vaccination. For women of childbearing age, regardless of birth year, routinely determine rubella immunity and counsel women regarding congenital rubella syndrome. Do not vaccinate pregnant women or those planning to become pregnant in the next 4 weeks. If pregnant and susceptible, vaccinate as early in the postpartum period as possible (7).

¶¶Varicella vaccination. Recommended for all persons who do not have reliable clinical history of varicella infection, or serologic evidence of varicella zoster virus (VZV) infection who might be at high risk for exposure or transmission. This includes HCWs and family contacts of immunocompromised persons, those who live or work in environments where transmission is likely (e.g., teachers of young children, day-care employees, and residents and staff members in institutional settings), persons who live or work in environments where VZV transmission can occur (e.g., college students, inmates and staff members of correctional institutions, and military personnel) adolescents and adults living in households with children, women who are not pregnant but who might become pregnant in the future, and international travelers who are not immune to infection. Do not vaccinate pregnant women or those planning to become pregnant in the next 4 weeks. If a woman is pregnant and susceptible, vaccinate as early in the postpartum period as possible. Approximately 95% of U.S.-born adults are immune to VZV (8,9).

***Meningococcal vaccine (quadrivalent polysaccharide for serogroups A, C, Y, and W-135). Consider vaccination for persons with medical indications: adults with terminal complement component deficiencies or with anatomic or functional asplenia. Other indications: travelers to countries where meningitis is hyperendemic or epidemic (e.g., the "meningitis belt" of sub-Saharan Africa, Mecca, or Saudi Arabia). Revaccination at 3–5 years may be indicated for persons at high risk for infection (e.g., persons residing in areas in which disease is epidemic). Counsel college freshmen, particularly those who live in dormitories, regarding meningococcal disease and the vaccine so that they can make an educated decision about receiving the vaccination (10). The American Academy of Family Physicians recommends that colleges provide education on meningococcal infection and vaccination and offer it to those who are interested. Physicians need not initiate discussion of the meningococcal quadrivalent polysaccharide vaccine as part of routine medical care.

References
1. CDC. Diphtheria, tetanus, and pertussis: recommendations for vaccine use and other preventive measures. Recommendations of the Immunization Practices Advisory Committee (ACIP). MMWR 1991;40(No. RR-10).
2. CDC. Prevention and control of influenza: recommendations of the Advisory Committee for Immunization Practices. MMWR 2003;52(No. RR-8).
3. CDC. Using live, attenuated influenza vaccine for prevention and control of influenza: supplemental recommendations of the Advisory Committee on Immunization Practices (ACIP). MMWR 2003;52(No. RR-13).
4. CDC. Prevention of pneumococcal disease: recommendations of the Advisory Committee on Immunization Practices (ACIP). MMWR 1997;47(No. RR-8).
5. CDC. Hepatitis B virus: a comprehensive strategy for eliminating transmission in the United States through universal childhood vaccination. Recommendations of the Immunization Practices Advisory Committee (ACIP). MMWR 1991;40(No. RR-13).
6. CDC. Prevention of hepatitis A through active or passive immunization: recommendations of the Advisory Committee on Immunization Practices (ACIP). MMWR 1999;48(No. RR-12).
7. CDC. Measles, mumps, and rubella—vaccine use and strategies for elimination of measles, rubella, and congenital rubella syndrome and control of mumps: recommendations of the Advisory Committee on Immunization Practices (ACIP) MMWR 1998;47(No. RR-8).
8. CDC. Prevention of varicella: recommendations of the Advisory Committee on Immunization Practices (ACIP). MMWR 1996;45(No. RR-11).
9. CDC. Prevention of varicella: updated recommendations of the Advisory Committee on Immunization Practices (ACIP). MMWR 1999;48(No. RR-6).
10. CDC. Prevention and control of meningococcal disease and meningococcal disease and college students: recommendations of the Advisory Committee on Immunization Practices (ACIP). MMWR 2000;49(No. RR-7).
11. *MMRW Morb Mortal Wkly Rep* 52, 2003.

V

TABLE 5-15, B   Recommended Adult Immunization Schedule for Adults with Medical Conditions—United States

Medical condition	Tetanus-diptheria (Td)*	Influenza†	Pneumococcal (polysaccharide)§¶	Hepatitis B**	Hepatitis A††	Measles, mumps, rubella (MMR)§§	Varicella¶¶
Pregnancy		A					
Diabetes, heart disease, chronic pulmonary disease, and chronic liver disease, including chronic alcoholism		B	C		D		
Congenital immunodeficiency, leukemia, lymphoma, generalized malignancy, therapy with alkylating agents, antimetabolites, radiation, or large amounts of corticosteroids			E				F
Renal failure/end-stage renal disease and patients receiving hemodialysis or clotting factor concentrates			E	G			
Asplenia, including elective splenectomy and terminal complement-component deficiencies		H	E,I,J				
Human immunodeficiency virus (HIV) infection			E,K			L	

Legend:
- ▢ For all persons in this group
- ▨ For persons with medical/exposure indications
- ▩ Catch-up on childhood vaccinations
- ▮ Contraindicated

From *MMWR Morb Mortal Wkly Rep* 52, 2003.

A. For women without chronic diseases/conditions, vaccinate if pregnancy will be at second or third trimester during influenza season. For women with chronic diseases/conditions, vaccinate at any time during the pregnancy.

B. Although chronic liver disease and alcoholism are not indicator conditions for influenza vaccination, administer 1 dose annually if the patient is aged >50 years, has other indications for influenza vaccine, or requests vaccination.

C. Asthma is an indicator condition for influenza but not for pneumococcal vaccination.

D. For all persons with chronic liver disease.

E. For persons aged <65 years, revaccinate once after ≥5 years have elapsed since initial vaccination.

F. Persons with impaired humoral but not cellular immunity may be vaccinated (9).

G. For hemodialysis patients use special formulation of vaccine (40 μg/mL) or two 1.0 mL 20 μg doses administered at one site. Vaccinate early in the course of renal disease. Assess antibody titers to hepatitis B surface antigen (anti-HBs) levels annually. Administer additional doses if anti-HBs levels decline to ≤10 mIU/mL.

H. No data have been reported specifically on risk for severe or complicated influenza infections among persons with asplenia. However, influenza is a risk factor for secondary bacterial infections that might cause severe disease in asplenics.

I. Administer meningococcal vaccine and consider *Haemophilus influenzae* type b vaccine.

J. In the event of elective splenectomy, vaccinate >2 weeks before surgery.

K. Vaccinate as close to diagnosis as possible when CD4 cell counts are highest.

L. Withhold MMR or other measles-containing vaccines from HIV-infected persons with evidence of severe immunosuppression.
   Please refer to Table 15-5A for footnote explanations.

TABLE 5-16   Immunizations during Pregnancy

IMMUNO-BIOLOGIC AGENT	RISK FROM DISEASE TO PREGNANT WOMAN	RISK FROM DISEASE TO FETUS OR NEONATE	TYPE OF IMMUNIZING AGENT	RISK FROM IMMUNIZING AGENT TO FETUS	INDICATIONS FOR IMMUNIZATION DURING PREGNANCY	DOSE SCHEDULE	COMMENTS
Live Virus Vaccines							
Measles	Significant morbidity, low mortality; not altered by pregnancy	Significant increase in abortion rate; may cause malformations	Live attenuated virus vaccine	None confirmed	Contraindicated (see immune globulins)	Single dose SC, preferably as measles-mumps-rubella*	Vaccination of susceptible women should be part of postpartum care
Mumps	Low morbidity and mortality; not altered by pregnancy	Probable increased rate of abortion in first trimester	Live attenuated virus vaccine	None confirmed	Contraindicated	Single dose SC, preferably as measles-mumps-rubella	Vaccination of susceptible women should be part of postpartum care
Poliomyelitis	No increased incidence in pregnancy, but may be more severe if it does occur	Anoxic fetal damage reported; 50% mortality in neonatal disease	Live attenuated virus (oral polio vaccine [OPV]) and enhanced-potency inactivated virus (e-IPV) vaccine†	None confirmed	Not routinely recommended for women in U.S., except persons at increased risk of exposure	*Primary:* Two doses of e-IPV SC at 4-8 wk intervals and a third dose 6-12 mo after the second dose *Immediate protection:* One dose OPV orally (in out-break setting)	Vaccine indicated for susceptible pregnant women traveling in endemic areas or in other high-risk situations
Rubella	Low morbidity and mortality; not altered by pregnancy	High rate of abortion and congenital rubella syndrome	Live attenuated virus vaccine	None confirmed	Contraindicated	Single dose SC, preferably as measles-mumps-rubella	Teratogenicity of vaccine is theoretic, not confirmed to date; vaccination of susceptible women should be part of postpartum care
Yellow fever	Significant morbidity and mortality; not altered by pregnancy	Unknown	Live attenuated virus vaccine	Unknown	Contraindicated except if exposure is unavoidable	Single dose SC	Postponement of travel preferable to vaccination, if possible

Continued

V

TABLE 5-16 Immunizations during Pregnancy—cont'd

IMMUNO-BIOLOGIC AGENT	RISK FROM DISEASE TO PREGNANT WOMAN	RISK FROM DISEASE TO FETUS OR NEONATE	TYPE OF IMMUNIZING AGENT	RISK FROM IMMUNIZING AGENT TO FETUS	INDICATIONS FOR IMMUNIZATION DURING PREGNANCY	DOSE SCHEDULE	COMMENTS
Inactivated Virus Vaccines							
Influenza	Possible increase in morbidity and mortality during epidemic of new antigenic strain	Possible increased abortion rate; no malformations confirmed	Inactivated virus vaccine	None confirmed	Women with serious underlying diseases; public health authorities to be consulted for current recommendation	One dose IM every year	
Rabies	Near 100% fatality; not altered by pregnancy	Determined by maternal disease	Killed virus vaccine	Unknown	Indications for prophylaxis not altered by pregnancy; each case considered individually	Public health authorities to be consulted for indications, dosage, and route of administration	
Hepatitis B	Possible increased severity during third trimester	Possible increase in abortion rate and prematurity; neonatal hepatitis can occur; high risk of newborn carrier state	Recombinant vaccine	None reported	Preexposure and postexposure for women at risk of infection	Three- or four-dose series IM	Used with hepatitis B immune globulin for some exposures; exposed newborn needs vaccination as soon as possible
Inactivated Bacterial Vaccines							
Cholera	Significant morbidity and mortality; more severe during third trimester	Increased risk of fetal death during third-trimester maternal illness	Killed bacterial vaccine	None confirmed	Indications not altered by pregnancy; vaccination recommended only in unusual outbreak situations	Single dose SC or IM, depending on manufacturer's recommendations when indicated	
Plague	Significant morbidity and mortality; not altered by pregnancy	Determined by maternal disease	Killed bacterial vaccine	None reported	Selective vaccination of exposed persons	Public health authorities to be consulted for indications, dosage, and route of administration	
Pneumococcus	No increased risk during pregnancy; no increase in severity of disease	Unknown	Polyvalent polysaccharide vaccine	No data available on use during pregnancy	Indications not altered by pregnancy; vaccine used only for high-risk individuals	In adults, one SC or IM dose only; consider repeat dose in 6 yr for high-risk individuals	

Immunobiologic agent	Risk from disease to pregnant woman	Risk from disease to fetus/neonate	Type of immunizing agent	Risk from immunizing agent to fetus	Indications for immunization during pregnancy	Dose schedule	Comments
Typhoid	Significant morbidity and mortality; not altered by pregnancy	Unknown	Killed or live attenuated oral bacterial vaccine	None confirmed	Not recommended routinely except for close, continued exposure or travel to endemic areas	*Killed; Primary:* Two injections SC at least 4 wk apart. *Booster:* Single dose SC or ID (depending on type of product used) every 3 yr. *Oral; Primary:* Four doses on alternate days. *Booster:* Schedule not yet determined	
Toxoids							
Tetanus, diphtheria	Severe morbidity; tetanus mortality 30%, diphtheria mortality 10%; unaltered by pregnancy	Neonatal tetanus mortality 60%	Combined tetanus-diphtheria toxoids preferred: adult tetanus-diphtheria formulation	None confirmed	Lack of primary series, or no booster within past 10 yr	*Primary:* Two doses IM at 1-2 mo interval with a third dose 6-12 mo after the second. *Booster:* Single dose IM every 10 yr, after completion of primary series	Updating of immune status should be part of antepartum care
Specific Immune Globulins							
Hepatitis B	Possible increased severity during third trimester	Possible increase in abortion rate and prematurity; neonatal hepatitis can occur; high risk of carriage in newborn	Hepatitis B immune globulin	None reported	Postexposure prophylaxis	Depends on exposure; consult Immunization Practices Advisory Committee recommendations	Usually given with HBV vaccine; exposed newborn needs immediate postexposure prophylaxis

Continued

V

TABLE 5-16 Immunizations during Pregnancy—cont'd

IMMUNO-BIOLOGIC AGENT	RISK FROM DISEASE TO PREGNANT WOMAN	RISK FROM DISEASE TO FETUS OR NEONATE	TYPE OF IMMUNIZING AGENT	RISK FROM IMMUNIZING AGENT TO FETUS	INDICATIONS FOR IMMUNIZATION DURING PREGNANCY	DOSE SCHEDULE	COMMENTS
Specific Immune Globulins—cont'd							
Rabies	Near 100% fatality; not altered by pregnancy	Determined by maternal disease	Rabies immune globulin	None reported	Postexposure prophylaxis	Half dose at injury site, half dose in deltoid	Used in conjunction with rabies killed virus vaccine
Tetanus	Severe morbidity; mortality 21%	Neonatal tetanus mortality 60%	Tetanus immune globulin	None reported	Postexposure prophylaxis	One dose IM	Used in conjunction with tetanus toxoid
Varicella	Possible increase in severe varicella pneumonia	Can cause congenital varicella with increased mortality in neonatal period; very rarely causes congenital defects	Varicella-zoster immune globulin (obtained from the American Red Cross)	None reported	Can be considered for healthy pregnant women exposed to varicella to protect against maternal, not congenital, infection	One dose IM within 96 hr of exposure	Indicated also for newborns of mothers who developed varicella within 4 days before delivery or 2 days after delivery; approximately 90%-95% of adults are immune to varicella; not indicated for prevention of congenital varicella
Standard Immune Globulins							
Hepatitis A	Possible increased severity during third trimester	Probable increase in abortion rate and prematurity; possible transmission to neonate at delivery if mother is incubating the virus or is acutely ill at that time	Standard immune globulin		Postexposure prophylaxis	0.02 ml/kg IM in one dose of immune globulin	Immune globulin should be given as soon as possible and within 2 wk of exposure; infants born to mothers who are incubating the virus or are acutely ill at delivery should receive one dose of 0.5 ml as soon as possible after birth
Measles	Significant morbidity, low mortality; not altered by pregnancy	Significant increase in abortion rate; may cause malformations	Standard immune globulin		Postexposure prophylaxis	0.25 ml/kg IM in one dose of immune globulin, up to 15 ml	Unclear if it prevents abortion; must be given within 6 days of exposure

From *ACOG Technical Bulletin*, No 160, Oct 1991.
PO, Orally; *SC*, subcutaneously.
*Two doses necessary for adequate vaccination of students entering institutions of higher education, newly hired medical personnel, and international travelers.
†Inactivated polio vaccine recommended for nonimmunized adults at increased risk.
From *ACOG Technical Bulletin*, No 160, Oct 1991.
ID, Intradermally; *IM*, intramuscularly.

TABLE 5-17 **Immunizing Agents and Immunization Schedules for Health-Care Workers (HCWs)***

GENERIC NAME	PRIMARY SCHEDULE AND BOOSTER(S)	INDICATIONS	MAJOR PRECAUTIONS AND CONTRAINDICATIONS	SPECIAL CONSIDERATIONS
Immunizing Agents Strongly Recommended for Health-Care Workers				
Hepatitis B (HB) recombinant vaccine	Two doses IM 4 wk apart; third dose 5 mo after second; booster doses not necessary.	**Preexposure:** HCWs at risk for exposure to blood or body fluids.	Based on limited data no risk of adverse effects to developing fetuses is apparent. Pregnancy should *not* be considered a contra-indication to vaccination of women. Previous anaphylactic reaction to common baker's yeast is a contraindication to vaccination.	The vaccine produces neither therapeutic nor adverse effects on HBV-infected persons. Prevaccination serologic screening is not indicated for persons being vaccinated because of occupational risk. HCWs who have contact with patients or blood should be tested 1-2 mo after vaccination to determine serologic response.
Hepatitis B immune globulin (HBIG)	0.06 ml/kg IM as soon as possible after exposure. A second dose of HBIG should be administered 1 mo later if the HB vaccine series has not been started.	**Postexposure** prophylaxis: For persons exposed to blood or body fluids containing HBsAg and who are not immune to HBV infection—0.06 ml/kg IM as soon as possible (but no later than 7 days after exposure).		
Influenza vaccine (inactivated whole-virus and split-virus vaccines)	Annual vaccination with current vaccine. Administered IM.	HCWs who have contact with patients at high risk for influenza or its complications; HCWs who work in chronic care facilities; HCWs with high-risk medical conditions or who are aged ≥65 yr.	History of anaphylactic hypersensitivity to egg ingestion.	No evidence exists of risk to mother or fetus when the vaccine is administered to a pregnant woman with an underlying high-risk condition. Influenza vaccination is recommended during second and third trimesters of pregnancy because of increased risk for hospitalization.
Measles live-virus vaccine	One dose SC; second dose at least 1 mo later.	HCWs† born during or after 1957 who do not have documentation of having received two doses of live vaccine on or after the first birthday **or** a history of physician-diagnosed measles or serologic evidence of immunity. Vaccination should be considered for all HCWs who lack proof of immunity, including those born before 1957.	Pregnancy; immuno-compromised persons‡, including HIV-infected persons who have evidence of severe immunosuppression; anaphylaxis after gelatin ingestion or administration of neomycin; recent administration of immune globulin.	MMR is the vaccine of choice if recipients are likely to be susceptible to rubella and/or mumps as well as to measles. Persons vaccinated during 1963-1967 with a killed measles vaccine alone, killed vaccine followed by live vaccine, or with a vaccine of unknown type should be revaccinated with two doses of live measles virus vaccine.

Modified from *MMWR Morb Mortal Wkly Rep* 46(RR-18), 1998.
HBsAg, Hepatitis B surface antigen; *HBV,* hepatitis B virus; *HIV,* human immunodeficiency virus; *IM,* intramuscular; *MMR,* measles, mumps, rubella vaccine; *SC,* subcutaneous.
*Persons who provide health care to patients or work in institutions that provide patient care (e.g., physicians, nurses, emergency medical personnel, dental professionals and students, medical and nursing students, laboratory technicians, hospital volunteers, and administrative and support staff in health-care institutions).
†All HCWs (i.e., medical or nonmedical, paid or volunteer, full time or part time, student or nonstudent, with or without patient-care responsibilities) who work in health-care institutions (e.g., inpatient and outpatient, public and private) should be immune to measles, rubella, and varicella.
‡Persons immunocompromised because of immune deficiency diseases, HIV infection, leukemia, lymphoma or generalized malignancy or immunosuppressed as a result of therapy with corticosteroids, alkylating drugs, antimetabolites, or radiation.

V

TABLE 5-17 Immunizing Agents and Immunization Schedules for Health-Care Workers (HCWs)*—cont'd

GENERIC NAME	PRIMARY SCHEDULE AND BOOSTER(S)	INDICATIONS	MAJOR PRECAUTIONS AND CONTRAINDICATIONS	SPECIAL CONSIDERATIONS
Mumps live-virus vaccine	One dose SC; no booster	HCWs† believed to be susceptible can be vaccinated. Adults born before 1957 can be considered immune.	Pregnancy; immunocompromised persons‡; history of anaphylactic reaction after gelatin ingestion or administration of neomycin	MMR is the vaccine of choice if recipients are likely to be susceptible to measles and rubella as well as to mumps.
Hepatitis A vaccine	Two doses of vaccine either 6-12 mo apart (HAVRIX), or 6 mo apart (VAQTA)	Not routinely indicated for HCWs in the United States. Persons who work with HAV-infected primates or with HAV in a research laboratory setting should be vaccinated.	History of anaphylactic hypersensitivity to alum or, for HAVRIX, the preservative 2-phenoxyethanol. The safety of the vaccine in pregnant women has not been determined; the risk associated with vaccination should be weighed against the risk for hepatitis A in women who may be at high risk for exposure to HAV.	
Meningococcal polysaccharide vaccine (tetravalent A, C, W135, and Y)	One dose in volume and by route specified by manufacturer; need for boosters unknown	Not routinely indicated for HCWs in the United States.	The safety of the vaccine in pregnant women has not been evaluated; it should not be administered during pregnancy unless the risk for infection is high.	
Typhoid vaccine, IM, SC, and oral	*IM vaccine:* One 0.5-ml dose, booster 0.5 ml every 2 yr. SC vaccine: two 0.5 ml doses, ≥4 wk apart, booster 0.5 ml SC or 0.1 ID every 3 yr if exposure continues *Oral vaccine:* Four doses on alternate days. The manufacturer recommends revaccination with the entire four-dose series every 5 yr	Workers in microbiology laboratories who frequently work with *Salmonella typhi*	Severe local or systemic reaction to a previous dose. Ty21a (oral) vaccine should not be administered to immunocompromised persons† or to persons receiving antimicrobial agents.	Vaccination should not be considered an alternative to the use of proper procedures when handling specimens and cultures in the laboratory.
Vaccinia vaccine (smallpox)	One dose administered with a bifurcated needle; boosters administered every 10 yr	Laboratory workers who directly handle cultures with vaccinia, recombinant vaccinia viruses, or orthopox viruses that infect humans	The vaccine is contraindicated in pregnancy, in persons with eczema or a history of eczema, and in immunocompromised persons† and their household contacts.	Vaccination may be considered for HCWs who have direct contact with contaminated dressings or other infectious material from volunteers in clinical studies involving recombinant vaccinia virus.

*Persons who provide health care to patients or work in institutions that provide patient care (e.g., physicians, nurses, emergency medical personnel, dental professionals and students, medical and nursing students, laboratory technicians, hospital volunteers, and administrative and support staff in health-care institutions).

†All HCWs (i.e., medical or nonmedical, paid or volunteer, full time or part time, student or nonstudent, with or without patient-care responsibilities) who work in health-care institutions (e.g., inpatient and outpatient, public and private) should be immune to measles, rubella, and varicella.

‡Persons immunocompromised because of immune deficiency diseases, HIV infection, leukemia, lymphoma or generalized malignancy or immunosuppressed as a result of therapy with corticosteroids, alkylating drugs, antimetabolites, or radiation.

Continued

TABLE 5-17 **Immunizing Agents and Immunization Schedules for Health-Care Workers (HCWs)*—cont'd**

GENERIC NAME	PRIMARY SCHEDULE AND BOOSTER(S)	INDICATIONS	MAJOR PRECAUTIONS AND CONTRAINDICATIONS	SPECIAL CONSIDERATIONS
Other Vaccine-Preventable Diseases				
Tetanus and diphtheria (toxoids [Td])	Two IM doses 4 wk apart; third dose 6-12 mo after second dose; booster every 10 yr	All adults	Except in the first trimester, pregnancy is not a precaution. History of a neurologic reaction or immediate hypersensitivity reaction after a previous dose. History of severe local (Arthus-type) reaction after a previous dose. Such persons should not receive further routine or emergency doses of Td for 10 yr.	Tetanus prophylaxis in wound management‡
Pneumococcal polysaccharide vaccine (23 valent)	One dose, 0.5 ml, IM or SC; revaccination recommended for those at highest risk ≥5 yr after the first dose	Adults who are at increased risk of pneumococcal disease and its complications because of underlying health conditions; older adults, especially those age ≥65 who are healthy	The safety of vaccine in pregnant women has not been evaluated; it should not be administered during pregnancy unless the risk for infection is high. Previous recipients of any type of pneumococcal polysaccharide vaccine who are at highest risk for fatal infection or antibody loss may be revaccinated ≥5 yr after the first dose.	
Rubella live-virus vaccine	One dose SC; no booster	Indicated for HCWs,† both men and women, who do not have documentation of having received live vaccine on or after their first birthday **or** laboratory evidence of immunity. Adults born before 1957, **except women who can become pregnant,** can be considered immune.	Pregnancy; immunocompromised persons†; history of anaphylactic reaction after administration of neomycin	The risk for rubella vaccine–associated malformations in the offspring of women pregnant when vaccinated or who become pregnant within 3 mo after vaccination is negligible. Such women should be counseled regarding the theoretic basis of concern for the fetus. MMR is the vaccine of choice if recipients are likely to be susceptible to measles or mumps, as well as to rubella.
Varicella zoster live-virus vaccine	Two 0.5-ml doses SC 4-8 wk apart if ≥13 yr of age	Indicated for HCWs† who do not have either a reliable history of varicella or serologic evidence of immunity	Pregnancy, immunocompromised persons,‡ history of anaphylactic reaction following receipt of neomycin or gelatin. Avoid salicylate use for 6 wk after vaccination.	Vaccine is available from the manufacturer for certain patients with acute lymphocytic leukemia (ALL) in remission. Because 71%-93% of persons without a history of varicella are immune, serologic testing before vaccination is likely to be cost-effective.

Modified from *MMWR Morb Mortal Wkly Rep* 46(RR-18), 1998.

V

TABLE 5-17   Immunizing Agents and Immunization Schedules for Health-Care Workers (HCWs)*—cont'd

GENERIC NAME	PRIMARY SCHEDULE AND BOOSTER(S)	INDICATIONS	MAJOR PRECAUTIONS AND CONTRAINDICATIONS	SPECIAL CONSIDERATIONS
Varicella-zoster immune globulin (VZIG)	Persons <50 kg: 125 μ/10 kg IM; persons ≥50 kg: 625 μ§	Persons known or likely to be susceptible (particularly those at high risk for complications, e.g., pregnant women) who have close and prolonged exposure to a contact case or to an infectious hospital staff worker or patient		Serologic testing may help in assessing whether to administer VZIG. If use of VZIG prevents varicella disease, patient should be vaccinated subsequently.

BCG Vaccination

GENERIC NAME	PRIMARY SCHEDULE AND BOOSTER(S)	INDICATIONS	MAJOR PRECAUTIONS AND CONTRAINDICATIONS	SPECIAL CONSIDERATIONS
Bacille Calmette Guérin (BCG) vaccine (tuberculosis)	One percutaneous dose of 0.3 ml; no booster dose recommended	Should be considered only for HCWs in areas where multi-drug tuberculosis is prevalent, a strong likelihood of infection exists, and where comprehensive infection control precautions have failed to prevent TB transmission to HCWs	Should not be administered to immunocompromised persons,‡ pregnant women	In the United States tuberculosis-control efforts are directed toward early identification, treatment of cases, and preventive therapy with isoniazid.

Other Immunobiologics That Are or May Be Indicated for Health-Care Workers

GENERIC NAME	PRIMARY SCHEDULE AND BOOSTER(S)	INDICATIONS	MAJOR PRECAUTIONS AND CONTRAINDICATIONS	SPECIAL CONSIDERATIONS
Immune globulin (hepatitis A)	**Postexposure**—One IM dose of 0.02 ml/kg administered ≤2 wk after exposure	Indicated for HCWs exposed to feces of infectious patients	Contraindicated in persons with IgA deficiency; do not administer within 2 wk after MMR vaccine, or 3 wk after varicella vaccine. Delay administration of MMR vaccine for ≥3 mo and varicella vaccine ≥5 mo after administration of IG	Administer in large muscle mass (deltoid, gluteal).

§Some experts recommend 125 μ/10 kg regardless of total body weight.

TABLE 5-18   Recommendations for Persons with Medical Conditions Requiring Special Vaccination Considerations

CONDITION	TD	MMR	VARICELLA	HBV	HAV	PNEUMOVAX[a]	INFLUENZA[b]	HbCV	MENINGOCOCCAL	IPV	OTHER LIVE VACCINES[c]	OTHER KILLED VACCINES[d]
HIV infection	Rou	Rou/Contr[e]	Contr[f]	Rou[g]	Rou	Rec	Rec	Cons	Rou	Rou	Contr	Rou
Severe immuno-compromise[h]	Rou	Contr	Contr[f]	Rou[g]	Rou	Rec	Rec	Rou[i]	Rou	Rou	Contr	Rou
Renal failure	Rou	Rou	Rou	Rec[g]	Rou	Rec	Rec	Rou	Rou	Rou	Rou	Rou
Diabetes	Rou	Rou	Rou	Rou	Rou	Rec	Rec	Rou	Rou	Rou	Rou	Rou
Chronic liver disease	Rou	Rou	Rou	Rou	Rec	Rec	Rec	Rou	Rou	Rou	Rou	Rou
Cardiac disease	Rou	Rou	Rou	Rou	Rou	Rec	Rec	Rou	Rou	Rou	Rou	Rou
Pulmonary disease	Rou	Rou	Rou	Rou	Rou	Rec	Rec	Rou	Rou	Rou	Rou	Rou
Alcoholism	Rou	Rou	Rou	Rou	Rou	Rec	Rec	Rou	Rou	Rou	Rou	Rou
Functional/anatomic asplenia	Rou	Rou	Rou	Rou	Rou	Rec[j]	Rec	Rec[j]	Rec[j]	Rou	Rou	Rou
Terminal complement deficiency	Rou	Rou	Rou	Rou	Rou	Rou	Rou	Rou	Rec	Rou	Rou	
Clotting factor disorders	Rou	Rou	Rou	Rec	Rec	Rou	Rou	Rou	Rou	Rou		Rou

Modified and updated from *MMWR Morb Mortal Wkly Rep* 42(RR-4):16 and 17, 1993.

Cons, Consider vaccination; *Contr*, contraindicated; *Rec*, recommended; *Rou*, routine as outlined for all adults.

[a]Pneumovax should be repeated in 5 years for patients in whom vaccine is recommended.

[b]Influenza vaccine should also be given to caregivers and household members.

[c]Includes bacille Calmette-Guérin, vaccinia, oral typhoid, yellow fever (if exposure cannot be avoided, persons with HIV can be given yellow fever vaccine; see text).

[d]Includes rabies (check postvaccination titers in HIV or severely immunocompromised persons), Lyme, inactivated typhoid, cholera, plague, and anthrax.

[e]For asymptomatic, nonseverely immunocompromised persons with human immunodeficiency virus (HIV), MMR can be considered in symptomatic HIV patients without severe immunocompromise.

[f]Varicella can be given to household members and caregivers, but if varicella-like rash develops after vaccination, contact should be avoided.

[g]Recommended for persons with severe chronic renal failure approaching or already receiving dialysis, and higher doses should be given. Antibody titers should be measured after vaccination in these patients and in those with HIV or severe immunocompromise (who may require higher doses) to ensure adequate response. Yearly titers should be measured in dialysis patients.

[h]Severe immunocompromise can result from congenital immunodeficiency, leukemia, lymphoma, malignancy, organ transplant, chemotherapy, radiation therapy, or high-dose corticosteroids.

[i]Only for persons with Hodgkin's disease.

[j]Give at least 2 weeks in advance of elective splenectomy.

V

TABLE 5-19, A   Recommended and minimum ages and intervals between vaccine doses[a]

VACCINE AND DOSE NUMBER	RECOMMENDED AGE FOR THIS DOSE	MINIMUM AGE FOR THIS DOSE	RECOMMENDED INTERVAL TO NEXT DOSE	MINIMUM INTERVAL TO NEXT DOSE
Hepatitis B1[b]	Birth-2 mo	Birth	1-4 mo	4 wk
Hepatitis B2	1-4 mo	4 wk	2-17 mo	8 wk
Hepatitis B3[c]	6-18 mo	6 mo[d]	—	—
Diphtheria and tetanus toxoids and acellular pertussis (DTaP)1	2 mo	6 wk	2 mo	4 wk
DTaP2	4 mo	10 wk	2 mo	4 wk
DTaP3	6 mo	14 wk	6-12 mo	6 mo[d,e]
DTaP4	15-18 mo	12 mo	3 yr	6 mo[d]
DTaP5	4-6 yr	4 yr	—	—
Haemophilus influenzae, type b (Hib)1[b,f]	2 mo	6 wk	2 mo	4 wk
Hib2	4 mo	10 wk	2 mo	4 wk
Hib3[g]	6 mo	14 wk	6-9 mo	8 wk
Hib4	12-15 mo	12 mo	—	—
Inactivated poliovirus vaccine (IPV)1	2 mo	6 wk	2 mo	4 wk
IPV2	4 mo	10 wk	2-14 mo	4 wk
IPV3	6-18 mo	14 wk	3.5 yr	4 wk
IPV4	4-6 yr	18 wk	—	—
Pneumococcal conjugate vaccine (PCV)1[f]	2 mo	6 wk	2 mo	4 wk
PCV2	4 mo	10 wk	2 mo	4 wk
PCV3	6 mo	14 wk	6 mo	8 wk
PCV4	12-15 mo	12 mo	—	—
Measles, mumps, and rubella (MMR)[i]	12-15 mo[h]	12 mo	3-5 yr	4 wk
MMR2	4-6 yr	13 mo	—	—
Varicella[I]	12-15 mo	12 mo	4 wk[i]	4 wk[i]
Hepatitis A1	≥2 yr	2 yr	6-18 mo[d]	6 mo[d]
Hepatitis A2	≥30 mo	30 mo	—	—
Influenza[j]	—	6 mo[d]	1 mo	4 wk
Pneumococcal poly-saccharide (PPV)1	—	2 yr	5 yr[k]	5 yr
PPV2	—	7 yr[k]	—	—

From *MMWR Morb Mortal Wkly Rep* 51 (RR-2), 2002.

[a]Combination vaccines are available. Using licensed combination vaccines is preferred over separate injections of their equivalent component vaccines (Source: *MMWR* 48[RR-5]:5, 1999). When administering combination vaccines, the minimum age for administration is the oldest age for any of the individual components; the minimum interval between doses is equal to the greatest interval of any of the individual antigens.

[b]A combination hepatitis B-Hib vaccine is available (Comvax(r), manufactured by Merck Vaccine Division). This vaccine should not be administered to infants aged <6 weeks because of the Hib component.

[c]Hepatitis B3 should be administered ≥8 weeks after Hepatitis B2 and 16 weeks after Hepatitis B1, and it should not be administered before age 6 months.

[d]Calendar months.

[e]The minimum interval between DTaP3 and DTaP4 is recommended to be ≥6 months. However, DTaP4 does not need to be repeated if administered ≥4 months after DTaP3.

[f]For Hib and PCV, children receiving the first dose of vaccine at age ≥7 months require fewer doses to complete the series (see *MMWR* 40[RR-1]:1-7, 1991 and *MMWR* 49[RR-9]:1-35, 2000).

[g]For a regimen of only polyribosylribitol phosphate-meningococcal outer membrane protein (PRP-OMP, PedvaxHib(r), manufactured by Merck), a dose administered at age 6 months is not required.

[h]During a measles outbreak, if cases are occurring among infants aged <12 months, measles vaccination of infants aged ≥6 months can be undertaken as an outbreak control measure. However, doses administered at age <12 months should not be counted as part of the series (Source: *MMWR* 47[RR-8]:1-57, 1998).

[i]Children aged 12 months-13 years require only one dose of varicella vaccine. Persons aged ≥13 years should receive two doses separated by ≥4 weeks.

[j]Two doses of inactivated influenza vaccine, separated by 4 weeks, are recommended for children aged 6 months-9 years who are receiving the vaccine for the first time. Children aged 6 months-9 years who have previously received influenza vaccine and persons aged ≥9 years require only one dose per influenza season.

[k]Second doses of PPV are recommended for persons at highest risk for serious pneumococcal infection and those who are likely to have a rapid decline in pneumococcal antibody concentration. Revaccination 3 years after the previous dose can be considered for children at highest risk for severe pneumococcal infection who would be aged <10 years at the time of revaccination (see *MMWR* 46[RR-8]:1-24, 1997).

TABLE 5-19, B   Guidelines for spacing of live and inactivated antigens

ANTIGEN COMBINATION	RECOMMENDED MINIMUM INTERVAL BETWEEN DOSES
≥2 inactivated	None; can be administered simultaneously or at any interval between doses
Inactivated and live	None; can be administered simultaneously or at any interval between doses
≥2 live parenteral*	4-week minimum interval, if not administered simultaneously

From *MMWR Morb Mortal Wkly Rep* 51(RR-2), 2002.
*Live oral vaccines (e.g., Ty21a typhoid vaccine, oral polio vaccine) can be administered simultaneously or at any interval before or after inactivated or live parenteral vaccines.

TABLE 5-19, C   Guidelines for administering antibody-containing products* and vaccines

SIMULTANEOUS ADMINISTRATION

COMBINATION	RECOMMENDED MINIMUM INTERVAL BETWEEN DOSES
Antibody-containing products and inactivated antigen	None; can be administered simultaneously at different sites or at any time between doses
Antibody-containing products and live antigen	Should not be administered simultaneously,† if simultaneous administration of measles-containing vaccine or varicella vaccine is unavoidable, administer at different sites and revaccinate or test for seroconversion after the recommended interval

NONSIMULTANEOUS ADMINISTRATION

PRODUCT ADMINISTERED		
FIRST	SECOND	RECOMMENDED MINIMUM INTERVAL BETWEEN DOSES
Antibody-containing products	Inactivated antigen	None
Inactivated antigen	Antibody-containing products	None
Antibody-containing products	Live antigen	Dose-related‡
Live antigen	Antibody-containing products	2 weeks

From *MMWR Morb Mortal Wkly Rep* 51(RR-2), 2002.
*Blood products containing substantial amounts of immunoglobulin, including intramuscular and intravenous immune globulin, specific hyperimmune globulin (e.g., hepatitis B immune globulin, tetanus immune globulin, varicella zoster immune globulin, and rabies immune globulin), whole blood, packed red cells, plasma, and platelet products.
†Yellow fever and oral Ty21a typhoid vaccines are exceptions to these recommendations. These live attenuated vaccines can be administered at any time before, after, or simultaneously with an antibody-containing product without substantially decreasing the antibody response.
‡The duration of interference of antibody-containing products with the immune response to the measles component of measles-containing vaccine, and possibly varicella vaccine, is dose-related.

V

TABLE 5-20 **Suggested intervals between administration of antibody-containing products for different indications and measles-containing vaccine and varicella vaccine***

PRODUCT/INDICATION	DOSE, INCLUDING MG IMMUNOGLOBULIN G (IGG)/KG BODY WEIGHT*	RECOMMENDED INTERVAL BEFORE MEASLES OR VARICELLA VACCINATION (MO)
Respiratory syncytial virus immune globulin (IG) monoclonal antibody (Synagis™)†	15 mg/kg intramuscularly (IM)	None
Tetanus IG	250 units (10 mg IgG/kg) IM	3
Hepatitis A IG		
Contact prophylaxis	0.02 mL/kg (3.3 mg IgG/kg) IM	3
International travel	0.06 mL/kg (10 mg IgG/kg) IM	3
Hepatitis B IG	0.06 mL/kg (10 mg IgG/kg) IM	3
Rabies IG	20 IU/kg (22 mg IgG/kg) IM	4
Varicella IG	125 units/10 kg (20-40 mg IgG/kg) IM, maximum 625 units	5
Measles prophylaxis IG		
Standard (i.e., nonimmuno-compromised) contact	0.25 mL/kg (40 mg IgG/kg) IM	5
Immunocompromised contact	0.50 mL/kg (80 mg IgG/kg) IM	6
Blood transfusion		
Red blood cells (RBCs), washed	10 mL/kg negligible IgG/kg intravenously (IV)	None
RBCs, adenine-saline added	10 mL/kg (10 mg IgG/kg) IV	3
Packed RBCs (hematocrit 65%)‡	10 mL/kg (60 mg IgG/kg) IV	6
Whole blood (hematocrit 35%-50%)‡	10 mL/kg (80-100 mg IgG/kg) IV	6
Plasma/platelet products	10 mL/kg (160 mg IgG/kg) IV	7
Cytomegalovirus intravenous immune globulin (IGIV)	150 mg/kg maximum	6
Respiratory syncytial virus prophylaxis IGIV	750 mg/kg	9
IGIV		
Replacement therapy for immune deficiencies§	300-400 mg/kg IV§	8
Immune thrombocytopenic purpura	400 mg/kg IV	8
Immune thrombocytopenic purpura	1000 mg/kg IV	10
Kawasaki disease	2 g/kg IV	11

From *MMWR Morb Mortal Wkly Rep* 51(RR-2), 2002.

*This table is not intended for determining the correct indications and dosages for using antibody-containing products. Unvaccinated persons might not be fully protected against measles during the entire recommended interval, and additional doses of immune globulin or measles vaccine might be indicated after measles exposure. Concentrations of measles antibody in an immune globulin preparation can vary by manufacturer's lot. Rates of antibody clearance after receipt of an immune globulin preparation might vary also. Recommended intervals are extrapolated from an estimated half-life of 30 days for passively acquired antibody and an observed interference with the immune response to measles vaccine for 5 months after a dose of 80 mg IgG/kg (Source: Mason W. Takahashi M, Schneider T. Presented at the 32nd meeting of the Interscience Conference on Antimicrobial Agents and Chemotherapy, Los Angeles, Calif., October 1992).

†Contains antibody only to respiratory syncytial virus.

‡Assumes a serum IgG concentration of 16 mg/mL.

§Measles and varicella vaccination is recommended for children with asymptomatic or mildly symptomatic human immunodeficiency virus (HIV) infection but is contraindicated for persons with severe immunosuppression from HIV or any other immunosuppressive disorder.

TABLE 5-21 Guide to contraindications and precautions[a] to commonly used vaccines

VACCINE	TRUE CONTRAINDICATIONS AND PRECAUTIONS[a]	UNTRUE (VACCINES CAN BE ADMINISTERED)
General for all vaccines, including diphtheria and tetanus toxoids and acellular pertussis vaccine (DTaP); pediatric diphtheria-tetanus toxoid (DT); adult tetanus-diphtheria toxoid (Td); inactivated poliovirus vaccine (IPV); measles-mumps-rubella vaccine (MMR); *Haemophilus influenzae* type b vaccine (Hib); hepatitis A vaccine; hepatitis B vaccine; varicella vaccine; pneumococcal conjugate vaccine (PCV); influenza vaccine; and pneumococcal poly-saccharide vaccine (PPV)	**Contraindications** Serious allergic reaction (e.g., anaphylaxis) after a previous vaccine dose Serious allergic reaction (e.g., anaphylaxis) to a vaccine component **Precautions** Moderate or severe acute illness with or without fever	Mild acute illness with or without fever Mild to moderate local reaction (i.e., swelling, redness, soreness); low-grade or moderate fever after previous dose Lack of previous physical examination in well-appearing person Current antimicrobial therapy Convalescent phase of illness Premature birth (hepatitis B vaccine is an exception in certain circumstances)[b] Recent exposure to an infectious disease History of penicillin allergy, other nonvaccine allergies, relatives with allergies, receiving allergen extract immunotherapy
DTaP	**Contraindications** Severe allergic reaction after a previous dose or to a vaccine component Encephalopathy (e.g., coma, decreased level of consciousness; prolonged seizures) within 7 days of administration of previous dose of DTP or DTaP Progressive neurologic disorder, including infantile spasms, uncontrolled epilepsy, progressive encephalopathy; defer DTaP until neurologic status clarified and stabilized **Precautions** Fever of >40.5° C ≤48 hr after vaccination with a previous dose of DTP or DTaP Collapse or shock-like state (i.e., hypotonic hyporesponsive episode) ≤48 hr after receiving a previous dose of DTP/DTaP Seizure ≤days of receiving a previous dose of DTP/DTaP[c] Persistent, inconsolable crying lasting ≥3 hr ≤48 hours after receiving a previous dose of DTP/DTaP Moderate or severe acute illness with or without fever	Temperature of <40.5° C, fussiness or mild drowsiness after a previous dose of diphtheria toxoid-tetanus toxoid-pertussis vaccine (DTP)/DTaP Family history of seizures[c] Family history of sudden infant death syndrome Family of history of an adverse event after DTP or DTaP administration Stable neurologic conditions (e.g., cerebral palsy, well-controlled convulsions, developmental delay)
DT, Td	**Contraindications** Severe allergic reaction after a previous dose or to a vaccine component **Precautions** Guillain-Barré syndrome ≤6 wk after previous dose of tetanus toxoid-containing vaccine Moderate or severe acute illness with or without fever	
IPV	**Contraindications** Severe allergic reaction to previous dose or vaccine component **Precautions** Pregnancy Moderate or severe acute illness with or without fever	
MMR[d]	**Contraindications** Severe allergic reaction after a previous dose or to a vaccine component Pregnancy Known severe immunodeficiency (e.g., hematologic and solid tumors; congenital immunodeficiency; long-term immunosuppressive therapy,[e] or severely symptomatic human immunodeficiency virus [HIV] infection) **Precautions** Recent (≤11 mo) receipt of antibody-containing blood product (specific interval depends on product) History of thrombocytopenia or thrombocytopenic purpura Moderate or severe acute illness with or without fever	Positive tuberculin skin test Simultaneous TB skin testing[f] Breast-feeding Pregnancy of recipient's mother or other close or household contact Recipient is child-bearing-age female Immunodeficient family member or household contact Asymptomatic or mildly symptomatic HIV infection Allergy to eggs
Hib	**Contraindications** Severe allergic reaction after a previous dose or to a vaccine component Age <6 wk **Precaution** Moderate or severe acute illness with or without fever	

V

TABLE 5-21   Guide to contraindications and precautions[a] to commonly used vaccines— cont'd

VACCINE	TRUE CONTRAINDICATIONS AND PRECAUTIONS[a]	UNTRUE (VACCINES CAN BE ADMINISTERED)
Hepatitis B	**Contraindication** Severe allergic reaction after a previous dose or to a vaccine component **Precautions** Infant weighing <2000 g[b] Moderate or severe acute illness with or without fever	Pregnancy Autoimmune disease (e.g., systemic lupus erythematosus or rheumatoid arthritis)
Hepatitis A	**Contraindications** Severe allergic reaction after a previous dose or to a vaccine component **Precautions** Pregnancy Moderate or severe acute illness with or without fever	
Varicella[d]	**Contraindications** Severe allergic reaction after a previous dose or to a vaccine component Substantial suppression of cellular immunity Pregnancy **Precautions** Recent (≤11 mo) receipt of antibody-containing blood product (specific interval depends on product) Moderate or severe acute illness with or without fever	Pregnancy of recipient's mother or other close or household contact Immunodeficient family member of household contact[g] Asymptomatic or mildly symptomatic HIV infection Humoral immunodeficiency (e.g., agammaglobulinemia)
PCV	**Contraindication** Severe allergic reaction after a previous dose or to a vaccine component **Precaution** Moderate or severe acute illness with or without fever	
Influenza	**Contraindication** Severe allergic reaction to previous dose or vaccine component, including egg protein **Precautions** Moderate or severe acute illness with or without fever	Nonsevere (e.g., contact) allergy to latex or thimerosal Concurrent administration of Coumadin or aminophylline
PPV	**Contraindication** Severe allergic reaction after a previous dose or to a vaccine component **Precaution** Moderate or severe acute illness with or without fever	

From *MMWR Morb Mortal Wkly Rep* 51(RR-2), 2002.

[a]Events or conditions listed as precautions should be reviewed carefully. Benefits and risks of administering a specific vaccine to a person under these circumstances should be considered. If the risk from the vaccine is believed to outweigh the benefit, the vaccine should not be administered. If the benefit of vaccination is believed to outweigh the risk, the vaccine should be administered. Whether and when to administer DTaP to children with proven or suspected underlying neurologic disorders should be decided on a case-by-case basis.

[b]Hepatitis B vaccination should be deferred for infants weighing <2000 g if the mother is documented to be hepatitis B surface antigen (HbsAg)-negative at the time of the infant's birth. Vaccination can commence at chronological age 1 month. For infants born to HbsAg-positive women, hepatitis B immunoglobulin and hepatitis B vaccine should be administered at or soon after birth regardless of weight. See text for details.

[c]Acetaminophen or other appropriate antipyretic can be administered to children with a personal or family history of seizures at the time of DTaP vaccination and every 4-6 hours for 24 hours thereafter to reduce the possibility of postvaccination fever (Source: American Academy of Pediatrics, In Pickering LK, ed, *Red Book: Report of the Committee on Infectious Diseases,* 25th ed. Elk Grove Village, IL, 2000, American Academy of Pediatrics.

[d]MMR and varicella vaccines can be administered on the same day. If not administered on the same day, these vaccines should be separated by ≥28 days.

[e]Substantially immunosuppressive steroid dose is considered to be ≥2 weeks of daily receipt of 20 mg or 2 mg/kg body weight of prednisone or equivalent.

[f]Measles vaccination can suppress tuberculin reactivity temporarily. Measles-containing vaccine can be administered on the same day as tuberculin skin testing. If testing cannot be performed until after the day of MMR vaccination, the test should be postponed for ≥4 weeks after the vaccination. If an urgent need exists to skin test, do so with the understanding that reactivity might be reduced by the vaccine.

[g]If a vaccinee experiences a presumed vaccine-related rash 7-25 days after vaccination, avoid direct contact with immunocompromised persons for the duration of the rash.

TABLE 5-22 Vaccinations for International Travel

DISEASE*	AREAS AFFECTED†	PROPHYLAXIS RECOMMENDED	IDEAL TIME BETWEEN LAST VACCINE DOSE AND TRAVEL
Tetanus	All	All travelers; vaccine series/booster.	Probably 30 days for series Anamnestic response to booster
Measles	All	Born after 1956; ensure immunity by antibody titer, diagnosed measles, or two doses of vaccine.	As MMR, 7-14 days
Rubella	All	Born after 1956 and any female of childbearing age; rubella titer or one dose of vaccine.	As MMR, 7-14 days
Mumps	All	Born after 1956; ensure immunity by antibody titer, diagnosed mumps, or one dose of vaccine.	As MMR, 7-14 days
Varicella	All	All travelers; antibody titer, reported illness, or vaccine series.	7-14 days
Hepatitis B	5%-20% of population are carriers in Africa, Middle East except Israel, all Southeast Asia, Amazon basin, Haiti, and Dominican Republic; 1%-5% of population are carriers in south-central and southwest Asia, Israel, Japan, Americas, Russia, and eastern and southern Europe.	Travelers for more than 6 mo in close contact with population or for less time but with high-risk activities (close household contact, seeking dental or medical care, sex); vaccine series.	Probably 30 days
Hepatitis A	Developing countries.	Travelers to rural areas; eating and drinking in settings of poor sanitation; vaccine or pooled immune globulin (IG).	Vaccine, 30 days Pooled IG, 2 days
Influenza	Tropics throughout the year; southern hemisphere from April to September.	Travelers for whom vaccine is otherwise indicated; give current vaccine and revaccinate in fall as usual.	7-14 days
Meningococcus*	Sub-Saharan Africa "belt" (Senegal to Ethiopia) from December to June; required for pilgrims to Saudi Arabia during Haj; epidemics reported in other African nations, India, Nepal, and Mongolia.	All travelers; vaccine.	7-10 days
Rabies	Endemic dog rabies exists in Mexico, El Salvador, Guatemala, Peru, Colombia, Ecuador, India, Nepal, Philippines, Sri Lanka, Thailand, and Vietnam.	Travelers staying for more than 30 days or at high risk of exposure to domestic or wild animals; vaccine series/booster.	7-14 days
Poliomyelitis	Developing countries not in western hemisphere; at risk all year in tropics; in temperate zones, incidence increases in summer and fall.	All travelers; vaccine series/booster.	Parenteral vaccine series, 28 day (see text) Anamnestic response to booster

Continued

V

TABLE 5-22   Vaccinations for International Travel—cont'd

DISEASE*	AREAS AFFECTED†	PROPHYLAXIS RECOMMENDED	IDEAL TIME BETWEEN LAST VACCINE DOSE AND TRAVEL
Typhoid fever	Many countries in Asia, Africa, Central America, and South America.	Travelers with prolonged stay in rural areas with poor sanitation; vaccine series/booster.	Oral vaccine, 7 days Parenteral vaccine, probably 14 days
Yellow fever*	North and central South America, forest-savannah zones of Africa; some countries in Africa, Asia, and Middle East require travelers from endemic areas to be vaccinated.	All travelers; vaccine/booster at approved yellow fever vaccination center.	10 days
Japanese encephalitis	Seasonally in most areas of Asia, Indian subcontinent, and western Pacific islands; in temperate zones, incidence increases in summer and early fall; in tropics, year-round incidence.	Travelers staying for more than 30 days in high-risk rural areas; staying outdoors during transmission season; vaccine series.	10 days
Cholera*	Certain undeveloped countries.	If required by local authorities, one dose usually suffices; primary series only for those living in high-risk areas under poor sanitary conditions or those with compromised gastric defense mechanisms (achlorhydria, antacid therapy, previous ulcer surgery); booster every 6 mo.	Probably 30 days
Plague	Africa, Asia, and Americas in rural mountainous or upland areas.	Travelers whose research or field activities bring them in contact with rodents; vaccine series/booster; consider taking tetracycline (500 mg four times a day) for chemoprophylaxis (inferred from clinical experience in treating plague).	Probably 30 days

From Noble J: *Primary care medicine*, ed 3, St Louis, 2001, Mosby.
*Only yellow fever vaccine is required for entry by any country; cholera vaccine may be required by some local authorities; and meningococcus vaccine is required for pilgrims to Mecca, Saudia Arabia, during Haj. However, it is important to follow CDC recommendations for all vaccines to prevent disease. If a required vaccine is contraindicated or withheld for any reason, attempts should be made to obtain a waiver from the country's consulate or embassy.
†Because areas affected can change, and for more specific details, consult CDC's traveler's hotline.

TABLE 5-23   Recommended Schedule of Hepatitis B Immunoprophylaxis to Prevent Perinatal Transmission

POPULATION GROUP	VACCINE DOSE*	AGE OF INFANT
Infants born to HBsAg-positive mothers	First dose	Birth (within 12 hr)
	HBIG†	Birth (within 12 hr)
	Second dose	1 mo
	Third dose	6 mo‡
Infants born to mothers not screened for HBsAg§	First dose	Birth (within 12 hr)
	HBIG‡	If mother is HBsAg positive, administer HBIG to infant as soon as possible, not later than 1 wk after birth
	Second dose	1-2 mo‖
	Third dose	6 mo‡

Modified from *MMWR Morb Mortal Wkly Rep* 40(RR-13):12, 1991.
HbsAg, Hepatitis B surface antigen; *HBIG,* hepatitis B immune globulin.
*See Table 5-20 for appropriate vaccine dose.
†HBIG is given in a dose of 0.5 ml, administered intramuscularly at a site different from that used for vaccine.
‡If four-dose schedule (Engerix-B) is used, the third dose is administered at 2 mo of age and the fourth dose at 12-18 mo.
§First vaccine dose is the same as the dose for an HBsAg-positive mother (see Table 5-20). If mother is HBsAg positive, continue that dose; if mother is HBsAg negative, use appropriate dose from Table 5-20.
‖Infants of women who are HBsAg negative can be vaccinated at 2 mo of age.

TABLE 5-24   Recommended Doses of Currently Licensed Hepatitis B Vaccines

POPULATION GROUP	RECOMBIVAX HB* DOSE IN μG (DOSE IN ml)	ENGERIX-B* DOSE IN μG (DOSE IN ml)
Infants of HbsAg-negative mothers and children <11 yr	2.5 (0.25)	10 (0.5)
Infants of HbsAg-positive mothers; prevention of perinatal infection	5 (0.5)	10 (0.5)
Children and adolescents 11-19 yr	5 (0.5)	20 (1.0)
Adults ≥20 yr	10 (1.0)	20 (1.0)
Dialysis patients and other immunocompromised persons	40†	40‡

Modified from *MMWR Morb Mortal Wkly Rep* 40(RR-13):7, 1991.
*Both vaccines are routinely administered in a three-dose series at 0, 1, and 6 mo. Engerix-B is also licensed for a four-dose series administered at 0, 1, 2, and 12 mo.
†Special formulation.
‡Two 1.0-ml doses administered at one site in a four-dose schedule at 0, 1, 2, and 6 mo.

Endocarditis Prophylaxis

BOX 5-1   Cardiac Conditions Associated with Endocarditis

Endocarditis Prophylaxis Recommended
High-Risk Category

Prosthetic cardiac valves, including bioprosthetic and homograft valves
Previous bacterial endocarditis
Complex cyanotic congenital heart disease (e.g., single ventricle states, transposition of the great arteries, tetralogy of Fallot)
Surgically constructed systemic pulmonary shunts or conduits

Moderate-Risk Category

Most other congenital cardiac malformations (other than above and below)
Acquired valvar dysfunction (e.g., rheumatic heart disease)
Hypertrophic cardiomyopathy
Mitral valve prolapse with valvar regurgitation and/or thickened leaflets

Endocarditis Prophylaxis Not Recommended
Negligible-Risk Category (No Greater Risk Than the General Population)

Isolated secundum atrial septal defect
Surgical repair of atrial septal defect, ventricular defect, or patent ductus arteriosus (without residua beyond 6 mos)
Previous coronary artery bypass graft surgery
Mitral valve prolapse without valvar regurgitation
Physiologic, functional, or innocent heart murmurs
Previous Kawasaki disease without valvar dysfunction
Previous rheumatic fever without valvar dysfunction
Cardiac pacemakers (intravascular and epicardial) and implanted defibrillators

From Dajani AS et al: *JAMA* 277:1794-1801, 1997.

V

BOX 5-2 Dental Procedures and Endocarditis Prophylaxis

Endocarditis Prophylaxis Recommended*

Dental extractions
Periodontal procedures including surgery, scaling and
    root planing, probing, and recall maintenance
Dental implant placement and reimplantation of avulsed
    teeth
Endodontic (root canal) instrumentation of surgery only
    beyond the apex
Subgingival placement of antibiotic fibers or strips
Initial placement of orthodontic bands—but not brackets
Intraligamentary local anesthetic injections
Prophylactic cleaning of teeth or implants where bleed-
    ing is anticipated

Endocarditis Prophylaxis Not Recommended

Restorative dentistry† (operative and prosthodontic) with
    or without retraction cord‡
Local anesthetic injections (nonintraligamentary)
Intracanal endodontic treatment; postplacement and
    buildup
Placement of rubber dams
Postoperative suture removal
Placement of removable prosthodontic or orthodontic
    appliances
Taking of oral impressions
Fluoride treatments
Taking of oral radiographs
Orthodontic appliance adjustment
Shedding of primary teeth

From Dajani AS et al: *JAMA* 277:1794-1801, 1997.
*Prophylaxis is recommended for patients with high- and moderate-risk cardiac conditions.
†This includes restoration of decayed teeth (filling cavities) and replacement of missing teeth.
‡Clinical judgment may indicate antibiotic use in selected circumstances that may create significant bleeding.

BOX 5-3 Other Procedures and Endocarditis Prophylaxis

Endocarditis Prophylaxis Recommended
Respiratory tract

Tonsillectomy and/or adenoidectomy
Surgical operations that involve respiratory mucosa
Bronchoscopy with a rigid bronchoscope

*Gastrointestinal Tract**

Sclerotherapy for esophageal varices
Esophageal stricture dilation
Endoscopic retrograde cholangiography* with biliary ob-
    struction
Biliary tract surgery
Surgical operations that involve intestinal mucosa

Genitourinary Tract

Prostatic surgery
Cystoscopy
Urethral dilation

Endocarditis Prophylaxis Not Recommended
Respiratory Tract

Endotracheal intubation
Bronchoscopy with a flexible bronchoscope, with or
    without biopsy†
Tympanostomy tube insertion

Gastrointestinal Tract

Transesophageal echocardiography†
Endoscopy with or without gastrointestinal biopsy†

Genitourinary Tract

Vaginal hysterectomy†
Vaginal delivery†
Cesarean section
In uninfected tissue:
    Urethral catheterization
    Uterine dilation and curettage
    Therapeutic abortion
    Sterilization procedures
    Insertion or removal of intrauterine devices

Other

Cardiac catheterization, including balloon angioplasty
Implanted cardiac pacemakers, implanted defibrillators,
    and coronary stents
Incision or biopsy of surgically scrubbed skin
Circumcision

From Dajani AS et al: *JAMA* 277:1794-1801, 1997.
*Prophylaxis is recommended for high-risk patients; optional for medium-risk patients.
†Prophylaxis is optional for high-risk patients.

TABLE 5-25 **Prophylactic Regimens for Dental, Oral, Respiratory Tract, or Esophageal Procedures**

SITUATION	AGENT	REGIMEN*
Standard general prophylaxis	Amoxicillin	Adults: 2.0 g; children: 50 mg/kg orally (PO) 1 hr before procedure
Unable to take oral medications	Ampicillin	Adults: 2.0 g intramuscularly (IM) or intravenously (IV); children: 50 mg/kg IM or IV within 30 min before procedure
Allergic to penicillin	Clindamycin *or*	Adults: 600 mg; children: 20 mg/kg PO 1 hr before procedure
	Cephalexin† or cefadroxil† *or*	Adults: 2.0 g; children: 50 mg/kg PO 1 hr before procedure
	Azithromycin or clarithromycin	Adults: 500 mg; children: 15 mg/kg PO 1 hr before procedure
Allergic to penicillin and unable to take oral medications	Clindamycin *or*	Adults: 600 mg; children: 20 mg/kg IV within 30 min of procedure
	Cefazolin†	Adults 1.0 g; children: 25 mg/kg IM or IV within 30 min of procedure

From Dajani AS et al: *JAMA* 277:1794-1801, 1997.
*Total children's dose should not exceed adult dose.
†Cephalosporins should not be used in individuals with immediate-type hypersensitivity reaction (urticaria, angioedema, or anaphylaxis) to penicillins.

TABLE 5-26 **Prophylactic Regimens for Genitourinary/Gastrointestinal (Excluding Esophageal) Procedures**

SITUATION	AGENTS*	REGIMEN†
High-risk patients	Ampicillin plus gentamicin	Adults: ampicillin 2.0 g intramuscularly (IM) or intravenously (IV) plus gentamicin 1.5 mg/kg (not to exceed 120 mg) within 30 min of starting the procedure; 6 hr later, ampicillin 1 g IM/IV or amoxicillin 1 g orally (PO)
		Children: ampicillin 50 mg/kg IM or IV (not to exceed 2.0 g) plus gentamicin 1.5 mg/kg within 30 min of starting the procedure; 6 hr later, ampicillin 25 g/kg IM/IV or amoxicillin 25 mg/kg PO
High-risk patients allergic to ampicillin	Vancomycin plus gentamicin	Adults: vancomycin 1.0 g IV over 1-2 hr plus gentamicin 1.5 mg/kg IV/IM (not to exceed 120 mg); complete injection/infusion within 30 min of starting the procedure
		Children: vancomycin 20 mg/kg IV over 1-2 hr plus gentamicin 1.5 mg/kg IV/IM; complete injection/infusion within 30 min of starting the procedure
Moderate-risk patients	Amoxicillin or ampicillin	Adults: amoxicillin 2.0 g PO 1 hr before procedure, or ampicillin 2.0 g IV/IV within 30 min of starting the procedure
		Children: amoxicillin 50 mg/kg PO 1 hr before procedure, or ampicillin 50 mg/kg IM/IV within 30 min of starting the procedure
Moderate-risk patients allergic to ampicillin/amoxicillin	Vancomycin	Adults: vancomycin 1.0 g IV over 1-2 hr; complete infusion within 30 min of starting the procedure
		Children: vancomycin 20 mg/kg IV over 1-2 hr; complete infusion within 30 min of starting the procedure

From Dajani AS et al: *JAMA* 277:1794-1801, 1997.
*Total children's dose should not exceed adult dose.
†No second dose of vancomycin or gentamicin is recommended.

V

TABLE 5-27 **Recommended Daily Dosage of Influenza Antiviral Medications for Treatment and Prophylaxis**

		AGE GROUPS			
ANTIVIRAL AGENT	1 TO 6 YEARS	7 TO 9 YEARS	10 TO 12 YEARS	13 TO 64 YEARS	65 YEARS AND OLDER
Amantadine[a]					
Treatment	5 mg per kg per day up to 150 mg in two divided doses[b]	5 mg per kg per day up to 150 mg in two divided doses[b]	100 mg bid[c]	100 mg bid[c]	100 mg or less per day
Prophylaxis	5 mg per kg per day up to 150 mg in two divided doses[b]	5 mg per kg per day up to 150 mg in two divided doses[b]	100 mg bid[c]	100 mg bid[c]	100 mg or less per day
Rimantadine[d]					
Treatment[e]	NA	NA	NA	100 mg bid[c]	100 or 200[f] mg per day
Prophylaxis	5 mg per kg per day up to 150 mg in two divided doses[b]	5 mg per kg per day up to 150 mg in two divided doses[b]	100 mg bid[c]	100 mg bid[c]	100 or 200[f] mg per day
Zanamivir[g,h]					
Treatment	NA	10 mg bid	10 mg bid	10 mg bid	10 mg bid
Oseltamivir					
Treatment[i]	Dose varies by child's weight[j]	Dose varies by child's weight[j]	Dose varies by child's weight[j]	75 mg bid	75 mg bid
Prophylaxis	NA	NA	NA	75 mg per day	75 mg per day

From *MMWR Morb Mortal Wkly Rep* 50(RR-4):1, 2001.
NA, Not applicable.
[a]The drug package insert should be consulted for dosage recommendations for administering amantadine to persons with creatinine clearance of 50 mL or less per min per 1.73m^2.
[b]5 mg per kg of amantadine or rimantadine syrup = 1 tsp/22 lb.
[c]Children 10 yr of age or older who weigh less than 40 kg (88 lb) should be administered amantadine or rimantadine at a dosage of 5 mg per kg per day.
[d]A reduction in dosage to 100 mg per day of rimantadine is recommended for persons who have severe hepatic dysfunction or those with creatinine clearance of 10 ml or less per min. Other persons with less severe hepatic or renal dysfunction taking 100 mg per day of rimantadine should be observed closely, and the dosage should be reduced or the drug discontinued, if necessary.
[e]Only approved for treatment in adults.
[f]Elderly residents of nursing homes should be administered only 100 mg per day of rimantadine. A reduction in dosage of 100 mg per day should be considered for all persons 65 yr of age or older if they experience side effects when taking 200 mg per day.
[g]Zanamivir is administered via inhalation by using a plastic device included in the package with the medication. Patients will benefit from instruction and demonstration of correct use of the device.
[h]Zanamivir is not approved for prophylaxis.
[i]A reduction in the dose of oseltamivir is recommended for persons with creatinine clearance of less than 30 ml per min.
[j]The dose recommendation for children who weigh less than 15 kg (33 lb) is 30 mg bid; for children weighing 15 to 23 kg (33 to 50.6 lb), the dose is 45 mg bid; for children weighing 23 to 40 kg (50.6 to 88 lb), the dose is 60 mg bid; and for children weighing more than 40 kg (88 lb), the dose is 75 mg bid.

TABLE 5-28   Recommended Postexposure Prophylaxis for Exposure to Hepatitis B Virus

VACCINATION AND ANTIBODY RESPONSE STATUS OF EXPOSED WORKERS*	TREATMENT		
	SOURCE HBsAg POSITIVE	SOURCE HBsAg NEGATIVE	SOURCE UNKNOWN OR NOT AVAILABLE FOR TESTING
Unvaccinated	HBIG† × 1 and initiate HB vaccine series‡	Initiate HB vaccine series	Initiate HB vaccine series
Previously vaccinated			
Known responder§	No treatment	No treatment	No treatment
Known nonresponder‖	HBIG × 1 and initiate revaccination or HBIG × 2¶	No treatment	If known high-risk source, treat as if source were HBsAg positive
Antibody response unknown	Test exposed person for anti-HBs¶ 1. If adequate,§ no treatment is necessary 2. If inadequate,‖ administer HBIG × 1 and vaccine booster	No treatment	Test exposed person for anti-HBs 1. If adequate,‡ no treatment is necessary 2. If inadequate,‡ administer vaccine booster and recheck titer in 1-2 mo

Anti-HBs, Antibody to HBsAg; *HB*, hepatitis B; *HBIG*, hepatitis B immune globulin; *HBsAg*, hepatitis B surface antigen.
*Persons who have previously been infected with HBV are immune to reinfection and do not require postexposure prophylaxis.
†Hepatitis B immune globulin; dose is 0.06 ml/kg intramuscularly.
‡Hepatitis B vaccine.
§A responder is a person with adequate levels of serum antibody to HBsAg (i.e., anti-HBs ≥10 mIU/ml).
‖A nonresponder is a person with inadequate response to vaccination (i.e., serum anti-HBs <10 mIU/ml).
¶The option of giving one dose of HBIG and reinitiating the vaccine series is preferred for nonresponders who have not completed a second 3-dose vaccine series. For persons who previously completed a second vaccine series but failed to respond, two doses of HBIG are preferred.

TABLE 5-29   Recommended HIV Postexposure Prophylaxis for Percutaneous Injuries

EXPOSURE TYPE	INFECTION STATUS OF SOURCE				
	HIV-POSITIVE CLASS 1*	HIV-POSITIVE CLASS 2*	SOURCE OF UNKNOWN HIV STATUS†	UNKNOWN SOURCE‡	HIV-NEGATIVE
Less severe§	Recommend basic 2-drug PEP	Recommend expanded 3-drug PEP	Generally, no PEP warranted; however, consider basic 2-drug PEP‖ for source with HIV risk factors††	Generally, no PEP warranted; however, consider basic 2-drug PEP‖ in settings where exposure to HIV-infected persons is likely	No PEP warranted
More severe#	Recommend expanded 3-drug PEP	Recommend expanded 3-drug PEP	Generally, no PEP warranted; however, consider basic 2-drug PEP‖ for source with HIV risk factors¶	Generally, no PEP warranted; however, consider basic 2-drug PEP‖ in settings where exposure to HIV-infected persons is likely	No PEP warranted

HIV, Human immunodeficiency virus; *PEP*, postexposure prophylaxis (see Box 5-7).
*HIV-Positive, Class 1—asymptomatic HIV infection or known low viral load (e.g., <1500 RNA copies/ml). HIV-Positive, class 2—symptomatic HIV infection, acquired immunodeficiency syndrome, acute seroconversion, or known high viral load. If drug resistance is a concern, obtain expert consultation. Initiation of PEP should not be delayed pending expert consultation, and, because expert consultation alone cannot substitute for face-to-face counseling, resources should be available to provide immediate evaluation and follow-up care for all exposures.
†Source of unknown HIV status (e.g., deceased source person with no samples available for HIV testing).
‡Unknown source (e.g., a needle from a sharps disposal container).
§Less severe (e.g., solid needle and superficial injury).
‖The designation "consider PEP" indicates that PEP is optional and should be based on an individualized decision between the exposed person and the treating clinician.
¶If PEP is offered and taken and the source is later determined to be HIV-negative, PEP should be discontinued.
#More severe (e.g., large-bore hollow needle, deep puncture, visible blood on device, or needle used in patient's artery or vein).

V

TABLE 5-30 **Recommended HIV Postexposure Prophylaxis for Mucous Membrane Exposures and Nonintact Skin[a] Exposures**

EXPOSURE TYPE	INFECTION STATUS OF SOURCE				
	HIV-POSITIVE CLASS 1[b]	HIV-POSITIVE CLASS 2[b]	SOURCE OF UNKNOWN HIV STATUS[c]	UNKNOWN SOURCE[d]	HIV-NEGATIVE
Small volume[e]	Consider basic 2-drug PEP[f]	Recommend basic 2-drug PEP	Generally, no PEP warranted; however, consider basic 2-drug PEP[f] for source with HIV risk factors[g]	Generally, no PEP warranted; however, consider basic 2-drug PEP[f] in settings where exposure to HIV-infected persons is likely	No PEP warranted
Large volume[h]	Recommend basic 2-drug PEP	Recommend expanded 3-drug PEP	Generally, no PEP warranted; however, consider basic 2-drug PEP[f] for source with HIV risk factors[g]	Generally, no PEP warranted; however, consider basic 2-drug PEP[f] in settings where exposure to HIV-infected persons is likely	No PEP warranted

HIV, Human immunodeficiency virus; *PEP,* postexposure prophylaxis (see Box 5-7).
[a]For skin exposures, follow-up is indicated only if there is evidence of compromised skin integrity (e.g., dermatitis, abrasion, or open wound).
[b]HIV-Positive, Class 1—asymptomatic HIV infection or known low viral load (e.g., <1,500 RNA copies/mL). HIV-Positive, Class 2—symptomatic HIV infection, acquired immunodeficiency syndrome, acute seroconversion, or known high viral load. If drug resistance is a concern, obtain expert consultation. Initiation of PEP should not be delayed pending expert consultation, and, because expert consultation alone cannot substitute for face-to-face counseling, resources should be available to provide immediate evaluation and follow-up care for all exposures.
[c] Source of unknown HIV status (e.g., deceased source person with no samples available for HIV testing).
[d]Unknown source (e.g., splash from inappropriately disposed blood).
[e]Small volume (i.e., a few drops).
[f]The designation, "consider PEP," indicates that PEP is optional and should be based on an individualized decision between the exposed person and the treating clinician.
[g]If PEP is offered and taken and the source is later determined to be HIV-negative, PEP should be discontinued.
[h]Large volume (i.e., major blood splash).

BOX 5-4 **Situations for Which Expert* Consultation for HIV Postexposure Prophylaxis Is Advised**

- Delayed (i.e., later than 24-36 hr) exposure report
  — the interval after which there is no benefit from postexposure prophylaxis (PEP) is undefined
- Unknown source (e.g., needle in sharps disposal container or laundry)
  — decide use of PEP on a case-by-case basis
  — consider the severity of the exposure and the epidemiologic likelihood of HIV exposure
  — do not test needles or other sharp instruments for HIV
- Known or suspected pregnancy in the exposed person
  — does not preclude the use of optimal PEP regimens
  — do not deny PEP solely on the basis of pregnancy
- Resistance of the source virus to antiretroviral agents
  — influence of drug resistance on transmission risk is unknown
  — selection of drugs to which the source person's virus is unlikely to be resistant is recommended, if the source person's virus is known or suspected to be resistant to ≥1 of the drugs considered for the PEP regimen
  — resistance testing of the source person's virus at the time of the exposure is not recommended
- Toxicity of the initial PEP regimen
  — adverse symptoms, such as nausea and diarrhea are common with PEP
  — symptoms often can be managed without changing the PEP regimen by prescribing antimotility and/or antiemetic agents
  — modification of dose intervals (i.e., administering a lower dose of drug more frequently throughout the day, as recommended by the manufacturer), in other situations, might help alleviate symptoms

HIV, Human immunodeficiency virus.
*Local experts and/or the National Clinicians' Postexposure Prophylaxis Hotline (PEPline [1-888-448-4911]).

BOX 5-5 Occupational Exposure Management Resources

National Clinicians' Postexposure Prophylaxis Hotline (PEPline)

Run by University of California–San Francisco/San Francisco General Hospital staff; supported by the Health Resources and Services Administration Ryan White CARE Act, HIV/AIDS Bureau, AIDS Education and Training Centers, and CDC.

Phone: (888) 448-4911
Internet: http://www.ucsf.edu/hivcntr

Needlestick!

A website to help clinicians manage and document occupational blood and body fluid exposures. Developed and maintained by the University of California, Los Angeles (UCLA), Emergency Medicine Center, UCLA School of Medicine, and funded in party by CDC and the Agency for Healthcare Research and Quality.

Internet: http://www.needlestick.mednet.ucla.edu

Hepatitis Hotline

Phone: (888) 443-7232
Internet: http://www.cdc.gov/ncidod/diseases/hepatitis/
 index.htm
Phone: (800) 893-0485

Reporting to CDC: Occupationally acquired HIV infections and failures of PEP.

HIV Antiretroviral Pregnancy Registry

Phone: (800) 258-4263
Fax: (800) 800-1052
Address:
 1410 Commonwealth Drive
 Suite 215
 Wilmington, NC 28405
Internet:
 http://www.glaxowellcome.com/preg_reg/
 antiretroviral

Food and Drug Administration

Report unusual or severe toxicity to antiretroviral agents.

Phone: (800) 332-1088
Address:
 MedWatch
 HF-2, FDA
 5600 Fishers Lane
 Rockville, MD 20857
Internet: http://www.fda.gov/medwatch

HIV/AIDS Treatment Information Service

Internet: http://www.hivatis.org

V

BOX 5-6 Management of Occupational Blood Exposures

Provide immediate care to the exposure site:

- Wash wounds and skin with soap and water
- Flush mucous membranes with water

Determine risk associated with exposure:

- Type of fluid (e.g., blood, visibly bloody fluid, other potentially infectious fluid or tissue, and concentrated virus)
- Type of exposure (i.e., percutaneous injury, mucous membrane or nonintact skin exposure, and bites resulting in blood exposure)

Evaluate exposure source:

- Assess the risk of infection using available information
- Test known sources for HBsAg, anti-HCV, and HIV antibodies (consider using rapid testing)
- For unknown sources, assess risk of exposure to HBV, HCV, or HIV infection
- Do not test discarded needles or syringes for virus contamination

Evaluate the exposed person:

- Assess immune status for HBV infection (i.e., by history of hepatitis B vaccination and vaccine response)

Give PEP for exposures posing risk of infection transmission:

- HBV: See Table 5-28
- HCV: PEP not recommended
- HIV: See Tables 5-29 and 5-30
  - Initiate PEP as soon as possible, preferably within hours of exposure
  - Offer pregnancy testing to all women of childbearing age not known to be pregnant
  - Seek expert consultation if viral resistance is suspected
  - Administer PEP for 4 wk if tolerated

Perform follow-up testing and provide counseling:

- Advise exposed persons to seek medical evaluation for any acute illness occurring during follow-up

HBV exposures

- Perform follow-up anti-HBs testing in persons who receive hepatitis B vaccine
  - Test for anti-HBs 1-2 mo after last dose of vaccine
  - Anti-HBs response to vaccine cannot be ascertained if HBIG was received in the previous 3-4 mo

HCV exposures

- Perform baseline and follow-up testing for anti-HCV and alanine aminotransferase (ALT) 4-6 mo after exposures
- Perform HCV RNA at 4-6 wk if earlier diagnosis of HCV infection desired
- Confirm repeatedly reactive anti-HCV enzyme immunoassays (EIAs) with supplemental tests

HIV exposures

- Perform HIV-antibody testing for at least 6 mo postexposure (e.g., at baseline, 6 wk, 3 mo, and 6 mo)
- Perform HIV antibody testing if illness compatible with an acute retroviral syndrome occurs
- Advise exposed persons to use precautions to prevent secondary transmission during the follow-up period
- Evaluate exposed persons taking PEP within 72 hr after exposure and monitor for drug toxicity for at least 2 wk

HBIG, Hepatitis B immune globulin; *HBsAg,* hepatitis B surface antigen; *HBV,* hepatitis B virus; *HCV,* hepatitis C virus; *HIV,* human immunodeficiency virus; *PEP,* postexposure prophylaxis; *RNA,* ribonucleic acid.

BOX 5-7   Basic and Expanded HIV Postexposure Prophylaxis Regimens

Basic Regimen
- **Zidovudine (Retrovir; ZDV; AZT) and Lamivudine (Epivir; 3TC); available as Combivir**
  - ZDV: 600 mg per day, in two or three divided doses
  - 3TC: 150 mg bid

Advantages
  - ZDV is associated with decreased risk of HIV transmission in the CDC case-control study of occupational HIV infection
  - ZDV has been used more than the other drugs for PEP in HCP
  - Serious toxicity is rare when used for PEP
  - Side effects are predictable and manageable with antimotility and antiemetic agents
  - Probably a safe regimen for pregnant HCP
  - Can be given as a single tablet (Combivir) bid

Disadvantages
  - Side effects are common and might result in low adherence
  - Source patient virus might have resistance to this regimen
  - Potential for delayed toxicity (oncogenic/teratogenic) is unknown

Alternative Basic Regimens
- **Lamivudine (3TC) and Stavudine (Zerit; d4T)**
  - 3TC: 150 mg bid
  - d4T: 40 mg (if body weight is <60 kg, 30 mg) bid

Advantages
  - Well tolerated in patients with HIV infection, resulting in good adherence
  - Serious toxicity appears to be rare
  - Twice daily dosing might improve adherence

Disadvantages
  - Source patient virus might be resistant to this regimen
  - Potential for delayed toxicity (oncogenic/teratogenic) is unknown

- **Didanosine (Videx, chewable/dispersable buffered tablet; Videx EC, delayed-release capsule; ddl) and Stavudine (d4T)**
  - ddl: 400 mg (if body weight is <60 kg, 125 mg bid) daily, on an empty stomach
  - d4T: 40 mg (if body weight is <60 kg, 30 mg bid) bid

Advantages
  - Likely effective against HIV strains from source patients who are taking ZDV and 3TC

Disadvantages
  - ddl is difficult to administer and unpalatable.
  - Chewable/dispersable buffered tablet formulation of ddl interferes with absorption of some drugs (e.g., quinolone antibiotics, and indinavir).
  - Serious toxicity (e.g., neuropathy, pancreatitis, or hepatitis) can occur. Fatal and nonfatal pancreatitis has occurred in HIV-positive, treatment-naive patients. Patients taking ddl and d4T should be carefully assessed and closely monitored for pancreatitis, lactic acidosis, and hepatitis.
  - Side effects are common; anticipate diarrhea and low adherence.
  - Potential for delayed toxicity (oncogenic/teratogenic) is unknown.

Expanded Regimen
Basic regimen plus one of the following:

- **Indinavir (Crixivan; IDV)**
  - 800 mg every 8 hr, on an empty stomach

Advantages
  - Potent HIV inhibitor

Disadvantages
  - Serious toxicity (e.g., nephrolithiasis) can occur; must take 8 glasses of fluid per day
  - Hyperbilirubinemia common; must avoid this drug during late pregnancy
  - Requires acid for absorption and cannot be taken simultaneously with ddl in chewable/dispersable buffered tablet formulation (doses must be separated by at least 1 hr)
  - Concomitant use of astemizole, terfenadine, dihydroergotamine, ergotamine, ergonovine, methylergonovine, rifampin, cisapride, St. John's Wort, lovastatin, simvastatin, pimozide, midazolam, or triazolam is not recommended
  - Potential for delayed toxicity (oncogenic/teratogenic) is unknown

V

Continued

BOX 5-7   Basic and Expanded HIV Postexposure Prophylaxis Regimens—cont'd

- **Nelfinavir (Viracept; NFV)**
  - 750 mg tid, with meals or snack, or
  - 1250 mg bid, with meals or snack

Advantages

- Potent HIV inhibitor
- Twice dosing per day might improve adherence

Disadvantages

- Concomitant use of astemizole, terfenadine, dihydroergotamine, ergotamine, ergonovine, methylergonovine, rifampin, cisapride, St. John's Wort, lovastatin, simvastatin, pimozide, midazolam, or triazolam is not recommended
- Might accelerate the clearance of certain drugs, including oral contraceptives (requiring alternative or additional contraceptive measures for women taking these drugs)
- Potential for delayed toxicity (oncogenic/teratogenic) is unknown

- **Efavirenz (Sustiva; EFV)**
  - 600 mg daily, at bedtime

Advantages

- Does not require phosphorylation before activation and might be active earlier than other antiretroviral agents (NOTE: this might be only a theoretical advantage of no clinical benefit)
- One dose daily might improve adherence

Disadvantages

- Drug is associated with rash (early onset) that can be severe and might rarely progress to Stevens-Johnson syndrome.
- Differentiating between early drug-associated rash and acute seroconversion can be difficult and cause extraordinary concern for the exposed person.
- Nervous system side effects (e.g., dizziness, somnolence, insomnia, and/or abnormal dreaming) are common. Severe psychiatric symptoms are possible (dosing before bedtime might minimize these side effects).
- Should not be used during pregnancy because of concerns about teratogenicity.
- Concomitant use of astemizole, cisapride, midazolam, triazolam, ergot derivatives, or St. John's Wort is not recommended because inhibition of the metabolism of these drugs could create the potential for serious and/or life-threatening adverse events (e.g., cardiac arrhythmias, prolonged sedation, or respiratory depression).
- Potential for oncogenic toxicity is unknown.

- **Abacavir (Ziagen; ABC); available as Trizivir, a combination of ZDV, 3TC, and ABC**
  - 300 mg bid

Advantages

- Potent HIV inhibitor
- Well tolerated in patients with HIV infection

Disadvantages

- Severe hypersensitivity reactions can occur, usually within the first 6 wk of treatment
- Potential for delayed toxicity (oncogenic/teratogenic) is unknown

Antiretroviral Agents for Use as PEP Only With Expert Consultation

- Retonavir (Norvir; RTV)

Disadvantages

- Difficult to take (requires dose escalation)
- Poor tolerability
- Many drug interactions

- **Saquinavir (Fortovase, soft-gel formulation; SQV)**

Disadvantages

- Bioavailability is relatively poor, even with new formulation

Continued

BOX 5-7   Basic and Expanded HIV Postexposure Prophylaxis Regimens—cont'd

- **Amprenavir (Agenerase; AMP)**

Disadvantages

— Dosage consists of eight large pills taken bid
— Many drug interactions

- **Delavirdine (Rescriptor; DLV)**

Disadvantages

— Drug is associated with rash (early onset) that can be severe and progress to Stevens-Johnson syndrome
— Many drug interactions

- **Lopinavir/Ritonavir (Kaletra)**

— 400/100 mg bid

Advantages

— Potent HIV inhibitor
— Well tolerated in patients with HIV infection

Disadvantages

— Concomitant use of flecainide, propafenone, astemizole, terfenadine, dihydroergotamine, ergotamine, ergonovine, methylergonovine, rifampin, cisapride, St. John's Wort, lovastatin, simvastatin, pimozide, midazolam, or triazolam is not recommended because inhibition of the metabolism of these drugs could create the potential for serious and/or life-threatening adverse events (e.g., cardiac arrhythmias, prolonged sedation, or respiratory depression)
— May accelerate the clearance of certain drugs, including oral contraceptives (requiring alternative or additional contraceptive measures for women taking these drugs)
— Potential for delayed toxicity (oncogenic/teratogenic) is unknown

Antiretroviral Agents Generally Not Recommended for Use as PEP

- **Nevirapine (Viramune; NVP)**

— 200 mg daily for 2 wk, then 200 mg bid

Disadvantages

— Associated with severe hepatotoxicity (including at least one case of liver failure requiring liver transplantation in an exposed person taking PEP)
— Associated with rash (early onset) that can be severe and progress to Stevens-Johnson syndrome
— Differentiating between early drug-associated rash and acute seroconversion can be difficult and cause extraordinary concern for the exposed person
— Concomitant use of St. John's Wort is not recommended because this might result in suboptimal antiretroviral drug concentrations

V

Definitions of Complementary/ Alternative Therapies

Acupuncture Thin needles are inserted superficially on the skin at locations throughout the body. These points are located along "channels" of energy. Heat can be applied by burning (moxibustion), electric current (electroacupuncture), or pressure (acupressure). Healing is proposed by the restoration of a balance of energy flow called *Qi*. Another explanation suggests that, possibly, the stimulation activates endorphin receptors.

Alexander Technique A body work technique in which rebalancing of "postural sets" (i.e., physical alignment) is taught by mentally focusing on the way correct alignments should look and feel and through verbal and tactile guidance by the practitioner.

Antineoplastons Naturally occurring peptides, amino acid derivatives, and carboxylic acids are proposed to control neoplastic cell growth using the patient's own "biochemical defense system," which works jointly with the immune system.

Applied Kinesiology A form of treatment that uses nutrition, physical manipulation, vitamins, diets, and exercise to restore and energize the body. Weak muscles are proposed to be a source of dysfunctional health.

Aromatherapy A form of herbal medicine that uses various oils from plants. Route of administration can be through absorption in the skin or inhalation. The action of antiviral and antibacterial agents is proposed to aid in healing. The aromatic biochemical structures of certain herbs are thought to act in areas of the brain related to past experiences and emotions (e.g., limbic system).

Ayurveda A major health system that emphasizes a preventive approach to health by focusing on an inner state of harmony and spiritual realization for self-healing. Includes special types of diets, herbs, and mineral parts and changes based on a system of constitutional categories in lifestyle. The use of enemas and purgation is to cleanse the body of excess toxins.

Biofeedback A mind-body therapy procedure in which sensors are placed on the body to measure muscle, heart rate, and sweat responses or neural activity. Information is provided by visual, auditory, or body-muscle cell activation so as to teach either to increase or decrease physiologic activity which, when reconstituted, is proposed to improve health problems (e.g., pain, anxiety, or high blood pressure). In some cases, relaxation exercises complement this procedure.

Brachytherapy Ionizing radiation therapy with the source applied to the surface of the body or located a short distance from the treated area.

Bristol Cancer Help Center (BCHC) Diet A stringent diet of raw and partly cooked vegetables with proteins from soy; claimed to enhance the quality of life and attitude toward illness in cancer patients.

Cell Therapy Healthy cellular material from fetuses, embryos, or organs of animals is directly injected into human patients to stimulate healing in dysfunctional organs. May also include blood transfusions or bone marrow transplantations.

Chelation Therapy Involves the removal—through intravenous infusion of a chelating agent (synthetic amino acid ethylenediamine tetraacetic acid [EDTA])—of metal, toxins, lead, mercury, nickel, copper, cadmium, and plaque as a way to treat certain diseases (e.g., cardiovascular). Ancillary treatments include the use of vitamins, changes in diet, and exercise.

Cognitive Therapy Psychologic therapy in which the major focus is on altering and changing irrational beliefs through a type of "socratic" dialogue and self-evaluation of certain illogical thoughts. Conditioning and learning are important components of this therapy.

Craniosacral Therapy A form of gentle manual manipulation used for diagnosis and for making corrections in a system made up of cerebrospinal fluid, cranial and dural membranes, cranial bones, and sacrum. This system is proposed to be dynamic with its own physiologic frequency. Through touch and pressure, tension is proposed to be reduced and cranial rhythms normalized, leading to improvement in health and disease.

Dance Therapy A movement-based therapy that aids in promoting feeling and awareness. The goal is to integrate body, mind, and self-esteem. It uses different parts of the body such as fingers, wrists, and arms to respond to music.

Diathermy The use of high-frequency electrical currents as a form of physical therapy and in surgical procedures. The term *diathermy,* derived from the Greek words *dia* and *therma,* literally means "heating through." The three forms of diathermy used by physical therapists are shortwave, ultrasound, and microwave.

Dimethylaminoethanol (DMAE) Pharmacologic therapy that uses a natural substance found in certain foods and the human brain. It is a precursor to the transmitter

From Spencer JW: *Complementary/alternative medicine: an evidence-based approach,* St Louis, 1999, Mosby.

acetylcholine. It is proposed to have a stimulant effect on the central nervous system if used as a supplement.

Electrochemical Treatment (ECT) A method using direct current to treat cancer. It involves inserting platinum electrodes into tumors and applying a constant voltage of less than 10 V to produce a 40- to 80-mA current between the anodes and cathodes for 30 minutes to several hours.

Electroencephalographic Normalization Gross neural activity is recorded from the scalp as an electroencephalogram (EEG) to assist in "restoring a balance in health" by training patients to produce more uniform and consistent EEG frequencies throughout certain or all areas of the brain (occipital, frontal, temporal, and parietal).

Environmental Medicine A practice of medicine in which the major focus is on cause-and-effect relationships in health. Evaluations are made of factors such as eating and living habits and types of air breathed. Testing in the patient's own environment is performed to determine what precipitators are present that may be related to disease or other health problems. A treatment protocol is developed from this information.

Eye Movement Desensitization and Reprocessing (EMDR) A technique that proposes to remove painful memories by behavioral techniques. Rhythmic, multisaccadic eye movements are produced by allowing the patient to track and follow a moving object while imaging a stressful memory or event. By using deconditioning, including verbal interaction with the therapist, the painful memory is extinguished and health improved.

Feldenkrais Method A bodywork technique in which its founder used the integration of physics, judo, and yoga. The practitioner directs sequences of movement using verbal or hands-on techniques or teaches a system of self-directed exercise to treat physical impairments through the learning of new movement patterns.

Hallucinogens The use of lysergic acid diethylamide (LSD) to produce at certain doses anticraving for certain illicit drugs such as cocaine, or ibogaine, a stimulant, to assist in developing tolerance and decreasing symptoms of dependence.

Hatha Yoga The branch of yoga practice that involves physical exercise, breathing practices, and movement. These exercises are designed to have a salutary effect on posture, flexibility, and strength, and are intended ultimately to prepare the body to remain still for long periods of meditation.

Hellerwork A bodywork technique that treats and improves proper body alignment through the development of a more complete awareness of the physical body. The goal is to realign fascia for improvement in standing, sitting, and breathing using "body energy," verbal feedback, and changing emotions and attitudes.

Herbal Medicine Herbs are used to treat various health conditions. Herbal medicine is a major form of treatment for more than 70% of the world's population.

Homeopathy A form of treatment in which substances (minerals, plant extracts, chemicals, or disease-producing germs), which in sufficient doses would produce a set of illness symptoms in healthy individuals, are given in microdoses to produce a "cure" of those same symptoms. The *symptom* is not thought to be part of the illness but part of a curative process.

Hydergine A phytotherapeutic method that combines extracts from the ergot fungus. Originally proposed to be used as an antihypertensive agent.

Hydrazine Sulfate A pharmacologic treatment proposed to treat certain cancers.

Hyperbaric Oxygen A therapy in which 100% oxygen is given at or above atmospheric pressure. An increase in oxygen in the tissue is proposed to increase blood circulation and improve healing and health and influence the course of disease.

Hyperthermia The use of various heating methods (such as electromagnetic therapy) to produce temperature elevations of a few degrees in cells and tissues, leading to a proposed antitumor effect. This is often used in conjunction with radiotherapy or chemotherapy for cancer treatment.

Immunoaugmentative Therapy A cancer treatment that proposes that cancer cells can be arrested by the use of four different blood proteins; this approach is also proposed to restore the immune system. Can be used as an adjunctive therapy.

Jin Shin Jyutsu A bodywork technique that uses specific "healing points" at the body surface, which are proposed to overlie energy flowing (Qi). The therapist's fingers are used to "redirect, balance, and provide a more efficient energy flow" to and throughout the body.

Laetrile A pharmacologic treatment using apricot pits that has been proposed to treat certain cancers.

Light Therapy Natural light or light of specified wavelengths is used to treat disease. This may include ultraviolet light, colored light, or low-intensity laser light. The eye generally is the initial entry point for the light because of its direct connection to the brain.

Magnetic Therapy Magnets are placed directly on the skin, stimulating living cells and increasing blood flow by ionic currents that are created from polarities on the magnets. Both acute and chronic health conditions are suggested to be treatable by this procedure.

Manual Manipulation A group of therapies with different assumptions and, in part, different areas of treatment. The major focus includes both stimulation and body manipulation, which are proposed to improve health or arrest disease, or both. Includes soft-tissue manipulation through stroking, kneading, friction, and vibration. Types include *massage*, adjustment of the spinal column *(chiropractic)*, and tissue and musculoskeletal *(osteopathic)* manipulation.

Mediterranean Diet A diet that is thought to provide optimal distribution of daily caloric intake of different nutrients and includes 50% to 60% carbohydrates, 30% fats, and 10% proteins. The diet is derived from the eating habits of people in the Mediterranean area, who were shown to have reduced rates of cardiovascular disease.

Mind-Body Therapies A group of therapies that emphasize using the mind or brain in conjunction with the body to assist healing. Mind-body therapies can involve varying degrees of levels of consciousness, including *hypnosis,* in which selective attention is used to induce a specific altered state (trance) for memory retrieval, relaxation, or suggestion; *visual imagery,* in which the focus is on a target visual stimulus; *yoga,* which involves integration of posture and controlled breathing, relaxation, and/or meditation; *relaxation,* which includes lighter levels of altered states of consciousness through indirect or direct focus; and *meditation,* in which there is an intentional use of posture, concentration, contemplation, and visualization.

Muscle Energy Technique A manual therapy with components of both passive mobilization and muscle reeducation. Diagnosis of somatic dysfunction is performed by the practitioner after which the patient is guided to provide corrective muscle contraction. This is followed by further testing and correction.

Music Therapy The use of music either in an active or passive mode. Proposed to help allow for the expression of feelings, which helps to reduce stress. Other types of "vibratory" sounds can be used mainly to reduce stress, anxiety, and pain.

Native American Therapies Therapies used by many Native American Indian tribes, including their own healing herbs and ceremonies that use components with a spiritual emphasis.

Naturopathy A major health system that includes practices that emphasize diet, nutrition, homeopathy, acupuncture, herbal medicine, manipulation, and various mind-body therapies. Focal points include self-healing and treatment through changes in lifestyle and emphasis on health prevention.

Neuroelectric Therapy Transcranial or cranial neuroelectric stimulation (TENS), once called "electrosleep"; originally used in the 1950s to treat insomnia. In a typical TENS session, surface electrodes are placed in the mastoid region (behind the ear) and, similar to electroacupuncture, stimulated using a low-amperage, low-frequency alternating current. It has been suggested that TENS stimulates endogenous neurotransmitters such as endorphins that produce symptomatic relief.

Ornish Diet A life-choice program based on eating a vegetarian diet containing less than 10% fat. The diet is high in complex carbohydrates and fiber. Animal products and oils are avoided.

Orthomolecular Therapy A therapeutic approach that uses naturally occurring substances within the body, such as proteins, fat, and water, that promote restoration or balance (or both) by using vitamins, minerals, or other forms of nutrition to subsequently treat disease or promote healing, or both.

Oslo Diet An eating plan that emphasizes increased intake of fish and reduced total fat intake. Diet is combined with regular endurance exercise.

Pilates An educational and exercise approach using the proper body mechanics, movements, truncal and pelvic stabilization, coordinated breathing, and muscle contractions to promote strengthening. Attention is paid to the entire musculoskeletal system.

Piracetam A pharmacologic treatment proposed to be useful in the treatment of dementia. Uses a cyclic relative of the transmitter gamma-aminobutyric acid (GABA).

Prayer The use of prayer(s) that are offered to "some higher being" or authority to heal and/or arrest disease. May be practiced by the individual patient, by groups, or by other(s) with or without the patient's knowledge (e.g., intercessory).

Pritkin Diet A weight management plan that is based on a vegetarian framework. Meals are low in fat, high in fiber, and high in complex carbohydrates.

Qi Gong A form of Chinese exercise-stimulation therapy that proposes to improve health by redirecting mental focus, breathing, coordination, and relaxation. The goal is to "rebalance" the body's own healing capacities by activating proposed electrical or energetic currents that flow along meridians located throughout the body. These meridians, however, do not follow conventional nerve or muscle pathways. In Chinese medical training and practice this therapy includes "external Qi," which is energy transmitted from one person to another so as to heal.

Raja Yoga Yoga practice that includes all of the other forms of yoga practice. The practitioner is instructed to follow moral directives, physical exercises, breathing exercises, meditation, devotion, and service to others to facilitate religious awakening.

Reconstructive Therapy A nonsurgical therapy for arthritis that involves the injection of nutritional substances into the supporting tissues around an injured joint. The intent is to cause the dilation of blood vessels, which will allow fibroblasts to form around the injury and begin the healing process.

Reflexology A bodywork technique that uses reflex points on the hands and feet. Pressure is applied at points that correspond to various body parts, to eliminate blockages thought to produce pain or disease. The goal is to bring the body into balance.

Reiki Comes from the Japanese word meaning "universal life force energy." The practitioner serves as a conduit for healing energy directed into the body or energy field of the recipient without physical contact with the body.

Restricted Environmental Stimulation Therapy (REST) A procedure that uses a completely sensory-deprived environment to increase physical or mental healing through a nonreactive state.

Rolfing A bodywork technique that involves the myofascia. The body is realigned by using the hands to apply a deep pressure and friction that allows more sufficient posture, movement, and the "release" of emotions from the body.

Shark Cartilage A cancer therapy that proposes that shark cartilage can interrupt blood supply to a tumor(s) and subsequently "starve" it of any nutrients by using the antiangiogenic properties and other substances contained in the cartilage.

Shiatsu A bodywork technique involving finger pressure at specific points on the body mainly to balance "energy" in the body. The major focus is on prevention by keeping the body healthy. The therapy uses more than 600 points on the skin that are proposed to be connected to pathways through which energy flows. A Japanese form of acupressure.

T'ai Chi A technique that uses slow, purposeful motor-physical movements of the body to control and achieve a more balanced physiologic and psychologic state.

Therapeutic Riding A form of animal-assisted therapy in which either passive or active movements are produced to aid in approximating the human gait. In certain cases, physiotherapeutic exercises are performed.

Therapeutic Touch A body energy field technique in which hands are passed over the body without actually touching to recreate and change proposed "energy imbalances" for restoring innate healing forces. Verbal interaction between patient and therapist helps to maximize effects.

Traditional Chinese Medicine An ancient form of medicine that focuses on prevention and secondarily treats disease with an emphasis on maintaining balance through the body by stimulating a constant, smooth-flowing Qi energy. Herbs, acupuncture, massage, diet, and exercise are also used.

Trager Psychophysical Integration A bodywork technique in which the practitioner enters a meditative state and guides the client through gentle, light, rhythmic, nonintrusive movements. "Mentastics" exercises using self-healing movements are taught to the clients.

Transcranial Electrostimulation Pulsed electrical stimulation of 50 microamperes or less is applied between two electrodes attached to the ear. The stimulation is proposed to activate endogenous opioid activity, which may assist in the treatment of certain health problems such as substance abuse and physical pain.

Twelve-Step Program A program such as Alcoholics Anonymous that is based on a series of 12 steps, or tasks, that participants are asked to complete. As members progress through the 12 steps, they are expected to gain courage to attempt personal change and develop a greater acceptance of themselves. Programs emphasize the group process through the sharing of stories and experiences and through social interactions with other group members. Most 12-step programs incorporate a spiritual component and ask members to turn their lives over to a higher power.

The definitions listed above are not complete; for additional information, the interested reader should consult books such as Micozzi's *Fundamentals of complementary and alternative medicine* and Spencer JW: *Complementary/alternative medicine: an evidence-based approach.*

Commonly Used Herbals with Documented or Suspected Risks

Commonly Used Herbals with Documented or Suspected Risks

HERBAL	PLANT SOURCE	COMMON USE	COMMENTS
Aconite (Monkshood)	*Aconitum napellus*	Analgesic, antipyretic, wound healing	Side effects include cardiac arrhythmia and respiratory paralysis.
Aloe (internally)	*Aloe barbadenis, Aloe vera,* various Aloe species	Constipation, general tonic, wound healing	Side effects include gastrointestinal (GI) cramping, diarrhea, nephritis, hypokalemia, albuminuria, and hematuria with chronic use.
Borage	*Borago officinalis*	Antidiarrheal, diuretic	Contains low levels of pyrrolizidine alkaloids (lycopsamine, amabiline, thesinine) that are potentially hepatotoxic and carcinogenic.
Calamus	*Acorus calamus*	Antipyretic, digestive aid	Some calamus species contain beta asarone, which may be carcinogenic.
Chaparral	*Larrea tridentata*	Anticancer	Case reports of liver toxicity have been associated with use.
Coltsfoot	*Tussilago farfara*	Antitussive, demulcent	Contains pyrrolizidine alkaloids that are potentially hepatotoxic and carcinogenic.
Comfrey	*Symphytum officinale,* various Symphytum species	Bruises, sprains, wound healing	Contains pyrrolizidine alkaloids that are potentially hepatotoxic and carcinogenic.
Ephedra (Ma-huang)	*Ephedra sinica,* various *Ephedra* species	Appetite suppressant, bronchodilator, athletic performance enhancement (often combined with caffeine-containing herbals)	Side effects include insomnia, irritability, GI disturbances, urinary retention, and tachycardia. Misuse can lead to hypertension and arrhythmias.
Germander	*Teucrium chamaedrys*	Appetite suppressant	Contains diterpneoid derivatives that are potentially hepatotoxic.
Licorice	*Glycyrrhiza glabra*	Antiulcer, expectorant	Should only be used in small doses for short duration (<4 wk). With high doses, hypertension, hypokalemia, and sodium and water retention may occur.
Life root	*Senecio aureus*	Emmenagogue	Contains pyrrolizidine alkaloids that are potentially hepatotoxic and carcinogenic.
Pokeroot	*Phytolacca americana*	Anticancer, antirheumatic	Contains a saponin mixture, phytolaccatoxin, and PWM (a proteinaceous mitogen), which can cause gastroenteritis, hypotension, and diminished respiration.
Sassafras	*Sassafras albidum*	Antirheumatic, antispasmodic, stimulant	Contains the volatile oil safrole, which is potentially carcinogenic.
Yohimbe	*Pausinystalia yohimbe*	Impotence	Side effects include anxiety, nervousness, nausea, vomiting, and tachycardia.

From Novey DW: *A clinician's guide to complementary & alternative medicine,* St Louis, 2000, Mosby.

Commonly Used Herbal Medicines

HERBAL MEDICINE	SCIENTIFIC NAME	COMMON USE	POTENTIAL INTERACTIONS	POTENTIAL ADVERSE EFFECTS	CONTRAINDICATIONS
Aloe vera (external only)	Aloe barbendenis, Aloe vera, various Aloe species	External: first-degree burns, cuts, abrasions	None known	Contact dermatitis	May delay healing of deep vertical (surgical) wounds
Arnica (external only)	Arnica montana	External: wound healing, inflammation	None known	Contact dermatitis; can damage skin with prolonged use	None unknown
Astragalus (or Tragacanth)	Astragalus membranaceus	Colds, flu, minor infections; hyperlipidemia, hyperglycemia (unproven)	None known	None known	None known
Bearberry	Arctostaphylos uva-ursi	Urinary tract inflammation	Any substance that acidifies the urine	Nausea and vomiting	Pregnancy, lactation, children under age 12 yr
Bilberry	Vaccinium myrtillus	Atherosclerosis, bruising, diarrhea, local inflammation of mucous membranes	Anticoagulants and antiplatelet drugs (possible)	Excessive consumption of berries; constipation	None known
Black cohosh	Cimicifuga racemosa	Dysmenorrhea, menopausal symptoms, premenstrual syndrome	None known	Gastric discomfort, dizziness, nervous system and visual disturbances, hypotension, bradycardia, increased perspiration	Pregnancy, lactation
Blessed thistle	Centaurea enedictus	Appetite stimulant, dyspepsia	None known	Allergies	Allergies to blessed thistle
Blue cohosh	Caulophyllum thalictroides	Menstrual difficulties; uterine stimulant	None known	Hypertension, respiratory stimulation, stimulation of intestinal motility	Should not be used without medical supervision; pregnancy, lactation, in children
Calendula	Calendula officinalis	External: wound healing	None known	None known	None known
Cascara sagrada	Rhamnus purshiana	Constipation	With chronic use due to potassium loss: cardiac glycoside, thiazide diuretics, corticosteroids, licorice root	Abdominal cramps	Intestinal obstruction, acute intestinal inflammation
Cat's claw	Unicaria tomentosa, U. guianesis	Cancer (anecdotal)	None known	None known	None known
Cayenne (Capsicum)	Capsicum frutescens	External: muscle spasms, chronic pain associated with herpes zoster, trigeminal neuralgia, surgical trauma	None known	Local burning sensation, hypersensitivity reaction	Injured skin, allergy
Chamomile	Matricaria recutita (formerly M. chamomile, Chamomile recutita)	External: skin and mucous membrane inflammation; internal: GI spasm and GI inflammatory disease	May delay concomitant drug absorption from the gut	Allergies (rare)	Allergies to chamomile (and other herbs of the daisy family); avoid in pregnancy

Common name	Latin name	Uses	Drug interactions	Potential adverse effects	Contraindications
Cranberry	*Vaccinium macrocarpon*	Prevention of urinary tract infection	None known	Overuse: diarrhea	None known
Dandelion	*Tanaxacum officinale*	Appetite stimulant, dyspepsia	None known	Contact dermatitis, gastric discomfort	None known
Devil's claw	*Arpagophytum procumbens*	Appetite stimulant, supportive therapy for degenerative disorder of the locomotor system	None known	None known	Gastric and duodenal ulcers; gallstone (use only after consultation with health care provider)
Dong-quai	*Angelica sinensis*	CNS stimulant, suppression of immune system, analgesia, uterus stimulant (effectiveness is controversial)	Contains courmarin derivatives, monitor with warfarin; possible synergism with calcium channel blockers	Photosensitivity; lowers blood pressure, possible CNS stimulation; possible carcinogenic (contains safrole)	Pregnancy
Echinacea	*Echinacea angustifolia, E. pallida, E. purpurea*	Supportive therapy for colds and flu	None known	Local tingling and numbing sensation with fresh juice	Long-term use not recommended; progressive systemic illness such as tuberculosis, leucosis, collagenosis, multiple sclerosis, AIDS and HIV infection, and other autoimmune diseases; allergy to plants in the daisy family
Eleuthero	*Eleutherococcus senticosus*	Improvement in well-being	Digitalis glycosides	High doses: irritability, insomnia, anxiety; skin eruptions, headache, diarrhea, hypertension, pericardial pain in rheumatic heart disease	Similar to ginseng
Evening primrose	*Oenothera biennis*	Hyperlipidemia, atopic eczema	None known	Nausea, GI disturbances, headache	None known
Eyebright	*Euphrasia officinalis*	Topical: conjunctivitis, eye irritations	None known	None known; cannot be recommended because of risk of potential contamination with homemade, nonsterile preparations	See "Potential Adverse Effects"
Fenugreek	*Trigonella foenum-graecum*	External: inflammation; internal: appetite stimulant	None known	Skin reactions with repeated external application	None known
Feverfew	*Tanacetum parthenium*	Migraine prophylaxis	Anticoagulants, antiplatelet drugs, thrombolytics	Mouth ulceration with chewing leaves, oral irritation, GI disturbances, increase in heart rate	Allergy to feverfew and other plants in the daisy family; pregnancy
Fo-ti	*Polygonum multiforum*	Rejuvenation, decreased liver and kidney function, insomnia, hyperlipidemia, immunosuppression, antimicrobial	None known	None known	Pregnancy

Commonly Used Herbal Medicines—cont'd

HERBAL MEDICINE	SCIENTIFIC NAME	COMMON USE	POTENTIAL INTERACTIONS	POTENTIAL ADVERSE EFFECTS	CONTRAINDICATIONS
Garlic	Allium sativum	Hyperlipidemia; other uses: antibacterial, anticancer, antifungal, antihypertensive, antiinflammatory agent, hypoglycemic	Anticoagulants, antiplatelet drugs	GI disturbances, garlic odor; may increase insulin level, producing decrease in blood glucose; high dose: anemia	Pregnancy and lactation
Ginger	Zingiber officinale	Dyspepsia, prevention of motion sickness	Anticoagulants, antiplatelet drugs; calcium channel blocker (possible)	None; GI irritation and discomfort with high dose	Gallstones (use only after consultation with health care provider); pregnancy (controversial)
Ginkgo	Ginkgo biloba	Symptomatic treatment of age-related organic brain syndrome, peripheral arterial occlusive disease (stage II of Fontaine), SSRI-induced sexual dysfunction, tinnitus, vertigo	Anticoagulants, antiplatelet drugs, thrombolytics	GI upset, headache, allergic skin reaction; cases of spontaneous bleeding have been reported	None known
Ginseng	Panax ginseng, P. quinquefolia	Improvement in well-being	Anticoagulants, antiplatelet drugs, thrombolytics; may potentiate MAOIs; stimulants (including caffeine), antipsychotic drugs, hormone therapy	High dose: breast tenderness, nervousness, excitation; estrogenic effects in women, hypotension, hypertension	Chronic use (should use 2 wk on and 2 wk off); acute illnesses, any form of hemorrhage; pregnancy and lactation
Goldenseal	Hydrastis canadensi	Inflammation of mucous membranes (unproven); does not mask illegal drugs in urine drug screens	May interfere with the ability of colon to manufacture B vitamins and may decrease their absorption; heparin (possible)	Hypoglycemia	Pregnancy and lactation
Gotu kola	Centella asiatica (formerly Hydrocotyle asiatica)	External: wound healing	None known	Hypersensitivity	None known
Grape seed	Vitis vinifera	Antioxidant	None known	None known	None known
Hawthorn	Crataegus spp.	Congestive heart failure; stage II of NYHA	Cardiotonic drugs, antihypertensive drugs	High dose: hypotension and sedation; nausea, fatigue, sweating, rash; none	Pregnancy, lactation
Horse chestnut	Aeculus hippocastanum	Chronic venous insufficiency	None known	GI disturbances, nausea, pruritus	None known
Hyssop	Hyssopus officinalis	Pharyngitis, expectorant	None known	None known	None known
Kava-kava	Piper methysticum	Anxiety, restlessness, sleep induction	Potentiation of CNS depressants and alcohol	Chronic use: kavaism with dry, flaking, discolored skin and reddened eyes; numbness of mouth with chewing, CNS depression	Pregnancy, nursing, endogenous depression

Common name	Scientific name	Uses	Interactions	Side effects	Contraindications
Licorice	*Glycyrrhiza glabra*	Gastric/duodenal ulcers	Due to potassium loss; digitalis glycosides, thiazide diuretics, corticosteroids, licorice	With prolonged use and with high doses: mineralocorticoid effects including sodium and water retention, hypokalemia, myoglobinuria	Gall bladder disease, kidney disease, pheochromocytoma and other adrenal tumors, diseases that cause low serum potassium livers, fasting, anorexia, bulimia, untreated hypothyroidism
Marshmallow	*Althaea officinalis*	Ingestion, irritation of oral and pharyngeal mucosa	May delay absorption of other drugs taken simultaneously	None known	None known
Milkthistle	*Silbum marianum*	Dyspepsia, supportive therapy for toxic liver damage	None known	Mild diarrhea	None known
Passion flower	*Passiflora incarnata*	Anxiety, insomnia (unproven)	None known	None known; may have MAOI activity	None known
Pau d'arco	*Tabebuia impetiginosa*	Cancer	Vitamin K	Chronic use: anemia	Bleeding disorders
Peppermint	*Mentha X piperita*	External: myalgia and neuralgia; internal: GI spasms, nausea, inflammation of oral mucosa	External: irritation of mucous membranes; overuse: heartburn, relaxation of esophageal sphincter	External: contact dermatitis; internal: mouth irritation, muscle tremor, hypersensitivity reaction, heartburn, bradycardia	Obstruction of bile ducts, gallbladder inflammation, severe liver damage, pregnancy
Plantain	*Plantago major*	External: inflammation of skin; internal: cough, oral and pharyngeal mucosa inflammation	None known	None known	None known
Pygeum	*Pygeum africanum*	Benign prostatic hyperplasia	None known	GI disturbance	None known
Saw palmetto	*Serenoa repens*	Benign prostatic hyperplasia, stages I and II	Hormone therapy	GI disturbance	Pregnancy, lactation, children, breast cancer
Slippery elm	*Scutellaria lateriflora*	Pharyngitis, GI inflammatory disorders	None known	Contact dermatitis	None known
St. John's wort	*Hypericum perforatum*	External: oil preparation for mild wounds and burns; internal: mild to moderate depression	MAOIs; SSRIs and other antidepressants, sympathomimetics	Possible photosensitization, GI disturbance	Pregnancy and lactation
Stinging nettle	*Urtica dionica*	Benign prostatic hyperplasia	None known	Allergy	Pregnancy; cardiac and renal dysfunction
Tea tree	*Melaleuca alternifolia*	External: bacteriostatic	None known	Allergic contact dermatitis	None known
Tumeric	*Curuma longa*	Dyspepsia	None known	None known	Obstruction of bile passages
Valerian	*Valeriana officinalis*	Restlessness, sleeping disorders	Possible with CNS depressants and alcohol	Strong, disagreeable odor; headache, excitability, cardiac disturbances, rare morning drowsiness	None known
Vitex (or chaste tree berry)	*Vitex agnus-castus*	Menstrual disorders	May interfere with dopamine-receptor antagonists	GI disturbances, itching, urticaria	None known

AIDS, Acquired immunodeficiency syndrome; *CNS*, central nervous system; *GI*, gastrointestinal; *HIV*, human immunodeficiency virus; *MAOI*, monoamine oxidase inhibitor; *NYHA*, New York Heart Association; *SSRI*, selective serotonin reuptake inhibitors.

Drug/Herb Interactions

The table that follows lists known drug/herb interactions for herbs included in this book. The pharmaceuticals and drug classes that are known to interact with herbal products are listed in the first column in alphabetical order, beside the names of the herbs with which they interact.

The reader should not assume that an herbal product not included here may be taken safely with a given drug or class of drugs. Research into herbal products is changing constantly, and new interactions are becoming known every day. Caution is always necessary when using herbal products, particularly when the client is taking them concurrently with pharmaceuticals.

From Skidmore-Roth L: *Mosby's Handbook of Herbs & Natural Supplements*, St Louis, 2004, Mosby.

DRUG/DRUG CLASSES	HERB	INTERACTION
ACE inhibitors	Pill-bearing spurge	May ↑ hypotension, do not use concurrently
ACE inhibitors	Pineapple	May antagonize ACE inhibitor actions, do not use concurrently
ACE inhibitors	Yohimbe	May ↓ or block actions of these drugs, do not use concurrently
ACE inhibitors	St. John's wort	May lead to severe photosensitivity, do not use concurrently
Acetazolamide	Quinine	When used with acetazolamide may lead to toxicity, do not use concurrently
Adenosine	Guarana	May ↓ the adenosine response
Alcohol	Betel palm	⎪aa effects of alcohol
Alcohol	Catnip	May enhance the effects of alcohol
Alcohol	Chamomile	May ⎪aa the effects of alcohol
Alcohol	Clary	⎪aa the action of alcohol
Alcohol	Corkwood	May ⎪aa anticholinergic effect
Alcohol	Goldenseal	May ⎪aa the effects of alcohol
Alcohol	Hops	⎪aa CNS effects
Alcohol	Jamaican dogwood	⎪aa effects of alcohol, do not use concurrently
Alcohol	St. John's wort	May ↑ MAO inhibition, do not use concurrently
Alcohol	Lavender	↑ sedation when used with lavender, do not use concurrently
All medications	Fenugreek	May cause reduced absorption of all medications used concurrently
All medications	Glucomanan	May ↓ the absorption of all medications if taken concurrently; separate dosages by at least 2 hours
All medications	Kaolin	↓ absorption of all drugs
All medications	Karaya gum	↓ absorption of all drugs
All medications	Pectin	↓ absorption of all drugs, vitamins, and minerals if taken concurrently
All oral medications	Flax	Absorption may ↓ if taken concurrently
All oral medications	Ginger	May ↑ absorption of all medications taken orally
All oral medications	Guar gum	May ↓ the absorption of all oral medications
All oral medications	Marshmallow	May ↓ absorption of oral medications, do not use concurrently
All oral medications	Mullein	May ↓ absorption of oral medications
Alpha-adrenergic blockers	Yohimbe	May result in ↑ toxicity, do not use concurrently
Alpha-adrenergic blockers	Butcher's broom	May ↓ action of alpha-adrenergic blockers
Alpha-adrenergic blockers	Capsicum peppers	May ↓ the action of alpha-adrenergic blockers
Aluminium salts	Quinine	May cause ↓ absorption of quinine
Amantadine	Jimsonweed	↑ antocholinergic effects
Amphetamines	Eucalyptus	May ↓ the effectiveness of amphetamines
Amphetamines	Rauwolfia	May cause ↓ pressor effects, do not use concurrently
Amphetamines	St. John's wort	May cause serotonin syndrome
Amphetamines	Khat	↑ action
Analgesics	Cola tree	May ↑ the effect of analgesics
Anesthetics	Ephedra	Causes ↑ arrhythmias when used with halothane anesthetics
Antacids	Jimsonweed	↓ action of jimsonweed
Antacids	Buckthorn	May ↓ the action of buckthorn if taken within 1 hour of the herb
Antacids	Cascara sagrada	May ↓ the action of cascara if taken within 1 hour of the herb
Antacids	Castor	To prevent decreased absorption of castor, do not take within 1 hour of antacids
Antacids	Chinese rhubarb	May ↓ the effectiveness of Chinese rhubarb if taken within 1 hour of the herb
Antacids	Green tea	May ↓ the therapeutic effects of green tea
Antianginals	Blue cohosh	May ↓ the action of antianginals, causing chest pain
Antianxiety agents	Cowslip	May ↑ the effect of antianxiety agents
Antiarrhythmics	Buckthorn	Chronic buckthorn use can cause hypokalemia and enhance the effects of antiarrhythmics
Antiarrhythmics	Khat	↑ action
Antiarrhythmics	Broom	May ↑ the effect of antiarrhythmics
Antiarrhythmics	Cascara sagrada	Chronic cascara use can cause hypokalemia and enhance the effects of antiarrhythmics
Antiarrhythmics	Chinese rhubarb	Chronic use of Chinese rhubarb can cause hypokalemia and enhance the effects of antiarrhythmics
Antiarrhythmics	Figwort	May ↑ the effects of antiarrhythmics
Antiarrhythmics	Fumitory	May ↑ the effects of antiarrhythmics
Antiarrhythmics	Goldenseal	May ↑ the effects of antiarrhythmics
Antiarrhythmics	Horehound	↑ serotonin effect, do not use concurrently

DRUG/DRUG CLASSES	HERB	INTERACTION
Antiarrhythmics	Licorice	↑ cardiac effects of antiarrhythmics, do not use concurrently
Antiarrhythmics	Aconite	↑ toxicity
Antibiotics	Acidophilus	Do not use concurrently
Anticholinergics	Jaborandi tree	When taken internally may ↓ effects of anticholinergics
Anticholinergics	Butterbur	May enhance the effects of anticholinergics
Anticholinergics	Jimsonweed	↑ effects of anticholinergics
Anticholinergics	Pill-bearing spurge	May ↓ effects of anticholinergic, do not use concurrently
Anticoagulants	Agrimony	May ↓ clotting times
Anticoagulants	Alfalfa	May prolong bleeding
Anticoagulants	Angelica	May prolong bleeding
Anticoagulants	Bilberry	May ↑ action of anticoagulants
Anticoagulants	Black haw	↑ the action of anticoagulants
Anticoagulants	Bogbean	May ↑ risk of bleeding
Anticoagulants	Buchu	Can ↑ the action of anticoagulants, causing bleeding
Anticoagulants	Chamomile	May interfere with the actions of anticoagulants
Anticoagulants	Chondroitin	Can cause ↑ bleeding
Anticoagulants	Coenzyme q10	May ↓ the action of anticoagulants
Anticoagulants	Fenugreek	Risk of ↑ bleeding when used concurrently
Anticoagulants	Feverfew	May ↑ anticoagulant effects
Anticoagulants	Garlic	May ↑ bleeding when used concurrently
Anticoagulants	Ginger	May ↑ risk of bleeding when taken concurrently
Anticoagulants	Ginkgo	↑ risk of bleeding
Anticoagulants	Ginseng	May ↓ the action of anticoagulants
Anticoagulants	Goldenseal	May ↓ the effects of anticoagulants
Anticoagulants	Horse chestnut	↑ risk of severe bleeding, do not use concurrently
Anticoagulants	Irish moss	↑ effects of anticoagulants, do not use concurrently
Anticoagulants	Kelp	May pose ↑ risk of bleeding, do not use concurrently
Anticoagulants	Kelpware	May pose ↑ risk of bleeding, do not use concurrently
Anticoagulants	Khella	↑ risk of bleeding when used with anticoagulants, do not use concurrently
Anticoagulants	Lovage	May ↑ effects of anticoagulants, do not use concurrently
Anticoagulants	Lungwort	May ↑ effects of anticoagulants, do not use concurrently
Anticoagulants	Lysine	Use of large amounts of lysine causes ↑ aminoglycoside toxicity, do not use concurrently
Anticoagulants	Meadowsweet	May ↑ risk of bleeding, do not use concurrently
Anticoagulants	Motherwort	May cause ↑ risk of bleeding, do not use concurrently
Anticoagulants	Mugwort	May cause ↑ risk of bleeding, do not use concurrently
Anticoagulants	Nettle	May ↓ effect of anticoagulants, do not use concurrently
Anticoagulants	Parsley	Large amounts may interfere with anticoagulation therapy
Anticoagulants	Pau d'arco	May result in ↑ risk of bleeding, do not use concurrently
Anticoagulants	Pill-bearing spurge	May ↑ effects of anticoagulants, do not use concurrently
Anticoagulants	Pineapple	May ↑ bleeding time when used with anticoagulants, do not use concurrently
Anticoagulants	Poplar	May ↑ bleeding time when used with anticoagulants, do not use concurrently
Anticoagulants	Prickly ash	May ↑ bleeding time when used with anticoagulants, do not use concurrently
Anticoagulants	Quinine	May ↑ action of anticoagulants, do not use concurrently
Anticoagulants	Safflower	May potentiate anticoagulant action, do not use concurrently
Anticoagulants	Saw palmetto	May potentiate anticoagulant effect of salicylants, do not use concurrently
Anticoagulants	Senega	May ↑ bleeding time, do not use concurrently
Anticoagulants	Tonka bean	May result in ↑ risk of bleeding, do not use concurrently
Anticoagulants	Turmeric	May result in ↑ risk of bleeding, do not use concurrently
Anticoagulants	Wintergreen	May cause ↑ risk of bleeding, do not use concurrently
Anticoagulants	Yarrow	May result in ↑ risk of bleeding, do not use concurrently
Anticoagulants, oral	Dong quai	May ↑ the effects of oral anticoagulants
Anticonvulsants	Ginkgo	May ↓ the anticonvulsant effect
Anticonvulsants	Ginseng	May provide an additive anticonvulsant action when taken concurrently
Anticonvulsants	Sage	May ↓ action of anticonvulsants, do not use concurrently
Antidepressants	Hops	↑ CNS effects
Antidepressants	Sam-e	Combining with antidepressants may lead to serotonin syndrome, do not use concurrently
Antidepressants	St. John's wort	Combined with these drugs may lead to severe photosensitivity, do not use concurrently
Antidiabetics	Alfalfa	May potentiate hypoglycemic action
Antidiabetics	Aloe	When taken internally may ↑ effects of antidiabetics
Antidiabetics	Blue cohosh	May ↓ the action of antidiabetics
Antidiabetics	Burdock	↑ hypoglycemic effect can occur
Antidiabetics	Elecampane	May ↓ blood glucose
Antidiabetics	Ephedra	May ↑ blood glucose
Antidiabetics	Eyebright	May ↑ the effects of antidiabetics when taken internally
Antidiabetics	Glucosamine	May ↑ the hypoglycemic effects of oral antidiabetics
Antidiabetics	Goat's rue	May ↑ the hypoglycemic effects of oral antidiabetics
Antidiabetics	Gotu kola	May ↓ the effectiveness of antidiabetics
Antidiabetics	Horehound	Enhance hypoglycemia, do not use concurrently
Antidiabetics	Horse chestnut	↑ hypoglycemic effects
Antidiabetics	Jambul	↑ effects of antidiabetics, do not use concurrently

Continued

DRUG/DRUG CLASSES	HERB	INTERACTION
Antidiabetics	Myrrh	May cause ↑ hypoglycemic effects, do not use concurrently
Antidiabetics	Myrtle	May cause ↑ hypoglycemic effects, do not use concurrently
Antidiabetics	Senega	May ↓ effects of antidiabetics, do not use concurrently
Antidiabetics	Raspberry	May ↑ hypoglycemia, monitor blood glucose levels
Antidiabetics	Siberian ginseng	May ↑ levels of antidiabetics, do not use concurrently
Antidiabetics, oral	Bay	May ↑ hypoglycemic effects
Antidiabetics, oral	Bee pollen	↓ effectiveness of antidiabetics, ↑ hyperglycemia
Antidiabetics, oral	Bilberry	May ↑ hypoglycemia
Antidiabetics, oral	Coenzyme q10	Oral antidiabetics may ↓ the action of coenzyme Q10 and deplete endogenous stores
Antidiabetics, oral	Coriander	May ↑ the effects of oral antidiabetics
Antidiabetics, oral	Dandelion	May ↑ the effects of oral antidiabetics
Antidiabetics, oral	Eucalyptus	May alter the effectiveness of antidiabetics
Antidiabetics, oral	Fenugreek	Hypoglycemial is possible when used concurrently
Antidiabetics, oral	Garlic	Because of hypoglycemic effects of garlic, oral antidiabetic dosages may need to be adjusted
Antidiabetics, oral	Ginseng	May ↑ the hypoglycemic effects of oral antidiabetics
Antidiabetics, oral	Glucomanan	May ↑ the hypoglycemic effects of oral antidiabetics
Antidiabetics, oral	Gymnema	May ↑ the action of oral antidiabetics
Antidiarrheals	Nutmeg	May be potentiated, monitor for constipation
Antidysrhythmics	Aloe	When taken internally may ↑ effects of antidysrhythmics
Antidysrhythmics	Coltsfoot	May antagonize antidysrhythmics
Antidysrhythmics	Devil's claw	Use cautiously because of possible inotropic and chronotropic effects
Antifungals	Gossypol	Concurrent use may cause nephrotoxicity
Antifungals, azole	Goldenseal	May slow the metabolism of azole antifungals
Antifungals, azole	Licorice	May ↑ levels of azole antifungals, do not use concurrently
Antiglaucoma agents	Betel palm	↓ effects of antiglaucoma agents
Antihistamines	Lavender	↑ sedation when used with lavender, do not use concurrently
Antihistamines	Khat	↑ action
Antihistamines	Corkwood	May ↑ anticholinergic effect
Antihistamines	Hops	↑ CNS effects
Antihistamines	Jamaican dogwood	May produce ↑ effect, do not use concurrently
Antihypertensives	Khat	↑ action
Antihypertensives	Aconite	↑ toxicity
Antihypertensives	Astragalus	May ↑ or ↓ action of antihypertensives
Antihypertensives	Barberry	May ↑ antihypertensive action
Antihypertensives	Betony	May ↑ action of antihypertensives
Antihypertensives	Black cohosh	↑ action of antihypertensives
Antihypertensives	Blood root	May ↑ hypotensive effects
Antihypertensives	Blue cohosh	↓ the action of antihypertensives and ↑ blood pressure
Antihypertensives	Broom	May ↑ the effect of antihypertensives
Antihypertensives	Burdock	May ↑ hypotensive effects
Antihypertensives	Cat's claw	May ↑ the hypotensive effects of antihypertensives
Antihypertensives	Coltsfoot	May antagonize antihypertensives
Antihypertensives	Dandelion	May ↑ the effects of antihypertensives
Antihypertensives	Goldenseal	May ↑ the effects of antihypertensives
Antihypertensives	Guarana	May ↓ the effects of antihypertensives
Antihypertensives	Hawthorn	May ↑ hypotension when used concurrently
Antihypertensives	Irish moss	↑ effects of antihypertensives, do not use concurrently
Antihypertensives	Jamaican dogwood	↑ effects of antihypertensive, do not use concurrently
Antihypertensives	Kelp	↑ hypotensive effects, do not use concurrently
Antihypertensives	Khella	↑ hypotension when used with antihypertensives, do not use concurrently
Antihypertensives	Licorice	May cause ↑ hypokalemia, do not use concurrently
Antihypertensives	Mistletoe	May cause ↑ hypotensive effect of antihypertensives, do not use concurrently
Antihypertensives	Queen Anne's lace	↑ hypotension when used with antihypertensives, use together cautiously
Antihypertensives	Rue	May cause ↑ vasodilation, do not use concurrently
Antihypertensives	Yarrow	May result in ↑ hypotension, do not use concurrently
Antilipidemics	Glucomanan	May ↑ the action of antilipidemics
Antilipidemics	Gotu kola	May ↓ the effectiveness of antilipidemics
Antimigraine agents	Butterbur	May enhance the effects of antimigraine agents
Antineoplastics	Yew	May cause ↑ myelosuppression, do not use concurrently
Antiparkinson agents	Kava	↑ symptoms of parkinsonism, do not use concurrently
Antiplatelet agents	Bilberry	May cause antiaggregation of platelets
Antiplatelet agents	Bogbean	May ↑ risk of bleeding
Antiplatelet agents	Dong quai	May ↑ the effects of antiplatelet agents
Antiplatelet agents	Feverfew	May ↑ the action of antiplatelet agents
Antiplatelet agents	Ginger	May ↑ risk of bleeding when taken concurrently
Antiplatelet agents	Saw palmetto	May lead to ↑ bleeding, do not use concurrently
Antiplatelet agents	Ginkgo	↑ risk of bleeding
Antipsychotics	Hops	↑ CNS effects

DRUG/DRUG CLASSES	HERB	INTERACTION
Antipsychotics	Kava	May result in neuroleptic disorder
Antiretrovirals	St. John's wort	When taken PO in combination with indinavir may ↓ the antiretroviral action.
Ascorbic acid	Chromium	Both chromium and ascorbic acid absorption ↑ when taken concurrently
Aspirin	Bilberry	May ↑ the anticoagulation action of aspirin
Aspirin	Bogbean	May ↑ risk of bleeding
Aspirin	Horse chestnut	↑ risk of severe bleeding, do not use concurrently
Atropine	Black root	Forms an insoluble complex with atropine; do not use concurrently
Barbiturates	Eucalyptus	May ↓ the effectiveness of barbiturates
Barbiturates	Jamaican dogwood	↑ effects of barbiturates, do not use concurrently
Barbiturates	Kava	↑ sedation
Barbiturates	Pill-bearing spurge	May ↑ effects of barbiturates, do not use concurrently
Barbiturates	Lemon balm	May potentiate the sedative effects of bariturates
Belladonna alkaloids	Mayapple	May ↓ laxative effects of mayapple, do not use concurrently
Benzodiazepines	Coffee	↓ the effect of benzodiazepines
Benzodiazepines	Cola tree	May ↓ the effect of cola tree products
Benzodiazepines	Goldenseal	May slow the metabolism of benzodiazepines
Benzodiazepines	Kava	↑ sedation and coma, do not use concurrently
Benzodiazepines	Melatonin	May ↑ anxiolytic effects of benzodiazepines, use cautiously
Beta-blockers	Betel palm	↑ action of beta-blockers
Beta-blockers	Butterbur	May enhance the effects of beta-blockers
Beta-blockers	Coenzyme q10	Beta-blockers may ↓ the action of coenzyme Q10 and deplete endogenous stores
Beta-blockers	Coffee	Caffeine in coffee ↑ blood pressure in those taking beta-blockers
Beta-blockers	Cola tree	May ↑ blood pressure when used with beta-blockers
Beta-blockers	Ephedra	Causes ↑ hypertension when used with beta-blockers
Beta-blockers	Figwort	May ↑ the effects of beta-blockers
Beta-blockers	Fumitory	May ↑ the effects of beta-blockers
Beta-blockers	Goldenseal	May ↑ the effects of beta-blockers
Beta-blockers	Guarana	May ↑ the effects of beta-blockers
Beta-blockers	Jaborandi tree	When used internally may ↑ adverse cardiovascular reactions, do not use concurrently
Beta-blockers	Khat	↑ action
Beta-blockers	Lily of the valley	May ↑ effects, do not use concurrently
Beta-blockers	Motherwort	May cause ↓ heart rate, do not use concurrently
Bethanechol	Jaborandi tree	When used internally, cholinergic effects ↑
Bronchodilators	Coffee	Large amounts of coffee may ↑ the action of some bronchodilators
Bronchodilators	Green tea	Large amounts of green tea ↑ the action of some bronchodilators
Bronchodilators	Guarana	May ↑ the action of bronchodilators
Caffeine	Creatine	May ↓ the effects of creatine
Calcitonin	Yellow dock	May cause ↑ hypocalcemia, do not use concurrently
Calcium supplements	Shark cartilage	May lead to ↑ calcium levels
Calcium-channel blockers	Khat	↑ action
Calcium-channel blockers	Lily of the valley	May ↑ effects, do not use concurrently
Calcium-channel blockers	Burdock	May ↑ hypotensive effects
Calcium-channel blockers	Goldenseal	May slow the metabolism of calcium-channel blockers
Calcium-channel blockers	Khella	↑ hypotension when used with calcium-channel blockers, do not use concurrently
Calcium-channel blockers	Barberry	May ↑ effect of calcium-channel blockers
Calcium-channel blockers	Betel palm	↑ action of calcium-channel blockers
Carbamazepine	Plantain	May ↓ effects of carbamazepine, do not use concurrently
Carbidopa	Octacosanol	May cause dyskinesia when used with carbidopa/levodopa, do not use concurrently
Cardiac agents	Squill	May ↑ effect of cardiac agents, causing life-threatening toxicity, do not use concurrently
Cardiac agents	Plantain	May ↑ effect of cardiac agents, do not use concurrently
Cardiac agents	Rauwolfia	May result in ↑ hypotension, do not use concurrently
Cardiac glycosides	Khat	↑ action
Cardiac glycosides	Lily of the valley	May ↑ effects, do not use concurrently
Cardiac glycosides	Aconite	↑ toxicity
Cardiac glycosides	Aloe	When taken internally may ↑ effects of cardiac glycosides
Cardiac glycosides	Betel palm	↑ action of cardiac glycosides
Cardiac glycosides	Beth root	May ↓ effects of cardiac glycosides
Cardiac glycosides	Black root	Forms an insoluble complex with cardiac glycosides; do not use concurrently
Cardiac glycosides	Broom	May ↑ the effect of cardiac glycosides
Cardiac glycosides	Buckthorn	Chronic buckthorn use can cause hypokalemia and enhance the effects of cardiac glycosides

Continued

DRUG/DRUG CLASSES	HERB	INTERACTION
Cardiac glycosides	Cascara sagrada	Chronic cascara use can cause hypokalemia and enhance the effects of cardiac glycosides
Cardiac glycosides	Chinese rhubarb	Chronic use of Chinese rhubarb can cause hypokalemia and enhance the effects of cardiac glycosides
Cardiac glycosides	Condurango	Absorption of digitoxin and digoxin may be ↓ when taken concurrently
Cardiac glycosides	Figwort	May ↑ the action of figwort
Cardiac glycosides	Fumitory	May ↑ the effects of cardiac glycosides
Cardiac glycosides	Goldenseal	May ↓ the effects of cardiac glycosides
Cardiac glycosides	Hawthorn	May ↑ the effects of cardiac glycosides
Cardiac glycosides	Horsetail	↑ toxicity and ↑ hypokalemia
Cardiac glycosides	Licorice	May cause ↑ toxicity and ↑ hypokalemia, do not use concurrently.
Cardiac glycosides	Mistletoe	May cause ↓ cardiac function, do not use concurrently
Cardiac glycosides	Motherwort	May cause ↓ heart rate, do not use concurrently
Cardiac glycosides	Night-blooming cereus	May ↑ actions of cardiac glycosides, do not use concurrently
Cardiac glycosides	Oleander	May cause fatal digitalis toxicity, do not use concurrently
Cardiac glycosides	Queen anne's lace	May ↑ cardiac depression, do not use concurrently
Cardiac glycosides	Quinine	May ↑ action of cardiac glycosides, do not use concurrently
Cardiac glycosides	Rauwolfia	Will cause severe bradycardia, do not use together
Cardiac glycosides	Rue	May cause ↑ inotropic effects, do not use concurrently
Cardiac glycosides	Senna	Chronic use may potentiate cardiac glycosides
Cardiac glycosides	Siberian ginseng	May ↑ levels of cardiac glycosides, do not use concurrently
Cardiac medications	Kudzu	Enhance effects of cardiac medications, do not use concurrently
Central nervous system depressants	Yarrow	May cause ↑ sedation, do not use concurrently
Central nervous system depressants	Goldenseal	May ↑ the effects of central nervous system depressants
Central nervous system depressants	Hawthorn	May ↑ the sedative effects of central nervous system depressants
Central nervous system depressants	Kava	↑ sedation, do not use concurrently
Central nervous system depressants	Mistletoe	May cause ↑ sedation, do not use concurrently
Central nervous system depressants	Passion flower	May cause ↑ sedation, do not use concurrently
Central nervous system depressants	Peyote	May ↑ effect of other CNS drugs, do not use concurrently
Central nervous system depressants	Hops	↑ CNS effects
Central nervous system depressants	Lemon balm	May potentiate the sedative effects of CNS depressants
Central nervous system depressants	Rauwolfia	May cause ↑ CNS depression, do not use concurrently
Central nervous system depressants	Skullcap	May potentiate sedation of CNS depressants, do not use concurrently
Central nervous system depressants	Senega	May cause ↑ CNS effects, do not use concurrently
Central nervous system depressants	Valerian	May ↑ effects of CNS depressants, do not use concurrently
Central nervous system depressants	Poppy	↑ CNS depression when use with CNS depressants, do not use concurrently
Central nervous system depressants	Nettle	May lead to ↑ CNS depression
Central nervous system depressants	Pokeweed	May ↑ action of CNS depressants, do not use concurrently
Central nervous system depressants	Yerba mate	May produce antagonistic effect, do not use concurrently
Central nervous system depressants	Queen Anne's lace	↑ action of CNS depressants, use together cautiously
Central nervous system stimulants	Squill	May ↑ effects of CNS stimulants, do not use concurrently
Central nervous system stimulants	Yerba mate	May ↑ effects CNS stimulants, use together cautiously
Central nervous system stimulants	Yohimbe	May result in ↑ CNS stimulation, do not use concurrently
Cerebral stimulants	Horsetail	↑ CNS effects, do not use concurrently
Cerebral stimulants	Melatonin	May have a synergistic effect and exacerbate insomnia, do not use concurrently
Cholinergics, ophthalmic	Jaborandi tree	When used internally cholinergic effects ↑

DRUG/DRUG CLASSES	HERB	INTERACTION
Cholinesterase inhibitors	Pill-bearing spurge	May ↑ effects of cholinesterase inhibitors
Ciprofloxacin	Fennel	Affects the absorption, distribution, and elimination of ciprofloxacin; dosages should be separated by at least 2 hours
Clonidine	Capsicum peppers	May ↓ the antihypertensive effects of clonidine
Contraceptives, oral	Alfalfa	May alter action
Contraceptives, oral	Black cohosh	May ↑ effects
Contraceptives, oral	Chaste tree	May interfere with the action of oral contraceptives
Contraceptives, oral	St. John's wort	When combined with oral contraceptives, may lead to severe photosensitivity, do not use concurrently
Corticosteroids	Buckthorn	Hypokalemia can result from use of buckthorn with corticosteroids
Corticosteroids	Cascara sagrada	Hypokalemia may result from concurrent use
Corticosteroids	Chinese rhubarb	Chronic use of Chinese rhubarb can cause hypokalemia and enhance the effects of corticosteroids
Corticosteroids	Licorice	May ↑ effects of corticosteroids, do not use concurrently
Corticosteroids	Perilla	May augment the effects of corticosteroids, do not use concurrently
CYP2A6, drugs metabolized by	Condurango	Use condurango with caution
CYP3A4, drugs metabolized by	Wild cherry	May slow metabolism, do not use concurrently
CYP450, drugs metabolized by	Myrtle	Do not use concurrently
CYP450, drugs metabolized by	Pennyroyal	Do not use concurrently with drugs metabolized by CYP450
CYP450, drugs metabolized by	Hops	↓ CYP450 levels
CYP450, drugs metabolized by	Milk thistle	Should not be used together
CYP450, drugs metabolized by	Black pepper	Avoid concurrent use
CYP450, drugs metabolized by	Condurango	Use condurango with caution, especially in clients with hepatic disorders
Decongestants	Khat	↑ action
Dhea	Melatonin	May ↓ cytokine production, do not use concurrently
Disulfiram	Pill-bearing spurge	Do not use concurrently
Disulfiram	Senna	Do not use with disulfiram
Diuretics	Yellow dock	May cause ↑ hypocalcemia, do not use concurrently
Diuretics	Bearberry	Concurrent use may lead to electrolyte loss, primarily hypokalemia
Diuretics	Cucumber	May ↑ the diuretic effect of other diuretics
Diuretics	Dandelion	May ↑ diuresis, leading to fluid loss and electrolyte imbalances
Diuretics	Gossypol	Concurrent use may cause severe hypokalemia
Diuretics	Horsetail	↑ effects of diuretics, do not use concurrently
Diuretics	Khella	↑ hypotension when used with diuretics, do not use concurrently
Diuretics	Licorice	May cause ↑ hypokalemia, do not use concurrently
Diuretics	Nettle	May ↑ effects of diuretics, resulting in dehydration and hypokalemia, do not use concurrently
Diuretics	Queen Anne's lace	↑ hypotension, use together cautiously
Diuretics	Yerba mate	May ↑ effects of diuretics, do not use concurrently
Diuretics, loop	St. John's wort	May lead to severe photosensitivity, do not use concurrently
Diuretics, loop	Aloe	When taken internally may ↑ effects of loop diuretics
Diuretics, thiazide	St. John's wort	May lead to severe photosensitivity, do not use concurrently
Diuretics, thiazide	Aloe	When taken internally may ↑ effects of thiazide diuretics
Diuretics, thiazide	Buckthorn	Hypokalemia can result from use of buckthorn with thiazide diuretics
Diuretics, thiazide	Cascara sagrada	Hypokalemia may result from concurrent use
Diuretics, thiazide	Chinese rhubarb	Chronic use of Chinese rhubarb can cause hypokalemia and enhance the effects of thiazide diuretics
Econazole vaginal cream	Echinacea	May ↓ the action of this cream
Electrolyte solutions	Agar	↑ dehydration
Emetics	Horehound	Granisetron and ondansetron ↑ serotonin effect, do not use concurrently
Ephedrine	Rauwolfia	May cause ↓ pressor effects, do not use concurrently
Epinephrine	Rauwolfia	May cause ↓ pressor effects, do not use concurrently
Ergots	Horehound	↑ serotonin effect, do not use concurrently
Estrogens	Alfalfa	May alter action
Estrogens	Hops	↑ hormonal levels
Furoquinolones	Cola tree	May ↑ the effect of cola tree products
Glucocorticoids	Squill	May ↑ effects of glucocorticoids, do not use concurrently

Continued

DRUG/DRUG CLASSES	HERB	INTERACTION
Glucose	Creatine	May ↑ the storage of creatine in muscle tissue
Guanethidine	Ephedra	May ↓ the effect of guanethidine
Hepatotoxic agents	Black root	Avoid concurrent use
HMG-coa reductase inhibitors	Coenzyme Q10	HMG-coa reductase inhibitors may ↓ the action of coenzyme Q10 and deplete endogenous stores
Hormone replacement therapy	Black cohosh	May alter the effects of other hormone replacement therapies
Hormone replacement therapy	Dhea	DHEA may interfere with estrogen and androgen therapy
Hormones	Saw palmetto	May antagonize hormone therapy, do not use concurrently
Hormones (animal)	Cat's claw	May interact with hormones made from animal products
Hypnotics	Clary	↑ the action of hypnotics
Hypoglycemics, oral	Bitter melon	May ↑ effects of oral hypoglycemics
Immune serum	Safflower	May cause ↑ immunosuppression, do not use concurrently
Immunomodulators	Echinacea	May ↓ the effects of immunosuppressants; should not be used immediately before, during, or after transplant surgery
Immunostimulants	Cat's claw	Do not use concurrently
Immunosuppressants	Ginseng	May diminish the effect of immunosuppressants; do not use before, during, or after transplant surgery
Immunosuppressants	Schisandra	May ↓ effectiveness of immunosuppressants, avoid use before, during, or after transplant surgery
Immunosuppressants	Safflower	May cause ↑ immunosuppression, do not use concurrently
Immunosuppressants	Mistletoe	May stimulate immunity, do not use concurrently
Immunosuppressants	St. John's wort	Rejection of transplanted hearts has occurred when taken PO with cyclosporine. Other immunosuppressants may have same interaction in this and other transplants
Immunosuppressants	Saw palmetto	May ↑ or ↓ immunostimulant effects, do not use concurrently
Immunosuppressants	Skullcap	May ↓ effects of immunosuppressants, do not use concurrently
Immunosuppressants	Turmeric	May ↓ effectiveness of immunosuppressants, do not use concurrently
Immunosuppressants	Maitake	May ↓ effects of immunosuppressants, do not use immediately before, during, or after transplant surgery.
Insulin	Basil	May ↑ hypoglycemic effects
Insulin	Bay	May ↑ hypoglycemic effects
Insulin	Bee pollen	↓ effectiveness of insulin, ↑ hyperglycemia
Insulin	Bilberry	May significantly ↓ blood sugar levels—monitor carefully
Insulin	Cat's claw	May interact with insulin
Insulin	Dandelion	May ↑ the effects of insulin
Insulin	Eucalyptus	May alter the effectiveness of insulin
Insulin	Garlic	Because of hypoglycemic effects of garlic, insulin dosages may need to be adjusted
Insulin	Ginseng	May ↑ the hypoglycemic effects of insulin
Insulin	Glucomanan	May ↑ the hypoglycemic effects of insulin
Insulin	Guar gum	May delay glucose absorption when used concurrently; insulin dose may need to be decreased
Insulin	Gymnema	May ↑ the action of insulin
Interferon	Astragalus	May prevent or shorten upper respiratory infections
Interleukin-2	Astragalus	May ↑ or ↓ effect of drugs such as interleukin-2
Ipecac	Mayapple	May ↓ laxative effects of mayapple, do not use concurrently
Iron salts	Bilberry	Interferes with iron absorption
Iron salts	Chromium	↓ chromium absorption when taken concurrently
Iron salts	Condurango	Iron absorption may be ↓
Iron salts	Ground ivy	May ↓ the absorption of iron salts
Iron salts	Hawthorn	May ↓ the absorption of iron salts; separate dosages by at least 2 hours
Iron salts	Hops	↓ absorption of iron salts
Iron salts	Horehound	↓ absorption of iron salts
Iron salts	Horse chestnut	↓ absorption of iron salts
Iron salts	Lady's mantle	↓ absorption of iron salts
Iron salts	Lavender	↓ absorption of iron salts
Iron salts	Lemon balm	↓ absorption of iron salts
Iron salts	Marshmallow	May ↓ absorption of iron salts
Iron salts	Meadowsweet	May ↓ absorption of iron salts
Iron salts	Mistletoe	May ↓ absorption of iron salts
Iron salts	Motherwort	May ↓ absorption of iron salts
Iron salts	Nettle	May interfere with absorption of iron salts
Iron salts	Oak	May ↓ absorption of iron salts
Iron salts	Plantain	May ↓ absorption of iron salts
Iron salts	Poplar	May ↓ absorption of iron salts
Iron salts	Prickly ash	May ↓ absorption of iron salts
Iron salts	Raspberry	May ↓ absorption of iron salts
Iron salts	Sage	May ↓ absorption of iron salts
Iron salts	Slippery elm	May ↓ absorption of iron salts
Iron salts	Squill	May ↓ absorption of iron salts

DRUG/DRUG CLASSES	HERB	INTERACTION
Iron salts	Valerian	May interfere with absorption of iron salts
Iron salts	Witch hazel	May ↓ absorption of iron salts
Iron salts	Yellow dock	May ↓ absorption of iron salts
Isoproterenol	Rauwolfia	May cause ↓ pressor effects, do not use concurrently
Kanamycin	Siberian ginseng	May ↑ action of kanamycin
Laxatives	Flax	May ↑ the action of laxatives
Laxatives	Senna	Additive effect can occur, do not use concurrently
Laxatives	Squill	May ↑ effects of laxatives, do not use concurrently
Levodopa	Octacosanol	May cause dyskinesia when used with carbidopa/levodopa, do not use concurrently
Levodopa	Rauwolfia	↓ effect of levodopa, with ↑ extrapyramidal motor symptoms
Lithium	Coffee	↓ levels of lithium
Lithium	Cola tree	May ↓ the effect of cola tree products
Lithium	Dandelion	Toxicity may occur if used concurrently
Lithium	Goldenrod	May result in dehydration and lithium toxicity
Lithium	Horsetail	Dehydration and lithium toxicity
Lithium	Juniper	Dehydration and lithium toxicity
Lithium	Nettle	May result in dehydration, lithium toxicity
Lithium	Parsley	May lead to dehydration, lithium toxicity
Lithium	Plantain	May ↓ effects of lithium, do not use concurrently
Magnesium	Melatonin	↑ inhibition of N-methyl-D-aspartate receptors, do not use concurrently
Magnesium	Quinine	May cause ↓ absorption of quinine
MAOIs	Khat	↑ action
MAOIs	Betel palm	May ↑ chance of hypertensive crisis
MAOIs	Butcher's broom	May ↑ action of MAOIs and precipitate a hypertensive crisis
MAOIs	Cacao tree	May ↑ the vasopressor effect of MAOIs
MAOIs	Capsicum peppers	May precipitate hypertensive crisis
MAOIs	Coffee	Large amounts of coffee should be avoided; hypertensive actions may occur
MAOIs	Cola tree	May ↑ blood pressure when used with phenelzine and tranylcypromine
MAOIs	Ephedra	Hypertensive crisis can occur when used concurrently
MAOIs	Galanthamine	Hypertensive crisis may occur
MAOIs	Ginkgo	May ↑ action of MAOIs
MAOIs	Ginseng	Concurrent use may result in manic-like syndrome
MAOIs	Green tea	Large amounts of green tea taken concurrently with MAOIs can cause hypertensive crisis
MAOIs	Guarana	Large amounts of guarana taken with MAOIs can result in hypertensive crisis
MAOIs	Jimsonweed	↑ anticholinergic effects
MAOIs	Night-blooming cereus	May ↑ cardiac effects, do not use concurrently
MAOIs	Nutmeg	May be potentiated, do not use concurrently
MAOIs	Parsley	When used with tricyclics or SSRIs may lead to serotonin syndrome, do not use concurrently
MAOIs	Passion flower	May cause ↑ MAOI activity, do not use concurrently
MAOIs	Rauwolfia	May cause excitation and/or hypertension, do not use concurrently
MAOIs	St. John's wort	May ↑ MAO inhibition, do not use concurrently
MAOIs	Valerian	May negate therapeutic effects of MAOIs, do not use concurrently
MAOIs	Yohimbe	May ↑ effects of MAOIs, do not use concurrently
Methyldopa	Capsicum peppers	May ↓ the antihypertensive effects of methyldopa
Minerals	Allspice	May interfere with absorption of minerals
Minerals	Pipsissewa	Should be taken 2 hrs before or after pipsissewa
Mithramycin	Yellow dock	May cause ↑ hypocalcemia, do not use concurrently
Morphine	Oats	May ↓ effect of morphine, do not use concurrently
Neuromuscular blockers	Quinine	May ↑ action of neuromuscular blockers, do not use concurrently
Nicotine	Lobelia	↑ effects of nicotine-containing products, do not use concurrently
Nicotine	Oats	May ↓ hypertensive effects of nicotine
Norepinephrine	Rauwolfia	May cause ↓ pressor effects, do not use concurrently
NSAIDs	Bearberry	May ↑ effect of NSAIDs
NSAIDs	Bilberry	May ↑ action of NSAIDs
NSAIDs	Bogbean	May ↑ risk of bleeding
NSAIDs	Chondroitin	Can cause ↑ bleeding
NSAIDs	Gossypol	Concurrent use may result in gastrointestinal distress and gastrointestinal tissue damage
NSAIDs	St. John's wort	When combined may lead to severe photosensitivity, do not use concurrently
NSAIDs	Turmeric	May result in ↑ risk of bleeding, do not use concurrently
NSAIDs	Saw palmetto	May lead to ↑ bleeding time, do not use concurrently
NSAIDs, topical	Jaborandi tree	Jaborandi tree action ↓ when used with topical NSAIDs, do not use concurrently
Opioids	Lavender	↑ sedation when used with lavender, do not use concurrently
Opioids	Parsley	May cause serotonin syndrome, do not use concurrently
Opioids	Corkwood	May ↑ anticholinergic effect

Continued

DRUG/DRUG CLASSES	HERB	INTERACTION
Opioids	Jamaican dogwood	↑ effects of opioids, do not use concurrently
Oxytocics	Ephedra	Causes severe hypertension when used with oxytocics
Paroxetine	St. John's wort	↑ sedation
Phenothiazines	Coenzyme q10	Some phenothiazines may ↓ the action of coenzyme Q10 and deplete endogenous stores
Phenothiazines	Corkwood	May ↑ anticholinergic effect
Phenothiazines	Ephedra	Tachycardia may result if used concurrently
Phenothiazines	Evening primrose oil	May cause seizures
Phenothiazines	Jimsonweed	↓ action of phenothiazines
Phenothiazines	Yohimbe	May result in ↑ toxicity, do not use concurrently
Phenytoin	Yellow dock	May cause ↑ hypocalcemia, do not use concurrently
Phenytoin	Valerian	May negate therapeutic effects of meds containing phenytoin, do not use concurrently
Plasma, fresh	Cat's claw	May interact with fresh plasma
Potassium-wasting drugs	Aloe	When taken internally may ↑ effects of potassium-wasting drugs
Psychoanaleptic agents	Cola tree	May ↑ the effects of psychoanaleptic agents
Psychotropic agents	Nutmeg	May be potentiated, do not use concurrently
Radioactive isotopes	Bugleweed	Can interfere with the action of radioactive isotopes
Salicylates	Horse chestnut	↑ risk of severe bleeding, do not use concurrently
Salicylates	Chondroitin	Can cause ↑ bleeding
Salicylates	Cola tree	May ↑ the effect of cola tree products
Salicylates	Gossypol	Concurrent use may result in tissue damage
Salicylates	Irish moss	↑ risk of bleeding, do not use concurrently
Salicylates	Pansy	May ↑ actions of salicylates
Scopolamine	Black root	Forms an insoluble complex with scopolamine; do not use concurrently
Sedative/hypnotics	Lavender	↑ sedation when used with lavender, do not use concurrently
Sedative/hypnotics	Cowslip	May ↑ the effect of sedative/hypnotics
Sedative/hypnotics	Catnip	May enhance the effects of sedatives
Sedative/hypnotics	Chamomile	May ↑ the effects of sedatives
Sedatives/hypnotics	Black cohosh	May ↑ hypotensive effects
Sodium bicarbonate	Quinine	May lead to toxicity, do not use concurrently
SSRIs	St. John's wort	Serotonin syndrome and an additive effect may occur. Concurrent use may lead to coma, do not use concurrently
SSRIs	Yohimbe	May cause ↑ CNS stimulation, do not use together
Statins	Goldenseal	May slow the metabolism of statins
Stimulants	Ginseng	Overstimulation may occur with concurrent use
Stimulants	Siberian ginseng	Concurrent use is not recommended, overstimulation may occur
Succinylcholine	Melatonin	↑ blocking properties of succinylcholine, do not use concurrently
Sumatriptan	Horehound	↑ serotonin effect, do not use concurrently
Sympathomimetics	Ephedra	↑ the effect of sympathomimetics and causes hypertension
Sympathomimetics	Rauwolfia	Will ↑ blood pressure, do not use concurrently
Sympathomimetics	Yohimbe	↑ yohimbe toxicity, do not use concurrently
Systemic steroids	Aloe	When taken internally may ↑ effects of systemic steroids
Tannic acids	Agar	↑ dehydration
Thyroid hormones	Soy	May interfere with thyroid hormone absorption, do not use concurrently
Thyroid hormones	Kelpware	May ↓ effects of thyroid hormones, do not use concurrently
Thyroid hormones	Spirulina	High iodine content of spirulina may ↓ action of thyroid hormones, do not use concurrently
Thyroid preparations	Bugleweed	Can interfere with the action of thyroid preparations
Thyroid preparations	Agar	Avoid concurrent use because of high iodine content in agar
Tolbutamide	Angelica	May delay elimination of tolbutamide
Toxoids	Safflower	May cause ↑ immunosuppression, do not use concurrently
Trazodone	St. John's wort	May cause serotonin syndrome
Tricyclic antidepressants	Coenzyme q10	Tricyclic antidepressants ay ↓ the action of coenzyme Q10 and deplete endogenous stores
Tricyclic antidepressants	Jimsonweed	↑ anticholinergic effects when jimsonweed used with tricyclics
Tricyclic antidepressants	Yohimbe	May result in ↑ hypertension, doses may need to be ↓
Tricyclic antidepressants	Corkwood	May ↑ anticholinergic effect
Tricyclic antidepressants	Ephedra	Hypertensive crisis can occur when used concurrently
Urinary alkalizers	Ephedra	↑ the effect of urinary alkalizers
Urine acidifiers	Bearberry	May inactivate bearberry
Vaccines	Safflower	May cause ↑ immunosuppression, do not use concurrently
Vaccines (passive)	Cat's claw	May interact with passive vaccines composed of animal sera
Vitamin B	Goldenseal	May ↓ absorption of vitamin B
Warfarin	Acidophilus	↓ warfarin action
Warfarin	Anise	May ↑ action of warfarin

DRUG/DRUG CLASSES	HERB	INTERACTION
Warfarin	Valerian	May negate therapeutic effects of warfarin, do not use concurrently
Xanthines	Cacao tree	May ↓ the metabolism of xanthines such as theophylline
Xanthines	Coffee	Large amounts of coffee ↑ the action of xanthines such as theophylline
Xanthines	Cola tree	May ↑ the action of xanthines
Xanthines	Ephedra	Causes ↑ central nervous system stimulation
Xanthines	Green tea	Large amounts of green tea ↑ the action of xanthines
Xanthines	Guarana	May ↑ pulse rate, blood pressure, and arrhythmias when taken concurrently
Zinc	Chromium	↓ chromium absorption when taken concurrently
Zinc	Melatonin	↑ inhibition of NMDA receptors, do not use concurrently

Herbal Resources

The following is a sampling of online resources that provide current, reliable information about herbal products, their uses, and their health effects. Some are consumer oriented, and others are intended for health professionals. The names of the sponsoring organizations' home pages are arranged alphabetically. URLs are provided for each individual site, or for the Internet portal through which the site may be accessed.

AGRICOLA (AGRICultural OnLine Access):
http://www.nal.usda.gov/ag98/

Alternative Herbal Index: Provides alphabetized monographs for more than 100 commonly used herbs, including information on usage, chemistry, interactions, and dosage, as well as a symptom-to-herb checker.
http://onhealth.webmd.com/alternative/resource/herbs/index.asp

Alternative Medicine Home Page, from the University of Pittsburgh: A compendium of resources to herbal and other alternative medicine information, broken into several categories. Each category includes a brief description of the linked material. Categories include:
- Databases
- Internet resources (divided into subject areas)
- Mailing lists & newsgroups
- AIDS and HIV
- Practitioner's directories
- Related resources
- Government resources
- Pennsylvania resources
http://www.pitt.edu/cbw/altm.html

American Botanical Council:
http://www.herbalgram.org/

American Herbal Pharmacopoeia:
http://www.herbal-ahp.org/

American Herbalists Guild:
http://www.americanherbalistsguild.com/

American Society of Pharmacognosy:
http://www.phcog.org/

British Herbal Medicine Association:
http://www.ex.ac.uk/phytonet/bhma.html

From Skidmore-Roth L: *Mosby's Handbook of Herbs & Natural Supplements*, St Louis, 2004, Mosby.

Dr. Duke's Phytochemical and Ethnobotanical Databases, from the Agricultural Research Service: A database of medicinal plants that allows the user to search by either common or scientific name. Provides information about the individual phytochemical components in each species, their biological actions, and relevant references.
http://www.ars-grin.gov/duke/plants.html

European Scientific Cooperative on Phytotherapy (ESCOP):
http://www.escop.com/

Herb Research Foundation (HRF): Contains an herbal question-and-answer column, an interface that allows the user to submit questions to the HRF foundation staff, herb news, herb references, and information about setting up media outreach and public education programs about safe and appropriate herb use. The HRF is a nonprofit research and education organization whose stated mission is to improve world health through the informed use of herbs. Some services are available free of charge, while others, such as custom botanical literature research and document delivery, involve a fee.
http://www.herbs.org

Herbal Abstract Page: A compendium of links to Medline and other abstracts of articles about Western herbal and traditional Chinese medical therapies and their documented effects on human health.
http://www.seanet.com/?vettf/Medline4.htm

Medicine, from MedlinePlus:
http://www.nlm.nih.gov/medlineplus/herbalmedicine.html

Herbs for Health, from About.com: Offers a variety of consumer information about American Indian herbs, Ayurvedic medicinal products, Chinese herbs, ethnobotany, and Western herbs, along with daily updates on herbs and other alternative medicine issues in the news. Provides numerous links to other sites for information about herbs and alternative medicine.
http://herbsforhealth.about.com/

Rocky Mountain Herbal Institute: Provides searchable general information about Chinese herbalism; describes continuing education courses available in Chinese herbal sciences and environmental health to medical and health professionals. Provides a free, searchable database of 220 Chinese herbs and related sample course materials.
http://www.rmhiherbal.org/

RxList Alternatives, from allnurses.com: Provides searchable user monographs and frequently-asked-questions lists for commonly used Western herbs, Chinese herbal remedies, and homeopathic remedies.
http://www.rxlist.com/alternative.htm

Southwest School of Botanical Medicine: A comprehensive list of files containing botanical illustrations, including digitized photographs, color prints, lithographs, engravings, line drawings, and wood prints. Includes both .jpeg and .gif file formats.
http://www.swsbm.com/HOMEPAGE/HomePage.html

United States Pharmacopoeia (USP): Under "Dietary Supplements", includes detailed information on the status of USP-NF Botanical Monograph Development Project.
http://www.usp.org/

World Health Organization Herbal Monographs: Under "Development", see the entry for *Alternative Medicine Home Page, from the University of Pittsburgh*.
http://www.who.int/medicines/library/trm/medicinalplants/monographs.shtml

APPENDIX 5

Relaxation Techniques

Relaxation Techniques

RELAXATION TECHNIQUE	SUMMARY	FURTHER RESOURCES
Breathing exercise	This is the foundation of most relaxation techniques. Have patients place one hand on the chest and the other on the abdomen. Instruct them to take a slow, deep breath, as if they were sucking in all the air in the room. While doing this, the hand on the abdomen should rise higher than the hand on the chest. This promotes diaphragmatic breathing that increases alveolar expansion in the bases of the lungs. Have them hold the breath for a count of 7 and then exhale. Exhalation should take twice as long as inhalation. Repeat this for a total of five breaths, and encourage patients to do this three times a day.	*Conscious Breathing* by Gay Hendricks is one of many good resources on using breathing for relaxation and health.
Meditation Transcendental/The relaxation response	To prevent distracting thoughts, the subject repeats a mantra (a word or sound) over and over again while sitting in a comfortable position. If a distracting thought comes to mind, it is accepted and let go, with the mind focusing again on the mantra.	www.mindbody.harvard.edu or *The Relaxation Response* by Herbert Benson; www.tm.org for information on transcendental meditation
Mindful meditation	This represents the philosophy of living in the present or in the moment. The *body scan* is one technique where the subject uses breathing to obtain a relaxed state while lying or sitting. The mind progressively focuses on different parts of the body, where it feels any and all sensations intentionally but nonjudgmentally before moving on to another part of the body. A patient with back pain may focus on the quality and characteristics of the pain as if to better understand it and bring it under control.	*Full Catastrophe Living* by Jon Kabat-Zinn describes this technique in full and the program for stress reduction at the University of Massachusetts Medical Center.
Centering prayer	This is a form similar to transcendental meditation that has a more religious foundation. The subject repeats a "sacred word" similar to a mantra. As thoughts come to mind, they are accepted and let go, clearing the mind to become more centered on the spirit within, as if the mind's preoccupied thoughts are the layers of an onion that are peeled away, allowing better understanding of the spirit at the core.	www.Centeringprayer.com; look under "method of centering prayer" for a nondenominational discussion.

From Rakel RE (ed): *Principles of family practice,* ed 6, Philadelphia, 2002, WB Saunders.

Continued

Relaxation Techniques—cont'd

RELAXATION TECHNIQUE	SUMMARY	FURTHER RESOURCES
Progressive muscle relaxation (PMR)	A form of relaxation in which the subject is attuned to the difference in feeling when the muscles are tensed and then relaxed. In a comfortable position, start by tensing the whole body from head to toe. While doing this, notice the feelings of tightness. Take a deep breath in and as you let it out, let the tension release and the muscles relax. This is then followed by progressive tension and relaxation throughout the body. One may start by clenching the fists and then tensing the arms, shoulders, chest, abdomen, hips, legs, and so on, with each step followed by relaxation.	www.uaex.edu/publications/pub/ fshei28.htm is a good review of PMR as well as other relaxation exercises. It is sponsored by the University of Arkansas. *You Must Relax* is a book by the founder of this technique, Edmund Jacobson.
Visualization/ Self-hypnosis	The subject uses visualization to recruit images that create a relaxed state. For example, if a person is anxious, visualizing images of a place and a time that were peaceful and comforting would help induce relaxation. This is best used in conjunction with a breathing exercise.	There are many audiocassettes that can guide people through a visualization "script" that can result in relaxation. Emmett Miller is one well-known author.
Autogenic training	This induces a physiologic response by using simple phrases. For example, "My legs are heavy and warm" is meant to increase the blood flow to this area, resulting in relaxation. This is done progressively from head to toe with the use of deep breathing and repetition of the phrase. After completing this, focus attention on any body part that may still be tense, and then focus the breath and phrase to that area until the whole body is relaxed.	The British Autogenic Society at www.autogenictherapy.org.uk is a good resource for more information.
Exercise/Movement Aerobic	While performing an aerobic exercise, focus attention on a phrase, sound, word, or prayer and passively disregard other thoughts that may enter the mind. Some may focus on their breathing, saying to themselves, "In" with inhalation and "Out" with exhalation, or repeating "one-two, one-two" with each step they take with jogging. Doing this will help the mind focus, preventing other thoughts that may cause tension.	*Beyond the Relaxation Response* by Herbert Benson includes discussion of his research on inducing the relaxation response while exercising.
Yoga	This has been practiced for thousands of years in India. In America, it has been divided into three aspects: breathing (pranayama yoga), bodily postures or asanas (hatha yoga), and meditation to maintain balance and health. Regular practice induces relaxation.	For the following therapies, it is best to encourage your patients to take a class at a local community center or gym and to pick up an introductory book at a library or bookstore.
Tai chi	An ancient Chinese martial art that uses slow, graceful movements combined with inner mindfulness and breathing techniques to help bring balance between the mind and body.	See above.
Qi gong	A traditional Chinese practice that uses movement, meditation, and controlled breathing to balance the body's vital energy force, chi.	See above.

Index

Bolded page numbers indicate
principal textual treatment. Page
numbers followed by f indicate
figures; t, tables; b, boxes.